Plastic Surgery

Principles and Practice

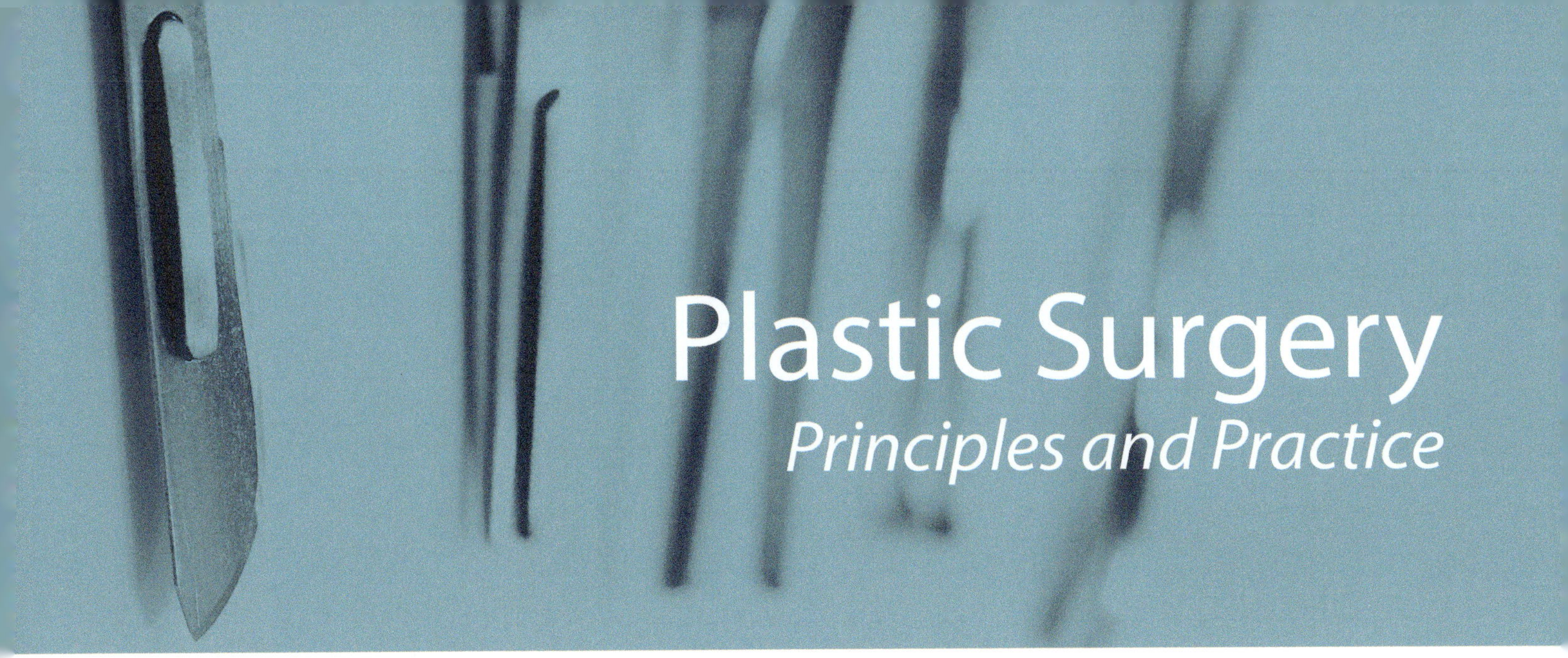

Plastic Surgery

Principles and Practice

Editor-in-Chief

Rostam D. Farhadieh BSc(Med)(Hons), MBBS, MD, EBOPRASF, FRACS(Plast), FRCS(Plast)

Consultant Plastic and Reconstructive Surgeon
Head of Department of Plastic Reconstructive and Hand Surgery
The Canberra and Calvary Hospitals, Canberra, ACT, Australia
Director, Panthea Clinics
Senior Clinical Lecturer
Sydney University Medical School
Sydney, NSW, Australia

Editors

Neil W. Bulstrode BSc(Hons), MBBS, MD, FRCS(Plast)

Consultant Plastic Surgeon and Lead Clinician for the Department of Plastic Surgery at Great Ormond Street Hospital
London, United Kingdom
Honorary Associate Professor, UCL Great Ormond Street Institute of Child Health
London, United Kingdom

Babak J. Mehrara MD

Plastic and Reconstructive Surgeon
Chief, Plastic and Reconstructive Surgical Service
Peter G. Cordeiro Endowed Chair in Plastic and Reconstructive Surgery
Memorial Sloan Kettering Cancer Center
New York, NY, United States

Sabrina Cugno MD, MSc, FRCSC, FACS, FAAP

Pediatric Plastic and Reconstructive Surgeon
Montreal Children's Hospital and Shriners Hospital
Assistant Professor, McGill University
Montreal Children's Hospital
McGill University Health Center
Montreal, QC, Canada

For additional online content visit ExpertConsult.com

ELSEVIER

Edinburgh London New York Oxford Philadelphia St Louis Sydney 2022

ISBN:
Print: 978-0-323-65381-7
E-book: 978-0-323-65382-4

Content Strategist: Belinda Kuhn
Content Development Specialist: Sharon Nash
Project Manager: Anne Collett
Design: Brian Salisbury
Illustration Manager: Anitha Rajarathnam
Multimedia Producer: Ramkumar Bashyam
Marketing Manager: Deborah Watkins

Printed in the United States of America

Last digit is the print number: 9 8 7 6 5 4 3 2

Dedication

"To inspirational mentors and dedicated apprentices everywhere"

Contents

Video Contents

Foreword

It is indeed a real honor to have been asked to write the *Foreword* to both the first and now the second edition of this very fine and updated state-of-the-art compilation of our plastic surgery specialty.

It is remarkable how things have changed just in one professional lifetime of a senior plastic surgeon still practicing: from an embryonic specialty fifty or so years ago, with limited knowledge and surgical techniques, to a specialty that has become, without doubt, a vital cornerstone for the effective functioning of all major medical centers. The plastic surgeon has evolved into the "go-to" problem solver, whose expertise can be called upon to help treat patients with a myriad of clinical problems. The plastic surgeon is consulted to treat all manner of wounds, congenital and acquired deformities and other challenging defects, oftentimes created by other specialists! These problem-solving skills have created synergies between plastic surgery and other surgical specialties which has allowed them to expand their therapeutic spectrum and tackle increasingly more difficult problems. Thus, they can focus on novel approaches for addressing the pathology at hand, without concern of how things will be put back together. The plastic surgeon has assumed the role of a "closer", who may have to use every asset in his or her "toolbox of tricks" and domain knowledge to adequately reconstruct the defect. And, when the tool does not fit the problem at hand, he or she must have a broad and creative background across domains to improvise and come up with novel solutions.

Today's plastic surgeon should be prepared to repair and reconstruct deformities and deficiencies of the skin and its content from head to toe. It is fair to say that plastic surgeons have become *the* new general-surgeons-of-today, or at least a "sophisticated" extension of what was once considered general surgery. The new, but still evolving mantra in today's medical establishments is: "if in doubt, call plastics." In this new role, it is imperative that the plastic surgeon remains up-to-date with the current state of expertise and techniques in the field. The volume of knowledge that trainees must acquire in plastic surgery today has grown exponentially, as is reflected in the length of the training process: from an extra two years tacked onto the end of a general surgery program back when I trained, to the new integrated model of plastic surgery that is at least six years in length and typically longer with additional fellowship training.

In the early days there were only a few classic plastic surgery texts, but now there are many multi-volume textbooks to cover the growing breadth of our specialty. However, there still exists a need for a convenient, single volume compendium that is succinct and practical but also comprehensive enough to give the student, resident, and seasoned practitioner a *vademecum* to help as a ready reference for everyday use. Although concise, the single volume text still needs to cover the essentials of plastic surgery, especially the principles of management and treatment that can be applied across the full spectrum of our ever-expanding specialty. I believe that this second edition of *Plastic Surgery: Principles and Practice* fulfills this need.

It has taken a major international collaborative effort, with an expanded editorial board, consisting of Ross D. Farhadieh (Australia), Neil Bulstrode (UK), Babak Mehrara (USA) and Sabrina Cugno (Canada), to produce this superb volume. They have recruited an international team of authors who have extensively revised this second edition with changes to most chapters, consolidation of several chapters and the addition of totally new chapters – all written by experts, who have updated the current status in their fields of interest, sharing many special pearls of wisdom. The chapters are all clearly set out and organized, providing an overview of core principles, the latest applicable basic science essentials, as well as clinical applications and techniques, and only the most pertinent bibliography for additional reading. Furthermore, the second edition has better graphics, colored illustrations, algorithms of management, embedded operative videos (especially in the Esthetic Section) and real clinical examples which are always better than line drawings in illustrating procedures. Though this text is aimed primarily at the trainee, I believe that it will also be useful as an excellent and quick resource for the experienced surgeon. It will be especially useful for residents and fellows preparing to take their board and fellowship exams.

I would again like to thank Dr. Ross Farhadieh for the honor of contributing the *Foreword* to this second edition of this excellent textbook, which I believe continues to nicely fulfill the tradition of passing down knowledge from one generation of problem solvers to the next. My hope is that that they can learn from what we have achieved and continue to push and expand the boundaries of our specialty, as they will no doubt tackle new and, assuredly, even more complex problems going forward. Again, my congratulations to the editors for recruiting such a world class group of distinguished plastic surgeons who have expertly summarized the current state-of-the-art of our specialty; and finally, to the publishers for producing this timely and comprehensive body of work.

Julian J. Pribaz, MBBS (Melbourne), FRCS (Edinburgh), FRACS (Plast)
Professor of Surgery, Morsani College of Medicine
Department of Plastic Surgery,
University of South Florida
Tampa, Florida

Preface

It is now a decade since I completed my formal plastic surgery training and six years since the publication of our first textbook. We embarked on the second incarnation of this textbook in the halcyon pre-COVID-19 days, substantially restructuring and rewriting large portions of the textbook to optimize the new edition. Like most plastic surgeons, I continue to find excitement in the art and variety of problems we are called upon to solve. That the body is the mission remains an alluring reason for most plastic surgical trainees and seasoned surgeons alike. It is the breadth, depth, variety, and scope of creativity that defines our craft. These can range from congenital hands differences, craniofacial syndromes, complex upper and lower limb traumas, head, neck, and breast cancer reconstructions, esthetic procedures across the body and the face, to the humble simple skin cancers. Like many of our colleagues, the variety of my own clinical practice, which includes complex microsurgical reconstructions, skin cancers, hand surgery, trauma reconstruction, as well as facial and body esthetic surgery, remains a source of immense professional satisfaction. The first rendition of this compendium came about because I found the single volume textbooks too broad-stroked and the classic multivolume behemoths, leaden and heavy. During the planning of this new edition it was clear that the aim of bringing together a perfect balance of detail and palatability remained a laudable aspiration. As I have continued to practice and teach plastic surgery with my own fair share of triumphs, failures, and challenges, it was self-evident that humility should be the cornerstone of any good surgical practice. Time and again it was clear that nothing is more valuable than good experience in this lifelong apprenticeship. So again, we set out to find the world's experienced and recognized authorities in their field for this edition, to add that most intangible element to any textbook, wisdom.

On this occasion, we were joined by my good friend and colleague Dr. Babak Mehrara from Memorial Sloan Kettering, who along with old bandmates, Mr. Neil Bulstrode from Great Ormond Street and Dr. Sabrina Cugno from Montreal Children's Hospital, brought the prefect blend of enthusiasm and sense of humour to compile this compendium. I am grateful to them for their time, their effort, and above all their friendship, which was after all, a prime motivator for the new edition. I also wish to thank all our colleagues who took time out of their busy schedules to make this volume possible. Personally, it was an incredible education and an opportunity to, on occasion, discuss my own clinical dilemmas with the masters. Our special and my own personal gratitude to Professor Julian Pribaz, who, despite the unprecedented times and heavy workload, was kind enough to take time to review this work and write the Foreword. My personal thanks to Professor Peter Neligan for his encouragement and advice early in the piece. We also wish to thank all the staff at Elsevier for their steadfast support of this project; Belinda Kuhn and Sharon Nash made this work possible and a fun project to navigate.

On a personal note, I wish to thank my mother Tadjvar, my brother Arash, my wife Yassi, and our children Dariush and Roxanna for their understanding, for all the time I spent away on this project, and for their unwavering support. My parents have been my guiding light in demonstrating the importance of strong work ethics and integrity. I also wish to extend my sincere thanks to my mentors, they are as important to a seasoned surgeon's career, as they are to a novice during training. Great surgeons and people can trace back to these fundamental influences and it remains a fabric of the narrative of who we become, the good, the bad, and the ugly. In plastic surgery, I wish to thank Mr. Bryan Mendelson who, during my extended visits, has always shown immense patience and generosity in teaching me the philosophy and techniques of facial esthetic surgery, and has shared many of his life experiences with me. My gratitude also goes to Mr. Stephen Flood, who illustrated by example a sensible approach to plastic surgery, kindness in mentorship, and leadership of a plastic surgery unit. As a plastic surgeon, I will be forever indebted to Professor Wayne Morrison, who has a curiosity, humility, dedication to teaching, generosity of will, and spirit that is tempered with a crisp sense of humor in equal inspirational measure. Since commencing practice I have always been fortunate enough to be able to seek his advice, guidance, and continue to learn from one of the greatest masters of our art. It was truly an honor and a privilege to serve as his registrar.

Rostam D. Farhadieh MBBS, MD, FRACS(Plast), FRCS(Plast)
Sydney, Australia
February 2021

List of Contributors

The editors would like to acknowledge and offer grateful thanks for the input of all contributors to the previous edition, without whom this new edition would not have been possible.

Jonathan Adamthwaite BA(Hons), MA(Oxon), FRCS
Consultant Plastic Surgeon
Department of Plastic Surgery
York Teaching Hospitals NHS Foundation Trust
York, United Kingdom

Nidal Farhan AL Deek, MD, MSc
Department of Plastic and Reconstructive Surgery
Chang Gung Memorial Hospital
Taoyun, Taiwan;
Chang Gung Medical College and Chang Gung University
Taoyun, Taiwan

Hanan Alhusainan, MD
Craniofacial Surgery Fellow
Montreal Children's Hospital
McGill University Health Center
Montreal, QC, Canada;
Craniofacial and Plastic Surgeon
Consultant, Plastic Surgery
King Abdullah Children's Specialist Hospital
Assistant Professor of Surgery
King Saud bin Abdulaziz University for Health Sciences
Riyadh, Saudi Arabia;
King Abdulaziz Medical City
National Guard Health Affairs
Riyadh, Saudi Arabia

Robert J. Allen Jr, MD
Assistant Attending
Plastic and Reconstructive Surgery
Department of Surgery
Memorial Sloan Kettering Cancer Center
New York, NY, United States

Rebecca Ayers, MBChB, FRACS
Department of Plastic Surgery
Dunedin Public Hospital
Dunedin, New Zealand

Gurdip Azad, MBBS, MRCP, FRCR, MD(Res)
Consultant Clinical Oncologist
Guy's and St Thomas's NHS Trust
London, United Kingdom;
Honorary Senior Clinical Lecturer
GKT Medical School and King's College London
London, United Kingdom

Alain J. Azzi, MD, MSc
Resident
Division of Plastic and Reconstructive Surgery
Montreal Children's Hospital
Montreal, QC, Canada

Alex Barnacle, BM, MRCP, FRCR
Consultant Interventional Radiologist
Department of Radiology
Great Ormond Street Hospital for Children
London, United Kingdom

Scott P. Bartlett, MD
Professor of Surgery
Department of Surgery
University of Pennsylvania
Philadelphia, PA, United States;
Chief, Division of Plastic Surgery
Department of Surgery
Children's Hospital of Philadelphia
Philadelphia, PA, United States

Irina Belinsky, MD
Clinical Assistant Professor of Oculoplastic Surgery
Director of Ocular Oncology
Department of Ophthalmology
NYU Langone Medical Center
New York, NY, United States

Oded Ben-Amotz, MD
Hand Fellow
Orthopedics
University of Pennsylvania
Philadelphia, PA, United States

Nathaniel A. Blecher, MD
Department of Plastic Surgery
University of Pittsburgh Medical Center
Pittsburgh, PA, United States

Kirsty Boyd, MD, FRCSC
Assistant Professor
Plastic Surgery
University of Ottawa
Ottawa, ON, Canada

Karl C. Bruckman, MD, DDS
Assistant Professor Surgery
Division of Plastic & Reconstructive Surgery
Stanford University School of Medicine
Stanford University Medical Center and
Lucile Packard Children's Hospital
Stanford, CA, United States

Donald W. Buck II, MD, FACS
Plastic & Reconstructive Surgery
St Louis, MO, United States

Neil W. Bulstrode, BSc(Hons), MBBS, MD, FRCS
Consultant Plastic Surgeon and Clinical Lead
Department of Plastic Surgery
Great Ormond Street Hospital for Children
London, United Kingdom;
Honorary Associate Professor
UCL Great Ormond Street Institute of Child Health
London, United Kingdom

Nicola Burr, MSc, Grad Dip Phys
Consultant Hand Therapist
Hand Therapy Department
Royal Free London NHS Trust
London, United Kingdom

Daniel P. Butler, MBBS, MRCS(Eng), MBA, FRCS
Plastic Surgery Senior Fellow
Plastic and Reconstructive Surgery
Charing Cross Hospital
London, United Kingdom

Marc A. Cohen, MD, MPH
Associate Attending
Head and Neck Service
Department of Surgery
Memorial Sloan Kettering Cancer Center
New York, NY, United States

Sydney R. Coleman, MD
Clinical Assistant Professor
Plastic Surgery
University of Pittsburgh Medical Center
Pittsburgh, PA, United States

Ryan Constantine, MD
Plastic Surgery Resident
Division of Plastic and Reconstructive Surgery
Department of Surgery
University of Colorado
Aurora, CO, United States

Michelle Coriddi, MD
Plastic and Reconstructive Surgery Service
Department of Surgery
Memorial Sloan Kettering Cancer Center
New York, NY, United States

Sabrina Cugno, MD, MSc, FRCSC, FACS, FAAP
Pediatric Plastic and Reconstructive Surgeon
Montreal Children's Hospital and Shriners Hospital
Montreal, QC, Canada;
Assistant Professor, McGill University
Montreal Children's Hospital
McGill University Health Center
Montreal, QC, Canada

David J. David, MD, FRCSE, FRCS, FRACS, FRCST
Professor of Craniomaxillofacial Surgery
Faculty of Medicine
University of Adelaide
Adelaide, SA, Australia;
Faculty of Medicine and Health Science
Macquarie University
Sydney, NSW, Australia

Kristen M. Davidge, MD, MSc, FRCSC
Plastic and Reconstructive Surgeon
Hospital for Sick Children
Toronto, ON, Canada;
Assistant Professor
Division of Plastic and Reconstructive Surgery
University of Toronto
Toronto, ON, Canada;
Associate Scientist
Child Health and Evaluative Sciences
Sick Kids Research Institute
Toronto, ON, Canada

Joseph Dayan, MD
Plastic and Reconstructive Surgery Service
Department of Surgery
Memorial Sloan Kettering Cancer Center
New York, NY, United States

Ilse Degreef, MD, PhD, FEBHS
Professor and Surgeon in Chief
Department of Orthopedic Surgery
University Hospitals Leuven
Leuven, Belgium

David J. Dunaway, MBChB, FDSRCS, FRCS
Consultant Craniofacial and Plastic Surgeon
Craniofacial Surgery
Department of Plastic Surgery
Great Ormond Street Hospital for Children
London, United Kingdom

Francesco M. Egro, MBChB, MSc, MRCS
Resident Physician
Department of Plastic Surgery
University of Pittsburgh Medical Center
Pittsburgh, PA, United States

Ebby Elahi, MD, MBA, FACS
Clinical Professor of Ophthalmology, Otolaryngology and Public Health
Icahn School of Medicine at Mount Sinai
New York, NY, United States;
Director
Fifth Avenue Eye Associates
New York, NY, United States

Dino Elyassnia, MD, FACS
Private Practice
Marten Clinic of Plastic Surgery
San Francisco, CA, United States

Kathryn Evans, BMedSci, BMBS, FRCS(Paed Surg)
Consultant Paediatric Urologist
St George's University Hospital
London, United Kingdom

Rostam D. Farhadieh, BSc(Med)Hons, MBBS, MD, EBOPRASF, FRACS, FRCS
Consultant Plastic and Reconstructive Surgeon
Head of Department, Plastic Reconstructive Surgery
The Canberra and Calvary Hospitals
Canberra, ACT, Australia
Director, Panthea Clinics
Senior Clinical Lecturer
Sydney University Medical School
Sydney, NSW, Australia

Michael W. Findlay, MBBS, PhD, FRACS, FACS
Supervisor of Plastic and Reconstructive Surgery Training
Division of Cancer Surgery
The Peter MacCallum Cancer Centre
Melbourne, VIC, Australia;
Plastic, Reconstructive and Hand Surgeon
Department of Surgery
The Canberra Hospital
Canberra, ACT, Australia;
Director, Program for Molecular and Cellular Innovation in Surgery
Department of Surgery
The University of Melbourne
Melbourne, VIC, Australia

Françoise Firmin, MD
Consultant Plastic Surgeon
Clinique Bizet
Paris, France

David M. Fisher, MB, BCh, FRCSC, FACS
Medical Director, Cleft Lip and Palate Program
Department of Plastic Surgery
Hospital for Sick Children
Toronto, ON, Canada;
Professor
Department of Surgery
University of Toronto
Toronto, ON, Canada

Stephen Flood, FRACS
Plastic and Reconstructive Surgeon
Department of Plastic and Reconstructive Surgery
Austin Hospital
Heidelberg, VIC, Australia

Antonio J. Forte, MD, PhD
Associate Professor and Consultant
Division of Plastic Surgery
Department of Orthopedic Surgery
Department of Neurosurgery
Mayo Clinic
Jacksonville, FL, United States

Adam C. Gascoigne, MBBS, PGDipAnat
Taylor Lab
Department Anatomy and Neuroscience
The University of Melbourne
Parkville, VIC, Australia

Mirko S. Gilardino, MD, MSc, FRCSC, FACS
Chief, Division of Plastic Surgery
McGill University Health Centre;
Associate Professor of Surgery & Pediatric Surgery
Director, H.B. Williams Craniofacial and Cleft Surgery Unit
Montreal Children's Hospital
Montreal, QC, Canada

Aina V.H. Greig, MA, PhD, FRCS
Consultant Plastic Surgeon
Department of Plastic Surgery
Guy's and St Thomas' NHS Foundation Trust
London, United Kingdom;
Honorary Adjunct Senior Lecturer
Kings College London, United Kingdom

Adriaan O. Grobbelaar, MBChB, MMed(Plast), FCS(SA)(Plast), FRCS(Plast), FRCS(ad eundem)(Eng)
Professor UCL Department of Surgery and Interventional Science
Consultant Plastic Surgeon
Department of Plastic Surgery
Great Ormond Street Hospital for Children
London, United Kingdom;
Inselspital
Bern, Switzerland

Geoffrey C. Gurtner, MD
Johnson and Johnson Professor
Department of Surgery
Stanford University
Stanford, CA, United States

Lucinda Gunn, BMBS, MRCP, PGDip Oncology, FRCR
Clinical Oncology Registrar
The Royal Marsden Hospital
London, United Kingdom

Bahman Guyuron, MD, FACS
Professor Emeritus, Plastic Surgery
Case School of Medicine
Zeeba Clinic
Lyndhurst, OH, United States;
Editor in Chief, *Aesthetic Plastic Surgery*

Elizabeth J. Hall-Findlay, MD, FRCSC
Private Practice
Banff Plastic Surgery
Banff, AB, Canada

Matthew M. Hanasono, MD
Professor and Fellowship Program Director
Department of Plastic Surgery
The University of Texas MD Anderson Cancer Center
Houston, TX, United States

John Harper, MBBS, MD, FRCP, FRCPCH
Honorary Professor of Paediatric Dermatology
UCL Great Ormond Street Institute of Child Health
London, United Kingdom

Kareem Hassan, MD
Resident Physician
Department of Plastic and
Reconstructive Surgery
University of Chicago
Chicago, IL, United States

Michael A. Henderson, MD, FRACS
Professor of Surgery
University of Melbourne
Head, Melanoma and Skin Service
The Peter MacCallum Cancer Centre
Melbourne, VIC, Australia

Geoffrey E. Hespe, MD
House Officer
Department of Surgery
Section of Plastic Surgery
University of Michigan
Ann Arbor, MI, United States

Tobias Heuft, Dr. med.
Consultant Department of Plastic Surgery
Dreifaltigkeits-Hospital
Wesseling, Germany

Stefan O.P. Hofer, MD, PhD, FRCS(C)
Wharton Chair in Reconstructive Plastic Surgery
Professor of Surgery
University of Toronto, ON, Canada;
Chief Division of Plastic Surgery
University Health Network
Toronto, ON, Canada

Steven E.R. Hovius, MD, PhD
Professor
Hand and Wrist Surgery
Xpert Clinic
Rotterdam, The Netherlands;
Professor
Plastic and Reconstructive Surgery
Radboudumc
Nijmegen, The Netherlands

Benjamin H.L. Howes, MBBS, PhD
Senior Plastic Surgery Registrar
Department of Plastic, Reconstructive & Hand Surgery
The Canberra Hospital
Canberra, ACT, Australia

Yun-Huan (Barry) Hsieh, MBBS, MS(PRS)
Plastic Surgery Registrar
Department of Plastic and Reconstructive Surgery
The Canberra Hospital
ACT, Australia;
Microsurgery Fellow
Department of Plastic and Reconstructive Surgery
Chang Gung Memorial Hospital
Taoyuan, Taiwan;
Laboratory Research Fellow,
Vascularized Composite Allotransplantation Centre,
Chang Gung Memorial Hospital
Taoyuan, Taiwan

Navid Jallali, BSc, MBCh(Hons), MD, FRCS
Consultant Plastic Surgeon
Department of Plastic Surgery
Charing Cross Hospital
London, United Kingdom

Barbara Jemec, MD, FRCS, EBOPRAS, FRCSC
Consultant Plastic Surgeon
Department of Plastic Surgery
The Royal Free NHS Foundation Trust
London, United Kingdom

Nikita Joji, MBChB, BSc(Hons), MRCS, PGCert(Med Ed)
Plastic Surgery Department
Royal Free Hospital
London, United Kingdom

Mazyar Kanani, PhD, FRCS
Cardiothoracic Surgeon
Cardiothoracic Unit
James Cook University Hospital
Middlesbrough, United Kingdom

Raghu P. Kataru, PhD
Senior Scientist
Department of Surgery
Memorial Sloan Kettering Cancer Center
New York, NY, United States

Julia L. Kerolus, MD
Assistant Professor
Facial Plastic and Reconstructive Surgery
University of Illinois at Chicago
Chicago, IL, United States

Veronica Kinsler, MA, MBBCh, MRCPCH, PhD
Professor of Paediatric Dermatology and Dermatogenetics
Genetics & Genomic Medicine Department
UCL Great Ormond Street Institute of Child Health
Department of Paediatric Dermatology
Great Ormond Street Hospital for Children
London, United Kingdom

Emily M. Krauss, MD, MSc, FRCSC
Assistant Professor
Division of Plastic Surgery, Department of Surgery
University of British Columbia
Victoria, BC, Canada

Jonathan I. Leckenby, MBBS, PhD
Assistant Professor
Division of Plastic Surgery, Department of Surgery
University of Rochester Medical Center
Rochester, NY, United States

Gordon K. Lee, MD, FACS
Professor
Plastic Surgery
Stanford Plastic Surgery
Stanford, CA, United States

Ben Levi, MD
Assistant Professor
Plastic Surgery
University of Michigan
Ann Arbor, MI, United States

L. Scott Levin, MD, FACS
Paul B. Magnuson Professor of Bone and Joint Surgery and Chairman
Department of Orthopedic Surgery
Professor of Surgery
Division of Plastic Surgery, Department of Surgery
University of Pennsylvania Health System
Philadelphia, PA, United States

Se Hwang Liew, MBBCh, MD, FRCS
Consultant Plastic Surgeon
Merseyside Regional Burns and Plastic Surgery Centre
Whiston Hospital
Liverpool, United Kingdom

Charles Y.Y. Loh, MBBS, MSc, MS, MRCS
Plastic Surgery Registrar
Plastic Surgery
St. Andrew's Centre for Plastic Surgery and Burns
Broomfield Hospital
Chelmsford, United Kingdom

Susan E. Mackinnon, MD
Minot Packer Fryer Professor of Surgery
Department of Surgery
Division of Plastic and Reconstructive Surgery
Washington University School of Medicine
St. Louis, MO, United States

Timothy J. Marten, MD, FACS
Founder and Director
Marten Clinic of Plastic Surgery
San Francisco, CA, United States

David W. Mathes, MD
Professor and Chief
Division of Plastic and Reconstructive Surgery
Department of Surgery
University of Colorado
Aurora, CO, United States

Gregory McCarten, MB, BS, FRACS, MA
Plastic and Reconstructive Surgeon
The Canberra Hospital
Canberra, ACT, Australia

Alan A. McNab, FRANZCO, FRCOphth, DMedSc
Head of Clinic
Orbital Plastic and Lacrimal Clinic
Royal Victorian Eye and Ear Hospital
East Melbourne, VIC, Australia

Babak J. Mehrara, MD
Plastic and Reconstructive Surgeon
Chief, Plastic and Reconstructive Surgical Service
Peter G. Cordeiro Endowed Chair
Plastic and Reconstructive Surgery
Memorial Sloan Kettering Cancer Center
New York, NY, United States

Bryan Mendelson, MBBS, FRCSE, FRACS, FACS, Diplomate American Board of Plastic Surgery
Plastic Surgeon
Aesthetic Plastic Surgery
The Centre for Facial Plastic Surgery
Melbourne, VIC, Australia

Shaun D. Mendenhall, MD
Assistant Professor of Surgery
Division of Plastic Surgery, Department of Surgery
University of Utah School of Medicine
Salt Lake City, UT, United States

Alexander F. Mericli, MD, FACS
Assistant Professor
Plastic Surgery
The University of Texas MD Anderson Cancer Center
Houston, TX, United States

Ximena Mimica, MD
Research Fellow
Head and Neck Surgery
Memorial Sloan Kettering Cancer Center
New York, NY, United States

Edwin Morrison, LLB, BComm(Hons Eco), MBBS, FRACS
Plastic and Reconstructive Surgeon
St. Vincent's Hospital
Melbourne, VIC, Australia;
The Peter MacCallum Cancer Centre
Melbourne, VIC, Australia

Wayne A.J. Morrison, MBBS, MD, FRACS, FRCSIre(Hon)
Professor
Department of Surgery
University of Melbourne
St. Vincent's Hospital
Melbourne, VIC, Australia;
Plastic Surgeon
Department of Plastic Surgery
St. Vincent's Hospital
Melbourne, VIC, Australia;
Adipose Tissue Lab Head
O'Brien Institute
St. Vincent's Institute
Melbourne, VIC, Australia;
Professor Honorary
Health Sciences
Australian Catholic University
Melbourne, VIC, Australia

Andrew Morritt, MBChB, MD, FRCS
Consultant Plastic Surgeon
Royal Hallamshire Hospital
Sheffield, United Kingdom

Afshin Mosahebi, MBBS, FRCS, PhD, MBA
Professor Plastic Surgery
Department of Plastic Surgery
UCL, Royal Free Hospital
London, United Kingdom

Peter M. Murray, MD
Professor and Chair
Department of Orthopedic Surgery
Mayo Clinic
Jacksonville, FL, United States;
Consultant
Department of Orthopedic Surgery and Neurosurgery
Mayo Clinic
Jacksonville, FL, USA;
Staff Physician
Department of Orthopedic Surgery
Nemours Children's Clinic
Jacksonville, FL, United States

Imran Mushtaq, MBChB, MD, FRCS(Glasg), FRCS(Paed)
Consultant Paediatric Urologist
Great Ormond Street Hospital for Children
London, United Kingdom

Nagarajan Muthialu, DNB, FRCSEd
Consultant Paediatric Cardiothoracic Surgeon
Cardiothoracic Unit
Great Ormond Street Hospital
London, United Kingdom

Simon Myers, MBBS, FRCS, FRCS(Plast), PhD
GAPS Professor of Academic Plastic Surgery
Queen Mary University
London, United Kingdom;
Honorary Consultant Plastic, Burn, Reconstructive and Aesthetic Surgeon
Barts & The London NHS Healthcare Trust
Blizzard Institute
London, United Kingdom

Paul S. Nassif, MD, FACS
Assistant Clinical Professor
Otolaryngology–Head and Neck Surgery
University of Southern California,
Los Angeles, CA, United States;
Facial Plastic Surgeon
Nassif MD, Inc
Beverly Hills, CA, United States

Tim H.J. Nijhuis, MD, PhD
Department of Plastic, Reconstructive and Hand Surgery
Radboudumc
Nijmegen, The Netherlands;
Plastic and Aesthetic Surgery
Velthuis Kliniek
Velp, The Netherlands

Dariush Nikkhah, BM, MSc, FRCS
Consultant Plastic and Hand Surgeon
Department of Plastic and Reconstructive Surgery
Royal Free London NHS Foundation Trust
London, United Kingdom

Niri S. Niranjan, MBBS, MS, FRCS, FRCS(Plast)
Consultant Plastic Surgeon
Plastic and Burn Surgery
St. Andrew's Centre for Plastic Surgery and Burns
Broomfield Hospital
Chelmsford, United Kingdom

Shelley S. Noland, MD
Assistant Professor
Plastic & Orthopedic Surgery
Medical Director
Peripheral Nerve/Brachial Plexus Clinic
Mayo Clinic College of Medicine
Mayo Clinic Arizona
Phoenix, AZ, United States

Chris Nutting, BSc(Hons), MD, PhD, FRCP, FRCR, MedFIPEM, FMedSCI
Consultant Clinical Oncologist
Radiotherapy
The Royal Marsden Hospital
London, United Kingdom

Adeyemi A. Ogunleye, MD, MS
Clinical Instructor, Plastic Surgery
Stanford Plastic Surgery
Stanford, CA, United States

Anne C. O'Neill MBBCh, MMedSci, FRCS, MSc, PhD
Associate Professor of Surgery
University of Toronto, ON, Canada;
Division of Plastic Surgery, University Health Network
Toronto, ON, Canada

Robert Pearl, BM, BSc, MD, FRCS, Dip Hand Surg
Consultant Plastic Surgeon
Department of Plastic Surgery
Queen Victoria Hospital
East Grinstead, United Kingdom

Grace Lee Peng, MD, FACS
Facial Plastic and Reconstructive Surgery
Beverly Hills, CA, United States

Olivia M. Perotti, BSc, MBBS, MS
Plastic Surgery Registrar,
Department of Plastic Reconstructive and Hand Surgery
The Canberra Hospital
Canberra, ACT, Australia

Mark Pickford, MBBS, MS, FRCS
Consultant Plastic and Hand Surgeon
Queen Victoria Hospital
East Grinstead, Sussex, United Kingdom

Hollie A. Power, MD, FRCSC
Clinical Lecturer
Division of Plastic Surgery, Department of Surgery
University of Alberta
Edmonton, AB, Canada

Krishna Rao, MCh, FRCS, FRACS
Consultant Plastic & Reconstructive Surgeon
Department of Plastic Reconstructive Hand Surgery
The Canberra Hospital Garran
Canberra, Australia

Aline Rau, MD
Plastic Surgery Resident
Division of Plastic and Reconstructive Surgery
Department of Surgery
University of Colorado
Aurora, CO, United States

Patrick L. Reavey, MD, MS
Assistant Professor
Surgery, Section of Plastic and Reconstructive Surgery
University of Chicago Medicine
Chicago, IL, United States

Dirk F. Richter, MD, PhD
Head of Department
Department of Plastic Surgery
Dreifaltigkeits-Hospital
Wesseling, Germany

Abigail M. Rodriguez, MD
Resident
Plastic Surgery
Baylor Scott & White Health – Temple
Temple, TX, United States

Carlo Riccardo Rossi, MD
Director, Surgical Oncology
Veneto Institute of Oncology (IOV)-IRCCS
Padua, Italy;
Full Professor
Surgical, Oncological and Gastroenteric Sciences
University of Padua
Padua, Italy

J. Peter Rubin, MD
Professor and Chair
Plastic Surgery
University of Pittsburgh
Pittsburgh, PA, United States;
Professor
Bioengineering
University of Pittsburgh
Pittsburgh, PA, United States

Michel Saint-Cyr, MD, FRCSC
Professor
Plastic Surgery
Baylor Scott & White Health – Temple
Temple, TX, United States

Donald Sammut, FRCS, FRCS(Plast)
Consultant Hand Surgeon
OneWelbeck Clinic
Marylebone, London, United Kingdom

Marlene See, MBBS, MSc, FRCS
Consultant Plastic Surgeon
Guy's and St. Thomas' NHS Foundation Trust
London, United Kingdom

Maria Z. Siemionow, MD, PhD, DSc
Professor of Orthopedics
Director of Microsurgery Research
University of Illinois at Chicago
Chicago, IL, United States

Bran Sivakumar, MBBS, BSc, FRCS
Consultant Hand, Plastic and Reconstructive Surgeon
Department of Plastic Surgery
Great Ormond Street Hospital for Children
London, United Kingdom

Oliver J. Smith, MBChB, BSc, MRCS
Specialist Registrar in Plastic Surgery
NIHR Academic Clinical Fellow
Department of Plastic Surgery
Royal Free Hospital
London, United Kingdom

Paul Smith, MBBS, FRCS
Honorary Consultant Plastic Surgeon
Department of Plastic Surgery
Great Ormond Street Hospital for Children
London, United Kingdom

Antonio Sommariva, MD
Unit of Surgical Oncology of the Esophagus and Digestive Tract
Surgical Oncology
Veneto Institute of Oncology IOV-IRCCS
Padua, Italy

Brian C. Sommerlad, MBBS, DSc(Med), UCL(Hon), FRCSEng, FRCSEd(Hon), FRCPCH, FRCSLT(Hon)
Honorary Consultant Plastic Surgeon
Department of Plastic Surgery
Great Ormond Street Hospital for Children
London, United Kingdom

Catherine Soufan, MBBS
Plastic and Reconstructive Surgery Registrar
The Peter MacCallum Cancer Center
Melbourne, VIC, Australia

Derek M. Steinbacher, MD, DMD, FACS
Professor of Plastic Surgery
Department of Surgery
Director Cleft and Craniofacial Program
Yale University School of Medicine
Yale New Haven Health
New Haven, CT, United States

Ajay R. Sud, MBChB, MSc
Plastic and Reconstructive Surgery
The Canberra Hospital
Canberra, ACT, Australia

Justine Victoria Sullivan, MBBS, MRCS
Research Fellow
Plastic Surgery
St. Andrew's Centre for Plastic Surgery and Burns
Broomfield Hospital
Chelmsford, United Kingdom

Marc C. Swan, DPhil, FRCS
Consultant Plastic Surgeon
Department of Plastic Surgery
Oxford University Hospitals NHS Foundation Trust
Oxford, United Kingdom

Jin Bo Tang, MD
Professor and Chair
Department of Hand Surgery
Affiliated Hospital of Nantong University
Nantong, Jiangsu, China;
Chair
The Hand Surgery Research Center
Affiliated Hospital of Nantong University
Nantong, Jiangsu, China

Ali Totonchi, MD
Associate Professor
Case Western Reserve University
Cleveland, OH, United States;
Medical Director Craniofacial Deformity Clinic
MetroHealth Hospital
Cleveland, OH, United States

William A. Townley, BM BCh, MD, FRCS
Consultant Plastic Surgeon
Plastic and Reconstructive Surgery
Guy's and St. Thomas' NHS Foundation Trust
London, United Kingdom

Lara S. van de Lande, MD
PhD Candidate
Craniofacial Surgery
Institute of Child Health University College London
London, United Kingdom;
Craniofacial Unit
Great Ormond Street Hospital
London, United Kingdom

Renata V. Weber, MD
Clinical Assistant Professor of Surgery
Rutgers New Jersey Medical School
Newark, NJ, United States

Fu-Chan Wei, MD, FACS
Distinguished Chair Professor
Department of Plastic Surgery
Chang Gung Memorial Hospital
Chang Gung University Medical College

Paul M.N. Werker, MD, PhD, FEBOPRAS, FEBHS
Professor and Chair
Department of Plastic Surgery
University Medical Centre Groningen
Groningen, The Netherlands

Jason Wink, MD, MSc
Plastic Surgery Resident
Plastic Surgery
University of Pennsylvania
Philadelphia, PA, United States

Simon Withey, MS, FRCS, FRCS(Ed), FRCS(Plast)
Consultant Plastic and Reconstructive Surgeon
Royal Free Hospital
London, United Kingdom;
Barts Heart Centre, St Bartholomew's Hospital
London, United Kingdom

Chin Ho Wong, MBBS, MRCS(Ed), MMed(Surg), FAMS(Plast Surg)
Plastic Surgeon
W Aesthetic Plastic Surgery
Singapore

Stacy Wong, MD
Plastic Surgery
Baylor Scott & White Health – Temple
Temple, TX, United States

Yasamin Ziabari, BSc(Hons), MBBS, FRCA
Clinical Fellow
Department of Anaesthesia
The Canberra Hospital
Canberra, ACT, Australia

Susan Zoltan, MD, FACS
Clinical Instructor
Ophthalmic Plastic and Reconstructive Surgery
Icahn School of Medicine at Mount Sinai
New York, NY, United States

Fatih Zor, MD
Associate Professor
Wake Forest Institute for Regenerative Medicine
Wake Forest University
Winston-Salem, NC, United States

1

Skin Structure and Function, Wound Healing and Scarring

JUSTINE VICTORIA SULLIVAN AND SIMON MYERS

Skin Structure and Function

The integument comprises the skin together with its appendages (Figs. 1.1 and 1.2). These include hair and hair follicles, sebaceous and sweat glands, and nails. The skin covers the entire body and is the largest organ of the body. It covers a surface area of more than 1.7 m^2, making up in total about 16% of normal body weight.[1] It has an array of functions. These include acting as a barrier to physical, biological and chemical agents, as well as to ultraviolet (UV) radiation. Skin barrier function also acts to control body hydration. Other functions include: sensory and thermoregulatory roles, vitamin D synthesis, immune surveillance, excretion of wastes through sweat glands, socio-sexual communication and reproduction, by virtue of its appearance and smell (e.g. hormones and pheromones).

Skin is divided into glabrous (covering the palms of the hands and soles of the feet) and hairy skin. The skin comprises of two layers, the outermost epidermis and the innermost layer, the dermis. Embryologically, these two layers of skin are derived from the ectoderm and mesoderm, respectively. The epidermis and dermis are firmly attached to each other, and together vary in thickness from around 0.5 to 4 mm or more depending on body site. At the point where the epidermis meets the dermis, invaginations that project into the dermis are formed, known as "rete ridges" or "pegs." Complementary projections of the dermis are called dermal papillae.

Epidermis

The epidermis is defined as a stratified squamous epithelium made up of several cell types. These include melanocytes (production of melanin pigment), Langerhans cells (immune function), Merkel cells (sensory function), and keratinocytes, of which the latter make up at least 80% of its cellular population.

The epidermis is arranged into distinct layers, each showing a pattern of keratinocyte proliferation, differentiation, and maturation. Four main layers exist. These are strata basale (germinativum), spinosum, granulosum, and corneum.[1] In thick skin, a fifth layer called the stratum lucidum is present and is found between the granular and the cornified layers. These layers reflect the sequential differentiation of keratinocytes as they migrate from the basal layer at the onset of terminal differentiation, having lost the ability to proliferate, to the outermost cornified layers where they are sloughed off. The process of terminal differentiation involves a series of biochemical and morphological changes, which result in the production of an anucleated cornified keratinocyte that forms the stratum corneum. Epidermal turnover takes on average 14–30 days.

The stratum basale is a single layer of cuboidal basal cells attached to the basement membrane by hemidesmosomes that contain integrins. Adjacent cells are attached by desmosomes that contain cadherins. The majority of the cells in this layer are mitotically active and are required for the continued renewal of the epidermis by upward displacement, replacing the cells of the outermost superficial layer that are lost during normal epidermal turnover.[2] These mitotically active cells derive from a population of putative stem cells that are thought to reside in the deep rete ridges of glabrous skin and at the tips of the dermal papillae in interfollicular epidermis or in the bulge region of the outer root sheath (ORS) of adult human hair follicles in hairy skin. Also arising from stem cells in the basal layer are transit amplifying cells and post mitotic cells which are displaced into the

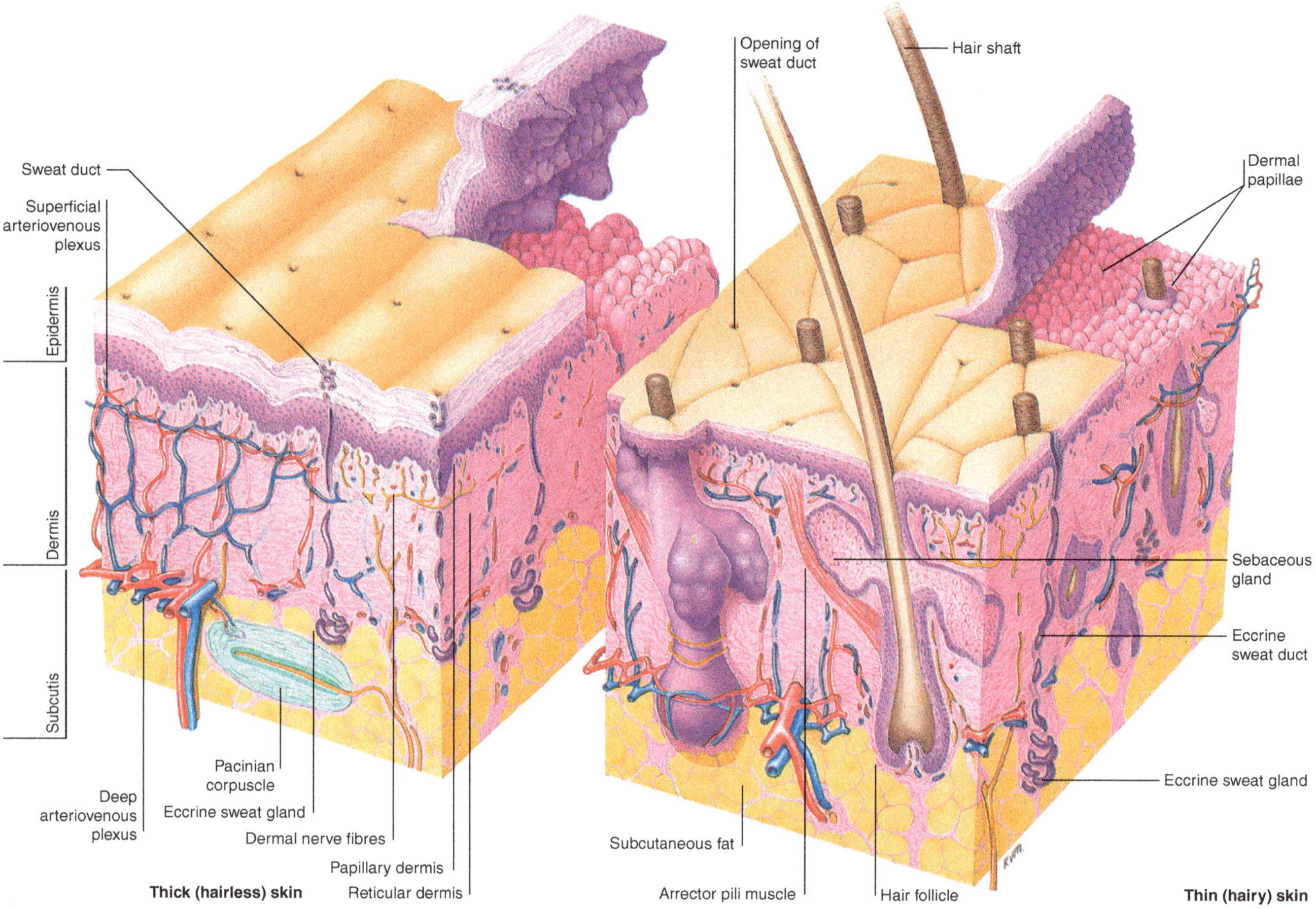

• **Fig. 1.1** Diagrammatic representation of the skin. (From Gawkrodger DJ, Ardern-Jones MR. *Dermatology: An Illustrated Colour Text*. 6th edn. Elsevier; 2017.)

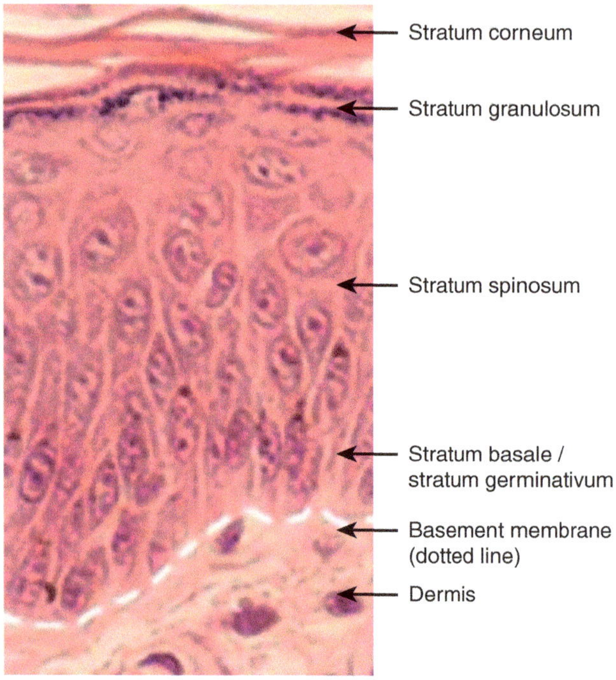

• **Fig. 1.2** Hematoxylin and eosin (H&E) histology of the skin.

suprabasal layers. Basal cells contain cytokeratins organized in bundles around the nucleus and insert into desmosomes peripherally.

Above this layer is the stratum spinosum, consisting of several layers of irregular, polyhedral shaped cells that display spiny projections. Cells from the previous layer lose contact with the basement membrane and are subsequently pushed up to form this one. Some cells in this layer are still mitotically active. Cells become progressively flattened as they move up towards succeeding layers. Cells contain lamellar granules (for the later provision of epidermal lipids responsible for the barrier properties of the stratified corneum) and more desmosomes for cell-to-cell adhesion.

The next layer, the stratum granulosum, comprises of three to five sheets of flattened cells. In this layer, as well as lamellar granules there are keratohyalin granules, which contain pro-filaggrin, a precursor of filaggrin that bundles the keratin filaments together.[2,3]

The stratum lucidum consists of several layers of flattened cells without nuclei and organelles, and a keratin-rich cytoplasm.

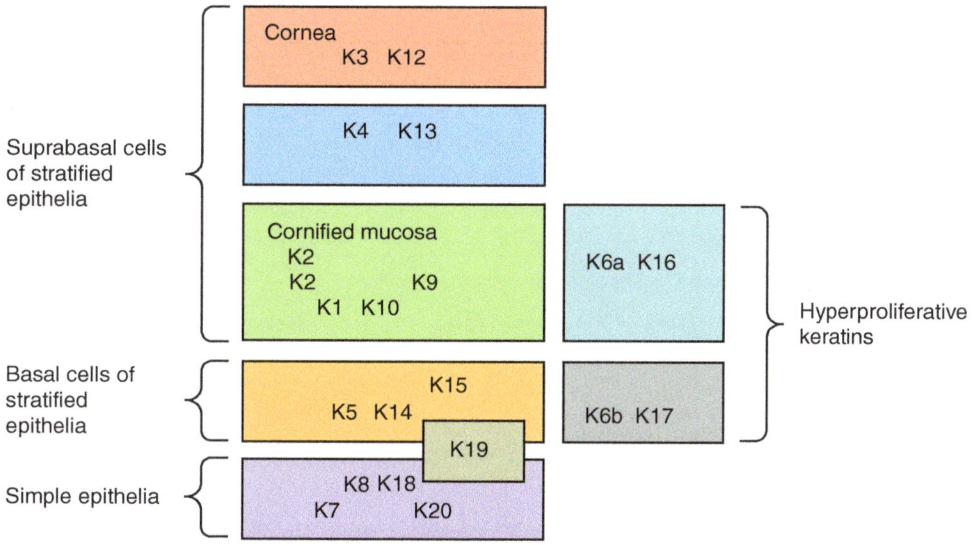

• **Fig. 1.3** Schematic representation of keratin expression in normal epithelia.

The cornified layer consists of dead, anucleated, highly keratinized cells called squames or corneocytes. Keratin filaments polymerize by forming strong disulphide bonds. Filaggrin, a protein component of the keratohyalin granule, is involved in this process. The cornified envelope forms due to the catalytic activity of the enzyme transglutaminase which crosslinks proteins such as involucrin (an insoluble 70–80 kDa cysteine rich protein) in the plasma membrane. Other proteins found as components of the cornified cell envelope include keratolinin, loricrin, small proline-rich proteins, the serine proteinase inhibitor elafin, filaggrin linker-segment peptide, and envoplakin. Lipids, discharged by lamellar granules, fill the intercellular spaces and contribute to the barrier properties of the epidermis. The lack of desmosomes in the cells that are closest to the outermost layer results in the loss or shedding of corneocytes from the skin.

Keratins

The cytoskeleton of all epithelial cells, including keratinocytes, is formed from the three groups of filaments, actin (microfilaments), tubulin (microtubules), and intermediate filaments. The keratins belong to the latter group, a multigene family of proteins that form filaments of 10 nm in diameter[4] in which keratins form the two largest groups. These groups, which comprise more than 30 members of the keratin family, have been designated as type I keratins (acidic), numbered 9–20, and type II keratins (basic), numbered 1–8. Usually, type I and type II keratin subunits pair up and the heterodimers formed are expressed according to epithelial type and in a differentiation-state specific manner. For example, in simple epithelia, keratin K8 and K18 are expressed. Cells in the basal layer of stratified epithelia express K5 and K14.[4] The differentiating suprabasal layers are characterized by the keratin pair K1 and K10. K6 and K16 are not found in normal epidermis except the outer root sheath of the hair follicle and junctional region. This keratin pair is also constitutively expressed in certain stratified squamous mucosal epithelia and the skin of the palm and sole. Expression of K6 and K16 is induced in wound healing epidermis, hyperproliferative epidermis such as psoriasis, squamous cell carcinomas, and hypertrophic scarring. Thus, keratin expression provides specific epithelial cell markers to assess epithelial proliferation and differentiation (Fig. 1.3).

The Dermo-Epidermal Junction (Basement Membrane Zone)

The basement membrane zone lies at the interface between the epidermis and the dermis and strongly attaches these layers to each other. It also serves as a support for the avascular epidermis. Four layers have been identified within the basement membrane zone. These layers are:

1. The plasma membrane of the basal keratinocyte, which is penetrated by hemidesmosomes.[3]
2. The electron-lucent lamina lucida that contains laminin, bullous pemphigoid glycoprotein, anchoring filaments and sub-basal dense plates.
3. The electron-dense lamina densa that contains collagen type IV and proteoglycans.
4. The collagen type VII rich-lamina fibroreticularis that contains anchoring fibrils (Fig. 1.4).

Fibroblasts or keratinocytes are capable of synthesizing many of the components of the basement membrane zone. However, the combination of both cell types leads to the correct assembly of the complex.

Dermis

The dermis is thicker than the epidermis and is a dense, irregular fibroelastic connective tissue composed of extracellular matrix (ECM). The dermis is composed mostly

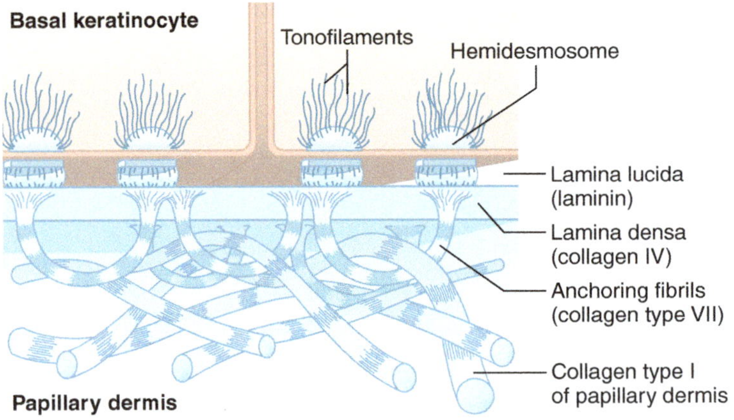

• **Fig. 1.4** The basement membrane zone.

of interwoven type I collagen with some type III collagen that provides the skin with its mechanical, tensile strength. It is subdivided into superficial papillary dermis that is in contact with the epidermis and deep reticular dermis.[1,3] The former is loosely woven and interdigitates with the epidermal ridges along the dermo-epidermal junction and contains thinner and more loosely arranged collagen and elastin fibers. It also contains more cells. The reticular dermis contains coarser and more tightly bound collagen fibers.[3] At the arbitrary plane of this division there is a subpapillary plexus of blood vessels. Other ECM components making up the dermis include the amorphous ground substance of glycosaminoglycans (GAGs), namely, hyaluronic acid, dermatan sulphate, chondroitin-6-sulphate, chondroitin-4-sulphate, and heparin sulphate. Skin appendages pass through the dermis and may extend into the underlying subcutaneous fat. The dermis also has a complex lymphatic and nerve network. The resident cell types of the dermis include fibroblasts, macrophages, and mast cells.[4]

Fibroblasts

The predominant cell type of the dermis is the fibroblast.[5] These cells synthesize and degrade connective tissue matrix proteins (dermal remodeling) and a number of proteins that provide the structural ECM and basement membrane framework. These cells migrate on and between the surfaces of collagen fiber bundles. They also promote the interaction between the epidermis and dermis by the synthesis of soluble markers that are important in the regulation of normal skin physiology as well as during wound healing. Some of these growth factors/cytokines include keratinocyte growth factors (KGF) 1 and 2, transforming growth factor-β1 (TGF-β1), platelet-derived growth factor-A (PDGF-A), vascular endothelial growth factor (VEGF), and granulocyte/macrophage colony-stimulating factor (GM-CSF), allowing fibroblasts to engage in paracrine and autocrine interactions. Fibroblasts also exist as a highly diverse population. For example, the papillary dermis and reticular dermis have distinct fibroblast subpopulations with different characteristics.

The Extracellular Matrix

The extracellular matrix (ECM), also known as the connective tissue or mesenchyme, is composed of a mixture of proteins and polysaccharides in which cells are embedded. In the dermis, the matrix macromolecules are secreted largely by fibroblasts that also help to orientate the matrix. For example, fibroblasts can bind to collagen and exert force along a fiber, re-aligning it. Both the dermis and the basement membrane of skin represent diverse forms of ECM. The ECM functions to provide structural support and tensile strength, for cell adhesion and migration, and to regulate cell behaviour, influencing their development, migration, proliferation, shape and function. The ECM is composed of two main classes of extracellular macromolecules:

1. *Structural proteins and the adhesive proteins*: among the structural proteins is collagen, the most abundant ECM component that provides tensile strength and helps to organize the matrix. Its deposition, degradation, and remodeling also appears to be tightly controlled. Elastin, another structural protein, functions to give resilience to the matrix. The adhesive proteins link components of the ECM both to one another and to the surfaces of cells. For example, laminin promotes the attachment of epithelial cells to the basement membrane, and fibronectin of fibroblasts and other cells to the ECM in the dermis.The major cell surface receptors responsible for the attachment of cells to the ECM are the transmembrane glycoproteins, integrins. The extracellular portion of integrins binds to collagens, laminins, and fibronectin; whereas the intracellular portion binds to the actin filaments of the cytoskeleton. This cytoskeleton-ECM linkage is responsible for the stability of cell–matrix junctions.
2. *Proteoglycans*: the proteoglycans are polymorphic macromolecules consisting predominantly of molecules with a core protein and glycosaminoglycan (GAG) side chain extensions with repeating disaccharide units. They are

divided into intracellular, membrane-bound, and extracellular groups. The extracellular molecules are relatively inflexible, taking up a spiral shape, and carry a negative charge, conferring hygroscopic and hydrostatic properties upon the ECM, and resist compressive forces. Proteoglycans regulate the function of several cellular processes, influencing cell proliferation and differentiation, and exert control over the behavior of the tissue as a whole under normal physiological conditions, during morphogenesis and during tissue repair processes. Some of these functions include organizing the ECM structure (GAGs and proteoglycans associate to form large complexes, for example aggregan; they can also associate with collagens and the basal lamina), ligand binding of potently active polypeptides modulating their bioactivity, cell adhesion, and transmembrane signaling.

Mesenchymal Stem Cells

The adult bone marrow contains mesenchymal stem cells (MSCs) (also known as marrow stromal cells) as well as hematopoietic stem cells (HSCs) (that generate all the blood cell lineages). MSCs are multipotent cells that have a high self-renewal capacity and give rise to many mesenchymal-derived tissues such as bone, cartilage, ligament, muscle tendon, adipose and marrow stroma. Human MSCs are fractionated from bone marrow aspirates by density centrifugation, collected from the density interface and cultured in the presence of fetal bovine serum specific for their expansion. The resulting cells in culture are a phenotypically homogeneous population. Human MSCs express surface antigens such as CD44, CD29, CD71 as analysed by flow cytometric analysis and are positive for the human MSC-specific antibodies such as SH-2 (for CD105) and SB-10 (for CD166). In vitro, these cells have been shown to undergo adipogenic, chondrogenic, and osteogenic differentiation depending on culture conditions.[6]

Epithelial/Mesenchymal Interactions

Evidence is accumulating that the mesenchyme plays a crucial role in epidermal homeostasis.[7] It is known that the epidermis, in turn, can influence the dermis with regards to structural remodeling, reinnervation, and vascularization. These epithelial/mesenchymal interactions are orchestrated by a complex network of communications between cell–matrix, cell–cell, and cell-diffusible factors.

The hair follicle provides a good system to study epithelial/mesenchymal interactions. For instance, the size and position of the developing hair follicles is determined by direct mesenchymal signals. Signaling between the dermal papilla and hair follicle epithelium is crucial for hair follicle development and function. The mesenchyme determines the fate of the epithelium. For example, the formation of epidermis and hair follicles is induced when cultured rabbit corneal epithelium is combined with embryonic hair-forming mouse dermis.

An understanding of the epithelial/mesenchymal interactions that takes place in skin arose from wound healing studies. Initially, Rheinwald and Green in 1975 showed the improved growth rates of keratinocytes grown on an irradiated mouse fibroblast feeder layer.[8] Since then, the importance of a dermal component for the improved clinical take of cultured epithelium has been well documented. In vitro skin models have been used to study the importance of epithelial/mesenchymal interactions.[9] Such organotypic cultures are composed of keratinocytes and mesenchymal cells grown in vitro on an extracellular matrix, and at an air–liquid interface to induce epidermal differentiation. They share similarities with wound healing, hyperproliferative and psoriatic skin, and have demonstrated the importance of epithelial/mesenchymal interactions in a number of processes including: epidermal homeostasis, production and deposition of basement membrane and ECM components, and secretion of diffusible factors.

Skin Aging

Aging occurs due to a combination of intrinsic and extrinsic causes. Intrinsic causes are due to less collagen and elastin being produced as a person ages, resulting in more fragile and thinner skin, thus forming wrinkles later in life. Dermatoporosis was first put forward as the name for chronic cutaneous fragility of the skin by Kaya and Saurat in 2007.[10] With aging the epidermis thins as it develops rete ridges due to keratinocytes losing the ability to proliferate effectively and the epidermal turnover is slower. The dermis loses volume due to loss of hyaluronic acid (HA) in the extracellular matrix and the collagen is more disorganized, seeing an increase in the ratio of type 3 compared to type 1 collagen. Delayed wound healing is a prominent feature of aging skin. The reduced HA leaves the skin more vulnerable to tears following minimal trauma. Extrinsic factors include: sun (UV radiation) and environmental damage, such as tobacco smoking. Several studies have shown that cigarette smoke furthers wrinkle formation, nicotine also induces expression of matrix metalloproteinases which degrade the extracellular matrix in human skin. Severe sun damage causes epidermal atrophy, which is histopathologically distinguished by solar elastosis (degraded dermal elastic tissue).

Type 1 – Classical Cutaneous Wound Healing

A wound, in the context of skin, is a breach in the barrier that distinguishes an organism from its environment. The process through which the organism works in order to address this breach is "wound healing," which, due to the important role the skin plays for the survival of the organism, is quite literally vital, and conserved through evolution. In the normal course of events, a lower species accepts tissue loss and heals a wound by exposure, licking, picking, and at the molecular level, scarring. The single most important

TABLE 1.1 A Revised Wound Classification Based on Clinical Management and Outcome

	Wound ± Intervention	Character Healing
Type I: Classical		
a) "Normal"/pimary incisional – incisional, no tissue loss	i) Closed early (<48 h)	Low risk of infection Minimal line scar
	ii) Closed late (>48 h)	Increased risk infection Increased risk chronicity More significant scar
	iii) Unclosed	Healing by granulation (similar to Type Ibii), but in absence of tissue loss) High-risk chronicity
b) "Normal"/secondary excisional – tangential tissue loss, no replacement	i) Above mid-dermis	Rapid re-epithelialization (<10 days) Minimal clinical scar
	ii) Below mid-dermis	Slow/absent re-epithelialization High risk of infection and chronicity Closure by scar
Type II: Neo-classical		
a) "Supranormal" by skin replacement	i) Early split- or full-thickness skin grafting of Type Ibii	Present gold standards Cosmetic and functional problems remain Donor defect
	ii) Biotechnological skin replacements (Cuono technique, in vitro composite grafts)	Ideally autologous and with viable cellular elements Opportunity to improve on Types Ibii and IIai
b) "Supranormal" with apparent acceptance of tissue loss	i) Type Ibi treated with CKAllo or vapour permeable membrane	Follicle recruitment by activated extended follicle units
	ii) Chronic full-thickness wound treated with CKAllo or vapour permeable membrane	Simulation of an acute wound environment

impact on wound healing by man has been the early closure of wounds, by apposition with sutures in incisional wounds, and skin replacement in excisional wounds. Humans can deny significant skin and composite tissue loss by a "like for like" replacement in the specialty of plastic and reconstructive surgery, and here we can boast a form of "supranormal wound healing."[11]

Wound Healing Classifications

There are many ways to classify wound healing. In simple terms, we can consider four phases – coagulation, inflammation, fibroplasia, and remodeling; four types – fetal, adult, acute, and chronic; four ages – young, plateau, regressing, atrophic; and two systems of healing – epidermal and dermal. We can also classify wound healing in terms of clinical features and their wound management (Table 1.1).

Phases of Wound Healing

Wound healing can be considered a process of four sequential but overlapping phases by which the body closes a breach in tissue continuity. There are many ways to define such a complex process. Key to understanding the standard classification of the process is a consideration of: the timing, the cellular activation or influx, and the chemical mediators.

Coagulation

This *immediate* response to cutaneous injury involves two cascades: the clotting cascade, with the formation of platelet clot which adheres to the collagen exposed following endothelial disruption; and the complement cascade and complement-mediated vasodilatation. Histamine released by mast cell degranulation, and kinins, contribute to vasodilatation and increased vascular permeability. The first cells involved then are platelets and mast cells, and the first mediators histamine, kinins, PDGF and TGF-β. The increasing interest in platelet-rich plasma (PRP) clinically in regenerative medicine is based on these early cascades.

Inflammation

Between the time of injury and around 4 days post injury, the clinical signs of inflammation develop. Classically these are redness, swelling, pain, and loss of function. These result from inflammatory mediators, and the capillary leak into the extracellular space that they coordinate. The next inflammatory cell type to arrive at the wound is the macrophage, followed by neutrophils, and then lymphocytes. Keratinocytes in the wound edge and follicle remnants migrate and proliferate, and fibroblasts are chemoattracted, and become activated.

Fibroplasia

From day 4, and for 2–4 weeks, the wound bed becomes vascularized, and type III collagen is laid down by fibroblasts to replace any dermal loss. In theabsence of epidermal cover, this appears clinically as granulation tissue. Closed wounds become red and raised for a while. Hydrated glycosaminoglycans form a ground substance for the collagen fibrils. This phase is characterized by fibroblast proliferation, but also by keratinocyte proliferation.

Remodeling

From a few weeks to 18 or more, the wound goes through a long phase of remodeling. Fibroblasts mature into myofibroblasts to contract the wound. Type III collagen is gradually replaced by type I collagen. Disorganized collagen becomes lamellar.

Repair vs. Regeneration

There are significant differences between the wound healing seen in fetal life and that seen in postnatal life. So-called scarless healing occurs for a period in the fetus, however this is not absolute but gestational age- and wound size-dependent.[12] In late fetal life scarring does occur, and before this point in time, a large enough wound will still result in scarring. In postnatal life, scarring is the inevitable and permanent consequence of a wounding beyond the epidermal basement membrane. An adult lower vertebrate like a salamander can regenerate an amputated limb, but won't aspire to climb Mount Everest! Whilst regenerative medicine attempts to harness the same plasticity seen in lower vertebrate regeneration, what is generally achieved is only "partial regeneration," and not replacement of like with like. The ongoing concern in manipulating adult/somatic stem cells to achieve true regeneration, is that of a loss of control and the risk of carcinogenesis.

Acute vs. Chronic Wound Healing

Acute wound healing is hard to distinguish absolutely from chronic wound healing, and the processes at a cell and molecular level may be similar. Chronic wound healing occurs when healing takes longer than might be anticipated in a fit healthy person, and is often associated with comorbidity. Such wounds seem to become stuck in the inflammatory or proliferative/fibroplastic phases. Local wound management can only usefully begin following an assessment and optimization of systemic comorbid conditions.

Epithelial/Epidermal vs. Mesenchymal/Dermal Wound Healing

The epidermis provides the ultimate barrier between the body and environment. The main cell type is the keratinocyte. Regeneration occurs from a population of follicle stem cells.[13] The dermis provides the structural support to the epidermis and other related adnexae. The main dermal cell type is the fibroblast. As in embryogenesis, there is ongoing "cross-talk" between the epidermis and dermis in somatic cutaneous wound healing, the epidermal element of which has been relatively underplayed. Even less consideration has given to the contribution of subcutaneous fat to cross-talk.

Wound Healing and Scarring

In many ways, wound healing and scarring are inseparable – the one leads to the other at some level, and over time. When does a wound become a scar? That will probably depend at a molecular level on very early wounding and wound management events. Whilst a scar is, again, the inevitable and permanent consequence of post-natal wounding beyond the basement membrane, and a compromise between regeneration and repair, at a clinical level, its significance is largely patient-related and subjective. This can now be captured clinically by the patient and observer scar assessment score (POSAS), which draws patients into their own management.[14]

Most patients would perceive a wound as a scar from the time that the wound is no longer open, and often that equates to the absence of exudate and any requirement for dressing care. Clinically, even a normotrophic scar will go through a natural progression to maturity. When young, it will be active. Most young scars exhibit features of hypertrophy. Most scars then go through a plateau period of relatively little clinical change in the absence of treatment. Most scars then go through a period of regression of inflammatory signs and symptoms, and eventually settle to a mature state. Some scars, after many months or years, and sometimes because of treatment, become very thin, pale, and atrophic.

When then does a normotrophic scar become a pathological scar? A normotrophic scar results from uneventful primary healing, but there is wide variation with age, site, and skin type, and a period of hypertrophy is not unusual. Hypertrophic scarring is classically seen in pediatric burn wounds that have struggled to heal. The scar becomes red, raised, painful, and itchy around 2–3 months following wound closure, particularly in wounds that have taken more than 3 weeks to heal. The scar settles over 18 months to 2 years, but often incompletely. Hypertrophic scars occur particularly in extreme Fitzpatrick skin types. Presumably, there is a bell curve distribution within the population, where those at the extreme end of hypertrophic scarring could be termed pathological. Hypertrophic scars do not spread outside the line of original tissue injury, being elevated and more visible scars characterized by excessive deposition of fibroblast-derived extracellular matrix proteins with persistent inflammation and fibrosis, containing mostly type III collagen orientated parallel to the epidermal surface. Over time they often spontaneously regress. Histologically, hypertrophic scarring shows a flattening of the epidermis and replacement of reticular dermis by scar tissue with prominent vertically oriented blood vessels. It is rare for the elderly to develop hypertrophic scarring, which is seen predominantly in 10–30-year-olds. Whilst a keloid scar shares many of the features of a hypertrophic scar, and may represent an extreme example of the same, it is defined by extension beyond the confines of the injury, by almost inevitable progression beyond 2 years, seldom regressing; by being refractory to most treatments, and recurring within 4–6 months of cessation of most treatments; behaving pathologically like a benign tumour. Keloid scars are predominantly composed of abnormal thick disorganized type I and typer III collagen bundles and overproduction of fibroblast proteins. They fail to downregulate wound-healing cells. Histologically, keloids show no flattening of the overlying epirdemis or scarring of the papillary dermis, with the presence of significant keloidal collagen. There is an absence of prominent vertically-orientated blood vessels with significant disarray of fibrocollagenous fascicles. Keloid scarring is more common in darker skin. There are a range of different treatment options but there is no definitive “best treatment.” Treatments range from surgical excision (but in keloids there is an increased risk of recurrence), pressure therapy, steroid treatments, laser and radiotherapy. Surgical excision alone has a high rate of recurrence of around 50%, it is improved slightly with use of intralesional corticosteroid injection into the newly excised scar. Intralesional steroids used alone usually require multiple treatments; they suppress inflammation and mitosis while increasing vasoconstriction of the scar; For example, triamcinolone acetonide will eventually flatten around 50–100% of keloids with a 9–50% recurrence rate.

Epidermal Wound Healing

Adult epidermal stem cell biology is relatively well understood. Keratinocyte stem cells reside primarily in the bulge region of the hair follicle, and, by asymmetric division, populate the interfollicular basement membrane with transit amplifying cells. These divide a number of times to provide the differentiating cells of the stratifying epidermis. A huge array of small peptides are involved in coordinating the response to epidermal wounding by autocrine, paracrine, and juxtacrine signaling. In a human model of epidermal healing, a number of phases of keratinocyte activity are suggested[15] (Fig. 1.5).

Acute Activation

Almost immediately following wounding, the epidermis expresses interleukin 1β [IL-1β] and interleukin 6 [IL-6], and the dermis transforming growth factor β1 [TGF-β1], committing transit amplifying cells to mitosis. Whilst TGB-β1 is antiproliferative, it is pro-migratory to keratinocytes.[16]

Early Activation

Towards 24 hours following wounding, keratinocyte proliferation and migration are clear. Epidermal expression of transforming growth factor α [TGF-α] and IL-6 is accompanied by dermal fibroblast keratinocyte growth factor [KGF] and IL-6 expression. A paracrine loop of epidermal IL-1β induction of the potent keratinocyte mitogen KGF from dermal fibroblasts seems likely.[17] TGF-α is both a keratinocyte mitogen and induces the migratory K6/K16 keratinocyte cytoskeletal phenotype in the suprabasal compartment. It may also recruit nearby follicles by juxtacrine signaling.[18]

Restitution

Over weeks, homeostasis is restored, with relatively late activation of the bulge to restore the transit amplifying population.

Dermal Wound Healing

Wound healing studies have concentrated far more on the dermis than epidermis, and particularly on macrophage production of TGF-β isoforms. This multifunctional growth factor appears to play a key role in dermal healing and scarring.[19] Whilst the TGF-β1 isoform promotes scarring, the TGF-β3 isoform appears to have the opposite effect.[20] TGF-β, however, remains a key pharmaceutical target.

A preoccupation with one growth factor, albeit a powerful, multifunctional factor with isoforms of different action, and for each a dose-dependent heterogeneity of responses, is arguably to ignore the complexity of wound healing cascades. There are many factors at play, often pleiotropic, and there is significant redundancy – so that many factors can contribute to the same outcome – i.e. rapid closure by scar. The growth factor that has shown most promise when delivered alone is platelet-derived growth factor (PDGF).[21]

The dermis is far more than an extracellular matrix populated by fibroblasts. It hosts a vascular network – arterial, venous and lymphatic, neural network, and supports the follicle and other adnexal stem cell niches. It must also, it seems, interact with the subcutaneous fat. One approach to tissue engineering to provide for wound tissue loss is to synthesize an appropriate nanotechnology scaffold for key cellular elements to populate and develop. This can be *biofunctionalized* by incorporating a latent growth factor.[22]

“Normal”/Primary Incisional Wound Healing (Type 1a)

Incisional wound healing occurs following surgical access, or “incisional” or lacerating trauma. In the former, the wound will begin sterile, and in the latter, some degree of contamination is usual. In neither instance is there significant tissue loss. Classically, in modern medical practice, these wounds are formally closed, although the timing of that closure will vary, and affect the quality of the healing processes, and the scar that results.

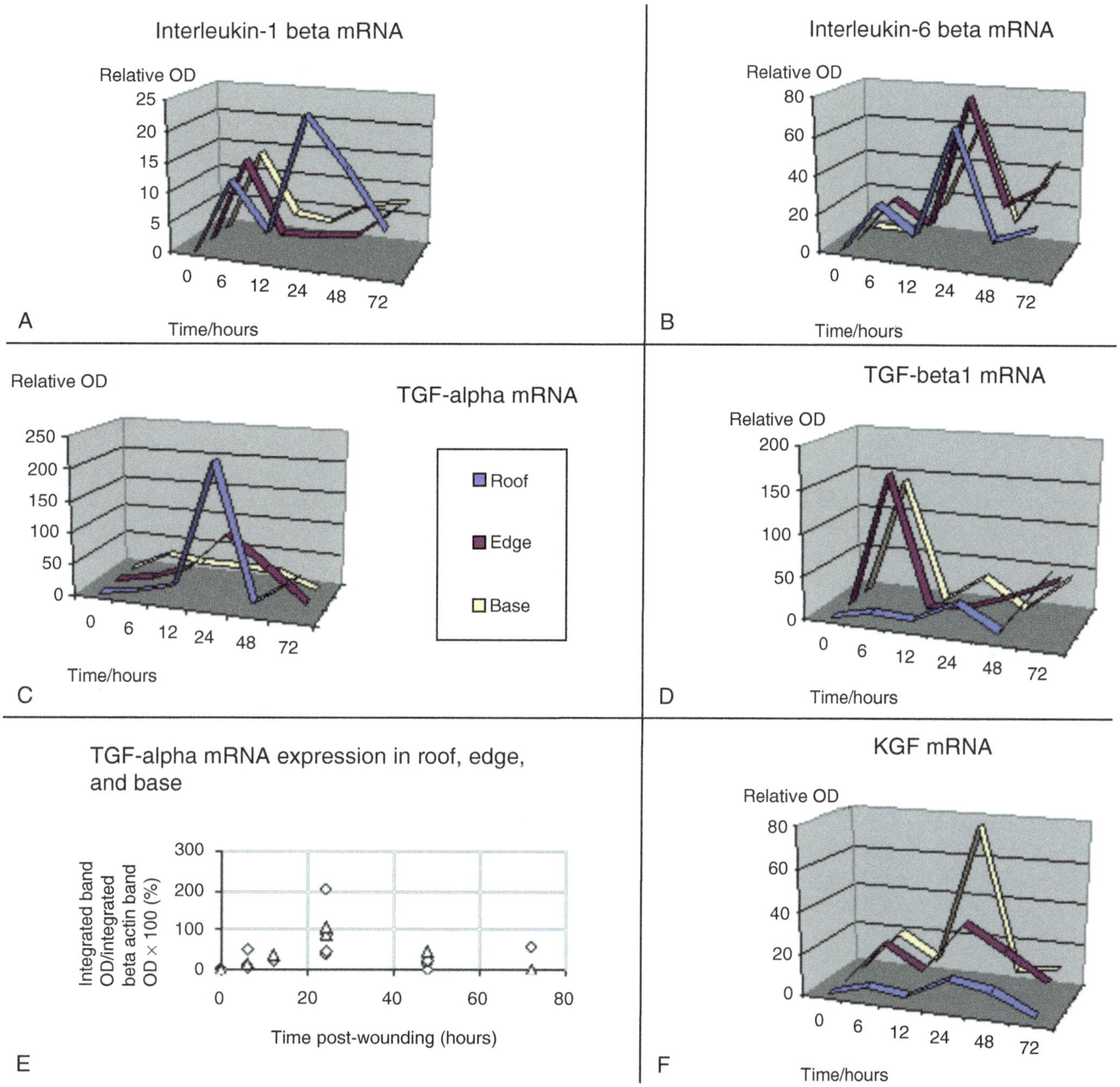

• **Fig. 1.5** Temporospatial cytokine and growth factor gene expression in human suction blister wound healing.

Early Closure (Type 1ai)

If an incisional wound is closed directly, the healing will tend to be optimal. Elective surgical wounds are closed at the end of the procedure performed under sterile conditions. Traumatic lacerating wounds will generally be cleaned and closed the same day, and before significant bacterial colonization occurs. A relatively arbitrary time limit to early closure has evolved in practice of 48 hours from injury. Beyond this, it is considered likely that colonization may be significant enough to deleteriously affect healing, and as a consequence the quality of scarring, which may become hypertrophic.

Late Closure (Type 1aii)

If a type 1a wound is sutured after 48 hours, wound colonization may result in infection, dehiscence, and delayed healing. Counter-intuitively, according to current dogma, if the wound is left open until day 4 or 5, as in "delayed primary closure," satisfactory results can be achieved at a stage when the inflammatory response has become established – although a recent Cochrane Review found no evidence for this.[23]

No Closure (Type 1aiii)

An incisional wound beyond the epidermal basement membrane that is left unclosed will gape and behave much like a deep excisional wound, healing by classical "secondary intent." The time to healing will be slow, because closure will rely on wound base contraction and edge re-epithelialization. As a consequence the quality of the scar will tend to "pathological."

"Normal"/Secondary Excisional Wound Healing (Type 1b)

Where surgery requires skin excision, or cutaneous trauma is tangential – e.g., burn injury, or friction loss – and the tissue loss is not replaced, then the time to healing and the scar quality will depend on the depth of the loss. Re-epithelialization and restoration of barrier function from adnexal remnants will be slower, the deeper the injury.

Above Mid-Dermis (Type 1bi)

Tangential tissue loss above the mid-dermis leaves a partial-thickness wound that will heal in around one week under ideal circumstances, and result in a "controllable" scar – as in the surgical split-thickness skin graft donor site. If a traumatic tangential injury clearly reaches the mid-dermis acutely, i.e. a mid-dermal burn injury, then optimal wound management is key to prevent extension of the tissue loss to type 1bii. In extreme Fitzpatrick types, even these type 1bi wounds can scar pathologically.

Below Mid-Dermis (Type 1bii)

Tangential tissue loss below the mid-dermis leaves a partial-thickness wound that will take 3 weeks or more to heal, and as a consequence will be more liable to chronicity and significant scarring. It is at this depth, or beyond, that intervention is considered. A full-thickness defect can only re-epithelialize from the wound edge, and will otherwise close substantially by scar contraction of the base.

Abnormal Wound Healing

Systemic and local factors may reduce the quality of the skin and/or affect wound healing adversely. These are important to recognize and optimize.

Systemic Factors

Systemic factors may be congenital or acquired. There are a handful of congenital conditions that affect the processes of healing, and in some instances the clinical quality of the skin and healing. A range of defects in collagen synthesis is seen in Ehlers–Danlos syndrome (EDS), Marfan's disease (MD) and epidermolysis bullosa (EB). EDS and MD are inherited multisystemic disorders primarily affecting the soft connective tissues with overlapping cutaneous features.

EDS is characterized by joint hypermobility, skin hyperextensibility, atrophic scarring, and general tissue frailty; There are many different subtypes. Patients with this condition have defects in collagen proteins and collagen-modifying enzymes. MD is autosomal dominant and affects an array of different systems in the body including the cardiovascular system and skeletal system (for example long bone overgrowth). A cutaneous feature is striae distensae occurring with no significant body size changes such as weight gain or pregnancy.

The skin is vulnerable, and healing slow in EB, a feature is minor trauma causing erosions and blister formation. This is due to mutation in the genes coding for proteins to the epidermis; for example, in the junctional variant, laminin 5 is deficient in the epidermal basement membrane zone. The premature aging condition, progeria, manifests many features of normal "acquired" aging. There are many different types, including: epidermolysis bullosa simplex (EBS), the commonest and often milder form where blistering occurs in the epidermis due to lack of adhesion of the skin directly to the basement membrane. It is an autosomal dominant condition and may be more localized (hands) or involve the whole body (generalized EBS). Dystrophic epidermolysis bullosa (DEB) blistering occurs in the lamina densa, which results in scarring of healed wounds causing joint contraction, digit fusion, contraction of mouth membranes and narrowing of the oesophagus. This form can be inherited in a recessive or dominant manner, often the recessive from being a more severe condition. This condition also increases the patient's risk of developing squamous cell carcinoma.

There have been some recent advances in treatment, such as a 7-year-old boy who received whole body grafting of genetically modified stem cells to treat EB. A virus was used as a vector to replace the defective gene "*LAMB3*" in a sample of the boy's skin, this was then used to grow large sheets of skin in the lab which was then skin grafted onto the child. Whereas the boy was previously in hospital, he was able to get back to the normal activities of daily living. So far this approach is only suitable for a subset of EB types.

With age, the changes in healing processes are fairly global, resulting in a delay in wound closure, and a reduction in wound strength. How much these changes are the result of increasing co-morbidities associated with age, rather than age itself, is not entirely clear. Other acquired, systemic factors include: nutrition, drugs, diabetes, and smoking. Vitamin C deficiency is the classic example of a nutritional factor, although scurvy is not likely with Western diets. Vitamin C is an essential cofactor for collagen synthesis. Vitamin A deficiency is again rare, but vitamin A can reverse steroid-induced collagenase activity. Zinc is important to many enzyme systems, and deficiency can be seen in large burn injury. In those same injuries, albumin can plummet to around 10g/L, and although this will delay healing, closure can be achieved.

Obesity is epidemic now in the Western world, and associated with many comorbidities and wound complications following surgery. Post-bariatric surgery plastic surgery reconstructions are challenging. Large blood vessels will have developed to support the tissue volume, and these may contribute to postoperative bleeding complications. Despite these hypertrophic vessels, tissue perfusion may be poor, and the tissue lymphedematous and critically colonized. Furthermore, closure after such excisional surgery is by definition under tension, so that infection and dehiscence are more common.

Antiinflammatory systemic glucocorticoids, nonsteroidal antiinflammatory drugs, and chemotherapy drugs globally suppress the cellular responses to wounding. Chemotherapeutic angiogenesis inhibitors, such as bevacizumab, a vascular endothelial growth factor neutralizing antibody fragment used in colonic cancer, cannot be prescribed 6 weeks before or after surgery to limit the wound healing risks.[24]

Diabetes mellitus may affect healing in a variety of complex ways, evident particularly at the lower limbs. Patients are susceptible to atherosclerosis in larger vessels, and tissue oxygen delivery is further reduced by the stiffness of the red blood cells, and the higher oxygen affinity of glycosylated hemoglobin. These effects are compounded by any neuropathy; and impaired cellular immunity, phagocytosis, and bacterial killing.

Smoking may affect wound healing in an immediate, and longer-term way. Nicotine causes sympathetic vasoconstriction, and carbon monoxide shifts the oxygen dissociation curve to the left. Long-term smoking accelerates atherosclerotic changes. Smoking appears to be a particular problem in surgery to superficial soft tissue planes, where wide skin undermining with the sacrifice of multiple perforators, and closure under tension are combined, as in abdominoplasty surgery.

Local Factors

One of the most controllable local factors for incisional wounds is surgical technique and the handling of tissue. Tissue handling within the specialty can be observed, *par excellence*, under the microscope during a microvascular anastomosis, where poor handling results in anastomotic thrombosis. Local factors often reflect systemic comorbidities, so that poor blood supply and oxygen delivery, and even critical bacterial colonization are more often than not a local manifestation of a systemic factor. Conversely, the radiotherapy that results in local thromboendarteritis obliterans and causes healing problems over time, may also have systemic effects. In terms of recurrence, radiotherapy is the most effective treatment for keloid scars, damping down the "overhealing" provided it follows extralesional excision directly. Breaches in the skin are inevitably colonized by commensals. With time and increasing bacterial number, the body mounts an inflammatory response, and the colonization is termed critical. Critical colonization is not anticipated until around 48 hours as a rule of thumb. Once 10^5 organisms are present per gram of tissue, the wound may be considered infected. Chronicity and some level of colonization go hand in hand. Bacterial biofilms are prevalent in chronic wounds, including anerobic organisms not isolated by standard culture systems, and this is an area of particular current interest in such wounds – and also, of course, in subcutaneous/cavity wounding and scarring, e.g. breast capsular contracture.

Mechanotransduction

There is a sense that the skin is constantly subclinically injured to some degree by sheer forces, and indeed even the force of gravity. That may drive the baseline turnover of the skin. The effects of physicomechanical forces on cell behavior, *mechanotransduction*, are becoming increasingly recognized and understood in wound healing.[25] In 1861, Karl Langer observed that the skin exhibits intrinsic tension,[26] and Langer's lines, defined by the direction in which circular excisional wounds will elongate to ellipses by anatomic site, are used today to orientate excisional surgery. *Tensegrity* describes the way in which mechanical forces regulate biological systems via perturbations in structural architecture — disruption of tensional integrity triggers cellular pathways that restore mechanical homeostasis.[27] Cells also actively generate intracellular tension, *cell traction forces*, as they interact with their environment during, for example, migration. A cell-centric view of mechanotransduction is, however, inadequate. Conformational changes in the extracellular matrix by mechanical forces can reveal cryptic binding sites, and expose growth factors. Nonstructural, extracellular, *matricellular* proteins, e.g. connective tissue growth factor, are increasingly implicated in the regulation of healing and scar formation.[28] Mechanosensing in the skin is a feature not just of fibroblasts, but keratinocytes and nociceptors. It is quite possible that physical cues during wound healing direct, in part, stem cell fate within that niche.

Any therapeutic effects of silicone gels, pressure garments, and linear taping, may work through mechanical offloading and mechanotransduction pathways. The use of Botox A to control tension across healing facial scars and improve scar quality is an interesting new approach.[29] Vacuum-assisted closure has become a common approach to complex wound management, and whilst poorly understood, must rely to a large extent on mechanotransduction.

Type 2 – Neoclassical Cutaneous Wound Healing

"Supranormal" Healing by Skin Replacement (Type 2a)

Classically, intervention to close a wound was sometimes considered "tertiary" wound healing. The great variety of techniques now available suggest a more structured classification.

Early Split-Thickness or Full-Thickness Skin Grafting of Type 1bii (Type 2ai)

Those tangential traumatic or excisional wounds that are unlikely to heal in a reasonable timescale, and therefore scar, are most commonly closed with split-thickness skin autograft. Where the wound is full-thickness, the environment optimal, and the defect limited in size, a full-thickness autograft will provide a superior reconstruction. Of course, any number of local and distant skin and fasciocutaneous flaps are considered for defects that have resulted in an ungraftable bed, and this category of skin replacement feeds into other classifications of flap reconstruction. Skin and fasciocutaneous free flaps are increasingly being used to close defects in hostile comorbid conditions, e.g. in "vasculoplastics" practice.

Biotechnological Skin Replacements (Type 2aii)

In recent years, products, often xenograft in nature, have been developed to provide the quality of a full-thickness graft reconstruction from a split-thickness skin graft donor site. "Dermal regeneration templates" like Integra engraft to provide a "neodermis" to support a thin autograft in two operative stages.[30] A single-stage Integra system has been available following the success of single-stage Matriderm grafting. Included here also is the Cuono system that combines allograft dermis with autologous cultured keratinocytes in the closure of full-thickness burn excision beds.[31] Cultured keratinocyte technology represents one of the most established forms of somatic stem cell therapy, and sits most coherently within plastic and reconstructive surgery.

"Supranormal" Healing with Apparent Acceptance of Tissue Loss (Type 2b)

When tangential tissue loss is accepted and no apparent attempt is made to replace like with like to the level of loss, then there are still interventions that seem to present some clinical advantage. George Winter presented his understanding of tangential wound healing in a porcine partial-thickness excisional model that included both edge and base contributions to restoration of epidermal barrier function, and introduced the world to the concept of "moist wound healing" that spawned a massive industry in moist wound healing dressing systems – initially vapour-permeable membranes. Whilst this transformed the "dry" wound management of the time, it has not proven a panacea, and far more sophisticated biological systems have evolved since (see below). The clinical evidence base for these, however, has been slow to evolve on a cost basis, and so marketplaces have yet to develop around economy of scale.

Type 1bi Treated with Cultured Keratinocyte Allograft or Biological Dressing (Type 2bi)

Cultured keratinocyte allografts have been used for decades to accelerate partial-thickness wound healing. Whilst they do not survive transplantation long term, they present a temporary and coordinated "growth factor factory." It may also be that they provide a juxtacrine mechanism for "discontinuous follicle recruitment" by bridging adnexal remnants separated by tangential partial-thickness wounding.[15] Biobrane is a conforming bilayer of porcine collagen and nylon. It is at least hemostatic, and adheres to a clean partial-thickness wound until shed when the epidermal barrier has been restored. The evidence for its efficacy and detail of any mechanism has never been established, but a role for the limitation of colonization of adherence seems likely.

Chronic Full-Thickness Wound Treated with Cultured Keratinocyte Allograft or Biological Dressing (Type 2bii)

Chronic full-thickness wounds are a huge financial burden to any healthcare system, and generally associated with comorbidity. Any comorbid condition should be optimized in the first instance. There then may be some further benefit from cell-based therapy or biological dressings. Both cultured keratinocyte allografts and autografts have been used to treat such wounds. It is suggested that even with poor clinical autograft take, a more acute healing picture is seen, at least clinically – healing is "kick-started." The wound bed can be modulated with, for example, hyaluronic acid, an important component of the embryonic extracellular matrix, to improve clinical take, perhaps by supporting a niche-like stem cell environment.[32]

Bone Healing

It is important to note there are two processes by which bone heals following trauma: direct intramembranous bone formation, which, in order to occur, requires anatomical reduction or the commonest type; and indirect fracture healing, which is a combination of both intramembranous and endochondral bone formation.

After trauma a hematoma is formed and acute inflammation causes this to coagulate around the fracture ends to form the foundation for callus formation. Inflammatory mediators involved include interleukin-6 produced by osteoblasts that promote production of primary cartilaginous callus and angiogenesis. Mesenchymal stem cells are then recruited and proliferate into osteogenic cells to create bony callus.

In endochondral bone formation the hematoma is replaced with fibrin-rich granulation tissue which then forms a soft cartilaginous callus to provide some stability to the fracture. This process takes about 8 days. At the same time the intramembranous ossification is occurring subperiosteally, adjacent to the fracture site, creating a hard callus to bridge the gap. This hard callus then undergoes mineralization, resorption, and subsequently revascularization, which occurs via two pathways; the angiopoietin-dependent pathway and the vascular endothelial growth factor (VEGF)-dependent pathway. The bone then remodels the hard callus into a lamellar bone structure with a central medullary cavity.

Fat

There has been a huge recent interest in fat grafting, not only for augmentation including following subcision of indented scars and scar-related fat atrophy, but also to improve healing and the quality of overlying scar. It is fascinating to reflect that Sir Harold Gillies may have used whole fat grafts in acute closure of craniofacial traumatic wounds with the same intent many decades ago.[33] It has been suggested that any effect on healing and scarring results not from the grafted fat directly, much of which is lost, but from stimulation of a local mesenchymal stem cell response. The current controversy is around the method of enrichment of autologous fat to provide safe augmentation long term, and the resolution of this will run parallel, with resolution of controversy around any effect on healing and scarring. A recent randomized controlled study in normal human volunteers demonstrated that enrichment of autologous fat with cultured autologous adipose-derived stem cells was significantly more effective, in graft survival terms, than a more standard approach.[34]

Lymphedema

Lower limb lymphovenous disease is a recognized cause of recurrent cellulitis and chronic wound healing. There is a newly recognized patient base in the morbid obese and post-bariatric population, and with the evolution of supra-microsurgical techniques, the promise of new therapies, e.g. lymphovenous anastomosis and lymph node transplantation.[35]

The Future

Modern genomic and proteomic techniques allow us to define the processes that control tissue volume and its nature in healing at a molecular level – broadly: migration, proliferation, differentiation, and apoptosis. Those techniques require very little material from biopsy, and we should expect to see more evidence from controlled longitudinal, human studies available to support our understanding of the different types of healing. The sheer complexity of the pathways and interactions within countless networks will require a systiomics, or systems biology, approach calling on applied mathematics and computer modeling. Resources to support controlled human studies of wound healing and interventions are limited in part by a perception that the area is mundane. There are, however, many gaps in our basic understanding of what are quite fundamental processes. Cell-based therapies are expensive, but will continue to offer the most rationale wound management solutions until our understanding is more complete. Longitudinal cost–benefit analyses of novel therapies remain few and far between.

References

1. Roger M, Fullard N, Costello L, et al. Bioengineering the microanatomy of human skin. *J Anat.* 2019;234(4):438–455.
2. Yousef H, Alhajj M, Sharma S. *Anatomy, Skin (Integument), Epidermis*; 2020. StatPearls [Internet]. PMID: 29262154.
3. Losquadro WD. Anatomy of the skin and the pathogenesis of nonmelanoma skin cancer. *Facial Plast Surg Clin North Am.* 2017;25(3):283–289.
4. Wang G, Zieman A, Coulombe PA. Skin keratins. *Methods Enzymol.* 2015;568:303–350.
5. Thulabandu V, Chen D, Atit RP. Dermal fbroblast in cutaneous development and healing. *WIREs Dev Biol.* 2018;7(2).
6. Song SJ, Jeon O, Yang HS, et al. Effexts of culture conditions on osteogenic differentiation in human mesenchymal stem cells. *J Microbiol Biotechnol.* 2007;17(7):1113–1119.
7. Blanpain C, Fuchs E. Epidermal homeostasis: a balancing act of stem cells in the skin. *Nat Rev Mol Cell Biol.* 2009;10(3):207–217.
8. Rheinwald JG, Green H. Epidermal growth factor and the multiplication of human epidermal keratinocytes. *Nature.* 1977;265:421–424.
9. Harrison CA, Dalley AJ, MacNeil S. A simple in vitro model for investigating epithelial/mesenchymal interactions: keratinocyte inhibition of fibroblast proliferation and fibronectin synthesis. *Wound Repair Regen.* 2005;13(6):543–550.
10. Kaya G, Saurat JH. Dermatoporosis: a chronic cutaneous insufficiency/fragility syndrome. Clinicopathological features, mechanisms, prevention and potential treatments. *Dermatology.* 2007;215(4):284–294.
11. Myers S. Keratinocyte Growth and Differentiation in Cutaneous Wound Healing and Cultured Keratinocyte Grafting. PhD thesis. University of London; 1999.
12. Longaker MT, Whitby DJ, Adzick NS, et al. Studies in fetal wound healing, VI. Second and early third trimester fetal wounds demonstrate rapid collagen deposition without scar formation. *J Pediatr Surg.* 1990;25(1):63–68; discussion 68–69.
13. Lavker RM, Sun TT, Oshima H, et al. Hair follicle stem cells. *J Invest Dermatol Symp Proc.* 2003;8(1):28–38.
14. Nicholas RS, Falvey H, Lemonas P, et al. Patient-related keloid scar assessment and outcome measures. *Plast Reconstr Surg.* 2012;129(3):648–656.
15. Myers SR, Leigh IM, Navsaria H. Epidermal repair results from activation of follicular and epidermal progenitor keratinocytes mediated by a growth factor cascade. *Wound Repair Regen.* 2007;15(5):693–701.
16. Jeong HW, Kim IS. TGF-beta1 enhances betaig-h3-mediated keratinocyte cell migration through the alpha3beta1 integrin and PI3K. *J Cell Biochem.* 2004;92(4):770–780.
17. Angel P, Szabowski A. Function of AP-1 target genes in mesenchymal-epithelial cross-talk in skin. *Biochem Pharmacol.* 2002;64(5–6):949–956.
18. Owen MR, Sherratt JA, Myers SR. How far can a juxtacrine signal travel? *Proc Biol Sci.* 1999;266(1419):579–585.
19. O'Kane S, Ferguson MW. Transforming growth factor beta s and wound healing. *Int J Biochem Cell Biol.* 1997;29(1):63–78.
20. Occleston NL, Laverty HG, O'Kane S, et al. Prevention and reduction of scarring in the skin by transforming growth factor beta 3 (TGFbeta3): from laboratory discovery to clinical pharmaceutical. *J Biomater Sci Polym Ed.* 2008;19(8):1047–1063.
21. Steed DL. Clinical evaluation of recombinant human platelet-derived growth factor for the treatment of lower extremity ulcers. *Plast Reconstr Surg.* 2006;117(7 Suppl):143S–149S; discussion 150S-151S.
22. Lim EH, Sardinha JP, Myers S, et al. Latent transforming growth factor-beta1 functionalised electrospun scaffolds promote human cartilage differentiation: towards an engineered cartilage construct. *Arch Plast Surg.* 2013;40(6):676–686.
23. Eliya-Masamba MC, Banda GW. Primary closure versus delayed closure for non bite traumatic wounds within 24 hours post injury. *Cochrane Database Syst Rev.* 2013;10:CD008574.
24. Lemmens L, Claes V, Uzzell M. Managing patients with metastatic colorectal cancer on bevacizumab. *Br J Nurs.* 2008;17(15):944–949.

25. Wong VW, Akaishi S, Longaker MT. Pushing back: wound mechanotransduction in repair and regeneration. *J Invest Dermatol.* 2011;131(11):2186–2196.
26. [No authors listed]. On the anatomy and physiology of the skin: conclusions by Professor K. Langer. *Br J Plast Surg.* 1978;31(4):277–278.
27. Ingber DE, Tensegrity I. Cell structure and hierarchical systems biology. *J Cell Sci.* 2003;116(Pt 7):1157–1173.
28. Eckes B, Nischt R, Krieg T. Cell–matrix interactions in dermal repair and scarring. *Fibrogenesis Tissue Repair.* 2010;3(4).
29. Ziade M, Domergue S, Batifol D, et al. Use of botulinum toxin type a to improve treatment of facial wounds: a prospective randomised study. *J Plast Reconstr Aesthet Surg.* 2013;66(2):209–214.
30. Loss M, Wedler V, Künzi W, et al. Artificial skin, split-thickness autograft and cultured autologous keratinocytes combined to treat a severe burn injury of 93% of TBSA. *Burns.* 2000;26(7):644–652.
31. Cuono CB, Langdon R, Birchall N, et al. Composite autologous–allogenic skin replacement: development and clinical application. *Plast Reconstr Surg.* 1987;80:626–635.
32. Myers SR, Partha VN, Soranzo C, et al. Hyalomatrix: a temporary epidermal barrier, hyaluronan delivery, and neodermis induction system for keratinocyte stem cell therapy. *Tissue Eng.* 2007;13(11):2733–2741.
33. Gillies HD, Millard DR. *The Principles and Art of Plastic Surgery.* Boston: Little, Brown, and Company; 1957.
34. Kølle S-F, Fischer-Nielsen A, Mathiasen AB, et al. Enrichment of autologous fat grafts with ex-vivo expanded adipose tissue-derived stem cells for graft survival: a randomised placebo-controlled trial. *Lancet.* 2013;382(9898):1113–11120.
35. Koshima I, Narushima M, Yamamoto Y, et al. Recent advancement on surgical treatments for lymphedema. *Ann Vasc Dis.* 2012;5(4):409–415.

2

Basic Skin Flaps and Blood Supply

EDWIN MORRISON AND WAYNE A.J. MORRISON

Introduction

Flap surgery is the commonest procedure in plastic surgery and is the essence of the discipline. Critical to its success is a sound understanding of soft tissue's blood supply, its compliance, and its mobility. As all flaps "rob Peter to pay Paul," it is also about conceptualizing the secondary defect and minimizing its consequences. The art and craft of plastic surgery necessarily requires an esthetic sense and experience.

Evolution of Flap Surgery

For almost a century, Manchot (1889)[1,2] and Salmon's (1936)[3] detailed studies of the skin's vascular design were unknown to clinicians. With limited understanding and the simplistic belief that the skin's blood supply was based on a random distribution in the horizontal plane, local flap surgery was unpredictable and its progress curtailed by an adherence to dogmatic rules such as length-to-width ratios and the superiority of proximal over distally-based flaps. A generation of surgeons failed to appreciate the simple observation that circumferentially incising large skin lesions in the process of their elevation and removal did not compromise their circulation. The explanation of course was that their blood supply was derived from the depths and not horizontally. Surgeons no doubt were aware of the circulation from below, but the reality was that sufficient numbers of these had to be divided to permit the flaps to transpose or rotate, and ultimately it was the base, fed by the horizontal input, that was the critical lifeline. Not until it would be shown that flaps could be completely islanded and still live was it possible to move flaps based on these deeper vessels. Milton (1970)[4] elegantly highlighted the fallacy of the length-to-breadth ratio using pig studies to demonstrate the existence of arterialized zones of the integument that would survive over extreme lengths, even if completely islanded, provided they retained their arterial source at their base. These exciting findings breathed life back into the clinical study of the soft tissue's blood supply. True to the adage that history is written by the victors, so too was the blinded acceptance of random pattern proposed by Gillies,[5] derived in part from the neglect of the publications of the Dutchman Johannes Esser (1917), Gillies' plastic surgery counterpart for the German army in World War I. Instead of the complex tube pedicle (Webster 1937),[6] Esser performed one-stage "arterialized biological island flaps" based on the palpable arteries of the head and neck region.[7] He clearly recognized the fundamental concepts of the flap's axial blood supply. Furthermore, Gillies was very aware of his work but publicly pronounced it "not up to the standards expected of the British and American people."

The first clinical application of the new "axial pattern" concept was the groin flap (McGregor 1972),[8] based on the superficial circumflex iliac branch of the femoral artery. The wide arc of rotation of this very long and narrow-based flap of like tissue expanded the single-stage reconstructive options for the regional wounds previously manageable only by multistage transfers requiring protracted immobilization and hospitalization.

What had been anecdotally reported in the early literature and had been empirically adopted in practice, the Indian forehead flap for nasal reconstruction and the epigastric flap in the lower abdomen (Shaw 1920),[9] now made sense. The former flap unwittingly captured the supratrochlear/supraorbital vessels and the latter the superficial epigastrics.

With this new awareness, omentum although not skin, was quickly recognized for its application as an arterialized flap by virtue of it wearing its blood supply on the outside of its surface. The vasculature could be pruned to critical arterial pedicles and tunneled from the abdominal cavity to cover far-flung defects and then skin grafted where needed (Fig. 2.1).

Other fundamental concepts of skin blood supply were soon elucidated. The myocutaneous flaps were described, where the skin relied for its blood supply on the multitude of small vessels perforating through the underlying muscle. Provided the muscle was raised on its blood supply, the overlying skin would survive, even when completely islanded. As muscles typically are vascularized often by a single source at their origin the muscle pedicle added even further length to the arc of flap rotation. The gracilis (Orticochea 1972)[10] and latissimus dorsi myocutaneous flap (Olivara 1976),[11],

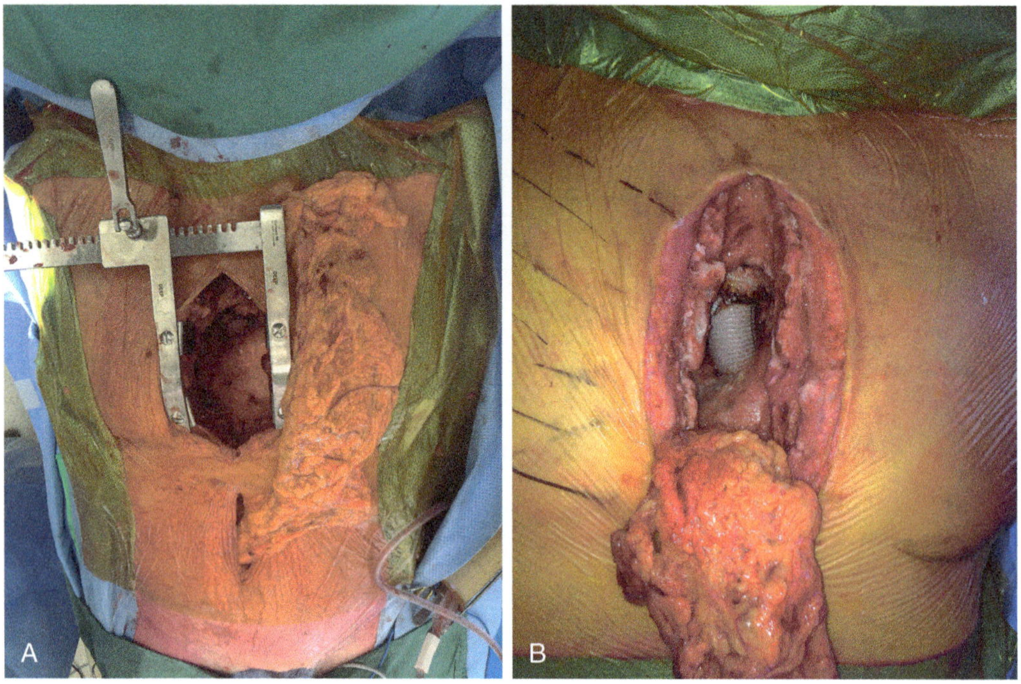

• **Fig. 2.1** Omental flap used for salvage of an infected aortic Dacron graft. (A) Omental flap raised and laid out before being tunneled into the thorax. Showing the reach of the omental flap. (B) Omental flap tunneled and wrapped around the infected Dacron aortic graft on the ascending aortic arch. (Courtesy Dr. Rostam D. Farhadieh)

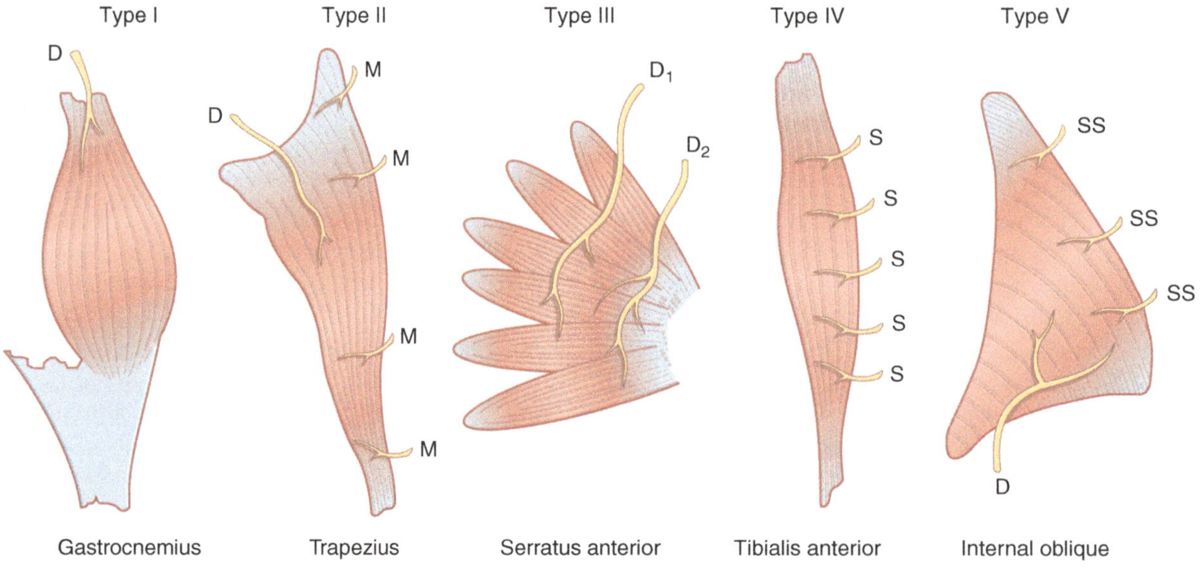

• **Fig. 2.2** Mathes and Nahai classification of muscle flaps. (From Hallock GG, Ahmadzadeh R, Morris SF. Classification of flaps. In: Wei F, Mardini S. *Flaps and Reconstructive Surgery.* 6th ed. Elsevier; 2017.)

reinventing the earlier findings of Tansini (1906),[12] were the first to be described and widely adopted. Muscle flaps without skin followed and the anatomical articulation of their vascular basis further expanded the options for one-stage locoregional reconstructions (Mathes and Nahai 1981) (Fig. 2.2).[13]

Fasciocutaneous flaps recognized for the first time that a significant contribution to skin blood supply was in the plane of the deep fascia and provided this fascia was included within the flap, large areas of previously unreliably vascularized skin would survive (Ponten 1981).[14] This particularly applies to the lower limb. Initially they were designed on the assumption their vascularity was in the plane of the fascia and in the limbs, flaps were based proximally to capture its source. It was soon clear that much of this fasciocutaneous blood supply derived from perforating branches of named deep vessels, emerging vertically between septofascial muscle planes from deep axial vessels and furthermore that these zones could be completely islanded from their proximal connections.

This led to the unifying concept of angiosome blood supply (Taylor and Palmer 1987),[15] where the tissue is considered as a three-dimensional territory or somite structure akin to vertebrate embryological development where not only skin, but whole mesenchymal somites including skin, muscle, and bone, have a vascular zone. This was supported by meticulous cadaver studies and expanded the earlier work of Manchot and Salmon.

Concurrent with this explosion in the understanding of the skin's blood supply, advances were being made in microvascular surgical techniques and instrumentation initially by the neurosurgeons, (Jacobson and Suarez 1962)[16] and quickly adopted for plastic surgery. Microsurgery was a technical disruptor of its time and had immediate application for replantation. Subsequently the transplantation of toes and territories of skin by anastomosing specific vessels flourished. The first such flap was an omental transfer to the scalp (McLean and Buncke Jr 1972).[17] Skin flaps soon followed (Taylor and Daniel, 1973;[18] O'Brien et al 1973[19]). More recently, supermicrosurgery has provided surgeons with greater confidence to explore free, pedicled, and 'freestyle' perforator flaps (Koshima 1997),[20] reappraise lymphatic surgery and the impetus to further examine the microvasculature anatomy (Saint-Cyer et al 2009[21]; Imanishi et al 2000[22]; Narushima et al 2018[23]).

Physiology and Anatomy of Skin Blood Supply

Flap surgery involves the transfer of tissue with its vascularity preserved. Necessarily this requires an understanding of the physiology and anatomy of the integument's blood supply.

The blood supply (15 mL/min per 100 cm^3) to the skin, greatly exceeds its metabolic needs because of its homeostatic role in thermoregulation and systemic circulation. This explains the relative robustness of skin flaps.

Perfusion of the skin's capillary beds is regulated by complex and incompletely understood local and systemic neurohumoral mechanisms. These act on precapillary sphincters and arteriovenous anastomoses influencing the filling and emptying of the dermal plexuses and in turn not just the circulation of the skin and subcutaneous tissue, but also insensible heat loss and venous return to the heart. Practically, it follows that the patient following flap surgery should be kept warm, well perfused, and pain-free to maximize the circulation to the peripheries. Technical factors largely underpin successful flap surgery. Clinical experience suggests that perforator flaps become hyperperfused following circumferential incision of the skin; leeching can temporarily alleviate venous congestion and topical vasodilators may beneficially alter the intrinsic blood supply of a flap. Smoking on the other hand is known to cause vasoconstriction in small vessels.

The circulation of the skin and its underlying structures consists of a non-uniform three-dimensional continuous vascular network. For the purposes of skin flap surgery, conceptualizing this vascular network as consisting of *horizontal* and *vertical* components is useful.

Running parallel with the skin, and constituting the horizontal component of the skin's blood supply, are the numerous vascular plexuses. Most important amongst these are the subdermal plexus and the deeper suprafascial plexus. Where no deep fascia exists an equivalent structure such as the panniculus carnosus (limited to the platysma, palmaris brevis, and the dartos muscles in man) serves a similar purpose. These are the vascular bases of (random) cutaneous and fasciocutaneous flaps.

Vessels arising vertically from their source arteries either *directly* supply the skin, or *indirectly* supply the skin after nourishing deeper structures such as muscle, tendon, and bone. These are known as "perforators" and they arise from the deep named vessels, axially in the limbs and perpendicularly in the trunk, and follow the dermatomes. They occur in their highest density over the less mobile soft tissue that is adherent to underlying septa; this is particularly evident in the limbs. Perforators anastomose initially with the prefascial plexus before continuing on to the subdermal plexus and are the *vascular pedicles on which islands of skin and other soft tissue components may be based.* It follows that separate islands of skin and fascia each based on a separate perforator but ultimately deriving from a common arterial axial vessel can be raised on this common axis and permit complex reconstructions with multiple independently oriented flaps.

Renewed interest in the hundreds of cutaneous perforators throughout the body has seen a renaissance in local flap surgery. Based on single perforators, perforator flaps offer greater flexibility to utilize the local tissues and achieve better like-for-like reconstructions all the while minimizing donor morbidity. Crucially, the size of the perforasome remains unknown. Relevant factors include perforator size, direction, density, orientation, and linkages with adjacent perforators and cutaneous nerves, as well as hyperperfusion of the skeletonized perforator[21,24] (Fig. 2.3). The blood supply of the skin and its underlying structures can also be divided into vascular territories, or *angiosomes,*[15] each one being interconnected with its adjacent territory by bi-directional arterioles, the direction interchangeable and determined by the relative pressure in each territory. *The angiosome is the vascular basis for composite flaps.*

Drainage of the skin is by a reciprocal three-dimensional venous network of avalvular bidirectional veins with a dominant subdermal component. This in turn drains into large caliber subcutaneous veins or venae comitantes that run with perforators. Superficial lymphatics follow subcutaneous veins and deeper lymphatics follow arteries.

Venous flaps[25] are generally transferred as free microvascular flaps where the flap is elevated superficially with only the venous system thereby obtaining a thin flap with little

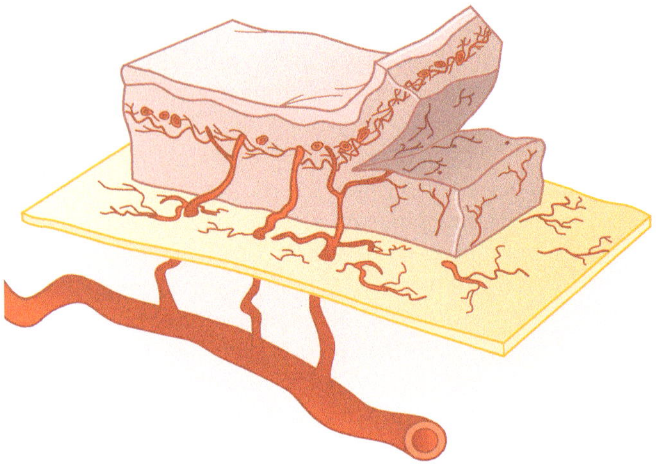

• **Fig. 2.3** Perforators arise from axial vessels in/directly to supply the overlying soft tissues. Connections between adjacent perforators are by direct connections within the subdermal plexus and indirect connections within the suprafascial plexus. (From Saint-Cyr M, Wong C, Schaverein M, et al. The perforasome theory: vascular anatomy and clinical implications. *Plast Reconstr Surg*. 2009;124(5):1529.)

morbidity. The flap is arterialized through its veins by anastomosing them to an artery in varying configurations, the tissue being nourished by retrograde perfusion. There is a small but significant body of work suggesting that these flaps may have a wider application than previously thought. Central to this modification of venous flaps to shunt restricted arteriovenous flaps. There are many classification systems based on efferent, afferent vessels, as well as shunt site.

Indications for Skin Flaps

Skin defects should ideally be repaired by replacement of what is missing and generally this will include fat, as well as skin. In many cases the local laxity of skin will allow direct closure and conversion of the deformity to a linear scar. This should be planned to lie within relaxed skin tension lines (RSTL) of Langer to minimize wound tension, optimize healing, and esthetic outcome. In some instances, although the wound may technically be closed directly, direct closure is undesirable. Excessive tension predisposes to unreliable healing and/or a contour "dish" deformity with dog ears; elliptical wounds tend to lengthen, as they are closed and may distort sensitive adjacent structures. This is a particular issue on the face, where numerous overlapping esthetic and functional subunits lie in close proximity to each other. In other instances, axially oriented linear scars predispose to joint contractures. Here, well designed local flaps from redundant areas can redistribute the tension so as to preserve available tissue, restore normal contour, and minimize the morbidity of the scar.

Though all wounds will eventually heal by secondary intention, infection risk, the need for prolonged wound care, and scar contracture limit this approach to only small convex defects. Defects that cannot be closed directly will need grafting or replacement with flaps. Skin grafts take by engaging with the vasculature of the underlying bed. They are inappropriate in avascular circumstances (exposed bone, tendon, fracture sites, irradiated tissue, and mobile beds) and here flaps are required as they possess an independent blood supply. Grafts often contract and may be a poor color match, and where the underlying fatty tissue is missing, result in contour defects and adherence to deeper tissues. Apart from burns and extensive injuries, where large areas of skin are required, it is generally accepted particularly with the wide range of flap options available, that skin grafts are inferior to flaps and are rarely the first choice. Other exceptions include the dorsum of the hand and foot where thin skin is required and few flaps meet these needs. Full-thickness skin grafts have an important place on the face where the tissues are thin with little subcutaneous fat (eyelids, inner canthus, proximal nose, and sometimes nasal tip). Flaps from adjacent regions to these sites are invariably too thick and may distort adjacent aesthetically sensitive subunits.

Elsewhere, flaps are generally indicated rather than grafts. Small defects are closed by local flaps from the immediate area and find their greatest expression in the head and neck region, particularly in association with skin cancer resection. Flaps may be in-continuity (transposition, rotation) or islanded (advancement) and their execution defines the quality of the plastic surgeon. Because of their near-perfect tissue match, the well-executed local flap may be difficult to spot. Larger defects will require locoregional flaps from a more distant site and are most likely transposed on their narrow base to maximize their reach (arc of rotation). Because their skin texture, color, and thickness may not match that of the original defect, they may require subsequent revision surgery. Such distant flaps may be fasciocutaneous, myocutaneous or muscle flaps with skin grafts. Composites of tissue may be included, muscle or tendon, fascia or bone, and allow functional reconstruction of complex defects. Their vascular basis will be on the vascular pedicle alone or together with their associated skin, muscle or fascial carrier respectively. Usually the secondary defect will closed directly.

Though beyond the scope of this chapter, very large skin or complex defects where a specialized tissue is needed, such as functional muscle or bone, innervated or hair-bearing skin, then free flaps are indicated. They are based on a vascular pedicle and require microvascular anastomosis. Prefabricated (arterialized zone of specialized skin created by the implantation of a vascular pedicle so as to render it transferable as a free flap suitable to match a specific defect) and prelaminated flaps (the neovascularization of composite tissue around a vascular pedicle for subsequent transfer) are more sophisticated free flap indications. Tubed pedicle flaps are now rare, but still find applications where there is an absence of recipient vessels at the defect site. The Indian forehead flap is a surviving example.

TABLE 2.1 Classification of Flaps Based on Movement and Blood Supply

Movement	Blood Supply
a. Local Skin Flaps	
Advancement	
In-continuity – rare	Random – intact skin base
Islanded – e.g., V–Y	Random – subcutaneous base
Keystone	Perforator base
Transposition	
In-continuity – e.g., rhomboid, bilobed, Z-plasty	Random – intact skin base
Islanded, e.g., propeller	Perforator base
Rotation, e.g., scalp	Random; arterialized
Combination	
b. Regional (Locoregional) Flaps	
Transposition	
Cutaneous, e.g., groin flap, forehead rhinoplasty, Abbe lip flap	Subcutaneous arterialized
Muscle/myocutaneous	Arterial pedicle
Fasciocutaneous	Septo(myo)fascial perforators
Neurovascular island flaps, e.g., digits	Neurovascular A–V pedicles
c. Distant Flaps	
Two-stage pedicle, e.g., cross finger, groin to hand	Random; arterialized
Multistaged 'waltzed' pedicle, e.g., tube pedicle	Random
d. Free Flaps	
Arterial	Arterial – microvascular anastomosis
Venous	Venous blood supply Arterialized
e. Prelamination and Prefabrication	

[a]Further class of flaps may be made for *allotransplantation* – opportunistic free flap allograft in patient simultaneously requiring organ transplant, e.g., abdominal wall with bowel transplant or what is currently in the realms of experimental surgery, *tissue engineering*, cell seeded artificial scaffolds, and or adipogenic matrices.

Design and Application of Flaps

Two concurrent considerations are critical to the successful planning of local flaps: (1) blood supply and (2) mobility of the adjacent tissue (laxity) (Table 2.1).

Flap Design and Blood Supply

The first consideration in designing a skin flap is to determine whether it will be viable. The vascular limitations on a flap's dimensions are not completely understood though the principles to follow are helpful. Some flaps in some sites seem more predictable than others, despite the principles and confidence in local flap surgery that comes with trial and error, and ultimately experience with what works and what does not.

The simplest skin flaps are based on the subdermal plexus, the richness of which varies around the body. Vague *length-to-breadth ratios* govern the size of these so-called *random flaps* with the only certainty being that a flap whose length equals its width will be viable anywhere on the body. Owing to the markedly increased vascularity of the face, such flaps can tolerate significantly higher length-to-breadth ratios. Apart from the native vascularity, caution needs to be taken when flaps are folded to repair complex defects or pass over convex surfaces. Similarly, tight closure when flaps are too small and failure to recognize previous scars in the region may compromise vascularity. Hematoma is perhaps the greatest enemy of local flaps due to increased tension and subsequent vascular compromise.

The area of conventional flaps can be increased by capture of an additional vascular component. Axial flaps which have a known arterial pedicle coursing along their axis in the superficial plane (e.g., groin, forehead or deltopectoral flaps) may be further enlarged in a random fashion, or by incorporating some of the skin supplied by the next cutaneous perforator in the adjacent angiosome.[26,27] Skin flaps elevated with the deep fascia and therefore with the suprafascial plexus intact create a *fasciocutaneous flap* which too can be elevated with significantly higher length-to-breadth dimensions (Fig. 2.4).

Length-to-breadth ratios of random flaps and the volume of tissue in axial flaps may also be increased by harnessing the delay phenomenon. Though its mechanism is incompletely understood *vascular delay* is a well-established surgical technique capable of improving the vascularity and reliability of a flap prior to its definitive elevation and inset.[28] It involves the strategic division of the flap's blood supply so as to deliver a sublethal ischemic insult. This is postulated to cause vessel dilatation, neovascularization, and ischemic preconditioning of the tissues at a metabolic level. It may also be beneficial in routine flap surgery on high-risk patients who are obese, smokers or have undergone previous irradiation.[18]

Flaps incorporating the horizontal component of the integument's blood supply are usefully classified as *flaps*

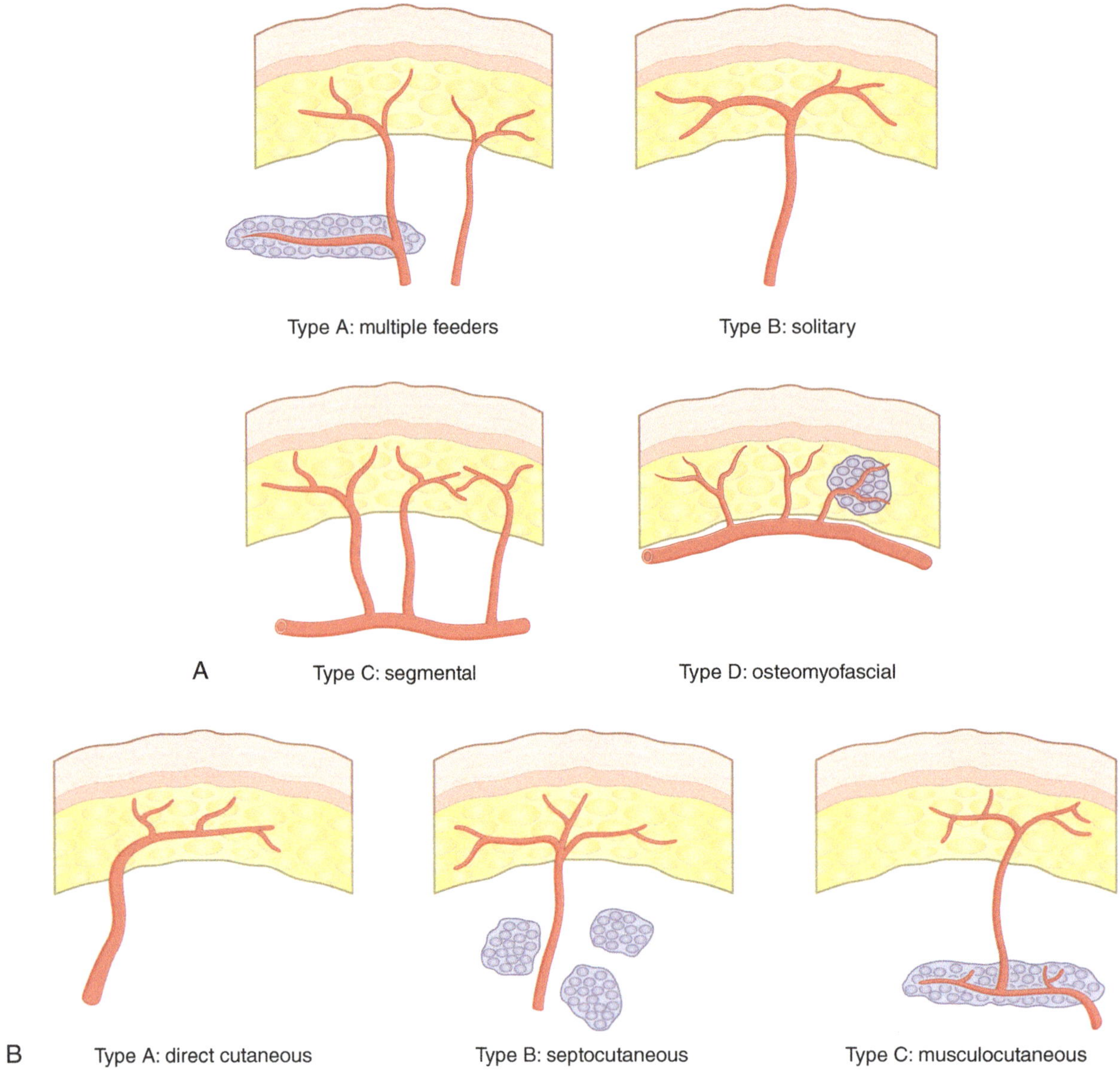

• **Fig. 2.4** (A) Fasciocutaneous flaps in Cormack and Lamberty's classification. (B) Mathes and Nahai's classification of fasciocutaneous flaps. (From Hallock GG, Ahmadzadeh R, Morris SF. Classification of flaps. In: Wei F, Mardini S. *Flaps and Reconstructive Surgery.* 6th ed. Elsevier; 2017.)

in-continuity. For similarly obvious reasons, flaps that are circumferentially incised through dermis or deep fascia (or its equivalent) are *island flaps* whose vascular basis are perforators.

Flap Design and Movement

Having determined that flap tissue is available and that it will be viable, the next question is how it can be moved to cover the defect. Flaps move by way of *transposition*, *rotation* or *advancement*, though in reality their movement usually involves some combination of all of these and is often aided by initial partial direct closure of the defect itself.

The first principle of local flap design is to pinch up the skin immediately adjacent to the defect and serially march around its perimeter until the zone of maximally lax skin is detected. It is from this tissue that the flap will be elevated. Because the tissue is lax it follows that the secondary defect should close directly.

Flaps In-continuity

Most local flaps are totally elevated from their bed but retain a critical skin base for their vascularity. This especially pertains to transposition and rotation flaps.

Transposition Flaps

Lax tissue immediately adjacent to the defect is elevated and transposed, sometimes across intact skin bridges. This creates a secondary defect that is usually closable directly because of the laxity.

The *rhomboid flap*[29] is a particularly useful example of such a flap commonly used in skin cancer surgery and the principles can be applied to all transpositions. The anticipated defect is conceived in the form of a rhomboid (unequal parallelogram with 60- and 120-degree angles) (Figs. 2.5 and 2.6). A diagonal across the rhomboid is extended the same distance as the length of an adjacent side of the defect

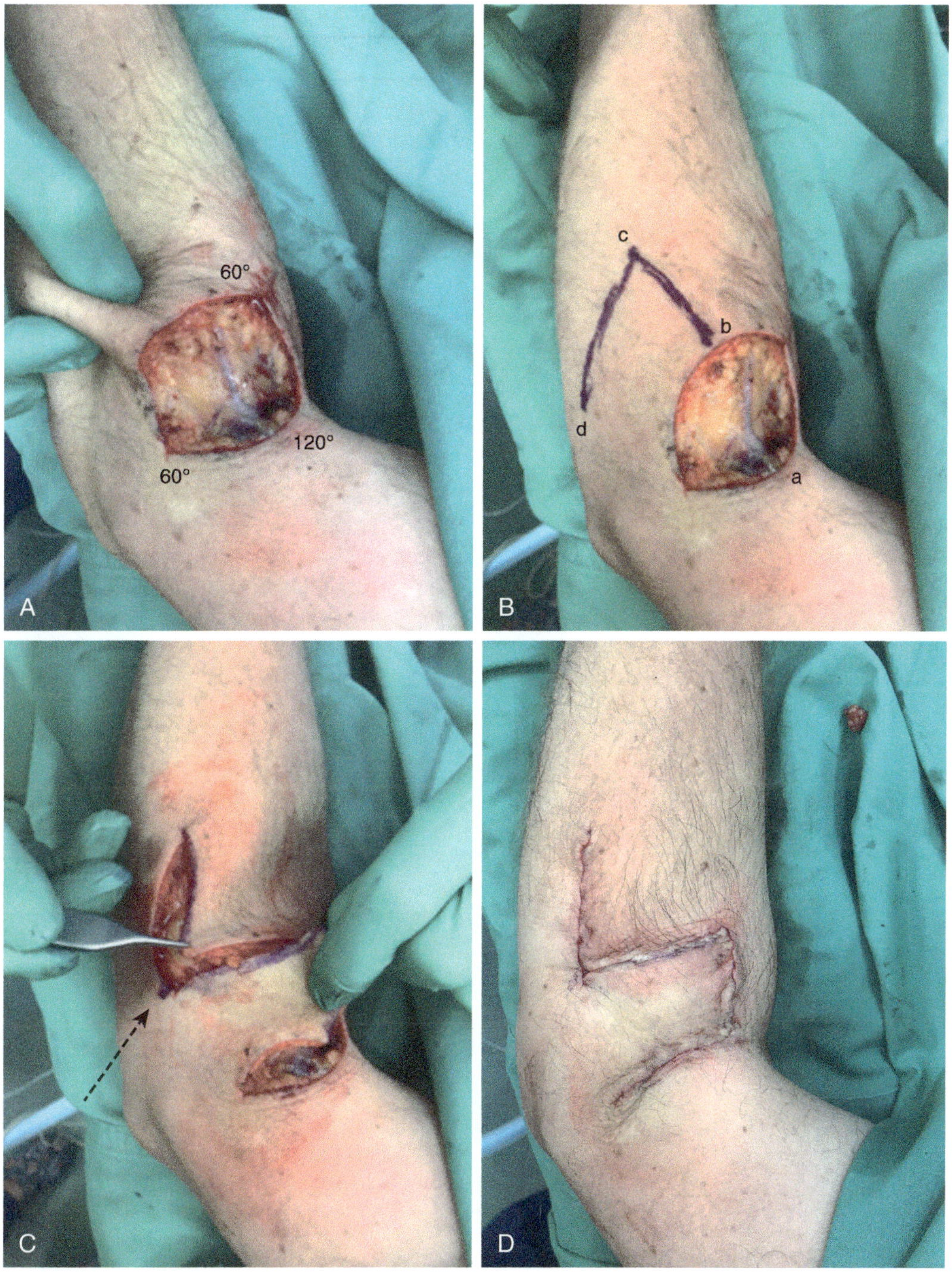

• **Fig. 2.5** Limberg's transposition flap designed with assessment of laxity for donor in the cubital fossa. (A) Showing the defect and the laxity of the surrounding tissues. (B) Flap design. (C) Transposition of the flap and closure of the defect. (D) Closure of the wound.

into the zone of laxity (*a* through *b* to *c*) A line is then directed backwards from the limit of this point (*c*) parallel with the side of the defect (*c–d*). The flap thus outlined is elevated and transposed into the defect. Preoperatively if point (*b*) is estimated to be able to approximate to point (*d*) then the secondary defect will close. Important elements of flap design include transposition of the flap around the more acute 60-degree angle which facilitates closure and the ability to orient the donor scar in skin creases or boundaries of cosmetic subunits. In some situations, the adjacent tissue has not enough laxity to permit direct closure of the secondary defect and a second flap from the more lax tissue adjacent to this defect is used creating a directly closable tertiary defect (bilobed flap). When flaps are used to cover exposed bone or other non-graftable defects, transposition flaps must be used even if the adjacent zone will not permit direct closure and here skin grafts are used for the secondary defect.

Z-plasty: The other common application of the transposition flap is in association with the Z-plasty, a fundamental design concept in plastic surgery. Z-plasties are used to release (lengthen) tight or webbed scars, redirect scars into a more favorable alignment and in combination with linear access incisions to prevent secondary linear contracture (e.g., Dupuytren's). The traditional Z-plasty design involves an axial incision along the course of the scar. A back cut extends from one end of the linear incision into the adjacent tissue at 60 degrees for the same length as the axial incision. A second back cut the same length is now made on the opposite side of the line commencing at the other end of the line and directed to the first. This creates an equal limbed Z incision with its diagonal in the axis of the original scar and flaps at 60 degrees (Fig. 2.7). By interdigitating (transposing) the two flaps created by the design across the midline the diagonal will now change at right-angles to the original axis (*B* and *C*). This way the scar is partially redirected and provided the planning is accurate it should ideally fall within an existing crease line. It is estimated that with a 60-degree transposition the original length of the scar axis will increase by 75%. To achieve maximum correction of tight scars it is essential to completely remove all of the underlying scar so that the contracture is fully released. Many times it is unrealistic to close 60-degree flaps and smaller angles are required at the expense of lesser lengthening. In fact, when there is not much contracture and the flaps are being used to redirect scars, then increasing length is undesirable as it will simply create redundant large dog ears. As with all flaps, tissue is borrowed from one place to give to another. Z-plasties lengthen at the expense of reduction in width. Z-plasties are no different to other local flaps in that if there is adjacent redundant tissue they work well. This is particularly so with contracted linear scars where the surrounding tissue is not involved. This tissue has been locked or gathered up in the scar but is not missing and on release it is available for transpositioning and scar lengthening. By contrast, where wide scarring has occurred such as burns, the Z-plasty is essentially cheating by taking tissue from one direction only to create tightness in another. Here imported skin is needed to replace what is lost either as a graft or more distant flap.

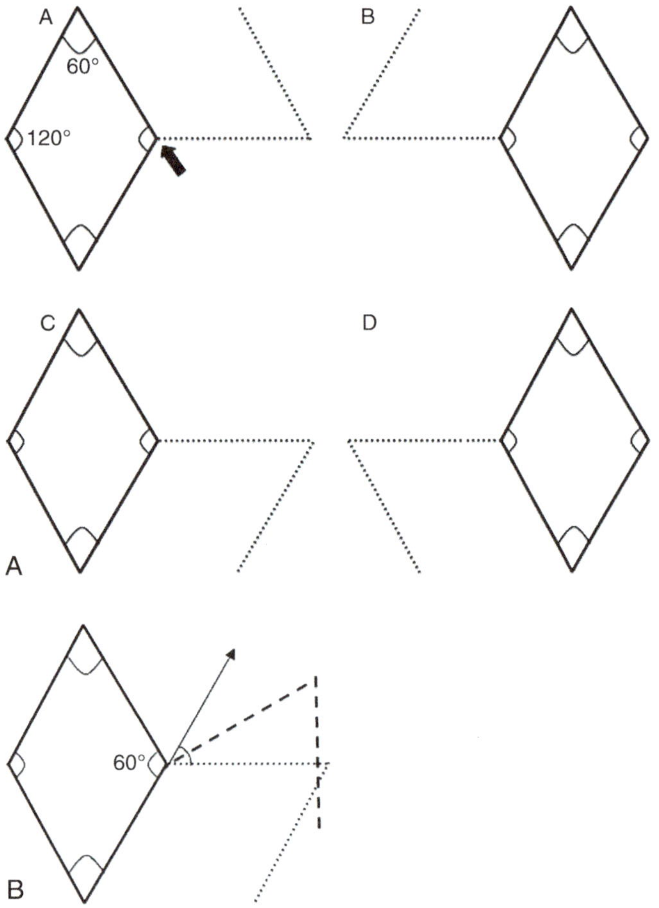

• **Fig. 2.6** (A) Schematic design of the rhomboid flap. (B) Dufourmentel flap variation. (From Chu EA, Byrne PJ. Local flaps I: bilobed, rhombic, and cervicofacial. *Facial Plast Surg Clin North Am.* 2009 Aug;17(3):349–60.)

Rotation Flaps

Are used in circumstances where there is no differential laxity in the immediate region of the defect. An exaggeratedly large flap is required extending well beyond the zone of the defect to recruit tissue progressively over a large distance. Rotation flaps are typically employed over the scalp and upper cheek zones. Generally, in designing these flaps it is essential to understand the concept of the pivot point. Their

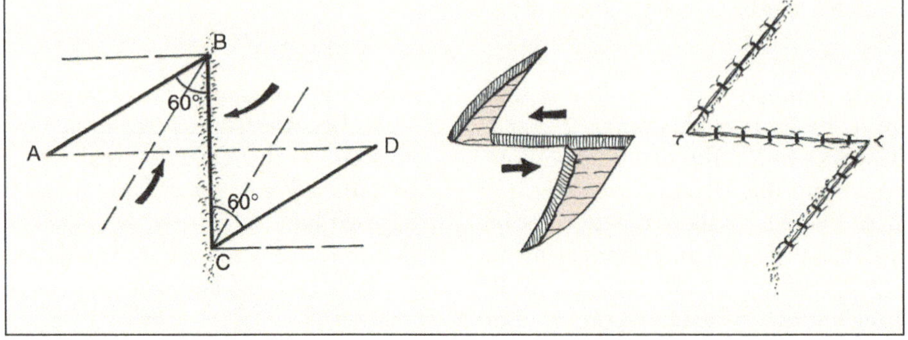

• **Fig. 2.7** Design and execution of 60-degree Z-plasty. (From Frodel JL, Sachin SP, Wang TD. Z-Plasty. In: Baker SR. *Local Flaps in Facial Reconstruction*. Philadelphia: Elsevier Saunders; 2014.)

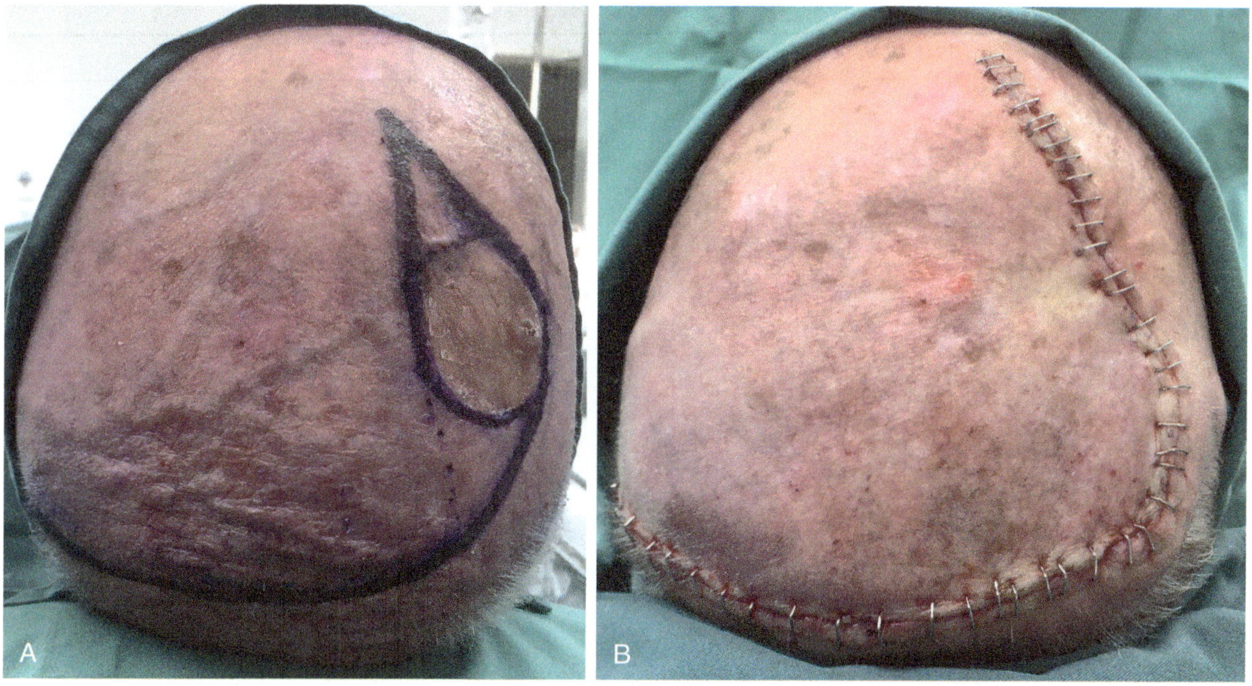

• **Fig. 2.8** Rotation flaps. (A) Preoperative marking of rotation flap of the scalp. (B) Immediate postoperative appearance. (Courtesy Dr. Cameron Keating.)

design involves triangulation of the defect, the shortest side being selected as the base (Fig. 2.8).

The side of the triangle that becomes the leading edge of the rotation flap will advance to meet its opposite side by mobilizing all that tissue beyond the defect sufficient to allow movement. This is achieved by a sweeping curvilinear incision extending from in line of the triangle base over a wide expanse until it encroaches into the zone of laxity. The whole of the large flap is elevated completely up to its base and rotated around its pivot point (until the incised edge of the flap rotates forward to close the defect). The base of the flap is that remaining bridge of tissue from the apex of the triangular defect to the point where the flap incision ceases. Most rotation flaps survive on a random blood supply but in the scalp known arterial axes should form the basis of the design and in these circumstances much narrower bases can be conceived.

Because of the spherical shape of the skull, skin flap design will need to accommodate for the changing lengths and mobility during flap rotation. The secondary defect should close directly by progressive recruitment of tissue along the whole course of the incision, or if a back-cut was done to relieve tension on the closure, tissue from the opposite axis should be chosen.

Pivot point: In both transposition and rotation flaps the pivot point is a crucial technical consideration. It always lies at the base of the flap furthermost from the defect and is the point at which the flap is tethered preventing further movement. Careful planning and oversizing of the flap design is necessary to avoid a flap being too small for the defect or becoming ischemic with closure under tension. *Planning in reverse* is a useful technique to determine the necessary dimensions of your flap preoperatively. A *back-cut* can reposition the pivot point somewhat closer to the defect but comes at the expense of the flap's vascularity.

Advancement Flaps

Lax adjacent tissue can be directly advanced into the defect. Realistically tissue will not advance much more than its capacity for direct closure and to gain real movement requires islanding of the advancement flap. Such flaps then become dependent on subcutaneous or perforator blood supply.

Island flaps are mostly advanced into the defect, though in some instances they may be transposed, as in perforator flaps. The classic island flap design is the *V–Y configuration.* In general, island flaps tend to be more mobile compared with those in-continuity. There are also varying degrees of islanding. Circumferential incision of the dermis alone leaves the deep fascia (or equivalent) intact and in the more mobile parts of the body such as the face, blunt dissection of the subcutis will usually suffice to achieve the desired amount of movement. Where the overlying skin is more adherent to the deeper structures, as occurs in the limbs and trunk, judicious release of the deep fascia is required to achieve meaningful movement. The keystone flap[24] owes much of its advancement to the mobility of the deep fascia after its release. This is variable around the body, but most pronounced in the limbs midway between joints, where longitudinal release of the deep fascia allows the overlying soft tissues to glide readily over the underlying muscles, effectively creating a bipedicled fasciocutaneous flap (Fig. 2.9). Selectively, the deep fascia may be further released distally then proximally to achieve yet more movement but this is theoretically at the expense of blood supply through complete division of the suprafascial plexus. The secondary skin defect is closed

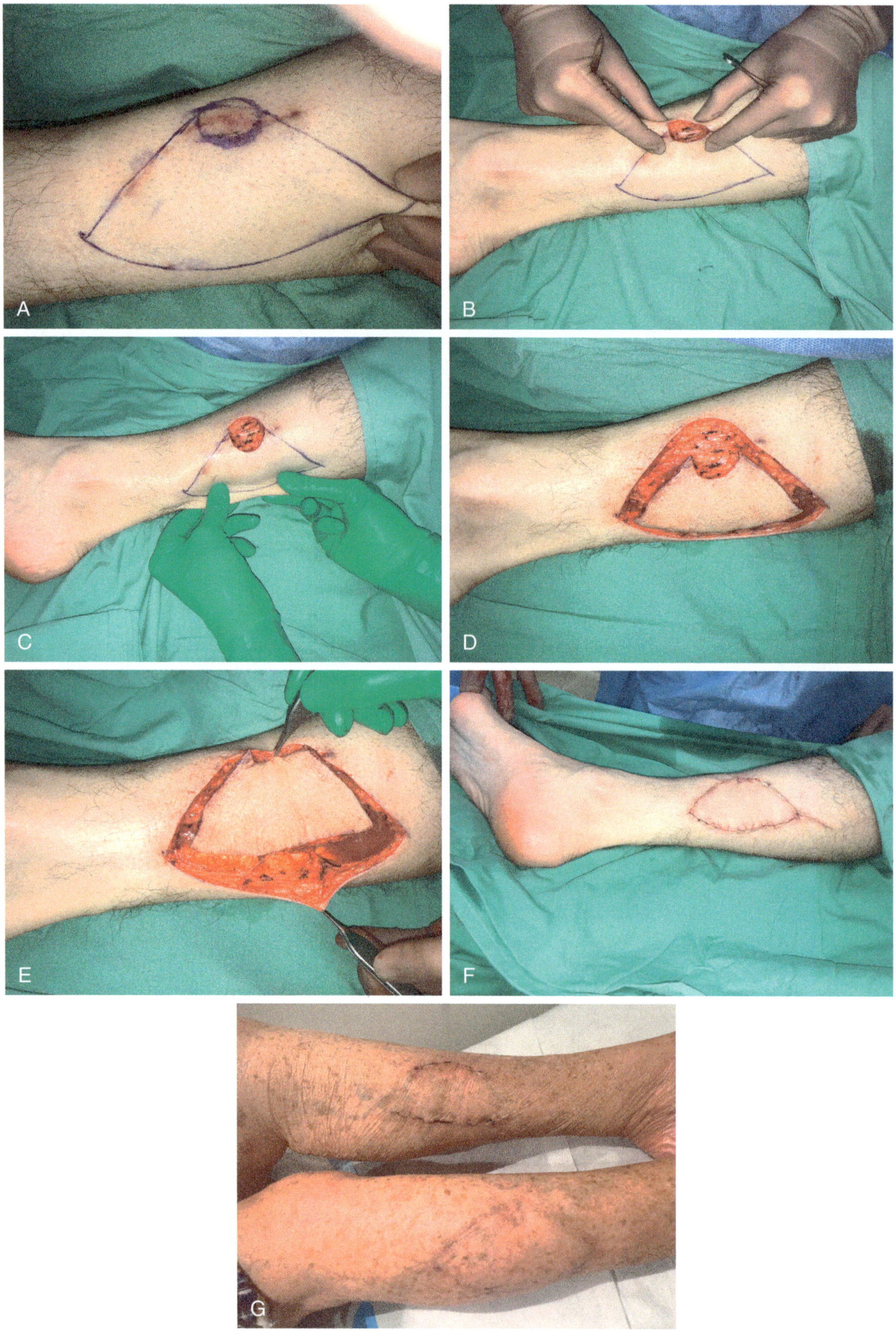

• **Fig. 2.9** (A) The design of the keystone flap. (B) Demonstration of lack of laxity at excision site. (C) Demonstration of laxity posteriorly. (D) Excision defect and flap elevation. (E) Transfer of the flap into the defect. (F) Closure of the defect. (G) Excellent long-term results from keystone flaps on both legs.

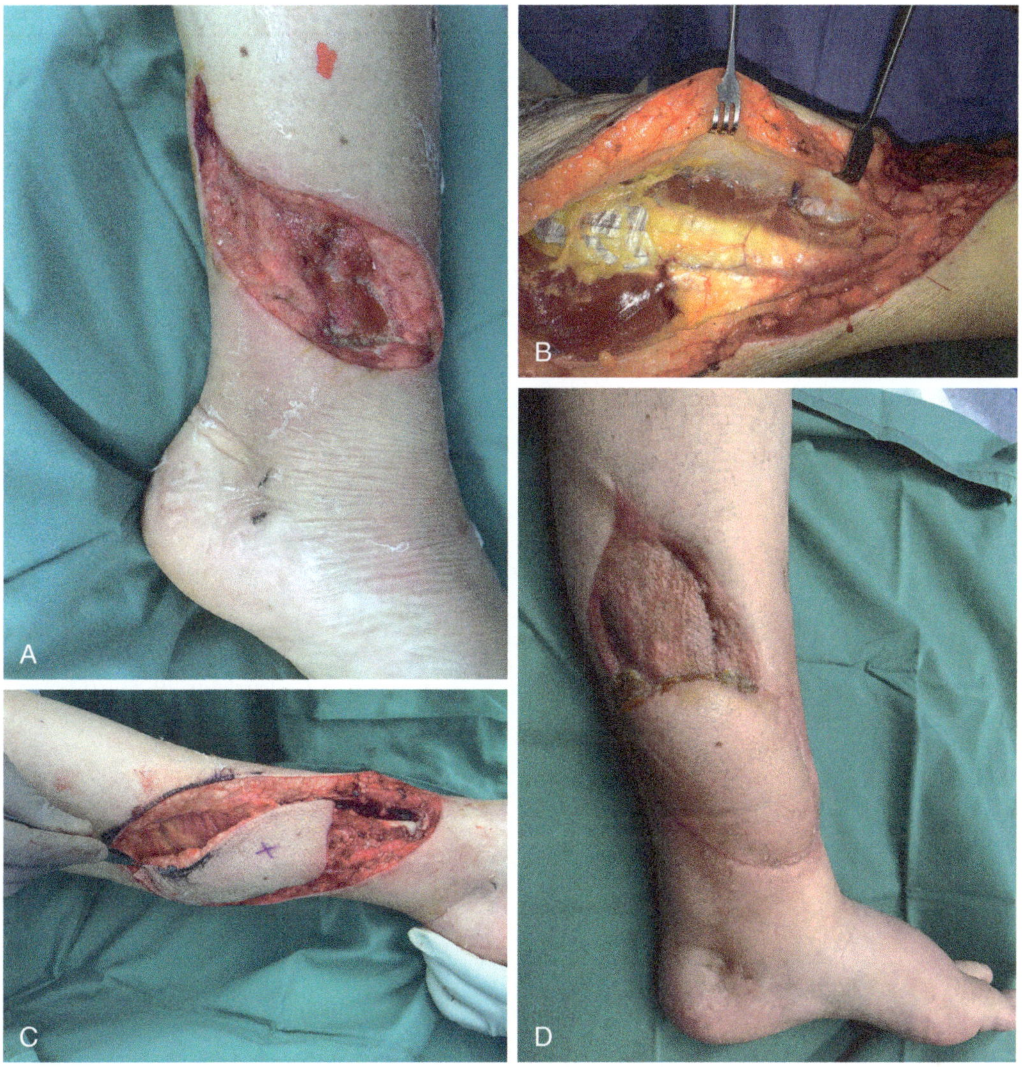

• **Fig. 2.10** Propeller flap design for traumatic lower limb reconstruction. (A) Defect, red dot indicating Doppler signal of perforator. (B) Subfascial dissection of the flap and perforator isolation. (C) Fully islanded flap. (D) Reconstruction results at 3 months. (Courtesy Dr. Rostam D. Farhadieh.)

typically in V–Y fashion oriented to maximally utilize the lax skin above and below the defect and not necessarily around prescribed angles. On occasions, creep and direct advancement of overtly lax tissue further around from the secondary defect will be adequate alone, and in some small defects this can be demonstrated by subcutaneous longitudinal release of the deep fascia alone, as in a limited fasciotomy. The *lateral pedicle island flap* on the limbs and the *horn flap* on the dorsum of the nose are variations on the above themes. A commitment to islanding requires certainty that a perforator lies at the base of the flap, hence larger flaps are preferable where no discrete perforator is identified. Where a sizeable perforator (0.5 mm) is identifiable, and meticulously dissected free of the deep fascia with its branches to the underlying muscle divided, even greater mobility through V–Y advancement or rotation ("propeller") of a skin island is possible. Indeed local flap surgery has been reinvigorated by a growing understanding and confidence in perforator anatomy resulting in better like-for-like and efficient reconstructions. The pivot point of a *propeller flap* is the perforator (Fig. 2.10).

Finally, consideration needs to be given to the insetting of the flap so as to camouflage its outline. To this extent, where possible the flap's axis and its margins should be parallel to crease lines and inset respecting cosmetic units. V–Y advancements along the nasolabial and glabella crease lines expound this concept. A flap design is less conspicuous with straight or gently curving margins than round flaps as circular lines are unnatural on the face and are instantly recognizable. Respecting this principle it is often better to resect a circular skin tumor as a square rather than simply as a circle. Taken further, consideration can be given to resecting and replacing whole cosmetic units to improve cosmetic outcomes. Well-designed larger flaps are often preferable to circular flaps which are prone to pin-cushioning as a result of cicatricial contracture. Scars crossing natural crease lines are conspicuous and across hollows will cause tenting or webbing. A further principle of flap repair is that a single flap cannot realistically repair a defect that transgresses two separate planes (e.g., cheek–alar base). In these cases two flaps from different axes or a flap and a graft will be required.

References

1. Manchot C. *Die Hautarterien des menschlichen Korpers*. Leipzig: Vogel; 1889.
2. Manchot C, Trans Ristic J, Morain WD. *The Cutaneous Arteries of the Human Body*. New York: Springer-Verlag; 1983.
3. Salmon M. *Artères de la Peau*. Paris: Masson et Cie; 1936.
4. Milton SH. Pedicled skin flaps: the fallacy of the length:width ratio. *Br J Surg*. 1970;57(7):502.
5. Gillies HD. The tubed pedicle in plastic surgery. *NY Med J*. 1920;111:1.
6. Webster JP. Thoraco-epigastric tubed pedicles. *Surg Clin North Am*. 1937;17:145.
7. Esser JF. Studies in plastic surgery of the face. *Ann Surg*. 1917;65:297.
8. McGregor IA, Jackson IT. The groin flap. *Br J Plast Surg*. 1972;25(1):3.
9. Shaw DT. Open abdominal flaps for repair of surface defects of the upper extremity. *Surg Clin North Am*. 1944;24:293.
10. Orticochea M. A new method of total reconstruction of the penis. *Br J Plast Surg*. 1972;25(4):347.
11. Olivara N. The latissimus flap. *Br J Plast Surg*. 1976;29(2):126.
12. Tansini I. Sopra il mio nuovo processo di amputazione della mammella. *Gazetta Medica Italiana*. 1906;57:141.
13. Mathes SJ, Nahai F. Classification of the vascular anatomy of muscles: experimental and clinical correlation. *Plast Reconstr Surg*. 1981;67(2):177.
14. Ponten B. The fasciocutaneous flap: its use in soft tissue defects of the lower leg. *Br J Plast Surg*. 1981;34(2):215.
15. Taylor GI, Palmer JH. The vascular territories (angiosomes) of the body: experimental studies and clinical applications. *Br J Plast Surg*. 1987;40(2):113–141.
16. Jacobson JH, Suarez EL. Microvascular surgery. *Chest*. 1962;41(2):220–224.
17. McLean DH, Buncke Jr HJ. Autotransplant of omentum to a large scalp defect, with microsurgical revascularisation. *Plast Reconstr Surg*. 1972;49(3):268.
18. Taylor GI, Daniel RK. The free flap: composite tissue transfer by vascular anastomosis. *Aust N Z J Surg*. 1973;41:1.
19. O'Brien BM, MacLeod AM, Hayhurst JW, et al. Successful transfer of a large island flap from the groin to the foot by microvascular anastomoses. *Plast Reconstr Surg*. 1973;52(3):271.
20. Koshima I. *Microsurgery in the Future: Introduction to Supramicrosurgery and Perforator Flaps*. Presented at First International Course on Perforator Flap and Arterialised Skin Flaps. Special Invited Lecture. Belgium: Ghent; 1997.
21. Saint-Cyr M, Wong C, Schaverein M, et al. The perforasome theory: vascular anatomy and clinical implications. *Plast Reconstr Surg*. 2009;124(5):1529.
22. Imanishi N, Nakajima H, Minabe T, et al. Angiographic study of the subdermal plexus: a preliminary report. *Scand J Plast Reconstr Hand Surg*. 2000;34:113.
23. Narushima M, Yamasoba T, Iida T, et al. Pure skin perforator flaps: the anatomical vascularity of the superthin flap. *Plast Reconstr Surg*. 2018;142(3):351.
24. Behan FC. The keystone design perforator island flap in reconstructive surgery. *Aust N Z J Surg*. 2003;73(3):112–120.
25. Nakayama Y, Soeda S, Kasai Y. Flaps nourished by arterial inflow through the venous system: an experimental investigation. *Plast Reconstr Surg*. 1981;67(3):328–334.
26. Cormack GC, Lamberty BGH. *The Arterial Anatomy of Skin Flaps*. Edinburgh: Churchill Livingstone; 1986.
27. Morris SF, Taylor GI. Predicting the survival of experimental skin flaps with a knowledge of the vascular architecture. *Plast Reconstr Surg*. 1993;92(7):1352.
28. Stelnicki EJ, Young VL, Francel T, et al. Blair, his surgical descendants, and their roles in plastic surgical development. *Plast Reconstr Surg*. 1999;103(7):1990.
29. Limberg AA. Design of local flaps. In: Gibson TA, ed. *Modern Trends in Plastic Surgery*. London: Butterworth; 1966:38.

3

Biomaterials and Structural Fat Grafting

NIKITA JOJI AND AFSHIN MOSAHEBI

General Principles

Living cells respond to physical and biochemical cues, e.g., hormones, cell–cell signaling molecules, and with the physical environment through the extracellular matrix (ECM), enabling them to adapt to changes in the physiological environment. Regulation of cell function (growth, migration, proliferation, and differentiation) is dependent upon contact or adhesion between cells and the substrate (ECM). ECM has three key components: collagen – the structural framework of ECM – proteoglycans, and adhesive matrix proteins (e.g., fibronectin, vitronectin). Initial contact of cells with a solid substrate is mediated by adsorbed adhesive proteins. Cell surface receptors subsequently form bonds leading to cytoskeletal reorganization and progressive spreading of the cell on the substrate. These receptors transduce biochemical signals to the nucleus by activating the same intracellular signaling pathways that are used by growth factor receptors. In addition to biochemical cues, mechanical forces play an important role in cell adhesion, growth, and possibly differentiation. These responses are mediated through internal cell receptors that respond to mechanical forces. Cell binding to ECM through specific cell–substrate contacts is critical to cell-growth control through mechanical forces resulting in alterations in cell shape and cytoskeletal tension.

A biomaterial is a nonpharmaceutical, nonviable material in intimate contact with living tissue in order to treat, augment, or replace any tissue, organ or function of the body. Ideal properties of a biomaterial include: biocompatibility, noncarcinogenicity, lack of allergenicity, cost-effectiveness, and ease of handling. Biomaterials or tissue engineering scaffolds contain chemical and structural information that may control tissue formation in a manner similar to cell–cell communication and cell–ECM interaction (Fig. 3.1). An appropriate 3D scaffold should facilitate normal cellular organization and behavior, define and maintain the desired tissue volume, whilst also promoting host integration and implant vascularization.

Ultimately, the scaffold should undergo nontoxic degradation as it is replaced by healthy host tissue, rendering a biodegradable scaffold ideal for use in tissue engineering. The cell–biomaterial interface also plays a significant role in the choice of scaffold due to the direct impact on cell adhesion, which is an important step in the survival of anchorage-dependent cells. Both cell proliferation and differentiation can be controlled by functionalization of the biomaterial surface; these interactions between cells and biomaterials have been shown to occur at the nanoscale.

With the advent of nanotechnology, nanoparticles are being merged with synthetic scaffolds to develop nanostructured biomaterials, enhance interaction of proteins that control cell adhesion and thus, tissue formation. Nanocomposites can be defined as multiphase solid materials where one of the phases has a dimension of less than 100 nm. Nanofibrous composite scaffolds are found to decrease immunogenicity, improve the capacity for cell interaction, and to harbor increased concentrations of fibronectin and vitronectin, the adsorption proteins that reduce apoptosis of transplanted cells. Biomaterials can be classified as bioinert, bioresorbable, or bioactive. A bioinert material does not induce a toxic response from the body on implantation and is usually associated with fibrous encapsulation, whereas a bioresorbable material undergoes degradation in the host by hydrolysis, enzymes or osteoclasts. Bioactive materials produce a biological response from the body that results in the formation of a bond between the material and host tissue. The type and site of biomaterial implantation governs a tissue response: hard tissues (bone, enamel, and dentin), soft tissues (breast and ocular implants), vascular implants (stents, heart valves, and vascular grafts) and connective tissue (cartilage, tendons, and ligaments).

A variety of possible scaffold biomaterials are available. Among these are biological polymers (e.g., collagen, elastin, chitosan, silk), biodegradable synthetic polymers (e.g., PGA, PLA, PDLA), synthetic biomimetic compounds (e.g., hydroxyapatite, calcium phosphates), allografts and xenografts or combinations of the above. Geometric variables such as porosity, pore size, and pore morphology are crucial. A porous scaffold provides a large surface area for neovascularization, nutrient and waste exchange, cell migration, and matrix deposition. Scaffolds can be made porous using several different methods. Porogens (i.e., salt or paraffin

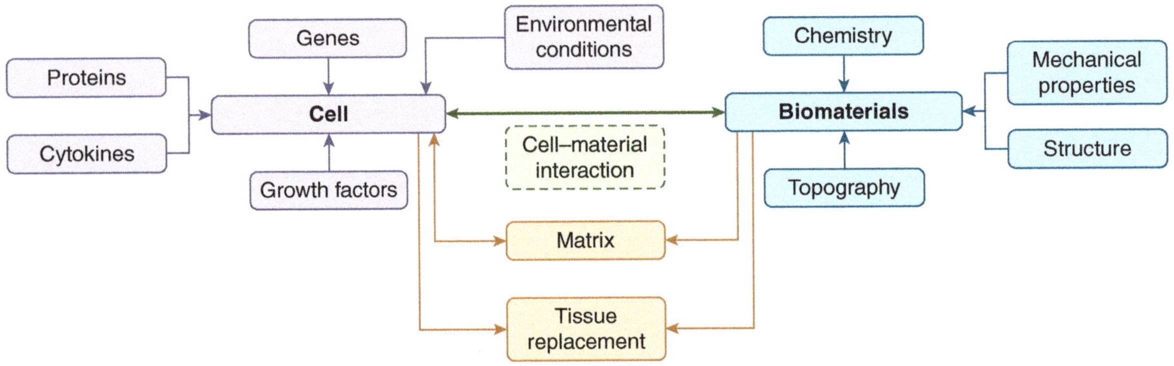

• **Fig. 3.1** Cell and biomaterial interactions and factors leading to tissue regeneration.

microspheres) can be incorporated in the polymer and subsequently leached out. Freeze drying of homogenized polymer solvents is another option, in addition to gel casting of organic scaffolds and sol-gel foaming. Surface properties, such as surface topography and chemistry, guide cellular behavior and control protein adhesion. If a biodegradable material is chosen for implantation, the rate of resorption should match the speed at which the body replaces the missing tissue and its degradation byproducts should be nontoxic. Finally, the biomaterial of choice ought to be economically viable and conform to the regulatory bodies.

Autologous Grafts

The word autologous means "related to self" and refers to tissue that has been derived or transferred from the same organism. Autologous grafts or "autografts" can be harvested and transferred from several different tissues in the body, e.g., skin, bone, tendon, cartilage. The focus of this section is on the autologous transfer of skin, adipose tissue, bone, and cartilage.

Skin Autografts

From superficial to deep, skin is composed of epidermis, dermis, and skin appendages. It has several functions, ranging from physical protection, prevention of fluid loss, protection against ultraviolet radiation, regulation of body temperature, sensation, immunological surveillance, to protection from microbiological organisms. Injured skin can heal itself through different phases of wound healing and epithelialization, whereby epithelium is reestablished across a wound. The different phases of wound healing consist of hemostasis, inflammation, proliferation, and remodeling, whereas epithelial repair consists of mobilization and migration of epithelial cells, followed by mitosis and differentiation into stratified squamous epithelial cells. If the injury to the skin is grave or the area of skin loss large, this process may take several months and result in significant scarring. In this instance the use of a skin autograft can aid the healing process. Skin grafts can either be split- or full-thickness. Split-thickness skin grafts (STSG) contain a variable amount of dermis and can be harvested from several sites (i.e., thigh, buttocks, and scalp). The donor site heals through epithelial repair and does not require closure. Full-thickness skin grafts (FTSG) contain the entire dermis and are usually taken from areas of the body with sufficient skin laxity to allow direct closure (i.e., groin, forearm, arm, postauricular and supraclavicular areas).

Skin grafts heal in four phases:

1. *Adherence* of the graft to its bed via immediately formed fibrin bonds.
2. *Serum imbibition.* Skin grafts swell in the first 2–4 days after application due to absorption of fluid.
3. *Revascularization* commences around the 4th day and is a consequence of new vessel formation along new and existing vascular channels in the graft.
4. *Remodeling* is the process whereby the histological structure of the graft returns to that of the normal skin.

Skin grafts can fail to "take" due to several reasons, e.g., hematoma, infection, excessive shearing, an inappropriate bed, or technical errors such as placing the graft upside down on its bed or allowing it to dry before application.

The main limitation of skin grafts is their tendency to contract. Contraction of grafts is more pronounced with split-thickness skin grafts compared to full-thickness skin grafts.

Adipose Tissue Autografting

Although autologous fat transfer has gained popularity over the past two decades, Neuber first described the technique in the medical literature in 1890s.[1] The injectable fat transfer was first described in the 1920s. In the 1950s Peer reported that fat grafts lose approximately 45% of their weight and mass per year.[2] He also emphasized the importance of a good vascular recipient bed combined with meticulous hemostasis to promote optimal graft survival. Autologous fat transfer can be regarded as the ideal filler. It induces neither host reaction nor a carcinogenic response. Being minimally invasive renders the procedure safe, and fat is also readily available and inexpensive. Limitations include the unpredictable and variable rate of absorption, the need for overcorrection, and the requirement for a surgical procedure.

Donor Site

The most common site is the abdomen due to availability and ease of access when the patient lies supine. Other sites include the flanks, extremities (inner thighs, inner knees, inner arms, trochanteric area) and gluteal area. A study investigating the viability of lipoaspirates in vitro using flow cytometry from three different anatomical sites – abdomen, flank, and thighs – found no difference in fat viability 12 weeks post transplantation.[3] Currently there is no consensus on the best donor site for autologous fat harvest.

Extraction Techniques

Vacuum extraction, syringe aspiration, and direct fat excision are well-described techniques in harvesting fat tissue. Although syringe aspiration is the most popular technique, there exists no current objective evidence to corroborate the benefit of this technique relative to other methods in terms of weight or volume of the fat grafts isolated. However, high negative pressure exerted on adipocytes in conventional liposuction has been reported to cause up to 90% adipocyte rupture.[4] Coleman popularized autologous fat transfer employing the syringe aspiration technique. A 3-mm cannula is connected to a 10-mL syringe and aspiration is achieved through manual suction by withdrawing the plunger.[5]

Infiltration with Local Anesthetic Agents

Some clinicians do not use local anesthetic during fat harvest but the majority inject the donor site with short-acting local anesthetic agents with or without epinephrine. The most commonly used agent is lignocaine with concentration doses ranging from 0.5% to 2% and doses of epinephrine ranging from 1:80,000 to 1:200,000. Coleman recommends using 0.5% lignocaine with 1:200,000 adrenaline. The main clinical advantage of infiltration with local anesthetic combined with epinephrine are reduction of potential donor site pain, blood loss and bruising.

It is uncertain whether the use of lidocaine adversely impacts fat graft survival. In a study by Moore et al[6] an inhibitory effect of lidocaine on adipocyte growth in cell culture was observed. In contrast, Keck et al[7] demonstrated that exposure to a variety of anesthetic solutions increased adipocyte viability in contrast to a dry technique. Furthermore, animal models pretreated with saline or lidocaine and epinephrine have demonstrated no significant effects on fat graft volumes or histological architecture.

Preparation

Centrifugation is a popular method of fat graft preparation. The process separates the nonviable components, including blood, oil, and lidocaine, leaving behind the adipocyte-rich segment for transfer. Coleman advocates 3 minutes of centrifugation of aspirated fat at 3000 rpm. This process separates the fat into a bottom layer of tumescent lidocaine and blood, a middle layer of usable fat graft and a top layer of oil from ruptured adipocytes. Other clinicians advocate the use of centrifugation at different spinning rates and duration.

Rohrich et al[8] have recently challenged the process of centrifugation and found no quantitative difference between the viability of processed and unprocessed fat graft viability. Similarly, Ramon et al[9] utilized a mouse model to demonstrate that fat cell survival after 16 weeks between centrifuged and noncentrifuged fat grafts in terms of weight and volume were comparable, whilst histological analysis showed noncentrifuged fat grafts exhibited less fibrosis.

Washing harvested fat grafts as a form of preparation has also been described, using lactate Ringer's solution to improve viability. The rational is to decrease levels of inflammatory mediators from the graft and minimize the immune response at the recipient site. However, there is a paucity of high-level evidence in the literature to affirm that washing harvested fat graft improves overall graft survival.

Application

To maximize graft survival the adipocytes must be in close vicinity to a blood supply. Studies have suggested that fat placed within 2 mm of an arterial supply will survive and greater distances risk necrosis and fibrosis. Thus the surface area of the fat graft in contact with a vascular recipient bed is essential to optimize graft survival. The "fanning out" technique is one method of injection that ensures small aliquots of fat graft are spread over a large surface area. Other commonly used injection methods, such as linear threading, serial puncture, and cross-hatching, can also be used to achieve the desired outcome. Slower injection speeds of 0.5–1 mL/s have resulted in greater fat graft survival rates compared to faster injection speeds of 3–5 mL/s. A curved microcannula 2–3 mm in diameter or blunt-tip needle 14–19 gauge is commonly used for autologous fat transfer.

Complications

In general, autologous fat transfer is a safe procedure with a low risk profile. However, patients must be warned about bruising, swelling, contour irregularity, and infection, in addition to fat necrosis and calcification. Rare cases of severe complications such as fat embolism of cerebral artery and retinal artery leading to stroke and blindness, respectively, have been reported in the literature during soft tissue augmentation of nasolabial fold and periorbital area.[10,11]

During the consent process it is important to ensure that the common and rare risks of fat transfer are made evident. Moreover, it important to discuss the limitations of the procedure, with emphasis on the unpredictability of the graft take in regard to partial and complete absorption over time.

The rise in popularity of autologous fat transfer in addressing contour deformity and volume restoration over the past few decades has propelled this technique to the forefront of reconstructive and aesthetic surgery. Despite its widespread adoption, there remains no consensus on the optimal donor site or most effective method of harvest and preparation. Further objective randomized clinical trials are required to guide current variations in practice. However, autologous fat transfer functions as a powerful tool in the armamentarium of plastic surgeons and practitioners must keep abreast of developments in order to ensure optimal graft outcome.

Bone Autografts

The success of bone autografts in the treatment of nonunions is well described. In the tibia, union rates of more than 90% have been reported using iliac crest bone graft at a mechanically stable site.[12] Bone grafting has also been effective in treating recalcitrant and infected nonunions as well as aiding the healing at the docking site of nonunions treated with distraction osteogenesis.[13] In addition to the mechanical properties and volume effect, the biological properties of bone autografts are also advantageous.

Autologous bone grafting has been considered as the gold standard in management of bone defects and nonunions. However, the introduction of a new generation of bone substitutes has challenged this notion, largely due to the morbidity associated with the harvesting procedure with reports of donor site pain, infection, and hematoma of varying incidences between 9% and 55%.[14]

Bone grafts heal by the following mechanisms: (1) adherence to the surrounding tissue, i.e., incorporation, (2) creeping substitution, also referred to as osseoconduction, a process whereby the bone graft acts as a scaffold along which angiogenesis occurs and new bone is formed by progenitor cells, and (3) osseoinduction, the differentiation of mesenchymal stem cells into osteocytes.

Autologous bone grafts possess biological advantages over allografts and synthetic bone grafts as they confer greater histocompatibility as well as an excellent combination of osteogenic, osteoinductive, and osteoconductive properties.

Autologous Cancellous Bone Grafts

The trabecular structure of cancellous bone generates a large surface area. This permits a greater incorporation of cellular components (mesenchymal stem cells and osteoblasts) and provides excellent osteogenic and osteoinductive properties. Additionally, the sizable trabecular surface area facilitates revascularization and integration of the graft at the host site. Conversely, a significant limitation of cancellous bone is its poor mechanical strength during the initial phase. However, increased stability is achieved within months due to the biological capacity of trabecular bone graft to induce new bone formation, once incorporated.

Autologous Cortical Bone Grafts

Cortical bone autografts have a different biological profile compared to cancellous bone autografts. In contrast to the low density of cancellous bone, the dense and highly organized structure of cortical bone provides initial mechanical strength and stability. However this structural integrity compromises the available surface area and constitutes a barrier to vascular in-growth and remodeling during graft incorporation. Furthermore, the subsequent lack of cellularity and growth factors diminishes the osteogenic potential of cortical bone grafts. The integration of cortical bone is mediated through osteoclastic activity resulting in resorption of the cortices and loss of bone. This results in transient weakness with reduction of mechanical strength of up to 75%.[15]

Autologous Vascularized Bone Grafts

Autologous vascularized cortical bone grafts have favorable biological attributes relative to standard autologous nonvascularized autografts. In addition, they are mechanically superior during the initial 6–12 months after the grafting procedure and offer a greater provision of nutrients to deep structures of the graft. Despite their many advantages, they carry an increased risk of donor site morbidity and can be more technically challenging during harvest and implantation, requiring both orthopedic input and microvascular skills. It has been proposed that more than 90% of the osteocytes may survive transplantation if patent vascular anastomoses and stability of the graft are achieved.[16] Osteoneogenesis by graft and host can lead to expeditious incorporation of the graft, whilst the residual weakness of the construct remains minimal.

Due to the advantageous and cost-effective combination of biological and mechanical properties, bone grafts continue to be important tools in the management of bone defects and nonunions.

Cartilage Autografts

Cartilage does not possess the regenerative capacity of bone or other connective tissues due to its lack of vascularity. Cartilage is composed of chondroitin sulphate, a gelatinous ground substance, into which collagen and elastic protein fibers are incorporated. It is flexible, very durable, and resistant to compressive forces. There are three types of cartilage: hyaline, elastic, and fibrocartilage. The most abundant type is hyaline, found in the nose, ear, trachea, larynx, smaller respiratory tracts, costal cartilages, and the articular surfaces of synovial joints. It is the precursor to bone in most of the embryonic skeleton. Injury to or congenital deformity of cartilage can result in pain, loss of mobility, and significant deformity. The management of moderate to severe cartilage defects is challenging due to the lack of intrinsic ability to self-repair.

Autologous Cartilage Grafts

Autologous cartilage grafts are commonly used in the reconstruction of congenital ear deformities, augmentation or revision rhinoplasty, and nipple reconstruction post mastectomy. They can be harvested from the costal cartilages, septum of the nose, and the ear. Autologous cartilage grafts can provide excellent results, but are associated with significant donor site morbidity and the final aesthetic result can be dependent on the carving skills of the operating surgeon.

Osteochondral Autograft Transfer

When reconstructing injured joint surface cartilage, transplants of cylindrical osteochondral plugs can be harvested from non-weight-bearing portions of the joint and transferred to the site of the defect. Osteochondral autograft transfer (OAT) offers the prospect of restoring the defect with true hyaline articular cartilage with greater wear characteristics and joint function. Furthermore, this technique can be performed in a single procedure using reusable equipment without the requirement of external laboratory assistance.

A recent 10-year follow-up study showed superior clinical results with OAT compared with microfracture in young athletes with focal osteochondral defects.[17] Several studies have corroborated similar improvements in both pain and function in patients with osteochondral defects of the knee.

One of the primary limitations is defect size, as the technique is best suited to small and medium-sized focal chondral defects . Much larger lesions up to 9 cm^2 require multiple osteochondral plugs and carry the risk of greater donor site morbidity. Other disadvantages include limited donor site availability and a size mismatch between the donor and recipient site.

Autologous Chondrocyte Implantation

Autologous chondrocyte implantation (ACI) aims to provide hyaline cartilage for repair of injured articular cartilage. This cell-based technique takes place in three stages: (1) 200–300 mg of cartilage is harvested arthroscopically from a lower weight-bearing area (intercondylar notch, superior ridge of the femoral condyles); (2) chondrocytes are isolated after enzymatic removal of the matrix, grown in vitro for 4–6 weeks, and then (3) applied to damaged areas during a second procedure.

ACI holds the advantage of treating larger lesions (up to 10 cm^2) with articular hyaline cartilage with minimal donor requirements. A clinical study of ACI demonstrated long-term improvement of symptoms in patients with isolated femoral condyle lesions and osteochondritis dissecans at 5–11 years after treatment.[18] Similar results were reported 10–20 years after ACI, where 74% of 224 patients described symptomatic improvement.[19]

Despite promising reports, ACI is technically more challenging and carries associated risks of graft failure, hypertrophy, and subsequent high reoperation rates of between 9% and 20%.[20] It is also dependent on in vitro expansion of chondrocytes, relying on external laboratories and higher costs. This theoretically also increases the chance of introducing infection, whilst also necessitating two operations.

Allografts and Xenografts

Allografts can be defined as graft tissue obtained from a donor of the same species as the recipient, but comprised of a different genetic make-up. The absence of donor site morbidity, general successful outcomes, and decreased surgical time render allografts a popular alternative to autologous grafts. In recent years, natural ECM have been procured, processed, and marketed for clinical use as patches to reinforce tissue repair.

Bone Allografts

Bone allografts can be applied to aid healing of bone injured either by trauma or secondary to iatrogenic causes. Survival of bone grafts depend on systemic factors that also affect wound healing, e.g., age, nutritional status, immunosuppression, diabetes, obesity. Scarring, infection, and previous radiotherapy at the site of the recipient bed can also adversely affect graft survival.

Allograft preparation requires treatment with ethanol in order to remove cellular material, followed by gamma irradiation for bacterial, fungal, and viral eradication. However, allografts lose some of their biological properties through the sterilization process and synthetic bone substitutes have only osteoconductive properties if combined with human growth factors or autograft.

Fascia Allografts

An engineered fascial device may be utilized for ligament repair, extension of rotational muscle transfers, grafting lacerated muscles, periosteal coverage, and wound healing. Fascia lata or fascia from the iliotibial tract are most commonly used and have several advantages: biocompatibility, ability to be replaced by the host tissue, good mechanical properties, and ease of handling.

An in vitro study comparing the histological features of allograft iliotibial bands with tibialis anterior tendons reported that they shared a similar structure composed of aligned collagen fibers.[21] Moreover, they observed that allograft iliotibial bands were superior in regard to creep, stress-relaxation, and viscoelastic properties. In addition, allograft iliotibial bands also demonstrated low cytotoxicity with a higher propensity to favor cell attachment and infiltration over time.

Dermal Matrices

Integra

Integra (Integra LifeSciences Corp., Plainsboro, NJ, USA) is a dermal regeneration matrix consisting of bovine collagen, chondroitin-6-sulphate and a silastic membrane. It has gained widespread use in the clinical treatment of deep partial-thickness and full-thickness burn wounds, full-thickness skin defects, and chronic wounds. The bovine collagen dermal component integrates with the host and the temporary epidermal silicone is peeled away as the dermis regenerates. A very thin autograft is then grafted onto the neodermis.

Integra has been successfully used in reconstructive surgery to augment soft tissue coverage over structures such as bone or tendon. However, it requires a two-stage procedure prior to sufficient defect coverage to allow for adequate vascularization of the template. Integra provides immediate donor site coverage independent of wound size. Additionally, it creates a smooth gliding surface between underlying structures, e.g., paratenon or nerves and STSG. Long-term outcomes after radial forearm flap donor site coverage with Integra and STSG show successful functional and aesthetic defect coverage.[22] A similar long-term study also reported improved scar cosmesis and skin elasticity after comparing Integra combined with STSG relative to STSG alone in acute burn treatment.[23] However, disadvantages to its use include cost, infection risk, and foreign body reaction.

AlloDerm

AlloDerm (LifeCell Corporation, Branchburg, NJ, USA) is fabricated by decellularizing cadaveric skin. After processing, the skin is reduced to a basement membrane and correctly aligned dermal collagen matrix that will theoretically not be rejected. During host integration, it is invaded by fibroblasts, and undergoes neovascularization and neoepithelialization, without evidence of rejection or adverse reaction to the implant from the host.

AlloDerm has been shown in clinical trials to be well tolerated. It has been used extensively in burns surgery to provide biological coverage of full-thickness burns and as a framework for split-thickness skin grafts[24] and for intraoral mucosa resurfacing after fistula repair.[25] Its ability to support neovascularization and tissue ingrowth permits persistent volume correction. This gives AlloDerm an advantage over other injectable forms of collagen. A significant drawback of AlloDerm sheets are the requirement for an incision for placement. An injectable form of AlloDerm (Micronized AlloDerm) has been created by homogenizing AlloDerm sheets cut into strips. The product comprises of injectable-sized particles of AlloDerm that maintain the ultrastructure of the dermis and can be introduced easily through a 26-gauge needle.

Several large published series of patients undergoing breast reconstruction utilizing acellular dermal matrices have reported low rates of capsular contracture.[26,27] In addition, animal studies have corroborated the absence of a capsule around implants where human acellular dermal matrix was placed, which was both observed clinically at the time of implant exchange and also confirmed histologically from biopsies.[28]

Strattice

Strattice (LifeCell Corporation, Branchburg, NJ, USA) is an acellular reconstructive tissue matrix derived from porcine dermis. It undergoes proprietary processing that removes cells and reduces the risk of xenogeneic rejection response. The presence of the α-Gal epitope on porcine tissues has been associated with rapid rejection. The enzymatic processing of Strattice significantly reduces the amount of α-Gal epitope in the absence of damage to the matrix integrity (collagen and elastin architecture).

Since its introduction in 2008, Strattice has been utilized in wide array of reconstructive procedures including primary breast reconstruction, breast revision surgery, and in abdominal wall reconstruction and hernia repair.

Performance of Strattice has been evaluated by implantation into the abdominal wall of a primate excisional repair model.[29] The animals tolerated the implants well and exhibited no clinical signs of inflammation, laxity, hernia or visceral tissue adhesion. Immunological evaluation of cell infiltration demonstrated an early, mixed cellular inflammatory response at 2 weeks, which was transient and diminished to baseline levels by 3 months. A study comparing three non-cross-linked, commercially available extracellular matrix scaffolds (Strattice, Veritas, and XenMatrix) showed that the intrinsic denaturation temperature for Strattice, Veritas, and XenMatrix was 51°C, 38°C, and 44°C, respectively. In addition, the susceptibility to collagenase degradation was increased in Veritas and XenMatrix. These findings suggest a greater number of extracellular matrix modifications in the Veritas and XenMatrix scaffolds.[30] In an in vivo primate model, Strattice permitted cell repopulation and was remodeled over 6 months. In contrast, Veritas was unstable at body temperature, absorbed rapidly and associated with moderate inflammation whilst XenMatrix caused severe inflammation.[30]

The use of Strattice for repair of incisional hernias in Yucatan pigs compared to primary closure demonstrated that primary closure resulted in greater scarring and bone hyperplasia along the incision line. In contrast, Strattice elastic modulus and tensile stress were similar to fascia and it facilitated a more complete wound healing response relative to primary closure.[31]

Clinically, Strattice may enhance soft tissue support in patients with poor quality mammary soft tissue support, especially in implant-based breast reconstruction post-mastectomy patients and in those undergoing augmentation mammoplasty. Furthermore, it has been associated with fewer implant-related complications, including capsular contracture, rippling, palpability, and malposition.

Alloplastic Materials

Metals

An ideal metal implant possesses the characteristics of biocompatibility, high tensile strength and resistance to corrosion. Advantages of metallic biomaterials include lack of donor site morbidity and widespread availability. Disadvantages include eliciting a host reaction and their considerable cost. Metals are routinely used in fracture fixation (plates, screws, and wires), cranial plates, and artificial joints. Most metals used as biomaterials are alloys. An alloy is a mixture of two or more metals into a single material. Commonly used alloys include the following.

Stainless Steel

Stainless steel is an alloy composed mainly of iron, chromium, and nickel. It is highly corrosion-resistant in the physiological environment compared to other formulations. Chromium forms a strongly adherent surface oxide layer which renders it resistant to corrosion. Despite the favorable anticorrosive properties of stainless steel, the leaching of metallic ions can lead to inflammatory reactions in surrounding tissues and cause pain.

Cobalt Alloys

Vitallium is an example of an alloy composed of cobalt, chromium, and molybdenum (Co–Cr–Mo). This alloy has similar strength to stainless steel but is lighter and less resistant to corrosion.

Titanium (Ti)

Titanium has the capacity to form direct chemical bonds with mineralized bone matrix. This "osseointegration" allows for robust incorporation between soft tissue as well as between implant and bone, and confers significant utility in prosthetic reconstruction. In the first stage the titanium implant is placed into bone and covered by periosteum or bone for a minimum period of 3 months. Subsequently, during the integration process the histological appearance shows calcified matrix in direct apposition to the metal surface without intervening fibrous tissue. It is this interaction which provides unparalleled stability and endows great mechanical strength to titanium implants.

Maxillofacial prosthetics largely rely on the support of titanium osseointegrated implants and titanium microplates are routinely use for bony internal fixation. Combined with aluminum and vanadium alloy, titanium becomes less malleable. There is also less scatter artifact on radiographic images compared to cobalt alloys and stainless steel.

Gold

Gold (Au) has limited applications in the field of plastic surgery. Although it is resistant to corrosion, it lacks sufficient mechanical properties and is costly. It still serves a purpose in facial palsy patients where it is utilized to create iatrogenic ptosis through gold loads placed on the upper eyelid to address lagophthalmos. However, a recent review reported fewer complications of infection and capsule formation with the use of platinum due to its higher biocompatibility relative to gold.[32]

Ceramics

Ceramics are solid materials composed of inorganic, nonmetallic substances. Chemically, they are formed through a combination of hybrid covalent and ionic bonds. The atomic repeating order can be short-range (e.g., glasses) or long-order (e.g., crystals). Advantages of ceramics are that they can be chemically inert in numerous environments or designed to be bioactive in the body with a composition that can mimic the mineral component of bone. They are excellent heat and electric insulators whilst also being corrosion-resistant. In addition, they are hard and brittle (fracture without deformation), strong in compression, but weak in shearing and tension. Examples of ceramic materials are porcelain, cements, pottery, and glasses (amporphous).

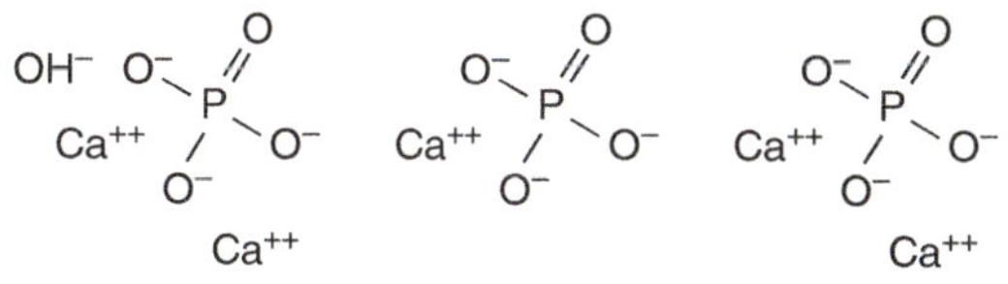

• **Fig. 3.2** Hydroxyapatite (HA).

Bioinert Ceramics

These include oxide ceramics (Al_2O_3, ZrO_2), silica ceramics, carbon fiber, and synthetic diamond. Alumina (Al_2O_3) and Zirconia (ZrO_2) are the two most commonly used structural bioceramics. They are primarily used as modular heads on femoral stem hip components, but can also be used for dental restorations including in crowns and bridges. They undergo less wear than metal components, and the wear particles generated are generally better tolerated. In addition, they have good mechanical and aesthetic properties.

Bioactive Ceramics

These include tricalcium phosphates, synthetic hydroxyapatite substitutes and bioactive glass (e.g., 45S5 Bioglass). Bioactive glass has osteoproductive characteristics and encourages bone cells to produce matrix. When implanted it binds to soft tissue and hard tissue to form a porous matrix that facilitates activation and infiltration of osteoblasts.

Bioglass (composition = 46.1% SiO_2, 24.4% NaO, 26.9% CaO, 2.6% P_2O_5 (mol %)) was the first material observed to form an interfacial bond with the host tissue. This bone-binding property is underpinned by accumulation of silicon ions upon implantation and the subsequent formation of a hydroxyapatite coating on the surface of Bioglass. The strength of the bond between Bioglass and cortical bone has been shown to mimic the strength of native host bone.

Hydroxyapatite (HA) and tricalcium phosphate are the most commonly used ceramics in plastic surgery. HA, the coral of genus *Porites*, has a calcium carbonate exoskeleton similar to bone. Through a hydrothermal exchange process of carbonate for phosphate, it adopts a structure identical to bone. The material is available in the form of blocks or granules and can bond to bone without evoking an inflammatory response. It provides a scaffold for bony ingrowth and is not resorbed (Fig. 3.2). A recent study evaluated a hybrid tissue-engineered bone construct of nanocrystalline HA.[33] The authors demonstrated that when the construct was seeded with osteoblasts, the scaffold with HA enhanced cell proliferation and promoted production of mineralized extracellular matrix greater than the plain scaffold.

Tricalcium phosphate (TCP) is a synthetic material, more porous than HA and prone to resorption. Its porosity ranges from 30% to 80% and is usually supplied in blocks or granules, similar to HA (Fig. 3.3). Calcium phosphate cement is a synthetic HA cement that forms a paste when mixed with water and a drying agent (sodium phosphate) and hardens to form microporous HA. The cement also improves contour adaptability and eliminates the need for prefabrication. It is biocompatible and associated with minimal reabsorption and inflammatory response.

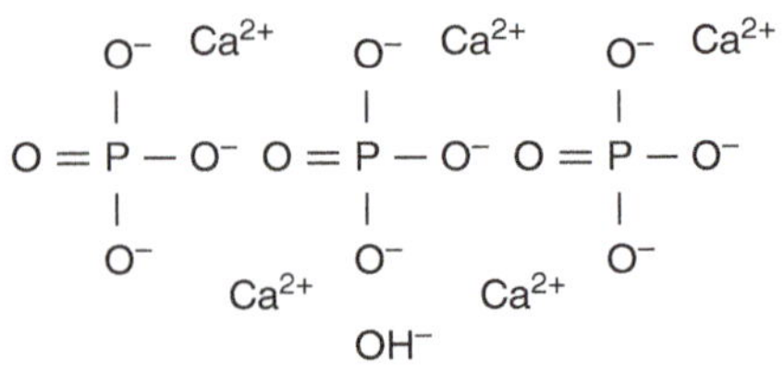

• **Fig. 3.3** Tricalcium phosphate.

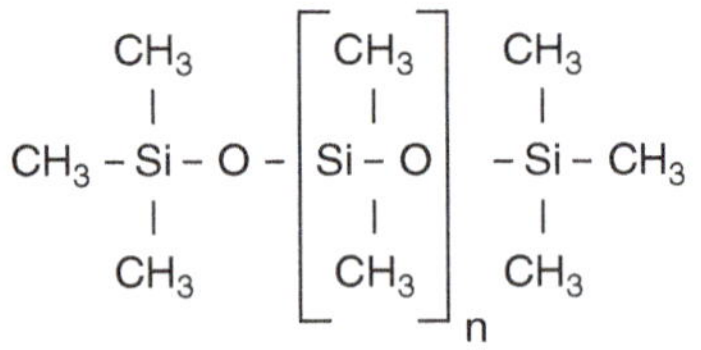

• **Fig. 3.4** Poly(dimethylsiloxane) (PDMS).

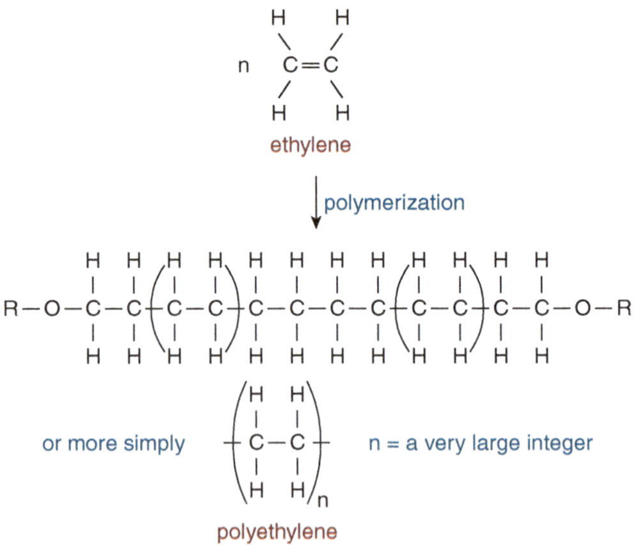

• **Fig. 3.5** Polyethylene.

Polymers

Polymers are long-chain molecules composed of small repeating units. Synthetic polymers can be found in facial implants, breast prostheses, sutures, implantable fabrics, and joint replacements.

Silicone

Silicone (Si), a semi-metallic element, found abundantly in nature in various forms, including silicone dioxide (silica) or silicates. Silicones are mixed inorganic–organic polymerized siloxanes. The basic repeating unit of silicone polymers is siloxane $(R_2SiO)_n$, where R is an organic group such as methyl, ethyl, or phenyl. The most commonly used formulation of silicone in medicine is poly(dimethylsiloxane) (PDMS) (Fig. 3.4). Silicone is available in various forms, including liquid, gel, or rubber, and is created by altering the length and cross-linking of the PDMS chains.

Medical grade silicone is biocompatible, nonallergenic and nonabsorbable, rendering it ideal for use in numerous medical devices ranging from catheters, prosthetic cardiac valves to intraocular lenses. In the field of plastic surgery, silicone implants have been used for malar and chin augmentation, whilst in hand surgery, silicone rods are routinely used for two-stage tendon reconstruction and as spacers for arthroplasty. In breast surgery, silicone has been used in prostheses since 1963 and the historic implants have been reported to still be in situ after 43 years.[34]

Silicone was initially regarded as a relatively inert biomaterial and thought to produce minimal inflammation. However, silicone induces capsule formation as part of a foreign body reaction. The cellular composition of the capsule has been examined extensively and suggests the role of the immune system in its pathogenesis. Capsular contraction of silicone implants can lead to pain, distortion, and hardness. However, the fibrous capsule that forms around the implant helps to maintain implant position and facilitates subsequent removal.

Alternatives such as porous polyurethane implants are reported to enable enhanced tissue fixation with a reduced incidence of capsule formation. Previous reports of carcinogenesis associated with polyurethane and its breakdown product 2,4-toluenediamine have been dispelled with epidemiological studies. However, they are perceived to feel unnatural and can be more technically difficult during implantation.

If silicone is subjected to repetitive loading and deformation, the resulting fragmentation into small particles can lead to the formation of silicone granulomas due to the ensuing immune reaction. However, there exists no evidence from numerous long-term epidemiological studies that silicone implants are associated with any autoimmune, connective tissue or neurological disorders. Although breast augmentation with silicone implants can result in damage to lactiferous ducts and glandular tissue, it is not a contraindication to breast feeding.

Polyethylene

This is the simplest carbon polymer – C_2H_4 – composed of a carbon backbone (Fig. 3.5). Pore sizes range from 100 μm to 250 μm and facilitate tissue ingrowth and stabilization during implant biointegration. High-density polyethylene (HDPE) (Medpore) is used for its properties of biocompatibility and high tensile strength. It is available in sheets and blocks that can be sculpted intraoperatively, and is commonly employed in orbital reconstruction and craniofacial augmentation. The porous nature of Medpore combined with its fibrovascular integration into host tissue permits an immune response to infection and is reported to possess overall low infection rates.

Polyethylene can be modified by adding a methyl group to each monomer to form poly(1-methylethylene) or polypropylene (Prolene). This material is commonly used as a nonabsorbable suture and can be woven into a fabric mesh, used for chest wall, pelvic floor, and abdominal wall reconstruction.

Replacement of the hydrogen atoms in polyethylene with fluorine yields polytetrafluoroethylene (PTFE,

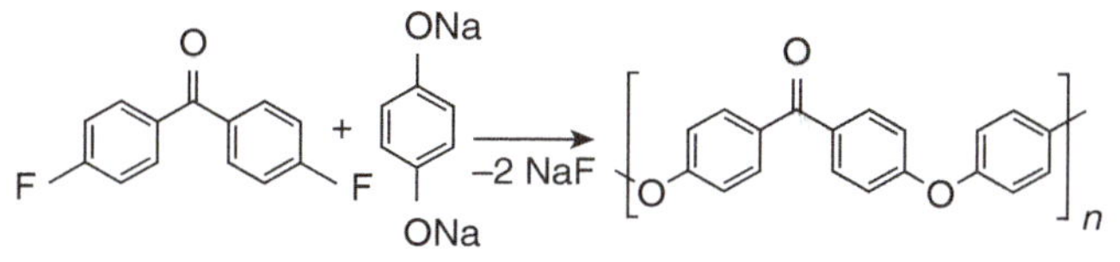

• **Fig. 3.6** Poly(aryl-ether-ether-ketone) (PEEK).

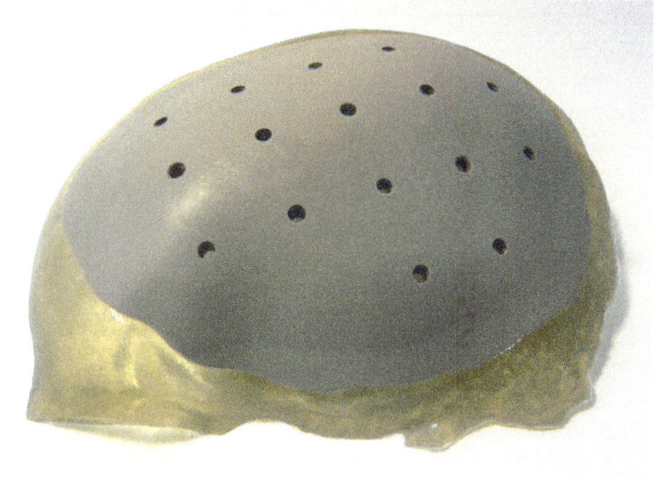

• **Fig. 3.7** PEEK implant applied in cranial vault reconstruction.

Teflon). PTFE is characterized by its soft macroporous surface which encourages adjacent tissue ingrowth and endows it with greater tensile strength, non-erosive nature and good biocompatibility. Rapidly stretching PTFE under certain manufacturing conditions results in the formation of a strong synthetic polymer known as expanded PTFE (ePTFE, Gortex). Its versatility has resulted in its extensive adoption as a medical implant in vascular grafting, in addition to chest wall, abdominal, and pelvic floor reconstruction. However, a limitation of PTFE vascular grafts is the high incidence of stenosis in small-caliber grafts secondary to thrombosis compared to autologous vein grafting.[35]

PEEK

Polyaryletherketone is a relatively new family of high-temperature thermoplastic polymers, consisting of an aromatic molecular chain backbone, interconnected by ketone and ether functional groups. The chemical structure of polyaromatic ketones confer resistance to chemical and radiation damage, whilst retaining the characteristics of biocompatibility, inertness and radiolucency. Polyetheretherketone (PEEK) has emerged as a highly promising candidate in the setting of orthopedic implants, as well as more recently in facial and cranial reconstruction. Its mechanical properties resemble native bone with similar biomechanical characteristics. However, PEEK lacks the bioactivity required for osseointegration and long-term stability of implants is directly dependent on screw fixation. As a radiolucent material, it produces minimal artifacts during imaging (Figs. 3.6 and 3.7).

Conclusion

A plethora of diverse biomaterials are available at the disposal of the practicing surgeon, each purporting unique benefits and limitations. They have gained widespread popularity and extensive use over the years due to their established clinical utility, ease of use, long "shelf life", safety and availability.

References

1. Kaufman MR, Bradley JP, Dickinson B, et al. Autologous fat transfer national consensus survey: trends in techniques for harvest, preparation, and application, and perception of short- and long-term results. *Plast Reconstr Surg*. 2007;119(1):323–331.
2. Peer LA. The neglected free fat graft. *Plast Reconstr Surg (1946)*. 1956;18(4):233–250.
3. Li K, Gao J, Zhang Z, et al. Selection of donor site for fat grafting and cell isolation. *Aesthetic Plast Surg*. 2013;37(1):153–158.
4. Kononas TC, Bucky LP, Hurley C, May Jr JW. The fate of suctioned and surgically removed fat after reimplantation for soft-tissue augmentation: a volumetric and histologic study in the rabbit. *Plast Reconstr Surg*. 1993;91(5):763–768.
5. Coleman SR. Facial augmentation with structural fat grafting. *Clin Plast Surg*. 2006;33(4):567–577.
6. Moore Jr JH, Kolaczynski JW, Morales LM, et al. Viability of fat obtained by syringe suction lipectomy: effects of local anesthesia with lidocaine. *Plast Reconstr Surg*. 1995;19(4):335–339.
7. Keck M, Zeyda M, Gollinger K, et al. Local anesthetics have a major impact on viability of preadipocytes and their differentiation into adipocytes. *Plast Reconstr Surg*. 2010;126(5):1500–1505.
8. Rohrich RJ, Sorokin ES, Brown SA. In search of improved fat transfer viability: a quantitative analysis of the role of centrifugation and harvest site. *Plast Reconstr Surg*. 2004;113(1):391–395; discussion 6-7.
9. Ramon Y, Shoshani O, Peled IJ, et al. Enhancing the take of injected adipose tissue by a simple method for concentrating fat cells. *Plast Reconstr Surg*. 2005;115(1):197–201; discussion 2–3.
10. Lee CM, Hong IH, Park SP. Ophthalmic artery obstruction and cerebral infarction following periocular injection of autologous fat. *Korean J Ophthalmol*. 2011;25(5):358–361.
11. Park SH, Sun HJ, Choi KS. Sudden unilateral visual loss after autologous fat injection into the nasolabial fold. *Clin Ophthalmol*. 2008;2(3):679–683.
12. Phieffer LS, Goulet JA. Delayed unions of the tibia. *J Bone Joint Surg Am*. 2006;88(1):206–216.
13. Biasibetti A, Aloj D, Di Gregorio G, Masse A, Salomone C. Mechanical and biological treatment of long bone non-unions. *Injury*. 2005;36(suppl 4):S45–S50.
14. Ebraheim NA, Elgafy H, Xu R. Bone-graft harvesting from iliac and fibular donor sites: techniques and complications. *J Am Acad Orthop Surg*. 2001;9(3):210–218.
15. Goldberg VM, Stevenson S, Shaffer JW, Davy D, Klein L, Zika J, et al. Biological and physical properties of autogenous vascularized fibular grafts in dogs. *J Bone Joint Surg Am*. 1990;72(6):801–810.
16. Tu YK, Bishop AT, Kato T, Adams ML, Wood MB. Experimental carpal reverse-flow pedicle vascularized bone grafts. Part II: bone blood flow measurement by radioactive-labeled microspheres in a canine model. *J Hand Surg Am*. 2000;25(1):46–54.

17. Gudas R, Gudaite A, Pocius A, et al. Ten-year follow-up of a prospective, randomized clinical study of mosaic osteochondral autologous transplantation versus microfracture for the treatment of osteochondral defects in the knee joint of athletes. *Am J Sports Med.* 2012;40(11):2499–2508.
18. Peterson L, Minas T, Brittberg M, Nilsson A, Sjogren-Jansson E, Lindahl A. Two- to 9-year outcome after autologous chondrocyte transplantation of the knee. *Clin Orthop Relat Res.* 2000;(374):212–234.
19. Peterson L, Vasiliadis HS, Brittberg M, Lindahl A. Autologous chondrocyte implantation: a long-term follow-up. *Am J Sports Med.* 2010;38(6):1117–1124.
20. Niemeyer P, Pestka JM, Kreuz PC, et al. Characteristic complications after autologous chondrocyte implantation for cartilage defects of the knee joint. *Am J Sports Med.* 2008;36(11): 2091–2099.
21. Delcroix GJ, Kaimrajh DN, Baria D, et al. Histologic, biomechanical, and biological evaluation of fan-folded iliotibial band allografts for anterior cruciate ligament reconstruction. *Arthroscopy.* 2013;29(4):756–765.
22. Wirthmann A, Finke JC, Giovanoli P, Lindenblatt N. Long-term follow-up of donor site morbidity after defect coverage with Integra following radial forearm flap elevation. *Eur J Plast Surg.* 2014;37:159–166.
23. Nguyen DQ, Potokar TS, Price P. An objective long-term evaluation of Integra (a dermal skin substitute) and split thickness skin grafts, in acute burns and reconstructive surgery. *Burns.* 2010;36(1):23–28.
24. Wainwright D, Madden M, Luterman A, et al. Clinical evaluation of an acellular allograft dermal matrix in full-thickness burns. *J Burn Care Res.* 1996;17(2):124–136.
25. Cole P, Horn TW, Thaller S. The use of decellularized dermal grafting (AlloDerm) in persistent oro-nasal fistulas after tertiary cleft palate repair. *J Craniofac Surg.* 2006;17(4):636–641.
26. Agarwal JP, Mendenhall SD, Anderson LA, et al. The breast reconstruction evaluation of acellular dermal matrix as a sling trial (BREASTrial): design and methods of a prospective randomized trial. *Plast Reconstr Surg.* 2015;135(1):20e–28e.
27. Mowlds DS, Salibian AA, Scholz T, Paydar KZ, Wirth GA. Capsular contracture in implant-based breast reconstruction: examining the role of acellular dermal matrix fenestrations. *Plast Reconstr Surg.* 2015;136(4):629–635.
28. Stump A, Holton 3rd LH, Connor J, Harper JR, Slezak S, Silverman RP. The use of acellular dermal matrix to prevent capsule formation around implants in a primate model. *Plast Reconstr Surg.* 2009;124(1):82–91.
29. Connor J, McQuillan D, Sandor M, et al. Retention of structural and biochemical integrity in a biological mesh supports tissue remodeling in a primate abdominal wall model. *Regen Med.* 2009;4(2):185–195.
30. Sun WQ, Xu H, Sandor M, Lombardi J. Process-induced extracellular matrix alterations affect the mechanisms of soft tissue repair and regeneration. *J Tissue Eng.* 2013;4:2041731413505305.
31. Monteiro GA, Delossantos AI, Rodriguez NL, Patel P, Franz MG, Wagner CT. Porcine incisional hernia model: evaluation of biologically derived intact extracellular matrix repairs. *J Tissue Eng.* 2013;4:2041731413508771.
32. Silver AL, Lindsay RW, Cheney ML, Hadlock TA. Thin-profile platinum eyelid weighting: a superior option in the paralyzed eye. *Plast Reconstr Surg.* 2009;123(6):1697–1703.
33. Wang M, Cheng X, Zhu W, Holmes B, Keidar M, Zhang LG. Design of biomimetic and bioactive cold plasma-modified nanostructured scaffolds for enhanced osteogenic differentiation of bone marrow-derived mesenchymal stem cells. *Tissue Eng Part A.* 2014;20(5–6):1060–1071.
34. Nahabedian MY. Explantation of 41-year-old implants following primary breast augmentation. *Ann Plast Surg.* 2007;58(1):91–94.
35. Johnson WC, Lee KK. A comparative evaluation of polytetrafluoroethylene, umbilical vein, and saphenous vein bypass grafts for femoral-popliteal above-knee revascularization: a prospective randomized Department of Veterans Affairs cooperative study. *J Vasc Surg.* 2000;32(2):268–277.

4

Local Anesthetics

YASAMIN ZIABARI

Introduction

Local anesthetic agents cause reversible blockade of the neuronal sodium (Na^+) channel, thereby blocking transmission of nerve impulses from nociceptive afferents.

Mechanism of Action of Local Anesthetics

In the un-ionized state, local anesthetics are varyingly lipid-soluble, thereby penetrating the phospholipid cell membrane into the axoplasm. Here, re-ionization of the molecule takes place. It is this re-ionized molecule that then enters and blocks sodium channels, preventing sodium influx into the neuron during depolarization, and thus halting propagation of an action potential.[1]

Local anesthetics have also been shown to exert far-reaching effects on other receptors, independent of their action on sodium channels. These include inhibition of the local tissue inflammation that results in nociceptor sensitization, leading to pain and hyperalgesia.[2] They may also be involved in the priming of descending inhibitory pain pathways, which could show clinical benefit in the reduction of neuropathic pain.[3] Furthermore, local anesthetics have been shown to have antithrombotic, antimicrobial, and neuroprotective actions.[4,5]

Nerve Fiber Characteristics and Differential Blockade

Local anesthetics show a greater affinity for receptors within sodium channels during their activated and inactivated states (i.e., during neuronal stimulation) compared to their resting states.[6] Hence neurons that fire more rapidly are more susceptible to local anesthetic block.

Other nerve fiber characteristics have been shown, in vitro, to govern the sensitivity of nerve fibers to local anesthetics.[7]

- Smaller nerve fibers with shorter axons are more easily blocked compared to larger never fibers with longer axons.
- Smaller diameter nerve fibers (e.g., 0.4–1.2 μm C-fibers, which transmit pain, temperature, and touch) are blocked at lower concentrations compared to larger diameter nerve fibers.
- Myelinated fibers (e.g., A-α fibers, which convey motor and proprioception) are more easily blocked than unmyelinated nerve fibers (e.g., C-fibers), as local anesthetic tends to pool within the myelin sheath.

The aforementioned principles do not, however, consistently correlate with the clinical observations. Nevertheless, when blocking peripheral nerves, there is usually an order in the disappearance of sensing modalities: autonomic, pain, temperature, deep pressure, and finally, motor function.

Physiochemical Properties of Local Anesthetics

Chemistry

Local anesthetics are weak bases.[1] Their basic molecular structure is comprised of a lipophilic aromatic moiety and a hydrophilic amino domain (Fig. 4.1).

Depending on the chemical linkage between the respective lipophilic and hydrophilic groups, local anesthetics can be classified as amides or esters. This linkage has implications on drug metabolism and allergenicity (Table 4.1).

Potency

The potency of local anesthetics correlates well with lipid solubility and molecular weight in vitro.[9]

Other factors affecting potency include tissue distribution and direct vasodilator actions of the local anesthetic.

Duration of Action

Local anesthetics are classed as "short-", "medium-", or "long-" acting.

The duration of action of local anesthetics positively correlates with the degree of protein binding; the more protein-bound a local anesthetic, the longer the duration of action, with the "unbound" portion of the drug being biologically active.[9] However, local anesthetic molecules remain bound to sodium channels for seconds only. Given such a high dissociation rate, of greater relevance are factors that maintain a high concentration of local anesthetic molecules around the nerve. These factors are:

- local anesthetic lipid solubility: there is a direct correlation between lipid solubility and protein binding
- tissue vascularity: this depends on regional blood flow and the addition of vasoconstrictors
- intrinsic vasodilatory properties of local anesthetics.

Local anesthetics generally cause vasoconstriction at very low concentrations and vasodilatation at higher, clinically useful, concentrations.[1] Considerable variability exists, however. Moreover, ester local anesthetics are more potent vasodilators compared to amides. The exception to this rule is cocaine, which causes vasoconstriction by blocking reuptake of norepinephrine at sympathetic nerve endings. The greater the intrinsic vasodilatory action of a local anesthetic, the more pronounced the effect of the addition of vasoconstrictors.

Onset of Action

The faster the diffusion of local anesthetic across a nerve sheath, the faster the onset of action. The rate of diffusion is determined by:

- the site of local anesthetic injection
- the concentration of local anesthetic used
- the degree of ionization of local anesthetic molecules.

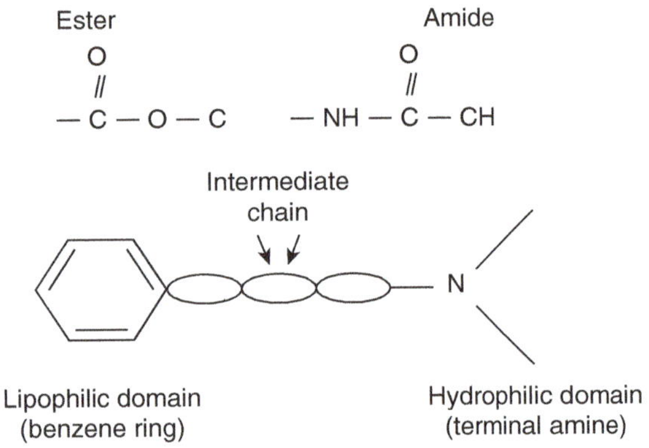

Fig. 4.1 Chemical structure of a local anesthetic.

The latter is related to a physiochemical property of a drug known as the pKa. The pKa is the pH at which 50% of the drug is present in an ionized form.[1] For basic drugs, such as local anesthetics, a greater proportion of drug is present in the ionized form at a pH below the pKa; at a pH above the pKa, a greater proportion of the drug will be un-ionized. The reverse is true for weak acids. Therefore, local anesthetics with a higher pKa will have a greater drug fraction present in the ionized state, resulting in a slow onset of action.[1] The most clinically relevant comparison is the faster action-onset of lidocaine (pKa 7.9) compared to bupivacaine (pKa 8.1).

Pharmacokinetics of Local Anesthetics

Absorption

Absorption of local anesthetics primarily depends on:

- the site of injection
- the addition of vasoconstrictors
- the physiochemical properties of the local anesthetic agent itself.

On reaching the systemic circulation, local anesthetics are taken up by distant organs according to vascular density.[10] Highly vascular organs such as the brain, heart, lung, liver, and kidneys, will have greatest exposure to the peak concentration of unmetabolized local anesthetic. Uptake is determined by the tissue-plasma partition coefficient.

Distribution

Local anesthetic molecules can be "free" or bound to plasma proteins.

Alpha-1 acid glycoprotein binds the weakly basic local anesthetic molecules with high affinity. However, albumin represents a greater fraction of plasma proteins, and as such has a high capacity (but comparatively low affinity) for binding to local anesthetic molecules.

Local anesthetic protein binding is pH-dependent and decreases as the pH decreases.[10] This has important

TABLE 4.1 A Comparison of the Main Characteristic Differences Between Amide and Ester Local Anesthetics

Class	Example	Allergenicity[a]	Pharmacokinetics	Stability
Amides	Lidocaine Mepivacaine Bupivacaine Ropivacaine Levobupivacaine	Rare[8]	Extensively protein-bound Hepatic metabolism by amidases; slower than ester metabolism thus potential for accumulation	Long shelf-life and heat-insensitive unless mixed with glucose
Esters	Procaine 2-Chloroprocaine Tetracaine (Amethocaine) Benzocaine Cocaine	Rare, but more common with the amides, especially with procaine Cross-reactivity may exist with other esters Implicated metabolite: *p*-aminobenzoic acid	Minimally protein-bound Hydrolysis by plasma cholinesterase and other esterases	Short shelf-life due to spontaneous hydrolysis

[a]Antioxidant additives, or preservatives such as metabisulfite or parabens may be implicated in causing non–anaphylactic reactions.

clinical relevance. For example, in local anesthetic systemic toxicity (see below), a metabolic acidosis may ensue secondary to tissue hypoxia. As the plasma pH decreases, the proportion of "free" drug increases, potentiating the toxicity. Furthermore, intracellular acidosis increases conversion of the local anesthetic molecule into the cationic state, rendering the molecule unable to cross the cell membrane. This "ion trapping" exacerbates the toxicity further.

Clearance and Metabolism

Esters (except cocaine) undergo rapid hydrolysis by plasma cholinesterases, and other non-specific esterases.[1] Their metabolites are inactive but may be associated with hypersensitivity reactions. Amides are metabolized in the liver by the action of amidases.[1]

Hepatic clearance is dependent on the hepatic blood flow, and the hepatic extraction ratio.

Hepatic extraction ratio depends on the ratio of unbound to protein-bound drug. Drugs that are comparatively less protein-bound (e.g., lidocaine) have a higher hepatic extraction ratio.[11] Clearance is thus only limited by hepatic blood flow. Hence, factors reducing hepatic blood flow may increase toxicity, e.g., heart failure.

Conversely, the clearance of drugs which are more protein-bound (e.g., bupivacaine) is more dependent on free drug concentration, as opposed to hepatic blood flow.[10] Intrinsic liver disease may, in turn, affect free drug concentration, e.g., a reduction in liver enzymes or reduced plasma protein production.

Patients with liver disease and cardiac disease can receive "normal dose" single-shot blocks. However, catheter infusions or repeated blocks should be given at a reduced dose.

Renal failure associated with severe uremia can be associated with reduced clearance and more rapid absorption of local anesthetic, leading to higher peak plasma concentrations.

Some local anesthetics may undergo first pass metabolism by lung extraction due to the lower pH of the lungs compared to the plasma, resulting in an "ion trapping" effect. This effect is lost in patients with right to left cardiac shunts, thus increasing the risk of toxicity.[12]

Local Anesthetics in Clinical Practice

Table 4.2 summarizes the pharmacokinetic and pharmacodynamic properties of the most commonly used local anesthetics.

Concentration of Local Anesthetics

A 1% solution of a drug contains 1000 mg of drug per 100 mL of solution. Thus a 1% solution of lidocaine contains 1000 mg of lidocaine per 100 mL (10 mg/mL). Similarly, a 0.5% solution of bupivacaine contains 500 mg of bupivacaine in 100 mL of solution (5 mg/mL).

Clinically Useful Adjuncts

Vasoconstrictors

Epinephrine is the most commonly used vasopressor. It slows the rate of absorption of local anesthetic, thereby prolonging the duration of action[13] and reducing the risk of toxicity. Furthermore, it can help decrease surgical blood loss, and may identify inadvertent intravascular injection. Absolute contraindications to use include injection close to tissues with inadequate collateral circulation (ankle, wrists, digits, and penis); as well as intravenous regional anesthesia. Relative contraindications to use include the presence or risk of tissue ischemia, cardiac disease, hypertension, and concomitant use of other sympathomimetic drugs (e.g., tricyclic antidepressants).

The maximum safe dose of epinephrine is 4 μg/kg; concentrations in excess of 1:200,000 should not be used (Table 4.3).

Sodium Bicarbonate

Sodium bicarbonate ($NaHCO_3$) raises the pH of the local anesthetic solution, thus increasing the fraction of unionized drug able to traverse the neuronal membrane.[13] It may also reduce the pain of injection.[14] Furthermore, the speed of onset of the local anesthetic is theoretically increased. However, the rise in pH seen is only modest, and limited by the solubility of the base form of the drug. This translates to only modest decreases in block onset time.[15]

The recommended dose is 1 mL of 8.4% sodium bicarbonate per 10 mL of local anesthetic.[13]

Topical Local Anesthetics

Topical local anesthetics are available in a variety of formulations and presentations. Their advantages include avoidance of first-pass metabolism, and avoidance of the risks of more invasive local anesthetic techniques.

The "ideal" topical local anesthetic formulation will maximize permeability and absorption via the stratum corneum, while limiting systemic absorption hence toxicity. As a general rule, drug delivery is enhanced by prior skin exfoliation and degreasing, as well as the application of a nonporous dressing (e.g., Tegaderm).

Disadvantages of topical local anesthesia include unpredictable absorption, uneven distribution or spread of the agent during application, and a failure of the occlusive dressings to stick to the skin. These agents should not be applied to broken, irritated, or infected skin.

Topical anesthesia lends itself well to procedures such as skin biopsy and removal, electrocautery, and superficial laser therapy. It also enables painless needle insertion.

Cutaneous Agents

The most commonly used topical agents are summarized in Table 4.4.

TABLE 4.2 Summary of Local Anesthetics Most Commonly Used in Clinical Practice

	Amides						Esters		
	Lidocaine	Mepivacaine	Prilocaine	Bupivacaine	Levobupivacaine	Ropivacaine	Procaine	Amethocaine	Cocaine
Onset of action	Fast	Fast	Fast	Medium	Medium	Medium	Slow	Slow	Medium
Relative potency	2	2	2	8	8	8	1	8	–
Duration of action)	Medium	Medium	Medium	Long	Long	Long	Short	Long	Short
Maximum dose (mg/kg)[a]	3	5	6	2	2.5	3	7	1.0	1.5
Maximum dose with epinephrine (mg/kg)	7	7	9	2.5	3	4	10	1.5	NA
Additional notes			Relative lack of vasodilatation Risk of methemoglobinemia	Greatest risk of cardiotoxicity Unpredictable block duration	*S*-enantiomer of bupivacaine; modestly less cardiotoxic and neurotoxic	Pure *S*-enantiomer Lower propensity for motor block compared to bupivacaine Marked vasoconstriction at low concentration		Local vasodilatory action Lower propensity for motor block compared to bupivacaine Marked vasoconstriction at low concentration	Moffat's solution: 2 mL 8% cocaine, 1 mL of 1: 10,000 epinephrine and 2 mL of 8.4% sodium bicarbonate Blocks reuptake of norepinephrine, thus can provoke hypertensive crisis and arrhythmias Potent vasoconstrictor

[a]Quoted maximum "recommended safe doses" vary. Most available data are extrapolated from animal studies. Other factors, including the site and speed of injection, are of greater relevance (see text).
NA, Not applicable.

Mucosal Agents

Examples of suitable ointments include cocaine 4%, benzocaine 5%–20%, and lidocaine 2%–5%. Lidocaine is also available as an aerosol preparation.

Transdermal Local Anesthetic Delivery

In order for a drug to passively diffuse across the stratum corneum, it must be lipophilic, non-ionized, and have a low molecular weight (<500 Daltons). Various technologies are evolving for further accelerate transdermal drug delivery.[16] The most relevant to plastic and reconstructive surgery are mentioned below.

TABLE 4.3 Equivalent Drug Concentrations for Standard Drug Solutions

Drug Solution	Drug Concentration (µg/mL)
1:10,000	100
1:100,000	10
1:200,000	5
1:400,000	2.5

Liposomal Drug Delivery

A liposome is a phospholipid vesicle comprised of at least one concentric phospholipid bilayer, enclosing an aqueous cavity. A liposome is thus able to transport both lipophilic and hydrophilic compounds, in the lipid bilayer and aqueous core, respectively.

Liposomes are currently the most common vehicles for targeted drug delivery, with the main advantages being potentially sustained and prolonged drug delivery by a physiochemically stable carrier.[17]

Liposomal bupivacaine (Exparel, Pacira Pharmaceuticals, Parsippany, NJ) is currently licensed only for use in the United States, for a limited albeit expanding number of clinical settings, which includes local infiltration in breast surgery. This drug utilizes DepoFoam technology, which involves encapsulating the bupivacaine within multivesicular liposomes.[17] These liposomes are comprised of multiple discontinuous internalized aqueous compartments, divided by biodegradable nonconcentric lipid bilayers (in contrast to unilamellar liposomes). This structure enables the bupivacaine to be released over time, enabling a much longer duration of action, and avoiding the need for local anesthetic catheter placement.

The current maximum dose of liposomal bupivacaine is 266 mg (20 mL). The drug volume can be expanded by dilution with either normal saline, or lactate Ringer's solution,

TABLE 4.4 Commonly Used Topical Local Anesthetic Preparations

Local Anesthetic	Trade Name (Pharmaceutical Company)	Formulation	Application Time (minimum–maximum)	Maximum Dose/Area	Particulars
Lidocaine 2.5% w/w + prilocaine 2.5% w/w	EMLA 5% (Astra Zeneca)	Cream + occlusive dressing	1–5 h	Adult: 60 g + 600 cm² Child: 6–11 years: 20 g + 200 cm² for 1–5 h 1–5 years: 10 g + 100 cm² for 1 h <2 months: 1 g + 10 cm² for 1 h	Not for use in pregnancy if <37 weeks' gestation Not for use in infants (<12 months) taking methemoglobin-inducing agents
Tetracaine 4% w/w	Ametop (Smith & Nephew)	Gel + occlusive dressing	30–45 min	Adult + child >5 years: maximum 5 tubes (1 tube = 1 g) at separate sites at single time	Not recommended for infants <1 month
Lidocaine 7% + tetracaine 7%	Pliaglis (Galderma)	Cream	30–60 min	1 mm layer (1.3 g of cream per 10 cm²)	Not recommended if age <18 years Apply with spatula only Peel off skin prior to procedure
Lidocaine 4% w/w	LMX 4 (Ferndale)	Liposomal + occlusive dressing	30 min – 5 h Child: 3–12 months: 4 h <3 months: 1 h	Adult + child >1 year: 2.5 g Child <1 year: 1 g	

up to a volume of 300 mL.[18] Furthermore, the drug can be admixed with bupivacaine solution, adding an additional 150 mg of bupivacaine to the drug mixture (either 60 mL of 0.25% bupivacaine or 30 mL of 0.5% bupivacaine).

Liposomal bupivacaine should be injected with a 25G needle, or larger, to avoid disrupting the liposomal structure. Any topical antiseptic skin preparations should be allowed to dry completely, as contact may cause the liposomes to disband, releasing toxic doses of bupivacaine into the plasma.[18] Liposomal bupivacaine tends not to spread or diffuse into surrounding tissues after injection. For this reason, small volume and frequent injections are required to cover the surgical site, ideally with 1–1.5 cm spacing intervals. The preparation should be injected slowly, and deeply, using a moving needle technique, and aspirating every 1–2 mL to avoid intravascular injection.[18]

Tumescent Anesthesia

Tumescent anesthesia involves the injection of a very dilute local anesthetic solution, coupled with epinephrine and sodium bicarbonate, into tissue until it becomes firm and tense (tumescent). The technique was initially pioneered in the 1980s for the purposes of liposuction, but its application has since expanded to cover a variety of surgeries. In the field of plastic and reconstructive surgery, this includes mastectomy, breast reduction, breast augmentation, and perhaps more controversially, breast reconstruction.

Standard tumescent solution is comprised of 500 mg lidocaine, 1 mg of epinephrine, and 12.5 mEq sodium bicarbonate added to a 1 liter solution of 0.9% normal saline. The epinephrine prolongs the duration of anesthesia, as well as reducing the incidence of bleeding.[19] The bicarbonate alkalizes the solution, thus accelerating the onset of anesthesia (see above).

The maximum recommended dose of lidocaine, with or without epinephrine, has not historically been applied to tumescent anesthesia. The American Society of Plastic Surgeons (ASPS) has endorsed higher doses of lidocaine in tumescent anesthesia based on available data. Additional studies have suggested that liposuction itself reduces systemic lidocaine absorption, as well as peak serum lidocaine concentrations. Peak serum concentrations typically occur 13–14 hours following initial infiltration.[19]

In summary, current recommendations are that lidocaine doses between 35 mg and 55 mg/kg can be used in tumescent anesthesia administered for liposuction. Best current evidence suggests reducing this dose to 28 mg/kg for tumescent anesthesia undertaken for other procedures.[19] Despite the relative excellent safety record for this technique, the same care and caution for minimizing the risk of local anesthetic toxicity (LAST) must be applied (see below).

Iontophoresis

Iontophoresis involves the application of a constant low-voltage direct current to actively transport drugs across a biological membrane.[16] Molecules which are hydrophilic and ionized, thus ordinarily being skin-impermeable, are ideal drugs for delivery by iontophoresis.

In the United States, the first FDA-approved iontophoretically delivered local anesthetic patch was LidoSite (lidocaine hydrochloride 10% and epinephrine 0.1%; Vyteris Inc, Fair Lawn, NJ, USA). Pretreatment with sonophoresis may work synergistically to enhance drug delivery.[16] This method of drug delivery is useful only for small surface areas and is limited by cutaneous irritation and mild patient discomfort.

Microporation

Microporation produces transient microchannels in the skin in order to form a conduit through which ordinarily impenetrable drugs may pass.[16] Examples include the P.L.E.A.S.E. (Pantec Biosolutions AG, Ruggell, Liechtenstein). High-velocity, high-pressure "needleless" "jet" sprays can deliver local anesthetic in a similar way.

Electroporation

Electroporation employs high-voltage (>100 volts) pulses for microsecond bursts, causing formation of aqueous channels within the stratum corneum, providing a conduit for the diffusion of molecules. The time between the high-voltage pulses allows the skin to depolarize, thus avoiding interference with current flow.[16]

Sonophoresis

Sonophoresis employs the use of low frequency (20–100 kHz) ultrasound waves to cause acoustic cavitation within the stratum corneum, resulting in the non-linear formation of acoustic microjets. The addition of surfactant material to the skin works synergistically to enhance the flux of hydrophilic molecules with large molecular weights that would ordinarily not traverse the skin membrane.[16] Ultrasound can have a thermal heating effect, and induce convective transport, both of which may contribute to enhancing lipid permeability of local anesthetics.[16]

Local Anesthetic Systemic Toxicity (LAST)

Local anesthetic systemic toxicity (LAST) is a spectrum of neurological and cardiovascular signs and symptoms, which result from the direct effect of local anesthetics on neuronal activity within the central nervous system, autonomic ganglia, and myocardium. The manifestation of these symptoms is related to the plasma concentration of the local anesthetic.

Symptoms and Signs

Raised plasma concentration of local anesthetics characteristically causes initial excitatory phenomena, secondary to suppression of inhibitory neuronal circuits. This is followed by nervous system and cardiovascular depression.

Central Nervous System Effects

The patient may complain of circumoral tingling, a metallic taste in the mouth, diplopia, dizziness, and tinnitus. They may appear confused, anxious or agitated; or show signs of muscle excitability and twitching. Convulsions may occur.[20,21] CNS depressant effects manifest as apnea and a reduced level of consciousness or coma.

Cardiovascular Effects

Cardiac toxicity often initially results in hypertension, and tachycardia. As plasma concentrations rise, this can rapidly evolve into ventricular arrhythmias: ventricular tachycardia, including polymorphic VT (torsade de pointes), and ventricular fibrillation.[20] Consequently, refractory hypotension, heart conduction blocks, or complete loss of cardiac output may occur.[20]

Importantly, current literature suggests that up to 50% of LAST presentations are atypical, presenting with cardiovascular signs only, and/or a delayed presentation.[20] Thus a high index of suspicion is paramount, and sufficient post-procedure monitoring is mandatory.

The propensity for cardiac toxicity varies between local anesthetics and can be quantified using the CC/CNS ratio; that is the ratio of the dose inducing cardiovascular collapse (CC) to the dose required to produce seizures. A lower CC/CNS ratio is associated with more cardiotoxic agents, and the more cardiotoxic agents are less likely to produce premonitory CNS signs, implying a narrower safety margin. Moreover, once malignant arrhythmias occur, they typically require prolonged resuscitation. However, less cardiotoxic drugs have been responsible for a significant number of LAST cases described in the literature,[20] demonstrating there is no room for complacency.

All local anesthetics are arrhythmogenic and, with the exception of cocaine, have direct myocardial depressant effects.

Prevention of LAST

Prevention of LAST is multifactorial, best achieved with a three-pronged approach[20]:

- Avoidance and recognition of inadvertent intravascular injection, achieved by:
  - use of real-time ultrasound guidance for performing nerve blocks
  - frequent aspiration during injections, repeated each time the needle is moved. A negative aspiration test does not exclude intravascular injection, particularly if the needle is placed in a small vessel, or a catheter technique is used
  - incremental injections based on patient's circulation time
  - use of a pharmacological marker, e.g., epinephrine, to aid detection of inadvertent intravascular injection.
- Limiting the systemic uptake of local anesthetic, best accomplished by:
  - using the lowest effective local anesthetic dose
  - prolonging drug clearance by the addition of epinephrine as an adjunct
  - adherence to maximum safe dosages, understanding that the concept of "maximum safe dose" is based mainly on extrapolations from animal data. It is clinically irrelevant unless the site, speed, and route of injection are taken into consideration.[20] It is vital that surgeons and anesthesiologists communicate the plan for local anesthetic administration during the presurgical pause, reducing the risk of additive toxicity.
- Knowledge of patient and operational factors that increase the risk of LAST.[20] These are summarized in Table 4.5. Where risk factors are identified, consideration must be given to lowering the total drug dosage and increasing the duration of monitoring post-procedure.

TABLE 4.5 Summary of Sensory Innervation of Important Branches of the Trigeminal Nerve

Trigeminal Nerve Division	Nerve	Branch	Sensory Supply (Ipsilateral Side)
Ophthalmic (V_1)	Frontal	Supraorbital nerve	Upper eyelid Forehead Scalp (until lambdoid suture)
		Supratrochlear nerve	Conjunctiva Lower medial forehead Skin of the upper eyelid Frontal sinus mucosa
Maxillary (V_2)	Infraorbital		Lower eyelid Side of nose Upper lip Facial gingiva, maxillary premolars, and anterior teeth
Mandibular (V_3)	Inferior alveolar	Mental nerve	Anterior chin Lower lip to mentolabial fold Lower teeth

Facilities, including "Local Anesthetic Toxicity Toolkit", together with local departmental algorithms for treatment of LAST, must be available in every operating room and recovery complex. All practitioners must be familiar with the location and usage of this apparatus.

Management of LAST

Management of LAST is underpinned by three principles:
- restoring the circulation to maintain tissue oxygenation
- controlling seizure activity to reduce oxygen consumption
- mitigating the systemic effects of local anesthetics.

Management requires an acute resuscitation team. All resuscitation team members, including surgeons, must be familiar with the resuscitation algorithm. The use of a cognitive aid/checklist is encouraged:

Stop injection of local anesthetic and call for help. If in doubt, call the Cardiac Arrest Team.

Start resuscitation (as per local cardiopulmonary resuscitation protocols):

Airway: maintain patency using chin lift/jaw thrust and airway adjuncts; intubate the trachea once skilled persons available.

Breathing: ventilate both lungs with 100% oxygen; hyperventilating the patient is not recommended.

Circulation: establish intravenous access, and control seizures by bolus administration of an intravenous benzodiazepines as first line. Simultaneously commence treatment.

Start Treatment

1. Start intravenous 20% lipid emulsion therapy **as soon as possible**:

   Give bolus over 2–3 minutes: 100 mL if patient >70 kg, or 1.5 mL/kg if patient <70 kg (ideal body weight).

   Start infusion over 15–20 minutes: 200–250 mL if patient >70 kg, or 0.25 mL/kg per minute if patient <70kg.

   Consider repeat bolus or increasing infusion to 0.5 mL/kg per minute until cardiovascular stability is restored.

   The infusion should continue for at least 10 minutes after cardiovascular stability is achieved.

   The maximum cumulative dose of 20% lipid emulsion should not exceed 12 mL/kg.
2. For seizures resistant to benzodiazepines, small propofol boluses may be administered; neuromuscular blocking agents may also be warranted.
3. Treat arrhythmias as per nationally endorsed resuscitation guidelines; amiodarone is normally the anti-arrhythmic of choice. Arrhythmias in LAST are typically refractory to treatment. Resuscitation may be prolonged.[20]
4. If cardiac arrest occurs, epinephrine should initially be given in small doses (≤1 μg/kg), to avoid exacerbating any arrhythmias.
5. Consider cardiopulmonary bypass in cases refractory to treatment.

Post-resuscitation Management

Patients must be managed in a high dependency unit.

Where 20% lipid emulsion has been administered, there remains a theoretical risk of acute pancreatitis for up to 48 hours. Regular clinical assessment, and serum lipase assays must be considered.

Methemaglobinemia

Methemaglobin is formed when the iron contained within hemaglobin is present in the ferric ($Fe3^{+}$) as opposed to the reduced ferrous ($Fe2^{+}$) state. The result is an inability to carry oxygen.[22]

Local anesthetics implicated in the development of methemaglobinemia are, namely, prilocaine (which is metabolized to o-Toluidine, which oxidizes hemoglobin to methemoglobin), benzocaine, and lidocaine.[22]

Methemoglobin levels exceeding 1% are deemed abnormal. Symptoms manifest with methemoglobin levels in excess of 10% and include a "slate-grey" discoloration of the skin, fatigue, shortness of breath, and generalized weakness, progressing to cardiac dysrhythmias and coma. Risk factors include preexisting congenital methemaglobinemia, the administration of drugs with a high oxidative stress (e.g., phenytoin, sulphonamides), and age <6 months.[1,22] The last mentioned is due to a reduced level of NADH reductase enzymes.[1]

Management of methemaglobinemia is with high concentration oxygen and the administration of a reducing agent such a methylene blue (1 mg/kg intravenously).

Sedation

A large volume of procedures carried out in plastic surgery lend well to topical anesthesia with or without patient sedation.

Sedation is a state encompassed within a spectrum, between "fully awake" and "anesthetized". Somewhere along this spectrum, the patient will become unable to maintain their airway and ventilate adequately. For this reason, "conscious sedation" is deemed the safest type of sedation. This is where the patient is able to verbally respond to the operator when prompted, signifying maintenance of the airway.

Basic Principles of Sedation

- As a general rule, the greater the number of drugs used to sedate patients, the greater the risk of drug synergy, and thus unpredictable pharmacodynamics. "Mixing" sedative agents should always be avoided.
- Children and elderly patients are at greater risk of idiosyncratic drug reactions.
- Sedation in obese patients with or without diagnosed obstructive sleep apnea (OSA), or obesity hypoventilation syndrome, must be approached with extreme caution and considered "high risk"; in many cases a general

anesthetic may be safer. This is due to the increased sedative sensitivity observed in this patient group, coupled with reduced sensitivity to hypercarbia.
- Sedation is not a surrogate for inadequate pain relief.
- Patients must always be consented for sedation, and be made aware that unlike a general anesthetic, awareness is an anticipated and "normal" part of the procedure.
- Fasting guidelines must be observed, as for a general anesthetic.

Discussion of different sedative agents is beyond the scope of this chapter.

Safety

It is the responsibility of the health professional administering sedation to ensure they are adequately experienced and qualified in dealing with the consequences of the drugs they administer. The safest setting within which to administer sedation is the hospital setting, with full patient monitoring (namely oxygen saturations, capnography, heart rate, and blood pressure), resuscitation facilities, and with the presence of an anesthetist.

Amongst surgeons, one of the most commonly observed misconceptions is that the presence of good oxygen saturations translates to an adequately maintained airway. It is imperative to understand that:
- adequate oxygenation does not always signify adequate ventilation; as such, the airway reflexes may also be absent or depressed, putting the patient at risk of aspiration;
- there is normally a 30-second lag between a fall in arterial oxygen saturation and its detection with pulse oximetry.

Based on current evidence, it is estimated that one-fifth of LAST cases occur outside the hospital environment. Furthermore, approximately one-half of cases occur in settings without the presence of an anesthetist.

Regional Techniques of Relevance to Plastic Surgery

There are many regional techniques that lend themselves well to plastic and reconstructive surgery. The advantage of successful regional techniques compared to local infiltration is a more predictable area of anesthesia, with minimal risk of tissue distortion.

The majority of regional techniques are carried out by anesthetists. The use of ultrasound-guided blocks has become increasingly popular.

The following criteria must be fulfilled prior to the commencement of any regional anesthetic technique:
- patient consent
- exclusion of contraindications to block
  - absolute contraindications: patient refusal, local anesthetic allergy (rare)
  - relative contraindications: localized infection; coagulopathy
- confirmation, both verbal and written, of the site and side to be blocked
- patient monitoring
- resuscitation equipment and drugs
- presence of a trained assistant
- an alternative management plan should the regional technique fail.

Intravenous Regional Anesthesia (Bier Block)

Indications

Surgery on the wrist or hand lasting less than one hour, e.g., foreign body removal; release of tendon contractures.

Principle

Local anesthetic is injected into the forearm previously exsanguinated by use of a tourniquet. Local anesthetic diffuses from the venous circulation into surrounding nerve endings, providing anesthesia below the level of the tourniquet.[23] Prior venous exsanguination prevents dilution of the local anesthetic, thus maintaining a sufficient concentration gradient for diffusion to occur.

The duration of the block is limited by tourniquet pain, which typically occurs after 30–45 minutes. Patients invariably require conscious sedation.

Technique

- An intravenous cannula is inserted into the opposite arm ("systemic circulation" access).
- A 22G intravenous cannula is also inserted into the hand of the limb to be blocked ("regional circulation" access).
- With the patient supine, the arm to be blocked is passively exsanguinated by elevation for 2 minutes.
- A double-cuffed tourniquet is placed proximal to the limb that is to be blocked. Adequate padding between the skin and the tourniquet is essential to prevent skin necrosis. It is imperative that both tourniquet cuffs are checked for leaks.
- An Esmarch bandage is applied to enhance limb exsanguination. At this point the distal cuff is inflated, followed by the proximal cuff. Once the proximal cuff is fully inflated, the distal cuff can be deflated. The cuffs are inflated to approximately 100 mmHg above systolic blood pressure.
- The Esmarch is removed, and the distal limb is checked for pallor and the absence of a distal pulse. Local anesthetic is then injected into the IV cannula of the exsanguinated limb. For the upper limb, 12–15 mL of 2% lidocaine or 30–40 mL of 0.5% lidocaine is a suitable regimen. Onset of anesthesia typically takes 5–10 minutes.

Complications

- Tourniquet pain: this typically occurs after 30 minutes. It is alleviated by inflating the proximal cuff, and deflating the distal cuff, which may afford a further 30 minutes of operating time.
- Local anesthetic toxicity: this can be avoided by ensuring correct function and application of the tourniquet, with

clear labeling of the "distal" and "proximal" cuffs. At the end of surgery, the tourniquet should be released in a graduated manner, preventing a sudden washout of local anesthetic into the systemic circulation.

- Hematoma: the smallest gauge IV line should be used. Should there be failed attempts at IV cannulation, pressure should be applied until bleeding stops, prior to limb exsanguination.
- Engorgement of the extremity: this occurs where arterial blood enters the limb in spite of the tourniquet, and venous blood is unable to escape. It can be avoided by ensuring good tourniquet function with a pressure of at least 100 mmHg above systolic.

Nerve Blocks for the Face

General Considerations

- All three anatomical landmarks discussed below can be identified by imagining a line drawn vertically parallel to the midline of the face, intersecting a centered pupil.
- The eyes must be protected from cleaning solutions.
- The needle should never be inserted directly into the relevant foramina, as this may cause damage to the neurovascular bundle. If immediate paresthesia is encountered on slow injection, the needle should be withdrawn and redirected.
- Topical anesthesia should be considered for intraoral blocks.
- Commonly used agents include 1% lidocaine or 1% mepivacaine.
- A 23G or 25G 25-mm intradermal needle attached to a 3-mL or 5-mL Luer lock syringe can be used.

For a detailed description of the relevant trigeminal nerve anatomy, please refer to an anatomy textbook.

Supraorbital Nerve Block

The supraorbital and the supratrochlear nerves can be blocked by a single injection technique.

Anatomy

The supraorbital nerve exits the supraorbital notch. At this junction, the nerve and its branches approximate with the orbital periosteum, underneath the obicularis and frontalis muscles. After giving off palpebral filaments to the upper eyelid, the nerve divides into medial and lateral branches, which fan out in a cephalad direction.

Landmark

The supraorbital notch (in a smaller percentage, closed to form a foramen), palpated at the junction of the lateral two-thirds and medial one-third of the inferior border of the supraorbital ridge, 2–3 cm lateral to the midline of the forehead (Fig. 4.2).

Technique

The needle is inserted 1 cm medial to 0.5 cm immediately superior to the supraorbital notch. The needle is then withdrawn a few millimeters and redirected medially towards the junction of the orbital rim with the nasal bone; 2–3 mL is injected.

Supratrochlear Nerve Block

Anatomy

The supratrochlear nerve exits the orbit 1 cm medial to the supraorbital nerve. It passes above the trochlea of the superior oblique muscle, and courses cephalad, giving off several small terminal branches.

Landmark

The supraorbital notch (see above), as the supratrochlear notch is difficult to palpate, or else absent in some people.

Technique

The needle is withdrawn a few millimeters and redirected (along the line of the supraorbital ridge) approximately 1 cm medially towards to the junction of the orbital rim with the nasal bone; 1–2 mL of local anesthetic is injected into the subcutaneous tissue in a fan-like distribution.

Application of mild pressure to the upper eyelid via a finger or roll of gauze while administering the aforementioned blocks may help to prevent palpebral edema and/or ecchymosis.

Infraorbital Nerve Block

Anatomy

The infraorbital nerve is the third branch of the maxillary (V2) division, which divides off within the pterygopalatine space, passing through the infraorbital fissure, along the floor of the orbit to enter the infraorbital canal. On exiting the canal, it gives off three terminal branches: the nasal, palpebral, and labial nerves.

Landmark

The infraorbital foramen, located along the inferior border of infraorbital rim.

Technique

The cheek is retracted and the infraorbital foramen is continually palpated (see Fig. 4.2). The needle is inserted into the mucosa directed approximately 0.5 cm above the upper second bicuspid tooth, aiming cephalad and laterally towards the lower border of the foramen; 2–3 mL of local anesthetic is injected.

Mental Nerve Block

Anatomy

The mental nerve is one of two terminal branches of the inferior alveolar nerve. It exits the mental foramen, an anterior opening of the mandibular canal. As it passes underneath the depressor anguli oris muscle, it divides into three further branches.

Landmark

The mental foramen, which is normally located between the two lower premolars in the adult, approximately 1 cm below

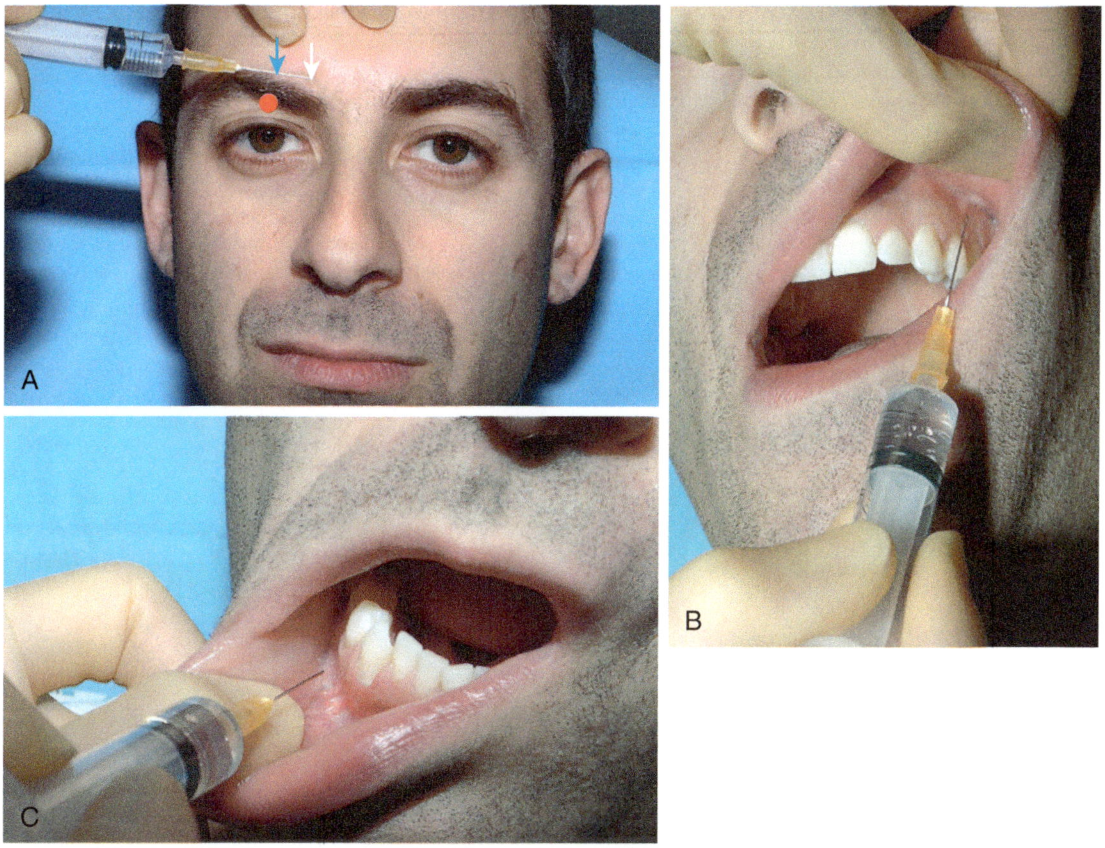

• **Fig. 4.2** (A) Supraorbital foramen (*red dot*); approximate positions of needle insertion for supraorbital (*blue arrow*) and supratrochlear (*white arrow*) nerve blocks. (B) Intraoral approach for infraorbital nerve block. (C) Intraoral approach for mental nerve block.

the gum-line. In children, the foramen is at the junction of the first and second primary molars.

There is some variability with the position of the foramen, however.

Technique (Intraoral Approach)

The cheek is retracted (see Fig. 4.2). The needle is inserted 0.5 cm above the mental foramen and directed caudally; 2–3 mL of local anesthetic is injected.

Where the foramen is not palpable, the nerve can be targeted by injecting the buccal mucosa at the junction of the two lower premolar teeth.

References

1. Peck TE, Hill S. *Pharmacology for Anaesthesia and Intensive Care.* 4th edn. New York: Cambridge University Press; 2014.
2. Kaba A, Laurent SR, Detroz BJ, et al. Intravenous lidocaine infusion facilitates acute rehabilitation after laparoscopic colectomy. *Anesthesiology.* 2007;106(1):11–18.
3. Toda S, Sakai A, Ikeda Y, et al. A local anesthetic, ropivacaine, suppresses activated microglia via a nerve growth factor-dependent mechanism and astrocytes via a nerve growth factor-independent mechanism in neuropathic pain. *Mol Pain.* 2011;7:2.
4. Hollmann MW, Gross A, Jelacin N, et al. Local anesthetic effects on priming and activation of human neutrophils. *Anesthesiology.* 2001;95(1):113–122.
5. Coghlan MW, Davies MJ, Hoyt C, et al. Antibacterial activity of epidural infusions. *Anaesth Int Care.* 2009;37(1):66–69.
6. Becker DE, Reed KL. Local anesthetics: review of the pharmacological considerations. *Anesth Prog.* 2012;59(2):90–102.
7. Gissen AJ, Covino BG, Gregus J. Differential sensitivities of mammalian nerve fibres to local anaesthetic agents. *Anesthesiology.* 1980;53:467–474.
8. Dewachter P, Mouton-Faivre C, Emala CW. Anaphylaxis and anesthesia controversies and new insights. *Anesthesiology.* 2009;111(5):1141–1150.
9. Butterworth J. Clinical pharmacology of local anaesthetics. In: Hadzic A, ed. *Textbook of Regional Anaesthesia and Acute Pain Management.* New York: McGraw-Hill; 2007. 105–1.
10. Burney RG, DiFazio CA, Foster JA. Effects of pH on protein binding of lidocaine. *Anesth Analg.* 1978;57(4):478–480.
11. Dillane D, Finucane BT. Local anesthetic systemic toxicity. *Can J Anesth.* 2010;57(4):368–380.
12. Kietzmann D, Foth H, Geng WP, et al. Transpulmonary disposition of prilocaine, mepivacaine, and bupivacaine in humans in the course of epidural anaesthesia. *Acta Anaesthesiol Scand.* 1995;39(7):885–890.
13. Shipton EA. New formulations of local anaesthetics, Part 1. *Anesthesiol Res Pract.* 2012;2012:546409. https://doi.org/10.1155/2012/546409.

14. Hanna MN, Elhassan A, Veloso PM, et al. Efficacy of bicarbonate in decreasing pain on intra-dermal injection of local anaesthetics: a meta-analysis. *Reg Anesth Pain Med.* 2009;34:122–125.
15. Chassard D, Berrada K, Boulétreau P. Alkalinization of local anesthetics: theoretically justified but clinically useless. *Can J Anaesth.* 1996;43(4):384–393.
16. Shipton EA. New delivery systems for local anaesthetics: Part 2. *Anesthesiol Res Pract.* 2012:289373.
17. Malik O, Kaye AD, Kaye A, et al. Emerging role of liposomal bupivacaine in anaethesia practice. *J Anaesthesiol Clin Pharmacol.* 2017;33(2):151–156.
18. EXPAREL. https://www.exparel.com/hcp/prescriptioninformation.pdf.
19. Holt NF. Tumescent anaesthesia: its applications and well tolerated use in the out-of-operating room setting. *Curr Opin Anaesthesiol.* 2017;30(4):518–524.
20. Neal JM, Barrington MJ, Fettiplace MR, et al. The Third American Society of Regional Anesthesia and Pain Medicine practice advisory on local anaesthetic systemic toxicity: executive summary 2017. *Reg Anesth Pain Med.* 2018;43(2):113–123.
21. Mather LE, Tucker GT, Murphy TM, et al. Cardiovascular and subjective central nervous system effects of long-acting local anaesthetics in man. *Anaesth Intensive Care.* 1979;7(3):215–221.
22. Guay J. Methemoglobinemia related to local anesthetics: a summary of 242 episodes. *Anesth Analg.* 2009;108(3):837–845.
23. New York School of Regional Anesthesia (NYSORA). Intravenous regional block for upper and lower extremity surgery. https://www.nysora.com/techniques/intravenous-regional-anesthesia/intravenous-regional-block-upper-lower-extremity-surgery/.

5

Lasers

SE HWANG LIEW

General Principles

LASER stands for Light Amplification by the Stimulated Emission of Radiation. Einstein first proposed the concept of stimulated emission in 1927. The first laser was developed in 1959 (ruby), and was first used on human skin in 1963.[1] The use of these early lasers was crude, and damage to cutaneous tissues and hence scarring was common.

It was the introduction of the concept of selective thermolysis by Anderson and Parrish in the 1980s[2] that saw the explosion of use in cutaneous medical lasers. This concept has led to the development of lasers that can act on specific targets or "chromophores" in certain layers of the skin, allowing for targeted therapy with minimal collateral damage in the form of scarring.

Laser Physics

Laser light is produced by the release of a series of coherent, unidirectional photons of light. These photons of light are generated by an external light source or electromagnetic field, which is used to excite a specific medium. Different mediums, which can be in solid, gaseous or liquid state, are selected to produce different lasers.

The atoms in the medium *absorb* the energy from the external source, thereby exciting some of their electrons into higher energy levels. Upon relaxation back into resting state, the energy lost is released as a photon of light in a process known as *spontaneous emission*. These photons are incoherent and go on to excite other electrons into higher energy levels resulting in multiple photons being spontaneously emitted throughout the material. This process continues until the number of electrons in the higher energy levels outnumbers those in the lower energy levels, resulting in a situation called *population inversion*. When this occurs, the high energy electrons will cause the photons to drop down into resting orbit, emitting a further photon of the same frequency and direction which is *in phase* with the incident photon without absorbing the incident photon. This process is called *stimulated emission* of photons and each photon released contains a specific amount of energy that is consistent throughout the material.

By placing the medium between two mirrors this process can amplify itself by allowing light that is produced at right-angles to the mirrors to pass back and forth through the medium producing increasing numbers of unidirectional, coherent photons which are then released, by transiently removing one mirror, as a laser beam.

Laser light has specific therapeutic properties, which are exploited in medical use. It is:

- Monochromatic: lasers have a specific wavelength and so have the ability to selectively target chromophores.
- Coherent: alignment of light waves allows high intensity to be focused over small area.
- Compressible: the high temporal coherence of waves allows for ultra-short pulses that deliver localized energy.
- Collimated: transmission of parallel rays of light without divergence allows for high localized intensity.

Laser Therapy in Cutaneous Treatment

Selective photothermolysis predicts that selective thermal damage of a chromophore will result when sufficient fluence (energy delivered per unit area – J/m^2), at a wavelength preferentially absorbed by that target, is delivered during a time (pulse duration) equal to or less than the thermal relaxation time of target.[2]

The use of laser in cutaneous treatment involves the selection of a specific wavelength, which is preferentially absorbed by a specific target or chromophore in the skin. This specific target can be oxyhemoglobin (vascular lesions), melanin (pigmented lesions) or water (skin resurfacing). Since the surrounding epidermis is spared, the treatment is specific, with little injury to normal skin.

The laser effect is influenced by a number of laser parameters including spot size, divergence/convergence of laser beam, wavelength, pulse duration, and fluence.

The first two factors are believed to be optimized in all modern lasers. The *spot size* of laser affects the optical penetration of light if its radius is equal or less than the distance for which light is free to diffuse within the tissues. Larger spot diameter will allow greater laser penetration due to greater internal reflection. Furthermore, a larger surface area can be treated faster. Most lasers therefore use a spot size that is greater than the penetrative depth of the laser (>4 mm).

The efficacy of laser treatment also depends on the *convergence* of incident light and the uniformity of irradiance.

Convergence of laser light allows for less external reflection from the skin surface and therefore deeper penetration and more selective target injury.

Different chromophores in the skin are targeted by lasers with different *wavelengths.* Wavelength also affects the depth of penetration, with laser light with a longer wavelength penetrating deeper into the dermis.

The most selective target heating is achieved when energy is deposited at a rate faster than the rate of cooling of the target chromophore. Longer *pulse duration* will achieve more efficient heating but if the pulse duration is too long there will be insufficient time for heat to dissipate, causing an undesirable temperature rise that will lead to damage to surrounding epidermis and dermis. These injuries could result in scarring or other cutaneous side effects. The time taken for heat to dissipate from a particular chromophore (the thermal relaxation time) in seconds is approximately equal to the square of the target's diameter in millimeters.[3] In treating vascular malformation where a variety of abnormal vessel diameters are present, at different depths under the epidermis, the setting of an ideal pulse duration for treatment becomes difficult.

In addition to pulse duration, sufficient *fluence* is also required to achieve a damaging temperature in a target chromophore (therapeutic threshold). The use of higher fluence will increase the risk of developing skin complications during treatment.

Laser Modality

A laser can be classified as either operating in continuous or pulsed mode. A *continuous* wave laser simply means that the laser emits a constant source of light without interruption, while a *pulsed* wave laser emits laser light at a predetermined duration and repetition rate. In a *Q-switched* laser, pulses are only emitted at peak intensity and for extremely short durations.

Most medical lasers are used in pulsed mode, as the targeting of chromophores becomes more specific, with less thermal damage to the surrounding tissues owing to the short thermal relaxation time of chromophores which allows for heat dissipation between pulses. A pulsed laser is used when the destruction of the target chromophore relies on heat denaturation or coagulation.

In a Q-switched laser, short pulses of high peak power laser light are emitted. Hence, it is used in conditions where a shattering effect is needed to destroy the target chromophores, i.e. pigmented lesions and tattoos (see below).

Laser Safety

Lasers can be broadly classified into four classes (Box 5.1). Most medical lasers used are Class 4 and hence suitable precautions need to be undertaken while undertaking laser procedures.

The MHRA (Medicines and Healthcare Products Regulatory Agency) has produced a guideline on the safe use of lasers.[4] All personnel who are associated with the purchase, supply, installation, use, and maintenance of medical lasers and intense pulsed light (IPL) systems should be familiar with the document.

Each hospital that undertakes laser treatment should have local safety rules, with a trained laser safety officer. The local safety rules should be specific to each clinical application and for each laser, and all personnel involved in laser use should be familiar with them. All staff should be appropriately trained for the use and maintenance of lasers, safety precautions, and adverse events reporting.

Specific safety precautions are:

- Eye protection: suitable eye protection should be used for each specific laser.
- Smoke/plume extraction: smoke plume may contain hair particles, viable cells, bacteria, viruses, prions, and other hazardous materials. Numerous toxic and carcinogenic gases will also be given off. It is therefore essential that precautions are taken to reduce such risks. A well-fitting, high filtration-efficiency face mask (e.g. particulate respirators that filter particles of 0.1 μm in size) should be used. A standard surgical face mask is not sufficient to act as the primary method of particle filtration. This should be supplemented by a dedicated smoke evacuator. A standard medical vacuum system (e.g., an operating theater wall suction system) is not suitable for smoke plume removal.
- Fire hazard: flammable substances such as alcoholic skin prep should not be used in areas where lasers are used. Fire extinguishing equipment should be readily available. Care should also be taken when performing laser treatments near nasopharyngeal or endotracheal tubes.

Types of Laser

The main types of laser used for cutaneous treatments are divided according to the chromophores they target – oxyhemoglobin (vascular lesions), melanin (pigmented lesions and hair removal lasers) or water (resurfacing lasers). *Ablative lasers* are the resurfacing lasers, such as CO_2 and erbium:YAG lasers, which remove the epidermis. *Nonablative lasers* selectively target the chromophores within the epidermis, or the dermis only. Most lasers that are used to treat vascular, pigmented lesions or hair, and the IPL systems fall into this group.

Commonly used lasers along with their wavelengths and target chromophores are listed in Table 5.1.

Fractionated Lasers

With the advance of laser technology, fractionated lasers have been developed in the past decade to improve the safety profiles of the traditional ablative lasers. First used in 2004,[5] fractionated lasers deliver laser beams that produce tiny columns of thermal injury called microthermal treatment zones (MTZs), interspersed with normal epidermis and dermis. As a result, healing is faster than the traditional ablative lasers, with fewer potential side effects. Both ablative and nonablative fractionated lasers are available. The advantage of this system is that it allows the resurfacing of nonfacial areas and also it allows deep penetration of the laser beam into the dermis thus encouraging collagen remodeling.

Ablative fractionated lasers can be based either on erbium:YAG for superficial treatments or CO_2 for deeper treatments (see below).

Intense Pulsed Light

Intense pulsed light (IPL) systems work on the same principle as the nonablative laser systems. The main difference is that the system delivers a range of wavelengths between 500 nm to 1200 nm in each pulse of light (non-laser) rather than just one wavelength.

IPL works well for vascular and pigmented lesions and also improves mild rhytids. The proposed mechanism of action is thought to be thermal denaturation of dermal collagen, leading to inflammatory changes and subsequent collagen synthesis and remodeling.

When IPL is used to treat vascular lesions, no postoperative purpura is seen owing to the longer wavelength resulting in more even heating of vessels. Its wide range of pulse width also allows treatment of large and small vessels.

• BOX 5.1 Classification of Lasers

Class 1 Lasers that are not capable of emitting hazardous levels of radiation under normal conditions.
Class 2 Lasers that have visible wavelength lasers with lower power output, which will not cause permanent damage to the eye in the 0.25 seconds it takes to blink.
Class 3 Lasers that, if viewed directly, can cause permanent damage to the eye.
Class 4 Lasers that produce a hazardous emission, either through direct or scattered radiation. Suitable eye protection must be worn. There is also a potential fire risk.

Cutaneous Side Effects of Laser Treatment

Temporary

Cutaneous blistering and serous crusting are common after laser treatment. These normally resolve within a few days, with no long-term sequelae. Patients are advised to keep the treated area clean.

Skin hyper- and hypopigmentation can occur and is more common in patients with darker skin types. The melanin in the skin competes with other chromophores in absorbing the laser energy, resulting in postinflammatory changes. If it occurs, it normally resolves with time, with or without application of topical skin depigmentation treatment.

Long Term

Scarring can occur in severe cases of burn due to laser treatment.

There is so far no indication that repeated laser treatment will result in any carcinogenic harmful effects to the skin.

To reduce the incidence of cutaneous side effects, it is common for most modern lasers to have an incorporated cooling device. This can be either cold air, cryogen spray, or contact cooling device.

In addition, clinicians have to ensure that patients' skin color is at its lightest when treatment is undertaken. This reduces the melanin load of the skin, which can compete with skin chromophores in absorbing laser energy. This can be accomplished by ensuring that patients undergoing treatments are not tanned at the time of treatment, or by temporarily depigmenting the skin before laser treatment with topical products such as hydroquinone.

Laser Treatment by Lesion Type

Vascular Lesions

Vascular lesions that are responsive to laser treatment include port wine stain, hemangiomas, facial telangiectasia,

TABLE 5.1 Commonly Used Medical Lasers

Medium	Laser	Wavelength (nm)	Chromophore
Solid	Alexandrite	755	Melanin Tattoo pigment
	Nd:YAG	1064 (deep lesions)	Melanin Tattoo pigment
	KTP	532 (epidermal lesions)	
	Copper vapor	578	Oxyhemoglobin
	Erbium:YAG	2940	Water
Liquid	Pigmented lesion dye	510	Melanin
Gas	Carbon dioxide (CO_2)	10,600	Water

KTP, potassium titanyl phosphate; YAG, yttrium–aluminum–garnet.

rosacea, spider nevus, cherry angioma, erythematous scars, and warts.

The gold standard *pulsed dye laser* has a wavelength of 585 nm, and causes vaporization of blood, local rupture of microvessels, and purpura.

The efficacy of treatment of vascular lesions depends on vessel size, depth, and wall thickness. Clinically, dark red or purple lesions tend to be larger and deeper, and respond less favorably than the more superficial, lighter-colored lesions. In treating port wine stain (PWS), a poorer response has been observed in lesions found on the extremities. The reason for this is unknown but it may be due to the effect of gravity or deoxygenation on the vasculature or possibly the increased vessel wall thickness of more distal vessels.

After treatment, purpura develops immediately and resolves in 1–2 weeks. Other side effects include scaling, crusting, and very rarely, scarring.

Technical Tips

- Always perform a test patch treatment before full treatment.
- If a smaller spot size is used then higher fluence is needed to achieve similar clinical results.
- The multipass technique has been shown to achieve better results.
- Tissue cooling is important to reduce the incidence of epidermal injury caused by stacking pulses (treating the same spot by firing two pulses sequentially).
- Avoid using 755 nm and 1064 nm lasers around the eyes without metal guards protecting the globe. As they have deeper penetration they can injure the eyes by targeting the retina and iris, and blindness has been reported.
- Larger spot size allows deeper tissue penetration.
- A range of other lasers are also helpful in treating vascular lesions:
  - *KTP* (frequency-doubled Nd:YAG laser): its longer pulse width avoids rupturing target vessels, hence avoiding purpura.
  - *V beam*: has a variable pulse width and a longer pulse width can be used to treat telangiectasia without as much purpura.
  - *Long pulsed Nd:YAG*: has a longer wavelength, with deeper penetration, and hence is more effective in deeper vessels, i.e., veins.
  - *Sequential lasers* (e.g., Cynergy): the first laser (pulsed dye) converts hemoglobin to methemoglobin, which is then targeted by the Nd:YAG laser; this allows the use of a lower fluence of Nd:YAG.
  - *Fractionated lasers*: can be used to treat resistant PWS that has very little chromophore left, as well as nodular PWS. They are helpful in flattening the PWS.

Pigmented Lesions

Q-switched lasers are most commonly used to treat pigmented lesions. They target melanosomes, causing rapid heating, expansion, and rupture.

Q-switched frequency-doubled Nd:YAG (532 nm) and the pigmented lesion dye (510 nm) lasers are most useful for superficial epidermal lesions such as freckles (ephelides) and solar lentigines while ruby (695 nm) and alexandrite (755 nm) lasers are of benefit in deeper lesions such as café-au-lait spots and nevi of Ota and Ito.

When using lasers to treat pigmented lesions, patients are always warned that sun exposure can cause the lesions to recur. This is because the melanocytes that produce the pigmentation are not destroyed by laser treatment. Posttreatment hyper- and hypopigmentation can occur.

Cautions should be taken when treating melasma and postinflammatory hyperpigmentation. These conditions generally get worse after treatment. Test patch treatment before a full treatment is important.

Tattoos

Q-switched lasers are used to treat tattoos. The laser energy is absorbed by pigment particles, leading to fragmentation of the particles which are then ingested by phagocytes. The pigment is then transported to the regional lymph nodes.

Black and blue ink absorb all wavelengths well and hence can be treated by a number of different lasers. Different colored inks absorb different colored wavelengths and thus different lasers are indicated to treat different colours: KTP – red; alexandrite – green; 510 nm pigmented dye – red, orange, purple, yellow

In general, 8–15 treatments are needed. Patients should be counseled that it may not be possible to completely clear the tattoos. This will result in a 'ghost tattoo' where only part of the tattoo is visible. Some patients may find this more unsightly than the actual tattoo itself.

Caution should be used in some circumstances when ink darkening (reduction of ferrous to ferric oxide or titanium oxide) can occur. This is especially important if the tattoo is of "flesh" color, or in cosmetic tattoos such as eyeliner, browliner, and lip liner.

Allergic reactions from laser-induced release of tattoo antigens, e.g., chromium-containing red or yellow inks, have also been reported.

Sun block should be removed prior to treatment as it may contain metal-containing oxides and salts (e.g., titanium dioxide) that may be flammable after exposure to high energy laser pulses.

To improve results, recently Q-switched lasers with shorter pulse duration (picoseconds) have been used with encouraging results. Such short pulses in high fluence are capable of generating a tremendous amount of pigment shattering.[6,7]

Esthetic Applications

There are three main factors that contribute to an aging face:

1. Gravitational effects that give rise to jowls and eyebrow ptosis, which are best dealt with by surgery.

2. Reduction in volume, which can be corrected by injection of synthetic fillers or autologous fat.
3. Photodamage.

Photodamage is a collective term to describe primarily the deleterious effect of sun on skin, resulting in damage to collagen and elastin. This leads to the formation of fine wrinkles (rhytids) and poor skin texture, and the formation of brown spots due to pigmentary dyschromia and facial red spots or thread veins due to damage to superficial blood vessels. Facial fine lines can be improved by removing the top layer of skin by chemical peel, dermabrasion or laser resurfacing. Laser resurfacing is superior as it gives precise depth of ablation and controlled thermal damage with the added benefit of skin tightening.

Laser Resurfacing

In laser resurfacing, CO_2 and erbium lasers are used. Energy is absorbed by intracellular water causing rapid heating and vaporization of tissue.

Most published series have reported an overall 90% improvement in rhytids. Most improvement can be expected in the perioral area and least in areas of dynamic wrinkling such as the glabella. The results decrease with time, probably due to delayed resolution of postoperative edema (down to 31% in glabella in 2 years in one study).

In acne scarring, the maximum improvement that can be expected after one treatment is 30%–50%. If resurfacing is used to treat pigmentary changes or lesions, there is a chance of recurrence.

CO_2 Lasers

The CO_2 laser has a wavelength of 10,600 nm and is highly absorbed by water. It was first introduced in 1964, in continuous mode for cutting and coagulating tissues. The development of a high energy pulsed mode in the 1990s expanded its use and made it the laser of choice in skin resurfacing.

A conventional CO_2 laser deposits energy in the upper 20 μm of skin (after 1 pass) due to strong water absorption. There can be 0.2–1 mm of residual thermal damage leading to prolonged downtime with long periods of wound healing. Re-epithelialization usually takes about 7 days with prolonged erythema that can last more than 6 weeks. Such thermal damage also leads to a high incidence of scarring and skin pigmentation changes. The thermal damage has an additional benefit of causing skin tightening.

In the mid-1990s, to reduce thermal damage and its associated side effects modification was made to the CO_2 lasers so that only pulses that are shorter than the thermal relaxation time (1 msec) were used. This was achieved by either the use of high energy, short pulsed (<1 msec) CO_2 lasers (Ultrapulse), or a focused beam with rapid scanning resulting in contact time of <1 msec (Silktouch/Feathertouch/Sharplan).

Erbium:YAG Lasers

The erbium laser was first used in 1996. It has a wavelength of 2940 nm and hence has 16 times higher water absorption compared to the CO_2 lasers. It penetrates 1 μm of skin (versus 20 μm for CO_2) and offers more precise skin ablation. It causes less thermal damage compared with the CO_2 lasers, and hence has a lower incidence of skin complications such as prolonged erythema and skin pigmentary changes. Due to the less significant thermal effect it offers poorer hemostasis and less skin tightening when used as a resurfacing tool.

Fractionated CO_2 Lasers

To minimize the thermal side effects of the CO_2 lasers, fractionated CO_2 lasers were recently developed. They deliver evenly spaced thermal injury, surrounded by healthy skin, which enables rapid epithelialization. Depending on the fluence used, re-epithelialization usually occurs after between 3 and 6 days, and the side effects associated with thermal injury such as prolonged erythema and skin pigmentary changes are less common than with non-fractionated lasers. In addition, because intact skin is interspersed with ablated skin, the depth of ablation can be increased without the fear of scarring. This is useful in upregulating skin collagen production, most useful in skin tightening,[8] and improving atrophic scars.[9] Histological examination of fractionated CO_2 laser-treated skin shows columns of thermally damaged skin, with immediate inflammatory response, followed by reorganization of dermal matrix and collagen induction.[10]

Fractionated CO_2 lasers also allow resurfacing of areas outside the face, which is not possible with traditional resurfacing lasers. They also allow treatment of darker skin types without a high risk of skin complications.

There is also evidence that fractionated CO_2 lasers improve both skin hypopigmentation and hyperpigmentation, as seen in conditions such as melasma. This is achieved by facilitating migration of melanocytes from neighboring skin, and changing the optical characteristic of skin by increasing production of collagen.[11]

The effects of fractionated CO_2 laser resurfacing depend on the depth of laser penetration, dermal coagulation, and spacing. Normally 2–4 treatments are needed, at intervals of 6–12 weeks.

For all the benefits mentioned above, fractionated CO_2 lasers are becoming the gold standard in esthetic resurfacing.

Preoperative Consultation

It is important to elicit the patient's expectation from treatment, as well as their acceptance of treatment down time and side effects before starting treatment. In preoperative history taking, the patient's skin type and scarring history must be noted. Roaccutane should be avoided for 9–12 months prior to treatment as it may compromise skin healing. If the patient has a history of cold sores, antiviral therapy should be started prior to laser resurfacing (aciclovir 400 mg t.d.s. 24 hours prior to treatment, and continued for 5 days afterwards). Treatment should ideally be offered when the patient has not had any recent significant sun exposure. Treatment while tanned may result in unfavorable pigmentation.

Patients should be warned of possible complications, which include acne flares, prolonged edema, erythema, postinflammatory skin hyperpigmentation, and skin hypopigmentation.

Test patch treatment is recommended before full treatment.

Postoperative Care

The author favors the open technique, where no dressing is used to the treated area. The patient is encouraged to wash the area as normal in the shower, and keep the area clean. Skin edema usually peaks at 48 hours, and resolves over 6–8 weeks. Elevation and application of ice will help. Some patients experience pruritus, usually in the first 5 days. A cold compress or emollients will help. Erythema usually resolves gradually over 2–5 months. Patients should be encouraged to use total sun block during this period of time.

Complications

Complications are uncommon if all the above precautions are taken. These include infection follicular occlusion leading to acne or milia, skin hyperpigmentation, and skin hypopigmentation

Laser Hair Removal

Laser hair removal is now the standard in long-term hair control.[12] Hair removal lasers with a wavelength of approximately 700 μm direct laser light precisely to each melanin-containing hair follicle. Several lasers are hence effective: the ruby laser (694 nm), alexandrite laser (755 nm), Nd:YAG laser (1064 nm), and the intense pulsed light source (590–1200 nm). Although the mechanism of follicular injury is likely to be thermal, the precise contributions of photomechanical damage or thermal denaturation to follicular injury are unknown. It is possible that after absorption of radiant energy, the large temperature difference between the melanosomes and their surroundings produces a localized rapid volume expansion, leading to microvaporization or "shock waves," which cause structural damage to the hair.

Studies on the efficacy of laser hair removal show that long hair-free periods are achievable with all of the above lasers. Several treatments are needed, usually at 4–6 weekly intervals when the hair has regrown. The hair-free period is variable after a course of 6–8 treatments, but usually ranges from 3 to 6 months. Permanent hair removal is rare. Complications from treatment are usually uncommon, especially if a test patch is performed prior to full treatment, and is more common in darker-colored skin. The most common complication is redness after treatment, which lasts a few hours. Less commonly patients can expect crusting of skin, and skin hyper- and hypopigmentation. Most of these complications are temporary, with skin pigmentation changes usually recovering in 6–9 months.

The use of the Nd:YAG laser is more beneficial in patients with darker-colored skin. The absorption of laser light by melanin is low at 1064 nm, and hence will cause less heating to the epidermal melanin. The low melanin absorption is somewhat counteracted by the deeper penetration of the laser light at longer wavelength, and the use of longer pulsed duration ensures the longer period of heating of the melanin in the hair follicles.

Other Indications for Laser Therapy

Resistant Warts. Flat warts can be treated with the pulsed dye laser. Thick warts can be treated with ablative lasers. In the case of recurrence, topical treatment or pulsed dye laser can be considered.

Keloid Scars. Erbium laser ablation, followed by regular Adcortyl injection.

Scar Resurfacing. Fractionated CO_2 laser as per esthetic resurfacing.

Cutaneous Malignancies and Premalignancies. Premalignant conditions such as actinic keratosis and Bowen's disease respond well to laser ablation, especially with the erbium laser. Erbium laser is also useful in treating superficial basal cell carcinoma, especially in patients with Gorlin syndrome, where repeated surgery can be disfiguring. The CO_2 or erbium lasers are useful in treating superficial in transit melanoma.

Kaposi's Sarcoma. Pulsed dye laser, photodynamic therapy (PDT), Nd:YAG and CO_2 lasers have been used with varying success to treat Kaposi's sarcoma.

Conclusion

The use of lasers for cutaneous conditions has become possible since the introduction of the concept of selective thermolysis by Anderson and Parrish in the 1980s. This has led to the development of lasers that can act on specific targets or "chromophores" in certain layers of the skin, allowing for targeted therapy minimizing collateral damage in the form of scarring.

References

1. Goldman L, Blaney DJ, Kindel DJ, Franke EK. The effect of the laser beam on the skin. *J Invest Derm.* 1963;40:121.
2. Anderson RR, Parrish JA. Selective photothermolysis: precise microsurgery by selective absorption of pulsed radiation. *Science.* 1983;220:524–527.
3. Anderson RR. *Selective Thermal Damage from Pulsed Laser Sources* MD thesis. Harvard Medical School; 1984.
4. Medicines and Healthcare Products Regulatory Agency. *MDA Document DB9602: Guidelines on the Safe Use of Lasers in Medical and Dental Practice.* British Standard BS EN60825; 1994, with 2002 amendment.
5. Manstein D, Herron GS, Sink RKH, et al. Fractional photothermolysis: a new concept for cutaneous remodeling using microscopic patterns of thermal injury. *Lasers Surg Med.* 2004;34(5):426–438.

6. Brauer JA, Reddy KK, Anolik R, et al. Successful and rapid treatment of blue and green tattoo pigment with a novel picosecond laser. *Arch Dermatol.* 2012;148(7):820–823.
7. Saedi N, Metelitsa A, Petrell K, Arndt KA, Dover JS. Treatment of tattoos with a picosecond alexandrite laser: a prospective trial. *Arch Dermatol.* 2012;148(12):1360–1363.
8. Hunzeker CM, Weiss ET, Geronemus RG. Fractionated CO_2 laser resurfacing: our experience with more than 2000 treatments. *Aesthet Surg J.* 2009;29(4):317–322.
9. Chapas AM, Brightman L, Sukal S, et al. Successful treatment of acneiform scarring with CO_2 ablative fractional resurfacing. *Lasers Surg Med.* 2008;40:381–386.
10. Hantash BM, Bedi VP, Kapadia B, et al. In vivo histological evaluation of a novel ablative fractional resurfacing device. *Lasers Surg Med.* 2007;39:96–107.
11. Goldberg DJ, Berlin AL, Phelps R. Histologic and ultrastructural analysis of melasma after fractional resurfacing. *Lasers Surg Med.* 2008;40:134–138.
12. Liew SH. A review of unwanted body hair and its removal. *Dermatol Surg.* 1999;25:431–439.

6

Tissue Expansion

DARIUSH NIKKHAH AND NEIL W. BULSTRODE

Background

The process of tissue expansion in reconstructive surgery was first reported by Charles Neumann, who described its application for auricular soft tissue reconstruction in 1957.[1] Neumann simply applied concepts found in both normal physiological as well as pathological processes of the human body. Examples of this phenomenon include pregnancy, where the abdomen increases in size to accommodate the enlarging fetus, and rapid neoplastic growth, which may result in soft tissue expansion, deformity, and eventual skin breakdown. African tribes have also adopted tissue expansion as part of their cultural background, enlarging facial structures such as the lip or the ear.[1]

Nearly half a century later, tissue expansion was repopularized by Radovan for use in postmastectomy breast reconstruction,[2] although its applicability soon became evident in other branches of plastic surgery. Tissue expansion enables soft tissue coverage of large defects secondary to burns, trauma, congenital malformations and cancer excision. It involves the insertion of an implant adjacent to a wound or defect that needs to be resurfaced. The implant is then incrementally enlarged by injection of isotonic saline, resulting in stretching of the overlying soft tissue. The expanded skin can then be used to resurface a defect or incorporate permanent prostheses, including those used for postmastectomy breast reconstructions. Tissue expansion exploits the principles of controlled mechanical skin overstretch in order to generate new tissues with ideal compliance and almost perfect skin color, texture match, and sensibility to the resurfaced defect.[3]

However, this useful tool on the reconstructive ladder does not come without its complications. In this chapter, we review the effects of tissue expansion on soft tissues and explore the tenets that govern its safe and effective use in the patient. We also discuss recent developments in tissue expansion such as external volume expansion and needleless expansion techniques with carbon dioxide.[4]

Viscoelastic Properties of Skin

The structural components of skin can be altered by expansion as demonstrated by several biomechanical studies. Its viscoelasticity means that the mechanical response to loading involves both a viscous (time-dependent) and an elastic (time-independent) component. Skin is mainly composed of dermis and epidermis. The predominant proteins in the dermal layer are collagen types I and III, which are produced by fibroblasts. In the relaxed state, their triple helical structure results in a wavy and convoluted alignment. Upon stretching, the collagen fibers straighten and realign parallel to each other.[3] The skin's elasticity, essential for joint movements, is due mainly to superficial thin bundles of microfibrils associated with progressively larger amounts of amorphous elastin to form elastic fibers. Once strain is released, elastin fibers return collagen to its relaxed coiled posture. If stretched excessively, elastin is prone to fragmentation, resulting in a loss of recoil. Viscoelastic properties change with age and repeated mechanical forces, resulting in skin laxity.

Skin is a dynamic organ and acclimatizes to constant mechanical forces applied to it due to its viscoelastic properties (Box 6.1). On a tissular and cellular level, constant mechanical stress induces changes termed *mechanical creep* and *biological creep*. These phenomena interact to restore resting tension of stretched tissues to baseline – stress relaxation (Fig. 6.1).[5] For example, a wound that was under tension intraoperatively but relaxed at outpatient follow-up is an example of stress relaxation.[3]

Creep is defined as the stretching of skin under a constant load over time. In order to explain the biomechanics of skin during the process of tissue expansion, a distinction was made between mechanical and biological creep. Mechanical creep describes the clinically observed elongation of skin beyond the original stretch when placed under sudden constant tension and is thought to be attributable to the morphological changes (stretching) of the dermal framework in response to stress. Upon stretching, the formerly convoluted collagen fibers straighten and realign parallel to each other, resulting in the extrusion of fluid from the collagen network and microfragmentation of elastic fibers, thus making the skin more viscous.

Biological creep occurs with the formation of new tissues as a result of a persistent chronic stretching force in an attempt to relieve the stress (stress relaxation). It underlies the mechanism of gap junctional disruptions, which results in cellular proliferation. Several studies have confirmed that the gain in skin surface area after expansion was caused by

• BOX 6.1 Summary of the Viscoelastic Properties of Skin

Mechanical Creep

The elongation of skin under a constant load over time
- Collagen fibers stretch out and become parallel
- Elastin undergoes microfragmentation
- Interstitial fluid is displaced (e.g., during intraoperative tissue expansion and skin suturing under tension)

Biological Creep

The generation of new tissue secondary to a persistent chronic stretching force (e.g., seen during pregnancy)

Stress Relaxation

The tendency for this resistance of skin to a stretching force to decrease when held at a given tension over time

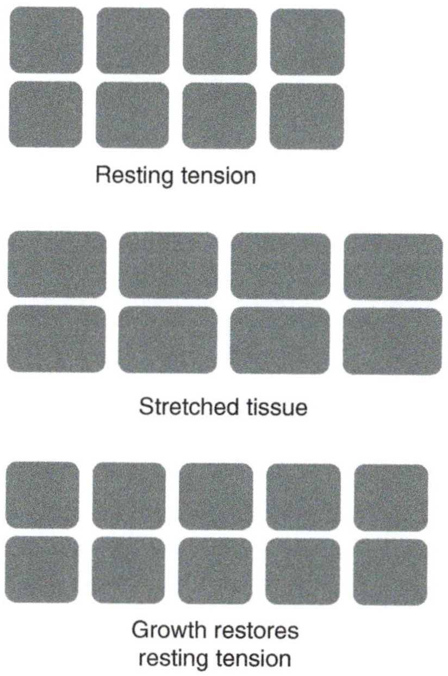

• **Fig. 6.1** Principle of tissue expansion. (Modified with permission of Lippincott Williams & Wilkins, from Sheng L, Yang M, Du Z, et al. Transplantation of stromal vascular fraction as an alternative for accelerating tissue expansion. *J Plast Reconstr Aesthet Surg*. 2013;66(4):551–557.)

new skin formation rather than simply stretching the preexisting skin. Over a period of 6–12 weeks, a multitude of growth factors, cytokines, adhesion molecules, and signal transduction proteins are induced to stimulate epidermal thickening, with concurrent dermal thinning and collagen fibril alignment of the newly expanded tissues (Figs. 6.2 and 6.3).[6] In fact, a study conducted by Vander Kolk et al demonstrated a significant increase in collagen production in expanded skins compared to control skins.[7] Additionally, growth factors, including epidermal growth factor (EGF), transforming growth factor beta (TGF-β), and platelet-derived growth factor (PDGF), are upregulated to stimulate

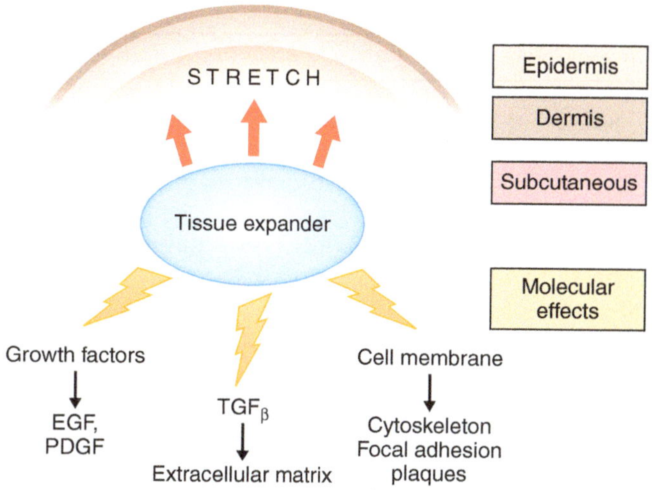

• **Fig. 6.2** Effects of tissue expansion on surrounding tissues. Stretching of surrounding tissues induces growth factors, which mediate cell proliferation and increased angiogenesis. Factors such as TGF-β influence extracellular matrix production while membrane-bound protein kinases, focal adhesion points and the cytoskeleton influence intracellular signaling cascades. (Reproduced with permission of Lippincott Williams & Wilkins, from Cherry GW, Austad E, Pasyk K, et al. Increased survival and vascularity of random-pattern skin flaps elevated in controlled, expanded skin. *Plast Reconstr Surg*. 1983;(5):680–687.)

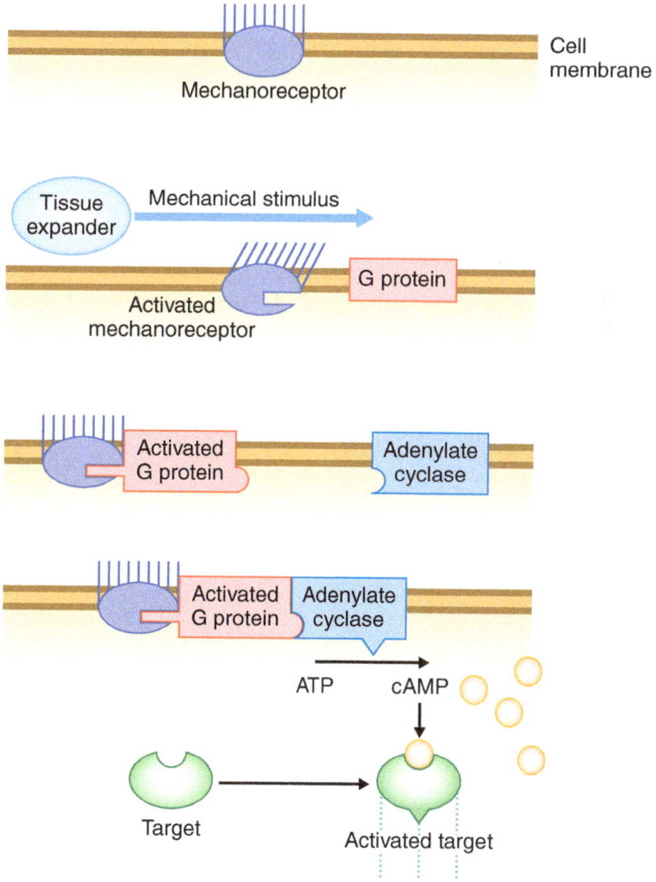

• **Fig. 6.3** Molecular cascade in response to tissue expansion resulting in cellular proliferation. (Reproduced with permission of Lippincott Williams & Wilkins, from Sheng L, Yang M, Du Z, et al. Transplantation of stromal vascular fraction as an alternative for accelerating tissue expansion. *J Plast Reconstr Aesthet Surg*. 2013;66(4):551–557.)

neoangiogenesis of the expanded tissues. Deformational forces acting on the cell membrane and disruption of integrins reduce cell–matrix adhesion and induce conformational changes of membrane proteins. Calcium channels open, leading to signal transduction and cytoskeletal microfilament contraction. The actin cytoskeleton then transmits mechanical forces intracellularly, resulting in increased gene expression and mitosis via interaction with protein kinases, second messengers, and nuclear proteins. Cellular proliferation then results in tissue enlargement.

Enhanced vascularity is among the most noticeable advantages of expanded tissues, exhibiting both higher vessel numbers and larger calibers compared to non-expanded counterparts. Enhanced vascularity is also seen in external volume expansion,[8,9] which was initially used by Khouri et al for non-surgical breast augmentation, and using some of the principles of tissue expansion.[8]

Similar to traditional tissue expansion techniques, external volume expansion devices use suction to mechanically stretch the skin.[9] They induce hypoxia, inflammation, and soluble mediators which in turn will result in cell proliferation and angiogenesis. The latter findings have been demonstrated in animal models. The high vessel density given by external expansion techniques has enabled better autologous fat graft take.

Pietramaggiori et al demonstrated that cyclic mechanical forces applied to the skin of living rats stimulated cell proliferation and vascular remodeling.[10] Additionally, a study by Erba et al supported the angiogenic role of vascular endothelial growth factor (VEGF) in cyclic dermal stretching.[11] Stretched skin presented with more densely packed vessels as well as a significantly increased thickening. However, the most important change during tissue expansion is tissue proliferation secondary to stress-induced cellular changes (biological creep). Sheng et al demonstrated that transplantation of angiogenic growth factor-secreting cells into expanding skins of rats resulted in accelerated tissue expansion, enhanced neovascularization of the expanded skin and promoted cell proliferation.[12] Expression of EGF, VEGF, and β-FGF were significantly enhanced in treated animals compared to control animals. Growth factor supplementation may well play an important role in the future of tissue expansion, both in reducing hospitalization times and flap retraction after expansion.

Tissue Changes during Expansion Techniques

In order to fully understand the mechanics involved in tissue expansion, we will first familiarize ourselves with the structural components of skin. Skin is a multilayered structure and has three well-defined anatomical regions. The outermost layer, the epidermis, forms a thin, uninterrupted and protective layer across most of the body's surface but contributes little to the skin's mechanical properties. The bottom layer, the hypodermis, is mainly made of fatty tissues

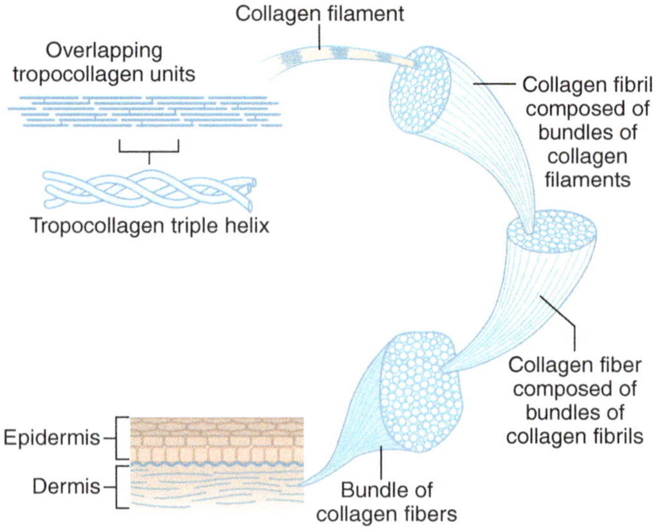

• **Fig. 6.4** Schematic illustration of the composition of collagen in the dermal matrix.

and serves as an insulating layer. The middle dermal layer holds most of the skin's adnexae, including nerve endings, sweat, and oil glands and consists of three main structural components that underlie the skin's strength and elasticity: collagen, elastic fibers, and extrafibrillar matrix. The dermis can be further divided into papillary and reticular layers. The papillary dermis contains thin collagen fibrils which are packed together into thicker collagen fibers (Fig. 6.4). Only about 15% of the dermis is type III collagen, most of which is found in the papillary layer. Collagen type I, the most abundant building block in vertebrates, is the principal protein providing tensile strength to the skin.

Johnson et al assessed the effects of tissue expansion on the mitotic activity in the epidermis in order to address the question whether there is a net gain in epidermal tissue.[13] Their studies confirmed that tissue expansion caused a marked increase in epidermal mitotic activity in a guinea-pig model. Studies on human volunteers supported this finding and demonstrated a significantly thickened epidermis of expanded human skin compared to non-expanded skin.[6] Although expanded tissues maintain their phenotypic characteristics, mechanical strain induces an increase in DNA synthesis and therefore cellular proliferation.[7] Biochemical pathways involved in this process include cytoskeletal, extracellular enzyme, membrane and cytosolic components that converge together to convert the pathway of mechanotransduction seen in tissue expansion into a cellular response, ultimately leading to cellular proliferation.[7] The dermis, in contrast, becomes thinner upon stretching, with hair follicles moving further apart. It may take up to 2 years for the thickness of this layer to return to normal.[6]

Subcutaneous fat tissues were also found to thin after expansion. Adipocytes were flattened, surrounded by fibrosis, or disappeared altogether during the expansion process. Similarly, skeletal muscles are known to undergo atrophy after expansion resulting in the so-called "bath-tub depression." Histologically, the atrophic muscle cells are

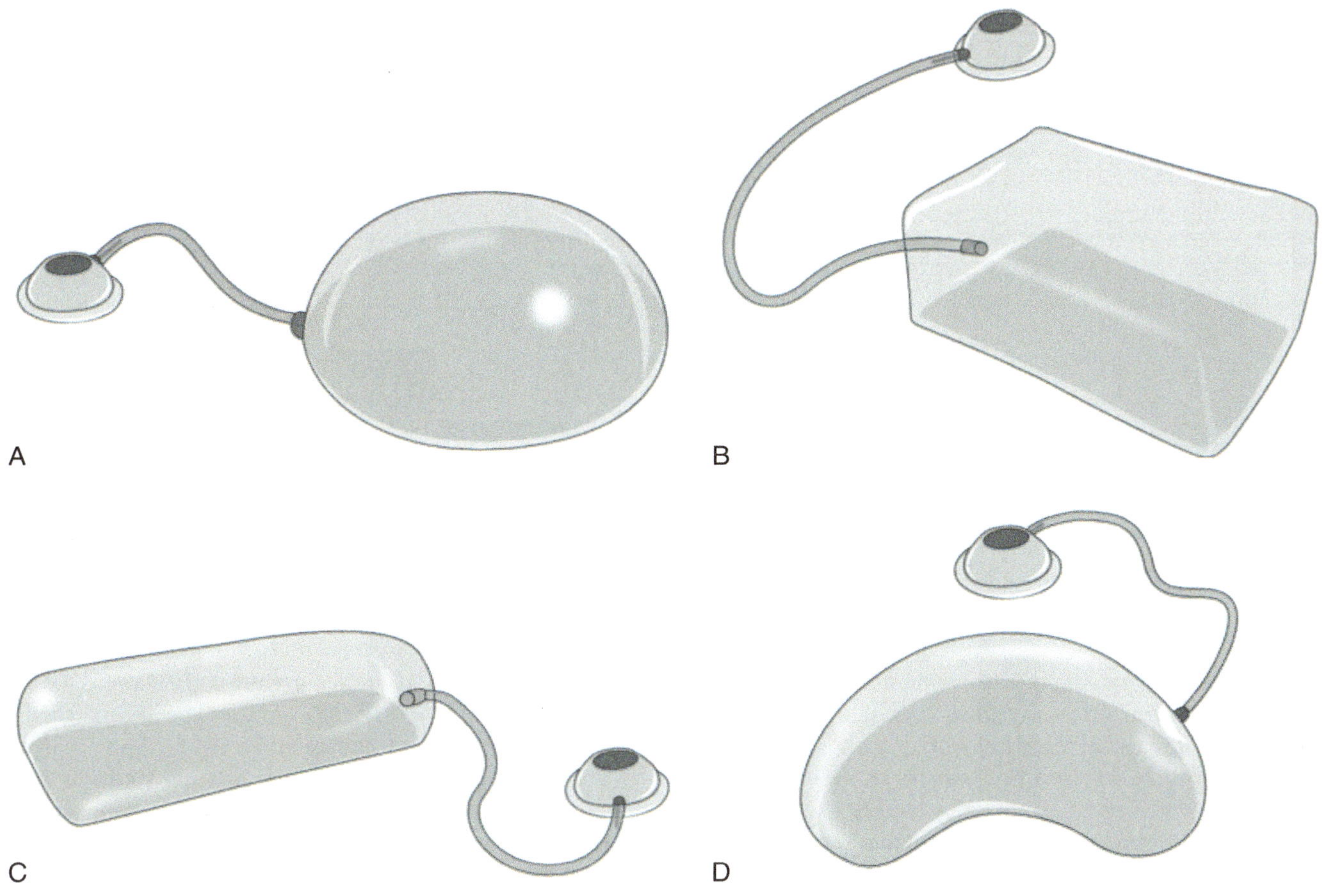

• **Fig. 6.5** Variation in shape of tissue expanders: (A) spherical; (B) rectangular; (C) cylindrical; (D) crescent.

surrounded by fibrous tissue and demonstrate abnormally arranged sarcomeres, large amounts of sarcoplasm, and also numerous large mitochondria.[6] As opposed to the changes in muscle tissues, the loss of subcutaneous fat is permanent.

Enhanced angiogenesis in expanded tissues versus non-expanded counterparts is of clinical significance and presents an advantage in flaps raised on such skin. Improved survival of flaps raised on expanded skin shows properties similar to a delay phenomenon. This was confirmed by Cherry et al, who, using a pig model, elevated random pattern flaps in expanded tissues or non-expanded tissue to determine whether these flaps survived for the same time intervals.[14] Flaps raised on expanded tissue had the greatest increase in surviving length, averaging 117% over control flaps, which was in large part due to an increased vascularity as well as vasodilatation in the angiograms of skins expanded over a period of 5 weeks. The pressure and mechanical stresses applied to expanding tissues resulted in tissue hypoxia, which induced the formation of an increased microcirculation in expanded tissues. Increased vascularity is thought to result from increased gene expression and significantly higher levels of angiogenic factors such as VEGF in expanded tissues compared to non-expanded controls.

Rapid rates of expansion have further been demonstrated to increase flap microvascularity compared to slowly expanded tissues. However, it should be noted that rapidly expanded tissues may become profoundly hypoxic up to 48 hours, which may compromise flap survival. In addition, significant patient discomfort accompanying rapid tissue expansion may limit the rate of expansion.

External volume expansion has broadly similar effects on tissues compared to conventional tissue expansion. Lancerotto and colleagues, in a murine model, demonstrated that the application of controlled non-invasive suction results in cell strain which in turn gives way to cell proliferation. Based on their results, after 48 hours of external volume expansion four factors, which include mechanical stimulation of cell, edema, and hypoxia, all contribute to cell proliferation in the epidermis and dermis as well as angiogenesis.[9] Chin and colleagues have also demonstrated in a mouse model that external volume expansion provides ischemic preconditioning of tissues via hypoxia/ischemia of tissues.[15]

Evolution of Tissue Expansion Devices

Each tissue expander needs to be carefully selected for its desired purpose, making tissue expansion a highly individualized procedure. Depending on the size and shape of the defect to be covered, different expander types may be selected (Fig. 6.5). The basic design is an inflatable silicone elastomer reservoir.[2] Isotonic saline is delivered in a controlled fashion via a valve port system which is either integrated into the expander

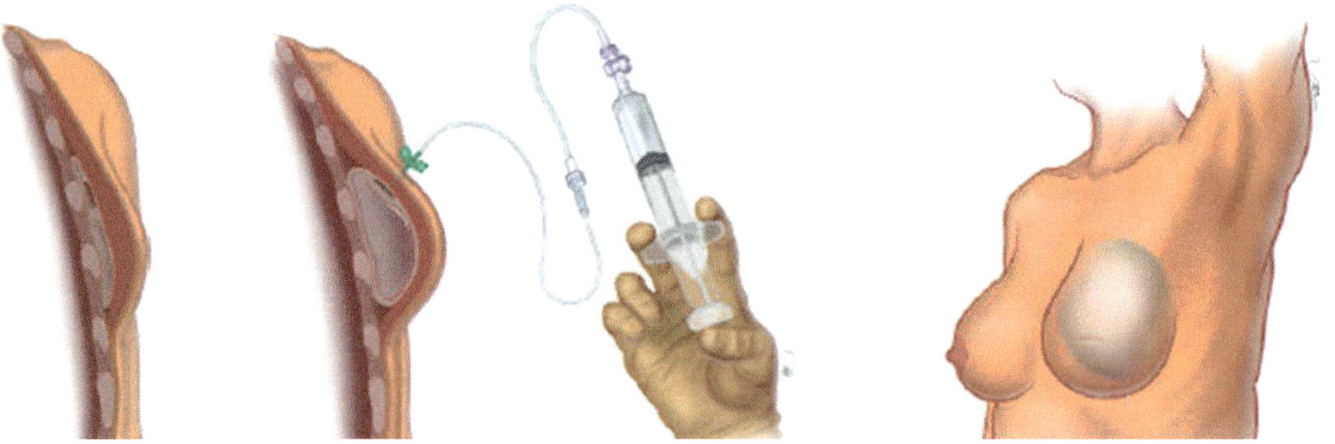

• **Fig. 6.6** Schematic illustration of submuscularly placed tissue expanders. An integrated injection port system allows saline injections directly into the expander. The permanent implant is then inserted. (From Adrada BE, Whitman GJ, Crosby MA, Carkaci S, Dryden MJ, Dogan BE. Multimodality imaging of the reconstructed breast. *Curr Prob Diagn Radiol.* 2015:44(6);487–495. Modified with permission from Reshaping You: Options for Breast Reconstruction ©2009. The University of Texas MD Anderson Cancer Center, Patient Education Office.)

or connected to the prosthesis via silicone tubing (Fig. 6.6). An integrated system offers the advantage of undermining a single pocket for expander placement, but also places the implant at risk of perforation by a misplaced needle. Internally placed remote ports remove the danger of expander perforation, but introduce potential complications, including kinking of the port, tube obstruction, and migration. To avoid these complications, the undermining for the port pocket is minimal, the port is placed over firm, supporting tissue and, if need be, the port position can be fixed with sutures. Externally placed portals have proved particularly useful in the pediatric population as they may alleviate pain and anxiety associated with frequent injections and the safety of such ports has been demonstrated repeatedly.

The shape of the expander is governed by the anatomical location and may, if necessary, be custom-made to fit any size or shape. Circular expanders are best suited to areas such as the breast, whereas crescentic and rectangular shapes have been described for the scalp and lower limbs, respectively.[2] A further parameter governing tissue expansion involves directional expansion in order to impart a certain contour to the expanded pocket. This may be of importance if a specific shape is required, such as for breast reconstructions.

In 1982, Radovan successfully applied a temporary tissue expander for postmastectomy breast reconstruction.[16] Such procedures, however, require a second surgical intervention to remove the expander and replace it with the final breast implant. Two years later, Becker described a permanent expander for breast reconstruction where a modified inflatable breast implant enables a reservoir to be attached and detached at a side-filling valve.[17] The implant therefore functioned both as a tissue expansion device and a permanent implant upon removal of the reservoir. In a more recent study, the Becker implant was compared prospectively to the two-stage expansion process in a randomized study and patient satisfaction was measured.[18] Seventy patients were randomized to receive either a round permanent Becker implant (n = 35) or undergo a two-stage reconstruction with a crescent-shaped expander (n = 35), later replaced by an anatomical implant. Thirty patients were excluded and therefore only 20 patients per group were evaluated. A significant 70% of patients in the Becker implant group underwent revision surgery secondary to upper pole fullness and poor ptosis. It was therefore concluded that a two-stage procedure achieves a better esthetic outcome.

There has been a gradual evolution and refinement in the two-stage expander to implant breast reconstruction. Many expanders for breast reconstruction now come with an integrated valve, selective lower pole expansion, textured anatomical expander, with suture tabs that allow the surgeon to fix the tissue expander to the chest wall. This provides stability to the expander and prevents migration, which was more common in non-tabbed expanders. Scott Spear identified that tabbed expanders lead to more predictability in the second stage of breast reconstruction in comparison to non-tabbed expanders.[19]

ADM has also been used as an adjuvant method for breast tissue expansion, instead of placing the implant submuscularly. ADM use by some surgeons is thought to improve lower pole projection and decrease the pain of expansion. However, ADM use has been reported to increase complications such as infection, skin flap necrosis, and explantation.

In an effort to minimize these traditional disadvantages of conventional tissue expanders, a new generation of pressure-sensitive self-expanding devices was first described in 1982. Austad and Rose created a permeable silicone balloon filled with a hypertonic NaCl solution which drew in body fluids down the osmotic gradient.[20] Despite being described as having some value for soft tissue reconstruction, these osmotic expanders are rarely in use nowadays due to major disadvantages.[21] First, there were relatively long inflation periods of 8–14 weeks. Second, high incidences of balloon rupture during the

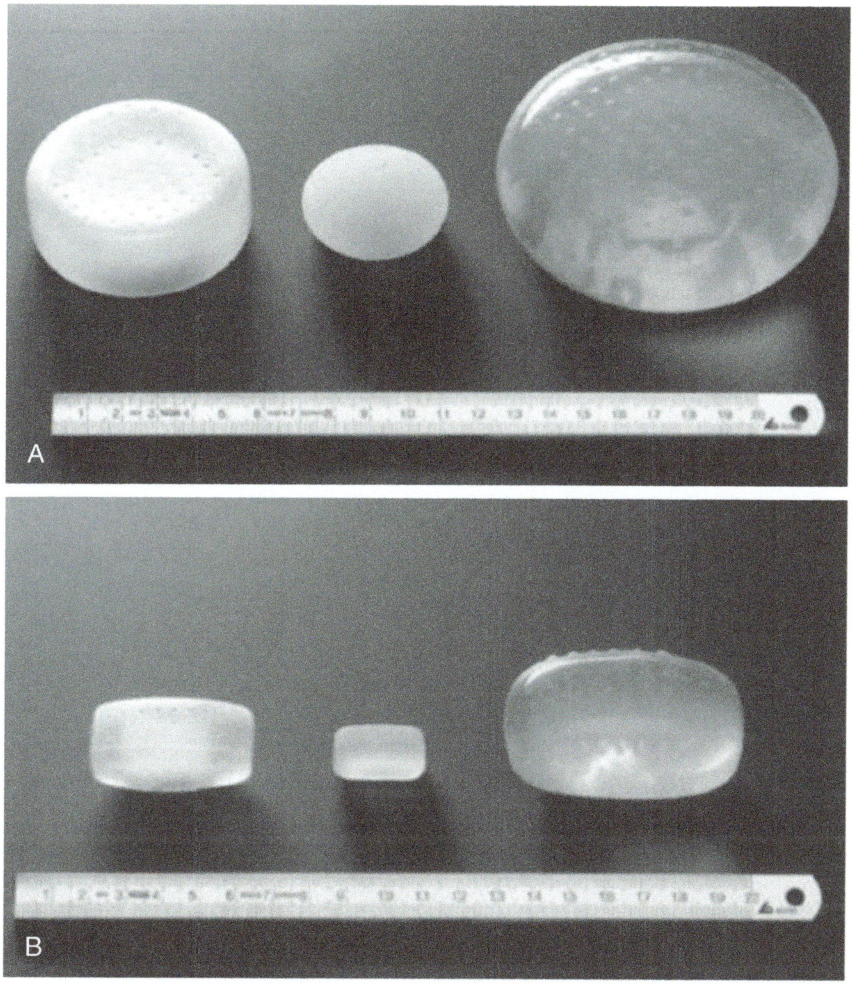

• **Fig. 6.7** (A) Round and (B) rectangular osmotic tissue expanders. The hydrogel (middle) is wrapped inside a loosely fitting silicone membrane (left) that contains pores for finely tuned water uptake.

early stages resulted in necrosis of the overlying tissues.[22] More than a decade after its initial conception, Wiese developed an osmotically active expander that was completely independent of the use of saturated saline. The implants exploited the osmotic forces of hydrogels, which consist of two components: a polymer network with constant quantity and an aqueous component that is variable. The gel is placed subcutaneously and absorbs body fluids from the extracellular space. Water uptake then causes gradual swelling of the hydrogel (Fig. 6.7). The theoretical advantages of self-inflating expanders, including less frequent hospital visits and injections as well as reduced anxiety and pain, led to their commercialization and distribution by Osmed (Ilmenau, Germany).

However, a recent case series using Osmed self-expanders conducted by Chummun et al demonstrated high incidences of expander infection among the pediatric population (2 out of 7; 28.5%), device migration and in some cases tissue ischemia and necrosis.[21] The fact that a small study population and single-center study was selected should be taken into account before prematurely dismissing self-expanding implants.

Further developments to reduce the clinical burden of the expansion process have been made with a carbon dioxide-based expander as an alternative to conventional and osmotic expanders. Its advantages include remote expansion without needles and a more rapid expansion time, in contrast to saline expansion, which needs multiple trips to outpatients with serial bolus injections that can be lengthy and disruptive to the patient. The osmotic self-expanders overcame these issues, however the major drawback was inability to control the rate of expansion. The gas-based system utilised an implantable tissue expander containing a reservoir of compressed carbon dioxide and an external hand held remote that would release a programmed increment of 10 mL and safety mechanism to prevent more than 30 mL being given in any day.[23]

Surgical Technique: Basic Incision and Design Plan

Tissue expansion requires meticulous preoperative planning, careful placement of the expander, and suitable incremental inflation. Without these sequential steps the final result would be compromised.[24] Placement is dictated by where the proximity of the defect is situated and this must be determined in advance after careful consideration of all possibilities. Easily recruitable sites of high tissue laxity should be determined before selecting skin of similar color, texture and hair-bearing quality to the recipient site. Tissue expansion may take up to 3–6 months depending on the anatomical site and the size of the expander.[2] Breast and abdominal tissues can tolerate large expansion volumes in one sitting, while forehead and scalp expand more slowly.[2] The characteristics common to ideal expander placement are: (a) easy accessibility through a small incision, (b) gradual enlargement over a relatively short time period, (c) no painful inflation spikes, (d) good long-term biocompatibility with the body, (e) resistance to infection and extrusion, and (f) no need for revision procedures.[25]

Selection of the ideal type, size, and shape of the expander requires some foresight in terms of the timetable for the inflation process, which must be individualized to the patient in question.[7] Radovan advised that the expander base should have the same size as the defect to be reconstructed as this allows for doubling of the surface area, enabling eventual coverage of both the donor and recipient sites.[3] In contrast, other investigators postulate the use of as large a tissue expander as possible, however without empirical evidence.[24]

In an effort to prevent arbitrary expander selection, several mathematical models have been developed to precisely calculate necessary dimensions. Early computational programs required the implant base diameter and the desired surface area gain to estimate the capacity of a spherical tissue expander. More sophisticated programs are able to calculate the volumes of rectangular tissue expanders after feeding the length and breadth of the lesion to be repaired, considering them the size of the base of the expander. Raposio and Santi incorporated a "correcting factor" by multiplying the surface requirements by 3/2 to account for potential tissue loss during tissue transfer.[26] However, software-based predictions of tissue expander size and shape are complicated by factors such as the surface on which the expander is placed upon. If placed over rigid flat surfaces, predicting the outcome of tissue expansion is straightforward. The difficulty occurs when expanders are placed over soft tissues with the tendency for inward compression or in areas of concavity, since the prediction of tissue expansion is less reliable. Due to such complexity, mathematical models failed to cross over to clinical routine where the trained surgeon's eye remains the ultimate, still arbitrary, judge.[17,18]

The primary incision is best placed perpendicular to the direction of expansion to avoid tension across the incision, which could result in wound dehiscence and broadening of the scar line. The ideal type of initial incision is still a matter of debate. However, no debate surrounds the issue of the ideal size; regardless of the type of incision, it should be as small as possible. Incisions can be made either at the junction of normal tissue and scarred area (i.e., paralesional incision) or remotely, so healthy tissue approximates healthy tissue. Paralesional incisions offer the advantage of minimal undermining of tissues for the insertion of expanders and their rates of infection, wound dehiscence and implant exposure do not seem to be statistically different to those in remote incisions. The latter, however, may offer better healing. There is, as yet, no final consensus as to which type of incision is definitely superior. This calls for controlled, randomized studies on site-specific expansions.

Another important consideration is the plane into which the expander is placed, as minimizing stress on overlying skin flaps aids during procedures such as mastectomies and increases the flexibility in choosing the final breast volume (see Fig. 6.7). Before placement of the expander into the pocket, meticulous hemostasis is warranted and a closed system suction drain is put in place. Irrigation with povidone-iodine and/or gentamicin/cefazolin is commonly performed to minimize the chance of infection, followed by intravenous administration of antibiotics effective against skin flora.[24]

After expander placement, the expansion process is usually delayed to allow the wounds to heal and reduce the chances of wound dehiscence. This also allows for any swellings to subside and problems with the skin flap to reveal themselves.[24] The expander is filled until the patient feels some discomfort or the overlying skin blanches, but excessive tension on the expander flap should be avoided as tissue necrosis may ensue. Finally it should be noted that despite meticulous planning and appropriate technique, expansion may not be successful. Success is also dependent on patient comorbidities, nutritional habits and local tissue factors.[2] Finally, patient cooperation in the expansion procedure is vital, as the process requires several interventions and involves many visits to the outpatient clinic.

Expanders can also be used to help facilitate free tissue transfer; they provide a thinner flap and increase the surface area of the flap beyond the defined anatomical boundaries of the blood supply of the flap.[27] The use of pre-expanded free flaps can be advantageous by minimizing donor site morbidity and reducing the need for split-thickness skin graft, leaving a concealed scar at the donor site.[27] Song and colleagues report the use of pre-expansion of scapular free flaps for neck burn reconstruction in 12 cases.[27] In terms of surgical technique the expander is placed below the deep fascia and above the tunica muscularis. Great attention is paid during dissecting over the superior border of teres major to prevent iatrogenic injury to the circumflex scapular artery.

External Volume Expansion with BRAVA

BRAVA is a form of external pre-expansion used prior to fat grafting. BRAVA (Brava LLC, Miami, FL, USA) is a well-established form of external breast expander. It applies a distractive mechanical force that induces the body to generate its own 3D vascularized scaffold[28] (Fig. 6.8). Like traditional tissue expansion, it expands the skin defect to generate a skin envelope but also stimulates angiogenesis in the native breast tissue. This form of external expansion allows for a more favorable recipient site for large volume fat transfer.

BRAVA has been applied for delayed and immediate breast reconstruction. Three weeks of pre-expansion is

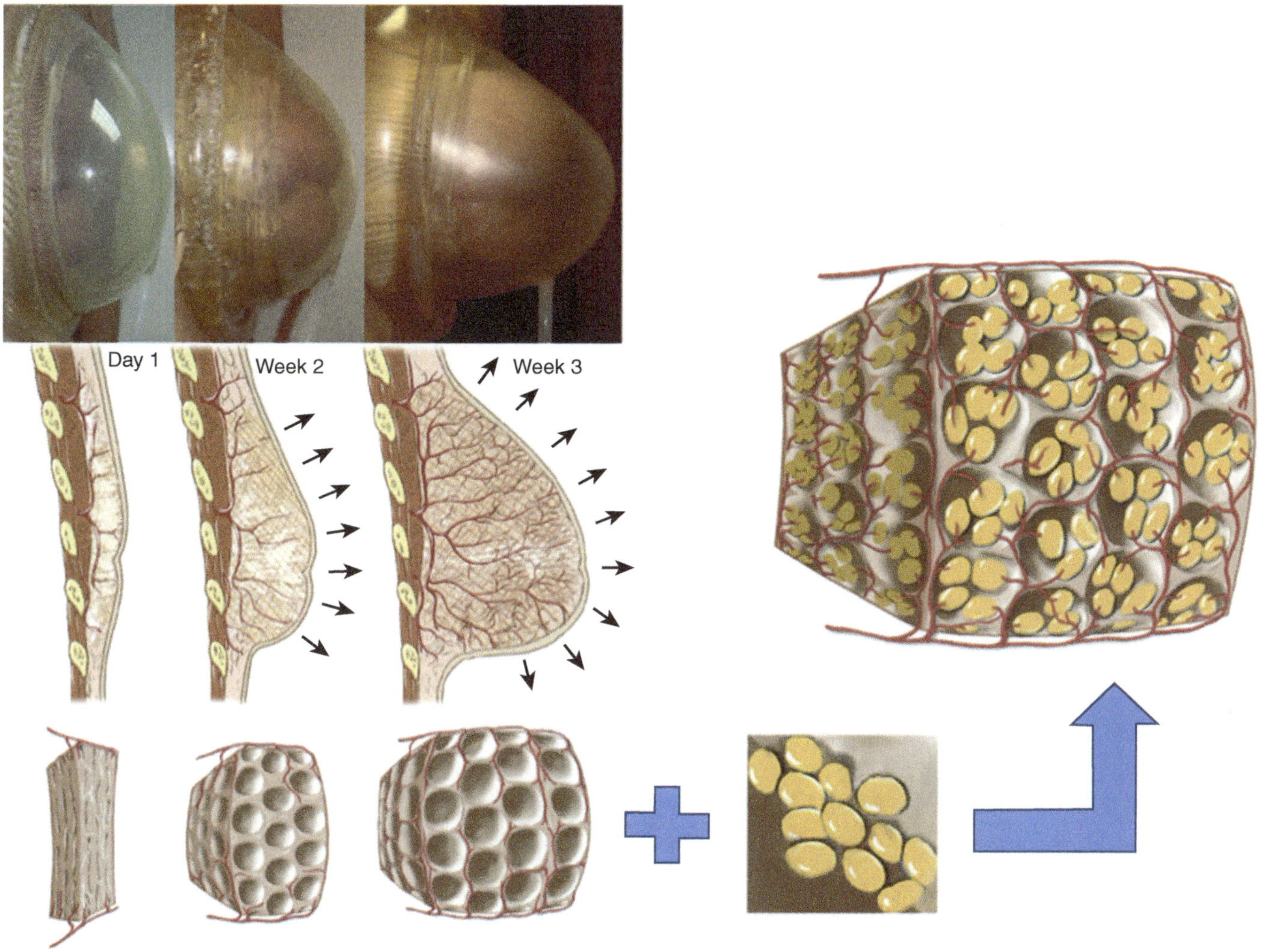

• **Fig. 6.8** BRAVA external volume expansion system. (Reproduced with permission from Kosowski TR, Rigotti G, Khouri RK. Tissue-engineered autologous breast regeneration with Brava®-assisted fat grafting. *Clin Plast Surg*. 2015;42(3):325–337, Fig. 1.)

performed. Patients are required to wear the BRAVA device at least 10 hours a day for 2–3 weeks before fat grafting of the mastectomy defect. In the authors' series 488 enrolled and only 87.5% completed reconstruction,[28] most likely due to the difficulty of wearing the external device for 10 hours per day, and the multiple sessions of fat grafting. Delayed radiated mastectomies required an average 4.9 procedures.

Although BRAVA and fat grafting is a labor-intensive procedure for both patient and surgeon, the complication rate is low, with a 2.9% reported incidence of skin necrosis and ulceration and 1% risk of pneumothorax. Like traditional tissue expansion, it preserves sensate native tissues, unlike insensate abdominal-based free flaps.

Advantages and Disadvantages of Tissue Expansion

Tissue expansion has many notable advantages to other plastic and reconstructive techniques. The expanded tissue usually provides sufficient soft tissue coverage for both the recipient as well as donor sites. Tissues from locally expanded sites allow same color, texture, sensation, and quality skin to be used in resurfacing a defect, thus avoiding the use of split-thickness skin grafts which are associated with more recipient and donor site morbidities[7] (Fig. 6.9). Additional advantages include the significantly higher vascularity of expanded tissues providing more robust skin coverage.

Disadvantages of tissue expansion include the long timeframe of up to several months for the expansion process to finish and multiple outpatient visits. Most commonly, a two-stage procedure is necessary – one to place the expander in and a second one to replace the temporary implant with a more permanent one. Significant complications may result in multiple interventions. Further disadvantages include the frequent outpatient visits for incremental tissue expansion, which can be particularly uncomfortable on the forehead and distal extremities. There is also a psychological impact of tissue expansion as there is a temporary disfigurement that can last for many months before the expander is removed.[2] However the recent development and use of AeroForm expanders eliminates this problem and makes

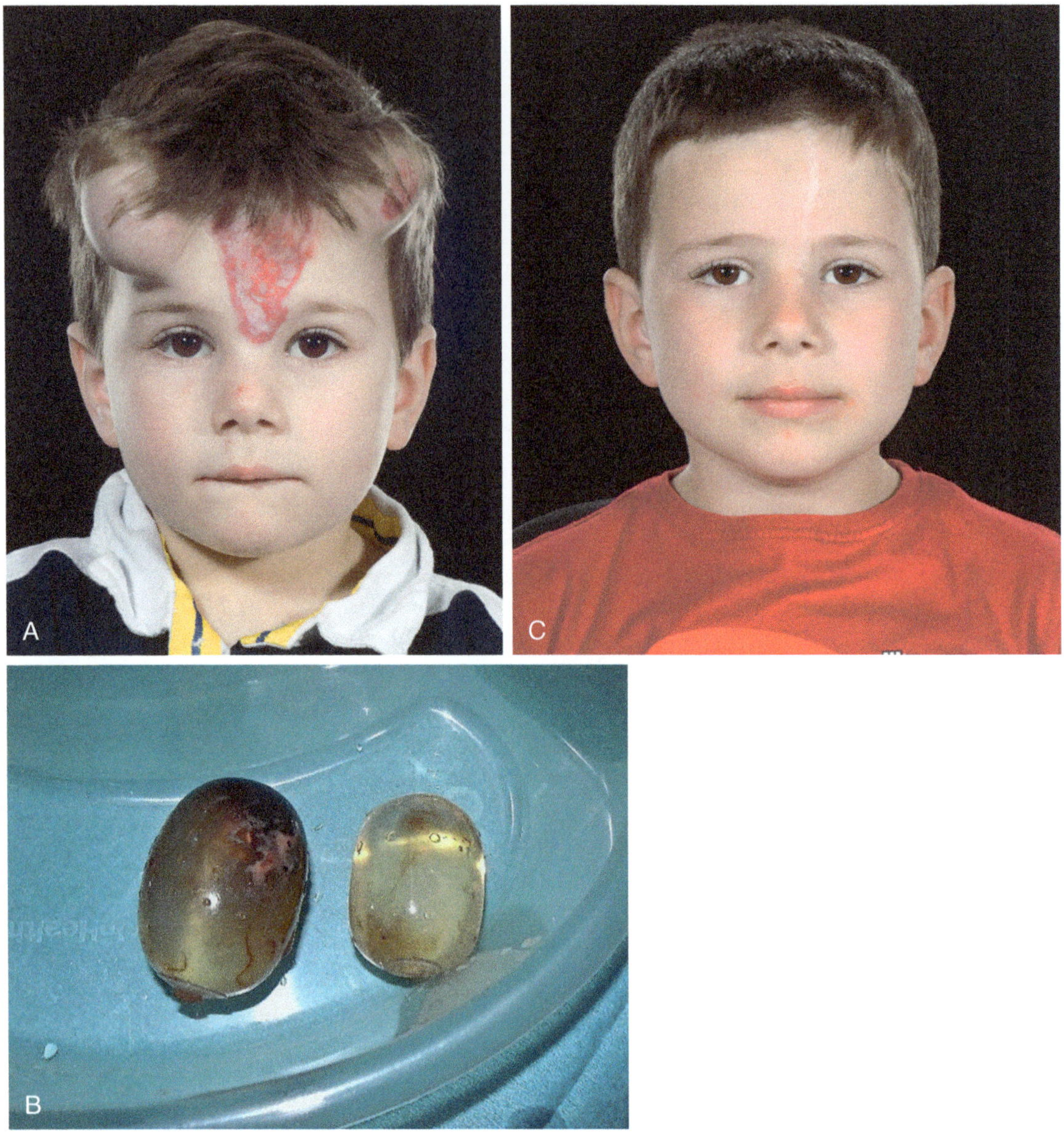

• **Fig. 6.9** (A) Expansion process used to reconstruct a large defect secondary to vascular malformation. (B) Explanted expanders in same patient. (C) Final result after advancing expanded tissues and excision of vascular malformation. An optimal color and skin quality match has been achieved.

tissue expansion less disruptive to the patient and reduces the expansion time compared to conventional saline expansion. Finally, tissue expansion is not without risks, and many large case series have noted major complications such as infection or implant exposure. A summary of associated complications is given below.

Complications

Tissue expansion, like any surgical procedure, comes with its own set of complications. In 1984, Manders et al summarized their experience with 41 expanders in 35 patients and divided the observed complications into major and minor categories.[29] Major complications include infection, implant extrusion and flap ischemia and may interrupt the expansion process. Minor complications, including seroma formation, scar widening, dog ear formation, transient pain, and neuropraxia, may resolve without failure of the procedure.

Antonyshyn et al performed a critical review of their results on tissue expansion over a 5-year period.[30] Sixty-six expansions were performed on 66 patients. Complications were identified and analysed based on their anatomical location, time of onset and detrimental results on the final outcome. Interestingly, the authors of this study noted some common sequelae of tissue expansion which, strictly speaking, were not complications. Transient pain following implant inflation was a commonly observed side effect, which was particularly associated with expansions of the distal extremities, dorsal trunk, and forehead. Clinically significant complications were most frequently observed with head, neck, and lower extremity expansion (39% in their case series) but generally did not affect the final outcome and excellent results were noted in 83% of cases. More serious complications tended to occur at the final stages of expansion with implant failure, neuropraxia, bone resorption, and late implant exposure being highlighted. Hematoma formation requiring prompt evacuation was observed in only one patient. Similarly, cellulitic infection of the skin covering the reservoir dome was observed in one patient only and was successfully treated with intravenous antibiotics. More severe complications, including infections involving the implant cavity and implant exposure secondary to incisional dehiscence, erosion through inadequate soft tissue cover, and pressure necrosis of soft tissues, were observed more frequently.

Pandya et al assessed complication rates of expansion at non-limb versus limb sites in a retrospective case series of 88 patients.[31] The overall incidence of complications was higher in the limb group (43%) compared to other sites (27%). Lower limb complications were also more frequently observed than upper limb complications (47% vs. 30%). They noted that exposure or infection of an implant on the extremity was not necessarily a sign of preceding failure. In these circumstances, expansion was suspended, appropriate antibiotics were administered and the area of exposure was allowed to heal. If the latter steps were successful, tissue expansion was restarted. The anatomical and physiological differences in the extremities could explain the higher complication rates. First, the extremities are in frequent motion and the underlying musculature can exert disruptive forces to the expander. Second, the flaps designed on the extremities are more difficult to encompass a curvilinear biconvex surface necessary for successful tissue expansion.

Fischer et al examined significant preoperative risk factors associated with failed tissue expander placement in breast reconstruction.[32] In their analysis they utilized the American College of Surgeons National Surgical quality improvement program datasets from 2005 to 2010 to determine perioperative risk factors associated with early expander loss. A multivariate regression analysis demonstrated several preoperative patient conditions that are associated with early device loss: age >55 years, obesity, and active smoking. Deep wound infection was the strongest predictor of loss (odds ratio (OR) 9.1, P <0.001). Patients with burns injuries have also been found to have greater complication rates during tissue expansion.[33]

Two-stage reconstruction – stage 1 (tissue expander), stage 2 (permanent implant) – is the commonest method of breast reconstruction. Lam and colleagues in a systematic review demonstrated that adjuvant radiotherapy post mastectomy increases the risk of capsular contracture and reconstruction failure.[34] Patients given adjuvant radiotherapy after tissue expansion had a high reconstruction failure rate of 22.9% compared to those given radiotherapy after stage 2 (5.9% failure). Irradiated patients were also found to have an inferior cosmetic outcome.[34]

Tissue expansion in the pediatric population has complication rates ranging from 13% to 30%.[35] In a large 12-year study (282 expanders in 94 patients) Gosain and colleagues noted that up to a third of families whose children undergo tissue expansion will have complications that may necessitate surgery or a modification of the initial reconstructive plan.[35] Families should be made aware of common complications, such as exposure, rupture, and infection, that would minimize delay to treatment.

Earlier versions of the AirXpander (AeroForm version 2) had significant device related problems with 10% of cases experiencing loss of communication and 27% of cases experiencing deflation and 4 cases experiencing over inflation.[4,23] The AeroForm version 2.5 had no reported incidences of loss of communication but still an 11% incidence of deflation. The device failure rate even in the new version (AeroForm v2.5) is still higher than conventional saline expansion.

Future of Tissue Expansion

Expansion of skin and subcutaneous tissues adjacent to the pathological skin to be replaced is probably the only method of reconstruction that creates almost normal structure, anatomy, and function in reconstructive surgery. This, however, may lead to the technique being restricted to patients with normal tissues surrounding the pathological defect. Furthermore, complications, especially in certain anatomical areas, are frequent, leading to further restrictions in terms of patient eligibility. In the future, as the underlying cell biology and molecular basis of tissue expansion is elucidated, former restrictions and complications may be overcome.

The field of regenerative medicine and tissue-engineering is yet to establish itself fully in clinical medicine. However, we have witnessed the use of BRAVA, which is a form of external tissue expansion that can generate an in situ biological scaffold that will accept fat graft for breast reconstruction. The authors state that it is a tissue-engineered method of autologous breast reconstruction. However, it is yet to take over from conventional methods of expansion as it is labor-intensive and involves multiple surgical procedures.

Alternate methods of expansion using an AeroForm CO_2-filled tissue expansion system instead of traditional saline, have shortened expansion times and improved patient comfort. Concerns were raised during earlier models of the AeroForm expander, mainly related to device failure resulting in premature deflation. Nonetheless the safety profile of these devices appears to be far superior to osmotic expanders, which have had high instances of infection and extrusion reported. However, it has yet to gain worldwide popularity to replace conventional saline expansion.

In summary, tissue expansion remains an important reconstructive tool in the armamentarium of plastic surgeons. It can overcome tissue shortages in challenging scenarios, providing an excellent color, quality, sensibility, and tissue match for the defect site. However, as discussed in this chapter it is not without its complications and patients undergoing this procedure should be appropriately consented about the timeframe and what to encounter during the process.

Ten Golden Rules of Expanders

1. Select a donor site where the consistency of the soft tissues are identical to those required to close the defect.
2. The access incision for the tissue expander should be placed at the margin of the defect and ideally through unscarred and non-radiated tissues.
3. Rectangular expanders give the most tissue expansion. Rectangular expanders increase surface area by 38% in contrast to round, which only give 25%.
4. The amount of fluid injected into the expander should be individualized to the patient and governed by tenseness, blanching of the overlying skin, and pain. Care in preventing overexpansion will reduce the chances of tissue ischemia and necrosis of the skin flaps.
5. The tissue expander should be sited on a base that resists mechanical deformation and directs the force of expansion outwards and towards the overlying soft tissues (e.g., bone).
6. The pocket which is dissected for tissue expander placement must be larger than the dimensions of the expander.
7. Delay implant inflation for approximately 2 weeks until sufficient time has passed for the wound to heal and edema to settle. This will reduce the chances of incisional dehiscence and will allow time for any problem with the flap to reveal itself.
8. One must recall that the capsule around the expander is highly vascular and capsulectomy can compromise the vascularity of the overlying skin.
9. Complication rates vary in tissue expansion depending on anatomical location. Extremity lower limb expansion has been shown to have higher rates of major complications in comparison to the scalp and the breast. In children one may consider exteriorizing the port to minimize discomfort and facilitate expansion. An exposed expander can be salvaged and expansion resumed in some cases.
10. Self-inflating expanders (Osmed) should be used with caution as the rate of expansion cannot be controlled. AeroForm carbon dioxide based expanders offer an alternative method of needleless expansion and have a comparable safety profile compared to conventional saline expansion.

References

1. Neumann CG. The expansion of an area of skin by progressive distention of a subcutaneous balloon; use of the method for securing skin for subtotal reconstruction of the ear. *Plast Reconstr Surg (1946)*. 1957;19(2):124–130.
2. Radovan C. Tissue expansion in soft-tissue reconstruction. *Plast Reconstr Surg*. 1984;74(4):482–492.
3. Shuter ML, Malata CM, Duffy JS, Sharpe DT. Determination of relative contributions of "mechanical" and "biological" creep in tissue expansion using in vivo pressure monitoring: a preliminary report. *Med Eng Phys*. 1994;16(1):24–28.
4. Ascherman JA, Zeidler K, Morrison KA, et al. Carbon dioxide-based versus saline tissue expansion for breast reconstruction: results of the XPAND prospective, randomized clinical trial. *Plast Reconstr Surg*. 2016;138(6):1161–1170.
5. De Filippo RE, Atala A. Stretch and growth: the molecular and physiologic influences of tissue expansion. *Plast Reconstr Surg*. 2002;109(7):2450–2462.
6. Takei T, Mills I, Arai K, Sumpio BE, et al. Molecular basis for tissue expansion: clinical implications for the surgeon. *Plast Reconstr Surg*. 1998;102(1):247–258.
7. Vander Kolk CA, McCAnn JJ, Knight KR, O'Brien BM. Some further characteristics of expanded tissue. *Clin Plast Surg*. 1987;14(3):447–453.
8. Khouri RK, Schlenz I, Murphy BJ, Baker TJ. Nonsurgical breast enlargement using an external soft-tissue expansion system. *Plast Reconstr Surg*. 2000;105(7):2500–2512; discussion 2513–2514.
9. Lancerotto L, Chin MS, Freniere B, et al. Mechanisms of action of external volume expansion devices. *Plast Reconstr Surg*. 2013;132(3):569–578.
10. Pietramaggiori G, Liu P, Scherer SS, et al. Tensile forces stimulate vascular remodeling and epidermal cell proliferation in living skin. *Ann Surg*. 2007;246(5):896–902.
11. Erba P, Miele LF, Adini A, et al. A morphometric study of mechanotransductively induced dermal neovascularization. *Plast Reconstr Surg*. 2011;128(4):288e–299e.
12. Sheng L, Yang M, Du Z, et al. Transplantation of stromal vascular fraction as an alternative for accelerating tissue expansion. *J Plast Reconstr Aesthet Surg*. 2013;66(4):551–557.
13. Johnson TM, Lowe L, Brown MD, et al. Histology and physiology of tissue expansion. *J Dermatol Surg Oncol*. 1993;19(12):1074–1078.
14. Cherry GW, Austad E, Pasyk K, et al. Increased survival and vascularity of random-pattern skin flaps elevated in controlled, expanded skin. *Plast Reconstr Surg*. 1983;(5):680–687.
15. Chin MS, Lujan-Hernandez J, Babchenko O, et al. External volume expansion in irradiated tissue: effects on the recipient site. *Plast Reconstr Surg*. 2016;137(5):799e–807e.
16. Radovan C. Breast reconstruction after mastectomy using the temporary expander. *Plast Reconstr Surg*. 1982;69(2):195–208.
17. Becker H. Breast reconstruction using an inflatable breast implant with detachable reservoir. *Plast Reconstr Surg*. 1984;73(4):678–683.
18. Eriksen C, Nordstrand Lindgren E, Frisell J, Stark B. A prospective randomized study comparing two different expander approaches in implant-based breast reconstruction: one stage versus two stages. *Plast Reconstr Surg*. 2012;130(2):254e–264e.
19. Spear SL, Economides JM, Shuck J, Patel KM. Analyzing implant movement with tabbed and nontabbed expanders through the process of two-stage breast reconstruction. *Plast Reconstr Surg*. 2014;133(3):256e–260e.
20. Austad ED, Rose GL. A self-inflating tissue expander. *Plast Reconstr Surg*. 1982;70(5):588–594.
21. Chummun S, Addison P, Stewart KJ. The osmotic tissue expander: a 5-year experience. *J Plast Reconstr Aesthet Surg*. 2010;63(12):2128–2132.
22. Ronert MA, Hofheinz H, Olbrisch RR. The beginning of a new era: self-filling tissue expander for defect coverage in a 3-year-old boy with a retroauricular nevus. *Plast Reconstr Surg*. 2003;112(1):189–191.
23. Ascherman JA, Zeidler KR, Jacoby A, et al. Carbon dioxide versus saline tissue expanders: does it matter? *Plast Reconstr Surg*. 2016;137(1):31–35.

24. Hudson DA, Grob M. Optimising results with tissue expansion: 10 simple rules for successful tissue expander insertion. *Burns*. 2005;31(1):1–4.
25. Mazzoli RA, Raymond WR 4th, Ainbinder DJ, et al. Use of self-expanding, hydrophilic osmotic expanders (hydrogel) in the reconstruction of congenital clinical anophthalmos. *Curr Opin Ophthalmol*. 2004;15(5):426–431.
26. Raposio E, Santi P. Computer-aided preoperative planning of tissue expansion. *Ann Plast Surg*. 1997;39(4):416–417.
27. Song B, Xiao B, Liu C, et al. Neck burn reconstruction with pre-expanded scapular free flaps. *Burns*. 2015;41(3):624–630.
28. Kosowski TR, Rigotti G, Khouri RK. Tissue-engineered autologous breast regeneration with Brava®-assisted fat grafting. *Clin Plast Surg*. 2015;42(3):325–337, (viii).
29. Manders EK, Schenden MJ, Furrery JA, et al. Soft-tissue expansion: concepts and complications. *Plast Reconstr Surg*. 1984;74(4):493–507.
30. Antonyshyn O, Gruss JS, Mackinnon SE, Zuker R. Complications of soft tissue expansion. *Br J Plast Surg*. 1988;41(3):239–250.
31. Pandya AN, Vadodaria S, Coleman DJ. Tissue expansion in the limbs: a comparative analysis of limb and non-limb sites. *Br J Plast Surg*. 2002;55(4):302–306.
32. Fischer JP, Nelson JA, Serletti JM, Wu LC. Peri-operative risk factors associated with early tissue expander (TE) loss following immediate breast reconstruction (IBR): a review of 9305 patients from the 2005-2010 ACS-NSQIP datasets. *J Plast Reconstr Aesthet Surg*. 2013;66(11):1504–1512.
33. Friedman RM, Ingram AE, Rohrich RJ, et al. Risk factors for complications in pediatric tissue expansion. *Plast Reconstr Surg*. 1996;98(7):1242–1246.
34. Lam TC, Hsieh F, Boyages J. The effects of postmastectomy adjuvant radiotherapy on immediate two-stage prosthetic breast reconstruction: a systematic review. *Plast Reconstr Surg*. 2013;132(3):511–518.
35. Gosain AK, Turin SY, Chim H, LoGiudice JA. Salvaging the unavoidable: a review of complications in pediatric tissue expansion. *Plast Reconstr Surg*. 2018;142(3):759–768.

7 Tissue Engineering

MICHAEL W. FINDLAY AND GEOFFREY C. GURTNER

Introduction

The reconstructive options for today's plastic surgeons are unprecedented in history. Despite this reality, the ideal reconstruction for many patients and defect types does not yet exist. The traditional paradigm of plastic surgery has centered around re-purposing existing tissues through grafting, locoregional or free flap transfer to replace "like with like" in keeping with the principles of Sir Harold Gillies. Re-purposing existing tissues is an elegant solution that serves us well and may be augmented through the use of prefabrication and prelamination techniques,[1] but the ideal reconstruction would replace "same with same" and thereby avoid donor site morbidity entirely. Recently, composite tissue allotransplantation (CTA) has demonstrated its ability to replace "same with same" through the use of tissue and organ donors for facial, limb, and other transplants. CTA is directly analogous to organ transplantation, a discipline that owes much of its origins to Dr Joseph Murray, a plastic surgeon and Nobel laureate, who pioneered live related organ donation over 60 years ago. Both organ transplantation and CTA patients carry a significant burden in terms of the sequelae of long-term immunosuppression including rejection, graft versus host disease, opportunistic infections, and increased incidence of certain cancers.[2]

Tissue engineering (TE) offers a means to grow replacement tissues and organs, thereby replacing "same with same" to restore form and function to the premorbid state. Patients with defects from trauma, cancer, burns, and often complex congenital conditions could all benefit immensely from advances in tissue engineering through the provision of improved and less morbid options for their management. In addition, tissue engineering has obvious benefits for esthetic surgery due to its potential to effect changes in skin texture, contour, tissue volume, and general appearance. Plastic surgeons already have significant expertise in the surgical manipulation of human tissues and organs. Tissue engineering builds on this foundation to form part of the present and future of plastic surgery.

Tissue engineering (TE) has been variably defined. The National Science Foundation in 1987 developed the following definition[3]: "Tissue Engineering is the application of the principles and methods of engineering and life sciences towards the fundamental understanding of structure-function relationships in normal and pathological mammalian tissues and the development of biologic substitutes that restore, maintain, or improve tissue function." More simply, tissue engineering is a discipline that utilizes cells, matrices, growth factors, and biomaterials to generate new tissues and organs for clinical use including multiple organ systems and tissues (Fig. 7.1). It is also used as a research tool to further our understanding of the interactions between these components in both health and disease states. Unfortunately, tissue engineering techniques are not yet able to replace organ transplants in transplantation surgery. However, the past decade has seen an exponential increase in the implementation of tissue engineering strategies in clinical practice. During this time, plastic surgeons have played a key role in the development and implementation of these techniques and various biomaterials in surgical practice.

Plastic surgeons may function as the primary drivers of advances in tissue engineering or they may partner with engineers and/or cell biologists to translate promising laboratory research from the bench to the bedside. Engagement of clinicians in research is vital to advancing the field of tissue engineering. It provides a means to address unmet clinical needs and it fosters the innovation that continues to expand our scope of practice in an age where our specialty is being undermined at the edges by other specialties. As tissue engineering becomes a more routine component of clinical practice, it is essential that every practicing plastic surgeon has a working knowledge of its principles. Here we outline tissue engineering as a discipline, describe its approaches, and highlight the emerging technologies that are likely to transform our specialty over the coming decades.

Experimental Tissue Engineering

Tissue Engineering as a Tool to Further Scientific Discovery

The common misconception about tissue engineering is that it is focussed solely on the production of new tissues and organs to replace lost or malfunctioning body parts. In practice, it is also used widely as a tool for scientific research. Tissue engineering techniques can recapitulate specific aspects

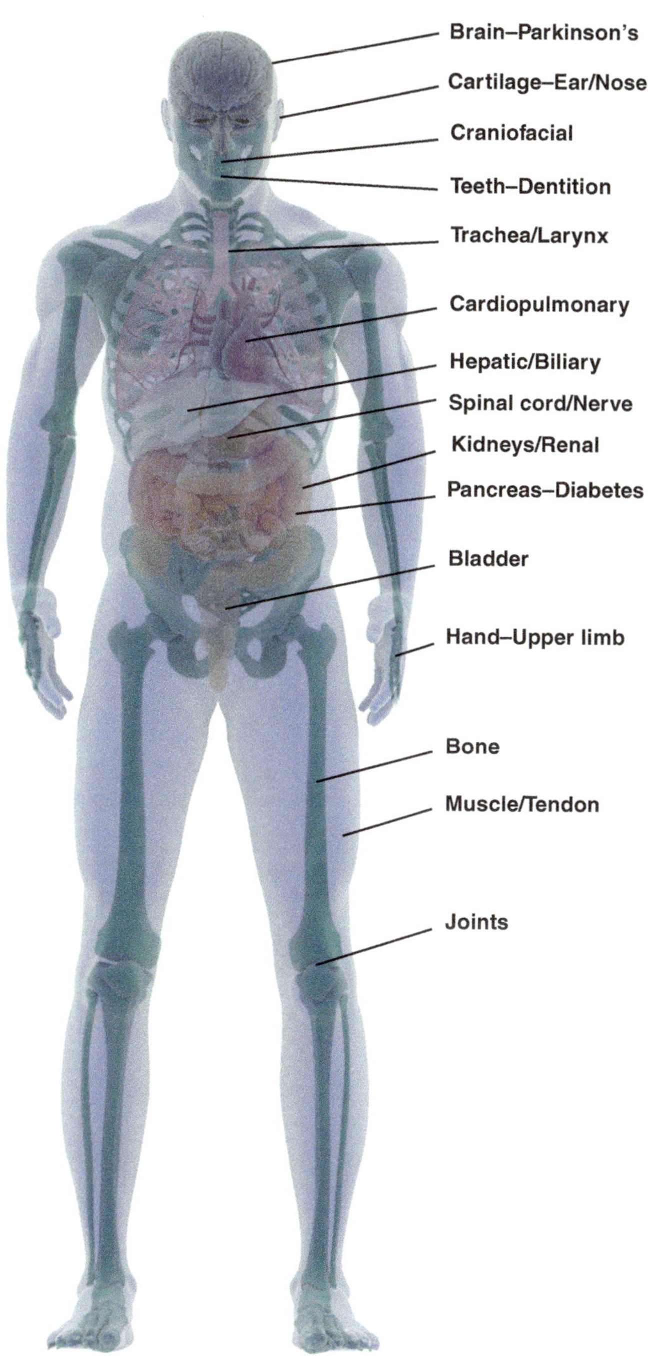

• **Fig. 7.1** Diagrammatic representation of the body showing examples of tissues and organs where tissue engineering research is close to or is already in clinical use.

of tissues and organs to permit the investigation of structure–function relationships and the testing of therapies such as new medicines. Both beneficial and maladaptive interactions between cell populations (including stem and progenitor cells) and their local environment can be studied across multiple different platforms (in vitro, ex vivo, and in vivo). There are manifold reasons that tissue engineering can be a useful research tool in plastic surgery. Conditions such as hypertrophic and keloid scarring do not occur in laboratory animals and therefore tissue engineering approaches are useful to approximate elements of these conditions and to develop and test novel therapies. Furthermore, many conditions that are treated in plastic and reconstructive surgery are not life-threatening and therefore it can be difficult to procure funding for expensive animal studies or human trials. Our management of human aging is difficult to replicate in experimental animals and therefore preclinical tissue and organ aging research requires suitable models to bridge the gap between basic research and human trials.

There are many tissue engineering techniques used experimentally to further plastic surgery including, three-dimensional (3D) cell culture/multicellular organotypic culture and tissue- and organ-on-a-chip technology where the local environment of multicellular constructs is tightly controlled. Worldwide, many laboratories use such techniques to examine conditions of relevance to our specialty, such as the effects of diabetes mellitus on wound healing, the survival of ischemic tissues, and Dupuytren's contracture amongst others.[4] An in vitro model of hypertrophic scarring was developed in our laboratory using tissue engineering principles. A collagen gel seeded with fibroblasts is placed under tension to replicate the conditions for human hypertrophic scar formation (Fig. 7.2). This model has provided invaluable insights into the interaction between cells and their matrix in hypertrophic scarring and facilitated the subsequent development of a murine model.[5] These models provide numerous opportunities for further study as they allow the use of technologies that are not readily used in humans, including gene editing, transgenic organisms, and viral transfection.

Applied Tissue Engineering – a Team-Based Discipline

Applied tissue engineering focuses on the translation of laboratory-based tissue engineering techniques into the clinical setting ("from bench to bedside"). Just as multidisciplinary teams are used for management of complex cancer cases, a team approach is often ideal for the development of new tissue engineering techniques in a clinically relevant manner. Plastic surgeons are well placed to partner with engineers and cell biologists to advise on such translational research and clinical trials based on the broad spectrum of our practice (both anatomically and in terms of subspecialty), skills in microvascular and peripheral nerve surgery, and our expertise in identifying unmet clinical needs. Without such partnership, much of fundamental cell science and biomaterials research does not translate appropriately into the clinical setting. Even highly publicized laboratory-based tissue engineering research can fail to translate to the clinical setting when the tissue engineered construct meets an intact whole organism, particularly when it has to interact with an intact immune system. Pioneering ear cartilage tissue engineering research by Langer and Vacanti excited the public and garnered both significant interest and funding for tissue engineering research but it did not directly translate in immune-competent animals, including humans[6] (Fig. 7.3). Such research outcomes emphasize the need for partnerships and team-based approaches in tissue engineering that

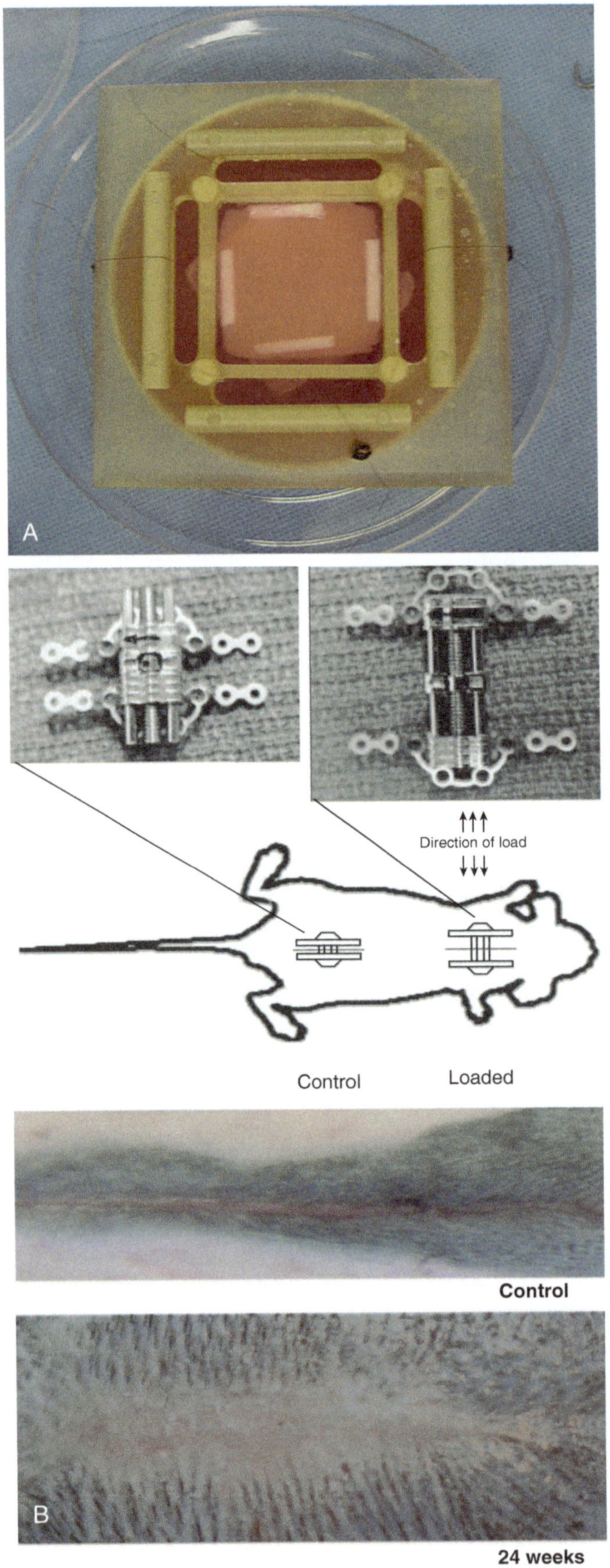

• **Fig. 7.2** (A) Tissue engineering of hypertrophic scar – the application of mechanical strain to a collagen matrix with admixed cells (center square) via sutures with small weights to replicate aspects of hypertrophic scarring in vitro permits the assessment of various cells and factors to help target hypertrophic scarring in humans. (B) The same concept used in vivo in a mouse to generate a hypertrophic scar response despite inability for common laboratory animals to produce hypertrophic scarring under normal conditions. This model permits the use of transgenic animals and various factors to gain improved insights into human hypertrophic scarring so that novel therapies may be developed. ((B) Reproduced with permission from Aarabi S, Bhatt KA, Shi Y, et al. Mechanical load initiates hypertrophic scar formation through decreased cellular apoptosis. *FASEB J*. 2007;21(12):3250–3261.)

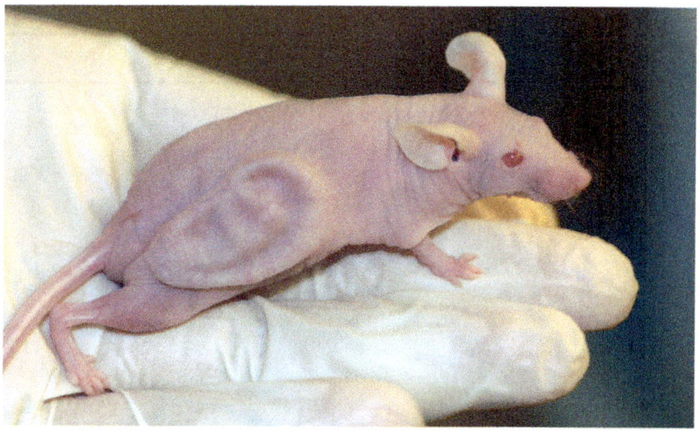

• **Fig. 7.3** Successful integration of a cartilage model grown in vitro into a subcutaneous pocket on the back of an immune compromised mouse. This pioneering research excited the public and increased the view that tissue engineering of whole new body parts was near to fruition. This approach could not be translated into immune competent animals, including humans, and demonstrates the need for clinicians with broad expertise in the response of whole organisms to various biomaterials. (Courtesy of Dr. Joseph P. Vacanti and the Laboratory for Tissue Engineering and Organ Fabrication, Massachusetts General Hospital, Boston, MA, USA.)

leverage the expertise of the group to achieve clinically relevant outcomes. Commercialization of successful research also requires a different, yet complementary skillset, but luckily there are improving pathways for commercialization through public and private institutions including universities, hospitals, and incubators. The current expertise in all of these fields makes tissue engineering an exciting and collaborative endeavor that can reap real rewards for patients.

Tissue Engineering in Plastic Surgery

The long history and problem-solving nature of plastic surgery has resulted in the development of a number of techniques that can be considered as forms of tissue engineering. Autologous fat grafting is a possible example. It has been used for over a century to address contour defects or provide additional volume. Our early understanding of its mode of action was that the adipocytes were simply being transferred and engrafted at the recipient site. A more nuanced understanding of this technique involves multiple overlapping processes that also include cell ischemia with chemokine signalling, inflammation, stem cell transplantation (adipose-derived stem cells– ADSCs) and recruitment of local and systemic stem cells. From a tissue engineering perspective, it involves the transfer of stem and progenitor cells within their native matrix along with parenchymal cells. A number of mechanistic studies demonstrate that both engraftment and adipogenesis occur to varying degrees depending on both local and systemic factors.[7] Yoshimura and colleagues proposed a more tissue-engineering-like approach through the addition of ADSCs to the lipoaspirate (cell-assisted lipotransfer) in an effort to improve engraftment and volume retention.[8] Whether this is beneficial is still uncertain. The addition of platelet-rich plasma (PRP) to lipoaspirate demonstrates some benefits over lipoaspirate alone for volume retention long term.[9] There is mounting evidence that autologous fat grafting may improve local vascularization and tissue quality in studies where it has been used underneath irradiated skin.[10,11] The exact mechanism for this effect is unknown but the data argue for a role for autologous fat grafting as a form of tissue engineering, despite ongoing debate as to whether de novo adipogenesis, simple engraftment or lipid cyst formation occurs in any given site or individual. Research to improve its reliability, long-term volume retention, and our understanding of its mechanism of action are ongoing.

Another clinical technique that uses tissue engineering principles involves the insertion of silicone rods (eponymously referred to as Hunter's rods) for the generation of a neo-sheath for secondary flexor tendon reconstruction in hand surgery.[12] Where a primary tendon repair has not been possible due to tendon shortening or contracture of the flexor tendon sheath, secondary tendon reconstruction with the use of a tendon graft becomes necessary. To achieve a functional reconstruction, it is necessary to reconstitute a glide plane for the tendon in the form of a neo-sheath. In this setting, a two-stage procedure is performed whereby a smooth, silicone rod with a roughly semicircular cross-section is inserted along the line of the required neo-sheath. Within weeks, encapsulation of the silicone occurs and once the silicone is removed, this forms a smooth tunnel for the tendon reconstruction to glide through during healing and active recovery.

There are now increasing numbers of commercially available tissue engineering products in plastic surgery. Some obvious examples include skin/dermal substitutes for burns and wound care, nerve conduits/wraps and acellular biomaterials for coverage of implants and hernia repairs. It is unsurprising that skin/dermal tissue engineering has one of the longest histories in plastic surgery due to the vital need for skin and dermal substitutes in acute and chronic burns patients and the relative ease of creating somewhat two-dimensional structures. Skin tissue engineering was one of the first published studies within the field.[13,14] Despite the commercial success of many of these products, there still does not exist an "off the shelf" substitute for a split-thickness skin graft, highlighting the ongoing need for translational tissue engineering research.

Irrespective of the type of technique, tissue engineering strategies share some common elements. They typically involve a cell source (either autologous or allogeneic) and a biomaterial of some sort (either exogenous or induced/endogenous) with the end result being new tissue or organ production. This may be achieved through the use of a mixture of cells and biomaterials and there remains significant overlap between tissue engineering, stem cell therapies, and the implantation of biomaterials.

From a regulatory perspective, tissue engineering strategies are stratified by whether they are cell-based or acellular and by whether they incorporate biological matrices and/or have synthetic components. Greater regulatory hurdles exist for cell-based applications and there are correspondingly

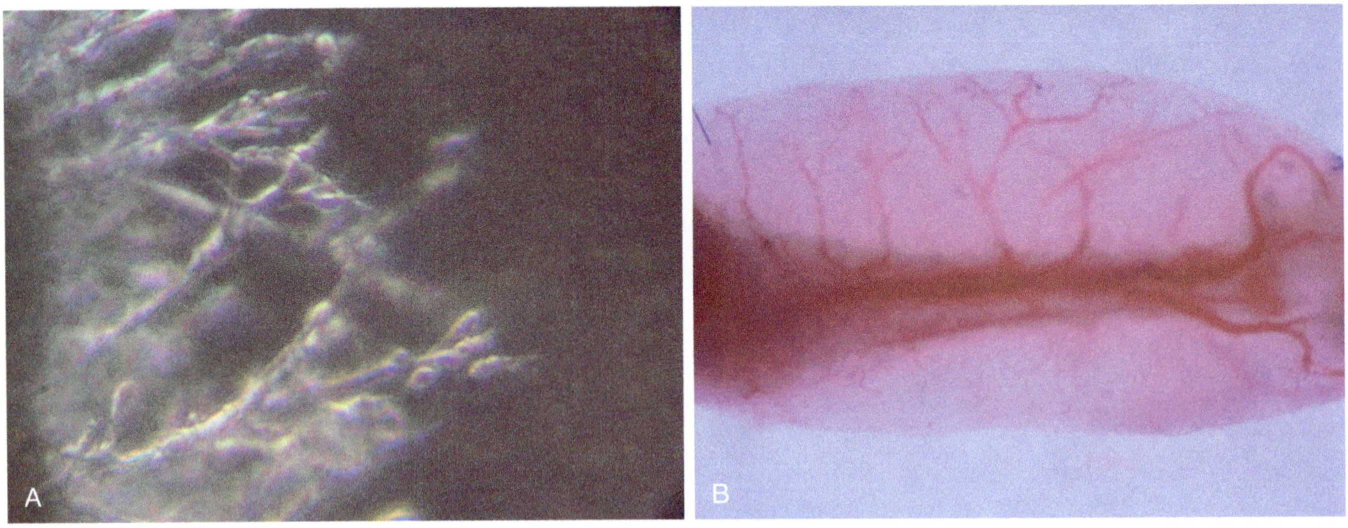

• **Fig. 7.4** (A) Angiogenesis appearing as sprouting of endothelial cells from the side of a vessel (appearance of leading edge at vessels at 5 days). (B) Profuse neovascularization from an arteriovenous pedicle into Matrigel within a tissue engineering chamber at 6 weeks post implantation. Note the arborization of vessels at the periphery of the specimen.

fewer cell-based products available for clinical use. Similarly, the use of materials that already have regulatory approval (e.g., components already used in clinical practice such as suture material or collagen) have an easier pathway to regulatory approval and are therefore found in more currently available products. Despite these hurdles, cell-based constructs can demonstrate excellent outcomes relative to non-cell-based applications, particularly when the patient or their recipient site have comorbidities (e.g., diabetes mellitus) that limit local recruitment of cells and/or the suitability of the recipient site. In practice, plastic and reconstructive surgeons have a wide range of clinical experience with tissue engineering products and therefore are well placed to take an active role in the development and implementation of new tissue engineering strategies in clinical practice. A thorough grounding in the basic principles of tissue engineering significantly helps us as a specialty to perform this role.

Targeted Tissue Engineering Strategies

Early attempts to grow specific tissues relied upon a subcomponent approach to tissue production. This empiric approach put together the subcomponents of tissues or organs in the hope that they might self-assemble into a useful structure in vivo. Sadly, this was rarely the case, but many useful insights were gained by considering the important subcomponents of specific tissues and organs and how they interact. Developmental studies examining cell interactions during tissue and organogenesis have improved our understanding of how new organs and tissues form naturally but they are of limited benefit for the production of new tissues clinically as adult stem cells demonstrate lineage restriction and it is difficult to replicate the fetal milieu ex utero. Tissue engineering researchers instead looked to fields where new 3D tissues grow in adult life. Tumorigenesis is probably the best example of this and many insights into tissue engineering have been gained by examining the process of tumor formation.

Neovascularization in Tumorigenesis and Organogenesis

There are numerous parallels between the study of solid tumors and the discipline of tissue engineering, with the exception that the goal of each of these fields is different (inhibit cancer growth versus stimulation of new organ growth). Much of our understanding of postnatal tissue growth owes its genesis to oncology researchers. Judah Folkman, a surgeon, established the need for new blood vessel growth (angiogenesis) for cancers to grow in three dimensions. Each cancer cell must remain in close contact with the blood supply, and the cells and the vasculature must form a mutually supportive ecosystem.[15]

New tissue growth requires new blood vessel formation (neovascularization). Two types of neovascularization have been identified. Vasculogenesis is the de novo formation of blood vessels from vessel progenitors. It is an in utero phenomenon, but it may make a small contribution to neovascularization in the postnatal setting under certain circumstances. Angiogenesis is predominantly a postnatal process where new blood vessels sprout from existing blood vessels under the influence of local factors (growth factors, chemokines, and physicochemical gradients) (Fig. 7.4). Angiogenesis is the predominant process in adult animals for new blood vessel formation and is one of the major targets of cancer therapies and tissue engineering strategies.

The vasculature of tissues changes under the influence of stimulators or inhibitors of angiogenesis. This process starts with signaling that increases vascular plasticity, typically under the influence of factors such as angiopoietin-1. The vasculature may then increase or decrease in branch points, vessel length, and vessel diameter, depending on the relative balance between pro-and anti-angiogenic signals. While new blood vessel formation is important, its regulation is just as important. Tissue engineering uses pluripotent and multipotent stem cells that are capable of forming multiple different types of tissue. The degree of vascularization within their microenvironment may influence their differentiation during the formation of tissue engineering constructs. For example, bone formation occurs readily in well-vascularized settings whereas cartilage formation is promoted in less vascular microenvironments. For this reason, pro- and anti-angiogenic signals must be tightly controlled both spatially and temporally during tissue engineering. Angiogenesis also supports tumorigenesis. Therefore, the stimulation of angiogenesis for tissue-engineering may pose a risk for tumorigenesis. For example, the stimulation of angiogenesis by adipose-derived stem cells (ADSCs) is one putative mechanism behind some reports of increased tumor recurrence following autologous fat grafting, particularly with c-MET-expressing breast cancer cell lines in animal models.[16] This has not been established in humans but such data remain a concern for tissue engineers in the long term.

At a stable tumor volume, tumor cells and endothelial cells send stimulatory signals to support each other, thereby maintaining total tumor volume. When tumor growth exceeds the ability of the vasculature to support it, focal tumor necrosis occurs. Normal tissues display co-regulation between the parenchyma and the vasculature with long-term maintenance of tissue or organ volume being dependent upon a stable vasculature. This is in contrast to wound healing responses where new blood vessels are formed to support tissue healing and scar formation but the new endothelial cells undergo apoptosis over months to years to return the site to a near pre-wounding vascular density and volume. For tissue engineering strategies to demonstrate their effectiveness, they have to be able to generate the required tissue and maintain that volume long term, rather than representing some form of aberrant wound healing response. The effectiveness of tissue engineering strategies must therefore be assessed over the long term and this is not often done effectively in experimental tissue engineering. Additional insights can be gained from such studies and can help direct studies in humans.[17] Inflammation is a potent source of pro-angiogenic factors but when excessive it may promote scar formation instead of the target tissue. There are numerous cells in the local microenvironment that contribute to the regulation of inflammation and their regulation is an important consideration in tissue engineering. The control of local inflammation will be discussed later in the chapter when we consider the local microenvironment for tissue engineering.

Seed versus Soil Hypothesis

Another parallel between oncology and tissue engineering is the 'seed versus soil' hypothesis. This was originally described by Stephen Paget as a way to understand tumor metastases. In the present context it refers to whether the "seed" (stem/progenitor cells) or the "soil" (the local microenvironment) is the most important factor in the generation of new stable tissue constructs.[18] The seed hypothesis focuses on the capacity of stem and progenitor cells to adapt to and alter their microenvironment to generate new vascularized tissue. The primacy of stem and progenitor cells in new tissue generation is well known but soil protagonists argue that the creation of a suitable microenvironment triggers the recruitment of endogenous stem and progenitor cells and provides the cues for them to replicate, differentiate and vascularize to generate a stable tissue construct. A composite view considers the needs of a stable stem cell niche and how this can be manipulated to facilitate the formation of new specific tissue in a controlled manner with reconstitution of a stable stem cell niche within the target tissue following completion of the necessary tissue growth. Where limitations to endogenous stem and progenitor cells may exist (patients with comorbidities including aging, diabetes mellitus, and irradiation), greater focus may be required on "seed" approaches that can compensate for deficits in stem/progenitor cell function and/or trafficking. Where normal stem and progenitor cell function is present, "soil" approaches can be very successful (e.g., young healthy animals). Both approaches rely upon the ability to temporarily bypass the normal control mechanisms that limit the formation of new tissues (and/or benign tumors). The control mechanisms that limit stem cell division and differentiation under normal physiological conditions are still incompletely understood. The risk of forming cancers remains a stigma for tissue engineering, despite little evidence to establish that tissue engineering techniques significantly increase the risk of cancer. As more is understood about these regulatory mechanisms, this uncertainty should decrease.

Stem and Progenitor Cells in Tissue Engineering

Stem cells are long-lived cells that are capable of a number of important functions, including the ability to form multiple different tissue types, encourage or participate in new blood vessel formation (neovascularization), immunomodulation and self-renewal.[19] Progenitor cells are usually daughters of stem cells that are already committed to a given cell fate (not multipotent) but are capable of both self-renewal and reconstituting their given cell/tissue type. Endothelial progenitor cells (EPCs) are a common progenitor cell type used in tissue engineering because of their putative ability to develop into vasculature/endothelial cells. Combinations of stem cells and endothelial progenitor cells are often used to support the coevolution tissues with their supporting vasculature.

Broadly, stem cells are divided into embryonic stem cells (totipotent or pluripotent), postnatal stem cells (multipotent), and induced pluripotent stem cells (iPSCs).[20] Embryonic stem cells are a valuable tool in the study of

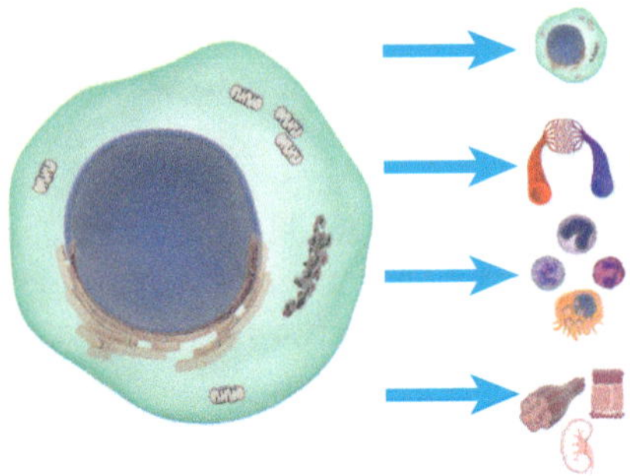

• **Fig. 7.5** Functional characteristics that define stem cells including self-renewal, support of new blood vessel formation, immune modulation, and differentiation capacity into multiple lineages. Early embryonic stem cells are totipotent (can form all three germ layers) and then undergo lineage restriction over time (pluripotency) until multipotent adult stem cells are formed (more restricted outcomes, e.g., mesenchymal stem cells that can differentiate into muscle, bone, cartilage or adipose tissue).

developmental processes and fundamental aspects of stem cell biology, but they have significant ethical issues as they need to be harvested from embryos, often secondary to the retrieval of the embryo from the uterus. This process is usually destructive of the embryo and therefore poses significant ethical problems and is not a readily available option for tissue engineering in conventional care settings. Postnatally, stem and progenitor cells are present in most tissues of the body and continue to have important roles in tissue homeostasis based on their support for cell turnover (with a more limited capacity to form multiple tissues), immunomodulation, vascularization, and self-renewal (Fig. 7.5).

Adipose tissue is a ready source of mesenchymal stem cells for tissue engineering and can be harvested by plastic surgeons as part of liposuction, abdominoplasty, and breast reduction techniques amongst others.[21] This gives plastic surgeons a ready source of patient-derived mesenchymal stem cells for tissue engineering research and clinical implementation. Adipose-derived mesenchymal stem cells are one of the most extensively studied and used stem cell populations in both research and clinical practice. Adult mesenchymal stem cells are multipotent. This means that they are already pre-committed to the following tissue types including adipose tissue, muscle, cartilage, and bone, although they can demonstrate additional lineages under specific circumstances.

Four key elements are necessary to generating tissue from them and any stem cell:

1. Vascularization/engraftment commensurate with stem cell survival;
2. stimulation of new tissue formation that occurs in parallel with the development of stable vascularization to support long-term tissue stability, particularly with tissues that are co-regulated with their vasculature, such as fat tissue;
3. control of differentiation to produce the desired tissue type rather than competing tissues or mixtures of different tissues (teratomas); and
4. reconstitution of a stable stem cell niche to support long-term tissue health and homeostasis.

Recent research by our group demonstrates that many patients have acquired defects in stem cell and progenitor cells with aging and conditions such as diabetes mellitus.[22,23] This can be through a combination of abnormal stem cell trafficking or impacts on specific important subpopulations of stem cells. Such research brings into question the feasibility of harvesting autologous stem cells directly from patients with comorbidities and may explain the variability in the success of translational tissue engineering research where these deficits have not been taken into consideration.

Induced Pluripotent Stem Cells (iPS Cells)

Induced pluripotent stem cells are adult cells that have been reprogrammed to an embryonic stem cell-like state and meet the relevant criteria for pluripotent stem cells including their expression of stem cell markers and the capacity to form cells from all three germ layers. Their reprogramming involves the introduction of genes for transcription factors that are important for the maintenance of pluripotency (Oct4, Sox2, Klf4, and c-Myc as originally described or Oct4, Sox2, Nanog, and Lin28 more recently).[20,24] iPSCs offer great promise for tissue engineering because of their pluripotent nature. They share a number of other features with embryonic stem cells in humans including the ability to form embryoid bodies, high telomerase activity, and similar methylation of their histones, but not all cell sources are equally able to generate iPS cells with this range of activity.[25] The surface marker profile of IPS cells is also similar to human embryonic stem cells (Nanog, Oct 3/4, Sox2, Tra 1-60 and Tra 1-81, and Ssea-3/4). Currently iPS cells are largely being used in vitro for mechanistic and feasibility studies but there are an increasing number of iPSC therapies being tested in clinical trials.[26] Most of these represent a form of stem cell-based therapy to target conditions where small numbers of functional cells are necessary, such as Parkinson's disease.

Concerns regarding the use of viral vectors to produce iPS cells has limited their clinical utility to date but as more gene editing techniques are developed, including the use of Crispr-Cas9 technology, it is anticipated that they will see increasing use in clinical studies in the near future, particularly where there may be issues with autologously-derived stem cells or where lineage restriction impairs the ability of native stem cells to generate the desired tissue or organ. Questions also remain as to their genetic stability, potential for teratoma formation, and the ability of them and their progeny to respond to microenvironmental cues like native stem cells. As they see increasing use in studies, it will become clearer as to whether these represent actual hurdles to widespread clinical implementation.

Crispr-Cas9, Gene Editing and Expression Technology

The ability to influence gene expression has been possible since the development of recombinant DNA technology.

This started with plasmids to facilitate the production of various proteins that could not be chemically synthesized. The development of viral vectors gave the ability to increase the expression of specific genes. Concerns over carcinogenesis due to viral DNA inclusion within the genome of the recipient prompted the transition from adenoviral to adenoviral-associated vectors but these have the setback of only transient expression. More recently, minicircle DNA and similar constructs have permitted the expression of various genes in a more controlled manner. While these approaches allow for targeted production of specific gene products, they do not overcome inherent limitations in the genes of the recipient.

Crispr-Cas9 technology provides a means to edit specific sequences within the genome of cells and was first recognized as part of the bacterial immune system that confers resistance to foreign genetic material that may be present in plasmids or bacteriophages. Its structure was adapted by Jennifer Doudna and Emmanuelle Charpentier in 2012 to facilitate its use for gene editing by fusing the four components of the *Streptococcus pyogenes* Cas9 endonuclease into a two-part system – the Cas9 endonuclease combined with a separate sequence-specific guide RNA.[27] A number of different versions of the Crispr-Cas9 system have now been generated based on various bacterial species. If applied to stem cells and combined with cell therapies and tissue engineering techniques, Crispr-Cas9 provides the means to address genetically-based diseases that affect specific tissues or organs. This gives the benefits of an autologously based solution to previously unsolvable genetically-based defects. It also provides a means to bypass aspects of immune surveillance in allogeneic cell-based constructs.[28] Crispr-Cas9 technology may herald the dawn of a new age of tissue engineering with increased opportunities for various clinical applications, including both congenital and acquired genetic defects.

Cell-Based Approaches

Cell-based approaches are centered around the introduction of cells into existing vascular beds or their engraftment to permit long-term survival, replication, and differentiation. These cells may be introduced through the use of cell suspensions, cells admixed with various matrices (including bioprinting/bioinks), and via multicellular aggregates referred to as organoids. While they may facilitate the recruitment of endogenous progenitors (both local and/or circulating), this is not the primary mechanism in cell-based approaches.

Cell suspensions are one of the most commonly used delivery methods as these are easy to prepare after the enzymatic digestion of tissues to generate single cell suspensions or via the mobilization of cultured cells. Co-culture techniques provide significant benefits relative to single-cell cultures as they more closely replicate the native state of the tissue and complementary cell types can facilitate cell survival and function (e.g., hepatocytes and endothelial precursor cells). Three-dimensional cultures such as spheroids are even better at replicating the native cellular microenvironment of tissues and organs and can provide additional benefits over co-cultures alone (Fig. 7.6). These may be dissociated into cell suspensions or delivered as small organoids but still require engraftment.

There have been a number of recent advances in 3D printing technology that facilitate implantation of cells admixed with supporting matrices. Bioink printers are now commercially-available and these combine cells and scaffold/matrix materials that form the bioink for additive manufacturing of 3D structures.[29] This permits control over the spatial orientation of functionally important tissues (e.g., the correct cellular arrangement for biliary drainage from hepatocytes within the liver constructs) but does not control the polarity of cells specifically. The most immediate problem in the clinical use of these 3D-printed constructs is their vascularization, particularly where large volume constructs are necessary (e.g., breast reconstruction or liver tissue engineering). An additional issue is the development of a stem cell niche that supports long-term survival and function of cells within the construct. It is essential to address these challenges before the use of bioinks to print 3D organs can be implemented clinically.

Vascularization and Use of Flaps in Tissue Engineering

The introduction of stem and progenitor cells into existing circulatory beds within the body has been an effective strategy for cell-based therapies but is limited by the ability of the body to produce sufficient neovascularization to support the survival of the cells. Implantation can be directly into tissues or via the circulation (e.g., introduction of pancreatic islet cells into the hepatic portal circulation) to address issues such as diabetes mellitus. Unfortunately, intravascular approaches have significant risks associated with them including portal venous thrombosis and portal venous hypertension, loss of 50%–70% of the transplanted islets, local ischemia/reperfusion injury in the liver and gut–liver axis inflammation amongst others.[30]

Injection or placement directly into tissues has a number of well-documented possible side effects including the risk of a local or systemic immune response, differentiation to a non-target tissue type, impaired engraftment and survival, impairment of local tissue/organ function (e.g., electrophysiological disturbance in the myocardium) and the risk of tumorigenesis longer-term.[31]

Heterotopic cell or construct engraftment (e.g., under the kidney capsule or in distant regions of the body) can limit the impact on local tissues following implantation but may not provide normal physiological control (e.g., contact with the portal and/or enteric circulation helps facilitate blood glucose control). Cell delivery may need to be fractionated so that the capacity for engraftment at each dose is not overwhelmed. Complex 3D structures have been developed over time in vivo with the help of tissue engineering chambers or scaffolds to provide support and space

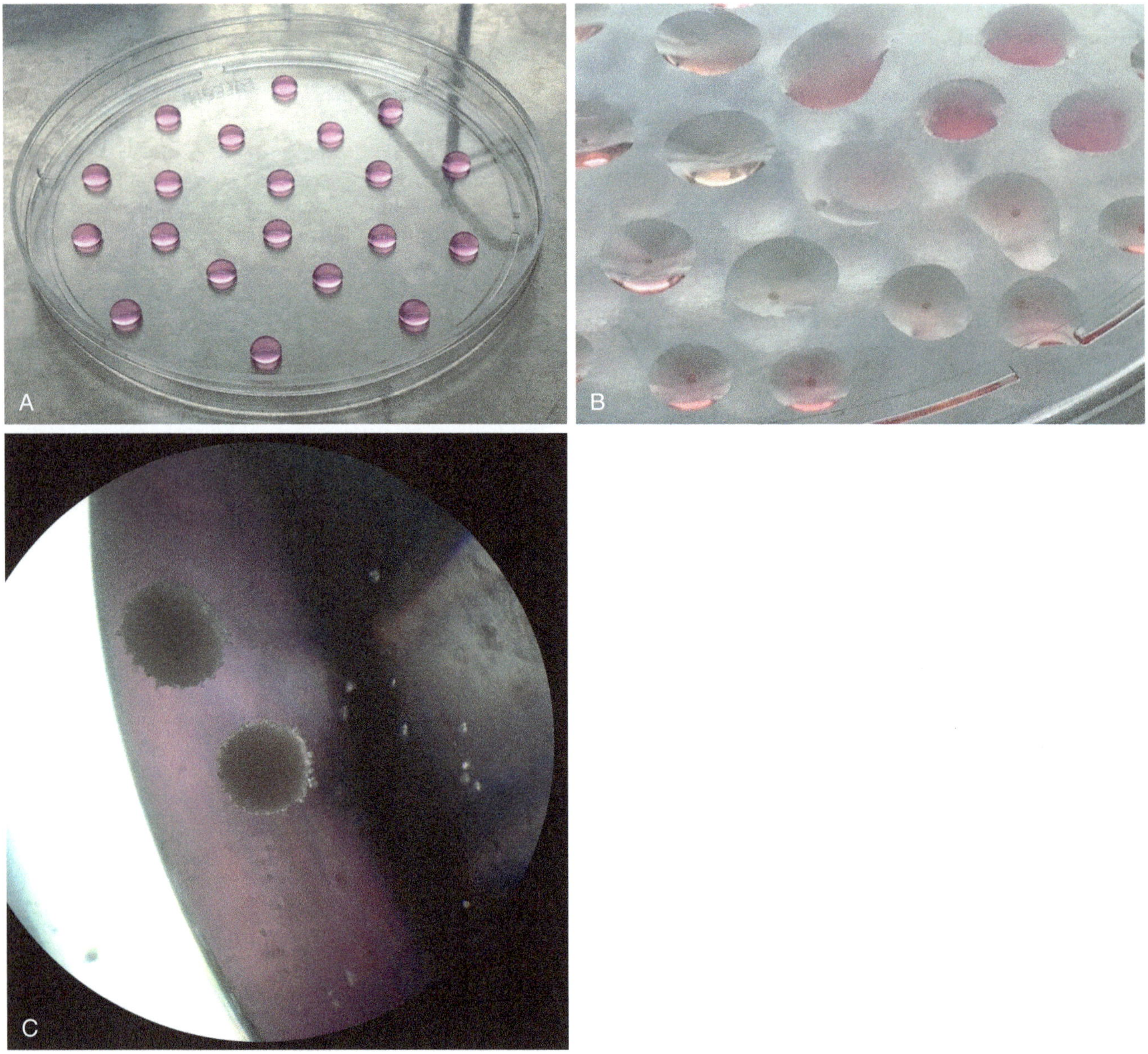

• **Fig. 7.6** Formation of 3D (organoid) cultures that more closely replicate the in vivo environment. (A) Single cell suspensions are aliquoted onto a petri dish lid. The lid is then inverted, leading to a hanging culture. (B) The spheroids self-assemble in the bottom of the culture drop and are visible (C) under light microscopy as 3D cellular aggregates ready for implantation or dissolution for cell-based therapies. Co-cultures may be used and differential labelling can be performed to assist in identification of the subcomponent cell types.

for subsequent tissue development. Plastic surgeons have a thorough working knowledge of how to isolate specific circulatory beds (as free flaps) and transplant them around the body. Free flaps have been used by our group and others as expendable microcirculatory beds for tissue engineering and to effect anticancer and antimicrobial effects through gene therapies including viral transfection and minicircle DNA technology.[32,33] Free flaps are a well-established platform for tissue engineering and provide an existing circulation and a supportive matrix for the development of constructs. The ability to isolate them from the circulation for a few hours permits the administration of cells and factors at concentrations much higher than can be given safely and when reimplanted in the body, they can be transferred to the needed site for them to have the best effect (Fig. 7.7).

Cell-Based Extracorporeal Support Devices and Extracorporeal Flap Perfusion Bioreactors

Extracorporeal support devices and bioreactors maintain perfusion within constructs that are separate from the body. Extracorporeal support devices are an alternative to cell transplantation and house parenchymal cells or other cell lines as required to bridge function for patients while they await definitive management in the form of organ or cell transplantation.[34] This can be particularly effective

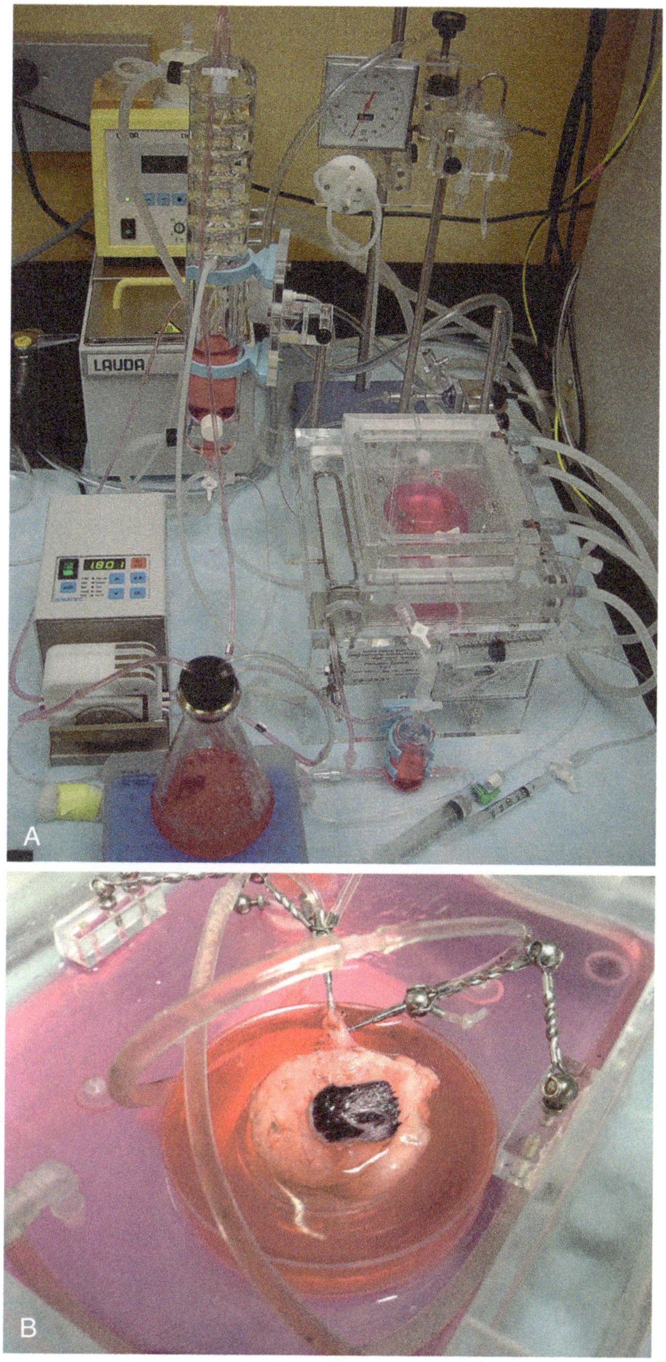

• **Fig. 7.7** (A) A controlled pressure oxygenating perfusion bioreactor for extracorporeal circulation of free flaps for tissue engineering and genetic manipulation. A perfusate is pumped into an oxygenating bell and passes into the arterial pedicle and is then collected from the venous side via a similar intravascular cannula. Cells can be administered and circulated ex vivo for extended periods. (B) A superficial inferior epigastric fasciocutaneous free flap cannulated and sitting in the perfusion chamber which is warmed via a water jacket.

to address acute exacerbations in conditions that show an acute-on-chronic pattern. Acute-on-chronic liver failure is a good example where cell-based extracorporeal support devices are being tested for their ability to sustain patients through acute episodes where non-cell-based artificial liver support systems do not demonstrate any survival benefit.[35]

The placement of tissue flaps on extracorporeal perfusion bioreactors permits a wide range of techniques to be applied to the explanted tissue before subsequent replantation. Explanted flaps represent an expendable microcirculatory bed (ECB) and can be perfused with factors, viral vectors, and cell populations at concentrations that could not be tolerated via systemic administration but when combined with extracorporeal perfusion bioreactors, it permits a longer time for administration of cells and other factors before reimplantation.[36,37] The un-incorporated factors or cells are washed out of the circulation prior to reimplantation. The main limitation of these devices is the limited amount of time that tissues or organs can be kept alive while explanted from the body which is generally no more than 48–72 hours. This limits the nature of interventions that can be performed and makes it difficult to develop true "off the shelf" flaps. Significant progress is being made in the vascularization of ex vivo grafts and the development of tissue engineered vessels. Phase 2 clinical trials of large vessel conduits for endstage renal patients are promising relative to currently available synthetic conduits (e.g., PTFE conduits) and submillimeter networks of fine vascular networks have been generated by co-culture experiments combined with 3D scaffolds for vessel formation but the reliable vascularization of large tissue constructs de novo and the formation of small caliber vessel constructs remains a significant challenge, particularly in immune-competent individuals.[38,39]

Bioreactors

Microenvironmental Approaches to Tissue Engineering

In simple terms, the "soil" must be fertile for new tissue growth but working out what ingredients are necessary to permit survival/recruitment, division and differentiation of stem and progenitor cells is not straightforward and requires manipulation of the stem cell niche. Niches can be manipulated to increase the likelihood of new tissue growth occurring. There are numerous ways to influence the stem cell niche, from the introduction of various matrices and scaffolds, the use of specific supporting cells, and the control of inflammation through wounding or pro- and anti-inflammatory agents.[40,41] Niche manipulation can be performed at the target site (local, in-vivo) and will generally produce locally matched tissue under the influence of paracrine factors and local cells. Niche manipulation in distant tissues for subsequent transfer (distant, in vivo) requires greater control over differentiation if the growth site has a different local microenvironment to the planned recipient site. Direct manipulation of the stem cell microenvironment in culture (in vitro) is relatively straightforward but requires subsequent engraftment and may not interact appropriately with the recipient immune system. A hybrid approach involves in vitro growth with support from devices to replicate the requisite conditions for tissue maintenance and growth including a circulation, gas exchange or mechanical forces such as shear or tension (ex vivo/bioreactor). Ex vivo approaches including the use of bioreactors have provided promising results for the formation of new tissues and cells that are morphologically and functionally more akin to their in vivo cousins, but it has been challenging to support new tissues long term ex vivo and the longer they are outside the body, the less likely they will survive reimplantation. As discussed above, it has been difficult to co-develop functional vascular networks on a large scale for clinical tissue engineering, thereby limiting the potential impact of ex vivo approaches. The elements shared by all of these microenvironmental approaches include: the use of local or recruited cells to support stem and/or progenitor cell function; matrices/scaffolds; and growth factors and control of inflammation to support an optimal local tissue response. Interestingly, stem cells can influence each of these factors themselves through interactions with the immune system and the ability to generate specific cells and secondary matrices. Therefore the "seed" and "soil" hypotheses are closely interlinked. We will examine each of these aspects of the microenvironment.

Supporting Cells in Tissue Engineering

Parenchymal cells and endothelial cells and their progenitors have been demonstrated to be highly supportive of stem cells and can help direct differentiation towards locally matching tissue. Adipose tissue is a good example, with multiple studies demonstrating that adipocytes secrete paracrine and endocrine factors (e.g., adiponectin, leptin) that support adipogenesis as a form of site-directed differentiation[17] and that endothelial cells and adipocytes secrete mutually supportive paracrine factors.[41] On this basis, adipose tissue autografts and xenografts have been demonstrated to support adipogenesis in vascularized matrices within tissue engineering chambers where the absence of adipose tissue resulted in little or no new adipose tissue production despite the development of a vascular network within the chamber.[41,42] There are numerous examples of local cell populations that support the survival and differentiation of stem cells towards a given phenotype including bile duct epithelial cells in the liver and mesenchymal cells for basal keratinocytes of the skin. These supportive cells should be actively considered in tissue engineering strategies and can be incorporated through the use of numerous methods including conventional or layered 2D co-culture or their combination in 3D-cultured organoids/spheroids.

Matrices and Scaffolds in Tissue Engineering

Matrices and scaffolds form the supporting structure around cells and are fundamental to numerous aspects of cell survival and function. Scaffolds are generally considered to provide the structural support as their principal function. Such support is necessary in tissue engineering for a number of reasons, including maintenance of a dedicated space for new tissue formation and protection from deformational forces such as compression. Matrices can also act as reservoirs for various growth factors and provide both sustained local release of these factors and co-factors that regulate growth factor function and interaction with cells.

The 3D structure of biomaterials can have a profound effect on tissue growth and function. Features such as pores can facilitate cellular in-growth, engraftment, and patterned cell development. The careful study of pore geometry in these microporous matrices has facilitated the generation of biomaterials that readily support neovascularization and/or tissue in-growth. However, it has been difficult to control the spatial orientation between specific cell types as required for functional neo-organ production. To achieve such organization, it has been necessary to refine biomaterials on a much smaller scale. So-called "smart" scaffolds have been functionalized by surface modifications that add binding sites for specific cell types to aid in the establishment of patterned cell development and the support of specific structure–function relationships. This has now been refined further by the use of nanotechnology to target individual cells at a level that controls their orientation and polarity relative to other cells and the surrounding matrix.

Practically, matrices and scaffolds fall into two categories: those that are tissue conductive and those that are tissue inductive. Tissue conductivity is the process whereby a matrix or scaffold supports its own incorporation and replacement by the target tissue from existing tissue (e.g., growth of bone through a construct from one side of a bony defect to the other). Inductive matrices and scaffolds facilitate the recruitment, replication, and differentiation of stem cells and progenitors to form new tissue de novo.

Matrices can be biological in origin or synthetic and each has its relative merits. From a regulatory perspective there are a number of matrices that have seen widespread use in experimental tissue engineering but are not suitable for human use, including Matrigel, a basement membrane-rich extract from the Engelbreth–Holm–Swarm sarcoma in mice. In practice this has the benefit of being a liquid at 4°C yet forms a gel at body temperature. It would be a good option as an injectable for contour deformities and readily supports adipogenesis when injected subcutaneously. It can also support the growth of multiple other tissue types including muscle, liver, and endocrine and exocrine pancreas.[41,42] However, its derivation from a sarcoma prompts important questions of its safety for human use. Biologically-derived matrices from non-cancer-based sources have demonstrated similar adipogenic potential in the laboratory[43] but show variable results in the clinical setting, with further study necessary before a reliable injectable scaffold for adipogenesis is clinically available. The key factors to consider when deciding upon a matrix is whether it suits the physicochemical needs of the tissue, is safe in the tissues (nontoxic and noncarcinogenic), stable for sufficient time to permit tissue growth, vascularization and differentiation, and whether its breakdown products are nontoxic to the body.

Inflammation and the Role of the Immune System in Tissue Engineering

The introduction of cells into tissues produces a local inflammatory reaction. Prior to engraftment, cells display features of sublethal cellular injury including swelling and the release of chemokines to promote neovascularization. In immune-compromised animals, engraftment readily occurs, even when using xenotransplants. Nude and Severe Combined Immunodeficient (SCID) mice are some of the easiest animal models to achieve engraftment of cell constructs and with xenografts. There is usually survival of some of the cell mass and a surrounding reaction that supports the growth of native adipose tissue. When similar autografting and xenografting experiments are performed in immune competent animals, the rates of graft take are often significantly lower and there may be little adipogenesis. Recent studies argue for the need for immune modulation involving an initial proinflammatory stimulus that facilitates the recruitment of cells to support neovascularization but avoids excessive or prolonged inflammatory responses that typically result in fibrosis. This initial inflammatory reaction is necessary to recruit circulating progenitor cells, particularly when there is an absence of local progenitors.

Studies in sealed tissue engineering chambers with acellular fat autografts demonstrate sufficient inflammation to support adipogenesis despite a local paucity of preadipocytes and mesenchymal stem cells. This adipogenic response is not seen when no autograft is put within the sealed chamber, despite neovascularization.[41] The same adipogenic response can be achieved when an inflammatory mediator (Zymosan) is introduced in the chamber without an autograft, the putative mechanism of action being recruitment of circulating stem cells and progenitors to promote adipogenesis. The promotion of a marked cellular response to ischemia within adipose tissue grafts is one of the proposed mechanisms for de novo adipogenesis seen following xenotransplantation.

Adaptive neovascularization is strongly supported by local and recruited macrophages with secondary recruitment of mast cells that release mediators with potent effects on local blood vessels. Mast cells produce numerous growth factors that are pro-angiogenic. They also help to suppress the immune system and this combination makes them an important microenvironmental cell for tissue engineering.[44] Prolonged ischemia or inflammation can trigger a maladaptive response in mast cells such as ischemia reperfusion injury, prompting considerations about the control of inflammation.[45]

Paradoxically, excessive inflammation is counterproductive to directed new tissue formation. Indomethacin is one antiinflammatory agent that supports adipogenesis through abrogation of the inflammatory response. Endogenous agents such as melatonin may also be used locally to support adipogenesis through an antiinflammatory role along with other mechanisms including protection of stem cells from oxidative damage.[46] Refined control of the immune system to facilitate tissue engineering (both locally and systemically) is still an aspirational goal, but it is clear that the immune system plays an important role in facilitating and limiting new tissue production. The capacity of specific stem cell subpopulations to modulate the immune system is a current area of active interest in stem cell therapies and tissue engineering.

Growth Factors and Chemokines in Tissue Engineering

Growth factors directly influence neovascularization and new tissue production in tissue engineering. They may be added to matrices, typically in a slow release form, to stimulate neovascularization, stem cell replication and differentiation. Alternatively, growth factor release may be stimulated within the tissues by recruitment of suitable cell sources. Tissue hypoxia induces cells to release chemokines such as stromal-derived factor-1 to attract circulating stem cells to the site along with immune cells. Under the influence of local chemokine, pH, and hypoxic gradients, and local tissue injury, growth factors are released. Proangiogenic growth factors include vascular endothelial growth factors (VEGF) and platelet derived growth factor (PDGF), and fibroblast growth factor (FGF). Physiologically, numerous growth factors are present at relatively low concentrations and replicating this pattern through the use of exogenous growth factors is often more effective than single growth factors at higher concentrations as there is an increased risk of unwanted side effects from higher growth factor concentrations. For example, FGF-2 used at low to intermediate concentrations is effective at supporting neovascularization and adipogenesis but increases fibrosis at higher concentrations.[47] Studies of the temporal course of growth factor release during the production of various tissues permits their incorporation into slow release vectors and/or matrices to replicate the signature of new tissue production. This has been effective both in vitro and in vivo to foster growth and differentiation along various lineages.

Tissue Engineering in Practice: Tissue Engineered Breast Reconstruction

Taking adipose tissue engineering for breast reconstruction as an example that is of significant relevance to plastic and reconstructive surgery, there have been great advances in this discipline over the past two decades. Following the identification of mesenchymal stem cells within adipose tissue of adults in 2002,[21] a number of targeted studies were undertaken in our laboratories and others that sought to understand the adipogenic microenvironment and how tissue generation could be scaled to produce clinically relevant volumes of new tissue in humans[17,41] (Fig. 7.8). Through a series of experiments, we established that the production of neovascularization within an adipogenic environment that included access to native vascularized adipose tissue would promote de novo adipogenesis. What followed was the

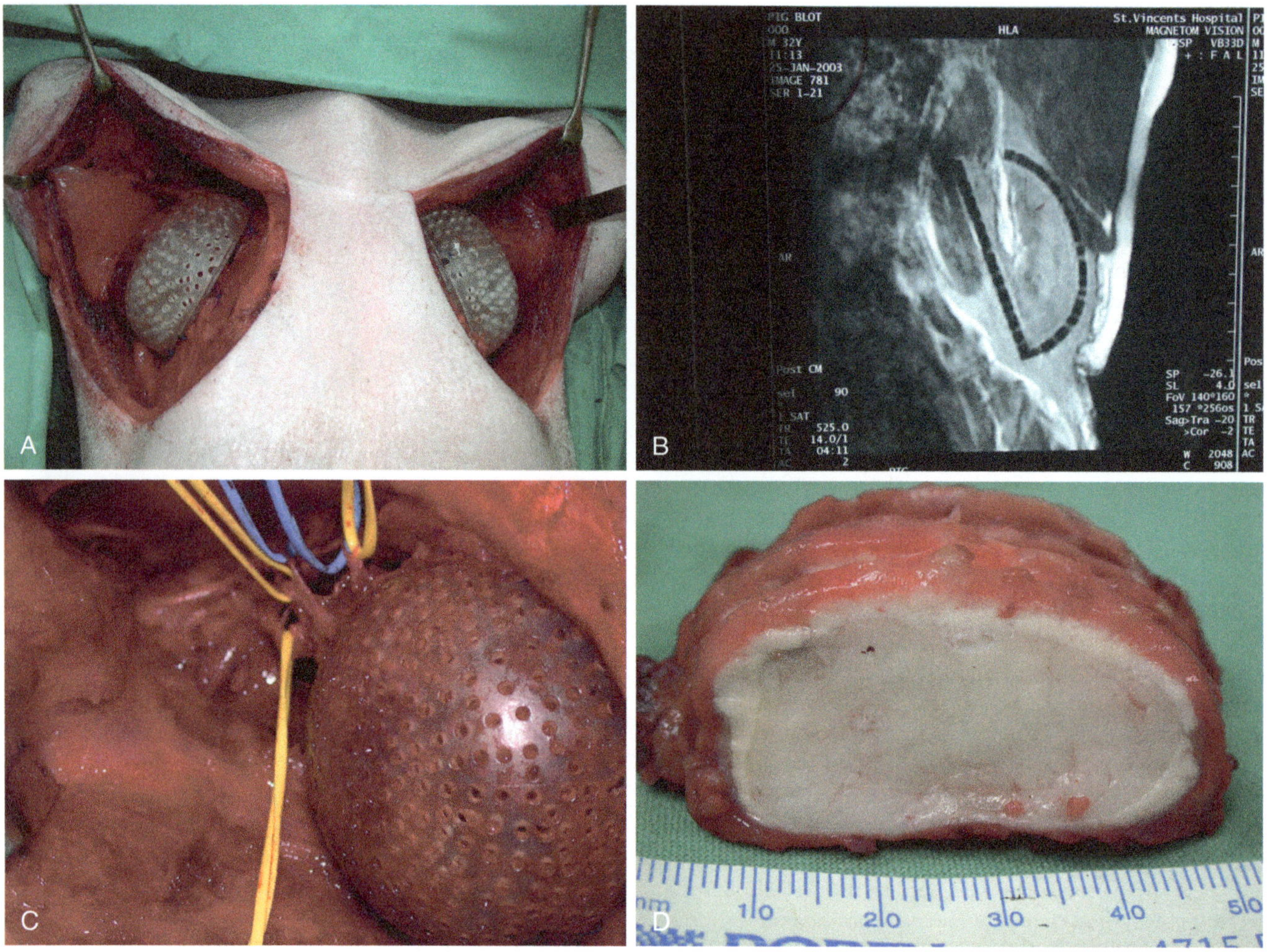

• **Fig. 7.8** (A) Bilateral perforated tissue engineering chambers are inserted into the breast area of a pig with or without a supporting poly-L lactic co-glycolic acid scaffold to replicate in situ tissue engineered breast reconstruction. Chambers could also be inserted in the groin area for distant growth and subsequent transfer. A small, pedicled adipose tissue flap is inserted through an opening in the chamber. (B) Magnetic resonance angiography is performed after 6 weeks to confirm new tissue growth and robust neovascularization similar to surrounding tissues. (C) At exploration of the chamber the pedicle can be identified and preserved to permit tissue transfer. (D) Almost complete replacement of the scaffold with new adipose tissue to create a functional, large volume tissue engineered adipofascial flap.

world's first large animal model for adipose tissue production. The tissue engineered breast flap was also transferrable on its vascular pedicle.[48] These studies led to human trials that demonstrated proof of principle that tissue engineered breast reconstruction is feasible in humans[49] but most breast cancer patients were not able to mount a sufficiently robust adipogenic response to effect their own breast reconstruction using existing techniques despite almost universal success of these techniques in animal models. These studies highlight some of the fundamental differences between healthy, young animal models in which the majority of tissue engineering research is undertaken and the gap to translate these into aged humans with comorbidities. There are numerous avenues of current exploration, including assessment of acquired stem cell subpopulation deficits secondary to comorbidities and aging and the augmentation of existing tissue engineering techniques through the incorporation of new techniques and technologies.

Regulation of Regenerative Medicine Therapies

Regulatory approval is necessary for the introduction of new regenerative medicine technologies for use in humans in most countries. Unfortunately, regulatory systems often lag behind the pace of change in the tissue engineering and regenerative medicine sector. In the United States, regenerative medicine technologies are termed HCT/Ps ("human cells, tissues, and cell-and-tissue-based products") and are regulated by the FDA under two pathways (sections) of the Public Health Services Act (PHSA). The 351 pathway regulates the introduction of HCT/Ps fundamentally the same as new drugs. The immense time and monetary cost of the 351 pathway has prompted many to investigate alternatives that provide earlier implementation of new regenerative medicine technologies. One approach is to base new HCT/Ps on materials with existing FDA-approval by repurposing them or using them in a novel manner. These include biologic agents (e.g., hyaluronic acids, collagen, and silk fibroin) and synthetic materials (e.g., lactic and glycolic acid polymers as used in absorbable sutures). As a group, these have been very widely implemented in regenerative medicine and the regulatory framework explains the increased interest in the use of these materials over novel ones.

The other main approach for navigating the regulatory systems is the 361 pathway. It was introduced in 2001 to limit the risk of infectious disease transmission from HCT/Ps and provides little to no regulation for these materials as long as they meet four criteria:

1. Homologous use (the use in patients is substantively similar to the function in the donor);
2. minimal manipulation or processing;
3. does not combine the cells or tissues with other materials/agents except water, crystalloids or preservatives/sterilizers; and
4. has no systemic effect and is not reliant on the metabolic activity of living cells for its primary function, and if allogenic, must be for use in a first- or second-degree blood relative.

Under the 361 pathway, there is no requirement for data to support the claims of the manufacturer and little oversight as to the consistency of the manufactured product. The result has been an explosion of new products, including acellular dermal matrices through to forms of stem cell therapy. Unfortunately, while many companies have put forward well-conceived, safe, and efficacious products that took advantage of the pathway to ease clinical implementation, many have little or no sound data upon which to base clinical decision-making. In some cases, the products simply do not meet all four criteria of the pathway.

Patients and clinicians often do not understand the differences between the two pathways and may mistakenly equate the FDA-notified 361 pathway HCT/Ps (where the FDA has made no substantive assessment as to their efficacy or quality control) with the more rigorous FDA-approved 351 HCT/Ps. Recently, the FDA has put in place "new" policies that seek to address these issues. By the FDA's own reporting, very few companies to date are proactively collaborating with the FDA to address the lack of compliance of their product(s) with the 361 pathway criteria. The end result is a need for significant scrutiny by clinicians with regard to the use of these products and improved regulatory mechanisms that strike an appropriate balance between patient safety/product efficacy and unnecessarily prohibitive regulatory hurdles.

Conclusion

We live in a time of unparalleled access to information and technology. Despite hundreds of years of clinical practice, there are still defects in plastic surgery and other surgical disciplines that cannot be addressed adequately by existing techniques. Tissue engineering is well developed as a discipline and the broad skillset of plastic and reconstructive surgeons makes us well placed to identify unmet clinical needs and to implement and test potentially impactful basic science research for the benefit of our patients and society as a whole.

References

1. Pribaz JJ, Maitz PK, Fine NA. Flap prefabrication using the "vascular crane" principle: an experimental study and clinical application. *Br J Plast Surg*. 1994;47(4):250–256.
2. Lantieri L, Grimbert P, Ortonne N, et al. Facial transplantation: facing the limits, planning the future. *Lancet*. 2017;389(10076):1293–1294.
3. Skalak R. *Tissue Engineering. Proceedings of a Workshop Held at Granlibakken, Lake Tahoe, California, February 26–29, 1988 (UCLA Symposia on Molecular and Cellular Biology)*. New York: Alan Liss; 1988.
4. Duscher D, Neofytou E, Wong VU, et al. Transdermal deferoxamine prevents pressure-induced diabetic ulcers. *Proc Natl Acad Sci U S A*. 2015;112(1):94–99.
5. Aarabi S, Bhatt KA, Shi Y, et al. Mechanical load initiates hypertrophic scar formation through decreased cellular apoptosis. *FASEB J*. 2007;21(12):3250–3261.
6. Cao Y, Vacanti JP, Paige KT, et al. Transplantation of chondrocytes utilizing a polymer-cell construct to produce tissue-engineered cartilage in the shape of a human ear. *Plast Reconstr Surg*. 1997;100(2):297–302; discussion 303–304.
7. Hong KY, Yim S, Kim HJ, et al. The fate of the adipose-derived stromal cells during angiogenesis and adipogenesis after cell-assisted lipotransfer. *Plast Reconstr Surg*. 2018;141(2):365–375.
8. Yoshimura K, Sato K, Aoi N, et al. Cell-assisted lipotransfer for facial lipoatrophy: efficacy of clinical use of adipose-derived stem cells. *Dermatol Surg*. 2008;34(9):1178–1185.
9. Kolle SF, Fisccher-Nielsen A, Mathiasen AB, et al. Enrichment of autologous fat grafts with ex-vivo expanded adipose tissue-derived stem cells for graft survival: a randomised placebo-controlled trial. *Lancet*. 2013;382(9898):1113–1120.
10. Rigotti G, Marchi A, Galie M, et al. Clinical treatment of radiotherapy tissue damage by lipoaspirate transplant: a healing process mediated by adipose-derived adult stem cells. *Plast Reconstr Surg*. 2007;119(5):1409–1422; discussion 1423–1424.
11. Borrelli MR, Patel RA, Sokol J, et al. Fat chance: the rejuvenation of irradiated skin. *Plast Reconstr Surg*. 2019;7(2):e2092.
12. Hunter J. Artificial tendons. Early development and application. *Am J Surg*. 1965;109:325–338.
13. Bell E, Ehrlich HP, Buttle DJ, et al. Living tissue formed in vitro and accepted as skin-equivalent tissue of full thickness. *Science*. 1981;211(4486):1052–1054.
14. Bell E, Ehrlich HP, Sher S, et al. Development and use of a living skin equivalent. *Plast Reconstr Surg*. 1981;67(3):386–392.
15. Folkman J. Tumor angiogenesis: therapeutic implications. *N Engl J Med*. 1971;285(21):1182–1186.
16. Eterno V, Zambelli A, Pavesi L, et al. Adipose-derived mesenchymal stem cells (ASCs) may favour breast cancer recurrence via HGF/c-Met signaling. *Oncotarget*. 2014;5(3):613–633.
17. Findlay MW, Messina A, Thompson EW, et al. Long-term persistence of tissue-engineered adipose flaps in a murine model to 1 year: an update. *Plast Reconstr Surg*. 2009;124(4):1077–1084.
18. Langley RR, Fidler IJ. The seed and soil hypothesis revisited – the role of tumor–stroma interactions in metastasis to different organs. *Int J Cancer*. 2011;128(11):2527–2535.

19. Weissman IL. Stem cells: units of development, units of regeneration, and units in evolution. *Cell.* 2000;100(1):157–168.
20. Takahashi K, Yamanaka S. Induction of pluripotent stem cells from mouse embryonic and adult fibroblast cultures by defined factors. *Cell.* 2006;126(4):663–676.
21. Zuk PA, Zhu M, Ashjian P, et al. Human adipose tissue is a source of multipotent stem cells. *Mol Biol Cell.* 2002;13(12): 4279–4295.
22. Duscher D, Rennert RC, Januszyk M, et al. Aging disrupts cell subpopulation dynamics and diminishes the function of mesenchymal stem cells. *Sci Rep.* 2014;4:7144.
23. Rennert RC, Januszyk M, Sorkin M, et al. Microfluidic single-cell transcriptional analysis rationally identifies novel surface marker profiles to enhance cell-based therapies. *Nat Commun.* 2016;7:11945.
24. Yu J, Vodyanik MA, Smuga-Otto K, et al. Induced pluripotent stem cell lines derived from human somatic cells. *Science.* 2007;318(5858):1917–1920.
25. Narsinh KH, Plews J, Wu JC. Comparison of human induced pluripotent and embryonic stem cells: fraternal or identical twins? *Mol Ther.* 2011;19(4):635–638.
26. Zimmer K. Increasing number of iPS cell therapies tested in clinical trials. *Scientist.* 2018.
27. Jinek M, Chylinski K, Fonfara I, et al. A programmable dual-RNA-guided DNA endonuclease in adaptive bacterial immunity. *Science.* 2012;337(6096):816–821.
28. Abrahimi P, Qin L, Chang WG, et al. Blocking MHC class II on human endothelium mitigates acute rejection. *JCI Insight.* 2016;1(1).
29. Hospodiuk M, Deey M, Sosnoski D, et al. The bioink: a comprehensive review on bioprintable materials. *Biotechnol Adv.* 2017;35(2):217–239.
30. Delaune V, Berney T, Lacotte S, et al. Intraportal islet transplantation: the impact of the liver microenvironment. *Transpl Int.* 2017;30(3):227–238.
31. Lukomska B, Stanaszek L, Zuba-Sturma E, et al. Challenges and controversies in human mesenchymal stem cell therapy. *Stem Cells Int.* 2019;2019:9628536.
32. Dempsey MP, Hamou C, Michaels J, 5th, et al. Using genetically modified microvascular free flaps to deliver local cancer immunotherapy with minimal systemic toxicity. *Plast Reconstr Surg.* 2008;121(5):1541–1553.
33. Ghali S, Bhatt KA, Dempsey MP, et al. Treating chronic wound infections with genetically modified free flaps. *Plast Reconstr Surg.* 2009;123(4):1157–1168.
34. Banares R, Catalina MV, Vaquero J. Liver support systems: will they ever reach prime time? *Curr Gastroenterol Rep.* 2013;15(3):312.
35. Lee KC, Baker LA, Stanzani G, et al. Extracorporeal liver assist device to exchange albumin and remove endotoxin in acute liver failure: results of a pivotal pre-clinical study. *J Hepatol.* 2015;63(3):634–642.
36. Chang EI, Bonillas RG, El-ftesi S, et al. Tissue engineering using autologous microcirculatory beds as vascularized bioscaffolds. *FASEB J.* 2009;23(3):906–915.
37. Michaels J, 5th, Dobryansky M, Galiano RD, et al. Ex vivo transduction of microvascular free flaps for localized peptide delivery. *Ann Plast Surg.* 2004;52(6):581–584.
38. Lawson JH, Glickman MH, Ilzecki M, et al. Bioengineered human acellular vessels for dialysis access in patients with end-stage renal disease: two phase 2 single-arm trials. *Lancet.* 2016;387(10032):2026–2034.
39. Miller JS, Stevens KR, Yang MT, et al. Rapid casting of patterned vascular networks for perfusable engineered three-dimensional tissues. *Nature Mater.* 2012;11(9):768–774.
40. Thomas GP, Hemmrich K, Habberton KM, et al. Zymosan-induced inflammation stimulates neo-adipogenesis. *Int J Obes.* 2008;32(2):239–248.
41. Kelly JL, Findlay MW, Knight KR, et al. Contact with existing adipose tissue is inductive for adipogenesis in matrigel. *Tissue Eng.* 2006;12(7):2041–2047.
42. Stillaert F, Findlay M, Palmer J, et al. Host rather than graft origin of Matrigel-induced adipose tissue in the murine tissue-engineering chamber. *Tissue Eng.* 2007;13(9):2291–2300.
43. Abberton KM, Bortolotto SK, Woods AA, et al. Myogel, a novel, basement membrane-rich, extracellular matrix derived from skeletal muscle, is highly adipogenic in vivo and in vitro. *Cells Tissues Organs.* 2008;188(4):347–358.
44. Karimi A, Shahrooz R, Hobbenhagi R, et al. Mouse bone marrow-derived mast cells induce angiogenesis by tissue engineering in rats: histological evidence. *Cell J.* 2018;19(4):578–584.
45. Bortolotto SK, Morrison WA, Han XL, et al. Mast cells play a pivotal role in ischaemia reperfusion injury to skeletal muscles. *Lab Invest.* 2004;84(9): 1103–1011.
46. Bonnefont-Rousselot D. Obesity and oxidative stress: potential roles of melatonin as antioxidant and metabolic regulator. *Endocr Metab Immune Disord Drug Targets.* 2014;14(3):159–168.
47. Toriyama K, Kawaguchi N, Kitoh J, et al. Endogenous adipocyte precursor cells for regenerative soft-tissue engineering. *Tissue Eng.* 2002;8(1):157–165.
48. Findlay MW, Dolderer JH, Trost N, et al. Tissue-engineered breast reconstruction: bridging the gap toward large-volume tissue engineering in humans. *Plast Reconstr Surg.* 2011;128(6): 1206–1215.
49. Morrison WA, Marre D, Grinsell D, et al. Creation of a large adipose tissue construct in humans using a tissue-engineering chamber: a step forward in the clinical application of soft tissue engineering. *EBioMedicine.* 2016;6:238–245.

8 Melanoma

CARLO RICCARDO ROSSI AND ANTONIO SOMMARIVA

Epidemiology

Over the past four decades, melanoma has shown a consistent increase in incidence in white populations, becoming one of the most frequent cancers in light skin populations. The incidence rate of this disease varies widely in relation to race, occurring much less commonly in black, Asian, or Hispanic populations. Although white and non-white populations have similar risks of developing plantar melanoma, non-white populations have a greater risk of developing noncutaneous melanomas (e.g., mucosal). Melanoma is now regarded as the fifth most common cancer in men and the sixth most common cancer in women in the United States. The highest recorded incidence of melanoma worldwide is in Australia and New Zealand, with an incidence of 27.3–55.8/100,000 for males and 23.4–41.1/100,000 for females. In the United States the incidence rate is 19.4/100,000 for men and 14.4/100,000 for women. In European countries the incidence rates are lower, being highest in Switzerland and Scandinavian countries. Moreover, they show a north to south gradient, with the highest rates in northern countries. This is probably related to both the increased protection against the sun's rays of the pigmented skin of southern Europeans and the different pattern of sun exposure (chronic in southern Europeans, intermittent in northern Europeans).[1] In many countries, early detection of primarily thin melanomas and improved survival rates have been observed, especially in young females. However, in most countries the incidence of thick melanomas remains constant or continues to increase, especially in the older age group. Melanoma occurs approximately 1.5 times more often in men than women, and prognosis is slightly better for women, considering other prognostic factors. The anatomic distribution of melanoma is sex-dependent, occurring more often on the trunk in males and on the arms and legs in women. Melanoma can occur at any age but is rare before the age of puberty. The median age at the time of diagnosis ranges between 45 and 55 years, with an increase in incidence after the age of 25 until 50 years.

Risk Factors

Current considerations in the epidemiology of melanoma have shown that melanoma results from an unidentified interaction between mutations in various genes and constitutional and/or inherited factors combined with environmental factors, mainly solar ultraviolet (UV) radiations.[2] Exposure to UV is the most important environmental factor predisposing to melanoma in susceptible populations. It is reported that people incurring severe burns in childhood appear to be at higher risk for the development of melanoma in later age.

Iatrogenic exposures, such as immunosuppressive agents and nonsteroidal antiinflammatory drugs, have been studied as additional environmental factors. Well-known host risk factors, such as melanocytic nevi on the skin, skin type, family history, and genetic susceptibility have been validated as risk factors in large-scale association studies. Patients with more than 100 nevi or giant nevi (>20 cm) have an increased risk of melanoma. In addition, genome-wide association studies have revealed genetic loci that underlie the genetic susceptibility of melanoma, some of which are related to known risk factors. Mutations or epigenetic silencing of the cyclin-dependent kinase gene (*CDK*) are linked to 20%–40% of familial melanoma. Other genes involved in familial melanoma carcinogenesis include *CDK4*, xeroderma pigmentosum genes and melanocortin 1 receptor gene (*MC1R*). Activating mutations in the *BRAF* gene have been discovered in over two-thirds of melanomas. Melanomas on skin without chronic sun-induced damage had frequent mutations in *BRAF*; in contrast, acral and mucosal melanomas as well as skin melanomas with chronic sun damage are frequently characterized by *KIT* mutations. These mutations are responsible for cancer cell behavior through mechanisms that are still undefined.

Clinical Diagnosis

Melanoma usually appears as an irregularly pigmented skin lesion with an irregular border and a tendency to grow or change over time. Melanomas arise mostly de novo, just occasionally within a congenital or acquired nevus. In the past, they were often diagnosed in advanced stages as large, ulcerated or vegetating lesions. The need to detect melanomas at an early stage of disease led to the development of the ABCDE criteria, an acronym for asymmetry, border irregularity, color alterations, diameter >6 mm, and evolution.

Not only are these simple criteria intended to allow both patients and nondermatologist healthcare professionals to differentiate common melanocytic lesions from suspicious pigmented lesions, they are also a useful tool for the dermatoncologist in guiding the decision to perform a biopsy. The sensitivity of clinical diagnosis by physicians with experience in differential diagnosis of suspected cutaneous lesions is about 70%. Dermoscopy, also known as epiluminescence microscopy, improves the diagnostic accuracy of melanocytic lesions. Dermoscopy, when adopted by experts, increases the sensitivity of clinical diagnosis up to 89%, reducing the number of negative biopsies. Since the diagnostic protocol of suspicious lesions includes a complete excision with safety margins, the problem of unnecessary scarring is significant. The real challenge in this case is to have a properly formulated diagnosis before acquiring a biopsy. Reflectance confocal microscopy is a currently available noninvasive technique that can be a reliable bridge between dermoscopy and histopathology.[3] In high-risk patients (e.g., with atypical mole syndrome), a follow-up examination with digital dermoscopy and total-body microphotography is also helpful in detecting early changes in lesions or in discovering new atypical lesions. In patients with a previous melanoma, the risk of harboring a second melanoma is significant and implies scheduled examinations of the skin at regular intervals for detecting second tumors or skin metastasis.

Biopsy

In the presence of a skin lesion with a clinical suspicion of melanoma, the patient is referred for an excisional biopsy. The biopsy of a suspected lesion is a simple procedure, practicable under local anesthesia on an outpatient basis. The procedure consists in complete removal of the lesion with about 1–2 mm of surrounding healthy skin up to the subcutaneous fat. During the procedure care should be taken to avoid causing trauma or injury to the specimen, which could compromise a correct histopathological analysis. The choice of incision lines of the biopsy must take into account the further excision of the skin involved, preferring longitudinal incisions in the biopsy of the limbs while trying to minimize as much as possible the need of skin grafts. Excisional biopsy allows an accurate histopathological diagnosis, providing all the histological parameters necessary to formulate a prognosis and to plan the best therapeutic strategy. However, excision of the whole lesion may not be indicated in some cases: for example, in the presence of a large lesion, or in the case of proximity of the lesion to difficult areas (subungual) or important structures (eye, nose, and ear). In these circumstances, punch or incisional biopsy should be considered. In the incisional or so–called "punch" biopsy, only a full-thickness portion or a pill of the most suspected portion of the lesion is removed. Superficial biopsies, "shave biopsy," and any type of laser or diathermocoagulation should be avoided, as they do not allow an accurate pathological staging and can lead to a significant delay in diagnosis of any potentially malignant lesions.

Histology

The histological diagnosis of cutaneous melanoma is not always easy and it would be desirable for an expert pathologist in the diagnosis of pigmented lesions of the skin to perform the analysis. In doubtful cases, morphology may indicate the use of immunohistochemical surveys (such as HMB–45, Ki–67, p16) and fluorescence in situ hybridization (FISH) techniques, the reading of which requires experienced operators.

Histologically, invasive cutaneous melanomas are divided into four major subtypes. These are based on growth pattern and location, and are categorized as:

- superficial spreading
- nodular
- lentigo maligna, or
- acral lentiginous.

A fifth subtype is also defined: desmoplastic melanoma. In general, the histologic subtype of melanoma is not a major factor in determining prognosis, but some histologic subtypes are more likely to be detected at an advanced stage, thus indirectly affecting prognosis.

Melanoma originates from the proliferation of melanocytes in the basal layers of the epidermis, which tend to expand radially and later invade deep into the dermis. Superficial spreading melanoma is the most common (70%), can occur in any location, and is characterized by a radial growth associated in the later stages to a pattern of vertical proliferation. Nodular melanomas, occurring in about 15%, are characterized by an exception to this pattern, with an exclusive vertical growth not accompanied by radial growth. Because of its invasiveness, it is usually diagnosed at a more advanced stage of invasion. Lentigo maligna accounts for about 10% of melanomas and is characterized by onset in old age, in chronically sun-exposed skin sites with a history of slow growth. These lesions are characterized by a long phase of intraepithelial growth and for this reason are considered a lesion with a better prognosis, though always remaining linked to the degree of invasion. Acral lentiginous melanoma is the less common type (5%); it is classified mainly for its site of origin (subnail bed and the palmar and plantar surfaces) rather than for histological features, which are similar to melanoma of the mucous membranes. Diagnosis is often delayed, especially for subungual forms often confused with posttraumatic hematoma. Among the rarer variants, desmoplastic melanoma has nontypical melanocytic cells and is characterized by a significant deposition of collagen, which hinders differential diagnosis with other fibrohistiocytic tumors or schwannomas.

The vertical growth phase is the tumorigenic phase in which the melanoma acquires the ability to metastasize. Morphologically, it is characterized by the presence of an expansive nodule larger than the intraepidermal component and/or by the presence of mitotic figures in the invasive component. In 1969, Clark formulated a histological classification with a prognostic value for melanoma based on the level of invasion in the anatomical layers of the skin, highlighting for the first time the prognostic significance of the degree of invasion (Table 8.1). However, the Clark system has proven to be a source of significant variability among pathologists, especially in stages III and IV, thereby losing its prognostic relevance in more recent years. In 1970, Breslow described a more objective method of classification, based on the measurement in millimeters of the vertical thickness of the tumor.[4] The Breslow thickness is measured from the granular layer or, if the lesion is ulcerated, from the bottom of ulceration, up to the point of maximum infiltration. This classification system has been shown to be more reproducible among pathologists, showing an excellent correlation with mortality. Prognosis tends to become progressively worse in logarithmic function, up to 8 mm, where it reaches a plateau. Among histological features assessed for their prognostic value, the presence of ulceration and mitosis are considered the most important, correlating in a totally independent way to the prognosis. Ulceration is defined as the absence of intact epithelium overlying the melanoma. Ulceration represents a phenotypic marker of aggressive tumor biology and predicts a greater propensity for invasion and metastasis.

TABLE 8.1 Melanoma Invasion Expressed as Clark Level

Level I	Confined to the epidermis
Level II	Invade but not fill or expand the papillary (superficial) dermis
Level III	Fill and expand the papillary dermis with extension to the papillary–reticular dermal interface
Level IV	Infiltrate into the reticular dermis
Level V	Infiltrate into the subcutaneous fat

Staging

To improve the outcomes of patients with melanoma, treatment based on accurate staging and patient stratification into stage groups is fundamental. The most widely used staging system for melanoma is based on the American Joint Committee on Cancer (AJCC), eighth edition (Tables 8.2 and 8.3). Today, 50%–70% of melanomas are diagnosed in an early stage (stage IA), with a very low risk of recurrence and distant spread. Therefore, it is important to identify which staging investigations are indicated in the different classes of risk. A meta-analysis performed comparing the usefulness of ultrasound, CT scan, PET, and PET–CT in the staging of patients with melanoma concluded that ultrasound is superior to the other methods in detecting metastasis to the lymph nodes, while PET–CT is superior in detecting distant metastases.[5] It is difficult to draw clear

TABLE 8.2 TNM Staging Categories for Cutaneous Melanoma

T Category	Criteria/Thickness	Criteria/Ulceration Status
TX	Primary tumor thickness cannot be assessed (e.g., diagnosis by curettage)	Not applicable
T0	No evidence of primary tumor (e.g., unknown primary or completely regressed melanoma)	Not applicable
Tis	Melanoma in situ	Not applicable
T1	≤1.0 mm	Unknown or unspecified
T1a	<0.8 mm	Without ulceration
T1b	<0.8 mm	With ulceration
T1b	0.8–1.0 mm	With or without ulceration
T2	>1.0–2.0 mm	Unknown or unspecified
T2a	>1.0–2.0 mm	Without ulceration
T2b	>1.0–2.0 mm	With ulceration
T3	>2.0-4.0 mm	Unknown or unspecified
T3a	>2.0–4.0 mm	Without ulceration
T3b	>2.0–4.0 mm	With ulceration
T4	>4.0 mm	Unknown or unspecified
T4a	>4.0 mm	Without ulceration
T4b	>4.0 mm	With ulceration

Continued

TABLE 8.2 **TNM Staging Categories for Cutaneous Melanoma—cont'd**

N Category	Number of Tumor-Involved Regional Lymph Nodes	Presence of In Transit, Satellite, and/or Microsatellite Metastases
NX	No regional metastases detected	No
N0	One tumor-involved node or in transit, satellite, and/or microsatellite metastases with no tumor-involved nodes	One tumor-involved node or in transit, satellite, and/or microsatellite metastases with no tumor-involved nodes
N1a	One clinically occult (i.e., detected by SLN biopsy)	No
N1b	One clinically detected	No
N1c	No regional lymph node disease	Yes
N2	Two or three tumor-involved nodes or in transit, satellite, and/or microsatellite metastases with one tumor-involved node	Two or three tumor-involved nodes or in transit, satellite, and/or microsatellite metastases with one tumor-involved node
N2a	Two or three clinically occult (i.e., detected by SLN biopsy)	No
N2b	Two or three, at least one of which was clinically detected	No
N2c	One clinically occult or clinically detected	Yes
N3	Four or more tumor-involved nodes or in transit, satellite, and/or microsatellite metastases with two or more tumor-involved nodes, or any number of matted nodes without or with in transit, satellite, and/or microsatellite metastases	Four or more tumor-involved nodes or in transit, satellite, and/or microsatellite metastases with two or more tumor-involved nodes, or any number of matted nodes without or with in transit, satellite, and/or microsatellite metastases
N3a	Four or more clinically occult (i.e., detected by SLN biopsy)	No
N3b	Four or more, at least one of which was clinically detected, or presence of any number of matted nodes	No
N3c	Two or more clinically occult or clinically detected and/or presence of any number of matted nodes	Yes

M Category	Criteria	LDH Level
cM0	No evidence of distant metastasis	Not applicable
cM1	Evidence of distant metastasis	Any
cM1a	Distant metastasis to skin, soft tissue including muscle, and/or nonregional lymph node	Not recorded or unspecified
cM1a(0)	Distant metastasis to skin, soft tissue including muscle, and/or nonregional lymph node	Not elevated
cM1a(1)	Distant metastasis to skin, soft tissue including muscle, and/or nonregional lymph node	Elevated
cM1b	Distant metastasis to lung with or without M1a sites of disease	Not recorded or unspecified
cM1b(0)	Distant metastasis to lung with or without M1a sites of disease	Not elevated
cM1b(1)	Distant metastasis to lung with or without M1a sites of disease	Elevated
cM1c	Distant metastasis to non-CNS visceral sites with or without M1a or M1b sites of disease	Not recorded or unspecified
cM1c(0)	Distant metastasis to non-CNS visceral sites with or without M1a or M1b sites of disease	Not elevated
cM1c(1)	Distant metastasis to non-CNS visceral sites with or without M1a or M1b sites of disease	Elevated
cM1d	Distant metastasis to CNS with or without M1a, M1b, or M1c sites of disease	Not recorded or unspecified

TABLE 8.2 **TNM Staging Categories for Cutaneous Melanoma—cont'd**

M Category	Criteria	LDH Level
cM1d(0)	Distant metastasis to CNS with or without M1a, M1b, or M1c sites of disease	Not elevated
cM1d(1)	Distant metastasis to CNS with or without M1a, M1b, or M1c sites of disease	Elevated
pM1	Evidence of distant metastasis, microscopically proven	Any
pM1a	Distant metastasis to skin, soft tissue including muscle, and/or nonregional lymph node, microscopically proven	Not recorded or unspecified
pM1a(0)	Distant metastasis to skin, soft tissue including muscle, and/or nonregional lymph node, microscopically proven	Not elevated
pM1a(1)	Distant metastasis to skin, soft tissue including muscle, and/or nonregional lymph node, microscopically proven	Elevated
pM1b	Distant metastasis to lung with or without M1a sites of disease, microscopically proven	Not recorded or unspecified
pM1b(0)	Distant metastasis to lung with or without M1a sites of disease, microscopically proven	Not elevated
pM1b(1)	Distant metastasis to lung with or without M1a sites of disease, microscopically proven	Elevated
pM1c	Distant metastasis to non-CNS visceral sites with or without M1a or M1b sites of disease, microscopically proven	Not recorded or unspecified
pM1c(0)	Distant metastasis to non-CNS visceral sites with or without M1a or M1b sites of disease, microscopically proven	Not elevated
pM1c(1)	Distant metastasis to non-CNS visceral sites with or without M1a or M1b sites of disease, microscopically proven	Elevated
pM1d	Distant metastasis to CNS with or without M1a, M1b, or M1c sites of disease, microscopically proven	Not recorded or unspecified
pM1d(0)	Distant metastasis to CNS with or without M1a, M1b, or M1c sites of disease, microscopically proven	Not elevated
pM1d(1)	Distant metastasis to CNS with or without M1a, M1b, or M1c sites of disease, microscopically proven	Elevated

Used with permission of the American College of Surgeons, Chicago, Illinois. The original source for this information is the AJCC Cancer Staging Manual, Eighth Edition (2017) published by Springer International Publishing.

guidelines for examinations that should be used for the staging of patients with melanoma. A general indication is to modulate the examinations in relationship with the risk and/or the presence of metastases. No examination staging should be performed in patients with melanoma in situ. For asymptomatic patients with T1 melanomas, clinical examination alone seems adequate for staging and follow-up. Careful skin and lymph node examination excludes other concomitant lesions and is considered sufficient for skin and lymph node metastasis. However, even in this lower-risk group, ultrasonography of the drainage basin (or basins) of the primary melanoma is advocated by some for its simplicity, high efficiency, low cost, and good tolerability, especially when the examination is performed by an experienced operator. In case of suspicious lymph node on ultrasound investigation, fine needle biopsy, combined with cytology, allows diagnostic confirmation in the vast majority of cases. Very controversial is the role of chest X-ray and abdominal ultrasound in the presence of intermediate risk (T2–T4a), while a certain consensus seems to emerge on the indication for total body CT scan or PET–CT in melanomas at high risk for distant metastasis (T4) and/or in the presence of lymph node metastases.

Wide Excision

Wide excision represents the standard treatment for primary melanoma and has the primary goal of achieving durable local control of disease, minimizing the risk of local recurrence and curing patients with clinically localized melanoma. Wide excision involves removal of a surrounding margin of normal skin, en bloc with subcutaneous tissue down to the muscular fascia, which should be excised only if clearly infiltrated. It is a simple surgical procedure, performed in most cases under local anesthesia, on an outpatient basis and less frequently under general anesthesia, especially when complex reconstruction techniques are required or a concomitant sentinel lymph node biopsy or

TABLE 8.3 Pathological Prognostic Stage Group (pTNM)

When T is ...	And N is ...	And M is ...	Then the Stage Group is ...
Tis	N0	M0	0
T1a	N0	M0	IA
T1b	N0	M0	IA
T2a	N0	M0	IB
T2b	N0	M0	IIA
T3a	N0	M0	IIA
T3b	N0	M0	IIB
T4a	N0	M0	IIB
T4b	N0	M0	IIC
T0	N1b, N1c	M0	IIIB
T0	N2b/c, N3b/c	M0	IIIC
T1a/b, T2a	N1a, N2a	M0	IIIA
T1a/b, T2a	N1b/c, N2b	M0	IIIB
T2b, T3a	N1a/b/c, N2a/b	M0	IIIB
T1a/b, T2a/b, T3a	N2c, N3a/b/c	M0	IIIC
T3b, T4a	Any N ≥N1	M0	IIIC
T4b	N1a/b/c, N2a/b/c	M0	IIIC
T4b	N3a/b/c	M0	IIID
Any T, Tis	Any N	M1	IV

Used with permission of the American College of Surgeons, Chicago, Illinois. The original source for this information is the AJCC Cancer Staging Manual, Eighth Edition (2017) published by Springer International Publishing.

lymphadenectomy is planned. The most important oncological principle is to preoperatively define the healthy margin that must be obtained for adequate surgical resection. The free excision margin should be measured radially from the edge of the lesion or the biopsy scar and should be adjusted according to the thickness of the primary tumor at histological examination. The width of excision margins has been investigated in several randomized controlled trials. Some meta-analyses show no differences in overall survival between large excisions (3–5 cm) and narrow excisions (1–2 cm), whereas they seem to highlight significant differences in disease-free survival.[6]

On the basis of currently available data, the appropriate excision margins should be tailored on the thickness of primary melanoma, as reported in Table 8.4. Although

TABLE 8.4 Recommended Excision Margin According to Melanoma Thickness

Thickness	Excision Margins
In situ melanoma	5 mm
Breslow ≤2 mm	10 mm
Breslow >2 mm	20 mm

melanoma in situ is considered a noninfiltrating lesion, in some cases a local recurrence can occur; in rare cases, it occurs as an infiltrative lesion with metastatic potential. A margin of 0.5 cm ensures excellent local control. In a particular form of melanoma in situ, lentigo maligna type, the lesion appears more extensive microscopically than upon clinical examination. For this reason, a 1-cm margin is advisable in the presence of lentigo maligna, due to the possibility of finding residual foci in the final pathologic assessment when conventional excision is adopted. Despite a close observation of these guidelines, some melanomas in situ require multiple excisions to achieve a safe margin, and occasionally split-thickness skin grafts or flaps are necessary for wound closure.

The surgical specimen, including skin and subcutaneous tissue, should always be sent for final histological analysis to detect residual tumor or satellite nodules. For this analysis, it is advisable to send an orientated specimen, which facilitates reexcision if margins are involved or are very close to the tumor. Primary closure can be obtained in the vast majority of cases, some time after mild mobilization of skin edge from the underlying fascia. Skin grafts or tissue flaps may be necessary for melanomas located in less mobilizable anatomical areas, such as the distal extremities and the scalp. In specific areas (nose, ears, eyelids), extensive demolition by removing portions of the cartilage may be necessary if clearly infiltrated. In these areas, if surgery involves disabling outcomes from an esthetic and functional point of view, the width of excision can be modulated based on the risk of recurrence. The reconstructive technique should be properly planned and all the cosmetic and functional factors should be discussed with the patient.

In these situations, some advocate Mohs micrographic surgery (MMS). MMS is a technique that involves sequential margin excision of skin around the tumor with immediate intraoperative histological margin assessment. MMS provides more a limited margin of excision and is performed, with favorable outcome, mostly in squamous cell and basal cell carcinoma. For melanoma, the presence of potential satellite microscopic disease discourages the use of MMS in infiltrating melanomas. A lower recurrence rate after use of MMS has been reported for melanoma in situ but, at this level of evidence, the technique should be performed in selected cases, preferably in the context of clinical trials. For melanoma of the nail bed and the distal phalanx, recommendations for treatment are not evidence-based. In general, for subungual or distal phalanx melanomas ≤2 mm thick, generally a 1-cm gross margin from the tumor can be obtained with amputation at the level of the distal phalanx. For more infiltrating melanomas, amputation is indicated at the level of the metatarsal/metacarpal phalanx. The function of the finger involved (first/second finger) can suggest more limited resection.

Sentinel Lymph Node Biopsy

The rationale for sentinel lymph node biopsy (SLNB) is based on the hypothesis that the lymphatic spread of metastatic cells from the primary melanoma to the regional lymph nodes is an orderly and definable process.

The first lymph node(s) that receives lymphatic drainage from the affected area is considered the sentinel lymph node (SLN), because it is the most likely to contain metastatic disease in that specific lymphatic basin. It follows that successful identification, surgical removal, and careful histological examination of all SLNs in a patient should provide a more accurate regional nodal staging. A significant percentage (15%–20%) of patients with a diagnosis of primary melanoma harbor undetectable metastasis (either clinically or with ultrasonography) in the regional lymph nodes. Micrometastases, if left untreated, will become clinically evident with time, thus motivating the need to discover this occult disease at an early stage. Nevertheless, the impact on survival of SLNB in melanomas remains unknown. In fact the Multicenter Selective Lymphadenectomy (MSLT–I) randomized trial designed to compare the outcome of melanoma patients who have undergone SLNB versus observation, showed nonsignificant improvement in survival after SLNB.[7] However, this surgical procedure is still considered the most accurate method for staging melanoma patients (see the AJCC cancer staging manual, eighth edition). According to the American Society of Clinical Oncology (ASCO), routine SLNB is not recommended for patients with thin melanomas that are T1a (nonulcerated lesion <0.8 mm in Breslow thickness). SLNB may be considered for thin melanomas that are T1b (0.8–1.0 mm Breslow thickness or <0.8 mm Breslow thickness with ulceration) after a thorough discussion with the patient of the potential benefits and risk of harms associated with the procedure. SLN biopsy is recommended for patients with intermediate-thickness melanoma (T2 or T3; Breslow thickness of >1.0–4.0 mm). SLN biopsy may be recommended for patients with thick melanomas (T4; >4.0 mm in Breslow thickness), after a discussion of the potential benefits and risks of harm.[8]

SLNB involves preoperative lymphoscintigraphy, obtained through the injection of a radiopharmaceutical (human albumin nanocolloid labeled with technetium ^{99m}Tc). The injection is intradermal, around the scar of the removed melanoma or close to the tumor if still present, and followed by early and late scintigraphic scans in the likely locations of lymphatic drainage.

Once the location of the sentinel node(s) has been identified, the cutaneous projection area of each single node is marked on the skin. SLNB is performed in the operating room, usually under local anesthesia associated with sedation or under general anesthesia according to the site of the lymphatic basin. Prior to sterile preparation of the patient, the primary site is further injected intradermally with 0.5–1 mL of a vital dye (Patent Blue), to increase the sensitivity of the method and to facilitate the finding of the lymph node. The use of the vital dye for SLNB should be avoided if the primary tumor is located on the face because of the risk of permanent tattooing, and in the case of a pregnant patient because of the low but not rare risk of reported allergic reactions (about 1% of cases). If the SLN is identified in the parotid or in a deep location, SLNB should be extensively discussed with the patient before surgery, because in these areas SLNB may require more extensive surgery and the patient is at a higher risk for potential complications.

The SLNB technique is very simple. Through a small skin incision, which takes into consideration the incision necessary for a subsequent radical lymphadenectomy, the district is entered and under the guidance of a radioisotope probe, tracing the blue lymphatic channels, the SLN(s) is identified and removed. Care should be taken to not disrupt or cauterize the lymph node capsule. Each SLN removed is checked ex vivo for radioactivity and the nodal basin is rescanned. In the case of potential background or shine radiation from the primary melanoma sites, concomitant wide excision can be performed beforehand to decrease radioactivity disturbance. All lymph nodes that are colored or that measure >10% of the radioactivity of the ex vivo count in the more radio-emitting sentinel should be considered sentinel nodes. Drains are infrequently required and most patients are discharged on the same day. The incidence of complications is low, mainly related to wound dehiscence/infection or lymphatic collection (seroma). The success of the procedure, which is related to a well-known learning curve, also depends on the location of melanoma and on the lymph node basin involved (95% in the axillary and inguinal regions and 85% in head and neck).

Histological examination of the SLN should be performed on thick sections cut from paraffin-embedded tissue. Intraoperative pathology evaluation is not recommended, because in frozen sections identification of single or small clusters of melanoma cells is more difficult and a potential loss of diagnostic tissue can occur during specimen sectioning. The histopathological analysis of the SLN needs multiple sections stained with hematoxylin–eosin for immunohistochemistry. Some standardized protocols define the number of histological sections, the interval between these and the type of immunohistochemical markers to use for histological examination of the SLN in melanoma, such as those proposed by the European Organisation for Research and Treatment of Cancer (EORTC) Melanoma Group. The percentages of positive sentinel nodes are affected by the type of protocol used, with a range between 18% and 33%.

Because of prognostic relevance, the histology report should specify the number of SLNs analysed, the number of positive lymph nodes, as well as the characteristics of the lymph node metastasis, reporting the maximum diameter, site (subcapsular, parenchymal or mixed), parenchymal invasion, and extracapsular extension. The presence of nevus cell clusters should be noted. In fact, the SLN is considered positive in the presence of isolated tumor cells only, even if these are displayed solely with immunohistochemical techniques. Histological status of the SLN is the most powerful independent predictor of survival in clinically node-negative melanoma patients. A negative SLNB is associated with a 5-year melanoma-specific survival rate of approximately 92%. Recurrence and death may occur in this group of patients due to a false-negative SLNB or a pure hematogenous pattern of metastases. A false-negative SLNB occurs in up to 10% of patients and is defined as the rate of development of clinical nodal disease in the same nodal basin. The reasons for a false-negative event after SLNB probably have multifactorial origins, related to an incorrect identification of the SLN during the procedure, to the presence of in-transit microscopic disease and, finally, to the presence of a very small burden of disease undetected at histological examination.

Lymphadenectomy

Lymph nodes are the most frequent site from metastases of melanoma. The lymphatic basin (or basins) at risk depend on the location of the primary; for melanomas of the head and neck, the laterocervical lymph nodes; for those of the trunk positioned above the Sappey line (extending from the navel to the iliac crest to the second lumbar vertebra), the axillary lymph nodes; and for those of the trunk below this line and the lower limb, the inguinal lymph nodes. Even the epitrochlear and popliteal lymph nodes, although rarely, may be the site of locoregional metastases. The main purpose of lymphadenectomy is to provide locoregional control of disease and it is indicated for patients with histo- and/or cytologically proven lymph node metastasis. Lymph node involvement is diagnosed in different ways, most frequently after SLNB, but a quota of patients may present clinically evident metastases at diagnosis or during follow-up. In the case of positive SLNB, 15%–20% of patients subjected to lymphadenectomy present additional lymph node metastases in the dissected basin. However, two randomized clinical trials have recently shown no advantage in survival for patients who have undergone a completion lymph node dissection (CLND) versus observation in cases of positive SNLB.[9,10]

Based on consideration of clinicopathological factors influencing the caseload composition of these clinical trials, at present ASCO recommendations are the following: in the case of a positive SLNB, CLND or careful observation are options for patients with low-risk micrometastatic disease, with due consideration of clinicopathological factors. For higher-risk patients, careful observation may be considered only after a thorough discussion with patients about the potential risks and benefits of forgoing CLND.[8] In order to help clinicians to select melanoma patients for CLND, a nomogram was recentely elaborated to predict non-sentinel nodes status in patients with positive SLNB (Fig. 8.1).[11]

The general principle in performing lymphadenectomy for melanoma is the en bloc excision of lymph nodes with surrounding fat tissue. Every attempt should be made to minimize morbidity through preservation of the motor nerves and muscle. The relative frequency of complications after lymphadenectomy has led some groups to consider more limited interventions, particularly in patients with positive SLNs in locations at risk of more significant complications. Axillary radical lymphadenectomy should include complete dissection of level I, II, and III lymph nodes, removing all fibro–fatty tissue around the axillary vein. A section of the pectoralis minor muscle is suggested by some for better access to level II–III lymph nodes or in presence of bulky level II and III nodes. During dissection, long thoracic and thoracodorsal nerves should be identified and sectioned only if directly involved by the tumor. In the case of metastasis to the inguinal lymph nodes, the standard approach involves the removal of the inguinal, external iliac, and obturator lymph nodes.[12]

In the classic description of inguinal dissection, a longitudinal skin incision is employed, extending 2–3 cm superomedial to the superior anterior iliac spine up to the apex of the femoral triangle. The skin flaps are created medially up to the pubic tubercle, the anterior margin of the gracilis and abductor muscles and laterally up to the superior anterior iliac spine and Sartorius muscle. The dissection continues deeply, through the incision of the fascia lata, over the underlining muscles and femoral vessels. The saphenous vein is sectioned at the apex of the femoral triangle and at the level of the saphenofemoral junction. Deep dissection (iliac and obturatory) involves sectioning of the oblique muscles and the inguinal ligament and through an extraperitoneal approach, access to the pelvic area of the iliac and obturator lymph nodes is achieved. Even if the use of inguinal lymphadenectomy is performed by some surgeons in selected cases (negative pelvic CT scan, negative lymph node of Cloquet, number of positive inguinal lymph nodes are ≤2, absence of a lymphatic drainage in deep pelvis views lymphoscintigraphy), evidence is too low to recommend this approach and a proper designed trial on this topic is desirable. For cervical lymph node metastastis, clear indications on the thoroughness of dissection are lacking and all the recommendations are supported by a low level of evidence and follow opinions of experts in this field. In the case of clinically evident cervical lymph node metastasis, surgery is aimed at the removal of all five levels of lymph nodes (submandibular, jugular, and supraclavicular). In the case of metastasis discovered after sentinel lymph node biopsy, selective lymphadenectomy, involving the removal of lymph nodes at different levels depending on the site of the primary tumor, the site of the sentinel node, and the lymphatic drainage highlighted at lymphoscintigraphy, is suggested. Removal of the superficial part of the parotid is recommended only if clinically involved, because of the high risk of nerve damage observed.

All lymphadenectomies are characterized by significant morbidity, which is variable depending on the site of

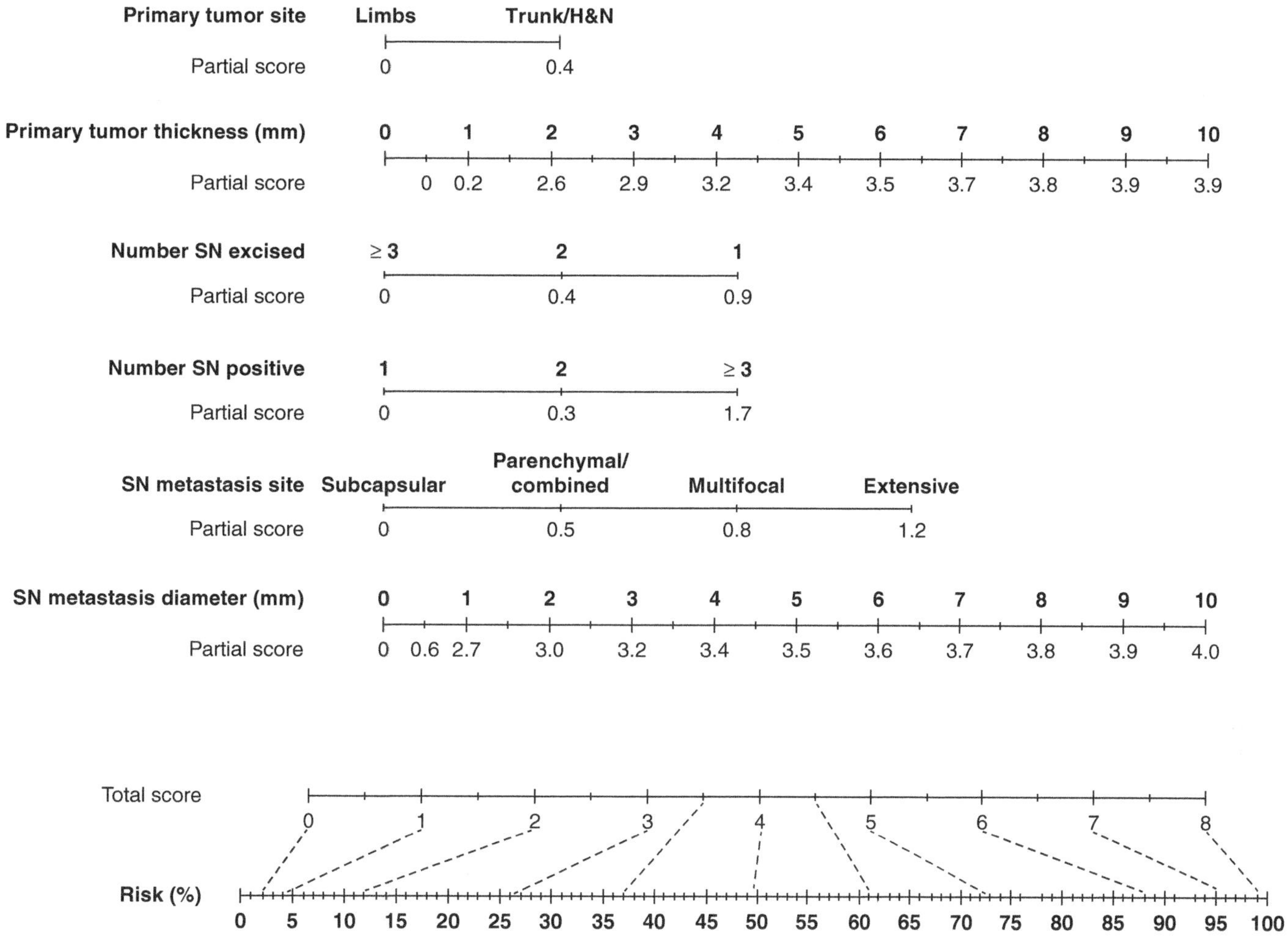

• **Fig. 8.1** Nomogram for the prediction of nonsentinel nodes status. For each patient, the risk of harboring metastatic melanoma in his/her nonsentinel nodes is estimated by calculating a total score, which is calculated by adding up the partial score for each of the six clinicopathological features.

dissection. Inguinal–iliac–obturator lymphadenectomy is the intervention burdened by the greatest number of complications by far (wound infection/dehiscence, lymphocele, lymphedema, and nerve damage), with an incidence that can reach up to 80%.[13] Aimed at reducing postoperative morbidity after inguinal lymphadenectomy, several variations have been proposed which consider skin-sparing techniques, sartorius muscle transposition and saphenous vein preservation. The benefits of these technical variants still remain uncertain, as no randomized trials have reported a clear reduction in postoperative morbidity. An interesting advancement to minimize surgical morbidity after inguinal dissection is videoendoscopic inguinal lymphadenectomy (Fig. 8.2).[14] After blunt dissection under the fascia of Camper, the working space is obtained using high-pressure CO_2 levels and three trocars are placed at a variable distance from the apex of the femoral triangle. The postoperative morbidity appears lower with respect to the open procedure, mainly for wound/skin-related complications, and the number of lymph nodes harvested seems comparable to that of conventional groin dissection. Nevertheless, before this technique is considered suitable for clinical practice, comparable oncological outcomes, lower postoperative morbidity, and better quality of life should be assessed in an appropriately designed randomized controlled trial.

In patients who undergo lymphadenectomy, the number of positive lymph nodes has an important prognostic value. If only one lymph node is micrometastatic, the 10-year survival rate is about 88%, dropping to 60% if 2–3 positive lymph nodes are found.[15] The 'N'-ratio (i.e., the ratio between the number of positive lymph nodes and total lymph nodes removed) seems to have a completely independent prognostic impact. Patients with a low N-ratio (less than 0.1 or including between 0.11 and 0.25) have a significantly better prognosis than patients with a high N-ratio (>0.25).[16]

For the prognostic importance of the number of lymph nodes and the N-ratio, the extension and quality of surgery becomes a primary factor in a patient's prognosis. Despite this evidence, shared parameters about quality control of lymph node dissections for melanoma are still lacking. The recommendations of the National Comprehensive Cancer

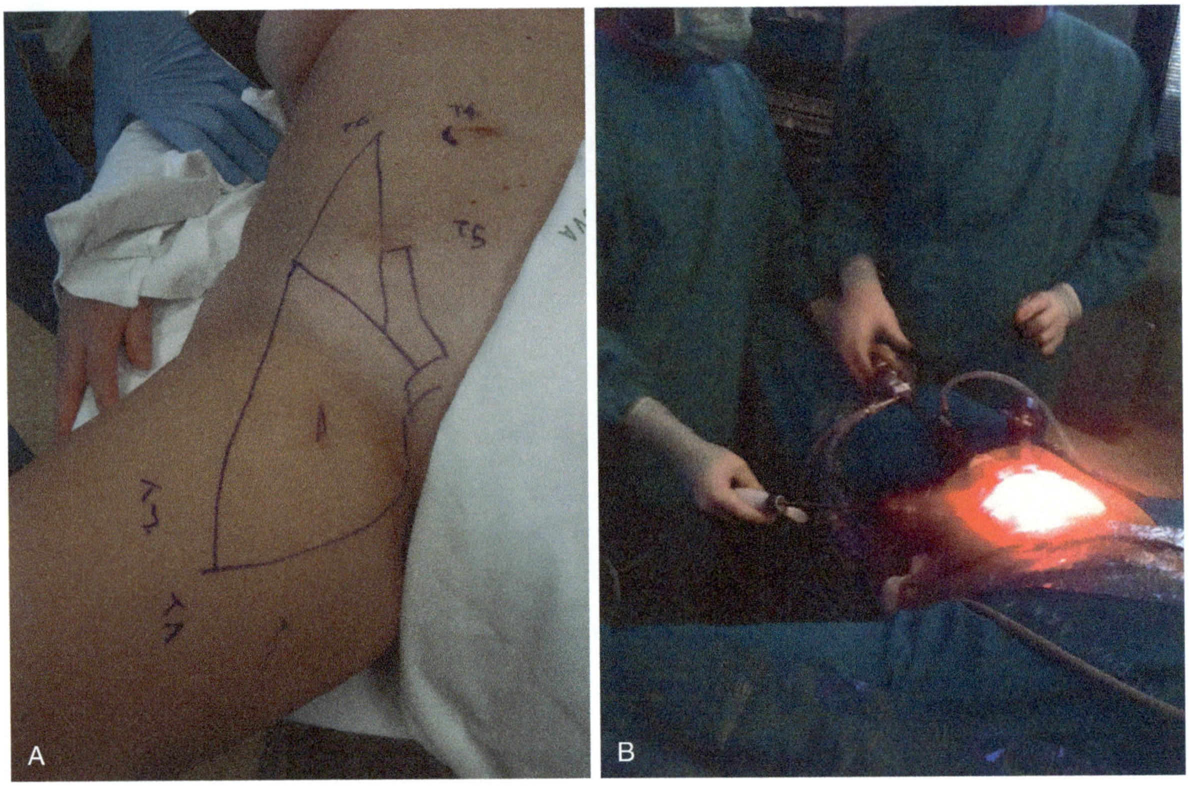

• **Fig. 8.2** Videoscopic groin dissection for groin metastasis. (A) Trocar positions; (B) intraoperative view.

Network (NCNN) require only a clear description of the anatomical limits of the dissection. The number of lymph nodes (with different limit values) and the N-ratio could be simple and objective parameters of quality, but no consensus on their use in clinical practice has been found.[16,17]

Adjuvant Therapy

Patients with lymph node metastasis are at high risk of recurrence and/or systemic metastases. For this reason, adjuvant (i.e., postoperative) therapy has been proposed to reduce the risk of death and recurrence in patients with high–risk melanomas. Interferon-alpha has shown some positive therapeutic effect.[18]

Recently the exciting survival benefits seen in patients with metastatic melanoma treated with immune targeted drugs have suggested their use in the adjuvant setting. Nivolumab and ipilimumab are immune checkpoint inhibitors that have been approved for the treatment of advanced melanoma. Adjuvant use of checkpoint inhibitors or combination therapy with the BRAF inhibitor dabrafenib plus a MEK inhibitor (trametinib) have also improved survival in patients with BRAF V600 mutations in the same clinical setting.[19–21]

The use of adjuvant radiotherapy after lymphadenectomy for melanoma remains controversial and no significant improvement of the overall survival has been observed. For patients at high risk for regional relapse (multiple affected lymph nodes or extracapsular spread), adjuvant radiotherapy after lymph node dissection seems to improve local control and should be considered in this group of patients.[22]

Locoregional Treatment

"In transit metastases" or "satellites" are defined as the locoregional spread in the lymphatic system between the site of the primary lesion and the main regional lymphatic basin. More than 20% of all recurrences for melanoma are in the form of in transit metastases or satellites. The 5-year survival rate of these patients stands at 25%–30%, with a better prognosis than other metastatic sites. In the presence of cutaneous and subcutaneous metastases, the therapeutic choices depend on the number, size, and location of the lesions. For a single or very few lesions, especially if the primary melanoma is associated with favorable prognostic factors, a simple radical excision represents the first-line treatment, possibly associated with SLNB, since the occurrence of occult metastases in regional lymph nodes is significant. Excluding these more favorable cases, the vast majority of patients present with multifocal and progressive lesions or bulky disease. In these cases, locoregional treatment should be proposed in absence of systemic metastases. For in transit lesions located in the limbs, hyperthermic isolated limb perfusion (HILP) represents the gold standard of treatment (Fig. 8.3).[23]

The rationale of HILP is the administration of a high dose of one or more chemotherapeutic drugs to the limb while avoiding systemic toxicity. During HILP, the femoral/axillary vessels are cannulated and the perfusion circuit is obtained through a specifically designed perfusion machine, which maintains an adequate blood flow under moderately hyperthermic conditions (39–41°C). Melphalan is the drug

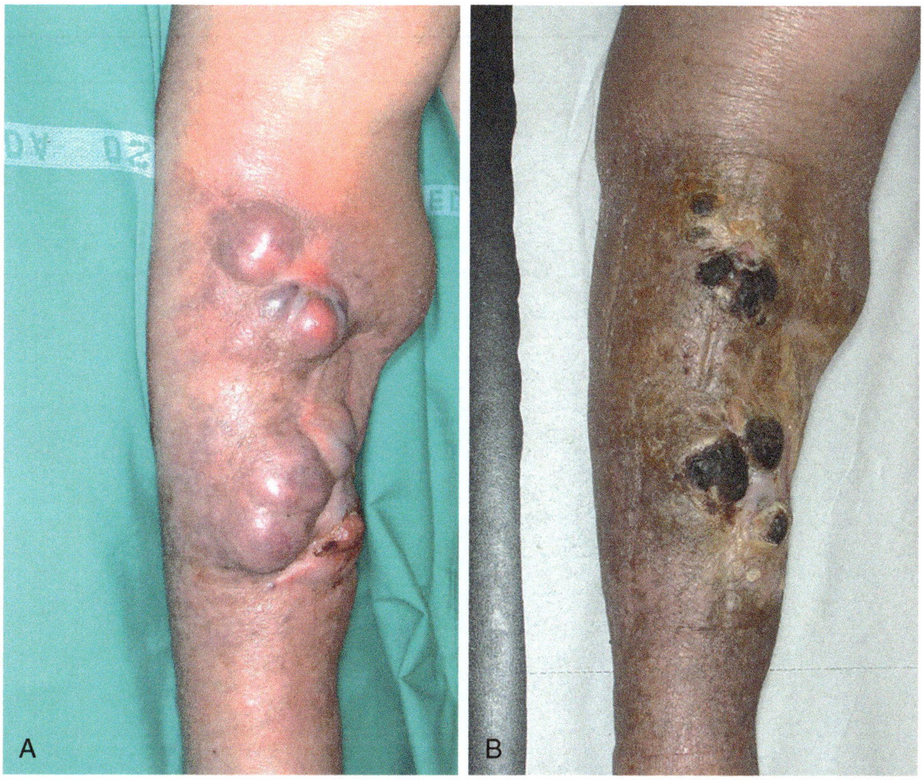

• **Fig. 8.3** Hyperthermic isolated limb perfusion (HILP) for bulky metastatic melanoma of the leg. (A) Before and (B) response after treatment.

of choice, with a complete response in around 50% of cases and a 5-year survival rate of 28.5%. In cases of no response, relapse or in the presence of a high tumor burden, the association of melphalan with tumor necrosis factor alpha (TNFα) provides a significant improvement in the complete response rate without an increase in toxicity. In patients with recurrence after HILP unfit for surgery, isolated limb infusion (ILI) can be used.[24] With respect to HILP, isolated limb perfusion is performed in absence of hyperthermia under hypoxic conditions (without oxygenation of the perfusate) and is considered less invasive since the catheters are placed percutaneously. The combination of melphalan and actinomycin–D achieves a complete response rate in 38% and a partial response rate in 46% of cases, with a 5-year survival rate similar to that for HILP. Recent evidence has suggested electrochemotherapy as a new therapeutic modality for patients with in transit metastases from melanoma (Fig. 8.4).

Electrochemotherapy is based on the physical and biological principle of electroporation (i.e., the ability of an external electric field applied on biological tissues to increase, by using a short and intense pulse, the permeability of cell membranes to various molecules). The use of electrochemotherapy in the presence of cutaneous and subcutaneous metastases has proved effective and the technique has recently been standardized. The European Standard Operating Procedures of Electrochemotherapy (ESOPE) classified the use of electrochemotherapy according to the type of tumor, the drug used (bleomycin or cisplatin), the route of administration (venous or intratumoral) and the type of electrode used.[25]

The main advantage is that electrochemotherapy is a minimally invasive procedure well accepted by patients. It is performed in a day hospital setting under local anesthesia and/or sedation, with limited side effects and very few contraindications. Electrochemotherapy has the considerable advantage, with respect to HILP and ILI, that it is easily repeatable in different sessions and can be applied to any region of the body. The complete response rate after a single session ranges from 9% to 100%, while the objective response varies from 62% to 100%, results that tend to increase after multiple sessions. A recent retrospective multicentric study shows a reported overall response of 74% with a complete response rate of 58%.[26]

Main prognostic factors identified as related to the tumor response are the nodule size and number. In conclusion, in the presence of in transit metastases, HILP remains the treatment of choice, as it ensures the highest rate of complete response, which is a factor that is able to influence both locoregional control and survival. ILI is a viable alternative, especially in frail patients with multiple comorbidities, for sites of disease distal to the middle third of the thigh. Electrochemotherapy is a promising technique that can be used in case of failure of HILP and isolated limb perfusion, as complementary treatment in combination with other locoregional therapies, or as an alternative where these are contraindicated or cannot be accomplished (metastases in the trunk, neck, and head).

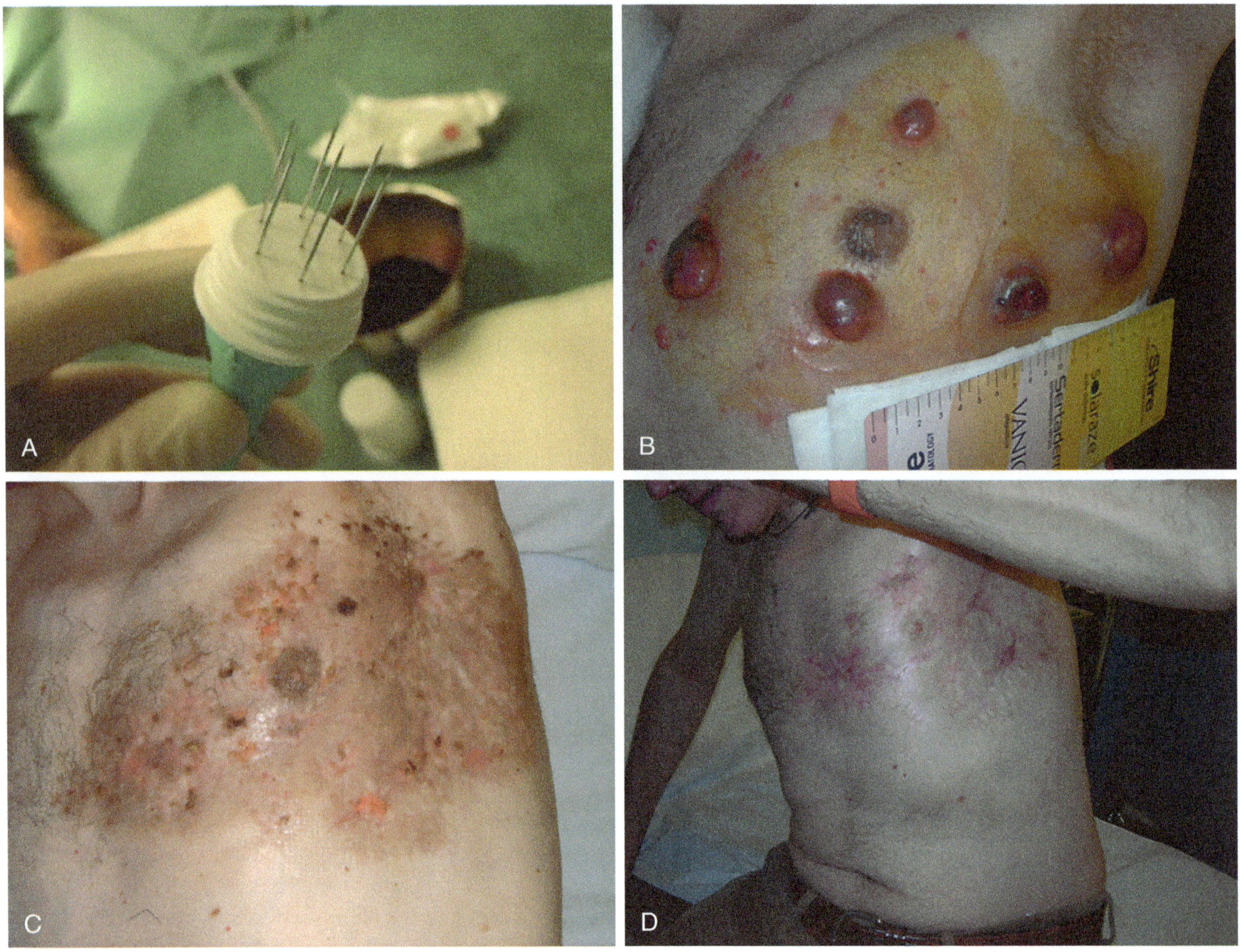

• **Fig. 8.4** Electrochemotherapy treatment for superficial metastases. (A) Hexagonal-array needle electrode for tumor electroporation; (B) cutaneous metastatic melanoma, baseline; (C) follow-up at 44 weeks; (D) follow-up at 60 weeks.

Distant Metastases

The most common sites of metastases from cutaneous melanoma are extraregional lymph nodes, the lung, the brain, the skin, and the liver, and less frequently, bone, adrenal glands, and gastrointestinal tract. In the presence of distant metastases, surgical treatment may have a dual purpose – palliative or curative. In the first case, surgery is mainly directed to treat a symptom that adversely affects the quality of life of a patient. For example, in selected patients with metastases to the gastrointestinal tract, surgery may offer good palliation for bleeding or intestinal occlusion. On the other hand, radical resection should be considered as first-line therapy whenever complete removal of all disease can be accomplished, since surgery with curative intent ensures 5-year survival of up to 30%, a result not obtainable with other systemic therapies.[27] For this reason, radical surgery should be considered in selected patients after multidisciplinary discussion, taking into consideration, as prognostic factors, the metastatic site (skin versus lung versus other sites), the number of metastases, the number of organs involved, the disease-free interval, the doubling time of the lesions, the LDH levels, and the performance status of the patient. However, for the majority of patients with stage IV disease, radical surgery remains contraindicated for the presence of unresectable, progressive or disseminated disease. These patients should be considered for systemic therapy or palliative care.

Until a few years ago, patients with metastatic melanoma had few treatment options. They had been treated with dacarbazine or other palliative chemotherapies, with poor results (median survival 6.2 months and only 25.5% of 1-year survival). Over the past decade, significant progress in understanding the molecular pathway of tumorigenesis and metastasis of melanomas, together with the definition of the regulatory role of the immune system in these mechanisms, led to the discovery of new drugs that have shown an encouraging clinical activity against metastatic melanoma. Among these, ipilimumab and nivolumab are immune checkpoint inhibitor anti-CTLA-4 and anti-PD-1, respectively, that promote antitumor immunity against melanoma, showing significant improvement in survival for patients with metastatic disease.[28,29] Another recent finding, closely linked to molecular biology of melanoma cells, was the discovery of the role of protein kinase pathway in tumor progression, which is regulated by the protein BRAF. Mutations in BRAF protein are found in half of patients with melanoma, resulting in constitutive activation of the kinase pathway, that can be specifically inhibited by the monoclonal antibody vemurafenib. Mutations in N-RAS protein can be inhibited by trametinib at MEK level. In these clinical setting, vemurafenib has been shown to improve tumor response rate and overall survival.[30] According to a recent meta-analysis the simultaneous inhibition of BRAF and MEK appears the most effective treatment for melanomas harboring BRAF V600 mutation, although anti-PD1 antibodies appear to be less toxic.[31] Despite the continuous improvement in target therapy for metastatic melanoma and new promising drugs under study, further trials evaluating combination therapies are essential to improve the results of treatment of stage IV melanoma in the near future.

Noncutaneous Melanomas

After cutaneous melanoma, ocular melanoma represents the second most common type and the most common primary intraocular malignant tumor in adults. The vast majority of ocular melanomas originate from uvea, whereas conjunctival melanomas are far less frequent. Incidence of uveal melanoma has remained stable over the past three decades. Patients with uveal melanoma are often asymptomatic and the tumor is diagnosed upon clinical examination with great accuracy. Fine needle biopsy is usually not suggested, as seeding of the needle tract has been reported. The choice of treatment takes into account many factors; among them, the size of the tumor is the most important. Historically, enucleation has been considered the definitive treatment of uveal melanoma, now restricted for large or symptomatic lesions. The alternative treatment most commonly adopted is radiotherapy. Among the radiotherapeutic strategies, the most common treatment is plaque brachytherapy, in which a small plaque with radioactive seeds is attached to the outside surface of the eye, overlying the tumor.[32] The plaque is left in place for a few days and then removed. After plaque radiotherapy, the survival results are the same as that after enucleation.

Despite an optimal local control, half of patients develop metastases within 15 years after treatment of the primary tumor. The most common site of metastasis for uveal melanoma is the liver, which is also the first site of metastasis for 80%–90% of all ocular melanoma patients. Other common sites of metastasis include the lung, bones, and the skin. The survival time after diagnosis of liver metastases depends on the extent of systemic spread. Recent findings in cytogenetics and genetics have allowed a better prognostic stratification and the determination of tumors with higher metastatic potential.[33] However, an effective systemic therapy is still lacking for primary mucosal melanomas arising from proliferation of melanocytes located in mucosal membranes of the gastrointestinal, respiratory, and urogenital tract.[34] More than half of mucosal melanomas originate from the mucosa of the nasal and oral cavity and the accessory sinuses. Less frequently, the sites of origin of mucosal melanomas are anorectum, vulva, and vagina. Mucosal melanomas can arise in almost any part of the mucosal membranes, with a reported 1% of cases of occult disease.

The lack of early and specific symptoms contributes to late diagnosis, and consequently to adverse prognosis. Because of their low incidence, no established protocols for treatment are available, and surgery represents the mainstay of therapy. More recently, more conservative surgery has been advocated, since a demolitive approach does not seem to show an advantage for survival. Adjuvant radiotherapy can provide better locoregional control in some locations, but did not show improvement in survival. Compared with cutaneous and ocular melanoma, mucosal melanomas have the lowest percent of 5-year survival. There is no effective systemic therapy for these aggressive tumors. Recent advances in molecular biology underlying mucosal melanomas have identified *KIT* as a potential marker for targeted therapy in around 25% of patients. Clinical trials with *KIT* inhibitors are ongoing.[35]

References

1. MacKie RM, Hauschild A, Eggermont AM. Epidemiology of invasive cutaneous melanoma. *Ann Oncol.* 2009;20(suppl 6): vi1–7.
2. Russak JE, Rigel DS. Risk factors for the development of primary cutaneous melanoma. *Dermatol Clin.* 2012;30:363–368.
3. Borsari S, Pampena R, Benati E, et al. In vivo dermoscopic and confocal microscopy multistep algorithm to detect in situ melanomas. *Br J Dermatol.* 2018;179(1):163–172.
4. Breslow A. Thickness, cross-sectional areas and depth of invasion in the prognosis of cutaneous melanoma. *Ann Surg.* 1970;172:902–908.
5. Xing Y, Bronstein Y, Ross MI, et al. Contemporary diagnostic imaging modalities for the staging and surveillance of melanoma patients: a meta-analysis. *J Natl Cancer Inst.* 2011;103:129–142.
6. Sladden MJ, Balch C, Barzilai DA, et al. Surgical excision margins for primary cutaneous melanoma. *Cochrane Database Syst Rev.* 2009:CD004835.
7. Morton DL, Thompson JF, Cochran AJ, et al. Sentinel-node biopsy or nodal observation in melanoma. *N Engl J Med.* 2006;355:1307–1317.
8. Wong SL, Faries MB, Kennedy EB, et al. Sentinel lymph node biopsy and management of regional lymph nodes in melanoma: American society of clinical oncology and society of surgical oncology clinical practice guideline Update. *J Clin Oncol.* 2018;36(4):399–413.
9. Leiter U, Stadler R, Mauch C, et al. Complete lymph node dissection versus no dissection in patients with sentinel lymph node biopsy positive melanoma (DeCOG-SLT): a multicentre, randomised, phase 3 trial. *Lancet Oncol.* 2016;17(6):757–767.
10. Faries MB, Thompson JF, Cochran AJ, et al. Completion dissection or observation for sentinel-node metastasis in melanoma. *N Engl J Med.* 2017;376(23):2211–2222.
11. Rossi CR, Mocellin S, Campana LG, et al. Prediction of non-sentinel node status in patients with melanoma and positive sentinel node biopsy: an Italian Melanoma Intergoup (IMI) study. *Ann Surg Oncol.* 2018;25:271–279.

12. Spratt J. Groin dissection. *J Surg Oncol.* 2000;73:243–262.
13. Chang SB, Askew RL, Xing Y, et al. Prospective assessment of post-operative complications and associated costs following inguinal lymph node dissection (ILND) in melanoma patients. *Ann Surg Oncol.* 2010;17:2764–2772.
14. Sommariva A, Pasquali S, Cona C, et al. Videoscopic ilioinguinal lymphadenectomy for groin lymph node metastases from melanoma. *Br J Surg.* 2016;103(8):1026–1032.
15. Gershenwald JE, Scolyer RA, Hess KR, et al. Melanoma staging: evidence-based changes in the American Joint Committee on Cancer, eighth edition cancer staging manual. *CA Cancer J Clin.* 2017;67(6):472–492.
16. Rossi CR, Mocellin S, Pasquali S, et al. N-ratio: a novel independent prognostic factor for patients with stage-III cutaneous melanoma. *Ann Surg Oncol.* 2008;15:310–315.
17. Bilimoria KY, Raval MV, Bentrem DJ, et al. National assessment of melanoma care using formally developed quality indicators. *J Clin Oncol.* 2009;27:5445–5451.
18. Mocellin S, Lens MB, Pasquali S, et al. Interferon alpha for the adjuvant treatment of cutaneous melanoma. *Cochrane Database Syst Rev.* 2013;6:CD008955.
19. Weber J, Mandala M, Del Vecchio M, et al. Adjuvant nivolumab versus ipilimubab in resected stage III or IV melanoma. *N Engl J Med.* 2017;377(19):1824–1835.
20. Maio M, Lewis K, Demidov L, et al. Adjuvant vemurafenib in resected BRAF-V600 mutation-positive melanoma (BRIM8): a randomized, double-blind, placebo-controlled, multicentre, phase 3 trial. *Lancet Oncol.* 2018;19(4):510–520.
21. Long GV, Hauschild A, Santinami M, et al. Adjuvant dabrafenib plus trametinib in stage III BRAF-mutated melanoma. *N Engl J Med.* 2017;377(19):1813–1823.
22. Burmeister BH, Henderson MA, Ainslie J, et al. Adjuvant radiotherapy versus observation alone for patients at risk of lymph–node field relapse after therapeutic lymphadenectomy for melanoma: a randomisedtrial. *Lancet Oncol.* 2012;13:589–597.
23. Kroon BB, Noorda EM, Vrouenraets BC, et al. Isolated limb perfusion for melanoma. *Surg Oncol Clin North Am.* 2008;17:785–794, (viii–ix).
24. Kroon HM, Thompson JF. Isolated limb infusion: a review. *J Surg Oncol.* 2009;100:169–177.
25. Mir LMGJ, Sersa G, Collins CG. Standard operating procedures of the electrochemotherapy: instructions for the use of bleomycin or cisplatin administered either systemically or locally and electric pulses delivered by the Cliniporator (TM) by means of invasive or non-invasive electrodes. *EJC Suppl.* 2006:14–25.
26. Kunte C, Letulé V, Gehl J, et al. Electrochemotherapy in the treatment of metastatic malignant melanoma: a prospective cohort study by InspECT. *Br J Dermatol.* 2017;176(6):1475–1485.
27. Ollila DW. Complete metastasectomy in patients with stage IV metastatic melanoma. *Lancet Oncol.* 2006;7:919–924.
28. Hodi FS, O'Day SJ, McDermott DF, et al. Improved survival with ipilimumab in patients with metastatic melanoma. *N Engl J Med.* 2010;363:711–723.
29. Weber JS, D'Angelo SP, Minor D, et al. Nivolumab versus chemotherapy in patients with advanced melanoma who progressed after anti-CTLA-4 treatment (CheckMate 037): a randomised, controlled, open-label, phase 3 trial. *Lancet Oncol.* 2015;16(4):375–384.
30. Chapman PB, Hauschild A, Robert C, et al. Improved survival with vemurafenib in melanoma with BRAF V600E mutation. *N Engl J Med.* 2011;364:2507–2516.
31. Pasquali S, Chiarion-Sileni V, Rossi CR, et al. Immune checkpoint inhibitors and target therapies for metastatic melanoma: a network meta-analysis. *Cancer Treat Rev.* 2017;54:34–42.
32. Collaborative Ocular Melanoma Study Group. The COMS randomized trial of iodine 125 brachytherapy for choroidal melanoma: V. Twelve-year mortality rates and prognostic factors: COMS report No. 28. *Arch Ophthalmol.* 2006;124:1684–1693.
33. Onken MD, Worley LA, Tuscan MD, et al. An accurate, clinically feasible multi-gene expression assay for predicting metastasis in uveal melanoma. *J Mol Diagnost.* 2010;12:461–468.
34. Patrick RJ, Fenske NA, Messina JL. Primary mucosal melanoma. *J Am Acad Dermatol.* 2007;56:828–834.
35. Minor DR, Kashani–Sabet M, Garrido M, et al. Sunitinib therapy for melanoma patients with *KIT* mutations. *Clin Cancer Res.* 2012;18:1457–1463.

9 Nonmelanoma Skin Cancer

MICHAEL W. FINDLAY AND CATHERINE SOUFAN

Introduction

Nonmelanoma skin cancer (NMSC) is the most common malignancy amongst Caucasians and occurs sporadically in all other populations.[1] NMSCs are comprised predominantly of basal cell (BCC) and squamous cell (SCC) carcinoma, among other rarer types of cutaneous malignancy. UV radiation exposure initiates approximately 90% of NMSCs, resulting in malignant transformation of keratinocytes. Despite improvements in public awareness and warnings of the harmful effects of excessive ultraviolet (UV) exposure, the incidence of NMSC has risen by 3%–8% per year since 1960 with an almost 300% increase in the past two decades in the United States.[2] This trend is predicted to continue as populations age worldwide. Fortunately, NMSC mortality is reducing due to a combination of earlier diagnosis and advances in treatment. While traditional treatment modalities once centered on surgical excision, there have been steady advances in nonoperative modalities, resulting in a broader spectrum of treatment options. As leaders in surgery of the skin and related tissues, it is essential that plastic surgeons have a thorough understanding of NMSC, including both current and future management options, so that the important trend of improved survival continues long into the future.

Basal Cell Carcinoma

Epidemiology

Keratinocyte tumors make up 90% of all malignant skin diseases and basal cell carcinomas comprise approximately 70% of keratinocyte tumors. BCC makes up over three-quarters of all NMSCs[3] and affects 1 million people in the United States each year. It is rarely metastatic, however it can cause significant morbidity via local invasion. While the pathogenesis is attributed to an interplay between patient exposure to environmental factors and patient-derived characteristics, most BCCs are sporadic. Environmental exposures are the major etiological factor, with a latency period of anywhere between 20 and 50 years from point of exposure to the development of the BCC. As such, most sporadic BCCs occur in older males (>50 years of age) with fair complexions, typically classed as Fitzpatrick skin types 1 and 2.

Risk Factors

BCCs can develop early in life, but age is an independent risk factor whereby the incidence rate doubles from 40 to 70 years of age. Intensive, intermittent UV exposure (particularly UVB rays) resulting in sunburn and blistering (particularly during childhood and adolescence) is a major risk factor for BCC. Fair skin types (Fitzpatrick skin types 1 and 2) and individuals in hot climates are at greater risk of incidental intermittent sunburn. In Australia, which experiences the greatest UV solar irradiation per area of any continent, these factors combine to produce the highest incidences of NMSCs and melanoma in the world. Additional environmental factors include tanning bed use, chronic inflammation (burns), ionizing radiation, arsenic and hydrocarbon exposure. Immunosuppression poses an elevated risk of BCC development, particularly among human immunodeficiency virus (HIV)-positive patients (fivefold greater incidence) and organ transplant recipients using photosensitizing antifungal prophylaxis such as voriconazole. The association between human papillomavirus and BCC is not yet clear.

Genetics

Multiple genes have been implicated in the development of BCC, including tumor suppressor genes, DNA repair genes, and genes involved in skin and skin appendage pigmentation. Approximately 90% of sporadic BCCs have activating mutations in the Hedgehog-signaling pathway, resulting in uncontrolled proliferation of epidermal basal cells. This pathway was identified by studying patients with basal cell nevus syndrome

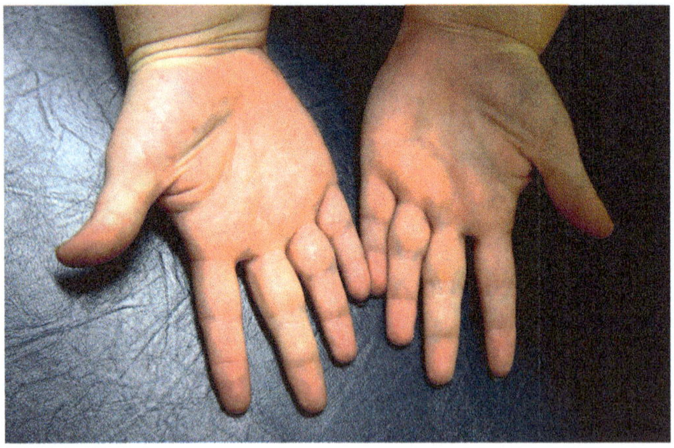

• **Fig. 9.1** Palmar pits in Gorlin syndrome. The patient's mother and brother were also both affected, with greater penetrance of phenotypic changes, but all three have palmar pitting.

(BCNS), also referred to as Gorlin syndrome, an autosomal dominant disease with constitutive mutations of the Hedgehog pathway. The specific gene involved in the majority of cases is the tumor suppressor *Patched* gene (*PTCH1*) (chromosome 9q), mutations of which lead to an increased risk of developing multiple BCCs from a young age, as well as a cluster of: keratocystic odontogenic tumors (KCOTs) in 75% of patients; palmar and plantar pits (Fig. 9.1); multiple skeletal abnormalities (e.g., bifid ribs, frontal bossing); and calcification of the falx cerebri. Approximately 10% of BCNS patients do not develop BCCs, indicating the involvement of multiple genes. The tumor-suppressor gene *p53* and melanocortin-1 receptor gene (*MC1R*) are also important for the development of BCC, but much less specific to this tumor. Those with pigment disorders and defects in DNA repair mechanisms, such as albinism and xeroderma pigmentosum, respectively, are also more susceptible to NMSC development.

Pathogenesis

BCC is a cutaneous malignant proliferation which is derived from basaloid cells. Basal cell carcinomas grow slowly, whereby the doubling time is 6–12 months. Individuals presenting with a BCC are at increased risk of having more lesions at the time of diagnosis and a 3-year cumulative risk for a second primary of 44% (10-fold increase over the general population).[4] They can be locally invasive, involving subcutaneous tissue, muscle, and bone (Figs. 9.2 and 9.3). Micronodular, morpheaform or infiltrative BCCs are more likely to recur after treatment. Long-term follow-up and annual skin examinations are warranted in those with a history of BCC, as they are also at an increased risk of developing other skin cancers. BCCs exhibit stromal dependence where tumor cells cannot engraft elsewhere without being transplanted along with adjacent stromal cells. Correspondingly, the incidence of metastasis is reported to be less than 0.55% and is associated with larger primary tumor size, greater depth of invasion, previous irradiation and central facial position rather than tumor subtype. When metastasis occurs, lymph nodes and lungs are the most commonly involved. Since 1981, 238 cases of metastatic BCC have been reported, most of which occurred in middle-aged men with an average tumor size of 7.5 cm and a median time of 9 years between primary tumor and first sign of metastasis.[5] Once metastasis does occur, the median survival is 10 months.

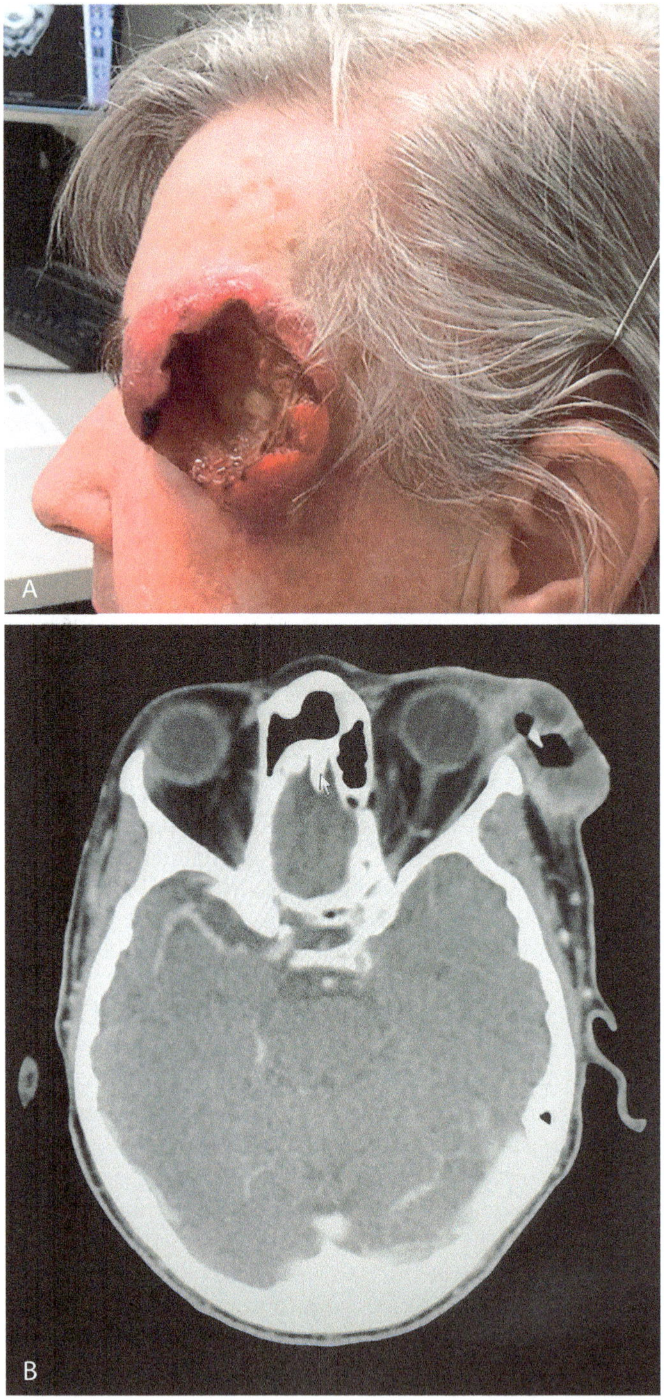

• **Fig. 9.2** (A) Local invasiveness of BCC of the left temple. Marked central tumor necrosis, chronic discharge and loss of ipsilateral forehead wrinkling consistent with locally advanced BCC destroying the frontal branch of the facial nerve and underlying temporal bone. The tumor had invaded the left orbit. (B) Axial CT scan demonstrating extension of the tumor into the left orbit, necessitating orbital exenteration for removal.

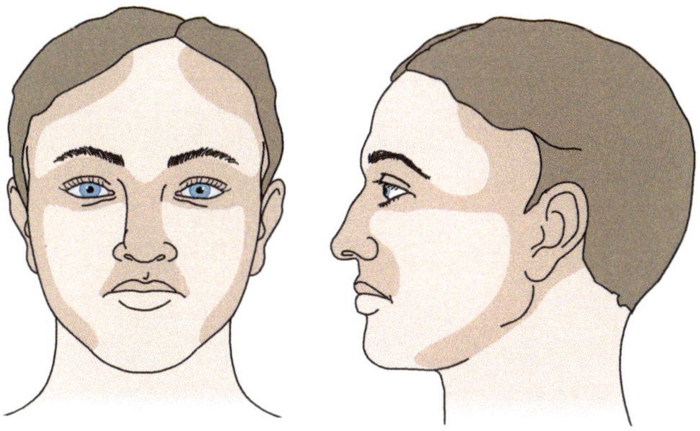

• **Fig. 9.3** High-risk zone for basal cell carcinoma. This corresponds to the regions of most benefit from Mohs micrographic surgery (MMS). It is important to note the involvement of skin near the hairline on the forehead and the region near the lateral jawline as these are distinct from the high-risk areas for cutaneous SCC (shown in Fig. 9.9), where there is relative forehead sparing but involvement of the lower lip and chin.

Clinical Presentation and Classification

BCCs usually present on sun-exposed areas, such as the head and neck, however they can occur in more occult photo-protected sites, particularly in the immunosuppressed. Due to its prevalence, multiple BCC classification systems have been developed, however a clinicopathological method is the most common in clinical use.

Commonly described subtypes include: superficial; nodular; micronodular; morpheaform/desmoplastic; infiltrating; pigmented and mixed (Table 9.1). A more simple, management-oriented approach is to classify BCCs as either discrete or diffuse, referring directly to how easy it is to judge their margins. This approach groups poorly circumscribed lesions (e.g., micronodular, morpheaform, infiltrative) on the basis that wider margins of excision are necessary to achieve clearance when compared with discrete lesions (such as superficial and nodular types). The anatomic location of BCCs may also favor the development of a particular subtype.

TABLE 9.1 Clinical and Histopathological Findings of BCC Subtypes

Subtype	Clinical Features	Histopathological Features
Superficial	Typically appear on the trunk as single or multiple well-defined erythematous finely-scaled patches or plaques with pearly rolled edges	Multifocal nests of atypical basiloid cells arising from basal layer of epidermis. These remain confined to the papillary dermis
Nodular	Typically a pearly papule or nodule with raised, rolled edges and telangiectasia. To assess: put lesion under tension to demonstrate pearling and then release to show refilling of telangiectasia. Ulceration occasionally present	Discrete nests of malignant basiloid cells in the dermis. Peripheral palisading. Mucoid stroma containing plump spindle cells
Micronodular	Multiple erythematous macule or thin papule/plaques most commonly found on the back. Nodules do not appear to be contiguous	Multiple small basaloid nests within the dermis. Individual nests are part of a complex network of intercommunicating tumor processes. May exhibit infiltration into surrounding tissues
Morpheaform/ Desmoplastic	Appear as depressed, scar-like, ill-defined, indurated plaques often with focal penetration of tissues. Direct perineural invasion can occur	Thin strands of basiloid cells surrounded by a sclerotic collagenous stroma
Infiltrative	Similar clinically to morpheaform subtype as are clinically diffuse, indurated and poorly defined. Can resemble a skin reaction or scar presenting as a depressed whitish plaque most commonly on upper trunk and face	Demonstrate nests and cords of tumor invading the surrounding tissues. Unlike morpheaform there is minimal to absent desmoplastic stromal response (the surrounding tissues can look relatively bland)
Pigmented	Pigmented variants of the other subtypes, including nodular, micronodular, multifocal and superficial BCC. Difficult to differentiate from seborrheic keratosis and malignant melanoma. The color varies from dark brown to black	Nests of basaloid cells, with an abundance of melanin and melanophages, and a moderate inflammatory infiltrate
Infundibulocystic	Well-defined pearly papule commonly on the head and neck	Anastomosing strands of basaloid cells with multiple infundibulum-like cystic structures
Basisquamous	Uncommon and unusual tumor that shares features of both basal cell and squamous cell carcinoma. Distinguished from BCC by their potential for metastasis and therefore clinically should be managed as though they are a SCC	Well-defined nodular or superficial BCC component overlying an invasive front showing BCC and SCC histological features

BCC, Basal cell carcinoma; SCC, squamous cell carcinoma.

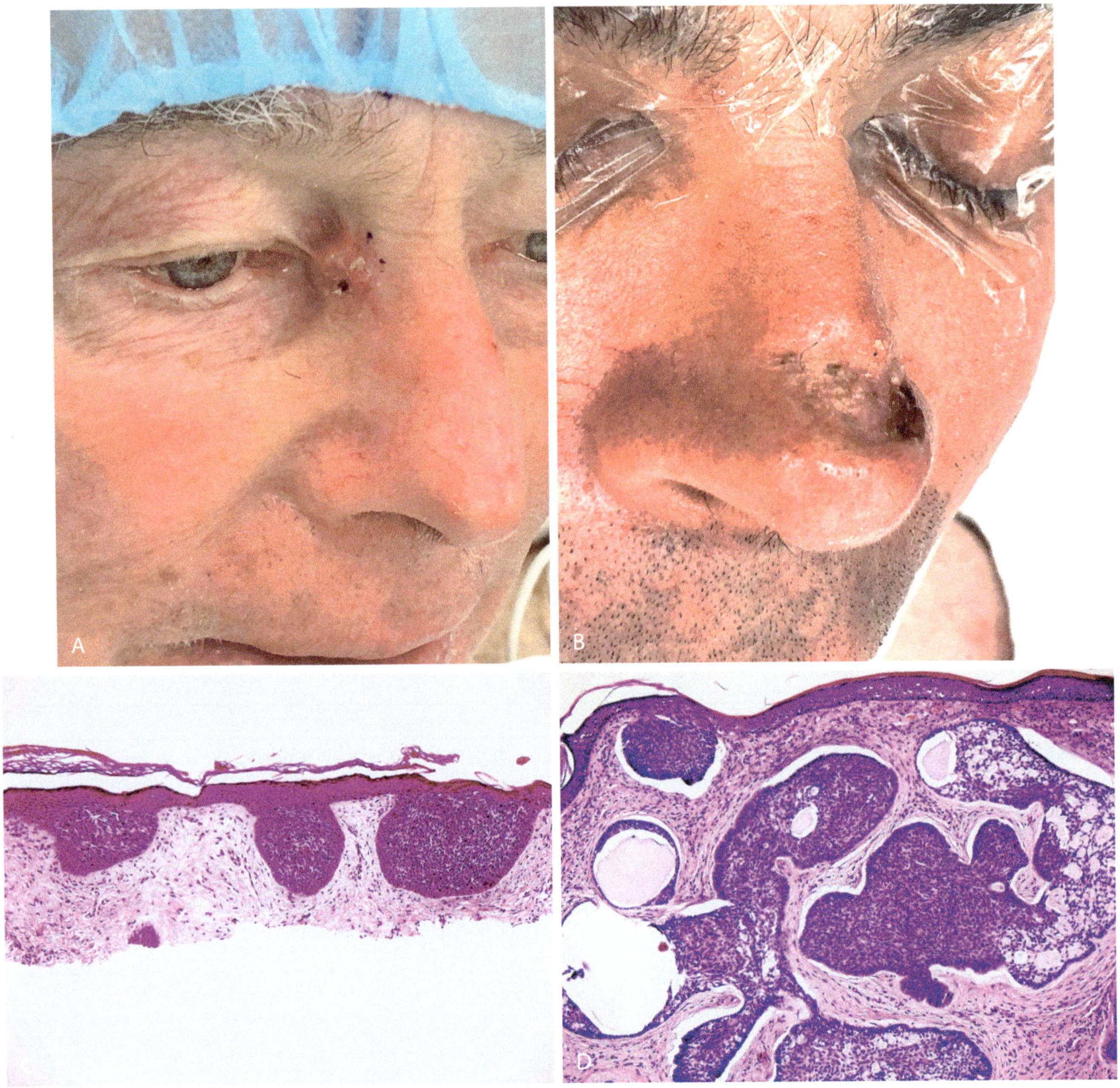

• **Fig. 9.4** (A) Superficial BCC near the right inner canthus. (B) An ulcerated nodular BCC on the nose demonstrating classic pearling and telangiectasia around an area of central ulceration. (C) Representative histopathology specimen for superficial BCC-small islets of basaloid tumor cells with peripheral palisading. Nests are well circumscribed and have effaced the dermo-epidermal junction without invading the papillary dermis. (D) Representative histopathology specimen for nodular BCC demonstrating islands of basaloid cells with peripheral palisading and peri-nest clefting from the surrounding specialized stroma (an artifact of processing). Note the relative basophilia of the tumor compared to the surrounding stroma. (C, D, Courtesy Dr. Alistair Robson, Consultant Dermatopathologist, St. John's Institute of Dermatology, London, UK.)

Diagnosis and Staging

Dermoscopy

Dermoscopy aids with evaluation of pigmented cutaneous lesions and can be used to help differentiate pigmented BCC from melanoma. Typical findings of BCC on dermoscopy include the absence of a pigment network and at least one of the following: ulceration, multiple blue-gray globules, leaf-like areas, arborizing vessels, large blue-gray ovoid nests, and spoke wheel areas.

Biopsy

Definitive diagnosis is made on histology following a punch, shave or excisional biopsy of the lesion. Histology of superficial BCC (Fig. 9.4C) usually reveals a basophilic tumor (blue) on standard hematoxylin and eosin staining. Buds of basaloid cells extend from the epidermal basal layer into the reticular dermis. Nodular BCCs (Fig. 9.4D) have nests of large basaloid cells with peripheral palisading in the papillary or reticular dermis. They may demonstrate peri-nest

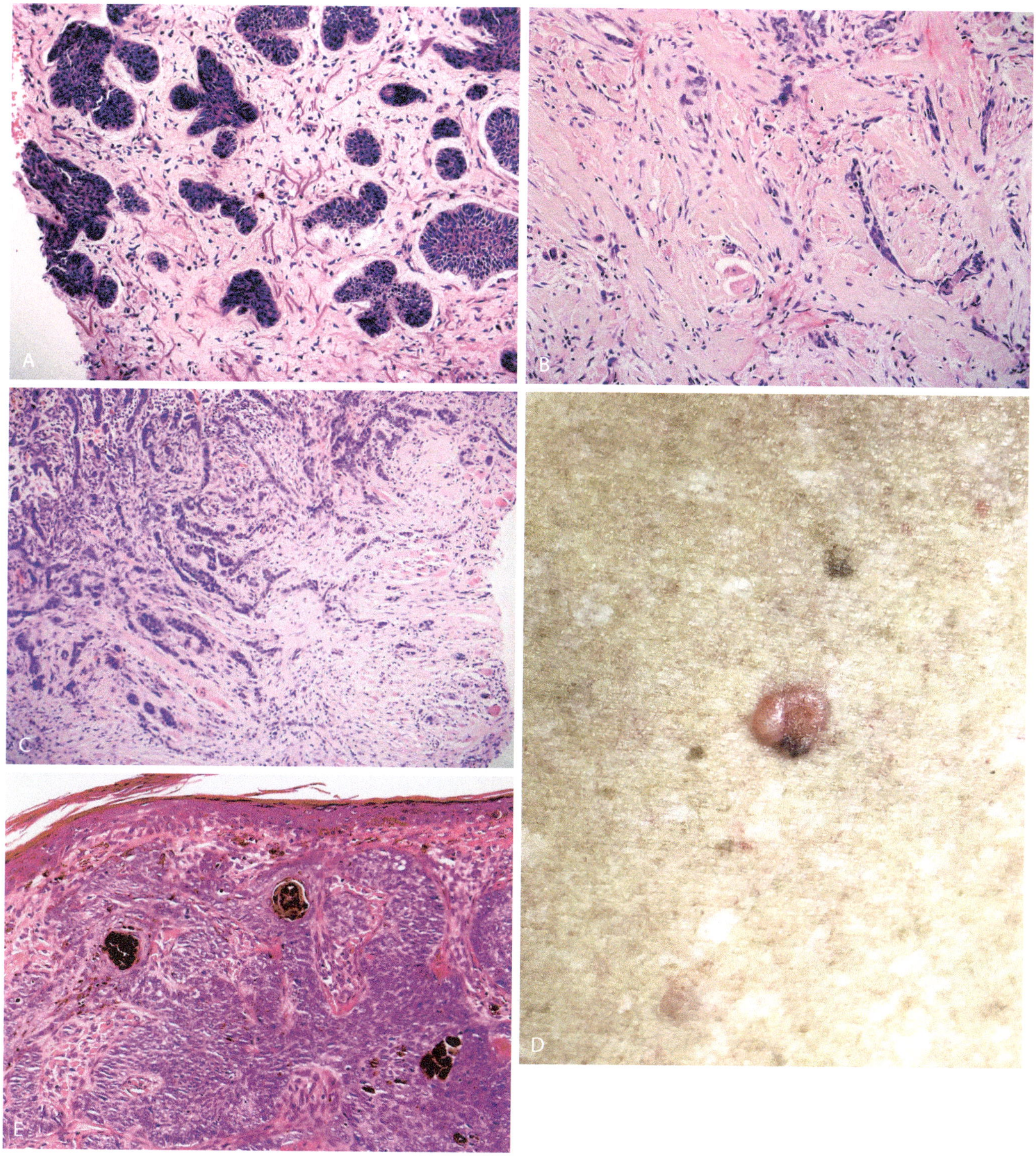

• **Fig. 9.5** (A) Representative histopathology specimens for a micronodular BCC: uniformly small nests of neoplastic basal cells with rounded peripheral contours extending widely throughout the dermis with surrounding specialized stroma. (B) Morpheaform BCC: strands of basaloid tumor cells extending deeply into the dermis embedded with a dense fibrous stroma. (C) Infiltrative BCC: long, thin strands of basaloid tumor cells penetrate deeply among the collagen fascicles. (D) A nodular BCC in the central field demonstrating a region of pigmentation that could easily be misdiagnosed as melanoma. (E) Pigmented BCC: numerous melanocytes are present amongst the basaloid tumor nests and there are occasional melanophages within the stroma. (A, B, C, E, Courtesy Dr. Alistair Robson, Consultant Dermatopathologist, St. John's Institute of Dermatology, London, UK.)

clefting consistent with retraction from surrounding stroma but this is usually a processing artifact. Micronodular BCC (Fig. 9.5A) is composed of multiple microscopic nodules smaller than 15 μm making it difficult to interpret tumor clearance when there are close margins. Tumors become infiltrative (Fig. 9.5C) when basaloid islands lose their epidermal connections and invade the underlying dermis, often as sheets or finger-like projections of tumor cells without much stromal reaction. In contrast, morpheaform BCC (Fig. 9.5B) consists of strands of tumor cells extending deeply into the dermis embedded within a dense fibrous stroma. Pigmented BCCs (Fig. 9.5E) have similar histology to the nodular subtype with numerous melanocytes among the tumor nests and melanophages in the stroma

Staging: TNM and Imaging

See below under Squamous Cell Carcinoma.

Management

Complete surgical excision with pathology confirmation remains the gold standard in the management of basal cell carcinoma. Their abundance in clinical practice, slow doubling time, stromal dependence, and significant rates of spontaneous regression (most studies demonstrate at least some degree of regression in around 20% of lesions[6]) have prompted the development of numerous treatment options, each with their relative merits. However, their potential to display a mixed clinicopathologic picture, variability in aggressiveness based on type, site, and patient factors and the fact that recurrent BCCs tend to demonstrate poorer prognosis, should prompt management based on the most effective modality in the individual to achieve complete removal or destruction of the tumor. As a result, treatment varies depending on anatomical location, BCC subtype, tumor size, depth of invasion, and patient co-morbidities (Table 9.2).

Nonoperative Management

Topical Therapies

Topical therapies provide a minimally invasive approach to BCC management in specific contexts. The success of this mode of therapy centers on the ability of the topical agent to reach the tumor in its entirety, the tumor response, and the compliance of the patient.

Cryotherapy utilizes liquid nitrogen to destroy superficial basal cell carcinomas. It requires a minimum of two freeze–thaw cycles achieving temperatures of −50°C to destroy the tumor with treatment of a margin of normal tissue to ensure destruction of subclinical extension. This method lacks histological tumor confirmation but cure rates are reported to be over 95%. Care must be taken when treating BCCs near the eye. Adverse outcomes include scarring, hypo- or hyperpigmentation and the possibility of obscuring tumor recurrence by scar tissue. Some have reported greater patient satisfaction with surgical excision compared to cryotherapy due to the superior cosmetic result.

Imiquimod 5% cream is an immune response modifier that increases the T-helper response by inducing interferon-α, tumor necrosis factor-α, and cytokines to destroy dysplastic keratinocytes by acting on Toll-like receptor 7 (TLR7). Although it is only FDA-approved for biopsy-confirmed nonfacial superficial BCCs <2 cm in size, some have shown efficacy in the treatment of nodular BCCs. However, care should be taken with off-label treatment due to reports of recurrences with increased subclinical extension due to

TABLE 9.2 Treatment Options for Basal Cell Carcinoma

Treatment Modality	Indication
Topical Cryotherapy Imiquimod[a] 5-Fluorouracil[a]	Small superficial BCC Biopsy-confirmed nonfacial superficial BCC <2 cm Nonfacial superficial BCC <2 cm
Oral Vismodegib	Locally advanced and metastatic BCC Neoadjuvant use prior to surgery to reduce surgical defect size of all subtypes
Photodynamic therapy	Multiple superficial or thin nodular BCCs
Radiotherapy	Primary BCCs in those unwilling or unable to undergo surgery; adjuvant therapy post-surgery for remaining positive margins
Operative standard excision	Workhorse. Surgical management of BCC, useful for all tumor types in all areas but clearest benefits in nonaggressive primary BCCs in non-high-risk locations
MMS	"Gold standard." Selective application: primary facial morpheaform or infiltrative BCC; recurrent BCC; any BCC in a high-risk location
Electrodessication and curettage	Nonaggressive primary BCCs <3 cm in low-risk locations; unable or unwilling to tolerate surgery
Pulsed dye laser[b]	Superficial and nodular BCCs <1.5 cm

BCC, Basal cell carcinoma; SCC, squamous cell carcinoma.
[a]Can be tried for the off-label use of small nodular BCC.
[b]Long-term follow-up outcomes still awaited.

selective clearing of superficial tumor. Furthermore, there is significant genetic variation in Toll-like receptors between individuals, with some individuals being unable to respond to imiquimod therapy as a result. Adverse reactions include local skin irritation (the severity may or may not correlate with histological clearance) and hence it should not be applied near the eye. 5-Fluorouracil has also been used for superficial and nodular BCCs. A systematic review found clearance rates of up to 90% for superficial BCCs. However, adverse reactions of erythema, pruritus, and pain limit its use. Imiquimod and 5-fluorouracil treatment should be restricted to small tumors in low-risk locations in patients who will not or cannot undergo treatment with more-established therapies of known long-term clearance rates.[7]

Oral Therapy

The FDA-approved oral Hedgehog pathway inhibitor vismodegib has shown efficacy in the treatment of locally advanced and metastatic BCCs[8] and in reducing the size of existing BCCs and development of new BCCs in those with BCNS.[9] The recent VISMONEO study[10] demonstrated its potential as a neoadjuvant therapy to reduce tumor size or provide a complete response (>50%) prior to surgery for inoperable (or functionally-inoperable) BCCs of all histologic subtypes. However, histologic changes to the tumor with the use of this drug may result in difficulty determining clear margins during Mohs surgery. In addition, the optimal duration of neoadjuvant treatment has not yet been determined as patients underwent surgery once vismodegib-related tumor changes plateaued. Adverse effects are the main limiting factor to continued use of vismodegib, including muscle cramps, hair loss, dysgeusia, weight loss and fatigue. With drug discontinuation the adverse events resolve but tumor regrowth occurs within months. Prolonged use may result in secondary acquired resistance.

Photodynamic Therapy

Photodynamic therapy (PDT) involves the topical application of a photosensitizing agent to the desired treatment area with subsequent activation of the drug by visible light to create reactive oxygen species which destroy neoplastic cells. Topical δ-aminolevulinic acid or methylaminolevulinate produce the photosensitizer protoporphyrin IX semi-selectively within tumor cells. In 2005, an international consensus on the use of PDT for NMSC recommended it as first-line treatment for superficial BCC. It is less effective in nodular BCC subtypes due to the thickness of the tumor limiting absorption of the topical medication into the dermis.[11] Although studies have demonstrated superior cosmetic outcomes of PDT compared to surgical excision, some tumors do not respond to treatment and it is associated with higher recurrence rates than surgery with long-term cure rates for superficial BCC of approximately 75%. Adverse reactions include erythema and pain. The inconvenience of multiple hospital visits makes it unsuitable for some patients. PDT should generally be reserved for those with tumors not amenable to other established-treatment methods or for those with multiple BCCs, such as BCNS patients.

Radiotherapy

Radiation therapy can be used for primary BCCs in those unwilling or unable to undergo surgery or as an adjuvant therapy post surgery for remaining positive margins. Control rates of over 90% have been reported, although there may be potential for aggressive recurrences post treatment. Disadvantages include lack of histologic verification of tumor removal, prolonged treatment course and poor cosmetic outcomes. Radiotherapy is contraindicated in patients with BCNS or xeroderma pigmentosum, as ionizing radiation can induce development of new BCCs within the radiation field.

Operative Management

Significant debate remains as to the most appropriate definitive treatment modality for BCC, especially whether standard surgical excision or Mohs micrographic surgery (MMS) is the most appropriate definitive surgical treatment. The two modalities use different processing techniques to determine margins, which can make direct comparison difficult. Compounding this in the literature is the variable use of clinical versus pathological margins, lack of direct comparison between these modalities in clinical trials and a paucity of appropriate outcome measures and suitable long-term follow-up. One example is the use of incomplete excision to suggest MMS provides better outcomes. Incomplete excision is an uncommon outcome following standard surgical excision using an appropriate margin. In specific instances, further resection may be halted and the defect dressed or skin grafted for definitive reconstruction once surgical clearance has been confirmed, referred to as a delayed reconstruction after pathology evaluation, or DRAPE procedure.[12] This minimizes the loss of important anatomical structures and has been referred to as "slow Mohs." If incomplete, then further resection is undertaken.

MMS provides the benefit of being able to undertake multiple cycles of resection and microscopic evaluation in real time, but the number of cycles is not generally included in statistics for comparison. While DRAPE procedures may be inconvenient for the patient, this approach provides excellent, cost-effective clearance while preserving important structures to aid the postoperative outcome and retains the histology blocks and sections for future review and additional tests such as immunohistochemistry should an atypical tumor be identified.

Standard Surgical Excision

Surgical excision for basal cell carcinoma produces cure rates in excess of 90%. A meta-analysis (89 studies and 16,000 lesions) identified that a 3-mm clinical margin for non-morpheaform BCC resulted in a cure rate of over 95% for lesions <2 cm in diameter. Incomplete excision in this study was associated with a 27% recurrence rate. While this is somewhat high, incompletely excised lesions often do not show any additional tumor on re-excision and such re-excision usually results in cure in this rarely metastatic tumor. Standard surgical excision is one of the most widely used and reliable approaches to achieve definitive tumor excision with confirmatory histopathology in a relatively cost-effective manner. However, incomplete excision rates for aggressive subtype primary BCCs or recurrent BCCs have been shown to be higher with this method compared to MMS, with over 10% incomplete excision rates in some reported studies. While this may reflect the clinical practice of staged excision/DRAPE, proponents of MMS correctly identify the capacity of MMS to produce equivalent or higher cure rates in a single visit. A wider radial margin (4–5 mm) is typically used for diffuse lesions up to 2 cm in diameter for this reason. This wider margin may increase the defect size relative to MMS with potential significance for esthetically or functionally sensitive areas such as in the central face. Reconstruction of these areas is commonly undertaken as esthetic units for improved postoperative appearance with

MMS demonstrating benefit if the excision can be contained within a specific subunit. Standard surgical excision remains the workhorse for definitive BCC excision and is one of the most cost-effective means to manage the millions of BCCs that occur worldwide every year.

Mohs Micrographic Surgery (MMS)

MMS is considered by many as the gold standard in BCC removal by providing equal or higher rates of tumor clearance when compared with other modalities. MMS involves histological analysis of tissue margins and therefore provides tumor clearance with maximal tissue conservation in areas of high risk for recurrence (periorbital, periauricular, and central face, see Fig. 9.3), resulting in smaller surgical defects compared to standard surgical excision. Five-year recurrence rates for primary and recurrent BCCs treated by MMS are approximately 1%–2% and 4–7%, respectively. Therefore it is especially useful for primary facial BCCs with aggressive clinicopathologic subtypes (morpheaform or infiltrative), recurrent facial BCCs and any BCC in a high-risk location. The use of MMS to treat the majority of BCCs is probably inappropriate however. The process can be lengthy for the patient and the Mohs practitioner as a number of cycles of excision, processing, and interpretation may be necessary to achieve clearance. The histology slides and blocks are not retained for subsequent review and this can be particularly problematic when an atypical tumor is identified within the lesion, thereby making diagnosis of the mixed tumor difficult. From a health economics perspective, MMS is significantly more expensive than standard excision and for nonrecurrent disease it has not been shown to produce better 5-year outcomes.[13] For these practical reasons, MMS is applied selectively in centers that offer it as a treatment modality. It is likely that formalized criteria for its use will be required into the future as populations age, rates of NMSC increase, and health budgets become tighter.

Electrodessication and Curettage

Electrodessication and curettage is an efficacious and cost-effective treatment modality, however, it is operator-dependent. Its use should be limited to small (<3 cm) non-morpheaform primary BCCs in low–moderate risk locations. Larger (>2 cm) and more aggressive tumors are associated with lower clearance (84%), when compared with the excellent clearance rate (98%) achieved in tumors <1 cm.

Pulsed Dye Laser

Pulsed dye laser (PDL) 595 nm has shown some efficacy for superficial and nodular BCCs. It targets the vascular network of these tumors leading to size reduction and complete regression in some cases. Clearance rates up to 90% with four treatments have been reported for small superficial and nodular BCCs (<1.5 cm). Cure rates were lower with larger tumors. The use of larger spot sizes and double-stacked pulses may allow single treatments to clear BCCs[14] but only a limited number of studies have been performed and the long-term effectiveness is unclear. Adverse events include hypopigmentation and scarring.

Squamous Cell Carcinoma

Epidemiology

Squamous cell carcinoma (SCC) is the second most common type of skin cancer, with an estimated annual incidence of 250,000 cases in the United States. It is the second most common cancer in the Caucasian population. Although less common than BCC, SCC has a greater potential for metastasis and is associated with a higher risk of mortality. Data from skin cancer studies external to national surveys have confirmed a high incidence of SCC at tropical and subtropical latitudes in Australia. According to the Cancer Council of Australia, the overall incidence rate of SCC in Australia is increasing, with an estimated 387 per 100,000 in people aged 14 years and over being affected – more than double the estimated incidence in 1985.

Risk Factors

In patients who received long-term therapy with psoralen and ultraviolet A (PUVA) for psoriasis, there is a 30-fold increased risk of NMSC, particularly SCCs. Additional risk factors include male gender, low Fitzpatrick skin type, albinism, epidermolysis bullosa, human papillomavirus (HPV) infection, smoking, previous ionizing radiotherapy treatment, chronic inflammation and irritation, and chemical carcinogens, such as arsenic and aromatic hydrocarbons. Immunosuppressed individuals, particularly organ transplant patients or those with leukemia and lymphoma, have a significantly increased risk of SCC, mainly in sun-exposed sites, with tumors typically developing 3–7 years after the onset of chronic immunosuppression. One-third of individuals with epidermodysplasia verruciformis develop SCCs due to chronic HPV infection. When SCC develops in an area of chronic inflammation and scarring, it is termed a Marjolin's ulcer. This diagnosis should be considered in any nonhealing wound as it carries a 50% risk of metastasis. SCC occurs commonly in xeroderma pigmentosum, a rare autosomal recessive genetic disorder characterized with marked hypersensitivity to ultraviolet rays appearing in early childhood. This results in a 10,000-fold increased risk of skin cancer on sun-exposed sites in this population. As such, these SCCs particularly involve the face, head, neck, and scalp.

Genetics

Increasing age and chronic UV exposure, including tanning bed use, are the most significant risk factors for SCC development, with a sharp increase in incidence over the age of 40. Approximately 90% of SCCs and over 75% of actinic keratoses have inactivation of the tumor suppressor gene *p53* secondary to UV damage. *p53* usually induces apoptosis of UV-damaged cells, thus preventing the development of dysplastic keratinocytes.

Mutational profiling of cutaneous SCC has evolved over the past decade in an effort to understand SCC biology and thus identify molecular targets for novel therapeutics. Mutations involving the family of *Ras* proto-oncogenes, which are commonly implicated in a variety of tumors, are one of the more common targets of therapy, specifically, *HRAS* and *KRAS*. Others include *TP53*, *CDKN2A*, *PIK3CA*, *MYC*, *FGFR3*, and *VHL*. Of note, the use of *Raf* inhibitors in melanoma patients has resulted in the development of cutaneous SCC with a strong association with *Ras* mutations and epidermal growth factor receptor (EGFR) mutations are present in over half of all aggressive SCC.[15]

Pathogenesis

Squamous cell carcinoma is a malignant neoplasm of suprabasal epidermal keratinocytes with full-thickness epidermal dysplasia. These may arise de novo or from precursor lesions such as actinic keratosis (AK), which have partial-thickness epidermal dysplasia. AKs are not considered to be a premalignant lesion, but rather as an important sign of UV-induced photo-damage that signals an increased risk of NMSC. Their estimated progression rate from AK to SCC is 0.025%–16% per year.

Bowen's disease is the eponymous name for squamous cell carcinoma in situ (SCCIS) and once the dysplastic keratinocytes have invaded the basement membrane, it becomes an invasive SCC. Although less common than BCCs, SCCs carry a risk of metastasis and death. Despite the rising incidence of SCC, there is a 20% reduction in mortality due to increased public awareness and more aggressive treatment of highly invasive tumors.

Clinical Presentation and Classification

Clinical Presentation

SCCs typically arise in sun-exposed sites, namely the head, neck, ears, dorsal hands, lips, and legs. The head and neck are the most common sites of occurrence for SCC in men, while the upper limbs followed by head and neck are the most common sites in females. In those with higher Fitzpatrick skin types, they may arise on both sun-exposed and protected sites. SCCs usually present as a changing solitary lesion developing from a pre-existing AK or Bowen's disease. AKs (Fig. 9.6A) appear as multiple ill-defined scaly erythematous macules, papules or plaques ranging in size from 2 mm to >2 cm, whereas Bowen's disease (Fig. 9.6B) is usually a well-defined solitary patch/plaque. Both of these precursor lesions can be confused with eczema or psoriasis, however they are typically asymptomatic and do not respond to topical steroids. The development of tenderness, increased size or scale and erosions may represent progression to SCC. In the setting of immunosuppression, multiple SCCs may develop in an eruptive fashion.

The most common appearance of an SCC is a firm, solitary, skin-colored or erythematous hyperkeratotic papule or plaque (Fig. 9.6C). It may also present as a pigmented lesion, chronic ulcer, smooth nodule, cutaneous horn or even a verrucous lesion (Figs. 9.6D and E). As the tumor progresses it invades and can become fixed to the underlying structures. Examination of regional lymph nodes is essential to exclude lymph node metastasis presenting as a nontender enlarged mass.

Genital and perianal SCC may develop in the setting of lichen sclerosus et atrophicus in both men and women. Similarly chronic evolving warty lesions in the perineal area and red velvety plaques on the penis are alternative presentations of SCC.

Keratoacanthomas (KA) (Fig. 9.6C) are rapidly growing nodules with a central keratotic crater that can increase to several centimeters within a few weeks followed by gradual spontaneous resolution. They typically arise in the sun-exposed extremities of elderly individuals. Due to the potential for local destruction and aggressive behavior they are regarded as a clinical subtype of SCC but do not metastasize and have a self-limiting course. Complete surgical excision to permit microscopic visualization of the junction between normal skin and the edge of the lesion is necessary to rule out well to moderately differentiated SCC and therefore surgical excision is usually warranted, particularly if the lesion has been present for some time at presentation.

Classification

While numerous subtypes of BCC have been described according to their microscopic appearance, they demonstrate little differences in biological behavior. Contrastingly however, SCCs demonstrate wide histopathological variability, which predict their markedly variable clinical behaviors. They range from indolent tumors with low metastatic potential, to remarkably aggressive tumors with high invasive potential. Thus, the capacity to distinguish between these variants microscopically is imperative in the clinical diagnosis and treatment of SCC, resulting in early accurate treatment of high-risk tumors and subsequent improved outcomes with a lower risk of tumor metastasis and recurrence.

Cutaneous SCC can be broadly divided into in situ and invasive disease. In situ SCC (SCCIS) or Bowen's disease has not crossed the basement membrane and therefore does not have metastatic potential. The overwhelming majority of invasive SCC (approximately 97%) are found in association with the malignant progression of an AK. Invasive SCC will frequently retain some resemblance to their precursor AK lesions, however they can be distinguished from the latter via the presence of infiltrative cells passing through the basement membrane into the dermis. Three broad histological grades of invasive disease exist based on their associated degree of nuclear atypia and keratinization:

- Well differentiated SCC: tumor cells containing only slightly enlarged, hyperchromatic nuclei with abundant amounts of cytoplasm. Often demonstrate classic hallmarks of squamous differentiation, including scaly hyperkeratosis and/or the presence of keratin horns. They are associated with very low malignant potential.

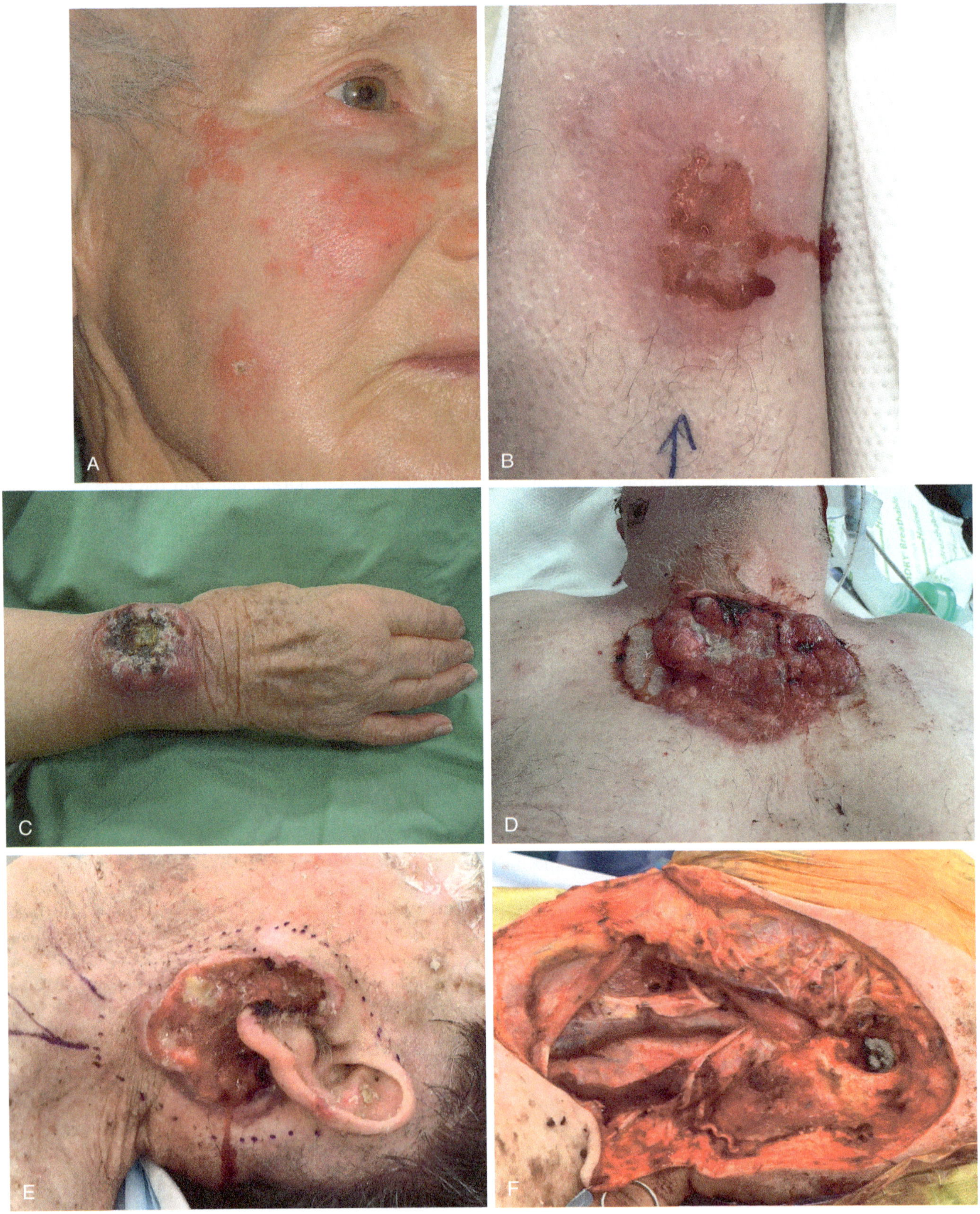

• **Fig. 9.6** (A) Actinic changes in the face of an elderly female. A crusty actinic keratosis (AK) is present on her lower cheek, Bowen's disease (SSCIS) is present over her right zygomatic arch. (B) Bowen's disease on the leg. (C) A keratoacanthoma (KA) developed quickly on the dorsum of the hand of this elderly woman that is clinically difficult to distinguish from well-to-moderately differentiated SCC. A central keratin plug is evident with surrounding elevated erythematous skin reaction. (D) Poorly differentiated squamous cell carcinoma of the upper chest showing a lack of keratosis consistent with the lack of differentiation. (E) Metastatic SCC of the scalp with ulceration involving the left parotid and upper (level 2) neck nodes demonstrating the metastatic potential of SCC. (F) The defect following surgical excision involving removal of the ear canal/middle ear, superficial parotidectomy, and modified radical neck dissection.

TABLE 9.3 High-Risk Factors for Squamous Cell Carcinoma Recurrence and Metastasis

Histological Features	Clinical Features
Poorly differentiated	Tumor size >2 cm diameter
Depth >2 mm or Clark level ≥4	Location: ear/lower lip/ temple/anogenital
Desmoplastic reaction surrounding infiltrating keratinocytes	Arising in prior scar
Perineural or intravascular invasion	Immunosuppression
	History of local recurrence

- Moderately differentiated SCC: subtype which shares features of both well differentiated and poorly differentiated tumors. Keratoacanthoma (KA) is considered to be a form of well to moderately differentiated SCC that typically occurs in the elderly
- Poorly differentiated SCC: Demonstrate greatly enlarged, pleomorphic nuclei and show a high degree of atypia and frequent mitoses with marked reduction in keratin production.

The other features used in SCC classification include size, location, lymphovascular or perineural spread and specific subtypes of SCC (see Table 9.3). Lesions under 2 cm in diameter arising within actinic keratosis or associated with human papilloma virus (HPV), that are well differentiated and do not demonstrate lymphovascular or perineural spread usually have the best prognosis amongst invasive forms of SCC. Immune suppression, anatomic location on the lower lip, the ear, temple or anogenital region or the development of invasive disease from an in situ SCC all carry a worse prognosis. Cutaneous SCC of the lower lip arises inferior to the wet–dry border of the vermilion and therefore is managed as a cutaneous SCC. SCC arising in chronic wounds and/or scars also pose a higher metastatic risk. There are a number of rarer subtypes of SCC with varying prognosis. Spindle cell SCC (if not associated with irradiation) is of lower risk. Adenoid (acantholytic) SCC poses a more intermediate risk and adenosquamous carcinoma is a higher risk tumor. Other subtypes can have varying degrees of risk, including SCC arising in adnexal cysts, clear-cell SCC, squamoid eccrine ductal carcinoma, follicular SCC, and papillary SCC.[16]

Diagnosis and Staging

Dermoscopy

On dermoscopy, SCCIS usually presents as irregular clusters of so-called "glomerular vessels" (coiled vessels) and/or globular vessels (small red clods). Nonpigmented in situ SCC can be difficult to diagnose on dermoscopy, however when compared to BCC, there is more scaling and the vascular pattern is glomerular/globular rather than branched. The hallmark of SCC is keratinization, thus white structureless areas are prevalent on dermoscopy. In well differentiated tumors, including keratoacanthoma, there may be a central area of superficial scale, horn or crust surrounded by a paler dull-white structureless zone. There may also be associated irregular groups of white perifollicular circles which are typical in SCC.[17]

Biospy

As with basal cell carcinoma, definitive diagnosis of SCC is made on histology following a punch, shave or excisional biopsy but clinical presentation with a hyperkeratotic or ulcerated lesion in actinic skin is often highly suggestive of SCC over BCC. The biopsy should be of sufficient depth to differentiate between in situ and invasive disease. For keratoacanthoma an excisional biopsy is recommended as the diagnosis depends on the overall architecture of the tumor. The presence of solar elastosis and marginal keratinocyte atypia suggests that the SCC is derived from a prior actinic lesion, whereas scar tissue may represent recurrent disease or SCC development within a prior scar. Immunohistochemical panels incorporating the cytokeratins and CD44 are often used to establish the diagnosis when lesions are poorly differentiated.

Histology usually reveals a predominantly eosinophilic (pink) tumor on standard H&E sections with a combination of normal and atypical squamous cells arranged as single cells, nests of cells or a single mass. Full thickness involvement of the epidermis indicates in situ disease (Fig. 9.7A), whereas dermal involvement represents invasive SCC (Fig. 9.7B). Subcutaneous involvement is unusual. Well differentiated tumors retain squamous features such as foci of keratinization in concentric rings of squamous cells, known as "keratin pearls." Keratin production is reduced with loss of differentiation.

Staging

The risk of recurrence and metastasis in poorly differentiated SCC is 28.6% and 32.8%, respectively, compared to that of well differentiated SCC being 13.6% and 9.2%, respectively.[18] When metastasis occurs it is usually to regional lymph nodes, and typically occurs 1–3 years following initial diagnosis and treatment. Recurrence of the primary lesion often precedes the development of metastasis. Features on histopathology associated with poorer prognosis include tumor arising in prior scar, tumor size >2 cm, depth of invasion >2 mm, desmoplastic reaction surrounding infiltrating keratinocyte islands, and perineural or intravascular involvement. High-risk sites for local recurrence and metastasis are the ear and lower lip, respectively (Table 9.3).[19]

Imaging

Imaging plays an important role in the evaluation and staging of locally advanced and metastatic BCC and SCC. Imaging is indicated if extensive disease in the form of bone or deep tissue involvement or perineurial spread is suspected; this may represent as T3, T4 or metastatic disease (Table 9.4).

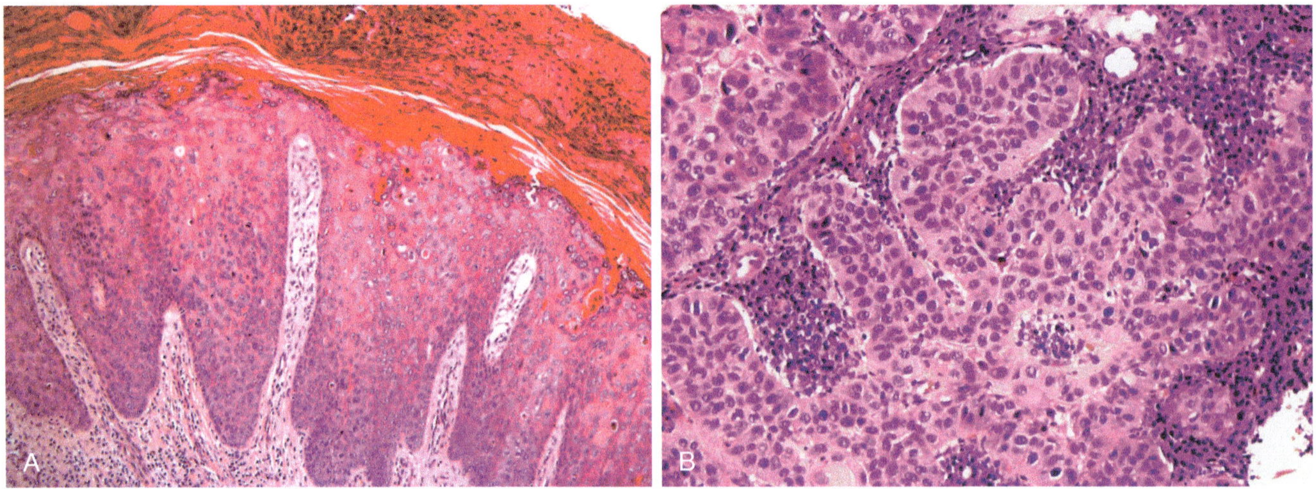

• **Fig. 9.7** Representative histopathology specimens of (A) Bowen's disease (SCCIS) demonstrating atypical cells arranged in nests or single cells involving the full thickness of the epidermis but not invading the dermis. (B) Moderately differentiated SCC with nests of atypical squamous cells infiltrating the dermis. (A, B Courtesy Dr. Alistair Robson, Consultant Dermatopathologist, St. John's Institute of Dermatology, London, UK.)

TABLE 9.4 Staging for Cutaneous Carcinomas

Component Grade	Tumor (T0–4)	Lymph Nodes (LN) (N0–3)[a]	Metastasis (M0–1)
0	No evidence of primary tumor	No spread to LN	No distant metastases
is	Carcinoma in situ (confined to the epidermis)		
1	≤2 cm in longest diameter	Spread to 1 ipsilateral LN and is ≤3 cm in diameter	Distant metastases
2	Tumor >2 cm but ≤4 cm in longest diameter	Spread to (a) 1 ipsilateral LN and is >3 cm but ≤6 cm in diameter and ECE(−) *or* (b) >1 ipsilateral LN, ≤6 cm in diameter and ENE(−) *or* (c) bilateral or contralateral LN ≤6 cm in diameter ENE(−)	
3	Tumor >4 cm in longest diameter or minor bone erosion or perineural invasion or deep invasion	Spread to (a) any LN >6 cm in diameter and ENE(−) *or* (b) any node with clinically overt ENE(+)	
4	Tumor with gross cortical or marrow invasion (T4a) or skull base or skull base foramen involvement (T4b)		

[a]NX is used where regional lymph nodes cannot be assessed. ENE, extranodal extension.

CT and CT/PET are both widely used in providing a baseline measure of metastatic disease and can be used to determine response to treatment. MRI is the modality of choice for assessing perineural invasion and is equivalent or superior in the assessment of bone involvement. CT is better able to detect central nodal necrosis, extracapsular spread, skull-base invasion, and cartilage involvement, however MRI sensitively detects neurotropic tumors, defines tissue planes, and distinguishes dense connective tissue from muscle. Both MRI and CT are useful in preoperative planning, especially with tumors suspected of involving lymph nodes or deep structures.

Sentinel lymph node (SLN) examination allows the identification of lymph node metastasis in clinically negative nodal basins. SLN biopsy is a minimally invasive staging procedure that may be used in identifying occult regional lymph node disease in selected high-risk patients.

TNM

The American Joint Committee of Cancer, AJCC (Table 9.4) has employed the TNM classification system to stage both basal cell and squamous cell carcinomas. This system combines grades within each of the T (primary tumor), N (degree of lymph node spread), and M (presence of distant metastasis) criteria to produce a classification of disease extent. Staging is divided by anatomic site and then into clinical (c) and pathology (p) stages. The eyelid, vulva, and penis have separate classification systems to the rest of the skin due to their thinner skin and proximity to the brain, urogenital system/pelvis, and large vascular structures respectively.

Regarding cutaneous neoplasms, the clinical stage (c) is the presumed staging based upon physical examination, medical imaging, and biopsy results from the primary tumor and/or fine needle aspiration (FNA) cytology (with or without ultrasound guidance) of clinically involved nodes. Pathology staging (p) is the staging based upon the "excisional" biopsy, including nodal basins if suspected of being involved. CT scanning with contrast is the most widely used imaging modality for advanced cases of NMSC. It provides good detail about the sites and size of involved nodal groups, provides definitive evidence of bone invasion and gross perineural involvement by demonstrating widening of foramina that transmit nerves.

The key points in the AJCC staging system are that stage and T level correlate, i.e., T4 lesions correspond to stage 4 lesions, unless an N or M level upgrades the stage. Stage 1 and 2 correspond to T1 and T2 lesions, respectively, with no nodal involvement or distant metastases. Stage 3 and above indicates a T3 lesion or any nodal involvement. Stage 4 is reserved for advanced T stage (T4), advanced nodal disease (N2 or above) or any distant metastases (M1).

The stage categories are grouped together to provide the overall tumor stage:

- Stage 0: T0/is, N0, M0
- Stage I: T1, N0, M0
- Stage II: T2, N0, M0
- Stage III: T3, N0, M0 or T1 to T3, N1, M0
- Stage IV: T1 to T3, N2, M0 *or* Any T, N3, M0 *or* T4, any N, M0 *or* Any T, any N, M1

Management

Staging permits an appropriate assessment of the severity of tumor invasion and also dictates whether a multidisciplinary team approach is necessary. Advanced skin cancers can present complex management and ongoing surveillance challenges that may necessitate a team approach. Luckily, the vast majority of cutaneous SCCs are low grade at the time of diagnosis. In general, those with in situ disease or circumstances that prevent definitive excision may be treated with topical therapies, whereas more invasive disease warrants surgical excision. The treatment of SCCs depends largely on the assessment of risk of tumor recurrence or metastasis (Table 9.5). Nonsurgical treatments can also be used as a neoadjuvant to reduce tumor size prior to definitive surgical excision. Close follow-up is necessary for all patients, as those who develop recurrence typically do so within 2 years of initial treatment.

TABLE 9.5 Treatment Options for Squamous Cell Carcinoma

Treatment Modality	Ideal Indication
Topical Cryotherapy Imiquimod 5-Fluorouracil Diclofenac[a]	SCCIS
Oral Capecitabine, cetuximab, erlotinib, gefitinib, interferon	Reduce incidence of SCC in organ transplant patients Locally advanced and metastatic BCC; neoadjuvant use prior to surgery to reduce surgical defect size of all subtypes
Photodynamic therapy	SCCIS
Radiotherapy	Primary SCCs in those unwilling or unable to undergo surgery; adjuvant therapy post-surgery for high-risk SCC; palliation; SCC of external auditory canal
Operative Standard excision MMS Electrodessication and curettage	Suitable for majority of cutaneous SCC, clearance may not be as good as MMS in high-risk SCC in head and neck High-risk SCCs in the head and neck[b] Low-risk, small (<1 cm), well differentiated primary SCCs, SCCIS

BCC, Basal cell carcinoma; SCC, squamous cell carcinoma; SCCIS, squamous cell carcinoma in situ.
[a]Long-term follow-up outcomes still awaited.
[b]High-risk: tumor diameter >1 cm, invasive (>6 mm deep) or aggressive histology, perineural, bone or muscle invasion, poorly defined clinical margins, prior site radiation or scarring, recurrent large SCC or immunosuppressed host.

Nonoperative Management

Topical Therapy

Cryotherapy is a quick and cost-effective method of treating SCCIS, with a single 30-second freeze achieving a clearance rate of 100% and a recurrence rate of 0.8% over a follow-up period of 6 months to 5 years in one large study. Overall, freeze times, number of cycles, clearance (50%–100%) and recurrence (0.8%–36.1%) rates are variable.[20] Adverse events include blistering, scarring, and hypopigmentation. This method should not be used to treat invasive SCC.

Topical imiquimod 5% cream used for SCCIS (5/week for 16 weeks) resulted in a 73% clearance rate, with no recurrence after 9 months of follow-up. 5-Fluorouracil once or twice daily demonstrated clearance in 69% and 93% of tumors after 4 weeks and 8 weeks, respectively, with a recurrence rate of 21% at 2 years.[20] Adverse events include erythema, pruritus, and pain. These agents cannot be used to treat invasive disease.

Topical diclofenac 3% gel has been approved for the treatment of actinic keratosis but only a few studies have demonstrated clearance of SCCIS lesions. Diclofenac inhibits cyclooxygenase-2, which is upregulated in NMSC lesions, therefore it inhibits angiogenesis and induces apoptosis. Further research is required to determine its long-term efficacy and optimal dosing regimen.

Oral Therapy

Capecitabine is an oral prodrug converted in the body to 5-fluorouracil (5-FU) and has demonstrated efficacy at low dose in reducing the incidence of SCC in patients with solid organ transplants. Adverse events include fatigue, nausea, gout, hand-and-foot syndrome, and poor renal function. Its optimal dosing regimen and use in non-organ transplant patients are yet to be established.

Approximately half of advanced SCCs contain epidermal growth factor receptor (EGFR) mutations, which may lead to a more aggressive phenotype. Activation of EGFR stimulates keratinocyte proliferation and leads to resistance to apoptosis. Cetuximab, a monoclonal antibody against the EGFR, is FDA approved for the treatment of recurrent or metastatic SCC of the head and neck. Additional treatments include interferon, erlotinib, and gefitinib, which have been employed with various results. These treatments may be indicated in high-risk SCCs, which may require formal staging with CT and MRI to detect perineural involvement and sentinel lymphadenectomy in cases where lymph node involvement is suspected.

Photodynamic Therapy

PDT can be used for SCCIS in patients with multiple lesions or in poor surgical candidates (either unable or unwilling to undergo surgery). Clearance rates for SCCIS range from 84% to 96%, and recurrence rates vary from 0.5% to 31%. PDT is not recommended for invasive SCC due to higher recurrence rates (up to 84% for invasive tumors) and risk of metastasis.

Radiotherapy

External beam therapy can be used for primary SCC treatment in those who are poor surgical candidates, as an adjunct treatment modality to surgery or as palliative treatment for symptomatic relief. Radiotherapy is useful in SCC because it semi-selectively targets rapidly dividing cells. Moderately to poorly differentiated (G3 and G4) tumors are often rapidly dividing and are more likely to demonstrate lymphovascular and perineural invasion and therefore radiotherapy helps control of the field and distant sites. However, when patients present late with advanced stage G1 and G2 tumors it can be challenging to treat them adequately with radiotherapy alone. Similarly, patients who do not complete their course of radiotherapy select for more radio-resistant clones within their tumors and thereby decrease the effectiveness of radiotherapy for further dosing should this be required into the future. The use of adjuvant radiotherapy in high-risk SCC reduces the risk of local recurrence and improves overall disease-free survival. Despite the risk of hearing loss, it is particularly useful for SCCs of the external auditory canal. Ionizing radiation should be avoided in those with BCNS and xeroderma pigmentosum.

Operative Management

Standard Surgical Excision

Standard excision is the most widely used treatment option for invasive SCC. A 5-mm clinical margin removes almost 95% of low-risk SCC lesions.[21] A wider margin up to 1 cm is used for more advanced lesions (e.g., >2 cm diameter, poorly differentiated SCC). DRAPE[12] is used when there is uncertainty about the margin so formal histopathology assessment is awaited (with the excision site being dressed or skin grafted) prior to formal reconstruction. In advanced cases, the additional margin can provide added safety due to the risk of missing noncontiguous/in-transit metastases or skip lesions indicative of hematogenous spread and often does not change the type of reconstruction used (as seen in Fig. 9.8).

Mohs Micrographic Surgery

Mohs surgery offers the potential to achieve complete tumor resection while preserving as much healthy tissue as possible. However, Mohs surgery is time and resource expensive, requires specialized equipment and training, and as such, is poorly suited to managing the vast majority of cutaneous SCCs in our aging populations. Case series demonstrate a lower local recurrence rate than with other modalities, with one series showing a cure rate of 92% at 4-year follow-up. MMS is considered by many to be the treatment of choice for high-risk lesions in the head and neck (Fig. 9.9), where there is an increased chance of recurrence (lip, ear, nasal tip, eyelid, nail bed, and anogenital area) but no controlled, clinical trial has been undertaken to permit direct comparison with standard surgical excision to date. Additional indications for MMS include tumor diameter >1 cm, invasive (>6 mm deep) or aggressive histology, perineural, bone or muscle invasion, poorly defined clinical margins, prior site radiation or scarring, recurrent large SCC or immunosuppressed host.

Electrodessication and Curettage

Electrodessication and curettage has been demonstrated to be as efficacious as standard surgical excision in the treatment of low-risk, small (<1 cm), well differentiated SCCs,[22] unless there is great concern over location risk and immune status. Recurrence rates vary with physician experience between 2% and 18.8% over 1 to 5 years of follow-up.

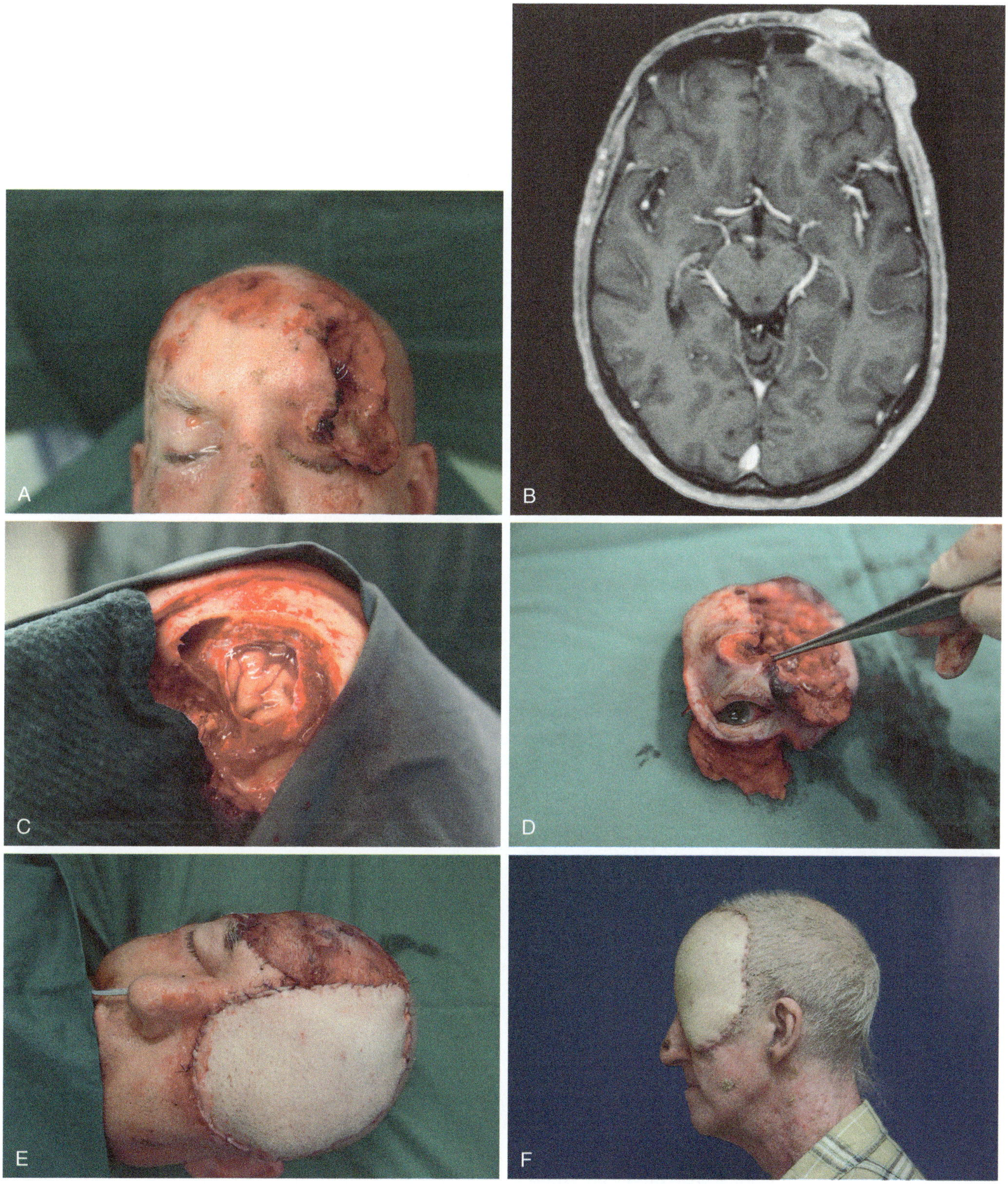

• **Fig. 9.8** (A) An advanced fungating SCC infested with maggots and invading the frontal bone and the dura of the frontal lobe of the brain. There was no systemic disease evident on imaging or clinical examination so using a multidisciplinary approach, the tumor was resected with the globe en bloc. (B) MRI demonstrates involvement of the dura over the left frontal lobe. (C) The remaining defect can be seen with exposed brain. (D) The resection specimen; the eye is evident. (E) Reconstruction performed in layers for dura through to a vertical rectus abdominus myocutaneous flap for defect coverage. (F) The patient had postoperative radiotherapy and continued to be followed up in a multidisciplinary setting (specialized nursing, ENT, neurosurgery, plastic and reconstructive surgery, radiation oncology, and opinions from specialist head and neck medical oncologists and radiologists).

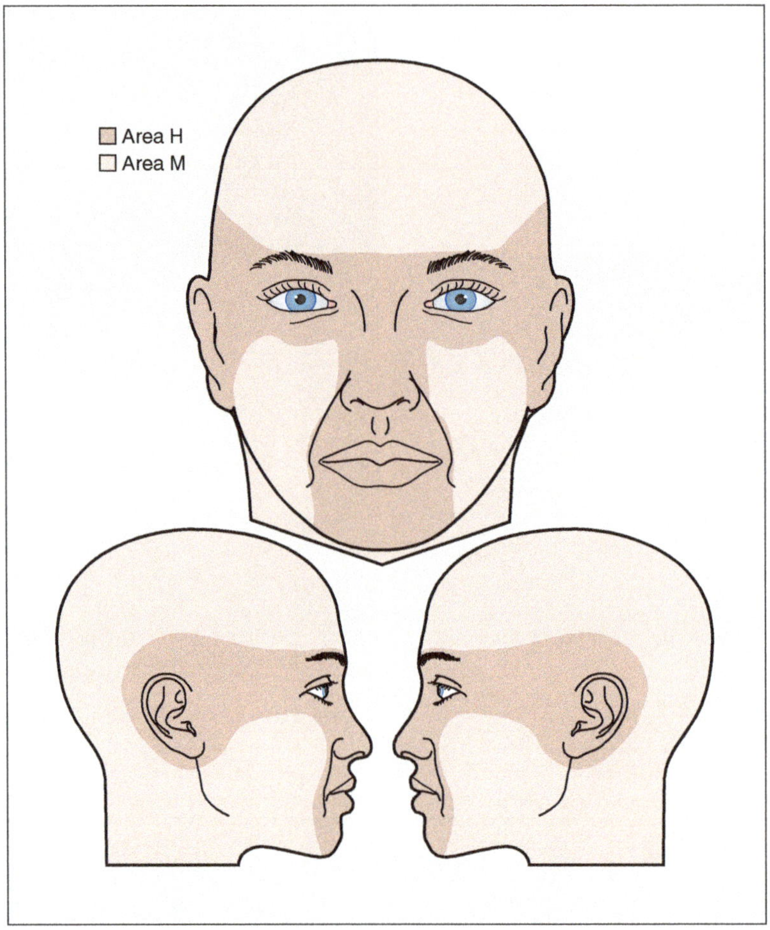

• **Fig. 9.9** High-risk zone for SCC, where MMS is most suitable. Area H represents the anatomic sites with the highest risk for recurrence and the greatest need for tissue sparing, followed by Area M. (From Lam C, Vidimos AT. Mohs micrographic surgery. In: Bolognia JL, Schaffer JV, Cerroni L, eds. *Dermatology*. 4th edn. Elsevier; 2017.)

Excision and Reconstruction, and the MDT

Appropriate management of nonmelanoma skin cancer should follow oncological principles, including the establishment of the definitive diagnosis through biopsy, adequate staging, identification of involved structures, and complete tumor clearance where this is the goal. At times curative resection is not possible, however surgical or adjunctive therapies are used to excise/reduce symptomatic tumor deposits as a "toileting" procedure. If a single treatment modality is believed to result in the most effective long-term outcome, then this modality is the treatment of choice in most cases, depending on a risk–benefit profile for the patient.

It is imperative that the individual goals of care are established and the subsequent treatment plan is tailored towards the individual prior to the initiation of any therapies. Patients in the following groups should be considered for discussion at the multidisciplinary team (MDT) to ensure appropriate work-up and treatment plans ensue[23]:

- All patients with high-risk cutaneous SCC, SCCs and BCCs that may involve the excision margins or are recurrent
- Patients suitable for Mohs surgery
- Immunocompromised patients or those with genetic predispositions who are presenting with skin cancers
- Patients with metastatic SCC or BCC diagnosed at presentation or on follow-up
- Patients who may benefit from radiotherapy
- Patients who may be eligible for entry into clinical trials
- Patients with specific management issues, such as cognitive impairment or medical comorbidities.

In the instance that surgical resection has occurred, the challenge of reconstruction remains. The principles of reconstruction center on restoring form and function (e.g., Fig. 9.8).

References

1. Stern RS. Prevalence of a history of skin cancer in 2007: results of an incidence-based model. *Arch Dermatol.* 2010;146(3):279–282.
2. Rogers HW, Weinstock MA, Harris AR, et al. Incidence estimate of nonmelanoma skin cancer in the United States, 2006. *Arch Dermatol.* 2010;146(3):283–287.

3. Griffin LL, Ali FR, Lear JT. Non-melanoma skin cancer. *Clin Med.* 2016;16(1):62–65.
4. Marcil I, Stern RS. Risk of developing a subsequent nonmelanoma skin cancer in patients with a history of nonmelanoma skin cancer: a critical review of the literature and meta-analysis. *Arch Dermatol.* 2000;136(12):1524–1530.
5. Wysong A, Aasi SZ, Tang JY. Update on metastatic basal cell carcinoma: a summary of published cases from 1981 through 2011. *JAMA Dermatol.* 2013;149(5):615–616.
6. Curson C, Weedon D. Spontaneous regression in basal cell carcinomas. *J Cutan Pathol.* 1979;6(5):432–437.
7. Love WE, Bernhard JD, Bordeaux JS. Topical imiquimod or fluorouracil therapy for basal and squamous cell carcinoma: a systematic review. *Arch Dermatol.* 2009;145(12):1431–1438.
8. Sekulic A, Migden MR, Oro AE, et al. Efficacy and safety of vismodegib in advanced basal-cell carcinoma. *N Engl J Med.* 2012;366(23):2171–2179.
9. Tang JY, Mackay-Wiggan JM, Aszterbaum M, et al. Inhibiting the hedgehog pathway in patients with the basal-cell nevus syndrome. *N Engl J Med.* 2012;366(23):2180–2188.
10. Mortier L, Bertrand N, Basset-Seguin N, et al. Vismodegib in neoadjuvant treatment of locally advanced basal cell carcinoma: first results of a multicenter, open-label, phase 2 trial (VISMONEO study). *J Clin Oncol.* 2018;36(15 Suppl):9509.
11. Arits AH, Mosterd K, Ab Essers K, et al. Photodynamic therapy versus topical imiquimod versus topical fluorouracil for treatment of superficial basal-cell carcinoma: a single blind, non-inferiority, randomised controlled trial. *Lancet Oncol.* 2013;14(7):647–654.
12. Behan FC, Rozen WM, Kwee MM, et al. Oncologic clearance with preservation of reconstructive options: literature review and the "delayed reconstruction after pathology evaluation (DRAPE)" technique. *ANZ J Surg.* 2012;82(11):780–785.
13. Smeets NW, Krekels GAM, JU O, et al. Surgical excision vs Mohs' micrographic surgery for basal-cell carcinoma of the face: randomised controlled trial. *Lancet.* 2004;364(9447):1766–1772.
14. Tran HT, Lee RA, Oganesyan G, Jiang SB. Single treatment of non-melanoma skin cancers using a pulsed-dye laser with stacked pulses. *Lasers Surg Med.* 2012;44(6):459–467.
15. Oberholzer PA, Kee D, Dziunycz P, et al. RAS mutations are associated with the development of cutaneous squamous cell tumors in patients treated with RAF inhibitors. *J Clin Oncol.* 2012;30(3):316–321.
16. Cassarino DS, Derienzo DP, Barr RJ. Cutaneous squamous cell carcinoma: a comprehensive clinicopathologic classification – part two. *J Cutan Pathol.* 2006;33(4):261–279.
17. Rosendahl C, Cameron A, Argenziano G, et al. Dermoscopy of squamous cell carcinoma and keratoacanthoma. *Arch Dermatol.* 2012;148(12):1386–1392.
18. Rowe DE, Carroll RJ, Day Jr CL. Prognostic factors for local recurrence, metastasis, and survival rates in squamous cell carcinoma of the skin, ear, and lip. Implications for treatment modality selection. *J Am Acad Dermatol.* 1992;26(6):976–990.
19. Schmults CD, Karia PS, Carter JB, Han J, Qureshi AA. Factors predictive of recurrence and death from cutaneous squamous cell carcinoma: a 10-year, single-institution cohort study. *JAMA Dermatol.* 2013;149(5):541–547.
20. Shimizu I, Cruz A, Chang KH, Dufresne RG. Treatment of squamous cell carcinoma in situ: a review. *Dermatol Surg.* 2011;37(10):1394–1411.
21. Schell AE, Russell MA, Park SS. Suggested excisional margins for cutaneous malignant lesions based on Mohs micrographic surgery. *JAMA Facial Plast Surg.* 2013;1–7.
22. Reschly MJ, Shenefelt PD. Controversies in skin surgery: electrodessication and curettage versus excision for low-risk, small, well-differentiated squamous cell carcinomas. *J Drugs Dermatol.* 2010;9(7):773–776.
23. Newlands C, Currie R, Memon A, Whitaker S, Woolford T. Non-melanomatous skin cancer: United Kingdom national multidisciplinary guidelines. *J Laryngol Otol.* 2016;130(suppl 2):S125–S132.

10

Atypical Skin Lesions

MICHAEL W. FINDLAY AND MICHAEL A. HENDERSON

Introduction

The atypical skin lesions are a diverse group of tumors that are uncommon but clinically important. They include a spectrum from benign lesions through to those that demonstrate local invasion and/or distant metastatic potential. Since these lesions are only seen infrequently during clinical practice, it is important to know the patterns associated with the more malignant of these tumors, how they may be discerned from common, benign lesions, and to understand the principles of their management so that clinically impactful mistakes are not made. For this reason, we cover some common surgically relevant lesions of the skin, including common types of cysts. We have divided the atypical lesions into benign or malignant and then by their cell/tissue of origin. Such a framework is not perfect due to our evolving understanding of the molecular and cellular bases of these tumors, but it provides a solid foundation for their study.

Benign Lesions

Benign lesions are clinically important for several reasons. They can be confused with malignant lesions, be symptomatic due to their size, appearance, location, irritation, and bleeding, or may undergo malignant transformation. Knowledge of the uncommon benign lesions can also provide a means to understand their malignant counterparts. Such knowledge is invaluable to the surgeon when examining the correlation between the clinical presentation and the histopathological diagnosis. Any discrepancy between these two should prompt the surgeon to seek clarification and/or a second opinion regarding the histopathological diagnosis. Good communication between the surgeon and the histopathologist is essential for good care.

Cysts

True cysts are defined as epithelial-lined "fluid-filled" spaces and are relatively common in clinical practice. There can be many names for various cysts, including a "wen," and often terms are incorrectly applied in general usage.

Epidermoid Cysts (Keratin Cysts)

These common cysts enlarge subcutaneously but maintain a connection to the overlying skin at their punctum. Lined by squamous epithelium, they produce soft keratin that fills the cyst with a waxy/cheesy material. Although often called sebaceous cysts, this is a misnomer as they do not contain sebum. True sebaceous cysts are uncommon, arising from the sebaceous glands. There are two types of epidermoid cyst. Epidermal inclusion cysts result from the inoculation of squamous epithelium into the dermis during trauma (e.g., body piercing). Infundibular cysts specifically arise at the infundibular portion of the hair follicle, but are otherwise clinically the same.

Management depends upon the state of the cyst at presentation. Patients typically present with cysts either as nontender lumps attached to the undersurface of the skin or when they become infected. Surgical excision in quiescence is ideal, but must include excision of the attachment to the overlying skin (the punctum) (Fig. 10.1). Significant compression can cause a release of keratin through the punctum, but this also increases the risk of infection. In infection, decompression of the cyst abscess, removal of the cyst material, and curettage of the cyst lining allows resolution of the infection and often reduces the size of the lesion down to a small scar. Curettage is associated with a significant risk of recurrence because of its inability to ensure complete removal of the lining of the cyst. Once the scar has settled appropriately, the scar, remaining cyst, and its punctum can be removed to stop recurrence. Uncommonly, they spontaneously resolve by becoming marsupialized and discharging.

Tricholemmal (Pilar) Cysts

Tricholemmal cysts are similar to epidermoid cysts except that they specifically arise from the outer root sheath of hair follicles. For this reason, they are sometimes referred to as isthmus-catagen cysts and are mobile and filled with keratin. They typically arise in the scalp as this has the highest density of hair follicles. They are usually multiple and the tendency to form tricholemmal cysts runs in families. Surgical excision is the treatment of choice and when excised with the overlying hair follicle, recurrence is unlikely. On histology, they can demonstrate areas of nuclear atypia,

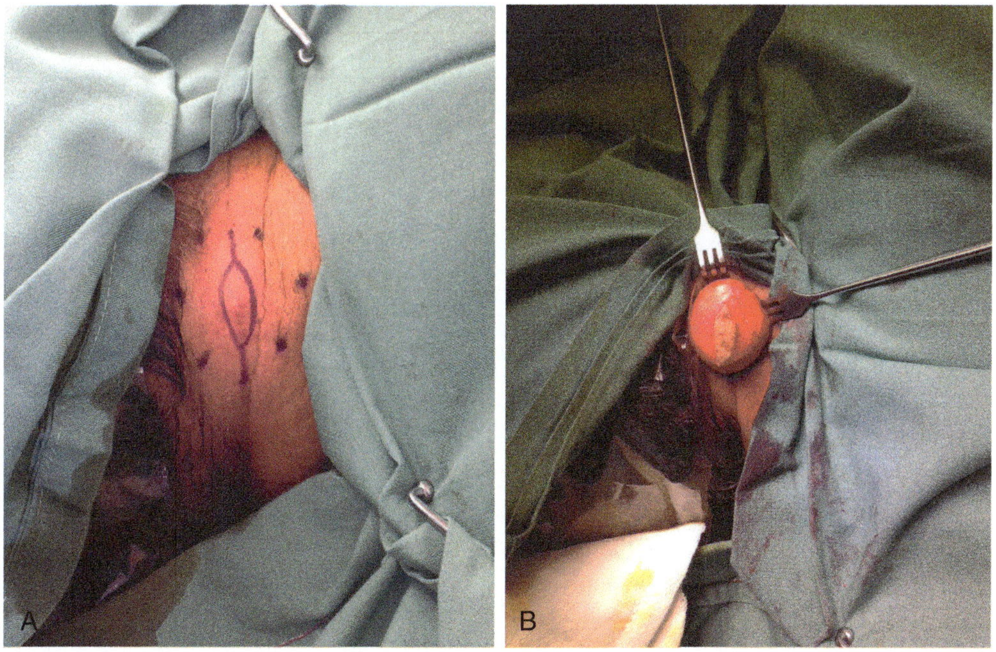

• **Fig. 10.1** (A) Epidermoid cyst of the posterior neck demonstrating a punctum where the skin communicates with the lumen of the underlying cyst. (B) Excision of the cyst with an ellipse of skin surrounding the punctum, demonstrating a very smooth cyst surface. (Photographs courtesy Michael W. Findlay, Charles Frewen, Andrew Ryan.)

mitotic figures, and dyskeratosis and therefore be confused with squamous cell carcinoma, but it is rare for them to undergo malignant transformation.

Dermoid Cysts

Dermoid cysts are hamartomas, often containing multiple epithelial derivatives (skin, hair etc.) and occasionally other tissues including fat, cartilage or bone/teeth. They are found in numerous organs and regions of the body. In the skin they are often near the midline or in the head and neck along tissue fusion planes. They can have intracranial, intraspinal, and other deep connections, including down to bone. As they are developmental in their origin and are present at birth, those with a superficial position and/or in the head and neck usually present at an early age, whereas dermoid cysts in other areas are more likely to be incidental findings or found following slow enlargement at any time in life. The key factors in their management are recognition of their potential to involve deeper structures (e.g., nasal dermoid with intracranial extension) and their potential to be associated with other conditions. Excision of the cyst with any communications to underlying structures is effective to prevent recurrence.

Benign Lesions Associated with Epidermis

Acrochorda

Acrochorda (*acrochordon* = singular) or skin tags are fibroepithelial polyps that appear as raised, smooth or irregular-surfaced pieces of skin on a small stalk called the peduncle. Nearly half of the adult population has at least one near skin creases in the neck, axilla, groin, breasts and eyelids. Shear forces of skin on skin are thought to be their underlying cause and therefore they are common in obesity. Female gender, human papilloma virus 6 and 11 and familial tendency are all thought to predispose to them. They may be symptomatic due to irritation from clothing or jewelry or when they bleed because of tractional injury. Acrochorda are usually small (2–5 mm) but occasionally larger. They are composed of a fibrovascular core and adipose tissue covered by normal skin. Numerous treatment modalities are available from ligation to cryotherapy and simple surgical removal, but the patient must be aware of the risk of further lesions.

Warts

Warts are focal (verrucous) keratinized lesions caused by human papilloma virus (HPV). The virus replicates in the stratum granulosum, inducing underlying basal keratinocytes to proliferate, causing a hyperkeratotic response. They may appear raised, flat, filiform, cauliflower or ingrown (e.g., plantar warts) and can also occur under or around the nails. Over 150 different types of HPVs have been characterized but, typically, only 1–2 strains cause each normal variant (verruca vulgaris HPV 2 and 4, cauliflower/Butcher's warts HPV 7, palmoplantar warts/myrmecia HPV 1, flat warts HPV 3 and 10).[1] These are distinct from the HPV strains associated with genital warts (HPV 6 and 8) and those producing an increased risk of intraepithelial neoplasia or invasive tumors affecting the vulva, penis, cervix or oral cavity (HPV 16 and 18).[2] Warts may be singular or multiple, with a predilection for the hands due to contact transfer. Wart infections are self-limiting and resolve once the host mounts an immune response to the virus. Surgical excision produces some release of HP virions, but topical therapies are a less invasive approach to induce an immune response.

Therapy is largely divided into management of the hyperkeratosis and induction of a suitable immune response. Hyperkeratosis management can be undertaken by multiple means, including use of salicylic acid (3%–60%, daily or twice/day), occlusive dressings, cryotherapy, and shaving by scalpel or sharp curette.

Topical therapies to promote an immune response include podophyllin (resin or toxin), formalin (3% solution), imiquimod (Aldara), retinoids such as tretinoin and 5-fluorouracil (5-FU). Podophyllin is available over the counter in most countries and can be applied without specific training. Other approaches that have been used include laser therapy, intralesional agents (bleomycin and interferon-alpha) and topical allergens or caustic agents. While usually successful, they have significant potential side effects not found with the mainstream therapies above. Patient education usually helps to avoid surgical intervention and scarring. Histologically warts demonstrate koilocytes (vacuolated cells with viral infection) and hypergranulosis with columns of parakeratosis and compact orthokeratosis. Typically, the marked hyperkeratosis and papillomatosis are associated with elongated rete ridges sloping inwards to the center of the lesion.

Malignant transformation is sometimes seen in longstanding immune suppression, but it is unclear to what degree HPV infection contributes because the patients already have increased risk of skin cancers. Epidermodysplasia verruciformis (Lewandowsky-Lutz dysplasia) is a rare autosomal recessive skin disorder that increases the susceptibility to HPV infections. These patients have a very high risk of skin cancer due to the increased risk of malignant transformation of their lesions.

Benign Lesions Associated with Hair Follicles

Pilomatrixoma

This benign appendageal tumor typically occurs in the head and neck region and demonstrates differentiation towards hair (follicular) cells. While considered tumors of children, they can occur in adults. They are associated with a mutation in the *CTNNB1* gene and while familial cases have been observed, the mode of inheritance has not yet been established. In addition to sporadic cases, they may be associated with Gardner syndrome (familial colorectal polyposis), myotonic dystrophy (especially if multiple lesions), and sarcoidosis. Pilomatrixomas present as firm nodules that are usually solitary and asymptomatic, but are occasionally associated with local pain if infected or inflamed. Usually slow-growing, they can be confused with other skin lesions, including nodular basal cell carcinoma, despite their deep position in the lower dermis or underlying adipose tissue. Lesions often contain calcium deposits that are visible on medical imaging. Pilomatrix carcinoma is well documented but very rare.

Histology demonstrates irregular islands of epithelial cells surrounded by a connective tissue capsule that produces a diffuse lesion in most cases. The epithelial cells are divided into basophilic (germinal) cells around the periphery and shadow cells (anucleated) centrally in keeping with a hair-like process. Chronic lesions have fewer basophilic cells and calcium deposits can be visualized through the use of special stains (von Kossa). The diffuse nature of most lesions leads to a greater risk of local recurrence unless a wide local excision is performed (1 cm or greater). Mohs micrographic surgery (MMS) has been trialed to minimize resection of uninvolved tissue, but its effectiveness remains unclear relative to standard surgical excision.

Trichoepithelioma

Trichoepithelioma is a tumor of the hair follicle and adnexae that is often confused with basal cell carcinoma (BCC). They typically arise as single or multiple small (<1 cm), firm round lesions on the face before or after puberty that may display pearling. The lesions form a basic hair follicle but no hair shafts and may have a different surface color depending on their site of origin. Solitary lesions are typically sporadic, but a familial (multiple) form of trichoepithelioma has been associated with mutations on chromosome16q21 (Brooke–Speigler syndrome).[3] Trichoepitheliomas are composed of nests of basophilic cells often arranged like a hair follicle but they do not display the surrounding myxoid stroma or perinest-clefting found in BCC. A desmoplastic variant commonly forms an annular shape that can be confused with BCC and has a marked desmoplastic surrounding response on histology (Fig. 10.2). Simple surgical excision of all forms without a significant margin is usually effective in preventing recurrence.

Trichofolliculoma

Trichofolliculomas arise directly from hair follicle tissue. They are uncommon small solitary nodules found around the face of adults. A central pore may express sebum and/or hair. They are thought to arise from hamartomatous rests of stem cells that show incomplete differentiation towards hair follicles as supported by the prominence of Merkel cells within the follicular epithelium in these lesions.[4] Their central follicle may have secondary or tertiary follicles and hair shafts may be present within the follicle lumen on histology, helping to distinguish them from trichoepitheliomas along with a prominent surrounding stroma. There is a sebaceous variant where the central follicle has well-differentiated sebaceous lobules emptying into it. They are considered benign with only a single case of perineural invasion ever reported.[5]

Tricholemmoma (Trichilemmoma)

Tricholemmoma is an uncommon benign tumor arising from the outer root sheath of hair follicles. It appears as a warty or smooth papule on the face and neck region, and when multiple lesions are present it is diagnostic of Cowden's syndrome (hamartomatous intestinal polyposis with multiple tricholemmoma lesions). Cowden's syndrome demonstrates autosomal dominant germline inheritance associated with mutations of the tumor suppressor gene *PTEN* (phosphatase and tensin homolog) located on chromosome 10q23.3[6] but other mutations are occasionally found (e.g., *BMPR1A*). PTEN is negative in sporadic tricholemmomas, but often

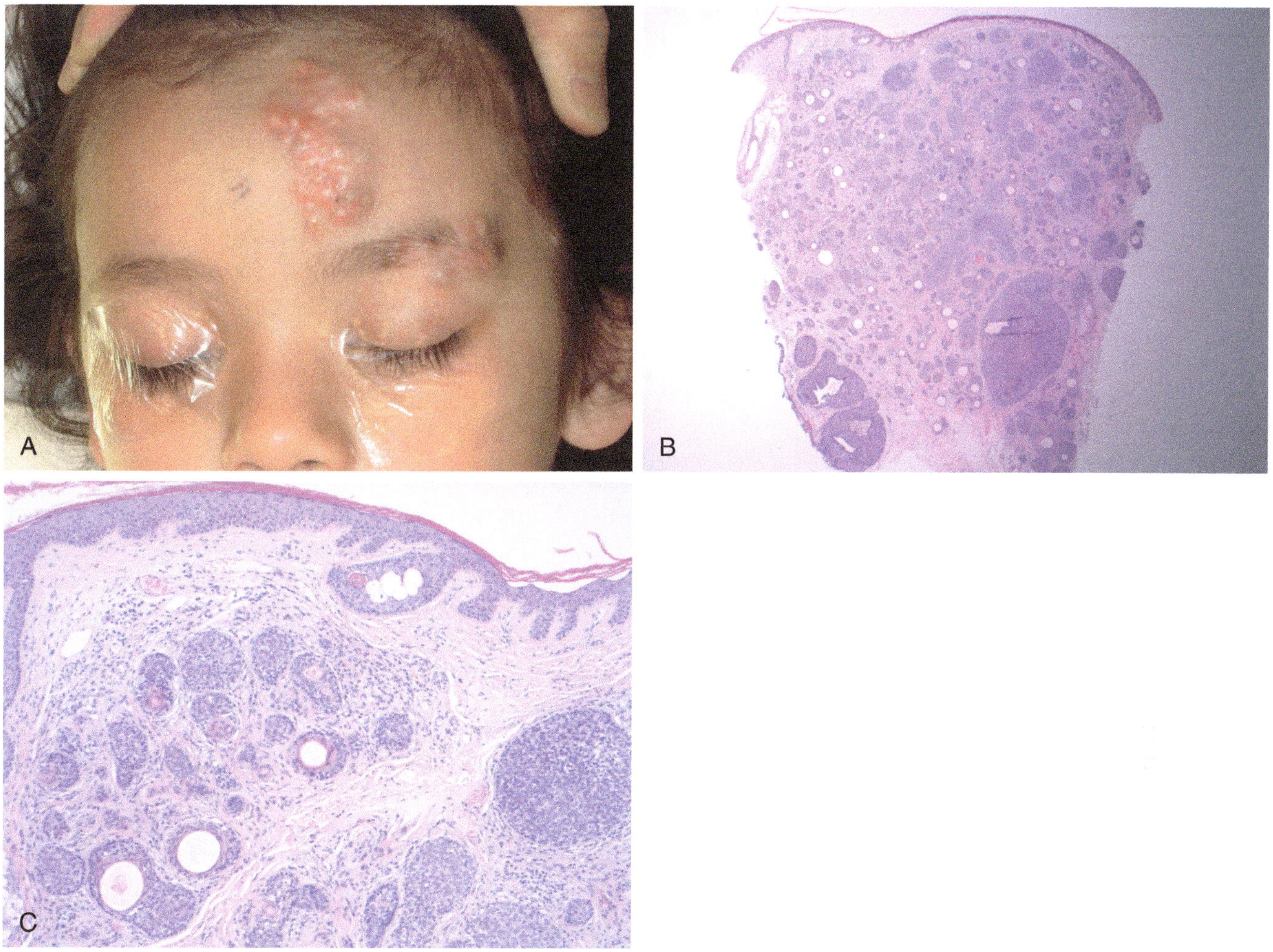

• **Fig. 10.2** (A) Six-year-old girl with multiple trichoepitheliomas within the V1 dermatome. No relatives had Brooke–Spiegler syndrome and therefore this may have been the result of a sporadic mutation. The main cluster was treated by simple excision. (B) Histopathology demonstrates nests of basaloid cells (without clefting) throughout the dermis with keratin microcysts. There is recapitulation of primitive hair bulbs, but no epidermal connection. (C) Desmoplastic trichoepithelioma demonstrating a "paisley-tie" pattern of strands and cords of basaloid cells, keratin microcysts, microcalcification, and stromal fibrosis. (Photographs courtesy Michael W. Findlay, Charles Frewen, Andrew Ryan.)

positive in Cowden's syndrome, presumably due to a loss of function mutation. On histology it appears as lobular downward growths of epidermis and is often surrounded by a hyaline band or thickened basement membrane. Clear cells or cells with prominent vacuoles are typically present (glycogen) and the lobules demonstrate peripheral palisading.

Benign Lesions Associated with Sebaceous Glands

Sebaceous Hyperplasia

Sebaceous hyperplasia is a common condition characterized by single or multiple soft small papules on the face, neck, and occasionally chest in middle-aged to elderly individuals. Most common on the forehead, nose, and cheeks, it presents with raised yellowish areas around a central follicular ostium. It can also affect the areola, penis, vulva, and oral mucosa.[7] Rhinophyma is considered by many to be a severe variant of sebaceous hyperplasia, but has closer linkages with acne rosacea. The pathophysiology relates to the effect of androgens on sebaceous glands. Androgens drive sebocyte turnover, and with advancing age androgen levels drop and sebocyte turnover slows down, resulting in over-crowding by primitive sebocytes that do not contain much sebum. As a result, the glands enlarge with a large number of immature cells. There is no malignant transformation potential, but they may be associated with skin cancer in transplant patients.[8] Sebaceous hyperplasia does not normally require any treatment, however patients may present due to esthetic concerns or because the lesions may be confused with BCC. Treatment options are manifold, including cryotherapy, photodynamic therapy, chemical peels, laser therapy (CO_2 or pulsed-dye), shave excision or formal excision, but all of these are associated with varying degrees of scarring and/or pigmentation changes. Oral retinoids (e.g., isotretinoin) have been used with some success, but sebaceous hyperplasia can recur upon cessation of therapy[9] therefore they are indicated only for severe disfiguring sebaceous hyperplasia.

Benign Sebaceous Adenoma

A benign neoplasm with a well-differentiated sebaceous pattern that presents as a slowly enlarging smooth, sometimes yellow papule with a central depression on the face and scalp. It can readily mimic BCC and is distinguishable from sebaceous hyperplasia histologically by a higher turnover of sebocytes, good differentiation of these cells, and because it is often mixed with other pilosebaceous components (e.g., hair). Benign sebaceous adenoma is the benign end of the spectrum of neoplasms involving sebaceous differentiation. Sebaceous neoplasms as a whole can show variable degrees of differentiation (from well to poorly differentiated) and a mixture of differentiation patterns based on the close proximity of the sebaceous gland with the pilosebaceous unit (hair, sebaceous, and apocrine sweat glands). Lesions can either be solitary or multiple, and when multiple may be associated with systemic conditions (e.g., Muir-Torre syndrome – internal malignancy with multiple sebaceous adenomas or sebaceous neoplasms).

Nevus Sebaceous of Jadassohn

A well-circumscribed benign congenital hamartomatous lesion presenting as a yellow to light brown velvety or papular plaque on the scalp and face of children or young adults. It was first described by Josef Jadassohn, a dermatologist, in 1895. Some lesions have a *PTCH* gene mutation, but most are considered to have a mosaic genetic abnormality. In addition to esthetic considerations, nevus sebaceous is important because it carries a risk of transformation to other tumors (approximately 24%) and can be associated with neurological phenomena as part of sebaceous nevus syndrome. Lesions may be present at birth, but typically get larger before or around puberty and malignant transformation typically does not occur in patients 10 years or younger. For these reasons, excision is considered optimal just prior to puberty (Fig. 10.3). Nevus sebaceous is relatively unique among the epidermal nevi because it often contains all skin components including epidermis, sebaceous, and apocrine glands, connective tissue and primitive hair follicles. Therefore, it is sometimes called an organoid nevus and can transform into numerous tumors both non-malignant (e.g., syringocystadenoma papilliferum, trichoblastoma or tricholemmoma) or malignant (8%–30% lifetime risk, BCC or other malignant tumors). Recent studies suggest that benign transformation is slightly more common than malignant transformation but the rates of these changes vary across studies. If a focal area of change develops within a sebaceous nevus, this should be biopsied to exclude malignant transformation and patients and their family should be advised to monitor the lesions for such changes. Rarely, patients with very large lesions can experience neurological disorders such as epilepsy. When these neurological disorders are more marked, including a combination of seizures, developmental delay, cranial nerve palsies, and/or hemiparesis and structural abnormalities of the brain, the constellation is referred to as nevus sebaceous syndrome. Nevus sebaceous is well circumscribed and therefore amenable to excision with a minimal margin and most practitioners would advise removal by teenage years or early adult life.

Benign Lesions Associated with Apocrine Glands

Hidradenoma Papilliferum

A benign cutaneous tumor derived from apocrine tissue that most commonly presents in the vulval region of middle-aged women, but can appear at extravulval sites in both sexes. Lesions appear as round, domed nodules that may ulcerate. On histology, they are identical to intraductal papillomas of the breast and therefore are considered to be ectopic breast tissue. They have a complex papillary structure showing an inner layer of PAS-positive columnar/cuboidal epithelium, a basal layer of myoepithelial cells that are S-100-positive, and a fine fibrovascular stroma.

Poroma

Benign adnexal neoplasms of epithelial cells that display ductal (usually distal) differentiation. While often described as "eccrine poromas," the majority are thought to be apocrine in origin. They present as solitary (<2 cm) skin-colored papules or nodules that may be mistaken for other lesions or develop within nevus sebaceous. They are typically asymptomatic, but can cause pain on ulceration or on the sole of the foot. Simple surgical excision is the treatment of choice because it is usually curative and provides suitable specimens for histopathology.

Benign Lesions Associated with Sweat Ducts

Syringoma

A benign adnexal tumor that typically presents as single or multiple small (<3 mm) skin or yellow colored dermal papules usually around the eyelids, penis or vulva. They affect 1% or less of the adult population and are usually the result of benign growth of eccrine sweat gland elements or eccrine differentiation of pluripotent stem cells. Four variants have been recognized[10]: (1) localized; (2) Down syndrome-associated; (3) generalized/multiple (including eruptive syringomas); and (4) familial variant.

On histology, they are a superficial dermal lesion characterized by abundant small ducts with a double-cuboidal epithelial lining and a sclerotic surrounding stroma. A PAS-positive secretion is present within the ductal lumen and the classic comma-shaped appearance of ducts on this lesion represent ducts that have elongated tails of epithelial cells upon sectioning. There are multiple management options from simple excision through electrocautery, cryotherapy, laser therapy, topical agents, topical or systemic retinoids. Simple excision with minimal margin achieves a definitive histopathology diagnosis (to exclude BCC) and can produce minimal scarring. Scar burden increases with the number of lesions present and therefore there is no perfect treatment for large numbers of lesions.

Cylindroma

Benign adnexal tumors (apocrine or mixed) that present as single or multiple lesions in the head and neck. When single, they are typically sporadic, occurring from middle age onwards as slow-growing, rubbery nodules that may

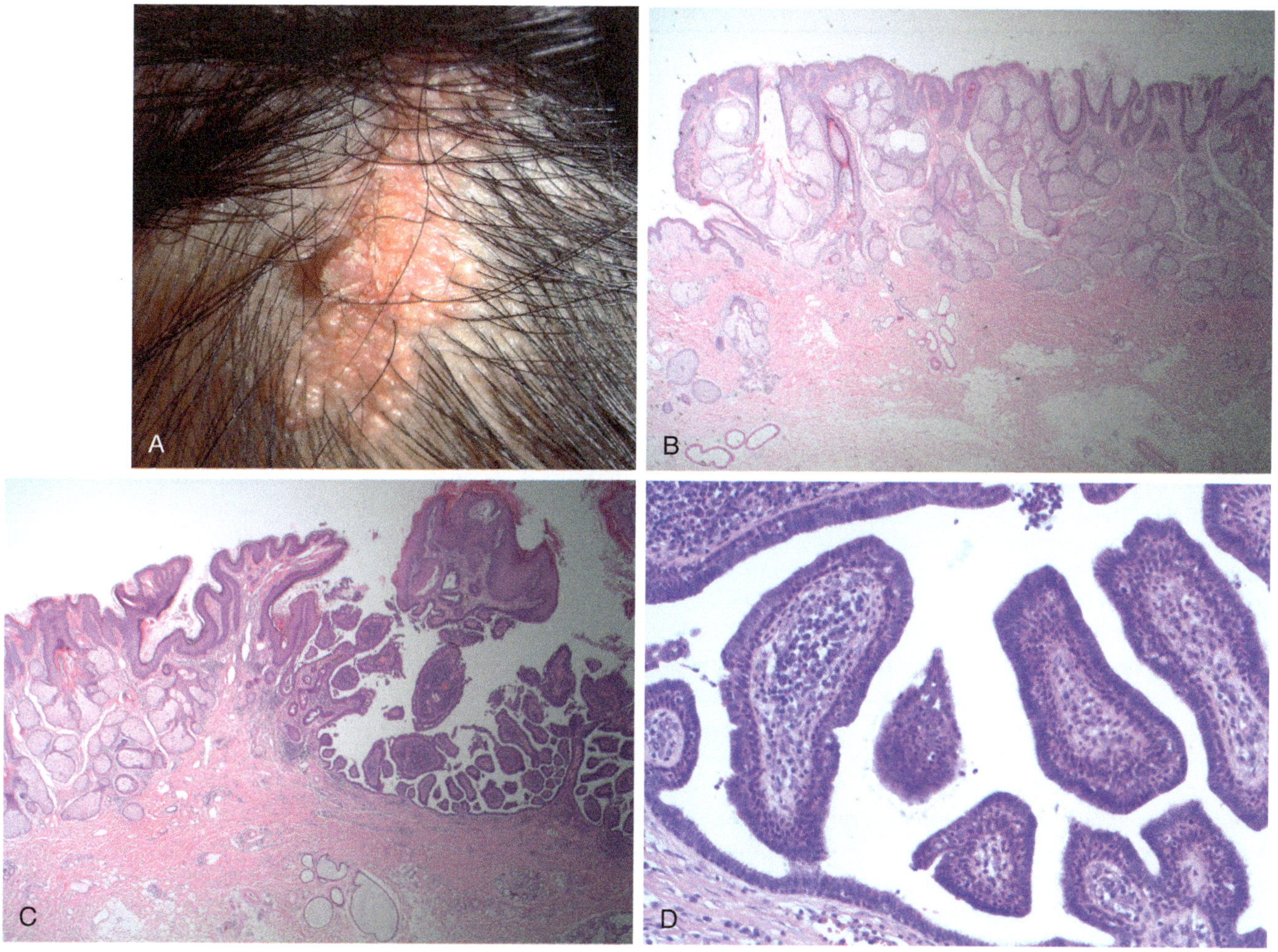

• **Fig. 10.3** (A) Nevus sebaceous on the scalp of an 11-year-old girl prior to simple excision. (B) Typical histopathology demonstrating epidermal nevus-like epidermal hyperplasia, ectopic apocrine glands in deep dermis and increased sebaceous glands associated with alopecia. (C–D) Syringocystadenoma papilliferum at the end of the same lesion (right), a benign apocrine neoplasm commonly associated with nevus sebaceous. (D) Typical appearance of "decapitation" secretions within the syringocystadenoma. (Photographs courtesy Michael W. Findlay, Charles Frewen, Andrew Ryan.)

reach up to 5–6 cm in size. Mutations in the *CYLD* gene (16a12-q13) are the principal cause of multiple cylindromas and may indicate familial inheritance (Brooke–Spiegler syndrome, an autosomal dominant syndrome with variable penetrance).[11] Cylindromas may have a similar origin to related tumors such as spiradenomas and trichoepitheliomas because mixed lesions have been reported. Definitive diagnosis is by biopsy. Histology demonstrates a dermal tumor with islands of basophilic cells demonstrating peripheral palisading, surrounding larger, more pale central cells. Lamina densa-like material (predominantly collagen IV) surrounds the islands and the nests to separate them from the dermal matrix and these often give the lesions a jigsaw-like pattern of polygonal or oval nest shapes. Spiradenomas are related lesions, but are distinct from cylindromas because they have lymphoid invasion. Management is typically through surgical excision, which is curative following complete excision.

Spiradenoma

These benign, solitary tumors that are thought to be of apocrine origin present on the upper, anterior half of the body as pink, red, purple or blue nodules up to 1 cm in diameter. They typically occur in 15–35-year-olds, although infantile cases (with superficial dermal nodules) have been reported. They can be episodically painful, and while most are sporadic, they can be associated with Brooke–Spiegler syndrome (with trichoepitheliomas, cylindromas, spiradenomas, and mixed lesions). Mutations in the *CYLD* gene on chromosome 9 have been associated with their development,[11] but spiradenomas also have increased expression of *p53*. Multiple, giant, linear, and grouped forms have all been described. Malignant transformation can occur, particularly in long-standing lesions. Surgical excision is usually curative, but when multiple, radiotherapy and hyperthermic limb perfusion chemotherapy have been used successfully to avoid widespread excision.

Benign Dermal Tumors

Dermatofibroma

Dermatofibroma (or superficial benign fibrous histiocytoma) is a common cutaneous nodule of the limbs that is typically asymptomatic, but has been reported to be the most common atypical lesion causing pain.[12] Their etiology remains unknown, but it may be trauma. Their prominent mast cells may release TGF-beta and other fibrinogenic factors to promote the fibrotic reaction seen histologically.[13] Syndecan 1 and fibroblast growth factor receptor 2(FGFR-2) have also been implicated in their formation.[14,15] Gene fusions have also been implicated in the formation of dermatofibroma, particularly the *ALK* gene (a receptor tyrosine kinase that has also been found in some malignancies such as anaplastic large cell lymphoma, neuroblastoma and non-small cell lung cancer. Lesions are usually solitary, but may be multiple. When numerous lesions are present (≥15) they may be associated with a systemic conditions, including immune suppression (e.g., HIV), autoimmune conditions (SLE, dermatomyositis, Graves disease, Hashimoto's thyroiditis, myasthenia gravis), malignancies (leukemia, myelodysplastic syndrome, cutaneous T-cell lymphoma, multiple myeloma), atopic dermatitis or Down syndrome.[16] Dermatofibromas can be PET-avid and may have a similar appearance to many other tumors. Dermoscopy can be useful to display an overlying peripheral pigment network with a central white area.[17] Ultrasound may show a solid hypoechoic nodule. A biopsy is warranted if there is any diagnostic uncertainty. Surgical removal is indicated if lesions are symptomatic, esthetically unacceptable or when diagnostic uncertainty remains. Excision of the tumor with minimal overlying skin is usually effective in preventing recurrence, but aggressive subtypes (aneurysmal, atypical, cellular, deep/subcutaneous) have a local recurrence rate of up to 20%.[16] Rare cases of metastasis have been described with these variants.

Unusual Malignancies of Skin

The malignant tumors described in this section are uncommon at best and hence there is a paucity of high-level evidence to guide treatment. Accurate histopathology evaluation is vital and given the complexity and the rarity of these tumors, referral for expert review may be considered. MMS has been reported for many of these tumors, particularly in sites where obtaining a wide margin may be problematic. In general, lesions successfully treated by MMS tend to be smaller and although results appear to be as good as standard wide surgical excision, the number of cases and/or length of follow-up are limited in most reported series. In cases where the completeness of excision is uncertain, DRAPE (delayed reconstruction after pathology evaluation)[18] should be considered.

Merkel Cell Carcinoma

Merkel cell carcinoma (MCC) is an uncommon aggressive cutaneous malignancy that is increasing in frequency. The cell of origin is unknown but is unlikely to be the Merkel cell, a mechanoreceptor found in skin. The mnemonic AEIOU has been proposed to summarize the most common clinical characteristics (asymptomatic, expanding rapidly, immune suppression, older than 50 years and UV-exposed site on fair skin).[19] Correspondingly, the lesion affects the sun-exposed areas of elderly males, is related to chronic UV exposure and immunosuppressed patients are over-represented (Fig. 10.4). Over 80% of cases are associated with Merkel cell polyomavirus (MCV or MCPyV), a double-stranded DNA virus that is classified as a class 2A (probably carcinogenic) human oncovirus by the International Agency for Research on Cancer. MCV is almost ubiquitous in the community after infection early in life. In some populations, it may be in as many as 97% of all MCCs. It inserts itself into the recipient cell genome without causing cancer and without the ability to replicate, therefore patients are not infectious with MCV when they develop MCC. The inserted viral genome requires a subsequent mutation to form a spliced variant capable for forming multiple different proteins (including large and small T antigens). These oncoproteins target tumor suppressor genes such as the retinoblastoma protein and thereby promote carcinogenesis. In studies from North America and Europe the incidence of Merkel cell polyoma virus-associated tumors is considerably higher than seen in Australia, where UV exposure may be more important.

The characteristic presentation is a rapidly growing firm non-tender flesh-colored nodule. The most common site is the face (25%), the head and neck, trunk, and limbs account for the remainder.[19]

The histological features are of a neuroendocrine tumor with three main patterns. Most common is the solid type – a densely blue (basophilic) tumor with pavementing of rapidly dividing tumor cells. The trabecular (cells arranged in cords or columns of invasive basophilic cells) and diffuse (poor cellular cohesion reminiscent of lymphoma-like tissue growth) patterns are less common. The potential for coexistence of MCC within BCC or SCC must always be considered and can be especially difficult to diagnose in desmoplastic NMSC variants. A further issue is potential confusion between a primary cutaneous MCC and a cutaneous metastasis from another neuroendocrine tumor, predominantly non-small cell lung cancer. The latter are commonly positive for thyroid transcription factor 1 (TTF-1) while MCC never do not react. The diagnosis of MCC is nearly always confirmed by immunohistochemical labeling with cytokeratin 20 (para-nuclear Golgi dot). A small proportion of MCCs however are CK-20-negative and in these cases the clinical scenario including imaging and the presence of other neuroendocrine immunohistochemical markers is usually confirmatory. Similarly immunohistochemistry can be of assistance in the occasional situation of MCC presenting as a lymph node mass or subcutaneous deposit with no known primary lesion.

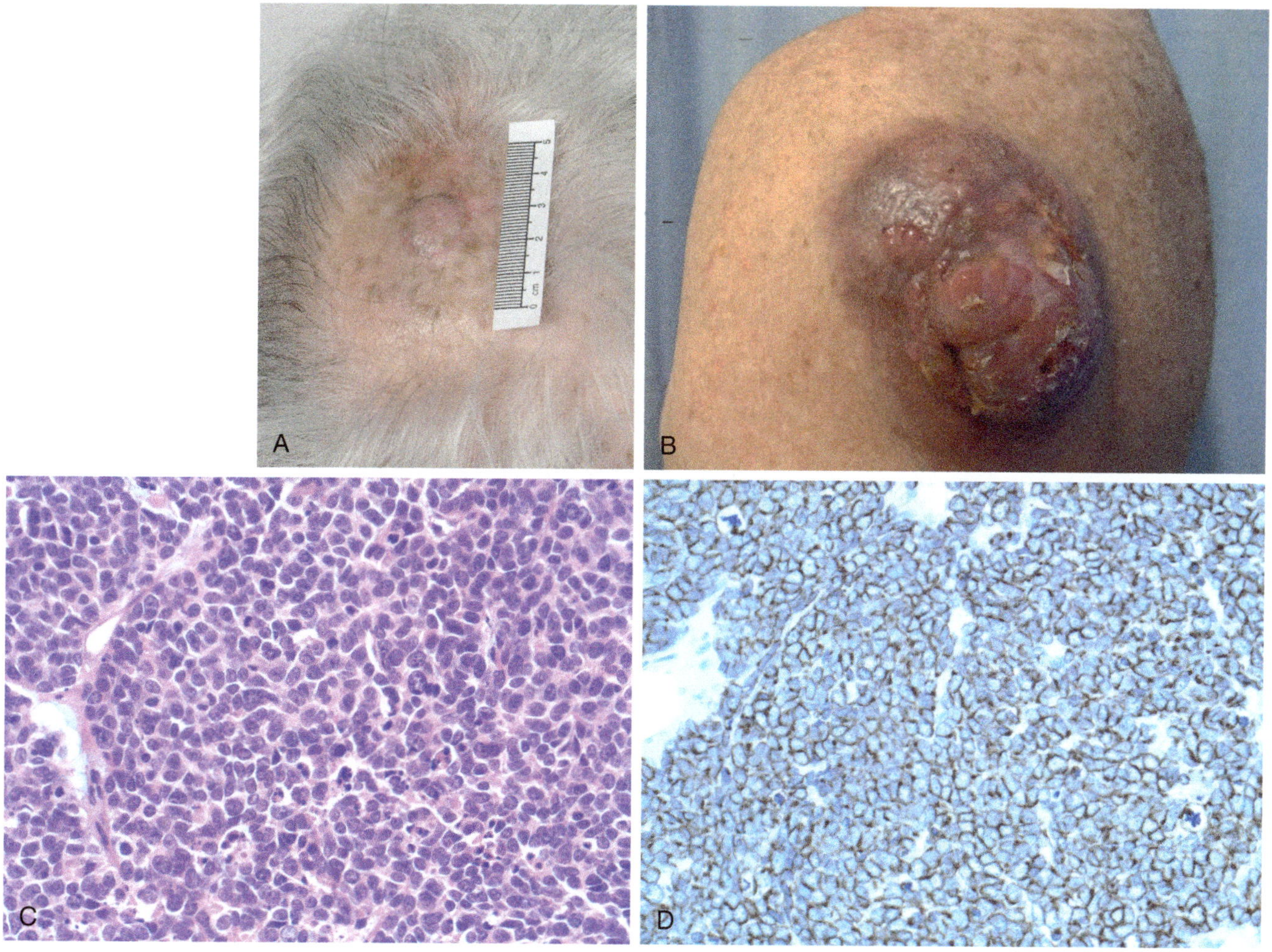

• **Fig. 10.4** (A) Merkel cell carcimoma arising in the anterior lower leg of a 72-year-old male. The lesion is raised and pink/purple in color. (B) A larger, neglected tumor on the shoulder of a 74-year-old male with evidence of recent bleeding from ulceration. (C) Histopathology showing an intensely basophilic, cellular dermal tumor with nuclear molding, minimal cytoplasm, numerous mitoses, and apoptosis consistent with a "small cell undifferentiated malignancy." (D) Cytokeratin 20 (CK20) immunolabeling shows the perinuclear "dot" of the Golgi apparatus and nuclear membrane. (Photographs courtesy Michael W. Findlay, Charles Frewen, Andrew Ryan.)

Staging

Prior to 2010, there were at least five competing staging systems in common use, limiting comparisons between centers worldwide. The current system is the TNM staging of the American Joint Committee on Cancer (AJCC), which focuses on the size and degree of invasion of the primary tumor, extent of in transit disease regional lymph node involvement and the presence and site of distant metastases, updated in 2016 to include information on pathology rather than clinical evaluation of regional lymph nodes and unknown primary lesions.[20] Five-year overall survivals were 51% for local disease only, 35% for regional lymph node involvement, and 14% for patients with distant spread. For patients with lymph node involvement, occult disease detected by sentinel node biopsy had superior survival compared to patients with clinically apparent regional lymph node involvement, 40% and 27%, respectively. For patients with clinically node-negative disease, the finding of lymph node involvement by sentinel node biopsy reduced the survival from 51% to 40%. Unknown primary MCC presenting clinically with lymphadenopathy had improved survival compared to patients with a known primary and regional lymph node involvement, 42% and 27%, respectively. Preoperative staging should include fine-slice CT scans of the chest, abdomen, and regional lymph node fields with PET scanning if available. Not all MCCs are PET-avid, especially if already irradiated.[21]

Other poor prognostic indicators include age >70 years, male sex, truncal or head and neck site (especially lip), organ transplant recipients, usually combined with immunosuppression, nodal or distant disease at presentation, and adverse histopathology features (small cell size, infiltrative pattern, high mitotic rate, depth of invasion, and lymphovascular invasion).[22]

Management

The management of the primary lesion and regional lymph nodes is an area of considerable controversy.[23] The data are limited by the rarity of the tumor, meaning studies are usually small, often from single institutions collected over a protracted time period so that patients are not treated in a similar fashion to more contemporary norms. In general, a wide excision of the primary lesion with a 1–2-cm margin down to deep fascia is recommended. Alternatively radiotherapy of the primary site after appropriate biopsy also offers reasonable results. There has been no successfully completed randomised study of these two treatment modalities. In North America surgical excision with adjuvant radiotherapy for patients with limited margins following definitive excision or high-risk larger tumors is more commonly undertaken compared to other regions, including Australia, where definitive radiation of the primary site, particularly if undertaken in association with regional lymph node basin treatment, is more common.

Approximately one-third of patients with clinically localized MCC will have occult lymph node involvement detected by sentinel node biopsy. For tumors less than 10 mm in size the risk of lymph node involvement is less than 10% and for lesions greater than 20 mm the risk may be 40% or higher.[24] Sentinel node biopsy should be strongly considered for all patients with clinically negative regional lymph node basins. Some authorities limit SNB for patients with MCC less than 10 mm to those with adverse prognostic features or the young, as overall the risk of a positive SNB is low(<10%). On the other hand, some centers recommend RT regardless of SNB status to patients with larger (>20 mm) lesions given the very high rate of lymph node involvement. Given the significant risk of developing distant disease in patients with lymph node involvement or tumors greater than 20 mm in size, adjuvant systemic chemotherapy (carboplatin and etoposide) concurrent with radiotherapy may be indicated, however this regime is not without toxicity, and as many patients are elderly it may not be appropriate.[25]

Most recurrences occur within 2 years of diagnosis. Locoregional recurrence is not uncommon. Palliative chemoradiotherapy may have limited benefit for locoregional and distant recurrence most commonly seen in liver, bone, lung, and soft tissue but rarely the brain. In recent years, it has become obvious that MCC are relatively responsive to immune checkpoint inhibitor therapy.[26] Early reports indicate response rates of over 60% with single agent anti PD-1 therapy. Given the rapidly changing landscape for immune-based therapies, strong consideration should be given to referring patients with disseminated MCC for participation in clinical trials. There is a suggestion based on early reports that patients treated previously with standard systemic therapy do not respond as well to immunotherapy. In view of the initial results in treating patients with disseminated disease, adjuvant checkpoint inhibitor therapy is currently an area of active investigation.

Adnexal Carcinomas

Malignant neoplasms of the pilosebaceous unit are very rare. They are classified with a bewildering array of terms, many of which are revised on a regular basis. The more common types include microcystic adnexal carcinoma, sebaceous carcinoma, and porocarcinoma. Overall survival is approximately 70% at 5 years.[27,28]

Microcystic Adnexal Carcinoma (MAC)

An infiltrative tumor usually of the head and neck (particularly central face) in older persons (Fig. 10.5A). The presentation is usually innocuous, as a slow-growing skin-colored plaque. Wide excision is indicated as the extent of the tumor is often considerably more than the clinical examination would suggest. Properly managed, local regional or distant recurrence is rare. Radiotherapy may have a role when surgical excision is compromised or not possible.[29]

Sebaceous Carcinoma

Occurs predominantly in the head and neck in older patients, with a predilection for the eyelid (Fig. 10.5B). If adequately excised, recurrence is rare.

MMS may have a role in managing this tumor, given its common involvement of the eyelid, but as with other unusual cutaneous malignancies, the evidence for its use is largely case series with few patients and/or relatively short follow-up.

Porocarcinoma

Arises not infrequently from a long-standing benign apocrine/eccrine poroma. Most involve the lower limbs in elderly persons as slow-growing lesions that increase their growth rate just prior to diagnosis. Lymph node involvement occurs infrequently. Sentinel node biopsy has been reported, however its use is still undefined. With wide excision, long-term survival is reasonable.[30]

Extramammary Paget's Disease

This rare tumor is classified as an adenocarcinoma of apocrine glands but considerable debate remains about the cell of origin. The typical histological appearance of Pagetoid spread is intraepithelial proliferation of large round, blue-staining basophilic cells, often with prominent nuclei extending throughout the dermis. The classic site is the perineum (vulva, penis, scrotum, and perianal area). In Caucasian populations females account for the majority of cases while males predominate in Asian populations. More rarely, the axilla and eyelid are affected. Up to one-third of affected patients have an occult malignancy (bladder, prostate, kidney, colon, and rectum). Approximately two-thirds of patients have in situ disease only.

The typical history is of a slowly progressive lesion (often mistaken for eczema or similar rash with consequent delay in diagnosis) in 70-year-olds (Fig. 10.6). The disease is frequently extensive at diagnosis and may be multifocal. Careful examination combined with punch biopsies to confirm

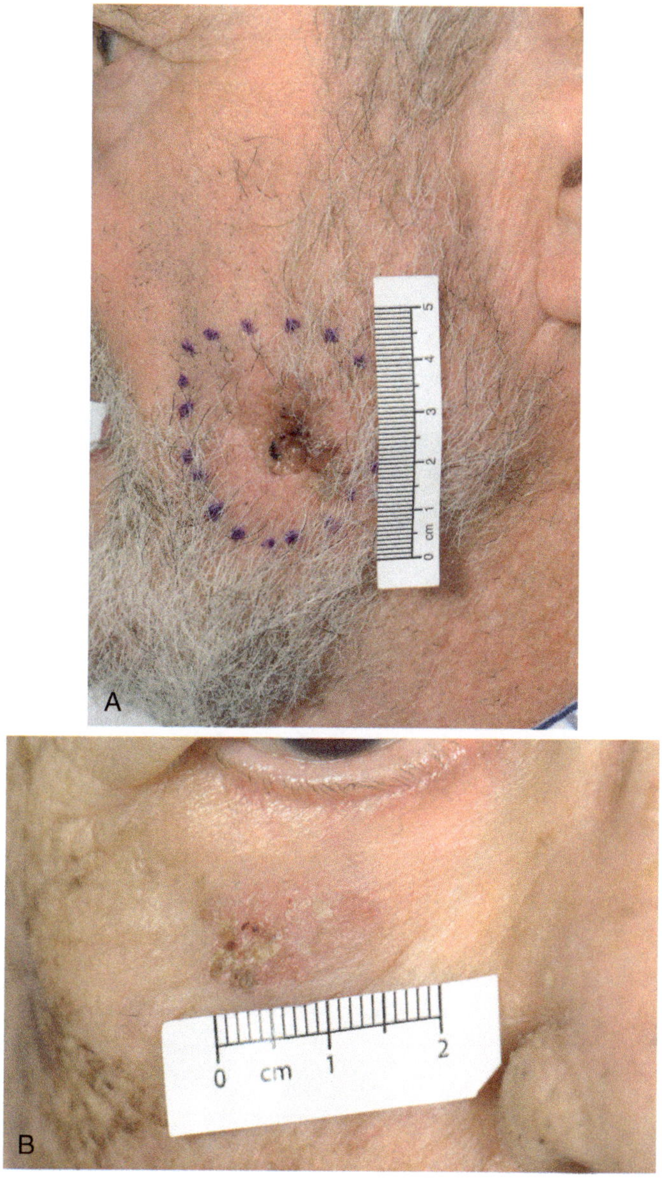

• **Fig. 10.5** (A) Microcystic adnexal carcinoma of the face in a 69-year-old male. The lesion extends subcutaneously to the dotted line on palpation and much further microscopically. (B) Sebaceous carcinoma of the right lower eyelid/cheek of a 76-year-old male, demonstrating a waxy/crust-like material amongst areas of ulceration, giving it a very different appearance from a seborrheic keratosis. (Photographs courtesy Michael W. Findlay, Charles Frewen, Andrew Ryan.)

the extent of the disease and the presence/absence of invasion are warranted for larger lesions. Exclusion of an underlying primary malignancy is appropriate.[31]

Wide surgical excision with clear margins is the treatment of choice. Local recurrence may occur in up to 50% of patients. Lymph node involvement occurs in up to two-thirds of patients with invasive disease. Sentinel node biopsy has been reported and in one small series over 40% of patients with invasive disease had lymph node involvement.[32] Lymph node involvement, dermal involvement and lymphatic, and/or vascular invasion are poor prognostic factors. The role of radiotherapy is controversial. Radiotherapy as monotherapy may be appropriate when surgery is contraindicated, however it is not clear if it is as effective as surgery. The literature is also unclear as to whether adjuvant radiotherapy after complete surgical excision offers major benefits. In patients with extensive in situ disease, topical imiquimod or photodynamic therapy (PDT) have been used with some success, but long-term outcomes remain undefined.[33]

Overall survival at 5 years is 60% for patients with invasive disease. Long-term follow-up is recommended due to the significant risk of locoregional recurrence.

Other Rare Adnexal Carcinomas

Pilomatrix carcinoma occurs in the head and neck of females, probably from a benign pilomatrixoma. Wide excision is indicated.

Malignant chondroid syringoma (malignant mixed tumor) occurs on the extremities and trunk, following an unpredictable course with spread to regional lymph nodes and distant sites. Wide excision is indicated.

Hidradenocarcinoma occurs in the head, neck, and extremities of elderly patients and pursues an aggressive course with regional and distant metastasis.

Malignant cylindroma is a very rare tumor probably arising from a benign cylindroma in older patients, which frequently metastasizes widely.

Eccrine spiradenocarcinoma develops in elderly patients, usually from a pre-existing benign spiradenoma. Wide excision is usually curative as lesions rarely metastasize.

Soft Tissue Sarcomas of Skin

Tumors of mesenchymal origin arising in skin account for less than 5% of all soft tissue sarcomas. Excluding Kaposi's sarcoma, dermatofibrosarcoma protuberans (DFSP) accounts for two-thirds of cases. Leiomyosarcoma of the skin and cutaneous angiosarcoma account for an additional 20%. Rare cases of fibrosarcoma, and myxosarcoma occur and should be managed as for these tumors elsewhere in the body. An unusual tumor of the skin is atypical fibroxanthoma (AFX). This term in the past has been used synonymously with the term malignant fibrous histiocytoma (MFH) of skin. MFH arising in other sites have subsequently been reclassified to other tumor types, i.e., fibrosarcoma and liposarcoma or where a specific tumor type cannot be identified as undifferentiated pleomorphic sarcoma (UPS). It is therefore a diagnosis of exclusion.[31] To further confuse matters, what was previously designated as MFH of skin is now classified as either AFX or pleomorphic dermal sarcoma (PDS). It should be pointed out, however, that UPS arising from structures deep to the skin and subcutaneous tissues may involve skin and should be managed as for high-grade sarcomas elsewhere around the body.

Compared to other soft tissue sarcomas, AFX and PDS are characterized by a low malignant potential but may have a significant risk for local recurrence.[32] Some authorities dispute whether AFX has any malignant potential whilst others see it as a continuum from AFX through PDS.

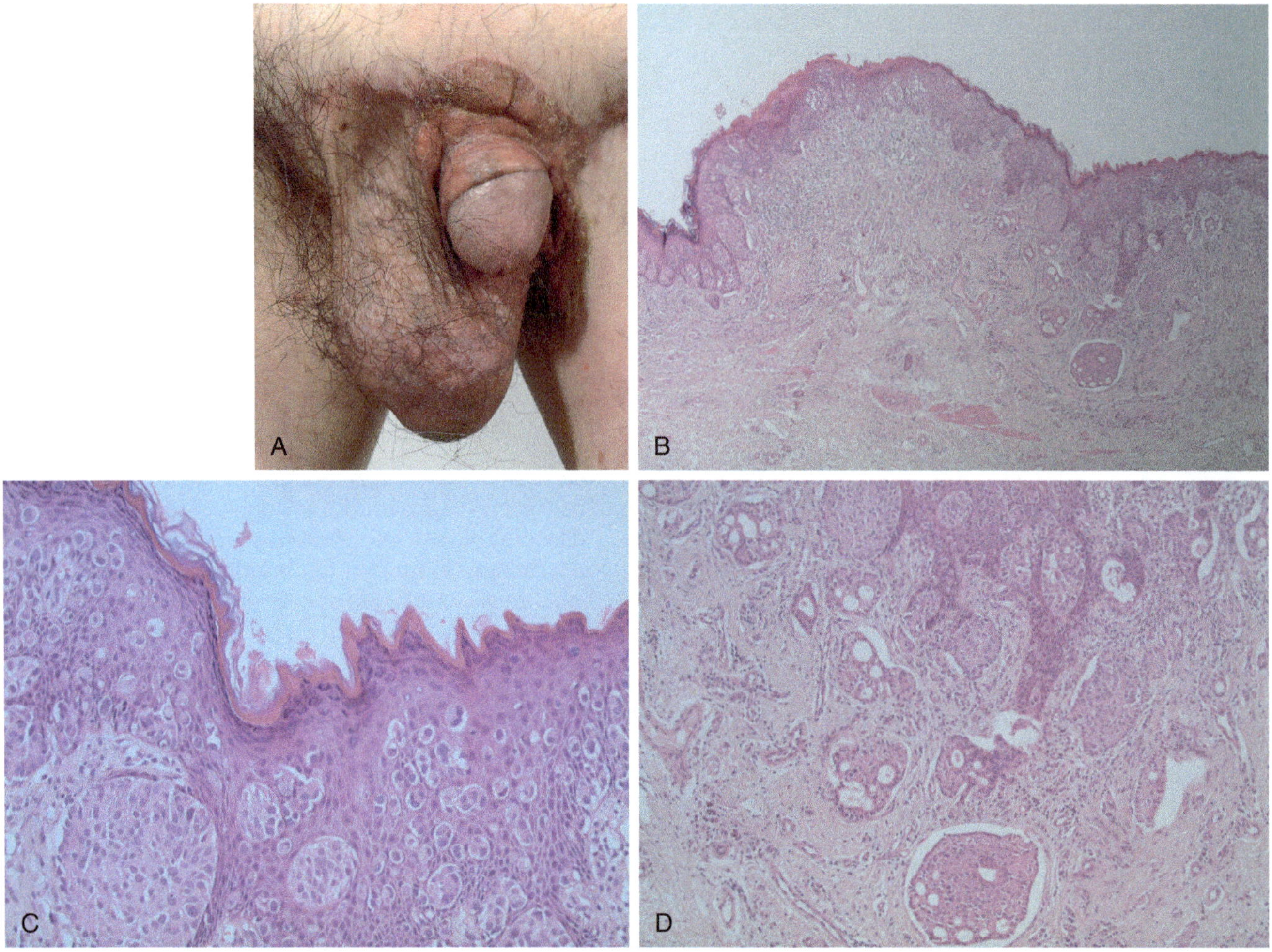

• **Fig. 10.6** (A) Extensive extramammary Paget's disease (EMPD) with invasive adenocarcinoma developing in a 70-year-old male. The patient had a long-standing "rash". No occult malignancy was found. (B) Histopathology demonstrates nested and single malignant cells in the epidermis, with malignant glands in the upper dermis (bottom right). (C) Nested and single malignant cells in "Pagetoid" distribution in the epidermis. (D) Invasive adenocarcinoma (bottom) with in situ EMPD in the epidermis above. (Photographs courtesy Michael W. Findlay, Charles Frewen, Andrew Ryan.)

The histological appearances of PDS and AFX are sheets of pleomorphic, bizarre-appearing epithelioid and spindle cells with abundant cytoplasm, hyperchromatic nuclei, and multiple nucleoli. Both multinucleated giant cells and atypical mitoses are commonly seen. Apart from invasion beyond the dermis, tumor necrosis and vascular and/or perineural infiltration are more commonly seen in PDS. There are no reliable histological or immunohistochemical features that distinguish the two tumors. Given the nonspecific histological features and absence of any specific markers, the role of immunohistochemistry is predominantly in excluding other differential diagnoses, including squamous cell carcinoma, melanoma, and leiomyosarcoma. The distinction that is made predominantly on the extent of the tumor is important, as tumors confined to the dermis or with minimal subcutaneous extension and now defined as AFX probably never or rarely metastasize, while more extensive tumors now categorized as PDS have a small but definite risk of metastasis and death. In support of a common etiology or continuum hypothesis, limited molecular studies have failed to identify any significant differences between the two tumors. The commonest finding is a TERT promoter mutation and most tumors have a UV signature.

Atypical Fibroxanthoma (AFX)

AFX occur predominantly in the head and neck (80%) and/or sun-exposed areas of elderly males (median age 70) (Fig. 10.7). AFX of the limbs occurs in younger patients (median age 40).

Management is by wide excision. Although most authorities recommend a 1–2-cm excision margin a meta-analysis could not detect any improvement with increasing margins over complete excision.[34] Local recurrence is uncommon (<10%), with adequate margins of excision and most recurrences occur within the first 2 years. Invasion beyond the dermis and local recurrence are associated with increased risk of both local and distant recurrence.[34] As noted above, metastatic disease is rare and some authorities argue that AFX that develop distant recurrence should be reclassified as PDS.

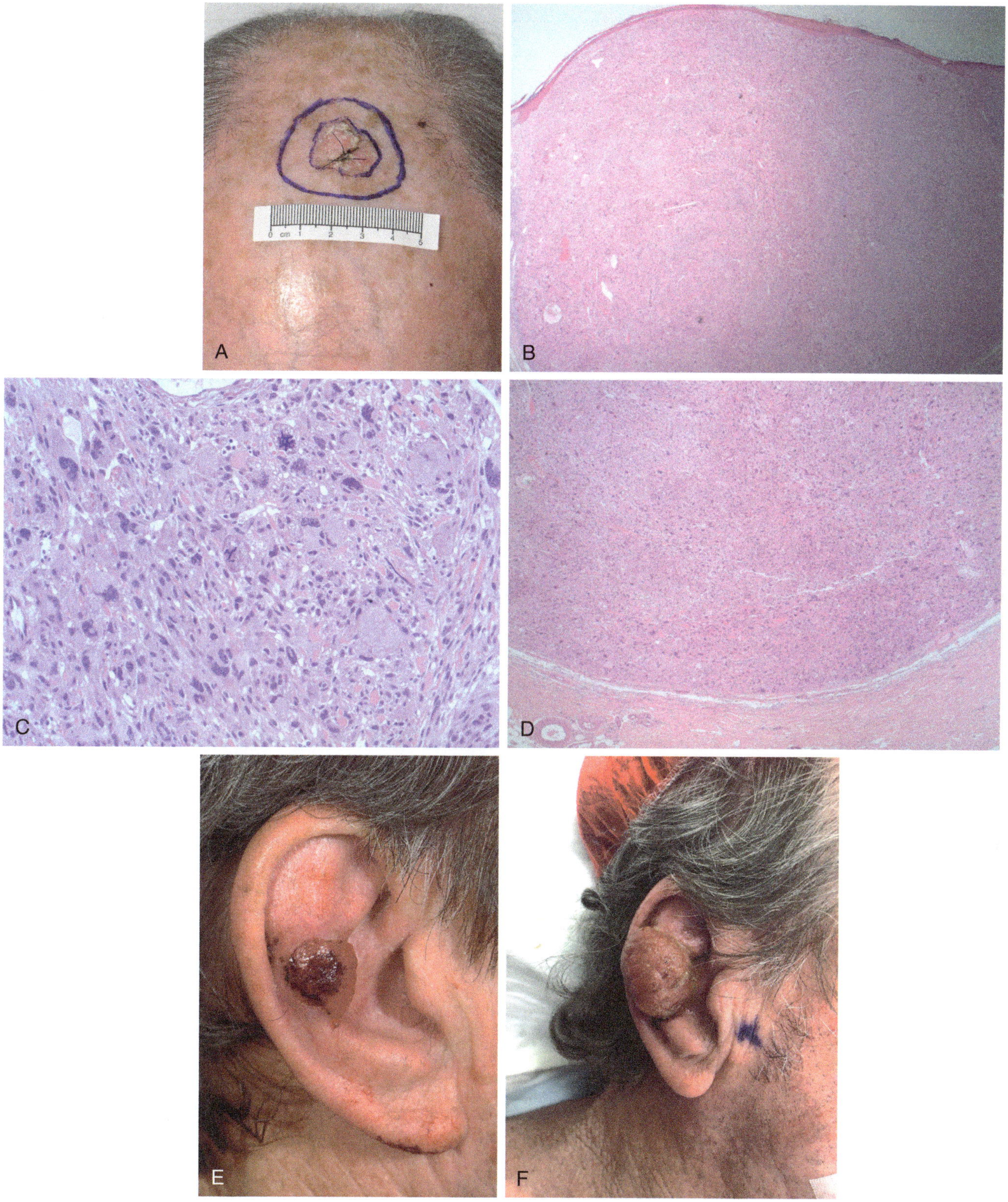

• **Fig. 10.7** (A) Atypical fibroxanthoma (AFX) on the scalp of a 72-year-old male. A raised pink lesion had grown slowly over at least 18 months. (B) Histopathology demonstrating a cellular dermal spindle cell tumor with attenuated overlying epidermis. (C) High-grade cytology with "pushing" appearance and circumscribed deep border in deep dermis (not subcutis). (D) AFX usually appears as a high-grade spindle cell malignancy, with tumor giant cells and atypical mitoses that are out of proportion to low-grade clinical behavior. (E) Biopsy-proven pleomorphic dermal sarcoma of the right antihelix of the ear. (F) The same lesion 3 weeks later demonstrating a significant increase in the tumor size and ongoing ulceration consistent with the aggressive nature of the tumor. (Photographs courtesy Michael W. Findlay, Charles Frewen, Andrew Ryan.)

Pleomorphic Dermal Sarcoma (PDS)

The presentation and appearance of PDS is remarkably similar to AFX. Given the issues with the definition of PDS as noted above, the reported rates of local recurrence and distant recurrence vary widely, with rates of up to 28% for local recurrence and 20% for distant recurrence. The optimal margin of excision is not defined, although many authorities recommend margins of 10–20 mm. Given that these tumors occur predominantly in the head and neck, in elderly and often frail patients, attaining wide margins may be difficult and for these patients, adjuvant radiotherapy may be recommended. In a series of 26 patients, 5% had evidence of metastatic disease at presentation. Overall, 5% had lymph node involvement at presentation or shortly after. Sentinel node biopsy has been described for PDS, but as the rate of lymph node involvement is low (<10%) the decision for sentinel node biopsy should be a nuanced one, based on patient and tumor factors if it is to be performed. Preoperative imaging to exclude the presence of metastatic disease would appear to be prudent in patients who are immunocompromised or have large tumors.

In the author's institution and another contemporary representative series, the rate of local recurrence was <5%. Similar results have been obtained with margin control surgery, i.e., Mohs micrographic surgery. The reported experience with MMS is limited by both the number of cases and length of follow-up, but it may be appropriate for small lesions, particularly in sensitive sites. The risk of distant recurrence in properly treated patients is low (<5%), with most occurring within 3 years of diagnosis.

Dermatofibrosarcoma Protuberans (DFSP)

This is an uncommon, dermally derived tumor[31] with a marked tendency to local recurrence. Hematogenous spread is uncommon (<5% of cases) and lymphatic spread is rare. Approximately 90% of tumors are low grade, however the remaining 10% display higher-grade sarcomatous transformation (most commonly fibrosarcoma). DFSP affects both sexes equally and is typically a tumor of the third and fourth decades, although pediatric cases have been described. Nearly half the tumors arise on the trunk, the proximal limbs approximately 40%, and the head and neck accounts for the remaining 10%–15%.[33]

Most present as small, slow growing, innocuous, indurated, skin-colored plaques that may become raised, pink, and eventually violaceous, with telangiectasia over time (Fig. 10.8). The lesion is attached to skin and advanced cases demonstrate the characteristic cutaneous nodules that give the tumor its name. Advanced lesions may ulcerate, bleed, and become fixed to underlying structures. The more malignant form of DFSP, with fibrosarcomatous transformation, presents in an identical fashion.[34] A less aggressive variant, the Bednar tumor more commonly seen in black persons, is an uncommon, pigmented form of DFSP (5% or less) where scattered melanosome-containing cells are seen in lesions that are otherwise indistinguishable from standard DFSP by histopathology. They have a slightly better prognosis than standard DFSP.

At least 10 histological subtypes of DFSP have been described. In general, DFSP demonstrates a monotonous population of spindle cells arranged in a typical storiform pattern with bland-appearing tumor projections invading away from the major tumor, which can be difficult to identify histologically and presumably explains the high rate of local recurrence seen following limited margins of excision. In most cases the diagnosis is straightforward with routine histology. Immunohistochemistry is useful to distinguish DFSP from other lesions but dermatofibroma, melanoma, leiomyoma, and leiomyosarcoma and atypical fibroxanthoma cannot always be excluded easily. Over 85% of DFSP label with CD34 but not factor XIIIa (labels the majority of dermatofibromas), vimentin or S100; however, DFSP with fibrosarcomatous transformation labels with CD34 in 50% of cases.

DFSP cells are characterized genetically by either a supernumerary chromosomal ring or linear translocation t(17:22)(q22;q13) in over 90% of cases. This alteration results in a fusion product involving platelet-derived growth factor B (PDGF-B) and the collagen 1A1 gene (*COL1A1*). This fusion protein leads to constitutive activation of the PDGF receptor, resulting in cell growth. More recent work suggests other novel molecular variants may be of importance in the development of these tumors.

The risk of distant or regional lymph node metastasis at presentation is very low, therefore preoperative imaging should be confined to evaluation of the primary tumor site by either MRI or CT scan. Planned margins of 2–4 cm usually result in tumor clearance and an acceptable rate of local recurrence (approximately 5% compared to rates >50% with incomplete/close margins).

DFSP with fibrosarcomatous change is reported to have a higher rate of local (38%) and distant (15% versus <5%) recurrence. In over 80% of cases involving fibrosarcomatous change, distant recurrence follows local recurrence, emphasizing the need for complete surgical excision.[35] Even with wide margins of excision, recurrent lesions have a subsequently higher rate of local recurrence (11%). In general, DFSP with fibrosarcomatous transformation should be managed as for high-grade sarcomas in other parts of the body.

DFSP is relatively radiosensitive but the role of adjuvant radiotherapy is currently undefined. In principle it should be reserved for cases where a complete excision is not possible or with extensive tumors. Specifically, patients with close margins should be managed by further excision if possible rather than adjuvant radiotherapy. Targeted therapies to address the constitutive activation of PDGF-B in DFSP are currently being assessed. Initial reports of imatinib (a tyrosine kinase inhibitor that inhibits the PDFG receptor) for advanced or recurrent disease indicate a response rate approaching 50%. The median survival of patients with advanced disease in one series was 19 months.[35] It may also have a role preoperatively to improve tumor resectability.

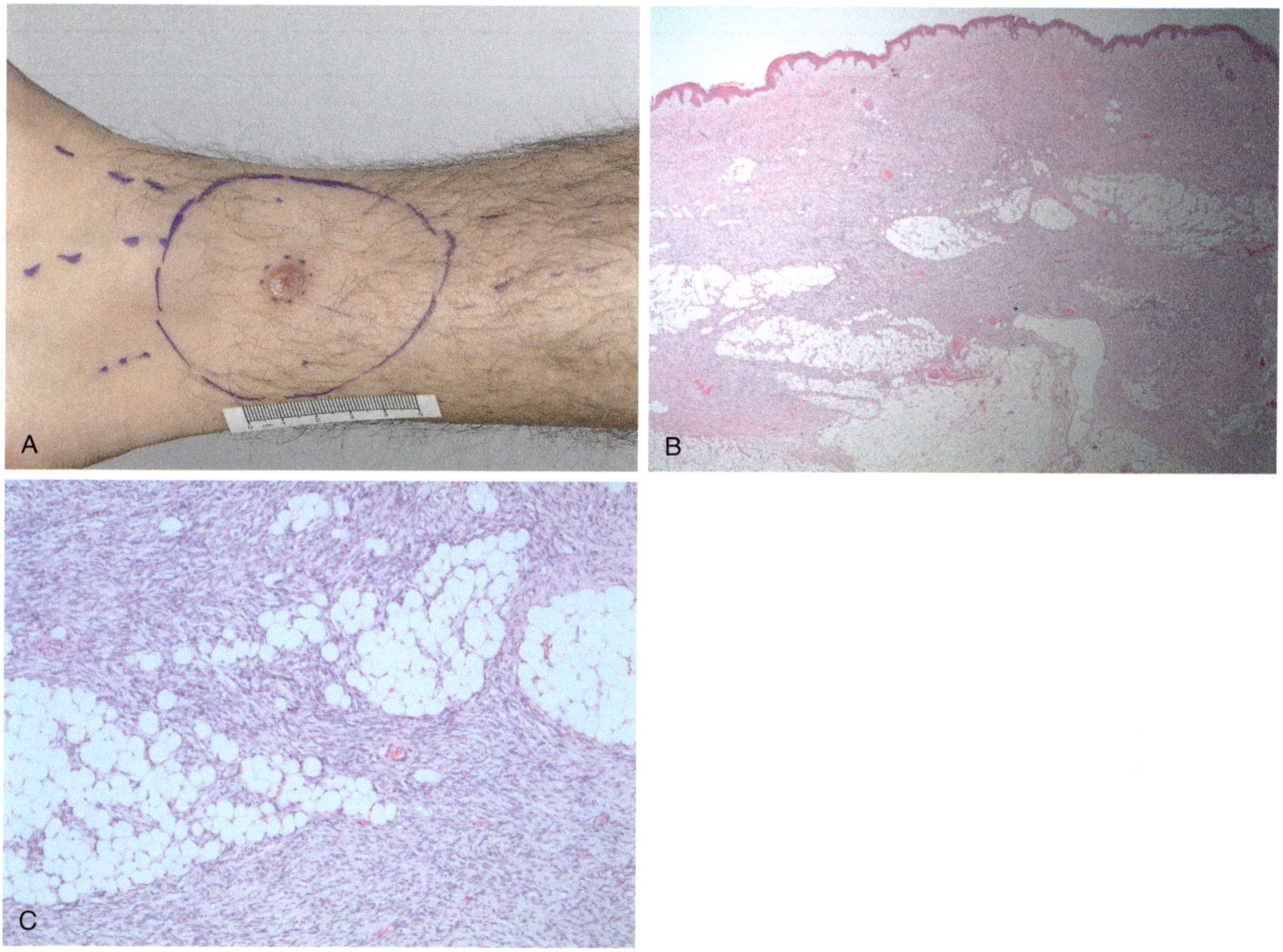

• **Fig. 10.8** (A) Typical pink thickened appearance of dermatofibrosarcoma protuberans (DFSP) seen in the initial stages. (B) Histopathology demonstrating cellular dermal and subcutaneous spindle cell proliferation with occasional storiform patterns (irregular whorl-like shapes) evident. Tumor is centered on the subcutis and appears to "lift" subcutis into dermis. (C) Bland spindle cells wrap around and entrap subcutaneous lobules. Note the low-grade cytology. (Photographs courtesy Michael W. Findlay, Charles Frewen, Andrew Ryan.)

Most recurrences occur within 3 years, however very late recurrences also occur. Follow-up by close physical examination and imaging of the primary site should be concentrated in the first 3 years. Ongoing annual follow-up after that time would seem reasonable.

Leiomyosarcoma (LMS)

Leiomyosarcoma of skin is also a tumor that has undergone review in recent years. Tumors arising in the dermis with minimal subcutaneous extension, probably from erector pili muscle, are classified as dermal LMS, while tumors arising from vascular smooth muscle in the subcutaneous tissue with minimal or no dermal or deep extension are classified as subcutaneous LMS (Fig. 10.9). The histological appearances are similar, although features such as necrosis and elevated mitotic rate are more common in subcutaneous LMS. The differentiation between dermal and subcutaneous LMS is therefore based predominantly on the site of origin. It may be impossible to distinguish the exact site of origin for larger tumors but as they behave in an aggressive fashion they are best considered as subcutaneous LMS. Subcutaneous LMS are larger and much more rapidly growing, with a significant risk of both local and distant recurrence. Dermal LMS, on the other hand, are usually small, slowly growing nodules in the skin, which if managed appropriately by wide excision rarely metastasize, if ever.

The median age of presentation for both tumors is the sixth decade. Males are overrepresented and the commonest site is the head and neck. Dermal LMS are considerably smaller at presentation than subcutaneous LMS (15 mm versus 50 mm). A recent contemporary series in our institution of 63 dermal and 19 subcutaneous LMS had similar rates of local recurrence (20% at 5 years). Similar to other series, no patients with dermal LMS developed metastatic disease however the five-year disease-specific survival for subcutaneous LMS was 80%. Adjuvant radiotherapy was used predominantly in the dermal LMS patients, particularly

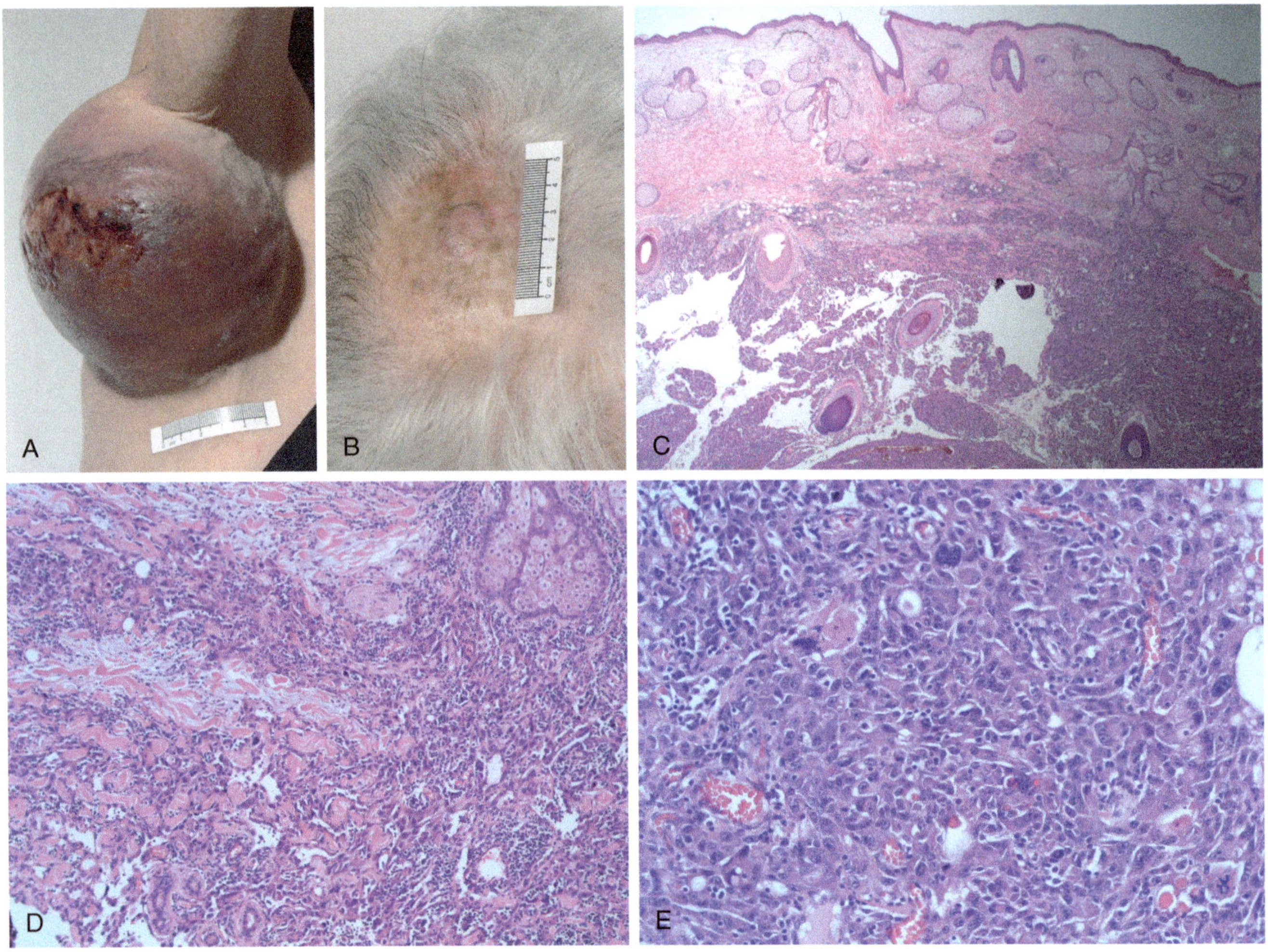

• **Fig. 10.9** (A) Advanced metastatic deposit of leiomyosarcoma involving the right axilla after a previous history of a primary lesion to the arm years earlier. (B) Typical appearance of an angiosarcoma developing in an 80-year-old female. The lesion is pink to purple in color and has surrounding vascular changes suggesting cutaneous extension over the scalp. (C) Low-power histopathology demonstrates a deep dermal, cellular, solid and partly cavitating spindle cell malignancy consistent with angiosarcoma. (D) Higher power demonstrates anastomosing and branching jagged slit-like vascular channels lined by atypical hyperchromatic endothelial cells. (E) A more solid component of the same tumor demonstrates high-grade malignant cytology, atypical mitoses and red blood cell extravasation. (Photographs courtesy Michael W. Findlay, Charles Frewen, Andrew Ryan.)

for larger tumors where wide margins of excision could not be achieved. For patients with a dermal LMS, a margin of at least 10 mm appears appropriate and for dermal LMS a margin of 20 mm has also been recommended, although there is little data to support these recommendations.[36] Preoperative staging with CT chest and abdomen would seem to be appropriate for larger subcutaneous LMS. Most recurrences occur within 3 years.

Cutaneous Angiosarcoma

This is a heterogenous condition that may arise de novo in the breast, in chronically lymphedematous or irradiated tissue, visceral sites, and the skin. The most common (>75%) cutaneous site is the head and neck (particularly scalp). Most patients are male, with a median age in the 70s. Most present as a small bruise becoming irregular, slightly raised with multifocal macules and papules that are purplish in color. One-third of patients have evidence of metastatic disease at presentation and work up with fine-cut CT chest and liver and whole-body PET scanning, where available, is appropriate. Very wide excision is indicated, but angiosarcoma is frequently multifocal, leading to a high (50%) local recurrence rate despite clear margins. There is limited data on the margins of excision but a 3 cm clearance appears reasonable. Wide field adjuvant radiotherapy incorporating draining lymph node fields reduces the risk of local recurrence and anecdotal evidence suggests it may prolong survival[37]; it should be strongly considered, particularly if the reported margins of excision are compromised. The role of sentinel node biopsy is undefined. Most recurrences (local, regional, and/or distant) occur within 2–3 years. The 10-year survival is approximately 20%–30%. Chemotherapy in the management of disseminated disease or inoperable locoregional recurrence is associated with reasonable response rates but unfortunately limited to only a few months' duration. The use of targeted therapies directed against vascular endothelial growth factor (VEGF) or its receptor (VEGFR), or tyrosine kinase inhibitors, is currently under evaluation.

Conclusion

The correct diagnosis and management of atypical tumors in clinical practice can be a daunting prospect. Revisions to tumor names, classifications and the emergence of mutational profiling has added to the challenge of managing patients with these lesions. In general, atypical lesions are a testament to the potential for any cell or stem cell type to develop benign tumors or to undergo malignant transformation. While not exhaustive, we have sought to cover some of the more important and clinically relevant lesions. These are provided so that the clinician will have sufficient information so as to critically appraise any histopathology diagnosis provided and thereby ensure the appropriate management of their patient. More common tumors such as melanoma are capable of mimicry and therefore the diagnosis of melanoma or other common mimics should always be entertained when there is any discrepancy between the clinical picture and the results of histopathology. The appropriate management of malignant atypical lesions may require a dedicated multidisciplinary team within a tertiary or quaternary health center. Careful consideration should be given to referring patients with atypical tumors that are at significant risk of recurrence and/or metastasis.

References

1. NIH. *National Cancer Institute. HPV and Cancer*, 2013. Available from: http://cancer.gov/cancertopics/factsheet/Risk/HPV.
2. Gillison ML. Human papillomavirus-associated head and neck cancer is a distinct epidemiologic, clinical, and molecular entity. *Semin Oncol.* 2004;31(6):744–754.
3. Layegh P, Sharifi-Sistani N, Abadian M, Moghiman T. Brooke–spiegler syndrome. *Indian J Dermatol Venereol Leprol.* 2008;74(6):632–634.
4. Wu YH. Folliculosebaceous cystic hamartoma or trichofolliculoma? A spectrum of hamartomatous changes inducted by perifollicular stroma in the follicular epithelium. *J Cutan Pathol.* 2008;35(9):843–848.
5. Stern JB, Stout DA. Trichofolliculoma showing perineural invasion. Trichofolliculocarcinoma? *Arch Dermatol.* 1979;115(8):1003–1004.
6. Liaw D, Marsh D, Li J, et al. Germline mutations of the PTEN gene in Cowden disease, an inherited breast and thyroid cancer syndrome. *Nat Genet.* 1997;16(1):64–67.
7. Hogan DJ. *Sebaceous Hyperplasia.* eMedicine; 2018. http://emedicine.medscape.com/article/1059368.
8. Salim A, Recce SM, Smith AG, et al. Sebaceous hyperplasia and skin cancer in patients undergoing renal transplant. *J Am Acad Dermatol.* 2006;55(5):878–881.
9. Yu C, Shahsavari M, Stevens G, et al. Isotretinoin as monotherapy for sebaceous hyperplasia. *J Drugs Dermatol.* 2010;9(6):699–701.
10. Friedman SJ, Butler DF. Syringoma presenting as milia. *J Am Acad Dermatol.* 1987;16(2 Pt 1):310–314.
11. Bowen S, Gill M, Lee DA, et al. Mutations in the CYLD gene in Brooke–Spiegler syndrome, familial cylindromatosis, and multiple familial trichoepithelioma: lack of genotype-phenotype correlation. *J Invest Dermatol.* 2005;124(5):919–920.
12. Naversen DN, Trask DM, Watson FH, Burket JM. Painful tumors of the skin: "LEND an EGG". *J Am Acad Dermatol.* 1993;28(2 Pt 2):298–300.
13. Yamamoto T. Dermatofibroma: a possible model of local fibrosis with epithelial/mesenchymal cell interaction. *J Eur Acad Dermatol Venereol.* 2009;23(4):371–375.
14. Sellheyer K, Smoller BR. Dermatofibroma: upregulation of syndecan-1 expression in mesenchymal tissue. *Am J Dermatopathol.* 2003;25(5):392–398.
15. Skroza N, Rotolo S, Ceccarelli S, et al. Modulation of the expression of the FGFR2-IIIb and FGFR2-IIIc molecules in dermatofibroma. *J Dermatol Sci.* 2008;51(1):53–57.
16. Pierson J, et al. *Dermatofibroma.* eMedicine; 2018. http://emedicine.medscape.com/article/1056742-clinical.
17. Zaballos P, Puig S, Llambrich A, Malvehy J. Dermoscopy of dermatofibromas: a prospective morphological study of 412 cases. *Arch Dermatol.* 2008;144(1):75–83.
18. Behan FC, Rozen WM, Kwee MM, et al. Oncologic clearance with preservation of reconstructive options: literature review and the "delayed reconstruction after pathology evaluation (DRAPE)" technique. *ANZ J Surg.* 2012;82(11):780–785.
19. Heath M, Jaimes N, Lemos B, et al. Clinical characteristics of Merkel cell carcinoma at diagnosis in 195 patients: the AEIOU features. *J Am Acad Dermatol.* 2008;58(3):375–381.
20. Harms KL, Healy MA, Nghiem P, et al. Analysis of prognostic factors from 9387 Merkel cell carcinoma cases forms the basis for the new 8th edition AJCC staging system. *Ann Surg Oncol.* 2016;23(11):3564–3571.
21. Miller SJ, Alam N, Andersen J, et al. Merkel cell carcinoma. *J Natl Compr Canc Netw.* 2009;7(3):322–332.
22. Tai PT, Yu E, Winquist E, et al. Merkel cell carcinoma of the skin. *J Cutan Med Surg.* 2000;4(4):186–195.
23. Bichakjian CK, Olencki T, Aasi SZ, et al. Merkel Cell Carcinoma, Version 1.2018, NCCN Clinical Practice Guidelines in Oncology. *J Natl Compr Canc Netw.* 2018;16(6):742–774.
24. Messina JL, Reintgen DS, Cruse CW, et al. Selective lymphadenectomy in patients with Merkel cell (cutaneous neuroendocrine) carcinoma. *Ann Surg Oncol.* 1997;4(5):389–395.
25. Poulsen M, Rischin D, Walpole E, et al. High-risk Merkel cell carcinoma of the skin treated with synchronous carboplatin/etoposide and radiation: a Trans-Tasman Radiation Oncology Group Study – TROG 96:07. *J Clin Oncol.* 2003;21(23):4371–4376.
26. Nghiem PT, Bhatia S, Lipson EJ, et al. PD-1 blockade with pembrolizumab in advanced Merkel-cell carcinoma. *N Engl J Med.* 2016;374(26):2542–2452.
27. Avraham JB, Villines D, Maker VK, et al. Survival after resection of cutaneous adnexal carcinomas with eccrine differentiation: risk factors and trends in outcomes. *J Surg Oncol.* 2013;108(1):57–62.
28. Crowson AN, Magro CM, Mihm MC. Malignant adnexal neoplasms. *Mod Pathol.* 2006;19(suppl 2):S93–S126.
29. Yu JB, Blitzblau RC, Patel SC, et al. Surveillance, Epidemiology, and End Results (SEER) database analysis of microcystic adnexal carcinoma (sclerosing sweat duct carcinoma) of the skin. *Am J Clin Oncol.* 2010;33(2):125–127.

30. Robson A, Greene J, Ansari N, et al. Eccrine porocarcinoma (malignant eccrine poroma): a clinicopathologic study of 69 cases. *Am J Surg Pathol.* 2001;25(6):710–720.
31. Hegarty PK, Suh J, Fisher MB, et al. Penoscrotal extramammary Paget's disease: the University of Texas M. D. Anderson Cancer Center contemporary experience. *J Urol.* 2011;186(1):97–102.
32. Ogata D, Kiyohara Y, Yoshikawa S, et al. Usefulness of sentinel lymph node biopsy for prognostic prediction in extramammary Paget's disease. *Eur J Dermatol.* 2016;26(3):254–259.
33. Nardelli AA, Stafinski T, Menon D. Effectiveness of photodynamic therapy for mammary and extra-mammary Paget's disease: a state of the science review. *BMC Dermatol.* 2011;11:13.
34. Polcz MM, Sebaratnam DF, Fernandez-Penas P. Atypical fibroxanthoma management: recurrence, metastasis and disease-specific death. *Australas J Dermatol.* 2018;59(1):10–25.
35. Ugurel S, Mentzel T, Utikal J, et al. Neoadjuvant imatinib in advanced primary or locally recurrent dermatofibrosarcoma protuberans: a multicenter phase II DeCOG trial with long-term follow-up. *Clin Cancer Res.* 2014;20(2):499–510.
36. Deneve JL, Messina JL, Bui MM, et al. Cutaneous leiomyosarcoma: treatment and outcomes with a standardized margin of resection. *Cancer Control.* 2013;20(4):307–312.
37. Shustef E, Kazlouskaya V, Prieto VG, Ivan D, Aung PP. Cutaneous angiosarcoma: a current update. *J Clin Pathol.* 2017;70(11):917–925.

11

Vascularized Composite Allotransplantation

MARIA Z. SIEMIONOW AND FATIH ZOR

"Losses must be replaced in kind."

Sir Harold Gillies

Historical Background

Advances in regenerative medicine have opened a new era and enabled reconstruction of devastating soft and bony tissue defects due to trauma, congenital deformities, and neoplastic conditions. Among the most promising advances within the realm of regenerative and restorative surgery is vascularized composite allotransplantation (VCA), which now allows for the reconstruction of defects that previously would have been treated with multistage flap reconstructions or prostheses. Similar to solid organ transplant (SOT), VCA involves transplantation of a vascularized graft, which is derived from different embryogenic origins and composed of a variety of heterogeneous antigenic tissues, across a genetic mismatch.[1]

Replacement of lost limbs and other organs is an old desire of humanity. The first historical mention of VCA dates back to Saints Cosmas and Damian (AD 286), who transferred an Ethiopian Moor's limb to a churchman. Later, successful solid organ transplantations constituted the initial milestones of VCA. The first successful human allograft was performed in 1957 by E. Peacock.[2] The allograft was composed of an en bloc digital flexor tendon mechanism. However, this transplantation did not contain skin. In the 1960s, immunosuppression was limited, which lead to the unfortunate rejection of the world's first hand transplant attempted by Robert Gilbert in 1964. Two weeks after the surgery, the graft was explanted and re-amputation was performed.[1] This complication delayed the next clinical hand transplantation, but studies about immunosuppression and experimental models continued to evolve to solve the problem. Once the clinical efficacy of cyclosporine (CsA) had been demonstrated in solid organ transplantation, studies were begun performing limb allograft transplantation in rats, dogs, and rabbits. In 1985, Hewitt reported the first successful rat limb allotransplantation. He also showed that transplanted bone marrow was functional and caused immune chimerism. During the same time period, Achauer mentioned the potential use of allografts for facial reconstruction. The first successful face transplantation in rats was performed by Maria Siemionow and colleagues.[3] Subsequently, many models of VCA were developed and reported in both small and large animals.[2,4] Pharmacological research continued during this time and new drugs were developed for immunosuppression. In 2003, Siemionow reported the first and the only rat transplant model of life-long donor-specific tolerance using a 7-day protocol of anti-alphabeta T-cell receptor monoclonal antibody and CsA.[5]

During the past 50 years, various clinical and experimental composite tissue allotransplantations have been performed, including: limb, trachea, flexor tendon apparatus, penis, nerve, knee, hand, face, abdominal wall, and uterus.[6,7]

Nomenclature

Autograft is a tissue that is transplanted from one location to another in the same individual. When the graft is transplanted from a genetically identical donor, such as transplants between syngeneic animals and human monozygotic twins, it is called *isograft*. *Allograft* is transplantation of tissues between genetically different individuals of the same species whereas *xenograft* is transplantation between different species.

Transplantation may also be described in terms of the site where the tissue is transplanted. *Orthotopic* transplantation means the recipient site is an anatomically similar site and *heterotopic* transplantation means the recipient site is different from the site of origin. In clinical practice, human kidney transplantation is performed to the groin region of the recipient, which is a heterotopic transplantation.

Despite the encouraging results, debate continues over the immunosuppression-related risks. Thus, the ultimate goal of allotransplantation is to obtain *transplant tolerance*, which is rejection-free acceptance of transplanted organs or tissues without the need for long-term immunosuppression. *Donor-specific tolerance* is defined as the state of donor-specific hyporesponsiveness in the recipient of allograft in the absence of immunosuppression. The state of tolerance to one organ or tissue (such as tendon) while simultaneously rejecting another (such as skin) is called *split tolerance*.[8] One of the best approaches to obtaining tolerance is hematopoietic stem cell chimerism. In *chimerism*, tissues from two genetically different organisms coexist in one organism. There are two types of chimerism: *macrochimerism* occurs when bone marrow is transplanted to a conditioned recipient, is engrafted, and produces all cell lineages; *microchimerism* arises from the migration of donor leucocytes from the allograft to the recipient and in microchimerism donor hematopoietic stem cells do not engraft, but are produced and migrated systemically.[9]

Basic Transplantation Immunology

Rejection is the major barrier to successful transplantation. During the immune response several interactions between the innate and adaptive immune system will lead to the rejection of transplanted cells, tissues, or organs unless the immune response is suppressed. The most important antigens contributing to allograft rejection are the major histocompatibility complex (MHC) antigens. The MHC proteins are encoded in chromosomes and have different nomenclature between species: human lymphocyte antigen (HLA) in humans, swine lymphocyte antigen (SLA) in swine, and RT1 in rat. There are two major classes of major histocompatibility complex (MHC) antigens. Class I antigens are expressed on nearly all nucleated cells and serve as the primary target for cytotoxic ($CD8^+$) T lymphocytes. Class II antigens are expressed primarily on vascular endothelium, antigen-presenting cells (APC), B cells, and activated T cells. Both class I and class II molecules have a specific site at which foreign peptide antigens can be presented after they have been processed by the cell. Innate immune system is activated as a result of ischemia–reperfusion injury, surgery, and trauma. Following this activation, foreign antigens are recognized by host T cells after being processed by host antigen-presenting cells (APC). This is called *indirect presentation*. In addition, host cells can recognize donor MHC antigens, which is called *direct presentation*.[10]

The allograft rejection or allorecognition is primarily regulated by T lymphocytes. The T cell lineage marker is called T-cell receptor (TCR) and there are two different types of T cells: alphabeta T cells, which are responsible for the allograft rejection, and gammadelta T cells, which are responsible for infections and antitumor activity. Mature alphabeta T cells are subdivided into two groups. T helper cells induce immune response and are CD4 positive. Cytotoxic T cells are responsible for cytotoxicity and are CD8 positive. Following allotransplantation, rejection begins with activation of T cells and T cells require a minimum of two signals for activation. The first step of T cell activation is recognition of foreign antigen by T cells (signal 1). The second step is activation of co-stimulatory signals (signal 2). The third step is T cell differentiation, which involves recreation of interleukin-2 following co-stimulatory signals (signal 3). Activated T cells are responsible for cell-mediated rejection of the allograft.[5,10]

Different types of allograft rejection may occur and are regulated by different mechanisms. Hyperacute rejection occurs within a few minutes after transplantation. This immune response is an antibody-mediated rejection process and the most frequent reason is the presence of presensitized antibodies against MHC antigens. Acute allograft rejection is a cell-mediated immune response and is observed in almost all composite tissue allotransplantation cases. The incidence of acute rejection exceeds 80% in hand and face transplants. It is primarily attributed to T cell activation. There is not enough data about antibody-mediated rejection (AMR) in VCA, although vascular rejection in solid organs is attributed to AMR.[10] Although not seen in the rat limb transplant model, there are several clinical case reports showing a B-cell-driven rejection episode with presence of donor-specific antibodies (DSA) and C4d positivity. However, it remains unclear whether these rejections were "truly" antibody-mediated or whether antibodies were bystanders of the rejection process.[11]

Chronic rejection is a common characteristic of solid organ transplantation; however, there are currently insufficient data available to define specific changes of chronic rejection in the VCA. The overall incidence of chronic allograft rejection in VCA recipients is low but has to be put in the context of the relatively short follow-up periods for most of the VCA transplants. Chronic rejection is characterized by fibrotic changes, myointimal proliferation of arteries and arterioles, loss of adnexa, skin, and muscular atrophy, and fibrosis of deep tissues,[10] which may be caused by non-immunogenic factors such as ischemia. Thus, the mechanisms of chronic rejection and its significance in VCA survival need further investigation.

In order to define and classify VCA rejection, various classification systems have been developed. The most accepted system for VCA rejection is the Banff 2007 Working Classification.[12] There are four grades of rejection: grade I mild, grade II moderate, grade III severe, and grade IV necrotizing acute rejection. In this system, the defining features to diagnose acute skin rejection include: inflammatory cell infiltration with involvement of epidermis and/or adnexal structures, epithelial apoptosis, dyskeratosis, and necrosis. This classification system is accepted by the International Society for Vascularized Composite Allotransplantation. Although, AMR and chronic rejection have not been implemented into the Banff 2007 classification, the Banff 2013 Meeting reported: "Current observations are that chronic VCA rejection is more similar than different from that in other organ transplants." The Banff 2013 Meeting Committee agreed to collect data for potential changes to the VCA–Banff system.[13]

Transplant immunology is the most important research area in the VCA field and many current studies attempt to define our knowledge and understanding of the rejection mechanisms, routine immunosuppressive regimes and tolerance-inducing strategies. Today, the only method of allograft rejection prevention is administration of chronic immunosuppression. There are several new drugs and protocols, which are used experimentally and clinically. However, the ultimate goal of transplant immunology is to provide donor-specific tolerance.

The practice of immunosuppressive administration can currently be divided into three phases: induction, maintenance, and rescue therapies. Induction immunotherapy is used as a means to overcome the ischemia–reperfusion injury and surgical trauma an allograft undergoes during the transplant procedure. Maintenance therapy is defined as immune suppression that is typically much lower in dose than induction therapy and therefore applicable in a chronic setting. Rescue therapy is similar to induction therapy in that it employs high-dose immune suppression and is usually given in response to a rejection episode. The efficacy of local immunosuppression in clinical VCA remains controversial. Topical treatments with steroid and tacrolimus ointments have achieved sufficient resolution of low-grade rejections. Immunosuppressive therapy has well-documented side effects which may give rise to conditions that shorten life. The incidence and severity of such side effects are well described, and this would allow for an informed decision to be made as to whether these side effects outweigh the potential benefit from VCA.

Experimental Models of VCA Transplantation

Experimental animal models constitute the workhorse of the VCA as they help to determine the technical feasibility and evaluate the effects of various immunosuppressive protocols and novel tolerance-inducing strategies.

Animal Models

During the past 20 years, many VCA models were developed to test the feasibility of transplantation of different body components as well as to assess the effects of various immunosuppressive protocols. The experimental models can be divided into two main categories, namely small and large animal models, including nonhuman primate models. Another classification of experimental models is based on the type and the content of the transplanted allograft:

- skin-containing VCA models (groin flap, abdominal wall, etc.)
- composite hindlimb allograft transplantation models (limb, groin–thigh osteomyocutaneous flap, knee allograft)
- composite facial allograft transplantation models (full face, hemiface, midface etc.)
- immunomodulatory VCA models (vascularized bone marrow, femur, sternum thymus).

The basic experimental models and their specific features are summarized in Table 11.1.

Skin and Soft Tissue VCA Models

These models include allografts containing skin, subcutaneous tissue, fat, and muscle (Fig. 11.1). The most frequently used skin-containing VCA model is the groin flap. This flap is also one of the first models used in allotransplantation research.[2] The groin flap model contains skin, fat, and lymphoid tissue harvested on the superficial epigastric vessels or femoral vessels. The groin flap is frequently used in immunological studies as it is technically simple and has low mortality. However, a disadvantage stems from the small size of the skin paddle. Other soft tissue flaps include both skin and various muscles, such as the semimembranous pectoralis flaps. Another soft tissue model is the total abdominal wall transplantation in which the entire abdominal wall skin is harvested on bilateral femoral vessels. This model was developed to investigate the effect of size of skin component on the development of chimerism. Fig. 11.1 presents examples of the skin and soft tissue models of VCA.

Hindlimb Allotransplantation Models

The rat hindlimb transplantation model was described in 1978.[14] In this model a circumferential skin incision at the mid-thigh level is made on the donor and next the superficial epigastric vessels, femoral vessels, saphenous nerve, and femoral nerve are dissected, and thigh muscles are sharply divided. During muscle transection, the sciatic nerve is dissected. Next, the femoral bone is cut with a saw. The recipient is prepared using the same technique. Following division of the donor femoral vessels the limb is transferred to the recipient. First, the femoral bone is fixed with an intramedullary rod and wire suture. The femoral vessels are subsequently anastomosed and the femoral, sciatic, and saphenous nerves are coaptated. Muscles and skin are closed anatomically. Hindlimb transplantation in the rat is a complex procedure involving connection of bone, muscles, nerves, vessels, and skin. The rat hindlimb allograft transplant is the most popular animal model tested in preparation for human hand transplantation. This underlies the importance of having a fast, simple surgical procedure (with short anesthesia) that provides good animal recovery and consequently robust data for statistical assessment. In order to obtain a fast and simple limb allotransplantation method, Chang et al described a groin–thigh osteomyocutaneous flap, which is composed of skin (groin), muscle (thigh), and bone (⅔ femur), based on the femoral vessels and superficial epigastric vessels.[15] The advantages of this model are shortened operative time, easy monitoring of graft rejection, decreased morbidity and mortality rates, and earlier postoperative ambulation.

Facial Allograft Transplantation Models

Since the face has many different anatomical structures and units, there are many facial allograft transplantation models,[4] developed to evaluate transplantation of different facial structures (Fig. 11.2). Siemionow et al were the first to develop a full-face scalp allotransplantation model.[3] This facial allograft transplant, which includes bilateral ear, neck,

TABLE 11.1 **Experimental Models of VCA and Their Specific Features**

Experimental Model	Tissues Included, Specific Features
Skin-containing VCA Models	
Groin flap as vascularized skin transplant model	Skin, fat, and lymphoid tissue. Simple, used in immunologic studies, small skin component
Semimembranosus muscle and epigastric skin transplant model	Skin, fat, muscle, and lymphoid tissue. Used for microcirculatory, physiologic, and immunologic studies
Total abdominal wall transplant model	Skin, fat, and lymphoid tissue. Contains large skin component
Hindlimb Models	
Rat hindlimb transplant model	Popular, but technically challenging animal model containing all tissue components including vascularized bone marrow
Groin–thigh osteomyocutaneous transplant model	Alternative model to hindlimb transplant. Less challenging technique, low mortality
Immunomodulatory VCA Models	
Vascularized femur transplant model	Femoral bone, bone marrow, cartilage and muscle. Applied for bone marrow induced chimerism studies
Bilateral vascularized femoral bone transplant model	Larger bone marrow content. Applied for tolerance induction studies
Composite vascularized skin/bone transplant model	Combination of groin flap with vascularized femur transplantation. Enables follow-up of rejection
Vascularized osteomyocutaneous iliac transplant model	Iliac bone, bone marrow, abdominal wall musculature, and wide skin island
Vascularized sternum transplant model	Sternum, skin, and muscles. Contains bone marrow
Thymus transplant model	Used for evaluation of effect of thymus on tolerance induction
Osteomyocutaneous sternum, ribs, thymus, pectoralis muscles, and skin transplant	Includes all three important immunological tissues (bone marrow, thymus, and skin) for immunology and tolerance studies
Facial Allograft Models	
Full face/scalp transplant model	Includes ear, neck, and facial skin without eyelids and nose. High mortality
Hemiface/scalp transplant model	Unilateral ear, neck, and facial skin. Used for immunological studies in facial transplantation
Hemiface calvarium transplant model	Temporal muscle and parietal bone included to hemiface scalp model. Contains bone marrow
Hemiface mandible tongue allotransplantation model	Mandibular bone and tongue are included into hemiface model. Contains bone marrow
Maxilla transplant model	Evaluation of response of maxillary bone to transplantation
Midface transplant model with sensory and motor units	First model to evaluate motor and sensory recovery after face transplantation
Total osteocutaneous hemiface transplant model	Includes entire hemiface: vascularized nose, premaxilla, eyelids, upper and lower lips, external ear and facial skin for immunological, histological, and biological evaluation of different facial tissues
Composite face and eyeball transplant model	Evaluation of optic nerve regeneration and evaluation of orbit content

and facial skin without eyelid and nose skin, is based on the bilateral common carotid artery and external jugular vein. However, the surgical procedure of full-face transplantation was challenging, with a high rate of mortality. Thus, a hemiface scalp allotransplantation model was developed in the Cleveland Clinic Laboratories. This model included the unilateral scalp, ear, neck, and facial skin – excluding eyelid and nose – and was based on the unilateral common carotid artery and external jugular vein. The hemiface scalp allotransplantation model is generally used for immunological studies assessing facial allograft transplantation. Yazici et al developed a hemiface calvaria model by including temporal muscle and parietal bone to the prior hemiface scalp model.[15] This model included parietal bone, with bone marrow cells, which were viable up to 100 days post transplant as confirmed by histology. The facial allograft model,

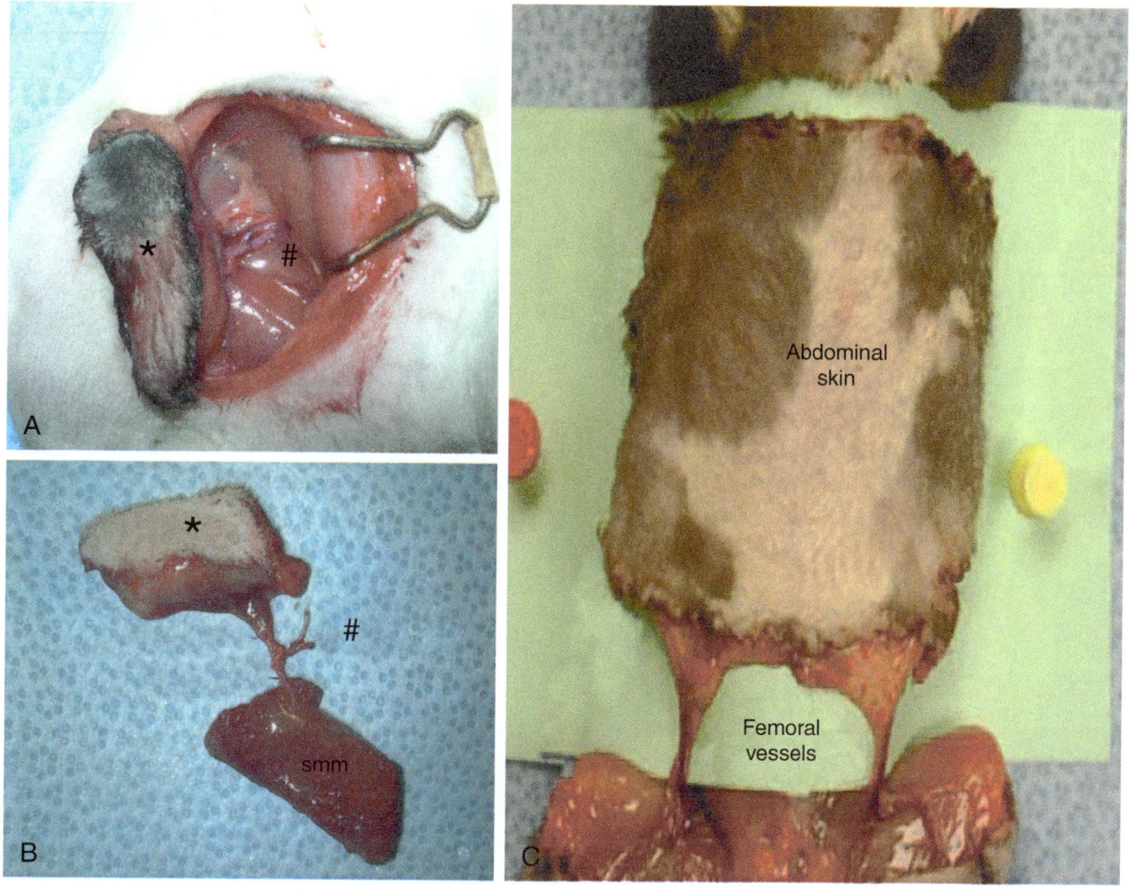

• **Fig. 11.1** Skin-containing VCA models. (A) Groin flap (*) raised on vascular pedicle (#) of the femoral artery and vein. (B) Semimembranosus muscle and epigastric skin flap model. * Epigastric flap; # vascular pedicle; *smm*, semimembranosus muscle. (C) Total abdominal wall transplant model harvested on the bilateral vascular pedicle of the femoral artery and vein.

containing mandible with bone marrow cells, was later described by Kulahci et al.[15] In this heterotopic allotransplantation model including hemiface mandible and tongue, Kulahci et al showed high levels of donor-specific chimerism. In the maxilla allotransplantation model, the maxilla was dissected along Le Fort II osteotomy lines based on the common carotid artery and external jugular vein and the harvested allograft was transplanted to the recipient. This model was developed to evaluate the maxillary response to allotransplantation. The first model that evaluated the motor and sensory recovery after facial allotransplantation was developed by Zor et al.[16] This composite midface transplant model with the sensory and motor neuromuscular units included premaxilla, mystacial pad, and nose with infraorbital and facial nerves. At 100 days post transplant, somatosensory evoked potentials (SSEP) and motor evoked potentials (MEP) tests revealed that sensory and motor recovery reached 67% of normal latency values for the infraorbital nerve and 70% for facial nerve latency values. Recently, a total osteocutaneous hemifacial allotransplantation model was developed in order to extend the application of the face/scalp transplantation in the rat model.[17] This model included all hemifacial structures, such as vascularized nose, premaxilla, eyelids, and upper and lower lips, external ear, and facial skin. This new model, including all the hemifacial soft tissues as well as the premaxillary bone segment with nose components, enabled immunological, histological, and biological evaluation of different facial tissues and structures in one complex composite allotransplantation scenario. The most recent advancement in facial allotransplantation models is the development of composite face and eyeball allotransplant model with the optic nerve.[18] This experimental model allows for evaluation of optic nerve regeneration and the effect of allotransplantation on composite facial tissues, including orbital content.

Immunomodulatory VCA Models

These models include vascularized bone and bone marrow transplantation, and immunological tissue transfers, such as thymus, in order to induce chimerism and immune tolerance (Fig. 11.3). Vascularized femur transfer is composed of femoral bone, bone marrow, periosteum, cartilage, and muscle tissues. This was initially described by Tai et al.[15] This model was used to investigate the effects of vascularized bone marrow transplantation on chimerism induction. Bilateral vascularized femoral bone transplantation model was then subsequently described by Agaoglu and Siemionow.[15] Bilateral femoral bones were harvested based upon the abdominal aorta and the inferior vena cava and after transfer connected to the same vessels in the recipient.

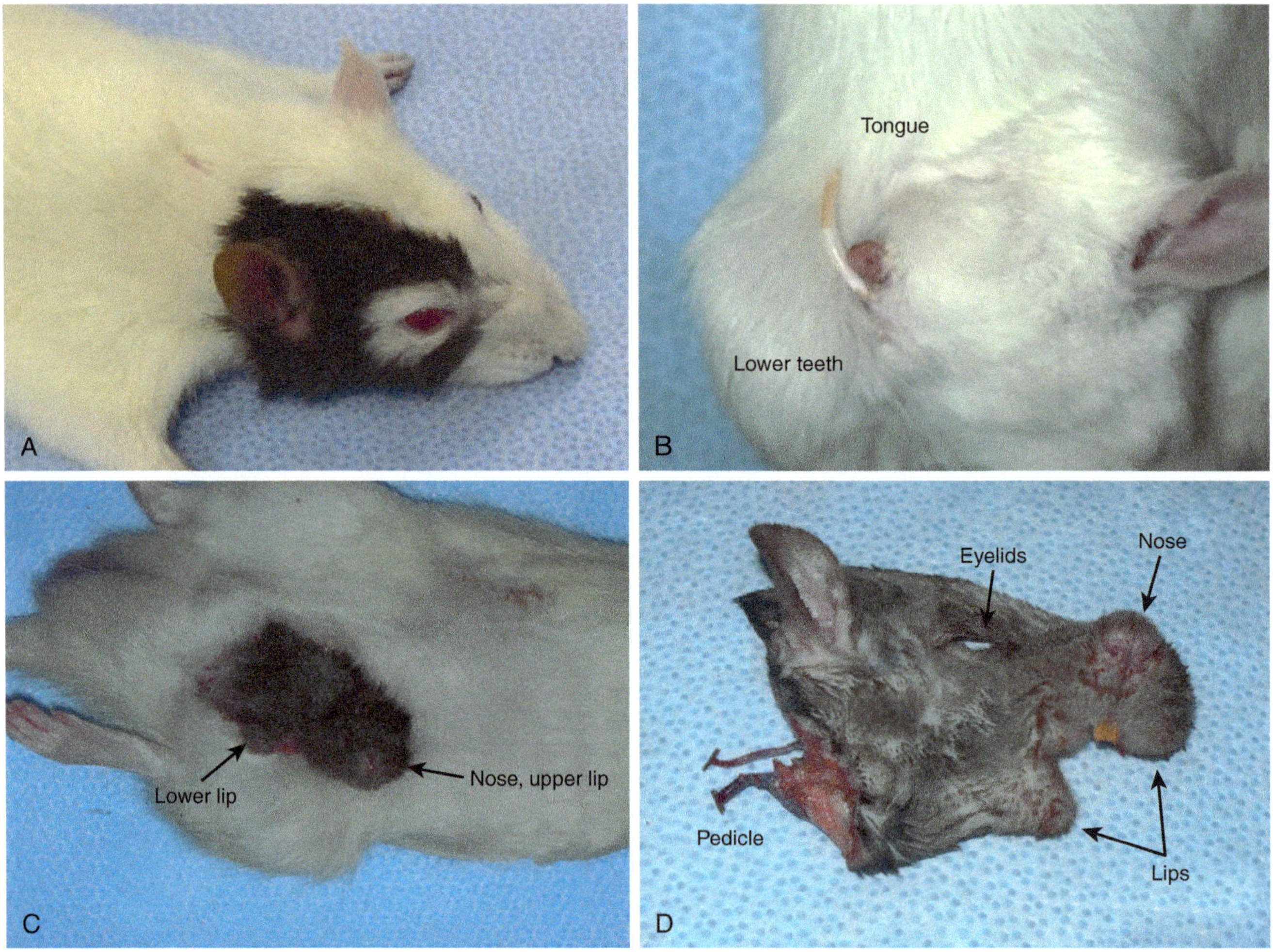

• **Fig. 11.2** Facial VCA models. (A) Hemiface and scalp allotransplantation model. (B) Hemiface mandible tongue allotransplantation model. (C) Midface transplant model with sensory and motor units. (D) Total osteocutaneous hemifacial allotransplantation model.

This model included the same tissue types but a larger bone marrow content, which allowed to induce higher levels of donor-specific chimerism in the recipient. Another vascularized bone marrow transplantation model was the composite vascularized skin/bone allograft model. This model was basically a combination of groin flap with vascularized femur transplantation. The allograft was carrying both – the skin component to assess skin flap rejection and bone marrow component to induce the chimerism. In order to reduce the morbidity and increase the allogenic load, a vascularized osteomyocutaneous iliac flap was described. This flap included iliac bone, abdominal wall musculature, and a large skin island, harvested on the iliolumbar artery and vein. This flap has a large skin island with bone marrow content, making this model almost an ideal composite tissue model. Unfortunately, it is technically a challenging model, and despite high bone marrow content the chimerism levels were reported to be low. Another bone marrow transplantation method is vascularized sternum transplantation. Sternum, including presternal skin and muscles, was first transplanted by Santiago et al.[15] The allograft was harvested on the thoracic aorta and superior vena cava.

When the bone marrow containing models are compared, it is seen that the limb model contains 48.75×10^6 bone marrow cells. On the other hand, iliac, femur, and sternum models contain 25, 50, and 7.5×10^6 bone marrow cells, respectively. The results of these experimental studies also revealed that chimerism levels are directly related to the amount of the transplanted bone marrow cells.

Another method of tolerance induction in experimental studies is to include thymus transplantation. The first thymus transplantation was described by Jiang et al in 1999.[15] Later, composite osseomusculocutaneous sternum, ribs, thymus, pectoralis muscles, and skin allotransplantation models were developed.[19] This model includes three important immunological tissues (bone marrow, thymus, and skin) and has the advantage of carrying bone marrow cells for chimerism induction, skin for monitoring of rejection as well as thymus for tolerance induction.

Large Animal Models and Other VCA Models

Large VCA animal models are accepted as valid, preclinical translational models and are developed for assessment of feasibility, to evaluate immune response to immunosuppressive

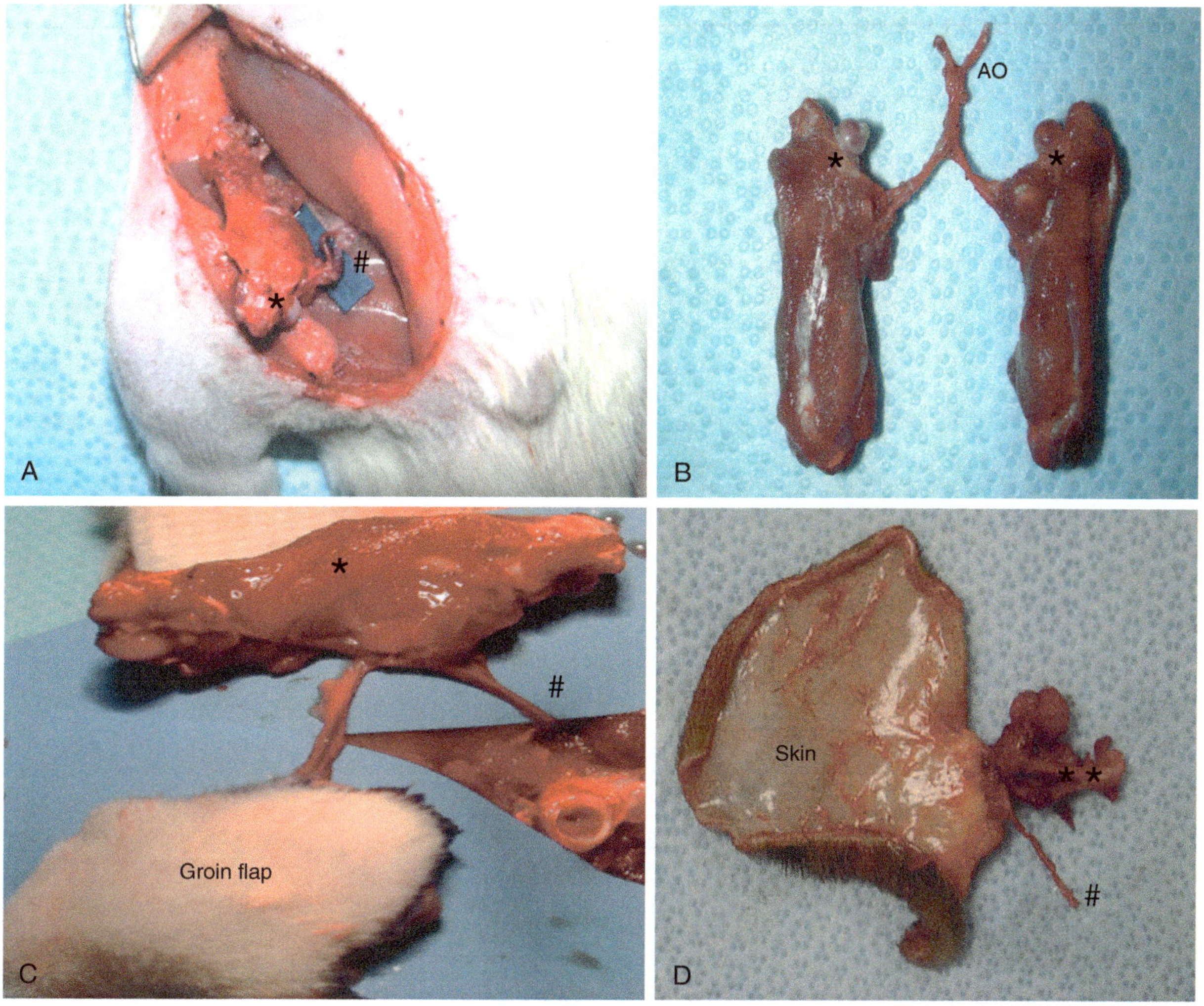

• **Fig. 11.3** Immunomodulatory VCA models. (A) Vascularized femur transfer: * femoral bone; # vascular pedicle of the allograft. (B) Bilateral vascularized femoral bone transplantation: * indicates the femoral bone; *AO*, abdominal aorta as the vascular pedicle of the allograft. (C) Composite vascularized skin/bone allograft model: * femoral bone; # vascular pedicle of the allograft. (D) Vascularized osteomyocutaneous iliac flap: ** iliac bone segment, # vascular pedicle of the allograft.

protocols in preparation for the clinical application of VCA transplantation. Facial allotransplantation models have been described in various large animal models, including dogs, rabbits, and swine.[20] A swine model of osteomyocutaneous radial forearm flap transplantation is described by Ren et al.[15] Nonhuman primate models of face transplantation were studied in cynomolgus monkeys.[21] Technical and immunosuppressive requirements for prolonged graft survival were tested in these models. Hand transplantation in nonhuman primates was described in baboons and Rhesus monkeys. Both partial and total hand transplantation and immunology related studies were assessed in these models. A preclinical swine model of whole eyeball transplantation has also been described by a group from the University of Pittsburgh.[22]

There are also other VCA models, which are developed for evaluation of changes occurring in different organs after transplantation. Of these, perhaps the most important is the cremaster muscle allotransplantation model, which was used for assessment of microcirculatory hemodynamics and leukocyte–endothelial interactions following allotransplantation. Laryngeal and penis allotransplantation models are examples of other VCA models that are tested and reported in the literature. However, these models are not clinically translational models.[23]

Cadaver Studies for VCA Transplantation

Allotransplantation potentially solves challenging reconstructive problems by allowing the surgeon to transfer the entire VCA organ, such as a human hand, in one procedure to the recipient. However, before clinical applications all technical aspects of VCA harvesting and transplantation have to be addressed and tested in cadaveric studies. For hand transplantation, the anatomic and technical challenges have been already determined by experience with hand replantation cases. But facial composite tissue allotransplantation has required extensive cadaver studies in order to determine time of surgery, recommended sequence and type of dissection, and pertinent anatomical structures.

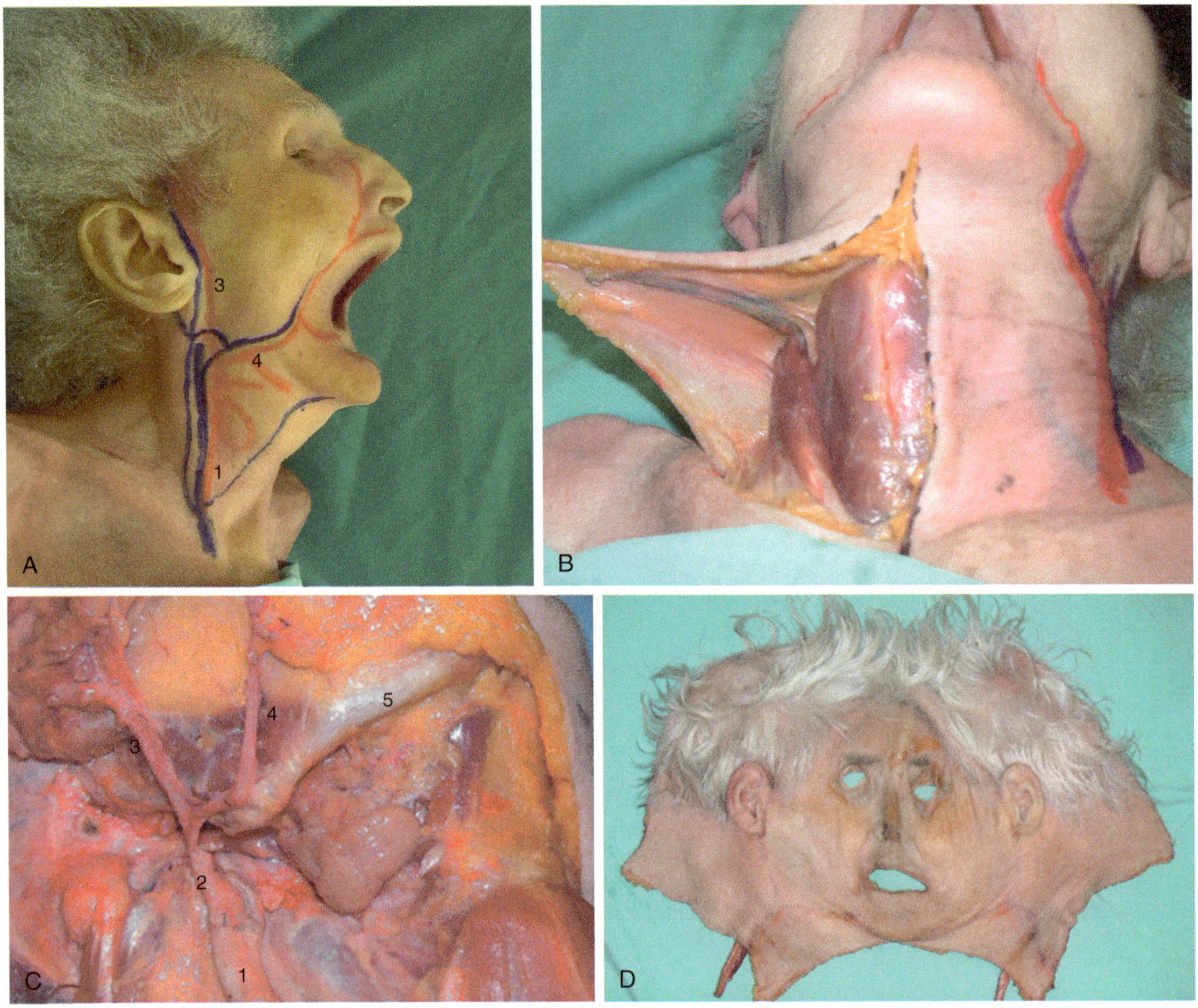

• **Fig. 11.4** Cadaver dissection of subplatysmal, sub-SMAS face/scalp flap. (A) The outline of the underlying vascular structures at the face and neck. (B) Following an anterior neck incision, dissection is performed at subplatysmal level. (C) The arterial network of the face/scalp flap after flap elevation: 1, common carotid artery; 2, external carotid artery; 3, superficial temporal artery; 4, facial artery; 5, mandible margin. (D) The harvested total face/scalp flap.

As a result, cadaver face transplantation studies have been performed in preparation for clinical application of face transplantation.

The technical feasibility of face/scalp transplantation was first confirmed in cadaver studies by Siemionow et al.[24] Briefly, a whole facial-scalp flap was elevated in the subplatysmal, sub-superficial musculoaponeurotic system (SMAS), and subgaleal planes within the neck, face, and scalp respectively. Siemionow et al have described the details of the surgical technique of facial-scalp flap harvesting in a cadaver study (Fig. 11.4). They also demonstrated the integrity of the vascular territories following facial flap harvest by methylene blue dye injection. As a continuation of this study, Siemionow et al performed a mock transplantation by harvesting a total face/scalp flap in one group of cadavers and transferring the flap to recipient cadavers.[24] During the donor flap inset, anatomical considerations of the flap anchoring sites and the length of arterial and venous pedicles and nerves incorporated in the flap were evaluated. The vascular pedicle was found to be suitable for microvascular anastomoses and nerve coaptation was feasible. The mean total time of facial flap harvesting was 235.62 ± 21.94 minutes. In this study, the sequence of procedures for mock facial transplantation was also described. Later, a coronal-posterior approach for facial-scalp flap harvesting from the donor cadavers was developed to prepare an extended length of the neurovascular pedicles used in composite facial allotransplantation. It is advocated that the extended length of the neurovascular pedicle will not only provide easier vessel anastomoses and nerve coaptation but also will allow for meticulous hemostasis after artery and venous anastomoses.

The face can be surgically divided into distinct anatomic and functional units. Reconstruction of each unit is unique. According to these anatomic principles, Lengelé described three main segmental face transplantation types that can be harvested based on one or more branches of the external carotid artery network and includes sensory and/or motor nerves specific for each region[25] representing: lower central facial allograft, midfacial allograft, and upper facial allograft.

Lower Central Facial Allograft (Type I)

The lower central facial allograft includes the donor's nose, lips, and chin. It is vascularized by bilateral facial vessels and contains all perioral muscles harvested under subperiosteal dissection. Motor innervation of these muscles arises from zygomatic, buccal, and mandibular branches of the facial nerve, whereas sensory nerves, the mental (V_3) and infraorbital (V_2) nerve, arise from the trigeminal nerve. If necessary, dissection can be extended deeper to include the middle part of the mandibular arch to restore bony support to the chin.

Midfacial Allograft (Type II)

The midfacial allograft contains the nose, upper lip, cheeks and the perioral muscles. It is harvested on both the right and left facial pedicles. Although it can include soft tissues only, it may also include the anterior part of maxilla and zygomatic arches and variable parts of the anterior palate. Graft sensitivity is restored by infraorbital nerves (V_2) with motor reinnervation relying on the zygomatic and buccal rami of the facial nerve. Another midfacial allograft, Le Fort II-based osteocutaneous face transplantation, was described by Yazici et al.[15] Using six cadavers, in combination with MRI and angiography, the authors showed the vascular territories in the masticatory space along with the internal maxillary artery's anterior pterygomaxillary extension.

Upper Facial Allograft (Type III)

The upper facial allograft includes the superficial planes of the forehead, eyelids, and base of the nose and the deeper planes of the frontalis, glabellar and orbicularis oculi muscles. It is raised on the bilateral superficial temporal artery pedicles and supraorbital sensory nerves (V_1). Motor innervation is provided by frontal and zygomatic branches of the facial nerve.

In addition to these three facial transplantation types, there are two more types proposed by Lengelé. Type IV is the total face transplantation, which combines all three described types; Type V is the total face and scalp transplantation.

Face transplantation is potentially indicated only for severe defects that either failed or cannot be repaired by conventional reconstructive techniques. Thus, face transplantation should be considered only in patients with massive facial defects. Since these massive defects often include bone deficits, the indications for face transplantation may be more rewarding when bone and soft tissue replacement is needed. Follmar et al carried out mock osteocutaneous face transplantation in the cadaver model.[15] The face was harvested in the subperiosteal plane and included the Le Fort III osseous segment. The allograft was inset by rigid internal fixation and soft tissue approximation. They showed that an osteocutaneous face transplant procedure was technically feasible. On the basis of their experiment and review of prior investigations, the authors have identified 10 points that present technical challenges specific to osteocutaneous transplantation of the face. These included: customization of the bony segment, sensory and motor innervation, extraocular movements, dentition, mastication, speech and swallowing, airway, vascular considerations, immunological considerations, and identity issues.

Baccarani et al presented two face-harvesting techniques in a fresh human cadaver model.[15] In the first technique, the skin and soft tissue of the face was harvested by dissections carried in subgaleal, sub-SMAS, and subplatysmal planes. In the second technique, the entire soft tissue and bony structures of the midface were harvested in a subperiosteal plane dissection combined with a Le Fort III osteotomy. Each face was harvested successfully as a bipedicled flap based on the external carotid arteries, the external jugular veins, and the facial veins. They showed that each technique was a theoretically viable approach to face harvest for facial VCA.

Baccarani et al compared two facial flap-harvesting techniques for alloplastic facial transplantation. They aimed to shorten donor-graft harvesting time and reduce warm ischemia time. Six paired SMAS plane-based composite facial-scalp flaps were harvested using either a superficial temporal artery (STA) or a facial artery (FA) pedicle technique or an external carotid artery (ECA) pedicle technique. They found that STA and FA pedicle-based flaps provide a shorter harvesting time and potentially safer dissection method for facial transplantation compared with previously reported total facial allograft harvesting techniques based on the ECA pedicle.

Later, Gordon et al applied orthognathic principles and practice to maxillofacial allotransplantation.[1] They planned the allotransplantation by either using dental cast models, cephalometric analyses, model surgery, and occlusal splint fabrication or using a mimic Gunning splint (an edentulous scenario). The results showed that functional and esthetic results are superior when using orthognathic principles. Brown et al later incorporated computer-assisted planning and intraoperative navigation to improve precision and efficiency in complex maxillofacial allotransplantation procedures.[15] Ten mock facial transplantations were performed, including: the facial skin, mimetic muscles, tongue, midface by means of a Le Fort III osteotomy, and mandible by means of the sagittal split osteotomies. They showed that preoperative computer planning, and intraoperative navigation provided precise osteotomies and a good donor–recipient skeletal match, which greatly reduced the need for intraoperative adjustments and manipulation.

More recently, allotransplantation of the orbital globe and periorbital tissues was studied by Siemionow et al.[26] In this cadaver model, they harvested the periorbital soft tissues, bony orbit, and orbital contents by performing a box osteotomy (Fig. 11.5). Both the external carotid artery and

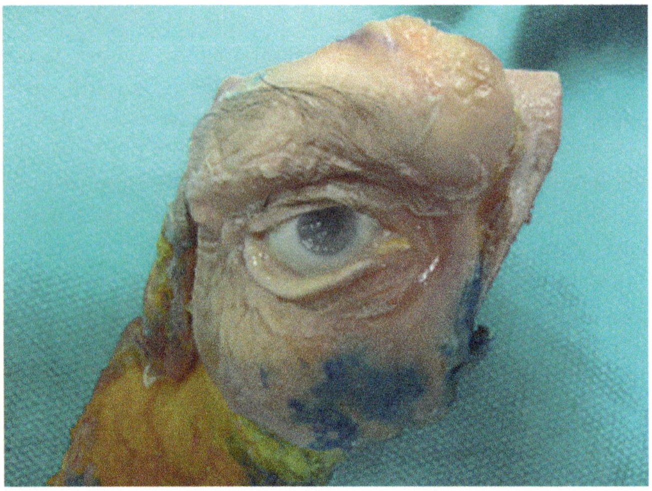

• **Fig. 11.5** The composite eye periorbital allograft is seen after harvest, based on external and internal carotid systems.

the ophthalmic artery were prepared and indocyanine was used to confirm perfusion of the flap.[27] As being the first human model of composite eyeball–periorbital transplantation, this study showed good perfusion of the osteocutaneous eye and periorbital flap and confirmed the feasibility of composite eyeball–periorbital transplantation in the clinical setting. Although harvesting of the flap required an intracranial approach, it introduced a new option for reconstruction of the periorbital region, including the eyeball.

Finally, cadaver studies have been performed to overcome some problems that have been confronted during the clinical application of face allotransplantation. The collected experience from prior facial allotransplantation has shown that the recovery of sensory function of the face allograft is unpredictable. The most frequent problem in the clinical setting is the lack of healthy donor nerves, especially in central face defects. In their study, Rodriguez-Lorenzo et al investigated the technical feasibility of transferring the supraorbital nerve to the infraorbital nerve in a model of central facial transplantation.[15] This study showed that supraorbital nerve to infraorbital nerve transfer is an anatomically feasible procedure in central facial allotransplantation and this procedure could be used to improve the restoration of midfacial sensation by the use of a healthy recipient nerve in cases where the recipient infraorbital nerves are not available.

Another nerve transfer study on allotransplantation was performed by Audolfsson et al and evaluated the technical feasibility of performing nerve transfers in facial transplantation for both sensory and motor neurotization.[15] The first part of this study evaluated the technical feasibility of nerve transfer from the cervical plexus to the mental nerve and the masseter nerve to the buccal branches of the facial nerve. The second part aimed to simulate the face transplantation scenario, focusing on sensory restoration of the midface and upper lip by neurotization of the infraorbital nerve, sensory restoration of the lower lip by neurotization of the mental nerve, and smile reanimation by neurotization of the buccal branches of the facial nerve. They concluded that all nerve transfer procedures are technically feasible and could be used in face transplantation either as a primary nerve reconstruction, or as a secondary procedure for enhancement of functional outcomes.

Clinical Applications of VCA Transplantation

VCA has considerable potential in reconstructive surgery. With a multidisciplinary, highly specialized surgical team and standard immunosuppression, almost any missing part of the human body can be restored using principles of reconstructive transplantation. Many clinical VCA applications have been reported and the golden principle of every procedure is the same: proper selection of the patient as well as the donor, a well-adapted VCA to the needs of the recipient, a multidisciplinary dedicated team, standard immunosuppression, and postoperative care. In this section, clinical applications of VCA are summarized.

Upper Extremity Transplantation

The loss of a hand, or both, is an important impediment for a patient and when replantation is impossible, and a prosthesis is not accepted, hand transplantation remains as the only viable solution for restoration of hand function. Since the first successful hand transplantation in Lyon in 1998, over 100 hand transplantation procedures have been performed all over the world.[2,28]

Owing to the many years of experience with hand replantation procedures, there were a limited number of anatomical and technical challenges encountered during hand transplantation. The time estimates, the recommended sequence of the transplant procedure, and the pertinent anatomical structures were already known. Today, bilateral forearm amputation is the worldwide-accepted indication for hand transplantation.

Certainly, patients with guillotine-type amputations at the level of the wrist joint and distal forearm are the best candidates. In order to reduce the warm ischemia time, two teams of surgeons working simultaneously are preferred. During the graft harvest, it is better to have an excess length of all donor structures, so they can be joined with the recipient tissues without any tension. This is especially important for neurovascular structures. Both teams must use a tourniquet to operate in a bloodless field for optimal identification of all available neurovascular structures, tendons, and muscles. Extensive incisions in the forearm must be made for better exposure of the neurovascular structures and to facilitate the dissection. Incisions are not placed directly above the nerves and vessels, as swelling may prevent direct closure, and the skin flaps must be prepared for Z-plasty transposition during closure. Skin incisions must be planned according to stump scarring and the possibility of creating a zigzag skin-flap closure. Dissection and identification of vital structures starts at the subcutaneous level and continues down to the bone. All available structures have to identified and tagged. After identification, the tourniquet is released to control bleeding. When preparation of all structures of the donor hand is completed, it is perfused with 500 ml of chilled University of Wisconsin (UW) solution through the brachial artery. The sequence of hand transplantation is as follows:

1. Osteosynthesis
2. Vessel repair (anastomosis of the one main artery and two veins)
3. Muscle–tendon repair/transfer
4. Definitive vessel and nerve repair
5. Skin closure and dressing.

During definitive vessel repair, the two main arteries and at least 4–6 veins must be anastomosed. It is important to anastomose not only the superficial veins but also deep venae comitantes. This guarantees the optimal venous return. All three main forearm/hand nerves (median, ulnar, and radial/superficial radial, depending on amputation level) must be repaired.

Following skin closure using the skin flaps in a Z-plasty manner, postoperative care and physical rehabilitation is started. The most important complications related to hand transplantation are infections and rejection episodes. Acute rejection episodes have a negative effect on the outcome of the upper extremity allotransplantation.

Immunosuppressive protocols of hand transplantation are similar to solid organ transplants and mainly include induction therapy with thymoglobulin or alemtuzumab combined with tacrolimus, mycophenolate mofetil, and prednisone. Maintenance therapy usually consists of tacrolimus with either mycophenolate mofetil or/and prednisone.

Face Transplantation

The first successful face transplantation was performed on November 27, 2005 in France.[29] Since 2005 there have been around 40 reports of facial composite tissue allotransplantation.[7] Perhaps one of the most important issues in face transplantation is selection of the recipient. Today, the only scoring system developed for recipient selection is the Cleveland Clinic's FACES score. This scoring system depends on the functional status, esthetic deficit, comorbidities, exposed tissues, and surgical history of the recipient which provides unique ability to objectively assess patients seeking face transplantation.

Matching the donor and recipient is essential to ensure compatibility for the major (ABO) blood groups, as well as a negative cross-match between the donor and recipient. Whether tissue matching for HLA confers a significant benefit on graft survival after facial transplantation is not known, however there are reports indicating that the number of the HLA mismatch may play a role in the number of acute rejection episodes. The cytomegalovirus immunization status of the donor and the recipient also must be taken into account.[30]

There are some screening issues unique to face transplantation. The transplanted tissue is visible and therefore must be cosmetically matched to the recipient. Broadly this means that the donor and recipient should be of the same sex, ethnicity, and also of similar age.

The surgery may begin simultaneously on the donor and the recipient but sometimes it is following removal of all scar tissues that the actual size of the facial defect of the recipient is determined and then the donor operation is started. The allograft is harvested based on a reliable pedicle, which generally includes either unilateral or bilateral facial and superficial temporal vessels. Depending on the reconstructive need, this allograft may contain soft and bony tissues and the level of dissection may be sub-SMAS or subperiosteal. The motor and sensory nerves are also prepared. The following steps can be summarized as: fixation of the allograft, microvascular vessel anastomoses, nerve coaptations, anatomical repair of the muscles, and other structures and skin closure.

Physiotherapy and speech therapy (if indicated) may begin as early as 48 hours following surgery. Generally, rehabilitation consists of supervised controlled passive and active motion exercises, assessment of mastication, smell, speech, swallowing, and facial expression. Gentle massage, sensory re-education, and education of new face acceptance are introduced. Psychological status (i.e., anxiety, depression), quality of life, and self-esteem of the patient are evaluated. Sensory and motor reinnervations are closely monitored.[30]

From an esthetic standpoint, the patients are satisfied with their results and have reported that they feel more comfortable in public, even knowing that multiple surgical revisions such as scar revision and redundant tissue excision are necessary in order to obtain an optimal esthetic outcome.

Other Clinical VCA Applications

Besides hand and face transplantation, there are other clinical applications of VCA, including: larynx, trachea, knee, femur, abdominal wall, peripheral nerve, tongue, scalp/external ear, penis, uterus, flexor tendon apparatus, lower extremity, and muscles.[31] However, most of these applications are still limited and supported by a small number of cases, except for uterus transplantation which has expanded significantly in recent years and babies have already been born after uterus transplantation.[32]

Laryngotracheal Transplantation

The first successful laryngo-tracheal allotransplantation was performed in the Cleveland Clinic in 1988. The allograft included the entire larynx, and adjacent tracheopharyngeal structures including thyroid and parathyroid glands. Functional results and patient satisfaction were excellent, with normal swallowing and speech restoration. Later, more than 20 laryngotracheal transplantations were performed. One of these transplantations also included the esophageal part, which is the first esophagus transplantation. Although the initial results are encouraging, the long-term success of laryngeal transplantation relies on proper surveillance of allograft rejection, prevention of chronic rejection, and appropriate rescue therapy in the case of graft failure.

Knee and Femur Transplantation

The first femur, knee, and surrounding soft tissue transplantation was performed by Hoffmann in 1996. The key problem of knee transplantation is monitoring of the acute rejection. The initial results were good, however; the long-term results were not satisfactory in most patients. Long-term results suggest that knee transplantation should be limited to cases with extensive composite tissue loss accompanied by cartilage and bone loss, deficient extensor mechanism and soft tissue and skin defects without any signs of infection. Transplantation should only be considered as the last option before above-knee amputation will be necessary in a young patient.

Lower Extremity Transplantation (LET)

There are only limited number of lower extremity transplantations reported and the results so far are discouraging.

To date, four cases of LET have been reported.[23] The first successful complete LET was performed between ischiopagus twins by Zuker and colleagues in 2006. In 2011, Cavadas and colleagues performed the world's first bilateral transfemoral allotransplantation of the lower extremities. During the long-term follow-up, at the 15th postoperative month the patient developed primary central nervous system posttransplant lymphoproliferative disease (PTLD). The immunosuppressive protocol was immediately discontinued, and both lower extremity allografts were removed, but despite the effort the patient died. The remaining two cases of lower extremity transplantation also resulted in extremity loss and the patient's death.

Abdominal Wall Transplantation

Abdominal wall allotransplantation was described by Levi and colleagues. Transplantation of abdominal wall allograft includes both rectus abdominis muscles, overlying fascia, subcutaneous tissue and skin, and is harvested based on the inferior epigastric vessels. The recipients of abdominal wall transplantation received simultaneous intestinal or solid organ transplantations (SOT) without alteration of the immunosuppressive protocol required for organ transplants. Despite mixed outcomes marked by graft failure and death of the patient in some cases, overall, the abdominal wall transplantation proved its feasibility in the tension-free closure of the abdomen after SOT and introduced the idea that the skin component of the abdominal wall graft may allow for early detection of solid organ rejection.

Peripheral Nerve Transplantation

Mackinnon was first to perform a successful peripheral nerve allotransplantation. The immunosuppressive protocol of peripheral nerve differs from other solid organ and VCA transplants. First, immunosuppression is needed only for the first 12–24 months and, second, it includes FK506, which is known to enhance nerve regeneration. The results of allogenic peripheral nerve transplantation show encouraging results.

Uterus Transplantation

Uterus transplantation has become a promising solution for patients with absolute uterine factor infertility. Brännström performed the first successful uterus transplant, showing that a live birth is possible after uterus transplantation. One of the key advantages of uterus transplant is that the immunosuppression is temporary because the organ can be removed after successful pregnancy. Deceased donor uterus transplantation with subsequent live birth is also possible.[32]

Penis Transplantation

From the reconstructive point of view, penile transplantation provides a unique technique to replace the missing corpora cavernosae, corpus spongiosum, urethra, glans, and skin with native structures. To date, there are 3 cases of penile transplantation worldwide, with encouraging results.[23] The first penile transplantation was performed in China in 2006.[33] Although the patient was able to void spontaneously at postoperative day 10, the transplanted penis was removed at day 14, due to psychological distress and at the request of the patient and his wife. The first successful penile transplantation was performed 8 years later, in South Africa. Later, the first US penis transplantation was performed in 2016. Despite these encouraging results, penile transplantation is far from being a routine clinical operation, and there are several challenges that must be overcome.

Pediatric VCA

The first pediatric bilateral hand transplantation was performed in 2015.[34] This case showed the surgical feasibility and restoration of functionality in pediatric VCA. There are, however, specific problems related to this patient population, such as growth of the allograft after transplantation, longer and possibly higher exposure to the immunosuppressive drugs, and the issue of noncompliance. Thus, the value of VCA in the pediatric population has still to be determined.

VCA Outcomes

Hand transplantation has become the most frequently performed VCA to date, with more than 100 upper limbs being transplanted in more than 70 patients worldwide.[35] The acute complications of upper extremity transplantation are related to vascular surgery and are similar to free tissue transfers. Patient survival in upper limb transplantation exceeds 98%. The overall graft survival exceeds 90% for patients who received antibody-based lymphocyte-depleting induction therapy and traditional triple-drug maintenance therapy.

According to International Registry on Hand and Composite Tissue Transplantation (IRHCTT) reports, patients with at least one year of follow-up have shown improvement in both the Hand Transplantation Scoring System (HTSS) and the Disabilities of the Arm, Shoulder, and Hand (DASH) score. According to the reports of the hand transplant programs, all recipients developed protective sensibility, 91% have tactile sensibility, and 82% regained partial two-point discrimination sensibility. Further, extrinsic motor function was sufficient in all patients to perform their daily activities. The majority regained independence after graft acceptance, enabling independent living and, in some cases, return to full-time occupation.[35] With a follow-up period of up to 21 years, it has been shown that immunosuppression-related complications include: serum sickness (3%), opportunistic infections (88%), acute rejection episode (85%), and metabolic complications, such as hyperglycemia, acute or chronic kidney disease, hypertension, Cushing syndrome, and avascular hip necrosis (70%). Despite the immunosuppression-related complications, the functional outcomes of upper extremity transplantation are good.

According to the literature for face transplantation, the estimated survival is 82.5%. As reported in 2016,[6] of 40 face transplant patients, seven had died due to perioperative problems and long-term complications of immunosuppression. In the clinical setting, all patients who received face transplantation accepted their new appearance without signs of psychological problems related to face transplantation. Good functional and esthetic results have been obtained following face transplantation. Sensory discrimination and hot–cold sensation returned between 8 and 12 months following transplantation. Different degrees of motor function return have been observed at between 12 and 24 months. Siemionow et al reported good functional outcomes of the first near-total face transplant (Fig. 11.6). However, in all reported cases, motor recovery was slower and less optimal compared to the sensory recovery.[31,36] The patient presented with return of breathing through the nose, being able to drink from a cup and eat solid foods. In addition, good sensory recovery was confirmed by restoration of sensation, which was close to normal. Also, motor recovery was satisfactory with return of essential facial functions such as pucker, smile, and pronunciation of the vowels "e," "i," "o."[30]

All face transplant recipients with at least 1 year of post-transplant follow-up experienced at least one episode of acute graft rejection, which was observed clinically and was confirmed histologically on skin and mucosa biopsies.

Wound healing problems, stenosis of Stenon duct, postoperative ptosis, and ectropion of eyelids were observed during the follow-up period and were treated surgically. Despite standard antibacterial and antiviral prophylaxis protocols the majority of recipients have experienced opportunistic bacterial, viral, and fungal infections. Insulin dependent new-onset diabetes mellitus, transient thrombocytosis, acute renal failure, thrombotic microangiopathy, transient steroid induced confusion, transient leukopenia, post-transplantation monoclonal B cell lymphoma, cervical dysplasia, severe rhabdomyolysis, acute respiratory distress syndrome, and diaphragmatic paralysis are the metabolic complications observed in face transplantation patients.[2,7,37]

Future VCA Perspectives

VCA have been shown thus far to be a viable option in a particular subgroup of patients who suffer from severe defects, not amenable to the modern-day reconstructive techniques. The long-term risks of current immunosuppressive protocols are the major concerns when debating VCA experimental surgery as a procedure that is improving "only"' quality of life. Thus, many experimental and clinical studies are currently focusing on safer immunosuppressive protocols and novel approaches such as tolerance-inducing strategies.

Transplantation of single functional units or new complex structures represents another topic for future development of VCA. Experimental studies of whole eye transplantation including the optic nerve have already been performed, as well as first cadaver studies testing the feasibility of composite periorbital eyeball transplant (CEPT), which may allow for clinical application in the near future. Reports on a whole head (allo-head and body) transplantation have been presented by the media, however there is a lack of reliable research or data.

Although much of this may sound like science fiction, in the future transplantation of the entire orbit for restoration of vision or transplantation of the cochlear apparatus for restoration of hearing function may become a clinical reality. We have to keep in mind that, just 10 years ago, VCA cases such as face transplantation were also considered as the stuff of science fiction.

Despite the expansion of clinical applications of VCA, the future of VCA depends on immunomodulatory and tolerance induction studies, which represent the holy grail of VCA transplantation. Better understanding of immunological responses (acute and chronic rejection), development of new less toxic immunosuppressive protocols, and tolerance-inducing modalities are needed, before all types of VCA transplants can be introduced to routine clinical practice.

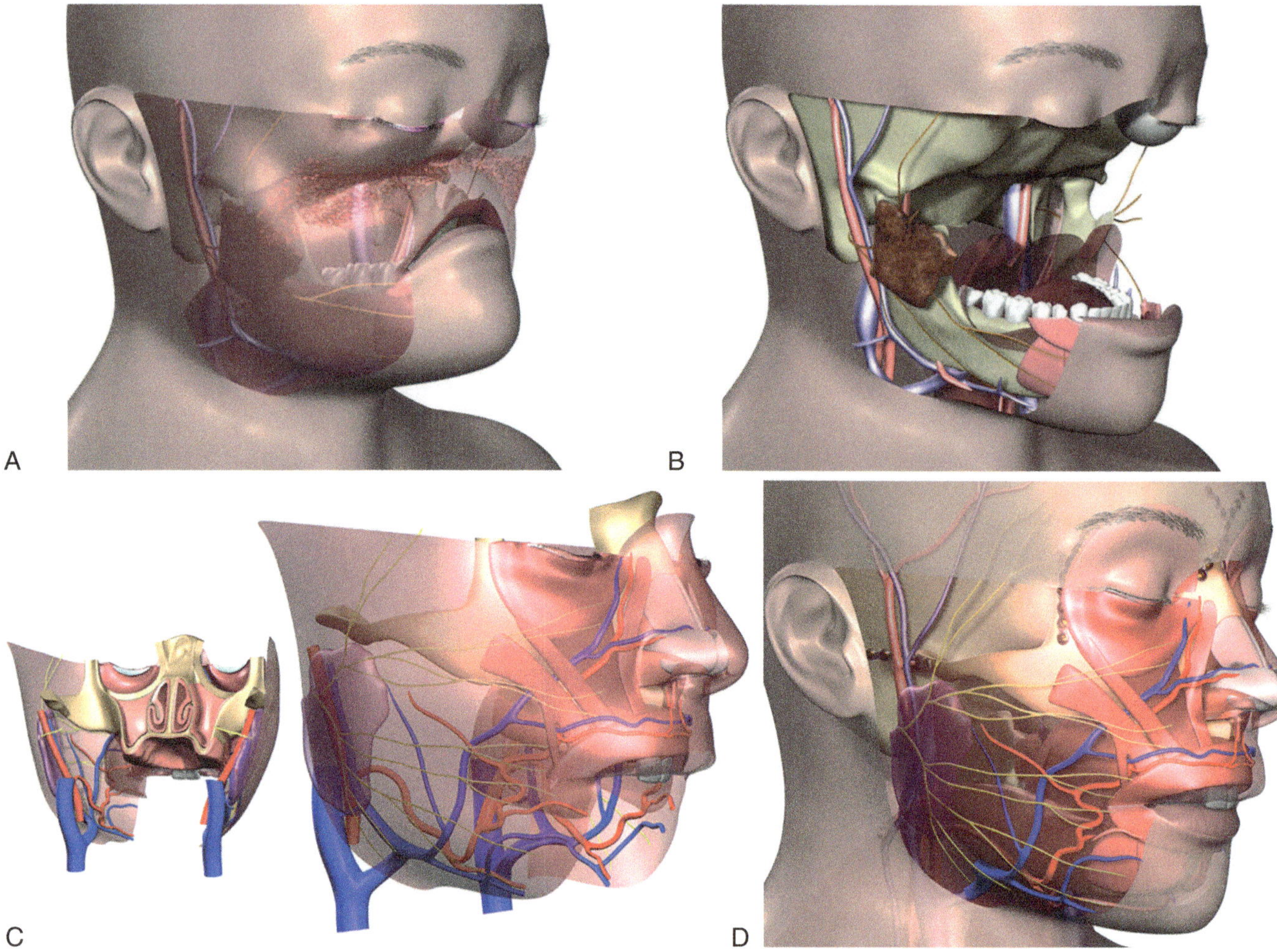

• **Fig. 11.6** Diagrams of the US first near-total face transplant, showing the sequence of the three-dimensional reconstruction that replaced 80% of the patient's face. (A) Patient deformity following gunshot injury and conventional reconstructive operations. (B) Following debridement of all scar tissues, the full facial defect is shown. (C) The face allograft (back view and right anterior view), included 535 cm^2 of facial skin, functional units of full nose with nasal lining and bony skeleton, lower eyelids and upper lip; underlying muscles and bones, including the orbital floor, zygoma, maxilla with teeth, hard palate and parotid glands, arteries, veins, and nerves. (D) Restoration of the craniofacial defect after face transplantation.

References

1. Gordon CR, Nazzal J, Lozano-Calderan SA, et al. From experimental rat hindlimb to clinical face composite tissue allotransplantation: historical background and current status. *Microsurgery*. 2006;26(8):566–572.
2. Siemionow MZ, Kulahci Y, Bozkurt M. Composite tissue allotransplantation. *Plast Reconstr Surg*. 2009;124:e327–e339.
3. Ulusal BG, Ulusal AE, Ozmen S, Zins JE, Siemionow MZ. A new composite facial and scalp transplantation model in rats. *Plast Reconstr Surg*. 2003;112(5):1302–1311.
4. Zor F. Facial vascularized composite tissue allotransplantation. *Gulhane Med J*. 2013;55(2):156.
5. Siemionow MZ, Izycki DM, Zielinski M. Donor-specific tolerance in fully major histocompatibility complex mismatched limb allograft transplants under an anti-alphabeta T-cell receptor monoclonal antibody and cyclosporine A protocol. *Transplantation*. 2003;76(12):1662–1668.
6. Sosin M, Rodriguez ED. The face transplantation update: 2016. *Plast Reconstr Surg*. 2016;137(6):1841–1850.
7. Siemionow M. The decade of face transplant outcomes. *J Mater Sci Mater Med*. 2017;28(5):64.
8. Siemionow M, Kulahci Y. Experimental models of composite tissue allograft transplants. *Semin Plast Surg*. 2007;21(4):205–212.
9. Siemionow M, Klimczak A. Advances in the development of experimental composite tissue transplantation models. *Transpl Int*. 2010;23(1):2–13.
10. Gorantla VS, Demetris AJ. Acute and chronic rejection in upper extremity transplantation: what have we learned? *Hand Clin*. 2011;27(4):481–493, (ix).
11. Kueckelhaus M, Fischer S, Seyda M, et al. Vascularized composite allotransplantation: current standards and novel approaches to prevent acute rejection and chronic allograft deterioration. *Transpl Int*. 2016;29(6):655–662.
12. Cendales LC, Kanitakis J, Schneeberger S, et al. The Banff 2007 working classification of skin-containing composite tissue allograft Pathology. *Am J Transplant*. 2008;8(7):1396–1400.
13. Schneider M, Cardones AR, Selim MA, Cendales LC. Vascularized composite allotransplantation: a closer look at the Banff Working Classification. *Transpl Int*. 2016;29(6):663–671.

14. Shapiro RI, Cerra FB. A model for reimplantation and transplantation of a complex organ: the rat hind limb. *J Surg Res.* 1978;24(6):501–506.
15. Siemionow M, Zor F. Allotransplantation. In: Farhadieh RD, Bulstrode NW, Gugno S, eds. *Plastic and Reconstructive Surgery: Approaches and Techniques.* Chichester: Wiley; 2015., Ch 12.
16. Zor F, Bozkurt M, Nair D, Siemionow M. A new composite midface allotransplantation model with sensory and motor reinnervation. *Transpl Int.* 2009;23(6):649–656.
17. Kulahci Y, Altuntas SH, Karagoz H, Cwykiel JM, Zor F, Siemionow M. A new total hemiface allotransplantation model in rats. *Microsurgery.* 2016;36(3):230–238.
18. Zor FP, Kulahci Y, Kurt B, Battal B, Gorantla V. Evaluation of immune responses following whole eye transplantation. *Transplantation.* 2018;102:S197–S198.
19. Bozkurt M, Klimczak A, Nasir S, Zor F, Krokowicz L, Siemionow M. Composite osseomusculocutaneous sternum, ribs, thymus, pectoralis muscles, and skin allotransplantation model of bone marrow transplantation. *Microsurgery.* 2012;33(1):43–50.
20. Kulahci Y, Bayram Y, Karagoz H, Sever C, Sahin C. Experimental craniofacial composite tissue allotransplantation (CCTA) models in rats. *Arch Clin Exp Surg (ACES).* 2012;1(3):181.
21. Barth RN, Bluebond-Langner R, Nam A, et al. Facial subunit composite tissue allografts in nonhuman primates: I. Technical and immunosuppressive requirements for prolonged graft survival. *Plast Reconstr Surg.* 2009;123(2):493–501.
22. Erbas VE, Sahin H, Oksuz S, et al. A preclinical swine model for whole eyeball transplantation. *Plast Reconstr Surg Glob Open.* 2016;4(45):42.
23. Kulahci Y, Karagoz H, Zor F. Experimental models of penile and lower limb transplantation: are they really translational? *Curr Opin Organ Transplant.* 2018;5(4):344–348.
24. Siemionow M, Unal S, Agaoglu G, Sari A. A cadaver study in preparation for facial allograft transplantation in humans: part I. What are alternative sources for total facial defect coverage? *Plast Reconstr Surg.* 2006;117(3):864–872.
25. Lengelé BG. Current concepts and future challenges in facial transplantation. *Clin Plast Surg.* 2009;36(3):507–521.
26. Siemionow M, Bozkurt M, Zor F, et al. A new composite eyeball–periorbital transplantation model in humans: an anatomical study in preparation for eyeball transplantation. *Plast Reconstr Surg.* 2018;141(4):1011–1018.
27. Siemionow M, Bozkurt M, Zor F, et al. A new composite eyeball-periorbital transplantation model in humans: an anatomical study in preparation for eyeball transplantation. *Plast Reconstr Surg.* 2018;141(4):1011–11018.
28. Dubernard J-M, Owen E, Herzberg G, et al. Human hand allograft: report on first 6 months. *Lancet.* 1999;353(9161):1315–1320.
29. Devauchelle B, Badet L, Lengelé B, et al. First human face allograft: early report. *Lancet.* 2006;368(9531):203–209.
30. Hashem AM, Djohan R, Bernard S, et al. Face transplantation for granulomatosis with polyangiitis (Wegener granulomatosis): technical considerations, immunological aspects, and 3-year posttransplant outcome. *Ann Plast Surg.* 2019;82(3):320–329.
31. Kollar B, Tasigiorgos S, Dorante MI, Carty MJ, Talbot SG, Pomahac B. Innovations in reconstructive microsurgery: reconstructive transplantation. *J Surg Oncol.* 2018;118(5):800–806.
32. Tardieu A, Dion L, Collinet P, et al. Uterus transplantation: questions and future prospects. *J Gynecol Obstet Hum Reprod.* 2019;48(1):1–3.
33. Hu W, Lu J, Zhang L, et al. A preliminary report of penile transplantation. *Eur Urol.* 2006;50(4):851–853.
34. Amaral S, Kessler SK, Levy TJ, et al. 18-month outcomes of heterologous bilateral hand transplantation in a child: a case report. *Lancet Child Adolesc Health.* 2017;1(1):35–44.
35. Shores JT, Malek V, Lee WPA, Brandacher G. Outcomes after hand and upper extremity transplantation. *J Mater Sci Mater Med.* 2017;28(5):72.
36. Siemionow MZ, Papay F, Djohan R, et al. First U.S. near-total human face transplantation: a paradigm shift for massive complex injuries. *Plast Reconstr Surg.* 2010;125(1):111–122.
37. Giatsidis G, Sinha I, Pomahac B. Reflections on a decade of face transplantation. *Ann Surg.* 2017;265(4):841–846.

12

Radiation Therapy and Soft Tissue Response

CHRIS NUTTING, LUCINDA GUNN, AND GURDIP AZAD

Radiation Principles

Radiotherapy is the medical use of ionizing radiation, generally as part of cancer treatment to control or kill malignant cells. Ionizing radiation is composed of particles that individually carry enough kinetic energy to liberate an electron from an atom or molecule. Directly ionizing radiation consists of alpha and beta particles. Indirectly ionizing radiation includes photon radiation which may be gamma radiation if produced by radioactive decay or X-rays if produced outside the nucleus.

Alpha Particle Radiation

An alpha particle is identical to a helium nucleus, containing 2 protons and 2 neutrons. Alpha particles are generally produced by a process of alpha decay. If ingested, inhaled or absorbed into the bloodstream, they can cause severe damage. Radium-226, radon-222, and polonium-210 are alpha emitters. Most alpha emitters occur naturally in the environment and are found in various amounts in almost all rocks, soils, and water. This form of radiation is rarely used for the treatment of cancer.

Beta Particle Radiation

Beta particles are high-energy, high-speed electrons or positrons emitted by certain types of radioactive nuclei. Cobalt-60, strontium-90 and iodine-131 are examples of some of the beta emitters. Iodine-131 is used in the treatment of benign and malignant thyroid disease. Strontium-90 is used in the treatment of metastatic bone cancer and has also been used for treating ocular melanoma. Beta particles are also a source of positrons used in positron emission tomography (PET).

Gamma Radiation

Gamma rays are produced by nuclear gamma decay and are emitted from a radioactive source, often following the emission of a beta particle. Gamma rays are less ionizing but more penetrating than alpha and beta rays and can be stopped by a few centimeters of lead. The commonly used gamma emitters are caesium-137, cobalt-60, and technetium-99m. Technetium is widely used for diagnostic studies, whereas caesium and cobalt are used in the treatment of cancer.

X-Rays

X-rays, like gamma rays, are part of the electromagnetic spectrum. They are emitted by electrons. X-rays of varying energies have many uses but are best known for their medical application. Low-energy X-rays (~10 keV) are used in diagnostic radiography to take images of part of a patient's body (e.g., chest or abdomen). The differential absorption of the X-rays by bone, air, and soft tissue generates a clear radiograph. High-energy X-rays (photons) are able to ionize atoms and disrupt molecular bonds, thereby causing potential damage to the tissues they pass through. The ionizing capability of X-rays is utilized in radiotherapy, which uses photons to kill malignant cells in the treatment of cancer. In radiotherapy the photons are generated by a machine called a linear accelerator (linac). The linac generates electrons and then speeds them up to almost the speed of light using electrical fields. As the electron is accelerated its kinetic energy is increased until such time as it collides with the target and the energy is released as a photon (Bremsstrahlung radiation).

Mode of Action in Malignancies

When radiation interacts with cells, ionization of DNA molecules takes place causing tumor cell death. The biological effect of ionizations is controlled by a number of factors, such as the number of ionizations that can cause DNA damage, free radical scavenging processes, and the degree of cellular repair. There are two mechanisms by which radiation causes cell damage: direct and indirect.

Indirect Effect

Approximately 60% of the human body is made of water; therefore the majority of ionizations generated by irradiation arise in the water molecules. When radiation interacts with water it breaks the bonds that hold the water molecule together, producing a positively charged hydrogen ion (H^{++}) and an uncharged hydroxyl radical (OH^{-}). The OH radical is often called a free radical as it has an unpaired electron and is highly reactive, causing cell damage. These free radicals may undergo further reactions to produce hydrogen peroxide, which also contributes to the destruction of the cells. Oxygen plays a key role in this process of radiolysis. Approximately two-thirds of the biological damage caused by X-rays or electrons is by indirect effect.

Direct Effect

If radiation causes ionization of the atoms that are part of the DNA molecule, or some other cellular component essential for the survival of the cell, then the cell may be destroyed directly by interference with its life-sustaining structure. This is referred to as the direct effect of radiation.

Biological Effect on the Cell Cycle

Cell cycle progression is vital for the growth and survival of a cell or organism (Fig. 12.1). The normal cell proliferation cycle goes through two main phases: mitosis (M phase) and DNA synthesis (S phase), which are separated by the G_1 (before cell division) and G_2 (after cell division) phases. G_0 is the resting phase before cell division begins. The average length of a cell cycle is 16 h; this is shorter for cancer cells. Cell cycle arrest normally occurs in response to events that threaten the integrity of the DNA. Cells are most sensitive to radiation in the M and G_2 phases and most resistant in the S phase of the cell cycle. After radiotherapy is delivered, cells may be in different phases of the cell cycle. Fractionating radiotherapy may allow resistant cells time to enter the sensitive phase of the cycle and be more amenable to cell kill. Following radiotherapy, DNA damage can also cause a progressive delay in G_1, S, and G_2 phases of the cell cycle. This delay gives the cells time to repair the damage.

Radiation Injury

Radiation kills actively dividing cancer cells efficiently; damage to cancer cells may occur immediately but may take months to take full effect. Along with the cancer cells, some rapidly dividing normal cells (skin, intestines, hair, and bone marrow) are also damaged in the process, leading to unwanted acute effects. Slowly dividing normal cells (nerves, brain, bone, vessels) exhibit radiation-induced damage later.

Radiation-related injury to the cells is divided into three main categories:

- *Lethal damage* is a complex, irreparable and irreversible mechanism leading to cell death. The cell is unable to repair the damage and gives rise to a linear component of cell killing.
- *Sublethal damage* following ionizing radiation can be repaired within hours of the injury taking place and would not lead to cell death, unless further radiation exposure was inflicted on the cells. Cellular repair mechanisms can protect them from further injury, which is important for normal tissues, as they are able to repair themselves between fractions of radiotherapy. The approximate time needed for half the sublethal damage to be repaired (half-life) is different for different tissues.

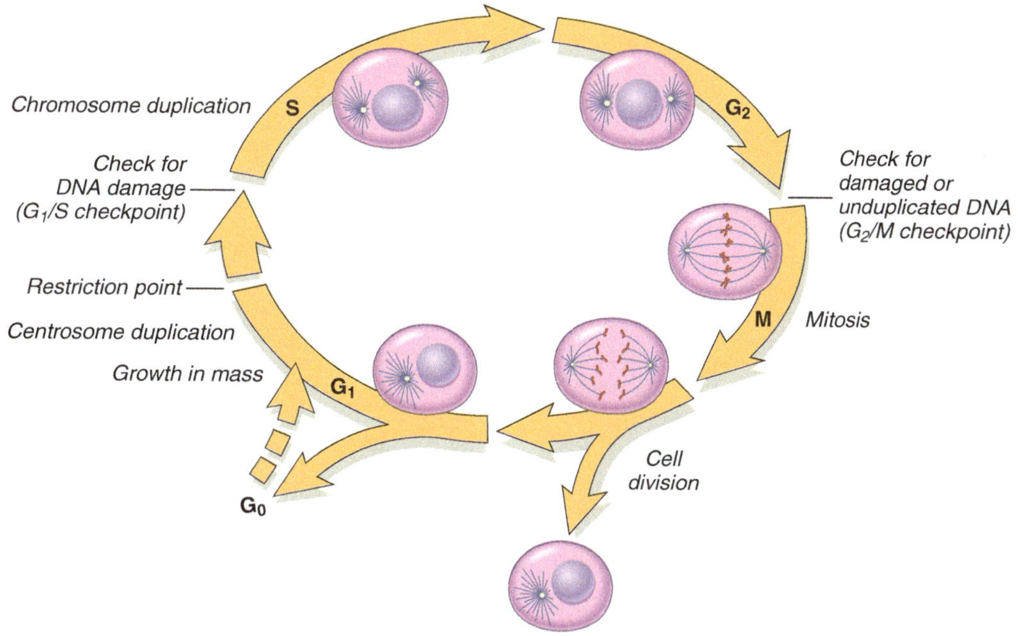

• **Fig. 12.1** The cell cycle. The figure shows the cell cycle phases (G_0, G_1, G_2, S, and M), the location of the G_1 restriction point, and the G_1/S and G_2/M cell cycle checkpoints. (From Mitchell RN. The cell as a unit of health and disease. In: *Robbins and Cotran Pathologic Basis of Disease.* 9th edn. Philadelphia: Elsevier Saunders; 2015. Modified from Pollard TD, Earnshaw WC. *Cell Biology*. Philadelphia: Elsevier Saunders; 2002.)

The recovery time is approximately 1 h and is thought to be complete by about 4 h in mammalian cells.

- *Potentially lethal damage* will inevitably kill the cells unless manipulated by repair-facilitated cell cycle arrest. Normal cells can readily be repaired in the S phase but not in the M phase. Tumor cells have defective cell cycle controls and therefore do not undergo cell cycle arrest required for repair, in contrast to the normal cells. A minimum of 6 h are required between fractions of radiotherapy to provide sufficient time for these repair mechanisms to work.

Modes of Delivery

Radiotherapy delivered by a machine is often referred to as external beam radiotherapy. It may also be delivered by placing a radioactive source inside the body, which is referred to as brachytherapy.

External Beam Radiotherapy

This is the commonest form of radiotherapy used for the treatment of cancer. Different machines are used for the delivery of varying energies.

The superficial machine produces X-rays that range from 50 to 150 kV (kilovolts) and is used for treating superficial skin lesions. It deposits most of its energy at the surface of the skin and 90% of the dose at a depth of approximately 5 mm from the surface of the skin.

The orthovoltage machine generates X-rays ranging from 150 to 500 kV energy, depositing maximum energy near the surface of the skin and 90% of the dose at a depth of approximately 2 cm from the skin surface. It is also used for treating superficial tissues, skin, and bone lesions.

The megavoltage machine produces X-rays of higher energies, usually 1 MV (megavolt) and above. A linear accelerator (linac) is commonly used for the delivery of these high-energy beams. The maximum dose of radiotherapy can be delivered to various depths depending on the energy of the beam used, aiding treatment of deep-seated tumors. Most linacs can also be adapted to treat superficial lesions, such as in cases of skin cancer. This treatment uses electrons instead of high-energy photons. Further technical advances in the design of the linac has permitted the use of intensity-modulated radiotherapy (IMRT); volumetric modulated arc therapy (VMAT); stereotactic radiotherapy (SBRT); image-guided radiotherapy (IGRT) and magnetic resonance imaging (MRI)-guided radiotherapy. All of these techniques allow shaping and modulation of the radiation beam to reduce radiation dose to normal tissues whilst intensifying dose to target.

Particle therapy using high-energy protons allows high doses of radiation to be delivered to a specific depth range with less entry and minimal exit dose. For this reason, proton beam therapy (PBT) has historically been used to target tumors that lie in close proximity to a critical organ at risk (OAR) that cannot be adequately spared using photons (e.g., paraspinal and skull base tumors). However, there is widespread interest in using protons in a variety of tumor sites where a significant reduction in the radiation dose delivered to normal tissues may be achievable.

Brachytherapy

Brachytherapy is a mode of delivering radiotherapy by using sealed radioactive sources that can be placed either inside a cavity containing the tumor (intracavitary) or directly in the tumor itself (interstitial). Other forms of brachytherapy include intraluminal, intraoperative, intravascular, and surface brachytherapy.

The main radioactive sources used for brachytherapy are iridium, caesium, and iodine.

The advantage of brachytherapy over external beam radiotherapy is the ability to deliver higher doses of radiation to the tumor and lower doses to the surrounding normal tissues. There tends to be a rapid fall-off in dose as the distance increases from the radioactive source, which restricts its use to the treatment of small and well-localized tumors.

Unsealed radioactive sources are also used for treatment and can be delivered either orally or intravenously. However, following treatment, limited-period precautions are necessary to avoid radiation exposure to individuals in close contact. Radioactive iodine-131 used in the treatment of thyroid cancer is an example of this form of treatment.

Fractionation

Curative treatment of cancer requires higher doses of radiation in order to produce sufficient cell killing. The total dose is delivered in small daily fractions over a period of time to minimize toxicity by allowing sufficient time for normal tissue recovery while inducing tumor cell kill. The efficacy of fractionation is based on the four Rs of radiobiology: repair of sublethal damage, redistribution of cells within the cell cycle, repopulation, and reoxygenation.

By splitting radiation into small daily fractions, normal cells with efficient repair mechanisms are able to repair sublethal damage in contrast to cancer cells, which have suppressed repair pathways. Both normal and malignant cells repopulate between fractions. Prolonging total treatment time over several weeks allows normal cell repopulation; however, some rapidly dividing tumors such as squamous cell carcinomas regenerate faster than the normal cells and exhibit accelerated repopulation. Fractionation increases damage to the tumor by allowing reoxygenation of the tumor environment and redistribution of the cells into radiosensitive phases of the cell cycle.

Conventional (standard) fractionation is the delivery of 1.8–2 Gy per day, given as five daily treatments a week over several weeks. Other fractionating regimens used are as follows:

- *Hyperfractionation:* The same total dose is delivered over the same time as in standard fractionation but more than one fraction is given per day at a lower dose per fraction. This reduces the late effects of radiotherapy.

- *Accelerated treatment*: The total dose is delivered over a shorter period of time compared with standard fractionation in order to overcome accelerated tumor repopulation.
- *Continuous hyperfractionated accelerated radiation therapy (CHART)* combines the above two approaches and is used in the treatment of rapidly proliferating tumors (e.g., lung cancer and some head and neck malignancies). It consists of three smaller fractions of radiotherapy per day, separated by 6 hours to allow recovery of normal tissues.
- *Hypofractionation:* Radiotherapy is delivered in a smaller number of fractions with a higher dose per fraction. There is potentially a higher risk of developing late effects in normal tissues with this regimen. It is used in the treatment of slow-growing tumors, which are generally resistant to standard fractionation schedules, and also in the palliative setting where development of late effects is less relevant.

Dose and Dose Rate

Dose is the general term used to determine the quantity of radiation. The energy imparted by ionizing radiation to matter at a specific point is defined as absorbed dose. The SI unit of absorbed dose is joule per kilogram (J/kg) also known as gray (Gy).

Dose rate is defined as the radiation dose delivered per unit time and measured in grays per hour. Radiation response decreases with decreasing dose rate and this is referred to as dose rate effect. The typical dose rate used in standard radiotherapy is 1 Gy/min.

Effects of Oxygen and Radiotherapy

Malignant cells are most sensitive to radiotherapy in the presence of oxygen. Hypoxic cells are radioresistant and are usually present in the core of the tumor, whereas the cells on the surface of the tumor have an abundant blood supply and are well oxygenated. As the tumor is exposed to radiotherapy, the outer, well-oxygenated layers of the tumor are rapidly destroyed and the hypoxic inner layers become oxygenated and thus radiosensitive between treatment fractions.

Treatment Parameters

Total Dose

Total dose refers to the total amount of ionizing radiation absorbed by the patient (expressed in Gy). Every tissue in the body has a tolerance dose beyond which the organ would be at risk of serious complications. Various dose/fractionation schedules can make it difficult to assess the total dose delivered to a particular organ. Therefore, a formula is applied to compare altered fractionation doses to standard 2 Gy per fraction doses to know the exact total dose delivered to an organ. This is referred to as a biologically equivalent dose.

Dose Fraction Size

Fraction size is a significant factor influencing the development of acute and late effects of radiotherapy. Large fraction sizes increase the severity of late normal tissue damage.

Volume Treated

The severity of acute and late normal tissue injury from radiotherapy depends on the volume of tissue irradiated. Tissues with a parallel organization, such as the lung and kidney, have a high functional reserve and exhibit a prominent volume effect. This means that the damage caused would depend on the dose distribution to the whole organ rather than to a small area. On the other hand, serial organs such as the spinal cord and gastrointestinal tract have little functional reserve and it is vital that radiation dose does not exceed tolerance at any point.

Time Elapsed

If the overall treatment time is increased, a greater amount of repopulation of the irradiated normal and tumor cells is permitted. This has an adverse effect on local tumor control, especially in rapidly proliferating tumors.

Radiation Effects

Acute Toxicity

The acute effects of radiotherapy are generally defined as those toxicities occurring up to 90 days from completion of treatment. Acute effects usually manifest in rapidly dividing cells in the area being treated and are thought to be due to depletion of stem cells. Common sites exhibiting early radiation effects are the skin (including hair follicles and sweat glands), mucous membranes of the gastrointestinal tract, and hematopoietic tissue.

If photon radiation is used it can take some weeks into the treatment course before erythema becomes evident, as initial dose is deposited in the deeper dermis. If a higher skin dose is required (e.g., when tumor involves the skin or in the treatment of a primary skin cancer), a tissue-equivalent bolus material may be applied over the treated field to increase the surface dose. Adjustments in radiation technique to use electrons or orthovoltage (less penetrating) radiation also increase the skin dose and result in the development of skin erythema within the first week of a fractionated course of radiotherapy.

The rates of onset of damage and recovery from it depend upon the turnover rate of epithelial cells. In a typical 6-week course of radical radiotherapy delivered with curative intent one would expect skin erythema and inflammation to develop at the treated site within the first 3 weeks. Epilation also occurs early and dry desquamation of the skin may follow as surface flaking of the stratum corneum. Towards the end of the course of radiotherapy moist desquamation of the skin is often seen, as exudate is released from the damaged skin cells. This is more commonly seen at the skin creases of the axillae and groins.

In radiotherapy to the head and neck, mucositis develops over the first few weeks, ranging from patchy isolated areas to confluent areas with ulceration. Taste disturbance is noted and salivary gland function is diminished. The latter results from acinar atrophy and chronic inflammation of the salivary glands.

Late Toxicity

The late effects of radiotherapy are generally the dose-limiting factor. High total dose, large fraction sizes, and large treatment volumes all contribute to a greater risk of late effects. The main mechanisms for the late effects of radiotherapy are believed to be damage to vascular and connective tissue and a reduction in the proliferative capacity of stem cells. Late effects tend to manifest in slowly proliferating tissues (e.g., lung, kidney, liver, heart, and nervous tissue).

Late normal tissue damage reflects a failure to regenerate functional tissue, whether through lack of stem cells or radiation-induced dysregulation of the normal healing process. This latter phenomenon is described as a result of recent research into radiobiology and molecular pathology of late radiotherapy effects. Cytokine cascades are activated early at the cell and tissue level after irradiation and remain active throughout the expression of late tissue damage. Skin atrophy, telangiectasia, necrosis, and fibrosis occur many months after radiotherapy. Skin atrophy is seen as shrinking and thinning of the skin in the irradiated field. Telangiectasia results from a failure in the regrowth of normal vasculature. It has been postulated that telangiectasia results from loss of smooth muscle cells in vessels, leading to a loss of capillary pressure control. Loss of endothelial cells as a result of radiotherapy may also contribute to its formation.[1] Necrosis is generally seen in atrophic skin, often developing as a result of trauma, and reflecting the impaired reaction of the vasculature to tissue injury. Many late effects of radiotherapy can be attributed to fibrinogenesis and excessive extracellular matrix and collagen deposition. Increased knowledge of the relevant cytokines and their actions has provided molecular targets for potential therapeutic intervention.

Osteoradionecrosis

Osteoradionecrosis (ORN) is defined as an area of exposed bone in a field of radiation that has failed to show any evidence of healing for 6 months with the absence of recurrent or residual tumor. The incidence of ORN is believed to have declined considerably over time; reported incidence ranges from 5% to 7%.[2]

The pathophysiology of ORN is described as a cumulative tissue damage induced by radiation. The 'three Hs' principle outlines how radiation results in a hypocellular, hypovascular, and hypoxic tissue environment. Tissue breakdown occurs as a result of cell death and collagen lysis exceeding cellular replication. The result is progression to a nonhealing wound.

A key event in the progression of ORN is the activation and dysregulation of fibroblastic activity that leads to atrophic tissue within a previously irradiated area. High-dose radiation leads to bone death via a combination of mechanisms described as progressive resorption of osteoclasts, periosteocyticlysis, extensive demineralization, and accelerated aging of bone.

Common sites for bone necrosis are the jaw (soft tissue tumors of the head and neck), ribs, and sternum (breast cancer), skull (brain tumors and soft tissue tumors of the scalp), and vertebral column (spinal cord tumors).

Advanced (stage III or IV) tumor/recurrent tumors, tumors invading bone, and tumors involving floor of mouth, tongue, and retromolar trigone have been shown to have a higher risk of ORN. Treatment-related factors contributing to the development of ORN include large treatment volumes, high radiation dose, and dose per fraction, with the highest incidence occurring with total radiation dose above 70 Gy. Modifiable risks include smoking, the use of bisphosphates, and poor dentition.[3] Patients should have a thorough dental assessment and extraction of any teeth in poor condition prior to commencing a course of radiotherapy to the head and neck in order to optimize oral health, though ORN has been seen in edentulous patients also.

The presentation of ORN varies with site. In cases of ORN of the mandible patients may present with pain, swelling, and trismus. ORN of the temporal bone can present with severe otalgia and offensive otorrhea. Exposed bone and pathological fracture may also be seen. Imaging with plain radiographs may highlight areas of local decalcification or sclerosis. Computed tomography (CT) or MRI scanning is used to delineate the affected area prior to definitive surgery. A deep biopsy of the lesion to rule out recurrent malignancy is generally recommended.

Treatment of ORN involves initial measures such as control of any superadded infection, gentle irrigation of the soft tissues, nutritional support, and analgesia. There is conflicting evidence regarding the use of hyperbaric oxygen therapy (HBOT) in the management of ORN, with some studies showing increased likelihood of attaining mucosal cover with HBOT. There remains no national or international guidelines and practice is dictated by local policy.[4]

Radiation Therapy and Wound Healing

The wound-healing capacity of irradiated skin may be severely impaired, with clinical implications for patients requiring treatment combining radiation and surgery. Approximately 60% of patients with solid malignant tumors receive radiotherapy as part of their treatment, either with curative or palliative intent. Radiotherapy is often used after surgery in malignant disease in cases of narrow or involved excision margins or to nodal basins post lymphadenectomy to reduce the risk of local disease relapse and improve overall survival. Radiotherapy may also be used before surgery to downstage a tumor prior to definitive resection (e.g., in preoperative radiotherapy for rectal cancer and extremity soft tissue sarcoma).

The process of wound healing is well described to occur in three phases: an inflammatory phase, which develops within days; a proliferative phase, which occurs over many days to weeks; and a remodeling/maturation phase, which extends from many weeks to years.

Unlike a surgical wound, however, fractionated radiotherapy results in repetitive injury to soft tissues. This results in an accumulation of inflammatory responses and dysregulation of the highly structured process of wound healing.

Cytokines known to be involved in the initial inflammatory response to tissue damage are transforming growth factor beta (TGF-β), vascular endothelial growth factor (VEGF), tumor necrosis factor alpha (TNF-α), interferon gamma (IFN-γ), and proinflammatory cytokines such as interleukin 1 and interleukin 8. These are all overexpressed following irradiation and lead to uncontrolled matrix accumulation and fibrosis.[5]

In the proliferative phase overexpression of additional cytokines (e.g., epidermal growth factor [EGF], fibroblast growth factor [FGF], and platelet-derived growth factor [PDGF]) leads to dysregulated granulation tissue formation, re-epithelialization, and neovascularization.

Matrix metalloproteinases (MMPs) are responsible for the remodeling phase and regulate extracellular matrix synthesis. Irradiation can lead to dysregulation of MMPs leading to disorganized collagen deposition by fibroblasts.

There has been much interest in the postoperative complication rates of reconstructive surgery after radiotherapy and the optimal timing of surgery and radiotherapy. Much of the published literature is in reconstructive head and neck surgery, breast surgery, and resection following preoperative radiotherapy for rectal cancer.

It is understood that previously irradiated patients have a higher risk of postoperative complications.[6] In cases of microvascular free flap transfer TGF-β1 has been shown to be over-expressed in free flaps for as long as 6 months after radiotherapy. Extracellular matrix remodelling has also been detected in the free flap for up to 5 months after radiotherapy completion.[7] The alteration in graft bed extracellular matrix organization after radiotherapy and prior to surgery has been shown to impact significantly on free flap survival in the pre-irradiated field.[8]

In head and neck reconstructive surgery, a large systematic review and meta-analysis combined data from 24 studies to compare outcomes for 2842 flaps performed in irradiated fields with 3491 flaps in nonirradiated fields. It was able to demonstrate that preoperative radiotherapy is associated with an increased risk of flap complications (RR 1.84, P <0.001), flap failure (RR 1.48, P <0.004), fistula formation (RR 2.05, P <0.001), and need for reoperation (RR 2.06, P <0.001).[9]

Where radiotherapy is required as multimodality therapy the timing of radiotherapy has been the subject of much debate with regards to the risk of delayed wound healing and reducing the success of microvascular free flaps when radiotherapy is used preoperatively.

This has been retrospectively investigated for sarcoma patients, where 119 patients with sarcomas of the head and neck, upper and lower extremities were reviewed, with approximately two-thirds receiving preoperative radiotherapy and one-third receiving postoperative radiotherapy. Free flap loss rates were significantly lower in the preoperative radiotherapy group (0% vs. 8.7%). Late recipient site complications also occurred less often in patients receiving preoperative radiotherapy (6.8%) compared to postoperative radiotherapy (26.1%).[10] A phase III Canadian study randomized 190 patients with soft tissue sarcoma of the extremities to either 50 Gy preoperatively or 66 Gy postoperatively. The study was closed early due to higher rates of wound complications in the preoperative group.[11] Subsequent follow-up, however, demonstrated higher rates of grade 2–4 late toxicity in the postoperative radiotherapy group, with equivalent local control. On balance it is now generally felt preferable to accept a higher rate of acute, reversible toxicity with preoperative radiotherapy in a bid to reduce the incidence of irreversible late effects observed following postoperative radiation.[12]

A review of 140 patients at the M.D. Anderson Cancer Center who underwent mandibular resection and reconstruction with a free fibular flap compared preoperative radiotherapy and immediate reconstruction, preoperative radiotherapy, and delayed reconstruction, postoperative radiotherapy, and no radiotherapy. Complications included orocutaneous fistula, osteoradionecrosis, and partial or complete flap loss. Forty-two percent of all patients studied had at least one complication, but the incidence of complications was relatively equal between the groups receiving pre- and postoperative radiotherapy.[13]

Our practice in cases of preoperative radiotherapy for head and neck malignancies is to recommend surgery takes place within 6 weeks of completion of radiotherapy. Published data supports this approach, showing an increase in flap loss, infections, and delayed wound healing when more than 6 weeks elapses from the last radiotherapy session and surgery.[14]

In breast cancer where there is a need for postmastectomy radiotherapy (PMRT), the optimal type and timing of reconstructive surgery also remains a controversial topic.[15] Reconstructive options include a prosthetic device (e.g., silicone or saline implants), autologous tissue (e.g., transverse rectus abdominis musculocutaneous flap) or a combination of both. Reconstruction can be immediate at the time of mastectomy, "immediate-delayed" as a two-stage procedure usually completed within a number of weeks, or delayed.

In those requiring PMRT, prosthetic implant-based reconstruction is generally discouraged due to risks of reconstruction failure. A large systematic review demonstrated implant-based reconstruction failure rates of approximately 20% irrespective of whether undertaken pre- or postradiotherapy.[16] Autologous flaps are also susceptible to radiation-related tissue damage, including fat necrosis, fibrosis, contracture, and loss of volume over time.[17]

Current National Comprehensive Cancer Network (NCCN) guidelines recommend that women undergoing implant-based reconstruction undergo initial reconstruction with a two-stage approach using a temporary tissue expander and that women planned for an autologous reconstruction are delayed until radiotherapy has been completed. Practice trends are evolving, however, and the optimal strategy will always need to consider patient suitability for reconstructive options and personal preference.[18]

In rectal cancer preoperative chemoradiotherapy is the current standard of care for T3–4 tumors and in selected patients with clinically node-positive disease, distal tumors or threatened mesorectal fascia involvement. The NCCN recommend surgical resection between 5 and 12 weeks post completion of radiotherapy, though optimal timing is yet to be determined. Surgical resection beyond 6 weeks may improve the proportion of patients achieving a pathological complete response (pCR) at resection, however delays risk tumor cell repopulation and may make surgical resection more difficult with an increase in postoperative complications. A large retrospective meta-analysis that included 3584 patients suggested that delaying surgery beyond 8 weeks increased the pCR rate by 6% but there was no evidence that long-term outcomes including overall survival were improved. Complication rates were similar.[19]

Supportive Management

Many of the early effects of radiotherapy are evident during a treatment course. Patients are given written advice on skin care management, which includes the use of a daily emollient applied after each fraction of radiotherapy. Avoidance of direct sunlight on the treated area is imperative, as is avoiding the use of potentially irritating chemical-containing compounds on the skin (e.g., body lotions, perfumes, talcum powders, etc.). If moist desquamation develops emollients are not helpful and paraffin gauze dressings may offer some comfort. Early detection and treatment of superadded skin infections with oral antimicrobials is recommended.

Oral mucositis often requires analgesia. Optimal pain control is essential to ensure patients are able to take adequate oral nutrition. Analgesia is given stepwise according to need using the World Health Organization (WHO) analgesic ladder. Analgesic mouthwashes can also be used. Early dietetic and speech and language assessment of these patients is important, and if necessary parenteral feeding may be used if there is insufficient oral intake.

Xerostomia can be experienced early in the treatment course and is a well-documented late effect of radiotherapy after treatment of the salivary glands in head and neck malignancies. There are limited satisfactory treatment options to ameliorate this symptom. Artificial saliva sprays and gels may offer some relief. Due to the potential significant consequences of xerostomia on quality of life, which include increased rates of dental caries and oral candidiasis, and difficulty chewing and speaking, parotid-sparing radiation techniques are now used such as IMRT.[20] Amifostine (a radioprotective agent) has also been shown to partially preserve parotid function after radiotherapy though it is not used in routine practice.[21]

The management of late radionecrosis involves optimal wound care: adequate debriding and cleansing, accurately assessing the wound, choosing the appropriate dressing based on the wound assessment, and encouraging granulation tissue formation and re-epithelialization. Alginates, foams, gauzes, hydrogels, hydrocolloids, and transparent films are the major moisture-retentive dressings available.[22]

HBOT can be used to treat osteoradionecrosis and radionecrotic wounds. Standard wound care should also be followed.

The aim of HBOT is to reverse the radiation-induced hypocellular, hypovascular and hypoxic tissue environment. HBO consists of exposing a patient to intermittent short-term 100% oxygen inhalation at a pressure greater than 1 atmosphere. HBO increases the oxygen concentration gradient so that the area around the necrosed hypoxic tissue has a high concentration of oxygen. This stimulates angiogenesis and reverses the hypoperfusion and hypoxia, giving tissues the propensity to heal. Initial reports of the benefit of HBO therapy were published as early as the 1970s. More recently a Cochrane Database Systematic Review concluded that for patients with late radiation tissue injury affecting the head, neck, anus, and rectum HBOT is associated with improved outcome.[4]

Early studies of pentoxifylline in combination with tocopherol have been shown to be efficacious in reversing radiation-induced fibrosis. Pentoxifylline may also have a role in the treatment of ORN. This oral drug has an anti-TNF effect and vasodilator action, which improves microcirculation and enhances oxygen delivery to tissues. Encouraging results have been shown in a small phase II study combining pentoxifylline with tocopherol (vitamin E) and clodronate for the treatment of ORN of the mandible, with all patients experiencing complete recovery within a median of 9 months.[23]

As the molecular basis of late radiation-induced tissue damage is now better understood, in particularly the specific cytokines central to the process, experimental molecular targets for therapeutic intervention are evolving. Fat grafting has been used in reconstructive surgery for years. There is now growing interest in the regenerative potential of adipose-derived stem cells (ADSCs) with their capacity for multilineage differentiation and ability to activate local stem cell niches.[24] Alongside injection of multipotent cells, topical administration of active substances to reduce the side effects of radiotherapy and the use of growth factors (e.g., TGF-β1, 2, and 3), basic FGF, PDGF, and VEGF are all areas for future development.[5]

Carcinogenesis

There is much evidence to support the carcinogenic property of ionizing radiation, namely studies from atomic bomb survivors in Japan, the Chernobyl nuclear accident, and people treated with high doses of radiation for cancer or other, benign conditions. In atomic bomb survivors the malignancies seen were leukemias and carcinomas of cells that line the body. There was no increase in the incidence of sarcomas (soft tissue tumors) in these patients. The risk of developing a radiation-induced malignancy varied significantly with age, with young children found to be 15 times as sensitive as middle-aged adults.

A contrast is seen with second malignancies induced by radiotherapy. These cancers are of cells lining the body but are often seen in tissues or organs not directly targeted and that therefore have received lower doses of radiation. Sarcomas are noted to arise in high-dose areas of radiation that lie within or immediately adjacent to the radiation fields (Fig. 12.2).[25]

Up to 10% of invasive cancers are caused by radiation, both ionizing and nonionizing radiation (ultraviolet, radiofrequency radiation). The probability of radiation causing a cancer is a stochastic effect, meaning the probability with which it occurs increases with effective radiation dose, but the severity of the cancer is independent of dose. The neoplastic transformation can be divided into three major independent stages: morphological changes to the cell, acquisition of cellular immortality (losing normal, life-limiting cell regulatory processes), and adaptations that favor formation of a tumor.

Those cancers that may develop as a result of radiation exposure are indistinguishable from those that occur naturally or as a result of exposure to other carcinogens. The impact of lifestyle factors such as smoking, alcohol consumption and diet significantly contribute to many of the same malignancies. There is some evidence that these effects may not simply be additive but multiplicative.[26]

The risk of developing a secondary malignancy following treatment for cancer is 17%–19%.[27] A UK study previously estimated that 1346 cases of cancer, or about 0.45% of the 298,000 new cancers registered in the UK in 2007, were associated with radiotherapy for a previous cancer.[28] The largest numbers of radiotherapy-related second cancers were lung cancer (23.7% of the total), esophageal cancer (13.3%), and female breast cancer (10.6%). The highest percentages of second cancers related to radiotherapy were among survivors of Hodgkin's disease and cancers of the oral cavity, pharynx, and cervix uteri. Following initial radiotherapy for breast cancer, excess risks were seen for cancers of lung, esophagus, bone, and soft tissue.[29] Cancers most strongly linked to radiation include bone and soft tissue sarcomas, but skin, brain, thyroid, breast, and stomach cancer can also occur. In most cases the risk of second malignancy is higher if the radiation exposure occurs earlier in life or during periods of rapid growth of a tissue, such as bone sarcomas during adolescence. Cells that have matured and are no longer proliferating appear to be less susceptible to the effects of radiation. Adolescent girls receiving mediastinal radiation therapy for Hodgkin's disease have been found to develop breast cancer more often than their adult counterparts.

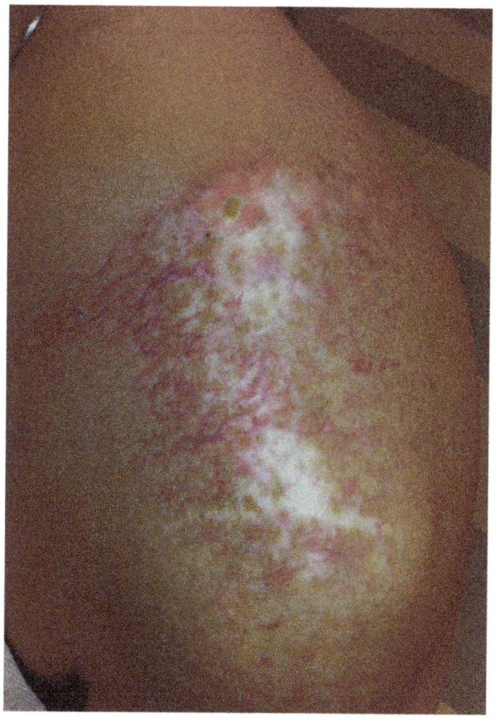

• **Fig. 12.2** A severe late skin reaction as a result of fast neutron therapy 22 years earlier following excision of a large dermatofibrosarcoma protuberans (DFSP) tumor from the shoulder. It demonstrates characteristic telangiectasia, hypopigmentation, subcutaneous fibrosis and, medially, delayed healing of a minor skin abrasion. (From Kane GM, Gurleen, D. Principles of radiation. In: Gurtner GC, Neligan PC, eds. *Plastic Surgery*, Vol. 1: *Principles*. Elsevier; 2018.)

Radiation-Induced Sarcoma

Radiation-induced soft tissue sarcoma is a rare malignancy with an overall incidence of less than 1% for patients with cancer who are treated with radiation and survive 5 years. Radiation-induced sarcoma has been defined as a lesion of different histology to that of a non-irradiated sarcoma, arising within a previous radiotherapy field, usually after a latency period of more than 4 years.[30] Although the threshold dose for radiation-induced sarcoma is not certain, most published data report a dose of 40–60 Gy. Dose–response relationships have been found between radiation dose and sarcomas. A 40-fold increase in the risk of bone sarcomas was observed following 60 Gy or more.[25] High-dose radiation appears not to increase the risk for leukemia and thyroid cancer. Stereotactic radiosurgery data support that there may be a lower risk for induction of a secondary malignancy because of a very high probability of complete cellular kill in the high-dose radiation field. Cells lose their ability to proliferate and, therefore, they are unable to sustain a malignant transformation.

Although advances in the delivery of radiotherapy appear to reduce the risk of late radiation toxicity, the newer technologies, such as intensity-modulated radiation therapy (IMRT), involve the use of more fields and consequently expose more normal tissue to low-dose radiotherapy. To deliver a specific dose to the center of the tumor, IMRT requires the accelerator to be energized longer, which results in higher radiation doses. Therefore, it has been estimated that the incidence of radiation-induced sarcoma may increase by 0.5% with IMRT.[31] In contrast there is reason to hope that the use of PBT may reduce dose to normal tissues and in turn reduce the risk of secondary malignancy compared to photons.[32]

Hereditary Cancer Syndromes

Genetic factors can predispose to a higher risk of developing radiation-induced second malignancy. About 5% of cancers are thought to arise in the context of a known hereditary cancer syndrome. Inherited gene mutations may lead to multiple tumors within the predisposed individual. Somatic cells may sustain transforming mutations following treatment with radiation and certain chemotherapeutic agents and lead to secondary cancers. Retinoblastoma and Li–Fraumeni syndrome are examples of such syndromes.

References

1. Denham J, Hauer-Jensen M. The radiotherapeutic injury – a "complex"' wound. *Radiother Oncol.* 2002;63:129–145.
2. Peterson DE, Doerr W, Hovan A, et al. Osteoradionecrosis in cancer patients: the evidence base for treatment-dependent frequency, current management strategies, and future studies. *Support Care Cancer.* 2010;18(8):1089–1098.
3. Caparrotti F, Huang SH, Lu L, et al. Osteoradionecrosis of the mandible in patients with oropharyngeal carcinoma treated with intensity-modulated radiotherapy. *Cancer.* 2017;123:3691–3700.
4. Bennett MH, Feldmeier J, Hampson NB, et al. Hyperbaric oxygen therapy for late radiation tissue injury. *Cochrane Database Syst Rev.* 2016;4:CD005005.
5. Haubner F, Ohmann E, Pohl F, et al. Wound healing after radiation therapy: review of the literature. *Radiat Oncol.* 2012;7:162.
6. Bourget A, Chang JT, Wu DB, et al. Free flap reconstruction in the head and neck region following radiotherapy: a cohort study identifying negative outcome predictors. *Plast Reconstr Surg.* 2011;127(5):1901–1908.
7. Lee S, Thiele C. Factors associated with free flap complications after head and neck reconstruction and the molecular basis of fibrotic tissue rearrangement in preirradiated soft tissue. *J Oral Maxillofac Surg.* 2010;68(9):2169–2178.
8. Mueller CK, Schultze-Mosgau S. Radiation-induced microenvironments – the molecular basis for free flap complications in the pre-irradiated field? *Radiother Oncol.* 2009;93(3):581–585.
9. Herle P, Shukla L, Morrison WA, et al. Preoperative radiation and free flap outcomes for head and neck reconstruction: a systematic review and meta-analysis. *Aust N Z J Surg.* 2015;85(3):121–127.
10. Chao AH, Chang DW, Shuaib SW, et al. The effect of neoadjuvant versus adjuvant irradiation on microvascular free flap reconstruction in sarcoma patients. *Plast Reconstr Surg.* 2012;129(3):675–682.
11. O'Sullivan B, Davis AM, Turcotte R, et al. Preoperative versus postoperative radiotherapy in soft tissue sarcoma of the limbs: a randomised trial. *Lancet.* 2002;359:2235–2241.
12. Miller ED, Xu-Welliver M, Haglund KE. The role of modern radiation therapy in the management of extremity sarcomas. *J Surg Oncol.* 2015;111:599–603.
13. Deutsch M, Kroll SS, Ainsle N, et al. Influence of radiation on late complications in patients with free fibular flaps for mandibular reconstruction. *Ann Plast Surg.* 1999;42(6):662–664.
14. Halle M, Bodin I, Tornvall P, et al. Timing of radiotherapy in head and neck free flap reconstruction – a study of postoperative complications. *J Plast Reconstruct Aesthet Surg.* 2009;62(7):889–895.
15. Ho AY, Hu ZI, Mehrara BJ, et al. Radiotherapy in the setting of breast reconstruction: types, techniques, and timing. *Lancet Oncol.* 2017;18(12):e742–e753.
16. Momoh AO, Ahmed R, Kelley BP, et al. A systematic review of complications of implant-based breast reconstruction with prereconstruction and postreconstruction radiotherapy. *Ann Surg Oncol.* 2014;21(1):118–124.
17. Tsoi B, Ziolkowski NI, Thoma A, et al. Safety of tissue/expander/implant versus autologous abdominal tissue breast reconstruction in postmastectomy breast cancer patients: a systematic review and meta-analysis. *Plast Reconstr Surg.* 2014;133(2):234–249.
18. National Comprehensive Cancer Network. *Breast Cancer*; 2018. Version 4.
19. Petrelli F, Sgroi G, Sarti E, et al. Increasing the interval between neoadjuvant chemoradiotherapy and surgery in rectal cancer: a meta-analysis of published studies. *Ann Surg.* 2016;263(3):458.
20. Nutting CM, Morden JP, Harrington KJ, et al. Parotid-sparing intensity modulated versus conventional radiotherapy in head and neck cancer (PARSPORT): a phase 3 multicentre randomised controlled trial. *Lancet Oncol.* 2011;12(2):127–136.
21. Rudat V, Muñter M, Rades D, et al. The effect of amifostine or IMRT to preserve the parotid function after radiotherapy of the head and neck region measured by quantitative salivary gland scintigraphy. *Radiother Oncol.* 2008;89(1):71–80.
22. Hom DB, Adams G, Koreis M, et al. Choosing the optimal wound dressing for irradiated soft tissue wounds. *Otolaryngol Head Neck Surg.* 1999;121:591–598.
23. Delanian S, Chatel C, Porcher R, et al. Complete restoration of refractory mandibular osteoradionecrosis by prolonged treatment with a pentoxifylline-tocopherol-clodronate combination (PENTOCLO): a phase II trial. *Int J Radiat Oncol Biol Phys.* 2011;80(3):832–839.
24. Bertozzi N, Simonacci F, Grieco MP, et al. The biological and clinical basis for the use of adipose-derived stem cells in the field of wound healing. *Ann Med Surg.* 2017;20:41–48.
25. Hall EJ, Wuu CS. Radiation-induced second cancers: the impact of 3D-CRT and IMRT. *Int J Radiat Oncol Biol Phys.* 2003;56:83–88.
26. Little JB. Ionizing radiation. In: Kufe DW, Pollock RE, Weichselbaum RR, et al., eds. *Cancer Medicine.* 6th edn. Hamilton, ON: B.C. Decker; 2000.
27. Morton LM, Onel K, Curtis RE, et al. The rising incidence of second cancers: patterns of occurrence and identification of risk factors for children and adults. *Am Soc Clin Oncol Educ Book.* 2014:e57–67.
28. Maddams J, Parkin DM, Darby SC. The cancer burden in the UK in 2007 due to radiotherapy. *Int J Cancer.* 2011;129(12):2885–2893.
29. Curtis RE, Freedman DM, Ron E, et al. *New Malignancies Among Cancer Survivors: SEER Cancer Registries. 1973–2000.* Bethesda, MD: National Cancer Institute; 2006:502.
30. Cahan WG. Radiation-induced sarcoma – 50 years later. *Cancer.* 1998;82(1):6–7.
31. Hall EJ. Intensity-modulated radiation therapy, protons, and the risk of second cancers. *Int J Radiat Oncol Biol Phys.* 2006;65:1–7.
32. Chung CS, Yock TI, Nelson K, et al. Incidence of second malignancies among patients treated with proton versus photon radiation. *Int J Radiat Oncol Biol Phys.* 2013;87(1):46–52.

13 Burns: Acute Care and Reconstruction

GEOFFREY E. HESPE AND BENJAMIN LEVI

Introduction

Burns can be a devastating injury that is nondiscriminatory, affecting individuals of all ages, races, and socioeconomic backgrounds. In the United States the incidence of burn injuries continues to rise, with approximately half a million individuals requiring medical therapy, 40,000 hospital admissions, and more than 3000 deaths annually.[1] The sequelae of burn injuries place a heavy financial burden on the national economy. As critical care management continues to improve, an increasing number of individuals with severe burns are surviving their initial injuries. Thus, there is an increasing need for plastic surgeons to provide appropriate acute burn care as well as reconstruction to help these individuals regain as much of their preinjury appearance and function as possible. This chapter will focus on the acute management of burn injuries, timing for surgical reconstruction, reconstructive options and anatomical considerations one must consider when managing patients with complex burn reconstruction needs.

Burn Assessment

When evaluating a new burn patient, it is important to initially manage the patient by the guidelines outlined in Advance Trauma Life Support (ATLS). Once this assessment is completed attention can be turned to determining the extent and depth of the burn. The extent of a burn injury is quantified by total burn surface area (TBSA). To calculate TBSA, one can use a Lund and Browder chart, which employs the rule of 9s (Fig. 13.1). There are slight variations between adults and children due to children's heads being larger and extremities smaller when compared to adults. TBSA can also be estimated by equating the area of a patient's hand to approximately 1% TBSA. The depth of burns can be broken down into superficial, partial thickness and full thickness. Superficial burns involve only the epidermis and do not result in blistering of the skin but are painful, with blanchable hyperemia. Partial-thickness burns are deeper burns that involve varying layers of the dermis and are classified as either superficial or deep depending on the extent of involvement. Superficial partial-thickness burns effect the papillary dermis and spare other skin appendages. This degree of burn presents with blistering of the skin and increased hyperemia but it is still blanchable. Deep partial-thickness burns involve all layers of the dermis (papillary and reticular) and physical examination will reveal decreased sensation and tissue that is pale in color. Full-thickness burns extend through the epidermis and dermis and down to subcutaneous tissue, muscle, and bone. These burns are insensate due to destruction of the nerves, nonblanchable, and typically have a leathery appearance. Additional ways to determine burn depth include examining tissue moisture, as superficial burns often appear moist whereas deeper burns appear dry. The surgeon can also look for the presence of hair follicle as deep burns will not have remnants of the hair follicle and/or the hair follicle can be removed easily upon attempt.

In our practice we typically wait approximately 3 days to allow burns to fully declare themselves as some burns may progress over time unless the patient has obvious large regions of full-thickness eschar. This thought process is in part due to the Jackson burn model, which describes the distinct zones within the burned area. The central aspect of the burn is classified as the zone of coagulation, which represents the most severely damaged portion of the wound. This area of the burn is nonsalvageable and should be treated with early excision and grafting. The tissue surrounding the zone of coagulation is the zone of stasis. This region represents damaged tissue and underlying vasculature and may be salvageable with appropriate fluid resuscitation. The outer region is the zone of hyperemia and represents tissue that should recover. The hyperemia is due to increased blood flow secondary to vasodilation. Similar to the zone of stasis, appropriate resuscitation is key to this tissue surviving. Once the extent of the patient's burns is evaluated, if the patient is not at a designated burn center it is important to determine whether transfer to a burn center is required.

% Total Body Surface Area Burn

Be clear and accurate, and do not include erythema

(Lund and Browder)

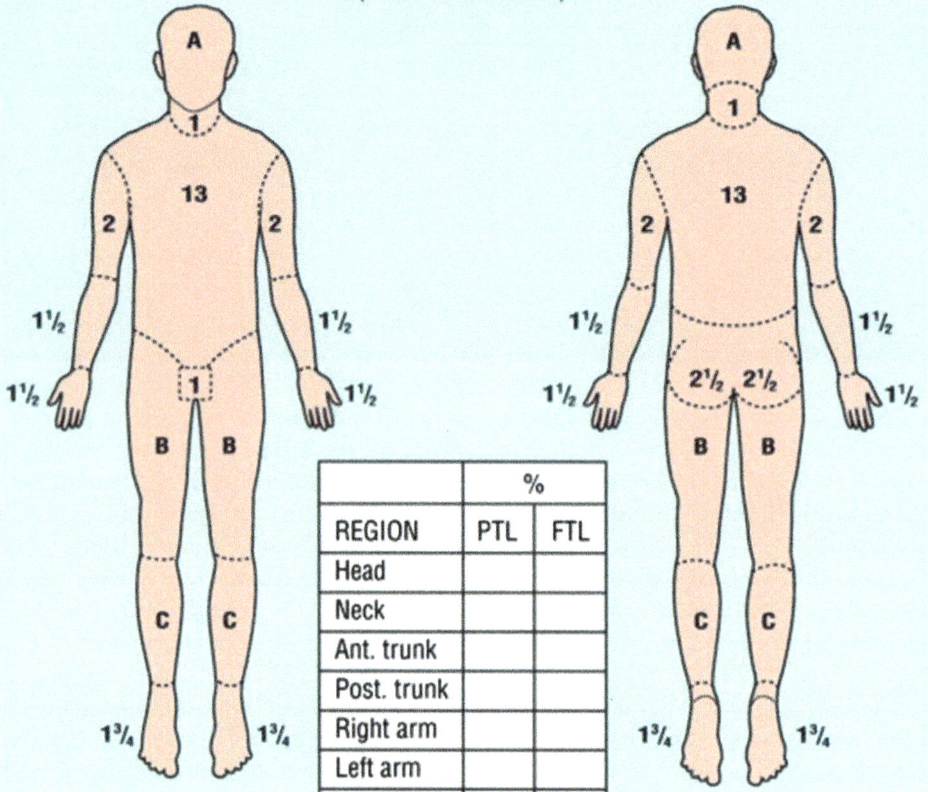

	%	
REGION	PTL	FTL
Head		
Neck		
Ant. trunk		
Post. trunk		
Right arm		
Left arm		
Buttocks		
Genitalia		
Right leg		
Left leg		
Total burn		

AREA	Age 0	1	5	10	15	Adult
A = ½ OF HEAD	9½	8½	6½	5½	4½	3½
B = ½ OF ONE THIGH	2¾	3¼	4	4½	4½	4¾
C = ½ OF ONE LOWER LEG	2½	2½	2¾	3	3¼	3½

• **Fig. 13.1** Lund and Browder chart. (Reproduced from Goutos I, Tyler M. Early management of paediatric burn injuries. *Paediatr Child Health*. 2013;23(9);391–396. Source: National Institute for Health and Care Excellence, http://www.cks.nhs.uk.)

Pathophysiology of Burn

Burns result in damage to varying degrees of the skin and subcutaneous layers as already mentioned. The depth of the burn depends on multiple factors such as the thickness of the tissue in that area, the mechanism of injury (thermal, electrical or chemical) and the duration of the resulting injury. Thermal injury results in damage to the blood vessels in the skin and subsequent thrombus formation in the vessels. There is also damage to the surrounding tissue leading to local release of inflammatory mediators such as tumor necrosis factor-alpha, interferon-gamma, and numerous interleukins with the development of subsequent edema.[2] The loss of proteins can lead to fluid shifts and fluid resuscitation is a key component of the acute resuscitative management. This will be discussed in detail later in this chapter. Loss of the skin, which is a protective barrier to the body, can also result in problems with thermoregulation.

Types of Burns

The mechanism of burns can typically be classified as thermal, chemical or electrical in nature. The majority of burns are thermal burns. These typically can be classified as either wet burns secondary to hot liquids or dry burns as a result of fire injury. Electrical burns are typically associated with work injuries, result in deeper tissue injury, and represent a small percentage of all burns that present to burn centers. Unlike thermal burns, TBSA does not always represent the extent of the patient's injury in electrical burns. When evaluating electrical burns, it is important to know the voltage involved, resistance, and type of current as well as determine the entrance and exit wounds. The extent of the injury depends on the resistance of the tissue involved. Electricity will pass through tissues with low resistance (i.e., nerves, vessels, muscle) resulting in less heating of the adjacent tissue but can lead to cell rupture due to electrical current driving water into cell membranes leading to electroporation. Bone, on the other hand, has high resistance and as a result electricity will not pass through it. Instead the electricity travels along the bone, which heats to a higher temperature then surrounding tissue causing tissue/muscle injury. Electrical burns do not only damage tissues but they can lead to cardiac arrhythmias, injury to solid organs and the gastrointestinal tract, and lead to possible compartment syndrome in extremities due to the deeper tissue/muscle injury as a result of the electricity traveling along the bone. Electrocardiogram monitoring is therefore important following electrical burns.

Due to the fact that TBSA may underrepresent the extent of damage sustained in an electrical burn, the Parkland formula may not provide adequate resuscitation. The Parkland formula can be used as a starting point but urine output (1 mL/kg per hour) should be used to evaluate resuscitation. When examining the current involved in an electrical burn this can typically be classified as either low voltage (<1000 V) or high voltage (>1000 V). Low voltage electrical burns typically occur within buildings and have more localized damage. High voltage injuries typically involve greater tissue damage and organ damage.

Due to the extensive thermal injury that can occur as the electrical current travels along the bone it is important to evaluate for compartment syndrome in affected extremities. Compartment syndrome is typically recognized by the 6 Ps: paresthesia, pain out of proportion, poikilothermia, pallor, pulselessness, and paralysis. Compartment pressures should be measured in limbs with concern and if the pressure is >30 mmHg, compartment release should be considered. Additionally, the extent of injury often progresses beyond the initial 3 days and thus we typically wait closer to 1 week before performing definitive closure with skin grafts to minimize graft loss following compartment release. Electrical injury frequently effects muscles and can lead to rhabdomyolysis. In patients with myoglobinuria it is important to check creatine kinase. The treatment for rhabdomyolysis is fluid resuscitation with a goal urine output of 2 mL/kg per hour. Increased excretion of myoglobin through the urine can also be done with mannitol or bicarbonate to alkalize the urine.

Chemical burns are the least frequent of burn injuries that present to burn centers. A majority of chemical burns occur at the workplace. The type of chemical determines the mechanism of injury as well as the treatment options. Most chemical injuries can be classified as acid, alkali, or organic compounds. When a patient presents to the emergency room with concern for a chemical burn it is important to remove any clothing on the patient that has been contaminated by the compound in order to prevent further injury. It is also very important to protect yourself from injury from the chemical so personal protective equipment is necessary. For the majority of chemical burns, once all clothing is removed it is important to thoroughly irrigate the burn to remove the inciting agent. This is true for most but not all agents. Potassium, sodium, and lithium can result in an explosion when these compounds come in contact with water and thus irrigation should be avoided.

Acid burns are typically limited to the area that was exposed and the resultant injury is caused by coagulation necrosis. Hydrofluoric acid, commonly used for glass etching, is a unique example as it is a weak acid but the fluoride ion is a noxious element. Hypocalcemia can occur due to the fluoride ions chelating calcium ions with serious consequences for the patient. Treatment of hydrofluoric acid burn is topical calcium gel to neutralize the fluoride ion.[3] Fertilizer, drain cleaners, and wet cement are examples of alkali compounds. Unlike acid burns which are usually self-limiting, alkali burns can effect deeper tissues as they will continue to denature proteins and cause liquefaction necrosis until the inciting agent is completely removed. Finally, organic compounds, such as petroleum or phenol, can affect cell membranes as well as have toxic effects on organs. Phenol should be wiped off with polyethylene glycol or ethyl alcohol soaked sponges as the agent is water-insoluble. Phenol is associated with liver toxicity and can lead to cardiac arrhythmias.

Inhalation Injury

During the initial evaluation of a burn patient it is important to determine the mechanism of injury. In patients who have sustained thermal injury, specifically as a result of fires in closed spaces, evaluation for inhalation injury is very important. Studies have shown that inhalation injury can increase the mortality associated with burn injuries by 20%.[4] Signs of inhalation injury typically include facial burns, singed nasal hairs, ashy sputum, and hoarseness. In patients where there is concern for possible inhalation injury it is important to perform early bronchoscopy to evaluate the patient's airway and to suction out any particulate matter. We often send quantitative cultures from each lung at the time of admission for intubated patients given the high incidence of community acquired pneumonia. Pneumonia in the setting of inhalation injury has been shown to increase mortality by 60%.[4] If there is evidence of airway injury, which can present as edema or erythema caused by superheated air or the presence of soot, it is important to intubate early to protect the airway. Multiple bronchoscopies with suction should be performed if large amounts of particulate matter remain. Intubation at the time of respiratory collapse can be extremely challenging.

In addition to physical injury due to inhalation of smoke and superheated air, there is also a risk of carbon monoxide poisoning. Patients will present with altered mental status and/or agitation and typically have hyperemic mucous membranes. This is due to carbon monoxide's higher affinity for hemoglobin than oxygen. More specifically, carbon monoxide has an approximately 200 times higher affinity for hemoglobin. It is important to check the patient's carboxyhemoglobin level to rule in or out carbon monoxide poisoning, the patient should be given 100% oxygen to help outcompete the carbon monoxide for binding sites on the hemoglobin as 100% oxygen substantially decreases the half-life of carboxyhemoglobin.

Cyanide poisoning is another complication of smoke inhalation. Hydrogen cyanide can be found in paints, plastics, and other household materials that can be combusted during a fire. Cyanide inhibits oxygen utilization in the electron transport chain due to it binding to the terminal cytochrome thus preventing cytochrome c oxidase function. Presentation is very similar to carbon monoxide poisoning, with patients having altered mental status in addition to alterations of the central nervous and circulatory system. There is no specific test for cyanide poisoning but decreased oxygen uptake can be calculated by measuring venous blood oxygen saturation compared to arterial blood oxygen saturation. A difference of greater than 10% suggests inadequate oxygen extraction. Treatment of cyanide poisoning is hydroxycobalamin, which chelates cyanide to cyanocobalamin. Empirical treatment of suspected cyanide poisoning is a reasonable option given the effectiveness and low toxicity of treatment.[5] Clinicians, however, should note that this treatment causes bodily fluids, including urine and wound exudate, to turn red.

Fluid Resuscitation

The key to the acute management of burn injuries is appropriate fluid resuscitation. Due to burn injuries damaging the protective epidermal layer, patients have extensive loss of proteins and fluid. As mentioned earlier in this chapter, during the initial phase of injury there is a substantial inflammatory response which can lead to increased capillary permeability during this period. It is important to restore interstitial volume to allow for proper organ perfusion and thus oxygenation. Fluid resuscitation is based on the Parkland formula (4 mL × %TBSA × weight (kg)), which calculates the amount of fluid that should be given in the first 24 hours. In elderly patients or patients with congestive heart failure, this formula should start closer to 2 mL × %TBSA × weight (kg). Half of this volume is given in the first 8 hours while the rest is given over the next 16 hours. When calculating TBSA, this should apply only to partial- or full-thickness burns. In adult patients the resuscitative fluid of preference is typically lactated Ringer's solution, but in children D5 ½ lactated Ringer's is used due to the risk of hypoglycemia given their small stores of glycogen. During the resuscitative effort, the patient's urine output is monitored to make sure that adequate resuscitation is occurring. In adult patients an optimal volume of urine output is typically 0.5 mL/kg per hour and in children it is higher, at 1 mL/kg per hour. This should be managed on an hourly basis to avoid under- or over-resuscitation as this can have negative effects on the injured tissues. Additionally, normalization of laboratory values can also be followed, for example lactate and pH. During difficult to resuscitate scenarios, monitoring of cardiac output is recommended. Additionally, newer protocols will advise switching from crystalloid to colloid resuscitation if, during the resuscitation, fluid has been increased above the protocol several times and it is estimated that the patient will receive 6 mL × kg × TBSA.

Systemic Effects

Although the majority of morbidity associated with burn injuries is due to damage to the skin, there are significant effects to other organ systems as well. Due to the loss of a protective barrier there can be alterations in core body regulation. It is important to closely monitor patient's temperature to maintain normothermia. Additionally, this loss of barrier function can also lead to bacterial and fungal infection. It is important to closely monitor for signs of infection and take quantitative cultures to help guide antibiotic therapy if indicated. Immediately after a burn injury there is an initial decrease in cardiac output and metabolism. This changes in the first 24–48 hours and switches to increased cardiac output and a hypermetabolic state. This produces an overall catabolic state, which necessitates increasing nutrition intake. In patients with TBSA totaling >40% it has been shown that their metabolic rates are doubled. This can remain elevated for up to 12 months following their initial injury.[2] In order to maintain body weight following substantial burns, calorie intake should be 40 kcal per % TBSA plus 25 kcal/kg of body weight.[6] In children suggested intake is 1800 kcal/m^2 in addition to 2200 kcal/m^2 for the area of burn.[7] Not only is calorie intake important, patients need a high protein diet in order to properly heal their wounds. It is suggested that in order to maintain their body mass patients must increase their protein intake to 1.5–2 g/kg of body weight. There is also damage to the gastrointestinal tract, which can result in translocation of gut bacteria.

Timing of Reconstruction

With an increasing number of individuals surviving their initial burn injuries and thus living longer, burn injuries can become a lifelong ailment. Determining the correct procedure and timing for burn reconstruction is important in order to provide these patients with the best possible outcome.

Whenever an injury is sustained to the skin, the body's natural response is to heal through scar formation and contracture. This is determined in part by the depth of injury and the amount of tension sensed across the wound. The greater the penetration of burn into the dermis, the more contraction that occurs due to higher populations of myofibroblasts as the wound heals.[8] Recent studies have also identified the fibroblasts involved in scar formation to be located in the deeper dermis.[9] Scar maturation can take at least 12 months if not longer to complete and the timing of reconstruction should take this into account. During the healing process, some patients will develop keloid or hypertrophic scars. In one study looking at military personnel who sustained burn injuries, the authors found that 80% of patients developed some extent of hypertrophic scarring during their healing.[10]

When planning reconstruction for a patient, the general mantra is to consider the reconstructive ladder: choosing the simplest option to produce an acceptable reconstruction while limiting donor site morbidity. Due to the complexity of burn reconstruction, this is not always the case. In many instances the extent and location of the burn will limit your reconstructive options and more complex operations may be indicated. Most superficial and superficial partial-thickness burns can be treated with local wound care and will heal without scar. Deep partial-thickness and full-thickness burns, however, will always form a scar regardless of the treatments: surgical or healing by secondary intention.

Acute Techniques to Limit Subsequent Reconstruction

In the acute setting, attention should first be directed to the resuscitative effort. During this period of time, burns of intermediate depth can progress to full thickness or remain at a more partial thickness injury level. Typically, burns are allowed to declare their depth over the first 3 days. An exception to this is in patients with large areas of full-thickness burn or eschar where early excision or escharotomies should be performed to prevent burn wound sepsis or compartment syndrome in circumferential burns of the extremities, chest or digits. Escharotomies can be performed at the bedside or in the operating room. Once the patient is stable, the next goal should be for excision of any dead tissue and coverage with autologous or homologous tissue. The first step is to tangentially excise dead and necrotic tissue to reveal healthy underlying tissue to create a wound bed that can successfully accept a graft. In order for a graft to survive, it requires underlying tissue with an adequate blood supply to support the graft. Excision of unhealthy damaged tissue can be performed using a Weck or Watson blade. The Versajet is an additional tool that can be used, though it is typically reserved for difficult areas such as the eyelids or hands. Once debridement is performed, meticulous hemostasis should be obtained. This can be done with thrombin spray and/or epinephrine-soaked non-stick gauze followed by compression.

Options for grafting are variable and will be discussed in detail later in this chapter. The optimal graft choice greatly depends on the quality of the underlying wound bed to allow for the best opportunity for the graft to survive and thus a successful reconstruction. Early coverage done in the acute setting is performed to decrease the need for further reconstruction in the future. The thickness of the grafts harvested and how much they are stretched or meshed will have a long-term effect on the final outcome. For example, the mesh appearance of the graft is almost impossible to completely eliminate. Additionally, hypertrophic scars are often more prominent in those with widely meshed and Meek grafts due to the need of the interstices to heal in secondarily (Fig. 13.2). We prefer sheet grafts for small areas or areas that are visible, especially in young healthy patients. In adults our practice is to typically harvest skin grafts that are 0.012 inches thick. If grafting to the face or hand, we use thicker grafts measuring 0.018 inches. In children, thinner grafts are used, measuring 0.008–0.010 inches.

When autografting is not a possibility either due to the quality of the recipient site or lack of donor sites there are several alternatives available to help bridge this period. Allografting/homografting is the use of human cadaveric skin which is a useful option when: (1) the burn surface area is too large to cover with autograft; (2) the wound bed is not ready for autograft as is the case in deep burns, elderly, diabetic, and debilitated patients. Allograft can serve as a test of the wound bed prior to harvesting a donor site and to allow for granulation tissue to grow in. For these patients, the allograft can be incorporated and then, after granulation tissue is established, the allograft can be removed and replaced with autograft with minimal additional debridement. This is especially useful in instances of malnourished or older, debilitated patients where debridement is down to adipose tissue. Xenografting is the use of graft from another species, usually porcine, which can be used in burns that are superficial partial thickness and would heal secondarily without needing an autograft. This additional layer can alleviate pain during dressing changes by serving as a layer between the painful skin and the wound dressing. Xenografts will begin to fall off 7 days after placement due to the lack of revascularization.

Biologic Skin Substitutes

It is also important to provide coverage for exposed vital structures such as vasculature, tendons, etc. In the acute setting, this can be accomplished by several different methods depending on the extent of the injury and quality of surrounding tissues. In healthy wound beds requiring coverage of vital structures, Integra (Integra LifeSciences, Princeton, NJ, USA) , a dermal substitute, can be used which consists of a bilayer configuration of bovine collagen and glycosaminoglycans from shark forming a decellularized matrix with a semipermeable silicone membrane. This allows for fibroblasts to infiltrate the matrix to begin to form a neodermis. Revascularization of the neodermis takes approximately 2–3 weeks at which point it can be covered with

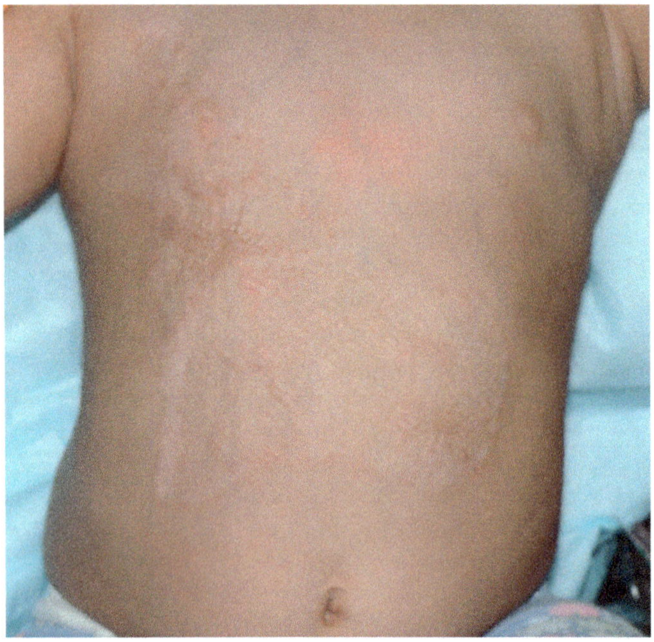

• **Fig. 13.2** Mesh skin grafting can result in unfavorable outcomes secondary to inadequacy of tissue and thus healing by secondary intention of the interstices.

a thin split-thickness skin graft (0.008–0.010 in). Integra is a useful temporizing dressing in traction or high energy burns where the depth is not yet known. Integra allows for surgeons to provide coverage over structures that would not typically accept a graft such as tendon without healthy overlying paratenon. In these cases, it is important to aggressively debride all necrotic tissue as well as a small rim of skin around the tendon (Fig. 13.3). Amniotic membrane-based tissue substitutes can also be used to treat exposed tendon and will be discussed in detail later in this chapter. Similar to Integra, the success of these biologics depends on adequate debridement.

Cultured Skin Substitutes

Recent advances in burn treatment have resulted in the addition of Epicel (Vericel, Cambridge, MA) and ReCell (Ativa Medical, Valencia, CA), which employ autologous cultured skin cells for grafting. Epicel is approved for patients with TBSA >30% which is comprised of deep dermal or full-thickness burns. A full thickness biopsy of the patient's skin is needed and in approximately 17 days 96 grafts can be generated. ReCell similarly uses autologous cultured skin cells in the form of a spray-on suspension that is indicated for acute partial-thickness burns or in adjunct with meshed autographs for full-thickness burns.

Adjacent Tissue Rearrangements

In areas where there is unaffected surrounding tissue, local flaps (i.e., V–Y advancement, island advancement, rotation flaps or rhomboid flaps) can be used to advance or rotate healthy tissue to cover exposed structures. However, in the acute period, the zone of injury is usually beyond the immediate wound and thus early grafting with subsequent adjacent tissue rearrangements is preferred. In instances where the wound bed is not amenable to dermal substitutes or local flap options, free tissue transfer can be considered to bring in healthy vascularized tissue. Though not common, this is often required for burns with exposed bone.

Occupational Therapy

Splinting is an important aspect of early reconstruction and grafting because it can help reduce contracture, secondary to wound healing. Working closely with occupational therapy to have customized splints created for the patient is key. Limiting contractions can help reduce the need for future surgeries. Neck and axillary contractures are the most common and need the most aggressive treatment. For full-thickness neck burns requiring grafting we will sometimes recommend a c-collar for up to 6 weeks. For axillary burns, a splint to keep the shoulder in abduction, especially at night is useful. For hand burns, intrinsic plus splints should be used at the time of graft placement but aggressive range of motion should be performed starting 4–5 days after graft placement. At that point splints should be used when the patient is resting or sleeping. In general, we recommend against aggressive passive elbow range of motion during the first week after injury to decrease the risk of heterotopic ossification. Elbows should be splinted in extension after graft placement.

Acute Reconstructive Needs

Acute reconstruction is important to help prevent local complications such as ectropion. Full-thickness burns in the periorbital region should be debrided and grafted either with homograft followed by thick split-thickness skin grafts (STSG) or full-thickness skin grafts (FTSG). Typically, FTSGs are useful for deep burns around the eyes. Grafts should be harvested from an area with light skin and without hair, such as the supraclavicular region or proximal inner arm. Concurrently, tarsorrhaphies should be performed at the time of grafting to alleviate the constant pull on the lower lid. For severe cases, permanent tarsorrhaphies are needed as temporary tarsorrhaphies will often pull through creating severe damage to the tarsal plate.

Intermediate and Late Reconstruction

Topical Scar Treatments

Conservative scar treatments focus on limiting the negative sequelae of scar maturation and to help prevent abnormal scar formation. During this period, which extends from the initial wound healing to complete maturation of scars, treatment consists of compression garments, silicone sheeting, steroid injections, massage, and topical treatments such as vitamin E and scar creams, with varying benefit. In a

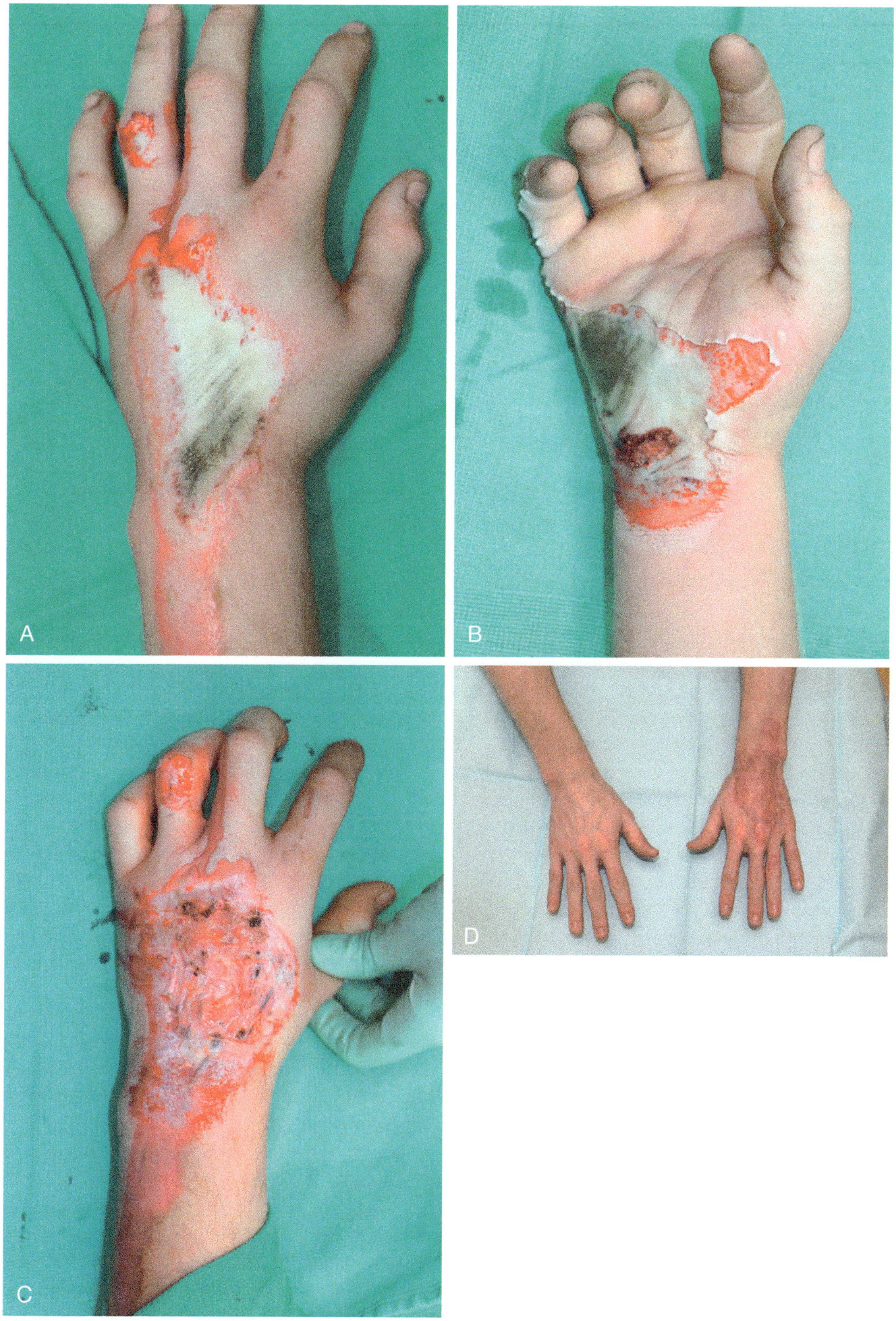

• **Fig. 13.3** (A,B) Showing full-thickness burns to the volar and dorsal surfaces of the left hand. (C) Debridement and application of primary Integra followed by secondary split-thickness skin graft. (D) Long-term follow up showing healed split-thickness skin graft on the dorsal aspect of the left hand.

meta-analysis by Anzarut et al, they found that global scar scores for burn injuries did not improve with pressure garment therapy.[11] In a randomized, double-blinded control trial examining the effects of silicone gel on burn scars, at 4 months all measures of the Vancouver Scar Scale (VSS) were improved in the silicone gel arm of the study.[12] Finally, in a recent systematic review investigating the efficacy of vitamin E in scar management, the authors concluded that at this point there is not enough evidence to support any significant benefit in scar management.[13] As one can see from this data, the available treatment options for burn scars have so far demonstrated mixed results and further research is likely needed.

Late reconstruction focuses on decreasing tension across wounds to help improve wound healing as well as dealing with the negative sequelae of wound healing, such as contractures. This will be discussed in greater detail later in this chapter.

Surgical Techniques for Reconstruction

Scar Release

There are many different techniques available for burn reconstruction, with each playing a unique role in the process. Each reconstructive challenge should be managed by the most effective approach to achieve an acceptable result. Scars are often hypertrophic in nature due to excessive tension, therefore release of this tension can turn an unfavorable scar into a favorable scar. As wounds heal through the formation of new collagen fibers, the resultant wound contracts. Scar contracture can result in significant morbidity when they occur at locations of articulation such as joints or the neck. To relieve tension and improve movement in the area of contracture, scar release can be utilized. An incision perpendicular to the area of maximal tension should be performed and taken down through scar to the healthy underlying tissue to allow for complete release. The ends of the release benefit from a fishtail incision to allow the release to completely open up (Fig. 13.4). Once the release has been performed, the defect should be assessed and covered. Depending on the location, the coverage can include a thick split-thickness skin graft, a full-thickness skin graft, a local or even free tissue transfer. Additionally, a temporizing biologic-like Integra can be used to help build up the wound bed prior to future grafting.

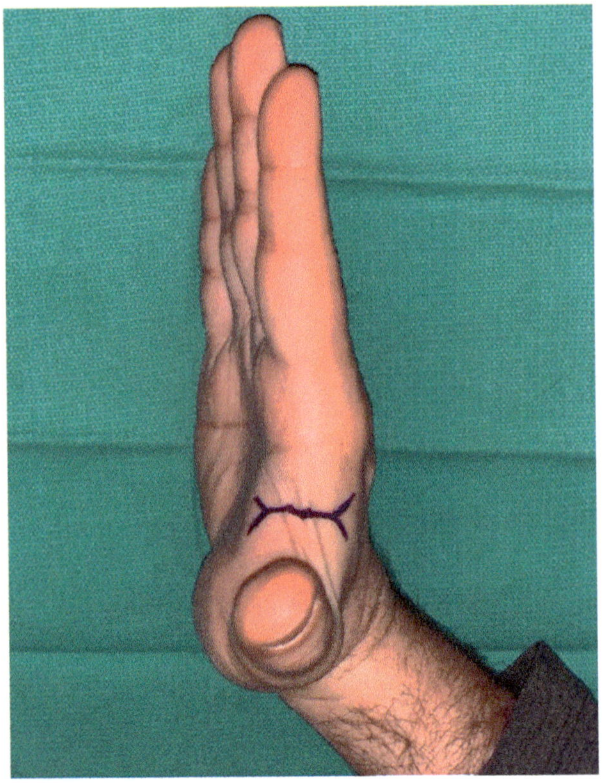

• **Fig. 13.4** Depiction of fishtail incision which can be used to increase release in areas of scar contracture.

Z-Plasty

Scar contractures on a smaller scale can be addressed with local tissue rearrangements. The most utilized technique for this is the Z-plasty. Z-plasties allow for one to reorient the tension of the scar as well as lengthen the scar. The central limb of the Z-plasty is directed along the length of the scar. Two equal length incisions are placed at equal angles of a given degree, which helps dictate the proportion of increased length that is gained by this maneuver (Table 13.1). The classic angle for a Z-plasty is 60 degrees, which allows for lengthening of the scar by 75%. Z-plasties can be constructed with different angles and thus different amounts of lengthening. In addition to altering the angle of the Z-plasty, multiple Z-plasties can be constructed in different configurations (i.e., double Z, 90-90, 5-flap jumping person) depending on the location and type of scar release one is looking for (Fig. 13.5). The 5-flap jumping person is useful in webspaces as it combines Z-plasties and a central V–Y, which depends on the webspace. Regardless of the angle of the limbs in a Z-plasty, the corner of each Z should be made at 90 degrees to improve blood flow to the tip of the random flap. In patients that have previous Z- plasties, we favor turning the Z flaps into a V–Y.

Grafting

As previously mentioned, in the acute management of burns, excision and grafting is the favored approach. There are several different grafting options following excision or scar release. When considering using the patient's own skin for autografting, one can consider split-thickness versus full-thickness skin grafting. Split-thickness skin grafts are harvested at depths that include the epidermis and varying degrees of the dermis, which allow for donor site healing via re-epithelialization and for the surgeon to harvest larger quantities for grafting. The papillary dermis is located just deep to the epidermis and is made up of the areas between the epidermal

TABLE 13.1 Z-Plasty Angles and Length Gained

Angle of Z-Plasty Lateral Limbs (Degrees)	Central Limb Length Gained (%)
30	25
45	50
60	75
75	100
90	120

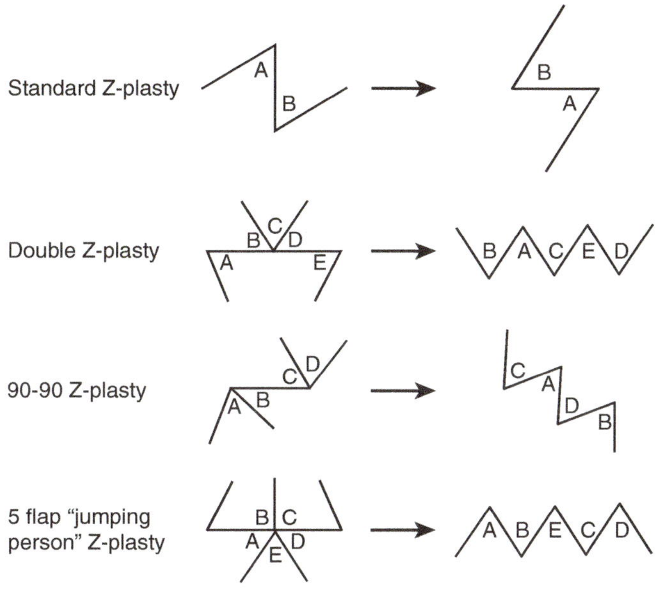

• **Fig. 13.5** Commonly used Z-plasty variations.

papillae. The reticular dermis is deep to the papillary dermis and makes up the majority of the dermal layer. This is the location of the majority of elastin fibers as well as sweat and sebaceous glands, hair follicles, and blood vessels. Grafts harvested at the deeper dermal layers have an increased risk of hypertrophic scarring. The surface area can be increased through meshing, whereby the skin is expanded and the interstices are allowed to heal in secondarily. Meshing is rarely used in burn reconstruction as scars form due to inadequate tissue so non-meshed thicker tissue should be used to prevent recurrent scarring and contracture. Full-thickness skin grafts include the epidermis and entire dermis and the donor defect is usually closed primarily. These grafts should be harvested without fat and if there is fat on the full-thickness graft it should be aggressively defatted prior to inset. The major difference between the two autografts is that split-thickness grafts have less primary contracture at the time of harvest but have greater secondary contracture over time, as compared to full-thickness skin grafts. Primary contraction is secondary to elastin found within the dermal layer. The thicker the dermis, the more elastin, which equates to increased contraction. Secondary contraction is attributed to myofibroblasts, which contract during wound healing to decrease the size of a wound. Thus full-thickness grafts are usually preferred for areas of esthetic importance and functional areas such as joints, hands, and the face.

Biologics

Another option for coverage after scar release is the use of Integra, which has been previously described. Integra allows for surgeons to provide coverage over structures that are typically not graftable, such as bone or tendon without healthy overlying periosteum or paratenon respectively. Dantzer and Braye examined Integra use in 31 patients (39 reconstructed sites) and demonstrated that it was an effective alternative for dermal reconstruction with only three patients demonstrating poor outcomes. They discuss that the disadvantages are the need for multiple surgeries, risk of infection and detachment of the silicone layer.[14]

Alloderm, a decellularized human cadaveric dermal matrix which created by first removing cellular components of the graft to make it immunologically inert while preserving the extracellular matrix is another option for grafting. In the setting of acute burn care it can be used as a dermal matrix for the revascularization and repopulation of skin cells.[8]

A more recent advance in alternative coverage options is the use of amniotic membranes (Fig. 13.6). The first use of amniotic membrane in the setting of burns was in 1913 by Stern.[15] Currently, EpiFix and EpiBurn are human amnion/chorion membranes which have been dehydrated and have been shown to contain cytokines and growth factors.[16] Studies have demonstrated that its use increased the rate of wound healing, decreased pain at the burn site, and the rate of infection.[16] Branski et al looked at its use in 100 patients in partial-thickness burns and was able to show a decrease in number of dressing changes and no significant difference in length of stay, rate of infection or rate of hypertrophic scar development when compared to topical antimicrobial therapy.[17] Reilly et al describe the use of amniotic membrane for both partial- and full-thickness burns.[18]

Tissue Expansion

Tissue expansion can be employed in burn reconstruction when there is healthy skin adjacent to an area of burn, or more commonly when the burn effects hair-bearing locations with resultant alopecia. Tissue expansion works through placement of an expansion device and gradually over time, usually 2–3 weeks, increasing the volume of the expander in order to stretch the skin. This technique allows for replacement of the damaged skin with similar adjacent tissue (Fig. 13.7). In the setting of scalp alopecia, tissue expansion can be used to replace hair-bearing skin when less

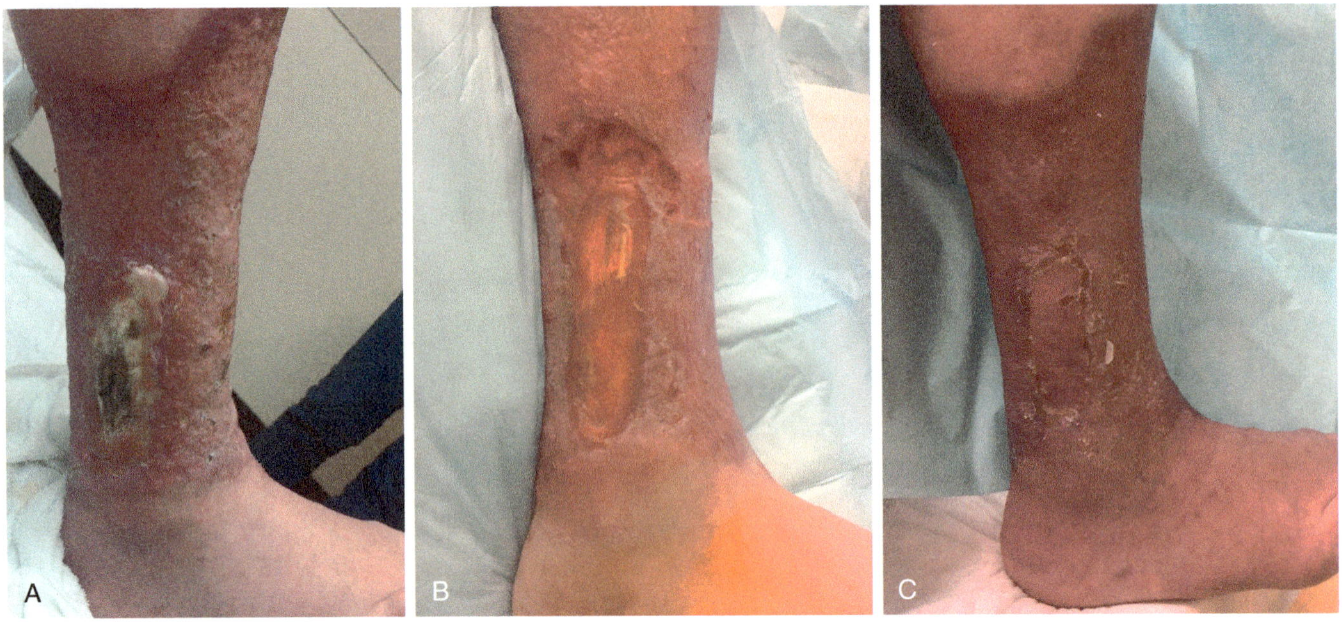

• **Fig. 13.6** (A) Preoperative depiction of a full-thickness burn to the right lateral leg with a nonhealing wound that (B) underwent debridement and EpiFix placement, (C) resulting in an acceptable reconstruction.

than 50% of hair loss is present. The disadvantages of tissue expansion though are the need for multiple operations, the contour deformity of the tissue expander when in place, and the risk of expander protrusion or infection. Additionally, hypertrophic scars are caused by excess tension on a wound closure, and after expansion scars are almost always closed under tension, recreating a new hypertrophic scar. Tension on the scar can also be deforming to surrounding structures, such as loss of the cervicomental angle.

Autologous Tissue Reconstruction

As one ascends the reconstructive ladder, when durable coverage of vital structures (nerve, vasculature, tendon) is required or there is a substantial soft tissue loss, one can consider local, region or free flap reconstruction. Local and regional flaps can sometimes be limited due to the extent of the sustained burn. In a study by Jabir et al, the authors demonstrated only 0.59% of patients required locoregional flaps.[19] In two large case series by Platt et al and De Lorenzi et al the number of burn patients requiring free flap reconstruction was 1.5% and 1.8% respectively.[20,21] When considering free flap reconstruction, options include but are not limited to supraclavicular flaps for neck reconstruction, latissimus dorsi, and anterior lateral thigh (ALT) flaps. The reconstructive requirements of a given situation can direct one to the appropriate flap. More specifically, when reconstructing the neck or axilla thinner flaps are utilized. In our practice we typically use supraclavicular for neck reconstruction and thoracodorsal artery perforator flaps for axillary reconstruction. Temporalis fascia flaps can be used when substantial hand coverage is needed along with a thin skin graft, which allows for a smooth surface for tendon movement. Based on this information, although flap coverage is not the mainstay of treatment it is still an important reconstructive option. When reconstructing lower extremity burns one can employ a similar algorithm to lower extremity trauma reconstruction. For wounds affecting the proximal third of the leg one can employ gastrocnemius flaps, for middle third defects one can use soleus muscle and for distal third wounds free tissue transfer should be considered (Fig. 13.8).

Nonsurgical Techniques

Lasers

Lasers have become an important aspect of long-term burn reconstruction. The advent of fractional CO_2 lasers has provided surgeons with a viable option for hypertrophic scarring. CO_2 lasers target water at a wavelength of 10,600 nm and help to break down collagen fibers (Fig. 13.9). As the collagen repairs itself, the desired effect is for them to reorganize in a more appropriate orientation. Fractional CO_2 lasers are effective at treating the firmness and texture abnormalities associated with hypertrophic burn scars.[22] Levi et al demonstrated that 96.7% of patients showed improved satisfaction of their burn scars following fractional CO_2 laser therapy. Additionally, they saw a decrease in neuropathic pain, pruritus, and contracture.[23] Pulse dye lasers (585 nm) can be used alone or in combination with CO_2 laser therapy to target the rubor associated with hypertrophic scarring as well as for treatment of symptoms such as pruritus. Pulse dye lasers target oxyhemoglobin and can be used to improve the color of scars. Most patients will require multiple sessions in order to achieve the desired results. Laser sessions can usually by spaced approximately 4–6 weeks apart to allow for appropriate recovery between treatments.

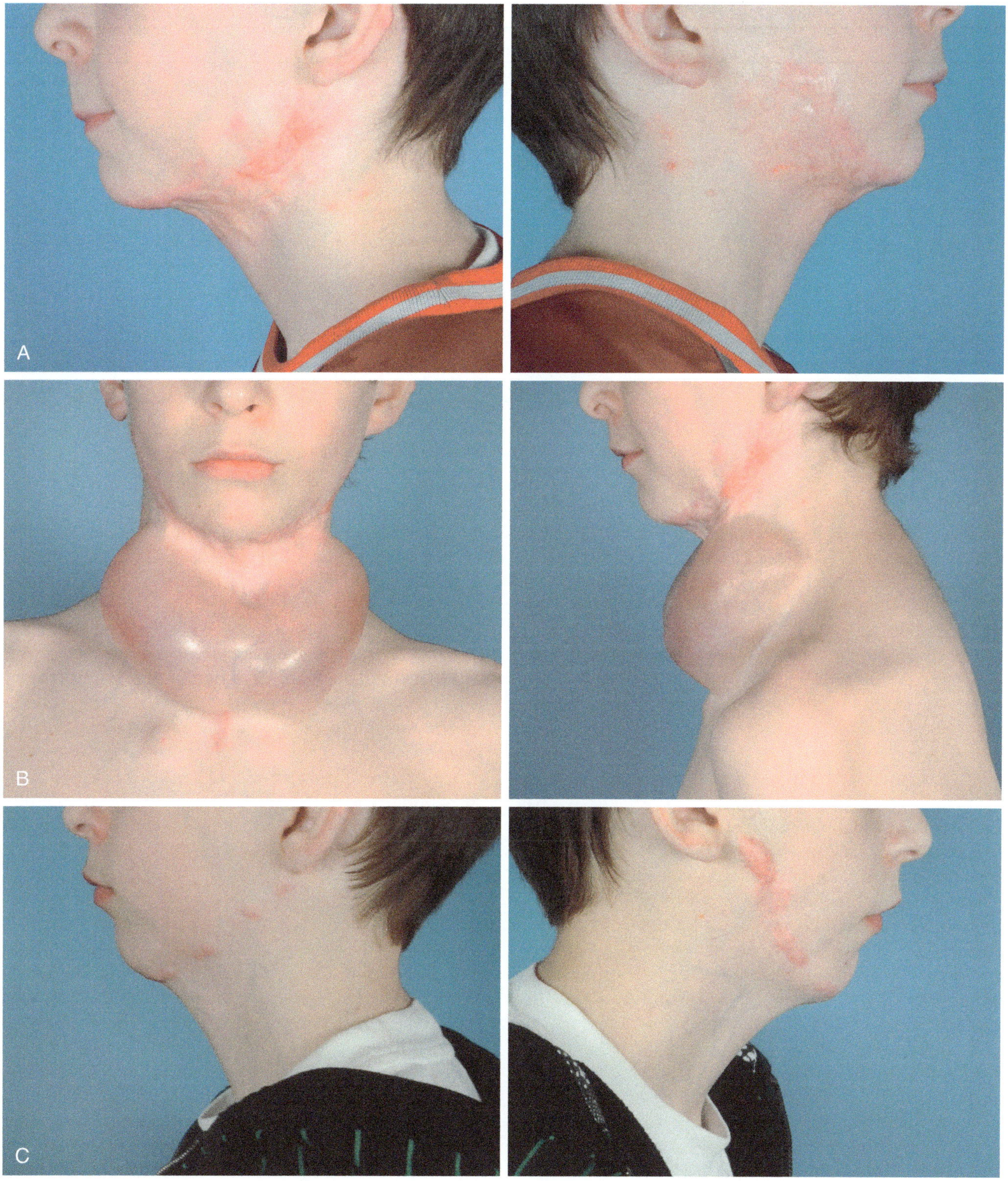

• **Fig. 13.7** (A) Preoperative appearance of a patient with significant scar contracture of the neck secondary to burn injury resulting in restriction of movement. (B) The patient underwent placement of tissue expanders. (C) Following scar excision and local tissue advancement the patient had a significant reduction in scar burden and significantly improved motion.

In a large prospective study, Hultman et al examined 147 patients with hypertrophic burn scars who underwent pulse dye and/or fractional CO_2 laser therapy for improvement of signs and symptoms from their hypertrophic burn scars. They reported a significant improvement in short-term follow-up (5 months) in the VSS (preop 10.43±2.37 to 5.1643±1.92 postop) and an improvement in UNC4P scores (preop 5.40±2.54 and 2.05±1.67 postop). Similar

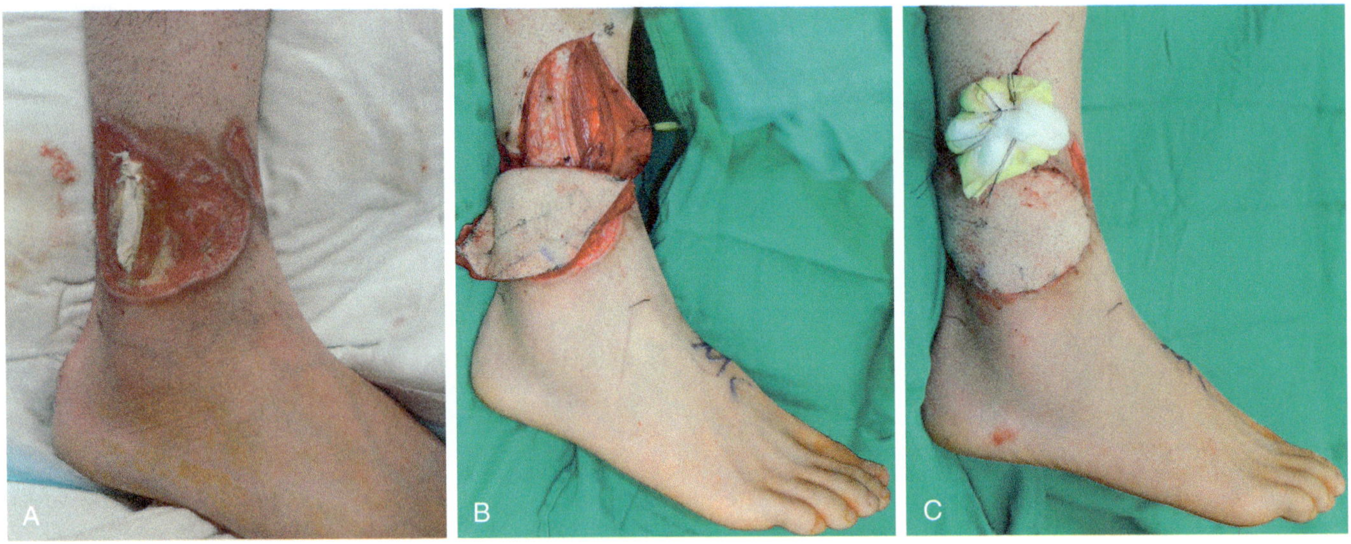

• **Fig. 13.8** (A) Preoperative views of a lateral lower extremity burn resulting in exposed tendon. (B) Intraoperative photograph following debridement and reconstruction with a free anterior lateral thigh flap, and (C) successful coverage of the exposed tendon.

results were seen at 30 months suggesting that laser therapy significantly improves signs and symptoms of hypertrophic scarring both subjectively and objectively.[24] Pulse dye lasers and fractional CO_2 lasers have also been shown effective in pediatric burn scars. Zuccaro et al retrospectively examined 125 pediatric patients with hypertrophic burn scars and found a significant improvement in the VSS preop versus postop after only a single treatment (7.37±2.46 vs. 5.76±2.29).[25]

Fat Grafting

There has been increasing interest recently in fat grafting for the treatment of numerous different ailments. Fat grafting has been shown to have positive wound healing effects as well as angiogenic capabilities.[26] This is in part due to the adipose aspirate containing immune cells, adipose stem cells, fibroblasts, preadipocytes and vascular endothelial cells.[27] Not surprisingly, fat grafting has been used in the context of burn reconstruction and is especially useful in situations of a soft tissue contour irregularity under the burned skin (Fig. 13.10). Several studies have demonstrated that fat grafting can improve the quality of burn scars but also improve pain associated with them. This is believed to be in part due to both a physical effect of introducing fat into these areas as well as the paracrine effects of cytokines associated with the transferred fat.[28] In a small retrospective study by Fredman et al fat grafting improved neuropathic pain associated with burn scars in 6 out of 7 patients.[29]

Anatomical Considerations

Face

When considering burn reconstruction options it is important to consider anatomical differences that should be taken into consideration. One of the most critical components of burn reconstruction is improving the appearance of the face. The approach to reconstruction of the face is dependent on the depth and location of the burn. There are many esthetic subunits with specific considerations that need to be appreciated. When evaluating the mouth, contracture of the oral commissure can lead to blunting and microstomia. In the acute setting, splinting can be used to prevent the development of microstomia. If scar contracture does occur, horizontal incisions can be made in the commissure and extended laterally, which should be closed in a Y–V fashion. It is important to preserve and properly orient the important landmarks of the lip such as the white roll and philtral columns when reconstructing the lip.

Eyebrow/Eyelid

Eyebrow reconstruction can be performed with a hair-bearing FTSG, tattooing or micrografts. It is helpful to use the contralateral eyebrow as a template, if available when performing eyelid reconstruction. Injury to the eyelids secondary to burns can be a very complex problem with numerous complications associated with it. Burn contracture can lead to ectropion due to inadequate soft tissue. In addition, eyelid injury can lead to corneal exposure and contracture of the canthi. Thus it is important to proceed with early debridement and grafting. When considering repair of ectropion it is important to consider the mechanism for its development. There are two main forces acting on the development of ectropion: extrinsic and intrinsic. Extrinsic forces are usually caused by scar contracture and are treated with release of the scar tissue and then FTSG can be used to graft open areas. Intrinsic forces act on the lamellae of the eyelid and each lamellae should be addressed individually. For repair of the upper eyelid repair one can consider Hughes or Cutler–Beard flaps. The lower eyelid can be addressed with

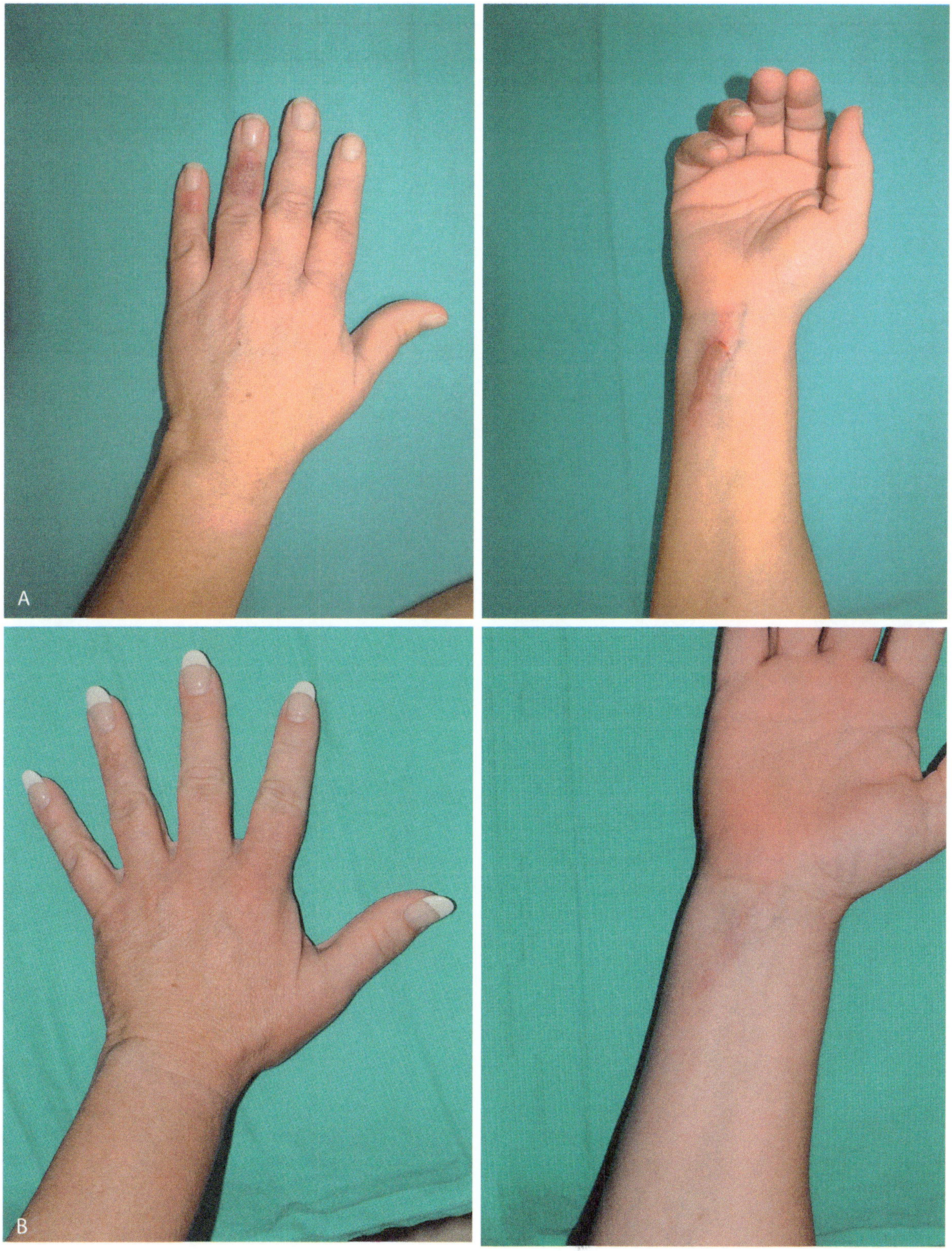

• **Fig. 13.9** (A) Preoperative appearance and (B) postoperative result following CO_2 laser resurfacing for hypertrophic scars following a contact burn.

Mustarde cheek advancement or pedicled temporoparietal fascial flap. Z-plasties can be used to release the medial canthi and local advancement flaps can be used for the lateral canthi. Finally, the inner and middle lamella can be augmented simultaneously using a palatal mucosal graft.

Nose

When evaluating the nose it is important to consider its different subunits and to reconstruct them in a manner that closely resembles the pre-burn appearance. This can

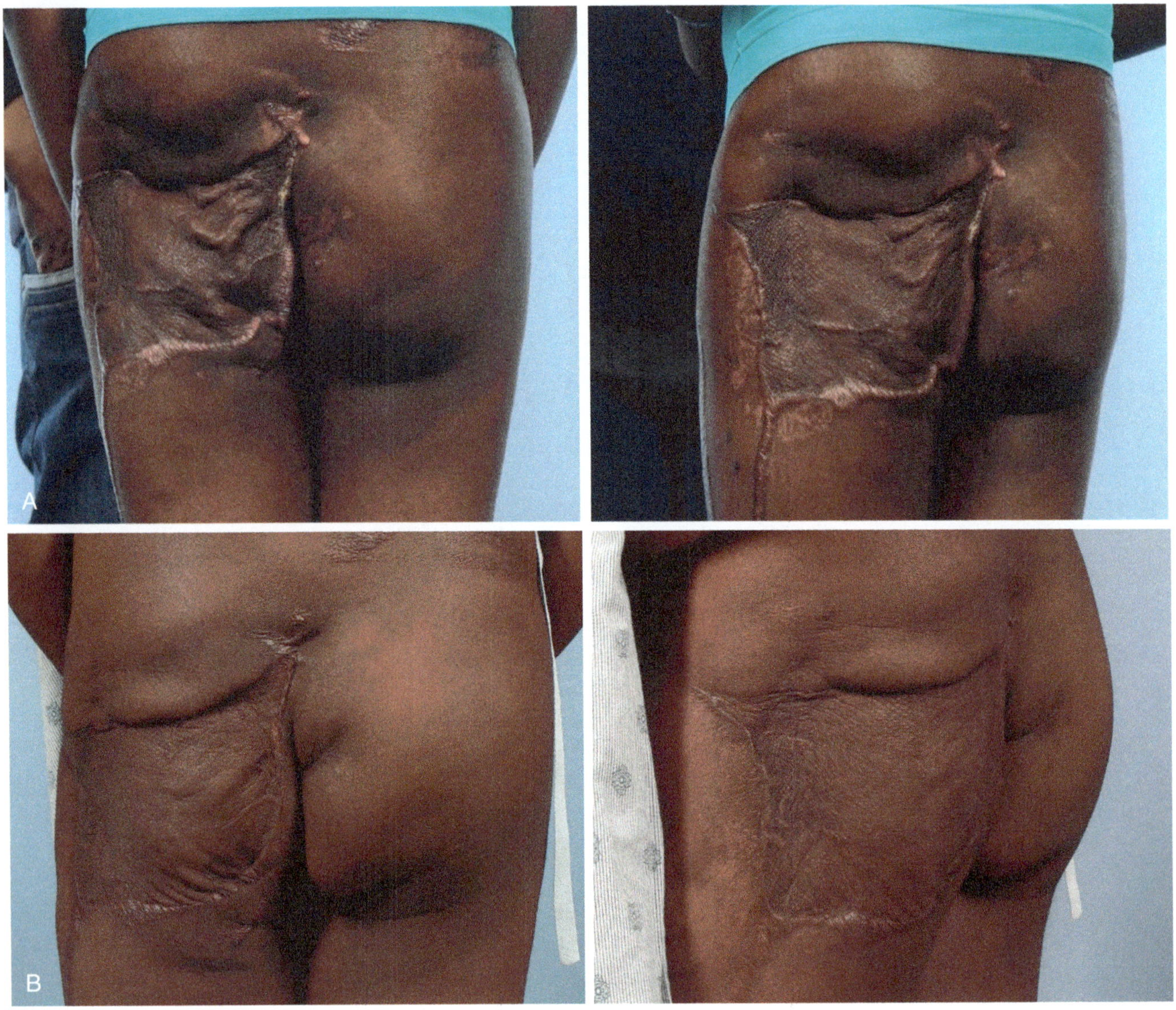

• **Fig. 13.10** (A) Preoperative and (B) postoperative views following fat grafting to a gluteal burn to improve volume and appearance.

be performed with FTSG or with dermabrasion along with STSG. For complete loss of nasal subunits, one can consider the use of a melolabial flaps, forehead flaps or bilobe flaps as done for Mohs reconstruction. Reconstruction of the nasal ala can be performed with a nasal turn-down flap, forehead flap or a composite graft from the ear if small.[30] For larger alar flaps, a free helical root flap can be used.[31,32]

Ear

Reconstruction of the ear incorporates standard advancement flap options. For small defects of the helical rim one can consider use of an Antia-Buch advancement flap or for larger defects a Davis conchal transposition flap. Complete ear reconstruction can also be performed with cartilage grafts from the ribs with a temporoparietal fascial flap or the use of an osseointegrated ear prosthetic.

Neck and Chin

Scar contracture of the neck and chin can lead to decreased mobility resulting in difficulty with mastication. It is a very common complication following burn injury to this region. Treatment typically involves release of scar contracture with FTSG of the resultant defect. When releasing the neck, the surgeon should keep in mind that in patients who have had previous tracheostomy they should consider bronchoscopic examination to ensure no residual tracheal fistula. When releasing the scar contracture, the incision should be taken down to the platysma. In severe contractures some surgeons will release part of the platysma. It is important in the postoperative period to institute aggressive range of motion exercises and physical therapy to prevent reoccurrence once allowing enough time for the skin graft to take, which is approximately 5 days. Alternatively, tissue expansion in the infraclavicular region can be performed if this area is unaffected and is thus a suitable donor site.

Scalp

Scalp reconstruction is important for the reconstitution of hair-bearing tissue. Small defects can be repaired with local rotational or advancement flap reconstruction. Defects that are less than 50% of the hair-bearing skin can usually be reconstructed using tissue expansion. In cases of extensive loss of the scalp with exposed bone, larger free flap reconstruction with latissimus dorsi muscle or omentum can be considered. Unfortunately, these procedures due not restore hair-bearing tissue but are necessary to salvage the underlying cranium.

Breast

As mentioned previously, the goal of burn reconstruction is to restore a patient's appearance to match their pre-burn state as much as possible. This is very important with regards to breast burns. Reconstructive options for the breast depend on the extent of the involvement. This can include tissue expansion, latissimus flap, free abdominal based flaps as well as nipple reconstruction. In children, it is important to make sure scar contractures in the breast are released to allow for proper breast development and expansion. Levi et al performed a retrospective study looking at tissue expander placement in burns involving the breast and found that endoscopic placement of the tissue expander resulted in lower complications, less time required to place the expander and shorter operative times.[33]

Axilla

When evaluating axillary burns, it is important to try to prevent contractures in the acute burn phase by maintaining the shoulder in an appropriate position; abducted approximately 90–120 degrees and flexed approximately 15–20 degrees. Axillary contracture management is guided by the classification of the contracture. Type I contractures spare the hair-bearing skin but involve the anterior and posterior axillary folds. Type II contractures involve the trunk and adjacent inner portion of the arm along with an axillary fold. Both type I and II contractures can be managed with surgical release of the scar contractures with subsequent skin grafting, either full thickness or split thickness depending on the extent. Finally type III contractures involve the trunk, upper arm, and complete axilla and are usually managed with flap reconstruction. Postoperatively having early occupational therapy and splinting can help prevent recurrence of contraction.

Elbow/Hand

The elbow can be a sensitive area due to the fact that contractures can limit arm mobility and is very commonly involved following burn injuries. The reconstructive options available for the elbow depend on the severity of the injury. Mild contractures of the antecubital fossa can usually be treated with local tissue rearrangements as previously described in this chapter. In addition, FTSG or unmeshed STSG can be used to resurface the antecubital fossa to help improve range of motion. For moderate contractures, more extensive procedures need to be performed, such as local or thin fascial flaps. For severe contractures, where there are not suitable surrounding tissues, one can consider the use of a free flap (ALT, contralateral radial forearm, gracilis).[34] Similarly, the hand requires special attention due to the fact that loss of function due to scar contracture can severely impact the quality of life of that patient. To prevent contractions, early splinting is important in hand burns. The wrist should be flexed to approximately 20–30 degrees, the metacarpal joints should be flexed to approximately 70–90 degrees with the interphalangeal joints in full extension and the thumb slightly opposed and abducted. Treatment of scar contractions can be managed by variations of Z-plasties to release tension such as jumping man plasties and V–Y advancement. FTSG should be utilized on the hands to prevent long-term secondary contracture. Fishtail incisions can be used for nailbed releases (Fig. 13.11).

Lower Extremity

Burn injury to the perineum can result in the formation of webs between the genitalia and the thigh. These webs can affect movement of the legs, impact hygiene, and distort the genitalia. Treatment should be performed early, with release of the scars and FTSG. Burn injury to the foot is similar in nature to the hand. The reconstructive approach is dependent on the extent and depth of the injury. Early treatment should be managed with splinting in extension to try to prevent contraction. For superficial and mild burns, Z-plasties can be used to release scar contracture. Deeper injuries can be treated with skin grafting. Severe foot burns with toe contractures will sometimes require tendon releases or K-wire fixation. Chang et al looked retrospectively at patients with toe burns and demonstrated that the more severe burns required more surgical treatments and were associated with higher complications.[35]

In summary, detailed initial assessment and fluid resuscitation using the Parkland formula as a guide are keys to improving survival in burn injuries. Understanding the pathophysiology of burn injuries, different types of burns (thermal, electrical and chemical) and common associated conditions (inhalation injury, carbon monoxide poisoning, compartment syndrome) all improve burn care. As more patients are surviving severe burn injuries, there is an increasing importance for appropriate burn reconstruction. Understanding the timing and appropriate reconstructive options available will hopefully improve patient long-term outcomes. In the acute burn period, adequate debridement and grafting (i.e., autograph, homograft, xenograft or other dermal substitutes) is important to limit the need for future reconstructive procedures. In late reconstruction, the emphasis is on reducing tension and contraction caused by the healing process. The options for

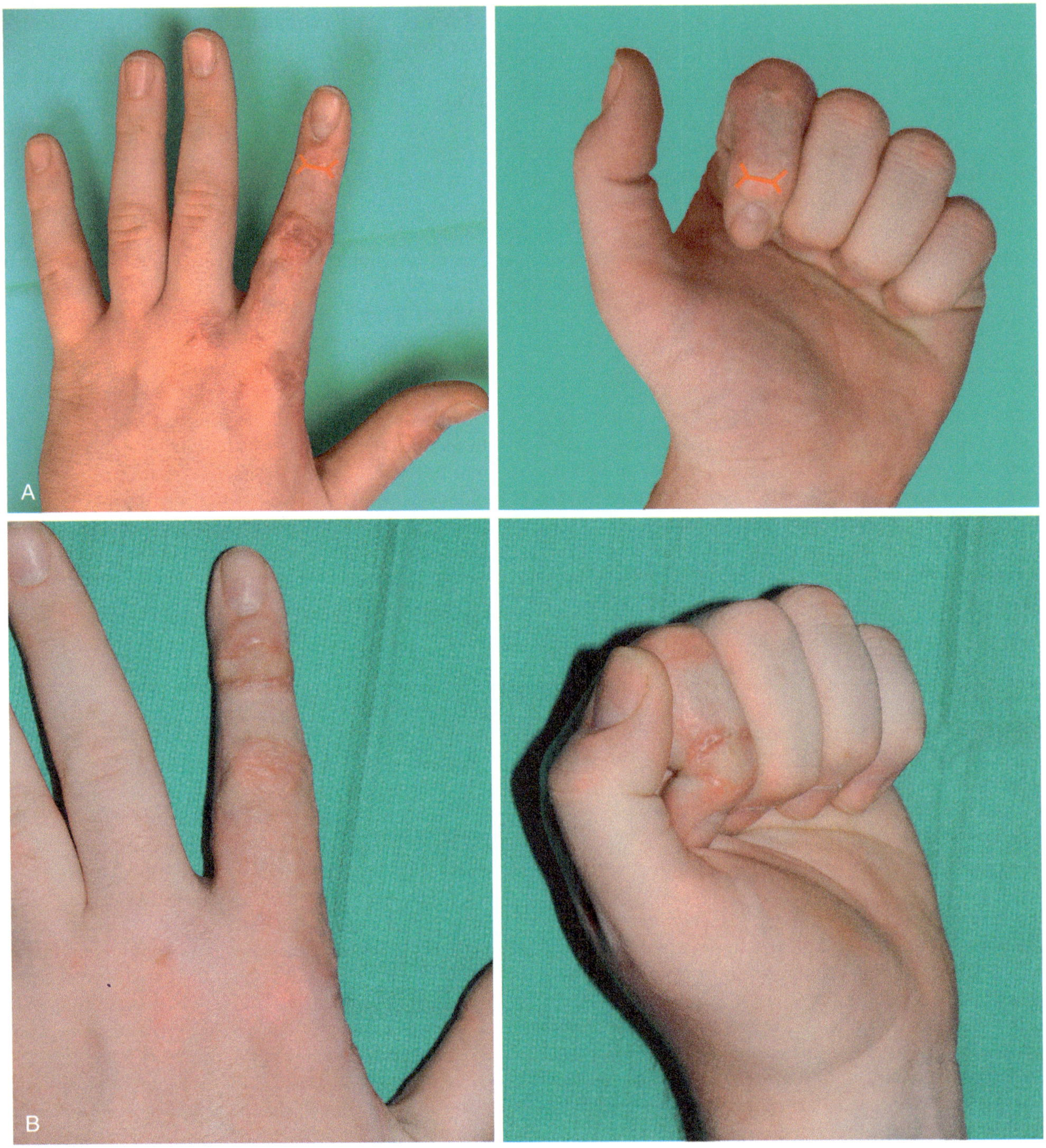

• **Fig. 13.11** (A) Preoperative appearance and (B) postoperative result of nailbed release for hand burn with decreased flexion at the DIP joint. Red lines in (A) mark where fishtail-releasing incisions were made.

reconstruction are numerous and can be tailored depending on a given situation. Not only is timing important but also the anatomical location of the burn. This chapter has described some of the nuances to specific body locations, hopefully contributing to improved understanding of acute burn management as well as burn reconstruction, and thus aiding the plastic surgeon in returning patients to pre-injury function.

References

1. Burn Incidence Fact Sheet. *American Burn Association*; 2018. [updated 2016]. Available from: https://ameriburn.org/who-we-are/media/burn-incidence-fact-sheet/.
2. Jeschke MG, Chinkes DL, Finnerty CC, et al. Pathophysiologic response to severe burn injury. *Ann Surg*. 2008;248(3):387–401.
3. Stuke LE, Arnoldo BD, Hunt JL, Purdue GF. Hydrofluoric acid burns: a 15-year experience. *J Burn Care Res*. 2008;29(6):893–896.

4. Shirani KZ, Pruitt Jr BA, Mason Jr AD. The influence of inhalation injury and pneumonia on burn mortality. *Ann Surg.* 1987;205(1):82–87.
5. Borron SW, Baud FJ, Barriot P, Imbert M, Bismuth C. Prospective study of hydroxocobalamin for acute cyanide poisoning in smoke inhalation. *Ann Emerg Med.* 2007;49(6):794–801, e1–2.
6. Curreri PW, Richmond D, Marvin J, Baxter CR. Dietary requirements of patients with major burns. *J Am Diet Assoc.* 1974;65(4):415–417.
7. Hildreth MA, Herndon DN, Desai MH, Broemeling LD. Current treatment reduces calories required to maintain weight in pediatric patients with burns. *J Burn Care Rehabil.* 1990;11(5):405–409.
8. Wainwright DJ, Bury SB. Acellular dermal matrix in the management of the burn patient. *Aesthet Surg J.* 2011;31(suppl 7):13S–23S.
9. Rinkevich Y, Walmsley GG, Hu MS, et al. Skin fibrosis. Identification and isolation of a dermal lineage with intrinsic fibrogenic potential. *Science.* 2015;348(6232):aaa2151.
10. Bombaro KM, Engrav LH, Carrougher GJ, et al. What is the prevalence of hypertrophic scarring following burns? *Burns.* 2003;29(4):299–302.
11. Anzarut A, Olson J, Singh P, Rowe BH, Tredget EE. The effectiveness of pressure garment therapy for the prevention of abnormal scarring after burn injury: a meta-analysis. *J Plast Reconstr Aesthet Surg.* 2009;62(1):77–84.
12. Momeni M, Hafezi F, Rahbar H, Karimi H. Effects of silicone gel on burn scars. *Burns.* 2009;35(1):70–74.
13. Tanaydin V, Conings J, Malyar M, van der Hulst R, van der Lei B. The role of topical vitamin E in scar management: a systematic review. *Aesthet Surg J.* 2016;36(8):959–965.
14. Dantzer E, Braye FM. Reconstructive surgery using an artificial dermis (Integra): results with 39 grafts. *Br J Plast Surg.* 2001;54(8):659–664.
15. Stern M. The grafting of preserved amniotic membrane to burned and ulcerated surfaces, substituing skin grafts: a preliminary report. *J Am Med Assoc.* 1913;60(13):973–974.
16. Herndon DN, Branski LK. Contemporary methods allowing for safe and convenient use of amniotic membrane as a biologic wound dressing for burns. *Ann Plast Surg.* 2017;78(2, suppl 1):S9–S10.
17. Branski LK, Herndon DN, Celis MM, Norbury WB, Masters OE, Jeschke MG. Amnion in the treatment of pediatric partial-thickness facial burns. *Burns.* 2008;34(3):393–399.
18. Reilly DA, Hickey S, Glat P, Lineaweaver WC, Goverman J. Clinical experience: using dehydrated human amnion/chorion membrane allografts for acute and reconstructive burn care. *Ann Plast Surg.* 2017;78(2, suppl 1):S19–S26.
19. Jabir S, Frew Q, Magdum A, El-Muttardi N, Philp B, Dziewulski P. Microvascular free tissue transfer in acute and secondary burn reconstruction. *Injury.* 2015;46(9):1821–1827.
20. Platt AJ, McKiernan MV, McLean NR. Free tissue transfer in the management of burns. *Burns.* 1996;22(6):474–476.
21. De Lorenzi F, van der Hulst R, Boeckx W. Free flaps in burn reconstruction. *Burns.* 2001;27(6):603–612.
22. Blome-Eberwein S, Gogal C, Weiss MJ, Boorse D, Pagella P. Prospective ealuation of fractional CO_2 laser treatment of mature burn scars. *J Burn Care Res.* 2016;37(6):379–387.
23. Levi B, Ibrahim A, Mathews K, et al. The use of CO_2 fractional photothermolysis for the treatment of burn scars. *J Burn Care Res.* 2016;37(2):106–114.
24. Hultman CS, Friedstat JS, Edkins RE, Cairns BA, Meyer AA. Laser resurfacing and remodeling of hypertrophic burn scars: the results of a large, prospective, before-after cohort study, with long-term follow-up. *Ann Surg.* 2014;260(3):519–529; discussion 29–32.
25. Zuccaro J, Muser I, Singh M, Yu J, Kelly C, Fish J. Laser therapy for pediatric burn scars: focusing on a combined treatment approach. *J Burn Care Res.* 2018;39(3):457–462.
26. Strong AL, Cederna PS, Rubin JP, Coleman SR, Levi B. The current state of fat grafting: a review of harvesting, processing, and injection techniques. *Plast Reconstr Surg.* 2015;136(4):897–912.
27. Bourin P, Bunnell BA, Casteilla L, et al. Stromal cells from the adipose tissue-derived stromal vascular fraction and culture expanded adipose tissue-derived stromal/stem cells: a joint statement of the International Federation for Adipose Therapeutics and Science (IFATS) and the International Society for Cellular Therapy (ISCT). *Cytotherapy.* 2013;15(6):641–648.
28. Fredman R, Katz AJ, Hultman CS. Fat grafting for burn, traumatic, and surgical scars. *Clin Plast Surg.* 2017;44(4):781–791.
29. Fredman R, Edkins RE, Hultman CS. Fat grafting for neuropathic pain after severe burns. *Ann Plast Surg.* 2016;76(suppl 4):S298–S303.
30. Taylor HO, Carty M, Driscoll D, Lewis M, Donelan MB. Nasal reconstruction after severe facial burns using a local turndown flap. *Ann Plast Surg.* 2009;62(2):175–179.
31. Pribaz JJ, Falco N. Nasal reconstruction with auricular microvascular transplant. *Ann Plast Surg.* 1993;31(4):289–297.
32. Ozek C, Gurler T, Uckan A, Bilkay U. Reconstruction of the distal third of the nose with composite ear-helix free flap. *Ann Plast Surg.* 2007;58(1):74–77.
33. Levi B, Brown DL, Cederna PS. A comparative analysis of tissue expander reconstruction of burned and unburned chest and breasts using endoscopic and open techniques. *Plast Reconstr Surg.* 2010;125(2):547–556.
34. Kung TA, Jebson PJ, Cederna PS. An individualized approach to severe elbow burn contractures. *Plast Reconstr Surg.* 2012;129(4):663e–673e.
35. Chang JB, Kung TA, Levi B, Irwin T, Kadakia A, Cederna PS. Surgical management of burn flexion and extension contractures of the toes. *J Burn Care Res.* 2014;35(1):93–101.

14 Congenital Melanocytic Nevi

SABRINA CUGNO, VERONICA KINSLER, AND NEIL W. BULSTRODE

Incidence of Phenotypic Classification

Congenital melanocytic nevi (CMN) are present at birth, or very occasionally arise in the first few years of life; tardive CMN. These lesions grow commensurate with the child, but tardive lesions can appear to grow more rapidly as the full extent of the CMN is often not initially apparent. The incidence ranges from 1% for small single CMN to approximately 1 in 20,000 for nevi projected to be greater than 20 cm in diameter in adulthood.[1] CMN are commonly classified according to maximum projected adult size and the total number of lesions at birth. The most recently proposed classification of size is small (CMN with an estimated diameter in adulthood of less than 1.5 cm), medium (M1, 1.5–10 cm and M2, 10–20 cm), large (L1, 20–30 cm, L2, 30–40 cm) and giant (G1, 40–60 cm, G2, >60 cm).[2] However, authors prefer not to employ the term *giant* as it is often unacceptable to patients and families. The estimates of projected adult size are determined in a variety of ways, none of which is accurate, but remain the most reliable methods currently available. Some clinicians use a scaling factor applied to the CMN diameter at birth. More specifically, a CMN on the head is predicted to enlarge by a factor of 1.7, on the trunk and upper extremity by a factor of 2.8, and on the lower extremity by a factor of 3.3.[3] This approach is not without fault, as CMN often affect more than one region of the body and it does not account for significant differences in growth between the sexes. Other clinicians therefore estimate the projected adult size by drawing the child's CMN onto an adult body map, and estimating the longest non-circumferential diameter. CMN can present as an isolated singular lesion or can be accompanied by a variable number of smaller discrete so-called *satellite* lesions. These lesions should be counted or estimated, as each satellite lesion represents an additional CMN.

Histological and Clinical Appearances of CMN

CMN consist of nests of nevus cells, which differ from normal melanocytes in their nondendritic morphology and proclivity to form nests. Melanocytic nests are present at the dermoepidermal junction, within the dermis and/or subcutaneous tissue, and nevus cells can be localized between collagen bundles and found surrounding dermal appendages, blood vessels, and nerves. Small and medium-sized CMN generally present clinically as homogenous pigmented lesions with well-delineated borders, an increase in skin surface markings, and variable hypertrichosis. Larger CMN express color variegation, are often asymmetric with irregular borders, can have a nodular surface, and are usually hypertrichotic (Fig. 14.1). Nodules are often appreciated to arise within the substance of the CMN or can be present at birth. Any such focal change within a CMN should be viewed with suspicion and reviewed by a pediatric dermatologist. Although malignancy should always be considered, the vast majority of nodules are benign and repeated excisions can thus be avoided.

The most common proliferations can be divided into classic proliferative nodules and neuroid overgrowths.[4] The classic nodules are well-defined, smooth, round or oval proliferations, are soft or firm, and occasiaonally have a shiny surface. The majority are 0.5–2 cm in diameter and often pink or less pigmented than the surrounding CMN. Although classic proliferative nodules have been suggested to be potential precursors to melanoma, definitive association is not supported in the literature. Histopathology and genetic investigations can assist in differentiating between benign proliferative nodules and melanoma, in particular array comparative genomic hybridization.[5] In contrast, neuroid overgrowths are poorly defined, round or ovoid, soft, and often pendulous. These can be several centimeters to >20 cm in diameter, and are lighter than the surrounding CMN or pink-red. Transformation of neuroid proliferations to melanoma has not been reported.[6]

Neurological Associations of CMN

Individuals with CMN can be divided into those with a cutaneous phenotype only (either single or multiple), and

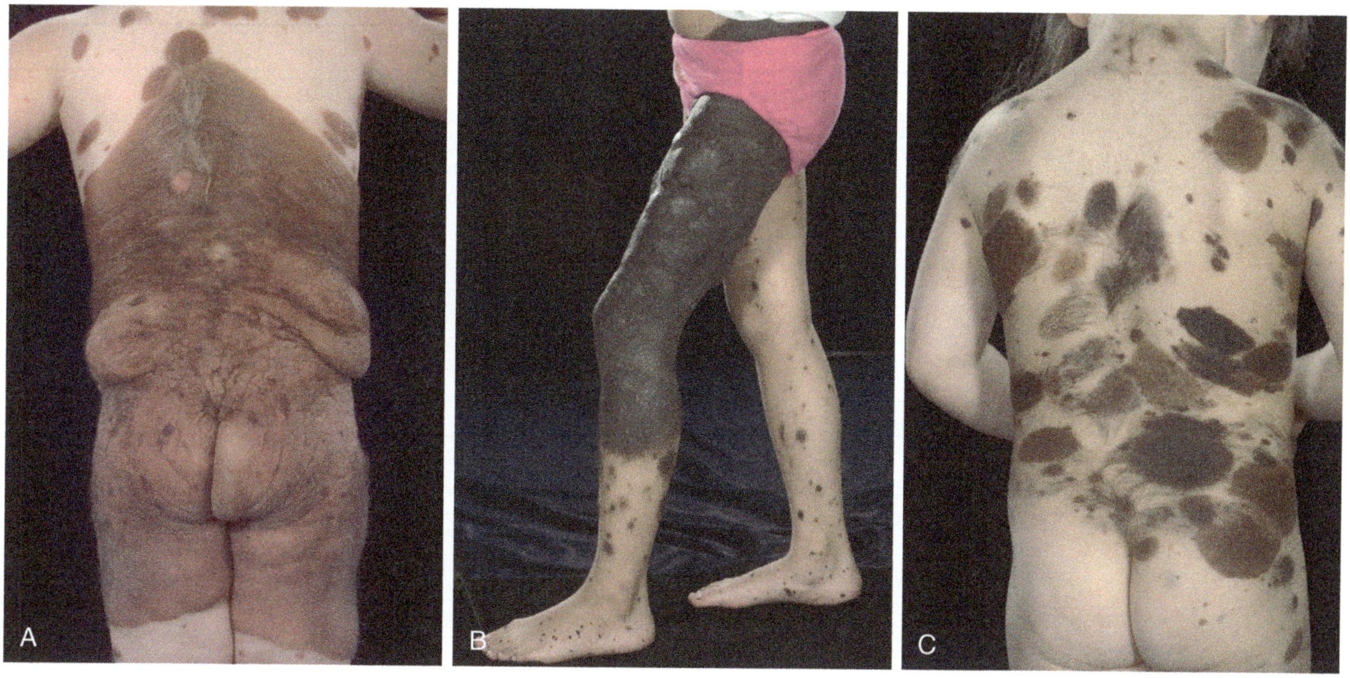

• **Fig. 14.1** (A–C) Clinical images of different cutaneous phenotypes of CMN.

those with extracutaneous features (either neurological or facial), the latter then termed *congenital melanocytic nevus (CMN) syndrome*. The projected adult size of the lesion, as well as the total number of CMN at birth, is known to be associated with adverse clinical outcomes. Neurological abnormalities are the most common complication of CMN, and this association has previously been known as *neurocutaneous melanosis*. The latter term has now been supplanted by *CMN syndrome*, as the neurological complications are not always melanotic in nature, and the literature has in the past been highly confusing by including both benign congenital neurological disease and primary melanoma of the CNS under the term neurocutaneous melanosis.[7]

The prevalence of neurological abnormalities increases with the size of the largest CMN and the total number of nevi.[8,9] CMN distribution, in particular lesions on the posterior axis, is not associated with an increased risk of neurological anomalies. The previously suggested connection between cutaneous distribution and neurological risk was confounded by the fact that the largest lesions are often located on the back. The most common neurological complication is intraparenchymal melanosis, where foci of melanin-producing cells are found within the brain parenchyma, most notably in the amygdala.[10] Intraparenchymal melanosis without other neurological abnormalities on MRI are benign congenital lesions and asymptomatic in approximately half of cases. The other half of cases can exhibit developmental delay and/or serizures. Developmental delay varies from mild speech delay to global developmental retardation or behavioral problems, such as attention deficit hyperactivity disorder or autistic spectrum disorder. Thus, when intraparenchymal melanosis is seen, authors suggest annual neurodevelopmental monitoring until school age, in an effort to detect developmental issues early. Even when symptomatic (delay or seizures), these lesions are not a sign of malignancy or of impending death, and should not be considered for biopsy or surgical resection. Although rare, progression to melanoma remains a possibility, however, this can arise in the central nervous system (CNS) even in the absence of visible intraparenchymal melanosis.

Other congenital neurological anomalies, such as Dandy–Walker malformation, hydrocephalus, and brain or spinal cord tumours, can occur, with or without leptomeningeal melanosis. These more complex neurological abnormalities are much more commonly symptomatic with manifestation of seizures and developmental delay, and therefore necessitate more rigorous management, with regular MRI, neurological assessments and, frequently, neurosurgical consultation.[11] This smaller (<10%) cohort of patients appears to be at highest risk of melanoma.[6] Interestingly, it has been shown that neurological symptoms in patients with CMN can be present in the absence of any perceptible radiological abnormality.[9,12] This finding has been proposed to be related to lesions that cannot be visualized with current imaging techniques.[13] Thus, the authors' current management protocol includes a gadolinium-enhanced MRI of the CNS (brain and whole spine) for any child with the onset of abnormal neurological signs or symptoms at any age (irrespective of a previously normal scan) and routinely for all children with two or more CMN at birth, independent of size or site, under the age of 1 year (ideally within the first 6 months of life) (Fig. 14.2). Follow-up of children with CMN or CMN syndrome depends on the severity of the cutaneous phenotype, the neurological presentation, and the risk of melanoma.[14] Patients should have access to a specialist pediatric dermatology clinic with input from a

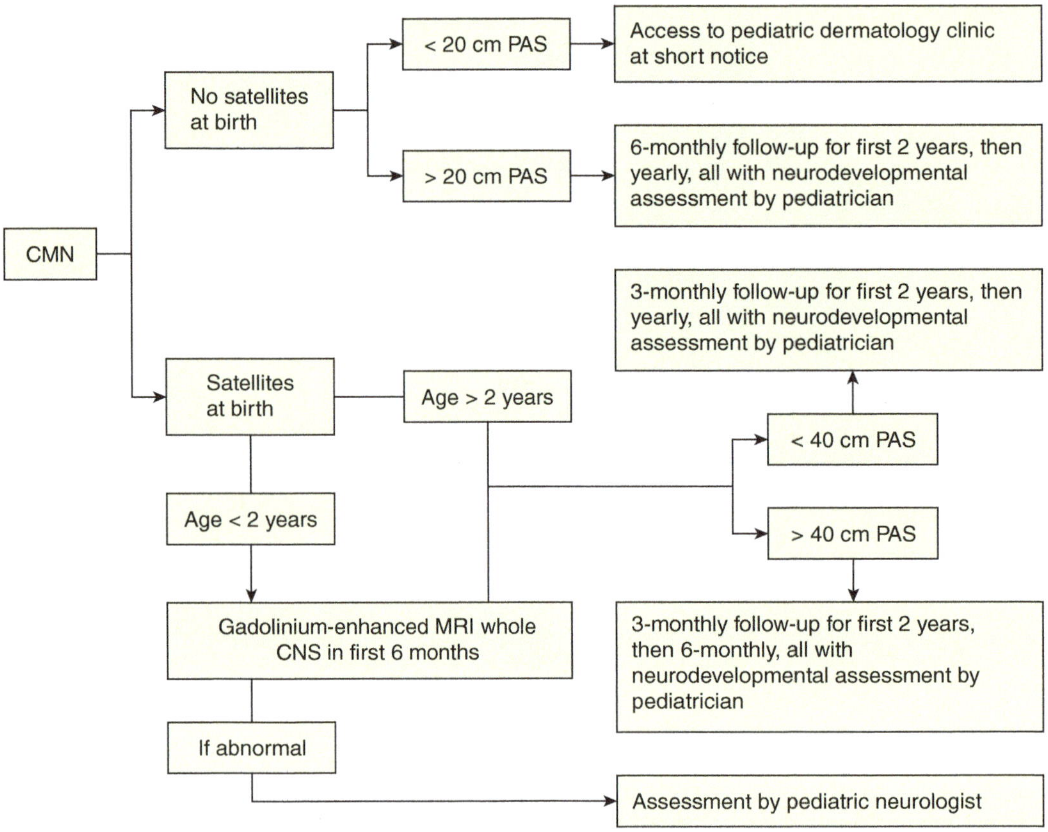

• **Fig. 14.2** Protocol for management of CMN in childhood. PAS, projected adult size.

multidisciplinary team, including pediatric plastic surgeon, neuroradiologist, neurologist, neurosurgeon, psychologist, and oncologist when necessary.

Other Associated Features of CMN

Characteristic facies in children with CMN has expanded the description of this condition (Fig. 14.3).[15] These typical features include a wide or prominent forehead, apparent hypertelorism, eyebrow variants, periorbital fullness, small/short nose, narrow nasal bridge, anteverted nares, broad nasal tip, broad or round face, full cheeks, prominent premaxilla, open mouth appearance, everted lower lip, and prominent or long philtrum[15] (Table 14.1). In support of the notion that children with CMN display a typical facies is the fact that aberration in neural crest development gives rise to melanocytic and facial development in humans. Indeed, a single genetic abnormality may be responsible for CMN, neurological abnormalities, and the typical facies of these children, by affecting the pluripotent cephalic neural crest cells that ultimately differentiate into diverse cell types, including melanocytes, neurons, glia, osteocytes, and chondrocytes. The genes on the RAS/MAPK pathway are known to be involved in facial development, and individuals with germ-line RASopathies have characteristic facies. This clinical finding is therefore consistent with *NRAS* mosaicism affecting neural crest or neuroectodermal structures, including pigment cells, cells of the CNS as well as bone and cartilage of the face. Furthermore, many RASopathies manifest abnormalities in growth and endocrine dysfunction, and a recent retrospective study[16] described metabolic and hormonal disturbances in children with CMN.

Thus, the term *congenital melanocytic nevus syndrome* is used to characterize and unite these aspects of the condition.[15] The following two criteria are included, both of which must be present: first, the presence of a CMN of greater than 5 cm projected adult size or more than one CMN of any size at birth; second, neurological involvement (clinical or radiological) and/or the presence of three or more typical facial features.

Melanoma and CMN

Primary melanoma of the skin or CNS is a rare complication of CMN in childhood. However, the incidence varies with the severity of the cutaneous phenotype. The cited estimates of the incidence of malignancy have been extremely variable, ranging from 0 to 40%. More recent and reliable data on the incidence of malignant melanoma and the clinical phenotype of CMN associated with its development have been published. Large studies have demonstrated that although there is an increased risk of melanoma in patients with CMN (especially during childhood and adolescence), as compared to the general pediatric population, it is in fact much lower than previously reported estimates, with the overall incidence for all sizes of CMN between 0.7%

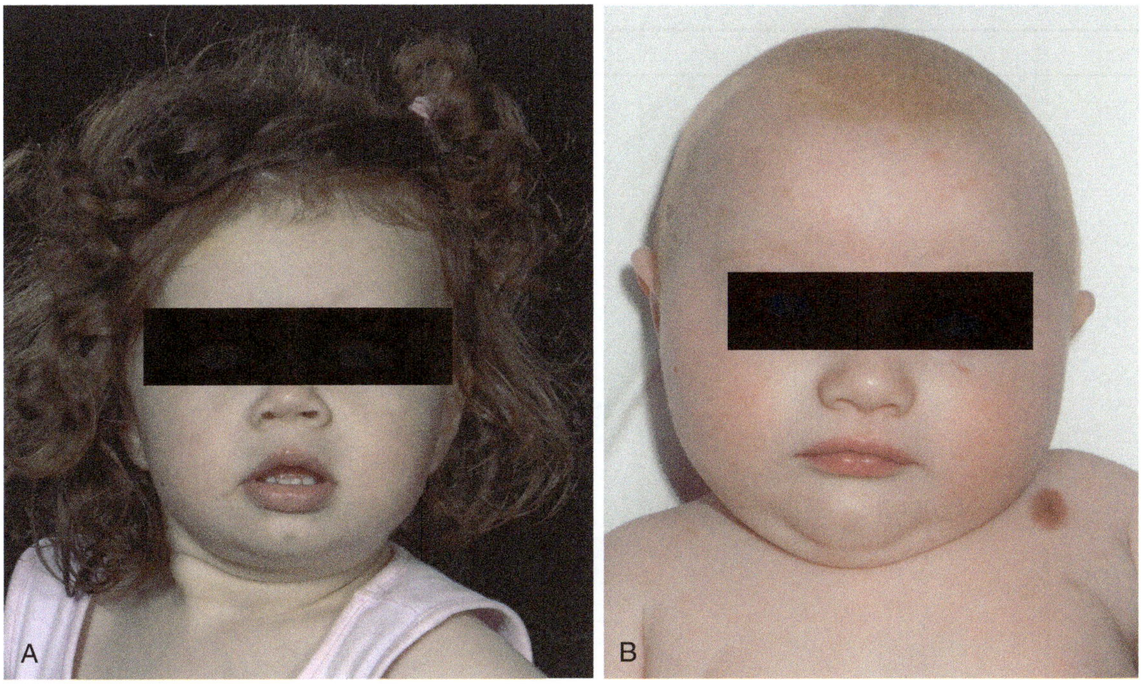

• **Fig. 14.3** (A, B) Facial appearances of children with CMN.

TABLE 14.1 List and Prevalence of Characteristic Facial Features of Children with CMN

Facial Feature	Prevalence (%)
Wide or prominent forehead	74
Apparent hypertelorism	12
Eyebrow variants	36
Periorbital fullness	27
Small/short nose	25
Narrow nasal ridge	18
Flaring nares	15
Broad nasal tip	34
Broad or round face	71
Full cheeks	55
Prominent premaxilla	10
Prominent everted lower lip	47
Prominent or long philtrum	20

The presence of three or more features is required to fulfill the facial criteria for congenital melanocytic nevus syndrome.

and 2.4%.[14,17,18] However, the risk of melanoma increases with CMN of projected adult size >40 cm and accompanied by multiple smaller CMN, and has been estimated at 10–15%.[9,17] In a substantial proportion of cases, the primary melanoma develops within the CNS rather than the skin.[14,17,19] A review of the literature concluded that primary CNS melanoma accounts for approximately one-third of melanoma occurring in patients with CMN.[19] However, a recent prospective study demonstrated CNS melanoma to be more common in childhood than cutaneous melanoma.[15] All cases were in children with multiple CMN (two or more at birth), and the majority occurred in those where either the largest CMN was >60 cm projected adult size or there were multiple CMN with no large nevus. Thus, the incidence of malignant transformation was estimated at 8% in children with CMN of projected adult size >60 cm, and 1% in children with any other cutaneous phenotype. However, recent data has revealed that the best predictor of risk for melanoma is not cutaneous phenotype, but rather the outcome of the screening MRI of the CNS, with a higher risk in children with complex congenital abnormalities of the CNS.[15] When melanoma does arise in these children, it is usually highly aggressive, refractory to therapy and rapidly fatal.[6,14,17] The median age of onset is estimated at 2 years.[4] Cutaneous melanoma arising in CMN usually presents as a new nodule, arising primarily in the deep dermis or subcutis. Primary CNS melanoma presents as either a solid intraparenchymal tumor or more commonly as leptomeningeal melanoma and is more common than cutaneous melanoma.[4]

Genetics of CMN and Implications for Treatment of Melanoma

The causative genetics of multiple CMN have been elucidated over the last decade. The majority (70%) of cases are caused by postzygotic mosaicism for oncogenic mutations in codon 61 of *NRAS*,[20] and CNM syndrome is therefore a mosaic RASopathy (genetic disorders of the

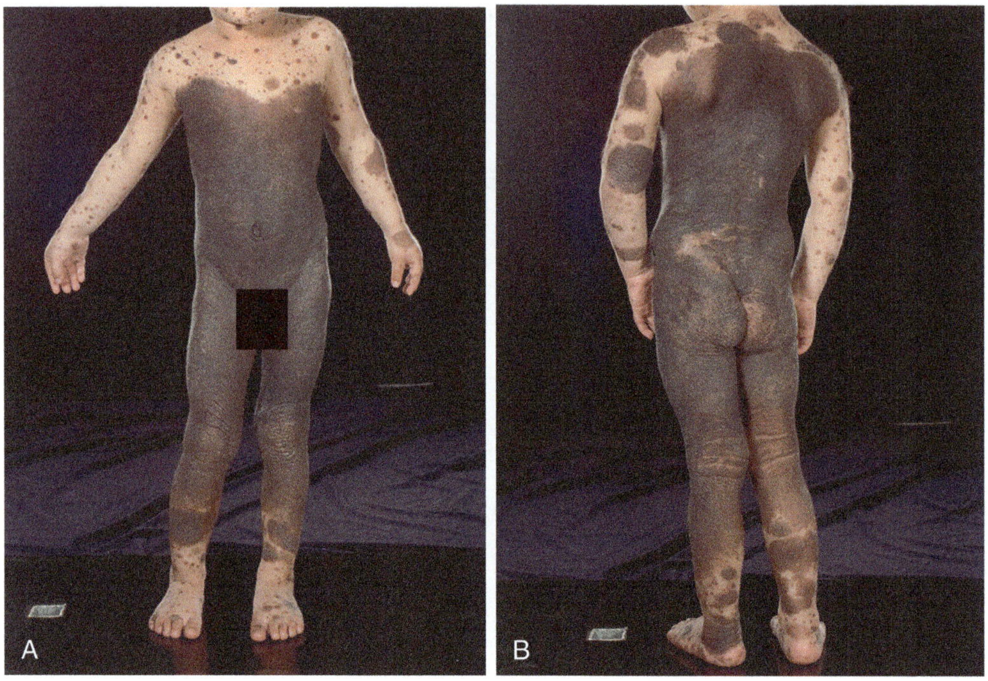

• **Fig. 14.4** (A, B) Child with a giant CMN and multiple smaller CMN, demonstrating the surgical impossibility of eradicating all lesions.

RAS/MAPK pathway).[21] Recently, mutations in *BRAF* have been described as a cause of multiple CMN in 7% of cases.[22,23] These developmental mutations predispose to melanoma in individuals with CMN syndrome by acting as the first insult in the subsequent occurrence of melanoma.[20]

Where melanoma does arise, genotyping of the tumor is relevant for therapy. The use of a MEK inhibitor (Trametinib), which targets the MAPK pathway, has been trialed on a compassionate basis for treating children with CMN melanoma associated with an underlying *NRAS* mutation,[24] resulting in clear symptomatic relief but not disease control. *BRAF* inhibitors would theoretically be appropriate in *BRAF*-mutant CMN with melanoma, although no cases have been published thus far. *BRAF* inhibitors would, however, be contraindicated in *NRAS*-mutant CNS.

Analysis of copy number is known to be highly contributory to CMN management. This has been demonstrated to differentiate between benign and malignant proliferations both in the skin[5] and more recently in the CNS.[7,25] If a suspected lesion (skin or CNS) is biopsied, some should be sent for histology, and some fresh for DNA extraction and ideally both *NRAS/BRAF* genotyping, and whole genome copy number (array CGH or SNP array).

Evidence is, however, suggestive of a germ line predisposition for the development of CMN, with a higher prevalence of smaller CMN in family members of affected individuals,[14,20] as well rare reports of large CMN in first-degree family members.[26,27] In one UK study, homozygosity and compound heterozygosity of variants in the melanocortin-1-receptor gene (*MC1R*) were found at a higher prevalence in individuals with CMN and certain variants were associated with a more severe cutaneous phenotype.[28]

Surgical Management of CMN

Irrespective of size, long-standing practice for treatment of CMN has been surgical removal. A commonly cited argument in favor of early surgical excision is to decrease or avert the potential for malignant degeneration to melanoma. However, *surgical excision has not been shown to reduce the risk of malignant melanoma formation in patients with CMN*. First, individuals at high risk for malignancy have very extensive CMN associated with numerous smaller CMN, which can total in excess of 400 CMN. *Complete* excision of a very large CMN and *all smaller nevi* remains an impossibility (Fig. 14.4). Second, there is some evidence that the behavior of nevus cells may in fact be altered by surgical intervention. In one study,[29] tissue expansion was associated with the development of new nevi, which was supported by individual case evidence from other centers (A Taieb, personal communication). The latter is thought to occur secondary to either non-nevus cell melanocytes that are activated by some aspect of treatment with tissue expanders or that treatment promotes the spread of nevus cells from the primary nevus, a type of benign metastasis known to occur in CMN and Spitz nevi. Moreover, an increased incidence of darkening of surgically treated areas of CMN and untreated areas of partially excised CMN was noted, and new CMN were

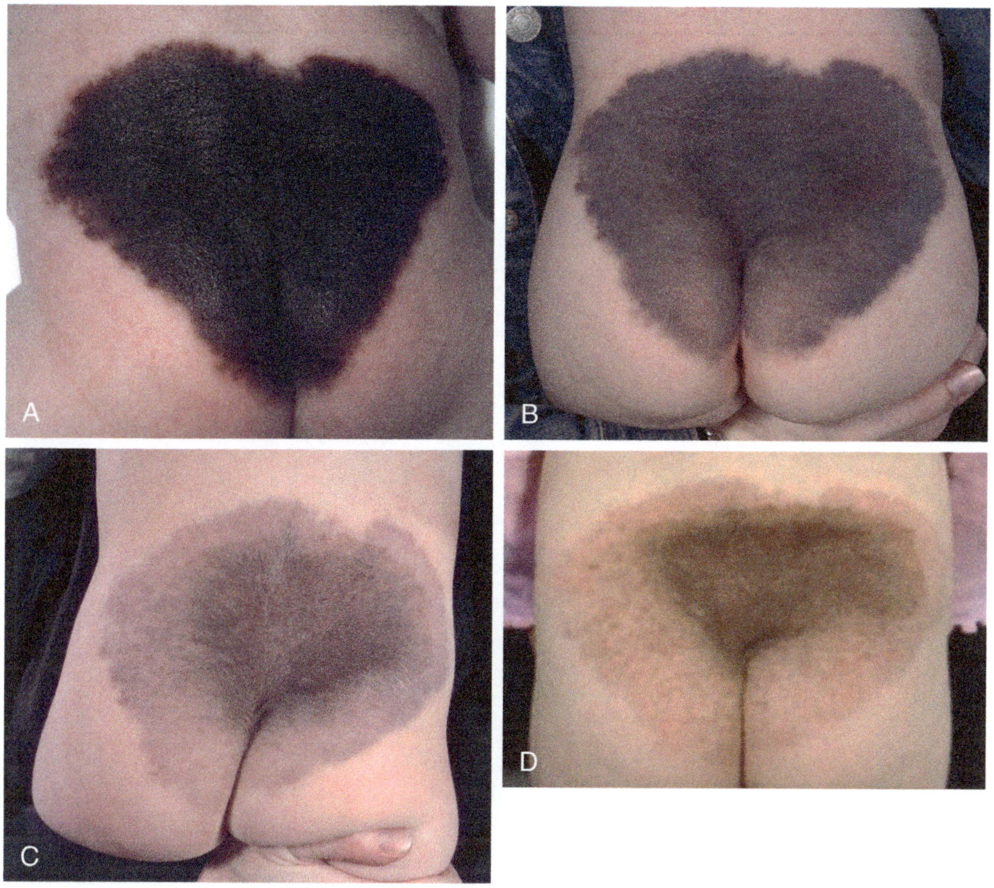

• **Fig. 14.5** Spontaneous lightening and regression of an untreated CMN. In this case, lightening became evident after 6 months of age. Images show the CMN at age (A) 2 months, (B) 1 year, (C) 2 years, and (D) 3 years. Of note, the last image (D) demonstrates CMN regression in addition to depigmentation.

found to appear at the edge of the treated area.[30] An additional important consideration is that the occurrence of *melanoma is not restricted to the CMN*, and thus surgical excision of the primary CMN does not preclude development of melanoma in the CNS or other extracutaneous location.

CMN can be esthetically displeasing and as such associated with considerable psychological morbidity. Thus, a secondary argument for surgical excision of CMN is esthetic concerns. However, there is evidence that untreated CMN often lighten over a period of years (Fig. 14.5). Thus, with the exception of tardive CMN, the color of CMN is darkest at birth. This phenomenon is related to the color of the normal skin, with more lightening in lighter skinned individuals. Serial photographs annually are excellent at assessing this spontaneous lightening which may otherwise not be noticed. Of note, scalp CMN appear to reliably display the most considerable amount of change. The latter is further supported by a recent series of spontaneous involution of scalp CMN in childhood.[31] Thus, removal of scalp lesions by tissue expansion is no longer advised, given the significant surgical intervention required and notable associated complication rate (e.g., alopecia). Often, however, these lesions extend into neighboring areas of face, which can be addressed surgically (Fig. 14.6). In fact, facial lesions, whether the primary CMN or a satellite lesion, are in the authors' practice routinely excised, as are CMN that can be completely removed by serial staged excision (Fig. 14.7). Plastic surgery is also routinely offered to patients with functionally troublesome or particularly prominent areas (e.g., large nodule) or areas suspect for malignancy. Clinical surveillance of CMN remains the principal treatment option for large or giant CMN or those in areas where excision would result in significant anatomic or functional compromise.

Earlier treatment modalities utilized in the surgical management of these lesions included curettage and dermabrasion. More recently, laser therapy has been introduced as an additional therapeutic option. One premise for these options has been the suggestion that superficial nevus cells bear the most malignant potential and therefore removal of these cells will effectively reduce the risk.[32] However, it is well documented that malignant transformation within CMN most often occurs within the deeper cells of the dermis and subcutaneous tissue.[33] Indeed, two-thirds of cutaneous melanoma within CMN develops below the dermoepidermal junction. Thus, the effects of superficial excision can mask

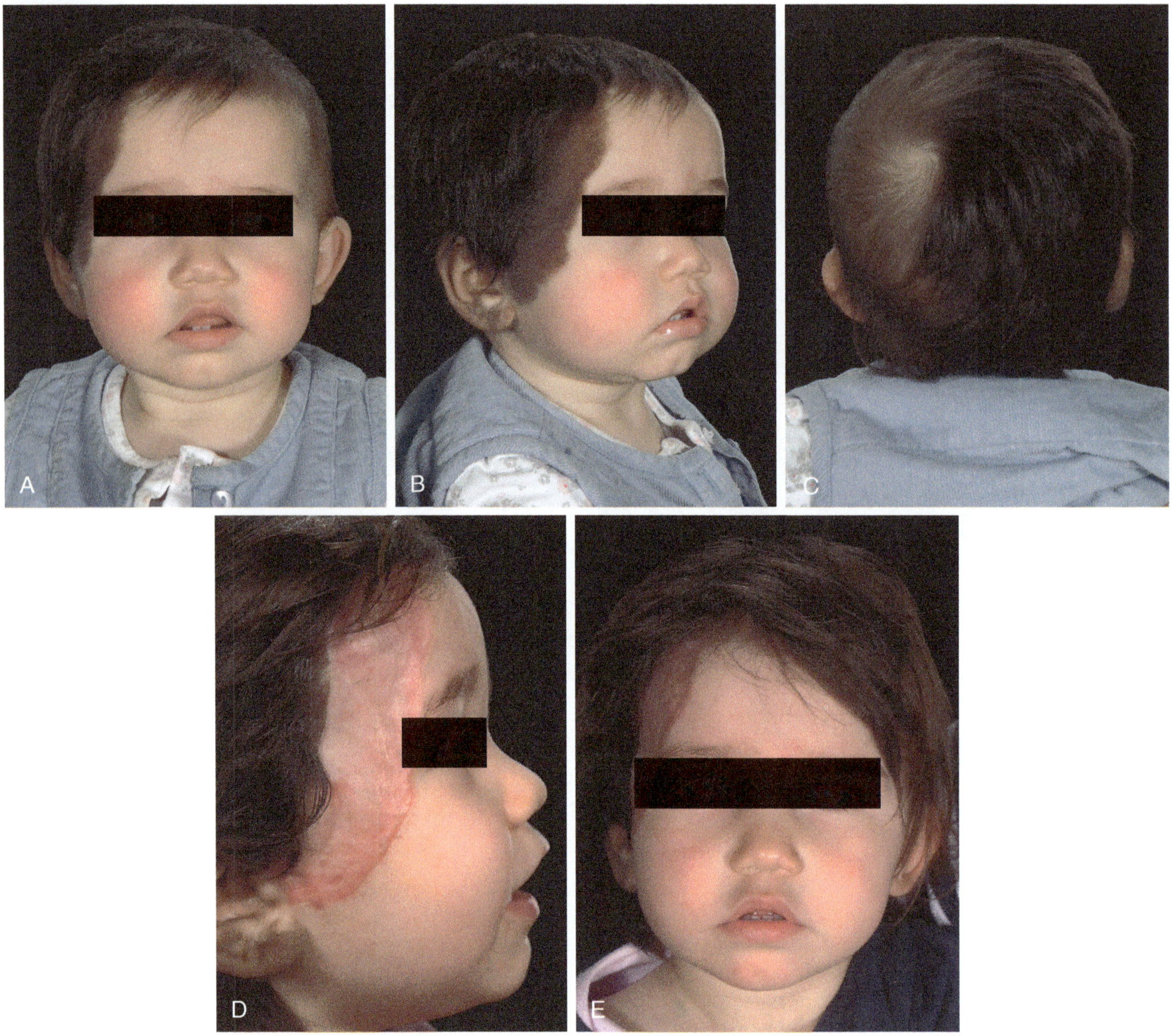

• **Fig. 14.6** (A–C) Child with a large CMN involving the scalp, forehead, temporal region, and lateral aspect of the cheek and ear. In this case, only the part of the CMN on the face was surgically excised. (D–E) The early result, at six months following excision, of the facial portion of CMN and resurfacing with a split thickness skin graft harvested from the scalp.

the appearance of a melanoma arising within the CMN. Moreover, these techniques are associated with significant morbidity, including bleeding, infection (sepsis), scarring, and recurrent folliculitis. Most importantly, all lesions treated with superficial removal re-pigment over time, at variable rates ranging from weeks to years. Large CMN extend through the entire dermis, often into subcutaneous tissue. Initially, after elimination of superficial nevus, there may be a noticeable decrease in pigmentation, as the deeper nevus cells do not produce melanin. However, once these deeper cells become more superficial they begin to produce melanin, resulting in re-pigmentation (Fig. 14.8). Recently, a large systematic study of digitally quantified colorimetric measurement of nevi has demonstrated unequivocally that superficial treatments (dermabrasion, curettage and laser) have no effect on final color of the CMN and may cause scarring.[34]

Currently, the primary measures in the surgical management of CMN include single stage excision with primary closure, serial excision, tissue expansion, and excision with either partial- or full-thickness skin grafting (with or without the use of dermal subsitutes). Any of the aforementioned techniques can be used alone or in combination, following consideration of the esthetic unit(s) to be addressed. While implemented by some clinicians, free or pedicled flap coverage (with or without tissue expansion) in an effort to eradicate large or giant CMN is not considered in the authors' surgical

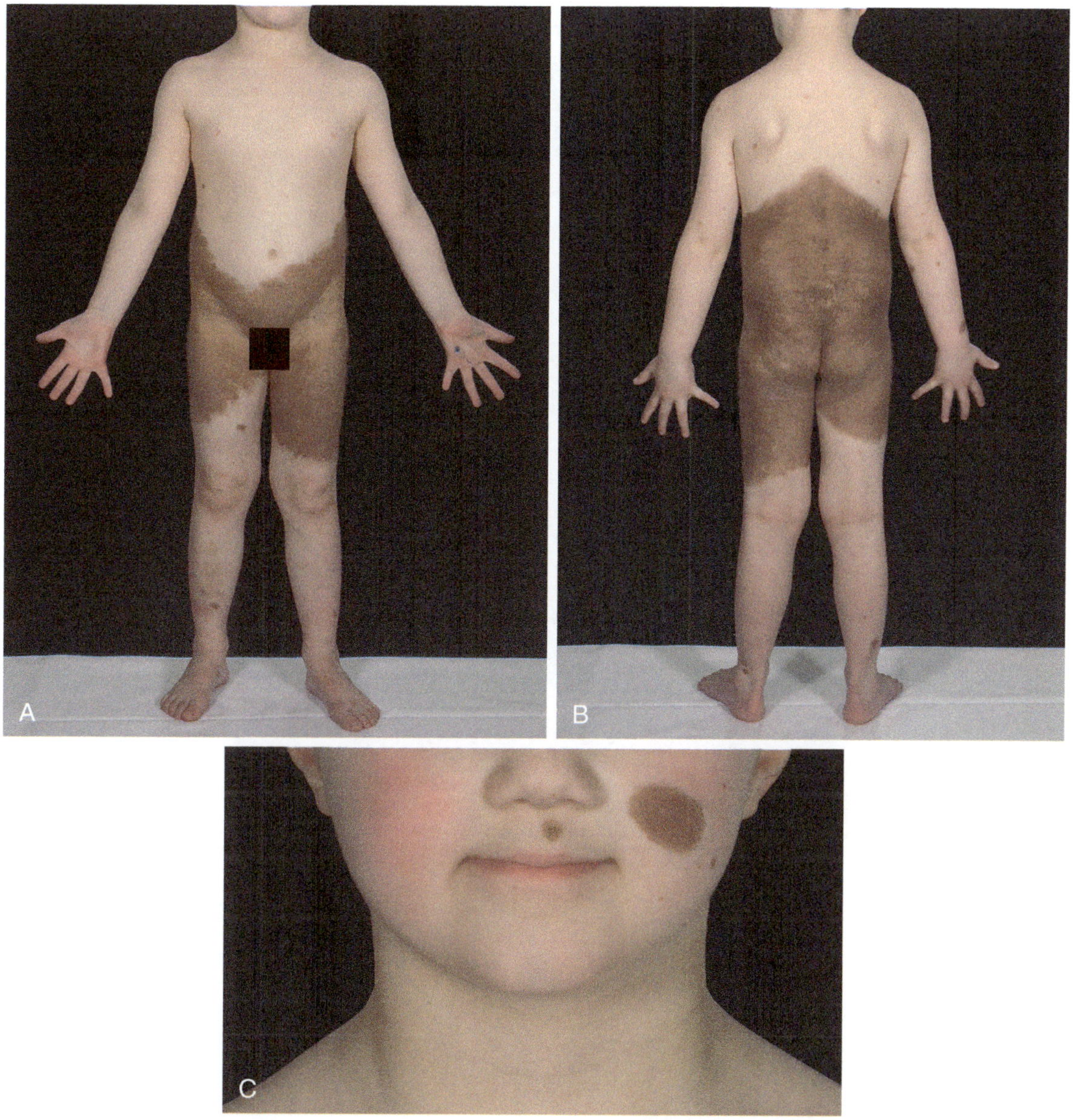

• **Fig. 14.7** (A, B) Child with a giant CMN and multiple smaller CMN. (C) Contrary to the child in Fig. 14.4, this patient would be offered the possibility of excising the two smaller CMN on his face.

armamentarium, given the previously stated points and in view of the considerable morbidity associated with these interventions. In general, unless there is a specific concern with regard to malignancy or functional issue, surgery is delayed until after 2 years of age. Occasionally, however, partial or complete excision with primary closure is effected earlier, taking advantage of skin laxity in infancy. It is important that the full thickness of the lesion be excised, and thus carried down to the subcutaneous tissue layer. In cases where excision and primary closure is not a practicable alternative, serial excision is considered if complete excision can be accomplished in two or three stages. In cases where closure with skin graft is planned, usually for CMN of the face or hand, either a split- or full-thickness skin graft is selected based on size and location of the excised lesion. For large areas where full-thickness skin graft coverage is planned, preexpansion of the donor skin prior to harvest minimizes the esthetic morbidity at the donor site.

As previously mentioned, in the authors' practice, facial lesions are routinely offered excision, sparing areas of nevi involving delicate facial structures that remain difficult to reconstruct without significant risk of iatrogenic deformity (e.g., alar rim, hair-bearing eyebrow). For facial lesions, where a split-thickness skin graft is selected, the scalp remains the donor site of choice. Full-thickness skin grafts are usually harvested from the postauricular area or supraclavicular fossa (with or without preexpansion of the area) depending on the size of the resulting defect. Tissue expansion of the area adjoining the CMN to be excised is generally avoided in the forehead. The latter usually does not give a superior esthetic result to skin grafting and is associated with

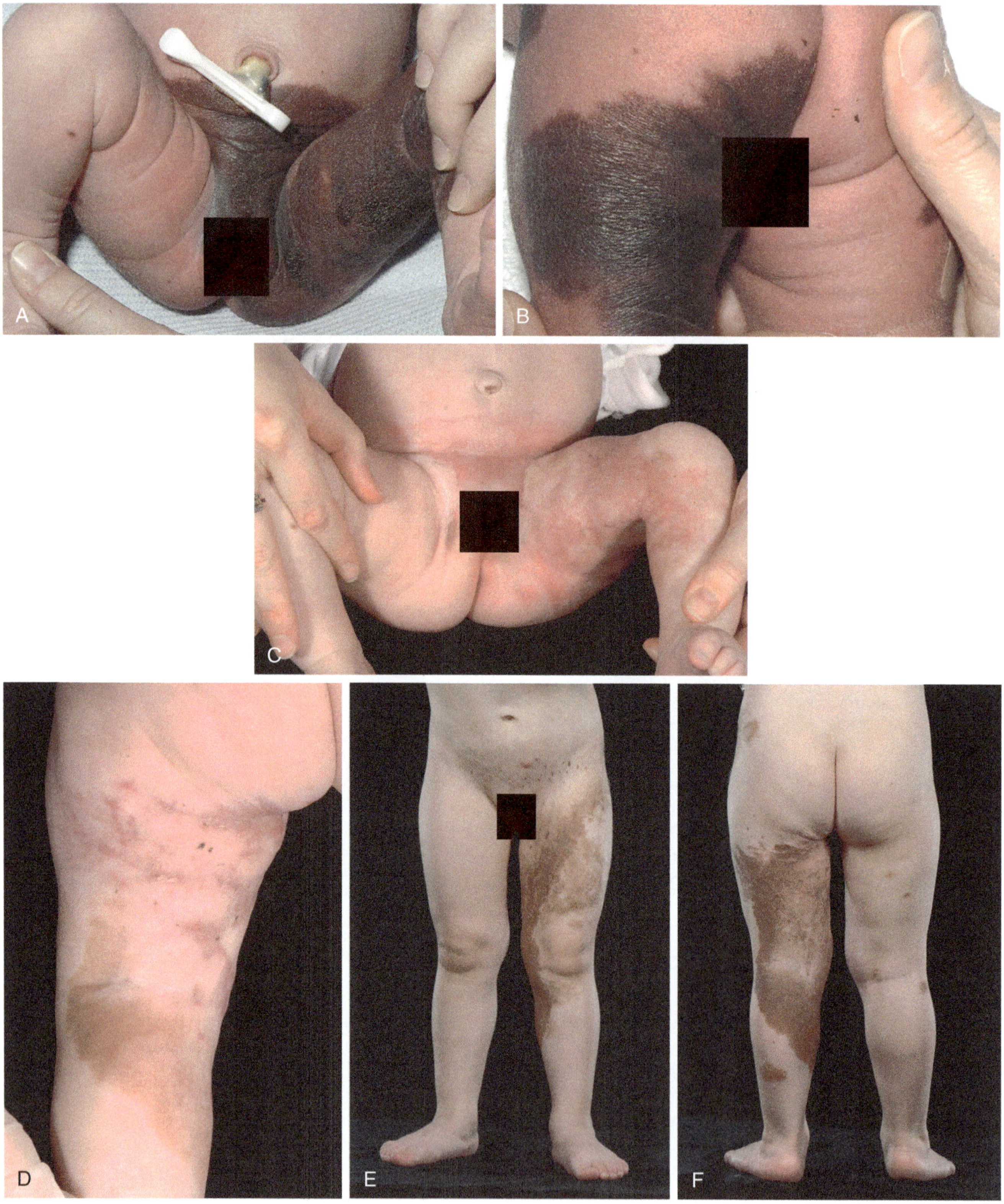

• **Fig. 14.8** CMN treated with superficial excision demonstrating re-pigmentation. (A, B) CMN at day 1 of life. (C, D) CMN 2 months following dermabrasion. (E, F) CMN 2 years following dermabrasion, which shows the return of pigment to all treated areas. Moreover, the CMN skin frequently has areas of scarring and recurrent folliculitis.

considerable risk for distortion of forehead musculature and unaffected neighboring cosmetic units (namely, the eyebrow and hairline).

Conclusion

CMN can be restricted to the skin or associated with neurological abnormalities and/or characteristic facial features (CMN syndrome). Management of children with multiple (>1) CMN or CMN syndrome necessitates a multidisciplinary approach involving the care of a pediatrician, dermatologist, plastic surgeon, neurologist, neuroradiologist, psychologist, and primary care physician. Children with more than one CMN at birth (irrespective of size or site) should have an MRI of the CNS and undergo routine neurodevelopmental assessment. Routine surgery with current techniques has not been shown to decrease the risk of malignancy in CMN. Moreover, there is no benefit to early intervention and some evidence suggests that surgery may adversely affect the behavior of CMN cells. Superficial removal techniques including laser are not recommended as they do not alter the final color of CMN. Serial photographs are taken at yearly intervals to assess spontaneous lightening. Surgical intervention is offered only to patients with CMN that are easily amenable to excision or those in esthetically highly sensitive areas, and is delayed at least for the first two years of life. Increasingly surgery is being delayed until patients can participate in the consent procedure.

References

1. Castilla EE, de Garça Dutra M, Orioli-Parreiras IM. Epidemiology of congenital pigmented naevi: I. Incidence rates and relative frequencies. *Br J Dermatol.* 1981;104:307–315.
2. Krengel S, Scope A, Dusza SW, et al. New recommendations for the categorization of cutaneous features of congenital melanocytic nevi. *J Am Acad Dermatol.* 2013;68:441–451.
3. Marghoob AA, Schoenbach SP, Kopf AW, et al. Large congenital melanocytic nevi and the risk for the development of malignant melanoma. A prospective study. *Arch Dermatol.* 1996;132:170–175.
4. Kinsler VS, O'Hare P, Bulstrode N, et al. Melanoma in congenital melanocytic nevi. *Br J Dermatol.* 2017;176(5):1131–1143.
5. Bastian BC, Xiong J, Frieden IJ, et al. Genetic changes in neoplasms arising in congenital melanocytic nevi: differences between nodular proliferations and melanomas. *Am J Pathol.* 2002;161:1163–1169.
6. Kinsler VS, O'Hare P, Bulstrode N, et al. Melanoma in congenital melanocytic naevi. *Br J Dermatol.* 2017;176:1131–1143.
7. Kinsler VA, Polubothu S, Calonje JE, et al. Copy number abnormalities in new or progressive "neurocutaneous melanosis" confirm it as primary CNS melanoma. *Acta Neuropathol.* 2017;133(2):329–331.
8. Marghoob AA, Dusza S, Oliveria S, Halpern AC. Number of satellite nevi as a correlate for neurocutaneous melanocytosis in patients with large congenital melanocytic nevi. *Arch Dermatol.* 2004;140:171–175.
9. Kinsler VA, Chong WK, Aylett SA, Atherton DJ. Complications of congenital melanocytic naevi in children: analysis of 16 years' experience and clinical practice. *Br J Dermatol.* 2008;159:907–914.
10. Barkovich AJ, Frieden IJ, Williams ML. MR of neurocutaneous melanosis. *AJNR Am J Neuroradiol.* 1994;15:859–867.
11. Waelchli R, Aylett SE, Atherton D, et al. Classification of neurological abnormalities in children with congenital melanocytic naevus syndrome identifies magnetic resonance imaging as the best predictor of clinical outcome. *Br J Dermatol.* 2015;173:739–750.
12. Ruiz-Maldonado R. Measuring congenital melanocytic nevi. *Pediatr Dermatol.* 2004;21:178–179.
13. Kinsler VA, Paine SM, Anderson GW, et al. Neuropathology of neurocutaneous melanosis: histological foci of melanotic neurones and glia may be undetectable on MRI. *Acta Neuropathol.* 2012;123:453–456.
14. Kinsler VA, Birley J, Atherton DJ. Great Ormond Street Hospital for children Registry for Congenital Melanocytic Naevi: prospective study 1988–2007. Part 1 – epidemiology, phenotype and outcomes. *Br J Dermatol.* 2009;160:143–150.
15. Kinsler VA, Shaw AC, Merks JH, Hennekam RC. The face in congenital melanocytic nevus syndrome. *Am J Med Genet.* 2012;158A:1014–1019.
16. Waelchli R, Williams J, Cole T, et al. Growth and hormone profiling in children with congenital melanocytic naevi. *Pediatr Dematol.* 2015;173:1366–1367.
17. Krengel S, Hauschild A, Schafer T. Melanoma risk in congenital melanocytic nevi: a systematic review. *Br J Dermatol.* 2006;155:1–8.
18. Bittencourt FV, Marghoob AA, Kopf AW, et al. Large congenital melanocytic nevi and the risk for development of malignant melanoma and neurocutaneous melanocytosis. *Pediatrics.* 2000;106:736–741.
19. Neuhold JC, Friesenhahn J, Gerdes N, et al. Case reports of fatal or metastasizing melanoma in children and adolescents: a systematic analysis of the literature. *Pediatr Dermatol.* 2015;32:13–32.
20. Kinsler VA, Thomas AC, Ishida M, et al. Multiple congenital melanocytic nevi and neurocutaneous melanosis are caused by post-zygotic mutations in codon 61 of NRAS. *J Invest Dermatol.* 2013;133:2229–2236.
21. Tidyman WE, Rauen KA. The RASopathies: developmental syndromes of Ras/MAPK pathway dysregulation. *Curr Opin Genet Dev.* 2009;19:230–236.
22. Etcheveers HC, Rose C, Kahle B, et al. Giant congenital melanocytic nevus with vascular malformation and epidermal cysts associated with a somatic activating mutation in BRAF. *Pigment Cell Melanoma Res.* 2018;31(3):437–441.
23. Polubothu S, McGuire N, Al-Olabi, et al. Does the gene matter? Genotype-phenotype and genotype-outcome associations in congenital melanocytic naevi. *Br J Dermatol.* 2020;182(2):434–443.
24. Kinsler VA, O'Hare P, Jacques T, Hargrave D, Slater O. MEK inhibition appears to improve symptom control in primary NRAS-driven CNS melanoma in children. *Br J Cancer.* 2017;116:990–993.
25. Kusters-Vandevelde HV, Kruse V, van Maerken T, et al. Copy number variation analysis and methylome profiling of a GNAQ-mutant primary meningeal analysis tumor and its liver metastasis. *Exp Mol Pathol.* 2016;102:25–31.
26. Danarti R, Konig A, Happle R. Large congenital melanocytic nevi may reflect paradominant inheritance implying allelic loss. *Eur J Dermatol.* 2003;13:430–432.

27. de Wijn RS, Zaal LH, Hennekam RC, et al. Familial clustering of giant congenital melanocytic nevi. *J Plast Reconstr Aesthet Surg.* 2010;63:906–913.
28. Kinsler VA, Abu-Amero S, Budd P, et al. Germline melanocortin-1-receptor genotype is associated with severity of cutaneous phenotype in congenital melanocytic nevi: a role for MC1R in human fetal development. *J Invest Dermatol.* 2012;132:2026–2032.
29. Kinsler VA, Bulstrode N. The role of surgery in the management of congenital melanocytic naevi in children: a perspective from Great Ormond Street Hospital. *J Plast Reconstr Aesthet Surg.* 2009;62:595–601.
30. Kinsler VA, Birley J, Atherton DJ. Great Ormond Street Hospital for Children Registry for Congenital Melanocytic Naevi: prospective study 1988–2007. Part 2 – evaluation of treatments. *Br J Dermatol.* 2009;160:387–392.
31. Strauss RM, Newton Bishop JA. Spontaneous involution of congenital melanocytic nevi of the scalp. *J Am Acad Dermatol.* 2008;58:508–511.
32. De Raeve LE, Claes A, Ruiter DJ, et al. Distinct phenotypic changes between the superficial and deep component of giant congenital melanocytic nevi: a rationale for curettage. *Br J Dermatol.* 2006;154:485–492.
33. Barnhill RL, Piepkorn MW, Busam KJ. *Pathology of Melanocytic Nevi and Malignant Melanoma.* 3rd edn. Berlin: Springer-Verlag; 2014.
34. Polubothu S, Kinsler VA. Final congenital melanocytic naevi colour is determined by normal skin colour and unaltered by superficial removal techniques: a longitudinal study. *Br J Dermatol.* 2020;182(3):721–728.

15 Vascular Anomalies

SABRINA CUGNO, ALEX BARNACLE, JOHN HARPER, AND NEIL W. BULSTRODE

Introduction

Vascular anomalies are disorders of the endothelium, which can be subclassified into vascular tumors and vascular malformations, distinguished by proliferating endothelium and quiescent endothelium, respectively[1] (Table 15.1). Vascular anomalies can present in individuals of any age and due to their varied subtypes and morphologies, patients present to clinicians in a wide variety of clinical specialties. These lesions often require significant diagnostic expertise and a multidisciplinary management approach. Arguably, in no area of pediatric medicine is incorrect terminology more pervasive than in the field of vascular anomalies. This is largely due to insufficient teaching on the subject for trainees, the wide variety of terms and labels used in the historic literature and the involvement of many different medical specialties, each with their particular interests and assumptions. Correct designation using the standardized classifications and terminology introduced by the International Society for the Study of Vascular Anomalies (ISSVA) is paramount for appropriate patient management.[2] In the majority of cases, the precise diagnosis can be made from a detailed history and physical examination. In instances where diagnostic ambiguity persists, imaging proves useful, with ultrasound sufficient in most instances. Rarely, is tissue biopsy required.

Vascular Tumors

The term *vascular tumor* encompasses a wide range of pathologies, including common infantile hemangiomas[3] and other rare lesions such as tufted angiomas and kaposiform hemangioendotheliomas. The majority of vascular tumors present in early childhood, have a rapid proliferative growth pattern, and are composed of solid tissue, forming focal soft tissue masses. In contrast, *vascular malformations* are made up of vascular channels or cysts and are often more diffuse. The most common vascular tumor is the *hemangioma*. Hemangiomas can be divided into infantile and congenital tumors. Infantile hemangiomas occur in approximately 3%–10% of infants, and in up to 30% of premature infants. These lesions are most common in Caucasian infants, with a lower frequency in infants of African or Asian descent, and are three- to fivefold more common in females than males.[4] In approximately 20% of infants, multiple hemangiomas may be present. Children with multiple infantile hemangiomas, usually five or more, may also have one or more hemangiomas in the liver. These are rarely of any clinical significance. Thus, when five or more infantile hemangiomas are noted, further investigation with abdominal ultrasound is mandatory to exclude the presence of hemangioma in the liver. The term *miliary hemangiomatosis* describes a rare condition in which a large number of small cutaneous hemangiomas, usually exceeding 20, are apparent soon after birth and recognized to be associated with internal lesions.

Infantile hemangiomas appear to arise from vasculogenesis, and more specifically, from multipotent derived stem cells, which have the potential to differentiate into multiple cell lineages and form human glucose transporter isoform 1 (GLUT1)-positive microvessels in immunodeficient mice.[5] During the proliferative phase, these cells produce vascular endothelial growth factor, an endothelial mitogen. Indeed, *GLUT1* is uniquely expressed on the endothelial cells of hemangiomas and provides a valuable marker for differentiation of hemangioma from other vascular tumors and vascular malformations. Hemangiomas have a characteristic evolution, appearing within the first few weeks of life, proliferating for several weeks to months, stabilizing between 6 and 12 months of age, and finally gradually regressing over a period of several years. At birth, the site of the future hemangioma is usually completely normal, with the median age of appearance at 2 weeks. However, in approximately 30% of cases, a nascent lesion may be present, such as an area of telangiectasia or pallor. Rapid growth then ensues, with approximately 80% of tumors attaining their maximal size by 3 months. After 12 months of age, the tumor usually begins the involuting phase. Classically, this stage is characterized by complete resolution of approximately 50% of lesions by 5 years of age, 70% by 7 years of age, and 90% by 9 years of age, which are estimates derived from the study of Bowers et al.[6] However, more recent clinical and histological work has demonstrated that involution is usually complete by age 4 years.[7] Following regression, infantile hemangioma can often leave residual telangiectasia, anetodermic cutaneous excess, fibrofatty residuum, scarring, and, rarely, significant structural deformity (Fig. 15.1).

TABLE 15.1 Current Classification of Vascular Anomalies

Tumors	Malformations	
	Slow Flow	Fast Flow
Infantile hemangioma (IH)	Capillary malformation (CM)	Arterial malformation (AM)
	Cutis marmorata telangiectatic congenital (CMTC)	Aneurysm
		Atresia
	Telangiectasias	Ectasia
		Stenosis
Congenital hemangioma (CH)	Lymphatic malformation (LM)	Arteriovenous malformation (AVM)
Rapidly-involuting congenital hemangioma (RICH)	Microcystic	Capillary malformation–arteriovenous malformation (CM–AVM)
Noninvoluting congenital hemangioma (NICH)	Macrocystic	
	Primary lymphedema	Hereditary hemorrhagic telangiectasia (HHT)
		PTEN-associated vascular anomaly (PTEN-AVA)
Hemangioendotheliomas	Venous malformation (VM)	Combined malformations
Kaposiform hemangioendothelioma (KHE)	Cerebral cavernous malformation (CCM)	Capillary–arteriovenous malformation (CAVM)
Other	Cutaneomucosal venous malformation (CMVM)	Capillary-lymphatic arteriovenous malformation (CLAVM)
	Glomuvenous malformation (GVM)	
	Verrucous hemangioma (VH)	
Pyogenic granuloma (PG)	Combined malformations	
	Capillary–venous malformation (CVM)	
	Capillary–lymphatic malformation (CLM)	
	Capillary–lymphatic–venous malformation (CLVM)	
	Lymphatic–venous malformation (LVM)	

From Greene AK. Current concepts of vascular anomalies. *J Craniofac Surg*. 2012;23:220–224.

The majority of hemangiomas are small and do not encroach onto anatomically sensitive areas, and as such, are clinically insignificant. These lesions are readily diagnosed in view of their characteristic appearance, including distinctive cherry-red color. Occasionally, deep-seated tumors, which do not alter the color of overlying skin, are encountered, often requiring ultrasound to confirm the diagnosis. With these hemangiomas, families should simply be reassured that the tumor(s) will resolve with time and the lesions followed only if there is cause for concern. Although infantile hemangiomas predictably undergo spontaneous involution, during their proliferative phase, they occasionally cause disfigurement and serious complications, including airway obstruction (subglottic hemangioma), amblyopia (periorbital or orbital hemangioma), cardiac failure, and/or hypothyroidism (hepatic hemangioma), ulceration and bleeding.[8] In the past, such lesions were treated with corticosteroids or laser therapy.[9] In 2008, Léauté-Labrèze et al[10] published a landmark paper where the unanticipated antiproliferative effect of propranolol on infantile hemangiomas was described. Propranolol has since proven to be highly effective and generally well tolerated,[11] and is now the systemic treatment of choice.[12] The therapeutic action of propranolol is secondary to vasoconstriction, inhibition of angiogenesis, and induction of apoptosis. According to a recently published national protocol,[13] the administration of propranolol requires some infants to be given their first dose in hospital and monitoring their heart rate and blood pressure over 2 hours. Adverse effects include bronchospasm, bradycardia, hypotension, hypoglycemia, seizures, hyperkalemia, and diarrhea. Evaluation with a baseline electrocardiogram and/or echocardiogram may be necessary for some infants. A history of asthma, blood glucose abnormalities, and congenital heart disease are considered contraindications for initiation

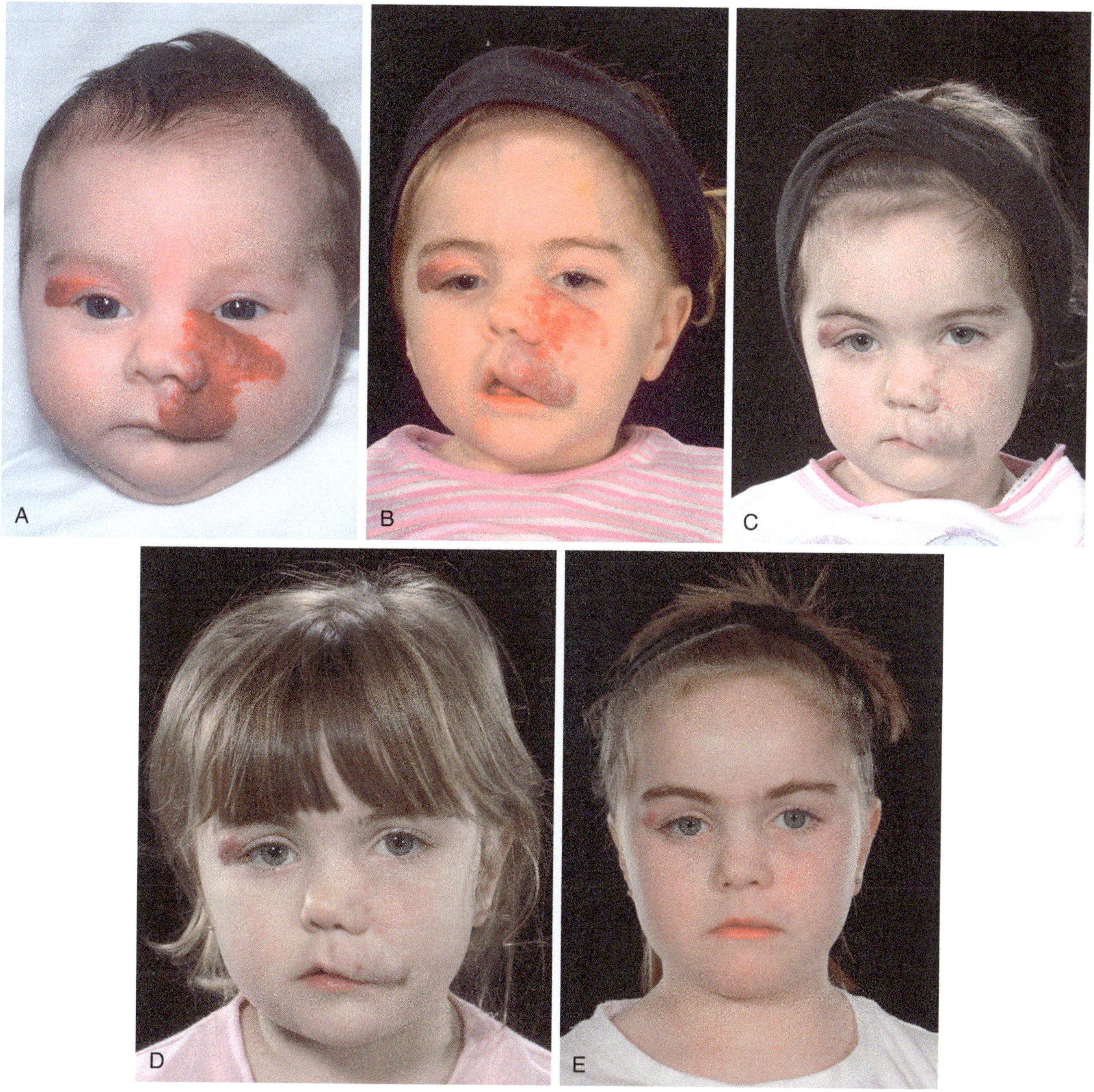

• **Fig. 15.1** (A) Hemangioma of the left cheek, lower eyelid, lateral nose, and upper lip in an infant. (B–E) Series of images at ages 3, 4, 5, and 10 years, which illustrate the natural regression of the hemangioma and resolution of the associated anatomical distortion.

of propranolol therapy. For small superficial hemangiomas, early use of the topical beta-blocking agent timolol, can be effective. The use of systemic corticosteroids is now reserved only as a second-line treatment, when propranolol is contraindicated.[14] There is no role for vincristine or interferon previously documented in the literature. The use of pulsed dye laser should be reserved for treatment of residual telangiectasia following tumor involution. Surgical excision is commonly performed for tumors that are in the involuting phase. This is considered when it is evident that surgical intervention will be necessary and the resultant esthetic outcome is predicted to be comparable to that anticipated during the involuted phase. Otherwise, resection is delayed until involution is complete. Serial excision or circular excision and purse-string closure can be utilized for surgical resection.[15] Occasionally, excision can be considered in the proliferative phase, if medical management is contraindicated or has failed, or as an emergency procedure, for instance a large hemangioma on the upper eyelid causing complete visual obstruction.[16]

Infantile hemangiomas can also occur in extracutaneous areas, most frequently in the liver. Internal organ

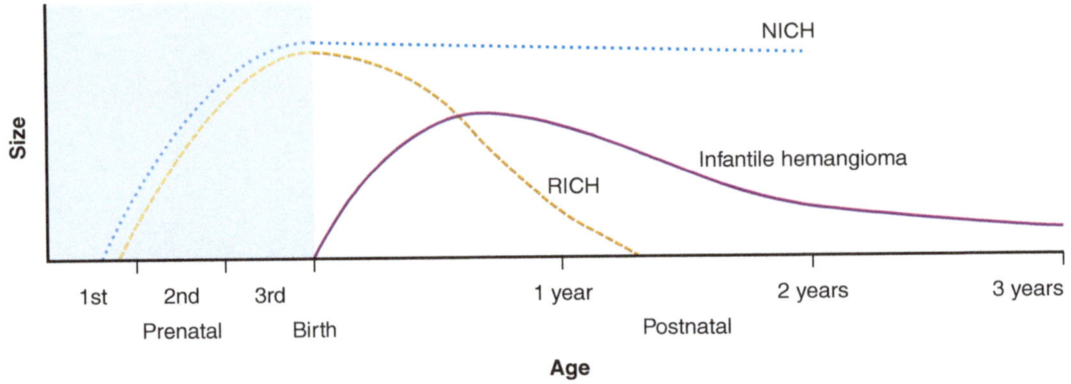

• **Fig. 15.2** Growth curves for rapidly involuting congenital hemangiomas (RICH), noninvoluting congenital hemangiomas (NICH), and infantile hemangioma (IH). (From Mulliken JB, Enjolras O. Congenital hemangiomas and infantile hemangioma: missing links. *J Am Acad Dermatol*. 2004;50:875–882.)

involvement is more common in infants with multiple cutaneous hemangiomas. These hypervascular hepatic lesions can lead to hepatomegaly and/or hypothyroidism. High output cardiac failure is more commonly associated with congenital liver hemangiomas.

The presence of a flat segmental facial hemangioma should prompt consideration of the associated diagnosis of *PHACES*. The term comprises *p*osterior fossa brain malformation, *h*emangioma, *a*rterial cerebrovascular anomalies (most common associated finding), *c*oarctation of the aorta and cardiac defects, *e*ye/endocrine abnormalities and *s*ternal clefting or supraumbilical raphe.[17] Evaluation of the brain and cerebral vasculature with MRI is important, although deciding which infants to image remains unclear. Similarly, segmental hemangiomas in the lumbrosacral region and perineum can be associated with ventral-caudal malformations, including omphalocele, imperforate anus, vaginal, and renal anomalies. Radiological investigation (ultrasound and/or MRI) is essential to exclude any associated abnormalities.

In contrast to infantile hemangiomas, congenital hemangiomas are almost always completely developed at birth and divided into *rapidly-involuting congenital hemangiomas* (RICH) and *noninvoluting congenital hemangiomas* (NICH), depending on their pattern of involution. Mulliken and Enjolras[18] have characterized the disparate growth curves for congenital compared with infantile hemangiomas (Fig. 15.2). Aside from the distinctive clinical presentation of these congenital lesions, as well as differing clinical course, negative GLUT1 immunohistochemical staining is an important characteristic to distinguish congenital tumors from their infantile counterparts. There are no distinctive imaging features that reliably differentiate between a RICH and a NICH, with both types appearing as well-defined, hypervascular, relatively homogeneous masses on ultrasound. For some RICH, involution may begin within the first week of life. In most infants with RICH, regression is complete within the first 7–14 months of life, with anetodermic cutaneous excess remaining. Interestingly, in a small proportion of patients with RICH, involution may be incomplete, resulting in a residuum clinically indistinguishable from NICH. A typical NICH forms a flat violaceous vascular plaque with coarse surface telangiectasia bordered by a blue-white rim. Unlike their infantile counterparts, congenital hemangiomas rarely require intervention in infancy. Given the clinical course of RICH, observation is the mainstay of treatment. Occasionally, very large RICH may cause high output heart failure due to their remarkable hypervascularity, in which case embolization may be considered to dampen the lesion's arterial supply until natural regression occurs. Acute cardiac failure is particularly common with hepatic RICH. Aside from their clinical behavior, hepatic RICH are typically unifocal, and are therefore readily distinguished from hepatic infantile hemangiomas, which are multifocal and usually clinically silent. Large RICH may also result in localized deformity requiring surgical intervention in later childhood. More specifically, these lesions may cause fat atrophy, resulting in contour deformity (in contradistinction to infantile hemangiomas, which often leave a fibro-fatty residuum) or excess anetodermic skin requiring excision. Moreover, regressed lesions can leave an unsightly bed of large, dysplastic veins, which respond well to sclerotherapy. Some lesions may be difficult to differentiate from other tumors, such as congenital fibrosarcoma or rhabdomyosarcoma, and as such may warrant early biopsy and/or surgical excision. NICH may necessitate excision for esthetic concerns as these lesions never involute.

Kaposiform hemangioendotheliomas (KHE) is a locally aggressive solitary vascular tumor, which is usually present at or soon after birth. This tumor often presents as a large violaceous soft tissue swelling (Fig. 15.3). Diagnosis can be confirmed with MRI, which shows a characteristic stranding of the surrounding fat, T2 hyperintensity, poorly defined margins and invasion of adjacent tissues. By 2 years of age, these tumors have usually undergone partial involution but complete involution does not occur. Kaposiform hemangioendothelioma is associated with Kasabach–Meritt phenomenon, characterized by thrombocytopenia $<25 \times 10^9$/L, petechiae, and bleeding. The other tumor related to this phenomenon is tufted angioma, which is more benign in nature and whose name derives from its histopathologic

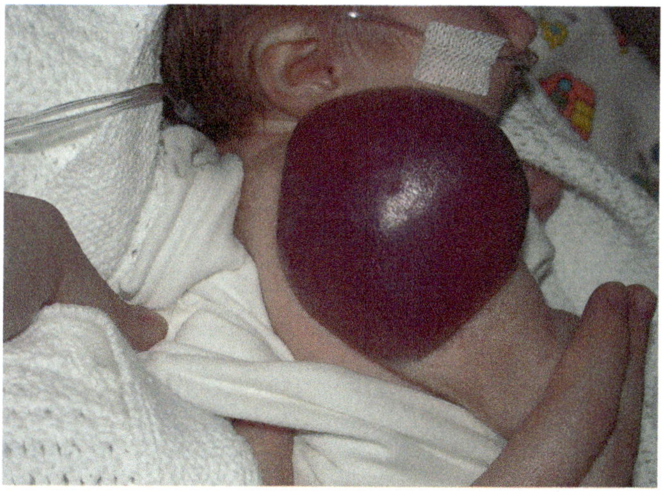

• **Fig. 15.3** Clinical image of an infant with a large violaceous edematous lesion typical of a kaposiform hemangioendothelioma.

appearance characterized by tufts of capillaries within the dermis. Tufted angioma and KHE share several clinical and histological features and are thought to be part of the same neoplastic spectrum. The treatment for KHE has traditionally been vincristine,[19] but recent reports of rapamycin (sirolimus),[20] have shown this drug to be highly effective. Platelet transfusion is contraindicated unless there is active bleeding or surgical intervention is planned. While the primary indication for therapeutic treatment is Kasabach–Meritt phenomenon, drug therapy is also considered for large asymptomatic tumors to minimize fibrosis and consequent pain and stiffness.

Pyogenic granuloma is a small, solitary pedunculated red papule that commonly occurs in childhood. The primary complications associated with this lesion are bleeding and ulceration. These tumors have been treated with laser, curettage, electrocautery, and shave excision, with a recurrence rate in excess of 40%. The latter is likely to be due to the fact that these lesions extend into the reticular dermis and therefore effective management requires full-thickness resection.

Vascular Malformations

Vascular malformations arise from abnormal development of vascular tissue during embryogenesis. Although present at birth, vascular malformations typically only become evident in childhood or occasionally, in adult life, do not undergo involution and grow commensurate with the child. Malformations are grouped into fast flow versus slow flow, with the former containing an arterial component. Genetic aberrations may give rise to vascular malformations, but the majority are nonsyndromic and nonfamilial. Gene mutations associated with arteriovenous malformations include mutations in endoglin (hereditary hemorrhagic telangiectasia type 1, HHT1), activin receptor-like kinase 1 (*HHT type 2*), *RASA1* (capillary malformation-arteriovenous malformation) or *PTEN* (PTEN-associated vascular anomaly). Capillary malformations giving rise to port wine stains and Sturge–Weber syndrome have been shown to be associated with a somatic mutation in *GNAQ* gene. Venous malformations can result from mutations in genes such as *TIE2* (sporadic venous malformations, cutaneomucosal venous malformation), glomulin (glomuvenous malformation), *CCM1/KRIT1*, *CCM2* or *CCM3* (cerebral cavernous malformations) genes. Mutations in *VEGFR3*, *FOXC2*, *SOX18* or *CCBE1* genes are linked to primary lymphedema.[2] Unlike infantile hemangiomas, vascular malformations tend to demonstrate an equal sex distribution.

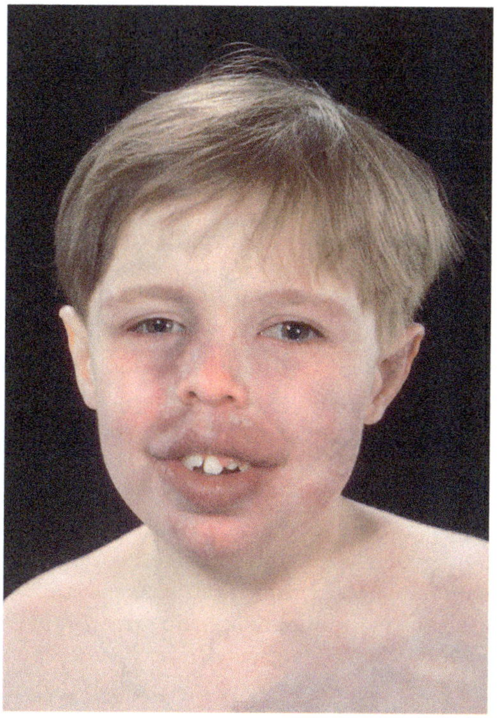

• **Fig. 15.4** Capillary malformation involving first, second, and third trigeminal nerve distributions bilaterally in a patient with Sturge–Weber syndrome.

Capillary malformations are caused by an excess of capillary-type vessels within the dermis. They commonly present at birth as a pink or red cutaneous discoloration. Over time, the color often deepens and the skin can thicken to eventually adopt a raised "cobblestone" appearance. A small proportion of lesions are associated with contiguous soft tissue and bony abnormalities. Traditionally, facial capillary malformations have been described as occurring in one of the three trigeminal nerve branch distributions (45%), with a greater proportion (55%) involving more than one dermatome or occurring bilaterally. However, there does not appear to be any pathophysiological relationship with the trigeminal nerve. With capillary malformations in the so-called first trigeminal nerve distribution, Sturge–Weber syndrome should be considered.[21] Sturge–Weber syndrome is a sporadic disorder, with an incidence of 1 in 50,000. The capillary malformation involves the first trigeminal nerve distribution, but may extend into the second and third (Fig. 15.4). The two other cardinal features of this syndrome are ocular anomalies (choroidal vascular abnormalities, glaucoma) and leptomeningeal involvement (capillary, venous or arteriovenous malformations). Ophthalmology consultation and intracranial MRI examination are mandatory in these patients. Midline capillary malformations are occasionally associated with central nervous system anomalies, such as encephalocele, occult spinal dysraphism, tethered spinal cord or arteriovenous malformations of the spinal cord (Cobb syndrome). Capillary malformations, particularly facial malformations, can result in significant psychological morbidity secondary to the disfigurement often associated with these lesions. Pulsed dye laser is now routinely offered as an early therapeutic modality. Laser treatment is highly beneficial in attenuating pigmentation of the capillary malformation and lessening the likelihood of developing secondary complications, including darkening, dermal thickening, and pyogenic granulomas. In later childhood, adolescence, and into adulthood surgical debulking may be required to correct any anatomical deformity.

Lymphatic malformations, historically referred to as "cystic hygromas" or "lymphangiomas," result from aberrant development of lymphatic tissue, and are not directly connected to the normal lymphatic system. They are commonly grouped into macrocystic or microcystic subtypes, depending on the size of the malformed channels (cysts) they contain. Microcytic malformations are usually defined as comprised of cysts less than 10 mm in diameter,[22] but in effect, they tend to be almost solid, containing a sponge-like tissue composed of stroma rather than cysts. Macrocystic lesions are the most common subtype of lymphatic malformation and typically arise in lymphatic-rich areas of the body, such as in the head and neck and axillae, although they occur in any anatomical region including the mesentery, orbits, and bladder wall. Lymphatic malformations can be apparent at birth, presenting as a soft, fluctuant swelling with normal overlying skin (Fig. 15.5). These lesions transilluminate and are usually non-tender. Some present following an acute intralesional bleed, with firm, tender, clot-filled cysts (Fig. 15.6). Lymphatic malformations are also prone to sudden expansion with concurrent, usually viral, illness, when the body produces more lymphatic fluid. Most lesions are easily diagnosed on ultrasound alone; however, MRI may be required to further define deep extension in complex lesions (Fig. 15.7). Microcystic lesions are more solid on palpation relative to their macrocystic counterparts. Moreover, the malformation may involve the contiguous skin and/or mucosa, presenting as vesicles, which may seep serous fluid or bleed. Microcystic lesions often have a large connective tissue component and on MRI demonstrate localized tissue overgrowth with a high T2 signal and a diffuse mild enhancement pattern. Lymphatic malformations are occasionally combined with cutaneous capillary malformations and with venous anomalies. Differentiation between lymphatic and venous malformations can be facilitated with thorough history and focused physical examination. While both types of malformations are soft and compressible, unlike venous malformations, lymphatic lesions do not expand with the Valsalva maneuver and cannot be "emptied" by compression or gravity. Morevoer, the overlying skin is often normal or displays only a subtle bluish hue. Large lymphatic malformations may cause significant morbidity secondary to mass effect, chylous effusions, recurrent infection (sepsis), bleeding, pain, and deformity. The first-line therapy for macrocystic or mixed (macro-/microcystic) lymphatic malformations is usually percutaneous sclerotherapy, which involves the injection of a sclerosing agent into the cysts to collapse and scar their walls and prevent their re-expansion (Fig. 15.8). Sclerotherapy can also be utilized to control recurrent infection and intralesional bleeds. Over the past three decades, various sclerosant agents including OK-432, sodium tetradecyl sulphate (STS), ethanol, bleomycin, and doxycycline, have been used in the treatment of lymphatic malformations. Doxycycline, STS, and bleomycin are currently the preferred sclerosants. Although microcystic lymphatic malformations tend to be less responsive to sclerotherapy, largely in view

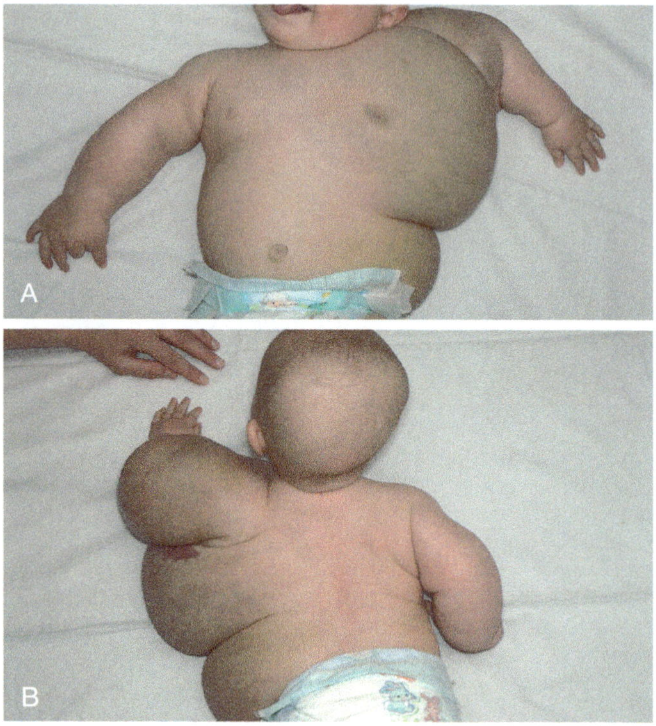

• **Fig. 15.5** Clinical images of a child with a large mixed macro- and microcystic lymphatic malformation involving the chest, axilla, and upper extremity; (A) anterior and (B) posterior views.

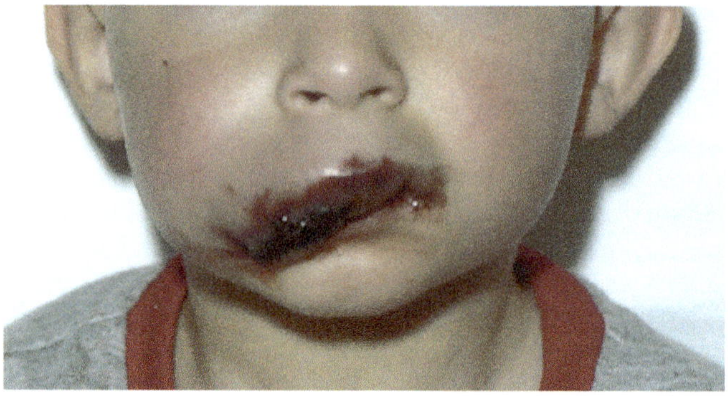

• **Fig. 15.6** Clinical image of a child with a microcystic lymphatic malformation of the right upper lip. This lesion was complicated by an episode of intralesional bleeding.

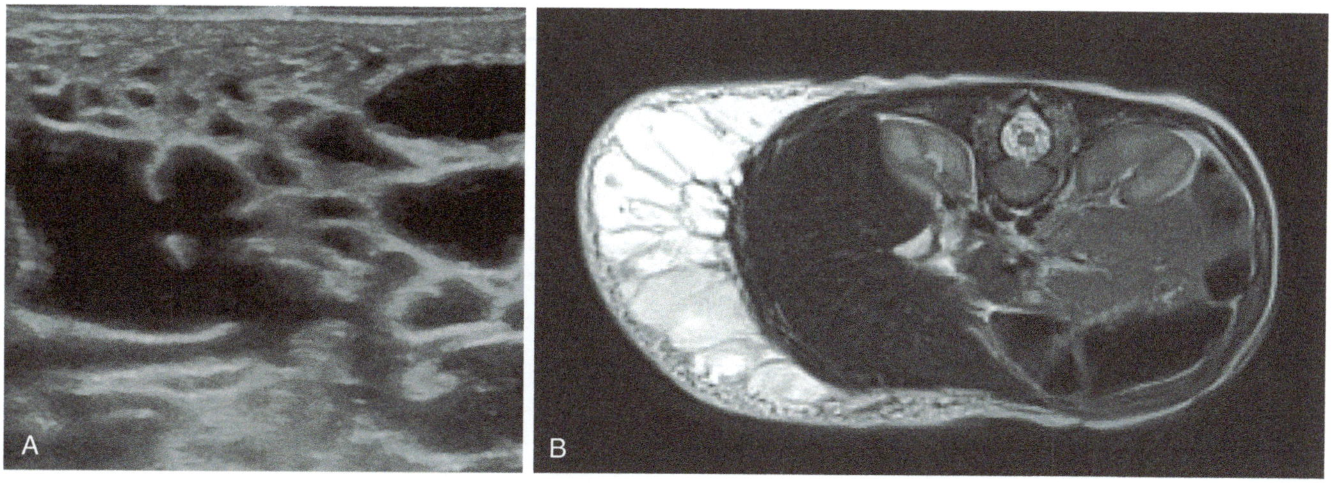

• **Fig. 15.7** (A) Ultrasound image of the lymphatic malformation of the chest wall in the child shown in Fig. 15.5. Cysts of varying sizes can be seen, separated by thin septae. (B) T2-weighted axial MRI image of the same lymphatic malformation. The majority of the macrocysts lie deep to the microcysts.

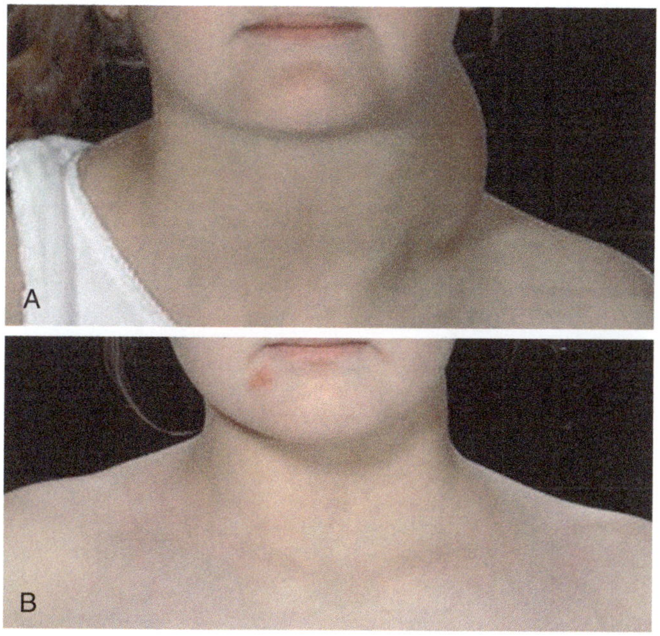

• **Fig. 15.8** Clinical images of a macrocystic lymphatic malformation of the neck (A) before and (B) after a single sclerotherapy treatment.

of the more solid nature of these lesions, some series have shown a good response rate with bleomycin. The most common complications associated with sclerotherapy are cutaneous ulceration and nerve injury, these potential risks varying according to the agent used. Lymphatic malformations that fail to respond to sclerotherapy can be considered for surgical resection. Seroma formation is the most common complication following surgical extirpation, and can be minimized by careful application of compressive dressings. Sclerotherapy can also be useful in the management of seromas. Complex and extensive lesions are associated with more significant morbidity, including infection, delayed healing, peripheral nerve injury, and deformity. Resection carries an important rate of recurrence, especially for lesions that involve multiple tissue planes where excision is usually incomplete (Fig. 15.9).

Venous malformations may present earlier than lymphatic malformations due to the associated discoloration of the overlying skin. However, many are deep-seated and are not problematic until they grow with puberty.[23] Venous malformations exhibit variable morphology, from focal round lesions (often mistaken for hemangiomas) to diffuse and ill-defined lesions involving multiple tissue planes, or clusters of dysplastic veins involving an entire limb. Most commonly, venous malformations are restricted to subcutaneous tissue and muscle (Fig. 15.10), though lesions may extend to deeper structures, such as bones and joints. In fact, venous malformations frequently occur around joints, particularly the knee, and as such can cause significant pain, restrictions in range of movement, synovitis, and occasionally hemarthroses. Lesions can be associated with pain, swelling, bleeding, and deformity (Fig. 15.11). Moreover, extensive venous malformations can be associated with localized intravascular coagulopathy and phlebothrombosis, due to widespread thrombosis of the very slow-flowing blood within the malformation, which consumes clotting factors and can lead to a coagulopathy in the normal circulating blood. On physical examination, these lesions are found to enlarge with dependent positioning and Valsalva maneuver. Calcified phleboliths can often be palpated within the mass, and are pathognomonic on imaging, appearing as rounded signal voids. Ultrasound is useful to confirm the slow-flow nature of the lesion. On MRI, these malformations are hyperintense on T2-weighted imaging and, in contrast to lymphatic malformations, enhance with contrast (often with a patchy distribution of enhancement due to the very slow flow of contrast through the malformation) (Fig. 15.12). Most malformations cause pain secondary to venous congestion and thrombus formation. For venous malformations of the extremities, the use of compression garments is recommended to reduce venous stasis, expansion, and localized intravascular coagulopathy. Like lymphatic malformations, sclerotherapy is usually the therapy of choice for treatment of symptomatic venous malformations,

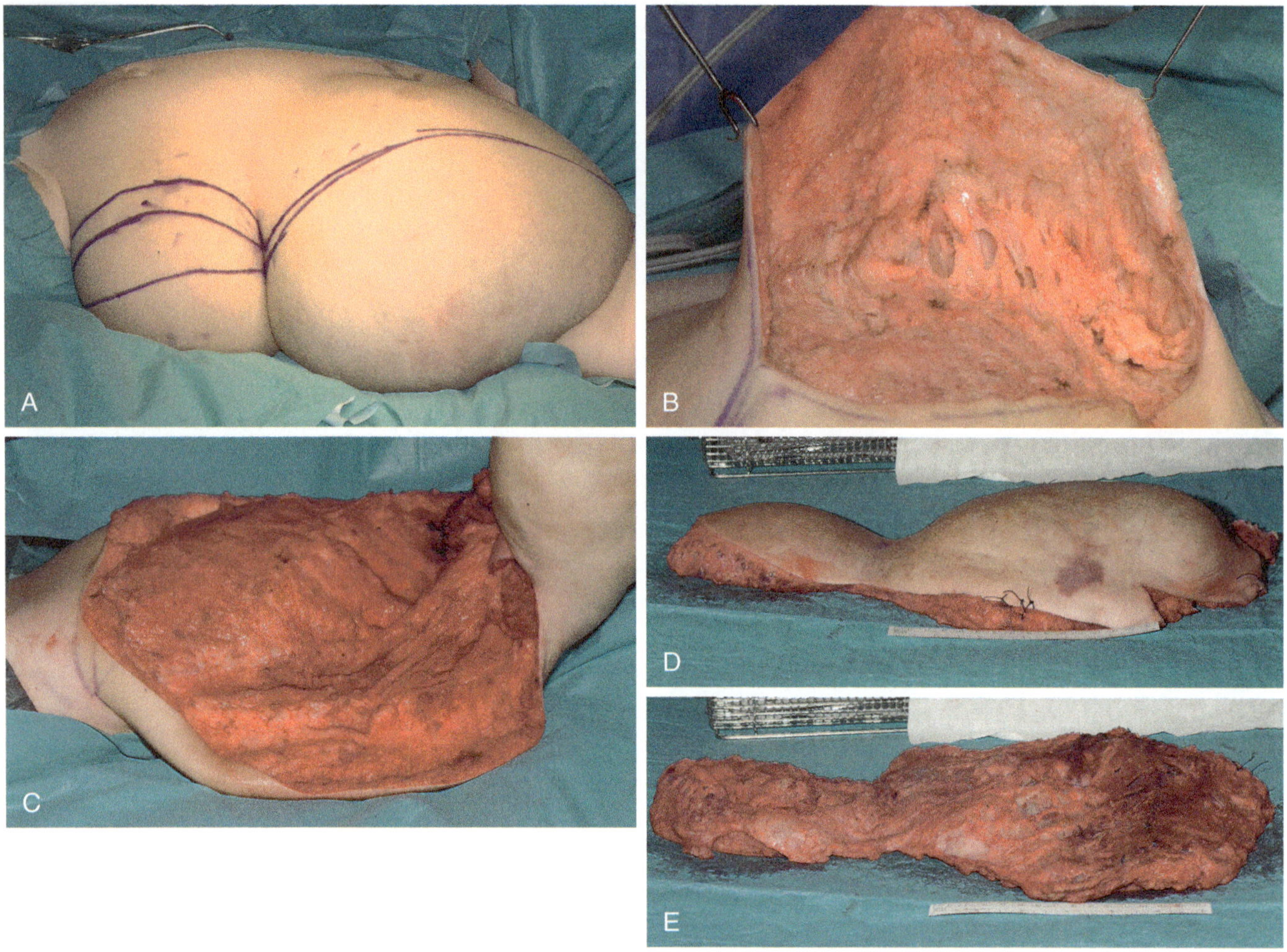

• **Fig. 15.9** The lymphatic malformation of the child in Fig. 15.5 was initially treated with sclerotherapy, following which surgical extirpation was undertaken in view of the extent of the lesion and associated disability it engendered. (A–E) Intraoperative photographs, including (A) marking of the malformation, (B) malformation in situ, (C) chest wall and axilla following excision of the lesion, and (D, E) specimen excised.

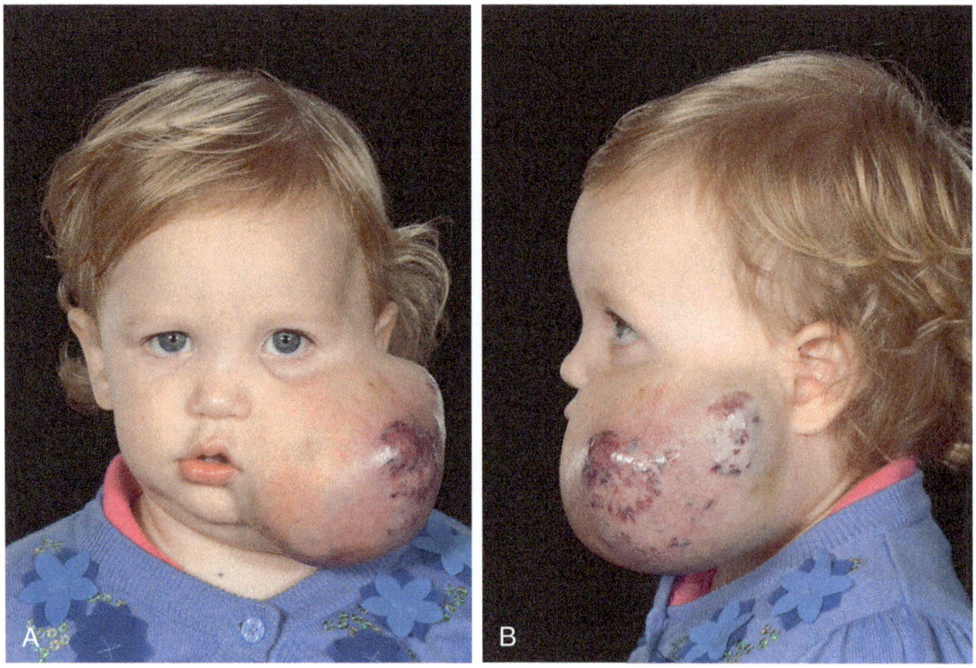

• **Fig. 15.10** Clinical images of a child with a venous malformation of the left cheek (A) anterior and (B) lateral views.

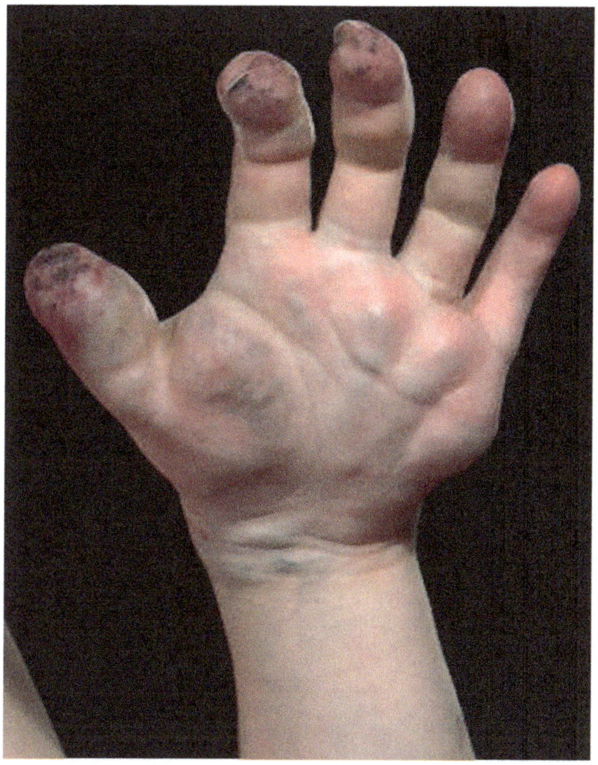

• **Fig. 15.11** Clinical image of a venous malformation of the hand. The significant anatomical deformity caused considerable functional impairment.

with resection reserved for well-localized lesions that can be removed completely or malformations that remain symptomatic or cause important residual deformity despite sclerotherapy. The therapeutic mechanism of sclerotherapy for venous malformations is the same as for lymphatic malformations, wherein the sclerosant induces fibrosis within the malformation, thereby shrinking the lesion, reducing venous stasis and mass effect. For these malformations, STS is usually the preferred sclerosing agent, although bleomycin and ethanol may have a role in selected cases. The complication rates are higher for venous sclerotherapy than for lymphatic lesions, partly due to the fact that the agent circulated in the bloodstream. Both STS and ethanol are associated with a potential for localized tissue necrosis, and both can cause nerve injury. When surgical resection is considered, caution must be exercised to avoid aggravating the existing deformity, and thus conservative resection is recommended, especially in view of the fact that complete removal is often unattainable and recurrence is high. Some centers advocate the use of prophylactic aspirin for recurrent pain secondary to phlebothrombosis and low molecular weight heparin in patients with significant coagulopathy, reducing the rate of thrombosis within the malformation and thereby decreasing the consumption of clotting factors.

Two syndromes commonly associated with venous malformations include *Maffucci syndrome* and *blue rubber bleb nevus syndrome*. The former is characterized by cutaneous venous malformations, with enchondromas and/or bony exostoses. The latter includes multiple, small (<2 cm) venous malformations localized to skin, subcutaneous tissues, and most particularly the gastrointestinal tract. The proposed treatment of blue rubber bleb nevus syndrome is rapamycin (sirolimus).[24]

Fibroadipose vascular anomaly (*FAVA*) is an underrecognized form of venous malformation that typically affects one or more muscles in a compartment of the forearm or calf.[25] Generally, it presents in childhood and patients usually report unexpectedly high levels of pain and contractures are common. It consists of dense fibrous tissue deposition within the muscle, often with one or two large caliber dysplastic veins. If recognized early, symptoms may be improved with percutaneous cryoablation. Advanced disease may require debulking of the muscle compartment.

Some low flow malformations are associated with considerable regional soft tissue and bony overgrowth. Certain forms of overgrowth have recognizable patterns and defined underlying genetic mutations, such as *CLOVES* syndrome; however, most are not part of a recognized syndrome and in such cases, inaccurate labels should be avoided. The term *Klippel–Trénaunay* syndrome has historically been used to label a wide range of overgrowth types with very little in common (Fig. 15.13). A significant proportion of overgrowth conditions are related to mutations of *PIK3CA* within the mTOR pathway and are part of a spectrum of diseases that for clarity and simplicity should be grouped as PIK3CA-related overgrowth spectrum (PROS).[26] mTOR inhibitors such as sirolimus may, in future, have an important role to play in modulating these conditions.

Arteriovenous malformations are the rarest form of vascular malformation, although clinically they usually attract the most attention.[27] These lesions arise from an error in vascular development during embryogenesis, where abnormal connections are created between arterial and venous system without intervening capillaries. The latter developmental aberration results in high velocity vascular shunting, usually leading to progressive enlargement of the feeding arteries and draining veins and increasing the complexity of the vascular anatomy at the center or nidus of the malformation. There appears to be a defect in the regional soft tissues that drives vasculogenesis and the recruitment of arterial supply. While some arteriovenous malformations remain small and inconsequential throughout life, others can demonstrate insidious growth, causing significant morbidity secondary to pain, bleeding, tissue necrosis (due to arterial steal), and high output cardiac failure. The majority are located within the musculoskeletal tissues of the trunk or extremities. Lesions localized to the head and neck often have complex deep connections (Fig. 15.14). Most malformations can be diagnosed on clinical examination, as a localized thrill and/or bruit are present and the soft tissues are typically warm and diaphoretic. Ultrasound can be used to confirm the diagnosis in deep-seated lesions. Dynamic cross-sectional imaging may help to define the extent of the lesion and highlight secondary complications, but is often unnecessary. Angiography should be reserved for those cases

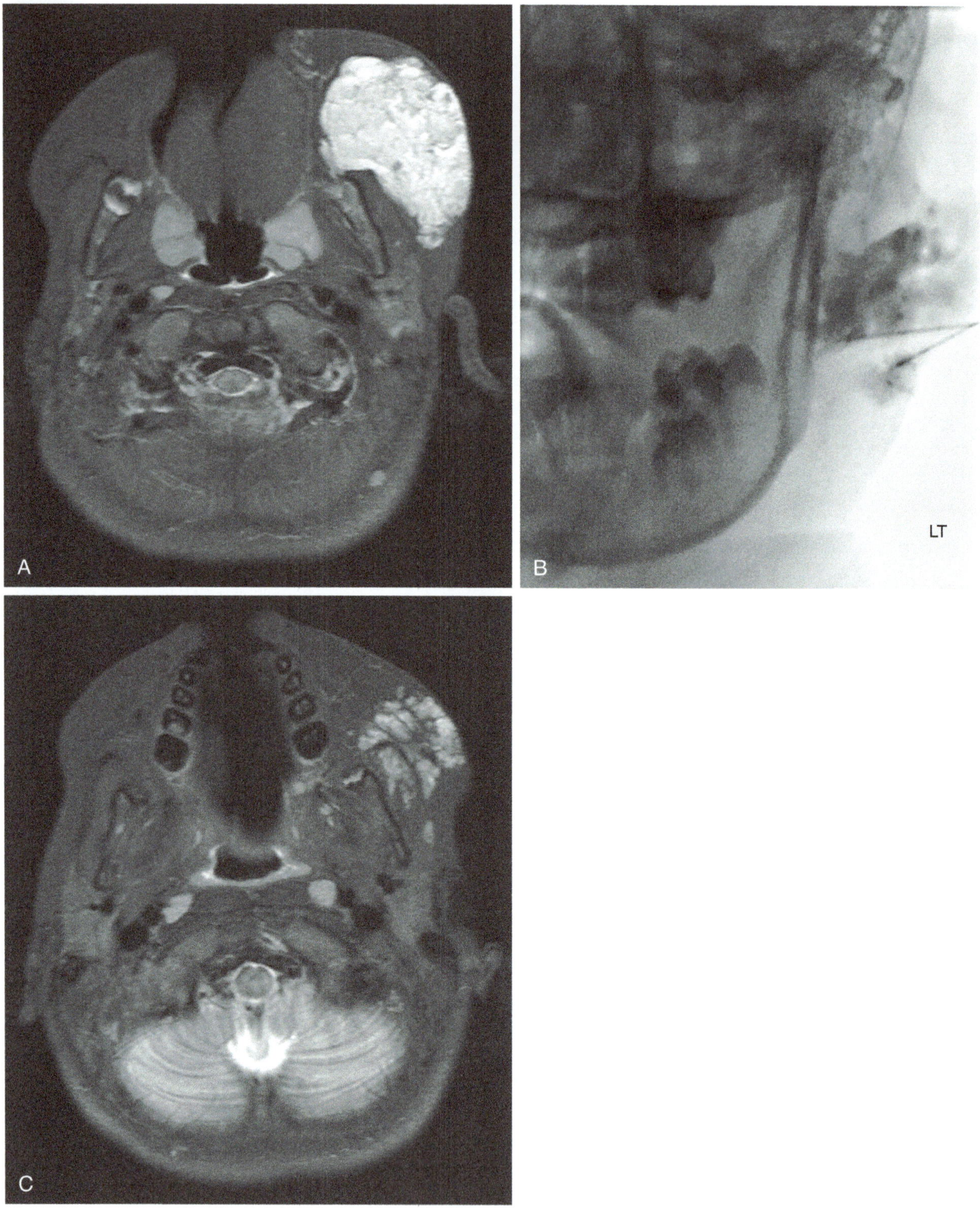

• **Fig. 15.12** (A) T2-weighted axial MRI image of a venous malformation of the left cheek in a child. The malformation is visualized as a lobulated, well-defined mass within the subcutaneous tissue. (B) Intraoperative fluoroscopic image of sclerotherapy of the lesion. A two-needle technique was used to instill opacified sclerosant into the malformation. (C) T2-weighted axial MRI image of the same venous malformation following four sclerotherapy treatments. The malformation was considerably reduced in size and the distortion of the adjacent soft tissues of the cheek was lessened. LT: Left side

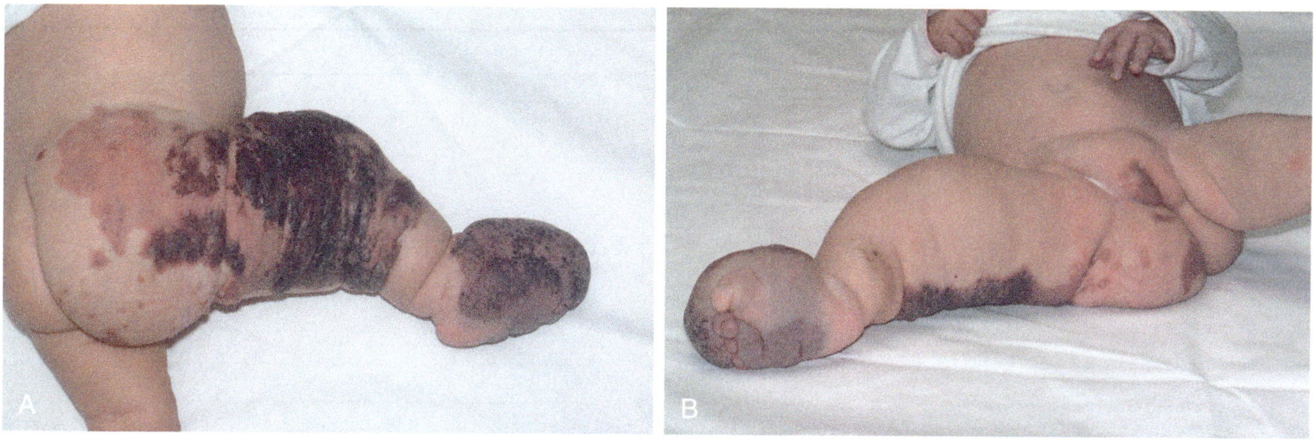

• **Fig. 15.13** Clinical images of a child with a capillary–lymphatic–venous malformation of the lower extremity, demonstrating considerable overgrowth and distortion of the limb, characteristic of Klippel–Trénaunay syndrome (A) lateral and (B) medial views.

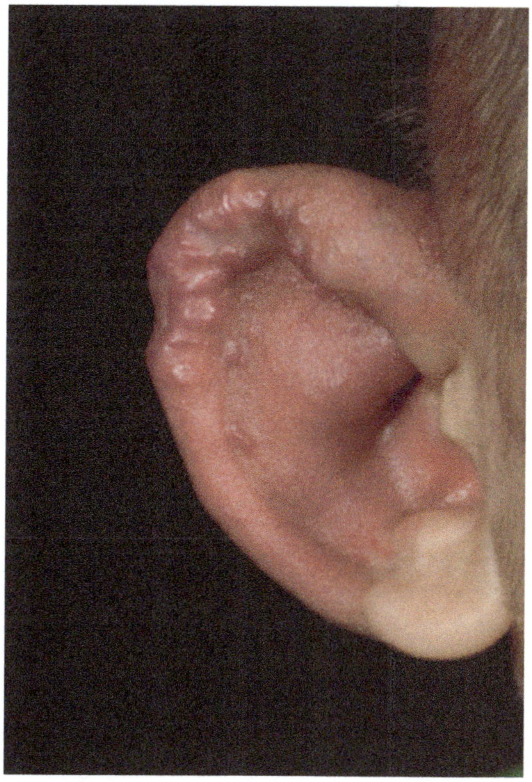

• **Fig. 15.14** Clinical image of an arteriovenous malformation of the ear.

where an interventional radiologist is planning to treat the lesion definitively. Schobinger proposed a classification system for arteriovenous malformations based on clinical characteristics, in an effort to guide decision-making in terms of intervention. Stage I (quiescence) describes a lesion that is warm and pink, and shunting is seen on color Doppler examination. In stage II (expansion), there is enlargement of the lesion, and a thrill or bruit may be noted. Stage III (destruction) is characterized by dystrophic skin changes, ulceration, bleeding, and pain. Finally, in stage IV (decompensation) congestive heart failure is present. Arteriovenous malformations remain the most challenging lesions to treat effectively. Management is complicated by the fact that these anomalies progress over time, complete extirpation is rarely possible, recurrence after treatment is high, and resection may be associated with significant morbidity and may result in more considerable deformity than the malformation per se. Liu et al[28] recommend resection for Schobinger stage I and II arteriovenous malformations in nonanatomically sensitive areas, where progression to a higher stage will render extirpation more difficult or if there is an aggravation of symptoms or deformity, for stages I and II lesions respectively. Intervention for stage III and IV lesions is dictated by degree of associated symptoms. Embolization should be considered as a first-line treatment for most lesions, as it is minimally invasive and can be injected directly to the point of shunting, traditionally called the nidus (Fig. 15.15). The latter can also be implemented prior to surgical extirpation to reduce the size of the malformation preoperatively and minimize intraoperative blood loss. Incomplete embolization or excision appears to stimulate the malformation to enlarge and become problematic. Thus, management of these complex lesions should remain the remit of an experienced multidisciplinary team. *Parkes–Weber syndrome* is characterized by small, diffuse, multifocal arteriovenous malformations with associated extremity overgrowth and an overlying pale capillary malformation. The *capillary malformation–arteriovenous malformation* is an autosomal dominant condition associated with *RASA1* gene mutation. Patients typically present with atypical capillary malformations that are small multifocal pink lesions surrounded by a pale halo, and can be associated with deeper-seated arteriovenous malformations.

Management of vascular anomalies necessitates interdisciplinary care by a dedicated team with expertise in plastic surgery, dermatology, interventional/diagnostic radiology, general pediatric surgery, orthopedic surgery, hematology/oncology, pathology, and vascular surgery. Moreover, allied health professionals such as psychologists, occupational therapists, and physiotherapists are also integral members of the team. In the majority of cases, the correct diagnosis can be made by thorough history and physical examination. Appropriate imaging and biopsy for histological analysis

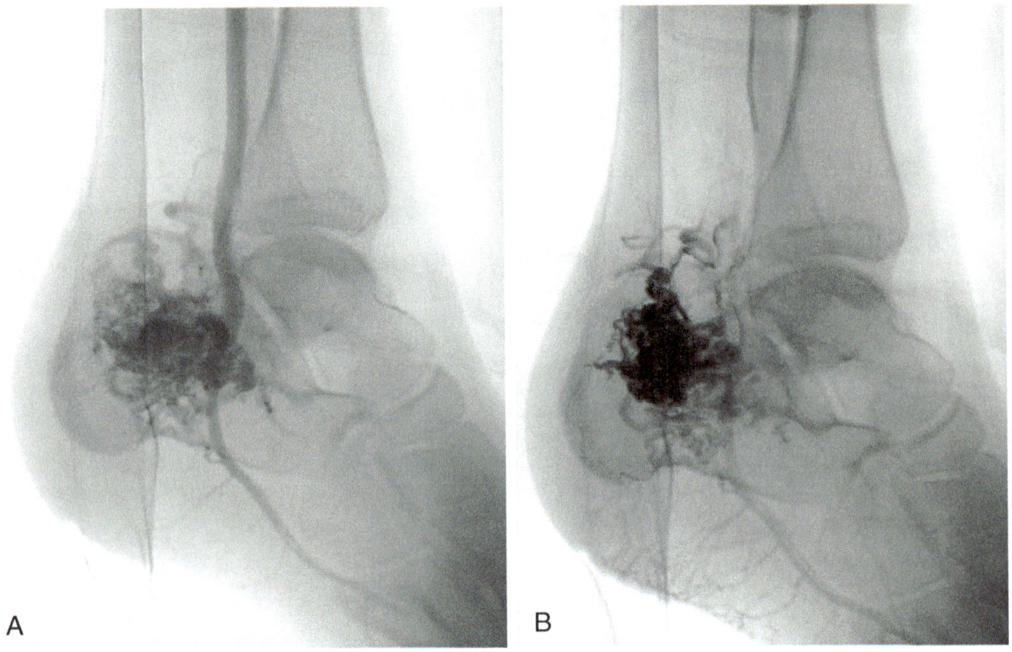

• **Fig. 15.15** (A) Angiography image demonstrating a focal high-flow arteriovenous malformation of the left ankle, which is supplied by the posterior tibial artery. (B) Angiographic image following embolization, demonstrating dense onyx material filling nearly the entire malformation while preserving the posterior tibial artery.

can assist where diagnostic ambiguity remains. Treatment depends on the nature, size, and location of the lesion, associated symptoms and anatomical deformity. Ultimately, management demands a holistic approach, which renders this field of medicine such a challenging and rewarding specialty.

References

1. Mulliken JB, Glowacki J. Hemangiomas and vascular malformations in infants and children: a classification based on endothelial characteristics. *Plast Reconstr Surg*. 1982;69:412–420.
2. Greene AK. Current concepts of vascular anomalies. *J Craniofac Surg*. 2012;23:220–224.
3. Léauté-Labrèze C, Harper JI, Hoeger PH. Infantile haemangioma. *Lancet*. 2017;390(10089):85–94.
4. Léauté-Labrèze C, Prey S, Ezzedine K. Infantile haemangioma: part I. Pathophysiology, epidemiology, clinical features, life cycle and associated structural abnormalities. *J Eur Acad Dermatol Venerol*. 2011;25:1245–1253.
5. Khan ZA, Boscolo E, Picard A, et al. Multi-potential stem cells recapitulate human infantile hemangioma in immunodeficient mice. *J Clin Invest*. 2008;118:2592–2599.
6. Bowers RE, Graham EA, Tomlinson KM. The natural history of the strawberry nevus. *Arch Dermatol*. 1960;82:667–680.
7. Couto RA, Maclellan RA, Zurakowski D, Greene AK. Infantile hemangioma: clinical assessment of the involuting phase and implications for management. *Plast Reconstr Surg*. 2012;130:619–624.
8. Léauté-Labrèze C, Prey S, Ezzedine K. Infantile haemangioma: part II. Risks, complications and treatment. *J Eur Acad Dermatol Venerol*. 2011;25:1254–1260.
9. Bennett ML, Fleischer AB, Chamlin SL, et al. Oral corticosteroid use is effective for cutaneous hemangiomas: an evidence based evaluation. *Arch Dermatol*. 2001;137:1208–1213.
10. Léauté-Labrèze C, de la Roque ED, Hubiche T, et al. Propranolol for severe hemangiomas of infancy. *N Engl J Med*. 2008;358:2649–2651.
11. Sans V, de la Roque ED, Berge J, et al. Propranolol for severe infantile hemangioma: follow-up report. *Pediatrics*. 2009;124:423–431.
12. Drolet BA, Frommelt PC, Chamlin SL, et al. Initiation and use of propranolol for infantile hemangioma: report of a consensus conference. *Pediatrics*. 2013;131:128–140.
13. Solman L, Glover M, Beattie PE, et al. Oral propranolol in the treatment of proliferating infantile haemangiomas: British Society for Paediatric Dermatology consensus guidelines. *Br J Dermatol*. 2018;179(3):582–589.
14. Chan H, McKay C, Adams S, Wargon O. RCT of timolol maleate gel for superficial infantile hemangiomas in 5 to 24 week olds. *Pediatrics*. 2013;131:1739–1747.
15. Mulliken JB, Rogers GF, Marler JJ. Circular excision of hemangioma and purse-string closure: the smallest possible scar. *Plast Reconstr Surg*. 202;109:1544-1554.
16. Weibel L, Hoey S, Syed S, et al. Periocular hemangioma: an eye-opening experience. *Arch Pediatr Adolesc Med*. 2007;161(10):1001–1002.
17. Frieden IJ, Reese V, Cohen D. PHACE syndrome: the association of posterior fossa brain malformations, hemangiomas, arterial anomalies, coarctation of the aorta and cardiac defects, and eye abnormalities. *Arch Dermatol*. 1996;132:307–311.
18. Mulliken JB, Enjolras O. Congenital hemangiomas and infantile hemangioma missing links. *J Am Acad Dermatol*. 2004;50:875–882.
19. Haisley-Royster C, Enjolras O, Frieden IJ, et al. Kasabach-Meritt phenomenon: a retrospective study of treatment with vincristine. *J Pediatr Hematol Oncol*. 2002;24:459–462.
20. Kai L, Wang Z, Yao W, Dong K, Xiao X. Sirolimus, a promising treatment for refractory Kaposiform hemangioendothelioma. *J Cancer Res Clin Oncol*. 2014;140:471–476.

21. Greene AK, Taber SF, Ball KL, et al. Sturge–Weber syndrome: frequency and morbidity of facial over-growth. *J Craniofac Surg.* 2009;20:617–621.
22. Greene AK, Perlyn C, Alomari AI. Management of lymphatic malformation. *Clin Plast Surg.* 2011;38:75–82.
23. Greene AK, Alomari AI. Management of venous malformations. *Clin Plast Surg.* 2011;38:83–93.
24. Yuksekkava H, Ozbek O, Keser M, Toy H. Blue rubber bleb nevus syndrome: successful treatment with sirolimus. *Pediatrics.* 2012;129:1080–1084.
25. Alomari A, Spencer S, Arnold R, Chaudry G, et al. Fibroadipose vascular anomaly; clinical-radiologic-pathologic featues of a newly delineated disorder of the extremity. *J Pediatr Orthop.* 2014;34:109–117.
26. Vahidnezhad H, Youssefian L, Uitto J. Klippel-Trenaunay syndrome belongs to the PIK3CA-related over-growth spectrum (PROS). *Exp Dermatol.* 2016;25:17–19.
27. Greene AK, Orbach DB. Management of arteriovenous malformations. *Clin Plast Surg.* 2011;38:95–106.
28. Liu AS, Mulliken JB, Zurakowski D, et al. Extracranial arteriovenous malformations: natural progression and recurrence after treatment. *Plast Reconstr Surg.* 2010;125:1185–1194.

16
Cleft Lip

MARC C. SWAN AND DAVID M. FISHER

For videos accompanying this chapter see ExpertConsult.com. See inside cover for access details.

Embryology

Between the 4th and 7th weeks of gestation, the two medial nasal prominences of the frontonasal process fuse to form the intermaxillary segment (Fig. 16.1), consisting of premaxilla and prolabium. In addition, the two maxillary prominences merge, from which the lateral lip and maxillary arch elements arise. By week 7 of gestation, mesenchymal confluence follows apoptosis of the epithelial seams between the medial nasal and maxillary prominences resulting in the formation a complete upper lip. Failure of fusion of the medial nasal prominence with the ipsilateral maxillary prominence results in a unilateral cleft lip and, if replicated bilaterally, a bilateral cleft lip results. The ratio of unilateral left, unilateral right, and bilateral cleft lip deformity is 6:3:1, respectively. The lateral nasal prominences form the alae of the nose and do not contribute to the upper lip. At the molecular level, several major signaling pathways, including *Bmp*, *Fgf*, *Shh*, and *Wnt*, are critical for midfacial morphogenesis, and subtle abnormalities in any one of these processes may lead to orofacial clefting.

Cleft lip is defined as a congenital abnormality of the primary palate. It may be complete or incomplete, unilateral or bilateral, and may be associated with a palatal cleft. The forme fruste cleft is qualified by a notch in the vermilion, a visible furrow extending from the edge of the lip to mid-nostril floor and subtle irregularity of the alae. A Simonart band occurs in approximately 30% of patients with a unilateral cleft lip and palate, and describes the small soft tissue bridge, most often devoid of orbicularis oris muscle, that spans the lateral and medial elements of a cleft lip. The integrity of the underlying alveolus is probably of greater clinical relevance than the magnitude of the soft tissue band, although the band will typically diminish the associated nasal deformity.

In the context of sporadic clefting, the risk of unaffected parents with one child with a cleft lip ± palate having a second affected child is approximately 4%, while with two affected children, the risk increases to 9%.[1] If one parent has a cleft lip ± palate, the risk of having an affected child is similarly around 4%, which increases to 17% for a second affected child. The anatomical severity of the cleft has a direct influence on the recurrence risk in first-degree relatives, with the type of cleft being predictive of the nature of the recurrence.[2]

Most obstetric units in the developed world now routinely offer a mid-trimester fetal anomaly ultrasound scan, with facial examination being advocated since 1984. Using 2D antenatal ultrasound, a Norwegian study detected up to 57% of cases of cleft lip ± palate, of which 43% had an associated anomaly; no cases of isolated cleft palate were diagnosed antenatally.[3] Diagnostic accuracy has improved with the advent of 3D sonography, which has led to a sensitivity of 95% and a specificity of 92.3%.[4] In high-risk populations (i.e., those with a positive family history of orofacial clefting), detection rates of 100% have been achieved. Antenatal magnetic resonance imaging offers no particular advantage over ultrasound for the diagnosis of cleft lip, but has significant potential in improving the diagnosis of cleft palate.[5]

Clinical Anatomy

The orbicularis oris is the highly complex sphincteric muscle of the lip that facilitates feeding, speech, and oral continence. It consists of four substantially independent

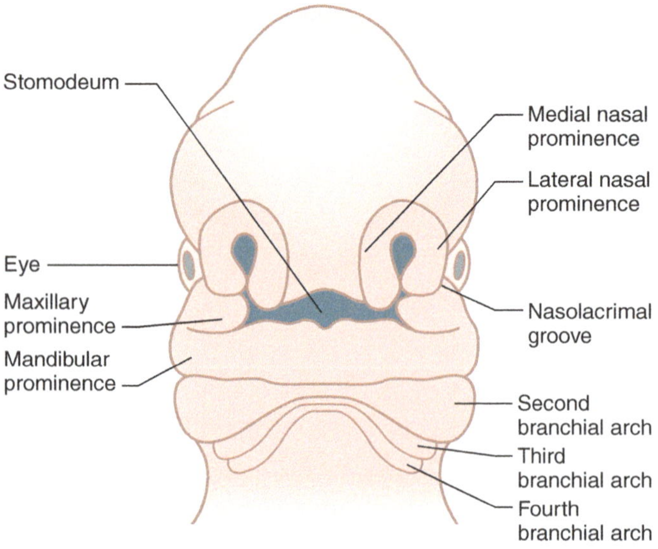

• **Fig. 16.1** Embryology of the primary palate. Failure of fusion of the medial nasal prominence and the ipsilateral maxillary prominence results in a unilateral cleft lip.

quadrants – upper, lower, left, and right – each of which contains a smaller pars marginalis and a larger pars peripheralis. The surface marking of the junction between the marginalis and peripheralis fibers is the border between the vermilion and skin. The pars peripheralis fibers fan out obliquely from the modioli to interdigitate with the other muscles of facial expression (including zygomaticus major superiorly and depressor anguli oris inferiorly) and terminate within the dermis. Their role is primarily one of articulation and facial expression.

The midline philtral dimple of the non-cleft upper lip is flanked by symmetrical philtral columns that arise from each peak of the Cupid's bow and curve gently cephalad to the base of the columella. The ridges of the philtral column are created by dermal insertions of the pars peripheralis fibers as they interdigitate in the midline, each crossing approximately 5 mm into the contralateral half of the upper lip. The Cupid's bow peaks are created by the pull of the levator labii superioris fibers inserting into the base of the ipsilateral philtral column. The cutaneous roll (alternatively, the "white roll" of Gillies or the "white skin roll" of Millard) is the mucocutaneous junction between the vermilion and skin. The cutaneous roll runs from commissure to commissure, but is most prominent centrally at the Cupid's bow and gradually attenuates laterally. It contains four to five rows of progressively superficially positioned pilosebaceous units containing tiny unpigmented silky vellus hairs, which by reflecting ambient light highlight the contour of the Cupid's bow. The vermilion has an associated midline tubercle caused by the eversion of opposing pars marginalis fibers. The vermilion–mucosal junction ("red line" of Noordhoff) represents an abrupt transition between the keratinized vermilion and thick nonkeratinized squamous epithelium of the oral mucosa.

In the unilateral cleft lip, the Cupid's bow is preserved in the medial lip element.[6] The lip height, as measured from the cleft side peak of Cupid's bow to the base of the columella, is characteristically deficient and the bow is sloped. The cutaneous roll of the entire length of the bow is well preserved. However, there is vermilion height deficiency below the cleft side half of Cupid's bow. The proposed peak of Cupid's bow on the lateral lip element has traditionally been less well defined. Noordhoff advocated preserving the proposed base of the philtral column as it is an anatomically determined landmark. He defined it as being located at the point where the cutaneous roll and the vermilion–mucosal junction begin to converge medially (Fig. 16.2). At "Noordhoff's point", there is adequate vermilion height (usually matching the height of the vermilion below the non-cleft side peak of Cupid's bow) and good quality cutaneous roll. Medial to Noordhoff's point, the quality of these features diminishes.

The height of the lateral lip element (as measured from the subalare to Noordhoff's point) is frequently different from the height of the non-cleft side (subalare to Cupid's bow peak). The latter is often excessive in incomplete clefts

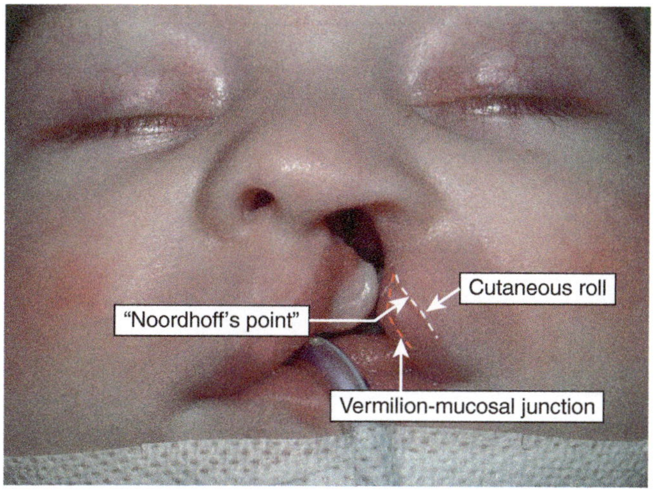

• **Fig. 16.2** Infant with a complete left cleft lip and palate. The cardinal position of "Noordhoff's point" is marked.

and usually shorter in complete clefts. The transverse length of the lateral lip element (Noordhoff's point to the commissure) is almost always shorter than that of the non-cleft side (Cupid's bow peak to the commissure). Lateral lip element hypoplasia, defined as combined height and transverse length deficiency, is present in almost two thirds of patients with a unilateral cleft.

The orbicularis oris muscle is misdirected by the cleft (Fig. 16.3). On the cleft side, the pars superficialis changes direction as it approaches the cleft to run almost vertically to find insertion to the cleft side nostril and periosteum of the piriform aperture. The pars peripheralis inserts into the lateral aspect of the alar and the nasolabial fold; contraction of the lateral lip element orbicularis produces a noticeable bulge in the lateral lip. On the non-cleft side, the orbicularis fibers insert into the base of the columella and nasal septum. Activation of orbicularis exacerbates the nasal deformity by splaying the alar cartilages, broadening the nasal tip, shortening the columella, and deviating the nasal septum to the non-cleft side. Successful correction of the unilateral lip deformity must address these aberrant muscular attachments.

In complete bilateral cleft lip and cleft palate, the prolabium and premaxilla are entirely separated from the lateral lip and maxillary arch elements. The dimensions of the prolabium will vary considerably between affected individuals, but there are some consistent findings. The cutaneous portion of the philtrum is devoid of the dimple and ridges that, in the non-cleft lip, define the shape and dimensions of the philtrum. The cutaneous roll of the prolabium is typically poorly defined when compared with the lateral lip elements, although it is usually better preserved in an incomplete bilateral cleft lip. The height of the prolabial vermilion is inadequate with the superior labial sulcus being shallow, and in some patients, entirely absent. Orbicularis muscle does not enter the prolabium; it therefore lies passively upon the premaxilla, which is protruded and may, in

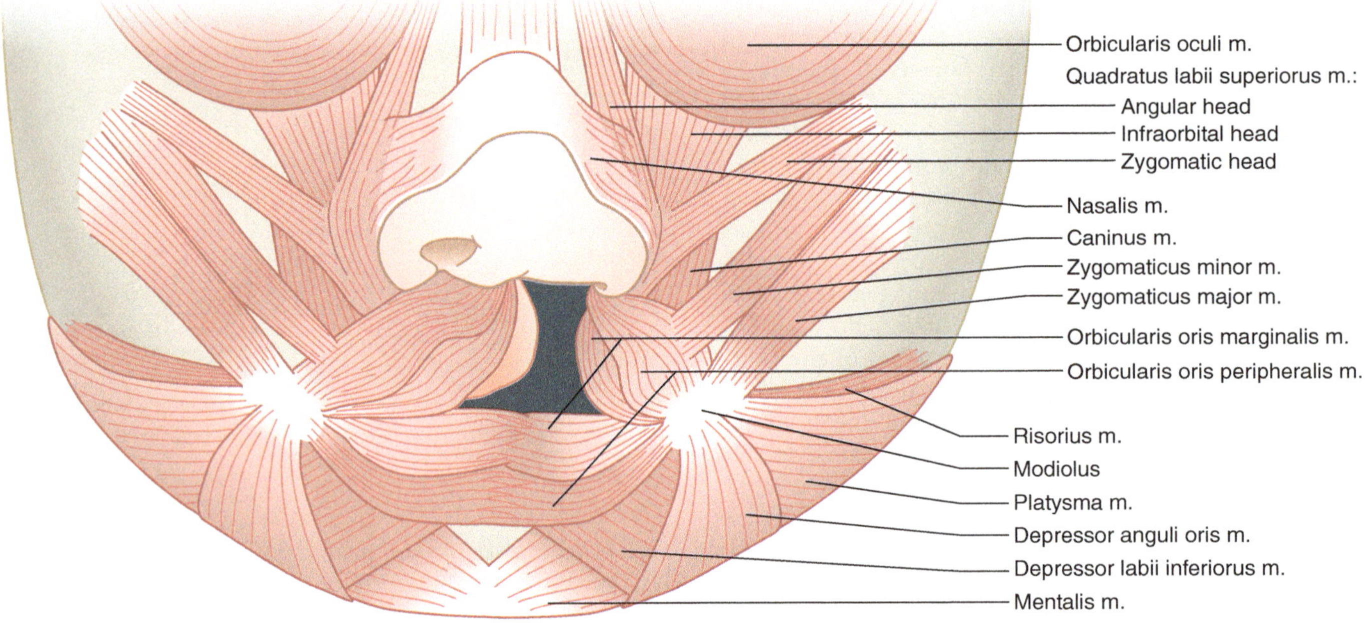

• **Fig. 16.3** Orientation of the orbicularis oris fibers in a patient with a complete left unilateral cleft lip. (Adapted from Millard RDJ. *Cleft Craft: the Evolution of its Surgery*. Boston: Little, Brown & Company; 1976.)

extreme cases, adopt a horizontal posture. The lateral lip elements in the bilateral cleft are similar to the lateral lip element of a unilateral cleft.

The inferior and superior labial arteries (which arise from the facial artery at the modiolus) are the primary blood supply to the lips (Fig. 16.4). They course close to the free border of the upper and lower lips, lying deep to the orbicularis muscle, juxtaposed to the mucosa, to anastomose with its fellow from the opposite side. The facial artery continues cranially along the line of the nasolabial fold, and after giving off the lateral nasal branch, becomes the angular artery, which then anastomoses with the dorsal nasal artery. The ascending septal branches of the superior labial artery nourish the columella and anastomose with the terminal branches of the anterior ethmoid artery and the lateral nasal artery.

In the unilateral cleft, the superior labial artery on the cleft side is unable to pass horizontally through the lip and therefore anastomoses with the ipsilateral lateral nasal artery. The resultant interruption of the upper lip arterial arcade is of little surgical importance in unilateral cases due to the density of collateral blood supply. However, in complete bilateral clefts, the prolabium receives no input from either the superior labial arteries or, indirectly, via the greater palatine arteries, and is therefore entirely reliant upon the terminal branches of the posterior septal artery (arising from the sphenopalatine artery), the anterior ethmoid artery and the lateral nasal artery.

The characteristics of the nasal deformity in the complete unilateral cleft were first described in 1931, and consists of a depressed cleft side nasal dome and splayed alar cartilages, with eversion of the alar rim and exposure of the nasal lining.[7] The cleft medial and lateral crura are not believed to be hypoplastic based on both cadaveric dissections and intraoperative observations. The cleft alar base is depressed due to the underlying maxillary hypoplasia. Furthermore, anomalous insertion of orbicularis oris into the alar base retracts it both laterally and inferiorly. The nasal spine, caudal nasal septum, and columella, together with the premaxilla, are deviated to the non-cleft side due to the unopposed action of the aberrant insertion of orbicularis oris. Nasal obstruction may result from septal deviation, turbinate hypertrophy, or obstruction of the external nasal valve by nasal webbing. In the bilateral cleft nose, the columella is typically short or nearly absent due to deficient soft tissue and the septum may be excessively broad.

Preoperative Assessment

It is essential to ensure that the infant is optimized prior to surgery; significant comorbidities are common in syndromic children and will inevitably require specialist pediatric input. Early liaison with the cleft anesthesia team is recommended, particularly if there are potential airway concerns. Failure to thrive is seen in approximately 40% of children with a palatal cleft and 9% of those with an isolated cleft lip, thus all cleft patients must be closely monitored preoperatively to ensure that they are gaining weight appropriately.[8] Close cooperation between the family and the cleft

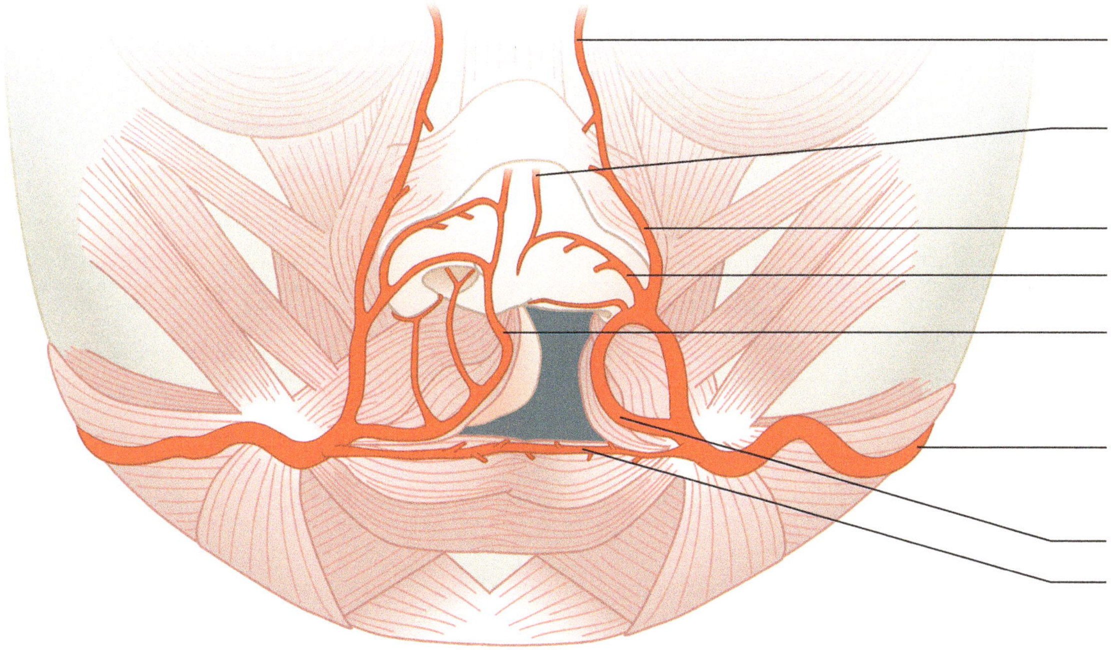

• **Fig. 16.4** Blood supply to the nasolabial complex in a patient with a complete left unilateral cleft lip. (Adapted from Millard RDJ. *Cleft Craft: the Evolution of its Surgery*. Boston: Little, Brown & Company; 1976.)

unit (via the clinical nurse specialist, dietician, and/or feeding specialist) is essential at this stage.

Although probably less controversial than the timing of palatal closure, currently no global consensus exists for the optimal timing for cheiloplasty. In 1966, Wilhelmsen and Musgrave proposed the "rule of tens" as a criterion for lip surgery: weight greater than 10 pounds (4.5 kg), hemoglobin over 10 g/dL and age over 10 weeks (which replaced a white cell count of less than 10×10^3 per mm^3 in their original iteration).[9] Millard observed that lip closure could occur at any time from birth to old age, and he advocated waiting until the child was 3 months of age as this achieved the best results in his opinion. Indeed, the majority of cleft centers defer surgery until the age of 3–6 months, since it allows the optimization of underlying medical issues, minimizes the anesthetic risks, and enables time for presurgical orthopedic treatment if indicated.

Straith performed neonatal lip repair under local anesthesia in the 1940s and many cleft centers continue to perform neonatal cleft lip repair (usually under general anesthetic) sometimes as early as 48 hours of age.[10] It has been argued that with modern specialist neonatal care and anesthetic support, the perioperative risks are minimized, and neonatal repair potentially facilitates improved integration of the child into the family network. There is little evidence to suggest that operating on neonatal cleft lips is unsafe. Although parents may express preference for earlier surgical intervention, there is no evidence of significant psychological morbidity in mothers when delaying repair until the age of 3 months.[11] The concept of an intrauterine cleft lip repair has garnered much interest due to the potential for scarless wound healing prior to 24 weeks' gestation. Furthermore, fetal repair might reasonably be expected to reduce the magnitude of the secondary "downstream" dentoalveolar and midfacial deformities. However, the technical challenges are vast, and although feasible in both small (murine and lapine) and large (ovine) animal models, albeit with guarded esthetic and functional results, the perceived benefits of fetal repair do not currently outweigh the significant risks of such early intervention.

The role of preoperative microbiological analysis in an attempt to predict the nasal and oropharyngeal flora at the time of cleft surgery is unhelpful, and culture results appear to have no influence on postoperative outcome regardless of whether antibiotics were used.[12] If children with an unrepaired cleft lip and palate undergo preoperative microbiological analysis (with swabs taken from the nasopharynx and oropharynx), approximately 30% will have positive cultures, with the predominant pathogen being *Staphylococcus aureus*, whilst beta-hemolytic streptococci were isolated in a small proportion of patients. The clinical significance of these results is unclear and debate continues as to whether preoperative microbiology analysis is justified. The evidence for cancelling an elective cleft procedure if a child has a concurrent upper respiratory tract infection remains ambiguous, although most cleft surgeons are cognisant of the increased postoperative risks, and would therefore be reluctant to proceed, favoring an honorable deferral for 4 weeks until the child has fully recovered.

TABLE 16.1 **Surgical Treatment Pathway for a Child with a Unilateral Complete Cleft Lip and Palate at The Hospital for Sick Children, Toronto, Canada, and the Spires Cleft Centre, Oxford, UK**

Patient Age	Hospital for Sick Children, Toronto	Spires Cleft Centre, Oxford
Prenatal diagnosis	Genetic counseling (if requested by family) Parental consultation with cleft surgeon	Genetic counseling (if requested by family) Parental consultation with cleft clinical nurse specialist
2 weeks	Presurgical orthopedics (if indicated)	Nil
3–6 months	Cleft lip repair and primary nasal correction	Cleft lip repair, vomerine flap closure of hard palate and primary nasal correction
9–14 months	Complete palate repair ± grommets	Soft palate repair ± grommets
≥3 years as required	Lip revision (if indicated)	Lip revision (if indicated)
≥4 years as required	Speech surgery (if indicated)	Speech surgery (if indicated)
≥7 years as required	Lobule rhinoplasty (if indicated)	Nil
8–10 years (mixed dentition)	Alveolar bone graft from iliac crest	Alveolar bone graft from iliac crest
≥7 years as required	Definitive septorhinoplasty (if indicated)	Nil
≥16–18 years (skeletal maturity) as required	Orthographic surgery (if indicated)	Orthographic surgery and/or Definitive cleft septorhinoplasty (if indicated)

A typical treatment pathway, from antenatal diagnosis to adulthood, for a child with a unilateral complete cleft lip and palate is outlined in Table 16.1; comparison is made between The Hospital for Sick Children in Toronto, Canada, and the Spires Cleft Centre in Oxford, UK. Whilst a child with an isolated incomplete cleft lip may require just the single operation, the burden of care in the case of a complete bilateral cleft of the lip and palate is far more substantial.

Presurgical Orthopedics

Historically, the first record of facial binding in order to realign the premaxilla in a complete bilateral cleft was in 1686. In the context of a complete unilateral cleft lip, presurgical orthopedics (PSO) is defined as the use of a device to improve the alignment of the maxillary arch segments in order to facilitate lip repair, and was first reported by McNeil in 1950, by utilizing a removable intraoral plate, and subsequently popularized by Burston. The principles have also been applied to the complete bilateral cleft lip in order to correct the protruded premaxilla.

PSO devices may be passive, such as a dental plate or facial strapping, or active, such as Latham's appliance, which is pinned to the child's maxilla, and is adjusted by turning an integral coaxial screw that gradually aligns the alveolar segments. In 1999, Grayson et al[13] introduced the concept of nasoalveolar molding (NAM), whereby the oral plate has nasal prong extensions that reposition the deformed nasal cartilages and lengthen the columella (Fig. 16.5). The resultant approximation of the alveolar segments allows the surgeon to perform a primary gingivoperiosteoplasty at the time of the lip repair, which is said to limit the need for secondary alveolar bone grafting in up to 60% of patients.[14]

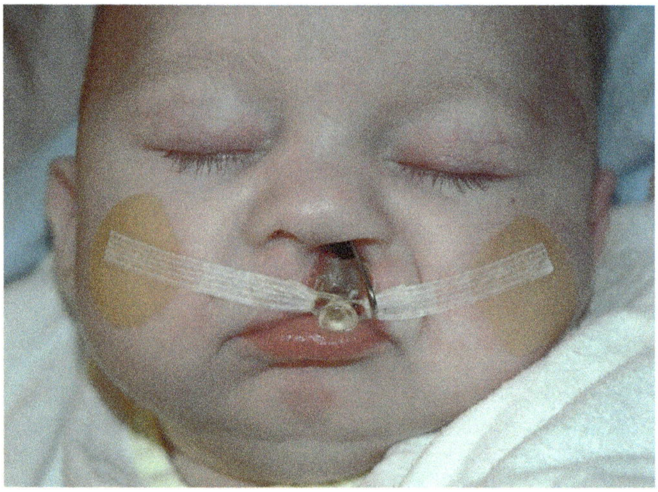

• **Fig. 16.5** Nasoalveolar moulding plate *in situ* with left nasal stent evident in a 3-month old infant with a complete unilateral cleft lip and palate.

In those institutions where PSO/NAM is not practiced, alternative strategies can be utilized to reduce alveolar cleft width, such as single-layer vomerine flap closure of the hard palate at the time of lip repair, with subsequent secondary bone grafting of the alveolus.

In spite of considerable enthusiasm for the deployment of PSO/NAM by its proponents, its adoption is by no means universal, with some units reserving its use for more severe deformities such as the wide unilateral cleft or asymmetrical bilateral cleft, while many units do not offer it as a treatment option. This may, in part, reflect concerns regarding the additional burden of care placed on families undergoing PSO/NAM treatment with the associated healthcare costs incurred. Moreover, robust evidence in support of the long-term positive effects of PSO or NAM is lacking; although as any surgeon who has struggled with a difficult primary lip repair may testify, the short-term benefits cannot be completely ignored. A recent systematic review of the literature failed to demonstrate a long-term benefit in the use of PSO.[15] While a systematic review examining the evidence for NAM reported that although there is a trend towards a positive effect, the results are inconsistent regarding long-term changes in nasal symmetry.[16] In 2013 Sommerlad presented the interim results of a randomized controlled study comparing PSO with controls in complete unilateral cleft lip and palate patients; no difference in esthetic or functional outcomes could be discerned at their 5-year and 10-year audit assessments.[17] The issue of PSO/NAM has a tendency to polarize opinion in the worldwide cleft community, a position that is unlikely to change until randomized controlled trial evidence with long-term follow-up becomes available for scrutiny.

Unilateral Cleft Lip Repair

The first recorded cheiloplasty was performed in China in AD 390. In renaissance Europe, Paré was extremely influential, with contemporaneous texts describing the scarification ("paring") of the cleft margins and approximation of the raw edges using needles and sutures. Husson first recognized that by creating curved incisions, a degree of lengthening of the lip repair could be achieved on wound apposition; a technique later refined by both Rose and Thompson. In 1844 Mirault identified that straight-line scars resulted in unsightly lip shortening, with the potential for notching, and introduced the concept of a triangular flap from the lateral lip element to both lengthen the lip and disrupt the scar. In 1949, LeMesurier recognized the importance of reconstructing the Cupid's bow using a quadrilateral flap from the lateral lip element, although it was Tennison who preserved the anatomy of the bow, and Randall who reduced the size of the triangular flap. Millard introduced his rotation-advancement technique in 1957, which has subsequently undergone numerous modifications. In 2005 Fisher published his anatomical subunit approximation technique, which utilizes the wound-lengthening principles of Rose and Thompson with the anatomic subunit approach of Berget and Mennick.

Principles of Surgical Repair

Regardless of the surgical technique employed, the principal goals of unilateral cleft lip repair remain constant. These include approximation of the medial and lateral lip elements at all levels (i.e., nostril sill, cutaneous roll, and vermilion–cutaneous junction) without loss of natural landmarks. Balance should be achieved by providing length where tissue is short and excision where height is excessive; poor quality tissue at the cleft margins should ideally be discarded. The scar of union should be placed along natural lines, with appreciation of the anatomical subunits of the nasolabial complex.

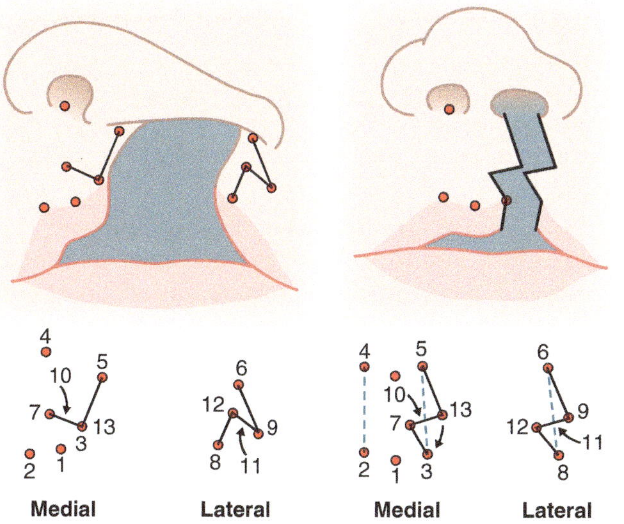

• **Fig. 16.6** The inferior triangle repair of Tennison as modified by Randall. (Modified with permission from Randall P. A triangular flap operation for the primary repair of unilateral clefts of the lip. *Plast Reconstr Surg Transplant Bull.* 1959;23:331–347.)

The nostril margins should be of equal circumference and the alar bases should be symmetric from the anterior view, with careful attention paid to reconstruction of a natural "nostril sill roll." Complete release of the aberrant attachments of the orbicularis oris muscle must be performed before undertaking a functional muscle reconstruction.

The height of the non-cleft side (i.e., the philtral column length from the lip–columellar crease to the Cupid's bow peak) provides the dimension that must be created by the cleft side reconstruction. The medial cleft side height (i.e., the philtral column length from the lip–columellar crease to the projected Cupid's bow peak) is short and will necessitate lengthening from the lateral cleft side lip height. The entire length of the Cupid's bow should be preserved in the medial lip element. In the lateral lip element, Noordhoff's point should be conserved and used to form the base of the philtral column incision. The cutaneous roll of the medial and lateral lip elements should be approximated in a side-to-side fashion (creating a "butt joint"). Vermilion height deficiency below the cleft side half of Cupid's bow should be augmented with attention paid to recreating a level vermilion-mucosal junction.

Operative Technique: Tennison–Randall Inferior Triangle Repair

The inferior triangle repair is a Z-plasty where the middle limb of the Z is shared by the incised medial and lateral cleft margins (Fig. 16.6). Whereas Tennison used a bent wire to stencil equal limbs of the Z-plasty scar, Randall refined the technique using calipers and geometric planning in order to minimize the size of the inferior triangle.[18] The "total lip height" of the non-cleft side is measured from a reference point in the nostril sill to the peak of the ipsilateral Cupid's bow. The "greater lip height" is measured on the medial cleft side from the proposed medial point of closure at the height of the lip in the nostril sill (symmetric with the reference point in the non-cleft side nostril sill) to the peak of the cleft side Cupid's bow. The difference between the total lip height and the greater lip height (i.e., the "lesser lip height") stipulates the base width of the inferior triangle required to level Cupid's bow.

There are a number of advantages of the inferior triangle repair. Firstly, nostril sill closure is accomplished by simple side-to-side approximation of the medial and lateral nostril sill elements, with resultant scarring at the base of the nose being kept to a minimum. Secondly, adequate lengthening of the medial lip height can be achieved even when the medial lip height is very short. Furthermore, the position of Noordhoff's point need not be compromised when the lateral lip height is short due to the lengthening effect of the Z-plasty. The repair may be criticized due to the non-anatomical alignment of the Z-plasty scar and the fact that secondary revisions may be hampered by the presence of the sizable triangular flap.

Operative Technique: Millard Rotation-Advancement Repair

The rotation-advancement technique is reported to account for the majority of lip repairs performed worldwide. The "rotation flap" is created by a curvilinear incision directed along the medial lip element such that it mirrors the non-cleft side philtral column in its lower half (Fig. 16.7).[19] The incision then gently arcs into the territory of the philtrum and approaches (but should never cross) the non-cleft side philtral column. This permits caudal rotation of the cleft side peak of Cupid's bow, and the resultant defect is resurfaced with a large triangular "advancement" flap from the lateral lip element. The triangular portion of pro-labial skin lateral to the "rotation flap" forms the "columella base flap," or "c flap," which rotates cranially to reconstruct the cleft side nostril sill. Millard noted that the rotation of Cupid's bow was often inadequate and subsequently introduced a "back-cut," which extends from the most cranial point of the rotation incision down the philtrum just medial to the non-cleft side philtral column. The resultant defect is now quadrilateral-shaped (rather than triangular) and can be filled by caudal rotation of the "c flap," however this risks lowering the transverse limb of the repair.

The main appeal of this repair is the "cut-as-you-go" approach and the preservation of the Cupid's bow and philtral dimple. In the lower portion of the lip, the scar mirrors the non-cleft side philtral column, however the esthetic result is compromised in the upper half of the lip as the scar fails to emulate a normal philtral column. Furthermore, excessive scarring is created at the base of the nose, and if the "c flap" is utilized to backfill the secondary defect created by the back-cut, it can no longer contribute to closure of the nostril sill, with the resultant risk of potential nostril stenosis. The cleft side alar base incision in Millard's original description produces a noticeable scar and is therefore

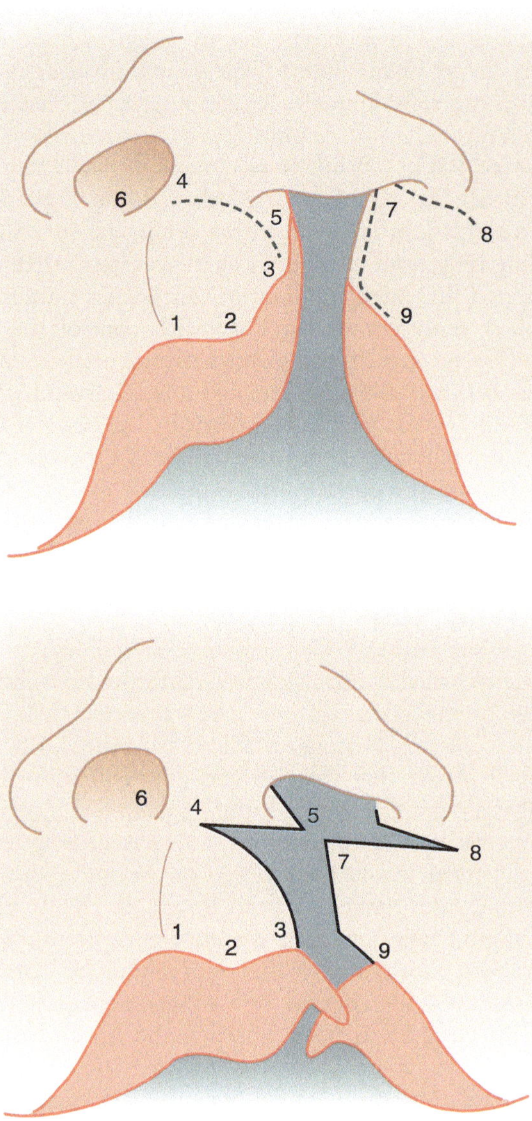

• **Fig. 16.7** Millard's original "rotation-advancement" technique of unilateral lip repair. (Modified with permission from Millard DR, Jr. Complete unilateral clefts of the lip. *Plast Reconstr Surg Transplant Bull.* 1960;25:595–605.)

best avoided, indeed many surgeons believe that such an aggressive alar base incision is unnecessary. The length of the marginal incision at the lateral lip must be of sufficient length to marry up with the full length of the corresponding rotation incision. In the case of a complete cleft with a vertically short lateral lip element, it may be necessary to extend the incision beyond Noordhoff's point in order to achieve adequate vertical height, which will further compromise the transverse length of the lateral lip. A criticism of the Millard technique, particularly in the wide cleft, is that it tends to produce a "short" lip; which can be "vertically short" if related to an inadequate rotation incision or back-cut, or "transversely short" if 'Noordhoff's point' is violated.

In 1987, Mohler published a modification to the standard rotation-advancement repair in an attempt to produce a scar that is more symmetric with the non-cleft philtral column in the upper half of the lip (Fig. 16.8).[20]

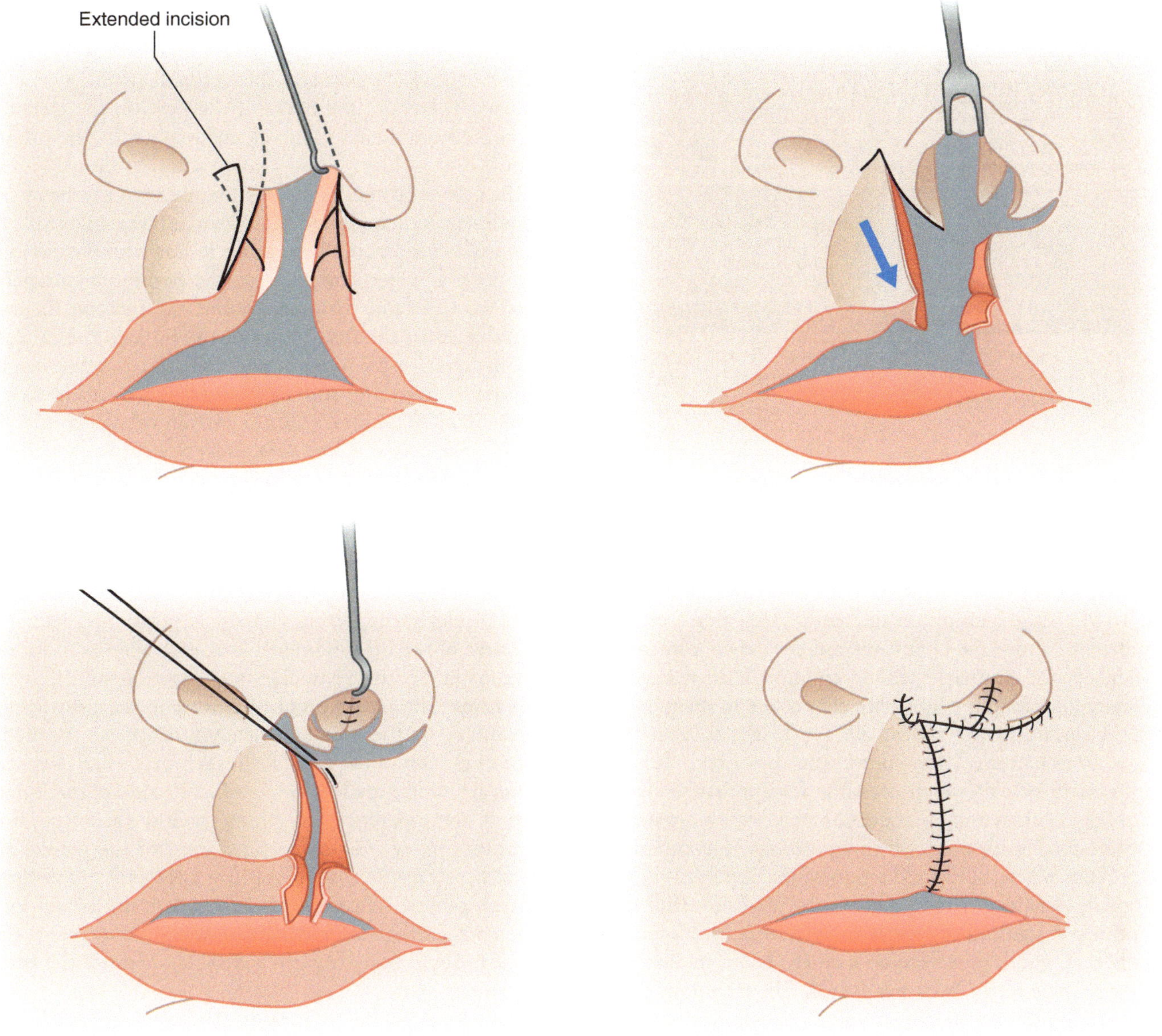

• **Fig. 16.8** Mohler's modification of the "rotation-advancement" repair with extension of the rotation incision into the columella and a right-angled back-cut to allow transposition of a Z-plasty into the lip. (Modified with permission from Mohler LR. Unilateral cleft lip repair. *Plast Reconstr Surg*. 1987;80:511–517.)

The curve of the rotation incision is straightened such that it extends into the columella base rather than towards the non-cleft philtral column. A 90° back-cut is created to the level of the labio-columella crease which allows the columella tissue to descend by transposing a Z-plasty into the lip such that the "advancement flap" is not required to encroach as medially, thus improving the lie of the scar. A relative contraindication to this approach is therefore a narrow columella. The resultant transverse limb of the repair is elevated such as to lie inconspicuously within the lip–nose junction. In common with all rotation-advancement repairs, the Mohler modification is prone to compromise of the transverse lateral lip length when the lateral lip is vertically short.

Noordhoff also modified Millard's original repair.[21] In the "Chang Gung repair," if rotation of Cupid's bow is inadequate, a small opening back-cut is created just above the cutaneous roll at the cleft side peak of Cupid's bow, into which is incorporated a small triangular flap from the lateral lip element. As well as providing additional height, the triangular flap also helps to accentuate the pout of the lip. Noordhoff also augmented the deficient vermilion below the cleft side Cupid's bow by means of a laterally based vermilion flap. Numerous additional modifications have been made to Millard's original "rotation-advancement" approach, with Stal et al providing a comprehensive account of the evolution of the technique.[22]

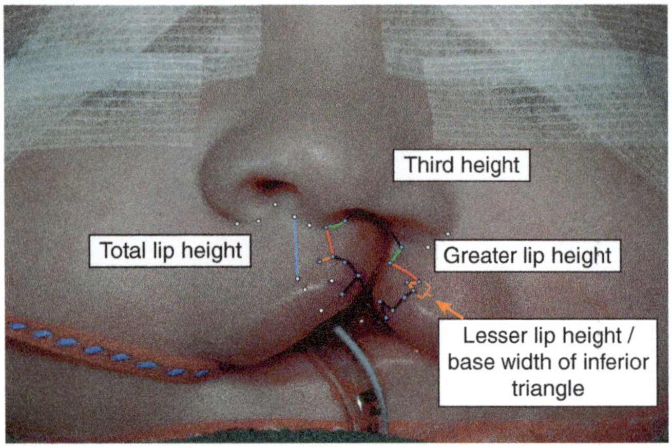

• **Fig. 16.9** The anatomical subunit approximation technique as described by Fisher. Key markings are shown, including the total lip height, greater lip height, lesser lip height, and the "third height."

Operative Technique: Fisher Anatomical Subunit Approximation Repair

The anatomical subunit approximation technique aims to produce a cutaneous scar along the "ideal line of repair" (Fig. 16.9).[23] The incision on the medial cleft side ascends from a point above the cutaneous roll such that it mirrors the ridge of the non-cleft philtral column. It then curves superolaterally along the lip–columellar crease to the medial point of closure in the nostril sill. Lip length is achieved by two mechanisms: the previously described Rose–Thompson principle (which accounts for approximately 1 mm of lengthening) and, if required, a small inferior triangle from the lateral lip element, which is positioned just superior to the cutaneous roll (a modification of the Tennison–Randall repair). The lengthening achieved by the Rose–Thompson principle significantly reduces the size of the inferior triangle that would otherwise be required had a traditional inferior triangle repair been performed. The technique also utilizes a Noordhoff's lateral vermilion triangle flap to augment the deficient vermilion height of the medial lip element on the cleft side.

This technique has a number of advantages over the inferior triangle and rotation-advancement repairs. In variance with the Millard technique, there is minimal scar at the base of the nose. The lip scar is positioned along the seams of anatomical subunits with the exception of, when required, a small triangle above the cutaneous roll. Tension is ideally positioned above the roll. Continuity of the cutaneous roll is achieved by side-to-side approximation of the roll elements. In common with the inferior triangle repair, lateral lip transverse length need not be compromised to achieve vertical height.

A summary of the skin markings for the anatomical subunit approximation technique is highlighted in Fig. 16.9. The Cupid's bow and philtral column heights are marked in the standard fashion, with the cleft side bow peak and philtral column heights being equidistant relative to the midline as the corresponding non-cleft side markings. Note that the non-cleft side Cupid's bow peak is not marked at the highest point of the curve of the lip, but rather where the straight portion of the non-cleft side half bow meets the convexity of the lateral lip element, as may be appreciated in Fig. 16.9. No such convexity exists on the cleft side of the medial lip element. Therefore, the curve of the bow on the cleft side will come from the lateral lip element lateral to Noordhoff's point.

The point of origin of the opening incision for the medial lip back-cut is then located just above the cutaneous roll (the "supra-white roll point") at a point in line with the cleft side bow peak and perpendicular to the vermilion–cutaneous junction. Caudally, from this point, the incision line will continue across the free border of the lip into the mucosa. The medial lip incision (equivalent to the greater lip height) will ascend from the "supra-white roll point" to the height of the cleft side philtral column (within the lip–columellar crease). The incision line then traverses superolaterally to the medial point of closure in the nostril sill (equivalent to the "third height").

The medial and lateral points of closure within the nostril sill are not distinct anatomical points and are arguably the hardest points to define in this repair. The medial point of closure in the nostril sill is positioned lateral to the curve of the lip–columellar crease. It will be positioned more medial in complete cases and more lateral in incomplete cases. The lateral point of closure in the nostril sill is then chosen on the lateral lip element, relative to the medial point of closure in the nostril sill, such that when these two points are approximated, two goals are accomplished: nares of equal circumference and symmetry of the alar bases from the anterior view. Gentle manipulation of the medial and lateral lip elements should confirm acceptable positioning of these points. In complete clefts where the lateral lip is tethered such that the medial and lateral lip elements cannot be brought together, it is advisable to release the lateral lip element first.

Calipers are used to measure the total lip height and greater lip height. The total lip height is measured with the lip at rest and is defined as the distance from the height of the non-cleft philtral column (at the lip–columellar crease) to the non-cleft side "supra-white roll point" (i.e., the non-cleft side equivalent to the point of origin of the opening incision for the medial lip back-cut). The greater lip height is measured with gentle downward traction on the lip to unfurl the medial lip and is defined as the distance from the height of the cleft side philtral column (at the lip–columellar crease) to the point of origin of the opening incision for the medial lip back-cut. The lesser lip height (equivalent to the base width of the small inferior triangle) is equal to the total lip height minus the greater lip height and less 1 mm (Fig. 16.10). The 1 mm accounts for the approximate length achieved by the Rose–Thompson principle. If an inferior triangle is required, the back-cut for the opening incision is drawn perpendicular to the greater lip height incision, and of a length equal to the lesser lip height (the inferior triangle being equilateral). The back-cut rotates the cleft side

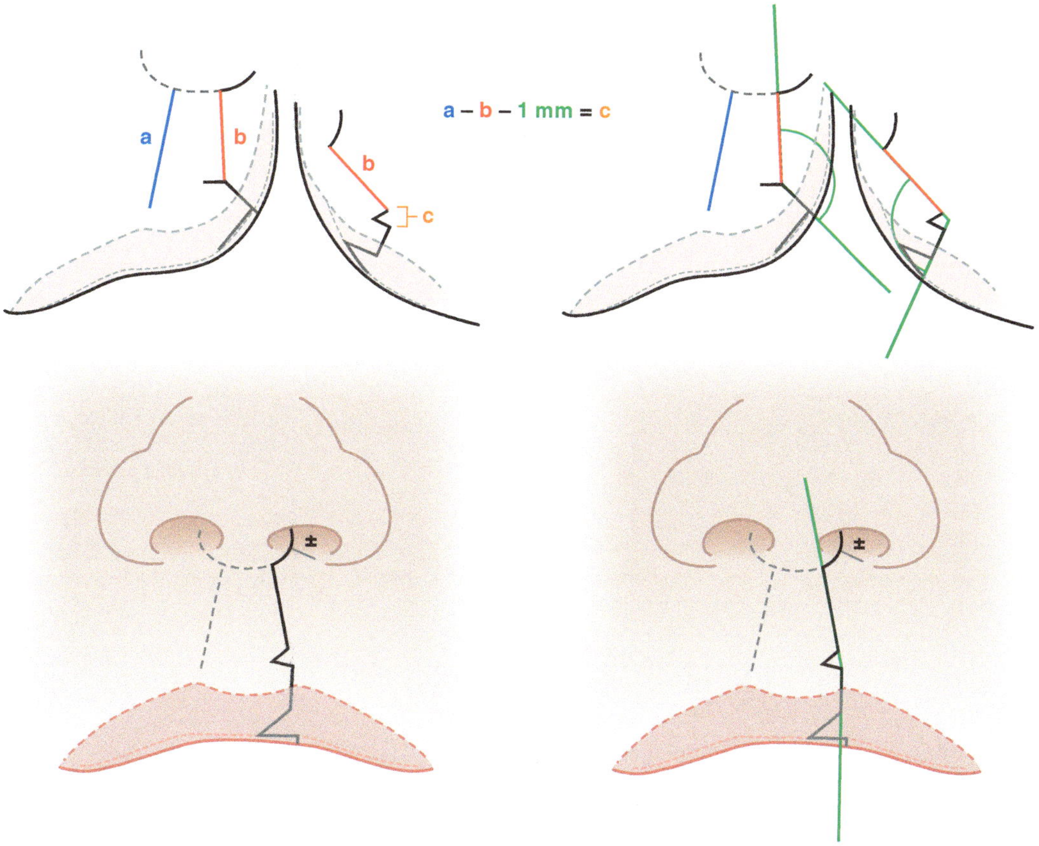

• **Fig. 16.10** The total lip height (*a*) and greater lip height (*b*) are measured from points just above the cutaneous roll (the "supra-white roll" point) at the bow peaks to the height of the ipsilateral philtral column in the lip–columellar crease. The base width of the inferior triangle (*c*) can then be calculated. Approximately 1 mm of lengthening occurs by the Rose–Thompson principle, thus reducing the size of the inferior triangle.

peak of Cupid's bow caudally. The lesser lip height is usually between 1 and 1.5 mm and never exceeds 2 mm. For incomplete clefts, an inferior triangle is often not necessary.

With respect to the lateral lip, Noordhoff's point is marked along the vermilion–cutaneous junction at the point where the cutaneous roll and red line begin to converge medially, as previously described (see Fig. 16.2). The natural convexity of the cutaneous roll lateral to Noordhoff's point is ideally suited for reconstruction of the cleft side curve of the bow. A "supra-white roll point" is marked above the cutaneous roll both in line with Noordhoff's point and perpendicular to the vermilion-cutaneous junction. Between the lateral point of closure in the nostril sill and the "supra-white roll point" on the lateral lip, three lengths must be accommodated: the greater lip height, the lesser lip height, and the "third height" (corresponding in length to the line connecting the height of the cleft side philtral column and the medial point of closure in the nostril sill). This is readily achieved by placing the greater lip height caliper on the lateral lip element such that its lower tip lies the lesser lip height distance away from the "supra-white roll point" and its upper tip lies the "third height" distance away from lateral point of closure in the nostril sill.

In the scenario of a complete cleft with a short vertical height to the lateral lip element, the angle of the greater lip height incision will be more horizontal and, in extreme cases, may be confluent with the upper limb incision of the inferior triangle (Fig. 16.11A). The contrary position is seen in an incomplete cleft with a relative excess of vertical height; the "third height" may be lengthened by lateralizing the medial and lateral points of closure within the nostril (Fig. 16.11B). If vertical height excess persists in spite of this maneuver, it may be necessary to perform a medially-based wedge excision of the upper lip below the lateral point of closure in the nostril sill (Fig. 16.11C). The lateral apex of this wedge excision should never extend laterally beyond subalare as this is unnecessary and leaves an unsightly scar. Care should be taken not to alter the vertical height of the lateral point of closure in the nostril sill as this will compromise the final vertical height of the alar insertion.

The vermilion deficiency below the cleft side half of Cupid's bow requires augmentation. An opening incision is created along the vermillion–mucosal junction below the cleft side half of Cupid's bow. This back-cut will receive a laterally based vermilion triangular flap from the lateral lip element as described by Noordhoff.

In incomplete clefts a wedge excision of the nostril sill above the medial and lateral points of nostril sill closure is performed (Fig. 16.12). The excision should be sufficient to balance the circumference of the nares with great care taken not to over-resect as the resultant nostril stenosis presents an unenviable reconstructive challenge. The mucosa of the

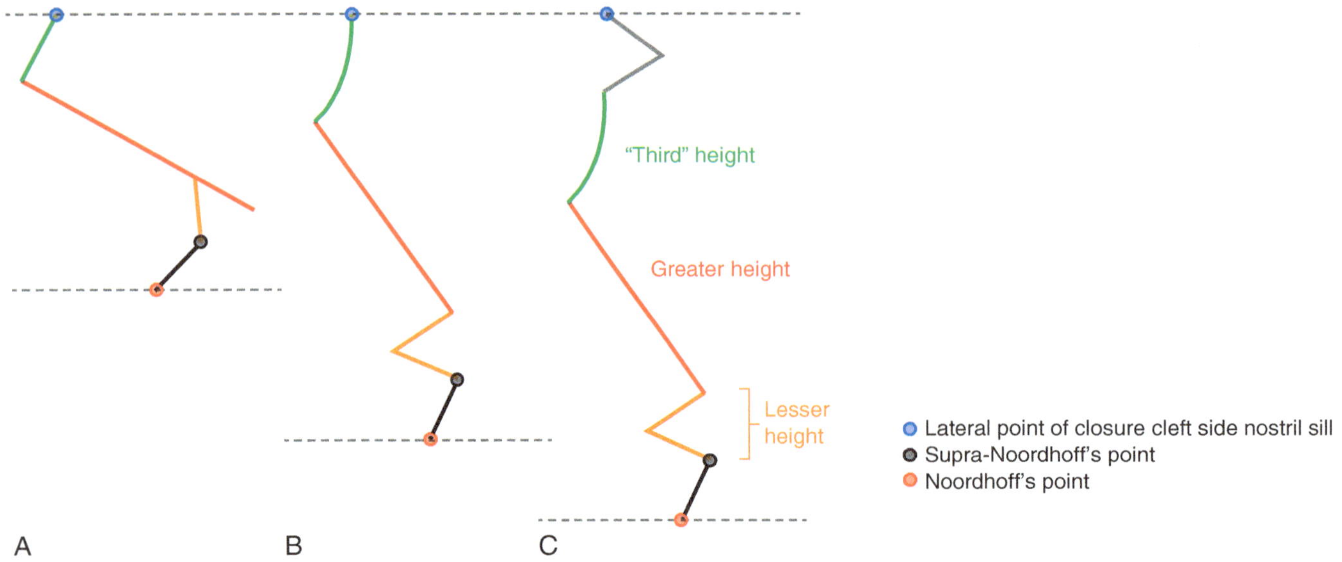

• **Fig. 16.11** Lateral lip markings vary depending on the vertical height of the lateral lip element. Note that the position of Nordhoff's point is not compromised regardless of the lateral lip height.

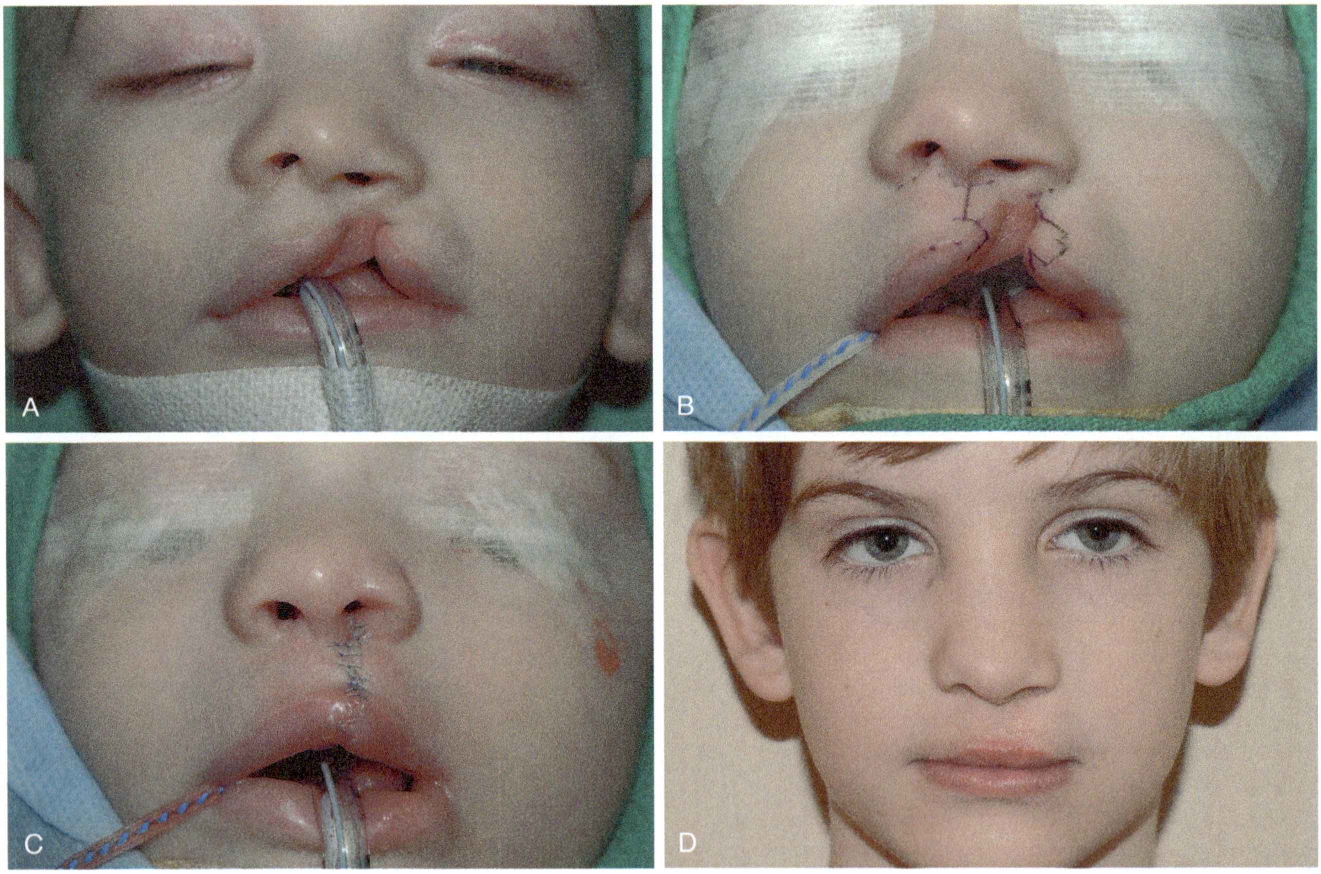

• **Fig. 16.12** Left incomplete unilateral cleft lip and palate: (A) preoperative view age 6 months; (B) intraoperative markings for the Fisher technique; (C) immediate postoperative view; (D) appearance at 9 years of age.

cleft margins is removed by wedge excision; a short lateral upper buccal sulcus advancement incision may be helpful on occasions.

In complete clefts, the mucosal incisions on the medial and lateral lip elements extend cranially to the points of attachment of each lip element to the greater and lesser alveolar segments, respectively. An upper buccal sulcus incision extending laterally from the point of attachment of the lateral lip element is made. From the medial point of closure in the nostril sill, the incision continues intranasally along the caudal margin of the septum for a distance of up to 12 mm to facilitate access for septal repositioning. The lateral free edge of the septal flap will receive the medial free edge of the lateral vestibular flap. The lateral vestibular flap is fashioned by incising from the lateral point of closure in the nostril sill to the attachment point of the lateral lip element to the alveolus and then along the piriform margin to allow supraperiosteal mobilization of the alar base. An anteriorly-based inferior turbinate flap may be required to augment nasal floor closure in clefts with a significant anteroposterior distance between the greater and lesser maxillary segments.

Bilateral Cleft Lip Repair

A fundamental advantage in bilateral cleft lip deformity is that of symmetry, however the philosophical approach to managing the premaxilla has evolved significantly over time. In 1556, Franco erroneously advocated primary excision of a protruding premaxilla – a practice now universally condemned. Fortunately, others subsequently recognized its importance and attempted to preserve it, often using quite elaborate devices to provide compression or traction in an attempt to correct its alignment. As the significance of the reconstructed orbicularis muscle in moulding the underlying premaxilla became recognized, the benefits of soft tissue closure over surgical setback on maxillary growth became evident.[24] The concept of a staged reconstruction by utilizing a temporizing lip adhesion has gained widespread acceptance. The destiny of the prolabium has provoked much debate, as techniques were devised to relocate it within the columella, the lip, or both. With a small prolabium, the importance of maintaining length of the frontonasal component was the motivation for using lateral lip skin flaps to augment below the prolabial component. In 1965 Manchester described a single-stage closure in which the prolabium is left attached to the premaxilla, the mucosa unrolled, and the lateral lip elements sutured to the sides of the prolabial component, without a muscle repair.[25] This technique therefore *preserved* the prolabial cutaneous roll and vermilion. Conversely, Millard's fundamental contribution was to *discard* the prolabial cutaneous roll and vermilion and introduce the lateral lip elements in order to achieve a single-stage bilateral lip closure. He also promulgated the concept of forked flaps to lengthen the columella.[26] Talmant favoured an unscarred Cupid's bow and, in a variant of the Manchester technique, preserved a large triangular mucosal flap from the prolabium to provide enhanced volume to the central tubercle.[27] Mulliken, in an adaptation of the Millard technique, also discards the prolabial cutaneous roll and vermilion.[28] He utilizes presurgical orthopedics by means of the Latham appliance and creates a narrow biconcave prolabial flap, establishes a median tubercle from the lateral labial elements, and aims to anatomically realign the alar cartilages.

The principles of bilateral cleft lip repair were outlined by Mulliken and include: the maintenance of symmetry (i.e., simultaneous bilateral lip repair), primary muscle reconstruction, adequate reduction of the prolabium, reconstruction of the median tubercle and Cupid's bow from the lateral lip elements, and primary rhinoplasty. PSO/NAM is commonly employed to control of the protruded premaxilla and to reduce the risk of the lateral alveolar segments collapsing medially thus creating a "locked out" premaxilla. A bilateral lip adhesion may be considered if PSO/NAM is either unavailable, not tolerated by the patient/family, or has been unsuccessful in correcting the premaxilla. The aim is to restore continuity to the upper lip such that it provides a physical constraint to the growth of the premaxilla. The incisions are designed so as to preserve the landmarks necessary for a subsequent definitive lip repair. Premaxillary setback is no longer recommended as a primary procedure due to the deleterious effects on midfacial growth.

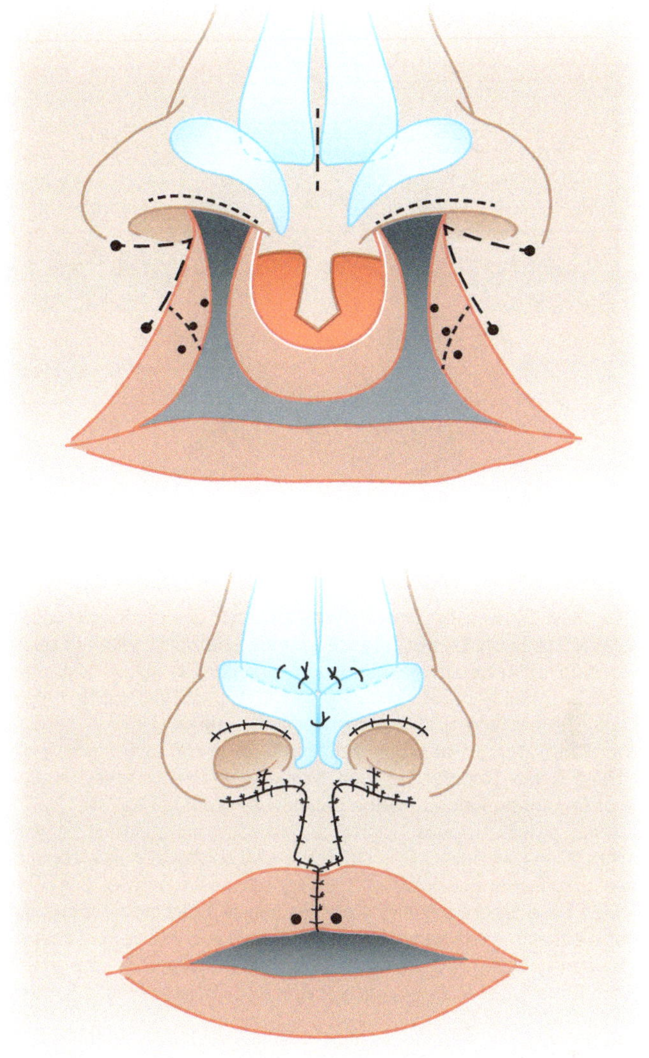

• **Fig. 16.13** Mulliken's method of single-stage bilateral complete cleft lip repair. (Modified with permission from Kohout MP, Monasterio-Aljaro L, Farkas LG, Mulliken JB. Photogrammetric comparison of two methods for synchronous repair of bilateral cleft lip and nasal deformity. *Plast Reconstr Surg.* 1998;102:1339–1349.)

Mulliken initially advocated a two-stage repair, however he subsequently abandoned the use of forked prolabial flaps

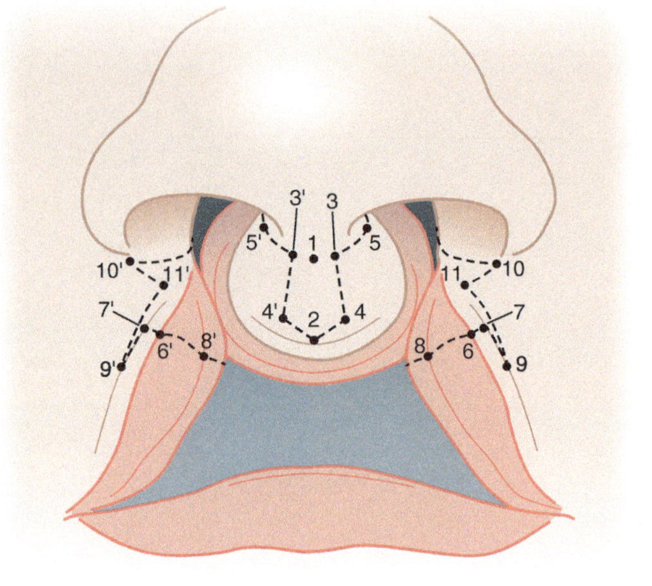

• **Fig. 16.14** Fisher's surgical markings for repair of a complete bilateral cleft lip. Points on the patient's left side are described, with the corresponding right-sided points assigned the prime (′) symbol. The corners of the prolabial skin are marked 3 and 4; 1 and 2 denote its height. Point 5 is just lateral to the lip–columellar crease. Point 6 denotes Noordhoff's point. Point 7 is the "supra-white roll" point, with point 8 being below Noordhoff's point on the vermilion–mucosal junction. Point 9 is made just above the cutaneous roll lateral to point 7. The distance between points 7 and 9 should equal the distance between points 2 and 4. Point 10 is placed medial to the alar insertion and meets point 5 at the height of the lip repair at the anterior nostril sill. Point 11 is positioned near the cleft margin at a distance from point 9 that is equal to the distance between points 3 and 4, and at a distance from point 10 that is equal to the distance between points 3 and 5. (From Bentz M, et al. *Principles & Practice of Pediatric Plastic Surgery*. Thieme NY. 2008.)

in favor of a single-stage repair (Fig. 16.13). He established that sufficient primary columellar lengthening and nasal tip projection could be achieved in a single procedure by manipulation of the alar cartilages (which are splayed and rotated caudally). He ceased creating an additional vertical nasal tip incision and accessed the alar cartilages via bilateral rim incisions alone. As the prolabial cutaneous roll and vermilion is of poor quality and should be discarded, Mulliken recommended a biconcave prolabial flap that is 2 mm wide at the lip–columellar angle and 4–5 mm wide between the bow peaks. The upper labial sulcus is invariably deficient in complete bilateral cleft lips and is usually augmented by a caudally-based prolabial mucosal flap that is draped over the premaxillary periosteum in order to reconstruct the posterior wall of the upper labial sulcus.

Fisher's method of bilateral lip repair utilizes a tie-shaped prolabial shield flap, although this may be modified depending on the ethnicity of the patient and the parental appearance (Fig. 16.14).[29] The dimensions of the prolabial flap in a 4–6-month-old child are typically 2.5–3 mm wide at the lip–columellar junction, 3.5–4.5 mm wide between the bow peaks, and 6–8 mm in height (Fig. 16.15). From the base of the prolabial flap at the lip–columella angle, the incisions pass superolaterally in a curvilinear fashion into each nostril sill. Noordhoff's point is marked on each lateral lip segment at the vermilion-cutaneous junction; in perpendicular orientation with the vermilion–cutaneous junction, and in alignment with Nordhoff's point, a "supra-white roll" point and a vermilion–mucosal junction point are marked. The incision along these three points is convex medially across the vermilion in order to replicate the median tubercle. A lateral back-cut is created from the "supra-white roll" point parallel with the vermilion–cutaneous junction, thus creating a cutaneous roll–vermilion flap whose geometry precisely corresponds to the caudal dimensions of the prolabial flap. Release of the lateral lip elements is performed via an upper lateral buccal sulcus incision in order to minimize the tension of the repair, with the soft tissues being freed from the underlying maxilla in a supraperiosteal plane such that the alar bases are completely mobilized. Aberrant insertions of the orbicularis oris muscle should be released from the lateral lip skin and the alar bases to allow descent of the cutaneous roll–vermilion flaps. The upper labial sulcus is recreated in a similar manner utilizing a prolabial mucosal flap. The interalar base width is reduced by means of an alar base cinch suture. A conservative primary rhinoplasty is advocated with the alar base dissection extending cephalad in order to release the attachments of the alar–accessory cartilage complex from the lateral piriform margin. The nasal tip is not routinely dissected and internal nasal valve plication sutures are employed.

Primary Nasal Correction

The timing of nasal correction may be considered to be primary (concurrent with cheiloplasty), intermediate (during the school years), or secondary (once facial growth is complete). The concept of primary repositioning of the alar cartilages was advocated by McComb and Coghlan, who disproved the belief that manipulation of the nasal cartilages might adversely affect growth.[30] The Tajima technique utilizes a reverse-U incision along the alar margin and redistributes the overhanging skin of the alar margin to augment deficient lining.[31] Open approaches, such as that described by Trott and Mohan, afford excellent visualization of the alar domes, but may compromise prolabial blood supply if adopted in complete bilateral cases, and carry a risk of nostril stenosis.[32] The goals of primary rhinoplasty include improving nasal contour, symmetry, and nasal tip projection, with relocation of the caudal nasal septum. Primary rhinoplasty may reduce the complexity of a definitive secondary rhinoplasty procedure. The potential risks of a primary rhinoplasty include iatrogenic deformity to the skin envelope and the introduction of scarring, which may complicate subsequent interventions.

Nasal splints, such as the commercially available silicone Koken conformers, are frequently used after primary rhinoplasty as they are believed to maintain the nostril contour postoperatively, and may reduce the risk of relapse.

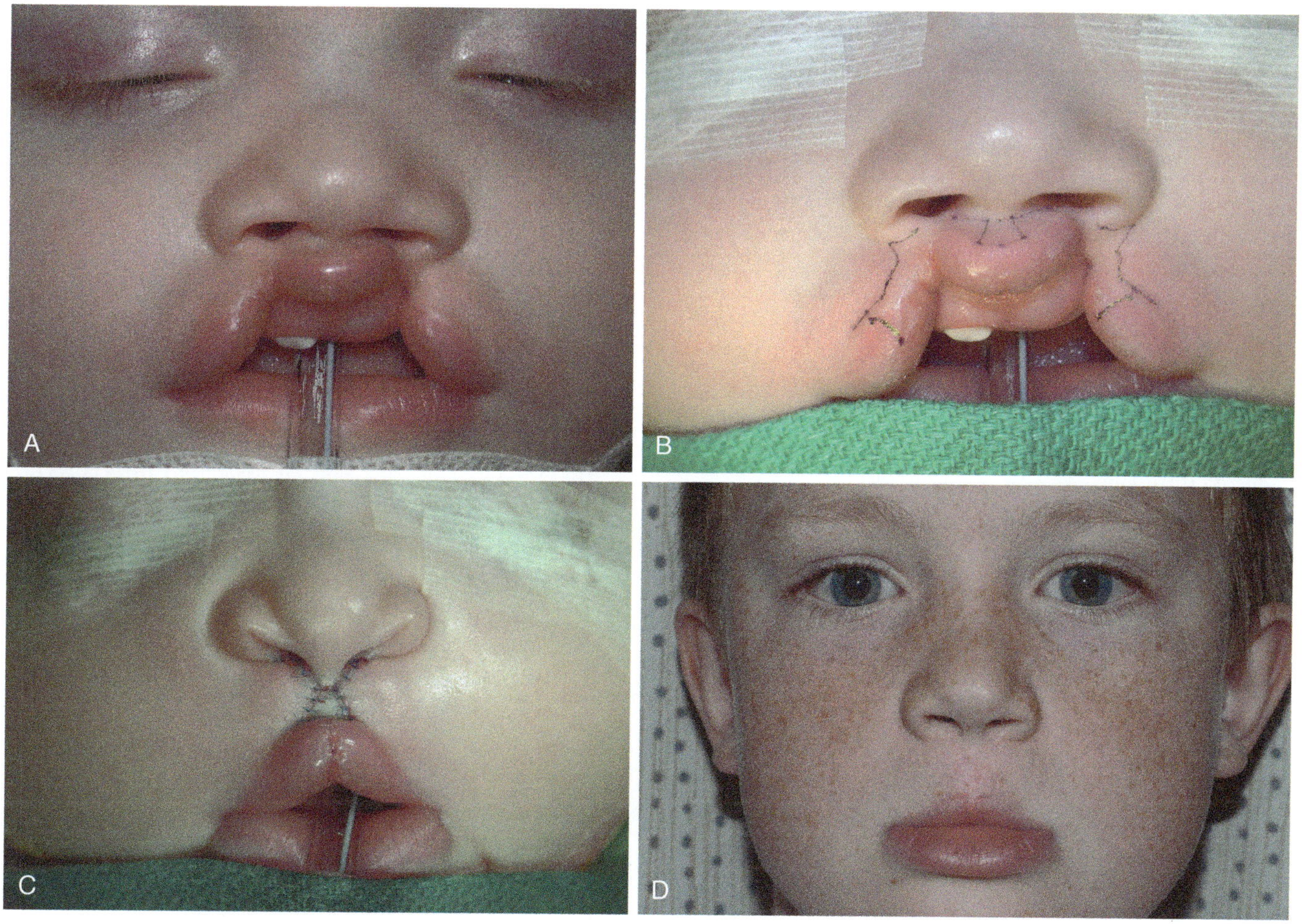

• **Fig. 16.15** Incomplete bilateral cleft lip and palate (no PSO necessary): (A) preoperative view age 5 months; (B) intraoperative markings for the Fisher bilateral technique; (C) immediate postoperative view; and (D) appearance at 10 years of age.

Evidence for their efficacy is largely anecdotal. The optimal duration of treatment is much debated, ranging from 5 days to many months or more. Moreover, patient–parental compliance is essential and is typically the rate-limiting step for their continued use.

Postoperative Care

The necessity for elbow restraints is much debated; at The Hospital for Sick Children in Toronto they are worn for 2 weeks postoperatively, whilst at the Children's Hospital in Oxford no splints are employed. Children may resume oral feeding immediately in the recovery room following surgery. Most units discharge patients the following day, although day-case repairs are becoming increasingly common in selected patients. If nonabsorbable sutures are used, removal is undertaken on the 5th–7th postoperative day, often under sedation or general anesthesia. Concerns regarding repeated anesthetics on the neurocognitive development of children, a desire to minimize the burden of care in this patient cohort, and to rationalize healthcare resources, has resulted in the use of absorbable skin sutures becoming increasingly widespread. Absorbable sutures may be associated with increased complications, including abscess formation or permanent suture marks, however, to date, the two closure methods have not been scientifically evaluated in the context of an adequately powered randomized controlled trial. Significant variance exists with regards to the need for a postoperative dressing. The preference at The Hospital for Sick Children in Toronto is for topical bacitracin–polymyxin B ointment, which allows adequate wound toilet to prevent excessive crusting; in Oxford the use of topical yellow paraffin is preferred. The use of intraoperative cyanoacrylate tissue adhesives (e.g., Dermabond) – often replacing the need for skin sutures when combined with deep dermal sutures – is becoming increasingly popular. In some centers a Logan bow may be employed to minimize tension across the lip repair, particularly in wider clefts.

Complications and Revision Surgery

Airways obstruction and anesthetic complications are rare in otherwise healthy infants. Rare potential complications include bleeding, infection, and wound dehiscence. A degree of scar contraction is inevitable, which will lead to a shortened lip at the early postoperative check. However, it invariably responds favorably to regular scar massage. Hypertrophic scars are less common, with keloid scars being extremely rare, even in darker skin types. Late inclusion dermoid cysts are occasionally seen.

Lip repairs performed with adherence to the defined principles are capable of producing reconstructions of excellent quality with minimal secondary deformity. Minor revisions, such as mucosal redundancy on the cleft side, can usually be deferred at least until the time of alveolar bone grafting. More significant deformities invariably warrant a complete lip revision. Timing is critical from the perspective of the child's psychosocial development; indeed the deformity may need addressing prior to commencing school. A secondary septorhinoplasty is commonplace in patients with a complete unilateral cleft lip and palate, and should be deferred until facial growth is complete.

Outcomes

Determining objective standardized outcome measures for cleft patients has been notoriously difficult to achieve. Indeed no international unanimity exists, although initiatives such as the International Consortium on Health Outcomes Measurement are attempting to address this shortfall. The 1992 Eurocleft study was the first international multicenter audit to compare treatment results in children with a unilateral cleft lip and palate.[33] Nasolabial esthetics were assessed by a panel using cropped 2D photographs, with significant differences in outcome noted between centers. Limitations exist with still photographs, with video analysis essential for the assessment of dynamic facial appearance and the quality of orbicularis oris reconstruction. Three-dimensional imaging is an exciting adjunctive tool in esthetic assessment. Quantitative measurement of nasolabial symmetry from 2D photographs is now possible using SymNose software.[34] A universally agreed objective method of facial esthetic assessment is vital if robust comparisons are to be made between centers.

The primary aim of cleft lip repair is to achieve a functional and esthetically acceptable nasolabial appearance by minimizing the visible stigmata of the cleft-related deformity. However, the psychological status of cleft patients, in particular their socioemotional functioning, is critical for their ability to fully integrate into society and lead content and fulfilling lives. Cleft patients achieve a similar level of educational and vocational attainment as controls, although economic achievement may be less marked; patients with cleft lip and palate have impaired psychological wellbeing with increased levels of anxiety and depression.[35] Many avoid positions that expose them to direct public contact; cleft patients are less likely to marry, particularly those with a bilateral deformity. These issues highlight the importance of the clinical psychologist as an integral member of the cleft service. The use of patient reported outcome measures (PROMs), such as CLEFT-Q, in the assessment of outcomes that matter to patients will become increasingly important.[36]

Conclusion

In 1937 Kilner stated, "there is no branch of surgery that offers greater fascination than that which concerns itself with the repair of congenital clefts of the lip and palate, and none in which successful results give greater satisfaction." He acknowledged that surgeons shoulder a tremendous responsibility for treating these children, although to achieve results of the highest standard requires the collective effort of every member of the multidisciplinary team and a sound relationship with the child and their family.

References

1. Curtis EJ, Fraser FC, Warburton D. Congenital cleft lip and palate: risk factors for counseling. *Am J Dis Child.* 1961;102:853–857.
2. Grosen D, Chevrier C, Skytthe A, et al. A cohort study of recurrence patterns among more than 54,000 relatives of oral cleft cases in Denmark: support for the multifactorial threshold model of inheritance. *J Med Genet.* 2010;47:162–168.
3. Offerdal K, Jebens N, Syvertsen T, Blaas HG, Johansen OJ, Eik-Nes SH. Prenatal ultrasound detection of facial clefts: a prospective study of 49,314 deliveries in a non-selected population in Norway. *Ultrasound Obstet Gynecol.* 2008;31:639–646.
4. Sommerlad M, Patel N, Vijayalakshmi B, et al. Detection of lip, alveolar ridge and hard palate abnormalities using two-dimensional ultrasound enhanced with the three-dimensional reverse-face view. *Ultrasound Obstet Gynecol.* 2010;36:596–600.
5. Descamps MJ, Golding SJ, Sibley J, McIntyre A, Alvey C, Goodacre T. MRI for definitive in utero diagnosis of cleft palate: a useful adjunct to antenatal care? *Cleft Palate Craniofac J.* 2010;47:578–585.
6. Mulliken JB, Pensler JM, Kozakewich HP. The anatomy of Cupid's bow in normal and cleft lip. *Plast Reconstr Surg.* 1993;92:395–403; discussion 4.
7. Blair V, Brown JB. Nasal abnormalities, fancied and real surgery. *Gynecol Obstet.* 1931;53.
8. Pandya AN, Boorman JG. Failure to thrive in babies with cleft lip and palate. *Br J Plast Surg.* 2001;54:471–475.
9. Wilhelmsen HR, Musgrave RH. Complications of cleft lip surgery. *Cleft Palate J.* 1966;3:223–231.
10. Straith CL, Pilling MA, Lewis JR. Repair of single cleft lip by the Hagedorn–Le Mesurier technic. *J Int Coll Surg.* 1950;13:394–401.
11. Slade P, Emerson DJ, Freedlander E. A longitudinal comparison of the psychological impact on mothers of neonatal and 3 month repair of cleft lip. *Br J Plast Surg.* 1999;52:1–5.
12. Thomas GP, Sibley J, Goodacre TE, Cadier MM. The value of microbiological screening in cleft lip and palate surgery. *Cleft Palate Craniofac J.* 2012;49:708–713.
13. Grayson BH, Santiago PE, Brecht LE, Cutting CB. Presurgical naso-alveolar molding in infants with cleft lip and palate. *Cleft Palate Craniofac J.* 1999;36:486–498.
14. Dec W, Shetye PR, Davidson EH, et al. Presurgical nasoalveolar molding and primary gingivoperiosteoplasty reduce the need for bone grafting in patients with bilateral clefts. *J Craniofacial Surg.* 2013;24:186–190.
15. Uzel A, Alparslan ZN. Long-term effects of presurgical infant orthopedics in patients with cleft lip and palate: a systematic review. *Cleft Palate Craniofac J.* 2011;48:587–595.
16. van der Heijden P, Dijkstra PU, Stellingsma C, van der Laan BF, Korsten-Meijer AG, Goorhuis-Brouwer SM. Limited evidence

for the effect of presurgical nasoalveolar molding in unilateral cleft on nasal symmetry: a call for unified research. *Plast Reconstr Surg*. 2013;131:62e–71e.
17. Sell D, Hay N, Chorbachi R, et al. *A Randomised Controlled Trial of Presurgical Orthopaedics: Outcomes at 5 Years and 10 Years of Age. 12th International Congress on Cleft Lip/Palate and Related Craniofacial Anomalies*; 2013. Florida: Orlando.
18. Randall P. A triangular flap operation for the primary repair of unilateral clefts of the lip. *Plast Reconstr Surg Transplant Bull*. 1959;23:331–347.
19. Millard Jr DR. Complete unilateral clefts of the lip. *Plast Reconstr Surg Transplant Bull*. 1960;25:595–605.
20. Mohler LR. Unilateral cleft lip repair. *Plast Reconstr Surg*. 1987;80:511–517.
21. Noordhoff MS. *The Surgical Technique for the Unilateral Cleft Lip-Nasal Deformity*. Taipei, Taiwan: Noordhoff Craniofacial Foundation; 1997.
22. Stal S, Brown RH, Higuera S, et al. Fifty years of the Millard rotation-advancement: looking back and moving forward. *Plast Reconstr Surg*. 2009;123:1364–1377.
23. Fisher DM. Unilateral cleft lip repair: an anatomical subunit approximation technique. *Plast Reconstr Surg*. 2005;116:61–71.
24. Friede H, Pruzansky S. Longitudinal study of growth in bilateral cleft lip and palate, from infancy to adolescence. *Plast Reconstr Surg*. 1972;49:392–403.
25. Manchester WM. The repair of bilateral cleft lip and palate. *Br J Surg*. 1965;52:878–882.
26. Millard DR. Bilateral cleft lip and a primary forked flap: a preliminary report. *Plast Reconstr Surg*. 1967;39:59–65.
27. Talmant JC. Current trends in the treatment of bilateral cleft lip and palate. *Oral Maxillofac Surg Clin North Am*. 2000;12:421–441.
28. Mulliken JB. Principles and techniques of bilateral complete cleft lip repair. *Plast Reconstr Surg*. 1985;75:477–487.
29. Fisher DM, Sommerlad BC. Cleft lip, cleft palate, and velopharyngeal insufficiency. *Plast Reconstr Surg*. 2011;128:342e–360e.
30. McComb HK, Coghlan BA. Primary repair of the unilateral cleft lip nose: completion of a longitudinal study. *Cleft Palate Craniofac J*. 1996;33:23–30; discussion 1.
31. Tajima S, Maruyama M. Reverse-U incision for secondary repair of cleft lip nose. *Plast Reconstr Surg*. 1977;60:256–261.
32. Trott JA, Mohan N. A preliminary report on open tip rhinoplasty at the time of lip repair in unilateral cleft lip and palate: the Alor Setar experience. *Br J Plast Surg*. 1993;46:363–370.
33. Shaw WC, Asher-McDade C, Brattstrom V, et al. A six-center international study of treatment outcome in patients with clefts of the lip and palate: Part 1. Principles and study design. *Cleft Palate Craniofac J*. 1992;29:393–397.
34. Pigott RW, Pigott BB. Quantitative measurement of symmetry from photographs following surgery for unilateral cleft lip and palate. *Cleft Palate Craniofac J*. 2010;47:363–367.
35. Ramstad T, Ottem E, Shaw WC. Psychosocial adjustment in Norwegian adults who had undergone standardised treatment of complete cleft lip and palate. I. Education, employment and marriage. *Scand J Plast Reconstructr Surg Hand Surg*. 1995;29:251–257.
36. Wong Riff KWY, Tsangaris E, Goodacre TEE, et al. What matters to patients with cleft lip and/or palate: an international qualitative study informing the development of the CLEFT-Q. *Cleft Palate Craniofac J*. 2018;55:442–450.

17 Cleft Palate and Velopharyngeal Dysfunction

SABRINA CUGNO AND BRIAN C. SOMMERLAD

For video accompanying this chapter see ExpertConsult.com. See inside cover for access details.

Embryology

The primary and secondary palates arise from the frontonasal process and palatal processes of the maxilla, respectively, separated by the incisive foramen. From the incisive foramen, fusion of these processes occurs, progressing anteriorly during weeks 5–6 for the primary palate and posteriorly in weeks 7–8 for the secondary palate. Aberration of this process results in clefts between these embryologically distinct regions. More specifically, a cleft of the primary palate occurs between the premaxilla and ipsilateral palatal process of the maxilla, while a cleft of the secondary palate occurs between the two palatal shelves, with each shelf united to the premaxilla.

Cleft palate can occur in isolation or in combination with cleft lip, unilaterally or bilaterally. A cleft of the lip involving the primary palate terminates at the incisive foramen, in keeping with the embryological origin of these structures as previously described. When a cleft of the lip and primary palate occurs in combination with a cleft of the secondary palate, the latter two malformations may be in continuity, resulting in the classic unilateral or bilateral cleft lip and palate or discontinuous (for example, cleft lip and primary palate with cleft of the soft palate or incomplete cleft lip and complete cleft of the secondary palate) (Fig. 17.1). An isolated cleft palate is subclassified as complete or incomplete, with the latter involving the soft palate with or without a portion of the posterior hard palate. In isolated cleft palate, the vomer is usually midline, vertically oriented, and attached to the palatal shelves as far back as the anterior extent of the cleft. The vomer also maintains a vertical orientation in complete bilateral cleft lip and palate; however, it may be laterally deviated contingent on the orientation of the premaxilla from which the vomer projects. This is in contradistinction to the morphology of the vomer in unilateral cleft lip and palate, where the cranial portion of the vomer is almost vertical with angulation (often at 90 degrees) of the caudal segment towards the palatal shelf to which it is attached on the non-cleft side. The point of attachment between vomer and palatal shelf can be discerned by the color variance of nasal and oral mucosa, respectively.

Isolated cleft palate is epidemiologically and etiologically distinct from cleft lip and palate. The incidence of cleft lip and palate varies by race, with approximately 2 in 1000 in Orientals, 1 in 1000 in Caucasians, and 0.4 in 1000 in Afro-Caribbean populations. Moreover, males are twice as likely to be affected than females. In contrast, isolated cleft palate occurs in 1 in 2000 live births across all ethnic backgrounds and more commonly in females, with a 2:1 predominance over males. Of all orofacial clefts, approximately 20% are isolated cleft lips, 35% isolated cleft palates, and 45% are clefts involving lip and palate. The etiology of clefting is multifactorial, including genetic factors, environmental factors and gene–environment interactions. Environmental risk factors include maternal obesity, diabetes mellitus, exposure to alcohol, smoke, diet, viral infections, drugs and various teratogenic agents, as well as physical and/or emotional stress. A strong association between the interferon regulatory factor 6 (*IRF6*) gene and nonsyndromic cleft lip and palate has been demonstrated. It has been reported that aberrations of *IRF6* comprise 12% of the genetic contribution to cleft lip and palate and increase the risk of recurrence threefold in families with one affected child.[1] The familial association for cleft palate is commonly cited as follows:

- If normal parents have a child with a cleft palate, the frequency of cleft palate in the next child is estimated at 2%
- If normal parents with a family history of cleft palate have a child with cleft palate, the risk for the next child is 7%
- If normal parents have two children with cleft palate, the risk for the next child is 1%
- If one parent has a cleft palate and no previously affected children, the risk for the next child is approximately 6%
- If one parent has a cleft palate and a child with cleft palate, the risk for the next child is 15%.

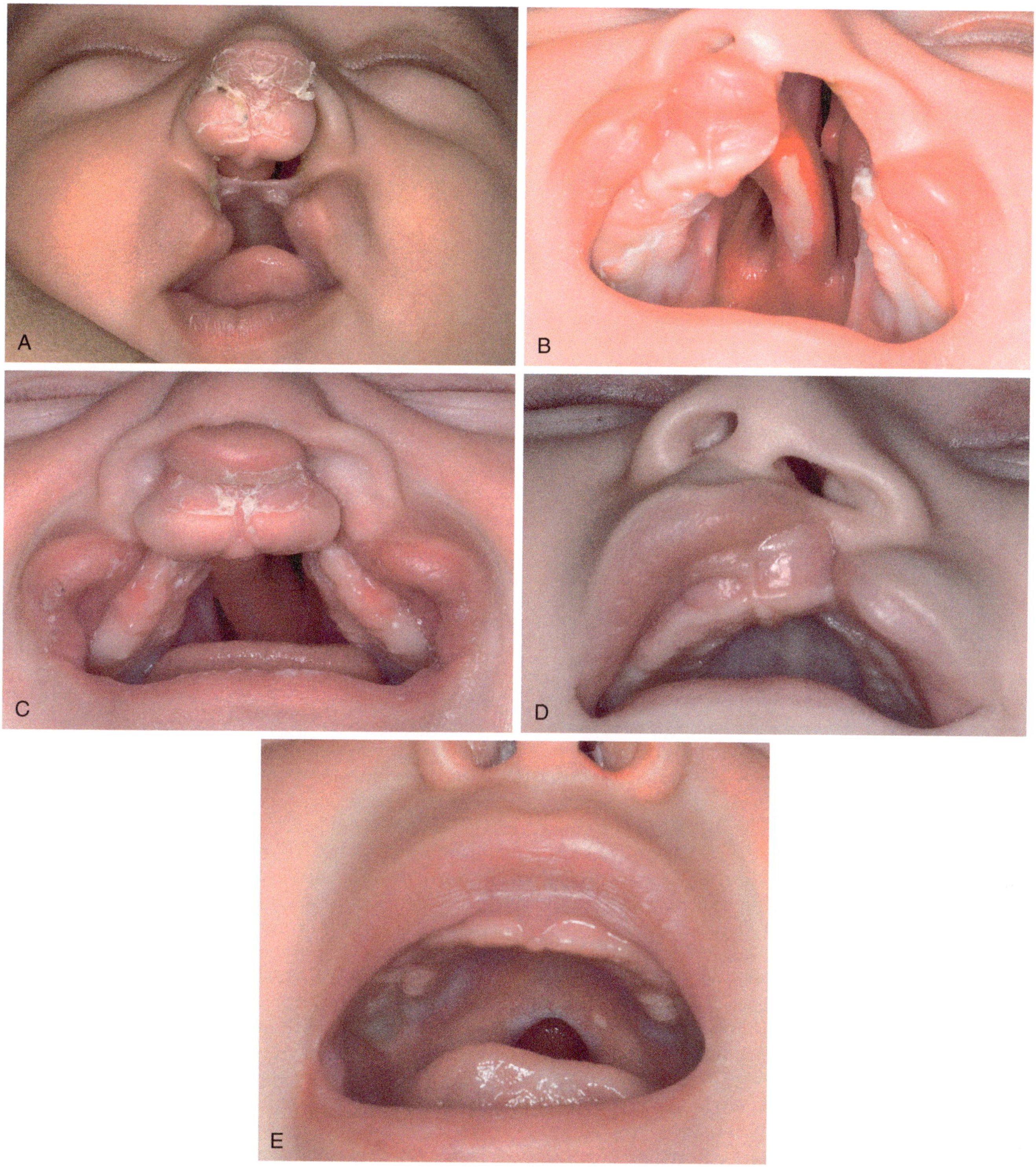

• **Fig. 17.1** Clinical images of permutations of the clefting process, given the distinct embryologic origin of lip and primary palate and of the secondary palate. (A) Complete bilateral cleft lip and primary palate. (B) Complete/incomplete cleft lip and primary palate and complete cleft of secondary palate. (C) Complete bilateral cleft lip, primary and secondary palates. (D) Incomplete cleft lip and primary palate. (E) Incomplete cleft of secondary palate.

Anatomy

The hard palate is composed of palatine processes of the maxilla and the palatine bone. The palate is supplied by the greater palatine vessels and nerves, which emerge through the greater palatine foramina in the posterolateral regions of the hard palate. The nasal mucosa of the hard palate is in continuity with the mucosa of the lateral nasal walls, and medially with the vomerine mucosa. The soft palate is the mobile palatal segment, with muscles that act synergistically

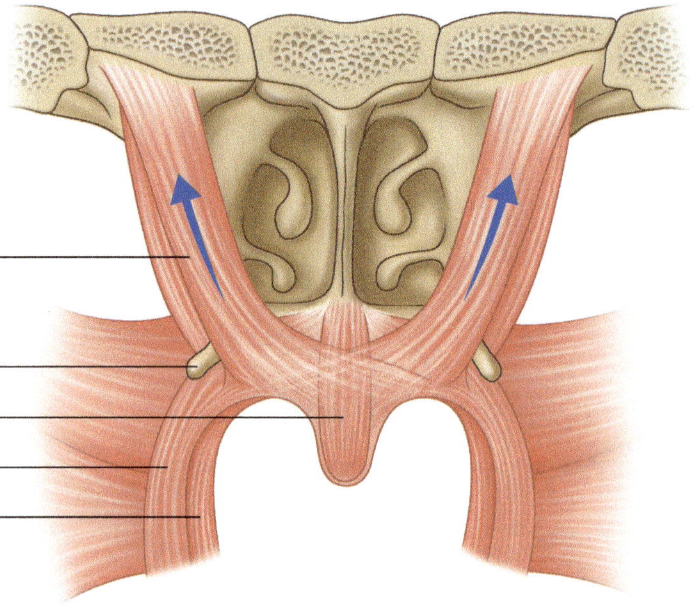

• **Fig. 17.2** A nasal view of dissected soft palate musculature, demonstrating the position of the levator veli palatini, which occupies the intermediate 40% of the soft palatal length. (From Kirschner RE, Baylis AL. Velopharyngeal dysfunction. In: Rodriguez ED, Losee JE, Neligan PC, eds. *Plastic Surgery*, Vol. 3: *Craniofacial, Head and Neck Surgery and Pediatric Plastic Surgery*. London: Elsevier; 2018.)

to effect velopharyngeal closure. The sensory supply of the soft palate is derived primarily from the lesser palatine nerves, which are comprised of several branches that extend from the lesser palatine foramina in the palatal process of the sphenoid through the palatal aponeurosis.

From a functional perspective, the levator veli palatini is considered the most important muscle of the soft palate. This muscle originates from the petrous temporal bone and the junction of bony and cartilaginous portions of the Eustachian tube. It then courses inferiorly, anteriorly, and medially to enter the velum and join the levator from the opposite side, forming the *levator sling*. The levator is found in the middle third (40%) of the velum,[2] between the two heads of the palatopharyngeus (Fig. 17.2). The levator is innervated by the pharyngeal plexus (motor branches of cranial nerves IX, X, and XI). Moreover, it has been suggested that the muscle also receives innervation from cranial nerve VII. This is supported by findings of hemipalatal palsy in patients with hemifacial microsomia.[3] The cumulative action of the levator is to pull the velum superiorly and posteriorly. In the cleft palate, the levator inserts into the cleft margin in the anterior half of the velum and *not directly into the posterior edge of the hard palate*, as is commonly cited.

The palatopharyngeus originates from the palatine aponeurosis, and then divides into vertical and transverse fibers. The vertical fibers, palatothyroideus, form the posterior faucial (tonsillar) pillars, course in the lateral pharyngeal walls and insert into the greater horns of the thyroid cartilage of the larynx. The transverse component, palatopharyngeus proper, courses posteriorly along the lateral pharyngeal walls and intermingles with the superior pharyngeal constrictor muscle. The palatopharyngeus is also innervated by the pharyngeal plexus. Although most of the literature supports the notion that the palatopharyngeus is more active during swallowing than speech, the palatothyroideus fibres are in an anatomical position to act as an antagonist to the elevating action of the levator muscle but as a synergist in stretching the velum backwards. The palatopharyngeus proper assists in the medial displacement of the lateral pharyngeal walls during velopharyngeal closure and contributes to the formation of *Passavant's ridge*. Further, muscular contraction of the palatopharyngeus stretches the velum inferiorly and laterally to increase the available velar surface area and optimize velar shape for contact with the posterior pharyngeal wall. In the midline of the cleft palate, the levator and palatopharyngeus fuse to form the "cleft muscle" as described by Veau.[4] However, in contradistinction to the levator veli palatini, the palatopharyngeus also inserts into the posterior border of the hard palate.

The palatoglossus is the most superficial (oral) muscle of the soft palate, traverses through the anterior tonsillar pillars and inserts into the tongue. As such, contraction results in tongue elevation, palatal depression, and narrowing of the pharyngo-oral isthmus. The muscle does not have an ascribed role in velopharyngeal closure per se. The levator, palatopharyngeus, and palatoglossus diverge anteriorly to insert into the margins of the cleft, aberrant palatal aponeurosis, as well as the oral and nasal mucosa.

The superior pharyngeal constrictor is a quadrangular muscle, which originates from the medial pterygoid plates and pterygomandibular raphe. The muscle courses around the pharynx, forming the lateral and posterior pharyngeal walls, enclosing the nasopharynx and upper oropharynx. The muscle fibres diverge superiorly and inferiorly as they

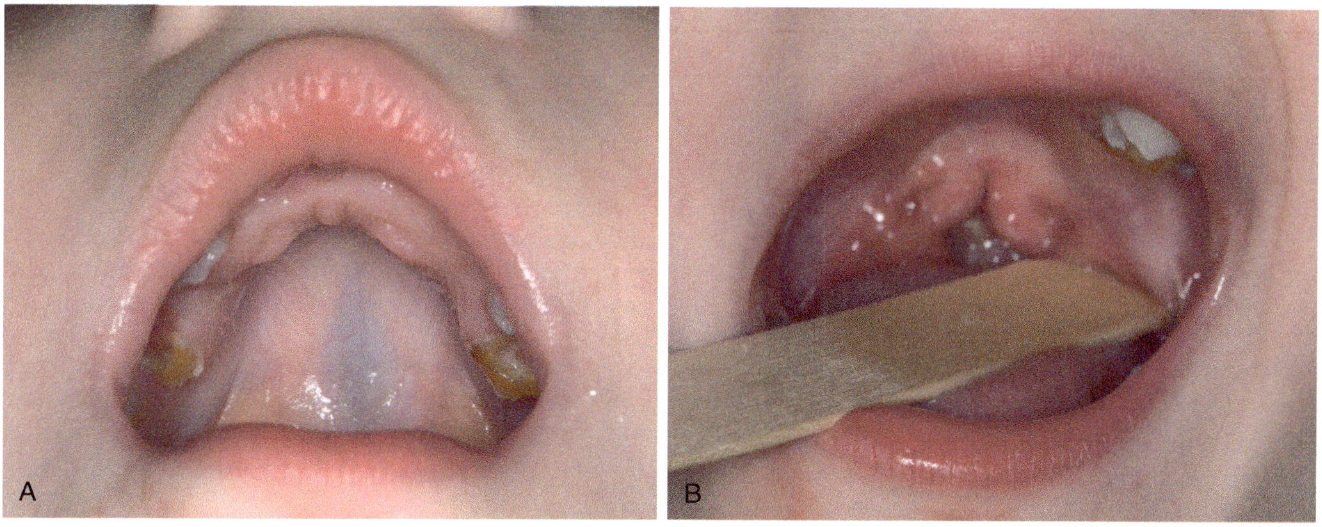

• **Fig. 17.3** (A) Clinical image of an overt submucous cleft palate, (B) demonstrating the zona pellucidum and bifid uvula.

approach the posterior midline to insert into the pharyngeal ligament. The space between the superior margin of the muscle and cranial base is occupied in the lateral nasopharyngeal wall by levator and Eustachian tube and in the posterior pharyngeal wall by the pharyngobasilar fascia. The muscle, innervated by cranial nerve X, causes medial excursion of the lateral pharyngeal walls and, along with palatopharyngeus, anterior displacement of the posterior pharyngeal wall. The latter accounts for the formation of Passavant's ridge. While historically considered a compensatory mechanism in patients with velopharyngeal insufficiency (VPI),[5] much evidence exists to challenge this assertion.[6] For instance, the ridge is often noted to be below and slower than palatal excursion.

The tensor veli palatini does not contribute to movement of the velum. The tensor originates from the scaphoid fossa of the greater wing of the sphenoid and membranous portion of the Eustachian tube. The muscle courses medially and inferiorly parallel to the levator and forms a tendon. The tendon hooks around the hamulus of the pterygoid plate (to which it is partially attached), assumes a horizontal orientation and inserts along the posterior border of the hard palate as the palatal aponeurosis, occupying the anterior third of the velum. In the cleft palate, the tensor palatini reaches the hamulus and appears to diverge into two components – a triangular tendinous insertion into the lateral posterior edge of the hard palate (does not form the palatal aponeurosis), in close proximity to the nasal mucosa, and a less substantial component, which passes toward the oral surface behind the greater palatine neurovascular bundle. Some authorities recognize a separate but closely related muscle, the dilator tubae, which rounds the middle third of the pterygoid hamulus without an insertion. There has been much debate as to whether the tensor (and/or dilator tubae), has a significant action on the velum and regarding the relative importance of the tensor (or dilator tubae) and levator in Eustachian tube function.

The musculus uvulae, thought to be supplied by the lesser palatine nerve, is a paired muscle located above the levator, attached to the palatal aponeurosis anteriorly and passing into the uvula posteriorly. The muscle is covered nasally and laterally by mucous glands. Contraction of the muscle may assist in velopharyngeal closure by adding to the bulk of the midline dorsal ridge over the levator eminence and also possibly by lifting the free border of the palate into deeper contact with the posterior pharyngeal wall.[7] Others argue that this muscle may not be of importance in velopharyngeal function.[8] In the cleft palate the presence of the musculus uvulae is controversial and rarely seen.

Finally, the salpingopharyngeus is a small muscle that originates from the torus tubarius and courses vertically along the lateral pharyngeal walls. While this muscle does not contribute to velopharyngeal closure, it may draw the lateral pharyngeal walls superiorly.

Submucous Cleft Palate

Submucous cleft palate is a form of cleft palate wherein the mucosa is intact but the underlying musculature is similarly abnormal to that of an overt cleft palate. In 1954, Calnan[9] qualified the overt submucous cleft palate with a classic triad, including bifid uvula, palpable notch in the posterior hard palate, and zona pellucidum. The zona pellucidum is a midline translucent zone that represents diastasis of the velar musculature (Fig. 17.3). Kaplan[10] described the *occult* subcumous cleft palate, where velar malfunction is observed, but the aforementioned or typical features are not apparent. Given evidence of velopharyngeal dysfunction (VPD), the diagnosis of occult submucous cleft palate is often made following evaluation with nasopharyngoscopy, where a midline groove or concavity is seen on the nasal surface of the palate. The latter is thought to represent hypoplasia or agenesis of the musculus uvulae, as well as velar musculature diastasis.[11] Sommerlad et al.[12] argued that there was a spectrum of severity in submucous clefting and described a scoring system based on the severity of each feature of the triad. In effect, Kaplan[10] postulated that isolated clefts of the secondary palate, overt, and occult submucous cleft palates are variations in expression of the same embryonic process. Diagnosis of submucous cleft palate is often delayed until speech development allows appreciation of VPD.

Associated Syndromes

While a syndrome occurs in approximately 10% of patients with cleft palate in association with cleft lip, associated syndromes are described in up to 50% of cases with isolated cleft palate.

Pierre Robin Sequence

The most commonly associated anomaly is Pierre Robin sequence, which occurs in approximately 1 in 8500–14,000 births. The condition typically occurs sporadically, but may be familial, with autosomal dominant mode of inheritance. The sequence includes micrognathia/retrognathia, glossoptosis, and respiratory distress.[13] While not a qualification of the sequence, a cleft palate occurs in approximately 60%–90% of cases. Indeed, in his original description of 1923, Pierre Robin, the French stomatologist credited for the identification of these infants, failed to include cleft palate as an associated feature, but later added cleft palate as an aggravating factor.[14] The cleft palate in the context of Robin sequence is typically U-shaped, as opposed to the classic V-shaped cleft palate, and implies a wider palatal gap. The theory for the occurrence of cleft palate in Robin sequence is that the posterior displacement of the mandible results in elevation and dorsiflexion of the tongue at approximately 9 weeks of gestation, preventing migration and fusion of the palatal shelves. The majority of cases (83%) present as a component of a named syndrome, including Stickler syndrome, velocardiofacial syndrome, Treacher Collins syndrome, fetal alcohol syndrome, Nager syndrome, oculo-auriculo-vertebral spectrum, Apert syndrome, ectrodactyly–ectodermal dysplasia clefting syndrome, Opitz-G/BBB syndrome, and orofacial digital syndrome. Thus, with the Robin sequence, the presence of other anomalous features should be considered (Fig. 17.4).

The glossoptosis in Robin sequence initiates a sequence of events including airway obstruction, increased energy expenditure, and impaired caloric intake from poor feeding. Thus, in the neonatal period, the primary objectives are to relieve airway obstruction and avert failure to thrive. However, glossoptosis is not the only contributor to upper airway obstruction in children presenting with Robin sequence. Acute angulation of the basicranium, pharyngeal, laryngeal and/or lingual anomalies, subglottic anomalies, hypotonia and central nervous system disorders may all cause or contribute to airway obstruction. Thus, microlaryngobronchoscopy is essential to determine the mechanism(s) of airway collapse and if obstruction can be relieved completely with treatment strategies that address tongue positioning alone. In effect, Sher et al,[15] based on endoscopic observations, demonstrated four patterns of pharyngeal collapse in patients with craniofacial anomalies, any of which can be found in Robin sequence.[16] In types 1 and 2, the retropositioned tongue is the primary etiologic factor responsible for obstruction, whereas in types 3 and 4 airway compromise is secondary to lateral pharyngeal wall collapse and pharyngeal stenosis, respectively. Thus, no single treatment will resolve respiratory obstruction in all patients, and management must be tailored to the specific underlying etiology. Airway compromise is assessed with oxygen saturation recordings and polysomnographic studies, the need for oxygen supplementation, and appropriate weight gain (with or without gavage feeding). Routine laboratory investigations and additional studies include serial blood gas analysis for elevated levels of carbon dioxide and serum bicarbonate, and pH recording for gastroesophageal reflux. As primary measures, management of airway compromise secondary to *glossoptosis* include prone or semiprone positioning and placement of a nasopharyngeal airway with or without continuous positive airway pressure. If the latter conservative treatment modalities fail to relieve airway obstruction, surgical intervention is warranted. Douglas[17] popularized the technique of glossopexy, originally described by Shukowsky in 1911. This procedure was later modified by Routledge[18] and various modifications were subsequently developed. The latter concept is based on the premise that airway obstruction is secondary to glossoptosis and surgical adhesion between tongue and lip can effectively mitigate the retrodisplacement of the tongue. In 1983 a French stomatologist, Viviane Epois,[19] asserted that the imbalance of the muscular insertion of the tongue on the mandible was responsible for the micrognathia, tongue elevation, and glossoptosis. More specifically, that the musculature of the floor of the mouth is under increased tension and impels the tongue superiorly and posteriorly, resulting in respiratory obstruction. The latter is the premise for the subperiosteal release of the floor of the mouth musculature for refractory cases of respiratory obstruction in the Robin anomalad.[20] Following release, the tongue can adopt a more anterior position. Mandibular distraction is now a well recognized and widely used surgical alternative in patients with obstruction refractory to conservative measures. With this method the tongue is indirectly pulled forward through muscular attachment to the lingual surface of the mandible.[21] In instances where the latter measures fail or in cases where other airway anomalies contribute to obstruction, tracheostomy is often required.

Stickler Syndrome

Stickler syndrome is a hereditary progressive arthro-ophthalmopathy with an estimated frequency of 1 in 10,000. It is an autosomal dominant connective tissue dysplasia characterized by cleft palate, degenerative joint changes, ocular manifestations, and progressive sensorineural hearing loss. Moreover, these patients often exhibit a characteristic flat facial appearance, secondary to hypoplasia of the midface and bridge of the nose (Fig. 17.5).

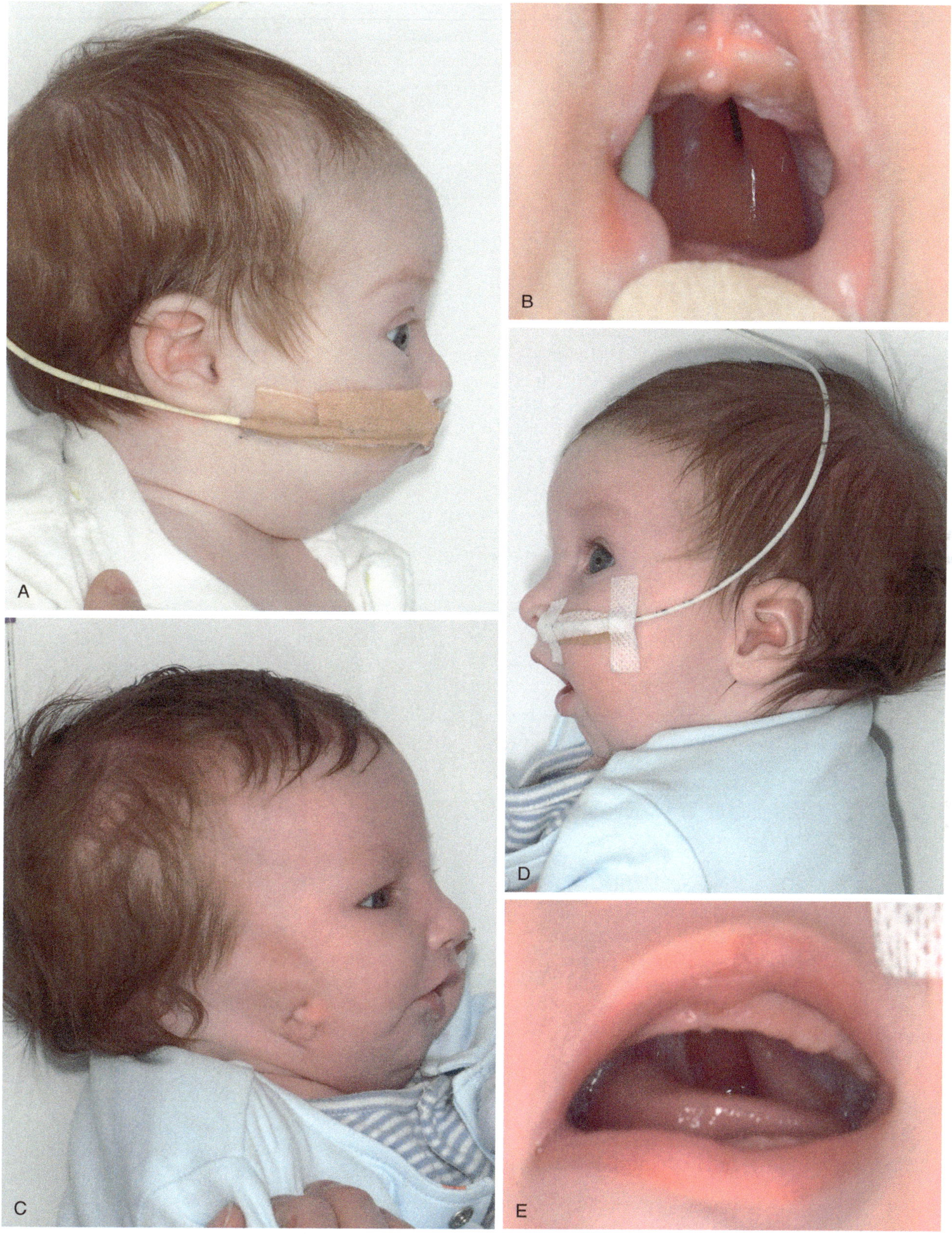

• **Fig. 17.4** Lateral photographs of infants with Pierre Robin sequence. (A) Nonsyndromic infant with severe micrognathia, nasopharyngeal airway and gavage tube in place. (B) A typical U-shaped cleft palate. (C, D) Infant with Pierre Robin sequence with right-sided craniofacial microsomia and microtia. (E) In this case, there is a cleft of the soft palate only.

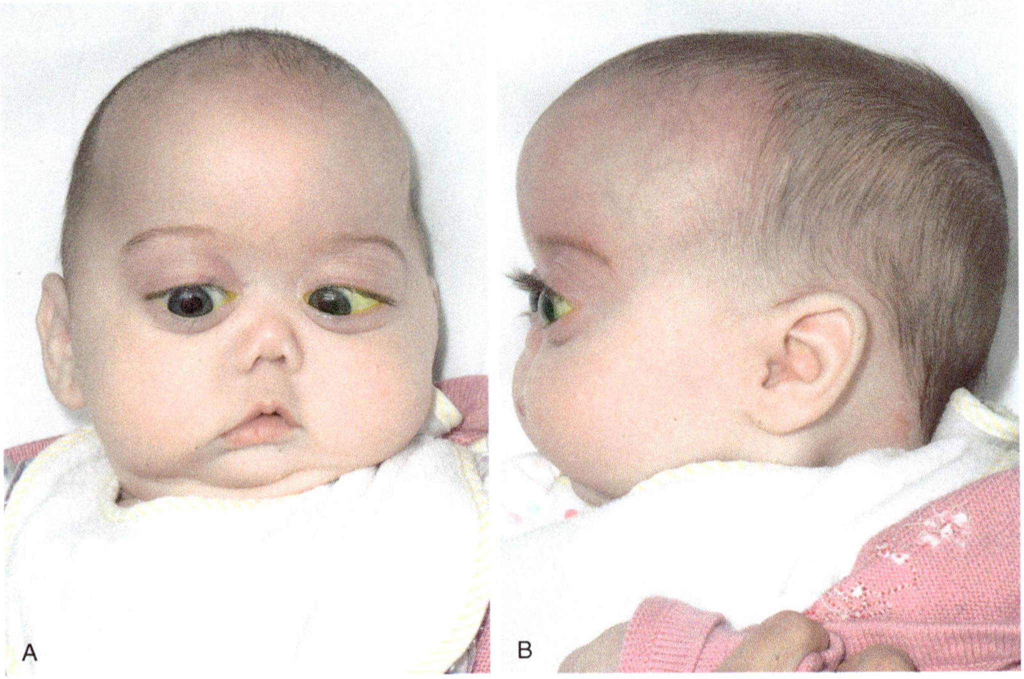

• **Fig. 17.5** Clinical image of infant with Stickler syndrome. Note the facial features characteristic of this syndrome, including prominent eyes, flat nasal bridge, anteverted nares, and mid-face hypoplasia. (A) anterior and (B) lateral views.

Van der Woude Syndrome

While rare (1 in 100,000), van der Woude syndrome is an autosomal dominant syndrome with variable expressivity also associated with cleft palate. Van der Woude syndrome is associated with *IRF6* mutations on chromosome 1q. Moreover, it is unique in that it may also be expressed as either cleft lip with or without cleft palate. A distinguishing feature of the syndrome is bilateral paramedian lower lip pits. *IRF6* mutations are also responsible for the popliteal pterygium syndrome, which is characterized by cleft lip and/or palate, lower lip pits and additionally qualified by the presence of bilateral popliteal webs, hypodontia, syndactyly, nail abnormalities, anomalies of the genitourinary system, and ankyloblepharon. Interestingly, as previously mentioned, the *IRF6* gene has been recognized to have the strongest genetic association with nonsyndromic cleft lip and palate. Indeed, some patients with van der Woude syndrome do not display the typical lower lip pits, and may be erroneously classified as nonsyndromic. Thus, *IRF6* mutations should be considered in those with affected parent–child and especially segregating cleft palate and cleft lip and palate.[22]

22q11.2 Deletion (Velocardiofacial) Syndrome

Although clinically under-recognized, velocardiofacial syndrome (VCFS) is the most common multiple anomaly syndrome in humans, with an estimated frequency of 1 in 2000–4000 live births and equal sex distribution. Microdeletions occur in the q11.2 region of chromosome 22, identified by fluorescence in situ hybridization (FISH) test. In these patients, the *TBX1* gene is always deleted, with 90% of patients having a deletion of the typical deleted region (TDR; common 22q11.2 deletion, size 3 Mb), while 10% have a smaller deletion of only the proximal 1.5 Mb of the TDR (proximal deleted region, PDR). Both TDR and PDR include the *TBX1* gene area. A few individuals with VCFS have shown unique 22q11.2 deletion intervals or a chromosome 10p14 deletion. In the majority of patients (>90%) 22q11.2 deletions occur as spontaneous events, with both parents unaffected. However, in approximately 10% of individuals, deletion is identified in a parent and thus there is autosomal dominant transmission with variable expression. There is phenotypic overlap between VCFS and DiGeorge, Sedlacková, conotruncal anomaly face and Cayler syndromes. Indeed, all these aforementioned syndromes are descriptions of the same entity, with over 180 separate anomalies or developmental sequences reported in association with VCFS covering nearly every organ and system. Notable among these are immune deficiency, hypocalcemia, conotruncal cardiac anomalies, short stature, learning difficulties, behavioral problems, psychiatric illnesses, and slender hands and digits. These patients also have a characteristic facial appearance, due to a combination of skeletal and soft tissue features. These include microcephaly, a long middle third of the face, flat zygomatic arches, mandibular retrognathia, broad nasal dorsum, narrow alar bases and bulbous nasal tip, hypotonic flaccid facies, narrow, downslanting palpebral fissures, and external ear anomalies (Fig. 17.6). Also reported in patients with VCFS are aberrant carotid and subclavian arteries. Indeed, it has been hypothesized that the large number of vascular anomalies in major vessels reported in patients with VCFS may result in a number of

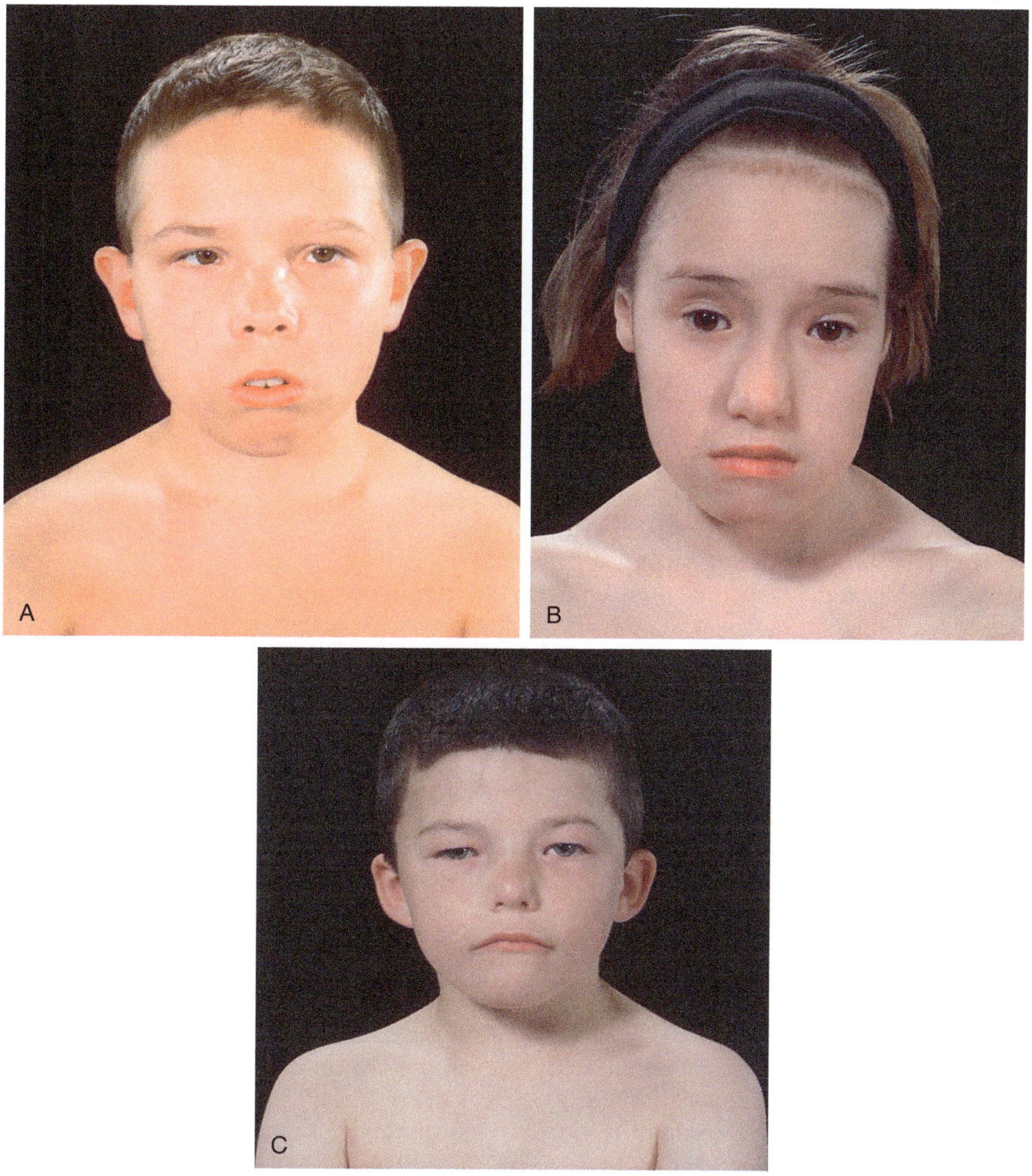

• **Fig. 17.6** (A–C) Clinical images of children with facies characteristic of velo-cardio-facial syndrome.

developmental sequences. The latter notion is supported by reports of Robin, DiGeorge, Potter, and holoprosencephaly sequences in individuals with VCFS. The phenotypic expression in this syndrome is markedly variable with no clinical feature occurring in all cases and no reported case with all or even most of the associated clinical findings.[23]

VCFS is now recognized as the most common syndrome associated with cleft palate and velopharyngeal insufficiency. The majority (approximately 75%) of children with VCFS have hypernasal speech and severe language impairment. Moreover, affected individuals commonly present with VPI, most often associated with overt or occult submucous cleft palate. While the frequency of VPI among individuals with nonsyndromic submucous cleft palate is approximately <9%, VCFS patients show VPI associated with submucous cleft palate in >70% of cases. In addition to overt or occult submucous cleft palate, there are several other factors that contribute to the high frequency of VPI in VCFS, including platybasia, congenitally short velum, palatopharyngeal disproportion, abnormalities of pharyngeal muscles with hypodynamic velopharynx, lymphoid tissue (adenoid) hypoplasia, and tonsillar hypertrophy. The latter anatomic and physiologic anomalies often render management of VPD in patients with VCFS a greater therapeutic challenge than in their non-syndromic counterparts, often necessitating a combination of palatoplasty and pharyngeal surgery. Despite the more extensive surgical correction required, speech outcomes are universally inferior when compared with those for non-syndromic patients.

Palatoplasty

Pathologic sequelae of cleft palate include feeding and nutritional difficulties, serous otitis media (with potential hearing loss), and abnormal speech development. Thus, the goals of cleft palate repair include improved feeding and normal speech, while minimizing the deleterious impact on maxillary growth and dental arch relationship.

In the neonatal period, feeding and adequate weight gain are a priority. Due to reduced ability to suck, and particularly to draw the nipple into the mouth, infants with cleft palate have difficulty feeding, and breastfeeding can only be achieved with considerable effort and modification of technique. In developed countries, most infants are bottle-fed, which allows a steady stream of milk, usually by a modified teat and soft bottle.

With regards to hearing, all patients with cleft palate should undergo a neonatal hearing assessment. Some argue that ventilation tubes should be inserted if there is a persistent conductive hearing loss of >45 dB on distraction testing or >35 dB on pure tone audiometry. However, given there is evidence that correction of the muscle abnormality in the cleft palate improves Eustachian tube function, others contend that insertion of ventilation tubes should be deferred.

Children with clefts generally do not have difficulties with swallowing and aspiration unless there is a coexisting intrinsic neuromuscular or anatomic abnormality of the tongue or pharynx. Evidence of the latter usually warrants further investigation with videofluoroscopy and endoscopy.

Timing of Repair

There is little debate that, in most situations, a cleft palate should be repaired. However, consensus is lacking on timing of repair. Restricted maxillary growth secondary to cleft palate repair has prompted some to promote two-stage palatoplasty, wherein the velum is repaired early in order to enable normal speech acquisition and hard palate closure delayed to facilitate maxillary development.[24] Delayed closure of the hard palate may benefit facial growth but most reports suggest detrimental effects on speech.[25] Irrespective, there is general agreement that soft palate repair should be effected before 12 months of age. The senior author aims to achieve complete palate closure by 6 months of age. There is evidence from a randomized controlled trial that speech outcome is superior following palatoplasty at 6 months as compared to 12 months.[26] In this study, children with clefts repaired at 6 months of age did not develop compensatory articulations, while those with palate repair delayed to 12 months of age did display abnormal articulation patterns. Further, no difference in maxillary arch development, soft tissue profile or velopharyngeal dysfunction was noted between the two groups at 4 years from surgery. There is currently an international randomized controlled trial, the Timing of Primary Surgery for Cleft Palate (TOPS trial), comparing palate closure at 6 and 12 months of age.

For submucous cleft palate repair, timing is similar to overt cleft palate repair for infants with obvious evidence of a submucous cleft and persistent feeding difficulties. Where feeding is not a considerable issue, repair is otherwise indicated if an infant is not producing pressure consonants (/d/, /b/) by 15–18 months. In the older child with submucous cleft palate, surgical treatment is *indicated only in the presence of consistent VPI* or persistent hypernasality, as the presence of submucous cleft palate does not ensure VPD.

Preoperative Assessment

Appropriate preoperative assessment is mandatory to ensure that there is no history of airway compromise or anemia and there is adequate weight gain. The main contraindications to palate repair are associated medial comorbidities, which may present an unacceptable increased anesthetic risk and suboptimal weight.

Controversy exists regarding the benefits of palate repair in older children and adults. Arguably, adults with unrepaired clefts have compensatory patterns of articulation that are so well embedded that palate repair is unlikely to make much difference to speech. However, there are reports of some improvement in speech even though normality is not achieved. An international task force has produced a report and recommendations on delayed palate repair.[27]

History of Palatoplasty

Before the development of general anesthesia, palate repair was performed on an awake patient. The first recorded repair was in France in 1819, when Roux repaired the palate of an Edinburgh medical student, John Stephenson, who went on to become professor of anatomy in McGill University, Montreal, Canada. In 1859, Bernhard von Langenbeck described bilateral bipedicled mucoperiosteal flaps for palate repair.[28] Lateral relaxing incisions are made at the junction of gingival and oral palatal mucoperiosteum lateral to the greater palatine neurovascular bundle, in addition to cleft marginal incisions (Fig. 17.7A). Further developments in technique by Victor Veau,[29] Thomas Kilner,[30] and William Wardill[31] were introduced to increase palatal length in an effort to aid in velopharyngeal closure (Fig. 17.7B). The three- or four-flap Veau–Wardill–Kilner pushback palatoplasty includes a V to Y incision and closure of the anterior hard palate. The resulting flaps are based on the greater palatine arteries posteriorly. Inherent in the pushback operation is release of the muscular attachments from the posterior edge of the hard palate. While the pushback palatoplasty lengthens the palate, theoretically retro-positioning the levator into a more favorable position, this has *not* been shown to be effective in improving speech. Moreover, by virtue of the fact that the bone is denuded anteriorly, this repair adversely affects maxillary growth and the single nasal mucosal layer anteriorly is associated with a higher rate of fistula. In effect, the latter procedure has been largely abandoned in modern era palatoplasty. The two-flap technique popularized by Janusz Bardach[32] does not aim to achieve pushback, but is believed by its proponents to improve exposure of the underlying velar musculature (Fig. 17.7C). Many surgeons simply return the flaps to their original position to avoid leaving raw areas of bone. Arguably, this may not avoid impairment of maxillary growth.

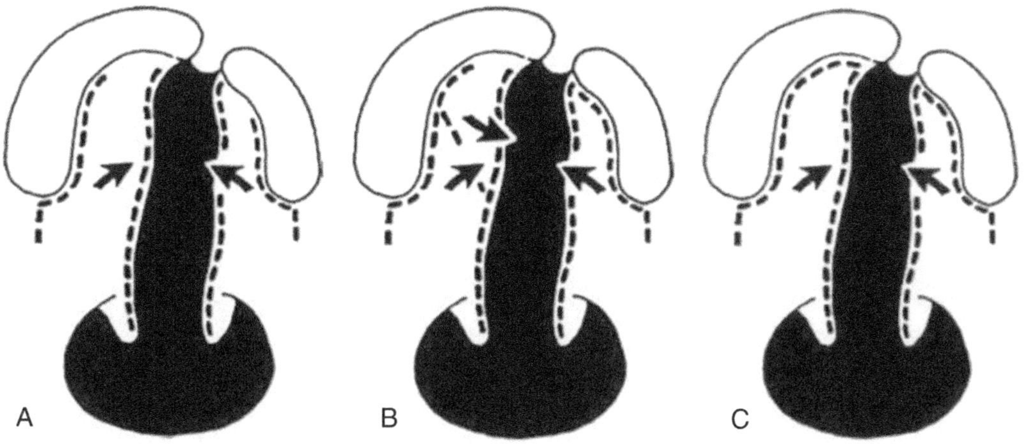

• **Fig. 17.7** Illustration of the (A) Von Langenbeck, (B) Veau-Wardill–Kilner, and (C) Bardach techniques. Dashed lines indicate incisions used. (From Losee JE, Kirschner RE. *Comprehensive Cleft Care*, 2009. Reproduced with permission of McGraw-Hill Medical.)

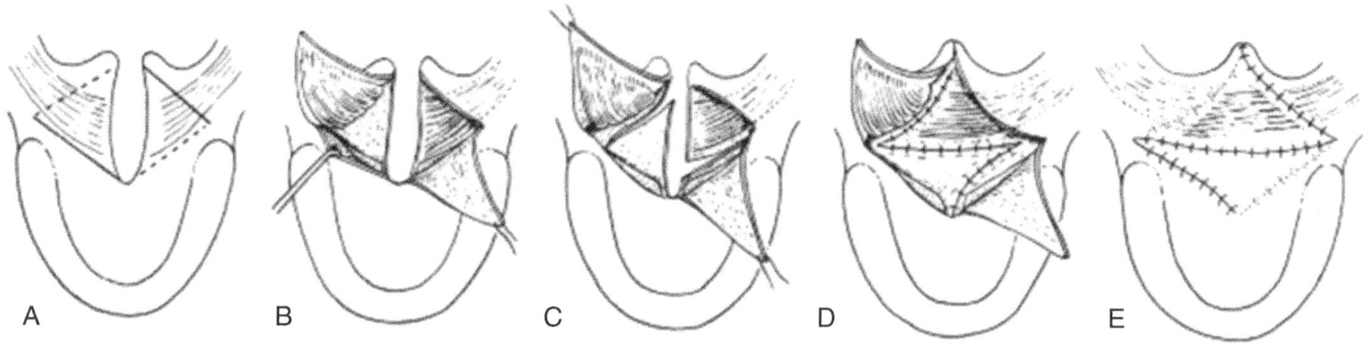

• **Fig. 17.8** (A–E) Diagrammatic illustration of key steps in the operative technique for velar closure as originally described by Furlow. (From Furlow LT. Cleft palate repair by double opposing Z-plasty. *Plast Reconstr Surg.* 1986;78:724–736. Reproduced with permission of Lippincott, Williams and Wilkins.)

In the early 20th century, Victor Veau[4] first described the anomalous cleft musculature and promoted the concept of suture approximation of the levator in a side-to-side fashion without any endeavor to address the aberrantly positioned muscle. Braithwaite[33] and Kriens[34] emphasized restoration of the levator sling by dissection of the abnormally positioned levator muscles prior to reapproximation. Edgerton and Dellon[35] suggested that, following dissection, the levator bundles should be rolled 180 degrees and sutured to the musculus uvulae near the uvular base. The double opposing Z-plasty technique, described in 1978 and later published in 1986 by Leonard T. Furlow Jr,[36] is often used for the primary repair of isolated clefts of the soft palate or submucous cleft palate, or as a secondary technique to lengthen the previously repaired palate. With this technique, 60-degree Z-plasties are outlined on both oral and nasal mucosa in opposite directions with the central limb placed along the cleft margin. The posteriorly based flap on each surface is composed of muscle (levator) and mucosa, and the anterior flap of mucosa only (Fig. 17.8). Possible advantages of this procedure include lengthening, increased vascularization of the muscle, and technical facility. Disadvantages are lateral tightening by Z-plasty closure, less anatomic reconstruction of the musculature, asymmetric velar excursion, and difficult closure with wide clefts. Cutting et al.[37] and Sommerlad[38] advocated more extensive dissection of the levator muscles and radical retropositioning of the velar musculature in their respective techniques of intravelar veloplasty. In an effort to facilitate closure, von Langenbeck incisions are often combined with Furlow's palatoplasty or radical intravelar veloplasty for palate repair.

There are several different protocols and techniques for repair, with variable sequences for closure of the lip, alveolus, hard and soft palates. In the senior author's practice, the operating microscope has been used for palate repair since 1991.[39] In clefts of the lip and palate, since 1993, a single-layer vomerine mucoperiosteal flap has been used for closure of the hard palate and nasal floor at the time of lip repair at 3 months of age. The vomer flap was first introduced by Pichler in 1926[40] and was originally described as an inferiorly based flap. This flap resulted in significant maxillary retrusion, presumably secondary to injury to the vomerime–premaxillary suture or due to its poor blood supply. However, long-term studies of the superiorly based vomerine flap have not demonstrated a similar deleterious effect on maxillary growth, likely due to the relatively more limited dissection.[41,42] In the case of unilateral cleft lip and palate, an incision is made at the junction of palatal and

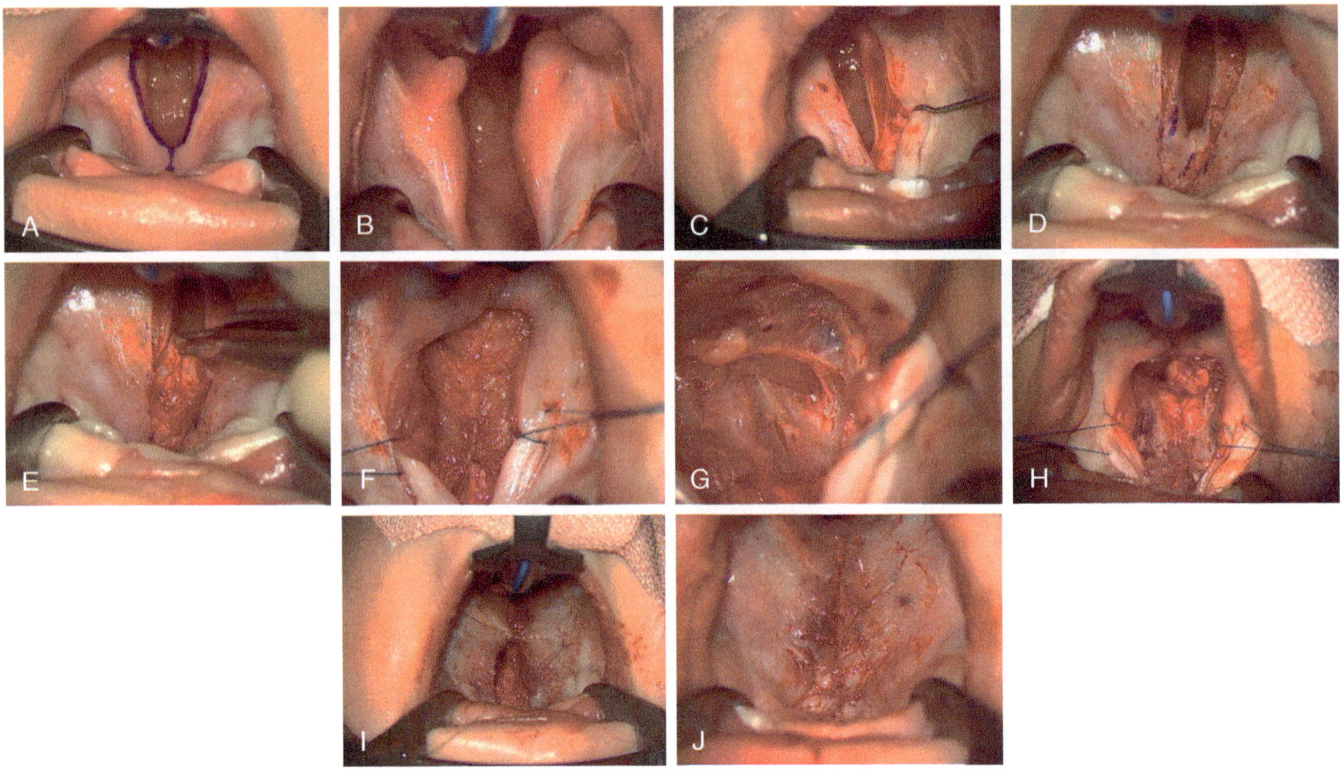

• **Fig. 17.9** Clinical images of key steps in the operative technique for velar closure by Sommerlad. (A) Marking of incision at junction of oral and nasal mucosa along cleft margin, with midline extension of the incision to allow elevation of oral mucoperiosteal flaps. (B) Junction of nasal and oral mucosa is distinguished by darker coloration of nasal mucosa. (C) Subperiosteal elevation of the oral mucoperiosteal flaps towards the posterior border of the hard palate. (D, E) Use of neomucosal vomerine flap for closure of the nasal layer of the soft palate. (F) Anteriorly oriented palatopharyngeus (and palatoglossus) fibers inserting into the posterior border of the hard palate. (G) Exposure and transposition of the levator muscle. (H) The levators are then united along with retro-displaced palatopharyngeus and tensor tendon. (I, J) Closure of oral layer with twisted loop mattress suture.

vomerine mucosa on the non-cleft side, extending posteriorly down the crest of the vomer and anteriorly around the side of the premaxilla to become continuous with the medial lip incision. The oral mucoperiosteum is incised along the margin of the cleft and elevated to allow the vomerine flap to be inserted underneath. In bilateral cleft lip and palate, one vomerine flap is elevated as previously described. As complete elevation of bilateral vomerine flaps may jeopardize the blood supply of the premaxilla and prolabium, the flap on the other side is elevated only to the prevomerine suture. In the interim period between cleft lip and anterior palate repair and soft palate repair, the exposed periosteal surface of the vomerine flap epithelializes to create an intact hard palate.

Sommerlad Technique for Palate Repair

A modified mouth gag is inserted followed by a gauze throat pack. The junction of the oral and nasal mucosa is marked with ink (Fig. 17.9A). The nasal mucosa is usually on the oral side of the edge of the cleft and darker than the oral mucosa (Fig. 17.9B). The palate is infiltrated with lidocaine with epinephrine, and the palate incised along the margin of the cleft at the junction of oral and nasal mucosa. The incision then extends from the midline at the anterior limit of the cleft anteriorly onto the posterior border of the hard palate to enable subperiosteal elevation of the oral mucoperiosteal flaps to expose the bony palatal shelves (Fig. 17.9C). Dimples are frequently seen on the oral side of the palate at a point where oral mucous glands are attached to the posterior border of the hard palate and tendinous nasal component of tensor palatini. Care must be taken to elevate these mucous glands intact with the oral flap (Fig. 17.9D). Dissection is facilitated with the use of a dental scaler or Freer's elevator. In wide clefts, where more extensive mobilization of the oral layer is necessary, dissection extends laterally to free the greater palatine neurovascular bundle, with incision of its surrounding periosteal sleeve when necessary. Elevation of the oral layer is continued posteriorly into the soft palate and laterally to the pterygoid hamulus, separating the oral mucosa and attached mucous glands from the underlying musculature, the palatopharyngeus, and palatoglossus. The nasal mucosa is mobilized from the nasal surface of the palatal shelves, if necessary, and sutured in the midline. For soft palate closure in patients with unilateral or bilateral cleft lip and palate, in whom a vomerine flap was used for closure of the hard palate at the time of unilateral or bilateral lip repair, a posteriorly based flap of the neomucosa from the epithelialized vomer may be raised and turned back to facilitate closure of the anterior nasal layer of the soft palate (Fig. 17.9E and F). Following closure of the nasal layer, the anteriorly oriented muscle fibres are seen inserting into the posterior border of the hard palate (Fig. 17.9G). For muscle dissection, an incision is started posteriorly approximately 4 mm from the midline and is extended anteriorly closer to the midline, just lateral to the nasal layer sutures, leaving the mucous glands in place centrally. The palatopharyngeus medially and the nasal component of the tensor tendon laterally are divided from the back of the hard palate and dissection proceeds in a plane between nasal mucosa and musculature. Vessels are seen on the nasal mucosa and are preserved where possible. The tensor tendon is then divided in an anteroposterior direction medial to the hamulus. The oral palatoglossus and palatopharyngeus fibres are then split to expose the levator, which is identified as a discrete cylindrical muscle within a defined fascial envelope (Fig. 17.9H), and is paler than the other palatal muscles. Dissection is continued until the muscle can be transposed to the posterior half of the velum. A stab incision is made in the nasal mucosa on each side, if a hole was not inadvertently created during muscle dissection. The latter permits draining in an effort to prevent hematoma formation. The levators are then united along with retrodisplaced palatopharyngeus and tensor tendon, which imparts strength to the repair (Fig. 17.9I). Finally, the oral layer is closed (Fig. 17.9J). First, one or two sutures are placed in the midline anterior to the muscle repair between oral mucosa and the nasal mucous glands. The latter occludes the dead space and assists in maintaining the muscle retropositioned. The oral layer is closed with a twisted loop mattress stitch. For repair of submucous cleft palate, a similar technique is used as described above, leaving the nasal layer intact and leaving, if possible, some mucous glands on the nasal layer in the midline.

The senior author aims to achieve velar closure without lateral releasing incisions (von Langenbeck). The need for lateral releasing incisions depends on the type, extent, and width of the cleft. Lateral releasing incisions are most often required in patients with Robin sequence with a wide U-shaped cleft, and anticipated if the width of the cleft at the back of the hard palate is in excess of 10 mm at an age of repair of 6 months. Hard palate closure without lateral releasing incisions depends on the "drawbridge effect" (where the sloping high-arched oral mucoperiosteal flaps are brought into greater proximity when mobilized into horizontal position), unfolding of the infolded areas of the flaps and division of the oral component of the tensor palatini insertion and/or the periosteal sleeve of the greater palatine neurovascular bundle.

Repair of Submucous Cleft Palate

In patients with submucous cleft palate, the extent of morphologic abnormality is not in direct proportion to the size of the velopharyngeal gap or severity of hypernasality. As previously mentioned, the latter is secondary to compensatory factors, including prominent adenoid pad and/or significant excursion of the pharyngeal musculature.[43] The authors' approach to the treatment of VPI in patients with submucous cleft palate is to optimize levator function with a radical dissection and retropositioning of the abnormally positioned velar muscles. Upon palate exploration, if the levators are deemed to be in a satisfactory location, then management favors a Hynes pharyngoplasty to augment the posterior pharyngeal wall.[44] Following reassessment at 6 months postoperative follow-up, the necessity for further surgery is determined. The latter may be either a modified Hynes pharyngoplasty or buccinator flap lengthening of the palate.

Complications of Palatoplasty

The complications commonly associated with cleft palate repair include acute airway obstruction, bleeding, infection, and partial or complete palatal dehiscence. The latter may result in fistula formation. Treatment of problematic fistulae depends on location and size. Associated symptomatology includes nasal regurgitation, as well as hypernasality and other manifestations of VPI. Corrective measures include repair with local mobilization of nasal and oral palatal tissue, with or without placement of interpositional tissue or material, such as a segment of pedicled buccal fat pad, cartilage graft or acellular dermal matrix, or formal palate re-repair. Other options include regional flaps (buccal mucosal or musculomucosal flaps, facial artery myomucosal flap, tongue flap) and rarely, free tissue transfer. When circumstances preclude surgical correction, an obturator can be utilized. Potential long-term sequelae of palatoplasty include maxillary retrusion and, most notably, VPI.

Velopharyngeal Dysfunction

The function of the velopharyngeal mechanism, which consists of the velum, lateral, and posterior pharyngeal walls, is to separate the oro- and nasopharynx during speech and deglutition. Normal velopharyngeal closure is necessary for proper consonant production and nasal resonance. In the English language, only three sounds – /m/, /n/, and /ng/ – do not require closure. The primary manifestations of ineffective closure of the velopharyngeal port are excessive nasal resonance or hypernasality and nasal air emission. Hypernasality results from abnormal coupling of the oral and nasal cavities during vowel production and nasal air emission is noted with consonant production.

Some authors have attempted to distinguish between *velopharyngeal insufficiency*, *incompetence* and *dysfunction*. Velophayngeal *insufficiency* refers to hypernasality and nasal air emission during speech secondary to anatomic aberration of the velopharyngeal sphincter. In contrast, velopharyngeal *incompetence* is employed to describe dysfunction of an anatomically intact velopharyngeal mechanism, usually secondary to neuromuscular discoordination. Finally, velopharyngeal *dysfunction* is a term used to describe all conditions that affect velopharyngeal closure, such that the valve does not achieve consistent and/or complete closure during oral sound production.

Irrespective of the nature of the VPD, in an attempt to overcome the inability to achieve velopharyngeal closure, children develop compensatory patterns of articulation (e.g., pharyngeal or nasal fricatives and glottal stops) and other secondary speech patterns, including hoarseness and low speech volume, which can significantly compromise speech intelligibility. Moreover, children may display behavioral idiosyncrasies such as nasal or facial grimace in an attempt to decrease nasal airflow. Causes of VPI include repaired cleft palate, palatal fistula, submucous cleft palate, maxillary advancement, congenital large pharynx or palatopharyngeal disproportion, adenoid regression, irregular adenoid pad and/or adenoidectomy. The influence of the adenoids on velopharyngeal closure merits more detailed description. Most children exhibit velo-adenoidal closure where the soft palate abuts the adenoid pad, which is positioned on the posterior pharyngeal wall in the area of usual velar contact. While adenoid regression does not affect velopharyngeal closure in children with a normal velum, in those with a previously repaired cleft palate, overt or occult submucous cleft palate, evidence or deterioration of existent VPI may be noted. In like manner, hypernasality or nasal air emission may occur following adenoidectomy in patients with no velar defect, but does not typically persist for more than 6 weeks postoperatively. Enduring VPI has been reported to occur in approximately 1 in 1500, more likely in patients with overt or occult submucous cleft palate, where removal of the space-occupying adenoids unmasks underlying palatal deficiency. Finally, in some patients, the shape of the adenoid tissue may in fact be detrimental to closure, wherein irregular surface morphology prevents a tight velopharyngeal seal. Velopharyngeal incompetence can occur in patients with generalized hypotonia (e.g., velocardiofacial syndrome), neurological conditions causing dysarthria (e.g., myotonic dystrophy, cerebral palsy, neurofibromatosis, Steinart's syndrome) or apraxia and cranial nerve defects (e.g., hemifacial microsomia).

Assessment of Velopharyngeal Function

Selection of the appropriate procedure for correction of VPD is based on speech evaluation by a trained speech and language therapist, direct physical examination of the palate, as well as instrumental assessment. On intraoral examination, static and dynamic palatal evaluation is assessed. Inspection for features of submucous cleft palate, as well as presence of palatal fistula and tonsillar hypertrophy, is completed. Normally, during production of "ah" presence of a simple midline palatal dimple is seen at the junction of the middle and posterior thirds of the soft palate. Presence of two lateral dimples, a single unilateral or complete absence of the dimple, as well as an anteriorly displaced dimple, are indicative of abnormal levator muscle insertion and functional compromise.[2]

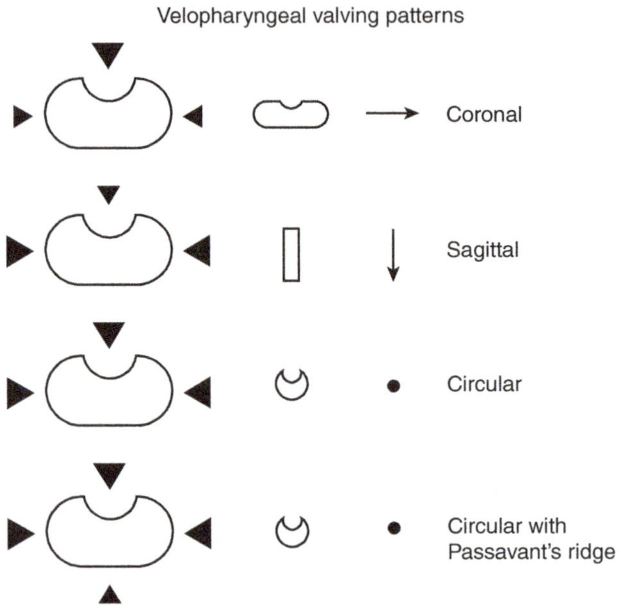

• **Fig. 17.10** Patterns of velopharyngeal valving. (From Croft CB, Shprintzen RJ, Rakoff SJ. Patterns of velopharyngeal valving in normal and cleft palate subjects: a multi-view videofluoroscopic and nasoendoscopic study. *Laryngoscope.* 1981;91:265–271.)

Nasoendoscopy allows direct visualization of the velopharyngeal mechanism from both anatomic and functional standpoints. With nasoendoscopy, the contribution of the velum, lateral and posterior pharyngeal walls (i.e., closure pattern) can be assessed, and in the presence of VPD, the size and location of the velopharyngeal gap as well as timing of velopharyngeal closure can be measured. Hypernasality is not necessarily related to the size of the velopharyngeal gap. Patients with a small velopharyngeal gap may present with severe hypernasality due to delayed time of velopharyngeal closure during speech. Velopharyngeal closure patterns, originally described by Skolnick et al[45] and Croft et al,[46] include coronal, sagittal, circular, and circular with Passavant's ridge. The most common pattern is coronal, where the velum approximates the posterior pharyngeal wall, while the lateral pharyngeal walls move medially to abut the lateral edges of the velum. In sagittal closure pattern, velopharyngeal competence is primarily a function of the lateral pharyngeal walls, which move medially posterior to the velum with the velum approximating the anterior edge of the abutted lateral walls. Circular closure involves equal contributions from velum and lateral pharyngeal walls, while circular closure with Passavant's ridge also includes forward movement of the posterior pharyngeal wall resulting in a true sphincteric closure pattern (Fig. 17.10). While nasoendoscopy is principally utilized as an investigative tool for elucidation of the underlying etiology of and treatment selection for VPD, some have implemented videonasopharyngoscopy as an instrument for visual biofeedback of the velopharyngeal sphincter during speech. Compensatory articulations may result in aberrant pharyngeal movements

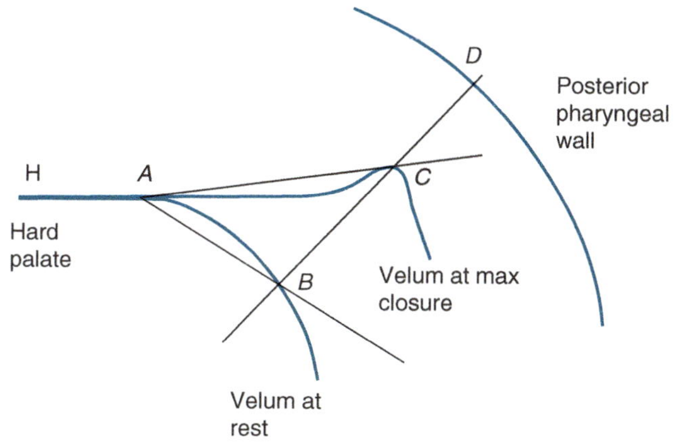

• **Fig. 17.11** Analysis of velar function. Measurements are made with the velum at rest in the nasal breathing position and at the point of maximum closure during production of the sound /i/. Levator function is best assessed during production of the sound /i/. *A*, Posterior edge of hard palate. *B*, Point on velum that forms the levator knee. *C*, Velar knee at the point of maximum closure. The levator knee is the bend in the soft palate formed by levator contraction. *D*, Projection of line *BC* onto the posterior pharyngeal wall, in the line of the levator action to identify the point on the posterior pharyngeal wall at which closure/contact would occur. *AB*, velar length at rest; *AC*, velar length at maximum closure or the functional length of the velum (extended length); *AC/AB*, extensibility; *BD*, velopharyngeal gap size at rest; *CD*, velopharyngeal gap at maximum closure; *BC*, velar excursion, distance traveled by velar knee from resting position to point of maximum closure; *BC/BD*, closure ratio (1 = complete closure).

and the latter method has been effectively used to alter velopharyngeal movements or valving pattern prior to surgery, improving prognosis for success. Others contend that correction of misarticulations with speech therapy alone can improve pharyngeal wall motion without the need for visual biofeedback. In general, nasoendoscopy cannot be performed in uncooperative children or those younger than age 4 years.

In contrast, multiview *videofluoroscopy*, with or without barium coating, also widely implemented to assess the above-mentioned parameters, can often be performed in children below 4 years of age. In the authors' practice, *lateral view* videofluoroscopy (without constrast) only is performed, as this view is deemed to provide the most anatomic and diagnostic information with regards to *levator* function, and its functional relation to the posterior pharyngeal wall.[47] Effective velar length refers to the portion of the soft palate that contributes to velopharyngeal closure, located between the posterior edge of the hard palate and levator knee or eminence (Fig. 17.11). The remaining portion of the velum extends below the contact region and therefore does not participate in closure. On lateral view videofluoroscppy, the effective velar length (*levator knee*), velar excursion, and the level of attempted palatal contact (velopharyngeal closure) can be ascertained. Moreover, posterior pharyngeal wall and Passavant's ridge displacement and direction of projection, as well as abnormal speech behaviors such as timing abnormalities and "tongue-backing" (where lingual movement is used to passively elevate the palate) can be seen during speech production. Both nasoendoscopy and videofluoroscpy also allow visualization of tonsillar and adenoid tissue, which may impede palatal excursion or present a limitation to appropriate placement of pharyngeal flaps, respectively. Of note, in the presence of a palatal fistula, velopharyngeal function should be assessed with the fistula covered, as velopharyngeal movements have been shown to improve or even normalize once an associated fistula is occluded. A limitation of videofluoroscopy is difficulty in distinguishing right and left palatal excursion. However, a "double levator knee" is usually apparent with asymmetric palatal movement.

A more objective measure of nasal resonance can be obtained with *nasometry*, where two separate measures of sound output from the nasal and oral passages are recorded during speech. A ratio of sound pressure energy generates a nasalance score. A high nasal score reflects a high degree of nasal emission, which is useful in cases where nasal air escape is inaudible in speech evaluation.

Static *magnetic resonance imaging* (MRI) may offer useful information regarding the position of the palate muscles. Dynamic real-time MRI scanning is a very promising future investigative tool, with the potential of providing three-dimensional visualization of the velopharyngeal port.

Upper airway assessment, including presence or absence of mouth breathing, snoring, obstructive sleep apnea or nasal airway obstruction, is essential prior to surgical management of VPI. Further, a Mueller test may be performed, in which lateral pharyngeal wall stability on deep inspiration against obstruction (with mouth and nose closed) is also examined. In the presence of symptomatology suggestive of obstructive sleep apnea on preoperative evaluation, a polysomnogram is requested. If indicated (i.e., structural impediment to flap harvest and/or inset), tonsillectomy and/or adenoidectomy is performed 3–6 months prior to surgery.

Surgical Management of Velopharyngeal Dysfunction

One of the primary principles of treatment for VPD is that *speech therapy will not correct VPI*. Following restoration of the structural elements to allow for velopharyngeal closure and correct nasal resonance, speech therapy is likely to be required to eliminate compensatory misarticulations and behavioral abnormalities (e.g., nasal grimace), as well as provide auditory reinforcement to promote closure. However, speech therapy can be applied if VPI is *intermittent* and therefore, although inconsistent, sphincteric closure can be achieved. Management of VPD aims to achieve satisfactory nasal resonance without inducing airway or nasal obstruction. Surgical management can be divided into palatal procedures and pharyngeal surgery.

Modifications to the velum include Furlow palatoplasty or palate re-repair with intravelar veloplasty. The former is implemented to lengthen the palate and re-establish the levator sling. Additionally, by performing a Z-plasty, recruitment of lateral pharyngeal tissue also results in tightening

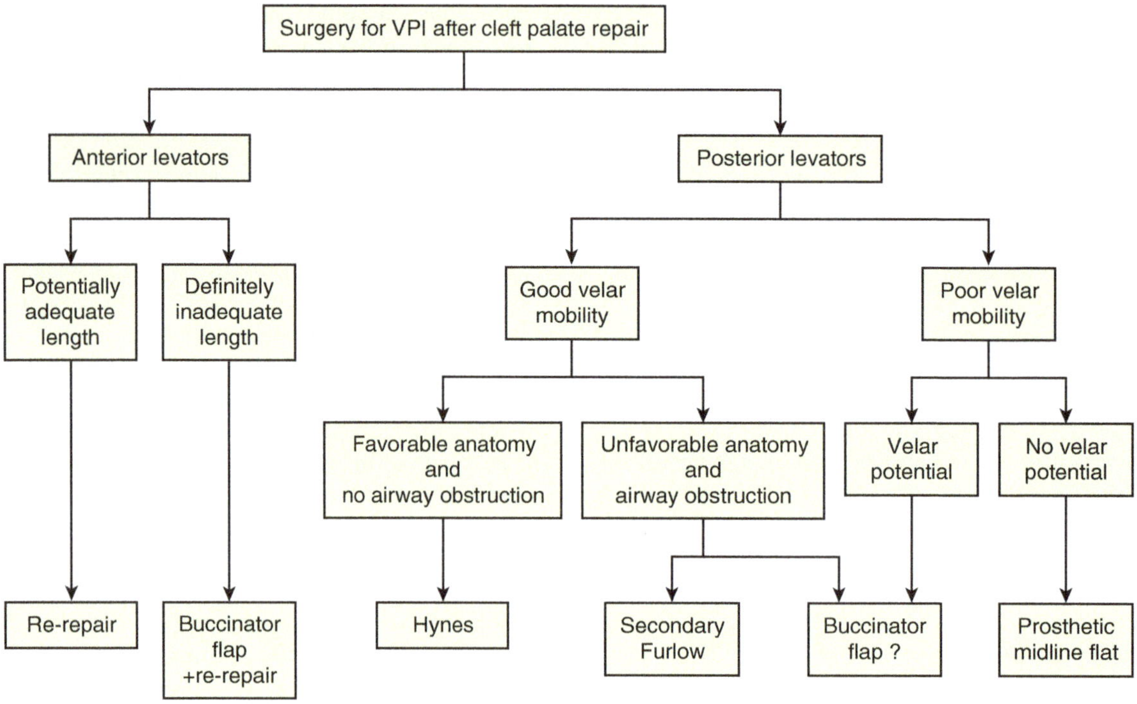

• **Fig. 17.12** Algorithm for the surgical management of VPI.

of the superior pharyngeal constrictor and consequently the velopharyngeal port. The premise for palate re-repair with intravelar veloplasty is to retroposition the palatal musculature in order to recruit the residual soft palate for velopharyngeal closure, thereby optimizing the position and function of the levator (i.e., increasing effective velar length).[48] Moreover, buccinator flaps can be interposed at the junction of hard and soft palates in a short velum with adequate motility and posteriorly positioned levator musculature in an effort to achieve palatal lengthening.[49] Pharyngeal procedures include pharyngeal flap, pharyngoplasty, and pharyngeal wall augmentation with either autologous or allogenic material. Fig. 17.12 outlines the senior author's algorithm for the surgical management of VPI.

Pharyngeal Flap

In 1865, Passavant described the original procedure for management of VPI in which adhesion between the soft palate and posterior pharyngeal wall was carried out, the forerunner of the pharyngeal flap. Later in 1875, Schoenborn introduced the inferiorly based pharyngeal flap,[50] which he later modified to a superiorly based flap.[51] Rosenthal[52] reported on the use of a pharyngeal flap in primary cleft palate repair, where a pharyngeal flap was combined with a von Langenbeck palatoplasty. The posterior pharyngeal flap was popularized by Padgett[53] as a salvage procedure in patients with failed primary cleft palate repair. The pharyngeal flap is designed to create a passive central obturator in the velopharyngeal sphincter, leaving two lateral ports (Fig. 17.13). Lateral gutters facilitate nasal breathing, nasal resonance, and mucous drainage. Hogan[54] later refined pharyngeal flap design with the introduction of the concept of lateral port control, in which the size of the lateral ports is carefully calibrated at the time of surgery with the use of catheters placed through the two ports. In 1979, Shprintzen et al[55] further advanced pharyngeal flap surgery with the advent of "tailor-made" pharyngeal flaps, wherein the width of the flap is determined by the degree of lateral wall motion as seen on preoperative nasoendoscopy and/or videofluoroscopy. Successful management of VPI with a pharyngeal flap necessitates satisfactory mesial movement of the lateral pharyngeal walls for lateral port occlusion,[56] and is therefore considered in patients with a sagittal closure pattern. If lateral wall motion is insufficient for lateral port closure (e.g., coronal closure pattern) or if the flap is too narrow (poor flap design) or attenuated (postoperative tubular contracture secondary to unlined flap undersurface), hypernasality may persist. In contrast, lateral port occlusion may result in airway compromise, hyponasality and mouth breathing. Interestingly, Karling et al[57] noted a correlation between flap width and adduction of the lateral pharyngeal walls. More specifically, patients with limited preoperative adduction demonstrated a greater increase in lateral wall excursion with a narrow flap than with a wide flap, while those with greater preoperative excursion showed a decrease in postoperative adduction in relation to flap width.[58] The latter "learning phenomenon" provides one possible explanation for those patients that retain a certain degree of velopharyngeal competence following surgical flap division or dehiscence. Other potential reasons for persistent velopharyngeal function following flap resection include augmentation of the posterior pharyngeal wall with the residual flap remaining as a pad or possibly anatomic changes in the pharynx secondary to the

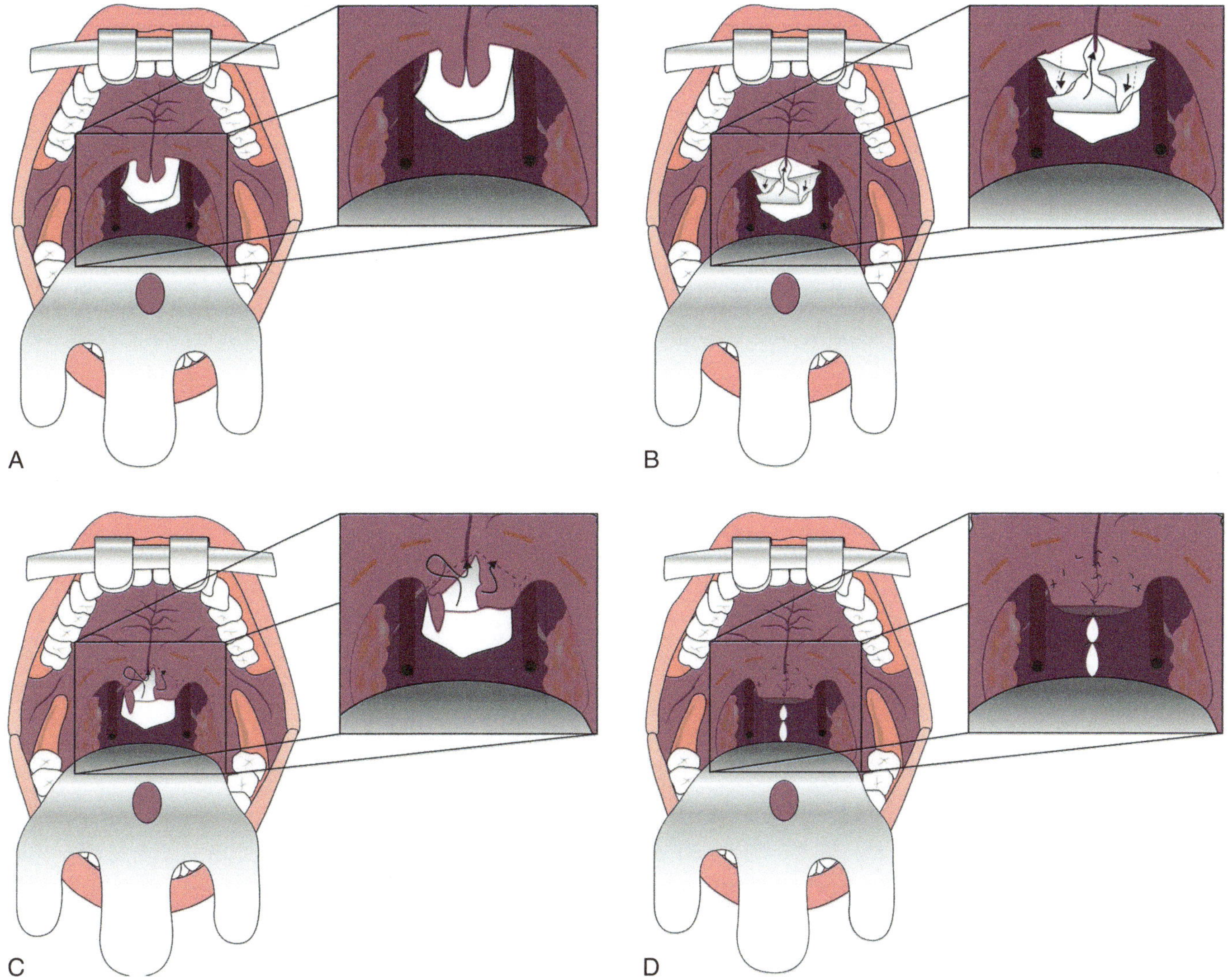

• **Fig. 17.13** Diagrammatic illustration of key steps in the operative technique for superiorly based pharyngeal flap harvest and inset. (A) Superiorly based flap is incised in the posterior pharyngeal wall and the soft palate is divided in the midline. (B) Posteriorly based flaps of nasal lining of the velum are elevated. (C) The pharyngeal flap is inset onto the nasal surface of the soft palate and the previously raised flaps from the nasal surface of the palate are used to line the raw (oral) surface of the pharyngeal flap. (D) The soft palate is closed in the midline, along with the donor defect in the posterior pharyngeal wall.

initial surgery, such as narrowing of the velopharyngeal port due to scar contracture at the donor site.

The most common complications of pharyngeal flap surgery include bleeding and airway compromise. The most notable complication is the potential for obstructive sleep apnea. There are a number of other factors that contribute to obstructive sleep apnea following pharyngeal flap harvest, in addition to the mechanical barrier of the flap per se at the level of the nasopharynx. Moreover, syndrome-specific features may aggravate any mechanical obstruction. More specifically, obstruction is often secondary to lateral wall collapse against a wide pharyngeal flap. The latter is especially notable in patients with velocardiofacial syndrome, in whom generalized muscular hypotonia presents a predisposition for pharyngeal wall collapse and obstruction. In addition, obstruction may occur as a result of flap harvest, which also narrows the lower portions of the pharynx, thus increasing resistance in the oro- and hypopharynx. The latter is secondary to the flap donor site that remains to heal by secondary intention thereby creating circular contraction. Other factors include posteriorly displaced tonsils that extend within the lateral ports and occlude the nasopharyngeal airway. Tonsillar hypertrophy may also compromise the oropharyngeal airway, as circular contraction brings them in closer proximity. Obstructive sleep apnoea occasionally necessitates division of the flap, when not amenable to nonsurgical management.

Caution should be exercised when selecting pharyngeal flap surgery in patients with VCFS, in view of the high prevalence of medial displacement of the internal carotid arteries. This poses significant risks in execution of this procedure given that the abnormal positioning of the vasculature in the pharynx is coincident with the region of pharyngeal flap harvest. Moreover, the danger of ectopic localization of the arteries is aggravated by the characteristically thin pharyngeal

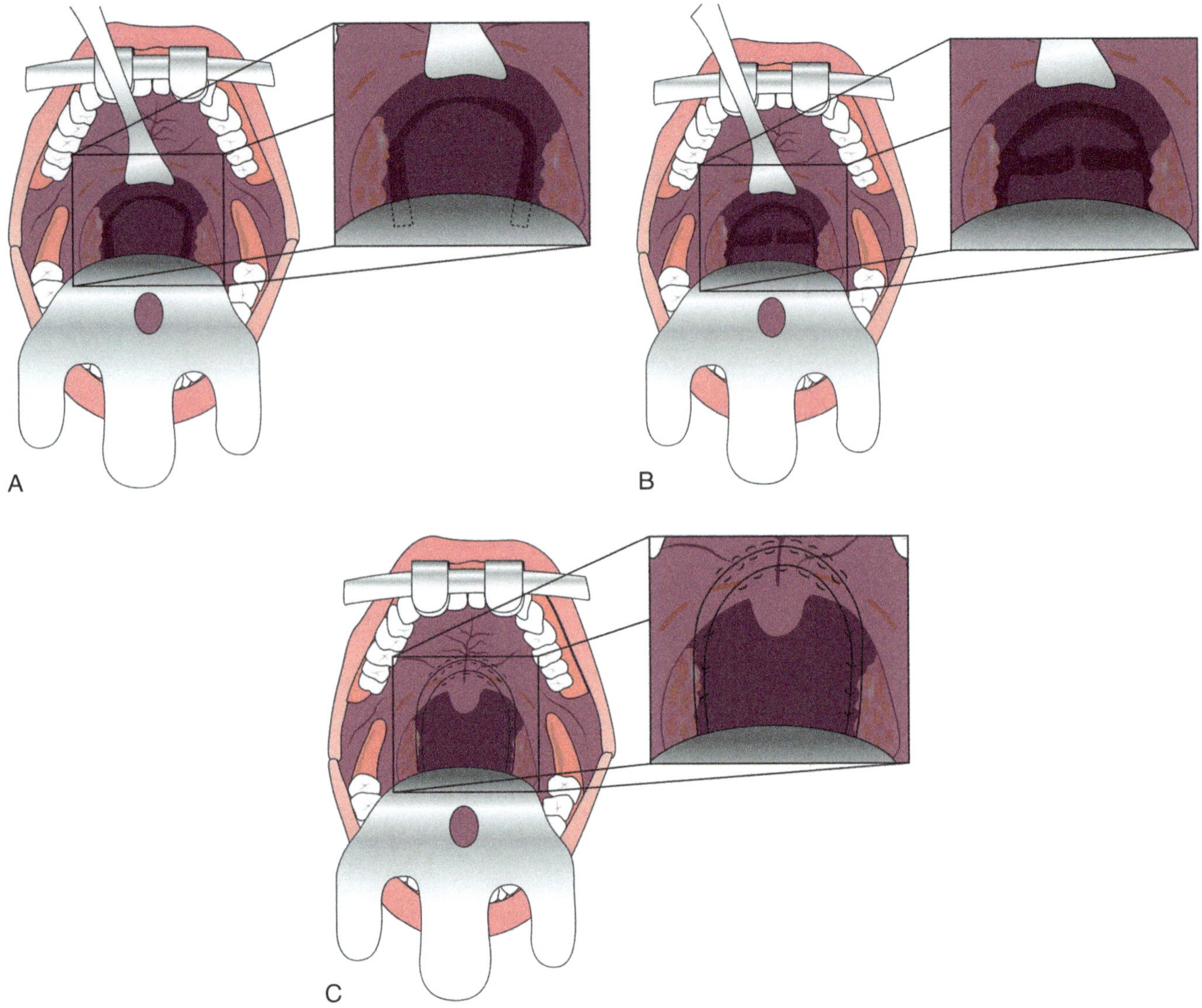

• **Fig. 17.14** Diagrammatic illustration of key steps in the operative technique for modified Hynes pharyngoplasty. (A) Bilateral palatopharyngeus muscle flaps are outlined. (B) Muscle flaps are elevated and transposed. (C) Flaps are sutured together end-to-end, as well as to the posterior pharyngeal wall.

musculature. Many favor evaluation of the cervical vasculature with MRI angiography prior to consideration of surgical velopharyngeal correction. However, the results obtained with more sophisticated imaging modalities cannot be extrapolated to the patient at the time of operation, where the internal carotids adopt a less median position with neck hyperextension. Thus, routine vascular imaging, even when aberrant pulsations are noted on preoperative nasoendoscopy, does not appear crucial or reliable. According to Mehendale and Sommerlad,[59] the most reliable measure is direct observation and palpation of the pharynx at the time of surgery. If necessary, the position and width of the pharyngeal flap can be modified to minimize the risk of artery exposure.

Pharyngoplasty

Hynes[60] described a technique for pharyngoplasty, where bilateral superiorly based musculomucosal flaps were elevated from the lateral pharyngeal walls and inset onto the posterior pharyngeal wall. Flaps included salpingopharyngeus and later modified to contain the descending fibres of the palatopharyngeus and a portion of the superior constrictor.[61] The elevated flaps, based at the level of the Eustachian cushions, are transposed 90 degrees and sutured to the posterior pharyngeal wall, which is incised transversely from the superior end of the posterior limb of one lateral flap to the other, at the level of attempted velopharyngeal closure or atlas (first cervical vertebra) (Fig. 17.14). The flaps are inset in overlapping fashion.[61] In his original description, Hynes described division of the soft palate in order to gain access to the nasopharynx and facilitate flap inset. Pharyngoplasty attenuates VPD by diminishing the central velopharyngeal space. This procedure is used in patients with a coronal or circular closure pattern and adequate palatal motion, or hypotonic velopharynx. In effect, these flaps are used to *augment the posterior pharyngeal wall*, thereby reducing the palatal movement necessary to achieve closure.

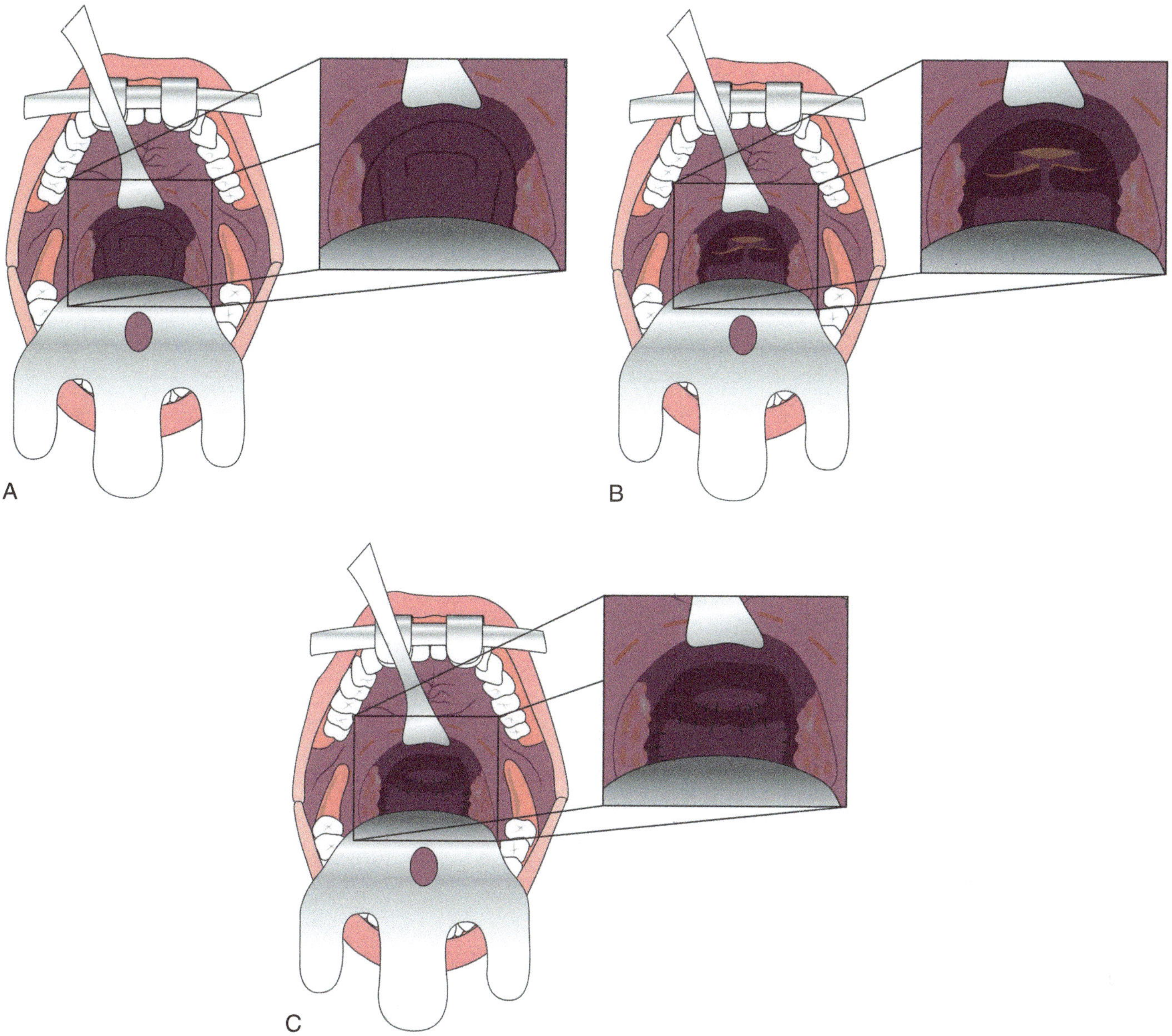

• **Fig. 17.15** Diagrammatic illustration of key steps in the operative technique for Orticochea pharyngoplasty. (A) Bilateral flaps from the posterior tonsillar pillars and an inferiorly based flap on the posterior pharyngeal wall are outlined. (B) Flaps are elevated and transposed. (C) Flaps are inset into the posterior pharyngeal flap.

Orticochea[62,63] described a pharyngoplasty, which is quite distinct from the Hynes pharyngoplasty despite the two procedures being often confused. In this operation, the flaps are raised from the posterior tonsillar pillars, based superiorly and containing palatopharyngeus muscle. The flaps are transposed and inset into a short but wide inferiorly based posterior pharyngeal flap *below* the level of attempted closure in the oropharynx and below that of the Hynes pharyngoplasty as previously described (Fig. 17.15). Jackson and Silverton[64] modified this procedure by altering the inferiorly based flap to a superiorly based flap in an effort to bring the flaps closer to the level of attempted closure, but later eliminated the supplementary posterior pharyngeal flap. Orticochea proposed the notion of *dynamic pharyngoplasty*, claiming that the transposed flaps of palatopharyngeus maintain intrinsic contractile function and therefore produce an active sphincter that assists in velopharyngeal closure (hence the term "sphincter pharyngoplasty"). However, many would argue that the dynamic nature of this procedure is questionable. Moreover, despite initial optimism that it would produce less airway compromise than a posterior pharyngeal flap, evidence suggests it is equally obstructive.

Prosthetic Management

Nonsurgical management is indicated in patients with a completely hypodynamic velopharyngeal mechanism (e.g., neuromuscular disorder), in those for whom surgical intervention is contraindicated or those with severe or persistent airway obstruction that is recalcitrant or not amenable to conservative management. Nonoperative treatment consists of placement of a prosthetic device, either palatal lift and/or pharyngeal obturator. The palatal lift device is used to reposition the palate to a location where minimal excursion is required to effect closure, while the pharyngeal obturator acts to occlude the defect in the velopharyngeal sphincter.

Management of Unilateral or Asymmetric VPI

Management of unilateral or asymmetric VPI includes pharyngeal bulb, skewed pharyngeal flap, unilateral pharyngoplasty, and unilateral adhesion of the adynamic hemi-velum to the posterior pharyngeal wall. Mehendale and Sommerlad[65] described the use of a *unilateral* Moore pharyngoplasty flap to support the nonfunctioning or poorly functioning side of the velum, thereby assisting the active contralateral levator to elevate the entire velum. As originally described, the Moore pharyngoplasty involves bilateral posterolateral pharyngeal flaps that are inset into a transverse incision at the junction of the middle and posterior thirds of the nasal surface of the velum.[66] Goals of this procedure include obliteration of the lateral pharyngeal recesses, increased tissue bulk on the nasal surface of the velum at the point of potential contact of the velum with the posterior pharyngeal wall, and possibly velar lengthening. Moreover, the flaps are thought to augment the action of the levator by forming an active muscular sling. As previously mentioned, unilateral or asymmetric VPI is a common finding in patients with oculo-auriculo-vertebral spectrum.[67]

References

1. Zucchero TM, Cooper ME, Maher BS, et al. Interferon regulatory factor 6 (*IRF6*) gene variants and the risk of isolated cleft lip or palate. *N Engl J Med.* 2004;351:769–780.
2. Boorman JG, Sommerlad BC. Levator palati and palatal dimples: their anatomy, relationship and clinical significance. *Br J Plast Surg.* 1985;38:326–332.
3. Dellon AL, Claybaugh GJ, Hoopes JE. Hemi-palatal palsy and microtia. *Ann Plast Surg.* 1983;10:475–479.
4. Veau V, Ruppie C. Anatomie chirurgicale de la division palatine. *J Chir.* 1992;20:1–30.
5. Glaser ER, Skolnick ML, McWilliams BJ, et al. The dynamics of Passavant's ridge in subjects with and without velopharyngeal insufficiency – a multi-view videofluoroscopic study. *Cleft Palate J.* 1979;16:24–33.
6. Calnan JS. Modern views on Passavant's ridge. *Br J Plast Surg.* 1957:89–113.
7. Huang MHS, Lee ST, Rajendran K. Structure of the musculus uvulae: functional and surgical implications of an anatomic study. *Cleft Palate Craniofac J.* 1997;34:466–474.
8. Boorman JG, Sommerlad BC. Musculus uvulae and levator palati: their anatomical and functional relationship in velopharyngeal closure. *Br J Plast Surg.* 1985;38:333–338.
9. Calnan JS. Submucous cleft palate. *Br J Plast Surg.* 1954;6:264–272.
10. Kaplan EN. The occult submucous cleft palate. *Cleft Palate J.* 1975;12:356–368.
11. Lewin ML, Croft CB, Shprintzen RJ. Velopharyngeal insufficiency due to hypoplasia of the musculus uvulae and occult submucous cleft palate. *Plast Reconstr Surg.* 1980;65:585–591.
12. Sommerlad BC, Fenn C, Harland K, et al. Submucous cleft palate: a grading system and review of 40 consecutive submucous cleft palate repairs. *Cleft Palate Craniofac J.* 2004;41:114–123.
13. Robin P. La chute de la base de la langue considérée comme une nouvelle cause de gene dans la respiration naso-pharyngienne. *Bull Acad Natl Med (Paris).* 1923;89:37–41.
14. Robin P. Glossoptosis due to atresia and hypotrophy of the mandible. *Am J Dis Child.* 1934;48:514–547.
15. Sher AE, Shprintzen RJ, Thorpy MJ. Endoscopic observations of obstructive sleep apnea in children with anomalous upper airways: predictive and therapeutic value. *Int J Ped Otorhinolaryngol.* 1986;11:135–146.
16. Sher AE. Mechanisms of airway obstruction in Robin sequence: implications for treatment. *Cleft Palate Craniofac J.* 1992;29:224–231.
17. Douglas B. The treatment of micrognathia associated with obstruction by a plastic procedure. *Plast Reconstr Surg.* 1946;1:300–308.
18. Routledge RT. The Pierre Robin syndrome: a surgical emergency in the neonatal period. *Br J Plast Surg.* 1960;13:204–218.
19. Epois V. Anatomie et evolution du squelette facial dans les fentes labio-maxillo-palatines. *Chir Pediatr.* 1983;24:240.
20. Delorme R-P, Larocque Y, Caouette-Laberge L. Innovative surgical approach for the Pierre Robin anomalad: subperiosteal release of the floor of the mouth musculature. *Plast Reconstr Surg.* 1989;83:960–964.
21. Tahiri Y, Viezel-Mathieu A, Aldekhayel S, et al. The effectiveness of mandibular distraction in improving airway obstruction in the pediatric population. *Plast Reconstr Surg.* 2014;133:352–359.
22. Stuppia L, Capogreco M, Marzo G, et al. Genetics of syndromic and nonsyndromic cleft lip and palate. *J Craniofac Surg.* 2011;22:1722–1726.
23. Shprintzen RJ. Velo-cardio-facial syndrome: 30 years of study. *Dev Disabil Res Rev.* 2008;14:3–10.
24. Schweckendiek W, Doz P. Primary veloplasty: long-term results without maxillary deformity – a twenty-five year report. *Cleft Palate J.* 1978;15:268–274.
25. Bardach J, Morris HL, Olin WH. Late results of primary veloplasty: the Marburg project. *Plast Reconstr Surg.* 1984;73:207–218.
26. Ysunza A, Pamplona C, Mendoza M, et al. Speech outcome and maxillary growth in patients with unilateral complete cleft lip/palate operated on 6 versus 12 months of age. *Plast Reconstr Surg.* 1998;102:675–679.
27. Sommerlad BC. International Confederation for cleft lip and palate and related craniofacial anomalies task force report – "palatoplasty in the speaking individual with unrepaired cleft palate". *Cleft Palate Craniofac J.* 2004;51:122–128.
28. Langenbeck B von. Die uranoplastik mittles ablosung des mucrosperiostalen gaumenuberzuges. *Arch Klin Chir.* 1986;2:205.
29. Veau V. *Division palatine.* Paris: Masson & Cie; 1931.
30. Kilner TP. Cleft lip and palate repair technique. In: Maingot R, ed. *Postgraduate Surgery.* Vol. 3. London: Medical Publishers; 1937.
31. Wardill WEM. Technique of operation for cleft lip and palate. *Br J Surg.* 1937;25:97.
32. Bardach J, Salyer KE. Cleft palate repair. In: Bardach J, Salyer KE, eds. *Surgical Techniques in Cleft Lip and Palate.* St Louis, MO: Mosby; 1991:224–273.

33. Braithwaite F, Maurice DG. The importance of the levator palatini muscle in cleft palate closure. *Br J Plast Surg*. 1968;21:60–62.
34. Kriens O. An anatomical approach to veloplasty. *Plast Reconstr Surg*. 1969;43:29–41.
35. Edgerton MT, Dellon AL. Surgical retrodisplacement of the levator veli palatini muscle. *Plast Reconstr Surg*. 1971;47:154–167.
36. Furlow LT. Cleft palate repair by double opposing z-plasty. *Plast Reconstr Surg*. 1986;78:724–736.
37. Cutting C, Rosenbaum J, Rovati L. The technique of muscle repair in the cleft soft palate. *Oper Tech Plast Reconstr Surg*. 1995;2:215–222.
38. Sommerlad BC. A technique for palate repair. *Plast Reconstr Surg*. 2003;112:1542–1548.
39. Sommerlad BC. The use of the operating microscope in cleft palate repair and pharyngoplasty. *Plast Reconstr Surg*. 2003;112:1540–1541.
40. Pichler H. Zur operation der doppelten lippen-gaumenspalten. *Dtsch Z Cir*. 1926;195:104.
41. Abyholm FE, Borcgrevink HC, Eskeland G. Cleft lip and palate in Norway. III. Surgical treatment of CLP patients in Oslo 1954–75. *Scand J Plast Reconstr Surg*. 1981;15:15–28.
42. Agrawal K, Panda KN. Use of vomer flap in palatoplasty: revisited. *Cleft Palate Craniofac J*. 2006;43:30–37.
43. Shprintzen ML, Croft CB, Shprintzen RJ. Velopharyngeal insufficiency due to hypoplasia of the musculus uvulae and occult submucous cleft palate. *Plast Reconstr Surg*. 1980;65:585–591.
44. Mehendale FV, Birch MJ, Birkett L, et al. Surgical management of velopharyngeal incompetence in velocardiofacial syndrome. *Cleft Palate Craniofac J*. 2004;41:124–135.
45. Skolnick ML, McCall GN, Barnes M. The sphincter mechanism of velopharyngeal closure. *Cleft Palate J*. 1973;10:286–305.
46. Croft CB, Shprintzen RJ, Rakoff SJ. Patterns of velopharyngeal valving in normal and cleft palate subjects: a multi-view videofluoroscopic and nasoendoscopic study. *Laryngoscope*. 1981;91:265–271.
47. Birch M, Sommerlad BC, Bhatt A. Image analysis of lateral velopharyngeal closure in repaired cleft palates and normal palates. *Br J Plast Surg*. 1994;47:400–405.
48. Sommerlad BC, Mehendale FV, Birch MJ, et al. Palate re-repair revisited. *Cleft Palate Craniofac J*. 2002;39:295–307.
49. Hens G, Sell D, Pinkstone M, et al. Palate lengthening by buccinator myomucosal flaps for velopharyngeal insufficiency. *Cleft Palate Craniofac J*. 2013;50:84–91.
50. Schoenborn K. Ueber eine neue Methode der Staphylorrhaphie. *Verh Dtsch Ges Chir*. 1875;4:235–239.
51. Schoenborn K. Vorstellung eines falle von Staphyloplastik. *Verh Dtsch Ges Chir*. 1886;15:57–68.
52. Rosenthal W. Pathologie und Therapie der Gaumendefekte. *Fortschr Zahnheilk*. 1928;4:55–56.
53. Padgett EC. The repair of cleft palates after unsuccessful operations, with special reference to cases with an extensive loss of palatal tissue. *Arch Surg*. 1930;20:453–472.
54. Hogan VM. A clarification of the goals in cleft palate speech and the introduction of the lateral port control (LPC) pharyngeal flap. *Cleft Palate J*. 1973;10:331–345.
55. Shprintzen RJ, Lewin ML, Croft ML, et al. A comprehensive study of pharyngeal flap surgery: tailor made flaps. *Cleft Palate J*. 1979;16:46–55.
56. Argamaso RV, Shprintzen RJ, Strauch B, et al. The role of lateral wall movement in pharyngeal flap surgery. *Plast Reconstr Surg*. 1980;66:214–219.
57. Karling J, Henningson G, Larson O, et al. Adaptation of pharyngeal wall adduction after pharyngeal flap surgery. *Cleft Palate Craniofac J*. 1999;36:166–172.
58. Shprintzen RJ, McCall GN, Skolnick ML. The effect of pharyngeal flap surgery on the movements of the lateral pharyngeal walls. *Plast Reconstr Surg*. 1980;66:570–573.
59. Mehendale FV, Sommerlad BC. Surgical significance of abnormal internal carotid arteries in velocardiofacial syndrome in 43 consecutive hynes pharyngoplasties. *Cleft Palate Craniofac J*. 2004;41:368–374.
60. Hynes W. Pharyngoplasty by muscle transplantation. *Br J Plast Surg*. 1950;3:128–135.
61. Hynes W. Observations on pharyngoplasty. *Br J Plast Surg*. 1967;20:244–256.
62. Orticochea M. Construction of a dynamic muscle sphincter in cleft palates. *Plast Reconstr Surg*. 1968;41:323–331.
63. Orticochea M. A review of 236 cleft palate patients treated with dynamic muscle sphincter. *Plast Recontr Surg*. 1983;71:180–191.
64. Jackson IT, Silverston JS. Sphincter pharyngoplasty as a secondary procedure in cleft palates. *Plast Reconstr Surg*. 1977;59:518–525.
65. Mehendale FV, Sommerlad BC. Unilateral Moore pharyngoplasty in the treatment of unilateral or asymmetric velopharyngeal incompetence. *Cleft Palate Craniofac J*. 2003;40:262–268.
66. Moore FT. A new operation to cure nasopharyngreal incompetence. *Br J Surg*. 1960;47:424–428.
67. Shprintzen RJ, Croft CB, Berkman MD, et al. Velopharyngeal insufficiency in the facio-auriculo-vertebral malformation complex. *Cleft Palate J*. 1980;17:132–137.

18

Congenital Ear Anomalies

SABRINA CUGNO AND NEIL W. BULSTRODE

For videos accompanying this chapter see ExpertConsult.com. See inside cover for access details.

Ear Development

The intricate contours of the external ear are attributed to delicate elastic cartilage covered with a thin layer of subcutaneous tissue and skin. The ear develops around the first branchial cleft, which is the groove between the first (mandibular) and second (hyoid) pharyngeal arches. Auricular development begins during the fifth week of gestation. At the sixth week of embryogenesis six tubercles, the auricular hillocks of His, appear on the first and second branchial arches. The three anterior hillocks of the mandibular arch give rise to the tragus, root of the helix, and superior helix, respectively, while the three posterior hillocks of the hyoid arch form the remaining components of the auricle (Fig. 18.1). The development of the ear is usually complete by the fourth month of gestation.[1] The auricles are initially positioned on the embryonic neck, and progressively migrate from this anterocaudal location posterocranially as the mandible enlarges until it reaches its final anatomic location by week 20. As a result, remnants of the developing ear may be found at any point along this route, often localized to the preauricular region, so-called *preauricular skin tags*. Rarely polyotia may be encountered, considered an extreme form of the rudimentary skin tag, distinguished by both size and morphology. Polyotia bears resemblance to the normal external ear and is often termed *mirror ear*, with a conjoined conchal bowl in place of the tragus (Fig. 18.2). The middle ear structures are also derived from the first and second branchial arches, and external auditory meatus and canal from the first branchial groove. Thus, patients with microtia typically have atresia of the external auditory canal and tympanic membrane, as well as variable deformities of the middle ear ossicles. Before subtleties of congenital anomalies can be recognized, the topography of normal ear must be appreciated and is illustrated in Fig. 18.3.

While the ear has its definitive form at birth, the auricular cartilage of the neonatal ear retains distinct malleability due to enduring high levels of circulating maternal estrogen. Estrogen upregulates the production of hyaluronic acid, which increases the pliability of cartilage. Estrogen levels are highest in the first 3 days after birth and decrease to a level comparable to older children at 6 weeks of age.[2] During this privileged period, *deformational* anomalies of the auricle can be corrected by nonoperative means with external moulding devices. Authors have reported

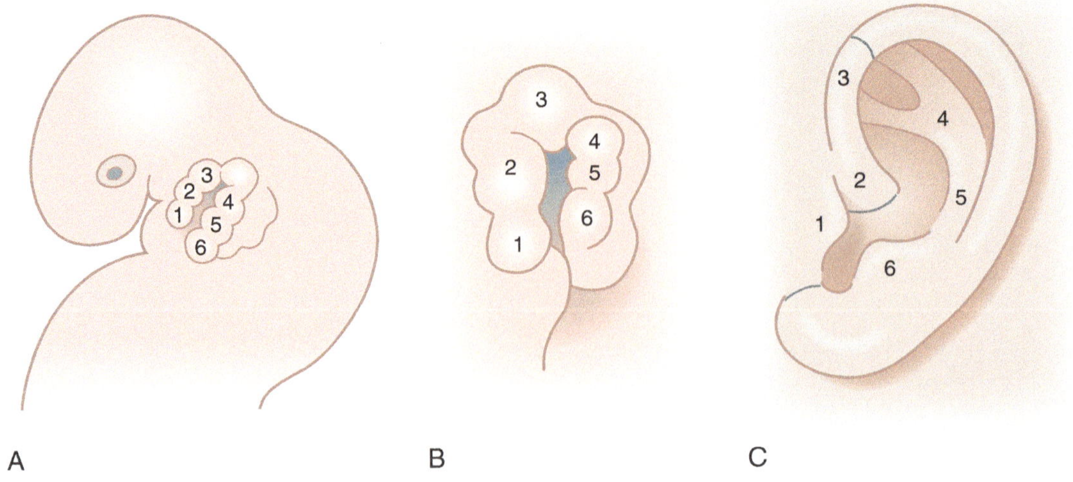

• **Fig. 18.1** Embryology of the external ear. Hillock formation in an 11-mm human embryo. Hillock configuration at 6 weeks' gestation in a 15-mm embryo and hillock derivations in the adult auricle. 1, tragus, 2, root of helix, 3, helical rim, 4, superior and inferior crus, 5 antihelix, 6, anti-tragus (Modified from Beahm EK, Walton RL. Auricular reconstruction for microtia: Part I. Anatomy, embryology and clinical evaluation. *Plast Reconstr Surg*. 2002;109:2473–2482.)

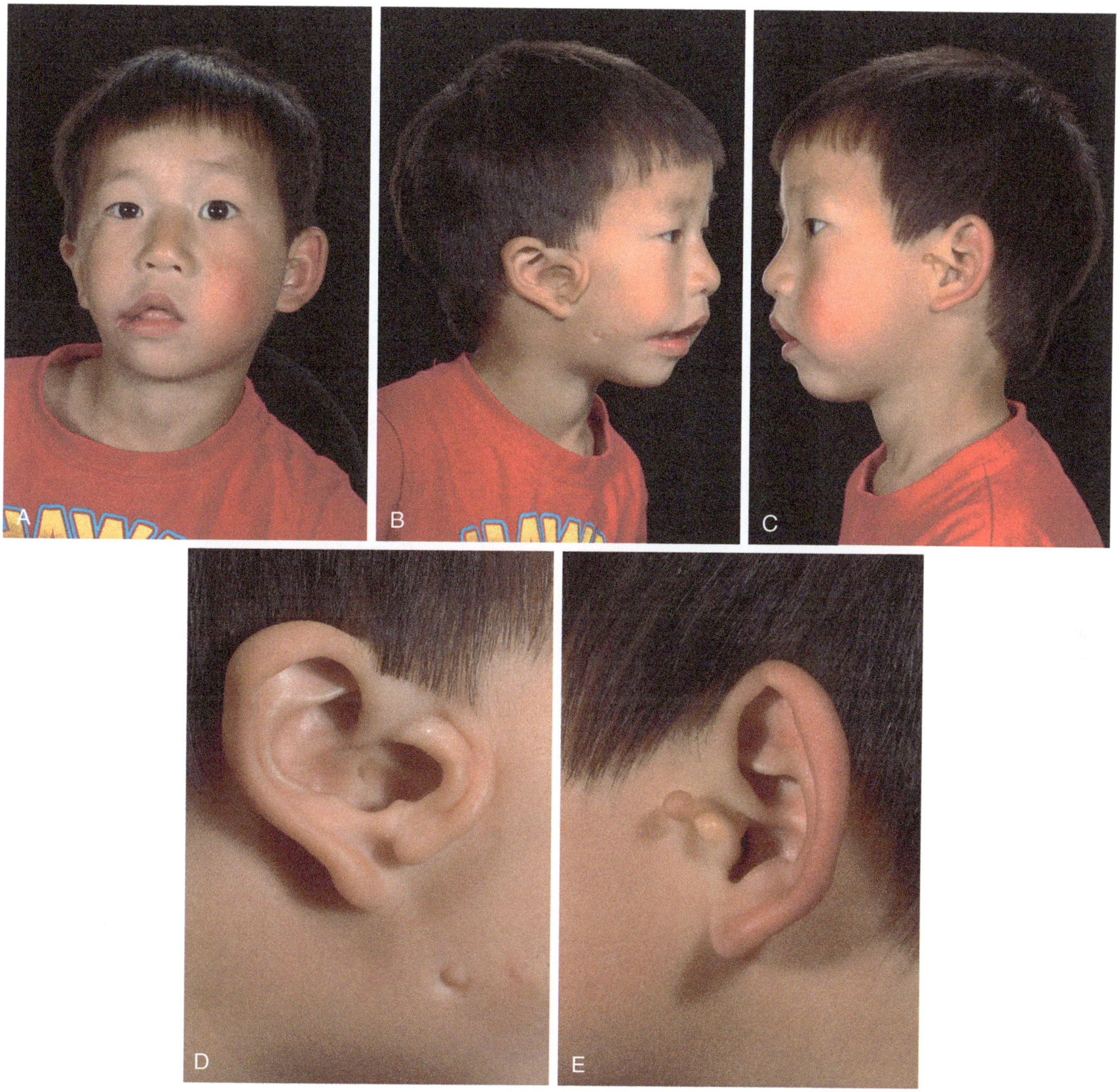

• **Fig. 18.2** (A–E) Patient with oculo-auriculo-vertebral spectrum who presented with simple preauricular skin tags on the left ear (E) and classic mirror ear on the right ear (D).

excellent results when correction is initiated within 3 days of birth.[2] Thereafter, alteration of deformational irregularities, like auricular malformations, must be effected by surgical means. There is no consensus as to the upper age limit that splinting therapy can be considered, nor reliable evidence on the length of time needed for auricular moulding.

There is marked variability in the phenotypic expression of congenital deformities of the ear, challenging classification of these anomalies. The classification system proposed by Tanzer in 1978[3] is still commonly used (Box 18.1). Congenital auricular anomalies can be categorized as either malformations or deformations. The malformed ear presents hypoplasia of cartilaginous and cutaneous constituents and gross morphological aberrations, whereas the deformed auricle has a normal chondrocutaneous component but irregular architecture. Further, while malformational anomalies arise from a combination of genetic and environmental factors, deformational abnormalities are deemed to result from external forces applied to the developing or neonatal ear and/or abnormal morphology or function of the three extrinsic and/or six intrinsic auricular muscles. The intrinsic musculature is mainly vestigial at birth but during auricular morphogenesis has an integral role in folding of the ear.

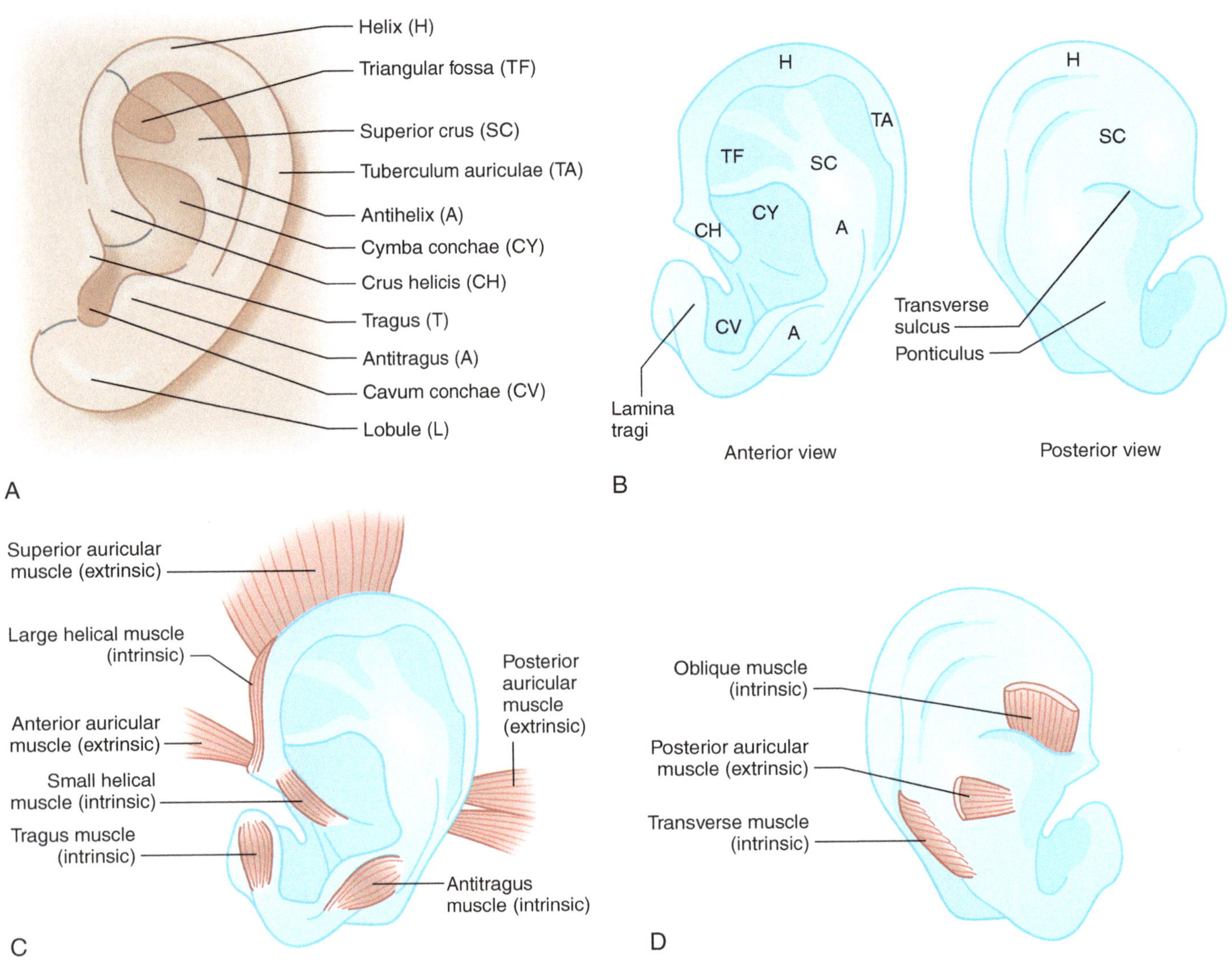

• **Fig. 18.3** External ear anatomy, including illustration of anterior and posterior views of ear cartilage anatomy, as well as extrinsic and intrinsic auricular muscles. (Modified from Beahm EK, Walton RL. Auricular reconstruction for microtia: Part I. Anatomy, embryology and clinical evaluation. *Plast Reconstr Surg*. 2002;109:2473–2482.)

• BOX 18.1 Ear Deformity Classification System of Tanzer[3]

Type 1: Anotia
Type 2: Completely hypoplastic ear (microtia)
  a. With atresia of the external auditory canal
  b. Without atresia of the external auditory canal
Type 3: Hypoplasia of the middle third of the auricle
Type 4: Hypoplasia of the superior third of the auricle
  a. Constricted (cup or lop) ear
  b. Cryptotia
  c. Hypoplasia of entire superior third
Type 5: Prominent ear

At birth, the normal auricle is approximately 66% of its adult size. The superior aspect of the helix is at the level of the tail of the eyebrow and the inferior aspect of the lobule corresponds to the base of the columella, with the long axis of the auricle inclined posteriorly at approximately 20 degrees from vertical. At 5 years of age, the ear has grown to within 8 mm of its full adult vertical height (approx. 5.5–7 cm), and is therefore approximately 87% complete. Ear length reaches its mature size at age 13 in males and age 12 in females. In contrast, ear width at age 5 years has attained approximately 97% of its adult size. The width of the ear continues to grow until age 7 and 6 in males and in females, respectively (width is approximately 55% of the length, 3–4.5 cm).[4] This has important implications regarding timing of operative correction.

Prominent Ears

Ideal projection of the normal external ear is often cited as 1.5–2 cm from the scalp, and the projection of the helix from the mastoid as 10–12 mm in the superior portion, 16–18 mm and 20–22 mm in the middle and inferior portions, respectively.[5] The auricle is considered as prominent if on frontal view it projects beyond these limits.

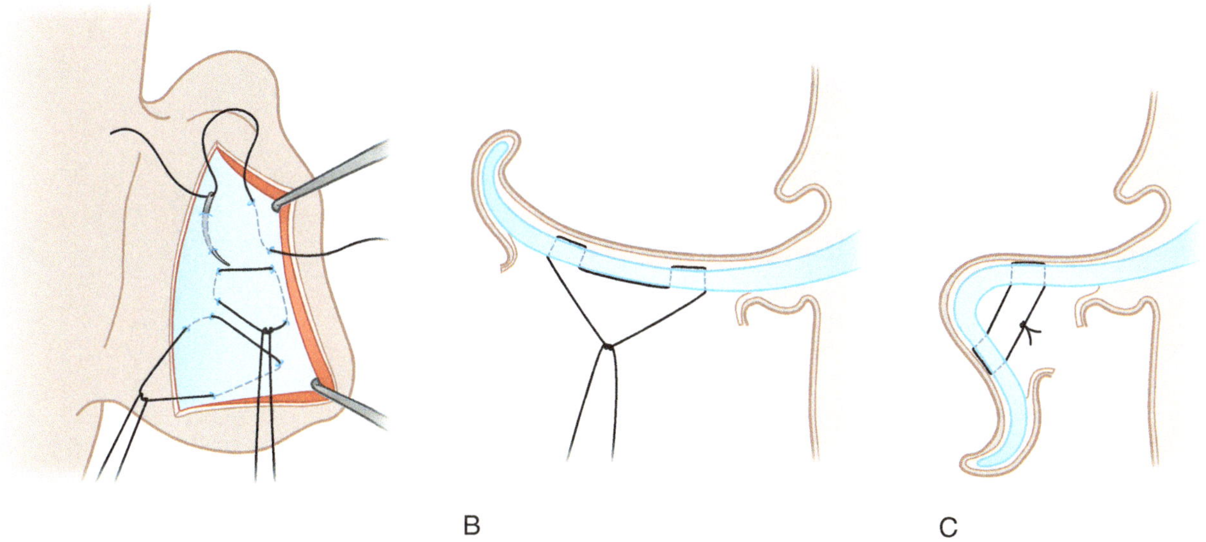

• **Fig. 18.4** (A–C) Diagrammatic illustration of Mustardé mattress suture placement for creation antihelical fold. (Modified from Mustardé JC. The correction of prominent ears using simple mattress sutures. *Br J Plast Surg*. 1963;16:170–176.)

Prominent ears or *prominauris* is the most common congenital abnormality of the ear. It is associated with an autosomal dominant inheritance pattern with variable penetrance. This deformational anomaly is qualified by one or a combination of the following features:

1. Effacement or reduced definition of the antihelical fold
2. Prominence of the concha (overdevelopment of the posterior wall of the concha and/or increased angle between mastoid and concha)
3. Prominence of the lobule.

Other commonly associated features include excessive angulation of the helical root from the temple, absence of the helical roll (*shell ear* deformity), and macrotia. There is no consensus regarding the optimal age at which to perform correction (otoplasty), and it may be considered as early as age 4 years. Ideally, the authors' preference is to delay correction until at least age 6 years. At this age the ear has nearly attained its final adult size and, although anecdotal, the increased rigidity of the auricle at age 6 appears to decrease the occurrence of inadvertent damage to the cartilage, which can result in irregularities in auricular form.

Numerous techniques have been described for correction of each of the three above-mentioned features of the prominent ear. Methods to recreate the antihelical fold are classified as cartilage suturing, cartilage scoring, and cartilage breaking. Cartilage breaking, initially proposed by Luckett in 1910,[6] involves placing a full-thickness cartilage incision or excision along the curve of the antihelix and superior crus, which permits the cartilage on either side of the incision to fold into position. As an alternative to this technique, some surgeons made a pair of incisions parallel to the desired antihelical fold and placed sutures between the two. The latter technique was modified by Converse[7] to obviate the sharp fold of the antihelix that often results. Mustardé is credited for creation of the antihelical fold with suture fixation, wherein at least three full-thickness mattress sutures are placed on the posterior surface of the cartilage to span the antihelix, with each suture purchase including cartilage and both perichondrial layers (Fig. 18.4).[8] Interestingly, Luckett in his original paper[6] suggested that the antihelical fold could be created by appropriate suture placement, although he did not explore the concept. Cartilage scoring techniques, as popularized by Stenström[9] and Chongchet,[10] are based on the principle of Gibson and Davis[11] that cartilage tends to warp away from the abraded perichondrial surface. Some authorities contend that so-called conchal excess is in fact secondary to a lack of antihelical fold, and once the fold is restored any apparent "excess" will be corrected. In fact, both Mustardé and Stenström addressed conchal protuberance by rolling back the posterior conchal wall, such that it is integrated into antihelix formation. Alternatively, conchal hypertrophy can be corrected with excision of a crescent-shaped cartilage segment (with or without overlying skin), through either an anterior or posterior approach, with care taken to avoid violation of the antihelix. Conchal mastoid sutures, elaborated by Furnas,[12] may be added to effect desired conchal setback, where the concha is sutured to the mastoid fascia and/or periosteum (Fig. 18.5). This maneuver effectively rotates the concha forward and outward, thereby increasing the protrusion of the angular ledge that marks the junction of the concha with the external auditory canal. Thus, when this procedure is carried out one must be cautious to avoid narrowing of the external auditory meatus. On the basis of cadaveric studies, Goulian and Conway[13] described the cartilage of the helix and concha as two discrete components, separated by a distinct fissure, and advocated relocation of the cauda helicis (helical tail) onto the cavum conchae to reposition the lobule. The latter is based on the commonly advanced premise that lobular protrusion is due to a displaced cauda helicis.[14] Many surgeons have subsequently adopted this

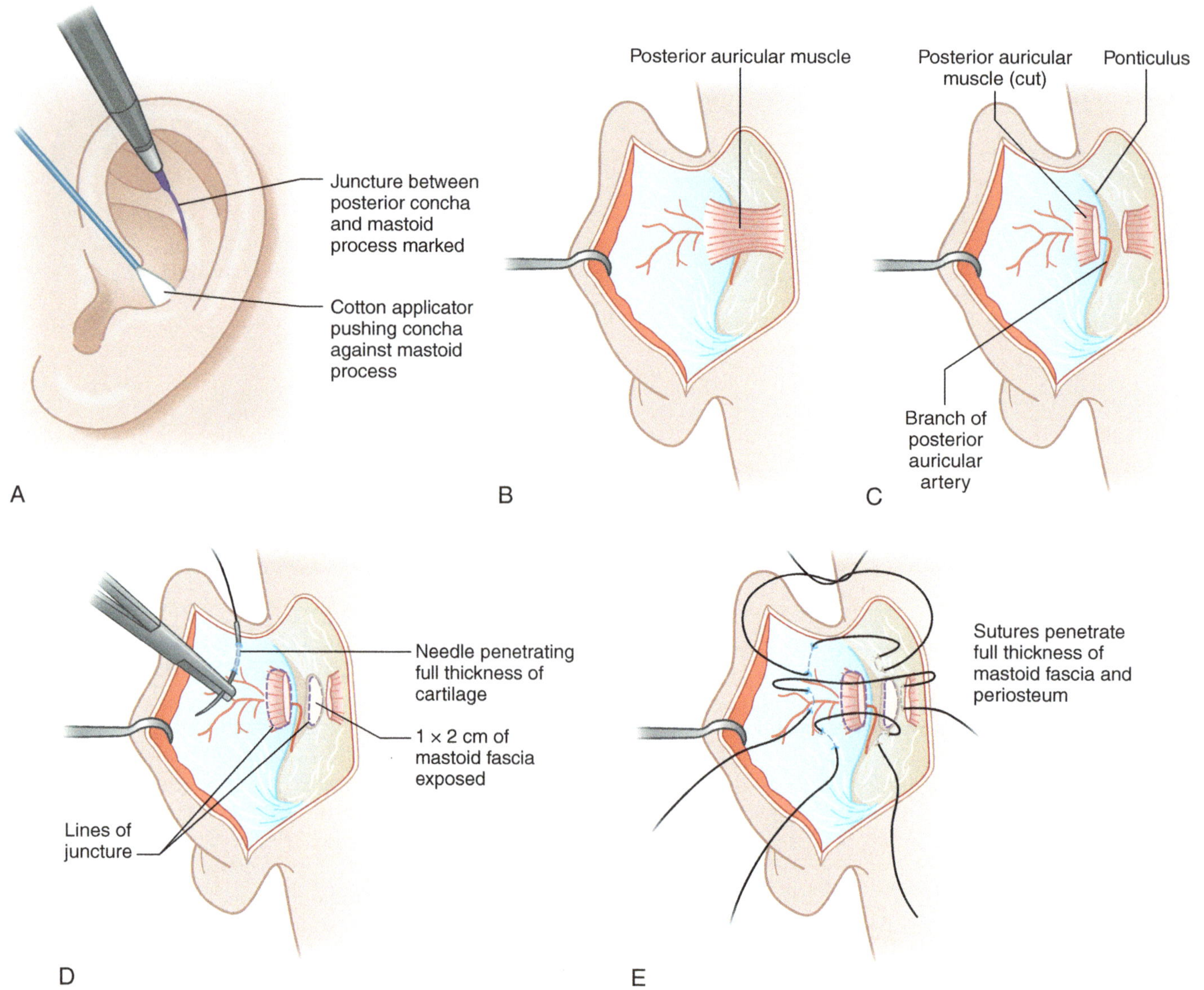

• **Fig. 18.5** (A–E) Diagrammatic illustration of key steps in the operative technique for placement of concha–mastoid sutures as originally described by Furnas. (Modified from Furnas DW. Correction of prominent ears by concha–mastoid sutures. *Plast Reconstr Surg.* 1968;42:189–193.)

approach and developed various technical modifications to retroposition the helical tail. Various other methods to address lobule prominence have been illustrated, such as fishtail excision of skin on the posterior surface of the lobule, wedge resection of the medial aspect of the lobule, and suture fixation of the lobule to the mastoid fascia.

There a number of complications associated with otoplasty, which differ depending on the technique used. With cartilage suturing, suture extrusion and granuloma formation may occur, necessitating suture removal and resulting in recurrence of ear prominence. Cartilage irregularities and/or deformity are more likely to occur with cartilage scoring and/or breaking techniques. Hematoma and infection are two early complications that can occur with any technique and merit more detailed mention. With regards to hematoma formation, rapid recognition and appropriate management is essential. In the early postoperative period, onset of severe often unilateral pain should prompt the immediate removal of the head dressing and if hematoma is confirmed, sutures released to drain the collection. Infection is another potentially devastating complication of prominauris correction, which mandates aggressive management with repeated washouts and intravenous antibiotics, as chondritis and cartilage deformity may ensue if not effectively controlled. Either of the latter two complications can result in significant cartilage destruction, for which correction may involve formal ear reconstruction.

The authors' preferred method for prominent ear correction is a modified Mustardé technique for antihelix formation with or without Furnas' method for conchal setback. In the majority of cases, otoplasty is performed under general anesthesia. The procedure begins with design for a conservative dumbbell-shaped outline for skin excision on the posterior (medial) side of the auricle. Following infiltration of local anesthesia to the posterior auricular surface in the subcutaneous plane, skin excision is performed and the posterior auricular skin is dissected off the perichondrium. If placement of Furnas sutures is anticipated, dissection is extended to the ponticulus (conchal ridge, site of muscle insertion) and an area of mastoid fascia for suture placement is exposed. Many often use a needle charged with methylene blue to mark the points for recreation of the antihelix. The needle is passed from the anterior (lateral) side and thus tattoos the exposed posterior cartilaginous surface at the desired location for suture placement. The authors do not utilize the latter technique, relying instead on familiarity with the architecture of the cartilage as viewed from the medial surface, to identify the conchal border, triangular fossa, and scapha, as underscored by Rubin et al.[15] A nonabsorbable braided suture is used for cartilage fixation. Following antihelical fold formation, conchal prominence is assessed. If deemed excessive, Furnas sutures are placed with no conchal cartilage excision, in an effort to reduce the distance between concha and mastoid prominence. In his original technical description, Furnas divided the posterior auricularis muscle fibers and posterior auricular ligament, which extend from the ponticulus to mastoid fascia, prior to suture placement.[12] Given that sutures are placed posterior to the muscle insertion on the concha and that great auricular nerve fibers span this area, the authors prefer to not divide these structures, ensuring rather that the posterior auricularis muscle is not strangulated with suture positioning. The latter is thought to avert the postoperative pain that may ensue following placement of conchomastoid sutures. If the lobule requires retropositioning, dissection is extended into the lobe such that a deep suture is placed from both the tail of the helix and the subcutaneous lobular tissue to the floor of the concha. The latter is an effective means to address lower third prominence and avoids tissue excision in and scar on the earlobe. Once hemostasis is assured, the incision is closed with a running horizontal mattress suture with absorbable suture and a head dressing is applied for 5 days. Once the dressing is removed, the patient is instructed to wear a headband at night for 3 months.

Other Auricular Anomalies

While prominauris often presents bilaterally, other auricular deformities are often unilateral. For unilateral correction, irrespective of the auricular anomaly, a template of the contralateral *normal* ear is made and the abnormal or missing part on the ear requiring correction is then addressed based on its contralateral counterpart.

In *Stahl's ear* deformity, a third tangential crus projects from the antihelix toward the helical rim at an approximate right-angle, flattening the helical rim and widening at the scapha. Aberrant insertion of the intrinsic transverse muscle has been postulated as the etiological origin of this anomaly.[16] For correction of Stahl's ear various techniques have been described, including wedge excision of the auricular segment occupied by the third crus, excision of the abnormal cartilage with reshaping to approximate the scaphal concavity, and removal of the anomalous cartilage section and substitution in a reversed position (Fig. 18.6).

Cryptotia is a congenital auricular anomaly seldom seen in the Caucasian population, but is common among peoples of East Asian origin, with a reported incidence of approximately 1 in 400 among the Japanese. It occurs when the superior pole of the auricle is buried beneath the scalp skin resulting in a lack of superior auriculocephalic sulcus, as well as associated distorted cartilage architecture (Fig. 18.7). It has been suggested that the invagination of the upper portion of the auricle is attributable to aberrant insertion of superior auricularis muscle into the upper portion of the helix, which normally extends from the epicranial aponeurosis to the dorsal protuberance of the triangular fossa.[17] The deformity of the cartilage results from anomalous auricular musculature, namely, intrinsic transverse and oblique muscles, which mold the auricle into its characteristic shape.[18] The transverse muscle, which extends from the conchal eminence to the scapha, forms the body of the antihelix and superior crus. The oblique muscle, between the eminence of the concha and triangular fossa, shapes the inferior crus. Although numerous techniques have been described for correction of this abnormality, the underlying principles of correction are similar. That is, cartilage plasty depending on the degree of cartilaginous deformity. and local tissue rearrangement to fill the gap created in the superior portion of the retroauricular sulcus and posterior aspect of the ear once the superior pole of the ear has been distracted from the scalp and fibrous soft tissue adhesions released. Methods to address the cutaneous defect include Z-plasty, V–Y plasty, advancement flap, a combination of local flap and skin graft, or tissue expansion.

The terms *constricted*, *cup*, and *lop ear* are often used interchangeably to describe variants of a similar auricular anomaly. Tanzer proposed a classification for constricted ears, which is valuable for reconstructive management of this deformity.[19] Group 1, involves the *helix only*, where the superior portion of the helix is folded, also referred to as *lop ear*. The latter can often be addressed with simple excision of the excess skin and cartilage, as auricular height is usually adequate. Alternatively, for cases with a characteristically angulated superior helical rim, the involved portion of rim can be detached and repositioned. The deformed segment of cartilage can be dissected from the scapha and transposed to the posterior surface of the scapha as either a pedicled flap or free graft. In group 2A, the *helix and scapha* are involved, lidding is more significant with increased constriction of the helical rim. Further, features of the prominent ear may be present, including ill-defined superior crus and enlarged conchal cavity. However, the cutaneous envelope is adequate, such that correction of the malformed cartilaginous structure can be redraped with the existing skin. The latter often qualifies the *classic lop ear*. The authors' preferred method of correction for this group is the technique described by Musgrave[20] (Fig. 18.8). This approach involves complete degloving of the superior pole cartilage. Thereafter, radial full-thickness incisions are made in the lidded segment of cartilage, which allows the cartilage to unfurl in a posterosuperior direction thereby restoring auricular height and width. Scoring of the anterior surface of the cartilage can be effected to assist with transposition of the multiple segments created. A conchal cartilage graft is harvested from

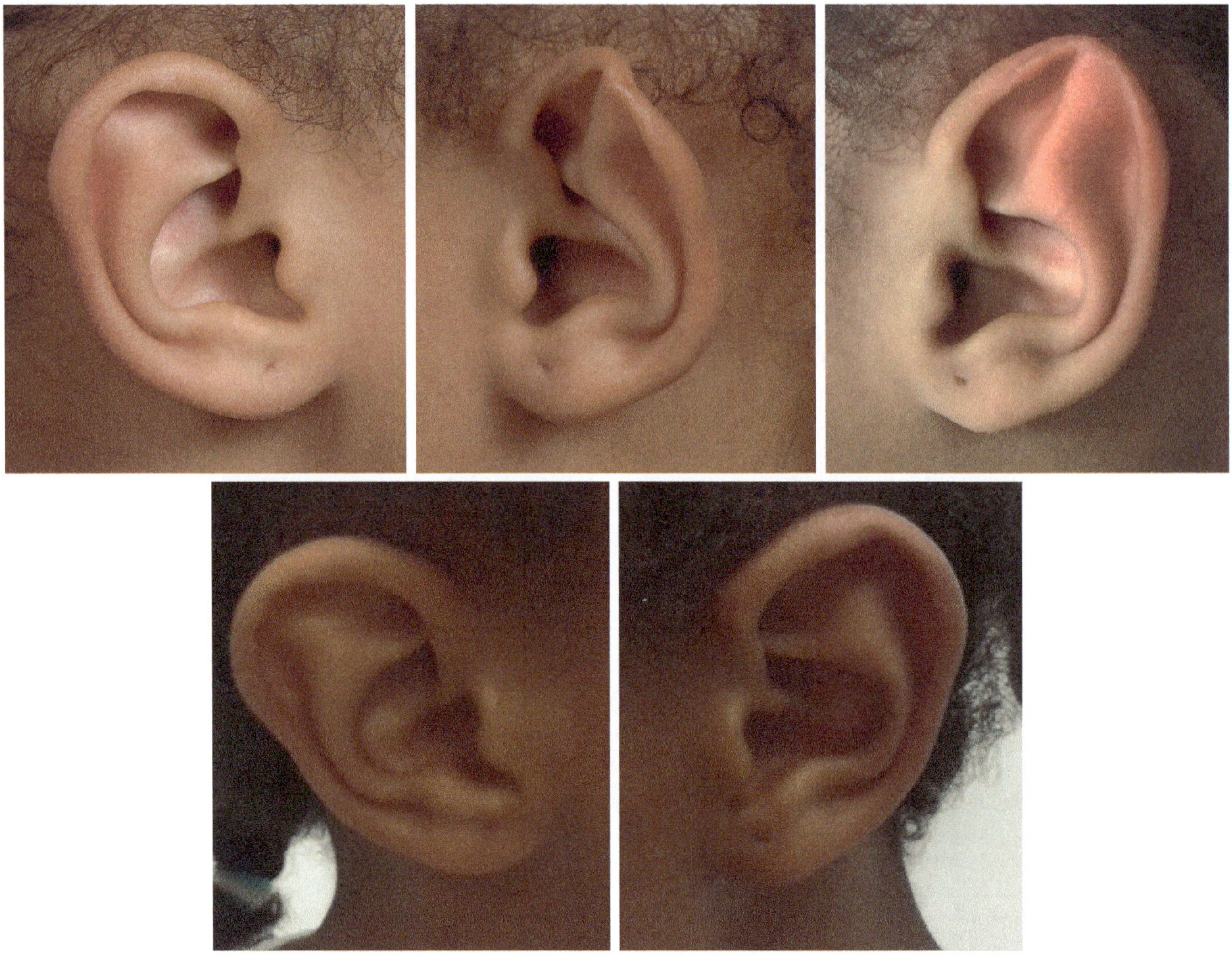

• **Fig. 18.6** Stahl's ear deformity, with normal contralateral ear. Correction of the deformity with excision and reshaping of the abnormal cartilage.

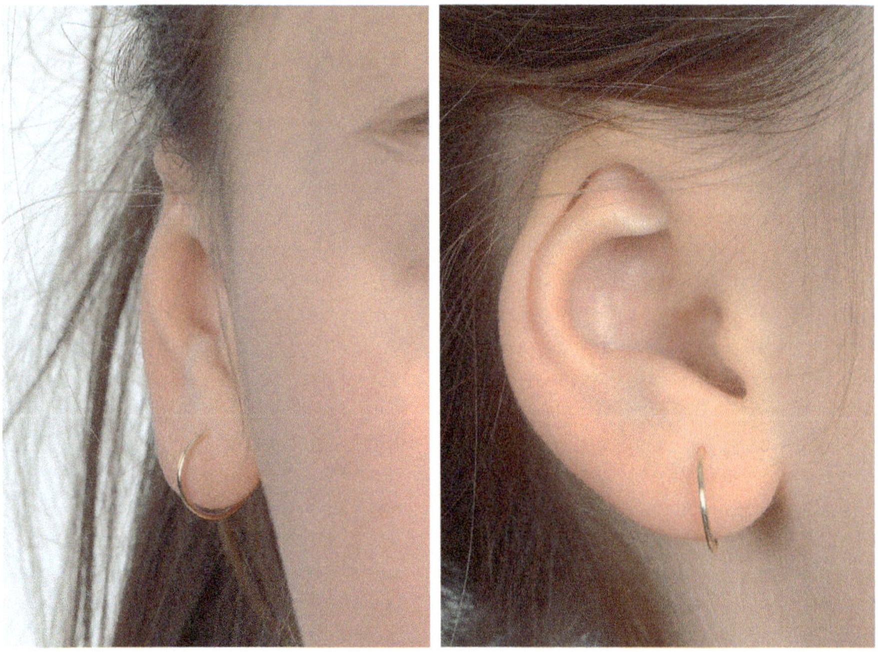

• **Fig. 18.7** Cryptotia ear deformity.

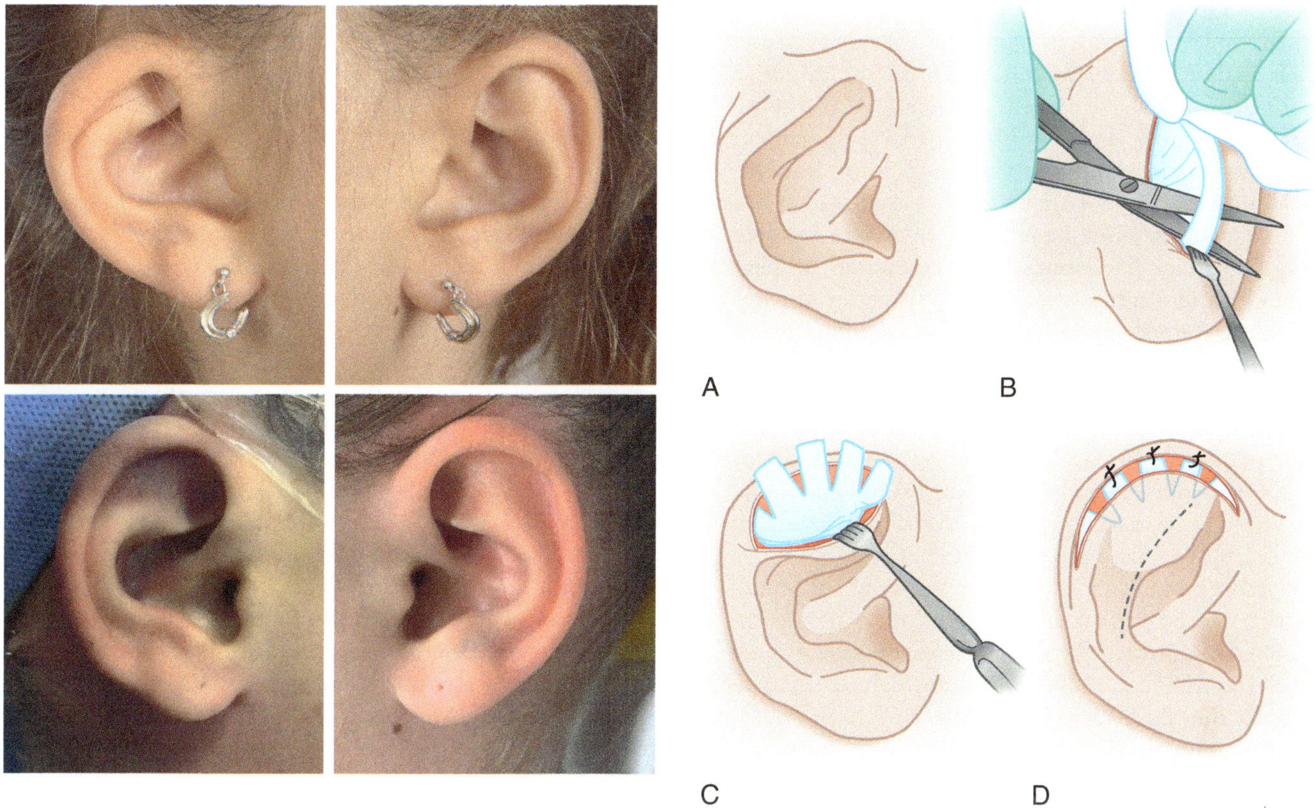

• **Fig. 18.8** Pre- and perioperative photographs of unilateral lop ear deformity corrected with the method described by Musgrave. (A–D) Diagrammatic illustration of key steps in the operative technique as illustrated by Musgrave. (A–D, Modified from Musgrave RH. A variation on the correction of the congenital lop ear. *Plast Reconstr Surg.* 1966;37:394–398.)

either the contralateral or ipsilateral (as originally described by Musgrave) ear and used as a curved strut to maintain the expanded cartilaginous segments in place and bridge the gaps in the expanded helical rim. The cutaneous envelope is redraped over the refashioned cartilage framework and the reconstruction supported with bolsters placed in the scapha beneath the helical rim and on the posterior surface of the ear. If necessary, a posterior skin approach can be added to address auricular prominence. Namely, placement of Mustardé sutures for recreation of the antihelical fold. The primary distinguishing feature between group 2A and 2B is *skin deficiency* in the latter subgroup. In this case, the constriction is more significant and the malformed ear has characteristics of both lop and prominent ears, including an overdeveloped concha, deficient superior helical margin, antihelical crura and antihelical body, and diminished auricular height (to which the term *cup ear* is usually applied). Group 3 is not unlike a conchal-type microtia deformity. As groups 2B and 3 involve deficiency of both skin cover and underlying cartilage, reconstruction necessitates framework fabrication with costal cartilage and recruitment of regional skin, as described in the following section for microtia reconstruction.

Microtia

The pathogenesis of microtia remains elusive, with phenotypic expression ranging from preauricular skin tags to *anotia*, or complete absence of the auricle. Microtia is a developmental malformation of the external ear with an estimated prevalence between 0.83 and 17.4 per 10,000 births.[21] The incidence of microtia differs among ethnic groups, being greatest among Asians (especially Japanese). Microtia occurs 20%–40% more commonly in males, involves the right side in nearly 60% of unilateral cases and bilateral deformity accounts for approximately 10% of cases.[22] The genetic and cellular mechanisms responsible for the normal morphogenesis of the external ear remain incompletely defined. Microtia appears to be associated with single gene mutations in syndromic and familial cases, whereas in sporadic cases a combination of genetic and environmental factors or polygenic causes are involved. The genetic contribution to microtia is supported by the higher concordance in monozygotic versus dizygotic twins, familial cases with autosomal dominant and recessive modes of inheritance, as well as the more than 18 microtia-associated syndromes for which chromosomal aberrations or single gene defects have been elucidated. Current theories for microtia development include high altitude, neural crest cell disturbance, and vascular disruption.[22] Evidence in support of the role of neural crest cells is derived from recent studies on the causative mechanisms of various teratogens on microtia, including retinoids and diabetic embryopathy. The development of microtia following localized vascular insult during embryogenesis is primarily supported by studies of Poswillo,[23] in which unilateral ear and mandibular anomalies resulted following ipsilateral hematomas at the junction of pharyngeal and hyoid arteries when monkeys were exposed to thalidomide and mice to triazine. This longstanding theory has been challenged by evidence of bilaterality in isolated microtia, as well as the occurrence of noncraniofacial anomalies frequently seen in the *oculo-auriculo-vertebral spectrum*. Johnston and Bronsky[24] disputed Poswillo's original experiments and contended that the development of hematomas was delayed in relation to drug exposure and that significant branchial arch hypoplasia preceded hemorrhage.

While more commonly an isolated unilateral abnormality, microtia can be present as a component of more complex craniofacial disorders. Most notable are those associated with aberration of first and second branchial arch derivatives, namely the oculo-auriculo-vertebral spectrum. Microtia may also constitute an important diagnostic feature of various other craniofacial syndromes, including Treacher Collins, Nager, Townes–Brocks, Kabuki, CHARGE, Meier–Gorlin syndrome, branchio-oto-renal and branchio-otic syndromes. Indeed, approximately 20%–60% of patients with microtia have associated anomalies or an identifiable syndrome.[22] Extracranial abnormalities include renal anomalies, cardiac defects, oral clefts, microphthalmia, polydactyly, and vertebral irregularities. Thus, clinical assessment of these patients must include observation for these commonly associated features.

Patients with microtia should be treated by a specialist multidisciplinary team, including plastic and reconstructive surgeon, otolaryngologist, audiologist and psychologist. Initial assessment should include formal audiology evaluation, with either auditory brainstem response testing in the newborn or audiogram in the child, which are mandatory to determine the degree and type of hearing loss. Microtia with aural atresia is associated with conductive hearing loss, although a small minority may exhibit sensorineural hearing loss despite the discrete embryonic origin of the internal ear. In the presence of an atretic external auditory canal, middle ear deformity and presence of cholesteatoma must be assessed. More advanced radiological examination may be indicated to investigate anomalous temporal bone (middle ear/ossicles) and facial nerve anatomy, to provide the anatomical detail essential for any projected otological surgery. More recent evidence has shown that patients with unilateral hearing loss benefit with regards to academic and career attainment from auditory rehabilitation with an amplification device, as functionally these patients have difficulty with localization of sound and understanding in noisy environments.[25] Patients with bilateral microtia and conductive hearing loss require early fitting with a bone-conduction hearing device to avert impairment of speech development. Current options for hearing rehabilitation include osseointegrated bone-anchored hearing aid (BAHA) and middle ear implants. Ideally, this device should be placed 65–70 mm posterior to the external auditory meatus to minimize scarring near the site of future placement of the ear construct. Authors do not currently advocate surgical restoration of the external auditory conduit (canaloplasty) and middle ear due to the associated postoperative morbidity, including infection, desquamation, meatal restenosis, and inconsistent results in hearing improvement. Canaloplasty should only be considered in patients with stenosis of the external auditory canal with risk of cholesteatoma.

Reconstruction

Although Sir Harold Gillies is credited as the first to propose the use of autogenous costal cartilage for auricular framework fabrication, the modern era of ear reconstruction began in 1959, when Tanzer reintroduced the use of rib cartilage for autologous microtia reconstruction, which is still recognized as the gold standard reconstructive option.[26] Brent[27,28] later refined autogenous reconstruction with the introduction of his four-stage technique. The primary advance contributed by Brent was placement of the cartilaginous framework in ideal position *prior to* transposition of the lobule, which is the reverse of Tanzer's sequence. In 1993, Nagata published his modified two-stage approach to autologous microtia reconstruction, wherein the lobule is transposed in the *same stage* as framework fabrication (including the tragus) and placement.[29,30] Thus, Nagata's first stage combines the first, second, and final stage of Brent's technique. In addition, both authors proposed their own respective classification systems to describe the variable appearance of the microtia deformity. A detailed comparison of the latter two classifications and techniques is provided in Table 18.1.[27–31]

In the authors' practice, auricular reconstruction is realized as a two-stage procedure, as initially described by Nagata and later modified by Firmin.[32] Autologous reconstruction is offered from the age of 9 years, depending on the physical and psychological maturity of the child. At this age, there is usually sufficient costal cartilage for framework fabrication and most children have the requisite level of understanding to be an active member in the treatment plan and postoperative rehabilitation and care.

For the first stage of reconstruction, following induction of general anesthesia, preoperative markings are made. On the unaffected side, two distances are outlined and transposed onto the side with microtia: the distance between the lateral canthus to the most anterior point of the helix and between the lateral commissure to the lowest point of the lobule. The latter two measures determine the ideal anterior- and inferior-most points for placement of the reconstructed ear. Next, the angle between the axis of the nasal dorsum and the normal ear is ascertained and the former

TABLE 18.1 Comparison of Two Classifications and Techniques for Microtia Reconstruction

	Brent[27,28,31]	Nagata[29,30]
Microtia Classification		
Types	1. Classical microtia (sausage-shaped vestige, usually with absent external auditory meatus) 2. Atypical microtia (concha, antihelix, tragus, antitragus, with absence of upper portion of ear, with or without presence of external auditory canal)	1. Lobular microtia (ear remnant with malpositioned lobule, without concha, external acoustic meatus and tragus) 2. Conchal microtia (lobule, concha, with or without external acoustic meatus, tragus, antitragus with incisura tragica, present to variable degrees) 2a. Small type, or 2b. Large type (depending on degree of conchal development)
Operative Technique		
Number of stages	Three (stage 2 and 3 combined) or four: 1. Cartilage framework fabrication/placement 2. Transposition of lobule 3. Elevation of ear construct and creation of auriculocephalic sulcus 4. Tragus construction, conchal excavation and contralateral otoplasty, if indicated	Two: 1. Cartilage framework fabrication (with tragal component)/placement and transposition of lobule (Brent stage 1, 2, and 4) 2. Elevation of ear construct and creation of auriculocephalic sulcus
Age at reconstruction	4–6 years	10 years (or chest circumference at xiphoid 60 cm)
Skin incision	Small incision anterior to vestige	W-shaped skin incision
Costal cartilage	Contralateral ribs, 6–8	Ipsilateral ribs, 6–9
Framework fixation	Clear nylon sutures	Wire sutures
Dressing	Closed suction drains	Bolsters
Tragus construction	Chondrocutaneous graft from contralateral ear	Rib cartilage
Elevation of ear construct and creation of auriculocephalic sulcus	Occipitalis turnover flap and skin graft with cartilage wedge	Temporoparietal or posterior auricular fascial flap and skin graft with cartilage wedge

two are marked on the abnormal side and used to determine the inclination of the ear construct. Finally, the course of the superficial temporal artery is marked using a Doppler probe. An outline of the normal ear is drawn onto X-ray film, which serves as the template for fabrication of the auricular framework. Once the location of the future ear on the abnormal side is determined, the outline of the normal ear is drawn, potential adaptations of the microtic vestige are assessed and then the appropriate skin approach is selected (Fig. 18.9).

The costal cartilage segments of ipsilateral ribs 6–8 are harvested through a 5-cm horizontal (or oblique) incision along the costal margin, preserving the posterior perichondrium in situ. The cartilaginous base block is fashioned from the synchondrosis of ribs 6 and 7. The helix and antihelix are shaped from the 8th rib. The tragus, antitragus, tragal bar, and cartilage block for framework elevation (second stage) are carved from remaining cartilaginous segments, and fixed in place with 38G wires (Fig. 18.10). During the carving of the auricular framework, cartilage shavings and unusable cartilaginous fragments are collected, morcelized, and placed in a Vicryl mesh sleeve that is then used to reconstitute the costal margin.[33] Intercostal nerve blocks (chirocaine, 2.5 mg/mL) are carried out for postoperative analgesia prior to inset of the mesh, and the cartilage block for the second stage is banked in a subcutaneous pocket along the inferior margin of the chest incision.

Based on the morphology of the microtia, Firmin[32] proposed a classification system, perhaps more useful than those of her contemporaries, based for the type of skin incision required for framework placement. Originally, type 1 skin incision was used for typical lobular microtia and involved lobular transposition with Z-plasty. However, Firmin has now abandoned type 1 skin incision in favor of type 2, transfixion, skin incision. The transfixion incision is indicated for both lobular and conchal type microtia, where the inferior portion of the auricle is sufficiently developed to accept the lower extremity of the framework. The latter approach consists of a full-thickness transverse incision of the remnant auricle, thereby creating two skin edges. The posterior skin edge is sutured to the inferior skin edge of a corresponding transverse incision in the mastoid skin, and the anterior skin edge is sutured to the edge of the superiorly-based skin flap that covers the

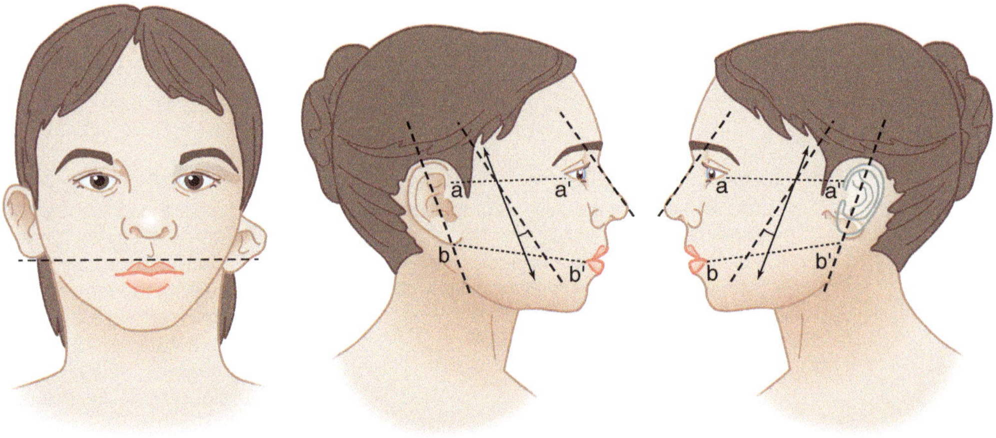

• **Fig. 18.9** Preoperative measurements and markings for assessment of ideal location for the reconstructed ear, as outlined in text.

cartilage framework. Type 3 skin incision is subclassified into type 3a, which is used when the ear is malformed but similar in size to the contralateral side, such that the deformed cartilage can be dissected from the skin envelope and the framework placed into the cutaneous pocket (sulcus is preserved, single-stage reconstruction), and type 3b, which is implemented for cases of anotia or where the microtic remnant cannot be used (e.g., significant auricular dystopia). Once the appropriate skin incision is made and the amorphous remnant cartilage is removed, the auricular pocket is dissected in the plane deep to the subdermal vascular plexus, with dissection extended beyond the limits of intended framework placement (marked auricular outline) to recruit sufficient skin to adequately cover the contours of the construct without undue tension. The cartilage framework is placed in the subcutaneous pocket over two suction drains.

If a temporoparietal fascial flap is required for partial or complete coverage of the cartilaginous framework (e.g., low temporal hairline or inadequate skin envelope in, for instance, cases of secondary reconstruction), it is harvested following dissection of a subcutaneous pocket through a 4-cm chevron-type incision placed at the apex of the temporal fossa, centered over the superficial temporal artery. The fascial flap is then covered with a split-thickness skin graft harvested from the contralateral scalp. Reconstruction for cases of bilateral microtia are executed simultaneously, with each step of this operative sequence performed in tandem. No dressings are applied to the reconstructed ear(s) to enable constant surveillance of the skin envelope and underlying construct. Patients are admitted to hospital for 4 nights, where the ear(s) is monitored and the vacutainer drains are changed every 4 hours to maintain the skin maximally applied to the contours of the framework. On day 4, the drains are removed and patients are discharged from hospital. Patients are placed on a 24-hour course of intravenous antibiotics, followed by oral antibiotics for a total of 1 week.

The second stage, framework elevation and sulcus formation, is routinely performed 6 months later, or after 12 months if a temporoparietal fascial flap was used for coverage of the construct. The framework is released through a perihelical incision extending to fascia. Elevation of the ear construct is buttressed by placement of the previously banked cartilage block behind the antihelix, positioned to form the posterior conchal wall. While a temporoparietal fascial flap is commonly used for coverage of the framework and cartilage block, authors prefer a random pattern galeal fascial flap. The retroauricular skin is advanced toward the sulcus and the posterior surface of the ear, auriculocephalic sulcus, and mastoid region are surfaced with a split-thickness skin graft harvested from the ipsilateral scalp before ear framework elevation (Fig. 18.11). Following the second stage, patients are admitted overnight to complete a 24-hour course of intravenous antibiotics, and then discharged on oral antibiotics for 7 days. The dressing remains in place until the first postoperative visit at 1 week. At 2 weeks, the auriculocephalic sulcus is fitted with an elastomer ear splint. The second stage presents an opportunity to carry out other refinements to the ear construct and/or additional reconstructive procedures to enhance facial form and/or symmetry. This combined reconstructive approach has become the authors' routine practice, with complementary procedures including contralateral prominauris correction, ear piercing, fat transfer for soft tissue augmentation, as well as genioplasty and malar augmentation to camouflage any associated bony deficiency.[34]

Oculo-auriculo-vertebral Spectrum

Microtia can be an integral component of a number of syndromes, including the *oculo-auriculo-vertebral spectrum* (more commonly referred to as *craniofacial microsomia*). In

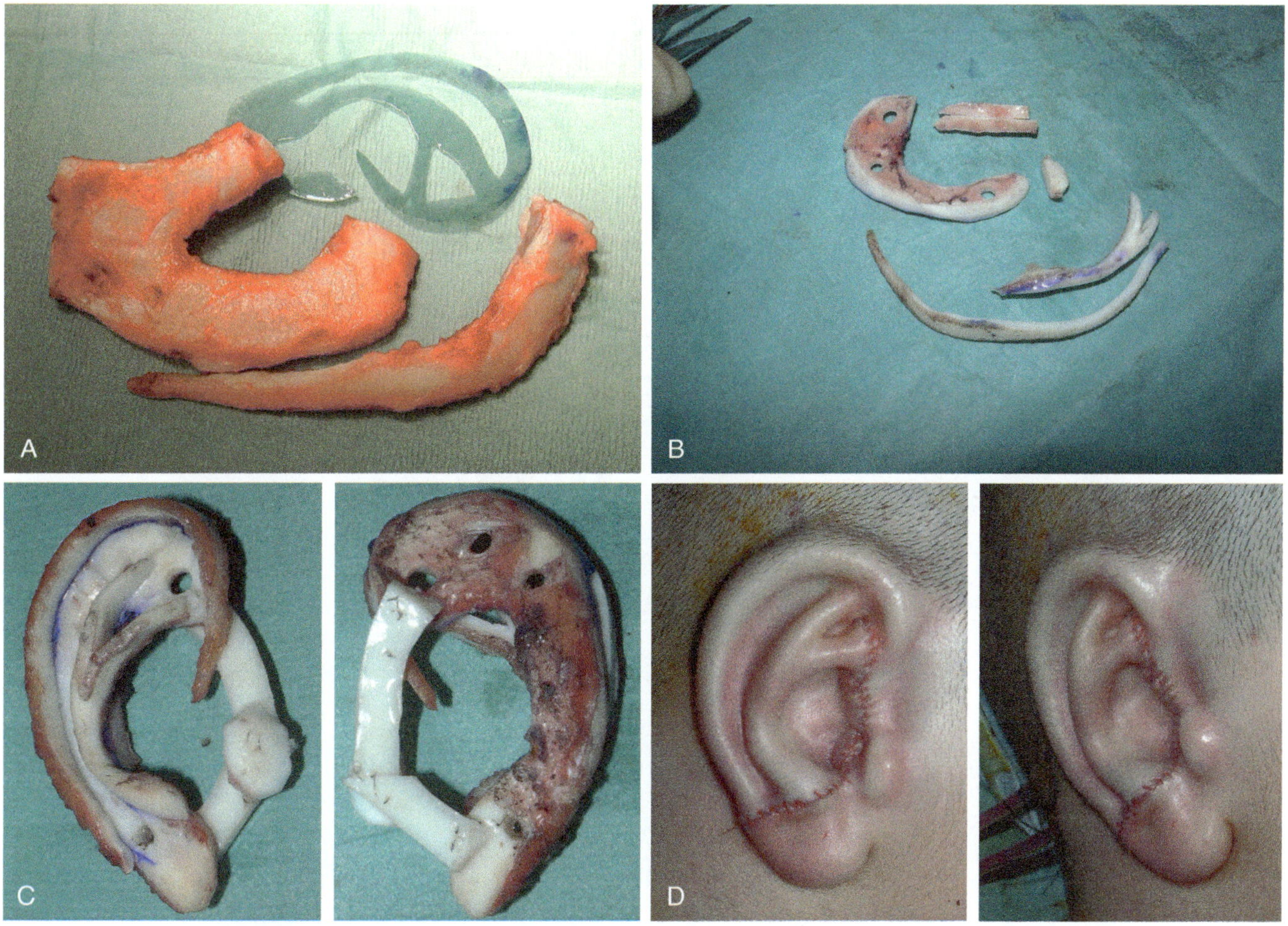

• **Fig. 18.10** Framework fabrication. The cartilage segments of ribs 6–8 (A) are harvested and (B) the framework fashioned as described in the text. The senior author has modified framework fabrication and no longer sculpts the antihelix, tragus, and antitragus segments as a single unit. (C) Instead, the antihelix and antitragus are shaped as a single component and a cartilaginous strut is made to span the base block, on which the tragus is placed. (D) This improves the projection of the tragus and depth of the concal bowl.

effect, microtia is considered a forme fruste of the craniofacial malformation sequence associated with craniofacial microsomia. However, all structures derived from the first and second branchial arches may be affected, unilaterally or bilaterally to different degrees. Moreover, other extracranial malformations may be present, including vertebral, renal, and limb anomalies. In these patients, significant dystopia of the vestige secondary to underlying deficiency of the craniofacial skeleton, notably the temporal bone, as well as soft tissue hypoplasia, renders selection of appropriate location for construct placement difficult. In addition, the external auditory meatus and canal may be in an ectopic position necessitating transposition. Thus, achieving a symmetric reconstruction presents a particular reconstructive challenge, especially when auricular reconstruction is one of several elements in the reconstructive sequence for facial dysmorphism (Fig. 18.12). Moreover, craniofacial deficiency is often associated with an insufficient skin envelope for framework coverage, as well as a low temporal hairline resulting in hair extending onto the skin that will drape the superior portion of the ear construct. Tissue expansion has been suggested to address the former and temporoparietal flap harvest for framework cover is generally used to deal with the latter. While more detailed description of reconstructive modifications in the presence of these features is beyond the scope of this chapter, these general points are mentioned for completeness.

Complications

There are a number of complications associated with autologous auricular reconstruction, related to both donor site and the site of reconstruction. With regards to donor site, the most notable complication is chest wall depression, often cited by proponents of synthetic reconstruction as a primary argument against costal cartilage harvest for framework fabrication. Leaving the posterior perichondrium in situ may potentially lessen chest wall morbidity by promoting cartilage regeneration at the donor site. In our practice, we have found that reconstitution of the costal margin as previously described minimizes potential contour deformity. During rib harvest, one may inadvertently create a breach in the

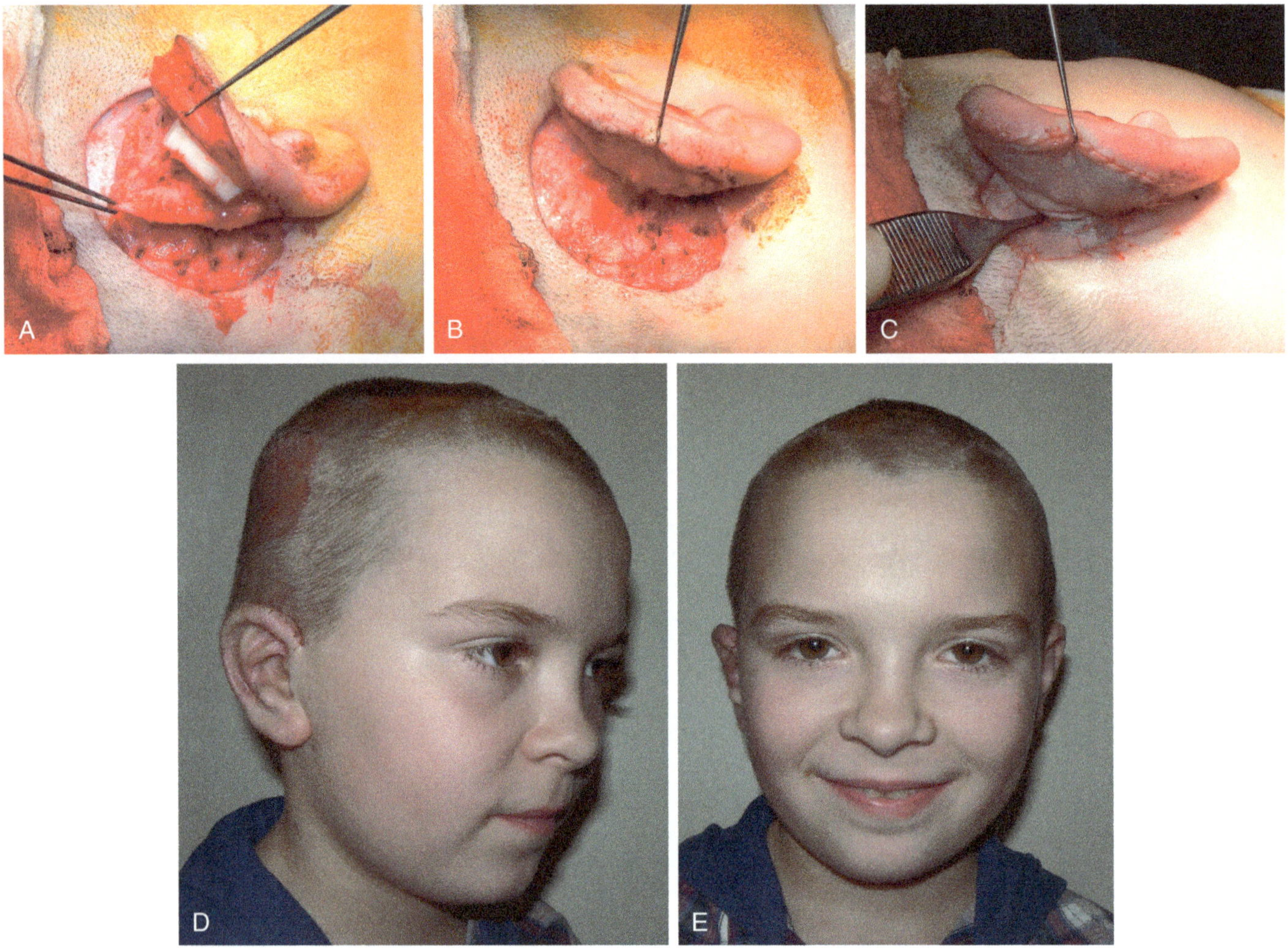

• **Fig. 18.11** Second stage of reconstruction. (A) The framework is released through a perihelical incision extending to fascia and elevation of the ear construct is buttressed with a cartilage block. (B) A random pattern galeal fascial flap is used for coverage of the framework and cartilage block. (C) The retroauricular skin is advanced toward the sulcus and the remaining areas surfaced with a split-thickness skin graft. (D, E) Early postoperative result achieved following completion of two-stage reconstruction in a patient with unilateral isolated microtia.

parietal pleura, resulting in pneumothorax. This is typically identified during the procedure and the pleural defect promptly repaired.

At the level of the reconstructed ear, the most common complication is exposure of the cartilage framework, which may occur as a result of extrusion of suture/wire material or vascular compromise of the overlying skin envelope. The latter mandates early recognition and appropriate treatment as cartilage resorption and distortion of the final form of the ear construct may result. In general, areas of exposure >10 mm^2 require surgical management with debridement and cutaneous or fascial flap coverage, depending on the location relative to the contours of auricle and adjacent tissue mobility (Fig. 18.13). Smaller defects can usually be addressed conservatively with local wound care. The most significant complication is infection with consequent cartilage resorption. Infection, usually secondary to *Pseudomonas*, most often occurs in the presence of a vestigial external auditory canal. Infection may also ensue following construct exposure. Additional complications include hematoma or seroma formation, cartilage framework resorption or fracture.

Alternative Reconstructive Options

The poor results achieved with autogenous cartilage in early reconstructive efforts incited others to find alternative options for framework fabrication. Silastic was used as a preferred implant material for auricular reconstruction for over two decades. However, high rates of implant extrusion necessitating explantation limited its continued use and costal cartilage, accredited largely to Tanzer, became the preferred framework material.

While autogenous reconstruction is now considered the primary reconstructive option in the pediatric population, two other alternative options should be

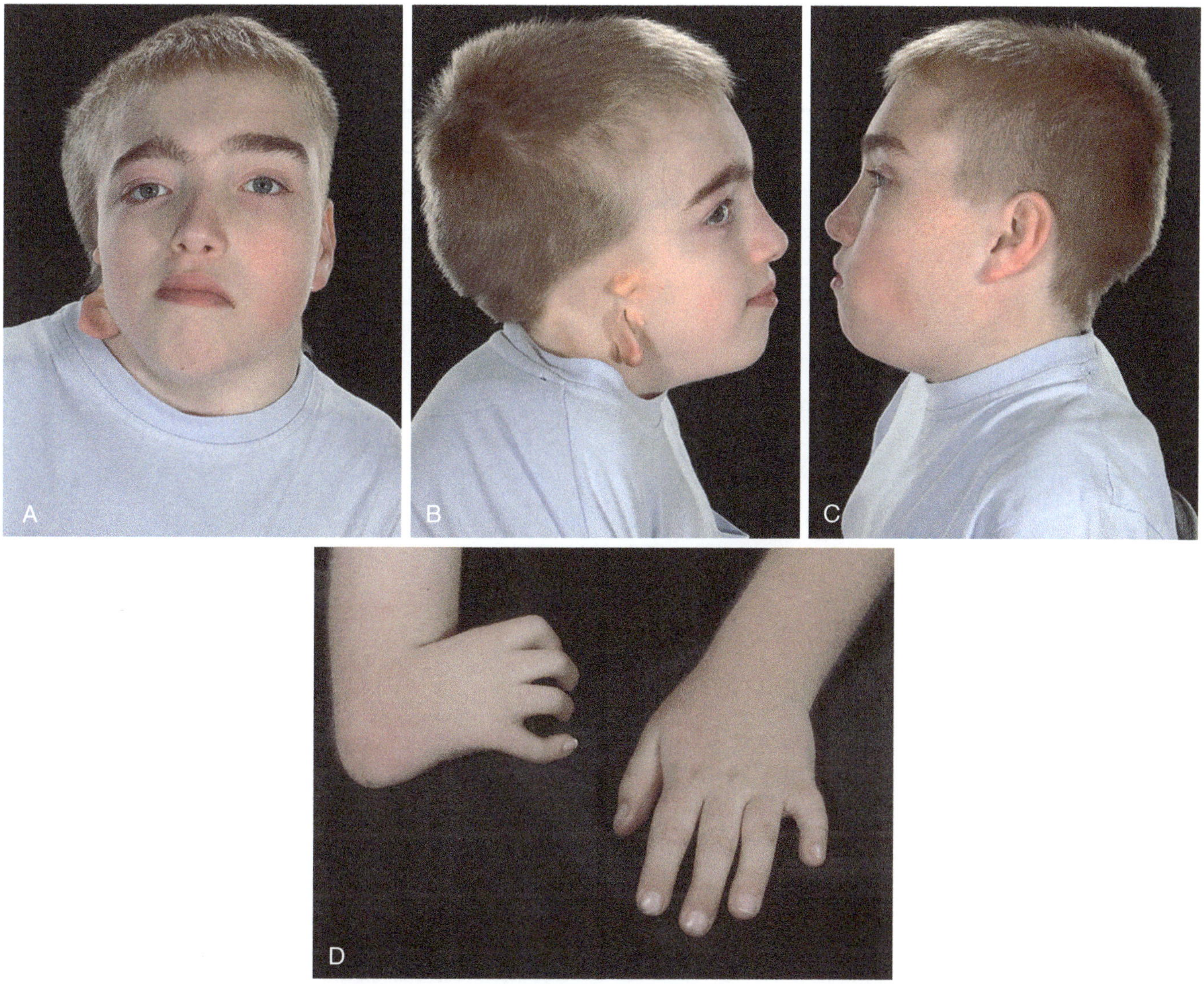

• **Fig. 18.12** (A–D) Patient with severe manifestation of the oculo-auriculo-vertebral spectrum who presented with significant dystopia of the auricular remnant.

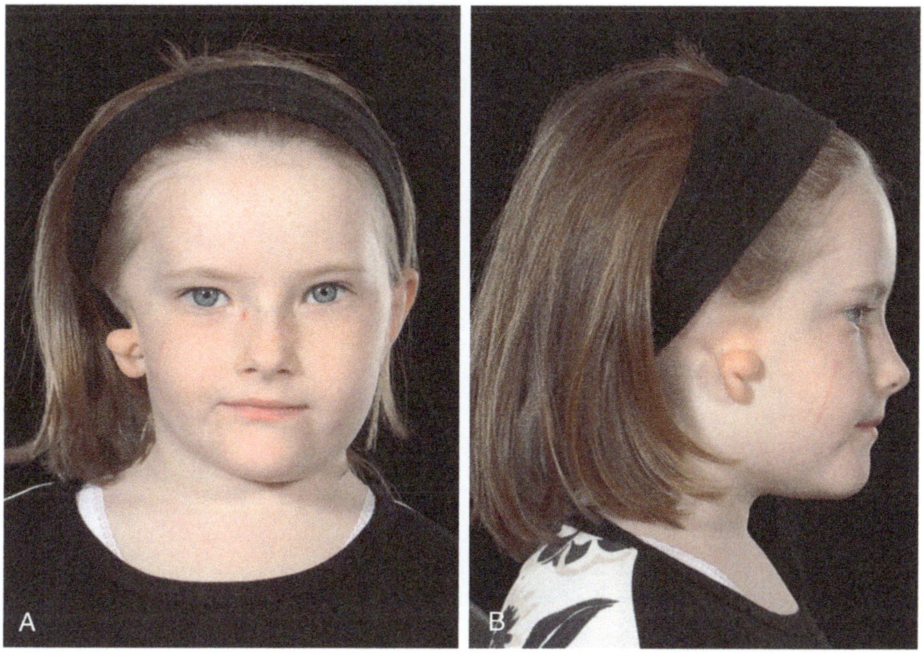

• **Fig. 18.13** (A–C) Patient with oculo-auriculo-vertebral spectrum who presented with right unilateral lobular microtia. (D) Twenty-nine days following the first stage of reconstruction, she presented with total necrosis of skin overlying the concha. (E–H) Coverage of the area of exposed cartilage graft was restored with harvest of a random superficial mastoid fascial flap, which was tunnelled beneath the cartilaginous ear construct to reach the distal extent of the defect. The fascial flap was then grafted with a split-thickness skin graft, harvested from the scalp (skin graft donor site shown).

Continued

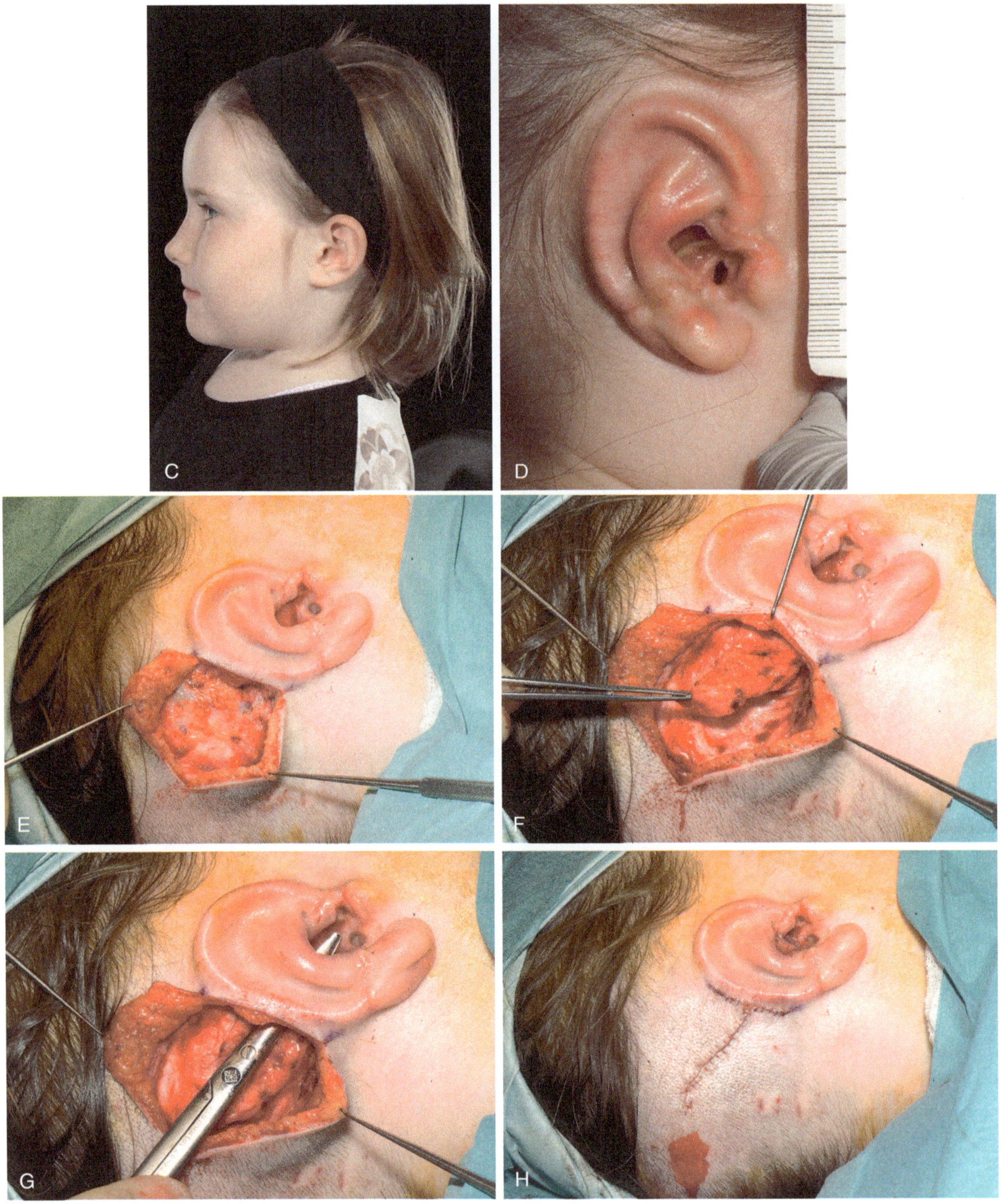

• Fig. 18.13 cont'd

mentioned, which also preclude harvest of costal cartilage for auricular framework construction. Namely, composite autogenous/alloplastic reconstruction and prosthetic reconstruction. The former consists of framework fabrication with porous polyethylene (Medpor) and coverage of the framework with a temporoparietal fascial flap, as popularized by Reinisch.[35] The porous structure of this material has proved a major advantage over smooth silicone implants, providing improved adherence to surrounding tissues. Further, fascial flap coverage has decreased the rates of implant extrusion, providing more robust soft tissue support. Prosthetic reconstruction in children is considered a salvage option following failed secondary autologous reconstruction where costal cartilage or soft tissue coverage remains insufficient for consideration of additional autogenous or alloplastic reconstruction. The latter option involves retention of the silicone auricular prosthesis with osseointegrated titanium implants. Finally, further advances in stem cell and tissue engineering to obtain a cartilaginous scaffold, may, in future, obviate the need for costal cartilage harvest and prove the ideal solution for framework fabrication.

References

1. Beahm EK, Walton RL. Auricular reconstruction for microtia: part I. Anatomy, embryology and clinical evaluation. *Plast Reconstr Surg*. 2002;109:2473–2482.
2. Tan ST, Abramson DL, MacDonald DM, Mulliken JB. Molding therapy for infants with deformational auricular anomalies. *Ann Plast Surg*. 1997;38:263–268.
3. Tanzer RC. Microtia. *Clin Plast Surg*. 1978;5:317–336.
4. Farkas LG, Posnick JC, Hreczko TM. Anthropometric growth study of the ear. *Cleft Palate Craniofac J*. 1992;29:324–329.
5. Tolleth H. Artistic anatomy, dimensions, and proportions of the external ear. *Clin Plast Surg*. 1978;5:337–345.
6. Luckett WH. A new operation for prominent ears based on the anatomy of the deformity. *Surg Gynec Obstet*. 1910;10:635–637.
7. Converse JM, Wood-Smith D. Technical details in the surgical correction of the lop ear deformity. *Plast Reconstr Surg*. 1963;31:118–128.
8. Mustardé JC. The correction of prominent ears using simple mattress sutures. *Br J Plast Surg*. 1963;16:170–176.
9. Stenström SJ. A "natural" technique for correction of congenitally prominent ears. *Plast Reconstr Surg*. 1963;32:509–518.
10. Chongchet V. A method of anti-helix reconstruction. *Br J Plast Surg*. 1963;16:268–272.
11. Gibson T, Davis W. The distortion of autogenous cartilage grafts: its cause and prevention. *Br J Plast Surg*. 1958;10:257.
12. Furnas DW. Correction of prominent ears by concha-mastoid sutures. *Plast Reconstr Surg*. 1968;42:189–193.
13. Goulian Jr D, Conway H. Prevention of persistent deformity of the tragus and lobule by modification of the Luckett technique of otoplasty. *Plast Reconstr Surg*. 1960;26:399–404.
14. Webster GV. The tail of the helix as a key to otoplasty. *Plast Reconstr Surg*. 1969;44:455–461.
15. Rubin LR, Bromberg BE, Walden RH, Adams A. An anatomic approach to the obtrusive ear. *Plast Reconstr Surg*. 1962;29:360–370.
16. Yotsuyanagi T, Nihei Y, Shinmyo Y, Sawada Y. Stahl's ear caused by an abnormal intrinsic auricular muscle. *Plast Reconstr Surg*. 1999;103:171–174.
17. Elsahy NI. An alternative technique for correction of cryptotia. *Ann Plast Surg*. 1989;23:66–73.
18. Hirose T, Tomono T, Matsuo K, et al. Cryptotia: our classification and treatment. *Br J Plast Surg*. 1985;38:352–360.
19. Tanzer RC. The constricted (cup and lop) ear. *Plast Reconstr Surg*. 1975;55:406–415.
20. Musgrave RH. A variation on the correction of the congenital lop ear. *Plast Reconstr Surg*. 1966;37:394–398.
21. Luquetti DV, Leoncini E, Mastroiacovo P. Microtia–anotia: global review of prevalence rates. *Birth Defects Res (Part A)*. 2011;91:813–822.
22. Luquetti DV, Heike CL, Hing AV, Cunningham ML, Cox TC. Microtia: epidemiology and genetics. *Am J Med Genet Part A*. 2011;158A:124–139.
23. Poswillo D. The pathogenesis of the first and second branchial arch syndrome. *Oral Surg Oral Med Oral Pathol*. 1973;35:302–328.
24. Johnston MC, Bronsky PT. Prenatal craniofacial development: new insights on normal and abnormal mechanisms. *Crit Rev Oral Biol Med*. 1995;6:368–422.
25. Bouhabel S, Arcand P, Saliba I. Congenital aural atresia: bone-anchored hearing aid vs. external auditory canal reconstruction. *Int J Pediatr Otorhinolaryngol*. 2012;76:272–277.
26. Tanzer RC. Total reconstruction of the external ear. *Plast Reconstr Surg*. 1959;23:1–15.
27. Brent B. The correction of microtia with autogenous cartilage grafts: I. The classic deformity. *Plast Reconstr Surg*. 1980;66:1–12.
28. Brent B. The correction of microtia with autogenous cartilage grafts: II. Atypical and complex deformities. *Plast Reconstr Surg*. 1980;66:13–22.
29. Nagata S. A new method of total reconstruction of the auricle for microtia. *Plast Reconstr Surg*. 1993;92:187–201.
30. Nagata S. Modification of the stages in total reconstruction of the auricle: Parts I–IV. *Plast Reconstr Surg*. 1994;93:221–266.
31. Brent B. Technical advances in ear reconstruction with autogenous rib cartilage grafts. Personal experience with 1200 cases. *Plast Reconstr Surg*. 1999;104:319–334.
32. Firmin F. State of the art autogenous ear reconstruction in cases of microtia. *Adv Oto-Rhino-Laryngol*. 2010;68:25–52.
33. Fattah A, Sebire NJ, Bulstrode NW. Donor site reconstitution for ear reconstruction. *J Plast Reconstr Aesth Surg*. 2010;63:1459–1465.
34. Cugno S, Farhadieh RD, Bulstrode NW. Autologous microtia reconstruction combined with ancillary procedures: a comprehensive reconstructive approach. *J Plast Reconstr Aesthet Surg*. 2013;66:1487–1493.
35. Reinisch JF, Tahiri Y. Polyethylene ear reconstruction: a state of the art surgical journey. *Plast Reconstr Surg*. 2018;141:461–470.

19

Rare Craniofacial Clefts

HANAN ALHUSAINAN, SCOTT P. BARTLETT, AND
MIRKO S. GILARDINO

Craniofacial clefts include a complex and heterogenous group of deformities that affect the face, causing significant functional and appearance-related issues for affected patients. The term "rare" craniofacial cleft is used to differentiate them from the more "typical" clefts of the lip and palate. Fortunately, atypical facial clefts are exceptionally rare, with a reported incidence of 1.4–4.9 for every 100,000 births.[1]

Etiology

Two theories predominate in establishing a cause of these deformities: the classic theory and mesodermal penetration theory.[2] Whereas a failure of fusion of the developing facial processes is proposed by the former, the role of neural crest cells in the development of the mesoderm and its failed penetration is the central tenet of the mesodermal penetration theory.[2]

There is increasing evidence that genetic predisposition plays a role in the pathogenesis of these rare craniofacial clefts.[2,3] The genetic component is more clearly evident in true midline clefts, further emphasizing the role of neural crest cells during embryogenesis.[2,4] Hu and Helms have demonstrated the critical role played by SHH (Sonic Hedgehog) signaling in regulating the pattern of neural crest cell migrations as well as the development of the facial primordium.[5] The transient loss of SHH signaling during the initial phases of neural plate patterning has been linked to abnormalities of craniofacial morphogenesis, leading to anomalies resembling cleft lip/palate defects, hypotelorism, and holoprosencephaly.[5] Excessive SHH signaling has been linked to mediolateral increment in the frontal process as well as hypertelorism.[5]

Classification

The complexity and heterogeneity of facial clefts pose a challenge to classification. Two main classifications are currently utilized: Van der Meulen's embryonic classification and the more widely used anatomical classification proposed by Tessier.[6,7] The latter delineates 14 locations for clefts, with the palpebral fissure as a central landmark, much like a wheel with spokes. Facial clefts extending downwards from the palpebral fissure are assigned the numbers 1 to 7, starting at the midline with Tessier 0 and each subsequent number representing a facial cleft more laterally positioned. Cranial clefts extending cephalad from the palpebral fissures are numbered 8 to 14, where Tessier 8 is the most lateral and extends into the corner of the orbit and each sequential cranial cleft is more medial than the last.[6] Facial and cranial clefts may exist separate from one another or combined, at which point they become true "craniofacial clefts." In such cases, the representative cleft numbers usually sum to 14 (e.g., 0,14; 3,11; 4,10) (see Fig. 19.1).[8,9] A number 30 cleft of the midline mandible is also included in the Tessier classification (Fig. 19.1).

When clinically classifying facial clefts, a number of important anatomical distinctions should be identified to assist in the proper diagnosis. For example, nasal structures are involved only in clefts nos. 0–3, while no. 4 is the first to avoid the nose. Radiologically, no. 4 is visualized medial to the infraorbital foramen, while no. 5 is localized lateral to this structure (Table 19.1).

The earliest documented history of facial clefts was first reported by Merkel and Trendelenburg, where they described facial clefts.[10] However, Tessier illustrated a more detailed and systematic classification for craniofacial clefts that is widely accepted today. Tessier's classification is unique given that it highlights the relationship between soft tissues and the underlying bone, stating that "a fissure of the soft tissue corresponds, as a general rule, with a cleft of the bony structure."[6] The converse is also possible. In addition, Tessier proposed the adoption of the term "cleft" for all craniofacial anomalies that fall along these lines, noting that there may be "excess" and/or "deficiency" clefts. Indeed, many surgeons consider both craniofacial microsomia and Treacher Collins syndrome as rare craniofacial clefts with variable amounts of soft tissue and bony involvement of the implicated Tessier cleft. For example, in craniofacial microsomia there may be a no. 7 cleft of the soft tissue associated with variable hypoplasia of the mandible whereas in Treacher Collins syndrome there may be a soft tissue cleft

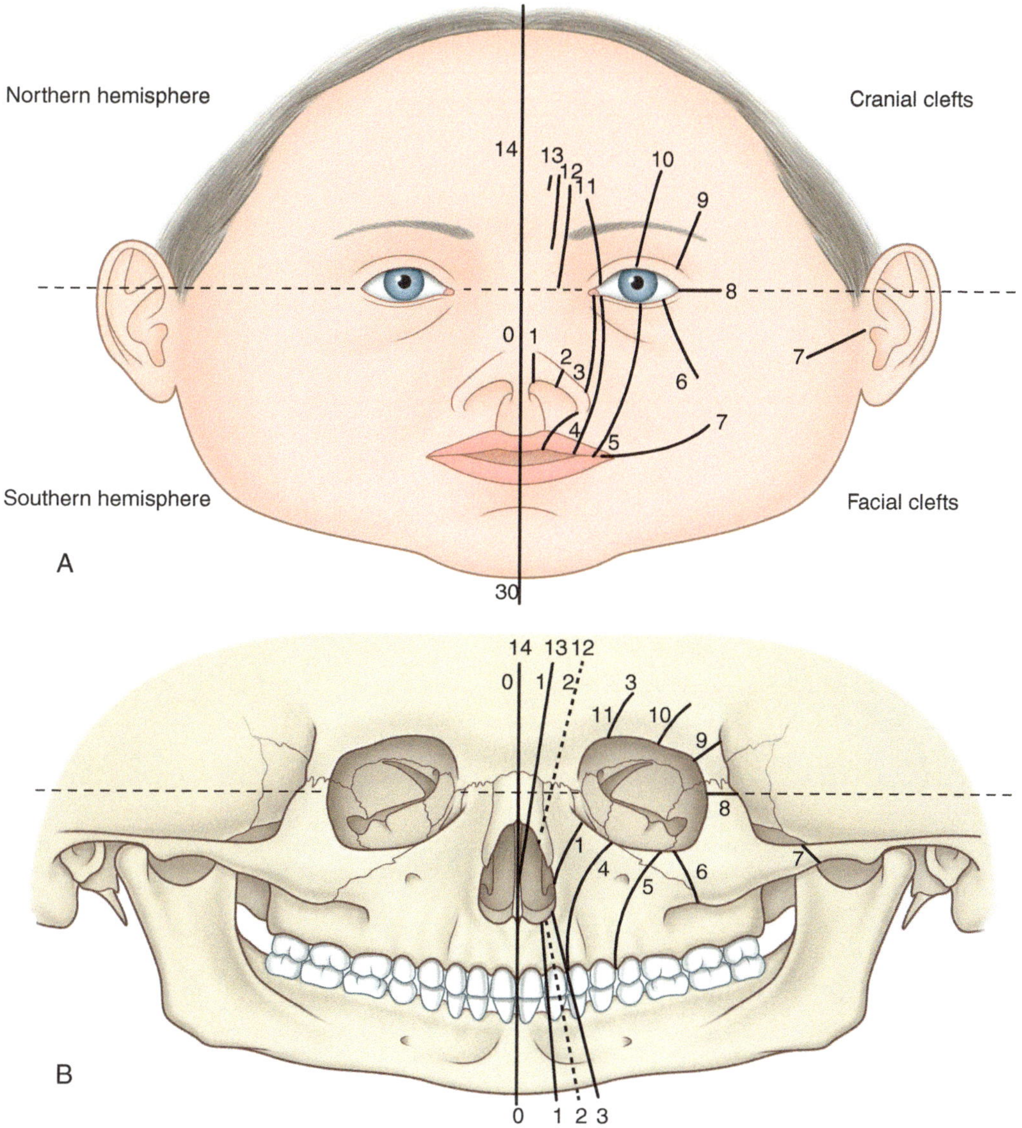

• **Fig. 19.1** (A, B) Tessier's classification (see text for number identification). (From Arnaud E, Paternoster G, James S. Orbital hypertelorism. In: Rodriguez ED, Losee JE, Neligan PC, eds. *Plastic Surgery*, 4th edn. Volume 3: *Craniofacial, Head and Neck Surgery and Pediatric Plastic Surgery*. Elsevier; 2018. Fig. 30.1.)

of nos. 6 or 7 and a hard tissue cleft of nos. 6, 7, and 8 or a combination thereof.

The main drawback of the Tessier classification is that it does not explain why clefts can occur at nonembryonic sites of fusion. While other authors have modified Tessier's original classification, it continues to be the most widely utilized.[11]

Van der Meulen's embryological classification is considered by some to be more comprehensive as it attempts to explain why some clefts occur in areas unrelated to embryologic fusion. In this system the term "dysplasia" is used since not all malformations are true "clefts." The dysplasias are classified according to time and location of developmental arrest (e.g., orbito-zygomatic dysplasia).[7] Hypoplasia of the mandible is graded according to the Pruzansky classification and as adapted by Kaban et al.[12,13]

Management

The management of facial clefts necessitates a multidisciplinary approach due to the involvement of multiple facial structures. Priorities remain airway and globe protection, followed by functional concerns such as the separation of nasal, orbital, and oral spaces, lip competence and eating. Furthermore, the treatment of craniofacial clefts necessitates the reconstruction of soft tissue and skeletal hypoplasia to obtain optimal esthetic improvement. It is important to note that there is no known, standardized "one-size fits all" surgical approach that can be constantly followed. This is because the majority of patients present with unique facial deformities within characteristic patterns of facial clefts. Even in extremely rare facial anomalies, the goal of the craniofacial surgeon is to get the desired result with fewest numbers of corrective surgeries.

TABLE 19.1 **Description of the Tessier Clefts: Course and Presentation[a]**

Cleft No.	Soft Tissue	Skeletal
0 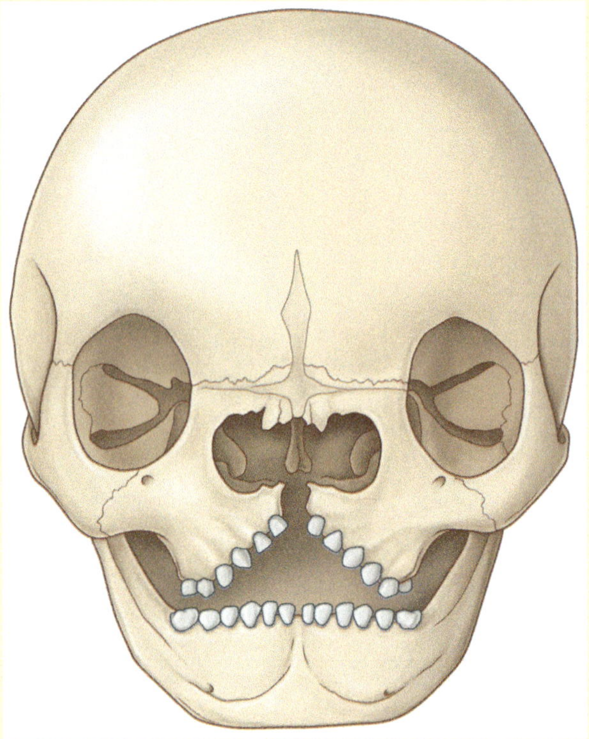	Starts in the midline, traverses the lip, alveolus and nasal components **A: Hypoplasia** Deficiencies of philtral columns Deficiencies of nasal structures (columella and septum) Arhinia may exist **B: Hyperplasia** Separated philtral columns Frenulum duplication Septal duplication Displaced alar cartilage Broad columella Clefted dorsum	Cleft travels between alveolus, maxilla and the nasal bones Central incisors laterally displaced V shape maxillary teeth Broad nasal bones and maxilla Broad body of the sphenoid The pterygoid plates are displaced laterally
1 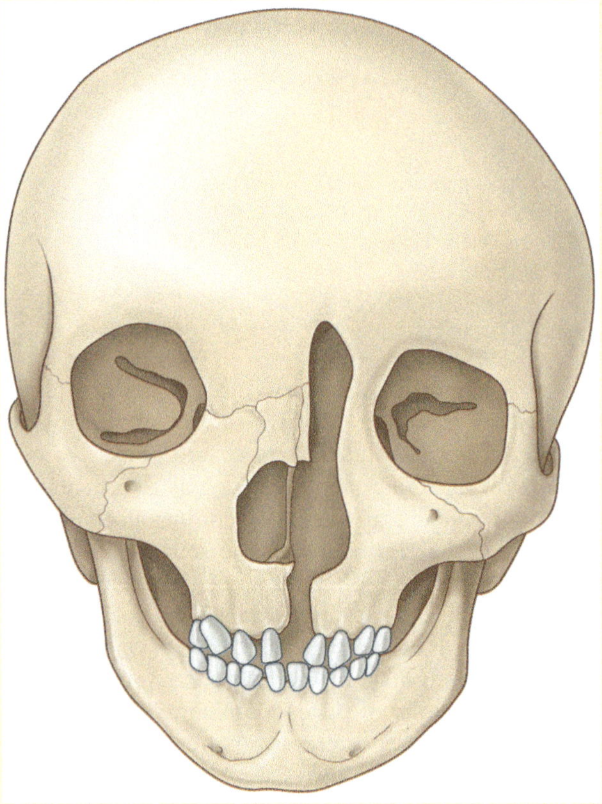	Starts at Cupid's bow and ascends through the soft triangle of the nose to the dome Cleft lip Notching of the soft triangle Deviation of the nasal tip Columella may be widened	Passes between the central and lateral incisors and through the alveolar process The central incisor may be missing The piriform aperture is violated lateral to the anterior nasal spine The nasal septum is spared Keel-shaped maxilla

TABLE 19.1 Description of the Tessier Clefts: Course and Presentation[a]—cont'd

Cleft No.	Soft Tissue	Skeletal
2 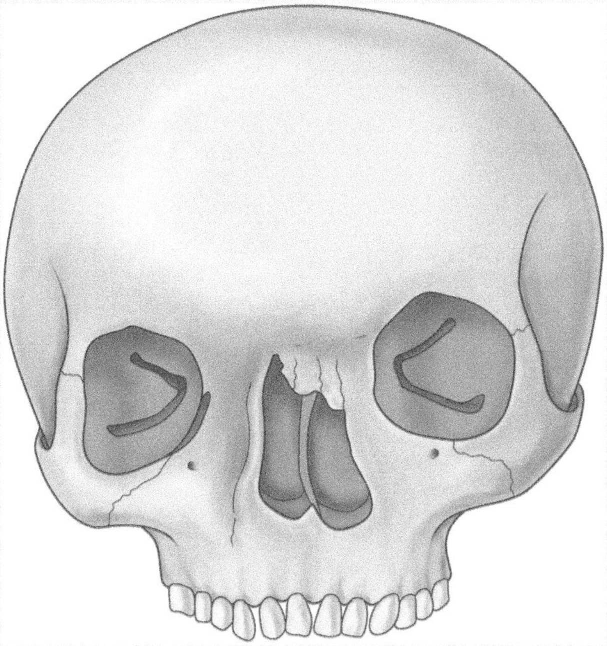	Begins at Cupid's bow (like no. 1 cleft), but courses through middle third of nostril (not dome) Travels medial to the palpebral fissure Cleft lip Disruption of the nostril The medial canthus displaced inferiorly The eyelid and lacrimal system are not disturbed	Crosses the alveolus between the lateral incisor and canine, into pyriform aperture The lateral incisor may be missing Nasal septum remains intact Enlarged ethmoid (hypertelorism)
3 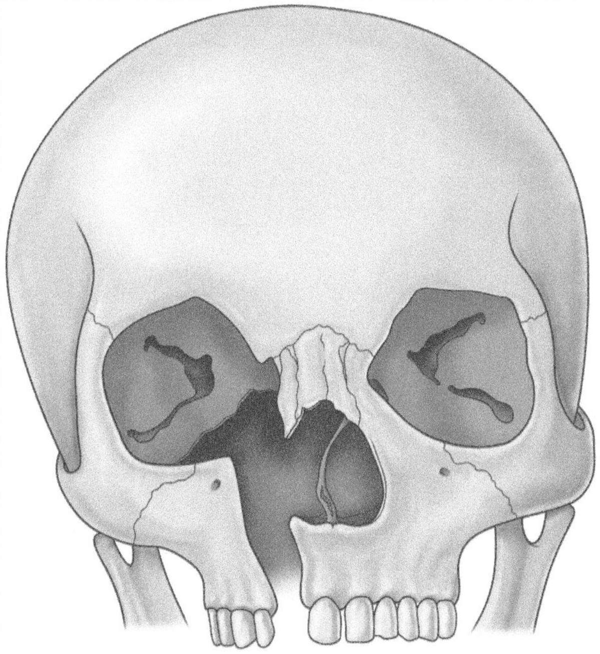	Known as the oro-naso-ocular cleft Cleft lip through Cupid's bow peak (similar to clefts no. 1 and 2), through alar base and medial canthus, separating nose from cheek Nasolacrimal disturbance (the cleft passes between the medial canthus and the inferior lacrimal punctum) Disruption of the nasal ala Blockage of the nasolacrimal duct and recurrent infections of the lacrimal sac are common Microphthalmia or anophthalmia in some cases The globe is displaced inferiorly and laterally	Starts at alveolus between lateral incisor and canine, involves lateral border of pyriform, into lacrimal groove Absence of the medial wall of the maxillary sinus Disruption of the frontal process of the maxilla Direct osseous communication of the oral, nasal, maxillary sinus and orbital cavities

Continued

TABLE 19.1 Description of the Tessier Clefts: Course and Presentation[a]—cont'd

Cleft No.	Soft Tissue	Skeletal
4 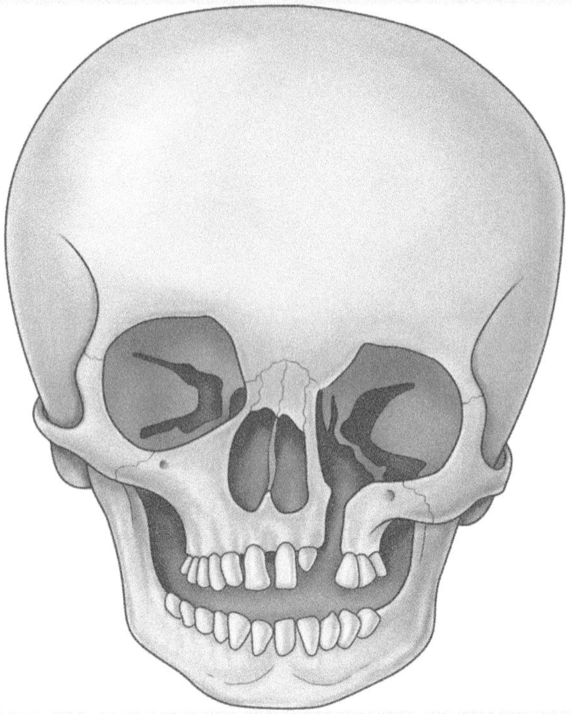	Known as *meloschisis* (separation of cheek) Through lip lateral to Cupid's bow, lateral to ala, through cheek, medial to infraorbital nerve, through the punctum Cleft lip The nasal ala is displaced superiorly The medial canthal tendon is displaced laterally and inferiorly The nasolacrimal system is affected	Through alveolus between the lateral incisor and canine, lateral to pyriform, into medial orbital rim and the floor May travel posteriorly to disrupt the palate and choanae Dystopia Extrophy of the maxillary sinus might be present
5 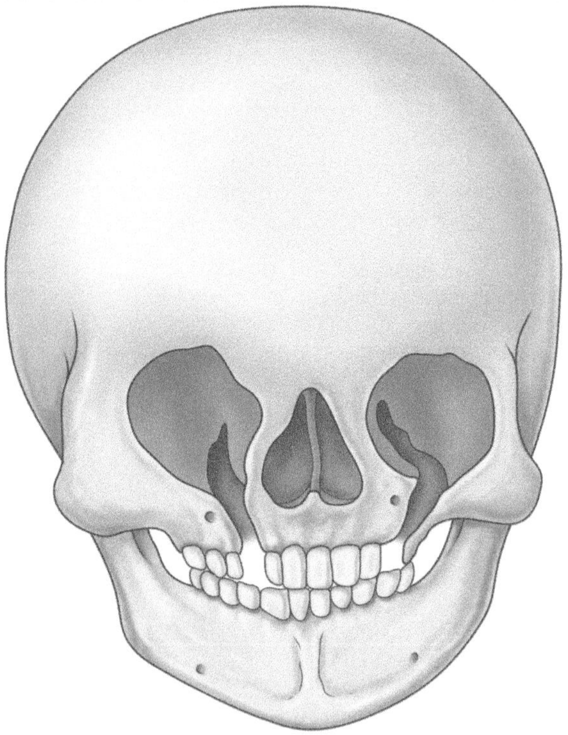	Cleft lip just medial to lateral commissure, through cheek, into the middle third of the lower eyelid Microphthalmia may be present	Posterior to cuspid, lateral to the infraorbital foramen, through the inferolateral orbital rim and orbital floor

TABLE 19.1 Description of the Tessier Clefts: Course and Presentation[a]—cont'd

Cleft No.	Soft Tissue	Skeletal
6 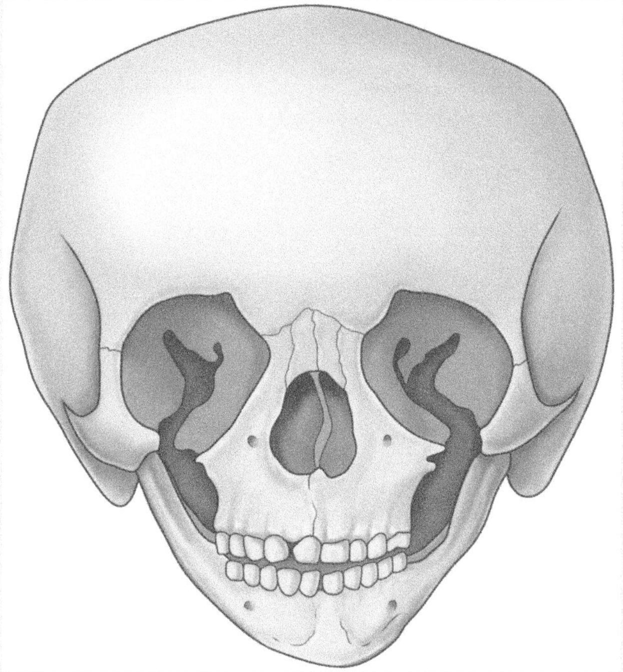	Extends from oral commissure towards lateral lower lid May produce: antimongoloid slant palpebral slant, lower lid coloboma, lateral canthal tendon displacement laterally Ear malformations May present with nos. 7 and 8 clefts in Treacher Collins syndrome	Travels from posterior maxilla to the zygomaticomaxillary suture through the inferior orbital fissure Hypoplastic malar bone (but still present) There is no alveolar cleft, but a short posterior maxilla may result in an occlusal tilt Commonly associated with choanal atresia
7 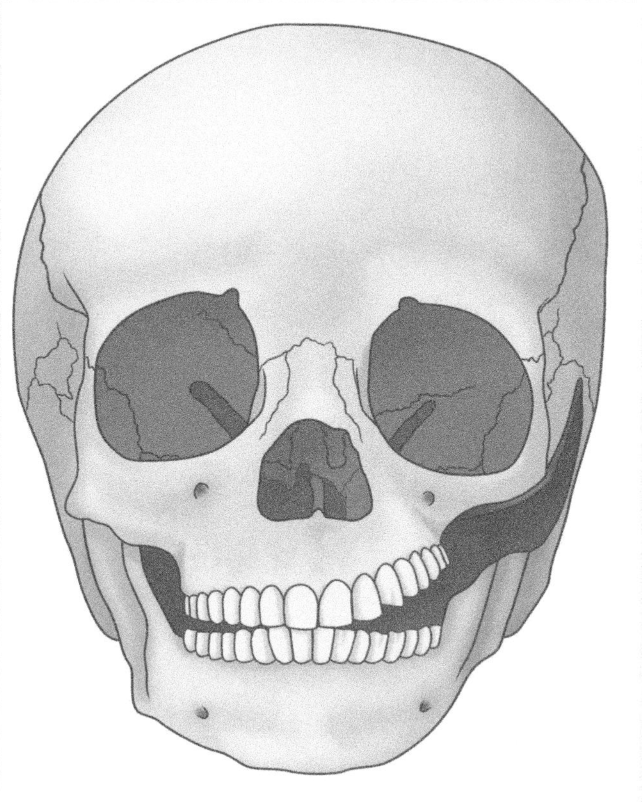	The most common of the atypical craniofacial clefts Begins at the oral commissure and varies from a mild broadening to a complete cleft Extends laterally towards the ear and may involve masseter Macrostomia Hypoplasia of soft palate and tongue Parotid abnormalities, atrophic temporal muscle Ear malformations The lateral canthal tendon is inferiorly displaced Cranial nerves V and VII may be affected	Cleft passes through the pterygomaxillary junction Posterior maxilla and ramus are hypoplastic (causing orbital dystopia) The zygomatic arch is clefted Condyle and coronoid can be present Open bite or crossbite is seen Hypodontia of the upper maxillary can be present Associated with craniofacial microsomia (graded using the Pruzansky Kaban classification for mandibular component)

Continued

TABLE 19.1 **Description of the Tessier Clefts: Course and Presentation[a]—cont'd**

Cleft No.	Soft Tissue	Skeletal
8 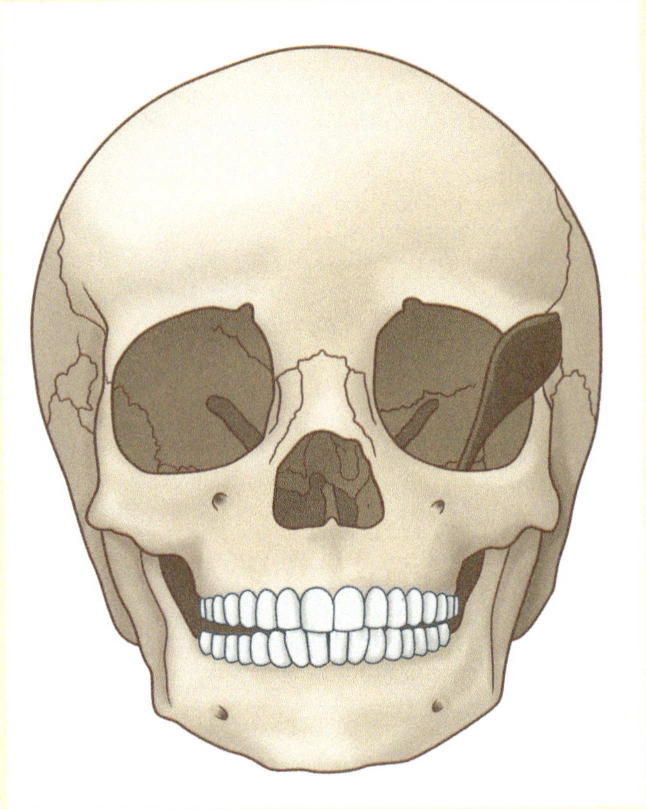	May present with a no.7 cleft Cleft through the lateral canthus and towards the temporal region Lateral canthal colobomas Epibulbar dermoid (associated with Goldenhar syndrome)	Centered at the frontozygomatic sutures Sesamoid bones may present in the temporalis–masseteric aponeurosis
9 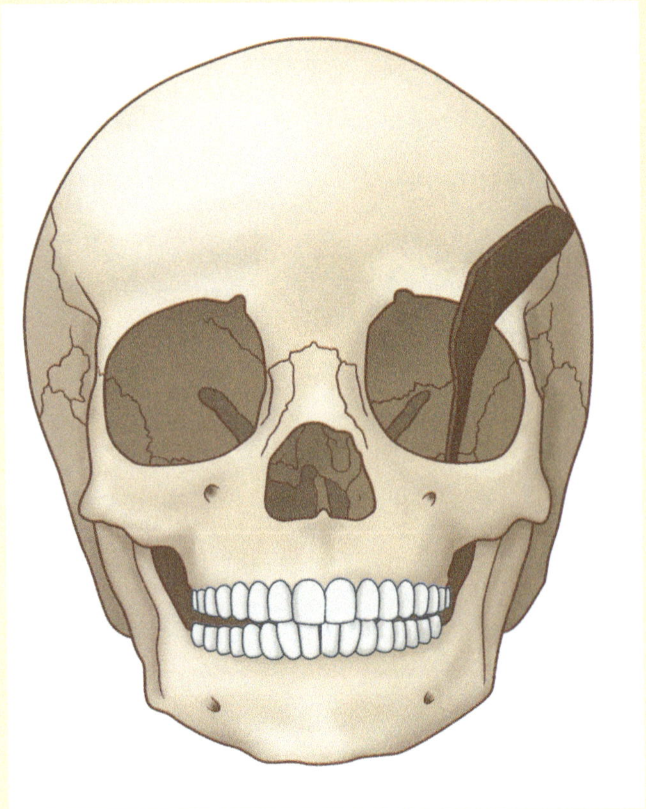	The rarest of the craniofacial clefts Cleft through the superolateral third of the lid, brow, and into temporal hairline The lateral canthal tendon is not affected The hairline is disrupted Microphthalmia may be present	Through the superolateral angle of the orbit Cleft of the greater wing of the sphenoid The lateral orbital rim is rotated posterolaterally

TABLE 19.1 Description of the Tessier Clefts: Course and Presentation[a]—cont'd

Cleft No.	Soft Tissue	Skeletal
10 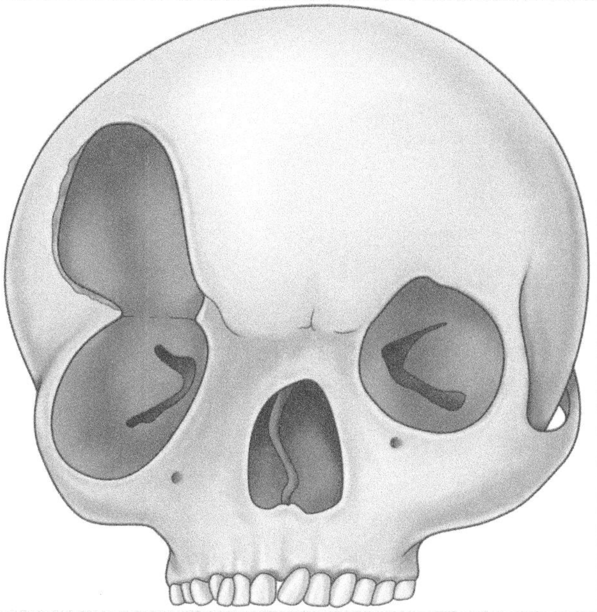	Cleft through the middle third of upper eyelid, brow, and into hairline Upper eyelid coloboma (middle third) Ablepharia can be seen	Travels through the midportion of the superior orbital rim lateral to the supraorbital nerve, extends to the orbital roof, and into frontal bone A fronto-orbital encephalocele is commonly present The orbit is rotated laterally and inferiorly
11 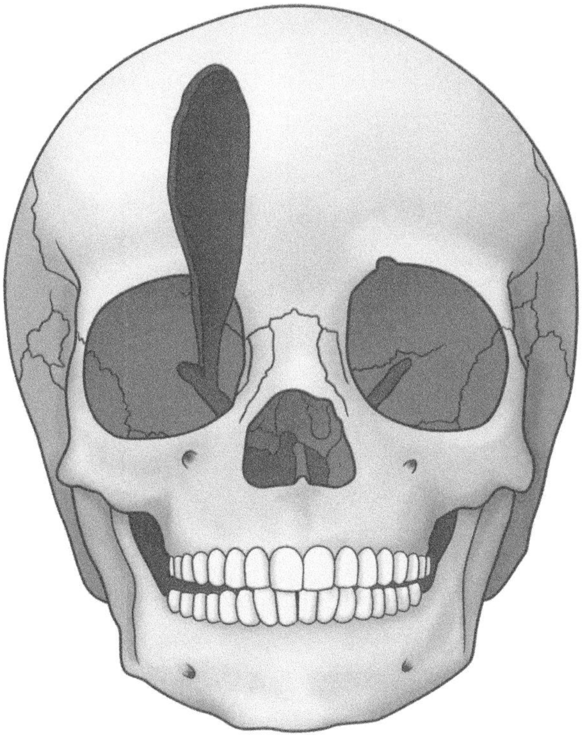	Through the medial third of the upper eyelid and eyebrow, into the frontal hairline	Passes through the medial side of the supraorbital rim and orbital roof Can pass through the ethmoid labyrinth Hypertelorism can occur

Continued

TABLE 19.1 **Description of the Tessier Clefts: Course and Presentation[a]—cont'd**

Cleft No.	Soft Tissue	Skeletal
12 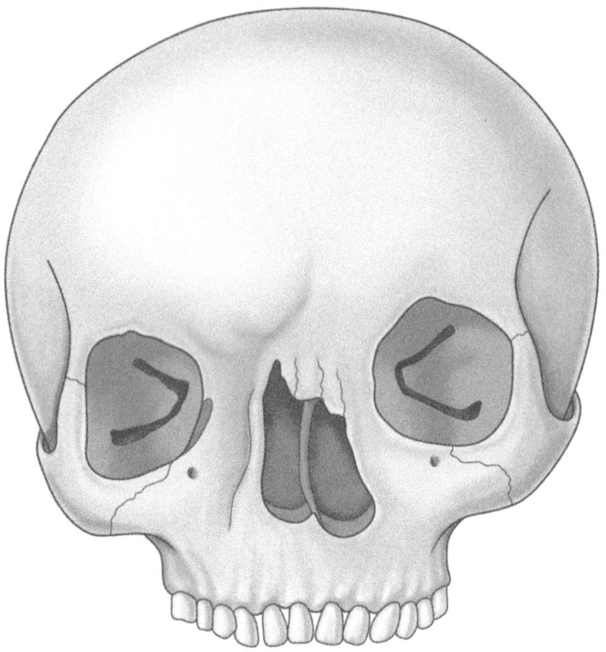	Starts just medial to the medial canthus, through the root of the eyebrow The medial canthal tendon is displaced laterally The eyelid is not disrupted Hair loss of the medial portion of the eyebrow	Travels through the ethmoid labyrinth, towards the frontal bone Olfactory groove lies medial to the cleft Normal cribriform Hypertelorism The frontal process of the maxilla is broadened and flattened
13 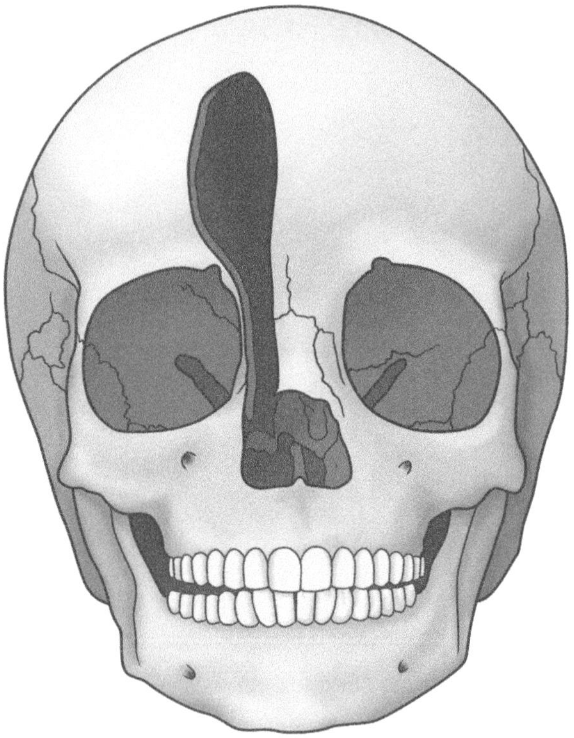	Extends from the dome of nostril cephalad, medial to the eyelids and eyebrow Can extend to the hairline May involve the medial canthus	Extends from the piriform aperture through nasal bone or between nasal bone and frontal process of maxilla Hypertelorism

TABLE 19.1 Description of the Tessier Clefts: Course and Presentation[a]—cont'd

Cleft No.	Soft Tissue	Skeletal
14 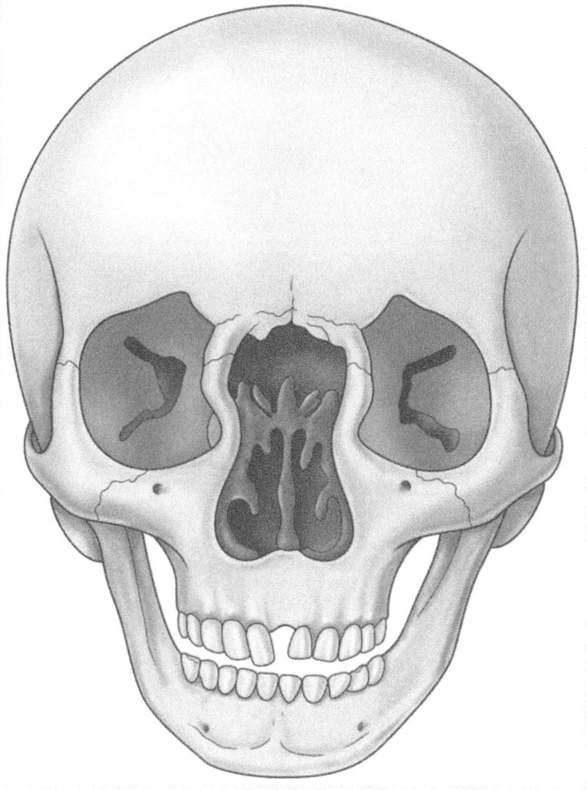	The cranial extension of no. 0 cleft **A: Hypoplasia** Holoprosencephaly (cyclopia, ethmocephaly, cebocephaly and primary palate agenesis) **B: Dysraphia** Encephalocele **C: Hyperplasia** Orbital hypertelorism	Travels through the frontal bone Broad crista galli and frontal sinus Hypotelorism or hypertelorism
30 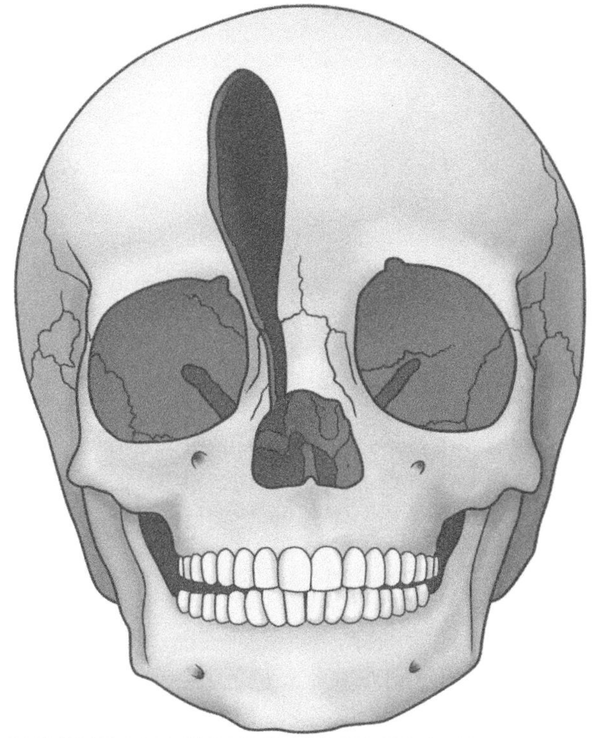	Cleft through the midline tongue, lower lip, and chin A bifid tongue	Midline, through the mandibular symphysis, hyoid, and possibly sternum of varying degrees

[a]It is important to note that this table serves as a guide, and that the features described for each Tessier cleft classification may be present to a greater or lesser degree. Not all features noted need be present for each particular cleft.

Illustrations for clefts 0, 1, 2, 3, 4, 5, 6, 10, 12, and 14 from Bradley JP, Kawamoto HK. Craniofacial clefts. In: Rodriguez ED, Losee JE, Neligan PC, eds. *Plastic Surgery*. 4th edn. *Volume 3: Craniofacial, Head and Neck Surgery and Pediatric Plastic Surgery*. Elsevier; 2018.

Skin

Facial cleft deformities usually involve shortening of the facial dimensions along the cleft, leading to a "short oculo-oral distance."[14] The goal of soft tissue closure is to normalize the face's vertical height, as well as to achieve repositioning of critical structures such as canthi, lower eyelids, lips and nose using traditional soft-tissue transposition techniques such as Z-plasties, back-cuts and/or rotation-advancements. Such repositioning must also incorporate excision of scarred tissues associated with the cleft.

Another important concept is the placement of scars to avoid the violation of anatomical facial units. In cases where the facial cleft involves a single-facial unit such as Tessier nos. 1, 2 or 5, a Z-plasty can be employed to provide esthetically acceptable lengthening and correction[15] (Fig. 19.2).

In facial clefts involving more than one facial unit, such as Tessiers 3 or 4, a midface rotation-advancement flap may provide superior esthetics to traditional interdigitating flaps or Z-plasties by limiting scars along the lines dividing subunits, as espoused by Chen et al.[16] The authors also describe the importance of the realignment and repair of facial muscles, noting that it provided more natural facial expression and animation, as well as progressive lengthening of the initially vertically-deficient midface[16](Box 19.1 and Fig. 19.3).

Attention must also be given to the mucosa at the time of skin repair as a significant portion of facial clefts are full-thickness. As in the more common clefts of the lip and palate, the mucosa is similarly closed using interdigitating flaps, Z-plasties, back-cuts, etc. Due to tissue deficiency which may be present, one may repair these defects initially with local flaps (rotation/advancement, back-cuts, Z-plasties), and then later in life transpose the scars to the boundary of the esthetic subunits with additional soft tissue flaps and/or tissue expansion to recruit additional tissue.[17]

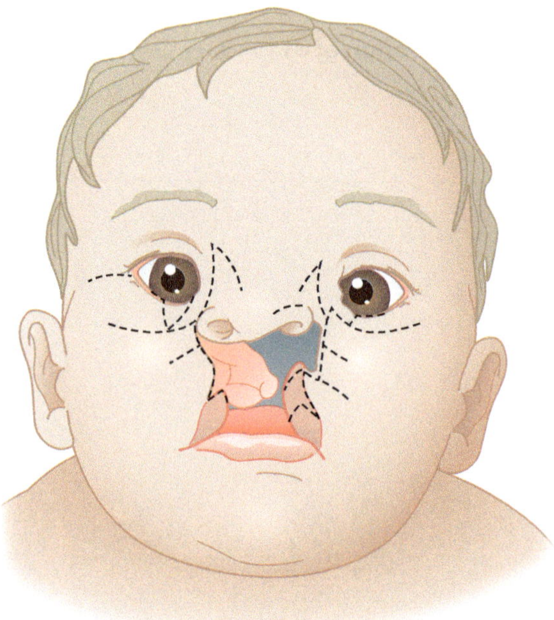

• **Fig. 19.2** Z-plasties.

• BOX 19.1 Key Elements of Repair for Tessier Clefts Nos. 4–7

- Advancement of a laterally-based cheek flap
- A lateral canthotomy to gain more length and advance tissues medially toward the medial canthus, nose, and lip
- Rotation of a medially-based nasal flap
- Medial canthopexy
- Periosteal relaxing incisions lateral to infraorbital bundle to facilitate medial advancement of the cheek
- An orbicularis oculi flap is an integral component within the flap
- Repositioning and repair of the clefted facial expression muscles
- Placement of scars along the lines of the facial units

Eyelids

Colobomas are commonly associated with facial clefts involving the eyelids, characterized by a partial- or full-thickness defect.[18] One of the key aims in determining the most appropriate type of reconstructive surgery is ensuring corneal protection. Artificial tears and ointments can be utilized, in addition to patching prior to surgical intervention for the eyelid reconstruction. Eyelid reconstruction can range from a simple repair or a minor modification procedure, to multiple complex surgical procedures involving flaps or grafts to achieve restoration of the anterior, middle, and posterior lamellae of the eyelid. It is often necessary to reposition the medial canthus either using a transnasal wiring technique or reattachment to the periosteum and is a crucial step in eyelid reconstruction. Sturdy reconstruction of the medial canthal complex is essential for appropriate lower eyelid support and to avoid inferior displacement. Lateral canthotomy can be used to assist medial translocation of the lid in cases where advancement is limited. Identification of the appropriate site is facilitated in unilateral cases by matching the unaffected side. Positioning is conversely more complex in bilateral cases, where estimation can be based on the relative position of the lateral canthus. Lastly, the planned medial canthal position should be 2 mm higher than the desired final location due to the tendency for inferior migration following skin repair. Appropriate assessment of the nasolacrimal system is required as it is often compromised in clefts involving the medial orbit.[19] Dacryocystorhinostomy or a similar procedure at an interval may be required to restore appropriate lacrimal function.[19]

Nose

Midline clefts can be accompanied by a nasal duplication, or alternatively an absence or excess of nasal structures.[2,20] Paramedian and/or oblique clefts frequently involve alar rim deformities, ranging from minor notching to malposition

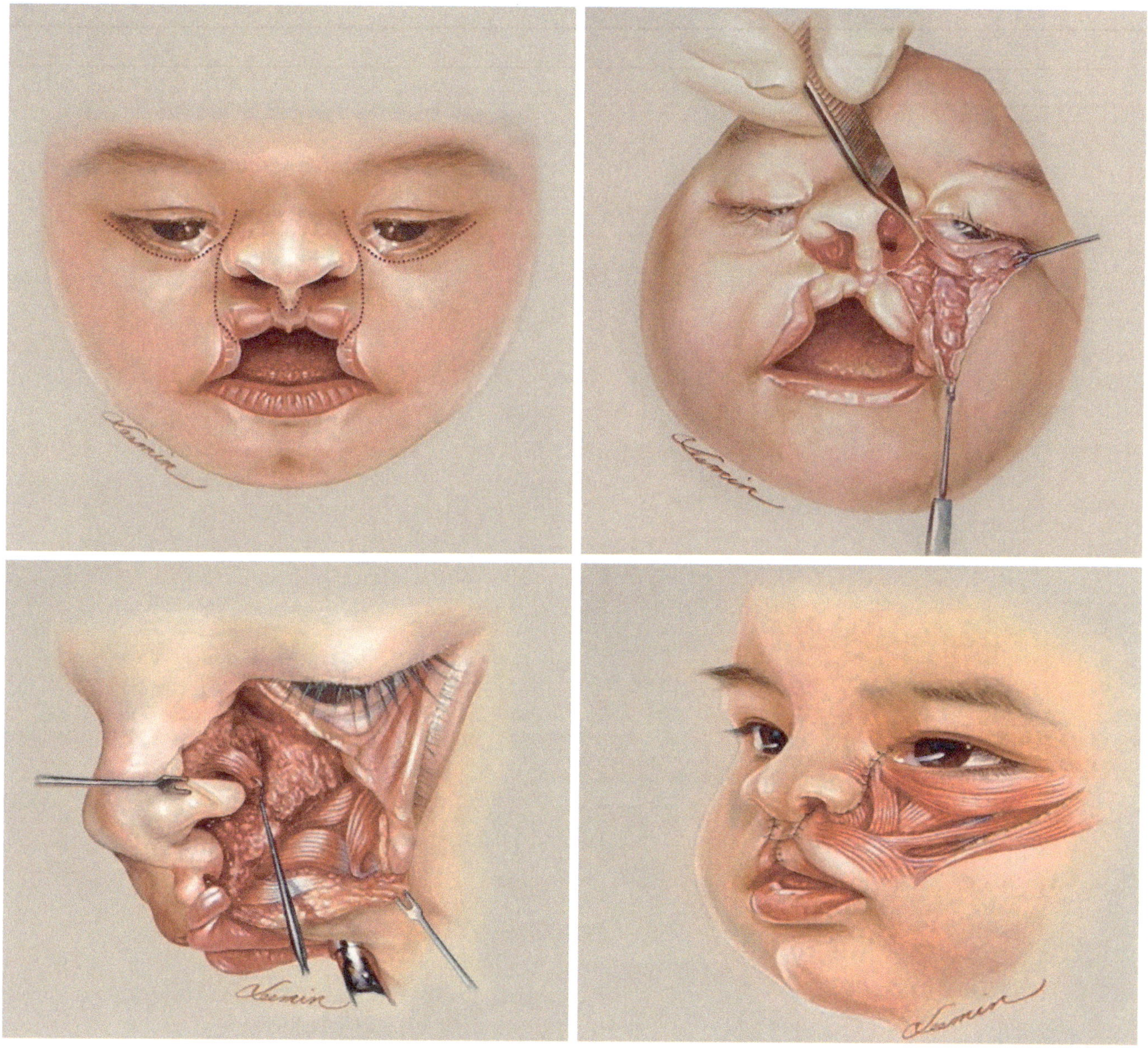

• **Fig. 19.3** Midface rotation advancement flap.

of the lateral crura, to total hypoplasia.[6] Another variant, the proboscis, represents an embryonic remnant of a tubular nasal appendage.[21] An encephalocele – also known as cranium bifidum – and hypertelorism can also be present.[2,20]

Nasal reconstruction must encompass three-dimensional reconstruction of missing or deformed structures as well as preservation or reestablishment of nasal airway function. Evaluation of all nose components should be done in both a qualitative and quantitative manner in accordance with three aspects: skin, lining, and availability of cartilaginous or bony support. Prudent planning and careful assessment of all surgical options is necessary. Some defects require skeletal and soft tissue repairs before other anomalies can be addressed. This is especially true in nasal reconstruction, where correcting skeletal, soft tissue and orbital abnormalities often takes precedence to provide a stable platform for eventual nasal reconstruction. In other situations, such as midline or paramedian clefts involving orbital hypertelorism (e.g., frontonasal dysplasia) may undergo simultaneous correction of hypertelorism (four-wall osteotomy or facial bipartition) associated with cantilever bone grafting for reconstruction of the nasal dorsum and/or soft tissue excess excision.

Bony defects can be present along the cleft from the alveolus to the orbit. Autologous bone graft is the preferred material, in particular from rib, split calvarial or iliac crest donor sites. Midline and paramedial clefts may have nasal dorsum deformities or instability due to absent or deformed septal cartilage or splayed/absent nasal bones. Provided that a patient has septal nasal cartilage, it can be utilized as a graft for reconstruction of the caudal septum or nasal dorsum. Otherwise, costal cartilage can be harvested for more substantial and stable material. A composite chondromucosal flap based on the septal branch of the superior labial artery can also be

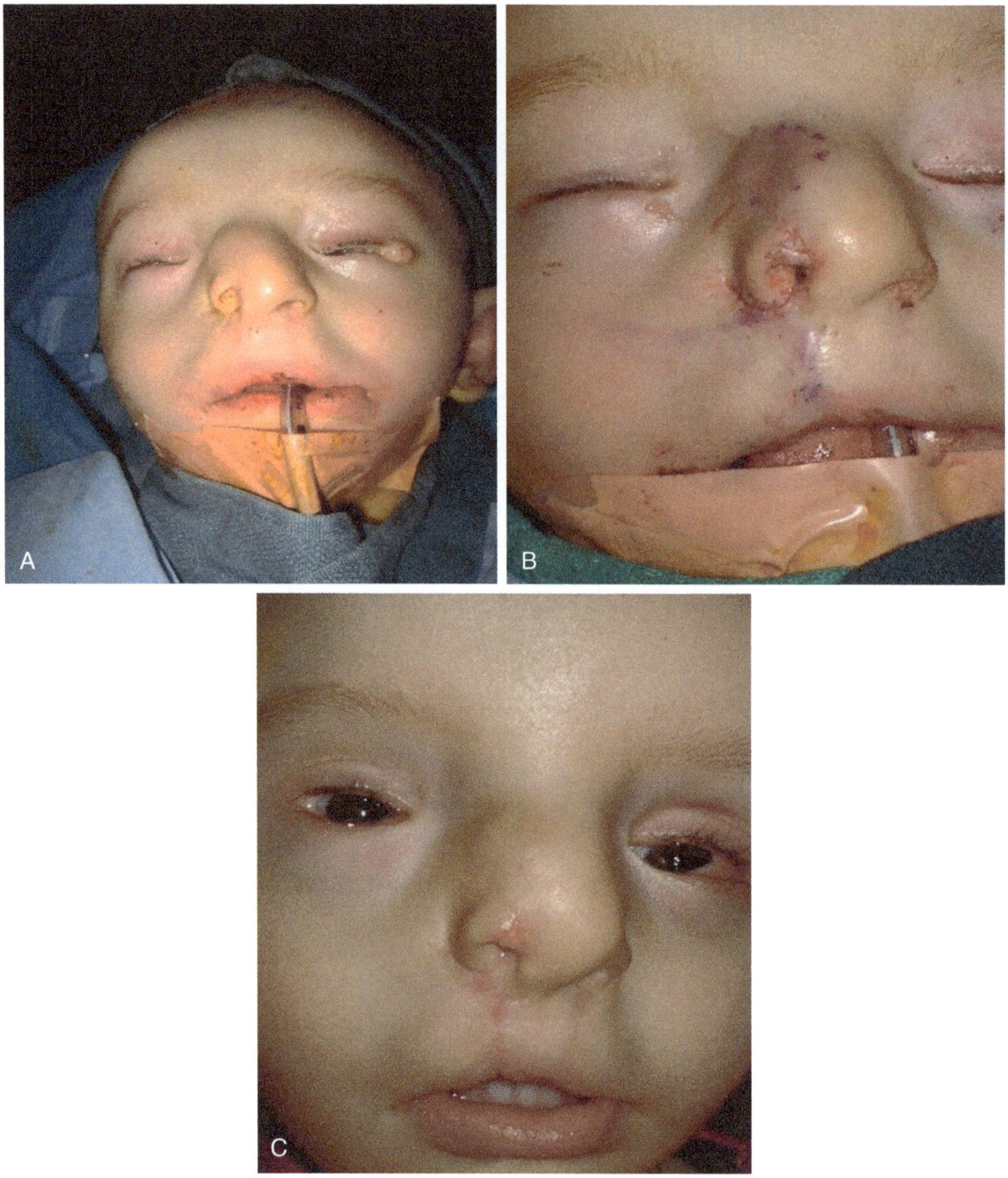

• **Fig. 19.4** (A) Preoperative photograph of Tessier cleft no. 2/12 showing typical notching of nasal ala and vertical malposition. (B) Postoperative photograph showing inferior repositioning of alar base and composite helical ear graft to reconstruct deficient alar tissue. (C) Three months postoperatively with improved nasal symmetry with healed composite graft.

utilized.[22] The workhorse for bony nasal vault reconstruction remains a cantilever split cranial bone graft, combined often with osteotomies to medialize displaced nasal bones in cases of bifidity. Traditional cartilaginous tip suturing and support techniques, with or without grafts, for tip reshaping can be done simultaneously or at a later stage.

Minor deficiencies of the tip and alar rim can be addressed with the use of cartilage grafts or composite grafts (e.g., conchal) for deficient or notched alars (Fig. 19.4). Alar repositioning is also essential and should be inferiorly overcorrected by 2 mm to account for the tendency for superior displacement.

Esthetically acceptable outcomes require reconstitution of the nasal lining to minimize the risk of developing secondary contractures. Adequate lining in case of minor nose defects can be achieved with local transposition flaps, while mucoperichondrial grafts can provide larger-scale lining from the adjacent nasal septum, if available.[22] For the skin deficiencies, midline and paramedian clefts that involve the nose, the techniques of repair for the skin defect are similar to those of the standard cleft lip – straight line, rotation/advancement or Z-plasty.[23,24] Sizable and complex defects could be approached with a number of workhorse flaps for the head and neck such as the frontonasal flap and forehead flap.[25,26] In addition, modification to these flaps such as prefabrication, tissue expansion or inclusion of cartilage, is also a viable option. This would enable the surgical team to reconstruct defects utilizing flaps that closely resemble the rest of the facial esthetic units in terms of color and texture.[25]

Cheek

Macrostomia is the most common of the atypical facial clefts and can occur in isolation or often associated with craniofacial microsomia[27] (Box 19.2). This transverse facial cleft ablates the oral commissure and results in a reduced distance between the oral commissure and the tragus.[6,27] Due to its higher incidence compared to other atypical clefts, more can be found in the literature detailing repair techniques.

In newborns diagnosed with macrostomia, it is recommended to commence an early repair at 3 months of age so as to have the infant's feeding patterns improved.[28] However, there is no clear impact on speech development. The aim of the surgical procedure is to restore the normal anatomy of the face along with the labial function. Here, various surgical procedures can be used depending on the patient's condition and the severity of the abnormality. For instance, a straight-line closure, Z-plasty, triangular flap and W-plasty may be considered in restoring normal mouth anatomy.[29,30]

One of the most commonly employed approaches is the Z-plasty, first described by Longacre. The major shortcoming of this method is unfavorable scarring of the oral commissure and cheek. Another option is a straight-line closure with incorporation of triangular flaps. The benefit of this technique is a more symmetrical oral commissure, as well as the repair of the orbicularis oris muscle. Vermilion transposition techniques such as that proposed by Eguchi et al, have the advantage of preservation of the continuity of the vermillion at the commissure, leading to normal thickness and color[31] (Box 19.3). In addition, this approach avoids placing the suture line in the mouth corner, and results in the better functioning of the oral sphincter[31] (Figs. 19.5 and 19.6).

Skeletal Reconstruction

Orbit

Facial clefts can occur with orbital anomalies such as orbital dystopia, hypertelorism, and microophthalmia or anophthalmia.[6] Orbital dystopia is a vertical displacement of the orbits which can occur in facial clefts where the maxilla and/or the orbital floor is involved.[32]

For dystopias with a small orbital defect, a bone graft is often sufficient to reestablish vertical support for the globe and improve facial appearance. However, if orbital dystopia is severe or associated with visual problems a more significant procedure, such as a four-wall box osteotomy, is likely warranted (Fig. 19.7). Moderate to severe hypertelorism is treated using the same technique. Unlike bone grafting alone which can be performed in young patients, box osteotomies generally need to be delayed until 6 years of age to minimize injury to unerupted teeth.[33] Patients with encephalocele are generally repaired within the first few months of life to minimize risks of meningitis. Some authors advocate for concomitant repair of associated hypertelorism with medial wall osteotomies while others delay orbital repositioning surgery to a later date, as discussed previously.[34] Lastly, facial bipartition can be considered for patients with significant hypertelorism and a V-shaped maxilla[33] (Figs. 19.8 and 19.9).

Maxilla

Skeletal deficiencies involving the maxilla are often associated with facial clefts, especially those involving the orbits and oblique facial clefts.[6] Generally speaking, for facial clefts involving the maxilla, treatment principles for bony reconstruction follow those of typical clefts of the lip. Despite having some strong proponents, the use of primary bone grafting in maxillary reconstruction has been limited. This is mostly due to its effect on midfacial growth, poor arch forms, and inadequate alveolar bone formation.[8] Bone grafting (iliac bone or otherwise) of the defect is usually performed in the phase of mixed dentition followed by orthodontic management in preparation of Le Fort I, II or III (or segmental) osteotomy for definitive bony repositioning at skeletal maturity.

Typically, corrective osteotomies are deferred until skeletal maturity to minimize the risk of midface growth disturbance. However, in severe cases with respiratory insufficiency, early surgical intervention may be warranted.[35] In order to adequately restore occlusion in maxillary hypoplasia, a Le Fort I osteotomy may be indicated. This procedure may also help in restoring alveolar relationships if

• BOX 19.2 Anatomical Pathology of Macrostomia

- Malposition of the oral commissure inferolaterally
- Interruption of the facial expression muscles, specifically orbicularis orbis
- Clefting of the oral mucosa

• BOX 19.3 Surgical Steps of Vermilion Transposition Flap

- Mark normal commissure site and determine distance between oral commissure and Cupid's bow on the unaffected side
- Elevate vermilion flap from lower lip, medially based
- Raise buccal mucosal flap
- Release of aberrant soft tissues
- Freeing of orbicularis oris muscle
- Transposition of orbicularis muscle: the superior limb of the orbicularis oris is sewn on the top of the lower muscle limb to re-establish a modiolus
- Transposition of vermilion flap upper lip over lower lip
- Closure of the skin with a straight or Z-plasty technique

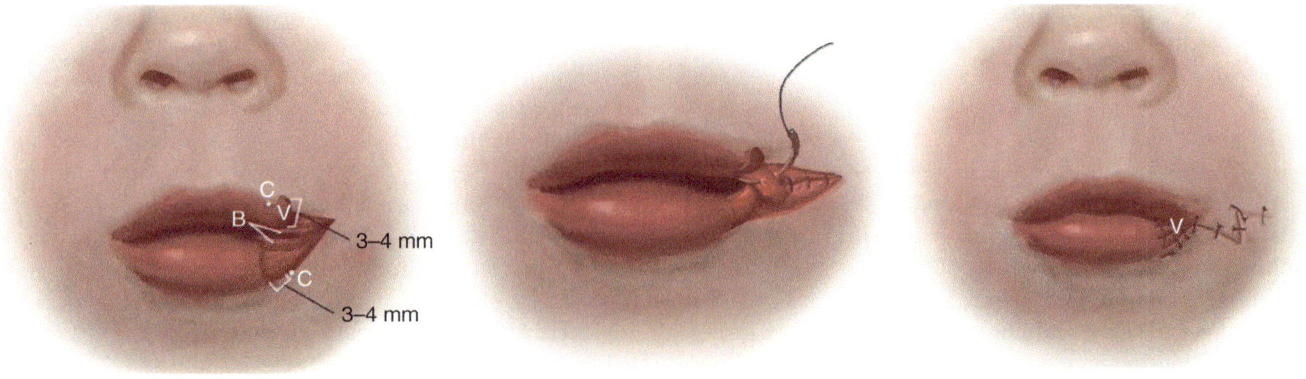

• **Fig. 19.5** Vermilion transposition flap.

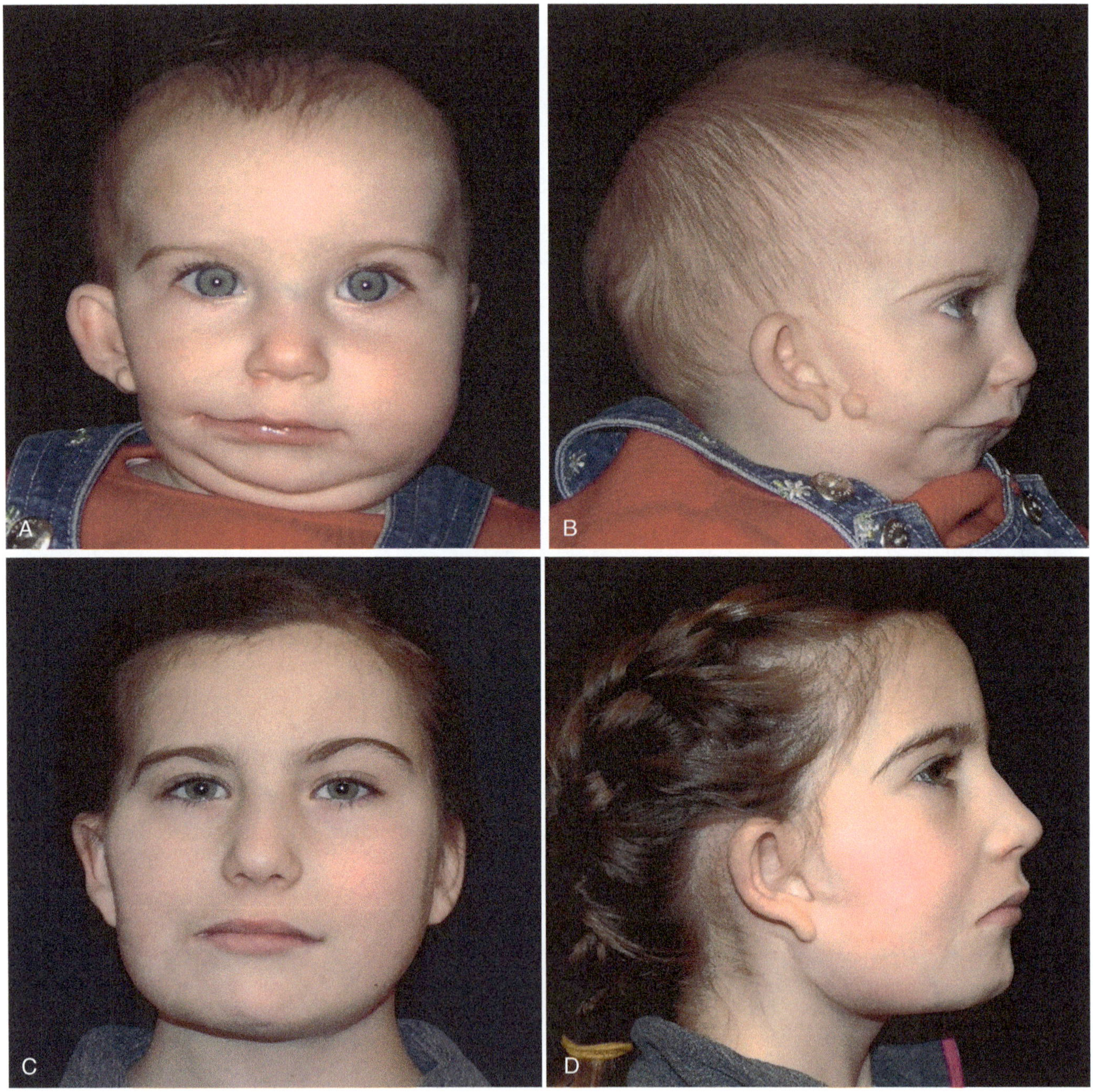

• **Fig. 19.6** (A, B) Preoperative and (C, D) postoperative photographs of a patient with a Tessier cleft no. 7. Initial macrostomia repair was followed by costochondral rib graft to right mandible, mandibular distraction, right-sided facial fat grafting, and setback otoplasty.

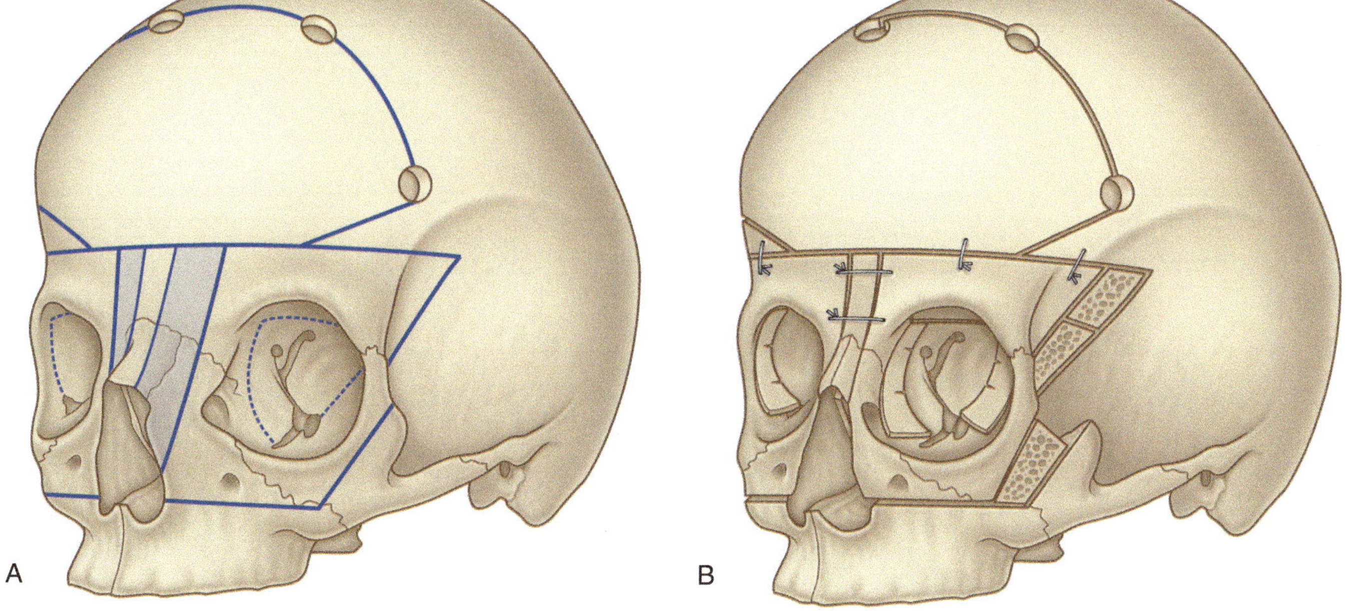

• **Fig. 19.7** (A, B) Box osteotomy. (From Arnaud E, Paternoster G, James S. Orbital hypertelorism. In: Rodriguez ED, Losee JE, Neligan PC, eds. *Plastic Surgery*. 4th edn. *Volume 3: Craniofacial, Head and Neck Surgery and Pediatric Plastic Surgery*. Elsevier; 2018. Fig. 30.2.)

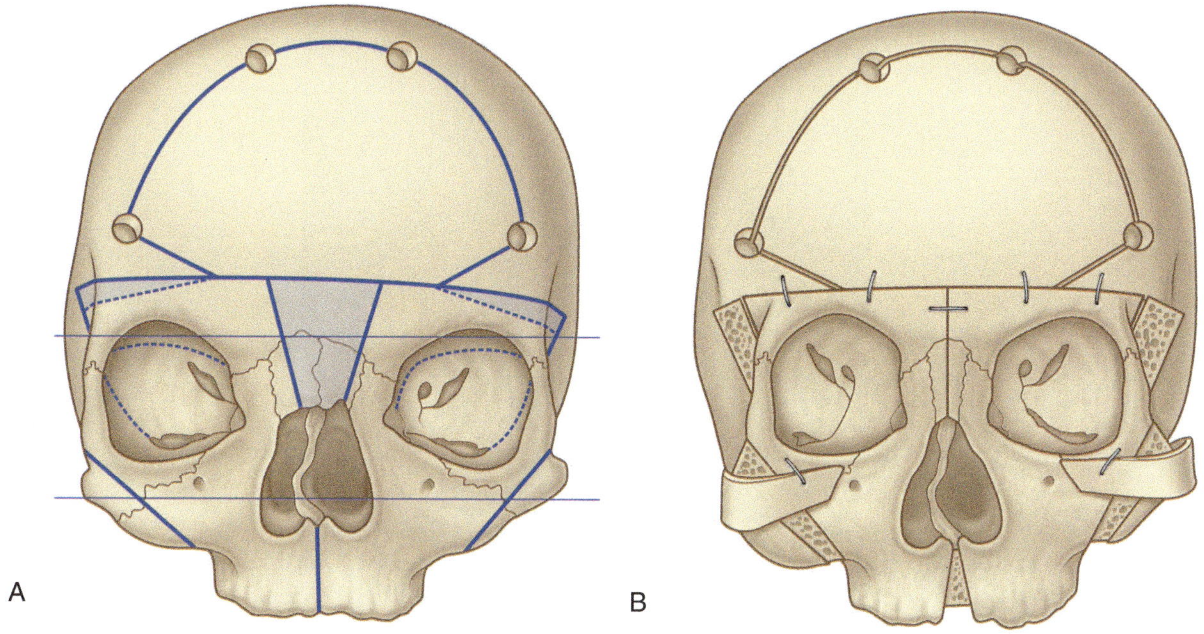

• **Fig. 19.8** (A, B) Facial bipartition. (From Arnaud E, Paternoster G, James S. Orbital hypertelorism. In: Rodriguez ED, Losee JE, Neligan PC, eds. *Plastic Surgery.* 4th edn. *Volume 3: Craniofacial, Head and Neck Surgery and Pediatric Plastic Surgery*. Elsevier; 2018. Fig. 30.3.)

dentition is intact. In cases where nasomaxillary retrusion is present, a Le Fort II may be more appropriate to avoid exacerbating the associated nasal recession.[36] On the other hand, extensive and significant hypoplasia affecting the malar complexes, orbits, and the maxilla would indicate utilizing an approach based on Le Fort III. This approach may produce abnormality with overprominent cheeks and an overprojected nasal bridge, hence segmental osteotomies may be considered.

Distraction osteogenesis can be considered for severe cases with significant midface hypoplasia that requires an advancement of more than 30 mm.[37] Maxillary canine eruption represents a reasonable indicator of timing for when this approach could be utilized with minimal risk to

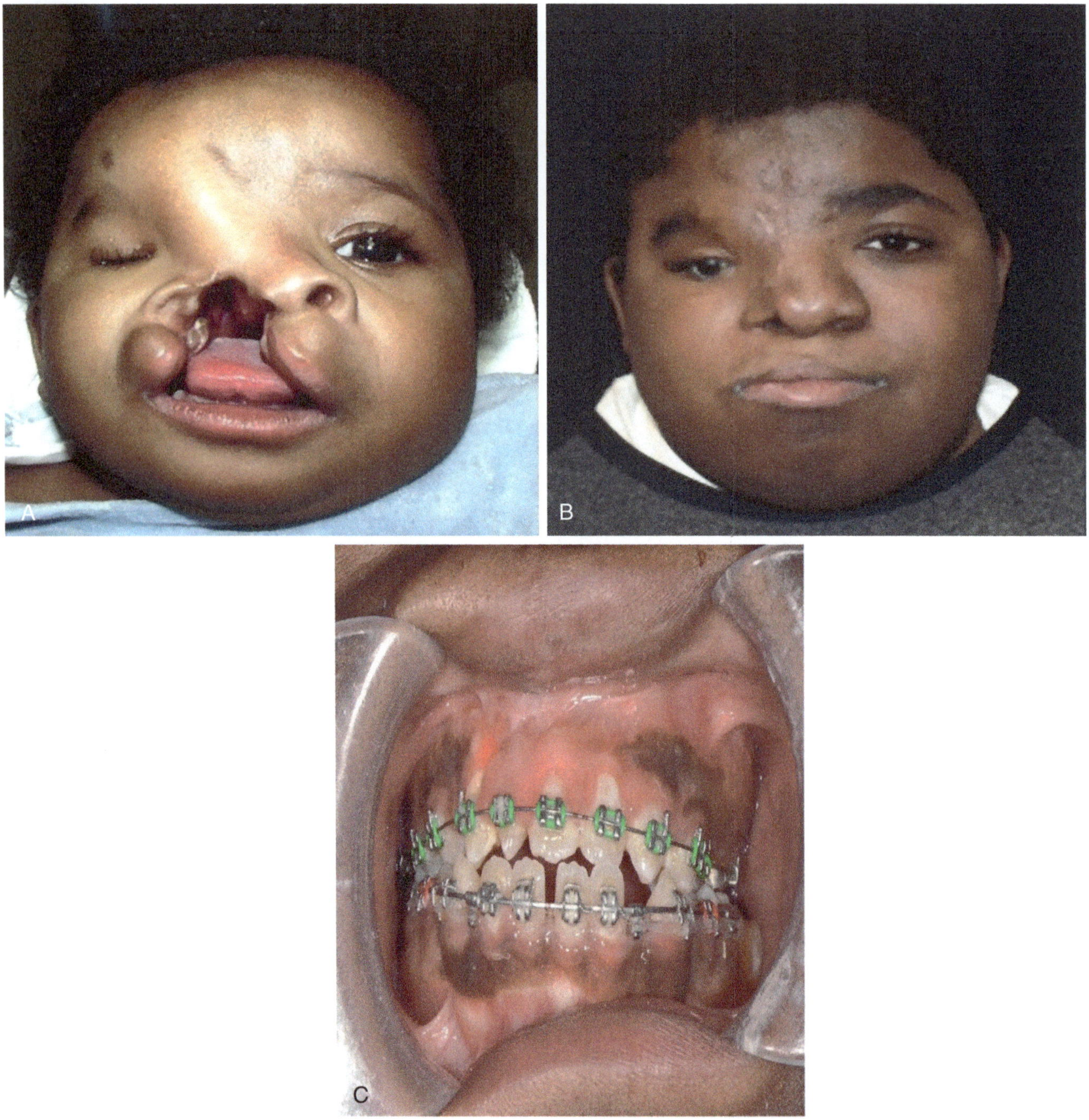

• **Fig. 19.9** (A) Patient with a Tessier cleft no. 3/11 demonstrating microphthalmia, orbital dystopia, and hypertelorism as well as severe involvement of the nose and cheek. (B) Result after an initial repair utilizing rotation advancement of soft-tissues and palate repair, followed later by hemifacial bipartition for improvement of globe positioning, and finally nasal revision with placement of ocular prosthesis. (C) Oral view showing occlusion.

permanent dentition.[37] The overarching goals of such procedures are to improve airway compromise if present, and to minimize facial asymmetry by normalizing maxillary dimension and/or levelling any associated occlusal cant.

Mandible

A true cleft of the mandible (type 30) is extremely rare.[6] It is generally combined with a midline cleft of the lower lip and involves adherence of the tongue to the floor of the mouth (Fig. 19.10). The mandible is hypoplastic on one or both sides. Usually such clefts are managed early in life with repair of the mucosal lining, osteosynthesis or bone grafting of the mandible and closure of the lip/chin skin defect by local soft tissue rearrangement. Further secondary mandibular surgery may be needed as the child matures. So far, there is no consensus on the appropriate age to undergo mandibular surgery.

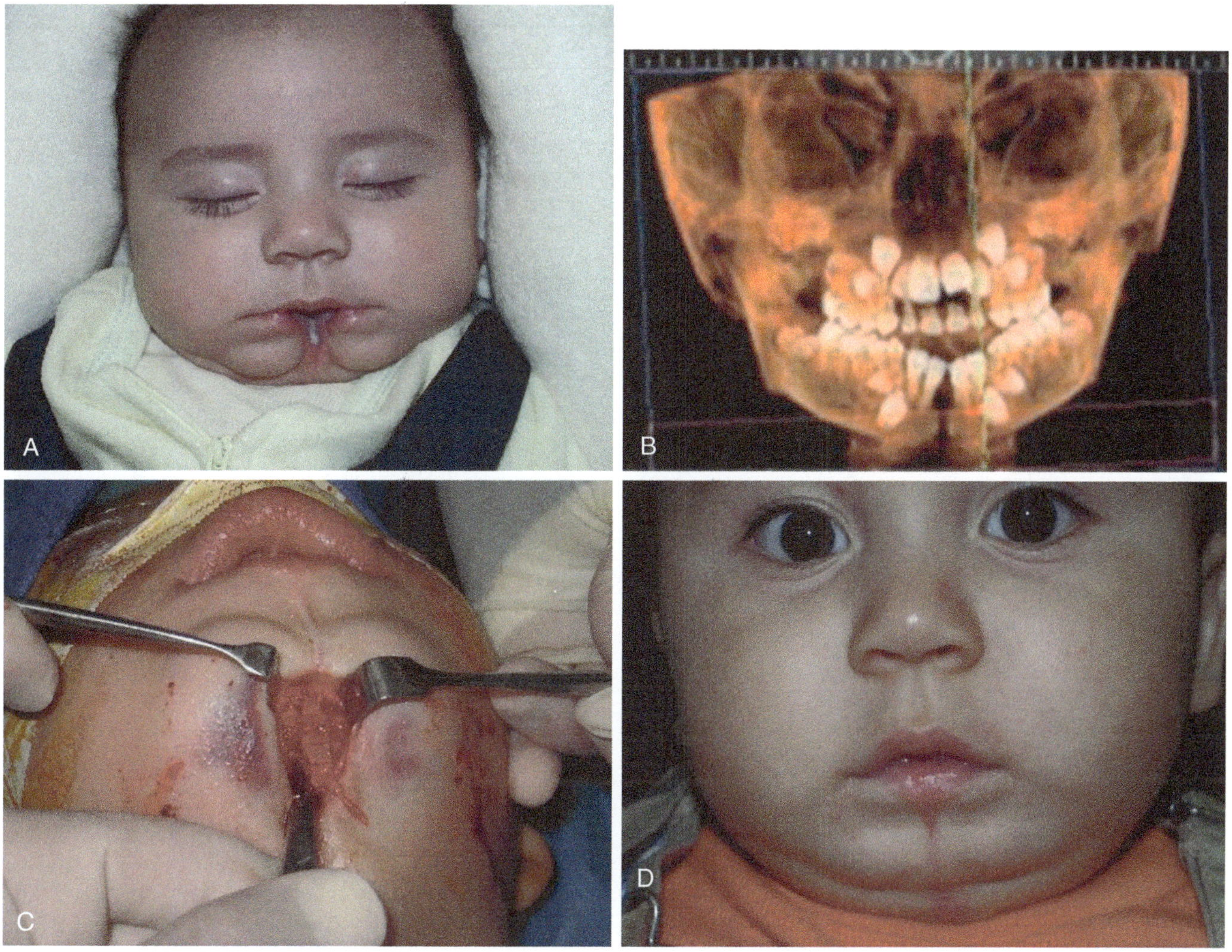

• **Fig. 19.10** (A) A patient with a Tessier cleft no. 30. (B) Preoperative CT scan demonstrating the bony mandibular midline cleft. Soft tissue repair was performed via excision and interdigitating flaps, followed at a second stage (C) by bony defect reconstruction with iliac bone graft. (D) The patient following reconstruction.

Prevention

The causes of facial clefts are still not fully understood. What is known is that folic acid supplementation during pregnancy has been linked to a lower risk of developing facial clefts.[38]

Conclusion

Rare craniofacial clefts present a challenge due to their infrequent presentation and high degree of variability. Their correction thus needs to be customized to suit the deformity. The priority remains the protection of vital functions such as oral competence, vision, and airway stability, followed later by esthetic concerns such as symmetry and optimal scar positioning. Optimal outcomes rely on the full gamut of plastic surgical techniques, stepwise correction, and thorough and thoughtful planning.

References

1. Kalantar-Hormozi A, Abbaszadeh-Kasbi A, Goravanchi F, Davaiet NR. Prevalence of rare craniofacial clefts. *J Craniofac Surg*. 2017;28(5):e467–e470.
2. Hunt JA, Hobar PC. Common craniofacial anomalies: facial clefts and encephaloceles. *Plast Reconstr Surg*. 2003;12(2):606–615. quiz 616,722.
3. Hunt JA, Hobar PC. Common craniofacial anomalies: the facial dysostoses. *Plast Reconstr Surg*. 2002;110(7):1714–1725.
4. Mishina Y, Snider TN. Neural crest cell signaling pathways critical to cranial bone development and pathology. *Exp Cell Res*. 2014;325(2):138–147.
5. Hu D, Helms JA. The role of Sonic hedgehog in normal and abnormal craniofacial morphogenesis. *Development*. 1999;126(21):4873–4884.
6. Tessier P. Anatomical classification of facial, cranio-facial and latero-facial clefts. *J Maxillofac Surg*. 1976;4:69–92.

7. Mazzola R, Mazzola R, Vermey-Keers C, Stricker M, Raphael B. A morphogenetic classification of craniofacial malformations. *Plast Reconstr Surg.* 1983;71(4):560–572.
8. Losee J, Kirschner R. *Comprehensive Cleft Care.* Maidenhead: McGraw–Hill Education; 2008.
9. Rodriguez ED, Losee JE, Neligan P, eds. *Plastic Surgery,* 4th Ed. Volume 3: Craniofacial, Head and Neck Surgery and Pediatric Plastic Surgery. Elsevier; 2018: see esp. ch. 31.
10. Port G, Kaposi H. *Chirurgie der Mundhohle*; 1906.
11. Richards A Dafydd H. *Key Notes on Plastic Surgery.* 2nd ed. Oxford: Wiley–Blackwell; 2014.
12. Kaban L, Mulliken J, Murray J. Three-dimensional approach to analysis and treatment of hemifacial microsomia. *Cleft Palate J.* 1981;18(2):90–99.
13. Pruzansky S. Not all dwarfed mandibles are alike. *Birth Defects.* 1969;5:120–129.
14. Alonso N, da Silva Freitas R, Azor de Oliveira e Cruz G, et al. Tessier no. 4 facial cleft: evolution of surgical treatment in a large series of patients. *Plast Reconstr Surg.* 2008;122(5):1505–1513.
15. da Silva Freitas R, Alonso N, Shin JH, et al. The Tessier number 5 facial cleft: surgical strategies and outcomes in six patients. *Cleft Palate-Craniofacial J.* 2009;46(2):179–186.
16. Chen PK, Chang FC-S, Chan F-C, et al. Repair of Tessier no. 3 and no. 4 craniofacial clefts with facial unit and muscle repositioning by midface rotation advancement without Z-plasties. *Plast Reconstr Surg.* 2012;129(6):1337–1344.
17. Menard RM, Moore MH, David DJ. Tissue expansion in the reconstruction of Tessier craniofacial clefts: a series of 17 patients. *Plast Reconstr Surg.* 1999;103(3):779–786.
18. Tessier P. Colobomas: vertical and oblique complete facial clefts. Simultaneous operation of the eyelid, inner canthus, cheek nose and lip orbitomaxillary bone graft. *Panminerva Med.* 1969;11(3):95.
19. Whitaker LA, Katowitz JA, Randall P. The nasolacrimal apparatus in congenital facial anomalies. *J Maxillofac Surg.* 1974;2:59–63.
20. Losee JE, Kirschner RE, Whitaker LA, Bartlett SP, et al. Congenital nasal anomalies: a classification scheme. *Plast Reconstr Surg.* 2004;113(2):676–689.
21. David LR, Sanger C, Fisher D, Argenta LC. Proboscis lateralis: a rare craniofacial anomaly, reconstruction, and long-term evaluation. *J Craniofac Surg.* 2008;19(4):1107–1113.
22. Burget GC, Menick FJ. Nasal support and lining: the marriage of beauty and blood supply. *Plast Reconstr Surg.* 1989;84(2):189–202.
23. Ortega J, Flor E. Incomplete naso-ocular cleft. *Plast Reconstr Surg.* 1969;43(6):630–632.
24. Thomson H, Sleightholm R. Isolated naso-ocular cleft: a one-stage repair. *Plast Reconstr Surg.* 1985;76(4):534–538.
25. Menick FJ. Nasal reconstruction: forehead flap. *Plast Reconstr Surg.* 2004;113(6):100e–111e.
26. Burget GC, Menick FJ. Nasal reconstruction: seeking a fourth dimension. *Plast Reconstr Surg.* 1986;78(2):145–157.
27. Powell WJ, Jenkins HP. Transverse facial clefts. *Plast Reconstr Surg.* 1968;42(5):454–459.
28. Boo-Chai K. The transverse facial cleft: its repair. *Br J Plast Surg.* 1969;22(2):119–124.
29. Chen K, Noordhoff S. Congenital macrostomia – transverse facial cleft. *Changgeng yi xue za zhi.* 1994;17(3):239–247.
30. Schwarz R, Sharma D. Straight line closure of congenital macrostomia. *Indian J Plast Surg.* 2004;37(2):121.
31. Eguchi T, Asato PH, Takushima A, Takato T, Harii PK. Surgical repair for congenital macrostomia: vermilion square flap method. *Ann Plast Surg.* 2001;47(6):629–635.
32. Edgerton MT, Jane JA. Vertical orbital dystopia – surgical correction. *Plast Reconstr Surg.* 1981;67(2):121–138.
33. Marchac D, Sati S, Renier D, Deschamps-Braly J, Marchac A. Hypertelorism correction: what happens with growth? Evaluation of a series of 95 surgical cases. *Plast Reconstr Surg.* 2012;129(3):713–727.
34. Macfarlane R, Rutka JT, Armstrong D, et al. Encephaloceles of the anterior cranial fossa. *Pediatr Neurosurg.* 1995;23(3):148–158.
35. Morovic CG, Monasterio L. Distraction osteogenesis for obstructive apneas in patients with congenital craniofacial malformations. *Plast Reconstr Surg.* 2000;105(7):2324–2330.
36. Henderson D, Jackson I. Naso-maxillary hypoplasia — the Le Fort II osteotomy. *Br J Oral Surg.* 1973;11(2):77–93.
37. McCarthy JG. *Craniofacial Distraction.* Cham: Springer International; 2017.
38. Wilcox A, Lie RT, Solvoll K, et al. Folic acid supplements and risk of facial clefts: national population based case-control study. *Br Med J.* 2007;334:433–434.

20

Craniosynostosis

LARA S. VAN DE LANDE, AINA V.H. GREIG, AND
DAVID J. DUNAWAY

History

Hippocrates provided the first description of what is now called craniosynostosis in 100 BC and noted the variation of skull deformities and correlated it with the pattern of cranial suture involvement. There are many historical descriptions of people with unusual head shapes. The Greek statesman and General Pericles had an unusually long, narrow head shape and was nicknamed "Squill head," and he might have had sagittal synostosis. Aristophanes and Galen both used the term oxycephalus for "tower head." The term craniosynostosis was first used by Otto in 1830 to describe the entity of premature suture fusion. Virchow described how in medieval Saxony, people believed that such children were thought to be changelings or monsters and that it was the devil who made them deaf, dumb, and blind. Virchow examined skulls from various museums and published a classification where he correlated synostosis of specific cranial sutures with head shape. What has become known as Virchow's law is that premature fusion of a cranial vault suture (craniosynostosis) inhibits skull growth perpendicular to the fused suture and compensatory overexpansion takes place at patent sutures. The general direction of growth after synostosis is parallel to the fused suture. For example, when synostosis of the sagittal suture occurs, growth proceeds in an anteroposterior direction, leading to scaphocephaly and a long, narrow, boat-shaped skull (Fig. 20.1).

Skeletal Development

The developing skull is divided into the neurocranium, which surrounds the brain, and the viscerocranium, which develops into the facial bones. The neurocranium is made up of bones that ossify directly, the membranous neurocranium, which forms the skull vault, and bones that undergo endochondral ossification and form the skull base. The flat bones of the skull grow by the deposition of new bone material at their margins. In their growth phase, these bones do not fuse but remain separated by specialized structures, the cranial sutures. Skull growth is needed to accommodate the size of the growing brain and depends on an exchange of signals between mesenchyme, the osteogenic front, and the dura mater.

Normal Calvarial Growth

Normal growth of the calvarium is complete at about age 2 years, the orbit at age 6 years, and the rest of the facial skeleton at about age 16–17 years. Brain growth drives the enlargement of the skull in infancy. The expanding brain doubles in size in the first 6 months of life and then doubles again in the second 6 months and doubles again between 12 and 24 months. The expanding brain creates separating tensional forces in the cranial sutures. The cranial sutures allow for skull deformation during birth and expansion during brain growth. The metopic suture normally starts to close at the age of 2 years. The sagittal suture begins to close after the age of 22 years, the coronal suture after 24 years, and the lambdoid after 26 years. It is within the normal range for them not to fully close until the age of 40 years.

Craniosynostosis

The prevalence of craniosynostosis ranges from 3.1 to 7.2 in 10,000 live births.[1] Fusion can occur in one or in multiple sutures and in 21% of the cases fusion is caused by a known gene mutation.[2,3]. In nonsyndromic craniosynostosis one suture is fused without additional birth deficits and can affect any cranial suture. Sagittal synostosis is the commonest, with a prevalence of 40%–60%. Overall, the incidence of craniosynostosis has increased, but especially a rise of metopic synostosis has been reported (25% of nonsyndromic craniosynostosis), currently the second most common type, followed by unicoronal synostosis (<15%) – an unexplained change that occurred in Europe and the United States.[4,5] The rarest type is lambdoid synostosis (1% of all craniosynostosis and 3% of nonsyndromic craniosynostosis). Craniosynostosis usually occurs as an isolated condition, but has been reported to be associated with more than 200 syndromes.[6] In syndromic craniosynostosis one or multiple sutures are fused with the presence of other congenital anomalies. Associated phenotypical features can include calvarial and facial hypoplasia and dysmorphology, hydrocephalus, deafness, blindness, mental retardation, and extremity anomalies. Craniosynostosis can have functional consequences.

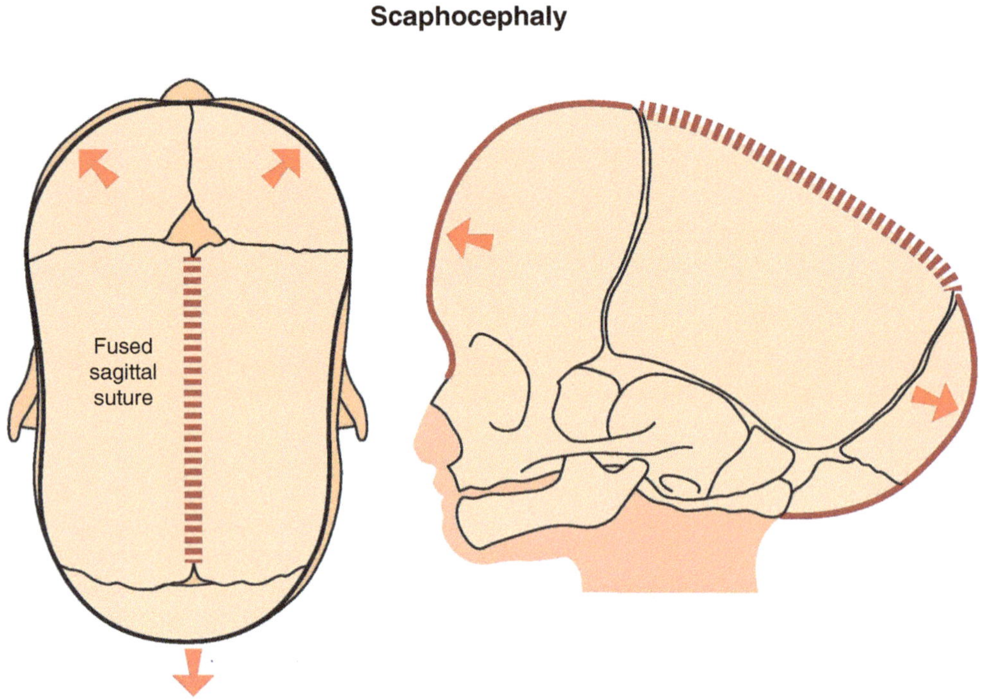

• **Fig. 20.1** Skull growth in sagittal synostosis causes scaphocephaly.

Classification of Craniosynostosis

Primary

- Nonsyndromic: sagittal, metopic, coronal, multisuture, lambdoid, frontosphenoidal
- Syndromic: e.g., Muenke, Crouzon, Pfeiffer, Apert, Saethre–Chotzen.

Secondary

- Metabolic disorder (e.g., hyperthyroidism, hypercalcemia, hypophosphatasia, sickle cell disease and thalassemia, vitamin D deficiency, renal osteodystrophy)
- Malformations (e.g., holoprosencephaly, microcephaly, shunted hydrocephalus, encephalocele)
- Exposure of fetus to teratogenic drugs (e.g., sodium valproate, phenytoin, retinoic acid)
- Mucopolysaccharidosis (e.g., Hurler syndrome, Morquio syndrome).

Molecular Mechanisms Involved in Craniosynostosis

Genes and Clinical Presentation: Nonsyndromic Craniosynostosis

Nonsyndromic craniosynostoses, capturing 60% of all craniosynostosis, are mainly sporadic, however due to advances in genetic diagnostics, nonsyndromic single suture patients are increasingly recognized as syndromic patients. An example of this is the discovery of the *FGFR3* P250R mutation in patients with (bi)coronal synostosis resulting in Muenke syndrome. Moreover, an increasing incidence among first-degree relatives (2%–10% of the patients) is seen, mostly in patients with metopic synostosis followed by multi-, sagittal, lambdoid and coronal suture.[7] Sagittal synostosis is thought to be the most isolated. Multisuture synostosis without known genetic cause has the highest frequency of associated symptoms, such as ear infections, palatal abnormalities, and hearing problems.[7]

The genetic causes of nonsyndromic craniosynostosis remain largely unknown. Mutations in the genes causing syndromic craniosynostosis and chromosomal abnormalities are not a common cause of nonsyndromic craniosynostosis. Nonsyndromic craniosynostosis as a ‘developmental pathway disorder’ has been suggested. On the latter, a stronger influence of genetic factors in the etiopathogenesis of nonsyndromic craniosynostosis has been implied. The *SMAD6* mutation was found in 7% of patients with midline (sagittal and/or metopic) nonsyndromic craniosynostosis and in 25% of the patients with familial occurrence of midline craniosynostosis.[8] Moreover, mutations such as *ALX4*, *BBS9*, *BMP2*, *EFNA4*, *IGF1R*, *RUNX2*, *SMURF1*, *SPRY1*, *SPRY4* are thought to be responsible for the fusion of a specific single suture.

Genes and Clinical Presentation: Syndromic Craniosynostosis

The best understood skull developmental cascades include bone morphogenetic proteins (BMP)/transforming growth factor beta (TGFβ), fibroblast growth factor (FGF), hedgehog (HH), eph-ephrin and wingless-type MMTV integration site family (WNT) signaling pathways. Most of these pathways are known to play a role in neural crest development, hence driving the morphogenesis of the craniofacial complex. There is good evidence that the primary pathology in craniosynostosis is within the dura mater and not within the bone. Cranial suture fusion and maintenance of patency are dependent on the interplay of transcription factors, cytokines, growth factor receptors, and extracellular matrix molecules.

The majority of craniosynostosis syndromes are caused by mutations in genes encoding FGFR-1, FGFR-2, and FGFR-3, and the transcription factors TWIST1 (upstream regulator of FGFRs), MSX2, and ALX4. Gain-of-function mutations are associated with the human genes *MSX2*, *ALX4* and *FGFR*, whereas loss of function is associated with the TWIST1 gene *EFNB1*. In 2016, *SIX2* was found in patients with syndromic complex or sagittal synostosis. *ZIC1* is among the latest identified craniosynostosis-associated genes. New mutations are expected to be found in the future, on account of which the number of syndromic craniosynostoses will increase. After the discovery of P250R *FGFR3* mutation, Muenke syndrome is the most frequent syndromic craniosynostosis, followed by Crouzon syndrome and Pfeiffer syndrome. Apert syndrome (*FGFR2*) has the lowest frequency. A complete list of genetic causes of craniosynostosis can be found in the OMIM database.[6]

Syndromic craniosynostoses exhibit variable clinical and genetic heterogeneity. Crouzon and Pfeiffer both have their mutation on *FGFR2*. These syndromes can occur clinically identical regarding facial features, but in Pfeiffer also broad and short big toes and thumbs are seen. This distinction can be difficult and even irrelevant.

Diagnostics

Targeted *FGFR1*, *FGFR2*, *FGFR3*, and *TWIST1* genetic testing is appropriate as a first-line test for patients with coronal, complex nonsyndromic, and syndromic craniosynostosis. Mutation analyses of *TCF12* and *ERF* are justified in all patients with coronal synostosis who are negative for *FGFR* and *TWIST1* mutations. The value of these tests for patients with sagittal and lambdoid CS is minimal, if any.

Most Common Syndromes

Muenke Syndrome

Genetics

- F*GFR3* Pro250Arg mutation
- Autosomal dominant or de novo
- Birth prevalence 1:30,000, 8% of the craniosynostosis cases.[9]

Clinical Features

- Brachycephaly due to fused (bi)coronal ± other sutures
- Various minor anomalies
  - Mild midface hypoplasia, downslanting palpebral fissures, mild ptosis, high arched palate, strabismus.

Minor anomalies of hands and feet, e.g., brachydactyly, clinodactyly, can occur. Almost all patients have hearing loss. Typically, females are affected more severely. In general, Muenke patients have a normal intellect, although developmental delay occurs in approximately one-third (Fig. 20.2).

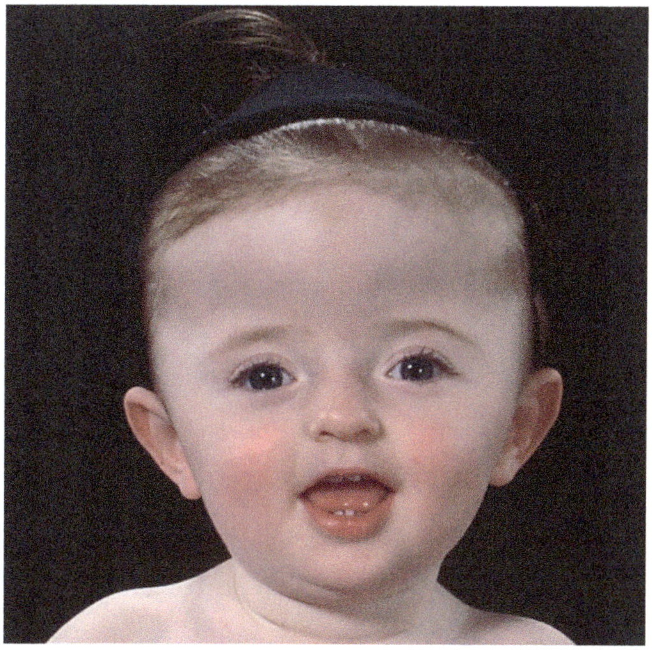

• **Fig. 20.2** Unoperated Muenke patient, female, age 1.3 years.

Crouzon Syndrome

Genetics

- *FGFR2* mutations
- *FGFR3* mutations Crouzon with acanthosis
- Autosomal dominant or de novo (increased risk with older paternal age)
- 16.5 per million births, 4.8% of the craniosynostosis cases.

Clinical Features. Brachycephaly due to fusion of bicoronal ± sagittal and lambdoid sutures (can be absent or delayed)

- Maxillary hypoplasia
- Hypertelorism due to short, wide anterior cranial base
- Exophthalmus with retruded supraorbital, infraorbital, and lateral orbital rims
  - Orbital dystopia and strabismus can occur
  - 20% develop optic atrophy
- Class III malocclusion.

Up to 30% present with hydrocephalus. Some have a reduced nasopharynx, which can contribute to obstructive sleep apnea (OSA). Also raised intracranial pressure (ICP) and hearing loss can be observed (Fig. 20.3).

Pfeiffer Syndrome

Genetics

- *FGFR1* mutation (8p11.2-p11)
- *FGFR2* mutation (10q26.13)
- Autosomal dominant or de novo (increased risk with older paternal age)
- 1 in 100,000 individuals.[10]

Clinical Features

- Brachycephaly due to fused bicoronal sutures
- Maxillary hypoplasia
- Broad radially deviated thumbs and big toes

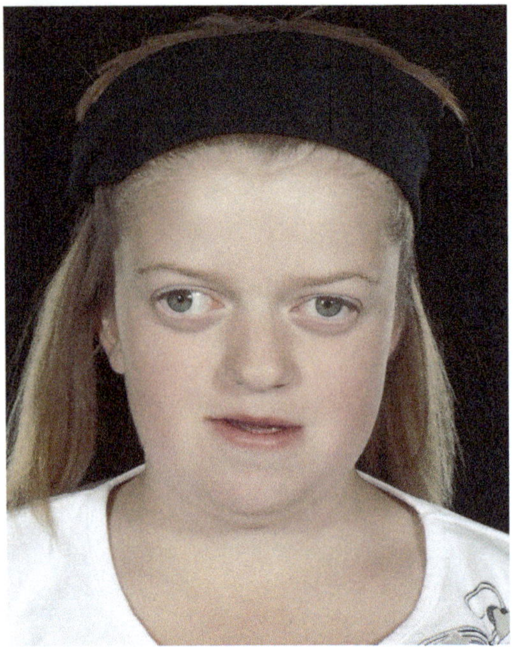

• **Fig. 20.3** Unoperated Crouzon patient, female, age 7 years.

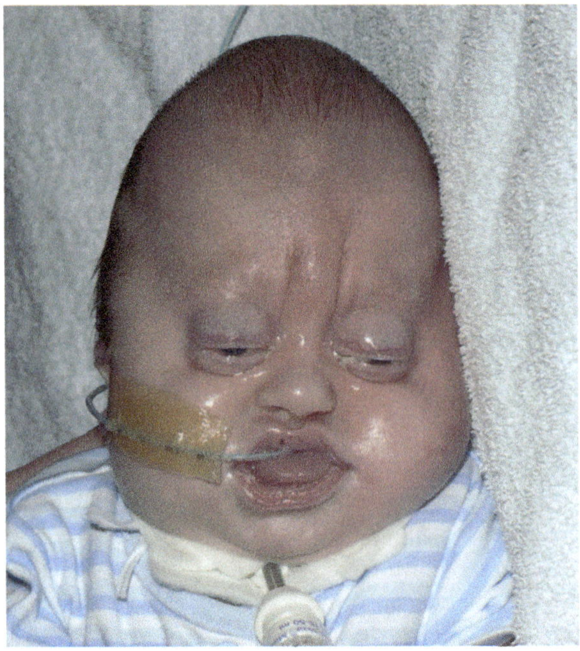

• **Fig. 20.4** Unoperated Pfeiffer patient, male, age 30 days.

- Exorbitism due to shallow orbits.

Partial syndactyly of fingers and toes is seen; additional anomalies can include ankylosis of the elbow and other joints, congenital airway malformations, deafness and neurodevelopmental abnormalities (Fig. 20.4).

Apert Syndrome

Genetics

- *FGFR2* (10q26.13) mutations
  - Amino acids Ser252Trp and Pro253Arg
  - Deletion exon IIIc
  - Alu insertion exon IIIc
- Autosomal dominant or de novo (increased risk with older paternal age)
- Birth prevalence 15.5 per 1 million births, 4.5% of craniosynostosis cases.[11]

Clinical Features

- Turribrachycephaly due to fused bicoronal sutures
- Hypertelorism
- Exorbitism due to shallow orbits
- Downslanting palpebral fissures
- Complex syndactyly of the hands and feet (Upton classification, see Table 20.1)
- Maxillary hypoplasia
- Wide-open calvarial defect from the root of the nose to the posterior fontanelle in the midsagittal plane
- Class III malocclusion, anterior open bite and dental crowding
- Cleft palate with high arched palate can occur.

Additional anomalies can include fusion and malformation of other joints, e.g., the elbows and shoulders, cervical vertebral fusions, congenital airway malformations, deafness, and neurodevelopmental abnormalities. Also, globe subluxation can occur. The quality of the skin frequently varies from normal, to dermal problems such as acne and hyperhidrosis (Fig. 20.5).

Saethre–Chotzen Syndrome

Genetics

- *TWIST1*
- *FGFR2*
- Autosomal dominant or de novo.

Clinical Features (see Fig. 20.6)

- Brachycephaly due to fused (usually) uni- or bicoronal (sometimes metopic) sutures
- Facial asymmetry
- Hypertelorism
- Maxillary hypoplasia
- High forehead and low frontal hairline, and late closing fontanelle
- Strabismus, ptosis, lacrimal duct stenosis, deviated nasal septum
- Small low-set posteriorly rotated ears with prominent crus
- Limb anomalies including: radioulnar synostosis, brachydactyly, cutaneous syndactyly and hallux valgus
- Congenital heart defects
- Ptosis
- Small ears with prominent horizontal crurae.

Rare Syndromes

Craniosynostosis occurs in over 200 known syndromes and the majority occur extremely rarely. A few examples are: craniofrontonasal syndrome, *ERF*, *TCF12*, Antley–Bixler syndrome with or without genital anomalies and disordered steroidogenesis, Baller–Gerorld syndrome, Beare–Stevenson syndrome, Carpenter syndrome, Jackson–Weiss

TABLE 20.1 Upton's Classification of the Apert Hand (1991)

Deformity	Type I	Type II "Mitten Hand"	Type III "Hoof Hand"
Thumb radial clinodactyly	Present	Present	Present
Index radial clinodactyly	Absent	Present	Present
First web syndactyly	Simple (nonosseous)	Simple (nonosseous)	Complex (osseous)
Complex 2–3–4 syndactyly and symbrachyphalangism	Present	Present	Present
4–5 syndactyly	Simple, incomplete	Simple, incomplete	Simple, complete

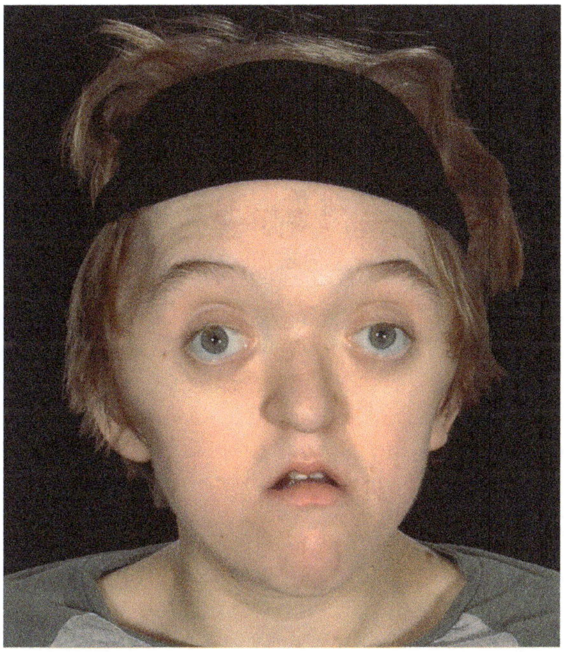

• **Fig. 20.5** Unoperated Apert patient, male, age 17 years.

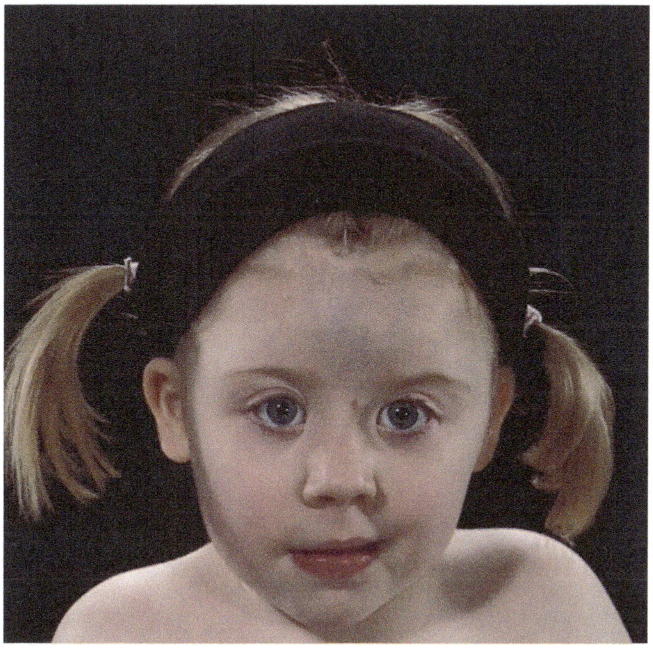

• **Fig. 20.6** Unoperated Saethre–Chotzen patient, female, age 3 years.

syndrome, Loeys–Dietz syndrome, and Shprintzen–Goldberg syndrome.

Parameters of Care for Craniosynostosis

Over the years, a multidisciplinary approach for children with craniosynostosis has evolved.[12–14] Various specialties are involved for optimal diagnosis, management, and treatment. Interdisciplinary craniofacial teams are commonly composed of members with expertise in anesthesia, craniofacial surgery, dentistry, genetics, hand surgery, intensive care, neurosurgery, nursing, ophthalmology, oral and maxillofacial surgery, orthodontics, otolaryngology, pediatrics, prosthodontics, psychology, public health, radiology, social work and speech-language pathology. Care for patients with craniofacial anomalies is best provided in a Craniofacial Team because of the complexity of the cases. Patients with craniosynostosis can have and develop significant problems and might need timely management. Therefore, it is important to assess a child with craniosynostosis as early as possible.

Craniofacial Assessment

Prenatal Diagnosis

Most patients with craniosynostosis are not detected during pregnancy. From the start of formation of cranial sutures at about 16 weeks' gestation and the antenatal ultrasound at 20 weeks' gestation there has not been enough time for growth distortion of the skull to have occurred, except in the most severe cases.[15]

Initial History and Examination from Birth to Age 3 Months

In the case of a patient suspected for craniosynostosis, craniofacial assessment should be performed. The most common presentation is an unusual head shape. The head may be long and narrow (scaphocephaly, dolichocephaly), triangular at the front (trigonocephaly), broad and flattened (brachycephaly) or skewed (plagiocephaly). The aims of a craniofacial assessment are to determine: (1) whether craniosynostosis is present; (2) whether there are additional features suggesting an associated syndrome; and (3) to assess whether urgent or elective management is required. The management of craniosynostosis varies because the cause and presentation of craniosynostosis is very heterogeneous. Most isolated nonsyndromic cases present electively, but a minority of syndromic cases present acutely and require immediate intervention.

During this assessment, information should be gathered on possible identifiable causes: (1) intrauterine constraint, e.g., primiparity, multiple pregnancy, abnormal lie, oligohydramnios; (2) teratogenic exposure, e.g., maternal use of oral retinoids, sodium valproate or phenytoin during pregnancy; (3) family history of abnormal head shape and genetic abnormalities. Moreover, information should be collected on: the conception (normal or assisted), pregnancy, birth history, and birth weight of the patient and their growth. Possible functional issues should be addressed and questions must be asked on the airway (breathing difficulties), feeding (choking, vomiting on feeds), eye protection (failure of eyelids to cover eyes during sleep or irritability), and raised ICP, because these problems might be an indication for early and acute intervention.

On examination, the skull should be examined from the front, back, sides, and top as well as palpation of the sutures for ridging (associated with suture fusion), assessment of the size, shape, and tension of the fontanelles, and head circumference measurements. The cephalic index (ratio of maximum breadth to length of skull, normally between 0.76 and 0.83 (in boys) or 0.84 (in girls)) provides an objective measurement. Moreover, signs for other congenital anomalies should be looked for in areas, such as the face, including mouth, e.g., hyper- or hypotelorism, exorbitism, midface hypoplasia, facial asymmetry, ear size, ear position and shape, cleft palate and malocclusion; hand and feet, e.g., syndactyly, longitudinally split nails, deviated thumb or big toe.

Other examinations should include:

- Eye evaluation (funduscopic examination and visual evoked potentials)
- ENT and hearing assessment
- Genetics assessment
- General assessment by a pediatrician (e.g., cardiovascular system)
- Speech and language evaluation
- Photography: clinical 2D (and if possible 3D) photographs
- Radiological image: X-ray/CT/MRI as necessary
- Assessment of parents for suggestive features of craniosynostosis.

Deformational Posterior Plagiocephaly

Craniosynostosis must be differentiated from deformational plagiocephaly that can occur due to prenatal, perinatal, and/or postnatal external causes.

Prenatal. Deformational plagiocephaly can occur due to prematurity, or intrauterine constraint, such as twin pregnancy.

Perinatal. Deformational plagiocephaly can occur due to assisted delivery with, for example, the use of a forceps.

Postnatal. Deformational plagiocephaly has become increasingly common after the "Back to Sleep" campaign. In 1992, the American Academy of Pediatrics (AAP) Task Force on Infant Positioning and Sudden Infant Death Syndrome (SIDS) recommended a back or side position of the infant when laid to sleep to reduce the incidence of SIDS. The incidence decreased from 1.2/1000 live births in 1992 to 0.56/1000 in 2001.[16,17] However, this resulted in a deformation of the normal skull. The skull of a newborn is malleable and due to pressure on the side the infant lies, changes in head shape can occur, including occipitoparietal flattening on the side where the child tends to lie, ipsilateral frontal bossing and ipsilateral anterior displacement of the ear and contralateral occipital bossing (Fig. 20.7).

If a child has a deformational plagiocephaly, the skull is often parallelogram-shaped when viewed from above, whereas a child with a unilateral synostosis has a failure of growth on one side of the head and so the head shape will tend to be trapezoidal (Fig. 20.8). Moreover, the distance from the lateral canthus to the root of the helix will be the same on both sides in a child with deformational plagiocephaly. In a child with a unicoronal synostosis, this distance will be shorter on the affected side due to a lack of growth.

In clinical practice, it is most difficult to distinguish positional plagiocephaly from lambdoid synostosis. In unicoronal synostosis the orbital shape and forehead symmetry are quite distinctive. An anterior–posterior and lateral skull X-ray can be helpful to exclude a closed cranial suture. Referral to a craniofacial unit is recommended if doubt remains or when premature fusion is detected.

Children with deformational plagiocephaly can be initially managed with physical therapy and/or repositioning. Physical therapy is recommended over repositioning alone in the infant older than age 7 weeks because even though physical therapy is as effective as repositioning, the infant should remain in a safe sleeping environment in compliance with the AAP. While the child is awake repositional treatment can be done by turning the head using supportive pillows and advice about spending at least 30 minutes per day of "tummy time." The child should not remain in one position for a long time, for example in a car seat or carry cot. When improvement fails with repositioning by 6 months of age or when severe deformity remains, a molding helmet or cranial orthosis can be considered. The use of molding helmets is controversial and expensive. There is a fairly substantive body of nonrandomized evidence that demonstrates

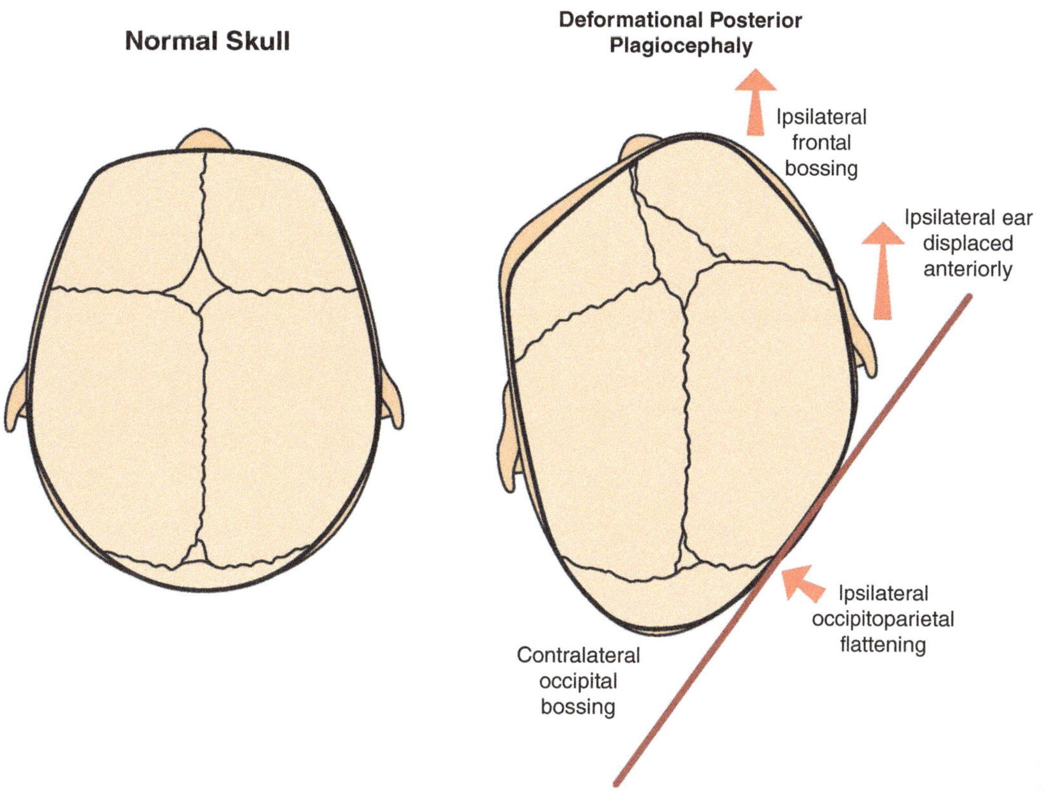

• **Fig. 20.7** Deformational posterior plagiocephaly.

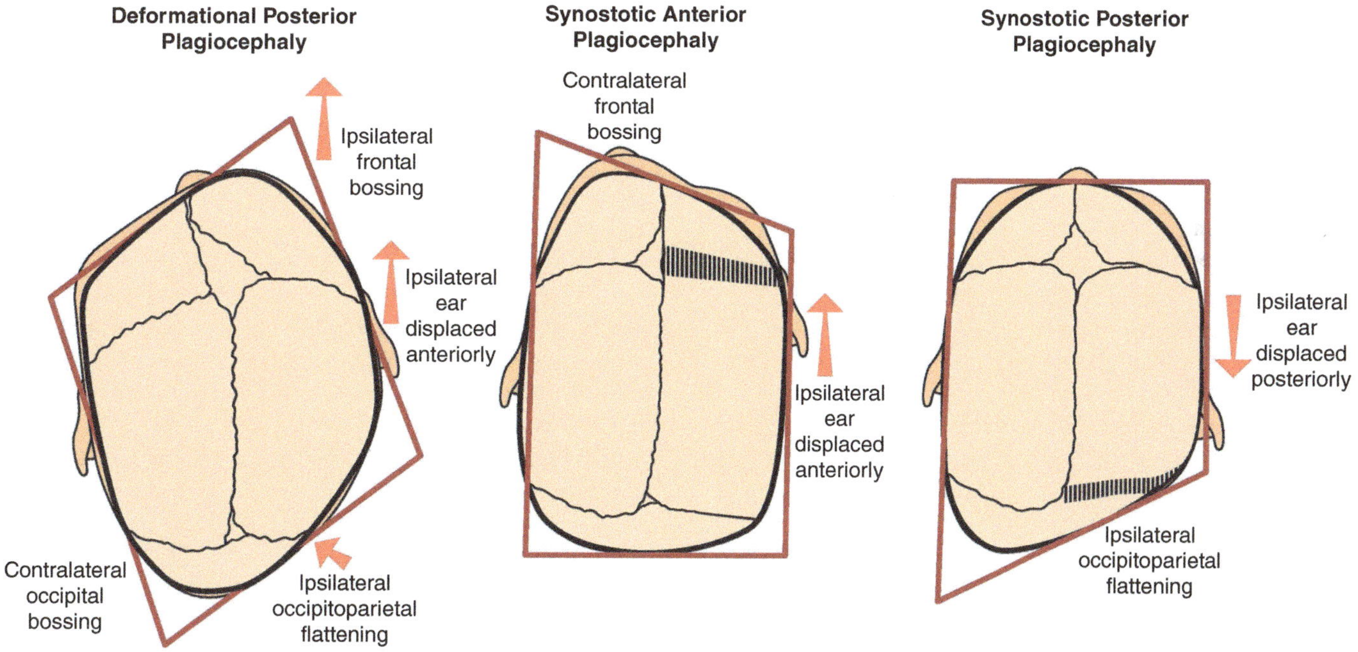

• **Fig. 20.8** Comparison of deformational posterior plagiocephaly and unicoronal craniosynostosis, which causes synostotic anterior plagiocephaly, and unilateral lambdoid synostosis, which causes synostotic posterior plagiocephaly.

more significant and faster improvement of cranial asymmetry treated with a helmet than with conservative treatment, especially if the asymmetry is severe and provided that the helmet therapy is applied during the appropriate period of infancy. In general, children with more severe positional plagiocephaly and infants who are helmeted early tend to have a better normalization of head shape.[18]

A systematic review of deformational plagiocephaly and developmental delay showed evidence of an association between the two: mild developmental delay in motor and some in language development. Most studies reporting developmental delay were in infants less than 2 years old, with associations not as strong in older children. The longevity of this relationship beyond age 2 years old is unclear from the available literature. The Congress of Neurological Surgeons has issued guidelines for the management of positional plagiocephaly.[19] Prompt referral for early management, such as physiotherapy, may ameliorate motor delays and identify those with needs for the long term.

Deformational plagiocephaly is not caused by craniosynostosis and must be differentiated from plagiocephaly due to craniosynostosis, e.g., anterior synostotic plagiocephaly due to unicoronal synostosis or posterior synostotic plagiocephaly due to lambdoid synostosis (see Fig. 20.8).

Radiographic Imaging

In cases of single-suture synostosis and nonsyndromic craniosynostosis, CT scanning and 3D reconstruction is the most useful investigation to examine the patency of each cranial suture.[20] In patients with complex multisuture craniosynostosis or syndromic craniosynostosis, an MRI, additionally to CT, can be useful to examine the intracranial anatomy in more detail to look for anatomical abnormalities (e.g., ventriculomegaly, Chiari malformation, syrinx, and agenesis of the corpus callosum) and craniocerebral disproportion.

Sagittal Synostosis

Premature fusion of the sagittal suture is the commonest of the craniosynostoses (40%–60%) with a prevalence of 1/5000 children. Nearly 80% of the sagittal synostoses are nonsyndromic and 6% are autosomal dominant. Males are more affected (3.5:1). Typically, a boat-shaped head (scaphocephaly) is seen due to growth inhibition in a perpendicular direction to the affected suture leading to a skull shape that is elongated in an anteroposterior direction. There is sagittal ridging, frontal bossing, and a wide interorbital distance due to the unrestricted growth of the patent coronal and metopic sutures. The unrestricted growth at the lambdoid suture causes occipital bulging. The skull base is not involved. Patients with scaphocephaly can present with other clinical signs, such as cerebral palsy, psychomotor retardation, or neurological signs. Elevated ICP is seen in 7%–13% of the cases. Radiographic imaging shows suture absence, which may be focal or generalized. Sagittal craniosynostosis can be associated with fusion of the metopic suture (see Fig. 20.1).

Metopic Synostosis

Normal metopic suture closure starts in the third trimester at the level of the glabella moving upwards towards the anterior fontanelle and is usually fused by the 9th month, but it may take up to 2 years. Premature fusion of the metopic suture causes a triangular-shaped head (trigonocephaly) (Fig. 20.9). There usually is associated hypotelorism. On axial CT an omega-shaped notch is commonly seen. Patients with metopic synostosis can also have midline and

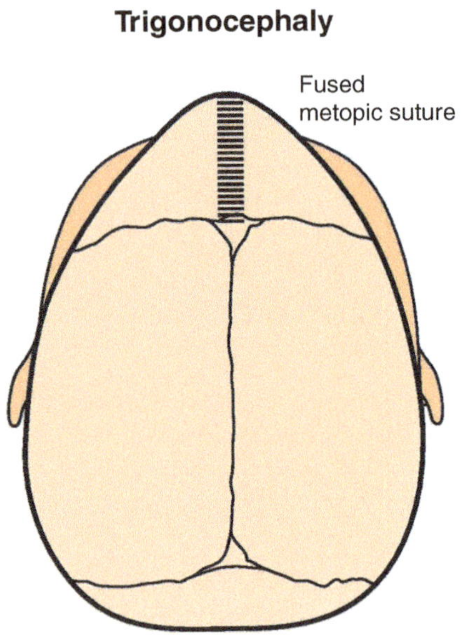

• **Fig. 20.9** Metopic synostosis causing trigonocephaly.

forebrain abnormalities. Nearly 75% of the cases identified postnatally are isolated, with 25% being syndromic. Associated syndromes include Jacobsen/11q23 deletion, chromosome 9p deletion, and Opitz C syndrome.

Coronal Synostosis

This is the second most occurring type of craniosynostosis and can be divided into unicoronal and bicoronal synostosis.

Unicoronal Synostosis

Unilateral fusion of the coronal suture accounts for approximately 20%–30% of craniosynostoses and occurs slightly more often in girls than boys. Association with *TWIST1* and *FGFR3* (pro250arg) gene mutations has been discovered in some cases. A reduced growth on the affected side results in flattening of the ipsilateral frontal and parietal bones. Also, a "Harlequin" deformity of the orbit is seen due to posterior displacement of the calvarium and resultant superior displacement of the ipsilateral orbital roof, the lesser wing of the sphenoid bone, and petrous ridge. There is compensatory bulging of the frontal and temporal regions contralaterally (see Fig. 20.8).

Bicoronal Synostosis

Bilateral fusion of the coronal suture is commonly seen in syndromic craniosynostosis. These patients present with brachycephaly and in the majority due to a *FGFR3* (pro-250arg) gene mutation, where it presents as an isolated feature. The forehead is large and flat. In other types of syndromic craniosynostosis, bicoronal synostosis is commonly found in association with midfacial hypoplasia and additional sutural fusions.

Lambdoid Synostosis

Lambdoid suture synostosis is a rare form of craniosynostosis, with a prevalence of <5% of all craniosynostoses.

Unilateral lambdoid synostosis needs to be carefully differentiated from posterior plagiocephaly, as the management of the two conditions is completely different. On imaging there is obliteration or sclerosis of the lambdoid suture. Unilateral lambdoid synostosis creates a trapezoid-shaped head (see Fig. 20.8). There is ipsilateral occipitoparietal flattening and compensatory growth causing contralateral parietal and frontal bossing, and also ipsilateral occipitomastoid bossing. The ipsilateral ear may be posteriorly displaced.

Multisuture Synostosis and Cloverleaf Skull

Most multiple suture synostoses are associated with syndromes. Common combinations include bilateral coronal with bilateral lambdoid synostoses or bilateral coronal synostoses with sagittal synostoses. When there is pansynostosis, the membranous bones of the calvarium expand between the sutures and give the appearance of a cloverleaf skull or Kleeblattschädel.

Treatment of Nonsyndromic Craniosynostosis

The philosophy of care is to employ a multidisciplinary team approach to correct anatomical deformity in a single stage and monitor for postoperative elevated intracranial pressure.

Functional Problems

Most patients with an isolated single suture craniosynostosis have few problems, once this is corrected. However, depending on the suture involved, functional problems can be seen.

Neurosurgical Problems

Depending on the suture involved, patients have increased risk of raised ICP: scaphocephaly 12%, trigonocephaly 9%, plagiocephaly 10%, and bilateral coronal synostosis 37%.[21] At Great Ormond Street Hospital (London, UK) these patients receive eye evaluation to look for signs for raised ICP preoperatively and annually postoperatively.

Neurodevelopmental Problems

The relationship between nonsyndromic craniosynostosis and learning difficulties remains controversial. An association between nonsyndromic craniosynostosis and neurocognitive deficits has been suggested.[22] In general, observed neurocognitive problems are mild. It is also uncertain if surgery for single-suture synostosis improves neurodevelopmental outcome.

Psychological Problems and Social Function

Contrasting results have been reported on the incidence of behavioral problems. Some studies show no difference to siblings or the norm and other studies showed up to 35% of infants with behavioral problems in nonsyndromic craniosynostosis, as reported by the parents.[23] Moreover, normal emotional and social development is seen.

Surgical Treatment of Nonsyndromic Craniosynostosis

Indications for surgical treatment are prevention or treatment of raised ICP and/or appearance. The timing of intervention is debated and it depends on factors such as time of presentation, functional problems, and wish of parents. With the exception of sagittal synostosis, which is generally treated early, patients are usually treated between 6 months and 2 years of age. Various surgical techniques are described and timing plays a role in choice. In case of an "early" treatment, the technique relies on the plasticity of the bone; when performed "late," cranial vault remodeling is the technique of choice.

"Early" Treatment: Up to 6 Months of Age

Strip Craniectomy

In patients with scaphocephaly a strip craniectomy can be a technique of choice, but it requires intervention in the first 2 months of life. Over time, variations and minor modifications have been published.

Endoscopic-Assisted Suturectomy with or without an Orthotic Helmet Device

This relatively new technique is composed of a "minimally invasive" strip craniectomy using an endoscope and can be used for the treatment of unilateral coronal synostosis. At some craniofacial surgery units patients are treated with an orthotic helmet for several months afterwards. The benefits of this technique might lie in low morbidity, short hospital stay and low blood transfusion need in comparison with other techniques.

Spring-Assisted Cranioplasty

Especially when treatment is needed over one vector (when growth is restricted in one direction), cranioplasty with the use of springs might be a technique of choice. Ideally, this procedure is performed at age 3–6 months, however it has been performed up to 14 years old at Great Ormond Street Hospital. The commonest indication is sagittal craniosynostosis (Fig. 20.10). Two to four springs are inserted and removed 3–6 months later. At Great Ormond Street Hospital, not only scaphocephalic patients, but also patients indicated for posterior vault expansion undergo this treatment with satisfying results and increased intracranial volume. In the future, spring-assisted cranioplasty might be used for other head shape abnormalities too. The advantages include less invasive surgery than calvarial remodeling, shorter operation time, less blood loss, and shorter hospitalization (Fig. 20.11).

Distraction Osteogenesis

Distraction osteogenesis has been used for the treatment of scaphocephaly with equally good results as other techniques.

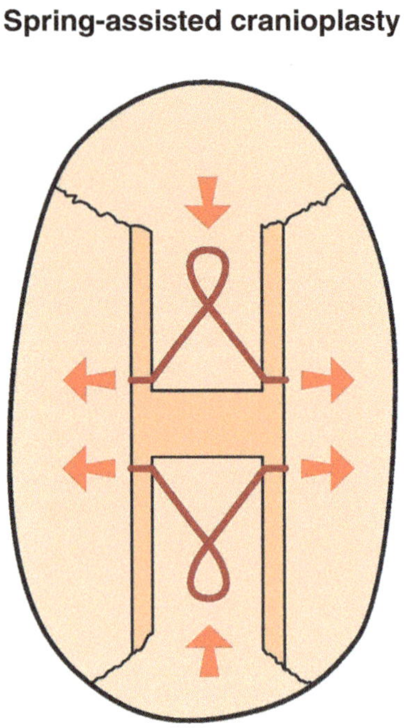

• **Fig. 20.10** Spring-assisted cranioplasty for sagittal synostosis.

A distraction device is placed on both sides of the craniotomy and fixed.

A period of distraction and consolidation follows, after which the device will be removed in a second procedure.

"Late" Treatment: Age 6 Months to 3 Years

Fronto-orbital Remodeling

Fronto-orbital remodeling (FOR) is indicated when the shape of the supraorbital and frontal region requires correction (Fig. 20.12). FOR is used in patients with metopic, unicoronal, and bicoronal synostosis and is usually carried out at approximately 9–18 months of age unless signs of elevated ICP are identified earlier. The goals are to provide improved morphology of the forehead and upper orbits and, where necessary, increased intracranial space in the anterior cranial vault for the brain and increased orbital volume, which allows the eyes to be positioned more normally for better protection from exposure.

Patients with metopic synostosis most commonly undergo a full reconstruction of the fronto-orbital bar (see Fig. 20.12). However, at Great Ormond Street Hospital we favor a limited procedure, which does not involve the entire fronto-orbital bar to limit orbital dissection. Routinely, a bicoronal incision is made and the anterior flap elevated with the temporal muscle. Then a frontal craniotomy is performed. This allows retraction of the brain so that any orbital osteotomies can be safely undertaken and harvests the frontal bone, which will be reshaped during the procedure. To undertake a traditional FOR, orbital osteotomies are completed across the orbital roof and superior aspect of the medial orbital wall, laterally through the lateral orbital wall and inferiorly just into the inferior orbital fissure. The three-quarters orbital osteotomy units are removed from the field and reshaped and then re-inset. The supraorbital bar is overcorrected. Fixation is generally achieved with resorbable sutures and plates and screws or stainless-steel wires. Calvarial bone is cut into segments, which are replaced as grafts to achieve a more normal appearance of the anterior cranial vault.

Calvarial Remodeling

Pi Procedure

In older patients with sagittal craniosynostosis (age 9–18 months) a more extensive surgery is needed, such as the Pi (Π) procedure (Fig. 20.13). The strips are resected at either side of the fused suture and anteriorly to the coronal suture. The sagittal suture itself is not resected. By this means the anteroposterior diameter can be shortened. The head is thus compressed and raised ICP due to this technique might be seen.

Posterior Cranial Vault Remodeling

Patients with unilateral or bilateral lambdoid synostosis benefit from posterior cranial vault remodeling. The procedure leads to an increased skull size and can help with the correction of a Chiari I malformation.

Total and Subtotal Calvarial Remodeling

When a child with sagittal synostosis presents after the age of 18 months a total calvarial remodeling is indicated. This technique includes a complete or almost complete remodeling of the calvarial vault.

Treatment of Syndromic Craniosynostosis

The philosophy of care is to employ a multidisciplinary team approach to maximize developmental potential, with staged operations and follow-up into adulthood.

Functional Problems

Syndromic craniosynostosis patients can have or develop problems with vision, airway, elevated ICP, hearing, nutrition, psychological, and social development (Fig. 20.14).

Neurosurgical Problems

Elevated ICP is a serious functional problem. It can have a slow onset and be difficult to recognize. Untreated craniosynostosis with elevated ICP will cause papilledema and eventually optic nerve atrophy and blindness. There is no consensus on what are normal levels of ICP in a pediatric population, as this is not routinely measured in healthy children. Elevated ICP results from a number of different factors, including craniocerebral disproportion, abnormalities of cerebrospinal fluid dynamics, impaired cerebral venous drainage secondary to generalized cranial base stenosis, and hydrocephalus. There is good evidence that obstructive sleep apnea secondary to upper airway obstruction and venous hypertension exacerbate elevated ICP in patients with syndromic craniosynostosis.[24] Hydrocephalus is common and is characterized by a progressive enlargement of

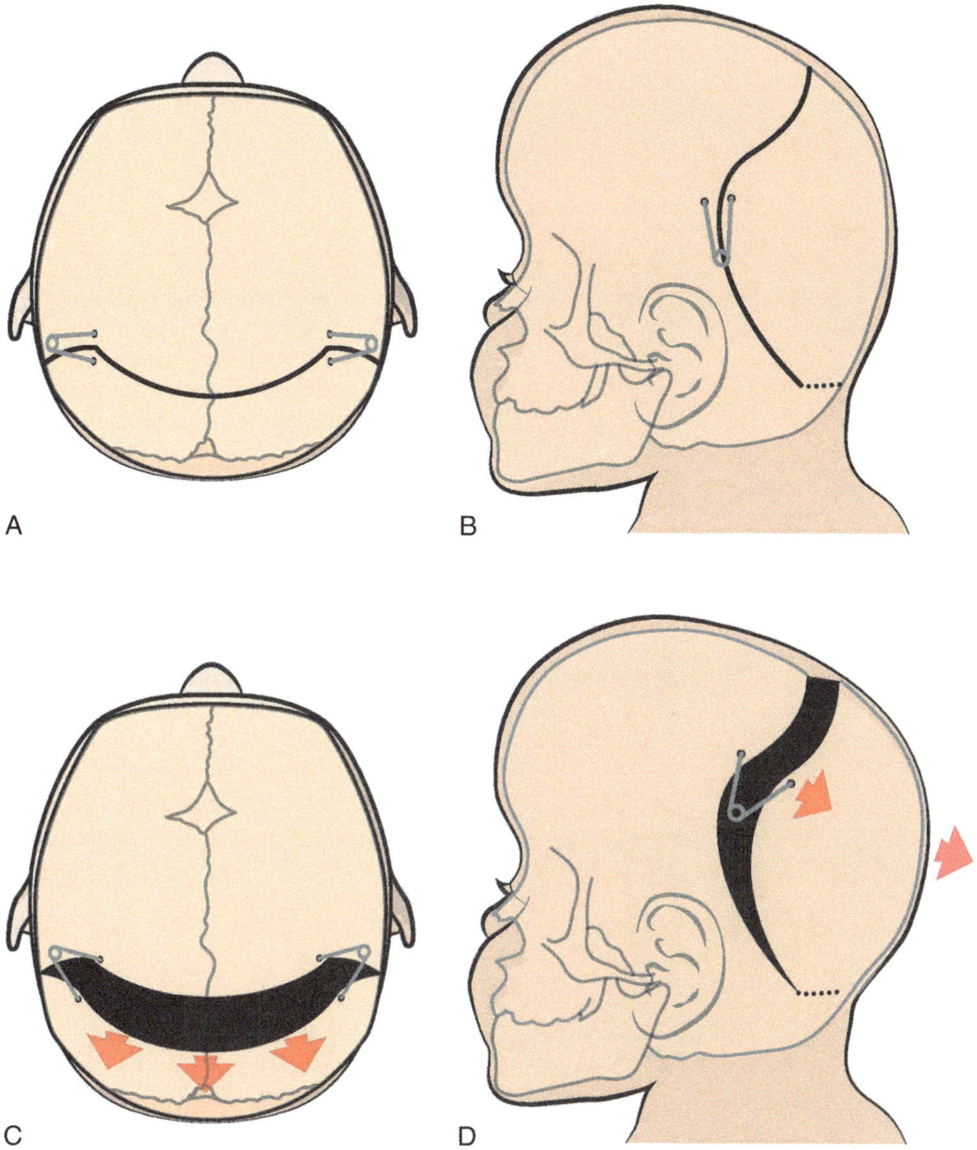

• **Fig. 20.11** Posterior spring-assisted cranioplasty.

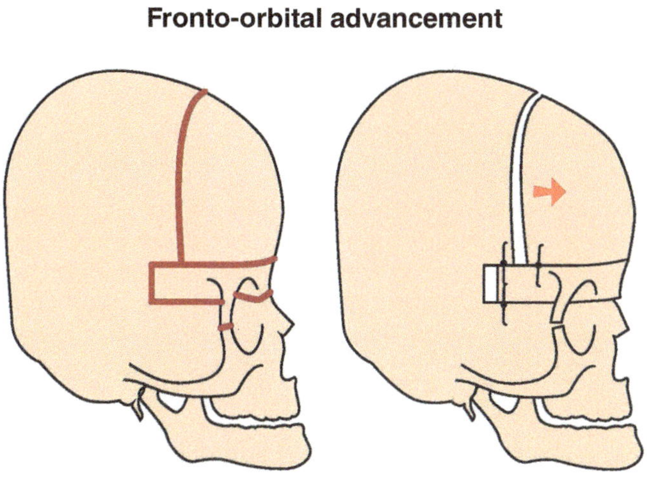

• **Fig. 20.12** Fronto-orbital advancement.

the ventricles over time, which is different from nonprogressive ventriculomegaly related to brain maldevelopment. The Chiari I malformation (cerebellar tonsillar herniation) is often found in patients with syndromic craniosynostosis and has a mechanical rather than developmental etiology and can be caused by a small posterior fossa (which in itself could be due to lambdoid suture fusion) or by venous congestion because of obstruction to venous outflow across the abnormal skull base. Brain anomalies that can occur include: defects of the corpus callosum, porencephalic cysts, mega cisterna magna, focal cortical tissue loss, and brain herniation through multiple areas of the skull base due to elevated ICP.

Ocular Problems

Primary ophthalmic findings in Apert, Crouzon, and Pfeiffer syndrome include exorbitism due to shallow orbits, increased interpupillary distance, strabismus, refractive

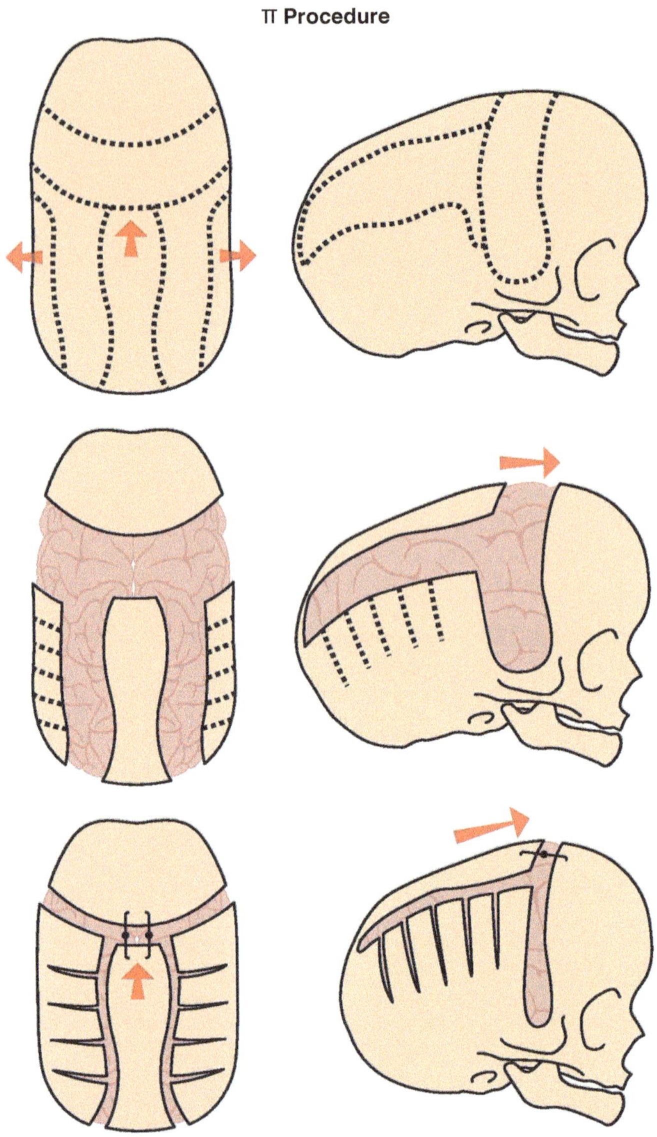

• **Fig. 20.13** Pi (π) procedure for the treatment of sagittal synostosis.

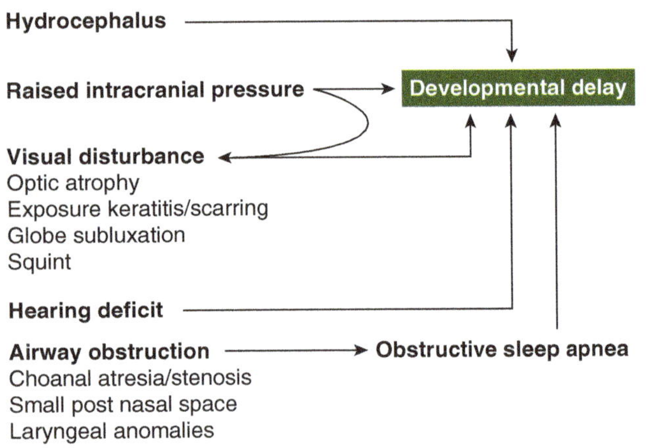

• **Fig. 20.14** Functional problems in syndromic craniosynostosis which contribute to developmental delay.

error, iris colobomata, cataracts, nasolacrimal duct obstruction, and ptosis. Secondary findings include amblyopia, corneal exposure, globe herniation, optic atrophy and papilledema. Major causes of visual loss are amblyopia, exposure keratopathy and optic atrophy, due to elevated ICP. Patients with syndromic craniosynostosis must undergo regular ophthalmological assessment.

Otological Problems

Hearing loss is common. External auditory canal anomalies can occur, with stenosis or atresia of either the bony or cartilaginous parts of the auditory canal, and malformations of the middle ear and ossicles, with concomitant conductive hearing loss. CT scanning can be helpful in defining the anatomical abnormalities. There is a higher incidence of middle ear effusions in patients with Apert syndrome, which may be related to the presence of a cleft palate.

Airway and Feeding Problems

Airway pathology can include midface hypoplasia, nasopharyngeal stenosis, choanal atresia or stenosis, and tracheal anomalies, and represents a significant source of potential morbidity and mortality.[25] Airway obstruction can cause failure to thrive, suboptimal neurological development, and developmental delay. Disruption of sleep states in OSA, particularly loss of sustained quiet sleep, has been shown to impair growth hormone release. There is a strong correlation between the presence of hydrocephalus requiring ventriculoperitoneal shunting and severe upper airway obstruction.

Many children with syndromic craniosynostosis need some form of airway support during infancy or childhood. A drop off the growth curve can be a useful predictor of the need for both airway and feeding intervention in children with craniosynostosis. A nasogastric tube or a gastrostomy tube may be required. Lymphoid hypertrophy occurs at approximately age 3–6 years and children whose airways become more obstructed at this age often benefit from tonsillectomy and adenoidectomy. Frequent monitoring for signs of upper airway obstruction is required. The use of nasopharyngeal airways, CPAP, and tracheostomy may be required to maintain an adequate airway.

Congenital Heart Defects

It is not uncommon for children with syndromic craniosynostosis to have congenital heart defects.[25] This leads to an increased risk when undergoing surgery or general anesthesia. Some children with congenital heart defects have the potential for either right to left or bidirectional shunts. Given that venous air embolism is common with craniosynostosis repair, the risk of coronary or cerebral air embolism is significant in these children.

Psychological Problems and Social Function

Syndromic craniosynostosis patients seem to have more behavioral problems, reported by the parents, particularly in Muenke and Apert.[26,27] These problems could be related to underlying cognitive impairment, QoL, and physical symptoms, such as OSA. In Apert and complex craniosynostosis an impact on emotional well-being and social function was reported by the parents. In young adults 33% of Crouzon patients reported periods of depressive mood; having or not having completed surgical treatment did not affect mean scores of emotional functioning.[26] Children with lower ID (<85) had 2–3 times higher risk of emotional problems than children with intelligence scores within the normal range.[26] Overall, in a review, all studies suggested a negative impact upon social experiences. There is repeated exposure to the social reaction of others, such as staring, comments, questions or teasing. Nonetheless, qualitative accounts of adults with Crouzon illustrate the ability to develop positive coping strategies.

Surgical Treatment of Syndromic Craniosynostosis

Most children with syndromic craniosynostosis require surgery to protect function, expand the cranial vault, advance the midface, and improve appearance. The management can be subdivided into "crisis interventions" for, e.g., threats to the airway, threats to vision, and raised ICP; "early interventions" for, e.g., hydrocephalus, visual disturbances, hearing deficit, obstructive sleep apnea, interventions in childhood to change appearance in order to support psychosocial development and wellbeing; and "late interventions" to improve esthetic appearance at the completion of growth (Table 20.2).

Management in Infancy

Management in infancy is generally directed towards the treatment and prevention of functional crises. Most commonly, cranial vault expansion is undertaken to treat craniocerebral disproportion and elevated ICP.

Broadly, there are two philosophies of surgical management at this stage:

1. Fronto-orbital advancement: proponents of this approach cite the advantages of the increased cranial volume achieved along with some degree of orbital protection (see Fig. 20.7). If the frontal advancement does not relapse, midfacial advancement can be achieved at a later stage with a subcranial Le Fort III osteotomy (age 4–10 years) thus avoiding the need for a second transcranial procedure (Fig. 20.15).
2. Posterior vault expansion (either an acute advancement with bone grafts, or gradual advancement using springs or distraction devices). Proponents of this approach believe it is a functionally better technique, because it can produce greater increases in cranial volume than frontal advancement and there is some evidence that the change in posterior cranial fossa anatomy treats Chiari malformations. This procedure leaves the forehead untouched, which is a great advantage from a technical point of view if a frontofacial advancement osteotomy is required at a later date.

TABLE 20.2 Sequence of Craniofacial Surgical Procedures in Syndromic Craniosynostosis

Age	Procedure
6 months to 3 years	Crisis intervention (ICP, orbital protection, airway), cranial vault expansion, midfacial or frontofacial advancement
4 to 8 years	Correction of midface deformities, primary and secondary cranial vault procedures, and adjunctive procedures
9 to 12 years	Correction of midface deformities, secondary cranial vault procedures, and adjunctive procedures
13 to 17 years	Late correction of midface deformities. Adjunctive procedures and orthodontic therapy
Over 17 years	Orthognathic surgery

In children with severe exorbitism, elevated ICP and upper airway obstruction, frontofacial advancement by distraction can be considered as early as 4 months of age.

Management of Midface Deformity in Childhood and Adolescence

Severe midfacial retrusion is usually corrected in childhood or adolescence. There are two commonly adopted strategies.

1. A frontofacial advancement, most commonly performed as a monobloc osteotomy (Fig. 20.16). Advancement of the monobloc segment increases intracranial volume, enlarges the orbits, increases upper airway volume and advances the midface. This procedure can be performed conventionally holding the advanced segment in position with bone grafts, plates, and screws, but is most frequently undertaken by internal or external distraction techniques. The procedure is effective and has been successfully adapted to deal with the anatomical facial flattening.[28]
2. A first stage forehead advancement (FOR, see Fig. 20.12) and a second (later) stage midface advancement (subcranial Le Fort III, see Fig. 20.15) in two operations. The Le Fort III can be performed conventionally or by distraction.

There is good evidence to suggest that a frontofacial advancement produces better functional outcomes and esthetic results than a two-stage forehead advancement and Le Fort III. The main disadvantage of this approach is its higher complication rate. The monobloc osteotomy results in a communication between the anterior cranial fossa and upper nasal spaces, which increases the risk of ascending infection, persistent CSF leaks, and mucocele formation. A separate forehead advancement and Le Fort III procedure reduces these risks. Opinion remains divided about the best approach.

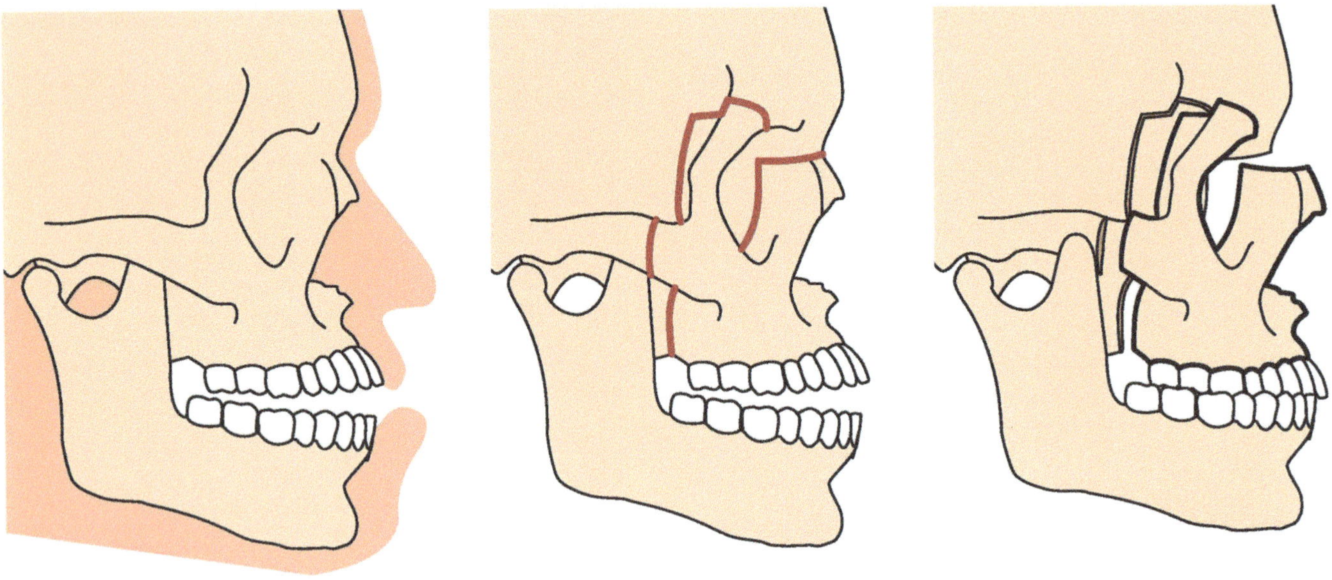

• **Fig. 20.15** Subcranial Le Fort III midface advancement.

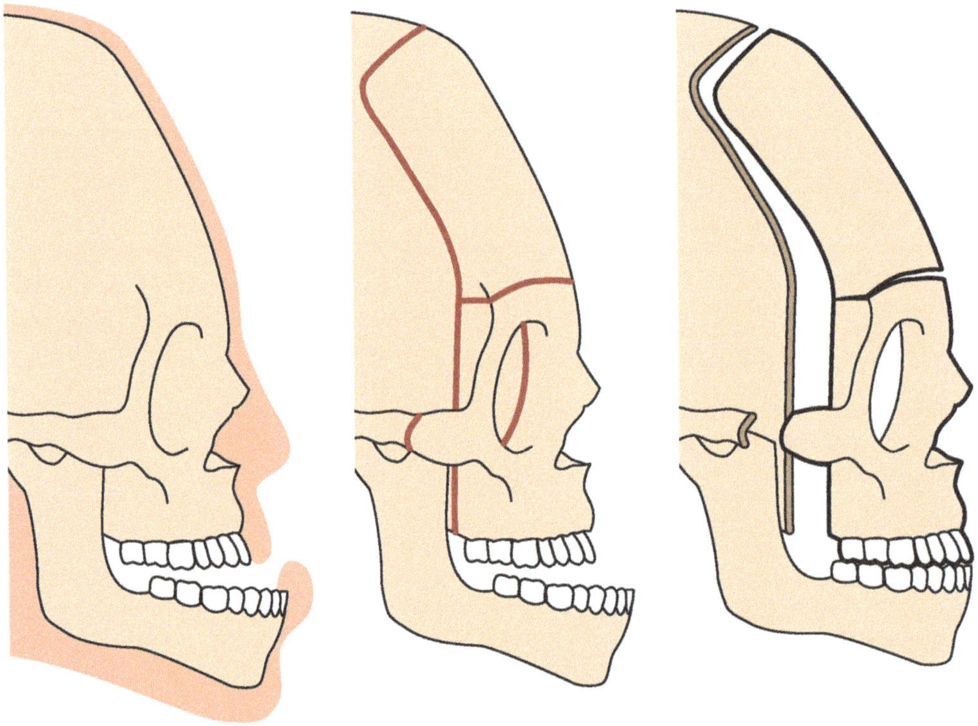

• **Fig. 20.16** Frontofacial advancement with monobloc osteotomy.

Orthognathic Procedures for Definitive Occlusal Correction

The mandible has normal growth potential in children with syndromic craniosynostosis, but the maxilla does not. This leads to a class III malocclusion, often with an anterior open bite. Although midface procedures performed in childhood and adolescence go some way to correcting this intermaxillary discrepancy, there is often a residual class III malocclusion. A Le Fort I osteotomy often combined with a mandibular ramus osteotomy (bimaxillary osteotomy) is generally required in combination with genioplasty. About 30% of patients with syndromic craniosynostosis require orthognathic surgery and this is carried out in conjunction with orthodontic treatment and planned for completion at the time of skeletal maturity (age 16–18 years).

Complications of Surgery for Syndromic Craniosynostosis

Early series looking at complications for all types of craniofacial surgery quoted mortality rates of between 1%

TABLE 20.3 Complications of Craniofacial Surgical Procedures

Early
Bleeding
Airway
Infection, e.g., meningitis
Neurosurgical, e.g., stroke, elevated ICP
CSF leak[30]
Intermediate
Bone loss, e.g., frontal bone[30,31]
Osteomyelitis/sequestrum
Plate infections
Late
Mucocele[30]
Late bone loss
Relapse
Seizures[28,30,32]
Premature aging[33,34]
Radiation exposure from multiple CTs[35]

and 2%. In a more recent multicenete review, the mortality had fallen to 0.1% for transcranial procedures and 0.3% for subcranial procedures.[29] These figures are similar to our own experience of a 0.11% mortality rate for all craniofacial procedures undertaken.[30] Higher mortality rates are seen in reviews quoting complications for frontofacial advancement, demonstrating the greater risks associated with major surgery.[29,30] The risk of death or significant morbidity most commonly arises from bleeding (either exsanguination or postoperative intracranial bleeding) or, less commonly, postoperative airway complications (Table 20.3).

Conclusion

Modern craniofacial surgery, despite the risks of serious complications, has transformed the lives and developmental potential of children with syndromic craniosynostosis. The treatment of craniosynostosis requires a dedicated multidisciplinary team because of the complex interrelated functional and anatomical problems caused by the condition. It is only with the help and advice of members of this team that craniofacial surgeons can make informed decisions about the timing of surgery and the use of different surgical techniques.

References

1. Cornelissen M, den Ottelander B, Rizopoulos D, et al. Increase of prevalence of craniosynostosis. *J Cranio-Maxillofac Surg.* 2016;44(9):1273–1279.
2. Wilkie AO, Byren JC, Hurst JA, et al. Prevalence and complications of single-gene and chromosomal disorders in craniosynostosis. *Pediatrics.* 2010;126(2):e391–400.
3. Sharma VP, Fenwick AL, Brockop MS, et al. Mutations in TCF12, encoding a basic helix-loop-helix partner of TWIST1, are a frequent cause of coronal craniosynostosis. *Nat Gene.* 2013;45(3):304.
4. Selber J, Reid RR, Chike-Obi CJ, et al. The changing epidemiologic spectrum of single-suture synostoses. *Plast Reconstr Surg.* 2008;122(2):527–533.
5. van der Meulen J, van der Hulst R, van Adrichem L, et al. The increase of metopic synostosis: a pan-European observation. *J Craniofac Surg.* 2009;20(2):283–286.
6. OMIM (Online Mendelian Inheritance in Man). http://www.ncbi.nlm.nik.gov/omim.
7. Greenwood J, Flodman P, Osann K, Boyadjiev SA, Kimonis V. Familial incidence and associated symptoms in a population of individuals with nonsyndromic craniosynostosis. *Gene Med.* 2014;16(4):302.
8. Timberlake AT, Choi J, Zaidi S, et al. Two locus inheritance of non-syndromic midline craniosynostosis via rare SMAD6 and common BMP2 alleles. *Elife.* 2016;5:e20125.
9. Morriss-Kay GM, Wilkie AO. Growth of the normal skull vault and its alteration in craniosynostosis: insights from human genetics and experimental studies. *J Anat.* 2005;207(5):637–653.
10. Vogels A, Fryns JP. Pfeiffer syndrome. *Orphanet J Rare Dis.* 2006;1:19.
11. Thompson DNP, Britto JA. Classification and clinical diagnosis. In: Hayward R, Jones B, Dunaway D, Evans R, eds. *The Clinical Management of Craniosynostosis.* London: MacKeith Press; 2004:12–44.
12. McCarthy JG, Warren SM, Bernstein J, et al. Parameters of care for craniosynostosis. *Cleft Palate Craniofac J.* 2012;49(suppl):1S–24S.
13. Warren SM, Proctor MR, Bartlett SP, et al. Parameters of care for craniosynostosis: craniofacial and neurologic surgery perspectives. *Plast Reconstr Surg.* 2012;129(3):731–737.
14. Vargervik K, Rubin MS, Grayson BH, et al. Parameters of care for craniosynostosis: dental and orthodontic perspectives. *Am J Orthod Dentofacial Orthop.* 2012;141(suppl 4):S68–S73.
15. Johnson D, Wilkie AO. Craniosynostosis. *Eur J Hum Genet.* 2011;19(4):369–376.
16. [No authors listed]. Changing concepts of sudden infant death syndrome: implications for infant sleeping environment and sleep position. American Academy of Pediatrics Task Force on Infant Sleep Position and Sudden Infant Death Syndrome. *Pediatrics.* 2000;105(3 Pt 1):650–656.
17. American Academy of Pediatrics Task Force on Sudden Infant Death Syndrome. The changing concept of sudden infant death syndrome: diagnostic coding shifts, controversies regarding the sleeping environment, and new variables to consider in reducing risk. *Pediatrics.* 2005;116(5):1245–1255.
18. Tamber MS, Nikas D, Beier A, et al. Guidelines: Congress of Neurological Surgeons systematic review and evidence-based guideline on the role of cranial molding orthosis (helmet) therapy for patients with positional plagiocephaly. *Neurosurgery.* 2016;79(5):E632–E633. Available at: https://tinyurl.com/y8t7owtv.
19. Flannery AM, Tamber MS, Mazzola C, et al. Congress of Neurological Surgeons systematic review and evidence-based guidelines for the management of patients with positional plagiocephaly: executive summary. *Neurosurgery.* 79(5):E623-E624. Available at: https://tinyurl.com/y8t7owtv.
20. Branson HM, Shroff MM. Craniosynostosis and 3-dimensional computed tomography. *Semin Ultrasound CT MR.* 2011;32(6):569–577.
21. Mathijssen IM. Guideline for care of patients with the diagnoses of craniosynostosis: Working Group on Craniosynostosis. *J Craniofac Surg.* 2015;26(6):1735–1807.
22. Kelleher MO, Murray DJ, McGillivary A, Kamel MH, Allcutt D, Earley MJ. Behavioral, developmental, and educational problems

in children with nonsyndromic trigonocephaly. *J Neurosurg.* 2006;105(suppl 5):382–384.
23. Becker DB, Petersen JD, Kane AA, Cradock MM, Pilgram TK, Marsh JL. Speech, cognitive, and behavioral outcomes in nonsyndromic craniosynostosis. *Plast Reconstr Surg.* 2005;116(2):400–407.
24. Hayward R. Venous hypertension and craniosynostosis. *Childs Nerv Syst.* 2005;21(10):880–888.
25. Greig AV, Wagner J, Warren SM, Grayson B, McCarthy JG. Pfeiffer syndrome: analysis of a clinical series and development of a classification system. *J Craniofac Surg.* 2013;24(1):204–215.
26. Maliepaard M, Mathijssen IM, Oosterlaan J, Okkerse JM. Intellectual, behavioral, and emotional functioning in children with syndromic craniosynostosis. *Pediatrics.* 2014;133(6):e1608–e1615.
27. Bannink N, Maliepaard M, Raat H, Joosten KF, Mathijssen IM. Obstructive sleep apnea-specific quality of life and behavioral problems in children with syndromic craniosynostosis. *J Dev Behav Pediatr.* 2011;32(3):233–238.
28. Greig AV, Britto JA, Abela C, et al. Correcting the typical Apert face: combining bipartition with monobloc distraction. *Plast Reconstr Surg.* 2013;131(2):219e–230e.
29. Arnaud E, Marchac D, Renier D. Reduction of morbidity of the frontofacial monobloc advancement in children by the use of internal distraction. *Plast Reconstr Surg.* 2007;120(4):1009–1026.
30. Dunaway DJ, Britto JA, Abela C, Evans RD, Jeelani NU. Complications of frontofacial advancement. *Childs Nerv Syst.* 2012;28(9):1571–1576.
31. Greig AV, Davidson EH, Grayson BH, McCarthy JG. Complications of craniofacial midface distraction: 10-year review. *Plast Reconstr Surg.* 2012;130(2):371e–372e.
32. McCarthy JG, Glasberg SB, Cutting CB, et al. Twenty-year experience with early surgery for craniosynostosis: II. The craniofacial synostosis syndromes and pansynostosis – results and unsolved problems. *Plast Reconstr Surg.* 1995;96(2):284–295; discussion 296–288.
33. Tulasne JF, Tessier PL. Long-term results of Le Fort III advancement in Crouzon's syndrome. *Cleft Palate J.* 1986;23(suppl 1):102–109.
34. Warren SM, Shetye PR, Obaid SI, Grayson BH, McCarthy JG. Long-term evaluation of midface position after Le Fort III advancement: a 20-plus-year follow-up. *Plast Reconstr Surg.* 2012;129(1):234–242.
35. Domeshek LF, Mukundan Jr S, Yoshizumi T, Marcus JR. Increasing concern regarding computed tomography irradiation in craniofacial surgery. *Plast Reconstr Surg.* 2009;123(4):1313–1320.

21

Orthognathic Surgery and Genioplasty

KARL C. BRUCKMAN AND DEREK M. STEINBACHER

ORTHOGNATHIC SURGERY

History

The term "orthognathic" stems from the Greek words *ortho*, which is to straighten, and *gnathic*, which describes the jaw. Orthognathic surgery is a subspecialty practiced by numerous disciplines, including oral and maxillofacial, plastic and reconstructive, and ear, nose, and throat surgeons. It is defined as osteotomies performed to the midface and mandible to reposition the tooth-bearing bony segments.

The concept of orthognathic surgery has its roots in rural America, with a long and storied history beginning in the mid-1800s.[1–3] After its inception, the subspecialty progressed in waves prior to and after the World Wars of the 20th century, as many surgeons developed new management strategies to care for wounded veterans.[4–7] The field of craniofacial surgery was also involved to a lesser extent with orthognathic procedures, comprising the work of Gillies and Tessier in the mid-20th century.[8–9] Without a doubt their approaches and techniques provided vital insight to the management of jaw deformities.

Modern orthognathic surgery is said to have been rooted in Europe in the 1950s, led by Hugo Obwegeser.[10] He went on to publish his techniques for the intraoral sagittal split osteotomy in 1955, followed by an extensive case series on Le Fort I osteotomies in 1969 and then his experience with concurrent bimaxillary surgery in 1970.[11,12] Obwegeser brought his techniques to the USA in the 1960s. In 1969, American plastic surgeon John Marquise Converse published numerous works with an orthodontist named Horowitz, further highlighting the importance of collaboration between the surgical and dental fields.[13]

American oral surgeons, who had recently separated from plastic surgery in the period following World War II, latched onto orthognathic surgery and began making further strides. The first known textbook dedicated to orthognathic surgery was written by oral surgeons Hines and Kent in 1972, followed by numerous other texts that focused on corrective jaw surgery in the 1980s by the likes of Bell, Profitt, White, and Epker, to name a few. Modern day advancements have continued within the subspecialty, led by both oral and plastic surgeons. Additional developments and clinical evolution has further advanced orthognathic surgery to a procedure with less morbidity, greater predictability, and is safe and reliable.[14]

Dentofacial Relationships and Terminology

A certain understanding of dental terminology is necessary in order to completely understand the concepts surrounding orthognathic surgery, as well as to communicate treatment plans efficiently and appropriately with orthodontic and other dental colleagues.

Beginning with the tooth, it is composed of various structures. The neurovascular component of it enters at the apex, an opening at the inferior portion of the tooth. These structures culminate at the dental pulp, which is surrounded by dentin. The dentin is subsequently encased by cementum, the outer tooth structure that provides attachments to the surrounding periodontal ligament and associated alveolar bone. Visible clinically, the enamel covers the superior portion of the dentin. The portion of the tooth including the enamel and dentin is considered the crown of the tooth, whereas the root of the tooth is comprised of the cementum, dentin, pulp tissue, and associated soft tissue attachments to the surrounding bone. The complete adult human dentition is composed of 32 teeth, 16 per jaw: 2 central incisors, 2 lateral incisors, 2 canines, 4 premolars, and 6 molars. The pediatric or deciduous dentition includes 20 teeth, 10 per jaw: 2 central incisors, 2 lateral incisors, 2 canines, and 4 molars.

Directionality within the mouth and relative to the teeth also uses a different nomenclature. Rather than anterior, posterior, medial, and lateral, the cardinal directions when discussing teeth include mesial (toward the dental midline), distal (away from the dental midline), lingual or palatal (toward the tongue or palate, relative to teeth on the mandible or maxilla, respectively), and buccal/labial (toward the soft tissue of the cheek and lip, respectively). The dental midline is that between the maxillary and mandibular central incisors (Fig. 21.1).

Dental relationships between the maxilla and mandible are also described in an organized fashion. The normal relationship of the maxillary to the mandibular teeth should include a slight buccal and labial displacement, with the lingual cusps of the maxillary teeth interposing with the buccal cusps of the mandibular teeth. A class I molar relationship is considered normal, and this is when the mesiobuccal cusp of the first maxillary molar is in occlusion with the buccal groove of the first mandibular molar. When this relationship is altered, and the maxillary molar is positioned mesially, this is termed class II occlusion, and when distally, is considered class III (Fig. 21.2). There should be approximately 2 mm of overlap with the maxillary to the mandibular incisors in both the anteroposterior and vertical planes, termed overjet and overbite (Fig. 21.3). When these relationships are reversed, the term crossbite is used, and it can be relative to an anterior or posterior location of the offending dentition. A crossbite can also be dental, skeletal, or a combination of both. This is relative to the position of the alveolar processes being centered over each other (skeletal) or the location of the teeth within these dental arches (dental). Also, crossbite can occur in a functional manner, whereas it is normal at rest and manifests with mastication.

An open bite, also termed apertognathia, is when teeth are not meeting along the occlusal plane. This can occur anteriorly, posteriorly, uni- or bilaterally. In certain occasions, often when the involved teeth are overly flared or impacted, these open bites can be corrected orthodontically. Oftentimes, though, this dental relationship is secondary to a skeletal abnormality, and must be corrected with a surgical intervention. It is important to note that when teeth are not meeting in occlusion, they will continue to over-erupt via appositional bone growth within the associated dental alveolus.

Another way to study the maxillary and mandibular dental relationships is to view them in both the sagittal and coronal planes. In the sagittal plane, the teeth should follow a gentle arc connecting from the mandibular condyle through the occlusal plane. This is referred to as the curve of Spee. In the coronal plane, a similar gentle arc can be drawn relative to the occlusal relationship created by the buccal inclination of the maxillary teeth with the lingual inclination of the mandibular teeth. This arc is termed the curve of Wilson (Fig. 21.4).

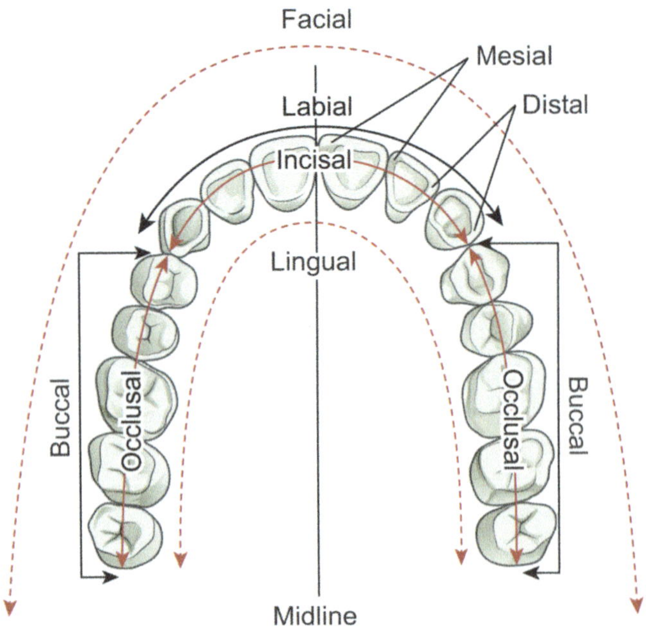

• **Fig. 21.1** Common terminology used to specify tooth surfaces: mesial/distal, facial/lingual, and occlusal/incisal. Dental terminology. This demonstrates the nomenclature used when discussing directionality within the oral cavity, relative to the dentition.

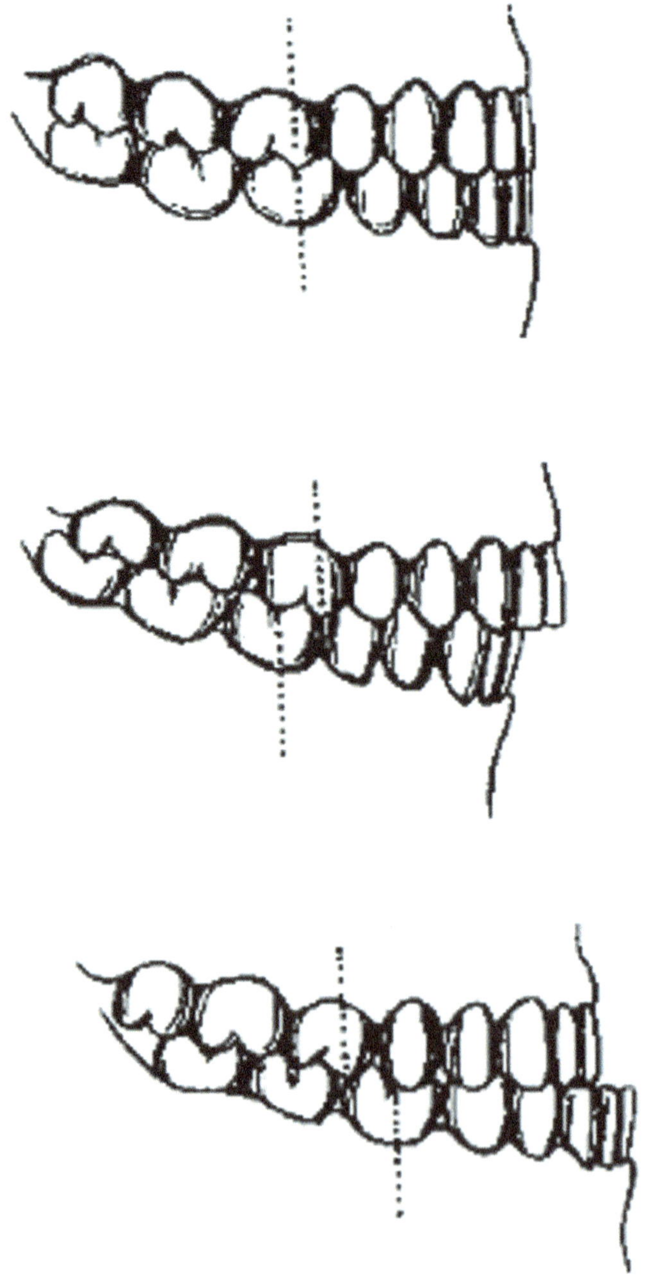

• **Fig. 21.2** Angle classification of occlusion. A, Class I normal occlusion. B, Class II, malocclusion. C, Class III, malocclusion.

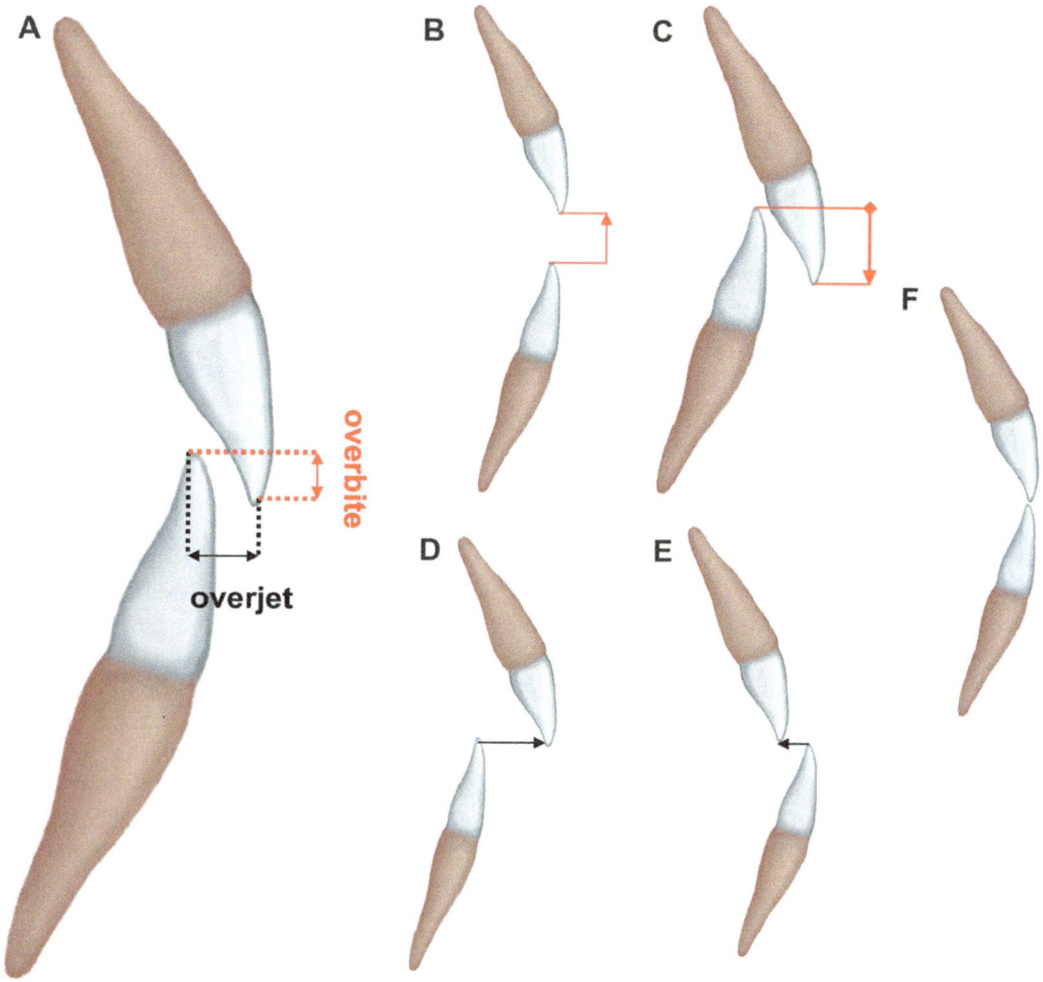

• **Fig. 21.3** Illustration of upper and lower incisor relationships. (A) Ideal overjet and overbite. (B) Open bite. (C) Deep bite. (D) Excessive overjet. (E) Reverse overjet or anterior crossbite or negative overjet. (F) Edge-to-edge relationship.

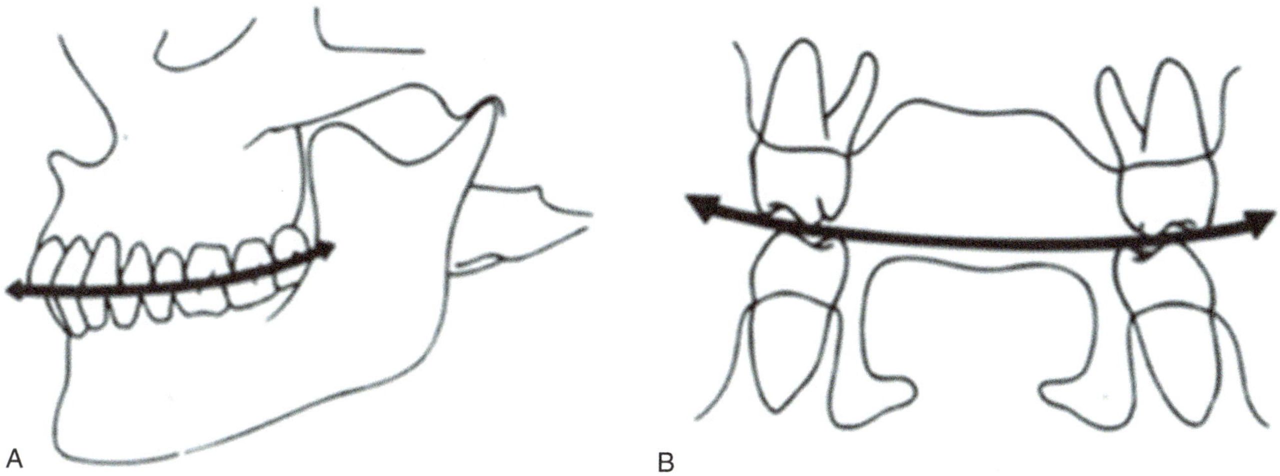

• **Fig. 21.4** Maxillomandibular relationships. (A) The curve of Spee, measured along the occlusal plane in the anteroposterior dimension. The curve of Wilson is shown in (B), which is a line drawn between the dentition in the frontal plane.

Lastly, there exist specific associations between the mandible and maxilla that also involve positioning within the temporomandibular joint. One such relationship is called centric relation. Centric relation is the reproducible maxillomandibular relationship whereby the mandibular condyles are seated within the anterior- and superior-most position of the glenoid fossa. It is independent of tooth contact. Centric occlusion, on the other hand, is the first tooth contact when in centric relation. Maximal intercuspation is the contact between the maxillary and mandibular dentition, independent of condylar position, and it may or may not coincide with centric occlusion.[15] This terminology is demonstrated on Poselts diagram (Fig. 21.5).

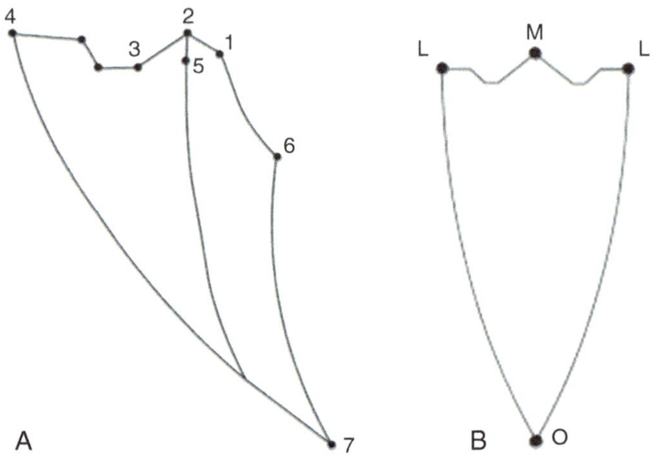

• **Fig. 21.5** Posselt's diagram. (A) The sagittal view: 1, centric relation; 2, maximal intercuspation; 3, edge to edge; 4, maximal protrusion; 5, resting position; 6, hinge axis terminating point; 7, maximal opening point. (B) The frontal view: M, maximal intercuspation; L, lateral deviation; O, maximal opening.

Clinical Evaluation

The evaluation of a patient who is appropriate for orthognathic surgery should always follow in a stepwise approach. There are two main reasons as to why a patient may be considering such a procedure, mostly to correct a functional or cosmetic abnormality. Functional issues can further be categorized based on dental malocclusion, masticatory difficulty, or an upper airway abnormality. Cosmetic abnormalities involve malposition of the maxilla or mandible causing facial disharmony and/or asymmetry.

Beginning with an overall appreciation of the facial form, the surgeon can view the face in the frontal plane by way of the vertical fifths. As such, the face is divided into fifths corresponding with the distance from medial canthus to medial canthus, medial canthus to lateral canthus (each side, respectively), and lateral canthus to helix of the ear (also, respective to each side of the face). These fifths should be equal. To further evaluate these measures, the distance between the medial canthi should coincide with the alar base, and the nasal dorsum width should be half of this value. The angle of the mouth should fall in line with the medial limbus of the eye, and the lateral canthus should coincide with the gonial angle. In the lateral view, the face can then be divided into horizontal thirds. The upper third is measured from trichion to glabella, middle third is glabella to subnasale, and lower third is subnasale to pogonion. These thirds should be equal. The lower third can further be subdivided into an upper third from subnasale to labii superioris, and a lower two-thirds from labii inferioris to pogonion[16–18] (Fig. 21.6).

Skeletal profiles are studied by evaluating the patient in the lateral view. A class I skeletal profile is considered the norm, with a slightly convex profile and a smooth transition from upper to middle to lower facial thirds. A class II

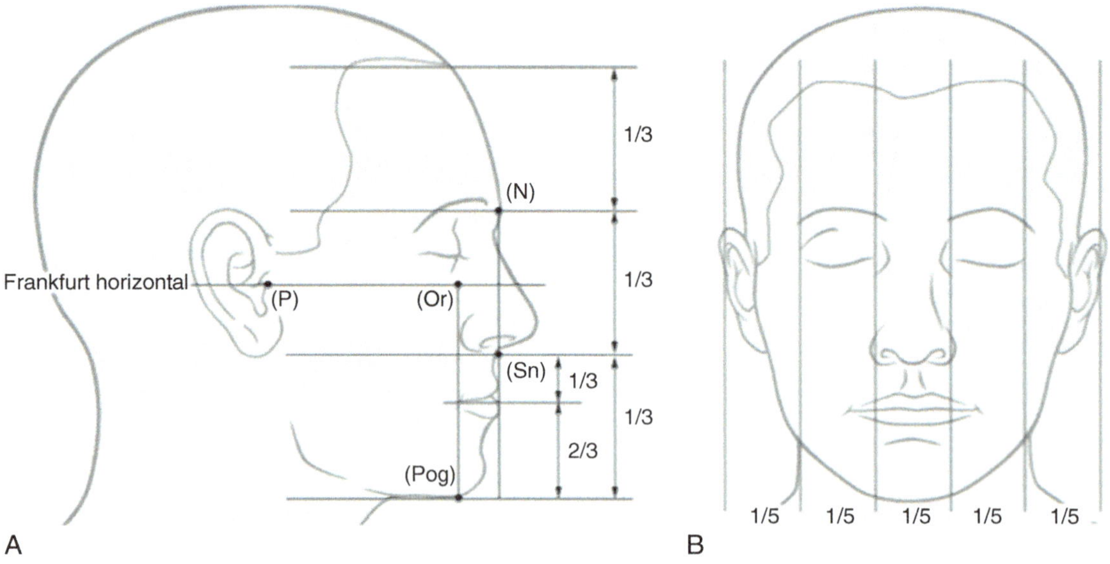

• **Fig. 21.6** Facial dimensions. (A) The proportionate facial thirds in the vertical dimension, while the facial fifths are shown in the horizontal dimension in (B).

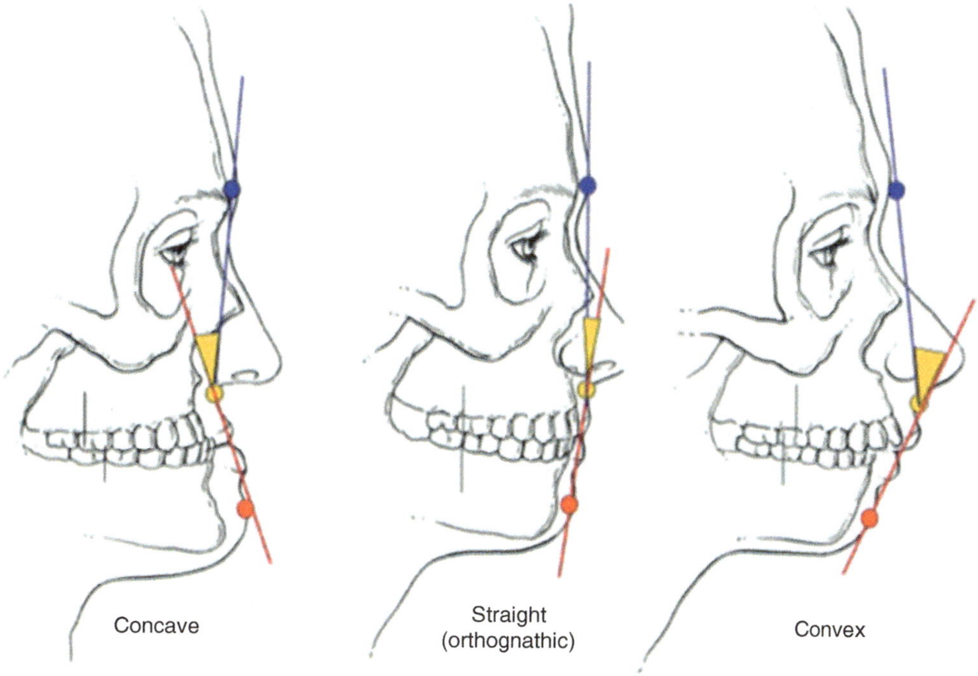

• **Fig. 21.7** Facial profile analysis. The facial profile can be classified as concave, convex, or straight.

skeletal profile is overly convex, whereas a class III profile is concave. Reasons for a class II profile can be due to a hyperplastic maxilla, or hypoplastic mandible, and a class III profile may be due to a hypoplastic maxilla or hyperplastic mandible (Fig. 21.7).

Individual measurements should be documented in the initial preoperative planning period. In the frontal view, the horizontal thirds and vertical fifths should be documented as described above. Interpupillary distance (65 mm ± 4), alar base width (32 mm ± 3), length of the upper lip (23 mm in males, 20 mm in females) and lower lip (40 mm in males, 44 mm in females), vermilion show, interlabial gap (2–4 mm), incisal show at rest (2 mm), tooth/gingival show upon smiling (gingiva should not be visible), chin point (relative to facial and dental midlines), and dental midline. In the profile view, a general comment on the skeletal profile should be documented as explained above. Presence of malar or perialar hollowing, nasal dorsum projection as per Goode's criteria (dorsal length 55%–60% greater than tip projection), nasolabial angle (90–95 degrees in males, 100–105 degrees in females), labiomental angle (120 degrees ±10, female more obtuse than male) and chin-to-throat distance (42 mm ± 6, or 4 fingerbreadths). The dental occlusion should then be closely evaluated, measuring overbite, overjet, Angle's classification, any discrepancy in centric relation – centric occlusion, maximal incisal opening, and any associated temporomandibular joint symptoms (clicking, crepitus, tenderness). The mandible should be viewed in animation with notice of any deviation on opening/closing, and the presence of any occlusal instability.

Upon completion of the measurements and record keeping, including a detailed medical/surgical/family history to determine whether the patient is fit to undergo such a procedure, a set of dental impressions should be taken. This is typically performed with an alginate material and appropriately-sized maxillary and mandibular impression trays. The entirety of the dentition, alveolar processes to the depth of the maxillary and mandibular buccal and lingual sulci, hard palate and maxillary tuberosity should be captured in the impression. A dental stone can then be poured into the tray, thus capturing a model of the maxillary and mandibular occlusal relationship for further study. A bite registration should also be taken in the patient's most reproducible occlusal pattern. The dental models and occlusal bite registration can then be combined with a facebow transfer (an apparatus used to accurately capture the relationship of the maxillary position relative to the skull base and Frankfort horizontal) to mount the exact dentofacial pattern on an articulator. This method is excellent for record keeping and can be used to perform traditional model surgery, although, with the advent of medical modeling and virtual surgical planning, it has become more of an educational tool used to allow trainees to formulate a better idea of the surgical treatment plan.

Radiography and Cephalometrics

Routine radiological examination is a necessary part of the orthognathic workup. In past times the standard was to perform a lateral cephalogram, as well as plain AP films. This was later supplemented with the panograph, and finally supplanted by the cone beam computed tomography (CT) scan. More so in the present day than previously, three-dimensional imaging has become the standard in many centers with the advent of cone beam CT scans. These cone beam scans subject the patient to a much lower dose of radiation than traditional CT imaging while maintaining adequate image quality. The three-dimensional scans also allow for virtual surgical planning to be performed, thus planning surgical movements expediently as compared to what was previously a time-consuming, multistep process of model surgery that was fraught with small errors that could further be amplified with each step of the process (Figs. 21.8 and 21.9). Virtual surgical planning has greatly streamlined the workflow process, eliminating the tedious steps involved with model surgery and allowing for preoperative visualization of each step in the surgical process. Osteotomies with subsequent bony movements can be planned and visualized in all dimensions, making fine-tuned adjustments to the yaw (i.e., rotation on the Z axis), pitch (rotation on the X axis), and roll (rotation on the Y axis) that were previously difficult to do with traditional model surgery. Intermediate

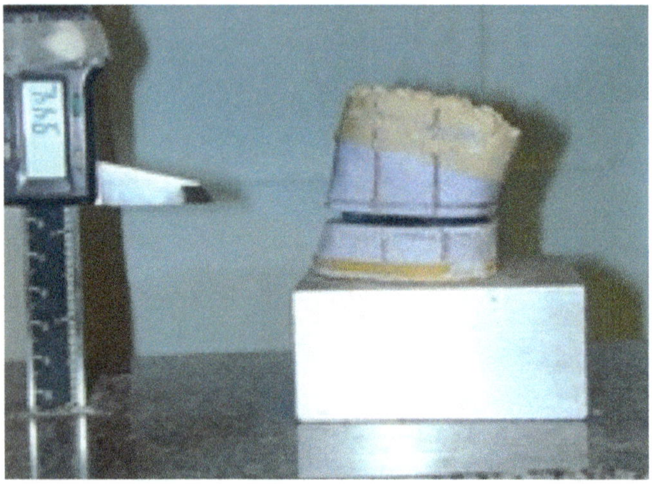

• **Fig. 21.8** Conventional model surgery. In this photo, an Erickson block is being used to take measurements of the mounted occlusal model. This type of device is used when performing model surgery in the traditional method prior to virtual surgical planning.

and final surgical splints are also fabricated during these planning sessions. Studies have also shown increased accuracy with virtual planning when compared to traditional methods (Fig. 21.10).

Radiographs are also useful when determining the appropriate time to operate on a growing, peripubertal patient. Serial cephalograms can be taken 6–12 months apart and compared for growth changes, as well as cervical spine radiographs (Fig. 21.11). AP hand and wrist films can be used to demonstrate whether the epiphyseal plate has closed, thus predicting cessation of maxillomandibular growth.

A baseline understanding of cephalometric analysis is also prudent for the operating surgeon. Various studies and analyses exist to examine the relationships of the maxilla, mandible, and skull base when viewing these structures on a lateral cephalogram. Looking at overall facial proportions, the upper facial height can be approximated measuring the distance from nasion to A point, whereas for lower facial height it is from A point from menton. The ideal facial plane is viewed by creating a vertical line, perpendicular to the Frankfort horizontal (orbitale to porion), from nasion to soft tissue pogonion. The anterior cranial base is identified as a line drawn between sella and nasion. The mandibular plane is a line drawn between gonion and menton, whereas the occlusal plane is created with a line between the maxillary and mandibular central incisors and first molars.

Other important cephalometric measurements can be evaluated when comparing the maxilla to the cranial base. This is best viewed with an angle created between the sella, nasion, and A point (SNA). The normal SNA value is 82 degrees ±3, with values greater than 85 degrees signifying a prognathic maxilla, and less than 79 degrees showing a retrognathic maxilla. The mandible is related to the cranial base by the angle between the sella, nasion, and B point (SNB). The normal SNB value is 79 degrees ±3, with a value

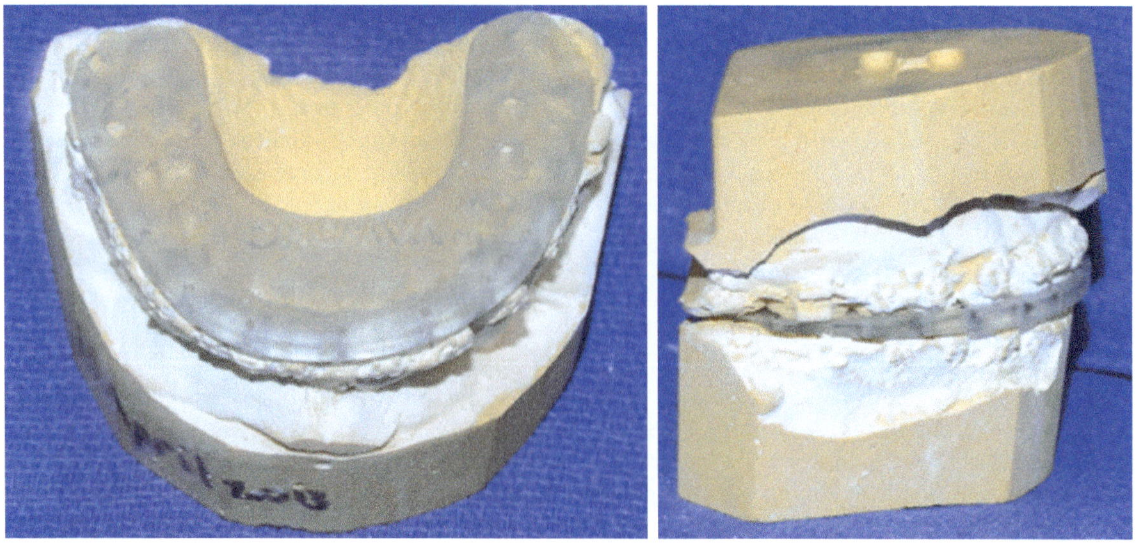

• **Fig. 21.9** Occlusal splints. These images demonstrate stone models that are used to create an acrylic occlusal surgical splint. The splints are fabricated for use intraoperatively when moving the maxilla and mandible into their new positions.

greater than 82 degrees being consistent with a prognathic mandible, and less than 76 degrees signifying a retrognathic mandible. Chin position is evaluated by looking at the angle between sella, nasion, and pogonion (SNPg). The normal value for SNPg is 80 degrees ±3, with a value greater than 83 degrees being consistent with a protruded chin, and less than 77 degrees showing a retruded chin. A relative measure of the positioning of the maxilla to the mandible is the angle between the A point, nasion, and B point (ANB). The normal ANB value is 1–5 degrees, thus often coinciding with a class I skeletal profile. An ANB value greater than 5 degrees often coincides with a class II skeletal profile, and less than 1 degree with a class III profile[19,20] (Fig. 21.12).

The upper airway can also be analyzed using cephalometric landmarks, and these values are useful when considering the potential for treating or creating obstructive airway issues with orthognathic surgery. The length of the soft palate is noted to be from PNS to P point, with a normal value of 37 mm. Values greater than this can be significant for a lengthened soft palate, and possibly naso-/oropharyngeal airway obstruction. Evidence of upper airway obstruction can also be elucidated when measuring

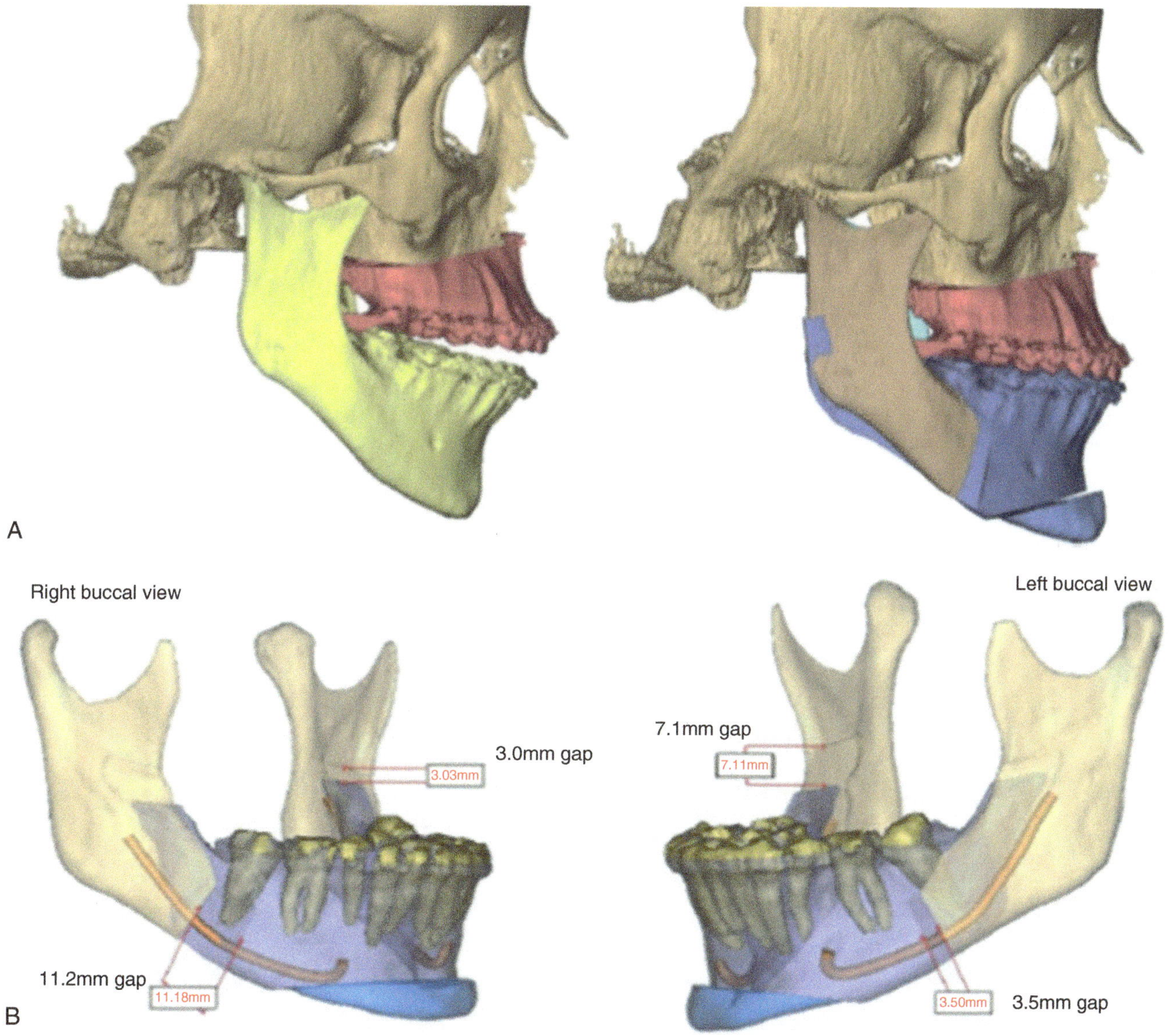

• **Fig. 21.10** Virtual surgical planning. Virtual surgical planning is performed after merging a computer rendering of the maxillary and mandibular dental aches with a computed tomography scan. Surgical movements can be simulated, showing precise measurements for each maneuver that is planned. Intermediate and final surgical splints are subsequently created from this session. (A) Shows movement of the maxilla via a Le Fort I procedure followed by bilateral sagittal split osteotomies to achieve counterclockwise rotation for closure of an anterior open bite. In a separate case, shown in (B), the surgeon can appreciate the amount of gapping and overlap that is created when performing yaw correction with bilateral sagittal split osteotomies.

the posterior airway space, which can be approximated with a line between the gonion to posterior pharyngeal wall (11 mm), as well as the distance from the mandibular plane to hyoid (15 mm). Lower than normal values for posterior airway space and higher than normal for mandibular plane to hyoid are consistent with airway obstruction[21,22] (Table 21.1).

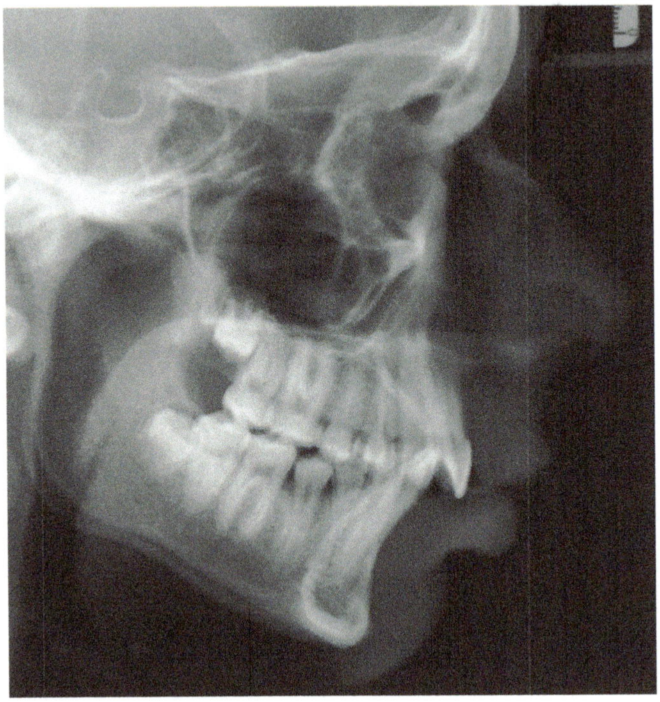

• **Fig. 21.11** Preoperative radiography. An example of a lateral cephalogram showing detailed craniofacial bony anatomy. The overlying soft tissue can often be identified when performing this imaging modality.

Orthodontics

It cannot be overstated the importance of developing a comfortable working relationship with an orthodontist who is well versed in surgical cases. Oftentimes the

TABLE 21.1 Common Cephalometric Measurements in Orthognathic Surgery

Cephalometric Landmarks	Normal Values (Range)
SNA	82 degrees (±3)
SNB	79 degrees (±3)
ANB	1-5 degrees
SN-MandP	32 degrees (±5)
OcclusalP-FH	9 degrees (±5)
Interincisal angle	135 degrees (±11)
SNPg	80 degrees (±3)
PNS-P	37 mm
PAS	11 mm
MP-H	15 mm

The left column lists common measurements that are made in the preoperative treatment planning for orthognathic surgery. The right column lists the normal values (including normative range). SNA, sella–nasion–A point; SNB, sella–nasion–B point; ANB, A point–nasion–B point; SN-MandP: sella–nasion–mandibular plane; OcclusalP-FH, occlusal plane–Frankfort horizontal; interincisal angle, angle created between the long axis of the maxillary and mandibular central incisors; SNPg, sella–nasion–pogonion; PNS-P, posterior nasal spine–P point; PAS, posterior airway space at the level of the gonion/mandibular plane; MP-H, mandibular plane to hyoid distance.

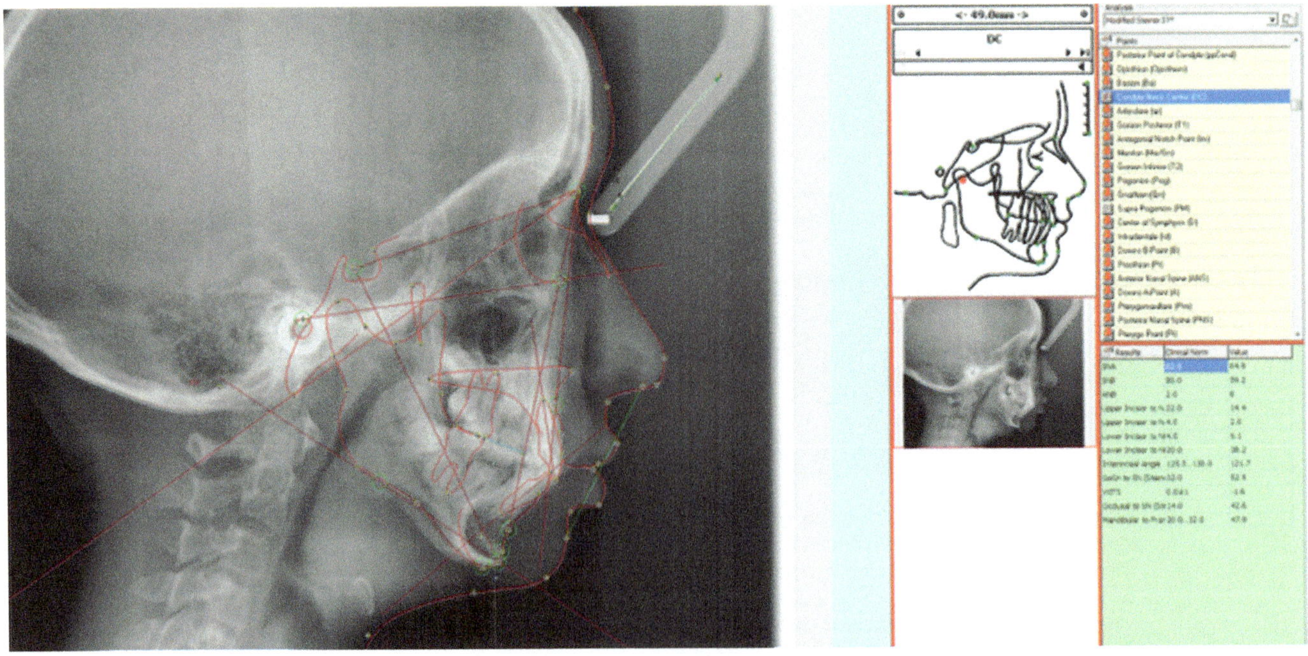

• **Fig. 21.12** Cephalometric tracings. Lateral cephalograms are used to plot specific anatomical landmarks that can further be analyzed using numerous software programs.

orthodontist will initiate the discussion with a patient about any potential surgical correction of their dentofacial deformity. Important points to note include the estimated length of presurgical orthodontics, or if it is possible to perform surgery prior to initiating orthodontic therapy. The concept of surgery first requires that the maxillary and mandibular dentition is in a position where it can be tripoded (anteriorly and posteriorly) into a stable condition after they have been repositioned. In this new postoperative relationship, the orthodontist must feel comfortable applying orthodontic movements to achieve an appropriate class I occlusal pattern.

Traditionally, an orthodontist will propose a treatment plan and alert the operating surgeon if any necessary teeth (often impacted or supernumerary) need to be removed to optimize the occlusal relationship. After this stage, the orthodontist will decompensate any previous misalignment of the dentition due to the pathological skeletal pattern present. The teeth are then leveled and aligned, often creating a malocclusion that appears worse to the patient than their premorbid condition. If interarch spacing is lacking to align the teeth appropriately, the orthodontist may plan for the surgeon to perform segmental osteotomies (traditionally of the maxilla) so that the arch form can be expanded. Once orthodontic movements are deemed appropriate by the orthodontist, a final surgical wire is often placed to maintain the teeth in their current position (as this dental pattern is used to create the surgical splints and final maxillomandibular relationship). After the surgery is performed, final orthodontic refinements are often necessary for a few months to fine-tune the new occlusal pattern. If third molars are present, it is often left to the discretion of the surgeon whether they will remove them at the time of surgery or prior. If removed prior, at least 6 months of bone healing and consolidation should be allowed prior to performing osteotomies, particularly of the mandible.[23]

Surgical Anatomy, Treatment Planning, and Operative Management

Performing orthognathic surgery necessitates a thorough understanding of head and neck anatomy. The focus of these procedures is on the midface and mandible, as the vast majority of these surgeries are initiated due to dentofacial deformities. With that being said, correction of any dental/occlusal pathology should be undertaken in a manner where a harmonious facial profile is also achieved.

Historically, orthognathic surgery involving the upper and lower jaw was considered a "bimaxillary" procedure. Upper jaw surgery is typically carried out with Le Fort-level osteotomies involving the maxilla. This bone is a paired, pyramidal structure with seven articulations with the frontal, ethmoid, nasal, zygomatic, palatine, vomer, and lacrimal bones. It supports numerous other structures, including the globes, sinuses, and muscles of mastication. Physiologically, the maxilla has an indirect role in ocular, olfactory, respiratory, and digestive functions. The maxilla also houses the upper dentition, so its form is central to correcting dentofacial discrepancies.

Postnatal midfacial growth is mainly appositional in nature. Secondary growth occurs at the cranial base and at the numerous facial sutures. Anteroposterior growth occurs at the temporozygomatic, nasomaxillary, and palatomaxillary sutures, as well as at the maxillary tuberosities. Growth in the vertical vector occurs at the frontozygomatic, frontomaxillary, and frontonasal sutures, as well as with bone deposition at the alveolar processes with tooth eruption and palatal remodeling. Facial growth in the transverse dimension is primarily at the midpalatal and zygomaticomaxillary sutures, with a lesser contribution from alveolar remodeling. Overall, midface growth can be simplified with the following equation: [(cranial base growth) + (sutural growth) + (appositional maxillary growth)] − (anterior maxillary resorption) = maxillary movement in the anterior and inferior vector (Fig. 21.13).

Relative to orthognathic surgery, the maxilla supports numerous muscles of facial expression and mastication. Each of these can be altered in various forms when performing upper jaw surgery. Regarding facial expression, the orbicularis oris, levator labii superioris alaeque nasi, buccinator, levator anguli oris, nasalis, and depressor septi. The masseter is involved with mastication and attaches to the maxilla, as well.

Vascularity to the maxilla is abundant, although can be compromised with Le Fort osteotomies. The major vascular inflow to the maxilla arises from the internal maxillary artery. This vessel is a takeoff from the external carotid artery, traversing posterior to the maxilla while giving off numerous branches to it, as well as the mandible. The main branches feeding the maxilla include the infraorbital, palatine, and alveolar branches. It is important to note that these branches are often transected after osteotomies are performed and maxillary down-fracture is completed. As such, additional vascular inflow in the form of the ascending pharyngeal artery, after branching from the external carotid, and ascending palatine branch of the facial artery are often the main source of perfusion to the maxilla during othognathic surgery.

Sensory innervation to the maxilla is mainly from the second branch of the trigeminal nerve. The infraorbital, superior alveolar, greater palatine, nasopalatine, and posterior nasal branches traverse small canals within the bony maxilla en route to soft tissue and dental innervation. Also, similar to the vascular inflow, these sensory branches are typically transected causing varying degrees of paresthesia and hypoesthesia after maxillary surgery.

As for the mandible, it is a paired bone that assumed a U-shape. Its articulations occur in the form of a joint with its two condylar heads and the opposing temporal bone, thus forming the temporomandibular joint. The main functions of the mandible are for mastication and speech. The bone can be further subdivided into numerous sectors: the condyle, neck, ramus, angle, body, parasymphysis, and symphysis.

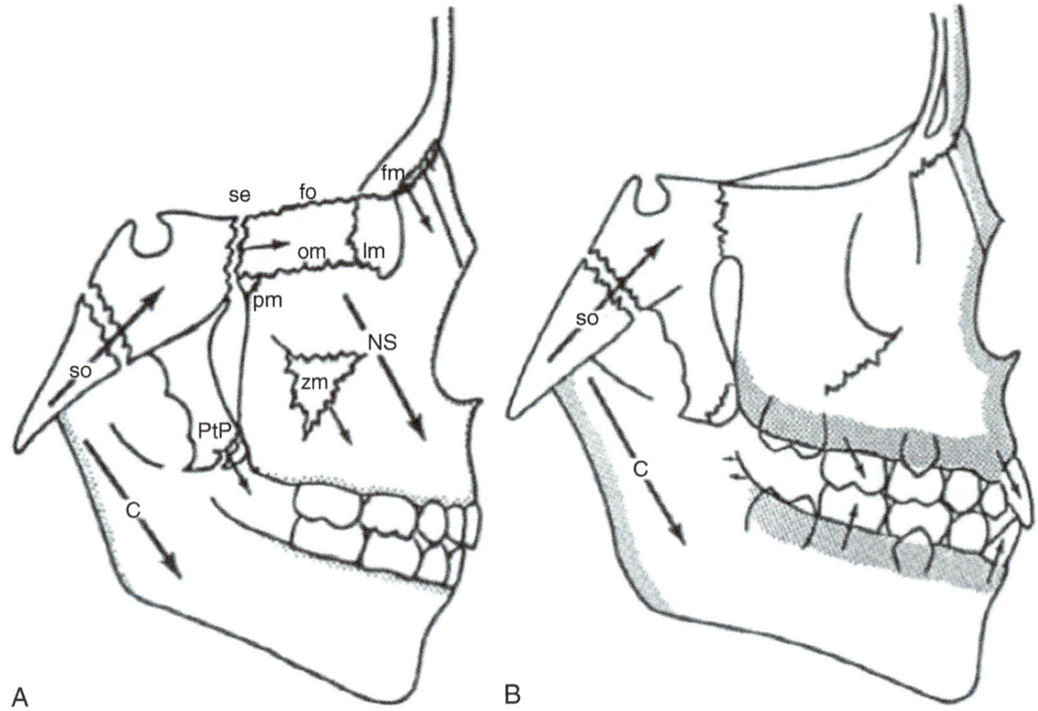

• **Fig. 21.13** Maxillary and mandibular growth. (A) shows the regions and directionality of postnatal maxillary growth, whereas postnatal mandibular growth is shown in (B). Cartilaginous growth: SO, spheno-occipital synchondrosis; C, mandibular condyle growth; NS, nasal septum; se, spheno-ethmoidal; PtP, pterygopalatine; fo, frontoorbital; om, orbitomaxillary; lm, lacrimomaxillary; pm, pterygomaxillary; fm, frontomaxillary; zm, zygomaticomaxillary; stippled area, appositional growth.

Mandibular growth occurs postnatally in a different manner than that of the maxilla. Numerous growth centers exist in the mandible, including the condylar cartilage, as well as the posterior ramus, alveolar process, and lingual tuberosity. Literature is variable on this topic, but transverse growth is typically completed prior to the adolescent growth spurt, whereas anteroposterior growth continues until approximately age 14–15 in females and 18–19 in males. The concept of the functional matrix, as described by Moss, is often discussed in concert with that of mandibular growth. Moss stated that form fits the function, whereas masticatory forces on the teeth stimulate alveolar bone growth, and actions of mastication via their associated musculature leads to subsequent bone growth at the areas of their attachment.[24] The masticatory muscles that attach to the mandible include the masseter, temporalis, and pterygoids, whereas the associated muscles of facial expression include the mentalis, platysma, depressor labii inferioris, buccinator, and depressor anguli oris. The mandible also acts as a means to support other soft tissues in the neck, including the geniohyoid, genioglossus, mylohyoid, and digastric muscles, as well as the mandibular retaining ligament. A fine line between aggressive muscle stripping and inadequate release exists when performing mandibular orthognathic surgery.

Vascular supply to the mandible is also primarily via the maxillary artery. The inferior alveolar arterial branch enters the mandible inferior to the lingula, a prominence of bone located mid-ramus on the lingual mandible, approximated at the level of the occlusal plane. It then traverses distally through a canal in the mandible, giving off numerous incisive arterial branches to supply blood to the teeth and periosteum before exiting the mental foramen.

Mandibular sensory innervation is by way of the third branch of the trigeminal nerve. After giving off buccal and lingual branches, the nerve follows a similar path to that of the alveolar artery whereby it enters the mandible via the same foramen just below the lingula. It then provides sensory innervation to the mandibular dentition prior to exiting via the mental foramen and innervating the soft tissue of the lip and chin. Temporary hypoesthesia is not uncommon during mandibular osteotomies, although complete, permanent nerve dysfunction is rare.

An understanding of the temporomandibular joint is essential when performing orthognathic surgery. The anatomy mainly involves the temporal bone and mandible, with a joint capsule being formed via numerous ligamentous structures spanning the temporal bone and connecting to the ramus of the mandible. The upper joint space along the temporal bone and lower joint space over the mandibular condyle is lined by an articular fibrocartilage, which produces a lubricating joint fluid and acts as a shock absorber for the forces of mastication distributed by the mandible. The intervening articular disc maintains this space, attaching anteriorly to the lateral pterygoid and assisting in mouth opening when this muscle activates, thus causing it to glide off the mandibular condyle.

It attaches posteriorly to the mandible. Maintaining this intricate disc/condyle relationship is necessary when performing mandibular movements, as significant temporomandibular disorders can ensue long term. This is a ginglymoarthroidal joint, thus allowing for hinging and sliding motions. The first 20 mm of mouth opening is a pure hinge axis rotation, followed by a translational movement of the articular disc over the eminence at the anterior aspect of the joint space. A resting position of 2–4 mm of mouth opening is maintained via numerous proprioceptive feedback mechanisms.

Physiologically, the mandible functions in concert with the maxilla to perform working movements in all cardinal directions. Protrusion of the mandible occurs with contraction of the lateral and medial pterygoids, and retrusion is carried out via posterior fibers of the temporalis, deep portion of the masseter, geniohyoid, and digastric muscle contraction. The mandible is elevated by the remaining temporalis, masseter, and medial pterygoid muscles, and depression occurs by action of the digastric, geniohyoid, and mylohyoid muscles. After the bony architecture changes with orthognathic surgery, the proprioceptive and functional nature of the muscles in their new anatomical position recovers rather quickly.[25,26]

Once all clinical information is gathered, a complete plan of care must be compiled. As discussed early in this chapter, the diagnosis is typically encompassing a functional pathology (due to a dentofacial deformity) and aesthetic concern. As with any surgical issue, the functional deficit must first be addressed. With orthognathic cases, this is likely due to a skeletal and dental discrepancy between the maxilla and mandible. Based upon the premorbid dental occlusal pattern, the surgeon will have an idea of what type of surgical technique is necessary to reposition the maxillary and mandibular dental arches, with the help of orthodontics, in order to achieve a class I dental occlusion. With the help of anthropometric and cephalometric normative values based upon clinical and radiographic examination, further information can be obtained to assist in the planning of which surgical techniques can be used to achieve an esthetic class I skeletal profile to complement the class I dental occlusion. When determining which operative procedures will be undertaken, it is prudent to understand the concept of postsurgical stability of the maxilla and mandible after performing orthognathic surgery. There are more stable and predictable movements that can be planned, those being (in order or more to less): maxilla up, mandible forward, maxilla forward and/or rotated, maxilla up plus mandible forward, maxilla forward plus mandible back, mandible rotated, mandible back, maxilla down, maxilla expanded transversely. This concept of stability and predictability of the movement is a function of bony contact (or lack thereof), and movements against opposing muscle vectors. Greater relapse can occur when unfavorable maneuvers are performed.

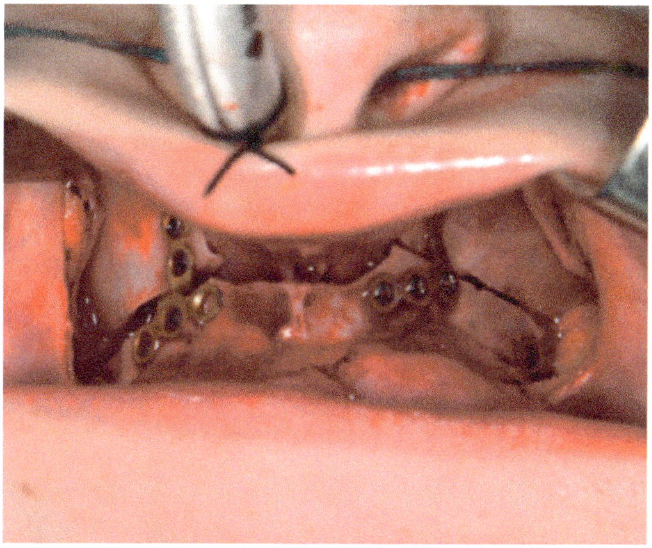

• **Fig. 21.14** Maxillary Le Fort I osteotomy. This intraoperative photograph shows an example of where the osteotomy is created at the Le Fort I level, including placement of internal fixation.

The use of maxillomandibular fixation after performing orthognathic surgery is also an important concept to consider, and this is often the personal decision of the operating surgeon. With stable movements, adequate postoperative dental occlusion and hardware placed soundly in good bone stock, it is often feasible to remove the final surgical splint and allow the patient to wear guiding elastics only. This will allow an easier time with oral hygiene, oral intake, breathing (given the potential for facial edema and nasal obstruction), as well as help prevent stiffness of the temporomandibular joint with immobility. Some surgeons, though, will opt to wire the final surgical splint into place with a combination of either guiding elastics or maxillomandibular fixation.

The first technique to discuss is the *Le Fort Iosteotomy* (Fig. 21.14). This procedure is based upon the studies of René LeFort who identified the three main levels of fracture that occur on the facial skeleton.[27] To review, the Le Fort I osteotomy is performed by creating transverse cut through the anterior and lateral maxillary walls and separating the nasal septum and pterygoid places from the distal segment, thus allowing the palate and dentoalveolar unit to move freely. The Le Fort II osteotomy traverses through the pterygoid plates, across the zygomaticomaxillary suture and inferior orbital rim, then through medial orbital wall and across the nasofrontal suture to create an inverted pyramid shape and allow complete movement of the entire maxilla. Le Fort III osteotomies allow the entire facial skeleton to be separated from the cranial base, whereby cuts are made across the nasofrontal junction, laterally across the medial orbital wall and through the inferior orbital fissure and sphenozygomatic suture, and then across the frontozygomatic and zygomaticotemporal junctions, while also separating the pterygoid plates. In the majority of orthognathic surgical cases dentofacial deformities are managed with conventional or high Le Fort I osteotomies.

To perform the Le Fort I osteotomy, surgical access is created by making an incision intraorally through the unattached mucosa beginning 5 mm cephalad to the mucogingival junction. Prior to incising, an adequate amount of vasoconstrictor ± local anesthetic should be injected and allowed ample time to take effect. The incision should be carried from first molar to first molar bilaterally, with a gentle "V" extending cephalad at the midline of the maxilla. Dissection proceeds sharply through the mucosa, submucosal tissue, and underlying musculature, keeping perpendicular to the initial incision so as to maintain the initial 5 mm cuff of mucosa and underlying soft tissue to reinforce the wound closure. The periosteum is then incised, and subperiosteal dissection is carried out cephalad along the anterior and lateral maxillary walls, as far posterior as the pterygomaxillary junction and anteriorly across the midline. Care should be taken in order to avoid injury to the infraorbital nerve as it exits its foramen in line with the pupil and maxillary canine. The nasal mucosa is then carefully lifted off of the maxillary antrum, medially off of the septum, and laterally off of the nasal sidewall. The surgeon's proposed osteotomy can then be inscribed across the anterior maxillary wall with a sterile pencil or marking pen. Using a reciprocating saw, the osteotomy is created starting at the lateral maxillary wall, working medially across the anterior wall of the maxilla until the cut is complete through the lateral nasal wall (a narrow malleable retractor should be placed within the antrum in order to protect the nasal mucosa). These osteotomies are performed bilaterally. A narrow osteotome and mallet can then be used to gently confirm completion of lateral nasal, anterior, and lateral maxillary wall osteotomies. Using a double-guarded, curved nasal septal osteotome, the nasal septum is then separated from the maxillary crest (no further posteriorly than 40 mm in order to avoid inadvertent injury to the internal maxillary artery). A curved osteotome is then inserted within the pterygomaxillary junction. One finger should be placed within the mouth along the palate, just posterior to the maxillary alveolus. That same individual will then direct the curved osteotome anteriorly, inferiorly, and medially while an assistant gently strikes the osteotome with a mallet. This will separate the pterygoid plates from the posterior maxilla, a maneuver that is necessary to appropriately mobilize the distal segment with minimal resistance. Prior to downfracture of the maxilla, it is important to alert the anesthesiologist that mean arterial pressure should be maintained at 65 mmHg. This will help to eliminate significant bony bleeding. Downfracturing can now be performed with either gentle manual downward pressure on the anterior maxilla, Rowe disimpaction forceps, or a Smith spreader. Tessier mobilizers can be placed along the posterior maxilla to gently advance the distal segment against the resistance of its soft tissue envelope. If bleeding ensues, attempts should be made to identify any larger vessels (such as the descending palatine artery and vein) and ligate them with vascular clips or ties. More prominent venous bleeding may be due to injury of the pterygoid venous plexus. If this is the case, packing the area and holding pressure is the appropriate tactic. If there is significant arterial hemorrhaging from posterior to the maxilla, the region should also be packed and interventional radiology should be alerted of the potential to embolize the offending vessel. Should there be no such service at the hospital, then proximal control must be obtained via clamping/ligating of the external carotid artery. The maxilla is now freely mobile and can be wired into maxillomandibular fixation or the intermediate/final surgical splint and then rigidly fixated with plates/unicortical screws at the nasomaxillary and zygomaticomaxillary buttresses.

In certain instances when there is either a transverse maxillary discrepancy (relative to the mandible) or an occlusal pattern with more than one plane, a *segmental Le Fort osteotomy* can be performed. It is oftentimes the decision of the orthodontist whether this adjunct to the Le Fort I is necessary. When a pure transverse discrepancy exists between the maxilla and mandible (i.e., the maxilla is constricted in its transverse direction), the orthodontist may be able to place a fixed appliance and slowly distract across the midpalatal suture (which may fuse as early as 11 years of age). In older patients with fused midpalatal sutures that only require transverse expansion of the maxilla, surgically assisted rapid palatal expansion can be performed. With this, an orthodontist places a transverse palatal distraction device that anchors to the molar teeth. The patient then undergoes Le Fort I osteotomy as per the standard technique, with the following alterations: the maxilla is not purposefully downfractured, and the midpalatal suture is osteotomized using a narrow osteotome. Confirmation of complete suture separation is performed in the operative theater by gently activating the distraction device. The patient can then begin distracting per the surgeon's protocol. Distraction typically commences on postoperative day 7 at a rate of 0.25–0.5 mm and rhythm of two sessions per day, for a total of 0.5–1 mm daily. Once the distraction is complete, typically overcorrecting slightly to allow for some relapse, a period of consolidation occurs for at least 8 weeks.[28,29]

When a patient has a transverse maxillary discrepancy as well as the need for movement in another vector, it is often best to perform a segmental osteotomy in one procedure. As such, once the maxilla is downfractured, a reciprocating saw can be used to carefully osteotomize the floor of the maxilla so that it can be expanded and leveled. This will involve the use of a surgical splint that can also stabilize the segments from collapsing back into their premorbid position prior to rigidly fixating the maxilla with plates/unicortical screws at the nasomaxillary and zygomaticomaxillary buttresses. Complications can occur specific to the Le Fort I osteotomy, including

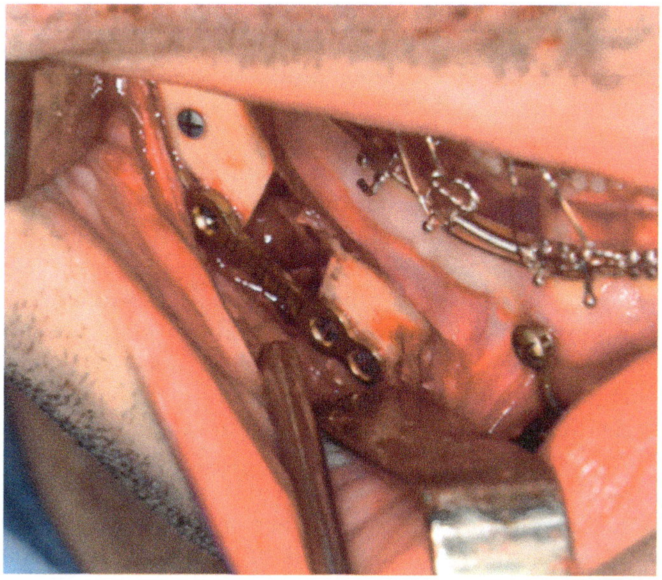

• **Fig. 21.15** Mandibular bilateral sagittal split osteotomy. This intraoperative photograph shows an example of where the osteotomy is created for a bilateral sagittal split, including placement of internal fixation.

neurosensory alteration to the infraorbital nerve. Other issues involve bony relapse or hardware malposition, malunion, nonunion, and infection, each of which can result from internal fixation during any orthognathic procedure. Maxillary sinusitis is a potential complication, as well as maxillary ischemia resulting from problems during the downfracture or positioning of the maxilla. Ischemic insult is more concerning, with segmentalization of the maxilla. Segmental maxillary osteotomies can also compromise the palatal soft tissue during the bone cuts and/or subsequent mobilization, which can persist in the form of an oronasal fistula.

The next procedure to discuss is the *mandibular sagittal split osteotomy* (Fig. 21.15). Vasoconstrictor ± local anesthesia is first injected intraorally along the external oblique ridge of the mandible. An incision is marked and created along the external oblique ridge cephalad as high as the maxillary occlusal table, gently tapering into the distobuccal line angle of the second molar (or third molar, if it is still present), continued as a sulcular incision buccally around the aforementioned tooth, and finally tapering laterally into the buccal mucosa to approximately the second mandibular premolar region. A cuff of unattached mucosa, approximately 5 mm, should be maintained when extending this incision anteriorly. The incision is then deepened through mucosa, submucosal tissue, and down to periosteum distal to the molar. Anteriorly, electrocautery can be used to complete the incision through mucosa, submucosal tissue, and minimally into underlying muscle. At this point, the incision should be directed immediately to the underlying buccal mandibular cortex, deep to the periosteum. The periosteum is then elevated off of the buccal cortex of the mandible cephalad to the level of the maxillary occlusal plane. At this point, attachments of the temporalis muscle may be adherent and necessitate sharp transection. A V-notch retractor is then placed along the anterior ramus of the mandible, and the soft tissue is elevated cephalad just enough to expose the lingula. The lingula is approximately at the level of the occlusal plane. Gentle dissection is carried out along the lingual aspect of the mandibular ramus to identify the lingula, just enough to safely insert a reciprocating saw. At this point, the lingual cortical osteotomy can be created with a reciprocating saw at the level of or just cephalad to the lingula. Working from posterior to anterior, the osteotomy should gently taper into the anterior cortex of the ramus where it is then carried caudally and just buccal to the molar teeth. If the dissection has not yet been completed, it is continued in a subperiosteal plane along the buccal cortex of the mandible as far anteriorly as the first mandibular molar/second premolar. The dissection should reach the inferior border of the mandible, where at this point a J-stripper can be used to elevate the periosteum in a region limited to where the anterior, vertical osteotomy will be performed (corresponding with the buccal groove of the mandibular first molar). Periosteal stripping should be limited along the posterior border of the mandible. At this point, the osteotomy can continue anteriorly along the superior aspect of the buccal mandibular cortex, just lateral to the dentition, gently tapering into the vertical cut at the level of the buccal groove of the first mandibular molar. Here, the vertical osteotomy is completed through the buccal cortex and inferior border of the mandible. Beginning with numerous small osteotomes and a mallet, the previously created osteotomy is confirmed to be complete, sequentially inserting larger osteotomes. Leaving the larger osteotomes in place within the sagittal cut, a Smith spreader can be used to gently separate the proximal and distal segments of the mandible. Care must be taken to gently separate the inferior alveolar nerve from the proximal segment so that it does not overly stretch with advancement of the distal segment. The distal mandibular segment can now be gently mobilized against the resistance of the overlying soft tissue envelope. Depending on the movements made (advancement versus setback versus rotation), any potential interferences should be removed with either a pineapple-shaped bur, or sagittal saw. The mandible can now be wired into maxillomandibular fixation or an intermediate/final surgical splint, and rigidly fixated with plates/unicortical screws, bicortical positional screws, or a combination of both.

The main complication of the sagittal splint osteotomy is injury to the inferior alveolar nerve, albeit typically transient. Other complications from this procedure include an unfavorable splint, temporomandibular joint dysfunction, and condylar resorption. Issues relative to the temporomandibular joint can best be avoided with careful positioning of the mandibular condyle during internal fixation and hardware placement.

An adjunct to orthognathic surgery that is usually for esthetic purposes is the *osseous genioplasty*. This procedure is often performed in conjunction with other mandibular osteotomies, as it can fine-tune placement of the chin point to correct midline asymmetries, adjust lower facial height, or anteroposterior projection. There are instances, though, where a functional benefit can be had with a genioplasty. The indications for genioplasty and surgical techniques are discussed fully in the section below. The main complications of osseous genioplasty include injury to the inferior alveolar nerve, as well as lip, and chin ptosis from inadequate soft tissue resuspension during wound closure.

Another procedure to correct mandibular misalignment is the *intraoral vertical ramus osteotomy*. This technique is particularly useful when correcting midline mandibular asymmetry relative to yaw/rotation, or for setting back the mandible. The approach is similar to that of the sagittal splint osteotomy, although the dissection must focus more on the ramus and less on the body of the mandible. An appropriate subperiosteal pocket is created on the buccal cortex of the mandible from the sigmoid notch to the inferior border. A Bauer retractor is placed within the notch and gentle caudal distraction is performed. At this point, a right-angle sagittal saw can be inserted intraorally and a bicortical osteotomy is created from the sigmoid notch caudally through the inferior border of the mandible. Care must be taken to direct this osteotomy posterior to the inferior alveolar canal. Identification of the antilingula can assist with this, although there may be some variation in the concordance of it with the lingula. Once the osteotomy is complete, the proximal segment is then directed lateral to the distal segment (as the distal segment maintains in continuity with the inferior alveolar nerve). Internal fixation is not typically applied, although maxillomandibular fixation is necessary for a period of bone healing. Certain nuances and complications with this procedure include widening of the bigonial angle, which may or may not be desired. Damage to the inferior alveolar nerve can certainly occur, although with an incidence of less than that with sagittal split osteotomies. The internal maxillary and masseteric vessels lie medial to the mandibular ramus at numerous points and can be injured during the bone cut. The proximal segment can be displaced medially with certain movements, thus leading to compression or transection of the inferior alveolar nerve between it and the distal segment. Another complication can be condylar sag, which is due to the proximal segment (which is in continuity with the mandibular condyle) undergoing aggressive muscle stripping and, thus, dropping caudally over time. This can lead to the development of temporomandibular joint disorders.

With the advent of distraction osteogenesis, cases requiring larger anterior movement of the mandible have been managed more reliably with regard to relapse and stability. Prior to its mainstream use, the *inverted-L osteotomy* was performed when mandibular advancements upward of 15–20mm were needed. The inverted-L is also indicated for patients with short posterior facial/ramus height, as well as anterior open bites. This is because the mandible can more readily be advanced in more than one vector with this osteotomy. The procedure often requires a transcutaneous approach, as larger hardware must be placed to span the bone gap, although with the use of virtual surgical planning, intraoral approaches have been documented. The mandible is dissected on its buccal cortex along the ramus and anteriorly beyond the angle. Muscles of the pterygomasseteric sling are gently reflected, and the temporalis muscle attachment is maintained on the proximal segment. A bicortical osteotomy is performed transversely from the anterior border of the ramus cephalad to and just posterior to the lingula/antilingula. The bone cut then continues caudally, perpendicular to the transverse one, through the inferior border of the mandible in the angle region. The distal segment is now free to be advanced in the appropriate anterior and/or caudal direction, and internal fixation with a spanning plate can be placed with uni- or bicortical screws. The determination of the period of maxillomandibular fixation is relative to the hardware placed (i.e., with the placement of a reconstruction plate and bicortical screws, guiding elastics will suffice). Complications associated with this procedure include damage to the inferior alveolar and facial nerves (if a transcutaneous approach is used), an unfavorable osteotomy, and bleeding from the vessels located medial and posterior (internal maxillary, masseteric, retromandibular) to the mandible, or within the facial soft tissue when accessing transcutaneously (facial).

Case Examples

Four case examples are illustrated on pages 297–304.

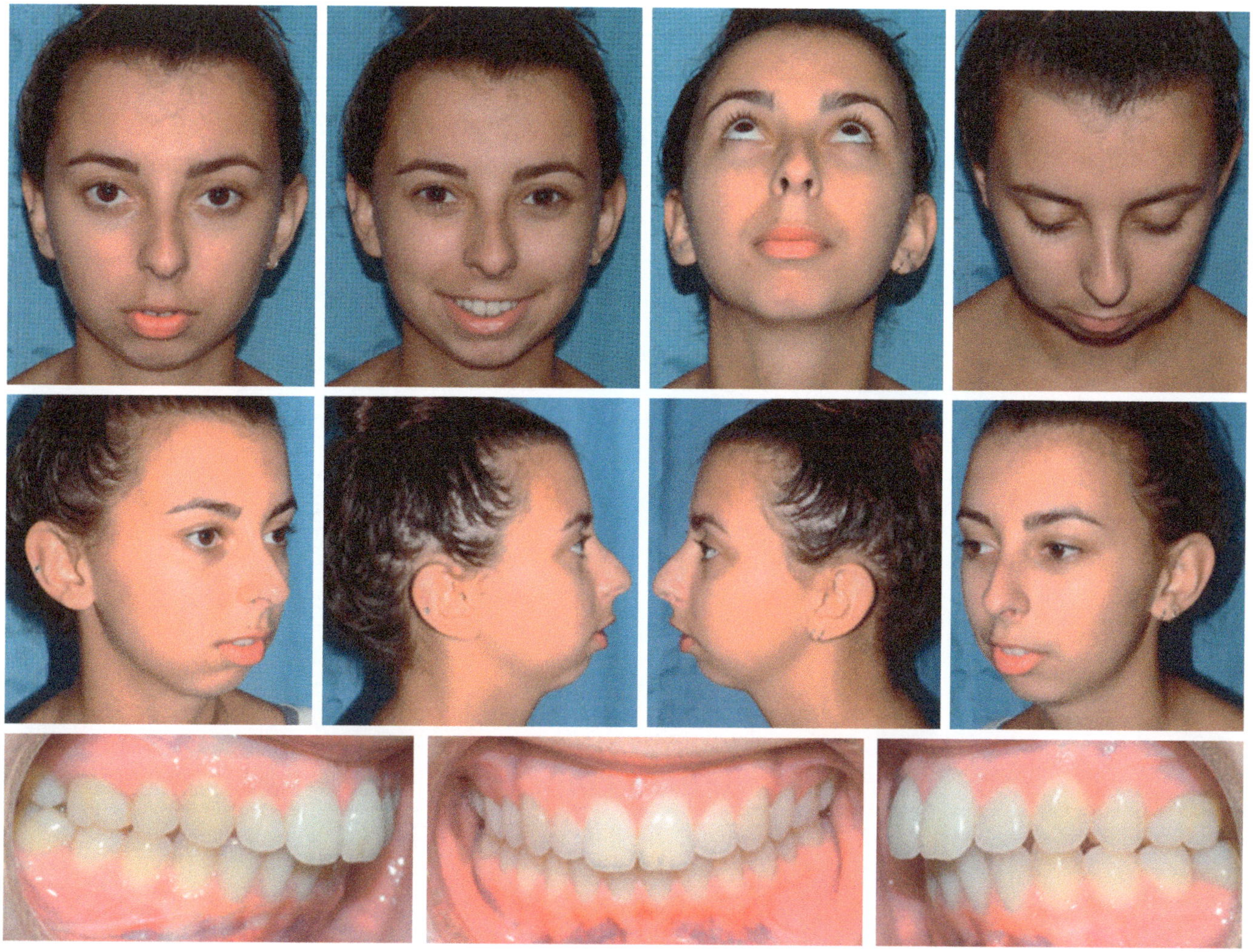

Case 1 Figure 1

Case 1: Mandibular Hypoplasia

This is an 18-year-old female with a significantly hypoplastic mandible who presented with complaints of having trouble chewing. Preoperatively, the patient is noted to have a short lower facial third, decreased anteroposterior mandibular length, and a prominent nasal dorsum. A class II molar relationship with excessive overbite and overjet is noted (Figure 1). One year postoperatively after undergoing yaw correction of the maxilla with a Le Fort I, mandibular advancement via bilateral sagittal split osteotomies, osseous genioplasty with advancement, fat grafting, and a staged septorhinoplasty, a much more harmonious facial profile is noted (Figure 2). The nasal dorsum is straighter with a subtle supratip break. There is a soft convexity to the facial profile with more proportionate facial thirds. Dental and facial midlines are coincident, and there is a class I molar relationship with a normal overbite and overjet.

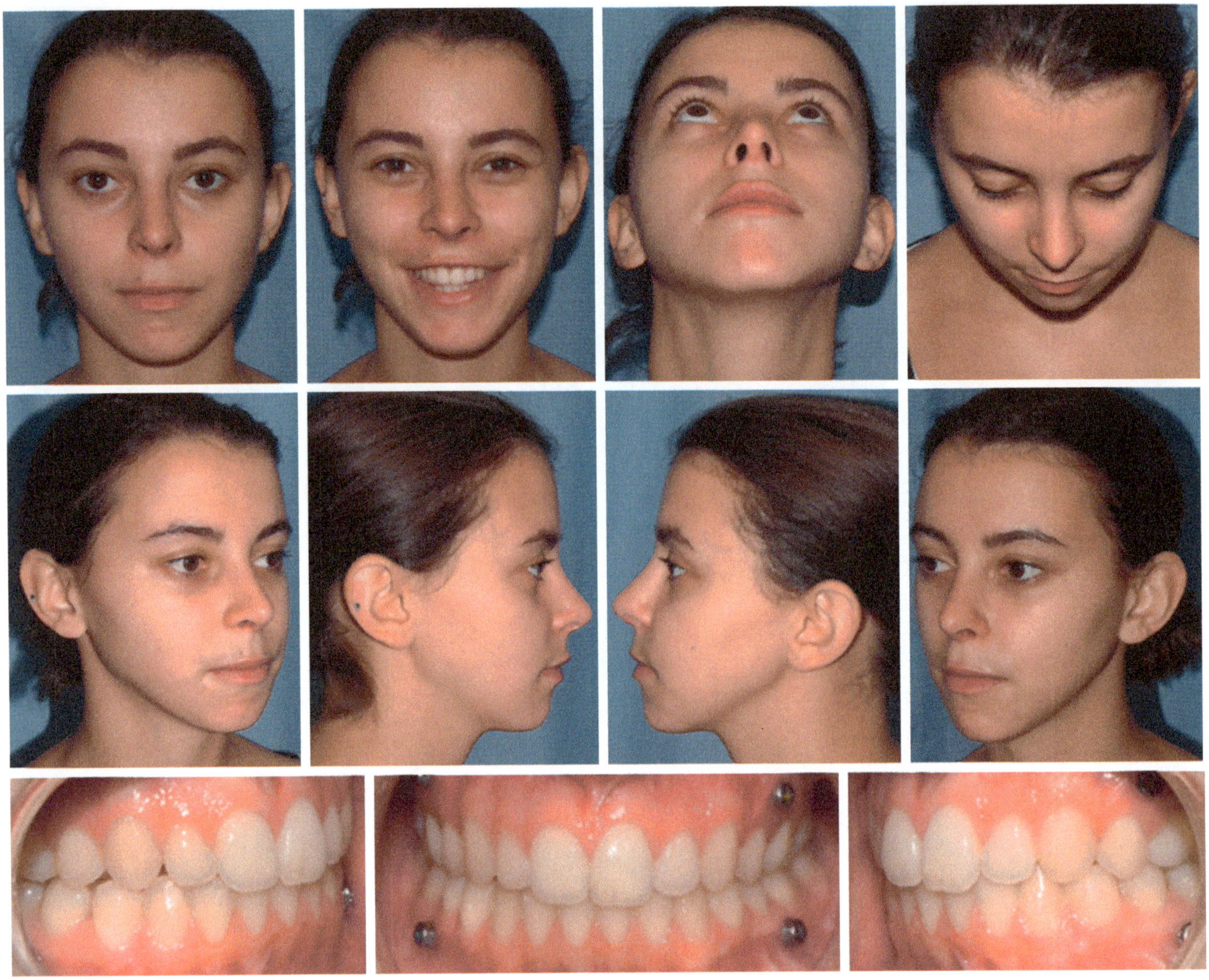

Case 1 Figure 2

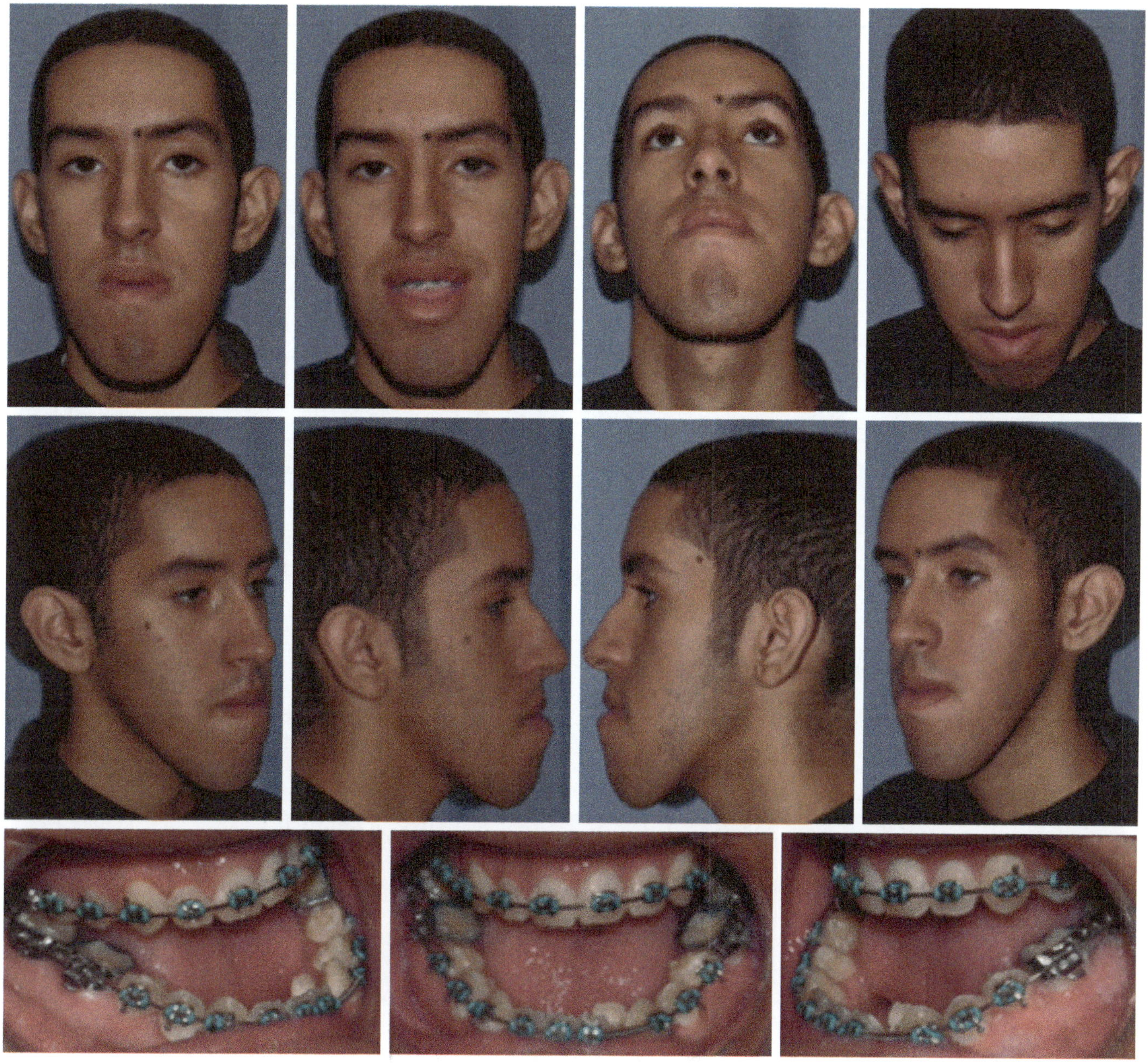

Case 2 Figure 1

Case 2: Mandibular Prognathism

This is a 23-year-old male who presented with an overly prominent mandible. Preoperative photographs show an elongated face in the frontal view with evidence of mentalis straining in order to close his mouth. There is a concave facial profile. The chin is long in the vertical dimension and wide transversely, with slight deviation to the left. There is a steep mandibular plane angle. The maxilla is relatively retrognathic with mild malar flattening. There is a class III molar relationship, significant anterior open bite, and the maxillary and mandibular midlines are not coincident (Figure 1). At one year postoperatively after undergoing Le Fort I for yaw correction, bilateral sagittal split osteotomies to set back the mandible, an osseous genioplasty with vertical shortening, and fat grafting, the vertical facial thirds are now more proportionate with a shorter facial length and less steep mandibular plane angle. The dentition is in a class I molar relationship, with dental and facial midlines now being coincident (Figure 2).

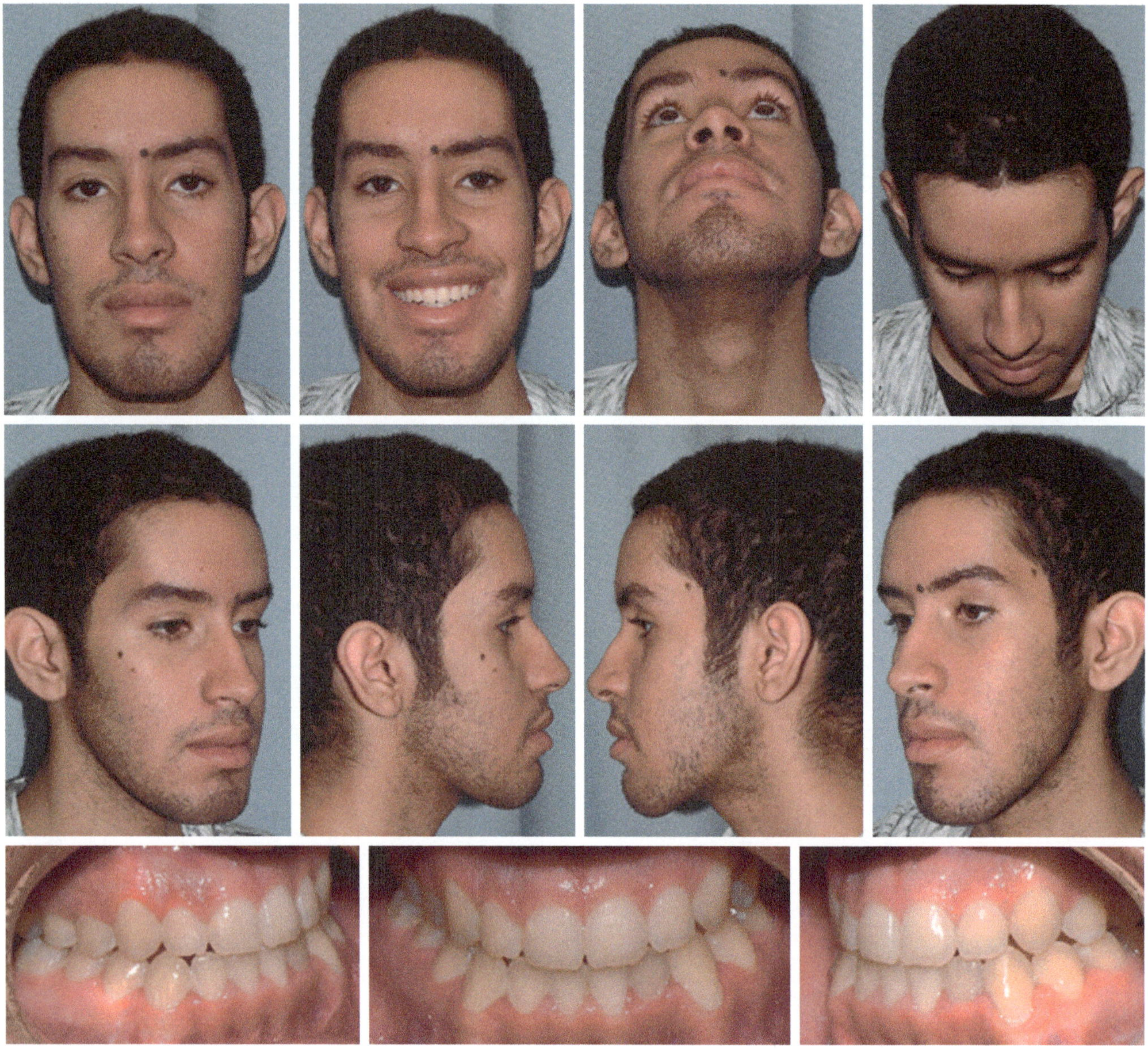

Case 2 Figure 2

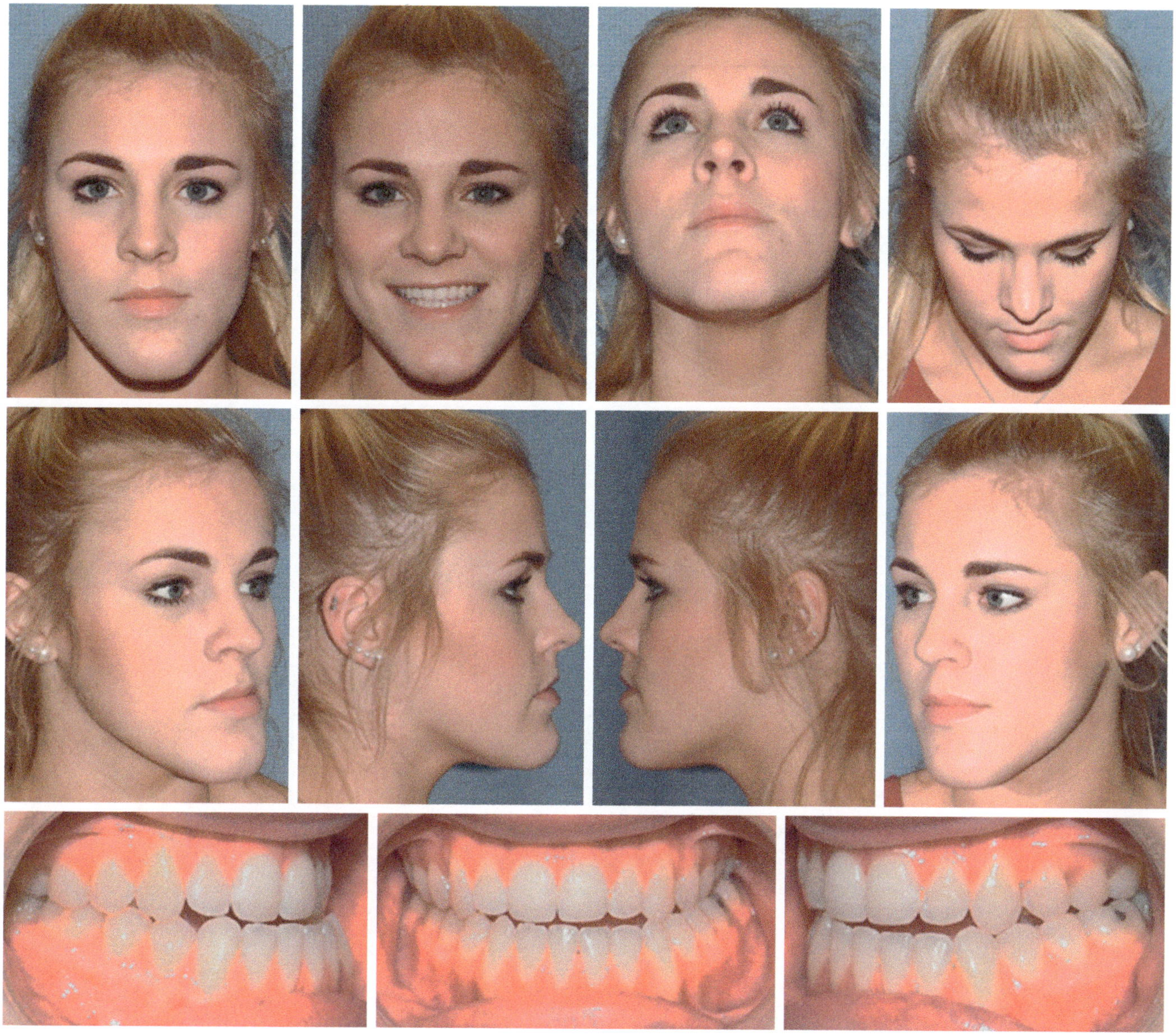

Case 3 Figure 1

Case 3: Mandibular Asymmetry

This is a 23-year-old female who presented with a prognathic, asymmetric mandible. In the preoperative clinical photographs there is a mild concavity to the facial profile, with an elongated and widened lower facial third and chin. The chin point is deviated to the left, as is the dental midline. The maxillary dental midline is also left of the facial midline. The left posterior dentition has a slight crossbite, and there is a negative overjet (Figure 1). The patient did not feel that the mandible was continually growing/deviating, and this was confirmed with a bone scan. Postoperatively at the one-year follow-up examination after undergoing Le Fort I advancement with yaw correction, mandibular setback via bilateral sagittal split osteotomies, osseous genioplasty with vertical reduction, and fat grafting, there are now proportionate facial thirds and fifths. There is a slight convexity of the facial profile with a shortened vertical height of the chin. The dental and skeletal midlines are now coincident, with a class I molar relationship. There is improved fullness in the malar region bilaterally. Appropriate overbite and overjet is now evident (Figure 2).

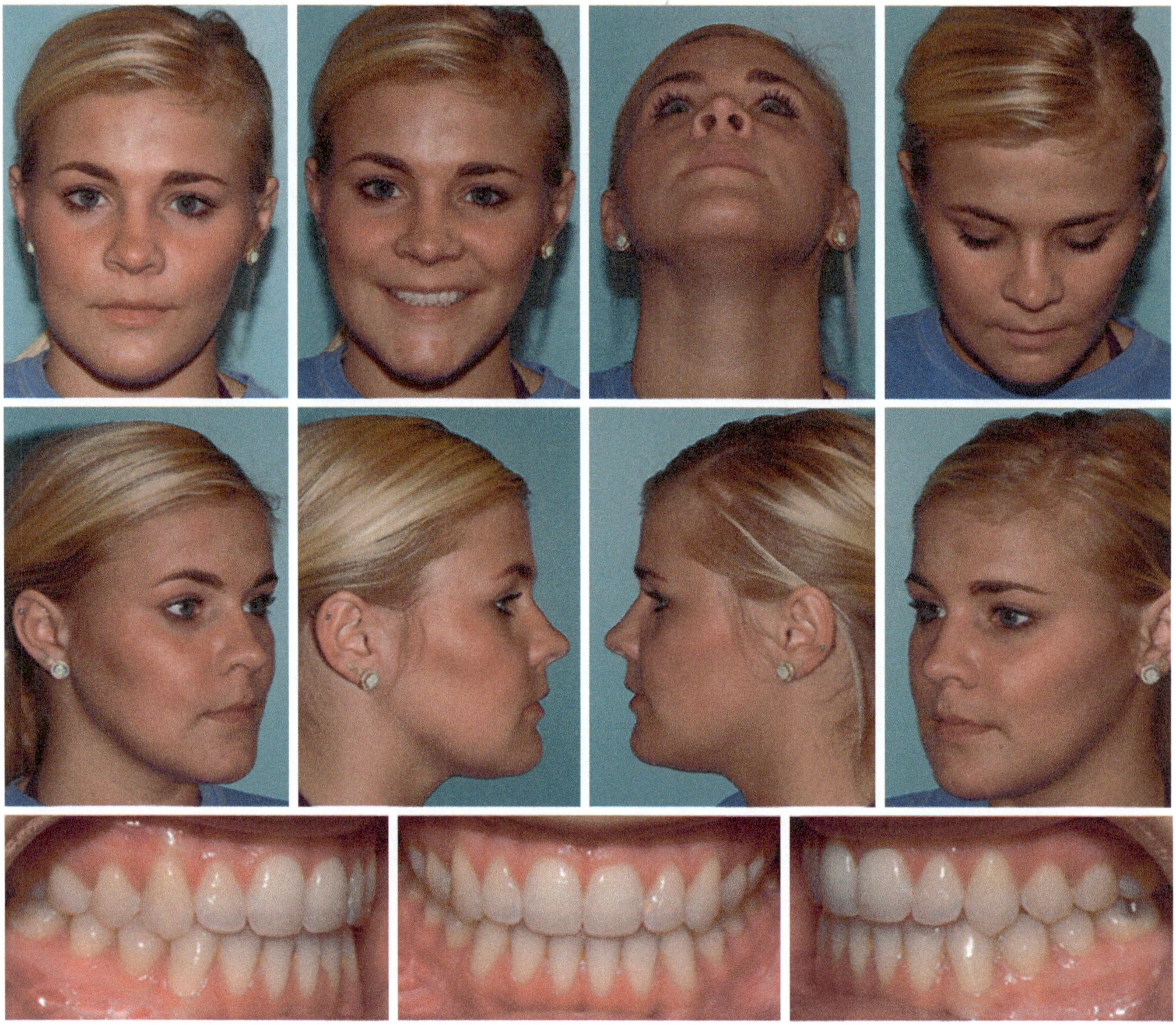

Case 3 Figure 2

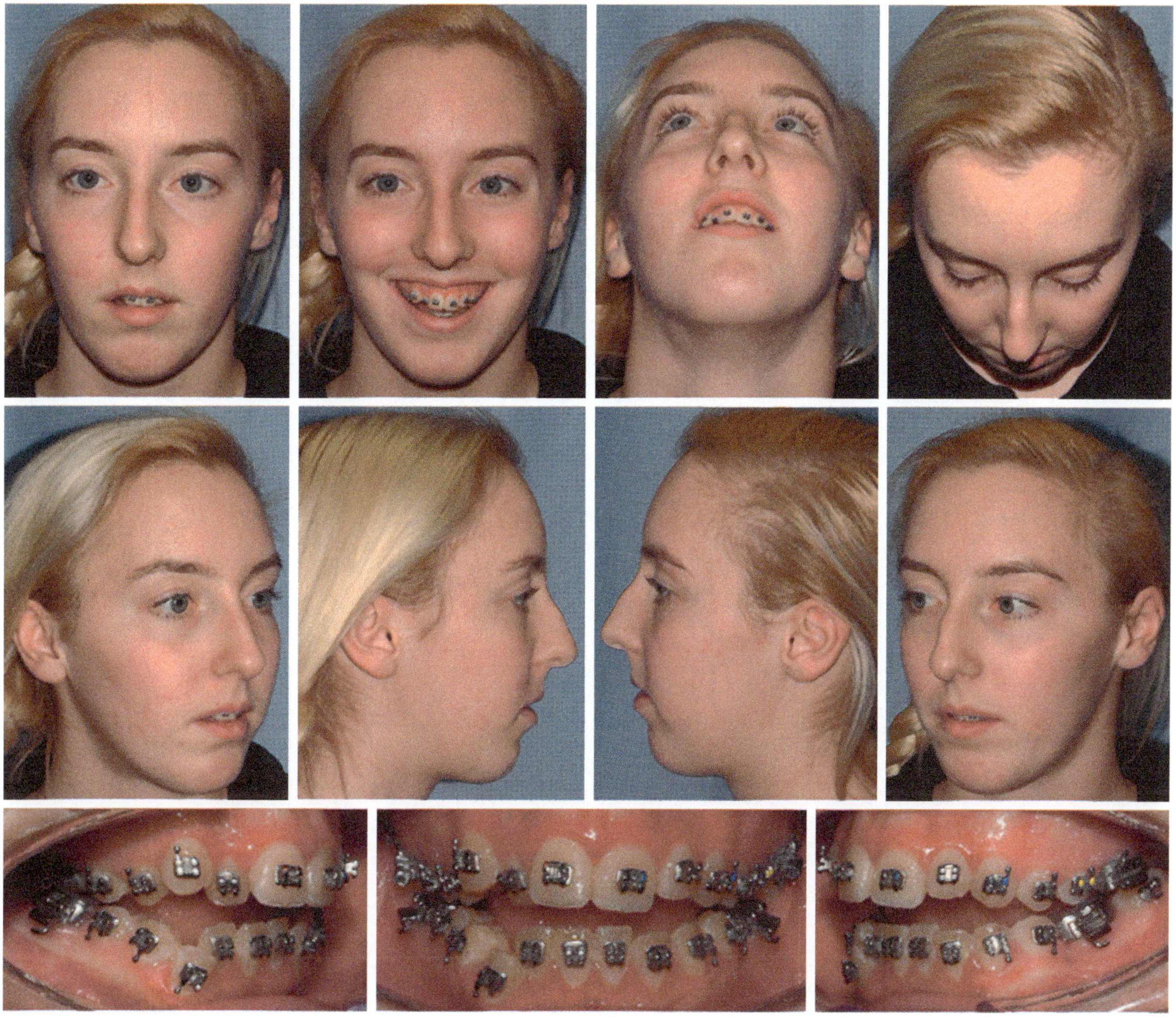

Case 4 Figure 1

Case 4: Maxillary Transverse Deficiency

This is a 17-year-old female who presented with complaints of difficulty with chewing and nasal breathing. Preoperative photos demonstrate an overall convex facial profile with mild vertical maxillary excess, an increased nasolabial angle, and a prominent nasal dorsum. There is excessive tooth show at rest and with smiling. The dental and facial midlines are coincident. Occlusal photographs display an anterior open bite, posterior cross bite, and class II molar relationship. There is crowding of the dental arch on the maxilla and mandible (Figure 1). At one year postoperatively from a segmental Le Fort I and bilateral sagittal split advancement, and genioplasty with fat grafting, as well as staged septorhinoplasty, you can appreciate a softer facial convexity with a smaller nasolabial angle. There is added fullness to the malar region, which was previously flat. The nasal dorsum is now straighter with a slight supratip break and symmetry of the dorsal esthetic lines. There is much less tooth and gingiva show at rest and with smiling. The maxillary and mandibular dental arches are well aligned and coincident with the facial midline, and there is a class I molar relationship (Figure 2).

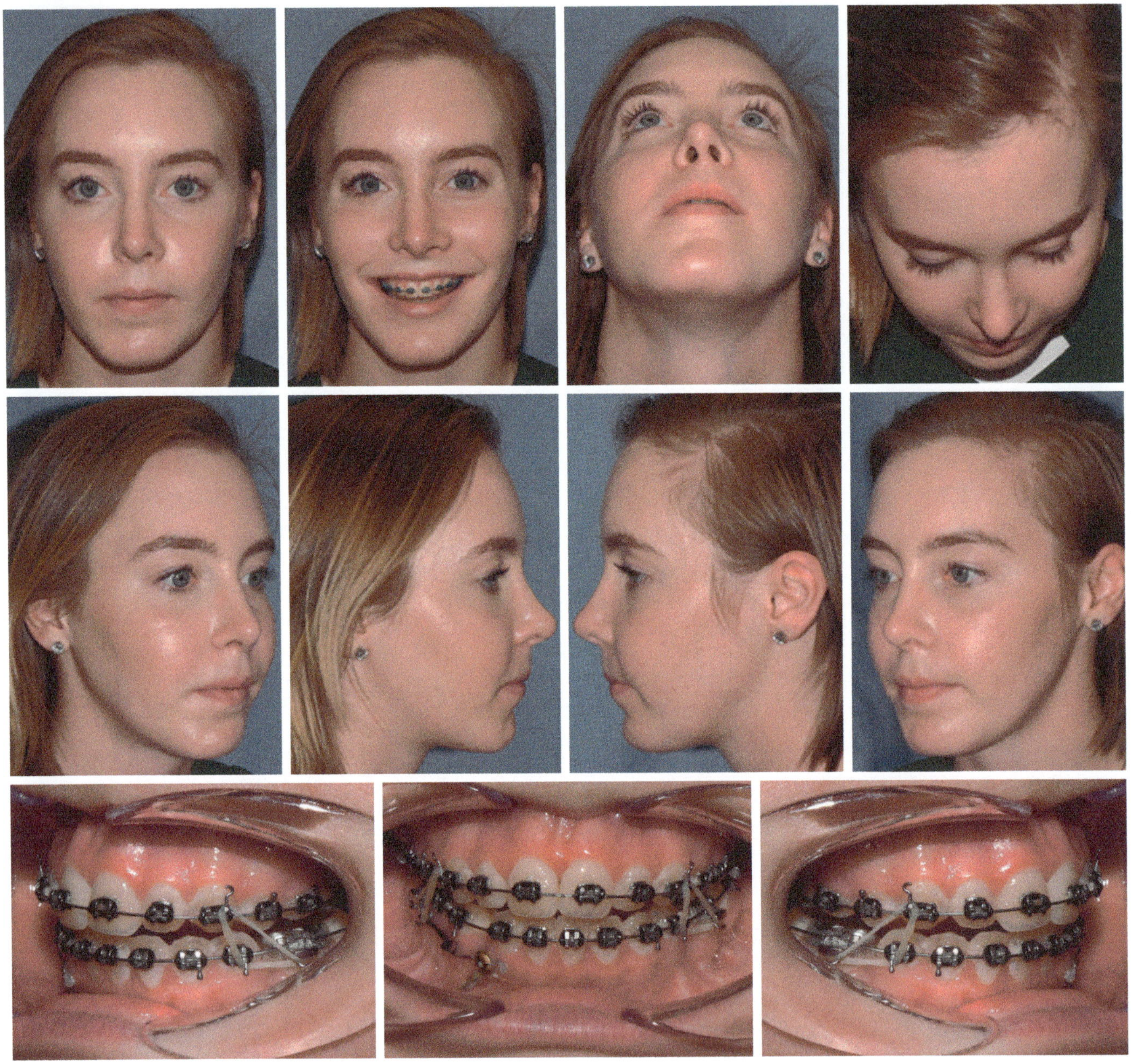

Case 4 Figure 2

Special Considerations

There are numerous physiological conditions other than dentofacial abnormalities that may require surgical correction with conventional orthognathic techniques. *Condylar hyperplasia* is a condition that causes asymmetric growth of the mandible. Condylar hyperplasia involves increased activity within the mandibular condyle growth center. This can cause deviation of the mandible, as well as development of an occlusal cant and open bite. The workup of this condition involves the conventional workup used for patients with dentofacial deformities, as well as a bone scan, or 99m-technetium scintigraphy[30] (Fig. 21.16). This scan can locate increased metabolic activity and uptake of the tracer within an overactive mandibular condyle, recording this value as a percentage that can be compared to the contralateral size. Within our group, a delta of greater than 10% between the condyles is an indication to perform a high condylectomy on the hyperactive side in order to cause cessation in growth prior to performing conventional orthognathic surgery for correction of the resultant dentofacial deformity. An alternative to high condylectomy is to simply wait for "burnout" of the overactive condylar growth center to occur and follow up with repeat bone scans.[31]

Patients diagnosed with *obstructive sleep apnea* are now being managed with orthognathic techniques as a first line treatment for severe symptoms. Many large academic centers evaluate these patients as part of a multidisciplinary team, and a polysomnogram is often ordered early in the workup of sleep apnea. The apnea–hypopnea index is a frequently referenced value when considering the severity of obstructive sleep apnea, with values ranging from 5 to 15 being mild disease,

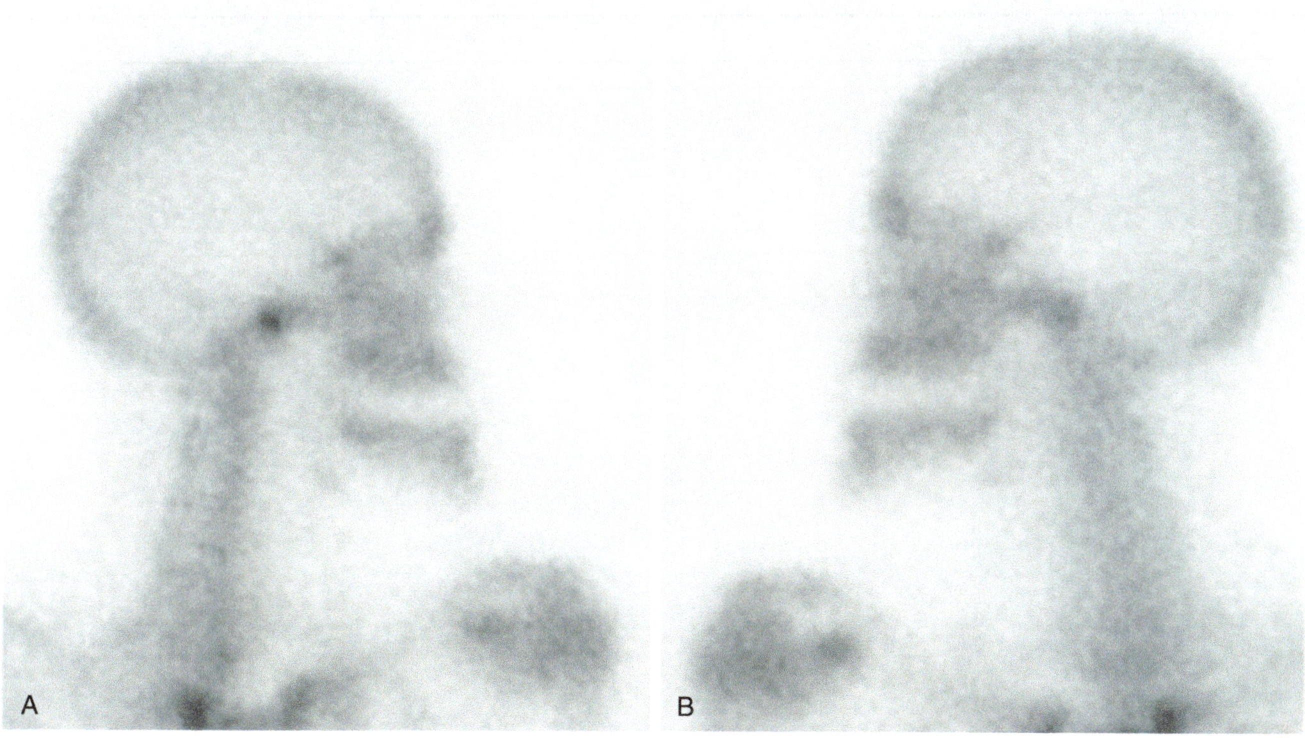

• **Fig. 21.16** 99m-Technetium bone scan. The right mandibular condyle demonstrates increased uptake (A) in comparison to the left side (B).

16 to 30 moderate, 31 and beyond being severe. Previously, patients diagnosed with obstructive sleep apnea underwent phased surgical treatment, with phase I protocols involving soft tissue procedures such as tonsillectomy, septoplasty, uvulopalatopharyngoplasty, and hyoid suspension, and phase II procedures involving maxillomandibular advancement and tracheostomy. Now, maxillomandibular advancement has become an initial surgical intervention for patients with severe obstruction. This is due to the demonstrable increase in airway volume that can be seen on postoperative three-dimensional volumetric analysis when advancing the maxilla and mandible anteriorly as a single unit.[32]

Cleft orthognathic surgery is another special consideration that must be managed in a manner separate from traditional jaw surgery. Patients with a previously corrected cleft lip and/or palate often have significant scarring that limits midfacial growth. Their common presentation is that of a retruded, hypoplastic maxilla with a subsequent class III skeletal profile. Orthognathic surgery with these patients is sometimes performed prior to cessation of skeletal growth for psychosocial regions, although relapse can certainly occur in a manner not different than that with non-cleft patients. Maxillary advancement within this cohort of patients can improve nasal tip and lip support, as well as correct their dental malocclusion. The alteration in airflow can sometimes be detrimental, though, as velopharyngeal incompetence can occur, resulting in hypernasal speech. It is also important to note if the patient has had a posterior pharyngeal flap in the past, as this can further limit anterior movement of the maxilla and may necessitate division prior to orthognathic surgery. Relapse rates have been shown to be more significant with cleft patients, especially with greater movements. In the rare event that a very significant anterior maxillary movement is necessary, distraction osteogenesis can be considered. Vascular compromise to the maxilla is also a concern, as the multiply-operated midface has aberrant vascular inflow that must be addressed cautiously.[33]

Rhinoplasty is an adjunct that can be considered with orthognathic surgery. Movements of the maxilla can alter the overall morphology of the nose. Anatomically, the caudal septum attaches to the anterior nasal spine. When performing osteotomies at the Le Fort I level, the caudal septum is first separated from its attachment to the anterior nasal spine, as well as the maxillary crest and vomer. After the distal segment of the osteotomized maxilla is moved into its new position, the septum should be reattached to the anterior nasal spine and passively seated on the maxillary crest and vomer. Formal rhinoplasty should be delayed until at least 6 months after maxillary orthognathic surgery is performed. It certain instances, such as mandibular surgery only, concomitant rhinoplasty can be performed to achieve a more esthetic, harmonious facial structure.[34,35]

GENIOPLASTY

Introduction

Genioplasty is a powerful tool in the surgeon's armamentarium. It is a procedure that can be used as an adjunct or a standalone treatment for refinement of the chin[36] (Fig. 21.17). The goals of this procedure are both functional and

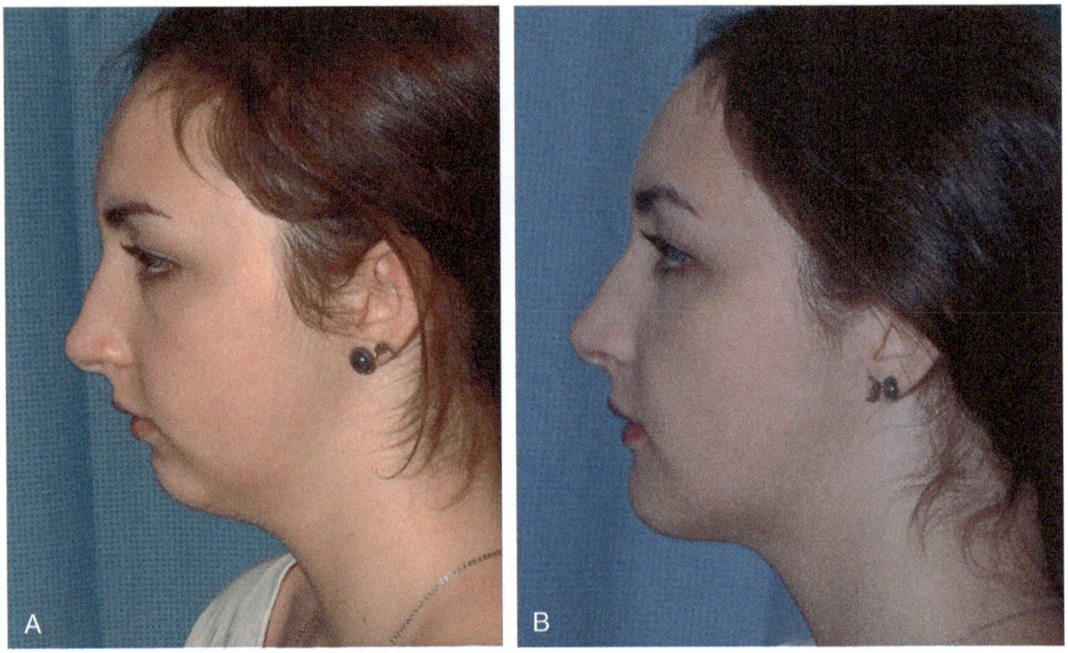

• **Fig. 21.17** (A) Preoperative and (B) postoperative photos in the lateral view of a patient with microgenia who underwent genioplasty as an adjunctive surgical procedure to augment the chin region.

esthetic, and the ramifications of each should govern the approach to surgical management of the mentum. This technique was first considered in the mid-20th century and has subsequently become a commonly performed procedure by facial surgeons. A thorough understanding of the surgical anatomy is paramount, as is an appropriate workup, including an evaluation of the bony foundation, dental occlusion, soft tissue overlay, and upper airway dimensions. Definitive surgical management of the mental region is then undertaken by way of either an osseous genioplasty, using osteotomies and/or contouring to reposition and reshape the chin, or placement of an alloplastic implant to augment the region. Appropriate patient selection and detailed surgical planning will lead to a satisfactory, long-lasting result.

Surgical Anatomy

The chin can be defined by its location in both the frontal and lateral views.[37] There are several cephalometric and anthropometric landmarks that define it when viewing from the lateral profile, beginning with the pogonion (most anterior projection of the mandible), menton (the most anterior, inferior aspect of the mandible), and gnathion (midpoint between the pogonion and menton). It is also defined by the labiomental sulcus (crease where the lower lip is at its most posterior, inferior point in the lateral view). The cervicomental (bisecting lines drawn that involve the anterior neck and inferior border of the mandible) and labiomental (bisecting lines drawn that involve the lower lip and anterior chin) angles can also be measured when studying the chin, as obtuse angles with these landmarks are often see in patients with a hypoplastic chin. In the frontal view, the height of the lower face is often measured when observing the length of the chin. This can be objectively measured when taking the lower facial third (subnasale to menton) and dividing it into the upper third (subnasale to labii superioris) and lower two-thirds (labii inferioris to menton).

There are numerous muscle attachments of clinical importance when observing the mental region and planning surgery. The numerous muscles important in the function and support of the tongue insert here, including the genioglossus, geniohyoid, and anterior belly of the digastric. The genial tubercle is a surgical landmark when determining the location of these attachments. The mylohyoid muscle inserts along the inferior border of the mandible and constitutes the structural support of the floor of the mouth. The platysma muscle, important for facial expression and tightening of the neck, inserts cephalically at the inferior mandibular border. Facially, the mentalis muscle is attached along the anterior aspect of the mandible in the chin region and functions with lower lip movement and oral competence. There is also a fat pad located medial to the mentalis muscle, and this structure provides additional volume/projection to the chin region. It is necessary to appropriately resuspend the mentalis and fat pad after genioplasty so as to avoid chin ptosis, a very complex esthetic deformity to correct.

Of clinical importance when planning genioplasty is the location of the sensory nerves of the mandible and the teeth. The mental foramen is a bony landmark that can be observed both clinically and radiographically, and this is where the mental nerve exits the mandible and enters the soft tissue overlying the chin. The nerve can loop anteriorly and inferiorly prior to exiting through this bony window, so it is important not to plan osteotomies directly along the margins of the foramen in these locations as it could put the nerve at risk for injury. The branches of the alveolar nerve that innervate the teeth also need to be preserved, as sectioning of them can lead to their compromise. Leaving approximately 5 mm between the apices of the teeth and the osteotomy should be sufficient to avoid and preserve the neurovascular bundle.

Indications for Genioplasty

Genioplasty is frequently considered for patients that have an overly deficient or prominent chin. The evaluation is performed by looking at the patient in all dimensions. From a frontal view, the chin width should transition smoothly from the body of the mandible to a gentle arc at the midline. Men tend to favor a wider, more angular jaw shape in this dimension, whereas women prefer a narrower, smoothly-tapering shape. The width of the chin can further be evaluated from the worm's-eye view. The midpoint of the chin should also be coincident with the facial midline (drawn as a perpendicular from the glabella and through a midpoint between the medial canthi, involving the nasal tip and trough of cupid's bow). Chin length can be appreciated in both the frontal and lateral views, and it should be considered with reference to the lower lip length. This dimension is approximately two-thirds of the lower facial third, measured from the stomion inferioris to the menton. Also visible from the lateral view is the chin position in the anteroposterior dimension. Numerous methods evaluate this, although a simplified way to view the chin in this dimension is a vertical line from the soft tissue nasion through the pogonion. Men tend to favor a more anterior position of the chin in this dimension, such as a flatter facial profile ensues, whereas women prefer a softer, convex curvature.

Also, when evaluating a patient for genioplasty, it is of vital importance to first determine if a dental malocclusion is present. If a patient has a dental malocclusion that is not correctable with orthodontics alone (i.e., maxillomandibular discrepancy that does not allow for dental compensation), then a patient should be considered for orthognathic surgery. Other than functional complications that can arise form an uncorrected malocclusion, the esthetic result can also be compromised when operating on the chin only when the entire jaw structure is misaligned. A good example of this is the patient with a convex, class II facial profile with microgenia. This is often accompanied by a nasal deformity that includes a downturned nasal tip and prominent dorsal hump. When the maxilla and mandible are left in a retruded position and only the chin is augmented/advanced/lengthened with or without a rhinoplasty to correct the aforementioned irregularities, the patient will still appear to have projection in the lower facial third. This is typically due to the lack of support from the retruded dentoalveolar units of the maxilla and mandible that could have been improved with maxillomandibular advancement. Methods to augment and provide lower facial/lip support (fillers, implants) in these circumstances are typically insufficient and do not provide a natural contour and result.

In line with the consideration of the occlusion and overall maxillomandibular relationship is an evaluation of the upper airway dimension relative to obstructive sleep apnea. Indications do exist where a patient may have an appropriate anteroposterior position of the maxilla and mandible, yet still have upper airway obstruction of clinical significance. Objectively, this can be identified on a lateral cephalogram with a below normal measurement of the posterior airway space (measured at the vertical level of the mandibular angle/inferior mandibular border), as well as on three-dimensional analysis of the upper airway with computed tomography showing a pattern on constriction at this level. In these instances, genioplasty can be performed to advance the genioglossal muscles, thus alleviating the upper airway obstruction.

Microgenia can be managed by two main modalities: osseous genioplasty with osteotomies to reposition the bone, or augmentation genioplasty with an alloplastic material. Osseous genioplasty is best performed via a transoral route. Osteotomies are created based upon the final position where the chin needs to be located. For example, when a straight anterior movement is necessary, a flatter, more horizontal osteotomy Is performed. If the chin needs to be advanced and shortened, a more oblique osteotomy can be developed. In instances where advancement and lengthening is needed, the osteotomy design is fashioned in a way so to minimize the final bone gap. With gaps less than 5 mm, the bone can be left to fill naturally or supplemented with bone allograft. With greater bone gaps, corticocancellous bone should be interposed. Titanium plates and screws are then used for fixation. When planning to use an alloplast, the most commonly used material is porous polyethylene.[38] Traditionally, silicone was used, although this has been shown to cause bone resorption and a tendency to shift over time. It is best to place the implant via an extraoral approach so that implant contamination (from oral flora) can be minimized. Alloplastic implants can provide appropriate augmentation in all dimensions, including width and anterior, vertical projection. They can also be further contoured with a knife or high-speed bur to customize them to the patient prior to fixating them with screws to the underlying bone.

Macrogenia is treated by performing osseous genioplasty with osteotomies to reposition the bone, contouring by way of resecting and shaving away gross amounts of bone, or a combination of the two. The osteotomy design is planned similarly to the aforementioned method for patients with microgenia. When a patient requires reduction that is mostly vertical, then a flatter, more horizontal osteotomy can be created. If reduction is needed in the vertical and anteroposterior dimension, then a more oblique osteotomy is used. The differential in length that needs to be reduced should be marked and the bone removed from the native mandible after the initial osteotomy is performed to separate the distal segment of bone. The distal bone can then be approximated to the native mandible and subsequently fixated with plates and screws. When there is excess width of the mandible in the frontal view, the excess bone can either be osteotomized and removed, or excised with a high-speed round bur. All of these maneuvers for reduction can also be performed by this method of bone excision and contouring without osteotomy and repositioning.

Surgical Technique

The intra/transoral approach to genioplasty is undertaken by first injecting local anesthesia with vasoconstrictor to the labial vestibule of the mandible. An incision is then designed approximately 5 mm into the unattached mucosa from canine to canine. This will allow for a 5-mm cuff of myomucosal tissue to remain for closure of the wound, as well as stay protected from injuring the mental nerve by incising between the mental foramen, respectively. A 15 blade followed by electrocautery is then used to incise and deepen the incision through mucosa and submucosa, down to the underlying mentalis muscle and associated fat pad. It is important to transect the mentalis in such a way as to leave a significant portion of muscle and fascia to anchor the resected mentalis to upon wound closure. Failure to do so can result in chin ptosis ("witch's chin deformity"). Once deep to the mentalis, the periosteum is incised and the subperiosteal plane is dissected from the anterior mandible. With the elevator positioned on the inferior border of the mandible (confirmed extraorally with the nonworking hand), subperiosteal dissection is continued posteriorly along the body. This dissection is then carefully extended cephalically as to identify the mental foramen bilaterally. The landmark for this is between the first and second mandibular premolars. Once located, the mental nerve can be found exiting each foramen and entering the buccal mucosa. Dissection can be performed cephalic to the foramen and connected to the caudal extent of the caudal dissection in this plane. While protecting the nerve, submucosal dissection can also be performed, and the incision can be safely lengthened, as needed. Once the surgeon can visualize the mental foramen and the anterior mandible is degloved to the inferior border of the mandible, the osteotomies can then be marked. The vertical midline is scribed into the mandible, as is the horizontal osteotomy. The bone cut is then made with a reciprocating saw, beginning laterally and working across the mandible. Once complete, the distal segment of bone will be freely mobile and attached to the genioglossal, mylohyoid, and platysma muscles. The bone can then be repositioned and secured with titanium plates and screws (Fig. 21.18). Additional osteoplasty can be performed, as needed, to optimize symmetry and contour. Through this access, further caudal dissection can also be undertaken to access the neck and perform platysmaplasty, should the case warrant it.[39] The wound is irrigated with normal saline. Bone graft is then placed within any bone gaps. The option to combine bone allograft with fibrin has also been described to provide excellent results.[40] The mentalis is carefully reapproximated with numerous absorbable braided sutures in a horizontal mattress or figure-of-8 fashion (Fig. 21.19). The mucosal layer is then closed with absorbable monofilament suture in a running fashion. A pressure dressing can be placed on the skin overlying the chin region to assist in maintaining the soft tissue in the appropriate vector for 3–5 days postoperatively.

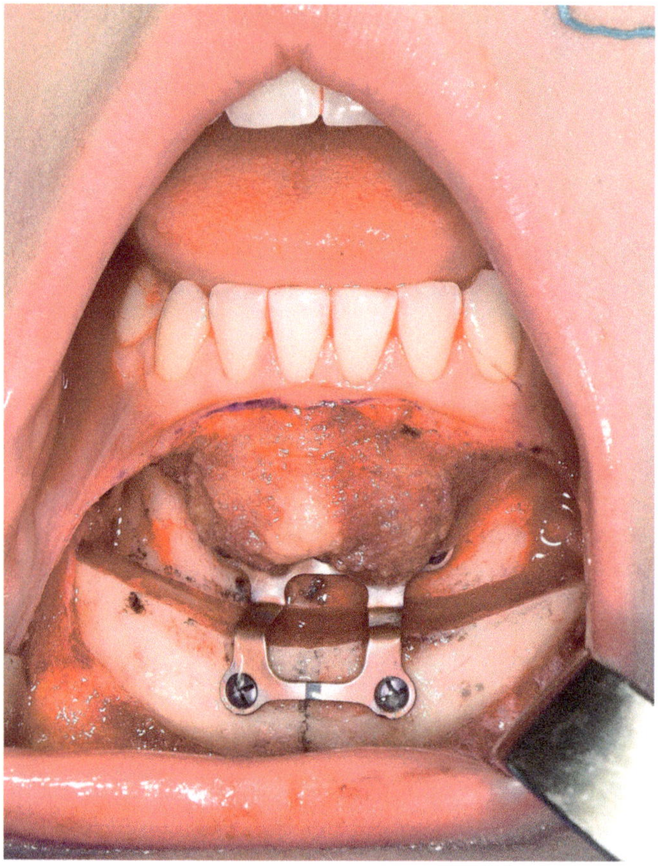

• **Fig. 21.18** Intraoperative photo of the chin after a traditional osteotomy to perform osseous genioplasty. The distal bony segment has been repositioned and secured in its new position with titanium plates and screws.

The extraoral approach is initiated by injecting local anesthesia with vasoconstrictor to the submental crease. A 15 blade is then used to incise through skin and subcutaneous tissue until the platysma is identified. Dissection is then continued in this suprafascial plane until the mandible is encountered. The periosteum along the inferior border is then incised down to bone, and subperiosteal dissection is carried out along the inferior border of the mandible, cephalad to the level of the mental foramen bilaterally. An alloplastic implant is then placed into this pocket, first soaking it in an antibiotic-infused solution. It is helpful to use porous polyethylene implants that allow the surgeon to separate them at the midline, thus facilitating placement of one half of the implant at a time. The skin can then be redraped temporarily, and the contours of the mandible can then be visualized. If necessary, modification of this type of implant can now be performed with a knife or high-speed round bur. Prior to final implant placement, the wound should be irrigated with normal saline. The implant is then secured to the mandible, typically with two screws per side. The pocket overlying the implant and deep dermal layers is

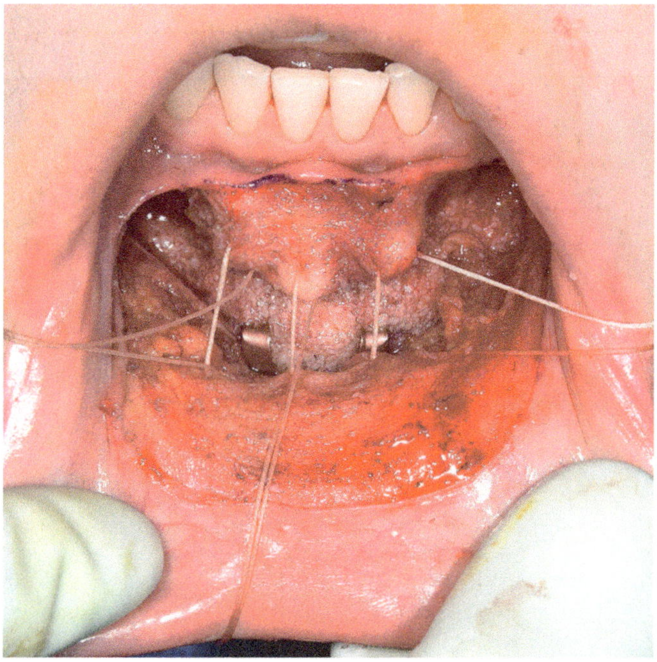

• **Fig. 21.19** Intraoperative photo of the genioplasty surgical site after the distal bony segment has been repositioned and secured with titanium plates and screws. Bone allograft mixed with fibrin has been placed in the bone gaps and used to further contour the chin. Absorbable, braided suture is placed in a mattressing-fashion to resuspend the mentalis muscle.

then closed with a resorbable braided suture, respectively, followed by a subcuticular absorbable monofilament suture. Similarly, a compression dressing can be placed on the skin as outlined in the prior section. A short course of antibiotics can be given postoperatively, in addition to a single intravenous dose prior to incision, when placing the alloplastic chin implant.

Complications

Complications that can occur with genioplasty include wound infection, bleeding (due to osteotomized bone, occasionally-injured attached musculature, and inferior alveolar vessels), hardware failure and/or infection, esthetic deformity (chin ptosis, contour irregularities at the site of the mandibular osteotomy), lip and chin numbness (stretch and/or transection of the mental nerve), and mentalis strain from excessive augmentation of the chin region.

References

1. Aziz SR, Simon P. Hullihen and the origin of orthognathic surgery. *J Oral Maxillofac Surg*. 2004;62:1303–1307.
2. Blair VP. Report of a case of double resection for the correction of protrusion of the mandible. *Dent Cosmos*. 1906;48:817–820.
3. Steinhauser EW. Historical development of orthognathic surgery. *J Cranio-Maxillo-Fac Surg*. 1996;24:195–204.
4. Wolfe SA. Gunther Cohn-Stock MS, D.D.S., father of maxillary orthognathic surgery. *J Cranio-Maxillo-Fac Surg*. 1989;17:331–334.
5. Kazanjian VH. Surgical treatment of mandibular prognathism. *Int J Orthodontia Oral Surg Radiogr*. 1932;18:1224–1239.
6. Dingman R. Surgical correction of mandibular prognathism, an improved method. *Am J Orthodont Oral Surg*. 1944;30:683–692.
7. Hofer O. Die vertikale Osteotomie des einseitig verkarzten aufsteigenden Unterkieferastes. *Z Stomat*. 1936;34.
8. Gillies H, Harrison SH. Operative correction by osteotomy of recessed malar maxillary compound in a case of oxycephaly. *Br J Plast Surg*. 1950;3:123–127.
9. Tessier P. The definitive plastic surgical treatment of the severe facial deformities of craniofacial dysostosis. Crouzon's and Apert's diseases. *Plast Reconstr Surg*. 1971;48:419–442.
10. Trauner R, Obwegeser H. Zur Operationstechnik bei der Progenie und anderen Unterkieferanomalien. *Dtsch Zahn Mund Kieferheilkd*. 1955;23:1–26.
11. Obwegeser H. The indications for surgical correction of mandibular deformity by the sagittal splitting technique. *Br J Oral Surg*. 1964;1:157–171.
12. Obwegeser HL. Surgical correction of small or retrodisplaced maxillae: the "dish-face" deformity. *Plast Reconstr Surg*. 1969;43:351–365.
13. Converse JM, Horowitz SL. The surgical-orthodontic approach to the treatment of dentofacial deformities. *Am J Orthod*. 1969;55:217–243.
14. Bell RB. A history of orthognathic surgery in North America. *J Oral Maxillofac Surg*. 2018;76:2466–2481.
15. Nelson SJ. *Wheeler's Dental Anatomy, Physiology, and Occlusion*. Philadelphia: Saunders; 2015.
16. Tolleth H. Concepts for the plastic surgeon from art and sculpture. *Clin Plast Surg*. 1987;14:585–598.
17. Powell N, Humphreys B. *Proportions of the Aesthetic Face*. Vol. 1. New York: Thième; 1984.
18. Legan HL, Burstone CJ. Soft tissue cephalometric analysis for orthognathic surgery. *J Oral Surg*. 1980;38:744–751.
19. Downs WB. The role of cephalometrics in orthodontic case analysis and diagnosis. *Am J Orthod*. 1952;38:162–182.
20. Steiner CC. Cephalometrics in clinical practice. *Angle Orthod*. 1959;29:8–29.
21. Farkas LG, Tompson B, Phillips JH, et al. Comparison of anthropometric and cephalometric measurements of the adult face. *J Craniofac Surg*. 1999;10:18–25; discussion 26.
22. Budai M, Farkas LG, Tompson B, et al. Relation between anthropometric and cephalometric measurements and proportions of the face of healthy young white adult men and women. *J Craniofac Surg*. 2003;14:154–161; discussion 162–153.
23. Proffit WR, Fields HW, Larson B, et al. *Contemporary Orthodontics*. St. Louis: Mosby; 2018.
24. Moss ML. A theoretical analysis of the functional matrix. *Acta Biotheor*. 1968;18:195–202.
25. Moore KL, Persaud TVN, Torchia MG. *The Developing Human: Clinically Oriented Embryology*. Philadelphia: Saunders; 2016.
26. Netter FH, Machado CAG, Hansen JT, et al. *Atlas of Human Anatomy*. Philadelphia: Saunders; 2018.
27. Le Fort R. *Revue Chirurgio*. Vol. 23. 1901:208.
28. Karp NS, McCarthy JG, Schreiber JS, et al. Membranous bone lengthening: a serial histological study. *Ann Plast Surg*. 1992;29:2–7.
29. McCarthy JG, Stelnicki EJ, Grayson BH. Distraction osteogenesis of the mandible: a ten-year experience. *Semin Orthod*. 1999;5:3–8.
30. Beirne OR, Leake DL. Technetium 99m pyrophosphate uptake in a case of unilateral condylar hyperplasia. *J Oral Surg*. 1980;38:385–386.

31. Wolford LM, Mehra P, Reiche-Fischel O, et al. Efficacy of high condylectomy for management of condylar hyperplasia. *Am J Orthod Dentofac Orthoped.* 2002;121:136–151.
32. Epstein LJ, Kristo D, Strollo PJ, et al. Clinical guideline for the evaluation, management and long-term care of obstructive sleep apnea in adults. *J Clin Sleep Med.* 2009;5:263–276.
33. Cheung LK, Chua HDP, Hägg MB. Cleft maxillary distraction versus orthognathic surgery: clinical morbidities and surgical relapse. *Plast Reconstr Surg.* 2006;118:996–1008.
34. Steinbacher DM. Nasal considerations and orthognathic surgery. In: Steinbacher DM, ed. *Aesthetic Orthognathic Surgery and Rhinoplasty.* New York: Wiley–Blackwell; 2019:421–445.
35. Steinbacher DM. Rhinoplasty and orthognathic surgery. In: Steinbacher DM, ed. *Aesthetic Orthognathic Surgery and Rhinoplasty.* New York: Wiley–Blackwell; 2019:447–487.
36. Walker ME, Sawh-Martinez R, Steinbacher DM. Osseous genioplasty. In: Steinbacher DM, ed. *Aesthetic Orthognathic Surgery and Rhinoplasty.* New York: Wiley–Blackwell; 2019:517–533.
37. May J, Steinbacher DM. Chin and submental aesthetics. In: Steinbacher DM, ed. *Aesthetic Orthognathic Surgery and Rhinoplasty.* New York: Wiley–Blackwell; 2019:289–329.
38. Shah A, Steinbacher DM. Alloplastic facial augmentation. In: Steinbacher DM, ed. *Aesthetic Orthognathic Surgery and Rhinoplasty.* New York: Wiley–Blackwell; 2019:559–572.
39. Wu RT, Timberlake AT, Bruckman KC, et al. Concurrent platysmaplasty and genioplasty using a novel intraoral approach. *Plast Reconstr Surg.* 2020;145(1):80–83.
40. Kim YA, Steinbacher DM. Demineralized bone–fibrin sandwich for genioplasty. *Aesthetic Plast Surg.* 2014;38(4):755–758.

22

Facial Reanimation

JONATHAN I. LECKENBY AND ADRIAAN O. GROBBELAAR

For videos accompanying this chapter see ExpertConsult.com. See inside cover for access details.

Introduction

Facial paralysis presents a complex challenge to the reconstructive surgeon. Since Sir Charles Bell first described the course of the facial nerve in 1821, our understanding has led to the development of the vast array of surgical options used to treat patients with facial paralysis.

Sir Harold Gillies stated in 1919 that the aim of surgical reconstruction is to restore the normal form; this primarily aims to preserve function and then subsequently address the esthetics. The fundamental problem when considering facial paralysis is that there is currently no conceivable way to restore the 17 muscles of facial expression successfully. The second challenge facing the surgeon is that no patient is the same as another. Not only the etiology behind facial paralysis dictates which operations are available, the age group, the anatomy available and, most importantly, what the patient wants all make the decision-making process vital.

The presentation of facial nerve paralysis also adds to the conundrum, ranging from an isolated marginal branch palsy to a complete bilateral palsy. The approach to the management of any patient with facial paralysis should be to break the face down into three units: the forehead, the eyes, and the mid- and lower face. In a young child, the skin quality is far superior to that of an elderly patient and thus problems encountered are different to the adult population. Frequently, there is minimal asymmetry at rest and therefore focus needs to be directed at restoring dynamic function. In the elderly patient, skin elasticity is poorer and asymmetry at rest may be strikingly obvious and static treatment options may yield the desired outcome.

What is the importance of facial palsy reconstruction? This is not cancer surgery and patient survival is not the main outcome being measured. The impact facial paralysis has on an individual can be devastating and can be broken down into functional and psychological factors. If a patient is unable to close their eye and the cornea is insensate, the globe will dry leading to ulceration and ultimately blindness. Diminished oral continence and poor speech are other functional problems encountered. A child who is unable to smile or convey emotion effectively may be subject to bullying and psychological trauma and an adult with profound asymmetry at rest make be mistaken for being angry by another individual, causing the patient to become socially reclusive.[1,2]

The aim of this chapter is to give the reader a strategy on how to tackle facial paralysis. The anatomy of the facial nerve and other important structures of the face will be reviewed as this provides the foundation on which the evolution of surgical techniques have been based. The information provided should enable a surgeon to have a methodical approach to patient management; however, it must be stressed that the information should be used as a guideline and that each patient will require a customized approach to a greater or lesser extent. This makes facial palsy surgery one of the most fascinating and challenging aspects of reconstructive surgery; not only are the technical aspects pushing the limits of modern surgery but the decision-making process is equally as difficult and one must select the correct tools from the surgeon's vast armamentarium to complete the task at hand. To the reconstructive surgeon it combines the epitome of what we seek to achieve: a functional outcome in which one has to consider the esthetic result, as the face is the center of human interaction.

Anatomy of the Facial Nerve

The facial nerve develops embryologically from the second pharyngeal branchial arch, the hyoid arch. The motor division derives from the basal plate of the embryonic pons whilst the sensory division arises from the cranial neural crest. The sensory portion, known as the intermediate nerve, is responsible for supplying taste to the anterior two-thirds of the tongue, secretory and vasomotor fibres to the lacrimal, submandibular, and sublingual glands, the mucous membranes of the nose and mouth, and finally, sensation over the external auditory meatus and posterior skin of the ear. The cortical fibers of the facial nerve arise from the lower third of the motor cortex, passing through the internal capsule and the middle third of the cerebral peduncle to supply the seventh nucleus in the lower pons and is closely related to the abducens and vestobulocochlear nerves. Of clinical importance, the supranuclear innervation is bilateral to the muscles of the forehead and eyes, but only contralateral to the muscles of the lower face; this accounts for the sparing of the forehead muscles in cases of supranuclear lesions in comparison to nuclear or infranuclear lesions. The course of the nerve can be simply divided as follows.

Intracranial Course

As the facial and intermediate nerves leave the brainstem, they course laterally towards the cranium, entering the petrous temporal bone through the internal auditory meatus. Here, within the facial canal, the intermediate nerve forms the geniculate ganglion. After a tortuous course it emerges through the stylomastoid foramen.

Greater superficial petrosal nerve is the first branch given off from the geniculate ganglion within the facial canal, and is responsible for the parasympathetic innervations of multiple glands. The second branch is the nerve to stapedius, providing motor innervations of the stapedius muscle. The final branch is the chorda tympani, responsible for taste sensation in the anterior two-thirds of the tongue.

Extracranial Course

After emerging from the stylomastoid foramen, the facial nerve passes through the parotid gland. The most immediate branch given off is the posterior auricular nerve that innervates the small muscles of the posterior ear and branches to the posterior belly of the digastric and stylohyoid muscles. The nerve divides into temporo-facial and cervico-facial divisions approximately 1.3 cm from the stylomastoid foramen. A useful clinical landmark for locating the trunk is at a point slightly anterior and inferior to the tip of the tragus[3]; the nerve typically lies between 1 cm and 1.5 cm deep to this. The nerve separates into the five principal branches at the pes anserinus.

The temporal branch courses cranially to cross the zygomatic arch within the superficial musculoaponeurotic system (SMAS), lying deep to frontalis but superficial to the deep temporalis fascia. The temporal branch is responsible for the innervation of frontalis, orbicularis oculi, and corrugators supercilii. An important efferent limb from this branch is responsible for the corneal reflex.

The zygomatic branch proceeds cranially, angled towards the lateral angle of the orbit. Here it supplies the orbicularis oculii.

The buccal branch is the largest branch and passes forward below the orbit and divides into deep and superficial divisions. The superficial branches lie superficial to the SMAS and supply procerus. The deep branches pass beneath zygomaticus and quadratus labii superioris, supplying them both. Further deeper branches go on to supply buccinator and orbicularis oris.

The marginal mandibular branch courses beneath the SMAS towards the chin, passing beneath depressor angulis oris (which it supplies). Here it branches to innervate the depressor labii inferioris and mentalis.

The cervical branch is the most inferior branch and passes towards the neck over the mandible beneath the SMAS. It primarily innervates the platysma.

There is much variability in the branching patterns of the facial nerve[4] and numerous interconnections between them, and caution must always be exerted when making a surgical approach to expose the nerve.[4–6]

There are 23 facial muscles, of which 17 are activated in facial expression. Broadly speaking, the musculature of the face can be divided into superficial and deep as described by Freilinger.[7] The most superficial layer consists of zygomaticus minor and orbicularis oris. The deepest layer consists of buccinator, mentalis, and levator anguli oris, and it is important to note that these three muscles are the only ones to be innervated via their superficial surface; the remaining muscles receive their supply from their deep surface.

Anatomy of Potential Donor Nerves for Facial Reanimation

Whilst discussing the anatomy of the facial nerve it is worth spending some time to consider other local nerves of the face. Frequently, another donor nerve is required when either there is absence of a functioning facial nerve or if it is inappropriate to consider its use. Here, three other potential donor nerves will be considered.

Masseteric Nerve

The masseter is one of the principle muscles of mastication. It arises from the zygomatic arch and the maxilla and inserts into the coronoid process and the ramus of the mandible. The muscle is divided into a superficial and deep portion and is innervated by a branch of the mandibular division of the trigeminal nerve. The masseteric nerve arises from the anterior division of the mandibular nerve which arises from the cranium through the foramen ovale. The masseteric nerve passes laterally in front of the temporomandibular joint lying deep to the temporalis tendon. It crosses the mandibular notch with the masseteric artery and enters the masseter on its deep surface and branches within the muscle, reaching the anterior border. The nerve can be found intraoperatively by delicately spreading the muscle fibres of the masseter which are oriented downwards and backwards superficially, then downwards and forwards in the deep portion of the muscle.[8,9] It is important to isolate suspected branches and use a nerve stimulator to confirm its function.

Hypoglossal Nerve

The hypoglossal nerve is the twelfth cranial nerve and its nucleus is located in the medulla oblongata. It passes through the cranium to emerge from the hypoglossal canal. The extracranial course is closely related to the vagus nerve and passes between the internal carotid artery and jugular vein, lying on the carotid sheath. It passes deep to the posterior belly of the digastric muscle and enters the submandibular region, coursing lateral to the hyoglossus muscle and inferior to the lingual nerve before it branches to innervate the tongue. It innervates all of the muscles of the tongue except palatoglossus, which is innervated by the vagus nerve. When considering using the hypoglossal nerve as a potential donor nerve, it is advocated that a terminal branch is used to minimize any loss of function.

Spinal Accessory Nerve

The spinal accessory nerve is the eleventh cranial nerve and is responsible for the innervation of the sternocleidomastoid and trapezius muscles. The nerve is unlike other cranial nerves in the fact it arises from the upper cervical spinal cord and enters the skull through the foramen magnum. Its intracranial course leads it to emerge from the jugular foramen. In the neck it crosses the internal jugular vein at the level of the posterior belly of digastric muscle and continues to travel caudally, piercing and supplying sternocleidomastoid and then terminating to supply trapezius.

Vascular Supply of the Face

The arterial supply of the face is predominantly via branches of the external carotid artery and the ophthalmic artery. The ophthalmic artery branches to give rise to the supraorbital and supratrochlear arteries to supply the forehead. Consideration here will be given to the branches that arise from the external carotid artery as these are of more practical use when free muscle transfer is proposed. The three main facial arteries most suitable for arterial anastomosis are the facial artery, the superficial temporal artery, and the transverse facial artery.

The facial artery arises in the carotid triangle just distally to the lingual artery behind the ramus of the mandible. It passes deep to the digastric and stylohyoid muscles and along the posterior border of the submandibular gland, superficial to the hypoglossal nerve. At the point of the anteroinferior angle of the masseter it crosses over the body of the mandible and proceeds tortuously towards the angle of the mouth. In the face it branches to give rise to the inferior and superior labial arteries and terminates as the angular artery and the lateral nasal artery.

The superficial temporal artery arises from the external carotid artery when it bifurcates to also give rise to the maxillary artery. The superficial temporal artery originates at the level of the parotid gland behind the neck of the mandible. It then courses cranially just anterior to the tragus, crossing superficially to the zygomatic process, and is covered by the auricularis anterior muscle and a dense fascia. The temporal and zygomatic branches of the facial nerve cross the artery and it is accompanied closely by the auriculotemporal nerve, which lies immediately posteriorly. It terminates by branching to form the parietal and frontal arteries.

The transverse facial artery arises from the superficial temporal artery before it emerges from the parotid gland. It travels transversely across the face, running between the zygomatic arch superiorly and the parotid duct inferiorly superficial to the masseter muscle.

When planning free functional muscle transfer good knowledge of the vascular supply is critical. Facial anatomy is by no means consistent and frequently secondary options are required[10]; in some cases even direct end-to-side anastomosis to the external carotid artery may have to be considered to prevent flap failure. Preoperative assessment with a Doppler can offer the surgeon some reassurance.

Etiology of Facial Paralysis

Congenital

Birth Trauma

There is an incidence of 1.8 out of every 1000 children born with facial nerve paralysis in Northern America.[11] Several factors increase the chance of facial nerve injury during childbirth, including instrumentation, birthweight over 3.5 kg and primigravida status. The exact mechanism of injury is unknown but likely to be caused by traction being placed on the nerve. The prognosis is excellent, with over 90% of children recovering completely without intervention.[12] In the rare case where complete transaction is suspected, surgical exploration may be beneficial.

Möbius Syndrome

Möbius syndrome is characterized by concomitant bilateral facial nerve and abducens nerve (CN VI) palsies. This leads to complete, bilateral facial paralysis leading to extreme difficulty in expressing emotion as well as oral incontinence and social ostracism.

CHARGE Syndrome

CHARGE association was first described in 1981 by Pagon et al[13] and may involve Coloboma, Heart anomalies, choanal Atresia, Retardation of growth and development, Genital and Ear anomalies. Although not all anomalies may be present, at either least four major features or three major and three minor features must be present. The major features are: coloboma, chonal atreisa, cranial nerve abnormalities, and auditory anomalies. The minor features include distinctive facial dysmorphology, facial clefting, tracheoesophageal fistula, congenital heart defects, genitourinary anomalies, developmental delay, and short stature.

Hemifacial Microsomia

Hemifacial microsomia covers a variety of congenital facial anomalies which arise as a lack of development of one side of the face. It is characterized by a hemifacial soft tissue deficiency, the poor development of the mandible, maxilla, and external ear.

With developmental facial palsy patients, the management is best looked after with a multidisciplinary approach. Individual cases may require the input of the cleft, ear or craniofacial surgeon whilst needing ongoing medical support. In these situations careful planning of the timing of procedures is required.

Infectious

Bell's Palsy

Bell's palsy represents 80% of the case load of a facial palsy surgeon. There is no known causative factor, however there is evidence herpes simplex virus plays a role. Incidence is around 30 cases per 100,000 per year, and is slightly higher in pregnant women (45 per 100,000).[14] Eighty percent of people will completely recover within 2 years. Of the 20% remaining, the problem ranges from having a complete dense facial paralysis to synkinesis.

Ramsay Hunt Syndrome

This syndrome is caused by varicella zoster virus involving the facial nerve. It is distinguished clinically from Bell's palsy by the presence of vesicles and pain in the ear, along with a myriad of other less common symptoms. Although far less common than Bell's palsy, the prognosis is worse and most patients do not recover from the facial paralysis and develop chronic neuralgia.

Otitis Media/Mastoiditis

An acute infection of the middle ear or mastoid bone can very rarely lead to facial nerve paralysis. This is likely to be secondary to localized inflammation and compression of the nerve in the facial canal. Prompt recognition and treatment yields favorable outcomes and in select cases mastoidectomy may be indicated.

Cholesteatoma

A cholesteatoma is a nonmalignant slow-growing skin cyst. It causes destruction of the inner ear through chronic infection and by local pressure effects as the cyst grows. Facial paralysis develops in less than 3% of cholesteatomas.

Lyme Disease

Lyme disease is caused by *Borrelia burgdorferi*, which is transmitted to humans by infected ticks. The symptoms are initially nonspecific, including headache, malaise, and fever; however, facial paralysis can develop in up to 11% of cases. The prognosis is excellent, with more than 99% of patients going on to full recovery without surgical intervention.[15]

Traumatic

Trauma to the face or cranium represents the second most common cause of acquired facial palsies. The type of injury is the most important prognostic factor. In blunt trauma with no associated bony involvement, the type of injury is likely to be a neuropraxia and full recovery is to be anticipated. A penetrating injury where there is a transaction of the nerve warrants urgent surgical exploration and an attempt at primary nerve repair within 3 days. When there is an injury of the temporal bone the prognosis is less favorable unless the onset of the facial palsy is delayed. In temporal fractures the incidence of associated facial nerve injury is between 5% and 10%, of which 40% will recover poorly. In this group of patients, the diagnosis of a facial nerve injury may be difficult due to other intracranial injuries, making the assessment difficult or impossible.[16]

Iatrogenic injuries may occur with soft tissue, bony or intracranial surgery. The injury may be unavoidable, however, prompt recognition and careful reconstructive planning is required.

Neoplastic

The facial nerve may be prone to compression at any point along its course by a space-occupying lesion. The most common cause is secondary to compression by an acoustic neuroma followed by glomus, facial neuromas, and carcinomas. Manipulation of the facial nerve is frequently required in the removal of these tumors which may lead to further injury.

Systemic and Neurological

A brainstem injury may result in permanent facial paralysis due to disruption of the motor nucleus. A central facial palsy may be caused by a lacunar infarct that affects the fibers of the internal capsule going to the facial nucleus. The nucleus itself may be prone to ischemic injury secondarily to an infarct of the pontine arteries.

Many systemic diseases may lead to facial paralysis as a consequence of disease progression. Conditions include multiple sclerosis, Guillain–Barré syndrome, autoimmune disease, and diabetes. Treatment of the underlying cause is the primary management in this category.

Clinical Examination

Clinical examination of the facial nerve is best undertaken in a logical routine, working from the top of the face downwards. Most pertinent information can be ascertained almost immediately by observing a patient as you greet them and they talk. Resting asymmetry may be difficult to assess in the pediatric population as the skin quality is superior to the more elderly patient group and therefore asymmetry may only become apparent during interaction with a child and attempting to get them to smile or speak. It is important to bear in mind that what a clinician views as being the major problem may not be perceived as such by the patient.

Simple examination of the face is usually sufficient to assess the facial nerve. Beginning at the brow, look for asymmetry of the wrinkles of the forehead at rest and then ask the patient to raise their eyebrows to exaggerate this. A particular area that requires close examination is the eye. Ask the patient to close their eyes as tightly as possible. Eye closure is predominantly achieved by the upper eyelid and the lower eyelid acts to maintain the lid margins in contact with the globe and assist tear drainage. Begin with assessing the condition of the globe; are there signs of epiphora, corneal irritation or ulceration? During the introductory period of the consultation it should be possible to see if the blink reflex is still intact and whether the Bell's reflex is effective. The height of the palpebral aperture should be compared between the two sides and measured during eye closure. When assessing the lower eyelid, the position of the lacrimal duct should be assessed as it normally should be lying pressed to the globe, however, when there is a moderate degree of ectropion it may be ineffective at lubricating the globe, leading to epiphora. The assessment of corneal sensation is paramount as an insensate eye that is unable to close effectively carries a high risk of corneal damage, ulceration, and scarring, which may ultimately result in blindness.

The midface must be examined at rest and during animation. At rest the position of the nose, alar symmetry, the presence of a nasolabial fold, the position of the philtrum and mouth must all be noted. This should be repeated whilst asking the patient to perform a closed mouth smile, an open mouth smile, and whilst attempting to show all their teeth. Internal examination of the mouth is prudent as it will give the surgeon a better idea of dental hygiene and the presence of dental caries. Functional assessment of speech should be performed by asking the patient to repeat labial sounds of "b," "p," and "m". The patient should be asked to pucker their lips and blow out their cheeks.

Not all patients will have a dense unilateral palsy and more subtle signs should be observed. The presence of synkinesis is particularly trouble for a patient and the most common symptom is involuntary eye closure during smiling. Dyskinesis may also be present and signs of involuntary muscle twitching must be observed.

An important part of the examination should be to examine other cranial nerves, particularly if they are to be considered as donor nerves in reanimation. The nerve to masseter can be examined by asking the patient to bite whilst palpating the muscles of mastication. Examination of the hypoglossal nerve is performed by asking the patient to protrude their tongue and observing that it does not deviate. Asking the patient to shrug their shoulders will confirm the function of the spinal accessory nerve.

A thorough discussion with the patient should then be performed if possible to illicit the symptoms they suffer from. Typically this will start with the patient listing the symptoms in order of severity. In the pediatric patient this discussion mainly involves the parents and what they have noticed. It is often useful to ask the parents to bring photos or videos of the child from home, as they may be somewhat apprehensive during the consultation. Parents can often feel negative emotions of guilt if their child has difficulty smiling; it is important to consider the psychological support a family may require before, during, and after treatment of their child. In the adult group, patients' primary concern may be with the eye with persistent watering or recurrent infections. With regard to the mouth, they may report function or psychological symptoms; drooling, difficulty eating or poor speech may be the primary concern. For some, the psychological implications of not being able to smile may be more concerning or the feeling that they are being perceived as angry or hostile may lead them to social isolation.

Once the clinical examination has been performed, discussion regarding the management with the patient or their parents is undertaken. It is important to ascertain the patient's or parents' expectations and modify this at an early stage if appropriate. A tailor-made approach that is patient-focused usually provides the most successful outcomes. After the consultation it is useful to ask the patient to have both photographic and video documentation. Each unit varies in their requirements, but this serves as a vital tool in assessing outcomes of intervention.

Many scoring systems have been proposed over time and the general consensus is that there is no ideal system. The most popularized is the House–Brackmann scale, originally described in 1985[17] and modified in 2009 to form the basis of the Facial Nerve Grading System 2.0.[18] It is a widely accepted system, simple, sensitive, accurate, and reliable, which grades facial function in six steps from normal (HB I) to total paralysis (HB VI). Multiple scoring systems are present and there is no universal opinion as to which is the most accurate.[11]

Diagnostic Studies

Diagnostic studies can play a critical role in the assessment of cranial nerves, either preoperatively, postoperatively, or during the monitoring nerve recovery. If there is any doubt regarding a facial nerve paralysis or a potential donor nerve paralysis, it is prudent to perform further testing.

Radiological imaging in the form of a computed topography (CT) scan or a magnetic resonance imaging (MRI) scan can be useful to exclude a space occupying lesion. Typically this has normally been performed prior to referral. Physiological MRI scans can be used to assess cortical remodeling for situations where relearning how to use a nerve to carry out a different function needs to be assessed.

Several electrophysiological tests can help guide the clinician. Electromyography (EMG) is most commonly used to assess the function of different branches of the facial nerve or potential donor nerve in comparison to the normal side. EMG is often combined with electroneurography (ENoG) which assesses nerve conductivity in comparison to muscle activity. The Nerve Excitability Test (NET) is used mainly to determine the prognosis of nerve recovery in unilateral facial nerve palsy. The facial nerve is stimulated at the angle of the jaw with increasing current until a barely perceptible twitch is seen in the face. This is compared with the normal side and a difference of more than 2–3.5 mAmp is considered abnormal. Due to the invasive nature of these tests, patients may not be able to tolerate the investigation, particularly in the pediatric group.

Management

When considering the management of facial paralysis the clinician must have a set of priorities to which they adhere. First, protection of the eye is paramount. Drying out of the globe can lead to corneal ulceration and ultimately blindness if untreated. Second, oral continence and speech should be restored. Third, facial symmetry should be restored to address the esthetic appearance of the patient and, consequently, the psychological impact of the paralysis.

Patients should be treated differently on age criteria. In the pediatric group the eye and forehead do not usually require surgical intervention and the focus of attention should be on smile restoration. In the aging patient, treatment options begin to become more limited as the ability of a nerve to regenerate diminishes with age, as does the chance of retraining the brain if a different nerve is used. The gold standard should be to recreate symmetrical spontaneous movement; this may not be possible in all cases, and many treatment options exist to help improve the circumstance.

Nonoperative Management

In cases where a spontaneous recovery is expected this represents the mainstay of treatment. In permanent partial or complete facial paralysis, this is a key adjunct to the operative management and is by no means exclusive. In patients complaining of the difficulty in eye closure at night, particularly in the absence of Bell's phenomenon, simple taping of the eyelids closed may be all that is required to relieve the symptom. Often, it is crucial to keep the eye hydrated and this may be achieved by using topical eye drops or lubricants.

Botulinum type A provides a reversible chemical method of denervation and may be used for two different patient groups; first, in patients complaining of asymmetry, and second, those complaining of synkinesis. When focusing on brow asymmetry or overactivity of the depressor, botulinum type A is often the initial first step in a patient's management as it is minimally invasive, provides rapid visual results, and is reversible. It is important to recognize that the dose is variable between patients and that it should be administered to the unaffected side. Typically, patients achieve a maximum response at 2 weeks and the dose should be repeated every 3 months and titrated as necessary. Botulinum A is effective in treating synkinesis, and the affected muscle groups may be directly injected to diminish their action. Dyskinesis is what a patient will complain of if there is involuntary twitching of muscle groups as they recover or fail to completely recovery. Botulinum type A is administered directly, typically requiring a lower dose, to the affected muscle groups and similarly repeated every 3 months and titrated as necessary. The key is to avoid paralyzing the muscle as this may increase asymmetry and lead to an unhappy patient outcome; if this arises it is important to reassure the patient that full recovery is expected.

Operative Management

Management is best approached by addressing the subunits of the face. In addition, some differences in treatment are preferred depending on the age of the patient, the etiology of the facial paralysis, as well as the degree of paralysis that exists.

Management of the Brow

The only management options available for the brow are static; resting symmetry is the goal of treatment. With a unilateral paralysis the drooping of the brow increases with age and decreased skin elasticity. All brow lifts are static, and currently there are no useful procedures that can provide dynamic forehead movement. Correction of brow ptosis may be approached surgically either directly or via an endoscopic approach.[19] Direct brow-lift incisions include brow, coronal or midforehead approaches. The direct brow lift through a superciliary brow incision is well recognized as the favored method in the setting of facial paralysis and can correct large discrepancies at the expense of a visible scar. An ellipse of skin and frontalis muscle is excised and pexy of orbicularis to the periosteum is performed for durability of the lift. The supraorbital nerve is at risk and must be carefully preserved, but even so, patients often complain of numbness. A coronal brow lift is approached through an incision in the scalp 4–6 cm posterior to the anterior hairline extending to the pinna. Elevation in the subgaleal plane is performed and 1–2 cm of scalp is removed by incising anterior to the initial incision. The scars are usually inconspicuous but the amount of lifting is much less than the direct brow incision and patients often complain of paresthesia posterior to the incision. A receding hairline, or family history of male-pattern baldness, may be a relative contraindication to a coronal brow lift, in which case a midforehead brow lift through a deep brow rhytid may be more appropriate.

Endoscopically-assisted brow lifts may be useful for small amounts of brow ptosis and are therefore not satisfactory in older individuals with significant ptosis. In contrast to the direct methods involving skin excision, endoscopic brow lift suspends the periosteum in an elevated position until adherence by healing is obtained. Elevation of both brows and the complete frontal region appears necessary to address the hyperfunction observed in the unparalyzed side, producing the best symmetry. An alternative is to weaken the contralateral normal frontalis muscle by frontal nerve denervation with or without frontalis muscle resection or chemodenervation with botulinum toxin A. Preservation of the supratrochlear and supraorbital nerves is also achieved by direct visualization endoscopically and incisions are smaller with less sensory disturbance and less alopecia.

Management of the Eye

The goal of corrective surgical procedures is to achieve complete eye closure, thereby providing corneal protection, with minimal ptosis in the open position. In principle, the upper eyelid needs to be lowered (unopposed action of levator palpebrae superioris) and the lower eyelid needs to be elevated. Standard static procedures include lid loading (upper lid) and tarsorrhaphy (upper/lower lid) as well as lower eyelid slings, whereas the palpebral spring implant (upper lid) and the temporalis muscle transfer (upper/lower lid) are classified as dynamic.

Lid loading was first described over 50 years ago and is well tolerated and highly efficacious. Gold and platinum have been the most widely used materials for implantation because of their high density and excellent side effect profile.[20] The amount of weight required for complete closure is frequently too large, and a large weight is more likely to detach and erode through the skin. Test weights attached to the upper eyelid with double-sided tape are used preoperatively to determine the lightest weight that will bring the eyelid within 2–4 mm of the lower lid. The most commonly selected weights are 1.0 g and 1.2 g, though standard sizes range from 0.6 g to 1.8 g. For the best results, they should be placed at least 4 mm above the lid margin (to decrease visibility). Care must be taken not to damage the levator insertion during the dissection for placement to avoid ptosis. Patients are advised that eyelid closure is a slow rather than a rapid blink and that they must practice holding the closure. Complications include a visible lump (capsule formation), ulceration, and/or extrusion, migration of the weight and irritation of the cornea. More recently, a flexible platinum chain has been described as an alternative to rigid gold weights, with multiple links allowing flexibility to adapt to the shape of the globe. Platinum has a better biocompatibility profile and a higher density compared to gold and can thus be made into a smaller implant with improved cosmesis. In terms of static support for the lower lid, the use of autologous conchal cartilage grafts can be an effective procedure to improve the function and appearance of the atonic lower eyelid.

A tarsorrhaphy results in support of the lower eyelid and decreases the amount of corneal exposure by lowering the upper lid. Mclaughlin's lateral tarsorrhaphy is a quick and simple procedure involving resection of the posterior lamellar of the upper lid (tarsal plate and conjunctiva) as well as an identical area of anterior lamellar of the lower lid (skin and muscle).[21] The two denuded areas are overlapped and both tarsal plates are sutured. It is especially indicated in older patients with concomitant senile ectropion but may result in the appearance of a smaller eye and difficulty when looking laterally. If this fails to achieve the desired result, then a fascial or palmaris longus tendon sling is used to support the lower lid with fixation points at the medial canthal ligament and supraorbital margin laterally. Proper placement of the tendon 1–2 mm below the lid margin is crucial as low placement will exacerbate an ectropion and high placement may result in an entropion. Canthoplasties are rarely performed as they tend to stretch over time in patients with facial paralysis.

The palpebral spring implant is a wire shaped by the surgeon in the form of an open safety pin. The lower arm is attached to the lid margin and the upper arm to the superior orbital rim. When the eye is opened by contraction of the levator muscle, the spring is compressed. When the levator is relaxed, the spring expands and forces the eyelid to a closed position. It has an advantage over upper lid weighting in that it will function equally well in the upright or supine position, but the results depend on the experience of the operator and the spring may loosen or fracture with time.[20]

The transfer of a strip of temporalis muscle was first described by Gillies to provide a dynamic closure of the eyelid using autologous tissue.[22] A 1.5-cm strip of temporalis muscle is detached superiorly, turned anteriorly, and extended with two strips of tendon or fascia, passed through the upper and lower eyelids, and fastened to the medial canthal ligament. Alternatively, a static sling can be placed in the lower lid as previously described and a dynamic temporalis transfer applied to the upper lid as this eyelid requires more movement. The temporalis muscle transfer is activated by closing the jaw and therefore frequent biting throughout the day results in frequent corneal lubrication. It does result in a bulge over the lateral orbital margin and a slit-like appearance to the eye, and is technically demanding to perform, but it can provide forceful and full eyelid closure, especially if the tension of the transferred muscle has been set correctly. It is also especially useful if sensibility of the cornea is diminished.

In order to restore the blink reflex, free functional muscle transfer (FFMT) must be considered. This should ideally be performed as part of a two-stage reanimation process where two cross-facial nerve grafts (CFNG) are harvested, one being attached to a functioning buccal branch, the other to a zygomatic branch of the contralateral side. At the second stage, a free platysma flap may be raised with its neurovascular pedicle, tunneled through the upper and lower lids and attached to the medial canthal ligament medially and temporal fascia laterally[23] (Fig. 22.1). The neurovascular pedicle is then typically joined to the CFNG from the functioning zygomatic branch and the superficial temporal vessels. This provides the patient with true spontaneous eye closure and restoration of the blink reflex.

A combination of lid loading, lateral tarsorrhaphies, and lower eyelid slings are the most frequently carried out procedures on the eyelids in facial paralysis patients.[24] In spite of this, treatment of epiphora is frequently unsatisfactory apart from ensuring that the lower lateral canaliculus is in association with the eye itself. Even with perfect position, however, epiphora can persist, possibly as a result of reduced inhibition on the lacrimal gland.

Management of the Mid- and Lower Face

Treatment in Children

Since the first description of a vascularized, innervated functional muscle transfer by Harii in 1976,[25] a two-stage reconstruction has become the gold standard, especially in children. In the first stage, a CFNG is connected to a functioning terminal branch of the facial nerve, typically a buccal branch, on the unaffected side and tunneled subcutaneously under the upper lip to the affected side. The donor nerve ideally should leave minimal deficit therefore a pure sensory nerve is used, usually the sural nerve from the leg; this leaves a small patch of numbness on the outside of the ankle and foot. The nerve graft is then allowed to regenerate across the face, which normally takes around

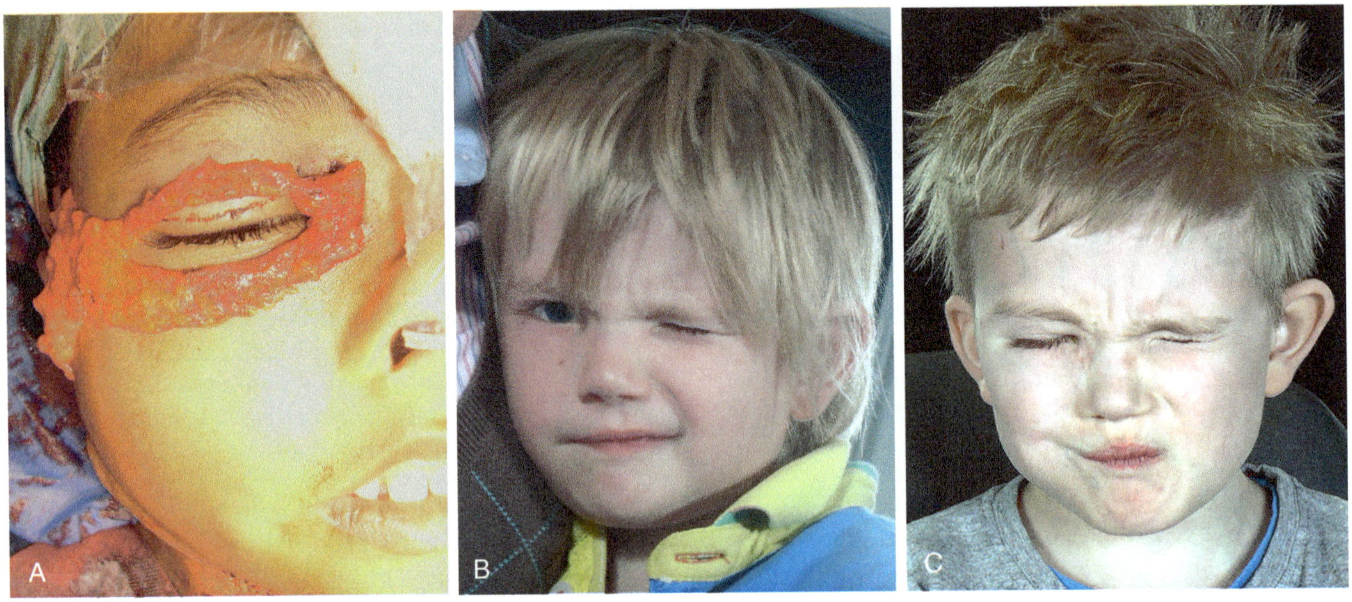

• **Fig. 22.1** Reanimation of the eye using a free functional platysma transfer. (A) Intraoperative photograph of the proposed inset of the muscle flap. (B) Preoperative and (C) postoperative photographs of a patient being treated with a functional platysmal transfer.

3–6 months and is monitored clinically with Tinel's sign. This may be unreliable in young children as they may not fully understand the test. Also, Tinel's sign is a more sensitive indicator of sensory nerve regrowth rather than motor nerve, therefore it is important educate the parents that this is not necessarily a sign of surgical failure. In the second stage of the surgery the patient receives a vascularized muscle flap that will be innervated by the CFNG over a 6–12-month period. Typical muscles used are the pectoralis minor, gracilis, and latissimus dorsi as these leave as little donor morbidity as possible.[26,27] At this stage the patient will slowly regain the movement on the affected side of the face.[28]

In bilateral congenital facial paralysis, the facial nerve is not available as a motor nerve to drive the new muscle, therefore a different cranial nerve may be used, e.g., V, IX or XII. A muscle must be chosen with an appropriate pedicle length and excellent results can be obtained using latissimus dorsi.[29] This operation can be performed in one stage, with the muscle flap being raised through an axillary approach by one surgical team, whilst the contralateral side of the face is dissected to raise an appropriate vascular pedicle and donor nerve by a second team before proceeding to the other side (Fig. 22.2). It is preferential to operate on these cases when they are young as the effect on cortical remodeling and relearning is beneficial.

When embarking on facial reanimation in children it is important to consider the impact the surgery and hospital appointments will have on a family and the child. The average time taken to complete the treatment is in the region of 2 years and this should ideally be completed before educational commitments become affected and before the child becomes fully aware of their palsy and the psychological implications begin to take hold. Surgery can be started from the age of 4 years and it is beneficial to allow time for the family to consider the surgical options in detail, therefore early referral is prudent.

Management in Adults

In elderly patients, or in cases where dynamic options are unavailable, the mainstay of treatment is with autologous grafts or synthetic materials. The use of synthetic grafts offers the benefit of no donor site morbidity at the risk of increased infection and extrusion of the material. Many examples of autologous grafts exist, ranging from palmaris longus to the Achilles tendon, however tensor fascia lata yields good to excellent results.[30] The graft can be easily harvested with two parallel incisions over the lateral thigh and provides sufficient graft length and breadth in comparison to others. The graft can be split into three distal slips, one being inserted at the midline of the upper lip, one just beyond the midline in the lower lip, and the last being inserted at the modiolus (Fig. 22.3). Over-tensioning of the graft is required in order to compensate for stretching over time. Due to the breadth of the graft, excellent support of the cheek is achieved which improves function and esthetic appearance of the midface. An adjunct static procedure, much akin to a lateral canthopexy in the eye, is to close the angle of the mouth. Although this reduces the aperture of the mouth, it helps to lift the lower lip to improve symmetry at rest and improve symptoms such as drooling.

Dynamic reanimation of the midface can be achieved with regional muscle transfers using the temporalis muscle, the masseter muscle or with a free microneurovascular (functional) muscle transfer. Use of the temporalis muscle to raise the lips is a very old technique. In 1934, Gillies folded the temporal muscle over the zygoma to the lip subcutaneously,

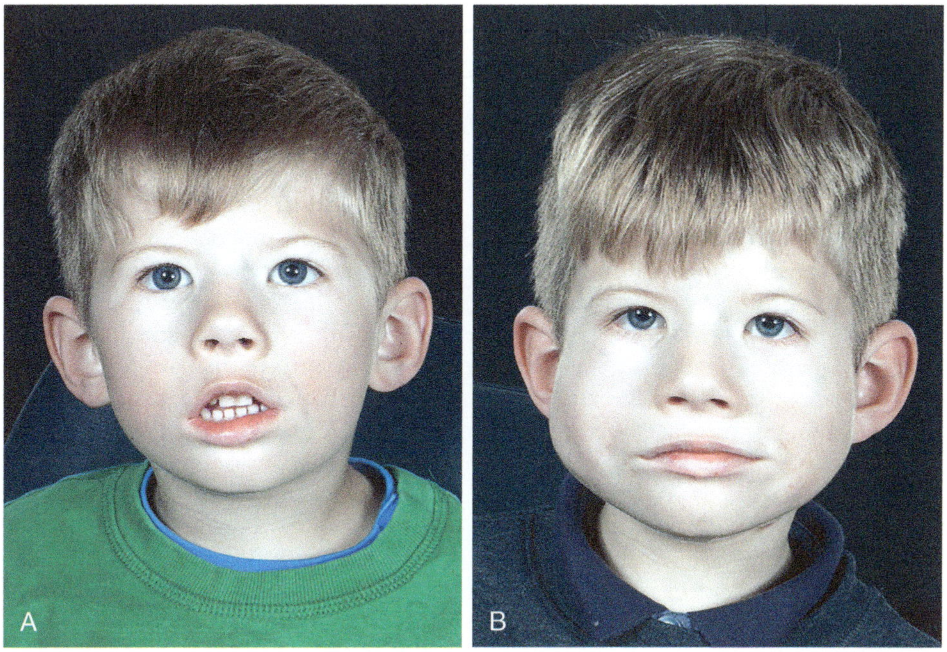

• **Fig. 22.2** Bilateral facial reanimation. (A) Preoperative photograph showing a bilateral facial paralysis (Möbius syndrome). (B) Postoperative photograph after facial reanimation using a bilateral latissimus dorsi free functional muscle transfer.

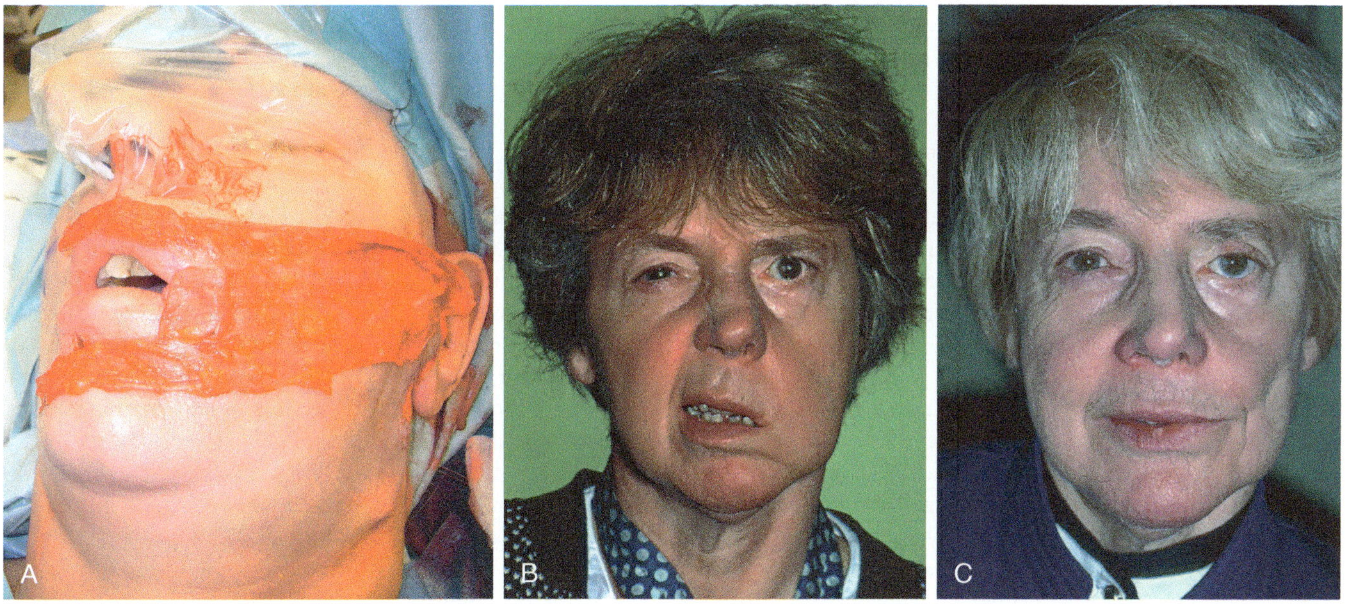

• **Fig. 22.3** Static support using tensor fascia lata graft. (A) Intraoperative photograph of the proposed inset of the graft at the upper lip, modiolus, and lower lip. (B) Preoperative and (C) postoperative photographs of a patient treated with a static sling for left-sided facial paralysis.

resulting in significant muscle bulging over the zygoma and a residual hollow in the temporal fossa. A masseter muscle transfer results in a hollow at the angle of the mandible from where the muscle has been removed. In 1997, Labbé modified this technique further by carrying out an osteotomy of the zygomatic arch, detachment at the coronoid process for insertion to the lips, and temporalis muscle repositioning/lengthening by detaching the posterior third resulting in a "temporalis slide." This procedure avoids contour problems and the routing provides good excursion but patients have to undergo intense physical therapy to relearn function. This is particularly useful in more elderly patients in whom FFMT is less effective and less reliable. Using local muscle transfers requires the brain to retrain in order to achieve truly spontaneous results; with age cortical plasticity diminishes and whether it is possible to achieve such a result remains to be seen. It has also gained popularity in children but the influence of division of the zygoma on midfacial growth has not been addressed.

Free functional muscle transfer was popularized by Harii and continues to be the gold standard of treatment for facial paralysis. It allows for a true spontaneous smile to be restored. The use of FFMT in adults has evolved over the years and different treatment modalities are available depending on age groups. When considering muscle choice, the clinician must take into account muscle bulk, pedicle length, and the size of the nerve. If a bulky muscle, such as latissimus dorsi, is used then adequate trimming of the muscle must be performed prior to inset. Pedicle length is vital if a one-stage procedure is to be considered.

For patients under the age of 20 years, a two-stage reconstruction is still advocated. Below this age, the ability of a nerve to regenerate along a cross-facial nerve graft is predictable and therefore favorable. In patients between 20 and 40 years, a one-stage procedure is performed. Normally latissimus dorsi is the chosen pedicle due to the length of the neurovascular pedicle. In this case, a small incision is made in the nasolabial fold of the functioning side of the face and a very distal buccal branch of the facial nerve is isolated. The paralyzed side of the face is then raised in a standard fashion and the thoracodorsal nerve from the muscle is tunneled to the contralateral side and coapted to the functioning distal buccal branch. The advantage this has over a two-stage procedure is that the nerve only has to cross over one neurorrhaphy in contrast to two in CFNGs and allows for a sufficient number of axons to reinnervate the muscle. For patients between the ages of 40 and 60 years, similarly a one-stage procedure is advocated using the latissimus dorsi muscle, however the donor nerve of choice is an ipsilateral branch of the masseteric nerve. The masseteric nerve is chosen due to the increased axonal counts which are sufficient to power a FFMT, compensating for the increased age. In patients over 60 years, FFMT is not suggested as the results are becoming increasingly unpredictable and fewer patients achieve good results.

Frequently a facial palsy patient may require multiple operations. This is in part due to the changes of an aging face but also to improve cosmesis. Static slings may stretch over time and require tightening or a FFMT may require revision due to the patient not being happy with the bulkiness. Although 80% of FFMT obtain either a good or excellent result, 20% gain no benefit and warrant another surgical option.

Isolated Marginal Branch Palsy

Lower lip deformity is due to lack of innervation of the depressor labii inferioris by the marginal mandibular nerve. This is more evident with speech when the paralyzed side remains elevated and the non-paralyzed side moves inferiorly. Nonsurgical management includes chemodenervation with botulinum toxin of the nonparalyzed depressor labii inferioris to improve symmetry. Surgical options include selective myectomy of the nonparalyzed depressor labii inferioris through the buccal surface of the lip, sectioning of the marginal branch of the contralateral facial nerve or transfer of the anterior belly of digastric muscle on the paralyzed side.[31] The digastric muscle consists of two muscle bellies, the anterior and posterior portions. Although the posterior belly is supplied by the digastric branch of the facial nerve, the anterior belly is supplied by the mylohyoid branch of the mandibular division of the trigeminal nerve, and thus is spared in facial paralysis. The anterior belly can be divided at the tendinous junction separating the two bellies and then transferred over the chin. It is secured to orbicularis oris at the lower lip and acts to recreate the downwards dynamic motion of the mouth and help symmeterize the position of the mouth, particularly during speech or eating. More recently there have been suggestions that combining the standard Conley transfer with a CFNG and an end-to-side neurorrhaphy in order to improve spontaneous independent muscle movement.[32] The size of the nerve to digastric and therefore the technical difficulties to do a adequate neurorrhaphy as well as the lack of physiological understanding and knowledge of nerve/endplate population in this clinical setting make this added complexity of the procedure of dubious value. In more complex congenital facial hypoplastic conditions such as second arch syndrome, or following extensive surgery in the digastric triangle, where the anterior belly of digastric may be absent or damaged an alternative is option is a free extensor digitorum brevis transfer. Other alternatives include the minihypoglossal nerve transfer or platysma transfer in patients with Bell's palsy patients with intact marginal mandibular nerve function.

Conclusion

The essential primary strategy when approaching the management of facial paralysis is to assess the patient in detail and to formulate a tailored plan for each individual. In general, early referral to a facial reanimation service is recommended, particularly in the pediatric patient group. A facial reanimation unit should be in a specialized center, which can cater for pediatric services and should be able to deliver all the treatment options available. Currently there is no standardized outcome measure for facial palsy surgery. The e-Face program has been validated and is probably the best objective assessment of unilateral facial palsy outcomes.[33] Recently an ICHOMS International Working Group published a treatment set for pediatric facial palsy patients.[34] The ultimate aim of facial reanimation surgery is to treat all the branches of the facial nerve affected and produce in addition to a symmetric spontaneous smile in response to emotion, an improvement functionally in all aspects.

The Future

Several new approaches to muscle/nerve interaction and reinnervation have appeared on the horizon. Endeavors are now being made to better understand the influence of the sensory axons on afferent feedback and motor input, but very little scientific data exist in the free functional muscle flap clinical setting. Selective neurolysis has been advocated by some authors as a treatment option for synkinesis and partially recovered facial nerve paralysis.[35] Contrary to early understanding of motor nerve, functional recent work suggests fine movements require an expectedly low number of motor neurons but a large convergence of afferent sensory input for feedback control.[36] The relevance of these findings for the facial reanimation surgeon remains to be seen.

References

1. Bradbury ET, Simons W, Sanders R. Psychological and social factors in reconstructive surgery for hemi-facial palsy. *J Plast Reconstr Aesth.* 2006;59(3):272–278.
2. Coulson SE, O'Dwyer NJ, Adams RD, Croxson GR. Expression of emotion and quality of life after facial nerve paralysis. *Otol Neurotol.* 2004;25(6):1014–1019.
3. Davies JC, Fattah A, Ravichandiran M, Agur AM. Clinically relevant landmarks of the frontotemporal branch of the facial nerve: a three-dimensional study. *Clin Anat.* 2012;25(7):858–865.
4. Davis RA, Anson BJ, Budinger JM, Kurth LR. Surgical anatomy of the facial nerve and parotid gland based upon a study of 350 cervicofacial halves. *Surg Gynecol Obstet.* 1956;102(4):385–412.
5. Dingman RO, Grabb WC. Surgical anatomy of the mandibular ramus of the facial nerve based on the dissection of 100 facial halves. *Plast Reconstr Surg Transplant Bull.* 1962;29:266–272.
6. Baker DC, Conley J. Avoiding facial nerve injuries in rhytidectomy: anatomical variations and pitfalls. *Plast Reconstr Surg.* 1979;64(6):781–795.
7. Freilinger G, Gruber H, Happak W, Pechmann U. Surgical anatomy of the mimic muscle system and the facial nerve: importance for reconstructive and aesthetic surgery. *Plast Reconstr Surg.* 1987;80(5):686–690.
8. Borschel GH, Kawamura DH, Kasukurthi R, Hunter DA, Zuker RM, Woo AS. The motor nerve to the masseter muscle: an anatomic and histomorphometric study to facilitate its use in facial reanimation. *J Plast Reconstr Aesthet Surg.* 2012;65(3):363–366.
9. Mundschenk MB, Sachanandani NS, Borschel GH, Zuker RM, Snyder-Warwick AK. Motor nerve to the masseter: a pediatric anatomic study and the "3:1 rule". *J Plast Reconstr Aesthet Surg.* 2018;71(1):54–56.
10. Henry FP, Leckenby JI, Butler DP, Grobbelaar AO. An algorithm to guide recipient vessel selection in cases of free functional muscle transfer for facial reanimation. *Arch Plast Surg.* 2014;41(6):716–721.
11. Niziol R, Henry FP, Leckenby JI, Grobbelaar AO. Is there an ideal outcome scoring system for facial reanimation surgery? A review of current methods and suggestions for future publications. *J Plast Reconstr Aesthet Surg.* 2015;68(4):447–456.
12. Laing JH, Harrison DH, Jones BM, Laing GJ. Is permanent congenital facial palsy caused by birth trauma? *Arch Dis Child.* 1996;74(1):56–58.
13. Pagon RA, Graham Jr JM, Zonana J, Yong SL. Coloboma, congenital heart disease, and choanal atresia with multiple anomalies: CHARGE association. *J Pediatr.* 1981;99(2):223–227.
14. Gilden DH. Clinical practice. Bell's palsy. *N Engl J Med.* 2004;351(13):1323–1331.
15. Jowett N, Gaudin RA, Banks CA, Hadlock TA. Steroid use in Lyme disease-associated facial palsy is associated with worse long-term outcomes. *Laryngoscope.* 2017;127(6):1451–1458.
16. Coker NJ, Kendall KA, Jenkins HA, Alford BR. Traumatic intratemporal facial nerve injury: management rationale for preservation of function. *Otolaryngol Head Neck Surg.* 1987;97(3):262–269.
17. House JW, Brackmann DE. Facial nerve grading system. *Otolaryngol Head Neck Surg.* 1985;93(2):146–147.
18. Vrabec JT, Backous DD, Djalilian HR, et al. Facial Nerve Grading System 2.0. *Otolaryngol Head Neck Surg.* 2009;140(4):445–450.
19. Adant JP. Endoscopically assisted suspension in facial palsy. *Plast Reconstr Surg.* 1998;102(1):178–181.
20. Terzis JK, Kyere SA. Experience with the gold weight and palpebral spring in the management of paralytic lagophthalmos. *Plast Reconstr Surg.* 2008;121(3):806–815.
21. McLaughlin CR. Permanent facial paralysis; the role of surgical support. *Lancet.* 1952;2(6736):647–651.
22. Deutinger M, Freilinger G. Transfer of the temporal muscle for lagophthalmos according to Gillies. *Scand J Plast Reconstr Surg Hand Surg.* 1991;25(2):151–154.
23. Guelinckx PJ. Blink restoration in long-standing facial paralysis: use of free neurovascular platysma transfer. *Plast Reconstr Surg Glob Open.* 2018;6(10):e1939.
24. Leckenby JI, Ghali S, Butler DP, Grobbelaar AO. Reanimation of the brow and eye in facial paralysis: review of the literature and personal algorithmic approach. *J Plast Reconstr Aesthet Surg.* 2015;68(5):603–614.
25. Harii K, Ohmori K, Torii S. Free gracilis muscle transplantation, with microneurovascular anastomoses for the treatment of facial paralysis. A preliminary report. *Plast Reconstr Surg.* 1976;57(2):133–143.
26. Harrison DH, Grobbelaar AO. Pectoralis minor muscle transfer for unilateral facial palsy reanimation: an experience of 35 years and 637 cases. *J Plast Reconstr Aesthet Surg.* 2012;65(7):845–850.
27. Gousheh J, Arasteh E. Treatment of facial paralysis: dynamic reanimation of spontaneous facial expression – apropos of 655 patients. *Plast Reconstr Surg.* 2011;128(6):693e–703e.
28. Harrison DH. Pectoralis minor for facial palsy. *Plast Reconstr Surg.* 1985;76(4):656–657.
29. Woollard AC, Harrison DH, Grobbelaar AO. An approach to bilateral facial paralysis. *J Plast Reconstr Aesthet Surg.* 2010;63(9):1557–1560.
30. Leckenby JI, Harrison DH, Grobbelaar AO. Static support in the facial palsy patient: a case series of 51 patients using tensor fascia lata slings as the sole treatment for correcting the position of the mouth. *J Plast Reconstr Aesthet Surg.* 2014;67(3):350–357.
31. Butler DP, Leckenby JI, Miranda BH, Grobbelaar AO. Botulinum toxin therapy versus anterior belly of digastric transfer in the management of marginal mandibular branch of the facial nerve palsy: a patient satisfaction survey. *Arch Plast Surg.* 2015;42(6):735–740.
32. Tzafetta K. Two-stage lower lip reanimation with cross-facial nerve graft and the anterior belly of digastric muscle transfer. *International Facial Nerve Symposium.* Los Angeles, USA: 2017.
33. Banks CA, Bhama PK, Park J, Hadlock CR, Hadlock TA. Clinician-graded electronic facial paralysis assessment: the eFACE. *Plast Reconstr Surg.* 2015;136(2):223e–230e.
34. ICHOM (International Consortium for Health Outcome Measurement. *Paediatric Facial Palsy: The Standard Set*; 2018. Available at: https://www.ichom.org/medical-conditions/paediatric-facial-palsy/.
35. Azizzadeh B, Frisenda JL. Surgical management of postparalysis facial palsy and synkinesis. *Otolaryngol Clin North Am.* 2018;51(6):1169–1178.
36. Gesslbauer B, Hruby LA, Roche AD, Farina D, Blumer R, Aszmann OC. Axonal components of nerves innervating the human arm. *Ann Neurol.* 2017;82(3):396–408.

23 Head and Neck Malignancies

XIMENA MIMICA AND MARC A. COHEN

Introduction

Head and neck cancers are the sixth most common group of malignancies worldwide.[1] In the United States, the estimated incidence is 65,000 new cases per year, which are most commonly diagnosed among adults older than 50 years of age.[2]

Geographic variations in the incidence and mortality rates of head and neck cancers are related to differences in patterns of exposure and behavior. Well-known risk factors include tobacco and alcohol consumption, betel chewing, and infection with high-risk human papillomavirus (HPV), specifically types 16 and 18, and Epstein–Barr virus (EBV).

Head and neck tumors can arise in the oral cavity, nasopharynx, hypopharynx, oropharynx, nasal cavity and paranasal sinuses, larynx, and salivary glands. Multiple histologies can be found in these sites, but more than 90% are squamous cell carcinomas (SCC). SCC is associated with aggressive behavior and high incidence of locoregional recurrence.

Several studies have reported an upward trend in the incidence of oropharyngeal cancer (OPC) worldwide. In the United States, HPV-related OPCs have risen since 1984.[3] The most affected population are younger men with a history of multiple lifetime oral sex partners and without a long history of tobacco and alcohol consumption. Clinical presentation differs from the classic stereotype and is characterized by small tumors with bulky lymph nodal disease at diagnosis.[4]

Evaluation of the Patient with Head and Neck Cancer

Patients diagnosed with head and neck cancers require a comprehensive evaluation by a multidisciplinary team consisting of head and neck surgeons, medical oncologists, radiation oncologists, plastic and reconstructive surgeons, dental surgeons, and speech pathologists.

Medical History

A complete medical history is collected, noting the onset and progression of symptoms and focusing on key risk factors that include tobacco and alcohol consumption, sun and environmental exposure, prior cancer history, number of sexual partners, immunosuppression, and other comorbidities. Family history and social circumstances are also recorded, as birthplace, ethnicity, and family support can play a role in treatment planning and rehabilitation. The rapid progression of symptoms suggests aggressive disease and may be an indication for emergency intervention.

Head and neck malignancies can have a major impact on patient´s activities of daily living, such as eating, speaking, swallowing, and breathing, which can affect performance status. Performance status is critical for assessing a patient's ability to tolerate treatment. A complete pretreatment assessment should include an evaluation of nutritional and dental status, focusing on the need for supplemental nutrition (orally or using a gastrostomy tube), eradication of periodontal disease, or dental extraction.

Clinical Examination

A comprehensive head and neck examination should be performed to address the primary tumor site and to search for second primaries, which can be present in 2%–5% of patients.[5,6] Examination should be performed with the patient sitting upright and begins with the evaluation of the skin of the scalp, face, and neck, followed by palpation of the thyroid, parotid gland, neck nodal basins, and abnormal masses. Testing of cranial nerve function should be included routinely, as well as rhinoscopy and external ear examination. The examination of the oral cavity should include observation of mucosal lesions, dental care, and palpation of the tongue, floor of mouth, base of tongue, and tonsils.

Endoscopic assessment can be done with a mirror or with a flexible fiberoptic endoscopy, which will include visualization of the nasal cavity, nasopharynx, oropharynx, hypopharynx, and larynx. Functional tests should be done to evaluate vocal cord mobility.

Imaging Examination

Modern imaging has dramatically enhanced diagnosis and staging of head and neck cancers.[7] Different modalities include ultrasound (US), computed tomography (CT), magnetic resonance imaging (MRI), and positron emission tomography (PET). Modality selection is affected by multiple factors, including availability, coverage, experienced radiologists, primary location of the tumor, and stage of the disease.

US is useful for the assessment of superficial or soft-tissue lesions located in the thyroid or parotid gland, it is sensitive for the detection of lymph node metastasis, but it is operator-dependent and requires expertise. CT is widely available, allows rapid image acquisition, and reduces artifacts related to respiration and swallowing; it is best suited for defining primary tumor and identifying bone invasion, and can be used for guiding tissue biopsy. MRI offers a superior soft tissue contrast and is preferred when the tumor needs to be differentiated from adjacent soft tissue structures, including tumors arising in the sinonasal region, oral cavity, and salivary glands.[8] PET/CT is frequently used to evaluate advanced head and neck cancers, regional and distant metastases, and post treatment response to chemoradiotherapy.[9]

Biopsy

Tissue confirmation of the diagnosis is necessary before any cancer treatment; samples can be obtained using fine needle aspiration, core needle, or surgical biopsy. Care must be taken to obtain representative tissue samples that allow accurate histological classification.

Staging

Correctly staging the disease is an essential component of the oncologic evaluation. It allows a universal understanding of the disease and influences decision making. The tumor–node–metastasis (TNM) staging system, developed by the American Joint Committee on Cancer (AJCC), is the most commonly used staging system. Information needed to stage patients is obtained from physical examinations, laboratory tests, imaging exams, pathology results, and surgical reports. T stage is based on the anatomic location and size of the primary tumor. N indicates regional disease and considers the number and location of regional lymph nodes. M indicates the presence of distant metastasis. These are translated to an overall stage classification ranging from I to IV. Early-stage disease includes stages I and II, and advanced stage disease stages III and IV.

The recent eighth edition of the AJCC staging manual introduces significant changes to the head and neck section.[10] The most significant updates are the creation of a separate staging classification for HPV-related OPC, the addition of depth of invasion (DOI) in the T category for oral cavity carcinoma, the incorporation of skin cancer staging (other than melanoma and Merkel cell carcinoma) in the head and neck chapter, the change in the T and N status in nasopharyngeal cancers, and the inclusion of the extranodal extension feature to the N category.

The T0 classification is used when the primary tumor is not known. More than 90% of unknown primary tumors are HPV- or EBV-positive, which is why T0 is only used for HPV-related OPCs and tumors located in the nasopharynx. T0 is not used for HPV-negative OPCs and other non-HPV-related cancers located in the oral cavity, larynx, hypopharynx, and paranasal sinus.

In this chapter, we will address staging by anatomical site, excluding tumors arising from the thyroid gland.

Oral Cavity

The oral cavity extends from the skin vermilion junction of the lips to the junction of the hard and soft palates superiorly, the circumvallate papillae inferiorly, and the anterior tonsillar pillars laterally. Different subsites in the oral cavity include the lips, alveolar ridge, buccal mucosa, retromolar trigone, hard palate, floor of mouth, and two-thirds of the anterior tongue. Table 23.1 summarizes the T stages for primary tumors of the oral cavity.

The main change in oral cavity clinical and pathological staging was the inclusion of DOI based on the results of a large international collaborative study of oral cavity cancer.[11] This study showed that DOI was significantly associated with disease-specific survival, supporting the relevance of this feature as a mark of biological behavior.

Clinical determination of DOI is challenging and requires the clinician to distinguish between a thick, exophytic tumor from one that is ulcerated and infiltrative; this information is used in conjunction with radiological features to plan treatment.

Of note, pathological DOI should be measured from the level of the basal membrane of the closest adjacent mucosa to the deepest point of tumor invasion.

Nasopharynx

The nasopharynx represents a transitional area between the nasal cavity and the oropharynx. It includes the vault, the lateral walls (formed by the orifices of the Eustachian tube superiorly and the superior constrictor inferiorly), the posterior wall, and the superior surface of the soft palate. Table 23.2 summarizes the T stages for primary tumors of the nasopharynx.

TABLE 23.1 T Stage for Primary Tumors of the Oral Cavity

T Category	T Criteria
Tis	Carcinoma in situ
T1	Tumor ≤2 cm with DOI ≤5 mm
T2	Tumor ≤2 cm with DOI >5 mm **or** tumor >2 cm but ≤4 cm with DOI ≤10 mm
T3	Tumor >2 cm and ≤4 cm with DOI >10 mm **or** tumor >4 cm with DOI ≤10 mm
T4a	Moderately advanced local disease Tumor >4 cm with DOI >10 mm **or** tumor invades adjacent structures only (e.g., through cortical bone of the mandible or maxilla, or involves the maxillary sinus or skin of the face)[a]
T4b	Very advanced local disease Tumor invades masticator space, pterygoid plates, or skull base and/or encases the internal carotid artery

[a]Superficial erosion of bone/tooth socket (alone) by a gingival primary is not sufficient to classify a tumor as T4.
From Amin MB, Edge S, Greene F, et al, eds. *AJCC Cancer Staging Manual*. 8th edn. New York: Springer International/American Joint Commission on Cancer; 2017.

TABLE 23.2 T Stage for Primary Tumors of the Nasopharynx

T Category	T Criteria
T0	No tumor identified, but EBV-positive cervical node(s) involvement
Tis	Carcinoma in situ
T1	Tumor confined to the nasopharynx or extension to the oropharynx and/or nasal cavity without parapharyngeal involvement
T2	Tumor with extension to parapharyngeal space and/or adjacent soft tissue involvement (medial pterygoid, lateral pterygoid, prevertebral muscles)
T3	Tumor with infiltration of bony structures at skull base, cervical vertebra, pterygoid structures, and/or paranasal sinuses
T4	Tumor with intracranial extension, involvement of cranial nerves, hypopharynx, orbit, parotid gland, and/or extensive soft tissue infiltration beyond the lateral surface of the lateral pterygoid muscle

Used with permission of the American College of Surgeons, Chicago, Illinois. The original source for this information is the AJCC Cancer Staging Manual, Eighth Edition (2017) published by Springer International Publishing.

TABLE 23.3 Clinical and Pathological T Stage for Primary HPV-Related OPC

T Category	T Criteria
T0	No primary tumor identified
T1	Tumor ≤2 cm in greatest dimension
T2	Tumor >2 cm but ≤4 cm in greatest dimension
T3	Tumor >4 cm in greatest dimension or extension to lingual surface of the epiglottis
T4	Moderately advanced local disease Tumor invades the larynx, extrinsic muscle of the tongue, medial pterygoid, hard palate, mandible, or beyond[a]

[a]Mucosal extension to lingual surface of epiglottis from primary tumors of the base of the tongue and vallecula does not constitute invasion of the larynx.
Used with permission of the American College of Surgeons, Chicago, Illinois. The original source for this information is the AJCC Cancer Staging Manual, Eighth Edition (2017) published by Springer International Publishing.

Oropharynx

The oropharynx includes the soft palate, tonsils, base of the tongue, and pharyngeal walls bounded superiorly by the nasopharynx and inferiorly by the pharyngoepiglottic fold. It extends from the level of the soft palate superiorly to the level of the hyoid bone inferiorly. Tables 23.3 and 23.4 summarize the T stages for primary HPV-related OPC and for primary non-HPV-related OPC, respectively.

The epidemiological transition in oropharyngeal disease led to one of the major changes in the staging system. The eighth edition adds the overexpression of the tumor suppressor protein p16, a surrogate biomarker for HPV infection, as an independent prognostic feature.[12] OPC is now staged based on the overexpression of p16. The Tis and T4b categories are no longer used for HPV-related OPC because they lack applicability to the disease.

Hypopharynx

The hypopharynx starts at the level of the hyoid bone and ends at the lower border of the cricoid cartilage. It is essentially a muscular line tube. Three areas can be distinguished: pyriform sinus, lateral and posterior pharyngeal walls, and postcricoid area. Table 23.5 summarizes the T stages for primary tumors of the hypopharynx.

Larynx

The larynx spans from vertebral level C3 to C6, suspended from the hyoid bone and continuous with the trachea. It is composed of six cartilages: three large, unpaired (cricoid,

TABLE 23.4 Clinical and Pathological T Stage for Primary Non-HPV-related OPC

T Category	T Criteria
Tis	Carcinoma in situ
T1	Tumor ≤2 cm in greatest dimension
T2	Tumor >2 cm but ≤4 cm in greatest dimension
T3	Tumor >4 cm in greatest dimension or extension to lingual surface of the epiglottis
T4a	Moderately advanced local disease Tumor invades the larynx, extrinsic muscle of the tongue, medial pterygoid, hard palate, or mandible[a]
T4b	Very advanced local disease Tumor invades lateral pterygoid muscle, pterygoid plates, lateral nasopharynx, or skull base or encases carotid artery

[a]Mucosal extension to lingual surface of the epiglottis from primary tumors of the base of the tongue and vallecula does not constitute invasion of the larynx.

Used with permission of the American College of Surgeons, Chicago, Illinois. The original source for this information is the AJCC Cancer Staging Manual, Eighth Edition (2017) published by Springer International Publishing.

thyroid, and epiglottis) and three paired (arytenoid, corniculate, and cuneiform). It is subdivided into three anatomic regions: supraglottis, glottis, and subglottis. Supraglottic subsites include the epiglottis, arytenoids, aryepiglottic folds, and false vocal cords. Glottic subsites include the true vocal cords and anterior and posterior commissures. Table 23.6 summarizes the T stages for primary tumors of the larynx.

Nasal Cavity and Paranasal Sinuses

Tumors of the nasal cavity and paranasal sinuses are grouped together in this category. The nasal cavity is limited by several bones. The superior boundary, or roof, is formed by the nasal bones, cribriform plate, and sphenoid bone. The floor is formed by the hard palate anteriorly and nasopharynx posteriorly. The lateral margins are the medial walls of the maxillary sinus.

Paranasal sinuses include the maxillary, frontal, ethmoid, and sphenoid sinuses. The maxillary sinus is a pyramidal cavity in the body of the maxilla. It is bounded superiorly by the orbital floor, inferiorly by the hard palate, posteriorly by the pterygoid plates and pterygopalatine fossa, and laterally by the pterygoid muscles. The frontal sinuses are located behind the superciliary arches and along and above the anterior aspect of the ethmoid sinus. The ethmoid sinus lies in the upper part of the nasal cavity between the orbits. The sphenoid sinus is posterior to the ethmoid sinus.

Tables 23.7 and 23.8 summarize the T stages for primary tumors of the nasal cavity and ethmoid sinus and for primary tumors of the maxillary sinus, respectively.

TABLE 23.5 T Stage for Primary Tumors of the Hypopharynx

Primary Tumor	T Criteria
Tis	Carcinoma in situ
T1	Tumor limited to one subsite of the hypopharynx and /or ≤2 cm in greatest dimension
T2	Tumor invades more than one subsite of hypopharynx or an adjacent site, or measures >2cm but ≤4 cm in greatest dimension, without fixation of hemilarynx
T3	Tumor >4 cm in greatest dimension or with fixation of the hemilarynx or extension to esophagus
T4a	Moderately advanced local disease Tumor invades thyroid/cricoid cartilage, hyoid bone, thyroid gland, or central compartment soft tissue[a]
T4b	Very advanced local disease Tumor invades prevertebral fascia, encases carotid artery, or involves mediastinal structures

[a]Central compartment soft tissue includes prelaryngeal strap muscles and subcutaneous fat.

Used with permission of the American College of Surgeons, Chicago, Illinois. The original source for this information is the AJCC Cancer Staging Manual, Eighth Edition (2017) published by Springer International Publishing.

Major Salivary Glands

There are three pairs of major salivary glands: the parotid, submandibular, and sublingual glands. Table 23.9 summarizes the T stages for primary tumors of the major salivary glands.

The parotid glands are bordered anteriorly by the masseter muscle and the mandibular ramus, superiorly by the external acoustic meatus and the condyle of the mandible, posteriorly by the mastoid process and the sternocleidomastoid muscle, and medially by the styloid process. Parotid tumors represent a challenge for the head and neck surgeon because of the intimate relation of the parotid glands with the facial nerve.

The submandibular glands are in the submandibular triangle, which has a superior boundary formed by the inferior ridge of the mandible and inferior boundaries formed by the anterior and posterior bellies of the digastric muscle. The submandibular glands are in close relation to the facial artery and vein, and the lingual and hypoglossal nerves.

The sublingual glands lie in the submucosal plate within the anterior floor of the mouth, superior to the mylohyoid muscle. The superior wall is the sublingual fold.

TABLE 23.6 T Stage for Primary Tumors of the Supraglottis, Glottis, and Subglottis

T Category	Supraglottis	Glottis	Subglottis
T1	Tumor limited to one subsite of supraglottis, with normal vocal cord mobility	T1 Tumor limited to the vocal cord(s) (may involve anterior or posterior commissure) with normal mobility T1a limited to one vocal cord, with normal mobility T1b involves both vocal cords, with normal mobility	Tumor limited to the subglottis
T2	Tumor invades mucosa of more than one adjacent subsite of the supraglottis or glottis or region outside the supraglottis (e.g., mucosa of base of tongue, vallecula, medial wall of pyriform sinus) without fixation of the larynx	Tumor extends to the supraglottis and/or subglottis, and/or with impaired vocal cord mobility	Tumor extends to vocal cord(s), with normal or impaired mobility
T3	Tumor limited to the larynx, with vocal cord fixation, and/or invades any of the following: postcricoid area, preepiglottic space, paraglottic space, and/or inner cortex of thyroid cartilage	Tumor limited to the larynx, with vocal cord fixation, and/or invasion of paraglottic space and/or inner cortex of the thyroid cartilage	Tumor limited to the larynx, with vocal cord fixation, and/or invasion of paraglottic space and/or inner cortex of the thyroid cartilage
T4a	Moderately advanced local disease Tumor invades through the outer cortex of the thyroid cartilage and/or invades tissues beyond the larynx (e.g., trachea, soft tissues of neck including deep extrinsic muscle of the tongue, strap muscles, thyroid, or esophagus)	Moderately advanced local disease Tumor invades through the outer cortex of the thyroid cartilage and/or invades tissues beyond the larynx (e.g., trachea, cricoid cartilage, soft tissues of neck including deep extrinsic muscle of the tongue, strap muscles, thyroid, or esophagus)	Moderately advanced local disease Tumor invades cricoid or thyroid cartilage and/or invades tissues beyond the larynx (e.g., trachea, soft tissues of neck including deep extrinsic muscles of the tongue, strap muscles, thyroid, or esophagus)
T4b	Very advanced local disease Tumor invades the prevertebral space, encases carotid artery, or invades mediastinal structures	Very advanced local disease Tumor invades the prevertebral space, encases carotid artery, or invades mediastinal structures	Very advanced local disease Tumor invades the prevertebral space, encases carotid artery, or invades mediastinal structures

N Staging for Tumors of the Head and Neck

Tables 23.10 and 23.11 summarize the clinical and pathological N staging, respectively, for primary tumors of the head and neck region, excluding the nasopharynx and HPV-related OPC, but including the oral cavity, hypopharynx, larynx, nasal cavity, and paranasal sinuses, and major salivary glands, as well as non-HPV-related OPC.

Table 23.12 summarizes the N staging for primary tumors of the nasopharynx. Tables 23.13 and 23.14 summarize the clinical and pathological N staging, respectively, for HPV-related OPC.

TNM Stage Grouping for Primary Tumors of the Head and Neck Region

Table 23.15 summarizes TNM staging for tumors of the head and neck region, excluding the nasopharynx and HPV-related OPC, but including the oral cavity, hypopharynx, larynx, nasal cavity and paranasal sinuses, and major salivary glands, as well as non-HPV-related OPC.

Table 23.16 summarizes TNM staging for tumors of the nasopharynx.

Tables 23.17 and 23.18 summarize the clinical and pathological TNM stage grouping for HPV-related OPC.

TABLE 23.7 T Stage for Primary Tumors of the Nasal Cavity and Ethmoid Sinus

T Category	T Criteria
T1	Tumor restricted to any one subsite, with or without bony invasion
T2	Tumor invading two subsites in a single region or extending to involve an adjacent region within the nasoethmoidal complex, with or without bony invasion
T3	Tumor extends to invade the medial wall or floor of the orbit, maxillary sinus, palate, or cribriform plate
T4a	Moderately advanced local disease Tumor invades any of the following: anterior orbital contents, skin of nose or cheek, minimal extension to anterior cranial fossa, pterygoid plates, sphenoid, or frontal sinuses
T4b	Very advanced local disease Tumor invades any of the following: orbital apex, dura, brain, middle cranial fossa, cranial nerves other than maxillary division of trigeminal nerve (V2), nasopharynx, or clivus

Used with permission of the American College of Surgeons, Chicago, Illinois. The original source for this information is the AJCC Cancer Staging Manual, Eighth Edition (2017) published by Springer International Publishing.

TABLE 23.8 T Stage for Primary Tumors of the Maxillary Sinus

T Category	T Criteria
T1	Tumor limited to maxillary sinus mucosa with no erosion or destruction of bone
T2	Tumor causing bone erosion or destruction, including extension into the hard palate and/or middle nasal meatus, except extension to posterior wall of maxillary sinus and pterygoid plates
T3	Tumor invades any of the following: bone of the posterior wall of maxillary sinus, subcutaneous tissues, floor or medial wall of orbit, pterygoid fossa, or ethmoid sinuses
T4a	Moderately advanced local disease Tumor invades anterior orbital contents, skin of cheek, pterygoid plates, infratemporal fossa, cribriform plate, sphenoid or frontal sinuses
T4b	Very advanced local disease Tumor invades any of the following: orbital apex, dura, brain, middle cranial fossa, cranial nerves other than maxillary division of trigeminal nerve (V2), nasopharynx, or clivus

Used with permission of the American College of Surgeons, Chicago, Illinois. The original source for this information is the AJCC Cancer Staging Manual, Eighth Edition (2017) published by Springer International Publishing.

Neck Dissections

The term "neck dissection" refers to the surgical removal of cervical lymph nodes for the management of metastatic nodal disease.

Cervical Lymph Node Levels

The current classification of cervical lymph node levels is based on the system proposed by Memorial Sloan Kettering Cancer Center in 1930, which originally divided the lateral neck into five anatomic levels: I, the submental and submandibular triangle; II–IV, the upper, middle, and lower jugular vein; and V, the posterior triangle group. Two more levels were added later: VI, the central compartment, and VII, the superior mediastinal group. Levels I, II, and V are further divided into sublevels IA, IB, IIA, IIB, VA, and VB (Fig. 23.1). Table 23.19 summarizes these cervical lymph node levels.

Patterns of Metastasis

The dissemination of tumors from primary sites in the head and neck to regional lymph nodes occurs in a sequential fashion along the various levels of lymph nodes in the neck.[13,14] This continuous pattern of dissemination significantly impacts the extent of surgery among patients without clinically evident nodal disease, as the surgeon will address only the lymph node levels at risk of harboring metastasis. Primary tumors of the oral cavity initially metastasize to lymph nodes in neck levels I–III; skip metastasis to levels IV or V are rare in the absence of metastatic disease at levels I–III. Primary tumors of the larynx, hypopharynx, and oropharynx initially metastasize ipsilaterally to lymph nodes in levels II–IV; primaries near the midline can metastasize both sides of the neck. Primary tumors of the thyroid frequently metastasize to level VI lymph nodes, followed by lateral neck levels II, III, and IV.

Indications for Neck Dissection

The most important prognostic factor for patients with SCC of the head and neck is the presence of nodal metastases. Lymph node involvement reduces survival by 50%.[15] Therefore, accurate assessment of the neck is necessary. The propensity for spread to regional lymph nodes is associated with many factors, such as T stage, histology, tumor subsite, and DOI. Tumors that frequently have bilateral lymphatic drainage (e.g., base of the tongue, supraglottic larynx,

TABLE 23.9 T Stage for Primary Tumors of the Major Salivary Glands

T Category	T Criteria
Tis	Carcinoma in situ
T1	Tumor ≤2 cm in greatest dimension without extraparenchymal extension[a]
T2	Tumor >2 cm but ≤4 cm in greatest dimension without extraparenchymal extension[a]
T3	Tumor >4 cm and/or tumor having extraparenchymal extension[a]
T4a	Moderately advanced disease Tumor invades skin, mandible, ear canal, and/or facial nerve
T4b	Very advanced disease Tumor invades skull base and/or pterygoid plates and/or encases carotid artery

[a]Extraparenchymal extension indicates clinical or macroscopic evidence of invasion of soft tissues. Microscopic evidence alone does not constitute extraparenchymal extension for classification purposes.

Used with permission of the American College of Surgeons, Chicago, Illinois. The original source for this information is the AJCC Cancer Staging Manual, Eighth Edition (2017) published by Springer International Publishing.

TABLE 23.10 Clinical N Stage for Primary Tumors Located in the Head and Neck Region (Excluding the Nasopharynx)

N Category	N Criteria
NX	Regional lymph nodes cannot be assessed
N0	No regional lymph node metastasis
N1	Metastasis in a single ipsilateral lymph node ≤3 cm in greatest dimension and ENE(−)
N2a	Metastasis in a single ipsilateral node > 3 cm but ≤ 6 cm in greatest dimension and ENE(−)
N2b	Metastases in multiple ipsilateral nodes, none >6 cm in greatest dimension and ENE(−)
N2c	Metastases in bilateral or contralateral lymph nodes, none >6 cm in greatest dimension, and ENE(−)
N3a	Metastasis in a lymph node >6 cm in greatest dimension and ENE(−)
N3b	Metastasis in any node(s) and clinically overt ENE(+)

Used with permission of the American College of Surgeons, Chicago, Illinois. The original source for this information is the AJCC Cancer Staging Manual, Eighth Edition (2017) published by Springer International Publishing.

TABLE 23.11 Pathological N Stage for Primary Tumors Located in the Head and Neck Region (Excluding the Nasopharynx and HPV-related OPC)

N Category	N Criteria
NX	Regional lymph nodes cannot be assessed
N0	No regional lymph node metastasis
N1	Metastasis in a single ipsilateral lymph node ≤3 cm in greatest dimension and ENE(−)
N2a	Metastasis in single ipsilateral node ≤3 cm in greatest dimension and ENE(+) **or** a single ipsilateral node >3 cm but ≤6 cm in greatest dimension and ENE(−)
N2b	Metastases in multiple ipsilateral nodes, none >6 cm in greatest dimension, and ENE(−)
N2c	Metastases in bilateral or contralateral lymph node(s), none >6 cm in greatest dimension, and ENE(−)
N3a	Metastasis in a lymph node >6 cm in greatest dimension and ENE(−)
N3b	Metastasis in a single ipsilateral node >3 cm in greatest dimension and ENE(+) **or** multiple ipsilateral, contralateral, or bilateral nodes, any with ENE(+) **or** a single contralateral node of any size and ENE(+)

Note: A designation of "U" or "L" may be used for any N category to indicate metastasis above the lower border of the cricoid (U) or below the lower border of the cricoid (L). Similarly, clinical and pathological ENE should be recorded as ENE(−) or ENE(+).

Used with permission of the American College of Surgeons, Chicago, Illinois. The original source for this information is the AJCC Cancer Staging Manual, Eighth Edition (2017) published by Springer International Publishing.

TABLE 23.12 N Stage for Tumors of the Nasopharynx

N Category	N Criteria
NX	Regional lymph nodes cannot be assessed
N0	No regional lymph node metastasis
N1	Unilateral metastasis in cervical lymph node(s) and/or unilateral or bilateral metastasis in retropharyngeal lymph node(s), ≤6 cm in greatest dimension, above the caudal border of cricoid cartilage
N2	Bilateral metastasis in cervical lymph node(s), ≤6 cm in greatest dimension, above the caudal border of cricoid cartilage
N3	Unilateral or bilateral metastasis in cervical lymph node(s), >6 cm in greatest dimension, and/or extension below the caudal border of cricoid cartilage

Used with permission of the American College of Surgeons, Chicago, Illinois. The original source for this information is the AJCC Cancer Staging Manual, Eighth Edition (2017) published by Springer International Publishing.

TABLE 23.13 Clinical N Stage for HPV-related OPC

N Category	N Criteria
NX	Regional lymph nodes cannot be assessed
N0	No regional lymph node metastasis
N1	One or more ipsilateral lymph nodes, none >6 cm
N2	Contralateral or bilateral lymph nodes, none >6 cm
N3	Lymph node(s) >6 cm

Used with permission of the American College of Surgeons, Chicago, Illinois. The original source for this information is the AJCC Cancer Staging Manual, Eighth Edition (2017) published by Springer International Publishing.

TABLE 23.14 Pathological N Stage for HPV-related OPC

N Category	N Criteria
NX	Regional lymph nodes cannot be assessed
N0	No regional lymph node metastasis
N1	Metastasis in ≤4 lymph nodes
N2	Metastasis in >4 lymph nodes

Used with permission of the American College of Surgeons, Chicago, Illinois. The original source for this information is the AJCC Cancer Staging Manual, Eighth Edition (2017) published by Springer International Publishing.

TABLE 23.15 TNM Staging for Tumors Located in the Head and Neck Region (Excluding the Nasopharynx and HPV-related OPC)

T/M1	N0	N1	N2	N3
T1	I	III	IVA	IVB
T2	II	III	IVA	IVB
T3	III	III	IVA	IVB
T4a	IVA	IVA	IVA	IVB
T4b	IVB	IVB	IVB	IVB
M1	IVC	IVC	IVC	IVC

Used with permission of the American College of Surgeons, Chicago, Illinois. The original source for this information is the AJCC Cancer Staging Manual, Eighth Edition (2017) published by Springer International Publishing.

TABLE 23.16 TNM Staging for Tumors of the Nasopharynx

T/M1	N0	N1	N2	N3
T0		II	III	IVA
T1	I	II	III	IVA
T2	II	II	III	IVA
T3	III	III	III	IVA
T4	IVA	IVA	IVA	IVA
M1	IVB	IVB	IVB	IVB

Used with permission of the American College of Surgeons, Chicago, Illinois. The original source for this information is the AJCC Cancer Staging Manual, Eighth Edition (2017) published by Springer International Publishing.

hypopharynx, and deep pre-epiglottic space involvement) and those approaching the midline should typically have both sides of the neck dissected.

A comprehensive neck dissection is indicated for patients with advanced nodal disease. Selective neck dissection is indicated for patients without clinical nodal metastases who have a risk of occult metastatic disease ranging from 15%–20% or for those with earlier stage nodal disease.[16] Neck dissection can be therapeutic or can be used to appropriately pathologically

TABLE 23.17 Clinical TNM Staging for HPV-related OPC

T/M1	N0	N1	N2	N3
T0	I	I	II	III
T1	I	I	II	III
T2	I	I	II	III
T3	II	II	II	III
T4	II	II	III	III
M1	IV	IV	IV	IV

Used with permission of the American College of Surgeons, Chicago, Illinois. The original source for this information is the AJCC Cancer Staging Manual, Eighth Edition (2017) published by Springer International Publishing.

TABLE 23.18 Pathological TNM Staging for HPV-related OPC

T/M1	N0	N1	N2
T0	I	I	II
T1	I	I	II
T2	I	I	II
T3	II	II	III
T4	II	II	III
M1	IV	IV	IV

Used with permission of the American College of Surgeons, Chicago, Illinois. The original source for this information is the AJCC Cancer Staging Manual, Eighth Edition (2017) published by Springer International Publishing.

stage the disease and determine the need for adjuvant treatment.

Types of Neck Dissection

There are four major types of neck dissection used for the surgical treatment of head and neck malignancies. They are classified as either comprehensive (radical, extended radical or modified neck dissection) or selective.

Radical Neck Dissection

Radical neck dissection (RND), first described by Crile in 1906,[17] is a block resection of all regional lymph nodes, including those in the internal jugular vein, sternocleidomastoid muscle, and spinal accessory nerve. RND does not include the removal of periparotid, occipital, retropharyngeal, or midline visceral nodes. This operative procedure has significant long-term morbidity, including cosmetic deformity, shoulder dysfunction, chronic neck and shoulder pain, cutaneous paresthesia, neck asymmetry, and edema. RND is reserved for patients with advanced head and neck cancer.

Extended Radical Neck Dissection

Extended RND includes the removal of additional lymph node groups and other nonlymphatic structures that should be documented separately. It is seldom indicated.

Modified Radical Neck Dissection

Modified RND (MRND) comprises the removal of lymph nodes at levels I–IV, while preserving one or more nonlymphatic structures that are routinely removed with RND. There are three subtypes of MRND:

MRND type I: selectively preserves the accessory spinal accessory nerve

MRND type II: preserves the spinal accessory nerve and sternocleidomastoid muscle

MRND type III: preserves the spinal accessory nerve, sternocleidomastoid muscle, and internal jugular vein

Selective Neck Dissection

Selective neck dissection refers to the selective removal of one or more lymph node groups at risk for metastasis, while sparing other lymph node groups that are routinely removed with RND. It is commonly indicated for patients with clinically negative nodal disease in which there is a high risk of micrometastasis and for patients with low nodal stage disease. The traditional nomenclature used for the various types of selective neck dissection – supraomohyoid neck dissection, anterolateral neck dissection, and central compartment dissection, among others – did not reflect the variation in lymph node levels and sublevels associated with these names. To avoid confusion and bring uniformity, in 2002, the American Academy of Otolaryngology–Head and Neck Surgery recommended that surgeons use the term "selective neck dissection" or "SND" followed by the specific lymph node levels or sublevels removed during surgery, in parentheses.[18]

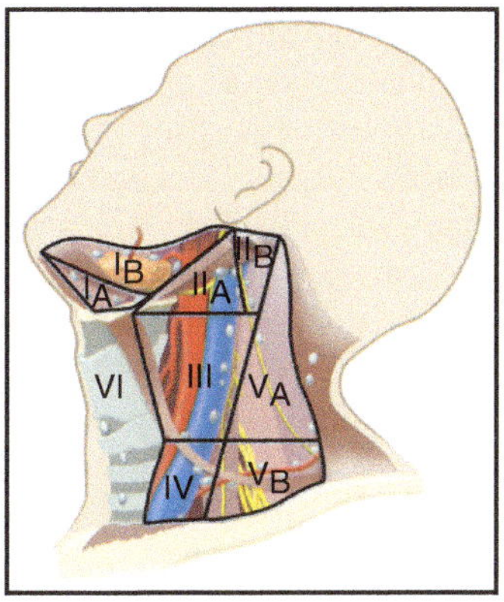

• **Fig. 23.1** The American Academy of Otolaryngology–Head and Neck Surgery modification of the system of assigning levels of cervical lymph nodes. (From Shah JP, Patel SG, Singh B, et al. Cervical lymph nodes. In: Shah JP, Patel SG, Singh B, et al. *Jatin Shah's Head and Neck Surgery and Oncology*. 5th edn. Elsevier; 2020: Fig. 11.6. Courtesy Memorial Sloan Kettering Cancer Center.)

Sentinel Lymph Node Biopsy

Sentinel lymph node biopsy (SLNB) is a minimally invasive surgery designed to identify and examine the primary draining lymph node for the presence of metastasis. It is hypothesized that SLN status correlates with the status of the whole lymphatic basin. In centers with expertise in this procedure, SLNB may be used as an alternative to the more invasive selective neck dissection to identify occult cervical metastasis in patients with N0 disease and early-stage oral cavity carcinoma (T1 or T2). According to the National Comprehensive Cancer Network Guidelines (version 2.2018),[19] patients with a positive SLN must undergo a completion neck dissection, and those with a negative SLN may be observed.

However, caution must be used when offering SLNB as an alternative to selective neck dissection. SLNB is a technically demanding procedure that includes preoperative injection of radiotracer, preoperative localization of radioactive

TABLE 23.19 Lymph Node Levels and Sublevels of the Neck

Level	Anatomic Landmarks	
IA	Submental: lymph nodes within the triangular boundary of the anterior belly of the digastric muscle and above the hyoid bone	
IB	Submandibular: lymph nodes within the area bounded by the anterior and posterior bellies of the digastric muscle and the inferior border of the mandible	
IIA	Upper jugular: anterior to the spinal accessory nerve	Lymph nodes extending from the upper third of the anterior of the internal jugular vein and adjacent spinal accessory nerve, from the skull base to the inferior border of the hyoid bone Anterior border: lateral border of sternohyoid muscle Posterior border: posterior border of sternocleidomastoid muscle
IIB	Upper jugular: posterior to the spinal accessory nerve	
III	Middle jugular: lymph nodes around the middle third of the internal jugular vein, from the inferior border of the hyoid bone to the inferior border of the cricoid cartilage Anterior and posterior borders: same as for level II	
IV	Lower jugular: lymph nodes around the lower third of the internal jugular vein, from the inferior border of cricoid cartilage to the clavicle Anterior and posterior borders: same as for levels II and III	
VA	Posterior triangle: above the inferior border of the cricoid cartilage	Lymph nodes in the triangle formed by the clavicle, posterior border of sternocleidomastoid muscle, and anterior border of the trapezius muscle
VB	Posterior triangle: below the inferior border of the cricoid cartilage	
VI	Central neck lymph nodes located between the carotid arteries from the suprasternal notch to the hyoid bone. This includes the pretracheal, prelaryngeal, and paratracheal lymph nodes	
VII	Superior mediastinal group lymph nodes in the anterosuperior mediastinum and tracheoesophageal grooves extending from the suprasternal notch to the innominate artery	

nodes via imaging, localization of radioactive nodes via gamma counting, intraoperative injection of blue dye, and localization and excision of the blue and radioactive nodes. Although SLN detection rates exceeding 95% have been reported,[20] they are dependent on the technical expertise of the center and the anatomical location of the disease.

Management of the Neck after Chemoradiotherapy

Assessing patients with advanced nodal disease who have received chemoradiotherapy for primary treatment represents a challenge, as they need to be followed up closely for recurrence. Image-guided surveillance is required to evaluate treatment response; the most accepted modality is PET/CT. The time to imaging follow-up of treatment response is an area of controversy; a minimum of 12 weeks after treatment is accepted to reduce false-positive rates.[9] If disease progression is noticed during treatment, a comprehensive neck dissection is recommended, whereas, in the case of complete radiological response, the neck can be observed. For persistent disease the extent of the surgery is determined by the extent of the disease.

Postoperative Complications

Complications can be classified as either acute or those that occur in the late postoperative period. Some acute complications can be life-threatening and require immediate intervention, such as carotid blowout and hematoma. Others, such as chyle leak and partial necrosis flap, can be managed conservatively in most cases. Late complications include seroma, facial edema, hypertrophic scar, and shoulder pain.

Carotid blowout syndrome is a severe complication and has been associated with the presence of a pharyngocutaneous fistula, prior radiotherapy, wound breakdown, and poor nutrition. Should this occur, the priority is ensuring a secure airway, compressing the site of bleeding, and ensuring adequate fluid resuscitation. Treatment is related to the patient's stability and the availability of interventional radiology; if that is not possible, consideration for transfer to a center with neuro interventional radiology should be make. Except in the immediate postoperative setting, surgery for vessel ligation is rarely indicated or performed as it is technically challenging and infrequently successful without significant morbidity.

Chyle leak can occur in 1%–3% of neck dissections,[21] and can be related to variations in anatomy, the fragile composition of the thoracic duct, the presence of bulky disease in the lower neck, and surgery after radiotherapy. Prompt diagnosis is needed because large-volume chyle leaks can impact the patient's nutritional status and electrolyte hemostasis.

Management of chyle leaks depends on drain output. Chyle leaks can be categorized as low-output (<500 mL/day) or high-output (>500 mL/day). A low-output leak can be treated conservatively with nonfat diet or medium-chain fatty acid diet, wound care, and, in some cases, octreotide. Surgical exploration should be considered in high-output fistulas when an identified thoracic duct can be ligated, covered with a muscle flap, and clipped with a thoracoscopy procedure or transabdominal embolization.

Radiotherapy

The fundamental goal of multimodality treatment is to maximize the probability of cure while minimizing the risk of toxicity that can compromise the patient's quality of life.

Radiotherapy is an essential part of the multidisciplinary management of head and neck malignancies, and it can be definitive, adjuvant, or palliative.

Definitive radiotherapy has a well-established role in tumors arising from the nasopharynx, oropharynx, hypopharynx, and larynx, and can be used in conjunction with chemotherapy (i.e., chemoradiotherapy) as an organ preservation approach.[22]

Indication for adjuvant radiotherapy is based on the presence of adverse prognostic features, such as positive and close margins, pathological positive lymph nodes, perineural invasion, lymphovascular invasion, and advanced T stage (T3 orT4).[19] The indication for systemic chemotherapy and radiotherapy is supported by two multicenter randomized trials that showed an improvement in locoregional control.[23,24] Long-term results of RTOG 9501 were published in 2012, and confirmed that the standard of care for patients with positive margins and extracapsular extension of positive nodes is concurrent chemoradiotherapy.

To diminish toxicities, radiotherapy techniques have evolved from 3D conformal radiation to intensity modulated radiotherapy (IMRT). New techniques such as image-guided radiotherapy and proton beam therapy (PBT) have been explored. IMRT is widely used; randomized studies showed reduced rates of xerostomia and improved quality of life.[25]

PBT may offer clinically relevant advantages in specific anatomical sites, sparing important at-risk organs. Multiple single-institution studies demonstrate the safety and efficacy of PBT,[26,27] but long-term results are still lacking.

References

1. Ferlay J, Soerjomataram I, Dikshit R, et al. Cancer incidence and mortality worldwide: sources, methods and major patterns in GLOBOCAN 2012. *Int J Cancer*. 2015;136(5):E359–E386.
2. Siegel RL, Miller KD, Jemal A. Cancer statistics. *CA Cancer J Clin*. 2018;68(1):7–30. 2018.
3. Chaturvedi AK, Engels EA, Pfeiffer RM, et al. Human papillomavirus and rising oropharyngeal cancer incidence in the United States. *J Clin Oncol*. 2011;29(32):4294–4301.
4. Hafkamp HC, Manni JJ, Haesevoets A, et al. Marked differences in survival rate between smokers and nonsmokers with HPV 16-associated tonsillar carcinomas. *Int J Cancer*. 2008;122(12):2656–2664.
5. Jain KS, Sikora AG, Baxi SS, et al. Synchronous cancers in patients with head and neck cancer: risks in the era of human

papillomavirus-associated oropharyngeal cancer. *Cancer.* 2013;119(10):1832–1837.
6. Sturgis EM, Miller RH. Second primary malignancies in the head and neck cancer patient. *Ann Otol Rhinol Laryngol.* 1995;104(12):946–954.
7. Antoniou AJ, Marcus C, Subramaniam RM. Value of imaging in head and neck tumors. *Surg Oncol Clin North Am.* 2014;23(4):685–707.
8. Juliano A, Moonis G. Computed tomography versus magnetic resonance in head and neck cancer: when to use what and image optimization strategies. *MRI Clin North Am.* 2018;26(1):63–84.
9. Mehanna H, Wong WL, McConkey CC, et al. PET-CT surveillance versus neck dissection in advanced head and neck cancer. *N Engl J Med.* 2016;374(15):1444–1454.
10. Amin MB, Edge S, Greene F, et al., eds. *AJCC Cancer Staging Manual.* 8th ed. New York: Springer International/American Joint Commission on Cancer; 2017.
11. Ebrahimi A, Gil Z, Amit M, et al. Primary tumor staging for oral cancer and a proposed modification incorporating depth of invasion: an international multicenter retrospective study. *JAMA Otolaryngol Head Neck Surg.* 2014;140(12):1138–1148.
12. Ang KK, Harris J, Wheeler R, et al. Human papillomavirus and survival of patients with oropharyngeal cancer. *N Engl J Med.* 2010;363(1):24–35.
13. Lindberg R. Distribution of cervical lymph node metastases from squamous cell carcinoma of the upper respiratory and digestive tracts. *Cancer.* 1972;29(6):1446–1449.
14. Shah JP. Patterns of cervical lymph node metastasis from squamous carcinomas of the upper aerodigestive tract. *Am J Surg.* 1990;160(4):405–409.
15. Leemans CR, Tiwari R, Nauta JJ, et al. Regional lymph node involvement and its significance in the development of distant metastases in head and neck carcinoma. *Cancer.* 1993;71(2):452–456.
16. Schmitz S, Machiels JP, Weynand B, et al. Results of selective neck dissection in the primary management of head and neck squamous cell carcinoma. *Eur Arch Oto-Rhino-Laryngol.* 2009;266(3):437–443.
17. Crile G. Excision of cancer of the head and neck with special reference to the plane of dissection based on one hundred and thirty-two operations. *J Am Med Assoc.* 1906;XLVII(22):1780–1786.
18. Robbins KT, Clayman G, Levine PA, et al. Neck dissection classification update: revisions proposed by the American head and neck society and the American Academy of otolaryngology-head and neck surgery. *Arch Otolaryngol Head Neck Surg.* 2002;128(7):751–758.
19. National Comprehensive Cancer Network. Head and Neck cancers. https://www.nccn.org/professionals/physician_gls/pdf/head-and-neck.pdf.
20. Civantos FJ, Zitsch RP, Schuller DE, et al. Sentinel lymph node biopsy accurately stages the regional lymph nodes for T1–T2 oral squamous cell carcinomas: results of a prospective multi-institutional trial. *J Clin Oncol.* 2010;28(8):1395–1400.
21. Genden EM, Ferlito A, Shaha AR, et al. Complications of neck dissection. *Acta Otolaryngol.* 2003;123(7):795–801.
22. Wolf GT, Fisher SG, Hong WK, et al. Induction chemotherapy plus radiation compared with surgery plus radiation in patients with advanced laryngeal cancer. *N Engl J Med.* 1991;324(24):1685–1690.
23. Cooper JS, Pajak TF, Forastiere AA, et al. Postoperative concurrent radiotherapy and chemotherapy for high-risk squamous-cell carcinoma of the head and neck. *N Engl J Med.* 2004;350(19):1937–1944.
24. Bernier J, Domenge C, Ozsahin M, et al. Postoperative irradiation with or without concomitant chemotherapy for locally advanced head and neck cancer. *N Engl J Med.* 2004;350(19):1945–1952.
25. Nutting CM, Morden JP, Harrington KJ, et al. Parotid-sparing intensity modulated versus conventional radiotherapy in head and neck cancer (PARSPORT): a phase 3 multicentre randomised controlled trial. *Lancet Oncol.* 2011;12(2):127–136.
26. Russo AL, Adams JA, Weyman EA, et al. Long-term outcomes after proton beam therapy for sinonasal squamous cell carcinoma. *Int J Radiat Oncol Biol Phys.* 2016;95(1):368–376.
27. Romesser PB, Cahlon O, Scher E, et al. Proton beam radiation therapy results in significantly reduced toxicity compared with intensity-modulated radiation therapy for head and neck tumors that require ipsilateral radiation. *Radiother Oncol.* 2016;118(2):286–292.

24

Oral Tongue and Mandibular Reconstruction

YUN-HUAN (BARRY) HSIEH, NIDAL AL DEEK, AND FU-CHAN WEI

Introduction

The oral tongue and mandible act as an inseparable functional unit of the lower face. Embryologically, tongue, mandible, and muscles of mastication share a common origin from the first branchial arch (BR). There is an interdependent developmental relationship between tongue and mandible, and the architectural malposition of one can lead to deformity of the other. The classic example is Pierre Robin Sequence, the syndromic condition that includes respiratory obstruction, glossoptosis, mandibular hypoplasia, and cleft palate.[1] The challenges of tongue reconstructions are chiefly due to its multidimensional roles in prehension, mastication, deglutination, speech articulation, and airway protection.[2] The optimal tongue reconstruction strategy depends on the size and the location of the defect, as the precise reconstruction goal varies from tip to base of the tongue. The complexity of mandibular reconstruction is to provide sturdy construction for its characteristic functions, including mastication, swallowing, speech, and smile. Esthetically, the mandible outlines the shape, contour, and height of the lower face. A well-defined jaw line is considered to be a sign of youth. The mandible reconstruction options are principally based on the location and tissue components of the defect (isolated bone, compound, composite, or extensive composite defects).[3] Simultaneous reconstruction of tongue and mandible may be required, and careful planning of relative anatomical positions is the key for satisfactory reconstruction. Oral tongue and mandible reconstruction signifies the classical indication for the "reconstructive escalator", where locoregional options are limited and free flaps are required.

Normal Anatomy and Function of Oral Tongue and Mandible

Anatomy of the Tongue

The tongue is a mass of skeletal muscle covered by mucous membrane, derived from two separate muscle halves that fuse into the midline fibrous septum. It is supplied by a pair of lingual arteries coursed above the greater horn of the hyoid bone, deep to hypoglossus. It branches into the dorsal lingual artery posteriorly and supplies the sublingual gland and floor of mouth anteriorly. Additional arterial supply comes from the tonsillar branch of the facial artery and the ascending pharyngeal artery.[2] The venous drainage of the lingual vein follows the course of arterial tributaries. Its dorsal branches drain directly into the internal jugular vein, whereas the tip of the tongue is drained by the sublingual vein and ends with the lingual, facial, or internal jugular vein.[2] Anatomical parts include the dorsum, tip, inferior surface (ventral tongue), and the base. The tongue is composed of both intrinsic and extrinsic muscle groups; each group consists of four muscles from each half of the tongue. The intrinsic muscle is comprised of superior longitudinal, transverse, inferior longitudinal, and vertical muscles. The multidimensional muscle fibres deliver great mobility as well as volume and shape transformability, thus allowing the tongue's performance of both gross and fine movements. The extrinsic muscle is comprised of genioglossus, hypoglossus, styloglossus, and palatoglossus, and each is attached to the mandible (and hyoid bone), hyoid bone, styloid process, and hard palate, respectively. Extrinsic muscles alter the relative position of the tongue and provide the stability of the intrinsic muscle. The orchestrated muscle function allows intelligibility of speech, and precise execution of the oral process and transport phases of swallowing. Based on functional and structural differences, the tongue can also be described as the anterior two-thirds (oral or presulcal), and posterior third (pharyngeal/postsulcal/tongue base), separated by sulcus terminalis. The mucosa appearances and function of these two parts are distinctive. The anterior two-thirds in general has a rougher surface covered by various forms of papillae (filiform, fungiform, and vallate) and taste buds within; this character assists the transportation and processing of the food bolus during mastication. The posterior third of the tongue is part of the oral pharynx; it has a smoother surface, with abundance of glandular tissues to facilitate swallowing.

To appreciate sensory and motor supply of the tongue is to understand their embryological derivations. The epithelial layer of the tongue derives from the first, third, and fourth BR. The epithelium of the presulcal part of the tongue derives from the midline tuberculum impar, and a pair of lateral lingual swellings (tongue primordium) from the first arch. The postsulcal part derives from the midline hypobranchial eminence of the third arch and, to a lesser extent, the fourth arch (vallecula). Respectively, sensory supply of first, third, and fourth arch are the lingual nerve (CN V_3 and chorda tympani nerve of CN VII), glossopharyngeal nerve (CN IX), and internal laryngeal nerve (CN X).The musculature, with the exception of palatoglossus, derives from suboccipital myotomes and migrates into the primordium, carrying its motor supply from hypoglossal nerve (CN XII) for voluntary movements. Palatoglossus, conversely, is part of the oropharynx and is supplied by the pharyngeal plexus from the vagus nerve. Lymphatics of the tongue drain into the floor of the mouth; the tip drains into sublingual nodes, the rest of the presucal part drains into submandibular nodes then to both the upper and lower cervical chain. The posterior part, on the other hand, drains directly into deep cervical nodes. Most clinically relevant feature of the tongue's lymphatic drainage is its bilateral drainage pattern, especially when the ipsilateral system is obstructed. This feature is more prominent in the posterior tongue, and prompts bilateral neck dissection in oncological resections. Although not part of the tongue, the floor of the mouth is its continuum and frequently involved in radical resection of the tongue. It contains a pair of sublingual glands in the sublingual folds, and is composed of a pair of mylohyoid muscles inferiorly and geniohyoids superiorly. The floor of the mouth is structurally analogous to the pelvic diaphragm; it separates the mouth from the neck, supports the weight, and thrusts the tongue.[2] The muscles attachment between mandible and hyoid bone further enhances the mobility of the tongue. Mylohyoid is supplied by the myohyoid branch of the inferior alveolar artery and the submental artery of the facial artery. It is innervated by the mylohyoid nerve from the inferior alveolar branch of CN V_3. Geniohyoid is supplied by the lingual artery and directly innervated by C1 fibres via the hypoglossal nerve.

Function of the Tongue

To understand the goals of tongue reconstruction, it is essential to appreciate its functions in deglutition, airway protection, and speech articulation. Deglutition has three distinct phases: oral, pharyngeal, and esophageal phases, where tongue movements are important for both the oral and pharyngeal phases. The oral phase is subdivided into: (1) stage I transport, (2) processing, (3) stage II transport, and (4) bolus formation. In stage I transport, it represents the moment of food reception, where the anterior third of the tongue surface is hollowed and the posterior third is sealed against the soft palate (posterior oral seal). In the processing phase, the anterior two-thirds of the tongue rotates at the posterior–anterior axis against a sealed posterior margin. This allows constant food bolus mixture with saliva, food grinding against hard palate, and continuous mastication. Stage II transport is defined by the movement of the food bolus through the posterior oral seal prior to the pharyngeal phase of deglutition. It starts with sealing of the anterior hard palate with the anterior third of the tongue and propulsion of the food bolus posteriorly in sequence into the oral pharynx by other parts of the tongue.[4] In the pharyngeal phase of the deglutition, the tongue base retracts then moves superoposteriorly, thus directing the food bolus toward the pharynx. The orchestrated movements of tongue, floor of mouth, and larynx protect the upper airway from aspiration. The closure of the velopharyngeal port by the tongue during food bolus propulsion prevents food or fluid regurgitation into nasal cavity.[5]

Tongue movements that are associated with speech and articulation can be categorized into four types based on the findings of Stone and Lundberg.[6] They are: (1) "front raising," where the anterior and middle tongue are raised ("t," "d"); (2) a complete midline groove with elevated lateral tongue margins ("she," "th"); (3) "back-raising," the reciprocal tongue movements of the first category ("k," "g"); and (4) "two-point displacement," where the tongue has an elevated anterior and posterior segment with a small central groove in the middle segment ("l"). The understanding of commonly used tongue movements during speech and articulation aids in preoperative patient assessments and consultation regarding the expected postoperative speech deficit.

Anatomy of the Mandible

The mandible is a strong, semicircular bone of the lower face. It is composed of two symmetrical halves that fuse at the symphysis, and a pair of condyles that articulate with temple bones.[4] Morphologically, the mandible is described in parts, including the processes (condylar, coronoid, and alveolar process), ramus, angle, body, and symphysis. The sophiscated design of the mandible offers a stable root for teeth, and a robust platform to withstand forces of mastication. Angle and ramus of the mandible consist of thick cortices and are designed to resist excessive unidirectional force, whereas trabeculae in the alveolar process and condylar head possess the ability to endure greater stress from multidirectional forces.[7] There are a total of 16 teeth on the mandible, providing opposing occlusion to the 16 teeth on the maxilla. The force on dentition is transmitted to the underlying trabecular bone in the alveolar process; this constant force serves as a remodeling stimulus to the mandible. Loss of dentition, altering mastication habits, and being edentulous thus alter or regress the mandibular strength and thickness. The mandible is supplied by a pair of inferior alveolar arteries with additional vascular tributaries from the periosteum and the attached muscles. The pair of inferior alveolar nerves supplies the sensation of the mandible and transmits sensation from the dentition, gingiva, and sulcus for protective feedback. The mandible also provides the attachments for the muscles of mastication, muscles of oral continence, and facial expression, floor of mouth, genioglossus, digastric muscle, and platysma.[2]

Etiology and Classification System

Etiology

The majority of oral cavity defects derive from oncological resections, and post-reconstruction complications. Oropharyngeal cancer is ranked 11th most common cancer worldwide, with incidence of 11.3/100,000 per year and 5-year survival of 64.8%.[8] Oral cancers are predominantly squamous cell carcinoma (86%), whereas verrucous carcinoma, sarcoma, melanoma, and lymphoma account for less occurrence. Prototypical risk factors are long-standing history of cigarette smoking and heavy alcohol consumption. Betel nut, in addition, is an established independent risk factor for oral cancer, with an adjusted odds ratio of 58.4%.[9] Statistically, there is a significant rise of human papilloma virus-associated oral tongue cancers affecting younger males and females less than 40 years old.[10] Similar to skin cancer, field cancerization in the oral cavity is common; it is associated with a complex defect, high incidence of recurrence, and second primary tumors. Reconstructive surgeons therefore need to have a close working relationship with the ablation team, and be prepared for repeated major reconstructions.

The majority of mandibular defects are the result of soft tissue tumor ablations. Odontogenic tumors represent uncommon heterogeneous lesions. Among them, ameloblastoma, a group of benign yet locally invasive tumors, is frequently associated with major mandibular resection and reconstruction. Segmental excision and vascularized bone reconstruction is considered the treatment of choice to achieve long-term successful tumor control. Osteoradionecrosis (ORN) of the mandible occurs uncommonly, with an estimated incidence of 8.2%. It is seen following radiotherapy of the oral cavity.[11] The risk of ORN increases in the presence of insufficient vascularized tissue coverage, aggressive muscle detachments, stripping of periosteum, marginal mandibulectomy, and mandibulotomy. Although conservative management is frequently employed, the definitive management of ORN remains segmental mandibular excision and free tissue transfer. A similar approach is recommended for other forms of osteonecrosis induced by infection, trauma, glucocorticoids, and high-dosage bisphosphonate. Trauma of the mandible is rarely associated with segmental mandibular loss, unless caused by ballistic wound or barotrauma. Patient stabilization should be the first priority prior to the consideration of mandibular reconstruction.

Classification of Oral Tongue Defects

Tongue reconstruction is defect-dependent, and a widely adopted classification system is currently unavailable. Most published classification systems are based on the defect percentage across the medial–lateral axis. The defects are generally subdivided into small glossectomy defect (less than one-third), hemiglossectomy, subtotal, and total glossectomy. Composite and compound defects involving the surrounding soft tissue and mandible are frequently incorporated in the classification to guide the reconstructive options.[12,13] These tongue classifications are useful in deciding simple reconstructions from complex options, but do not accentuate the regional anatomical differences for the guidance of reconstruction selections. The key deciding factors for complex reconstructive options of the tongue are the location (presulcal versus postsulcal), involvements of floor of the mouth, and the presence of bony defect. Thus, in addition to size, categorization of tongue defects into presulcal and postsulcal (tongue base) with or without involvements of floor of the mouth and mandible should be considered. These variants enhance clinical relevance of the classification, facilitate logistic defect reconstruction planning, and allow comparative studies to be conducted.

Classification of Mandibular Defects

The mandible is a semicircular structure that delivers unified and coordinated actions to its attached musculatures. Disruption of its continuity drastically reduces the power of mastication, speech articulation, deglutition, and protective mechanisms against upper airway obstruction and aspiration. Segmental bone defect is thus the most common indication for mandibular reconstruction. In contrast, marginal mandibulectomies are generally not reconstructed. Nevertheless, in the presence of insufficient residual mandibular height (less than 1 cm) and the necessity for mandibular height augmentation for dental rehabilitation, onlay nonvascularized or vascularized bone flap is recommended. In our practice, the classification system formulated by Daniel[3] is the most clinically relevant tool in dictating options for defect reconstructions. It accounts for soft tissue involvement and the need for its synchronous reconstruction. The system classifies the defect into: (1) isolated bone; (2) compound defect (bone, oral lining or skin); (3) composite defect (bone, oral lining, and skin); (4) extensive composite (bone, oral lining, skin and intervening soft tissues).[3] In dentulous patients, teeth are powerful landmarks to describe defect locations within teeth-bearing segments. On many occasions, defect distance can also be estimated based on the documented number of resected teeth. To simplify the descriptive terms for mandibular defects, Jewer's classification[14] is commonly used. The system signifies letter "L," "C," and " H" to correspond to lateral segments, central segments (between canines), and condylar defects. Combined use of the letters enables the description of complex and extended defects; for instance, using "LCL" represents an angle-to-angle defect of the mandible. Although soft tissue defects were added in the modified Jewer's classification, using "O," "M," and "S" to represent osseous, mucosa, and skin defects, this new addition does not distinguish small composite defects from extensive soft tissue loss.

Reconstruction Principles

Patient Evaluation

Detailed medical assessments including social status and reconstruction expectation should be evaluated. With best intention, both tongue and mandibular reconstruction can still have devastating outcomes due to the complexity of their respective functions and esthetic importance. Allowing sufficient consultation time for emotional response from both the patient and their family is essential. Presenting clinical photos of similar cases during the consultation decreases the risk of miscommunication and expectation disparity.

Multidisciplinary assessments are mandatory for surgical planning and streamlining the corresponding adjuvant therapies. It is indispensable to have a thorough understanding of the patient's present physical status, disease progression, and life expectancy. These factors can affect the final tactics of the reconstruction. Physical optimization and surgical risk minimization with emphases on cigarette cessation, anticoagulation management, and strategy of deep vein thrombosis prophylaxis reduce unnecessary complications for patients.

Reconstruction Preparation and Logistics

Surgical ablation and reconstruction are better done simultaneously, in a two-team model. The concept of a two-team approach needs to be utilized to shorten the anesthetic period, lessen physiological demand, and facilitate the recovery process. Nevertheless, a two-team approach is donor-site dependent, and inapplicable in locoregional reconstructions. Although preoperative assessments of the presumed defect provide guidance for the reconstructive approach, the ideal assessment occurs intraoperatively after ablative surgery. This allows the defect to be measured accurately, and permits the formulation of flap choice, flap design, vessel positions, and insets. Clear communication between the ablation and resection teams perioperatively is imperative; although a drastic change of intraoperative plan is unlikely, good communication permits a dynamic surgical approach to ensure ultimate reconstruction is achieved.

Tongue Reconstruction Goals and Surgical Pearls

Tongue reconstruction requires the restoration of both mobility and loss of tissue bulk against weakened native propulsive power of the tongue. Therefore, meticulous execution of surgical margins to retain maximum intrinsic and extrinsic muscles effectively reduces the loss of tongue function. Similarly, preservation of pharyngeal muscles and minimization of their use in regional reconstructions maximizes their coordinated intraoral functions with the tongue. The thickness of the flap should appropriately match the residual tongue. If the flap is thicker than the native tongue, the mobile part of the tongue (anterior two-thirds) may be overpowered. Conversely, if the flap is thinner than the native tongue, it results in tongue asymmetry. The length of neotongue should also match the native tongue if the tip is not affected. In the resected tip, the length of the neo-tongue should extend no shorter than the location of the incisors. If the length of the tongue is insufficiently reconstructed, the overall mobility is reduced and affects "front raising" speech articulation, as well as the process and transport II phases of oral deglutition. Insufficient length of the neo-tongue and inadequate tissue replacement at the junction between floor of mouth and mobile tongue (anterior two-thirds) can cause tongue tethering, and will be worsened post radiotherapy.

When the floor of the mouth is resected or neck dissection is performed, complete separation of the oral cavity from the neck is crucial. Complete separation of the oral cavity from the neck avoids fistula formation. Subsequent wound infection, necrosis, and abscess of the neck may develop, leading to delayed pedicle thrombosis of the free flap and possible arterial or venous blowout. In the posterior third of the tongue, volume replacement is the most important. As the tongue normally seals against the soft palate during the transport and process phase of oral deglutition, lack of volume replacement will, therefore, increase the risk of aspiration. The tongue base propulses fluid and food boluses towards the laryngopharynx during transport II phase to initiate pharyngeal deglutition. Failure of its superoposterior movements due to loss of its bulk post reconstruction, reduces overall swallowing efficiency and increases the likelihood of nasal regurgitation via the velopharyngeal port. The incomplete contact of the posterior tongue will increase the difficulties of "back raising" articulation as the result of insufficient volume replacement. In an extended defect that involves the floor of the mouth and buccal sulcus, the contouring of the flap is commonly inadequate to reconstruct the concavity of the buccal sulcus. The sulcus functions as a food reservoir during mastication and helps in directing the saliva and food toward the oropharynx during deglutition. To avoid bulkiness and formless reconstruction of the buccal sulcus, an origami technique can be utilized.[15] The steps of the procedure are: (1) pre-fixing the flap to the defect; (2) marking the area of concavity at the sulcus on the flap; (3) de-epithelialization of the triangulated concaved edge; (4) edge-to-edge repair of the deepithelialized skin.[15] However, the technique is restricted in bulky flaps or bulky insets, as skin-deep folding may be difficult.

Sensation is complementary to muscular function of the tongue for prehension, speech, and deglutition. The tongue possesses a significant portion of the cortical homunculus, and sensory feedback allows constant adjustments of the tongue position and movements. This coordinated function is the key to the high functioning tongue articulations that can be observed among trumpet players. Evidently, sensory preservation from surgical ablation and reinnervation is generally recommended. Tongue reconstruction with sensory reinnervation results in superior sensory recovery compared with those left with spontaneous resensitization. Coaptation to lingual and inferior alveolar nerve provides statistically superior sensory function than other nerves. The overall tongue function is enhanced in those with sensory recovery post reconstruction compared with those without.[16] However, sensory reconstruction of the tongue should proceed with caution. The potential development of hyperalgesia and allodynia during axon regeneration may outweigh its benefit, especially among those who are planned for postoperative radiotherapy. Motor innervation is sought after functioning muscle transfer, and the common donor nerve is the hypoglossal. Motor nerve reinnervation reduces the impact of muscular atrophy, and the reanimated flap provides much needed protective function of the neo-tongue.

Mandibular Reconstruction Goals and Surgical Pearls

The goal for mandibular defect reconstruction is both functional and esthetic. Specifically, it aims to restore sturdy continuum of the mandible, reinstate accurate occlusion, preserve or reestablish condylar articulation of the temporomandibular joint (TMJ), achieve sensory reconstruction, and provide adequate bone width and height for dental osseointegration and esthetics. To achieve functional and esthetically pleasing reconstruction of the mandible, adequate restoration of occlusion is crucial. Occlusion provides a platform for constant intraoral force transmission from mandible to maxilla. The force provides constant stimuli for mandibular remodelling, soft tissue positioning, and dentition alignments. Malocclusion induces unopposed force of the mandible, and is associated with dental caries, masticatory muscle contracture and shortening, mandibular recession, as well as dentition loosening and shift. It can lead to significant anterior subluxation of TMJ with mandibular swing, thus worsening the malocclusion and facial asymmetry. Sensory reconstruction is important, yet difficult to achieve in complex resections. Where possible, inferior alveolar nerve should be reinnervated with sural nerve graft to restore sensation of the lip, especially in benign cases such as ameloblastoma reconstructions. Protective mechanism of the oral cavity and maintenance of oral continence will be impaired if numbness and/or dysesthesia of the lip persists. The optimal segmental reconstruction of the mandible is with a free vascularized bone flap that has durable soft tissue. Alternatively, segmental defects can be reconstructed with vascularized soft tissue flap with/without a reconstruction plate. The second option is typically reserved for patients who present with advanced disease and short life expectancy. It is worth noting that a mandibular reconstruction plate with soft tissue coverage is associated with significant risk of plate-related complications, that include osteomyelitis, screw loosening, stress fracture of the plate, osteocutaneous fistula, and plate exposure. It is reported that up to 46% of these patients will present with plate exposure, most commonly in the combined lateral and central segments (L-C segment)[17] and patients who received postoperative radiotherapy.

Surgical Options

Tongue Reconstruction with Non-Flap Options

Primary closure can generally be achieved in small and isolated presulcal tongue defects up to a third of tongue resection. As a structure that consists of pure skeletal muscle, postoperative functional compensation of the tongue can be expected. Primary closure is contraindicated in similar defects that involve the floor of the mouth, particularly if the remaining floor of mouth mucosa is less than 1 cm away from the gingiva. Healing by secondary intention is indicated when the defect cannot be reconstructed by primary closure without substantial distortion, or as the result of postoperative dehiscence. Oncologically, the primary site of the tumor is more difficult to monitor for recurrence if allowed to heal secondarily. In small defects among suitable patients, primary closure or healing with secondary intention can be utilized; the resultant speech and swallowing is superior not only because more muscle was preserved but also due to the avoidance of the potential overpowering effect of the flap to the native tongue.

Full-thickness/split-thickness skin grafts and mucosa grafts are rarely used for tongue reconstruction. Within the narrow spectrum of skin graft application in tongue reconstruction, to ensure its success, maneuvers such as overgrafting and quilting technique can be used. Tie-over dressing, on the other hand, may be poorly tolerated, and is a potential risk of upper airway obstruction. These techniques should be reserved for candidates who are unfit for any other forms of reconstruction and present with a well-vascularized noninfected wound bed that is shallow and flat.

Tongue Reconstruction with Intraoral Flap Techniques

Intraoral local flaps, in theory, are the optimal donor tissues for tongue reconstructions. These options, however, are restricted due to limited donor tissue and potential risk of trismus at the donor sites. They are generally unable to provide the bulk that is required for tongue reconstruction; they are, nevertheless, important options for defects that are small and thin.

Facial artery myomucosal flaps (FAMM) and the buccinator myomucosal island flap resurface small to moderate size defects that require thin tissue for reconstruction among edentulous patients. FAMM flaps are based on the facial artery anterior to Stensen's duct, and can be based superiorly or inferiorly for anterior third tongue reconstruction.[18] In contrast, the buccinator myomucosal island flap is based on the buccal artery (from the internal maxillary artery) posteriorly, or branches of the facial artery anteriorly.[19] The buccinator myomucosal flap has wider flap reach, is comparatively more versatile, and able to cover the anterior two-thirds of the tongue. Flap orientation should be carefully designed, using the flap sparingly to prevent postoperative trismus.

Mandible Reconstruction with Nonmicrosurgical Techniques

Mandible reconstruction with nonmicrosurgical technique is generally reserved for small benign defects that do not require subsequent radiotherapy or patients who are unsuitable for prolonged microsurgical reconstructions. These techniques include the use of nonvascularized bone graft or bone substitutes, and prosthetic implants. Nonvascularized bone graft and bone substitute are suitable for small to moderate size bony defects up to 6 cm. They require both well-vascularized wound beds without pre- or postoperative radiotherapy. Durable vascularized tissue coverage is essential for eventual union to occur. These techniques are commonly used for enucleation procedures for benign lesions such as primary ameloblastoma, and usually covered by local gingival flaps. Nonvascularized bone has a more significant role in marginal defect reconstruction for height augmentation prior to dental osseointegration. It may still be indicated for segmental defects in biomechanically favorable locations such as body or ramus of the mandible. The durability of nonvascularized bone is frequently in doubt as it atrophies significantly compared with vascularized options. Alternatively, a mandibular reconstruction plate is used to replace the need of bony reconstruction. The use of a reconstruction plate invariably requires durable soft tissue reconstruction for its coverage with a pedicle flap.

Regional Flap Reconstruction for Oral Tongue and Mandibular Defects

In modern day reconstruction, regional flaps have a limited role, but remain valuable options, especially in critically ill patients or patients with a vessel-depleted neck.

Soft Tissue Regional Flaps

Submental Artery Flap

The submental artery (SMA) flap is a fasciocutaneous flap located in the submental region. The flap is based on submental artery located 5–6.5 cm from the origin of the facial artery. The artery courses deep to the submandibular gland via myelohyoid muscle inferior to the mandibular angle and extends medially deep to anterior digastric muscle. Once it reaches the mandible margin, it branches to supply platysma and overlying skin.[20] It is a reliable flap with pliable tissue; the pedicle length enables it to reach to ipsilateral tongue, floor of mouth, and oropharynx. Oncologically, this flap is raised over common regions of nodal metastasis. Therefore use of this flap should proceed with caution, and the flap is better dissected off the regional lymph nodes to prevent metastasis.

Pectoralis Major Myocutaneous Flap

The pectoralis major myocutaneous (PMC) flap is classified as a type V muscle flap by Mathes and Nahai, with one dominant artery and several secondary segmental arteries.[21] The dominant artery originates from the pectoral branch of the thoracoacromial artery, whereas secondary segmental arteries derive from the superior thoracic artery, clavicular branch of the thoracoacromial artery, lateral thoracic artery, and internal mammary artery.[21] A PMC flap is more commonly used as a salvage procedure in the modern reconstruction era. It is a thick flap with a bulky pedicle. The muscle is based on its axial blood supply, whereas the skin is based on a random pattern. A PMC flap typically requires larger tunneling to breach the oral cavity from the neck for intraoral reconstruction, which invariably produces an unsightly bulge at the recipient site, and is less suitable for anterior tongue and oral cavity reconstruction. It can also be raised as an island flap and the pedicle skeletonized to counteract the undesirable cosmesis. It is a durable flap to cover a mandibular reconstruction plate, and is applicable to cover vascularized or nonvascularized bony reconstruction of the mandible. A two-stage operation is frequently planned for mandibular coverage, where the pedicle is commonly divided after 3–4 weeks for superior contouring results. A major drawback of the PMC flap is donor site morbidity. Reduction in adduction and internal rotation of the arm is expected.[2] The bulk of the flap invariably shrinks as muscle atrophies, which can produce a sagging appearance and intraoral pooling. Surgical refinement or secondary operation may be needed for these corrections. Regaining protective sensation post reconstruction is unlikely.

Supraclavicular Artery Island Flap

Supraclavicular artery island flap is a recent addition to regional flap options for head and neck reconstruction. It is a fasciocutaneous flap over the tip of the shoulder and extends to midlateral deltoid muscle. The flap is based on the supraclavicular branch of the transverse cervical artery. Anatomical studies have revealed the flap is a combination of axial flap proximally and random pattern distally, demarcated at the origin of the deltoid muscle.[22] It provides thin sizable hairless skin with good reach up to 30 cm; distal necrosis may occur in flaps with reach greater than 20 cm. Level V neck dissection can damage the course of the supraclavicular pedicle, however, it is usually preserved and thus not contraindicated. It is advisable to use handheld Doppler intraoperatively to ensure the patency of the pedicle prior to its dissection. Flap prelamination with skin graft, and delayed procedure can be applied to extend its versatility.

Bone-Bearing Regional Flaps

Regional bone-bearing flaps are convenient options with creative use of regional osseous constructs and shapes. Nevertheless, none of the described options has achieved popularity due to poor bone quality, fragile osseous blood supply, inadequate cortical thickness, restricted flexibility in bone insetting, and significant donor site morbidity. Although general consensus recommends pedicle-based or downgraded reconstruction in failed primary microsurgery reconstructions, however, head and neck reconstruction with regional flap consists of higher subsequent complication rates than those who received second free flaps.[23] The success rate for a second free flap reconstruction was 94.1% in the published series. Regional options of bone-bearing flaps for intraoral reconstruction include the use of vascularized bone from the ribs, clavicle,[24] and scapula. They can be harvested with pectoralis major, sternocleidomastoid,[25] and trapezius, respectively, as pedicle osteomusculocutaneous flaps. In addition, a temporalis osteomuscular flap can also be used for simultaneous soft tissue and bony reconstruction of the intraoral cavity.

Pectoralis Major Osteomusculocutaneous Flap

Intergraded harvesting of fifth rib into a traditional PMC flap added further diversity to the flap for composite oromandibular defects.[21] The blood supply to the fifth rib is based on a vascular plexus derived from its periosteum and pectoralis muscle. The blood supply to the osseous component is small and occasionally unreliable. The drawback of this technique is the difficulty of inset, and insufficient cortical thickness for functional mandibular reconstruction and dental osseointegration. Hemothorax and pneumothorax are possible donor site morbidities. They should be actively monitored, and promptly treated. Similarly, sternum can be harvested in conjunction with a PMC flap. It shares similar drawbacks with ribs, and a long-term result is not yet available. There is also reported success of a latissimus dorsi flap incorporating rib for extensive mandibular reconstruction.

Microsurgical Reconstructions of Oral Tongue and Mandible

Microsurgical reconstruction for tongue and mandibular reconstruction comes with a greater than 95% success rate. Different from local regional flaps, free flaps are not restricted by defect size and location. The flexibility of free flap positioning is unrestricted from its pedicle, thus liberating the imagination and creativity of free flap inset and design. The phenomenon of mucosalization popularized the use of free fasciocutaneous flaps for intraoral reconstruction over intestinal flaps (jejunal flap). Muscle flaps can adequately replace the volume deficit, and may also enhance the overall function if reanimated. When using a muscle flap or flap with a muscle component, the operating surgeon needs to be mindful of total ischemia time; the completion of inset and arterial anastomosis should be kept within 4 hours to prevent irreversible muscular injury.

For head and neck reconstruction in general, the use of distant free flap donor sites such as lower extremities is preferred. This principle permits a two-team approach, and shortens overall operative time. An abdominal donor site is generally avoided as disruption of internal viscera may induce ileus, and possible bowel obstruction. This can significantly reduce the patient's nutritional status postoperatively, prolong healing time, and increase overall bed-bound related complications. In addition, increase in intraabdominal pressure and pain reduces inspiratory effort, increases atelectasis of the lung, and escalates the risk of postoperative pneumonia. Single free flap reconstruction is suitable for most tongue and mandibular reconstruction. In extended oromandibular defects, a combined technique of locoregional flaps with free flap may be necessary. If volume replacement is necessary, double free flap reconstruction should be considered. The commonly used recipient vessels are superior thyroid artery, transverse cervical artery, and facial artery. The lingual artery is uncommonly used for head and neck reconstruction, if preserved, however, it can be a reliable option. The following represent common soft tissue and bone-bearing free flap options in oral tongue and mandibular reconstructions.

Soft Tissue Free Flaps

Radial Forearm Free Flap

The radial forearm free flap (RFFF) is also known as the Chinese flap and was introduced in 1978. It is one of the most commonly used flaps in intraoral reconstruction today. It is easy to raise, provides thin and pliable tissue, allowing large skin paddle harvest with a lengthy pedicle, and good vascular caliber.[21] It is usually raised as a fasciocutaneous flap by suprafascial or subfascial dissection, however, it can also be harvested as an adipofascial flap, or osteocutaneous flap incorporating radius. It is a type C fasciocutaneous flap, based on the radial artery and its perforators. The artery is drained preferentially by a pair of accompanying venae comitantes, and cephalic vein to a lesser extent.[21] Allen's test should be performed in the case of a radial dominant forearm.

The flap planning starts with locating the radial artery by palpation; the skin paddle border should be designed within the radial border of the forearm without extending to the extensor surface. A tourniquet should be used to minimize bleeding while optimizing the surgical field to prevent unnecessary vascular injury. The dissection starts at the radial edge in the suprafascial plane as described by Wong et al.[26] The distal pedicle is ligated at the wrist, followed by careful dissection proximally preserving paratenons and superficial radial nerve. Once the dissection is completed, the tourniquet is released and flap and distal circulation is observed for 15–20 minutes. This is to ensure the integrity of the pedicle is preserved, circulation of the flap is adequate, and distal circulation of the hand and fingers is unaffected. If circulation of the hand is compromised, interposition vascular anastomosis should be performed to restore its perfusion. If innervation is planned for tongue reconstruction or as soft tissue coverage for mandibular reconstruction, antebrachial cutaneous nerve can be included during harvesting.

As there are nine fasciocutaneous branches of the radial artery in the forearm, multiple skin paddles can be designed for multiple defect reconstruction. This concept is commonly used for trismus release where two skin paddles were designed based on the same vascular system. Similarly, double skin paddle design is useful to separate the oral tongue from the floor of the mouth to prevent tethering of the tongue. If tissue volume is required, a proximally-based flap can be designed, however, this will significantly shorten the pedicle length. Alternatively, volume augmentation can be achieved by harvesting a flap with excess, and invaginating the excess flap for volume augmentation after de-epithelialization.

As an osteocutaneous flap, the quality of the radius is inadequate to replace segmental mandibular defects, as it lacks cortex thickness, is brittle, and unsustainable for osteotomies. It is an unsuitable option if full functional reconstruction is anticipated. It may be indicated for marginal mandibular defect reconstructions, nevertheless, the bone quality is inappropriate for subsequent osseointegration for full dental rehabilitation.

Donor site morbidity is the major drawback of the RFFF. The donor site is commonly closed with full- or split-thickness skin grafts. The donor site may present with contracture, stiffness of the wrist and fingers, recurrent wound breakdown and tendon exposure. These complications are predominately related to failure of the skin graft, representing integral disadvantages of skin graft reconstructions. Suprafascial technique reduces the incidence of tendon exposure, and lessens risk of graft failure. Preferentially using a thick split-thickness skin graft for a larger defect, and a full-thickness skin graft for a smaller donor site defect may reduce the contracture from the skin grafts. However, in selected cases, a proximally-based local flap may be used successfully for donor site closure and prevent the above mentioned complications. If an osteocutaneous flap is used, the risk of distal radius fracture is clinically significant. In high-risk patients, prophylactic plating may be necessary (Fig. 24.1).

Gracilis Flap

The free gracilis muscle flap is the most commonly used flap for functional muscle reconstruction. It can be harvested as a muscle flap or musculocutaneous flap. Gracilis muscle is a Mathes and Nahai type II muscle flap, and is supplied by a branch of the medial femoral circumflex artery or a direct branch from the profunda femoral artery.[21] The minor pedicles arise from either the superficial femoral or descending genicular artery. It is drained by two venae comitantes accompanying the artery. Both skin and muscle components of the gracilis provide the bulk for volume replacement. The pedicle length (7 cm) is relatively short, thus restricting its wider utilization for intraoral defect reconstructions. The maximum dimensions of both muscle and skin components are 8×30 cm.

The flap is raised based on its dominant artery pedicle and motor reinnervation is possible with inclusion of the anterior branch of the obturator nerve. The landmarks include the pubic tubercle and medial femoral condyle as well as the outline of adductor longus and gracilis muscle. Adductor longus is palpable when placing the patient in flamingo position, whereas gracilis is palpable when the lower limb is in full abduction with a straight leg. The patient is positioned supine, with a sandbag placed under the contralateral hip. Starting with distal dissection is preferred to avoid confusion of musculature, and avoid unnecessary vascular injury. The vascular pedicle is commonly found at 6–12 cm below the public tubercle, and divides into 3–6 branches into the muscle belly. The perforators to skin are found between gracilis and adductor longus, more commonly from the musculocutaneous course from the anterior aspect of the gracilis. This flap is useful for subtotal or total glossectomy. The muscle component is used for volume replacement at the tongue base, whereas the fasciocutaneous component can be used separately for presulcal tongue reconstruction.

The donor site is well tolerated with a hidden scar. Harvesting gracilis does not significantly affect the lower leg function. As the viability of the distal part of the skin is variable, placing the distal part of the flap anteriorly serves better inset planning. Any ischemic insult intra- or post-operatively will impede the muscular functional recovery. If perfusion insufficiency is detected postoperatively, some surgeons will deem the flap to be unsalvageable from the functional aspect. A second muscle flap may be needed for repeated reconstruction.

Anterolateral Thigh (ALT) Flap

The ALT flap is a highly diverse flap with wide range of applications. It is commonly used as a cutaneous or fasciocutaneous flap; it can also be raised as a musculocutaneous and osteomusculocutaneous flap. It is based on the descending and/or oblique branch of the lateral femoral circumflex artery, and drained by its accompanying vena comitans. Compared with the RFFF, the ALT flap delivers greater dimension and tissue volume. However, it is usually thicker and this is worse among patients with higher BMI. To counteract this disadvantage of the flap, several strategies were developed: (1) the flap can be thinned while perfused; (2) it can be raised by suprascarpa dissection; and (3) flap design can be shifted distally to raise a thinner flap.

The ALT flap has moderate pedicle length and is 12 cm on average. Eighty-five percent of its perforators submerge through a musculocutaneous course and 15% are septocutaneous. Unfortunately, 2% of the population perforators are not of adequate size or are absent in ALT territory. Intraoperative change of free flap planning may sometimes be necessary. Alternative plans to ALT in the absence of perforators include anteromedial thigh (AMT) flap, tensor fascia lata (TFL) flap, and profunda artery perforator (PAP) flap. Ultimately, changing to the contralateral site for another ALT harvesting can also be attempted, as the absence of the perforators is rarely symmetric. When additional volume is required, vastus lateralis can be incorporated into the flap and raised as a composite, or combined flap. The muscle can be motorized by the inclusion of posterior division of the femoral nerve, and a sensate flap can be raised if lateral femoral cutaneous nerve is preserved and contained within

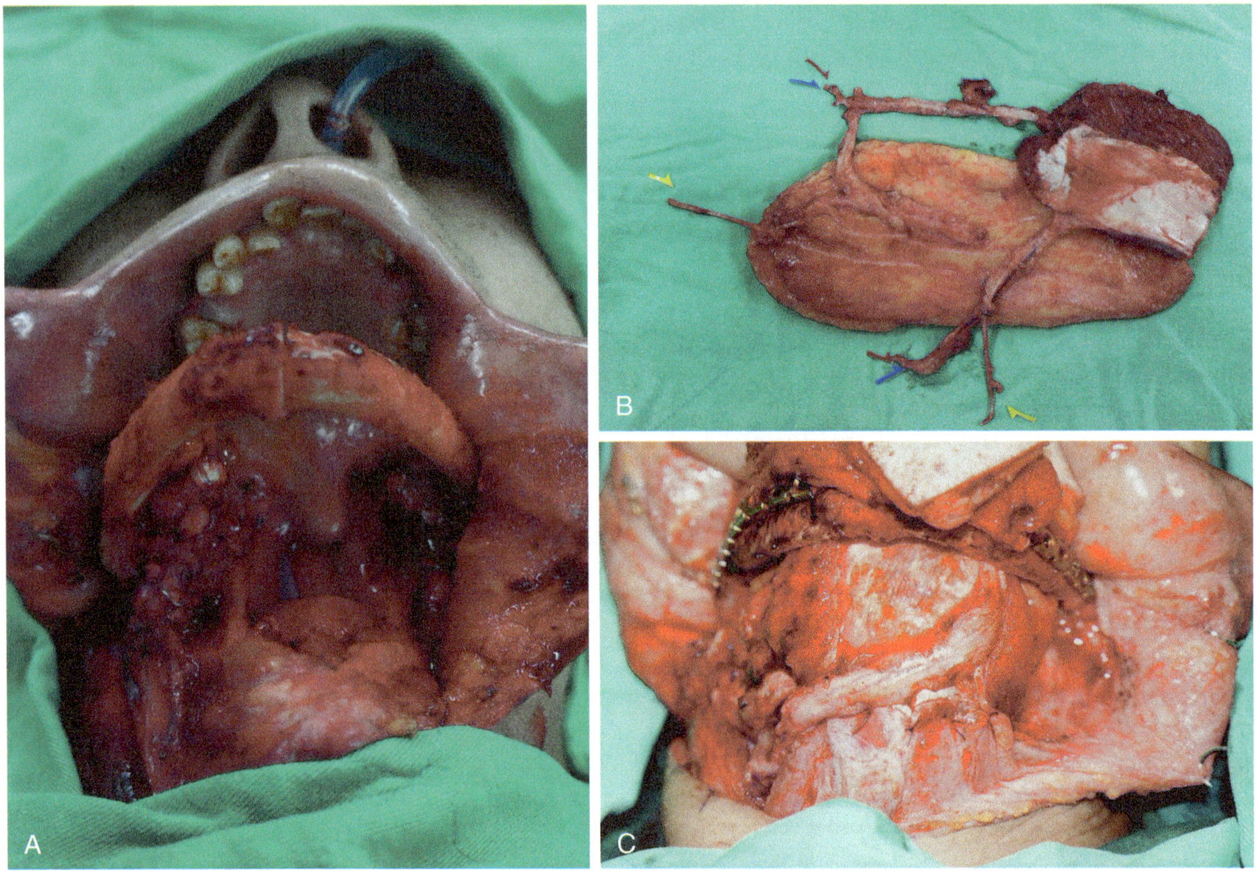

• **Fig. 24.1** (A) Total glossectomy and marginal mandibulectomy. (B) Anterolateral thigh combined with vastus lateralis muscle (yellow arrows, point at sensory and motor nerves). (C) The flap in place at the end of reconstruction before neck closure (adequate coverage of the mandible, and restoration of floor of the mouth).

the flap. In intraoral reconstructions, we prefer the use of a cutaneous flap with suprafascial dissection. It is a common option for presulcal tongue reconstruction, and for soft tissue coverage of the reconstructed mandible. Cutaneous only ALT flap is comparatively more pliable than its fasciocutaneous variant, and provides greater suitability for mobile tongue reconstruction.

In preparation for ALT flap harvest, the lower limb is kept in a neutral anatomical position. ALT flap marking consists of a line drawn between the anterior superior iliac spine (ASIS) and the midpoint of the lateral patella. This line represents the septum between rectus femoris and vastus lateralis. Hand-held Doppler is used for perforator localization and is concentrated within a 3 cm radius at the midpoint between ASIS and the lateral patella. The maximum flap size that allows direct closure is 8×22 cm^2. An initial exploratory medial incision is made for perforator identification and vessel preparation. A 1-cm back cut on both the proximal and distal edge of the medial incision is recommended. This step allows a greater angle of gentle lateral folding, utilizing gravity to assist the flap dissection. At this stage, a secured rolled towel should be placed beneath the partially dissected flap to prevent kinking and accidental avulsion of the perforators. During perforator and pedicle dissection, keeping a bloodless operating field is vitally important. This concept can significantly reduce iatrogenic injury to the perforators and pedicles, and enhances the survival rate of the free flap. Once the flap dissection is completed, all edges of the flap should be examined for its perfusion and drainage prior to the ligation of the pedicles. A suprafascial technique of ALT dissection is considerably more challenging, as the perforators are significantly smaller in the suprafascial plane and the perforator may be more subject to kinking and twisting. Extra attention is needed during the flap inset to prevent vascular adversities. The preservation of the fascia reduces the risk of muscle herniation of the donor site and may reduce subtle muscular weakness postoperatively. Split-thickness skin graft, dynamic suture techniques or delayed primary closure may be needed if primary closure is untenable.

Profunda Artery Perforator (PAP) Flap

The PAP flap is relatively new in head and neck reconstruction. It is typically raised as a nonsensate flap, and no case of motorized PAP has been reported. The flap is based on medial branches of the profunda artery, and supplies 10–12 cm of pedicle length with small to medium-size caliber (0.8–2 mm).[21] The perforators are generally bigger than those from ALT tributaries, and the course of the perforators is less torturous with less anatomical variations.

For a PAP flap, the patient is placed in the supine position with a roll of towel placed underneath the gluteal region of the operative side. This reduces the tension of adductor muscles while it medializes and flattens the posterior fasciocutaneous tissues of the thigh. The hip is externally rotated, abducted, and flexed and the knee is in full flexion (flamingo position). Alternatively, the lithotomy position can also be used for PAP harvesting. Surface marking of the PAP flap extends from the midpoint of the perineum to the insertion of semitendinosus, representing the midline of adductor magnus. Additionally, the outline of gracilis (palpable on hip abduction and knee flexion) is also drawn, indicating the anterior border of the flap. The flap is designed 8–10 cm distal to the groin crease where the first group of perforators are expected while avoiding undesirable scar placement in the perineum. Hand-held Doppler is used to ascertain the location of the perforators. The flap can be harvest transversely or longitudinally. In a transversely based flap, the scar is better concealed but widening of the scar is common; conversely, a longitudinally-based flap is more overt but scar widening occurs less commonly. The reported maximum diameter of the flap for primary closure is 8×6 cm^2; a longer flap can be harvested in practice with attainable primary closure. The greatest criticism of this flap is the flap harvesting ergonomics, and the ideal position is currently under investigation.

Medial Sural Artery Perforator (MSAP) Flap

The MSAP flap is an analogous flap to the RFFF. It is modified from the gastrocnemius muscle flap and was first introduced in 2001. It is raised as a fasciocutaneous flap and provides thin and pliable tissue. It is based on the medial sural artery and drained by its venae comitantes. The flap consists of a pedicle length up to 15 cm. It is useful for medium-size defect reconstruction up to 8×12 cm^2.[21] The vessels are small and prone to spasm; careful dissection and pedicle handling, constant warm saline irrigation, and generous topical application of lidocaine, propiverine, and magnesium sulphate on the vessels can reduce the risk of vasospasm and its arterial thrombosis sequela.

The patient is placed in the supine position with the hip joint abducted and knee joint flexed at 90 degrees for flap design. A line is drawn from the midpoint of the popliteal crease to the midpoint of the medial malleolus. The medial sural artery commonly gives rise to 1–2 cutaneous perforators located between 8 cm and 13 cm below the popliteal fossa. Although hand-held Doppler is routinely used to search for the perforators, their actual location constantly deviates significantly from the signal up to 2–3 cm. In the senior author's unit an endoscopic-assisted approach is routinely used to enhance the perforator localization and reduces the unnecessary shift of flap design. Based on Langer's line of the lower limb, the MSAP flap is designed obliquely to facilitate primary closure of the donor site. Under tourniquet control, an anterior skin incision is made deep to the deep fascia, followed by subfascial dissection in search of cutaneous perforators. Once the preferred perforator is selected, retrograde dissection is performed to identify the medial sural artery. The posterior boundary of the flap should be preserved at this point to prevent incidental traction, twisting, or kinking of the perforator during the intramuscular dissection of the perforators. The vascular pedicle is then dissected proximally until adequate pedicle length and appropriate vascular caliber is achieved, frequently in the popliteal fossa at the junction of where the medial sural artery bifurcates from the popliteal artery. The posterior border incision is made as the final step to complete the flap harvest. Similar to the PAP flap, the major drawback is the surgeon's operating posture and position. Donor site morbidity is minimal, and skin graft may occasionally be necessary.

Thoracodorsal Artery Perforator (TDAP) Flap

The TDAP flap is a modified flap based on the traditional latissimus dorsi myocutaneous flap. It is raised as a fasciocutaneous flap based on a medial or lateral branch of the thoracodorsal arteries, drained by two venae comitantes. The blood supply is constant and reliable. The flap consists of up to 15 cm of pedicle length. The TDAP flap is a thin flap and capable of resurfacing large defect areas (18×55 cm). It is not routinely raised as a sensate flap; the color of the flap matches well with the color of the head and neck region. The perforators of the medial branch are detectable at 4 cm below the scapular spine, whereas the lateral branch is detectable 10 cm below the axilla and 2 cm medial to the posterior axillary line. The patient is positioned in the lateral decubitus position and secured with a sandbag and lateral supports; the ipsilateral arm is prepped and left free. Hand-held Doppler is used to locate the perforators based on either the lateral or medial branch. The flap dissection starts with its superior border directly above the latissimus dorsi muscle to search for perforators. Once the perforators are identified, intramuscular dissection begins the search for parent vessels. In the inferior border, the flap is elevated off the latissimus dorsi muscle. Due to positioning of the flap, a two-team approach is difficult. The TDAP flap is not the first surgical option for head and neck reconstruction. However, it is a suitable option if a large flap is required for extended reconstruction.

Fibula Flap

The historical succession of free fibula flaps starts with the introduction of the concept in 1975 by Taylor et al.[27] Wei et al elucidated the possibility, reliability, and applicability of cutaneous inclusion to a free fibula flap. This anatomical study illustrated the consistent circulation of a lateral skin paddle of the leg from the peroneal artery through its septocutaneous perforators.[28] Though not included in the subsequent novel description of using a free fibula flap for mandibular reconstruction,[29] the added skin paddle to the free fibula flap undoubtedly increased its versatility, simplified complex mandibular reconstruction, and inspired subsequent development of its osteomusculocutaneous variant. Fibula is a desirable vascularized osteocutaneous flap for mandibular reconstruction due to: (a) the long straight bone (20–26 cm) with high cortical density and sturdy triangular construct; (b) the thickness of the bone is nearly uniform and consists of tridimensional flat surfaces, allowing flexible inset configurations as well as secured internal fixation and dental osseointegration; (c) the sturdiness of the bone allows multiple osteotomies for shaping and flap inset; (d) it has a long pedicle length and with sizable vascular calibers; (e) it is possible to harvest a reliable skin paddle; (f) it can be designed as a chimeric flap and used as a flow-through flap; (g) sural nerve harvesting is accessible through the donor site; (h) as a distant flap, it enables a two-team approach to the operation.

Before starting the procedure, a sterile tourniquet is applied at mid-thigh and incomplete lower leg exsanguination is performed prior to tourniquet inflation. The patient is placed in a supine position on the operating table with the knee flexed at 90 degrees and the hip internally rotated by placing a roll under the ipsilateral pelvic girdle. A stack of small size drapes is used for heel elevation, thus reducing the tension of muscular attachment to the fibula, and increasing accessibility during dissection. Based on the patient positioning, a free fibula flap can be raised through an anterior, posterior or combined approach. However, the anterior approach is preferred in the service of the senior author. The left fibula is the preferred donor bone, although there is no clinical evidence of a "dominant leg," the right donor site is generally avoided practically as the right foot is used for motor vehicle control and control of other heavy machineries. Routine use of an angiogram is not recommended unless there is an absence of pedal pulses on examinations, significant history of lower limb trauma, or detected peripheral vasculopathy during consultation.

Detailed surgical steps have been previously described;[28] only key points of free fibula harvesting are discussed in this chapter. A fibula flap is always raised as an osteoseptocutaneous flap with a maximum skin paddle up to 14 cm in width. In addition to concomitant soft tissue defect reconstruction with an osteocutaneous fibula flap, the skin paddle is also a valuable tool for postoperative flap monitoring, and facilitates tension-free soft tissue closure when soft tissue reconstruction is not essential. The skin paddle is based on the septocutaneous perforators, which are located at the junction of the middle and lower third of the leg, derived from the posterior crural septum. A single septocutaneous perforator enables supply to a large skin paddle. Suprafascial dissection anterior to the posterior crural septum is recommended for the preservation of superficial peroneal nerve and its branches. Skin graft is usually needed for donor site closure. If skin grafting is intended, preservation of paratenons is vital for successful grating. Conversely, if primary closure is intended, the maximal width should be kept within 4–6 cm. Careful intraoperative assessment of skin tension after primary closure is necessary to prevent compartment syndrome. In designing the fibula osteotomy site during flap harvest, it is indispensable to leave a 6-cm segment inferior to head of the fibula and 6 cm above the lateral malleolus. With this approach the stability of the knee and ankle joint can be preserved. High ankle shoes are recommended postoperatively to ensure the stability of the ankle on the operated side is maintained. Early intraoperative detection of the peroneal magnus artery is vital. Its detection is by observing the excessive arterial size of the peroneal artery once skeletonized, and clamping the distal end of the artery to inspect the maintenance of pedal pulses and absence of foot ischemia. With proper inspection and assessment, significant donor site morbidity can be avoided in the presence of the peroneal magnus artery. The most significant reported donor site morbidity is clawing of the big toe secondary to flexor hallucis longus (FHL) contracture. Meticulous preservation of the neurovascular bundle supply to FHL during flap harvest, and thorough reapproximation of muscle origin to the residual interosseous membrane with appropriate tension, are effective measures to prevent flexion contracture of the big toe.

Deep Circumflex Iliac Artery (DCIA) Flap

Iliac bone provides excellent bone stock, great width, and cortical thickness for bony reconstructions. It was first introduced as an osteocutaneous flap in 1979. Due to its natural curvature a free DCIA flap can be carved for mandibular reconstruction. This flap provides sturdy bony reconstruction with robust soft tissue coverage. The flap was initially described based on the superficial circumflex system, but the design has shifted to the more reliable deep circumflex vessels.[21] In addition, the ascending branch to internal oblique muscle can be included, forming a dual arterial supply system to enhance the reliability of the flap. The pedicle is relatively short with arterial length of 6 cm and 9 cm for the vein. The artery and veins are of large caliber, with diameter of 2.8 mm and 3.6 mm, respectively. The maximum dimension of the bone is $16{\times}4{\times}1\ cm^3$, $10{\times}8\ cm^2$ for the muscle, and $20{\times}20\ cm^2$ ($20{\times}12\ cm^2$ for primary closure) for the skin.[21] Designing the anterior cut more posterolaterally instead of ASIS can lengthen the pedicle effectively. This flap can be raised as a composite osteocutaneous flap or osteomusculocutaneous flap. Alternatively, the skin component can be harvested as a perforator flap over the iliac bone or based on the perforators of abdominal skin. Internal oblique muscle can be added into the flap to increase its reconstruction versatility through chimeric design. When designing DCIA, ASIS should be spared to preserve the integrity of the inguinal ligament; composite design of the flap is no longer routine as the size of the soft tissue and flexibility of the flap inset is restricted. Preferably, composite inclusion of muscle layers and perforator-based harvesting of skin components maximizes the applicability of the flap into complex reconstruction of the head and neck. The landmarks of the flap are ASIS, iliac crest, pubic tubercles, and inguinal ligaments. Expected locations of the perforators are located 5–11 cm posterior to the ASIS and 4 cm above the iliac crest.[21]

The patient is placed in a supine position, and a rolled towel is placed under the hip to improve the access of the donor site. The incision starts 2 cm above the inguinal ligament and iliac crest, down to external oblique muscle to identify skin perforators. Variable surgical approaches were described, and detailed description of the harvest is beyond the scope of this chapter. In mandible reconstruction (angle), ipsilateral harvest is favorable due to its natural shape. DCIA harvesting permits a two-team approach, and the donor site can be closed primarily. The good bone stock offered by ilium provides solid bony reconstruction and dental rehabilitation. However, the less frequent use of DCIA reflects its disadvantages. The DCIA vascular system is prone to spasm and its related higher failure rate. The breach of intraabdominal plane can lead to serious complications such as bleeding, visceral injury, and hernia. Gait disturbance may occur in large bony harvest, constant discomfort, and recurrent wound breakdown in low BMI patients have been reported.

Scapular Osteomusculocutaneous Flap

The scapular osteomusculocutaneous flap is based on the subscapular artery axis, and is a valuable option for complex mandibular reconstruction. The components of the flap consist of the lateral border of the scapula, scapular and/or parascapular skin, and latissimus dorsi muscle.[21] The flap can be harvested up to 14 cm. Alternative design with a medial border or bipedicled flap designs have also been described. The major drawbacks of the flap in mandibular reconstruction are the surgical positioning and bone stock quality. Lateral surgical positioning prohibits a two-team approach strategy, and this flap lacks cortical thickness for sturdy mandibular reconstruction. It is usually reserved as second-line option.

Defect-Directed Reconstruction

Tongue Reconstruction

Tongue defects are conventionally divided into hemiglossectomy, subtotal glossectomy, and total glossectomy. This division allows quick classification for clinical research, but does not reflect the differences in reconstruction goals based on regional anatomical needs. Functional partition of the tongue is to divide the tongue into anterior, middle, and posterior third (tongue base). Additional factors influencing reconstruction options are the involvement of the floor of the mouth and the presence of an extended compound defect involving the mandible. Acknowledgment of these factors in addition to defect size permits the formulation of defect-directed reconstruction of the tongue.

Tongue-Only Defect Reconstruction

Small Tongue Defects

These defects represent defects of the anterior third, glossectomy of less than a third, and small central/posterior defects. They usually present after benign lesion excisions. The tongue is a specialized skeletal muscle, and functionally irreplaceable. Small defects are best reconstructed by primary closure, healing by secondary intention, or rarely, a well-designed local tongue flap. In anterior third glossectomy, the tongue length invariably shortens, resulting in considerable functional deficit affecting the transport and process phases of oral deglutition. Similarly, the shortened tongue affects speech articulation and impairs speech intelligibility. The remaining mobile tongue can usually compensate the lost function sufficiently with adequate speech therapy and rehabilitation. One-third glossectomy reduces the width of the tongue; given the tongue is highly conformable, primary closure or healing by secondary intention are acceptable reconstruction options. However, if desired, intraoral flaps such as the FAMM flap, and buccinator myomucosal flap, may be used if tongue tethering would occur with primary closure. These local options provide thin and pliable tissues that do not overpower the remaining tongue by their bulk. Generally, the functional outcome is acceptable with simple reconstructions in this group; regional and free flap options are not indicated for small tongue defects.

Presulcal Glossectomies with No Tongue Base or Floor of Mouth Involvement

The presulcal region represents the anterior two-thirds of the tongue. Its anterior third is thin, agile, and flexible, and the middle third is bulkier, conformable, and useful for food bolus transport. It is involved in the oral part of the deglutition and articulates three out of four different types of speech, including "front raising," "middle groove," and "two-point displacement." The general principle for this defect reconstruction is the more anterior the defect, the thinner the flap needs to be. The reconstruction goals are to restore mobility, symmetry, and length while preventing excessive bulkiness. In hemiglossectomy defects, a thinner flap is ideal for its reconstruction. Reconstructing this defect with an excessively bulky flap will hinder the movement by the flap size, volume, and the weight. Free flap options for presulcal hemiglossectomy are the RFFF, suprafascial ALT, PAP, MSAP, and TDAP flaps. The smaller and more anterior the defect, the more favorable are the RFFF and the MSAP flap. Conversely, distally-based suprafascial ALT and PAP flaps are preferred for bigger and more posterior defects, whereas the TDAP flap is commonly reserved as a second-line option (Fig. 24.2).

Glossectomies Involving the Tongue Base

In defects involving the tongue base, volume replacement becomes vital. The base of the tongue is part of the oropharynx, where bulk forms the basis of its function. Tongue base (postsulcal or posterior third of the tongue) is responsible for the prevention of nasal regurgitation and aspiration. It initiates the pharyngeal phase of deglutition and produces "back raising" speech articulation. In hemiglossectomy that involves the tongue base, the goals of the reconstruction are volume reconstruction and restoration of length and width. Sensory reconstruction may not be essential, as spontaneous

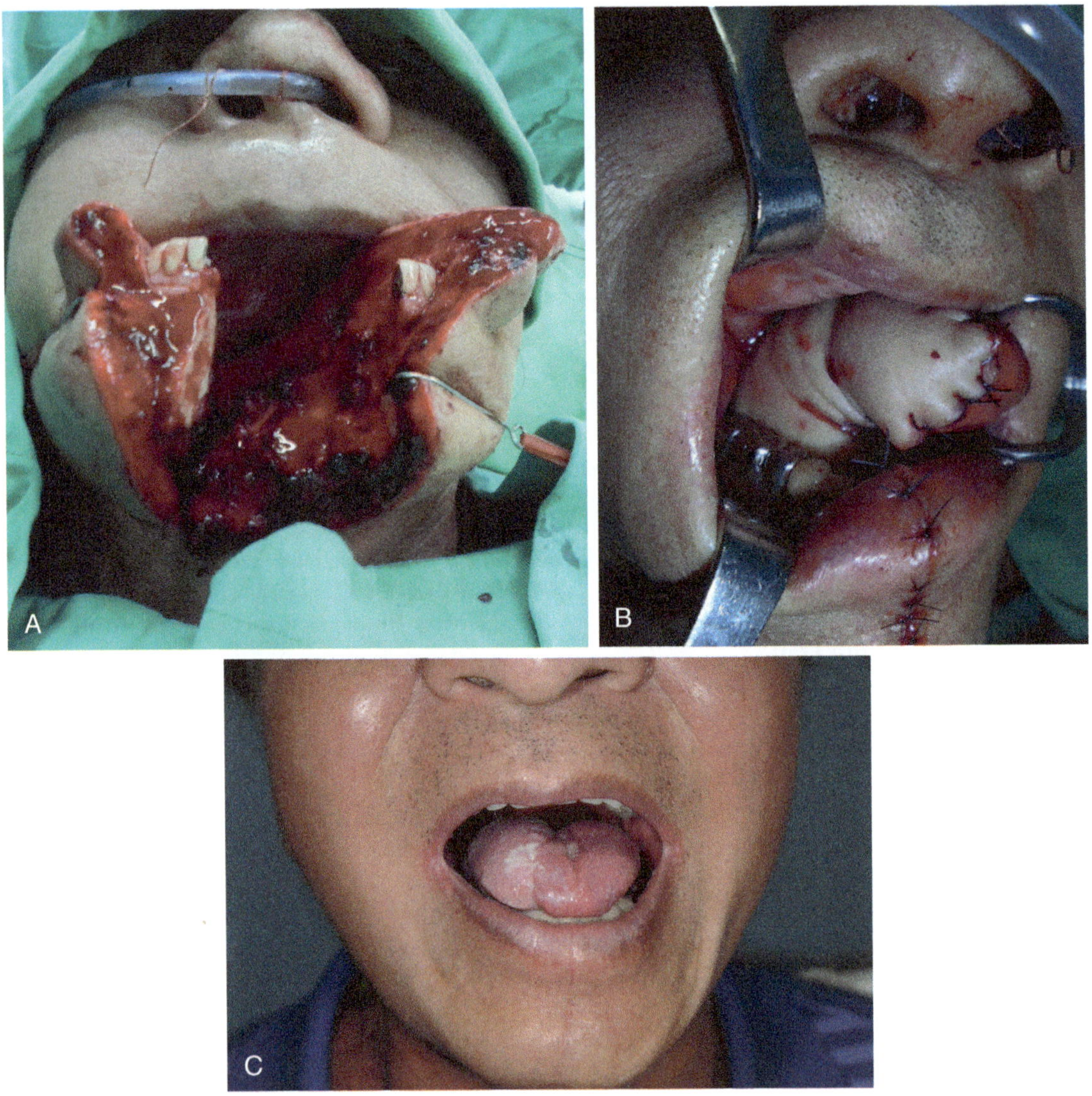

• **Fig. 24.2** (A) Hemiglossectomy defect. (B) Neotongue reconstruction with anterolateral thigh flap. (C) Outcome at 1 year post reconstruction.

resensitization can be expected, and the overall protective sensation of the tongue is preserved from the contralateral side.

Proximally-based ALT with or without vastus lateralis inclusion is the preferred option. A PAP flap with adductor magnus can be an alternative approach. A TDAP flap can be used in the absence of previous alternatives. The reconstruction approach to subtotal and total glossectomy involving tongue base is similar to the approach to hemiglossectomy. The expected outcome is poor, and patients may require lifelong nasogastric feeding with a permanent nonfunctional tongue despite our best reconstruction effort. The concept of an oversize flap should be employed as all flaps will eventually shrink with time; it is always easier to debulk and revise the size than volume and size reconstruction. Dynamic functional reconstruction may be achieved by using free gracilis. Sensory reinnervation with sural nerve graft can be recommended to restore protective sensation; motor reinnervation is vital if a functioning muscle flap is chosen. If the epiglottis is partially resected, utilizing local tissue for its reconstruction is important for functional preservation. Direct free flap inset to the epiglottis will significantly increase the risk of aspiration. When insetting the flap, the most reliable part of the flap is utilized for the reconstruction of the oropharynx. Laryngeal suspension should be considered as part of the reconstruction in large posterior tongue defects. Frequently, a lesion in the tongue base affects its surrounding soft and bony tissues and careful preoperative assessment and frequent discussion with the ablation team is important to prevent alteration of the surgical plan intraoperatively (Fig. 24.1).

Glossectomies Involving the Floor of Mouth

This group of defects derive from lesions of the ventral tongue with floor of mouth extension or vice versa. Simpler reconstruction tactics, including primary closure, healing by secondary intention, or skin graft, invariably result in tethering of the tongue. A tethered tongue impairs speech intelligibility, the oral phase of deglutition, pooling and drooling of the salvia. To prevent tethering of the tongue, flap reconstruction is preferred. If a full-thickness floor of mouth defect is present, the reconstruction goal is to separate the neck from the oral cavity, reconstruct the hyoid–mandible complex, and volume replacement for dead space obliteration. For isolated floor of the mouth defects, local or regional flaps can be used. For combined floor of the mouth and tongue or extensive floor of the mouth defects, RFFF or the MSAP flap can be considered. The fascial layer of the flap can be used for mandibular–hyoid complex reconstruction in replacement of the lost floor of mouth. Similar concepts apply as to hemiglossectomy, subtotal, and total glossectomy involving floor of mouth, but the amount of volume replacement is increased in ascending order. Flaps capable of providing large surface reconstruction and volume replacement are suitable in these situations. Proximally-based ALT, ALT with vastus lateralis muscle, PAP, and PAP flap with adductor magnus muscle are the preferred choice. Muscle flap such as gracilis may be considered for functional reconstruction, and TDAP flaps would be the second-line options (see Fig. 24.1).

Mandibular and Compound Mandibular–Tongue Defects Reconstruction

Free Flap Selection for Segmental Mandibular Reconstruction

Free vascularized bone flap incorporating soft tissue coverage with a low profile of donor site morbidity offers a good reconstruction choice for segmental mandibular defect. Although the segmental defect may be bridged successfully with nonvascularized bone in the short term, the high complication rate with infection, graft atrophy, and graft loss prohibits its long-term success and thus wider acceptance.[30] Compared to free fibula flap, DCIA has a relatively shorter pedicle, and the skin paddle of DCIA is relatively unreliable and less mobile than fibula. Although modified techniques are available to address these weaknesses, the thicker and less pliable skin texture provides less flexibility for inset and compliance for intraoral resurfacing. The donor site morbidity is significantly greater in DCIA than free fibula flap, it is reported to have greater incidence of postoperative donor site pain, protracted gait pain and gait disturbances, lateral femoral cutaneous nerve dysesthesiae, intraabdominal complications, and risk of pelvic fractures. Furthermore, despite being a thick and sturdy bone, iliac crest, in contrast to fibula, provides limited high-quality bone for mandibular reconstruction, and is less well tolerated for osteotomy. Osteocutaneous design of the RFFF may seem to have great potential. The osseous component, however, lacks solid bone stock, is unmalleable for osteotomies, too brittle to provide sturdy segmental mandibular reconstructions, and is associated with donor distal radius fractures requiring prophylactic plating or bone grafting. Scapula-based osteocutaneous flaps provide versatile soft tissue reconstruction to head and neck, but the osseous component is not robust enough for adequate segmental mandibular reconstruction. The location of the flap prohibits the two-team approach, thus it is not commonly used. Similar to osteocutaneous RFFF, scapula-based osteocutaneous flap may be suitable only for marginal mandibulectomy resections without intention of subsequent dental rehabilitation with osseointegration.

Other described but rarely used donor sites of vascularized bone include ribs, humerus, and metatarsus. They in general do not possess high-quality bone stock for consideration in segmental mandibular reconstruction, but may have a restricted role in augmenting a marginal defect. For these reasons, free fibula flap remains the unchallenged and widely acceptable option for segmental mandibular reconstruction. In our unit, left fibula is our first choice of vascularized bone, followed narrowly by the right fibula.

Technique of Mandibular Reconstruction with Free Fibula Osteoseptocutaneous Flap

For segmental reconstruction of the mandible, once the resection is completed, accurate occlusion position should be identified; the relative position can be secured by temporary maxilla–mandibular fixation to facilitate shaping and fixation of the reconstruction plate. A customized mandibular reconstruction plate, or generic pre-bent plate with various sizes, can be used. Miniplates in some instances can be selected instead. Once the occlusion relationship is set with internal fixation of the reconstruction plate, the maxilla–mandibular fixation is released, and TMJ position can then be verified. Recipient vessels are prepared, any branches of ipsilateral (and sometimes contralateral) external carotid arteries can be chosen, nevertheless, superior thyroid artery, transverse cervical, and facial arteries are used more commonly. Branches of internal or external jugular veins are routinely dissected as recipient veins. After confirming the adequate length of the pedicle, the pedicle is ligated and transferred to a side table. Ex vivo osteotomies and shaping is designed to gain maximum freedom and accuracy to conform the fibula into the desired arch, as opposed to in vivo osteotomies. This step will not compromise the viability of osteocytes, as prolonged ischemia time does not affect their survival.

On the side table, the pedicles are protected at all times. The shaping and osteotomy is guided by stacked wooden tongue depressors. These tongue depressors are stacked to match the height of the fibula. They are measured and marked against the reconstruction plate to formulate the osteotomy designs, and that design is then used as a template for guided osteotomy execution on the free fibula. The freedom to rotate the fibula permits instant feedback of osteotomy tomography to the operating surgeon, thus gaining greater appreciation of the angulation and articulation between each segments. This technique allows serial measurements and refinements of the osteotomy and permits trial insets for both soft tissue and bone, thus facilitating the best possible crafting of the neo-mandible. Each segment of the fibula should be designed longer than 3 cm post osteotomy to ensure adequate circulation to the bone is maintained. A sensible design is thus required to achieve

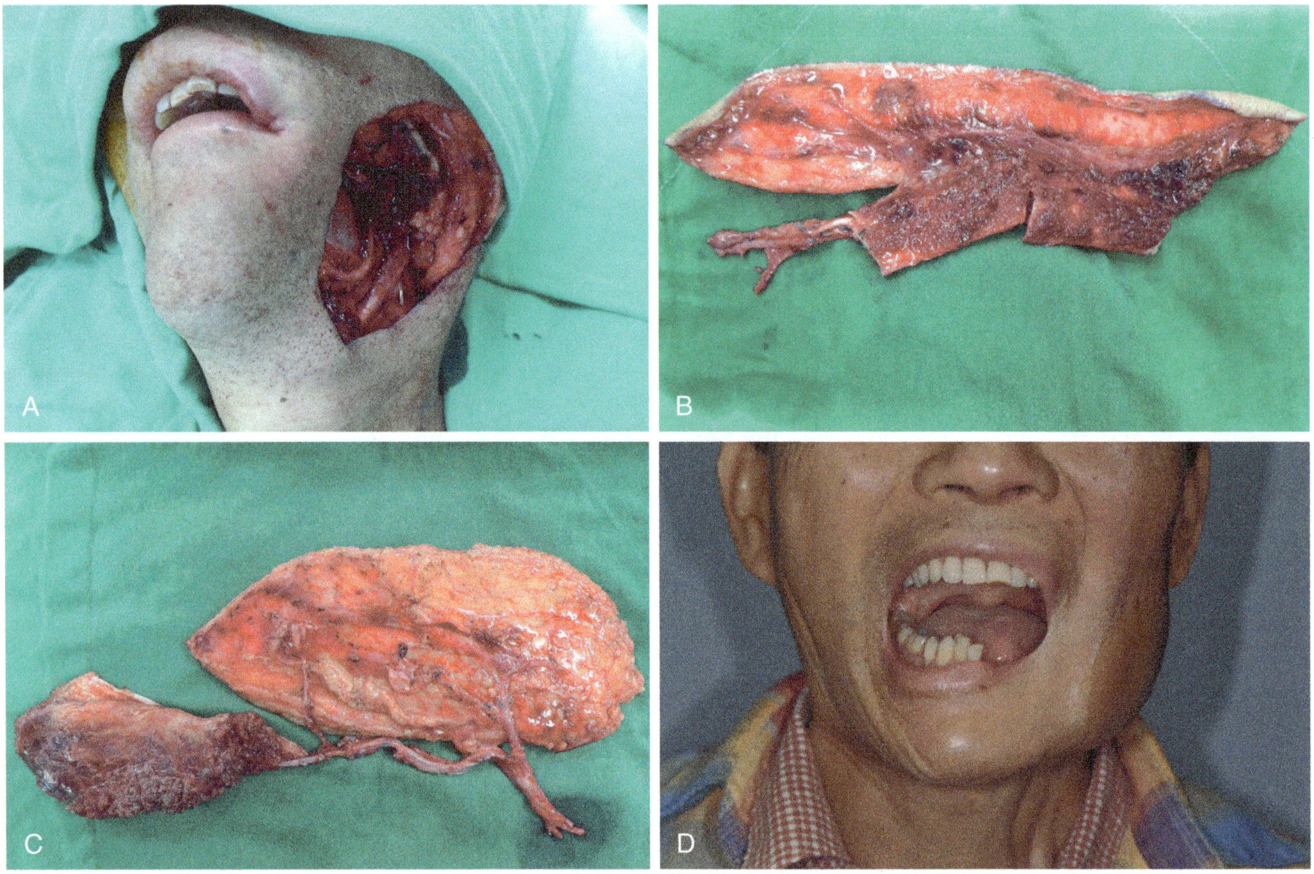

• **Fig. 24.3** (A) Extensive composite mandibular defect. (B) Two-strut fibula osteoseptocutaneous flap. (C) Anterolateral thigh flap combined with vastus lateralis. (D) Appearance at 1 year post reconstruction.

the balance between perfect mandibular shaping and viable fibula segments. In double-barrel design, a 3-cm bony segment should be removed subperiosteally at the folding hinge to prevent possible kinking, twist, or stretching of the pedicle between the two barrels. A double-barrel technique is commonly used for central mandibular defect ("C" defect); in this region both restoration of mandibular continuity and height of the mandible are necessary if dental rehabilitation is planned. Rigid bony fixation is needed, allowing direct bone healing for postoperative dental and TMJ rehabilitation. A monocortical screw is recommended to prevent pedicle injury. Performing microvascular anastomoses after both bony and soft tissue inset is advocated. Sensory reconstruction of inferior alveolar nerve should always be considered, as its reinnervation significantly enhances the reconstruction outcome, in particular in those who presented with benign mandibular lesions. In lateral segment defects ("L" defects), low placement bony fixation with a reconstruction plate, or plate-only reconstruction can be considered (Fig. 24.3).

Soft Tissue Reconstruction in Composite or Compound Mandibular Defects

Reconstruction of the soft tissue should be done meticulously. Regional characteristics of the oral cavity should be considered for appropriate reconstruction. Insufficient replacement of soft tissue volume in a gravity-dependent area such as floor of mouth and tongue base invites fluid accumulation and infection. Oral lining should always aim for watertight closure for the complete separation of the oral cavity from the neck. Failure to achieve this may result in saliva leakage through the neo-mandible into the neck, leading to delayed infection and pedicle thrombosis. Adequately resurfacing the mobile portion of the oral cavity concurrently with mandible reconstruction is equally important. In regions like the retromolar trigone, the junction between the ventral tongue and the floor of the mouth, insufficient surface replacement can result in trismus and tongue tethering. These can be considered as flaws of surgical design, requiring subsequent revision surgeries. In contrast to insufficient tissue replacement, excessive bulky flap due to design or flap choice can equally result in hindrance of functional recovery. Over-bulky reconstruction in the retromolar trigone region can result in repetitive dental trauma to the flap. As long-term soft tissue shrinkage is expected, and occurs more readily among muscular flaps than fasciocutaneous flaps, oversizing the flap is the secure option if optimal flap size is in doubt. It is always harder to replace than resect.

Marginal Mandibulectomy Reconstruction

Not all isolated, composite, or compound marginal mandibulectomies need synchronous bony and soft tissue reconstruction. The bony reconstruction is only indicated when the residual bone height is less than 1 cm, or there is a need for mandibular augmentation for dental osseointegration. If bony reconstruction is required, onlay nonvascularized bone graft, pedicled vascularized rib, clavicle, and scapula may be utilized. Nevertheless, apart from clavicle, the cortical thickness of all other options is suboptimal for dental rehabilitation. It is proposed, if the intention is functional reconstruction of marginal mandibulectomy defects, onlay inset of free fibula flap should be considered.

Reconstruction of Extensive Oromandibular Defect

The versatility of free fibula has been extensively reported. Apart from its standard design as an osteoseptocutaneous flap, it can also incorporate soleus and FHL in the situation of need. In the extended composite defects involving oral tongue and mandible, one flap would not sufficiently replace all components of the defects. Arguably, having one donor site may seem more appealing than two, however, extensive harvesting of a free fibula donor site may still be insufficient for synchronous reconstruction of mandibular defect and tongue. This results in trading considerable donor site morbidity for less optimal reconstruction outcome. Harvesting an independent fasciocutaneous flap specific for tongue and surrounding soft tissue reconstruction in addition to standard free fibula delivers greater freedom of inset, conformability, and superior soft tissue availability to satisfy all requirements of the reconstruction. The restraint in use of a double free flap is mostly due to the expected protracted operating time. With sufficient staff power, simultaneous workflow is attainable. With sound surgical logistics in place, the difference between single and double free flap reconstruction for extensive oromandibular defect is negligible.[31] The preferred free flaps are the combination of free fibula and ALT flap. With a double reconstruction team approach, the reconstruction sequence commonly starts with free fibula harvest during surgical ablation. The aim is to complete fibula harvest upon the completion of the surgical resection. The first reconstruction team would then start exploring the recipient vessels and work on mandibular plating and osteotomy of the fibula as well as revascularization, whereas the second reconstruction team would start harvesting the ALT flap after the defect size is confirmed and measured. ALT harvest would be expected to finish by the time of fibula completion, thus the second flap inset can start (see Fig. 24.3).

Osseointegration

Osseointegration represents the final step of completing functional reconstruction of the mandible. Free fibula osteoseptocutaneous flap delivers reliable high-density cortical bones with consistent diameters to withstand the fixation of osseointegration and the subsequent use of the dental implant. Dental osseointegration has three discrete stages: (1) setting the implant fixture into the bone with cover screws protecting the internal threat; (2) cover screws are removed, healing abutments are screwed into the fixtures, a palatal mucosal graft is harvested and secured around the abutments and protected with a removal stent; (3) dental prosthesis fitting. Osseointegration can be performed as a primary or secondary operation and in accordance with the timing of the stage one procedure. Double-barrel inset of fibula aims to correct the insufficient facial and alveolar process heights, achieving greater esthetic appearance and allowing subsequent osseointegration. This is commonly used in central mandibular segment reconstruction, and allows primary osseointegration. Similarly, to achieve mandibular height restoration, vertical distraction osteogenesis can alternatively be performed. It is associated with a higher rate of infection, and only permits secondary osseointegration.[32]

Postoperative Complications and Management Approach

In free flap reconstruction of the head and neck, the success rate is greater than the quoted 95%. Nevertheless, despite best efforts of meticulous planning and surgical execution, some free flaps fail. Once the flap is deem unsalvageable, general wound care management should be initiated on the ward. Different to microsurgery reconstructions to other regions, a failed free flap in head and neck reconstruction should prompt early replacement by another similar flap after identifying the reasons behind the failure. Local and systematic control of infection should be achieved with intravenous antibiotics, an appropriate dressing regimen and early surgical debridement. The defect size should be reassessed and the remnant of anatomical structures identified, and a surgical reconstruction plan should be discussed while the patient is being optimized. Furthermore, for intraoral reconstructions that are located in the gravity-dependent areas such as the floor of the mouth, partial necrosis of the flap is an alarm call for early repeated reconstruction, especially when floor of mouth integrity is compromised. Similarly, for free muscle reconstruction of the tongue with gracilis, any intraoperative or postoperative perfusion insufficiency will have a drastic effect on functional recovery; in this setting, replacement with a new free functioning muscle flap is recommended. For a failed fibula free flap, a contralateral fibula flap can be used for the subsequent reconstruction. Alternatively, a soft tissue flap and reconstruction plate could be considered, especially in poor prognosis patients. Any fluid collection in the neck due to wound dehiscence or flap edge necrosis from the intraoral reconstruction should be attended to for early washout to prevent pedicle infection and subsequent thrombosis. If neck dissection is performed, great care should be taken to ensure the great vessels are well protected to prevent rare but deadly complication with carotid artery or internal jugular vein blowout. Late complications include radiation-induced osteoradionecrosis, soft tissue shrinkage, and its associated trismus, tongue tethering, and sunken appearances. Metalware-related complications such as metal fatigue fracture, metal exposure, osteonecrosis, and orocutaneous fistula. Each one of these complications presents with great challenge to both the patient and the treating

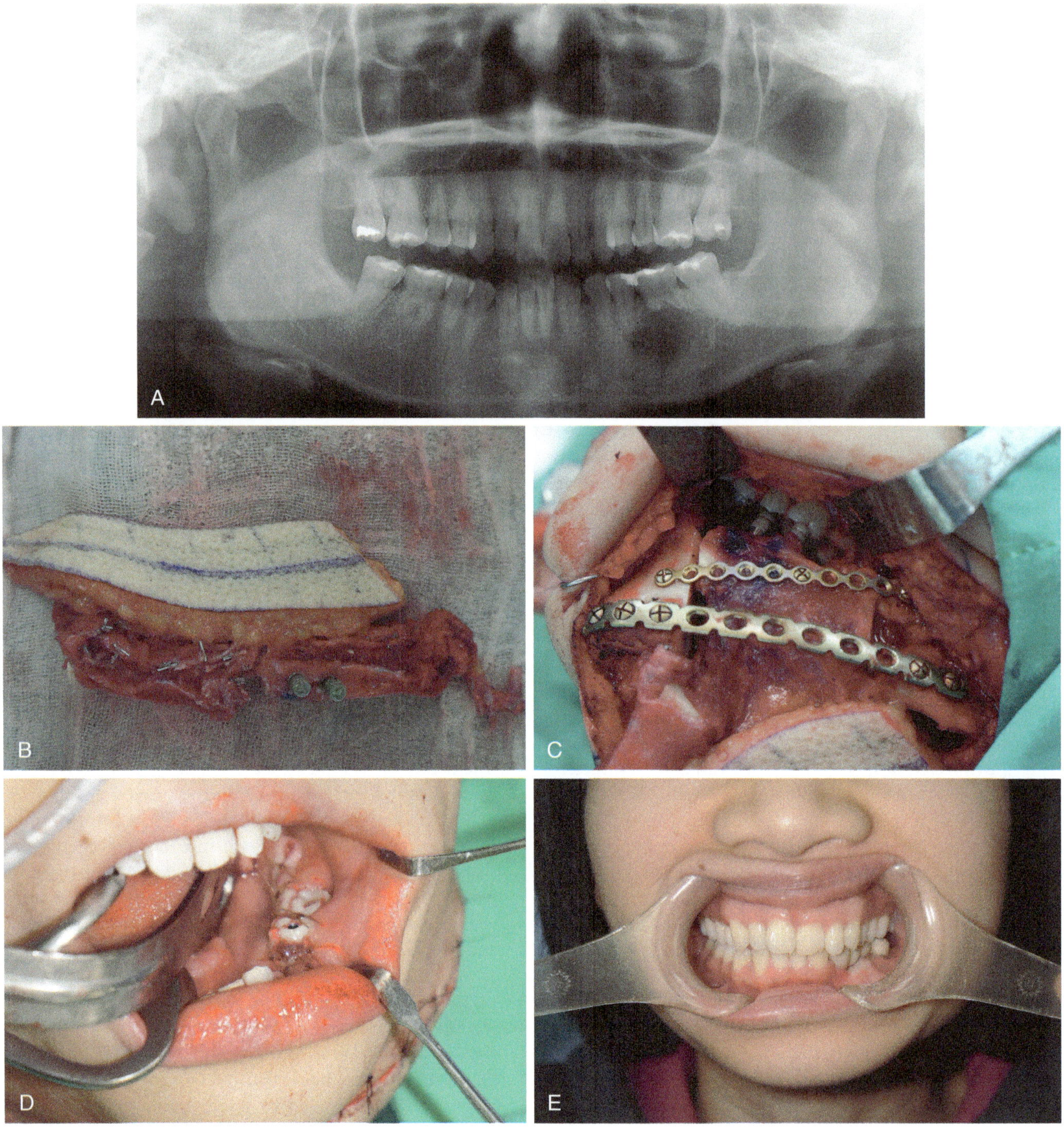

• **Fig. 24.4** (A) Ameloblastoma of the mandible body, on panoramic X-ray. (B) One-strut fibula osteoseptocutaneous flap with immediate dental implants. (C) Inset of the bone strut. (D) Appearance at the end of surgery with immediate crowns (jaw-in-a-day procedure). (E) Appearance at 2 years post jaw-in-a-day reconstruction.

surgeon. If patients remain physically fit, revision reconstruction is generally needed to resolve primary operation and adjuvant therapy-induced complications.

Computer-Assisted Surgery and Jaw-in-a-Day

Computer-assisted surgery, such as computer-aided design and computer-aided manufacture (CAD-CAM), and the concept of jaw-in-a-day are representative examples of recent integration of available technology into the world of reconstructive microsurgery. CAD-CAM was developed to enhance the precision and improve operation efficiency in executing segmental mandibular reconstruction through the application of virtual surgical planning. Similarly, jaw-in-a day utilizes the integrated data from a CT scan to prefabricate the precise angulation of a mandibular reconstruction plate, location of osseointegration fixture, and dental prosthesis (Fig. 24.4).[33] Despite their obvious advantages, these new technologies do not replace the training of free-hand mandibular reconstruction with free fibula flap. Any alterations of the surgical plan, such as advance of disease progression, deviated dental occlusions, or failed delivery of the free fibula flap at the premeasured site, will signify the loss of all preparatory work. Furthermore CAD-CAM does not account for the pedicle reach to the recipient vessels, multitargeted soft tissue reconstruction, anatomical variations, and cross-section topography of the osteoseptocutaneous fibula flap.[34] These technologies can thus be of hindrance if the reality fails to match the expectation. Case selection for use of these technologies is vital, and they are suitable mostly for benign lesions without extensive soft tissue involvements. Overdependence on these newly developed virtual planning tools may reduce the overall capacity of surgical skills; having a good foundation of free-hand segmental mandibular reconstructions increases the freedom of operation and adaptability to potential intraoperative change of the surgical plan which thus ensures the delivery of a reconstructed mandible.

Conclusion

Tongue and mandible reconstructions are inherently complex. A thorough understanding of regional anatomy, reconstruction options, and their respective limitations is crucial to achieve satisfactory functional and esthetic outcome.

The ideal reconstruction approach in general for both tongue and mandible is microsurgical reconstruction. Other options with simpler reconstruction approaches frequently compromise quality of life. Careful surgical planning and execution is the only means of any microsurgical success in reconstruction. Meticulous postoperative flap monitoring and prompt exploration and flap salvage should form the basis of microsurgical care. If inevitable partial or total flap failure occurs, swift arrangement of surgical debridements and subsequent reconstruction should be planned. Even if a second free flap is indicated, these principles shorten the hospital stay of the patient and prevent head and neck complications, and ensure improved quality of life.

References

1. Parada C, Chai Y. Mandible and tongue development. *Curr Top Dev Biol.* 2015;115:31–58.
2. Last RJ, McMinn RMH. *Last's Anatomy, Regional and Applied.* Edinburgh: Churchill Livingstone; 1994.
3. Daniel R. Mandibular reconstruction with vascularized iliac crest: a 10-year experience – discussion. *Plast Reconstr Surg.* 1988;82:802–803.
4. Hiiemae KM, Palmer JB. Tongue movements in feeding and speech. *Crit Rev Oral Biol Med.* 2003;14(6):413–429.
5. Pitts T. Airway protective mechanisms. *Lung.* 2014;192(1):27–31.
6. Stone M, Lundberg A. Three-dimensional tongue surface shapes of English consonants and vowels. *J Acoust Soc Am.* 1996;99:3728–3736.
7. Moon HS, Won YY, Kim KD, et al. The three-dimensional micro structure of the trabecular bone in the mandible. *Surg Radiol Anat.* 2004;26:466–473.
8. National Cancer Institute. SEER website. Available at: https://seer.cancer.gov/statfacts.
9. Lu CT, Yen YY, Ho CS, et al. A case-control study of oral cancer in Changhua County, Taiwan. *J Oral Pathol Med.* 1996;25:245–248.
10. Bleyer A. Cancer of the oral cavity and pharynx in young female: increasing incidence, role of human papilloma virus and lack of survival improvement. *Semin Oncol.* 2009;36:451–459.
11. Reuther T, Schuster T, Mende U, Kubler A. Osteoradionecrosis of the jaws as a side effect of radiotherapy of head and neck tumor patients: a report of a thirty year retrospective review. *Int J Oral Maxillofac Surg.* 2003;32:289–295.
12. Krishnakumar T, Kuriakose MA, Joseph ST, Shetty S, Iyer S. Options in glossectomy defect reconstruction: proposal for a classification system. *Oral Oncol.* 2013;49:S81.
13. Engel H, Huang JJ, Lin CY, et al. Strategic approach for tongue reconstruction to achieve predictable and improved functional and aesthetic outcomes. *Plast Reconstr Surg.* 2010;126(6):1967–1977.
14. Jewer DD, Boyd JB, Manktelow RT, et al. Orofacial and mandibular reconstruction with the iliac crest free flap: a review of 60 cases and a new method of classification. *Plast Reconstr Surg.* 1989;84:391–403.
15. Tsao C-K, Megias Barrera J, Loh C. From flat into concave shape in soft tissue free flaps in oral cavity reconstruction: the origami technique. *Oral Oncol.* 2016;55.
16. Baas M, Duraku LS, Corten EML, Mureau MAM. A systematic review on the sensory reinnervation of free flaps for tongue reconstruction: does improved sensibility imply functional benefits? *J Plast Reconstr Aesthetic Surg.* 2015;68(8):1025–1035.
17. Wei F, Celik N, Yang W, Chen I, Chang Y, Chen H. Complications after reconstruction by plate and soft-tissue free flap in composite mandibular defects and secondary salvage reconstruction with osteocutaneous flap. *Plast Reconstr Surg.* 2003;112(1).
18. Pribaz J, Stephens W, Crespo L, Gifford G. A new intraoral flap: facial artery musculomucosal (FAMM) flap. *Plast Reconstr Surg.* 1992;90(3):421–429.
19. Zhao Z, Li S, Yan Y, et al. New buccinator myomucosal island flap: anatomic study and clinical application. *Plast Reconstr Surg.* 1999;104(1):55–64.
20. Martin D, Pascal JF, Baudet J, et al. The submental island flap: a new donor site. Anatomy and clinical applications as a free or pedicled flap. *Plast Reconstr Surg.* 1993;92(5):867–873.
21. Wei FC, Mardini S. *Flaps and Reconstructive Surgery.* Amsterdam: Elsevier; 2016.
22. Ross RJ, Baillieu CE, Shayan R, Leung M, Ashton MW. The anatomical basis for improving the reliability of the supraclavicular flap. *J Plast Reconstr Aesthetic Surg.* 2014;67(2):198–204.
23. Wei FC, Demirkan F, Chen HC, et al. The outcome of failed free flaps in head and neck and extremity reconstruction: what is next in the reconstructive ladder? *Plast Reconstr Surg.* 2001;108:1154–1160.
24. Siekaly H, Calhoun K, Rassekh CH, Slaughter D. The clavipectoral osteomyocutaneous free flap. *Otolaryngol Head Neck Surg.* 1997;117:547–554.
25. Wei D, Liu J, Zhao W, et al. Use of the versatile sternocleidomastoid flap in oral and maxillofacial surgery: our experience. *Br J Oral Maxillofac Surg.* 2013;51(8):742–746.
26. Wong CH, Lin JY, Wei FC. The bottom-up approach to the suprafascial harvest of the radial forearm flap. *Am J Surg.* 2008;196(5):60–64.

27. Taylor IG, Miller GDH, Ham FJ. The free vascularized bone graft. *Plast Reconstr Surg.* 1975;55:533.
28. Wei FC, Chen HC, Chuang CC, Noordhoff MS. Fibular osteoseptocutaneous flap: anatomic study and clinical application. *Plast Reconstr Surg.* 1986;78:191–200.
29. Hidalgo DA. Fibula free flap: a new method of mandible reconstruction. *Plast Reconstr Surg.* 1989;84(1):71–79.
30. Moura LB, Carvalho PH, de A, et al. Autogenous non-vascularized bone graft in segmental mandibular reconstruction: a systematic review. *Int J Oral Maxillofac Surg.* 2016;45(11):1388–1394.
31. Wei FC, Demirkan F, Chen HC, Chen IH. Double free flaps in reconstruction of extensive composite mandibular defects in head and neck cancer. *Plast Reconstr Surg.* 1999;103:39–47.
32. Chang YM, Wallace CG, Hsu YM, Shen YF, Tsai CY, Wei FC. Outcome of osseointegrated dental implants in double-barreled and vertically distracted fibula osteoseptocutaneous free flaps for segmental mandibular defect reconstructions. *Plast Reconstr Surg.* 2014;134:1033–1043.
33. Qaisi M, Kolodney H, Swedenburg G, Chandran R, Caloss R. Fibula jaw in a day: state of the art in mandibular reconstruction. A report of 3 cases. *J Oral Maxillofac Surg.* 2016;74(6):1284.
34. Deek NF, Wei FC. Computer-assisted surgery for segmental mandibular reconstruction with the osteoseptocutaneous fibula flap: can we instigate ideological and technological reforms? *Plast Reconstr Surg.* 2016;137(3):963–970.

25 Midface Reconstruction

MATTHEW M. HANASONO

Introduction

Reconstruction of the midface, particularly of the maxilla, following tumor removal is a significant challenge because of its complex three-dimensional architecture and important role in facial esthetics and function. The goals of reconstruction include: (1) maintaining midfacial height, width, and projection; (2) creating a stable platform for mastication and dental restoration; (3) separating the oral cavity from the nasal cavity; (4) preserving a patent nasal airway; (5) supporting the soft tissues of the face, including the nose, lips, cheeks, and eyelids; and (5) restoring the bony orbit to avoid changes in orbital volume and globe position that may result in eye exposure or impaired vision, or provide stable wound closure for the exenterated orbit.

In the past, maxillary reconstruction mainly involved prosthetic obturation. This option results in immediate dental restoration without further surgery but, in larger defects, as well as in cases where radiation-associated tissue contracture occurs, instability, poor retention, and oronasal leakage of air, liquid, and food may occur.[1–3] Furthermore, results of prosthetic obturation are disappointing or unacceptable in extensive midfacial defects, such as those that involve the orbital floor. The advent of microsurgery has permitted primary single-stage reconstruction of these complex facial defects, avoiding the use of a prosthesis as well as various combinations of local and regional flaps that have poorer esthetic and functional results and higher complication rates.[4]

Reconstructive Approach

One of the biggest challenges associated with reconstructing the maxilla is that the defects created by oncologic resection are highly variable. Several classification systems have been proposed, each with its strengths and weaknesses.[5–10] According to Archibald et al,[11] the ideal maxillary treatment algorithm should "use a functional approach that defines the defect-related challenges, prioritizes the reconstructive goals, and identifies how and to what extent each of the microsurgical free flaps could meet these goals." Therefore, rather than memorizing a specific classification system, it is more important to understand the critical structures that need to be addressed during the reconstruction and base the surgical approach on these needs. These structures include: the palate and alveolus, the orbital floor, and the orbital contents.[7,10] This chapter will examine each of these areas.

Reconstruction of the Palate and Alveolus

Posterior Defects

Palatoalveolar defects that are unilateral and posterior to the canine tooth are well suited to reconstruction by a number of techniques. Prosthetic obturation can give excellent results for such defects.[1–3,7] The obturator is stabilized by both canine teeth, which have very long, stable roots, and the contralateral molars. An obturator is usually the simplest solution for these defects, requiring no further surgery, and, therefore, no donor site morbidity (Fig. 25.1). The maxillectomy wound is either packed or a temporary prosthesis is placed and secured to the wound. Once healed, an obturator is fabricated by a maxillofacial prosthodontist. Another advantage of obturation is that the maxillectomy cavity can be inspected for local cancer recurrence under direct vision by removal of the prosthesis. However, some patients experience problems with fit causing leakage of foods and liquids during eating or air during speech production due to tissue contracture, particularly those who have been irradiated. Periodic refitting and replacement is also required for the life of the patient, which is another relative disadvantage.

Posterior palatoalveolar defects can also be reconstructed with various autologous tissue flaps. The temporalis muscle pedicled flap can be transposed into the oral cavity to reconstruct these defects.[5,12] The muscle is harvested using a hemicoronal incision and removal of the mandibular condyle facilitates transposition into the oral cavity. The main disadvantage of this technique is that it often leaves a noticeable donor site depression, although this can be minimized by leaving the anterior one-third to one-half of the muscle in situ or by placing an implant (e.g., porous polyethylene) or filler (e.g., delayed autologous fat grafting) in the donor site. The temporalis muscle can also be used to reconstruct midpalatal defects that do not involve the alveolus at all.[7]

The majority of posterior palatomaxillary defects in the author's practice are reconstructed with soft tissue free flaps.[13] Bony free flaps are also suitable but do not offer

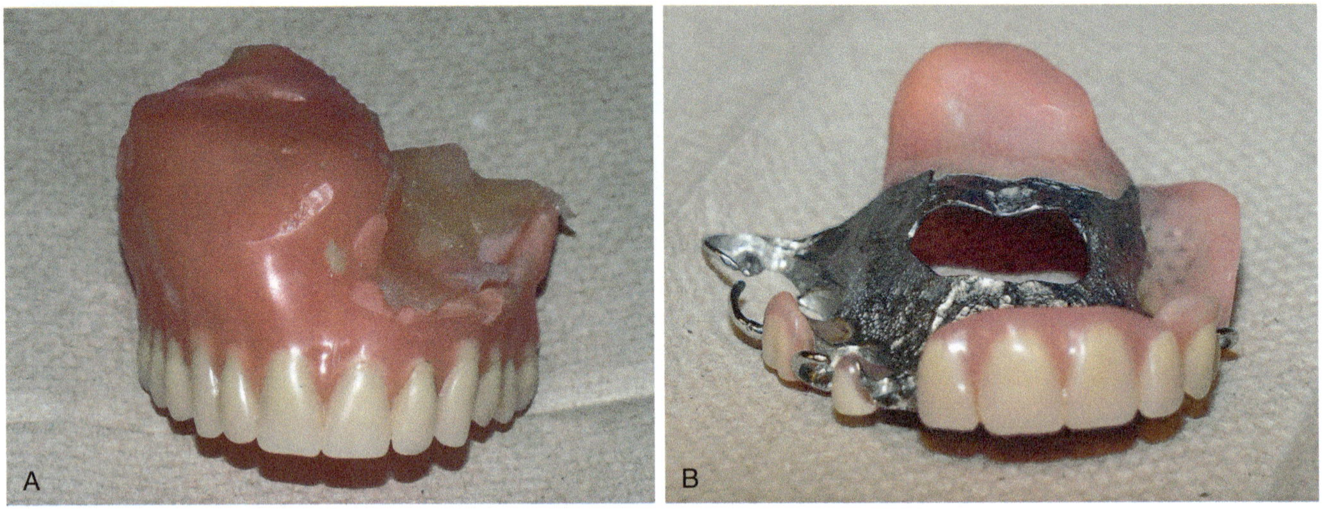

• **Fig. 25.1** Examples of palatal obturator prostheses. (A) Obturator created for a large right hemimaxillectomy defect, stabilized with adhesive to the remaining edentulous left maxilla. (B) Obturator created for a smaller left posterior palatoalveolar maxillary defect, stabilized using clasps that hook around the remaining teeth.

significant advantages for most patients, unless osseointegrated implants for dental restoration are desired. Most patients that are referred for flap reconstruction have rejected the idea of an obturator or have tried one and been unsatisfied. The anterolateral thigh (ALT) flap, rectus abdominis myocutaneous (RAM) flap, and radial forearm fasciocutaneous free flap (RFFF) have been most frequently described for soft tissue reconstruction of posterior palatoalveolar defects.[5,8,9,13] The ALT free flap is most commonly selected in the author's practice because of its long pedicle, minimal donor site morbidity, and ability to adjust flap thickness by inclusion of vastus lateralis muscle to increase thickness or microdissection to thin the flap (Fig. 25.2). The RAM flap is often excessively thick in most patients, while the RFFF is usually avoided because it is thin and does not obliterate the maxillary sinus, creating an air space superior and inferior to the flap, theoretically raising the risk for fistula formation.

The pedicle of the flap is tunneled from the oral cavity to the neck where a microvascular anastomosis is performed to the facial artery and vein, which are exposed with a short incision made 1–2 fingerbreadths below the inferior border of the mandible. When creating this tunnel, care is taken not to divide the parotid duct as a hole is made in the buccinator muscle and a 2–3 fingerbreadth-wide subcutaneous pathway to the recipient vessels is dissected. Alternately, the superficial temporal vessels can be used as recipient vessels. The ideal reconstruction is level with the remainder of the hard palate or slightly higher. This allows space for a prosthesis for dental restoration if the patient later desires one. A bulky or ptotic flap does not permit fitting of a dental prosthesis.

Hemipalatoalveolar Defects

A number of techniques have been advocated for maxillary defects that involve around half of the palate and alveolus. At many centers, patients are treated with a prosthetic obturator for these defects.[1] The difficulty with obturators for hemipalatoalveolar defects is that there is a limited amount of teeth and alveolar arch to create stable fixation of the prosthesis.[7] Metal clasps used for fixation of the prosthesis can eventually cause loosening of teeth because of the high torque forces exerted when masticating with an unstable obturator. Soft tissue contracture around the obturator can also cause distortion of the facial features, such as elevation of the upper lip and deviation of the nose toward the side of the defect. Fewer patients can be successfully treated with an obturator following hemipalatomaxillectomy than posterior maxillectomy.[1,4]

Some authors have advocated soft tissue free flap reconstruction, for example with a RAM free flap.[5,9] This flap is a highly reliable flap and will create a watertight seal between the oral and nasal cavities. The bulk of the flap is used to restore the shape of the cheek. However, in the author's experience, soft tissue flaps tend to contract and descend with time, particularly when postoperative radiation is given. This can result in unilateral loss of midfacial projection and facial symmetry. Additionally, the nose will start to deviate toward the side of the maxillectomy unless the portion of the maxilla adjacent to the external nose (sometimes referred to as the piriform rim) is preserved. Retention of a dental prosthesis following soft tissue reconstruction tends to not be stable for the same reasons obturators are often unstable.

The radial forearm osteocutaneous, scapula, iliac crest, and fibula free flaps have all been proposed for bony reconstruction of hemipalatomaxillectomy defects.[14–20] The bone portion of the radial forearm osteocutaneous flap is osteotomized and rigidly fixed with titanium miniplates to reconstruct the alveolar arch, restoring anterior maxillary projection.[14,15] The skin paddle is used to reconstruct the oral palatal side and can be wrapped around the bone so

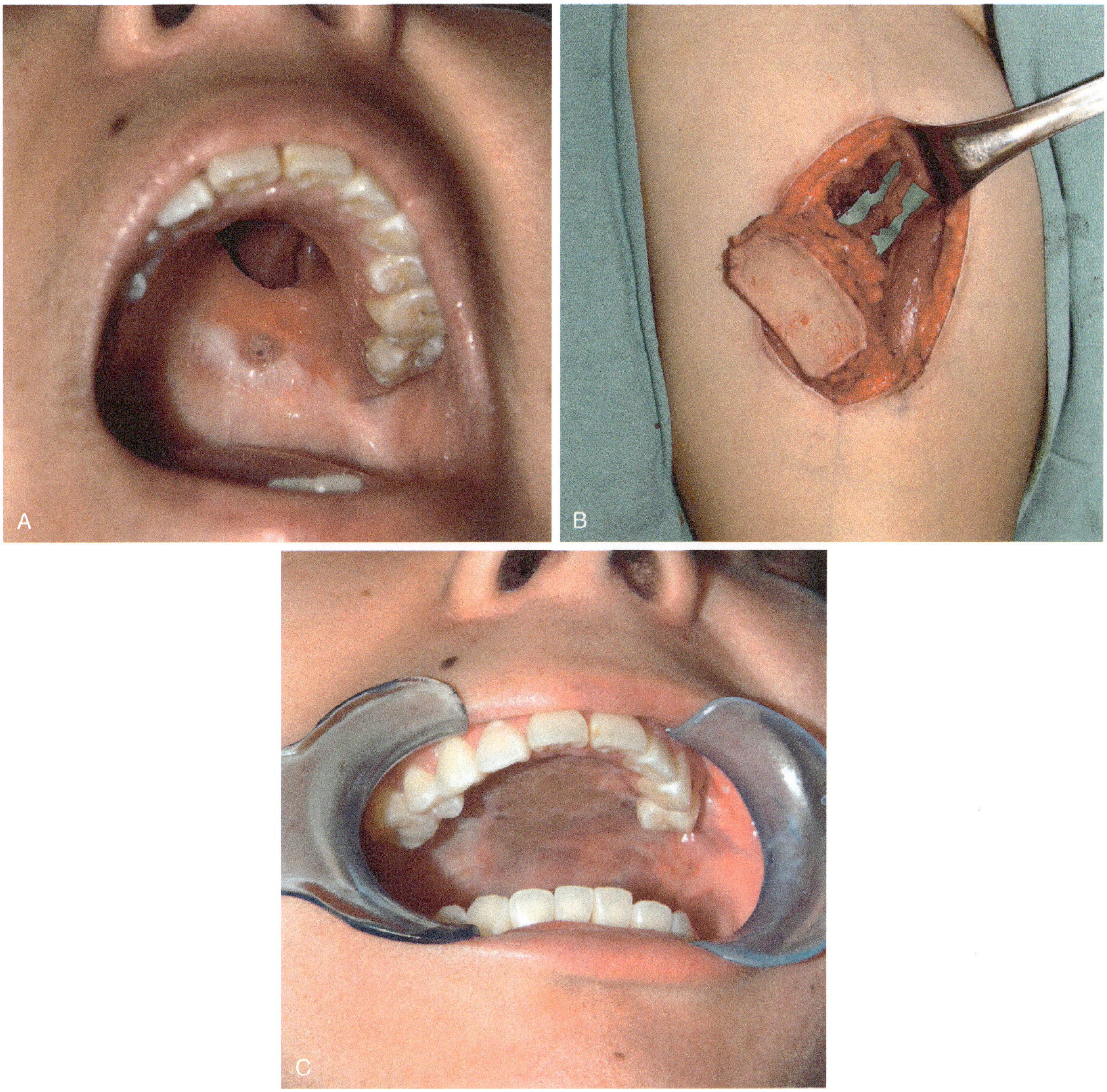

• **Fig. 25.2** (A) A left posterior palatoalveolar defect. (B) An anterolateral thigh (ALT) free flap after dissection, measuring approximately 5×5 cm. (C) Postoperative appearance several months following reconstruction with the ALT free flap.

that there is a skin paddle on the nasal side, de-epithelializing the intervening skin to which the lip is attached (so-called "radial forearm sandwich flap").[14]

The scapula is also a popular choice for hemimaxillectomy reconstruction.[16] In most descriptions the scapular bone, either perfused by the circumflex scapular artery or the angular branch of the thoracodorsal artery, is oriented such that the flat surface lies roughly in the coronal plane and the relatively lateral edge of the scapular bone rests inferiorly. One problem with this orientation is that it may be difficult to accurately restore the subtle nuances in maxillary shape. However, the lateral edge of the bone is often, though not always, thick enough to accommodate placement of osseointegrated implants for dental restoration. The bone can also be oriented transversely, taking advantage of the triangular shape of the scapular tip (scapular angle) to restore anterior maxillary projection, though the bone is usually not thick enough for osseointegrated implant placement in this orientation and rigid fixation is more challenging.

The iliac crest free flap, based on the deep circumflex iliac artery, in contrast provides ample thickness and height for osseointegrated implant placement.[17,18] The thick cortex of the bone also helps with implant retention, compared to the scapula, which tends to have a thin cortex and proportionately more medullary bone. In most cases, the bone is oriented vertically so that the flat surface faces roughly coronally, where the anterior maxillary wall was previously. The difficulty with the iliac crest is that, in many patients, the skin paddle is very thick and requires revision surgery for debulking. A very bulky flap can occlude the airway and require prolonged tracheostomy use. Alternately, the internal oblique muscle can be used to close the palatal defect, requiring either skin grafting of the muscle surface or allowing muscle to mucosalize spontaneously, or a thin fasciocutaneous free flap, such as the RFFF, can be used in combination with the iliac crest bone.

The author's preferred method for reconstruction following hemipalatomaxillectomy is to use the fibula osteocutaneous free flap.[19,20] The fibula osteocutaneous flap has a thin skin paddle such that most patients are not at risk for airway occlusion when that skin paddle is used to restore the palatal mucosa. The main advantages, however, are the long length of bone that can be osteotomized to mimic the complex shape of the maxilla and the height and width of the bone that make it a good substrate for placement of osseointegrated implants. Also, because the donor site is distant from the head, simultaneous flap harvest and bone shaping can be performed with the maxillary resection, saving considerable operative time.

The ipsilateral fibula is typically used for maxillectomy defects to orient the lateral surface of the fibula superficially for titanium plate fixation and the skin paddle inferiorly to reconstruct the palate while the pedicle of the flap comes to lie posteriorly and laterally (Fig. 25.3). A small amount of muscle is left adherent to the bone and the nasal surface is allowed to mucosalize spontaneously. If the resection is extended to include the malar eminence of the maxilla (superior portion of the maxilla), an additional segment of bone is used to restore this area.[19] The mean height of the lateral surface of the fibula is approximately 18 mm, which roughly corresponds to the height of the premaxilla (mean of 20 mm) and the malar bones (mean of 22 mm).[20] Because the premaxilla is inferior to the malar bones in the cranial–caudal dimension, the bones need to be offset from each other, either by angling a "single-barrel" reconstruction (Fig. 25.4) downward or positioning the fibular segments in a "double-barrel" configuration (Fig. 25.5).[20] The facial or superficial temporal blood vessels are used as recipient blood vessels. Vein grafts are commonly needed to reach the recipient blood vessels.[21]

Bilateral Palatoalveolar Defects

When both sides of the maxilla have been resected, including the anterior alveolar arch, osteocutaneous free flap reconstruction is usually necessary.[1] Prosthetic obturators are usually not stable because they do not have enough teeth and alveolus (if any) to attach to and they tend to be heavy when replacing sizable maxillary resections.[7] Soft tissue reconstruction will result in loss of midface projection, a stable surface for mastication, and support of the nose. The radial forearm osteocutaneous free flap and the iliac crest osteocutaneous free flap generally do not provide long enough segments of bone to restore any but the smallest of anterior maxillary defects. The scapula can be oriented transversely, such that the tip or angle of the scapula becomes the anterior-most point of the midface (i.e., the premaxilla), to restore the entire alveolus. However, as mentioned above, it is unlikely that the scapula can accommodate osseointegrated implants in this orientation. The scapula also does not have enough additional bone to restore the malar portion of the maxilla unless it is designed with more than one bone segment based on separate blood supplies (i.e., circumflex scapular and angular branch of the thoracodorsal arteries).

Therefore, for bilateral maxillary defects, the fibula osteocutaneous free flap seems to be the most commonly described flap in the literature.[10,13,19,20] Multiple osteotomies can be made to recreate the curvature of the anterior maxilla.[19] If only the hard palate and alveolus are removed, using a Le Fort I-type osteotomy, then the fibula is shaped like the letter "U."[20] For defects that include the malar portion of the bone, additional fibular segments are needed to restore this region, essentially mirror imaging the reconstruction described above for a hemimaxillectomy.[19]

Care needs to be exercised during fibula shaping for midfacial reconstruction because even minor inaccuracies in creation of osteotomies as well as positioning of the assembled fibula construct can result in a suboptimal esthetic and functional outcome. The author has found use of computer planning and three-dimensional (3D) printed models with computer-generated fibula cutting guides to be especially helpful in performing bony midfacial reconstruction (Fig. 25.6).[22–27] Use of this technology allows for accurate planning of the reconstruction preoperatively and facilitates creation of more precise osteotomies. More recently, the availability of 3D-printed titanium plates has added further accuracy to the reconstruction. Challenges to use of this computer-aided design and computer-aided manufacturing (CAD/CAM) technology include the need for adequate lead-time to generate the models, cutting guides, and plates, costs associated with design and manufacture of these items, and limited ability for intraoperative changes to the surgical plan.

Reconstruction of the Orbital Walls

The orbital walls, in particular the orbital floor and medial orbital wall, may be resected in combination with the palate and alveolus (often referred to as a "total maxillectomy") or only with the superior portion of the maxilla, sparing the palate and alveolus (a "suprastructure maxillectomy"). Failure to accurately reconstruct the bony orbit can have severe consequences with regards to the eye and vision. If the orbital floor is reconstructed at a different vertical height than the contralateral side (vertical dystopia), then diplopia may result. If the orbit is not fully reconstructed, then orbital contents will herniate through any remaining bony defects and enophthalmos may result. If the reconstructed orbital cavity is of smaller volume than the contralateral

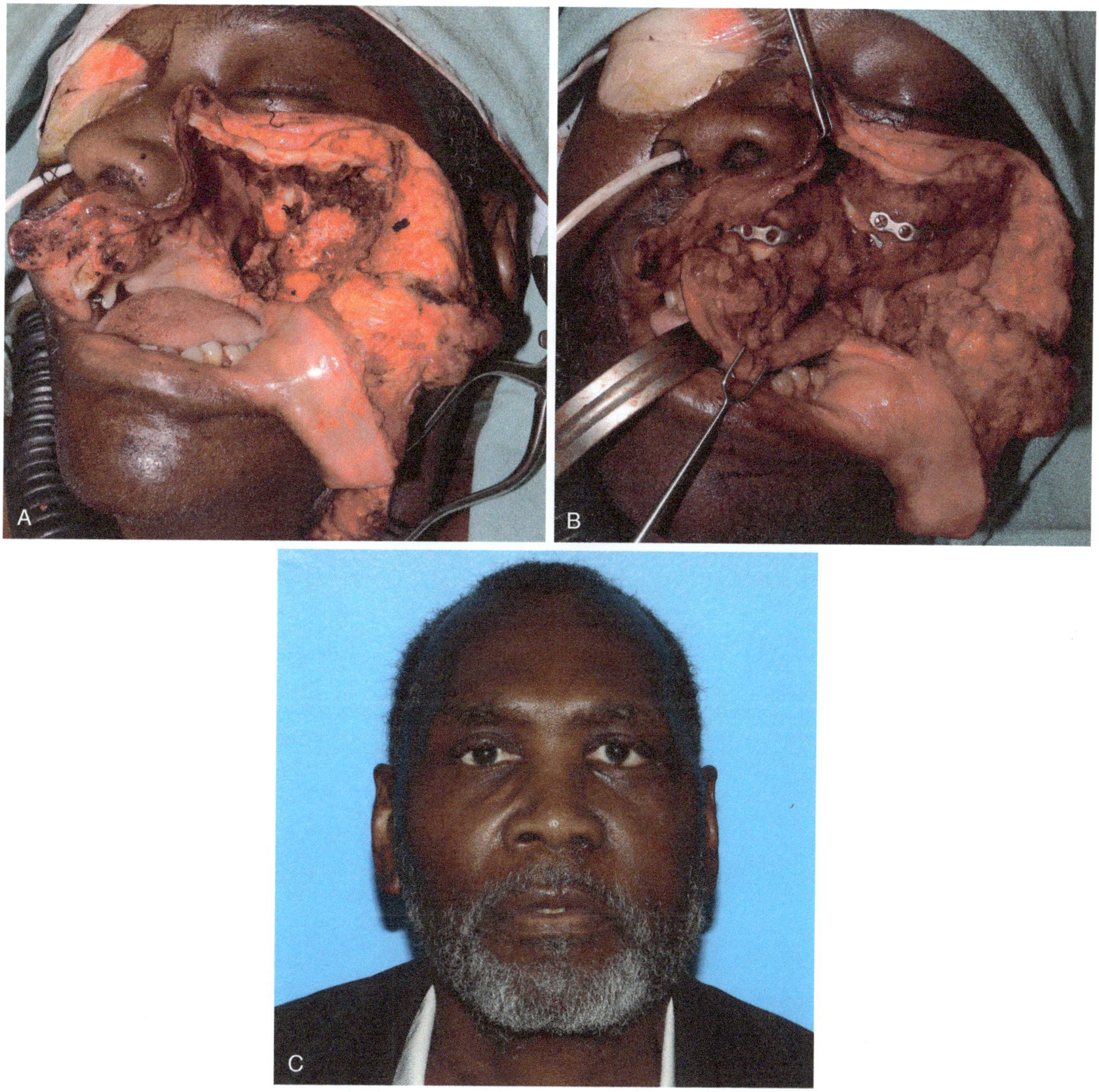

• **Fig. 25.3** (A) A left hemimaxillectomy defect, that extends to the midline. (B) Reconstruction of the hemimaxillectomy defect with a fibula osteocutaneous free flap. The fibula height is very close to the height of maxillary bone in the malar region as well as the height of the premaxilla. The fibula skin paddle is used to close the palatal mucosal defect. (C) Postoperative appearance demonstrating excellent facial symmetry.

side, then exophthalmos and, potentially loss of vision, can result. With either enophthalmos or exophthalmos, the eyelids may not fully close and problems with tearing and dry eyes severe enough to result in exposure keratitis may occur. Impingement of the extraocular muscles can also cause diplopia and impingement on the optic nerve can cause blindness. Prosthetic obturators are not an option when a total maxillectomy is performed because they do not provide appropriate support for the eye.

The author's experience suggests that, when supported by a soft tissue free flap, the orbital floor can usually be successfully reconstructed with bone grafts or alloplasts even when postoperative radiation therapy is administered (Fig. 25.7).[28,29] Many surgeons, however, feel that bone grafts are relatively more resistant to radiation-associated complications than are alloplasts.[30] In a review of orbital floor reconstruction for trauma, Kirby et al[31] found that autologous bone reconstruction was more likely to be complicated by orbital dystopia and enophthalmos compared to titanium mesh and porous polyethylene, possibly due to increased difficulty in shaping the reconstructed orbital floor, irregular thickness, and unpredictable resorption. Obviously,

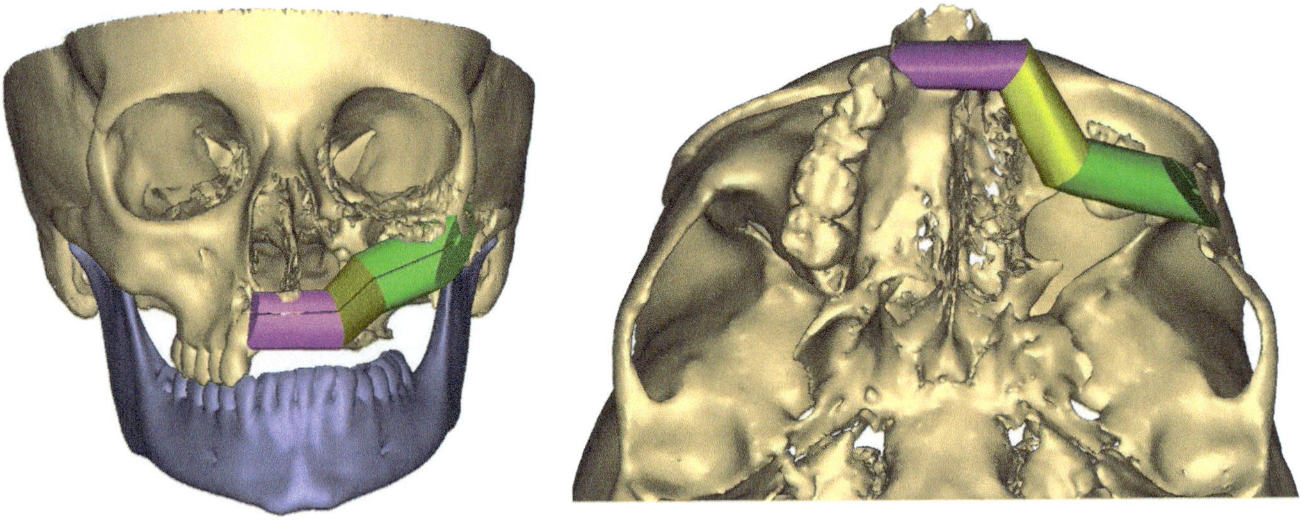

• **Fig. 25.4** Design of a "single-barrel" fibula free flap reconstruction for a left maxillectomy that extends slightly past the midline.

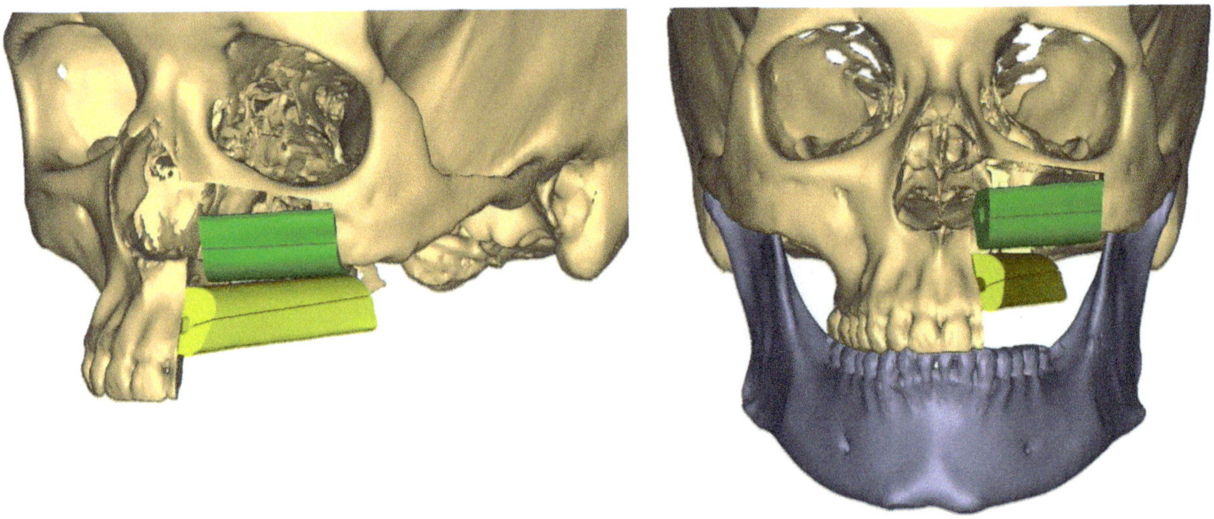

• **Fig. 25.5** Design of a "double-barrel" fibula free flap reconstruction for a left maxillectomy that does not fully extend to the midline. This configuration allows for a greater number of osseointegrated implants to be placed for dental restoration and also the more superior bone (green segment) supports the nose at the piriform aperture better.

alloplastic materials have the advantage of being available in unlimited quantities and carry with them no donor site morbidity.

When reconstructing the orbital floor, titanium mesh can be bent to fit the contours of the orbit once adequate surgical exposure has been achieved but prior to performing any osteotomies. This mesh can be used as the definitive reconstruction or used as a template for accurate bone graft reconstruction. It is important when reconstructing the orbital floor that no mesh or bone graft edges or other hardware impinge on the optic nerve, globe, or the extraocular muscles. Typically, a gap of a few millimeters in the orbital floor reconstruction is left in the region of the orbital apex as displacement or an excessively long graft or mesh can injure the optic nerve, causing visual loss. Here again, computer-generated 3D models can be of great assistance in creating a very accurate orbital floor reconstruction and 3D printed plates are becoming available to potentially make reconstruction simpler and more accurate.[32] It should be remembered that excessive retraction on the globe can stretch the optic nerve, causing vision loss (traumatic optic neuropathy) and excess pressure on the globe can cause bradycardia via the oculocardiac reflex.

Orbitomaxillectomy (Maxillectomy with Orbital Exenteration)

Orbital exenteration is defined as removal of the entire contents of the bony orbit, including the globe,

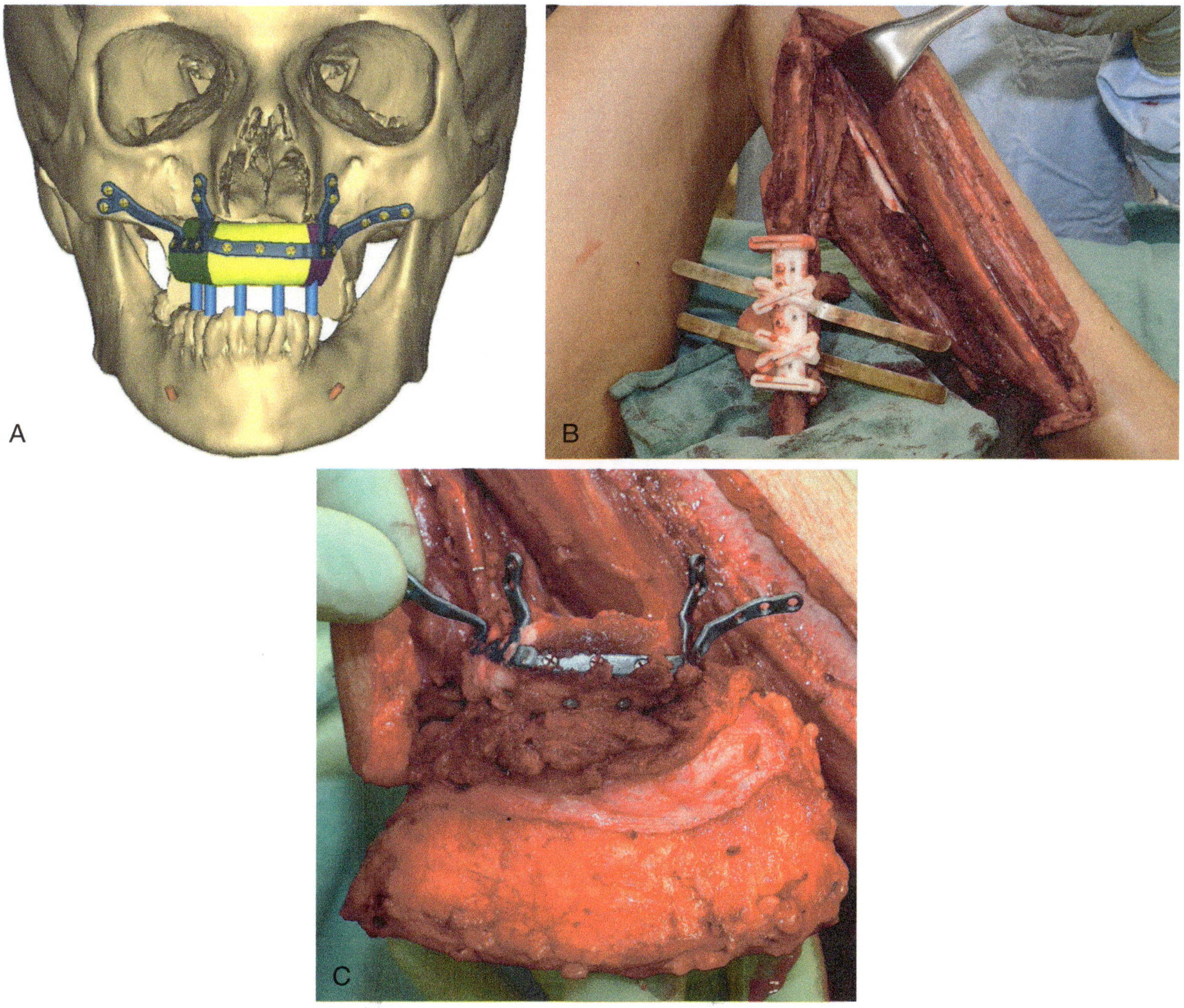

• **Fig. 25.6** (A) Computer-aided design for a "U-shaped" fibula osteocutaneous free flap to reconstruct a bilateral maxillectomy (total palatectomy) defect. (B) A computer-generated cutting guide helps the surgeon to make precise fibular osteotomies for shaping. (C) Fibula free flap following dissection, osteotomies, and rigid fixation with a custom 3D-printed titanium reconstruction plate.

extraocular muscles and periorbital fat, and many times includes the eyelids, in contrast to enucleation, which involves only removal of the globe. Orbital exenteration is indicated for tumors of the maxilla that penetrate the inferior and medial orbital walls and invade the contents of the orbit. Orbital exenteration is also performed for lacrimal gland cancers as well as periorbital skin cancers.

Skin grafts or even healing by secondary intention can be used to line the bony orbit following orbital exenteration if the patient is not irradiated. Healing by secondary intention is usually a slow process, and, for that reason, skin grafting is often preferred. When radiation is given preoperatively or postoperatively, well-vascularized flaps are indicated to cover the orbital bones because stable skin graft take or spontaneous healing is unlikely. In patients who are not suitable candidates for a free tissue transfer, a temporalis muscle flap or temporoparietal fascia flap covered by a skin graft can be utilized.[33] These flaps sometimes do not reach the medial orbit. In these cases, the lateral orbital wall can be removed, allowing the flaps to cover the medial orbit.

In all other patients, free flaps are the preferred reconstructive method following orbital exenteration.[33] Flap choice depends on patient body habitus and preference, surgeon experience, and the desire for an orbital prosthesis. If a prosthesis is planned, then a thinner, more pliable flap should be used that can create a concave surface to accommodate the prosthesis. A radial forearm fasciocutaneous free flap is a good choice because it provides thin supple tissue that can be contoured to the eye socket and has a very long pedicle that can reach either superficial temporal or facial vessels.[33,34] Osseointegrated implants can be placed in the infraorbital rim to further aid in prosthesis retention.

However, if the defect includes removal of one or more walls of the bony orbit, a bulkier flap is usually indicated. Bulky flaps are better suited for supporting the intracranial contents if the superior orbital bone has been removed or preventing a sino-nasal-orbital fistula if the medial or

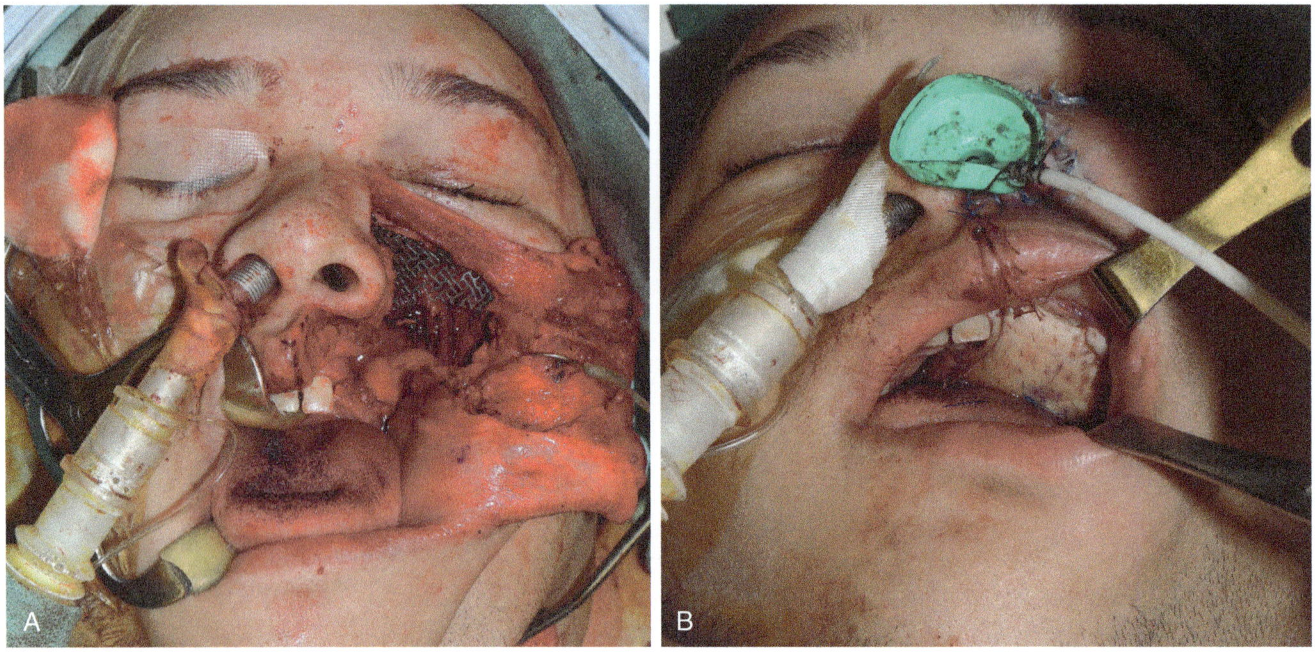

• **Fig. 25.7** (A) Left total maxillectomy including resection of the orbital floor. (B) The orbital floor was reconstructed with a titanium mesh implant. The mesh is supported by an ALT free flap, which is also used to close the palatal defect.

inferior orbital bones have been removed (Fig. 25.8).[33,34] The ALT free flap is again the author's preferred flap for such extended orbital exenteration defects.[34] This flap can be harvested to include some of the vastus lateralis muscle to place against the orbital apex and any skull base defects where it can help to seal off cerebrospinal fluid leakages if they occur. The RAM free flap can also be used provided the patient does not have too much subcutaneous abdominal fat. The superficial temporal blood vessels or the facial vessels are used as recipient blood vessels.

In some cases, an orbital exenteration is combined with a maxillectomy (i.e., orbitomaxillectomy). When the palate has been preserved, a slightly larger ALT or RAM free flap can be used to fill the combined maxillary sinus and orbital cavity.[5,13] The mucosa of the maxillary sinus should be completely removed to prevent later mucocele formation. When the defect also includes the palate, an ALT or RAM free flap with two skin paddles can be harvested with each skin paddle based on separate perforating blood vessels to independently close the orbital and palatal defects. The intranasal surface does not need to be lined with skin as the raw surface of these free flaps spontaneously mucosalize rapidly, usually within 2 weeks.

Complications

Most series have suggested that free flap failure rates are about the same for midface reconstruction as other types of head and neck reconstruction.[13] Because vein grafting and a relatively long course of the pedicle through subcutaneous tissues beneath the cheek skin are required for many maxillary and midface reconstructions, meticulous technique and attention to avoiding tension, compression, twisting, and kinking of the blood vessels is required to avoid flap vascular compromise.

Aside from complications associated with compromised flap perfusion, there are risks for a number of other complications. Soft tissue complications such as ectropion, nasal obstruction or deviation, and diplopia secondary to impingement of the extraocular muscles or inaccurate orbital floor reconstruction may require revision surgery. Following orbital floor reconstruction, a forced duction test should be performed while still in the operating room. Visual acuity checks and tests for diplopia should be performed as soon as the patient is awake and continued for several days. The use of hardware in midfacial reconstruction introduces other risks as well. When titanium plates or meshes are utilized for bony fixation or reconstruction of the orbital floor, there is a risk of implant infection or exposure, especially in patients who receive radiation therapy. Well-vascularized coverage of the hardware with soft tissue flap components minimizes the risk for hardware exposure and extrusion. To keep the nasal airway patent, a nasal trumpet is often inserted on the side of the defect at the time of surgery and left in place for 2 weeks when a soft tissue flap is used to reconstruct the maxilla.

Other challenges in midfacial reconstruction are the potential for fistula formation. An oronasal (i.e., palatal) fistula may require another flap in order to close the fistula if large and, especially, if not repaired immediately. Alternately, the fistula can be occluded with a palatal prosthesis that simultaneously addresses missing teeth. An even more difficult fistula to manage is a sino-naso-cutaneous fistula along a lateral rhinotomy

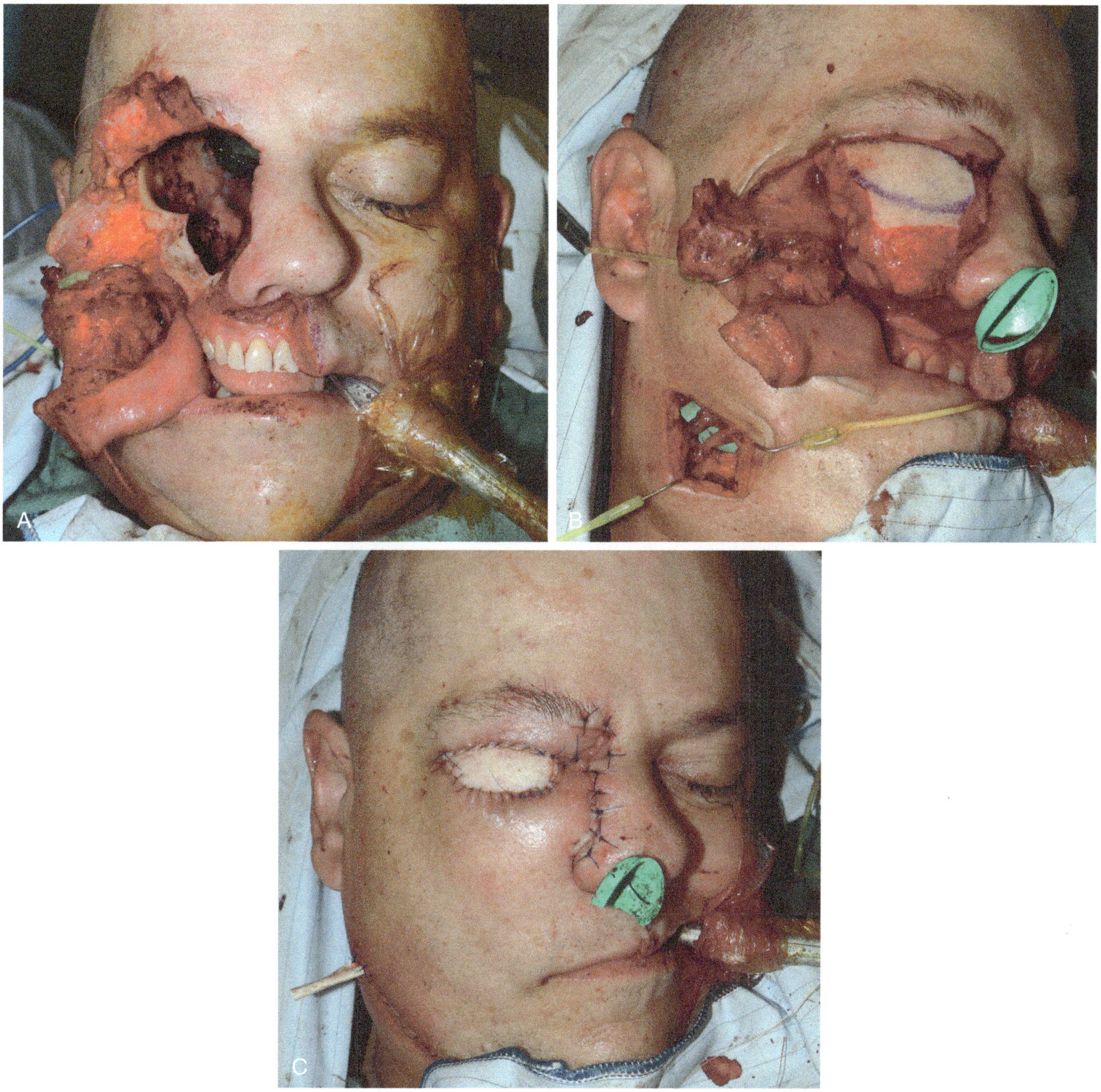

• **Fig. 25.8** (A) Reconstruction of an orbitomaxillectomy defect that includes orbital exenteration and resection of the orbital floor but preservation of the entire palate and alveolus. (B) ALT free flap inset, filling the maxillary sinus, which is denuded of mucosa, and the bony orbit (closed orbital cavity), minimizing the chance for developing a sino-naso-cutaneous fistula. (C) Immediate postoperative appearance.

or Weber–Fergusson incision. In the author's experience, such fistulae almost always require an additional free flap for reliable closure.

Outcomes and Conclusions

In our experience with 246 maxillary free flap reconstructions, free flap survival was about 97%.[13] Two of eight free flap losses were related to compression of the pedicle in the subcutaneous cheek tunnel connecting the free flap to the recipient blood vessels, underscoring the need to create a wide enough tunnel and avoid pressure over the cheek and neck.[13] Long-term complications included a 2.5% incidence of oroantral fistula and a 4.6% incidence of sino-naso-cutaneous fistula, emphasizing the need for design of reconstructive flaps to reinforce thin or radiated soft tissues of the cheek and meticulous closure of lateral rhinotomy and Weber–Fergusson incisions.[13] Orbital complications of diplopia and hardware infection or exposure did not seem to be related to choice of material (bone graft or alloplast) used to reconstruct the orbital floor in the limited number of cases studied.

Approximately 95% were judged to have good to excellent speech outcomes (80% or greater intelligibility).[13] Patients with poorer intelligibility had additional resection of either the soft palate or the tongue. Swallowing outcomes were also excellent, with 95% independent of tube feeding.[13] The few patients who had prolonged or permanent feeding tube dependence had other comorbid factors or additional oral cavity resections compromising the swallowing mechanism. Dental restoration was correlated with the appropriate use of bone for defects that involved hemipalatoalveolar and bilateral palatoalveolar resection. In those cases, osseointegrated implants were highly successful for providing stable fixation of a dental prosthesis.

In summary, appropriate flap selection, and careful attention to flap shaping and insetting is critical for restoring premorbid appearance and function. Avoidance of complications requires meticulous technique and highly accurate reconstruction. Computer planning and 3D-printed models and hardware have shown great promise in recent years for improving outcomes of bony reconstruction, including the palate and alveolus as well as the orbit. Factoring in dental restoration is important for achieving total functional and esthetic rehabilitation of patients with complex midfacial defects.

References

1. Moreno MA, Skoracki RJ, Hanna EY, Hanasono MM. Microvascular free flap reconstruction versus palatal obturation for maxillectomy defects. *Head Neck*. 2010;32(7):860–868.
2. Rieger JM, Tang JA, Wolfaardt J, Harris J, Seikaly H. Comparison of speech and aesthetic outcomes in patients with maxillary reconstruction versus maxillary obturators after maxillectomy. *J Otolaryngol Head Neck Surg*. 2011;40(1):40–47.
3. Chigurupati R, Aloor N, Salas R, Schmidt BL. Quality of life after maxillectomy and prosthetic obturator rehabilitation. *J Oral Maxillofac Surg*. 2013;71(8):1471–1478.
4. Andrades P, Militsakh O, Hanasono MM, Rieger J, Rosenthal EL. Current strategies in reconstruction of maxillectomy defects. *Arch Otolaryngol Head Neck Surg*. 2011;137:806–812.
5. Cordeiro PG, Santamaria E. Classification system and algorithm for reconstruction of maxillectomy and midfacial defects. *Plast Reconstr Surg*. 2000;105:2331–2346.
6. Brown JS, Rogers SN, McNally DN, Boyle M. A modified classification for the maxillectomy defect. *Head Neck*. 2000;22(1):17–26.
7. Okay DJ, Genden E, Buchbinder D, Urken M. Prosthodontic guideline for surgical reconstruction of the maxilla: a classification system of defects. *J Prosthet Dent*. 2001;86:352–363.
8. Brown JS, Shaw RJ. Reconstruction of the maxilla and midface: introducing a new classification. *Lancet Oncol*. 2010;11(10):1001–1008.
9. Costa H, Zenha H, Sequeira H, et al. Microsurgical reconstruction of the maxilla: algorithm and concepts. *J Plast Reconstr Aesthet Surg*. 2015;68(5):e89–e104.
10. Rodriguez ED, Martin M, Bluebond-Langner R, et al. Microsurgical reconstruction of posttraumatic high-energy maxillary defects: establishing the effectiveness of early reconstruction. *Plast Reconstr Surg*. 2007;120:103S–117S.
11. Archibald S, Jackson S, Thoma A. Paranasal sinus and midfacial reconstruction. *Clin Plast Surg*. 2005;32:309–325.
12. Dallan I, Lenzi R, Sellari-Franceschini S, Tschabitsher M, Muscatello L. Temporalis myofascial flap in maxillary reconstruction: anatomical study and clinical application. *J Craniomaxillofac Surg*. 2009;37:96–101.
13. Hanasono MM, Silva AK, Yu P, Skoracki RJ. A comprehensive algorithm for oncologic maxillary reconstruction. *Plast Reconstr Surg*. 2013;131:47–60.
14. Cordeiro PG, Bacilious N, Schantz S, Spiro R. The radial forearm osteocutaneous "sandwich" free flap for reconstruction of the bilateral subtotal maxillectomy defect. *Ann Plast Surg*. 1998;40:397–402.
15. Chepeha DB, Moyer JS, Bradford CR, Prince ME, Marentette L, Teknos TN. Osseocutaneous radial forearm free tissue transfer for repair of complex midfacial defects. *Arch Otolaryngol Head Neck Surg*. 2005;131:513–517.
16. Clark JR, Vesely M, Gilbert R. Scapular angle osteomyogenous flap in postmaxillectomy reconstruction: defect, reconstruction, shoulder function, and harvest technique. *Head Neck*. 2008;30:10–20.
17. Genden EM, Wallace D, Buchbinder D, Okay D, Urken M. Iliac crest internal oblique osteomusculocutaneous free flap reconstruction of the postablative palatomaxillary defect. *Arch Otolaryngol Head Neck Surg*. 2001;127:854–861.
18. Brown JS, Jones DC, Summerwill, et al. Vascularized iliac crest with internal oblique muscle for immediate reconstruction after maxillectomy. *Br J Oral Maxillofac Surg*. 2002;40:183–190.
19. Hanasono MM, Skoracki RJ. The omega-shaped fibula osteocutaneous free flap for reconstruction of extensive midfacial defects. *Plast Reconstr Surg*. 2010;125(4):160e–162e.
20. Chang EI, Clemens MW, Garvey PB, Skoracki RJ, Hanasono MM. Cephalometric analysis for microvascular head and neck reconstruction. *Head Neck*. 2012;34(11):1607–1614.
21. Maricevich M, Lin LO, Liu J, Chang EI, Hanasono MM. Interposition vein grafting in head and neck free flap reconstruction. *Plast Reconstr Surg*. 2018;142:1025–1034.
22. Hanasono MM, Jacob RF, Bidaut L, Robb GL, Skoracki RJ. Midfacial reconstruction using virtual planning, rapid prototype modeling, and stereotactic navigation. *Plast Reconstr Surg*. 2010;126(6):2002–2006.
23. Levine JP, Bae JS, Soares M, et al. Jaw in a day: total maxillofacial reconstruction using digital technology. *Plast Reconstr Surg*. 2013;131(6):1386–1391.
24. Seruya M, Fisher M, Rodriguez ED. Computer-assisted versus conventional free fibula flap technique for craniofacial reconstruction: an outcomes comparison. *Plast Reconstr Surg*. 2013;132(5):1219–1228.
25. Matros E, Albornoz CR, Rensberger M, Weimer K, Garfein ES. Computer-assisted design and computer-assisted modeling technique optimization and advantages over traditional methods of osseous flap reconstruction. *J Reconstr Microsurg*. 2014;30:289–296.
26. Zhang WB, Wang XJ, Liu C, et al. Reconstruction of maxillary defects with free fibula flap assisted by computer techniques. *J Craniomaxillofac Surg*. 2015;43:630–636.
27. Pang JH, Brooke S, Kubik MW, et al. Staged reconstruction (delayed-immediate) of the maxillectomy defect using CAD/CAM technology. *J Reconstr Microsurg*. 2018;34:193–199.
28. Nakayama B, Hasegawa Y, Hyodo I, et al. Reconstruction using a three-dimensional orbitozygomatic skeletal model of titanium mesh plate and soft-tissue free flap transfer following total maxillectomy. *Plast Reconstr Surg*. 2004;114:631–639.

29. Fu K, Liu Y, Gao N, et al. Reconstruction of maxillary and orbital floor defect with free fibula flap and whole individualized titanium mesh assisted by computer techniques. *J Oral Maxillofac Surg*. 2017;75:1791e1–1791e9.
30. Cordeiro PG, Chen CM. A 15-year review of midface reconstruction after total and subtotal maxillectomy: part II. Technical modifications to maximize aesthetic and functional outcomes. *Plast Reconstr Surg*. 2012;129:139–147.
31. Kirby EJ, Turner JB, Davenport DL, Vasconez HC. Orbital floor fractures: outcomes of reconstruction. *Ann Plast Surg*. 2011;66:508–512.
32. Tarsitano A, Battaglia S, Ciocca L, Scotti R, Cipriani R, Marchetti C. Surgical reconstruction of maxillary defects using a computer-assisted design/computer-assisted manufacturing-produced titanium mesh supporting a free flap. *J Craniomaxillofac Surg*. 2016;44:1320–1326.
33. Moyer JS, Chepeha DB, Prince ME, Teknos TN. Microvascular reconstruction of the orbital complex. *Facial Plast Surg Clin North Am*. 2009;17:225–237.
34. Hanasono MM, Lee JC, Yang JS, Skoracki RJ, Reece GP, Esmaeli B. An algorithmic approach to reconstructive surgery and prosthetic rehabilitation after orbital exenteration. *Plast Reconstr Surg*. 2009;123(1):98–105.

26 Pharyngeal Reconstruction

ROSTAM D. FARHADIEH, AJAY R. SUD, EDWIN MORRISON, AND WAYNE A.J. MORRISON

Introduction

The upper aerodigestive (UAD) tract is an intricate maze of alleyways, muscular tubes, and cords that allows humans to have a common functional pathway for oral intake and breathing, as well as harmonizing vibrations into speech. Articulation of speech is dependent on the symphony of functions of these passages, influenced by the larynx, epiglottis, pharyngeal walls, soft and hard palate, the tongue musculature, salivation, lip seal or oral competence and dentition as a tightly ordered orchestra. Many of these functional elements involve the pharynx. The posterior reaches and ramifications of the UAD tract coalesce into a continuous 15 cm-long muscular collecting tube, the pharynx, which begins in continuity with the nasopharynx superiorly and connects to the esophagus inferiorly. It extends from the skull base to the esophagus and comprises three parts: upper or nasopharynx behind the nose, middle or oropharynx behind the mouth, and lower or hypo- or laryngopharynx behind the epiglottis and larynx.

Pathology

Pharyngeal cancers are predominately squamous cell carcinoma (SCC) and are of two types: HPV+ related to human papilloma virus (better prognosis) and HPV− usually linked to alcohol and tobacco. Risk factors include alcohol and tobacco, exposure to Epstein–Barr virus, and Chinese ethnicity, especially for nasopharyngeal carcinoma. Organ preservation has become the main aim in the management of UAD tract malignancy. Fortunately, early stage disease can be effectively treated conservatively with radiotherapy or chemoradiation combination so that function can largely be preserved. Given the morbidity of surgery in this most sophisticated functional zone, its place is increasingly reserved for advanced stage disease or in salvage treatment after failure of nonsurgical protocols. Sadly, most patients present at advanced stages and are associated with poor overall survival. Between 70% and 85% have stage 3 or stage 4 disease at presentation and 5-year survivals are reported around 15%–35%.[1] The reality is that most surgery is palliative and although the prime focus here is inevitably on removal of the cancer and reduction in the risk of local recurrence, the overall focus must be on the quality of survival. By contrast, nasopharyngeal cancers have a better prognosis as they are mostly responsive to radiotherapy and rarely require surgical resection or reconstruction.

Anatomy

The nasopharynx is open to the nasal cavities anteriorly and extends from the base of the skull superiorly to the upper surface of the soft pallet where it becomes the oropharynx. The oropharynx communicates with the mouth anteriorly and includes the soft palate, the tonsils, and the tongue base posterior to the circumvallate papillae. The oropharyngeal tube extends from the soft palate above to the hyoid below. The hypopharynx is continuous below the oropharynx, extending from the level of the hyoid bone to the esophageal inlet. The larynx lies in close anterior proximity. The thyrohyoid membrane through which the internal branch of the superior laryngeal nerve gains access to the larynx is located superolaterally. The detailed anatomy of the UAD tract can be found in specialized texts. Anatomically, the area has a rich lymphatic drainage to the jugular chains as well as the retropharyngeal nodes and the node of Rouvière,[2] with frequent crossing of the midline. The pharyngeal muscular tube, which spans from the base of the skull to the C6 vertebra, comprises circular fibers that form constrictions to propel contents into the esophagus and longitudinal fibers that lift the walls of the pharynx during swallowing.

Indications for Surgery and Reconstruction

Most commonly, major UAD tract defects result from surgical ablation of malignancies. It is accepted that radiotherapy is just as effective as surgery for eradication of early disease, and because radiotherapy is less destructive to function, it is the preferred modality of treatment. Surgery is therefore reserved for advanced stage or recurrent cancers and will be inevitably destructive. The principles of wide oncological resection, the proximity of the vital structures and the protection of the upper airway patency, speech, and deglutition dictate the indications for reconstruction of any significant UAD tract defects. Many pharyngectomies for advanced disease are associated with combined laryngectomy. Thus most advanced neoplasms involving the oropharynx, hypopharynx or cervical esophagus will result in a pharyngeal defect requiring reconstruction.

Classification of Pharyngeal Defects

A useful classification of pharyngeal defects was previously devised by Disa et al,[3] however, this classification did not specify whether the defect involved the larynx or the base of the tongue. More recently, Urken et al,[4] proposed a new classification scheme that addresses this issue:

- Type 0: minimal defects of the pharyngoesophageal segment that are amenable to primary closure
- Type I: non-circumferential defect with a presence of a viable strip of mucosa, measuring a minimum of 2 cm in width
- Type II: circumferential defect extended no further cephalad than the level of the vallecula
- Type III: circumferential or noncircumferential defect extended cephalad to the level of the vallecula
- Type IV: any resection that extends caudal to the level of the clavicles.

Historical Perspectives

The first attempts at pharyngoesophageal reconstruction date back to the nineteenth century. These proved notoriously unreliable, with chronic aspiration, hemorrhage, and early death in the postoperative course, followed by stricture formation in those who survived the immediate aftermath of the surgery. This led to a loss of enthusiasm for reconstruction until Wookey rekindled interest in 1948 with a random pattern anterior neck skin flap to reestablish the UAD tract. His two-stage reconstruction included using the cervical skin raised as a random flap sutured to the upper and lower ends of the defect, but left open anteriorly thereby exteriorizing the pharynx and esophagus. The sulcus thus created was closed 5 weeks later at a second-stage operation. The next surgical leap came when Bakamjian described the more reliable axial deltopectoral flap, based medially on what has subsequently been shown to be the upper second and third internal thoracic artery perforating branches.[5] It was, however, still a two- or three-stage treatment and was not uniformly reliable.

In 1979, Ariyan's description of a tubed myocutaneous pectoralis major flap finally made possible a single–stage ablative reconstruction with a more predictable outcome.[5] Subsequently, both the trapezius and latissimus dorsi myocutaneous flaps were described as alternatives for a single–stage reconstruction, but not surprisingly did not achieve significant popularity.[2]

Parallel with these skin tube developments, more reliable pedicled interposition gastrointestinal reconstructions were being attempted as far back as the 1930s; their primary role, however, was in total esophagectomies. Adaptation of the Ivor–Lewis gastric pull-up to the cervical esophagus and pharynx was one such procedure, which has survived as a mostly reliable option into the modern era. In addition to the gastric pull-up, the spectrum of these pedicled flap reconstructions included the left colon and the seldom used pedicled jejunum.[5]

In 1959, Seidenberg[6] reported the first successful harvesting and transferring of a jejunal free flap using microsurgical techniques, reportedly with threaded 6–0 silk sutures under loupes magnification. His patient died 5 days postoperatively from a massive cerebrovascular accident, but the first successful human free flap was found to be viable at the time. The following year Hiebert and Cummings Jr[7] performed an uneventful gastro-antral free graft joining 2 mm-diameter gastroepiploic vessels to the superior thyroid artery end to side and facial vein end-to-end. They noted the report of Jacobson and Suarez, the acknowledged founders of microvascular technique that occurred subsequent to their procedure, recommending using a microscope. These feats were performed at least a decade before the tidal wave of microsurgery began, with the works of Buncke et al, Daniel and Taylor, and O'Brien et al,[5] and others who used other tissues, including omentum and skin. Soon, microsurgical free tissue transfer was to become a first-line mainstream reconstructive option.

Microvascular technique brought with it the promise of a reconstruction not bound by restraints of pedicle length or random proportions. The reliability of an axial flap transfer into the defect revolutionized the approach to major reconstructive challenges. Gastro-omental, gastric antral, ileocolic as well as colon free flaps have been described; however by far the most common visceral reconstruction is a free jejunal reconstruction.[7] The earliest significant clinical series of microsurgical jejunal reconstructions were those reported by Jurkiewicz.[5] But his daring and technical skill were not widely adopted for almost a further 20 years. The free jejunal flap, whether as a tube or patch, has since become one of the two most reliable reconstructive tools for laryngopharyngectomy and/or cervical esophagus reconstruction.

Tubed or patch fasciocutaneous flaps are the other main alternative reconstructive options for pharyngeal defects. The most common flaps used are the anterolateral thigh and radial forearm flaps.

Assessment and Planning

As with any operative surgery, planning remains the most important step in execution of the technique. This is best considered as part of a regular multidisciplinary (MDT) meeting, which includes, in addition to head and neck, oral maxillofacial and plastic surgeons, radiation oncologists, medical oncologists, pathologists, speech therapists, dieticians, physiotherapists, and social workers, as well as a radiologist specializing in head and neck malignancies. An estimation of the extent of the defect and the need for reconstruction is discussed at these meetings. The reconstructive team, in conjunction with the ablative team, can decide on the best reconstructive option and begin planning for surgery after assessment of all possible donor sites. Previous history of laparotomy and upper GI surgery is noted and the patient's forearms and thighs are assessed.

A decision is also made at these multidisciplinary meetings in relation to the need for perioperative radiotherapy and preoperative dental surgery, as well as nutritional needs. Most, if not all, patients requiring major reconstruction have either advanced disease or chemoradiation failure for relatively advanced disease and suffer from malnutrition. The need for nutritional supplementation is almost universal, including during the radiation therapy period. This may require percutaneous endoscopic gastric (PEG) tube insertion, depending on the surgical unit. Nutritional status will influence wound healing and reduce fistula formation. Uncomplicated healing streamlines the programming of radiation therapy in the shortest time window possible for the best therapeutic outcome.

Reconstruction

The broad principles of pharyngeal reconstruction are:

- maintaining or recreating a patent airway and protection from aspiration;
- reestablishing the integrity of the pharyngeal pathway to allow swallowing and adequate caloric intake; and
- voice and speech rehabilitation.

All of these endeavors have in common the creation of a patent tube. Salvage of all these functions is possible to various extents. The advent of microsurgery has made possible transfer of large amounts of tissue sculpted to more or less reconstruct the created defect. In addition, introduction of tissues with a new vascular supply into settings of advanced disease requiring major resections and radiotherapy or following chemoradiation failure, promotes better wound healing and discourages fistula formation.

The two key determinants that influence the nature of the reconstruction are the *surgery* (i.e., the defect created as well as donor availabilities) and the *patient's general status*. Many of these patients have life-long history of heavy smoking and drinking, with the attendant risk of cardiac or respiratory disease and malnourishment. These are all factors to be considered in the light of the length of surgery and the added morbidity from choice of donor sites. The added burden of a laparotomy or a chest flap on the respiratory reserves, the speed of skin flaps versus bowel in patients with poor cardiac reserve or malnourishment, and the benefits of donor sites that allow simultaneous access during the primary resection for two-team surgery are issues to ponder. Preoperative anesthetic, respiratory, and cardiac assessment is mandatory. Any reasonable optimization of the patient's status should be undertaken prior to surgery.

All patients require confirmation of continuity and integrity of the UAD tract at 7–10 days postoperatively, with a contrast study before removal of nasogastric tubes and resumption of oral intake.

Reconstructive Options

Local Flaps

In practical terms, these include surrounding cervical skin and soft tissue and they rarely provide a practical reconstructive option for major defects. Not only is the neck skin vasculature unreliable, especially after flap elevation and block dissection, but it is generally sacrosanct to ensure cover of vital structures such as the carotid vessels. Frequently, the neck skin has been or will be irradiated. The generalized devascularization associated with the treatment modalities greatly favors the importation of new, independently vascularized tissue, either from a regional source or more commonly now as a free flap transfer. Recently, the supraclavicular flap based on the transverse cervical vessels including a deltoid skin extension has been successfully used in lower level pharyngeal reconstructions.

Regional Flaps

Aside from the pectoralis major flap, other pedicled flaps described include gastric pull-up flap, the myocutaneous latissimus dorsi and trapezius flaps, as well as the traditional fasciocutaneous deltopectoral or its modification the internal mammary artery perforator (IMAP) flap. This is essentially a paramedian vertically oriented propeller flap based on the second or second and third internal mammary perforators. It can be rotated 180° and employed for some hypopharyngeal reconstructions.

Pectoralis Major

This type V Mathes and Nahai myocutaneous flap remains one of the most reliable reconstructive options for the head and neck.[3] With the advent of microsurgical reconstructions it has been increasingly relegated to a second choice or salvage reconstructive option. Some of the current indications for its use include:

- situations where general patient state and systemic disease dictate reduced operative time
- in combination with another flap or alone, where an external skin defect is present or has evolved after primary surgery
- in coverage and protection of major neck vessels
- in closure of pharyngostome
- wound dehiscence.

This flap is based on the pectoral branch of the acromiothoracic axis. It is most commonly raised as a myocutaneous flap with its skin island placed medially in women to reduce breast tissue inclusion. The skin component is rolled to form a tube to reconstruct circumferential defects. In order to avoid traction on the vascular pedicle a 3-cm cuff of muscle should be retained at the clavicular origin where possible. A so-called defensive incision for accessing the muscle without violating the potential deltopectoral salvage flap is made and the flap is raised and, where possible, tunneled through the neck into the defect. For partial defects the skin island can be designed as a patch and sutured into the remnant pharyngeal mucosa. Anchoring the remnant pharynx and cervical esophagus to the prevertebral fascia, interdigitating the lower flap inset with the esophagus, and de-epithelialization of the leading skin edge have also been described as means of reducing stricture and fistula formation. Others have advocated removal of the skin island and using only the myofascial component of the flap for repair to reduce bulk and to discard the least vascularized tissue component. Table 26.1 lists published outcome studies specific to pharyngeal reconstructions. Increased flap complication rates are reported with hypopharyngeal reconstructions, female patients, previous radiation therapy, obesity, patients >70 years old, and preoperative malnutrition (albumin <4.0 g/dL).[11]

Flap bulk often precludes meaningful voice rehabilitation using a tracheoesophageal puncture (TEP). In addition, recurrent descent and obstruction of the stoma may require surgical revisions.

Free Flaps

The most common arterial recipient vessel is the superior thyroid or facial and the most common veins are the internal and external jugular or facial veins. Free flap reconstructions are broadly divided into two groups: the *visceral free flaps*, the commonest being the jejunal transfer, and *fasciocutaneous free flaps*, from the radial forearm and anterolateral thigh.

Free Jejunum

For obvious reasons, jejunum is an ideal reconstructive option for pharyngeal and upper esophageal reconstructions. Previous laparotomy, although not absolute, is a relative contraindication to its use. Patients with minimal respiratory reserve should be considered with caution, given the additional morbidity of a laparotomy. A segment of proximal jejunum up to 25 cm length can be transferred as a free flap. The luminal diameter of the jejunal flap ranges between 3 and 5 cm. Despite its advantages, this flap has several technical shortcomings.

- It is exquisitely sensitive to hypoxia; any hypoxia beyond 3 hours will almost always result in flap death and subsequent potentially catastrophic fistula formations.[12]
- The vein is particularly thin and will not tolerate traction.
- The pedicle remains relatively short in comparison to its fasciocutaneous counterparts; the average length is described as 4–6 cm, with a maximum length of 10 cm based on superior mesenteric vascular axis.

An isolated segment of jejunum is measured under mild stretch to the length of the defect and is transferred in an isoperistaltic orientation. The loop is chosen as proximal to the duodenum as is feasible because here the mesenteric vessels are longest. The oropharyngeal inset can be technically difficult, not least due to usual size discrepancies. Either a slit in the antimesenteric border or closing suture of the oropharyngeal remnant may be used to readjust for size mismatches. Island jejunal patches based on the same vascular arcade can be reoriented and inset into a split in the upper end of the tube to accommodate wide oropharyngeal discrepancies. A nasogastric tube is passed through the jejunal segment, and the tube length is adjusted and anchored at either end, such that the pedicle trails without tension into the recipient vessel site field. Definitive repair of each end awaits microvascular anastomosis so as to reduce ischemic time. The lower inset is performed last. All bowel anastomoses are done using interrupted sutures rather than staples or continuous sutures. Any significant redundancy in bowel length will increase the postoperative swallowing difficulties and a common error is to design the segment too long. A survey of the reported outcomes in the literature, outlined in the next section, supports its reliability and low complication rate (Fig. 26.1).

Flap monitoring can be performed by visualizing the mesentery through a temporary window in the neck incision or externalization of a separate jejunal ring isolated separately on the same vascular arcade. High reconstructions may be visible through the mouth, otherwise by endoscopy.

Free Skin Flaps

Tubed Anterolateral Thigh Flap

The anterolateral thigh (ALT) flap, originally described as a type B fasciocutaneous flap by Song and colleagues, has been more recently shown to be mostly a type C fasciocutaneous flap.[13] The flap is based on the descending branch of the lateral circumflex artery. Often multiple perforators are noted, which can be harvested after dissection through their intramuscular course. This is a robust flap with a very long pedicle. The typical head and neck cancer patient is male and has lost weight, both favorable characteristics for ALT flap usage. This makes it the preferred skin flap for pharyngeal reconstructions. Its fascial layer can be taken beyond the limits of the skin edge and permits a double-layer repair without overlap of the suture lines, thereby reducing fistula and stricture formation. The long pedicle makes for easy anastomosis compared with bowel and the donor site can be closed directly. This flap has gained strong popularity in reconstruction of the hypopharynx[13] (Fig. 26.2).

Tubed Radial Artery Forearm Flap

Assessment and operative planning for the radial artery flap starts preoperatively with confirmation of a favorable Allen's test. This confirms viable perfusion of the hand after ligation of the radial artery. The radial forearm flap is a well-vascularized fasciocutaneous flap[11] based on the radial artery and its venae comitantes, a long, large-diameter pedicle that has ensured this flap's popularity. The subcutaneous venous tributaries can be taken as alternative or additional drainage. The perforating vessels penetrate the radial aspect of the thin septum separating the flexor carpiradialis (FCR) and brachioradialis tendons. The septocutaneous perforators are concentrated in the lower third of the forearm along the axis of the artery and the fascia lateral or medial to this cleft is not essential for its viability. As the flap vascularity is distal and the skin is favorably thinner distally, the flap design is correspondingly from this region. It should be noted that the forearm skin is less hairy on the ulnar side and the skin island is best harvested from this side, its vascular source being still adequate from the radial perforators carried via the fascial bridge. When the flap is designed distally it is necessary to trace the pedicle to the cubital fossa even if

TABLE 26.1 Pectoralis Major and Other Myocutaneous Flaps: Reported Outcomes

	Defect	No. of Patients	Successful Swallowing	Stricture (%)	Fistula Leak (%)	Flap Failure (%)	Medical Complication (%)	Immediate Mortality (%)	Patient Received Voice Prosthesis (%)	Functional Outcome (%)
Pectoralis Major										
Chan et al[8]	Pharyngeal (circumferential)	92	100	27.2	23.9					35.8
Clark et al[5]	Hypopharyngeal	68	81	12	35		15	3	44	100
Chan et al[9]	Hypopharyngeal	30	100	26.7	0					
Espitalier et al[5]	Hypopharyngeal	41		39	22	2.5		0	2	100
	Cervical									
	Esophageal									
Spriano et al[5]	Hypopharyngeal	37		0	13	0	10	3	24	100
Saussez et al[5]	Hypopharyngeal	12		17	33	0	0	0	50	83
Leite et al[10]	Oropharyngeal and hypopharyngeal	84			31	2				
Pectoralis Major + Trapezius + Sternocleidomastoid										
Carlson et al[5]	Cervical	45		27	78	2	0	0		
	Esophageal									
	Hypopharyngeal									
Range				0–39	0–78	0–2.5	0–15	0–3	24–50	35.8–100

Modified from Farhadieh RD, Morrison WAJ. Pharyngeal reconstruction. In: Farhadieh RD, Bulstrode NW, Cugno S, eds. *Plastic and Reconstructive Surgery: Approaches and Techniques*. Chichester: Wiley; 2015:352.

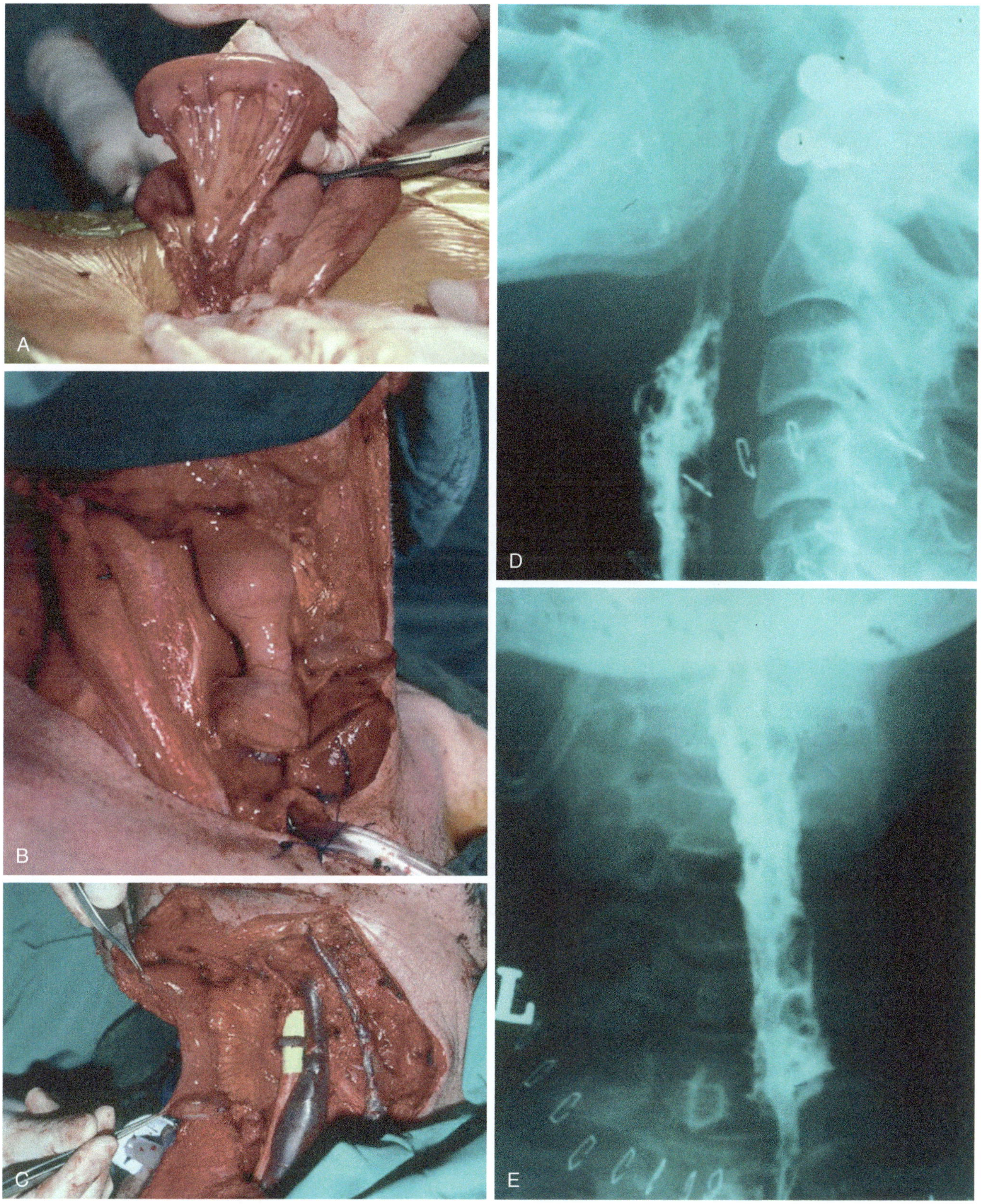

• **Fig. 26.1** (A) Jejunal loop harvest. (B) Inset of the jejunal reconstruction. (C) End-to-side venous microanastomosis with internal jugular vein. (D,E) Follow-up contrast swallow. (Courtesy Professor Wayne A. J. Morrison.).

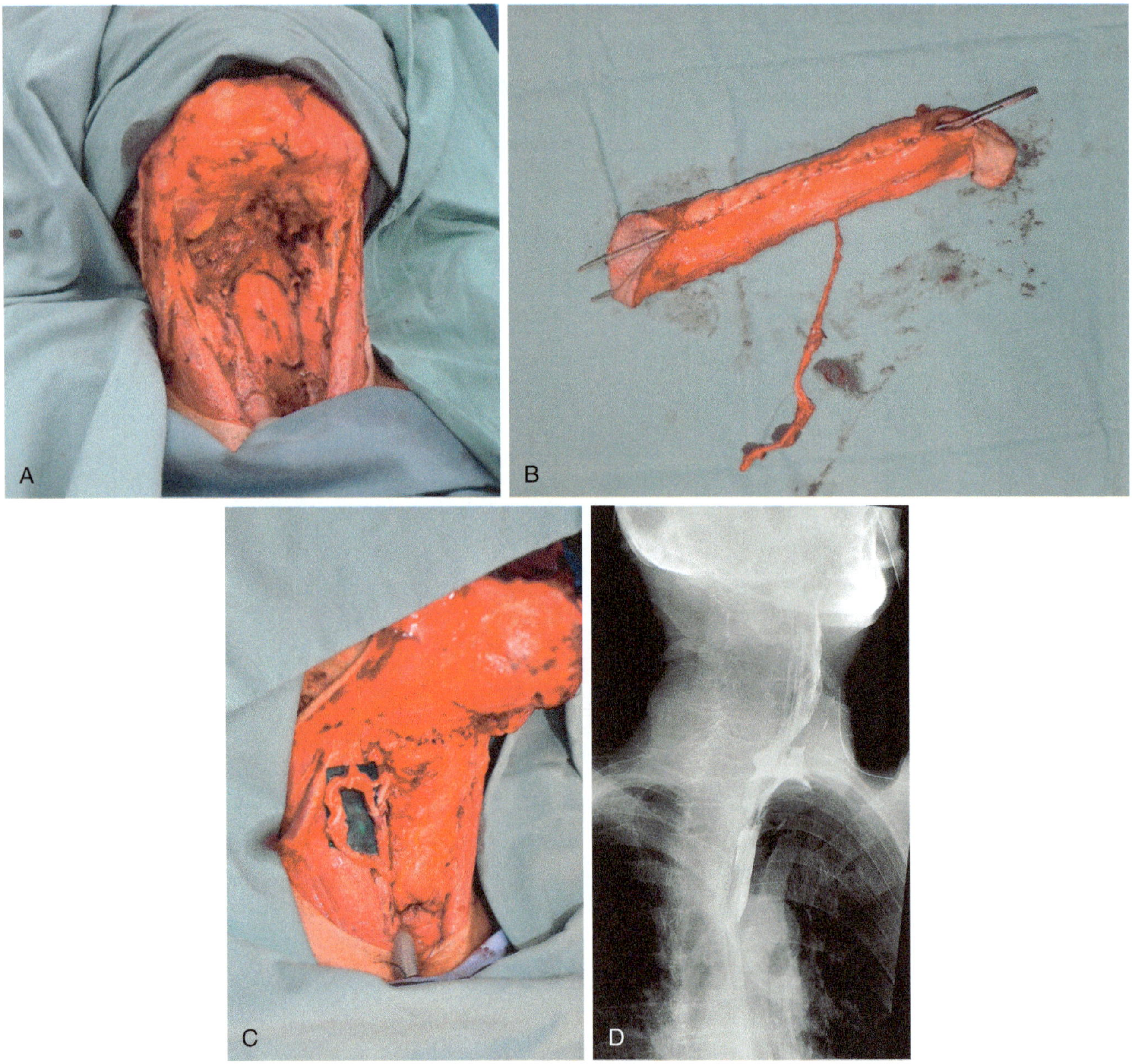

• **Fig. 26.2** Pharyngeal reconstruction following total laryngopharyngectomy with a tubed anterolateral thigh (ALT) flap. (A) Site of laryngopharyngectomy defect. (B) Tubed ALT flap. (C) Flap inset and microanastomosis with right superior thyroid vessels. (D) Contrast swallow at one week postoperatively. (Photos courtesy Dr. Rostam D. Farhadieh.)

pedicle length is not an issue, as the venae comitantes are of very small diameter until almost the level of the cubital fossa.

Miscellaneous Flaps

Lateral arm, ulnar, and even tensor fascia lata flaps have been described as fasciocutaneous options. Ileocolic segments using the ileocecal valve, free colonic segments, as well as gastro-omental flaps have also been described as visceral alternatives. These options represent third-line options and are beyond the scope of this text.

Complications

Pharyngeal reconstruction poses many challenges. In addition to existing patient comorbidities, prior radiation and ablative surgical resection are strong predictors of postoperative complications. Selber et al[14] published the overall complication rate for 349 patients receiving pharyngoesophageal over an 11-year period. Patients were grouped according to defect extent and location. Most were reconstructed with the anterolateral thigh flap (60%). There were 15.5% total esophagectomies, all of which received supercharged jejunal flaps. Of the 349 patients:

- 81 patients (23.2%) had recipient site complications and
- 51 patients (14.6%) had donor site complications.
- The fistula rate trended higher in circumferential defects (11% vs. 6%) and the stricture rate was significantly higher (9.3 vs. 3.8).
- In total, 302 patients (86.5%) had an oral diet after reconstruction, 64 (18%) of whom required supplemental tube feeds.

- Among 147 patients (42%) who received tracheoesophageal puncture (TEP), 19 (12.9%) eventually failed.
- Approximately 87% of patients with TEPs achieved fluent speech.
- The 5-year survival was low for all groups, ranging from 0 to 35%.

Radiotherapy

Benatar et al[15] reviewed 429 patients who received preoperative radiotherapy on free flap success, local and general complications, postoperative mortality, time of decannulation, duration of enteral nutrition, and length of stay was assessed in univariate and multivariate analyses. Preoperative radiotherapy was a significant risk factor for fistula formation and wound infection. Previous neck irradiation at doses of 60 Gy was associated with an increased risk of free flap failure, overall local complications, hematoma, and longer duration of enteral nutrition and hospital stay.

Flaps

Pectoralis Major

The reduced operative time, avoidance of the complications and morbidity related to abdominal surgery as well as inherent risks with microsurgical flap procedures are often cited as clinical grounds for use of the pectoralis major flap as a primary reconstructive option. Koh et al[16] reported a comparison of the average operating times for the pectoralis major, 76 + 7 min (54–105 min), and the free flap, 145 + 11 min (115–205 min), components of reconstruction cases. Leite et al[10] performed a retrospective analysis of 84 patients receiving a pectoralis major flap reconstruction. There were 15 cases of partial flap loss, two total flap losses, and 31 fistulae. The independent risk factors for fistula formation were preoperative serum hemoglobin <13 g/dL, preoperative serum albumin <3.4 g/dL, and hypopharynx reconstruction.

Free Jejunum Flaps

In addition to general medical morbidity and mortality related chiefly to cardiorespiratory embarrassment, flap–related complications include:

- total flap necrosis (0–13%)
- pharyngocutaneous fistula formation (0–22%)
- stricture formation (0–16%)
- abdominal complications (0–4.35%).[8,9,17]

In a recent series of 368 consecutive pharyngeal reconstructions the authors compared their results with a meta–analysis of published free skin flaps. They show that the jejunum was superior in all parameters (pharyngocutaneous fistula (8.2% vs. 18.7%), stricture formation (10.9% vs. 17.9%), and resumption of oral diet (91.6% vs. 90.7%).[18] More recently, Kurita et al[19] published a study demonstrating 243 successful jejunal transfers without any failures. The surgical site infections occurred in 15 cases (6.2%) and fistula formation in 9 cases (3.7%). The perioperative mortality rate was 0.4%. There were 7 cases (2.9%) with donor site morbidity.

Radial and ALT Flaps

Complications include:

- total flap failure (0–5%)
- pharyngocutaneous fistula (1%–27%)
- stricture formation (2%–30%)
- partial flap loss (0–5%).

Voice

At its most basic, voice represents increasing complex manipulation of a fundamental tone, which finds its origin at the larynx, before passing through the chambers above and exiting as voice. Speech is conversion of this sound by the tongue, the soft and hard palates, lips, pharynx and teeth. The vocal folds open and close in rapid succession, allowing air to form periodic sound waves. The movement theory behind vocal fold function is called myoelastic aerodynamic theory.[20] In simple terms, as the pressure rises below the vocal folds, this pressure leads to release of the air and forces the vocal cords apart, thereby generating vibration. As the pressure drops momentarily the vocal folds fall back into their midline position and the cycle continues.

Voice Rehabilitation Devices

There are many forms of vocal rehabilitation, basically divided into *nonsurgical* or surgical. The nonsurgical means include the electrolarynx and pneumatic artificial larynx. Surgical methods of reconstruction are themselves divided into neoglottis, TEP, and prosthesis, and visceral voice tube reconstruction.

Neoglottis

Using local tissues as flaps, a deliberate fistula is created between the trachea and the esophagus. The problem with this method is that there is a high rate of regurgitation and aspiration, as well as stenosis and fistula closure.

Tracheoesophageal Puncture and Prosthesis

In this method, a fistula is created between the posterior wall of the trachea and the esophagus. A prosthetic device with a one-way valve is then placed across the fistula. By occluding the tracheal stoma, air is forced through the fistula, vibrating sequentially up the esophagus and being articulated into speech on leaving the mouth. The one-way valve prevents regurgitation of food from the esophagus into the trachea. There are a variety of these prostheses on the market, including Blom–Singer, Provox, and Nijdam devices. There is debate as to whether TEP should be performed primarily or secondarily, some arguing that the incidence of stricture and fistula formation is higher in a primary setting although other studies disagree.[21] Despite their inherent advantage in application and functional outcome there are a number of associated disadvantages, which include: dilatation of the TEP and associated aspiration and regurgitation, stenosis, uncommonly esophageal perforation, colonization with fungus and bacteria, dislodgment of the prosthesis into the trachea leading to aspiration, and obstruction from secretions and food particles. This TEP procedure can be performed between the posterior tracheal wall as well as the neo-esophagus when constructed from pedicled or free tissue transfer.

Visceral Voice Tube Reconstruction

Where a free jejunum or ileocolon is used, a segment of jejunum or ileum can be used as a voice chamber. These are uncommonly used. The jejunal segment or ileum is used as a conduit for air to be transferred into the neo-esophagus and pharynx.[22]

Complications and Clinical Outcomes

Study Results

There are a large number of publications reporting functional outcomes, including swallowing, stricture and fistula formation, operative surgical outcomes such as flap failure, and medical complications as well as death, but there are no randomized trial studies comparing the various visceral and fasciocutaneous flap reconstructions. Many of the functional outcome measures are not consistent across the literature, making comparisons difficult. In general, it is thought the jejunal flap yields better swallowing with less chance of stricture, whereas fascio- or myocutaneous flaps, by the virtue of tubing inset and incisional closures, are more likely to stricture. Piazza et al[23] also more recently published data suggesting that free flaps have half the stricture rate of a pedicled pectoralis major flap.

The voice and thus speech quality associated with skin flaps, however, is thought to be superior to the wet quality of jejunum voice, but the evidence is weak. One small series reports most of the speech parameters were inferior with the jejunal reconstructions.[24] In a longer-term study of patients undergoing jejunal reconstructions, Sharp et al reported 73% of their series had no dysphonia and 89% had no or mild dysphagia.[25] In a large series, Deschler and colleagues reported a comparison between 919 jejunal flaps and 179 tubed forearm radial flaps. Flap losses were 7.5% versus 1.8%, whereas fistula and stenosis formation were 17% versus 23% and 9.1% versus 16%, respectively.[26]

The best speech is achieved with a TEP, although tracheal, jejunal as well as ileal conduits have been reported, but remain uncommon.[27] Other reports from data pooled from a large series of results suggest that the risk of stenosis or fistula formation is increased substantially with tubed fasciocutaneous radial forearm flaps when compared to jejunal reconstructions. Tables 26.2 and 26.3 summarize outcomes of some of the larger data series on pharyngeal reconstructions.[28]

Management Strategies for Major Flap Complications

Fistulae and Strictures

Fistulae are common complications of pharyngeal reconstructions. The literature, although varied, reflects a trend towards a higher rate in fasciocutaneous flaps, perhaps reflecting the additional seam suture line associated with tubing of the flaps, as well as, in pedicled flaps, the risk of tension on the most vital part of the flap. Various studies have sought to delineate specific predictive risk factors attributable to:

- tumour factor – extent of disease and extent of oncological resection; or
- patient factors – preoperative albumin, age, sex, weight, as well as radiation history among other parameters.

Stricture formation, which may be related to flap type or postoperative radiation therapy, could lead to dysphagia. This is often treated with repeated endoscopic dilatations.

The use of a salivary bypass stent (SBS) may also reduce strictures and fistulae. Piazza et al[23] recently published a study comparing 105 patients in the SBS group versus 89 patients, and had a fistula rate of 7% versus 26% in the group without SBS; the stricture rate was also favorable, at 3% versus 18%.

Flap Type

A recent report looked at early postoperative indicators for fistula formation. Postoperative fever during the first 48 hours, atrial fibrillation, and preoperative albumin could not be implicated. However, a persistent low postoperative albumin (as early as the third postoperative day) as well as elevated white cell count was shown to be an indicator of an early leak.[30] Most commonly, fistulae are managed conservatively, ideally directing drainage to the contralateral neck, away from the great vessels if a neck dissection has been performed. The great majority of small fistulae close spontaneously over the course of 1–2 weeks. Significant leaks will require judicious debridement of necrotic and infected tissues and importation of healthy vascularized tissue. Consideration of regional flaps such as pectoralis major, deltopectoral and latissimus dorsi are the likely best options. Clinical surveillance remains important as contrast studies may yield false-negative rates of up to 14%. Appropriate prophylactic antibiotics, antireflux medication (proton pump inhibitors or ranitidine) and meticulous surgical technique and tension-free closure help reduce infection and fistula rates. Late fistulae during or after radiation therapy are relatively rare, but should be considered with any patient who presents with evidence of infection in the neck during the late postoperative period.

Flap Failure

This is a serious setback for the patient and the surgeon. Luckily, with increased experience and better practices, failure rates continue to decline in major institutions. Monitoring is difficult, but early recognition of flap compromise may enable revision of the anastomoses and salvage of the flap. This is possible with skin flaps but unlikely with bowel. Acceptance of failure and early debridement may allow immediate redo reconstruction in the interests of obtaining healing in time for optimal scheduling of radiotherapy.

TABLE 26.2 Microsurgical Flaps: Reported Outcomes

	Defect	No. of Patients	Successful Swallowing	Stricture (%)	Fistula Leak (%)	Flap Failure (%)	Medical/ Other Surgical Complication (%)	Mortality (%)	Received Voice Prosthesis (%)	Functional Voice Prothesis (%)
Mixed Free Flaps										
Clark et al[5]	Hypopharyngeal	15 RFFF, 11 ALT, 30 jejunum	84	14	27	5	12		44	
Antohi et al[5]	Pharyngoesophageal	8 RFFF, 13 scapular + LD, 6 gastro-omental, 3 jejunum	81	19	25	2	15	3		
Tan et al[29]	Pharyngeal	14 RFFF, 21 ALT, 10 jejunum		16	17	1				
RFFF										
Azizzadeh et al[5]	Pharyngoesophageal	20	85	20	20	0		0	20	100
Disa et al[3]	Hypopharyngeal	52	95	2	1	4				
Murray et al[5]	Hypopharyngeal	242	66	18	14	1.5		1	22	87
ALT										
Murray et al[5]	Hypopharyngeal	67	98	11	16	2.3		1	52	88
Yu et al[5]	Pharyngoesophageal	26	95	15	8	4	0		52	88
Chan et al[8]	Pharyngeal	24	100	12.5	12.5	0	0	0		
Sagar et al[5]	Hypopharyngeal	20	65	30	25	0	10	0	100	40
Spyropoulou et al[13]	Hypopharyngeal	55	69	5	18	2	12			
Range			65–100	2–30	1–27	0–5	0–15	0–3	2–100	87–100

ALT, anterolateral thigh flap; LD, latissimus dorsi; RFFF, radial forearm free flap.
Modified from Farhadieh RD, Morrison WAJ. Pharyngeal reconstruction. In: Farhadieh RD, Bulstrode NW, Cugno S, eds. *Plastic and Reconstructive Surgery: Approaches and Techniques*. Chichester: Wiley; 2015:357.

TABLE 26.3 Jejunal Free Flaps: Reported Outcomes

	Defect	No. of Patients	Successful Swallowing	Stricture (%)	Fistula Leak (%)	Flap Failure (%)	Medical Complications (%)	Mortality (%)	Received Voice Prosthesis (%)	Functional Voice Prothesis (%)
Perez-Smith et al[18]	Pharyngolaryngeal	368	91.6	10.9	8.2	2.98	3.8	3.8	71	78.1
Chan et al[8]	Pharyngeal	86	100	2.3	4.6	3.4	0	0		
Schusterman et al[17]	Cervical	48	88	22	16	6	4	2		
Carlson et al[5]	Cervical	26	80	16	20	4	19	0		
Triboulet et al[5]	Cervical	77	98.4	12	12		7	5		
Uchiyama et al[5]	Hypopharyngeal	168				2				
Benazzo et al[5]	Cervical	126				10	15		68	
Disa et al[3]	Hypopharyngeal	29	100	10	10	3	3	0		100
Okazaki et al[12]	Pharyngoesophageal	90	88	7	7	0				
Pesko et al[5]	Pharyngoesophageal	20	90	0	0	0				
Sarukawa et al[5]	Pharyngoesophageal	6				4	33	17		
Kurita et al[19]	Pharyngoesophageal	243			9	0	15	1		
Yu et al[5]	Pharyngoesophageal	191	94	13	13	6		0	29	
Ferakose et al[5]	Cervical	31	98	7	7	7	16	0		22
Mardini et al[28]	Cervical	12	83	0	0	0	43	7		
Range		6–368	88–100	0–22	0–32	0–10	0–43	0–17	29–68	22–100

Modified from Farhadieh RD, Morrison WAJ. Pharyngeal reconstruction. In: Farhadieh RD, Bulstrode NW, Cugno S, eds. *Plastic and Reconstructive Surgery: Approaches and Techniques*. Chichester: Wiley; 2015:358.

But the wisdom of this secondary reconstruction is in part determined by the state of the patient as well as local cervical tissues. Where there is gross contamination and infection there is a real risk of repeat microsurgical failure, and a regional flap reconstruction should generally be considered, after debridement, external fistula formation, salivary diversion, and settling of infection. Onoda et al,[31] however, with experience of over 600 free jejunal transfers at their unit, report use of an immediate second jejunal flap where the first flap has failed, allowing adjuvant therapy to proceed quickly. The most important clinical sign of a jejunal flap failure is per oral bleeding.

Future Directions and Tissue Engineering

Current reconstructive techniques provide restoration of only the most primitive of functions. The great frontier for a reconstructive surgeon remains a nuanced reconstruction and return of function. Despite the use of acellular dermal matrix in other arenas of reconstruction, its application in laryngotracheal and pharyngeal reconstruction is limited to case reports, retrospective chart reviews and a single industry-funded prospective cohort study.[32]

Increasingly, tissue engineering is yielding promising results in regenerating various tissues and structural combinations. The three requirements are scaffold, cells, and *in vivo* regulatory growth factors. Rudimentary tracheal reconstruction for tracheal stenosis has already been performed using a combination of Marlex and bovine collagen-based scaffold.[33] Recent studies have been published demonstrating tissue-engineered tracheal graft based on 3D printing in animal models. Tissue-engineered tracheal graft has been created by stratifying tracheal mucosa decellularized extracellular matrix (tmdECM) hydrogel on the luminal surface of the scaffold and transferring human inferior turbinate mesenchymal stromal cell (hTMSC) sheets onto the tmdECM hydrogel layer. These graft have been anastomosed end-to-end to the native trachea and complete re-epithelialization was achieved on the entire luminal surface within 2 months in a rabbit model.[34]

This is of course a long way away from reconstructing a functional larynx. Although still in its infancy, the future is pregnant with hope that one day *like tissue* can in fact be replaced with *like tissue*, as Sir Harold Gillies, the founder of the discipline of plastic surgery, had set in stone as the ultimate aim of restoration surgery.

References

1. Wookey H. The surgical treatment of carcinoma of the hypopharynx and the oesophagus. *Br J Surg*. 1948;35(139):249–266.
2. Sabatier RE, Bakamjian VY. Transaxillary latissimus dorsi flap reconstruction in head and neck cancer. Limitations and refinements in 56 cases. *Am J Surg*. 1985;150(4):427–434.
3. Disa JJ, Pusic AL, Hidalgo DA, Cordeiro PG. Microvascular reconstruction of the hypopharynx: defect classification, treatment algorithm, and functional outcome based on 165 consecutive cases. *Plast Reconstr Surg*. 2003;111(2):652–660; discussion 661–653.
4. Urken M. *Atlas of Regional and Free Flaps for Head and Neck Reconstruction*. Vol VII edn. Philadelphia: Lippincott, Williams & Wilkins; 2011.
5. Farhadieh RD, Morrison WAJ. Pharyngeal reconstruction. In: Farhadieh RD, Bulstrode NW, Cugno S, eds. *Plastic and Reconstructive Surgery: Approaches and Techniques*. Chichester: Wiley; 2015:349–361.
6. Seidenberg B, Rosenak SS, Hurwitt ES, Som ML. Immediate reconstruction of the cervical esophagus by a revascularized isolated jejunal segment. *Ann Surg*. 1959;149(2):162–171.
7. Hiebert CA, Cummings Jr GO. Successful replacement of the cervical esophagus by transplantation and revascularization of a free graft of gastric antrum. *Ann Surg*. 1961;154:103–106.
8. Chan YW, Ng RW, Liu LH, Chung HP, Wei WI. Reconstruction of circumferential pharyngeal defects after tumour resection: reference or preference. *J Plast Reconstr Aesthet Surg*. 2011;64(8):1022–1028.
9. Chan JY, Chow VL, Chan RC, Lau GI. Oncological outcome after free jejunal flap reconstruction for carcinoma of the hypopharynx. *Eur Arch Oto-Rhino-Laryngol*. 2012;269(7):1827–1832.
10. Leite AK, de Matos LL, Belli M, et al. Pectoralis major myocutaneous flap for head and neck reconstruction: risk factors for fistula formation. *Acta Otorhinolaryngol Ital*. 2014;34(6):389–393.
11. Corten EM, Schellekens PP, Hage JJ, Kon M. Clinical outcome after pedicled segmental pectoralis major island flaps for head and neck reconstruction. *Ann Plast Surg*. 2009;63(3):292–296.
12. Okazaki M, Asato H, Takushima A, et al. Analysis of salvage treatments following the failure of free flap transfer caused by vascular thrombosis in reconstruction for head and neck cancer. *Plast Reconstr Surg*. 2007;119(4):1223–1232.
13. Spyropoulou GA, Lin PY, Chien CY, Kuo YR, Jeng SF. Reconstruction of the hypopharynx with the anterolateral thigh flap: defect classification, method, tips, and outcomes. *Plast Reconstr Surg*. 2011;127(1):161–172.
14. Selber JC, Xue A, Liu J, et al. Pharyngoesophageal reconstruction outcomes following 349 cases. *J Reconstr Microsurg*. 2014;30(9):641–654.
15. Benatar MJ, Dassonville O, Chamorey E, et al. Impact of preoperative radiotherapy on head and neck free flap reconstruction: a report on 429 cases. *J Plast Reconstr Aesthet Surg*. 2013;66(4):478–482.
16. Koh KS, Eom JS, Kirk I, Kim SY, Nam S. Pectoralis major musculocutaneous flap in oropharyngeal reconstruction: revisited. *Plast Reconstr Surg*. 2006;118(5):1145–1149;discussion 1150.
17. Schusterman MA, Shestak K, de Vries EJ, et al. Reconstruction of the cervical esophagus: free jejunal transfer versus gastric pull-up. *Plast Reconstr Surg*. 1990;85(1):16–21.
18. Perez-Smith D, Wagels M, Theile DR. Jejunal free flap reconstruction of the pharyngolaryngectomy defect: 368 consecutive cases. *J Plast Reconstr Aesthet Surg*. 2013;66(1):9–15.
19. Kurita T, Kubo T, Tashima H, Fujii T. Free jejunal flap transfer with multiple vascular pedicles for safe and reliable pharyngo-esophageal reconstruction. *Head Neck*. 2018;40(10):2210–2218.
20. Van Den Berg J. Myoelastic-aerodynamic theory of voice production. *J Speech Hear Res*. 1958;1(3):227–244.
21. Sinclair CF, Rosenthal EL, McColloch NL, et al. Primary versus delayed tracheoesophageal puncture for laryngopharyngectomy with free flap reconstruction. *Laryngoscope*. 2011;121(7):1436–1440.

22. Sakurai H, Nozaki M. Reconstruction of the pharyngoesophagus with voice restoration. *Int J Clin Oncol.* 2005;10(4):243–246.
23. Piazza C, Bon FD, Paderno A, et al. Fasciocutaneous free flaps for reconstruction of hypopharyngeal defects. *Laryngoscope.* 2017;127(12):2731–2737.
24. Mendelsohn M, Morris M, Gallagher R. A comparative study of speech after total laryngectomy and total laryngopharyngectomy. *Arch Otolaryngol Head Neck Surg.* 1993;119(5):508–510.
25. Sharp DA, Theile DR, Cook R, Coman W. Long–term functional speech and swallowing outcomes following pharyngolaryngectomy with jejunal flap reconstruction. *Ann Plast Surg.* 2010;64:743–746.
26. Deschler DG, Doherty ET, Reed CG, Anthony JP, Singer MI. Tracheoesophageal voice following tubed free radial forearm flap reconstruction of the neopharynx. *Ann Otol Rhinol Laryngol.* 1994;103(12):929–936.
27. Ahmad I, Kumar BN, Radford K, O'Connell J, Batch AJ. Surgical voice restoration following ablative surgery for laryngeal and hypopharyngeal carcinoma. *J Laryngol Otol.* 2000;114(7):522–525.
28. Mardini S, Salgado CJ, Kim Evans KF, Chen HC. Reconstruction of the esophagus and voice. *Plast Reconstr Surg.* 2010;126(2):471–485.
29. Tan NC, Lin PY, Kuo PJ, et al. An objective comparison regarding rate of fistula and stricture among anterolateral thigh, radial forearm, and jejunal free tissue transfers in circumferential pharyngo-esophageal reconstruction. *Microsurgery.* 2015;35(5):345–349.
30. Chan JY, Liu LH, Wei WI. Early prediction of anastomotic leakage after free jejunal flap reconstruction of circumferential pharyngeal defects. *J Plast Reconstr Aesthet Surg.* 2013;66(3):376–381.
31. Onoda S, Kimata Y, Yamada K, Sugiyama N, Sakuraba M, Hayashi R. The best salvage operation method after total necrosis of a free jejunal graft? Transfer of a second free jejunal graft. *J Plast Reconstr Aesthet Surg.* 2011;64(8):1030–1034.
32. Hui A, Hong P, Bezuhly M. Use of acellular dermal matrices in laryngotracheal and pharyngeal reconstruction: systematic review. *J Laryngol Otol.* 2017;131(7):585–592.
33. Kanemaru S, Hirano S, Umeda H, et al. A tissue-engineering approach for stenosis of the trachea and/or cricoid. *Acta Otolaryngol Suppl.* 2010;(563):79–83.
34. Park JH, Park JY, Nam IC, et al. A rational tissue engineering strategy based on three-dimensional (3D) printing for extensive circumferential tracheal reconstruction. *Biomaterials.* 2018;185:276–283.

27

Reconstruction of the Skull Base

ALEXANDER F. MERICLI AND MATTHEW M. HANASONO

Introduction

The skull base is a complex anatomic region through which the major blood vessels of the head and neck, cranial nerves, and spinal cord pass. A variety of congenital malformations and neoplasms can involve the skull base. As surgical techniques, instrumentation, and imaging technology have improved over recent years, many skull base lesions can now safely be resected using an endonasal approach, thus minimizing morbidity and obviating the need for extensive reconstruction.[1] However, many lesions still require an open resection in order to achieve clear margins. Reconstructive plastic surgeons thus play a major role in reconstructing the functional, anatomic, and cosmetic defects that such skull base resections often create.

The goals of skull base reconstruction include sealing dural leaks, dead space obliteration, separating the aerodigestive tract from the intracranial space, protecting the brain, and restoring cranial nerve function and appearance. Historically, reconstructive efforts were limited to skin grafts, pedicled flaps, and staged tubed flaps; such reconstructions were plagued by a variety of wound healing complications and significant cosmetic deformity. As such, skull base resections were associated with poor outcomes.

As is true for many aspects of reconstructive surgery, the advent of microsurgery brought about development of the tools necessary to reliably improve the cosmetic and functional results associated with skull base resections.[2–4] Presently, microvascular techniques are considered the gold standard for most skull base reconstructions, providing the means to transfer well-vascularized tissue wherever needed, thereby allowing for a watertight, durable partition between the central nervous system and external environment. In many cases, advances in reconstruction now permit treatment of lesions that were deemed unresectable in the past due to the morbidity associated with their removal.

Anatomy

The skull base separates the extracranial and intracranial anatomy. Located on the extracranial side of the skull base are the sphenoid sinuses, ethmoid sinuses, pterygopalatine fossae, infratemporal fossae, and orbits. On the intracranial side, the skull base forms the anterior, middle, and posterior fossae. Multiple classification systems have been introduced based on anatomic boundaries, pathology, and reconstructive requirements. The Irish classification system has emerged as the most popular, due to its simplicity and clinical utility.[5] Irish and colleagues[5] reviewed 77 cases and divided the skull base into three regions, based on the relationship of the tumor to the anterior, middle, and posterior cranial fossae (Fig. 27.1). In this classification, resections can involve removal of skull base bone with or without removal of the underlying dura.

Region I defects typically involve or arise from structures that abut the anterior cranial fossa, including the orbits and orbital contents, the nose, the paranasal sinuses, and the cribriform plate. The posterior boundary of Region I includes the clivus and foramen magnum, as tumors in this region are also approached anteriorly. We have further subdivided Region I into midline and lateral or paramedian regions.[6] Midline Region I tumors often originate from the ethmoid and sphenoid sinuses or the cribriform plate. These include esthesioneuroblastomas, for example. Lateral Region I tumors include those that arise from the orbit or periorbital structures, such as lacrimal gland tumors.

Region II extends from the posterior orbital wall to the petrous portion of the temporal bone. Region II defects result from tumors originating from the lateral skull base, primarily the infratemporal and pterygopalatine fossae, which can extend into the middle cranial fossa. Tumors that originate in this region include nasopharyngeal carcinomas, glomus jugulare tumors, sphenoid wing meningiomas, and clival chordomas, as well as parotid tumors that become deeply infiltrative and maxillary or cheek neoplasms with posterior spread. The latter usually occurs via the maxillary division of the trigeminal nerve (V_2).

Region III defects are usually associated with tumors arising from the ear, parotid, or temporal bone, and may extend intracranially into the middle or posterior cranial fossae. Region III tumors include cutaneous tumors involving the external auditory canal, such as squamous and basal cell

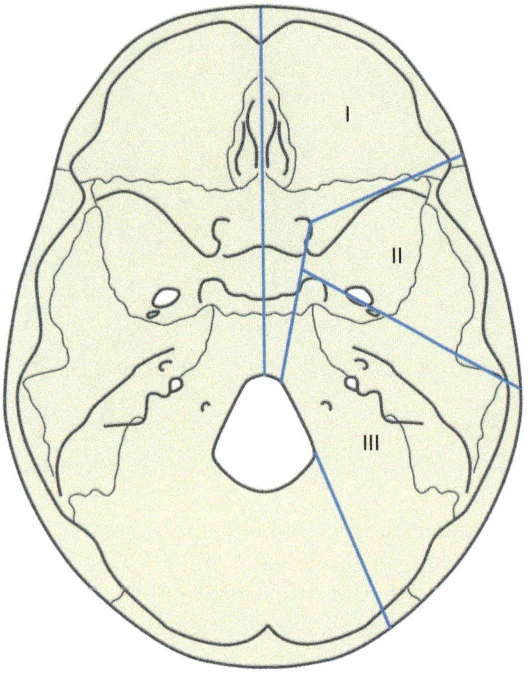

• **Fig. 27.1** Skull base regions. (Modified with permission from Irish JC, Gullane PJ, Gentili F, et al. Tumors of the skull base: outcome and survival analysis of 77 cases. *Head Neck.* 1994;16:3–10.)

carcinomas, as well as parotid malignancies and, occasionally, sarcomas that arise directly from the temporal bone.

Reconstructive Approach

The location of the tumor predicts the reconstructive needs. In the following sections, we will discuss flap selection and specifics of flap design and inset for each skull base region. Occasionally, defects will encompass more than one region and it will be necessary to modify flap design to address the reconstructive needs of two or more regions, or potentially perform a double free flap reconstruction. In addition to selection of the reconstructive flap, the possibility of needing grafts or implants should also be considered. For example, Region I defects of the orbital walls and frontal calvarium may require skeletal reconstruction in order to prevent change in eye position, pulsatile exophthalmos, and cosmetic deformity. Autologous bone grafts or manmade implants, such as titanium mesh, porous polyethylene, or polyetheretherketone (PEEK), can be considered for these applications.

Cranial nerve deficits should be anticipated based on the location of the tumor, as well as by a full preoperative physical exam of cranial nerve function, which should be documented in detail in the preoperative note. Various procedures to address facial nerve paralysis should be discussed with the patient preoperatively in any case where resection of the facial nerve is a possibility.[6,7] Such procedures include direct nerve repair, cable nerve grafting, dynamic reanimation with vascularized muscle transfer, anastomosis to other cranial nerves (e.g., masseteric nerve to facial nerve or hypoglossal nerve to facial nerve transfers), and static reanimation with a fascial graft and periocular procedures, such as gold eyelid weight placement, canthoplasty, lateral tarsorrhaphy, and browlift.[6,7]

Other functional deficits might include those arising from loss of glossopharyngeal (IX), vagus (X), spinal accessory (XI), and hypoglossal (XII) nerve function.[8] Resection of the glossopharyngeal nerve can result in uncoordinated swallowing and aspiration, which may be addressed with temporary or permanent gastrostomy tube placement as well as postoperative speech and swallowing therapy. Unilateral hypoglossal nerve deficits are generally well tolerated, but may also require speech and swallowing therapy. Vocal cord paralysis following transection of the vagus nerve can be addressed by an otolaryngologist postoperatively with vocal cord injection of various filler materials and/or medialization thyroplasty. Transection of the spinal accessory nerve results in shoulder drop that is best addressed with physical therapy.

A discussion of the patient's desire for an orbital or ear prosthesis, if loss of the eye or auricle is a possibility, should take place preoperatively since this may influence flap choice, particularly for an orbital prosthesis.[9] Both orbital and auricular prostheses can be secured either with adhesive or through the use of osseointegrated implants. If an osseointegrated implant is preferred, and postoperative radiation is a possibility, consideration should be given to placing the implant at the time of tumor resection; many have reported decreased implant reliability when placed after radiation is given.[2] Similarly, if the skull base resection includes removal of the middle ear components, an otologist should be involved preoperatively for placement of a bone-anchored-hearing aid (BAHA), which also requires an osseointegrated implant.[10] In many cases, placement of an osseointegrated implant is challenging after substantial resection of bone, since fairly thick bone stock must surround the implant in order for it to be stable. In such cases, an implant-retained prosthesis may not be possible.

Region I

Midline Region I tumors requiring an open extirpation are usually resected with an anterior craniofacial approach, resulting in communication of the nasal cavity with the intracranial space. Such a resection involves endonasal surgery or a lateral rhinotomy combined with a bicoronal incision followed by a frontal craniotomy. If the defect is small and limited to the upper nasal cavity, the intracranial space can be separated from the sinuses with a pedicled pericranial flap or galeafrontalis flap, both of which derive their blood supply from the supratrochlear and supraorbital vessels.[11–13] In situations where these blood vessels have already been transected, or in larger defects involving the external nose, forehead, and/or orbit, a free flap may be necessary. If there is no skin defect and the flap is needed as a watertight partition between the aerodigestive tract and intracranial space, then it may be buried and monitored with an implantable Doppler probe. Moderate size muscle free flaps, such as the

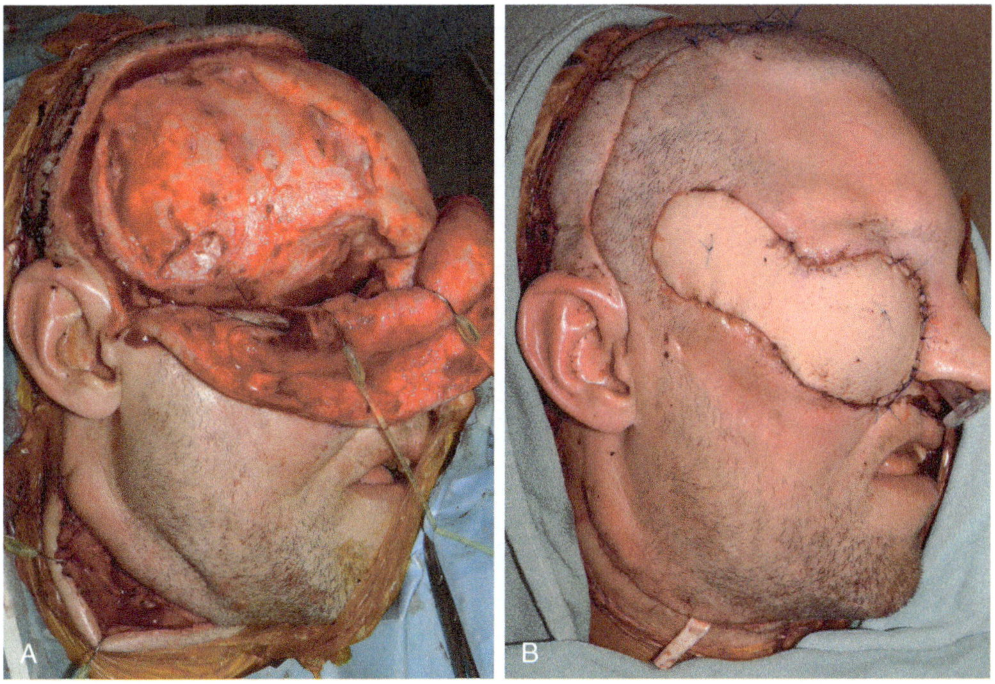

• **Fig. 27.2** (A) Zone I skull base defect following a right orbital exenteration with frontal craniotomy resulting in communication with the anterior cranial fossa. (B) Reconstruction with an anterolateral thigh (ALT) myocutaneous free flap anastomosed to the right facial artery and vein. The muscle (vastus lateralis) is placed against the dural patch to help prevent cerebrospinal fluid leaks and is also used to obliterate possible communication with the nasal cavity and paranasal sinuses.

rectus abdominis, vastus lateralis, and serratus anterior muscle free flaps, are good options in this situation.

Lateral Region I defects frequently involve orbital exenteration (Fig. 27.2). If the resection spares the medial and inferior walls of the orbit, it is well suited to the eventual use of a prosthesis. In order to accommodate a prosthesis, the orbit must be resurfaced with thin, pliable, well-vascularized tissue that will maintain the concave shape of the cavity. This can be achieved with a free radial or ulnar forearm fasciocutaneous free flap. A pedicled temporalis muscle or temporoparietal fascia flap with a skin graft may also be an option here, although removal of some of the lateral orbital bone is usually necessary to allow these flaps to reach the medial orbit. If the orbital exenteration results in communication with the sinuses or nasal cavity, then a bulkier free flap is preferred. The anterolateral thigh (ALT) and rectus abdominis myocutaneous (RAM) free flaps are highly customizable and allow for the design of flap with a variable amount of muscle, tailored to the defect's requirements. The muscle conforms to the complex geometry of the defect, sealing exposed dura and/or sinonasal cavities. This feature helps to minimize the occurrence of a sinonasocutaneous fistula; such fistulae are exceedingly difficult to heal owing to persistent pressure from the nasal airway.

Region II

Portions of the sphenoid and squamosal temporal bones make up Region II and include the infratemporal fossa and pterygopalatine fossa areas. Resection of Region II tumors is frequently performed through an anterior transmaxillary approach. After resection of the skull base bone in this region, the dura will be in direct communication with the nasopharynx (Fig. 27.3). The temporalis muscle may reach this area, but often does not provide adequate bulk to restore cheek contour if a substantial amount of the maxilla is resected. To reach this area, the coronoid process of the mandible is removed and a tunnel is created into the maxillary cavity. It will also help with exposure if the zygomatic arch is temporarily removed and then plated back into position after flap rotation.

In most cases, a moderately thick myocutaneous flap, such as the ALT or RAM free flaps, are best suited to reconstruction of maxillectomy defects and coverage of the skull base. When there is no oral mucosal, palatal, or external cheek defect, the skin paddle of the free flap can be deepithelialized and the entire flap buried. The adipofascial flap provides bulk, which is less prone to radiation atrophy than muscle; the muscle component serves as a seal against exposed dura mater. Persistent bulk and volume maintenance is important in these reconstructions in order not only to maintain facial contour, but also to adequately support the skull base so as to prevent herniation of the intracranial contents into the pharynx or oral cavity. In cases where postoperative radiation is planned, slight overcorrection of bulk may be considered in anticipation of radiation-associated atrophy. However, in obese patients such flaps

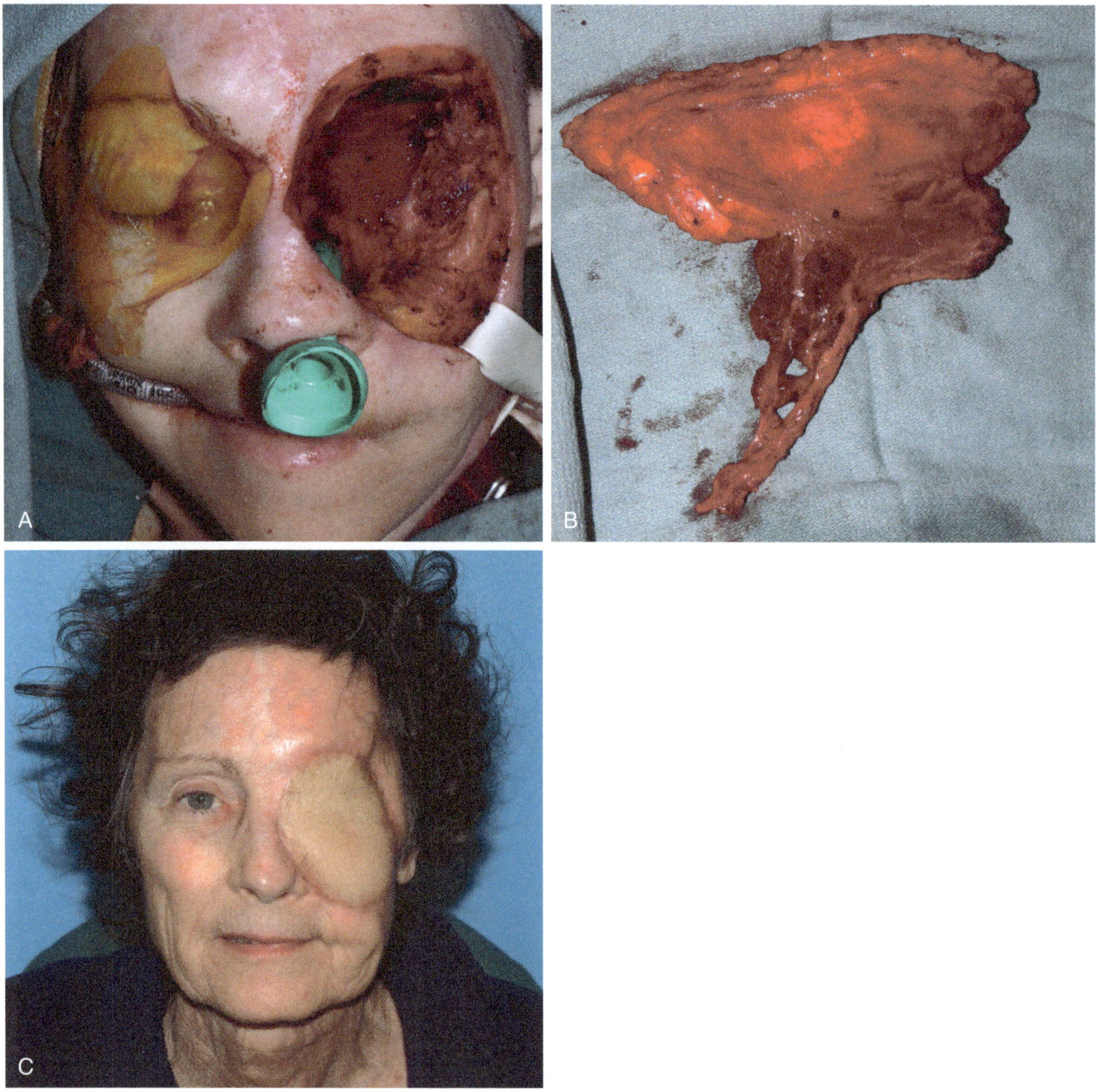

• **Fig. 27.3** Combined Zone I and Zone II skull base defect. (A) A left orbitomaxillectomy with removal of the roof of the orbit and posterior wall of the maxilla has been performed with exposure of the dura of the anterior and middle cranial fossae. (B) An ALT free flap including a portion of the vastus lateralis muscle for bulk was harvested for reconstruction. (C) Postoperative result.

may need to be thinned in order to fit within the confines of the maxillary space.

As in reconstruction of the maxillectomy defect, if the orbital floor is resected and the globe is spared, then skeletal reconstruction of the orbital floor is mandatory. Failing to reconstruct the orbital floor or performing an inaccurate reconstruction can result in enophthalmos, vertical dystopia, or diplopia. Various alloplastic materials are commercially available. Alternatively an autologous calvarial or iliac crest bone graft can be used. Although autologous grafts can be revascularized, our own experience does not support use of one material over another.[14] However, evidence supports covering the entire implant or graft with well-vascularized tissue if adjuvant radiation is anticipated. If the globe is removed as well as the bony orbit, as in an orbitomaxillectomy, then reconstruction of the floor is not necessary, nor is maintaining a concave orbital cavity. In these situations, the reconstructive priority is filling the volume of the resected orbit and maxilla with vascularized tissue, sealing the exposed dura, and replacing any missing skin.[14]

In other cases, Region II may be approached laterally, requiring a parotidectomy and possibly removal of the posterior portion of the mandible. An intraoral defect may result. In such cases, the ALT or RAM free flaps may be designed with two skin paddles, one for the intraoral wound and one for the external wound. If there is a limited mandibular defect restricted to the condyle and ramus, we have had satisfactory results with soft tissue reconstruction alone.[15] The flap is harvested with adequate bulk, usually by the inclusion of muscle, to prevent mandibular deviation. If a more sizable mandibular defect results from the skull base resection, then an additional bony or osteocutaneous free flap, such as the fibula free flap, may be needed for optimal restoration of function and appearance.

Region II tumors may arise from or spread to the parotid gland and facial nerve. In some cases, resection may also require division of one or more branches of the facial nerve even if not invaded by tumor. In all cases that may involve removal of the parotid and/or resection of the facial nerve, reconstruction of the facial nerve and adjunctive procedures are discussed with the patient preoperatively. Whenever possible, the first choice is direct repair of the nerve or cable nerve grafting, as long as proximal and distal ends of the nerve are identifiable (Fig. 27.4).[16,17] When the proximal end of the facial nerve is not available for grafting, coaptation to other donor nerves, such as the masseteric branch of the trigeminal nerve or an end-to-side coaptation to the hypoglossal nerve, are options.

When nerve repair or nerve grafting are not possible or facial paralysis has been longstanding and judged to be futile, then static as well as dynamic reanimation should be considered. While static procedures, including lower facial slings (Fig. 27.5), canthoplasty, lateral tarsorrhaphy, gold (or platinum) upper eyelid weight placement, and browlift can be performed at a secondary stage, we strongly consider performing them concurrently with oncologic resection and flap reconstruction whenever the odds of clinically meaningful facial nerve recovery are low or zero (e.g., when complete facial nerve paralysis has been present >12–18 months).[6,7] This spares the patient some of the morbidity of facial paralysis and does not delay adjuvant therapy to perform a second surgery in cancer cases. Static procedures do not interfere with recovery of grafted nerves and, in fact, we feel it is safer not to reopen wounds to perform reanimation procedures due to the risk of injuring intact or grafted nerves as well as incurring wound healing complications in radiated tissues.[6,7]

Evidence supports nerve repair and nerve grafting even in the settings of advanced age, preoperative nerve weakness (not longstanding complete paralysis), and postoperative radiation therapy.[16,17] While these remain risk factors for poor or non-recovery of motor function, in many cases meaningful recovery is possible and the morbidity of repair or grafting is low. What is not clear at this time is the role of immediate motorized free muscle transfer (e.g., gracilis, latissimus dorsi, serratus anterior, and pectoralis minor muscle free flaps) for lower facial reanimation at the time of oncologic resection. The benefit-to-cost ratio of performing functional free muscle transfer following a long skull base resection and free flap reconstruction of the resulting wound is debatable and the effect of postoperative radiation on both reinnervation and muscle contractility remains

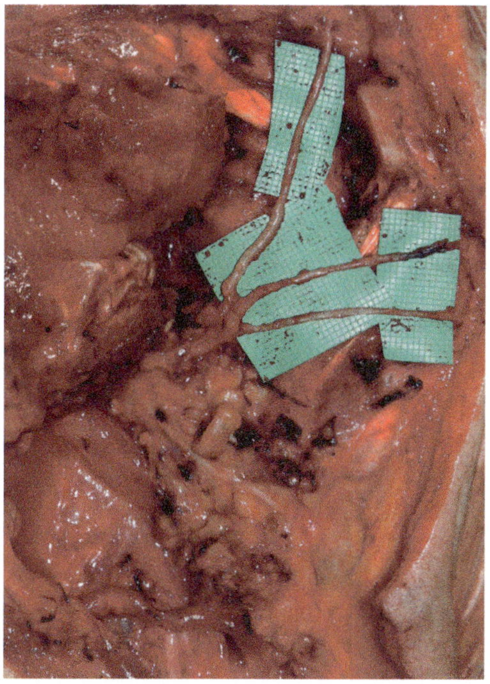

• **Fig. 27.4** Multistrand cable nerve grafting to restore facial nerve function to temporal, zygomatic, and buccal branches of the right facial nerve following radical resection of the facial nerve, temporal bone, and zygomatic bone. An epineural repair was performed under the operating microscope.

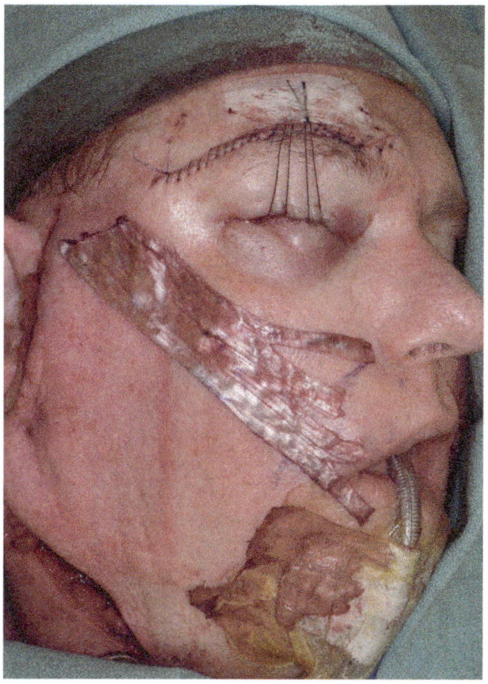

• **Fig. 27.5** Static facial nerve reanimation following right lateral skull base surgery, including a direct browlift, lateral canthoplasty, and fascial sling using a tensor fascia lata graft. The fascial sling was attached to the lateral nasal ala, nasolabial crease, oral commissure, and upper and lower lips through small counter incisions.

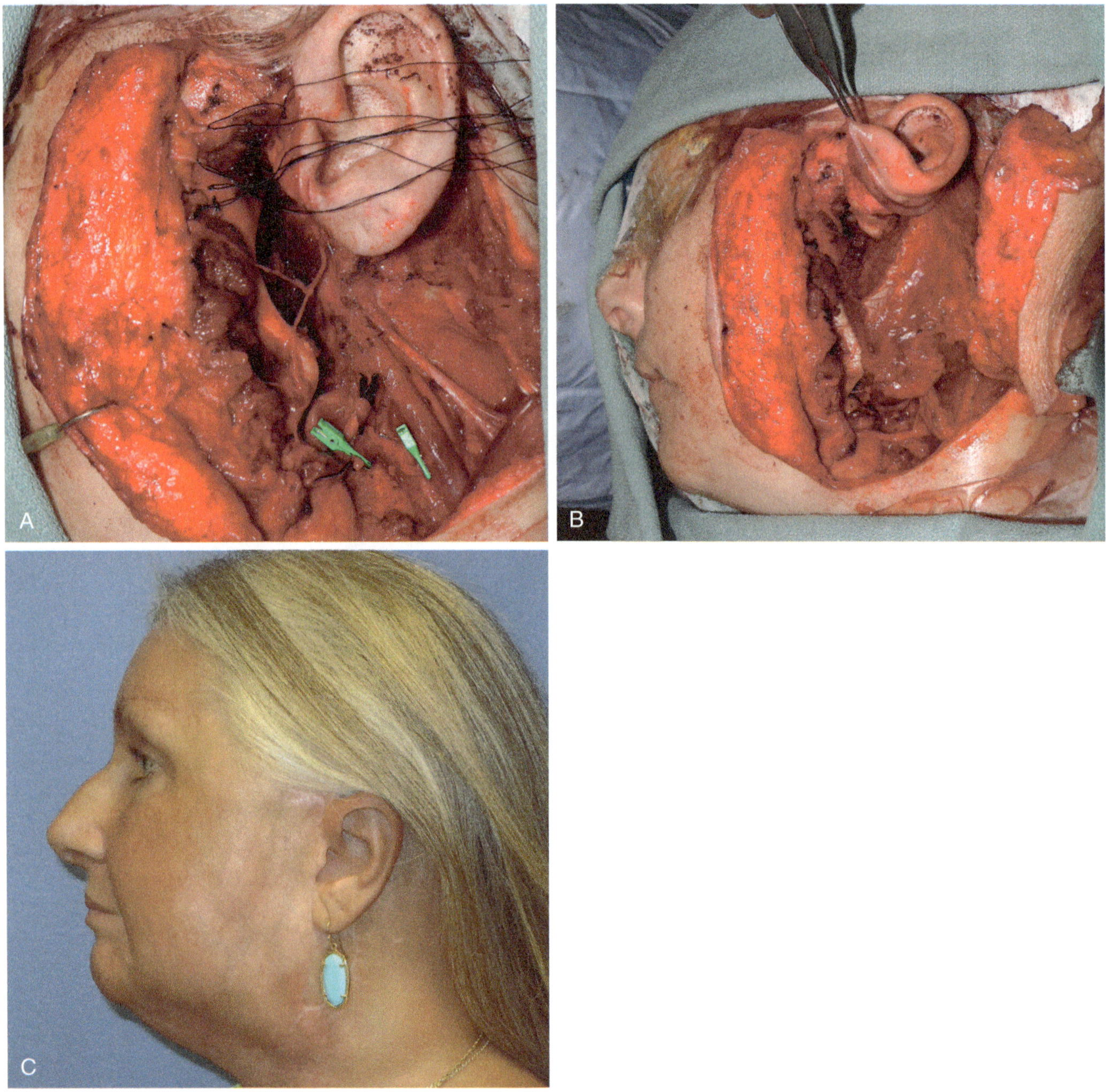

• **Fig. 27.6** (A) Zone III skull base defect following a left lateral temporal bone resection and total parotidectomy including division of the facial nerve. (B) Cable nerve grafts performed to restore facial nerve function. The defect is reconstructed with an ALT myocutaneous free flap, with muscle placed into the deepest portion of the defect and obliterates the Eustachian tube orifice. (C) Postoperative result demonstrating a small skin paddle from the ALT free flap. Note return of midfacial tone following cable nerve grafting, approximately 1 year after the reconstruction.

unknown or unpredictable, with very few reported cases in the literature.

Region III

Region III defects will often include a parotidectomy or temporal bone resection and may include removal of a portion of the posterior cranial fossa. Larger, bulky flaps, such as the ALT or RAM are frequently required.[7,18] If a lateral temporal bone resection and or mastoidectomy is performed, well-vascularized muscle is helpful to obliterate the Eustachian tube orifice, seal off any exposed dura, and/or cover an exposed sigmoid sinus (Fig. 27.6).[7,18]

If resection of the middle ear is anticipated, upfront BAHA placement should be considered.[9] If the external ear is resected, reconstruction is best addressed separately in a delayed manner. Prosthetic rehabilitation is the mainstay for oncologic auricular reconstruction; these prostheses can be secured with an adhesive or through the use of osseointegrated implants, provided adequate bone stock remains

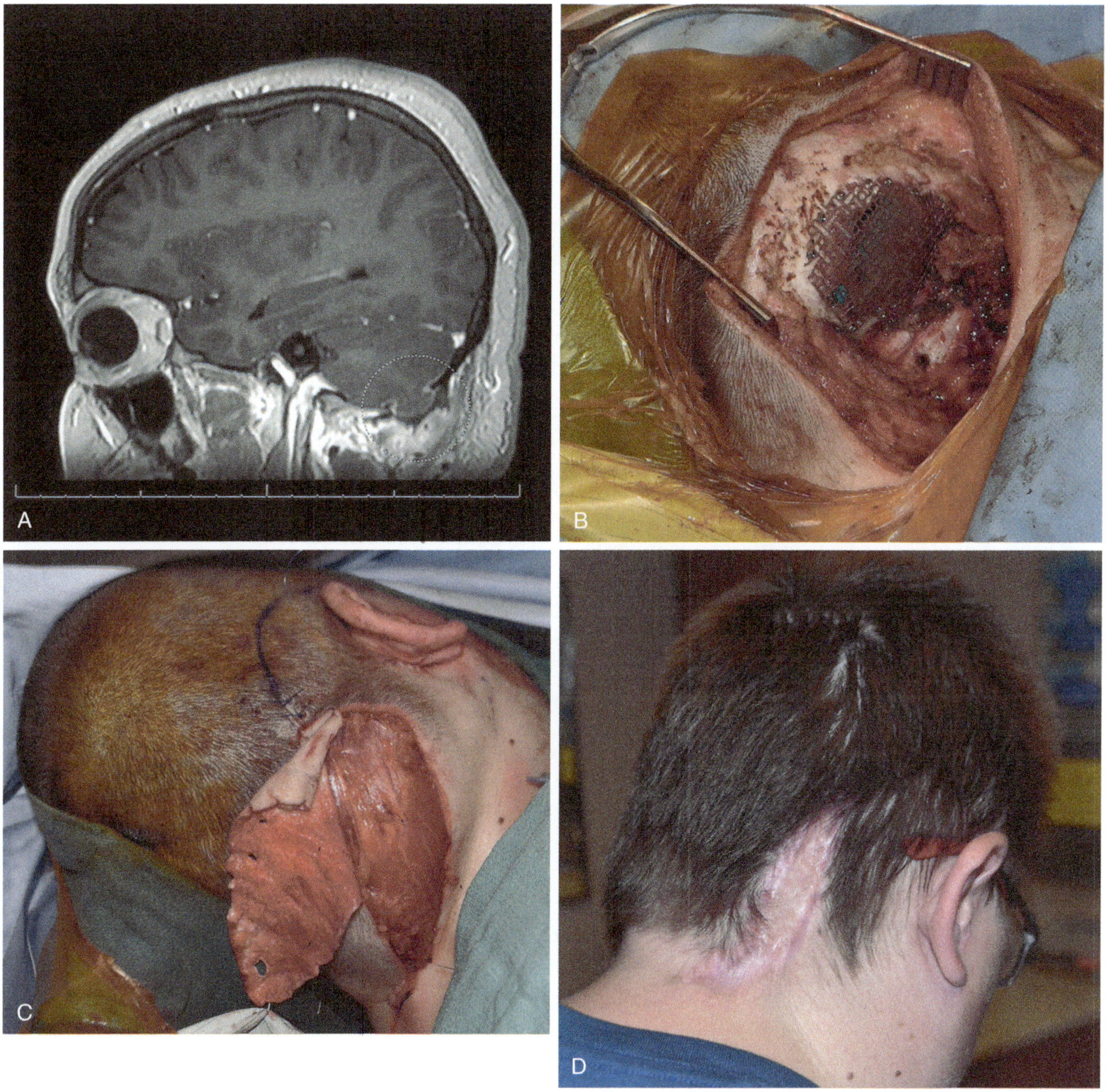

• **Fig. 27.7** (A) MRI demonstrating occipital sarcoma recurrence with encephalocele formation through prior craniectomy defect. (B) Defect after tumor resection, encephalocele resection, dural reconstruction, and skull base repair with titanium plate, abutting the foramen magnum. (C) Soft tissue reconstruction with free vastus lateralis muscle flap and skin graft (reflected). (D) One-year postoperative appearance.

available to stabilize the implants. In practice, loss of the auricle is usually well tolerated from a psychological standpoint and few patients are interested in undergoing an additional procedure for prosthetic or autologous restoration of the ear.

Region III defects limited to the occipital bone may require reconstruction for dead space management, skin replacement, and hardware coverage (Fig. 27.7). Cranioplasty may be needed for sizable calvarial defects. Titanium mesh is most commonly used but delayed reconstruction with custom-made PEEK implants may give superior contour and avoid any sharp edges that are prone to exposure over time.[19]

Technical Points

Flap inset is a particularly important technical consideration. Gravity will act to pull the flap away from the skull base. The fascial components of the flap are suspended to periosteum and other fascial or ligamentous tissues of the skull base. Insetting the flap under appropriate skin tension with the head in the neutral position will minimize postoperative ptosis. Slight flap volume overcorrection is desirable when postoperative radiation is anticipated. However, the flap must not be inset too tightly or so bulky that it compresses the brain or compromises flap perfusion.

The superficial temporal vessels are considered a first-line option for free flap reconstruction in Region I. Neck recipient vessels, such as the facial artery and vein, may be a shorter reach for Regions II and III defects. However, skull base defects are often a significant distance away from most suitable recipient vessels, making vein grafts a frequent necessity in these cases. In our own experience, vein grafting is highly reliable and should not be a deterrent from the free flap reconstruction when use of a free flap would lead to the best functional and esthetic outcomes.[20]

Postoperative Care and Management of Complications Specific to Skull Base Reconstruction

The principal goal of skull base reconstruction is to separate the aerodigestive tract from the brain and intracranial contents. The overall complication rate remains significant, ranging between 29% and 60%.[3,4,6,21] A more recent study from MD Anderson reports an overall complication rate of 30%.[6] As in all anatomic areas, free flap loss rates have decreased and now are 1.9%–4% for the skull base.[6,21] Meticulous isolation of the dura and brain by well-vascularized soft tissue flaps is necessary to prevent meningitis, cerebritis, brain abscesses, neurological injury, and death. Postoperatively, the patient should be maintained on prophylactic intravenous antibiotics with empiric coverage of normal sinonasal flora with antibiotics that can penetrate the blood–brain barrier.

In addition to flap monitoring, frequent neurological examinations should be conducted. Postoperative computed tomography (CT) or magnetic resonance imaging (MRI) scans are obtained according to the recommendations of a neurosurgeon. While it is not uncommon to see small amounts of intracranial air on imaging in the early postoperative period, increasing pneumocephalus or any change in the clinical neurological exam should trigger a prompt return to the operating room. Such neurological findings could suggest a number of complications, including infection, flap dehiscence, hematoma, or intracranial bleed.

Any concern for a cerebrospinal fluid leak (CSF) should be evaluated and confirmed with a beta-2 transferrin test. Most minor CSF leaks can be effectively treated conservatively with antibiotic prophylaxis and bed rest. Closed suction drains are taken off suction and allowed to drain by gravity. Compression dressings are usually contraindicated in free flap reconstruction because they may impede blood flow to the flap. Lumbar drains or reoperation for dural repair are more invasive options for recalcitrant leaks.

If a portion of the orbit has been reconstructed, visual acuity and extraocular muscle function should be frequently examined postoperatively. Any concern for decreased visual acuity should prompt an ophthalmological exam and imaging. Impingement of the optic nerve or entrapment of an extraocular muscle by the reconstruction usually requires a return to the operating room. Traumatic optic neuropathy can also occur secondary to traction during surgery and is usually treated with high-dose steroids.

Because use of either a regional or free flap may limit the utility of physical exam to detect local recurrence, serial imaging is mandatory for disease surveillance and should be incorporated into the survivorship plan.

References

1. Reyes C, Mason E, Solares CA. Panorama of reconstruction of skull base defects: from traditional open to endonasal endoscopic approaches, from free grafts to microvascular flaps. *Int Arch Otorhinolaryngol.* 2014;18:S179–S186.
2. Neligan PC, Mulholland S, Irish JC, et al. Flap selection in cranial base reconstruction. *Plast Reconstr Surg.* 1996;98:1159–1166.
3. Chang DW, Langstein HN, Gupta A, et al. Reconstructive management of cranial base defects after tumor ablation. *Plast Reconstr Surg.* 2001;107:1346–1355.
4. Teknos TN, Smith JC, Day TA, et al. Microvascular free tissue transfer in reconstructing skull base defects: lessons learned. *Laryngoscope.* 2002;112:1871–1876.
5. Irish JC, Gullane PJ, Gentili F, et al. Tumors of the skull base: outcome and survival analysis of 77 cases. *Head Neck.* 1994;16:3–10.
6. Hanasono MM, Silva A, Skoracki RJ, et al. Skull base reconstruction: an updated approach. *Plast Reconstr Surg.* 2011;128:675–686.
7. Hanasono MM, Silva AK, Yu P, Skoracki RJ, Sturgis EM, Gidley PW. Comprehensive management of temporal bone defects after oncologic resection. *Laryngoscope.* 2012;122:2663–2669.
8. Chiu ES, Kraus D, Bui DT, et al. Anterior and middle cranial fossa skull base reconstruction using microvascular free tissue techniques: surgical complications and functional outcomes. *Ann Plast Surg.* 2008;60:514–520.
9. Hanasono MM, Lee JC, Yang JS, et al. An algorithmic approach to reconstructive surgery and prosthetic rehabilitation after orbital exenteration. *Plast Reconstr Surg.* 2009;123:98–105.
10. Nader ME, Beadle BM, Roberts DB, Gidley PW. Outcomes and complication of osseointegrated hearing aids in irradiated temporal bones. *Laryngoscope.* 2016;126:1187–1192.
11. Kiyokawa K, Tai Y, Inoue Y, et al. A reconstruction method using musculopericranial flaps that prevents cerebrospinal fluid rhinorrhea and intracranial complications after extended anterior skull base resection. *Skull Base Surg.* 1999;9:211–219.
12. Siniscalchi EN, Angileri FF, Mastellone P, et al. Anterior skull base reconstruction with a galeal-pericranial flap. *J Craniofac Surg.* 2007;18:622–625.
13. Clavenna MJ, Turner JH, Chandra RK. Pedicled flaps in endoscopic skull base reconstruction: review of current techniques. *Curr Opin Otolaryngol Head Neck Surg.* 2015;23:71–77.
14. Hanasono MM, Silva AK, Yu P, Skoracki RJ. A comprehensive algorithm for oncologic maxillary reconstruction. *Plast Reconstr Surg.* 2013;131:47–60.

15. Reyes C, Mason E, Solares CA. Panorama of reconstruction of skull base defects: from traditional open to endonasal endoscopic approaches, from free grafts to microvascular flaps. *Int Arch Otorhinolaryngol.* 2014;18:S179–S186.
16. Iseli TA, Harris G, Dean NR, Iseli CE, Rosenthal EL. Outcomes of static and dynamic facial nerve repair in head and neck cancer. *Laryngoscope.* 2010;120:478–483.
17. Gidley PW, Herrera SJ, Hanasono MM, et al. The impact of radiotherapy on facial nerve repair. *Laryngoscope.* 2010;120:1985–1989.
18. Rosenthal EL, King K, McGrew BM, et al. Evolution of a paradigm for free tissue transfer reconstruction of lateral temporal bone defects. *Head Neck.* 2008;30:589–594.
19. Hanasono MM, Goel N, DeMonte F. Calvarial reconstruction with polyetherether ketone implants. *Ann Plast Surg.* 2009;62:653–655.
20. Maricevich M, Lin LO, Liu J, Chang EI, Hanasono MM. Interposition vein grafting in head and neck free flap reconstruction. *Plast Reconstr Surg.* 2018;142:1025–1034.
21. Kim K, Ibrahim AM, Koolen PG, et al. Analysis of morbidity and mortality in patients undergoing skull base reconstruction. *J Craniofac Surg.* 2015;26:135–140.

28 Cheek Reconstruction

ADAM C. GASCOIGNE AND ROSTAM D. FARHADIEH

Introduction

Defects of the cheek pose a challenge for the reconstructive surgeon. It is a mostly flat and relatively featureless terrain whose superficial appearance conceals a complex arrangement of fascia, arteries, and nerves. Its esthetic significance is associated with its contour, the preservation of which should be a priority for the reconstructive surgeon, though a carelessly-placed scar may also be disfiguring. Fortunately, it is also an area where the surgeon has a number of options for reconstructing defects with excellent functional and cosmetic results.

Anatomy

The cheek comprises one of the original esthetic units of the face as described by Gonzalez-Ulloa. It is bordered by the eye, nose, lips, chin, mandible, and ear. Functionally, it is important for mastication, swallowing, and speech. It forms a discrete esthetic unit of the face whose appearance was classically described by Menick as "a relatively flat, expansive surface, except for the soft roundness of the nasolabial folds and the cheek prominences," that acts as a "picture frame" for the central face. As such, its contour is of utmost importance.[1]

It is bordered by the infraorbital rim and zygomatic arch superiorly, the lower lid-cheek junction, nasofacial junction, nasolabial fold, marionette line, and labiomandibular crease medially, the mandible inferiorly, and the preauricular contours of the tragus and helix of the ear laterally.

Esthetic Subunits

Traditionally, the cheek may be divided into four subunits: medial, lateral, buccal, and zygomatic.[2,3] In some texts, infraorbital and parotidomasseteric subunits are described, which are roughly analogous to the medial and lateral subunits, respectively.[4] Taken together, the medial, zygomatic, and buccal subunits constitute the midcheek.

Work by Mendelson has redefined the midcheek by taking into account fascial spaces and retaining ligaments identified in anatomical studies (Fig. 28.1). He divides the midcheek, which is itself defined as the area between the lower eyelid and nasolabial junction, into the lid-cheek, malar, and nasolabial segments, separated by the palpebromalar groove and nasojugal groove.[5] This categorization more faithfully reflects the transition between the thin skin of the eyelid and the distinct contours of the malar and nasolabial segments, particularly in the aging face.

Skeletal

The facial skeleton underlying the cheek consists of zygoma, maxilla, and mandible.[6]

Layers

The layers of soft tissue in the cheek correspond to the basic five layers found in the scalp (Box 28.1). From superficial to deep, the layers are skin, followed by a layer of dense subcutaneous fat which is separated into lobules enclosed by fibrous septa. The third layer, the superficial musculo-aponeurotic system, or SMAS, was first described in 1976 by Mitz and Peyronie.[7] The SMAS is continuous with frontalis superiorly and platysma inferiorly, between which it envelops the muscles of facial expression. There is another, looser layer of fat between this and the fifth layer, that of the periosteum or deep fascia, which is often absent in the face where the tissues do not overlie bone or skeletal muscle.[8] In areas of the face not overlying bone, different layers are encountered. For example, in the parotid region this is represented by the parotid fascia, and in the buccal subunit of the cheek, the innermost layer is the buccal mucosa.

Fascia

Fascial structures provide an anchor between bone and skin and provide soft tissue contours throughout the body. Though there is no deep fascia in the face, the principle remains valid, with fascial condensations fixing the soft tissue of the face to the underlying facial skeleton. The retaining ligaments of the face were first examined by Furnas in 1989.[9] He described several groups of ligaments, that remain essential to our understanding of the soft tissue structure of the cheek, contributing to the formation of the contour of the face (Box 28.2). They have since been studied in some detail and are of particular relevance for esthetic plastic surgical procedures such as rhytidectomy.[8] In reconstruction, it may be necessary to disrupt intact retaining ligaments in

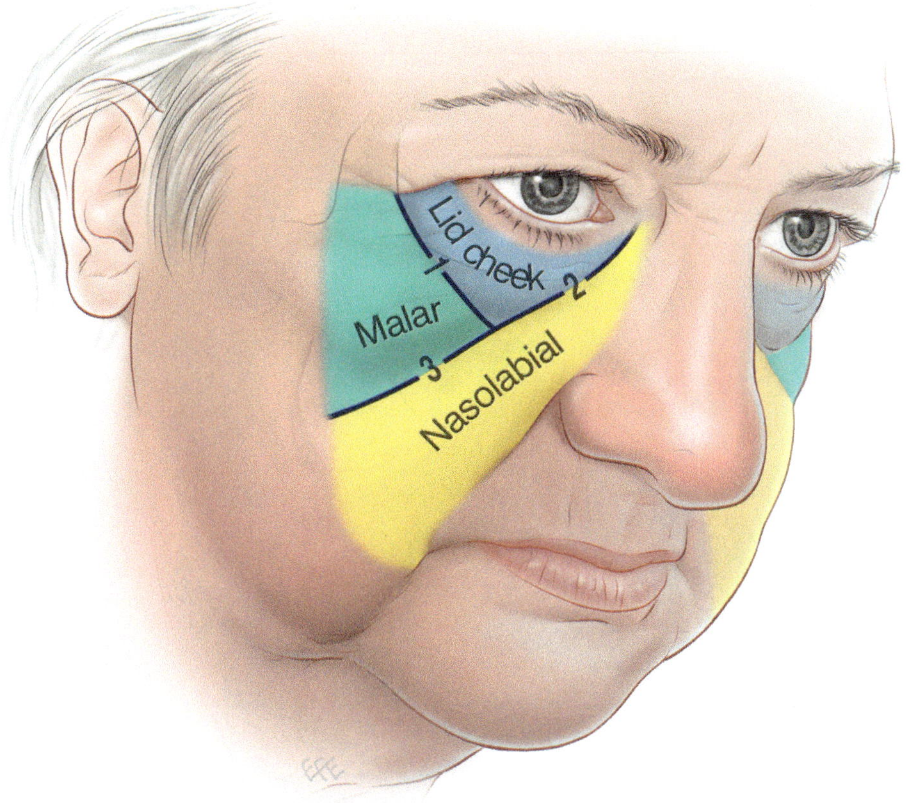

• **Fig. 28.1** Esthetic subunits of the cheek, separated by *1*, palpebromalar groove; *2*, nasojugal groove; *3*, midcheek furrow. (From Mendelson BC, Jacobson SR. Surgical anatomy of the midcheek: facial layers, spaces, and the midcheek segments. *Clin Plast Surg.* 2008;35(3):395–404.)

• BOX 28.1 Tissue Layers of the Face

1. Dermis
2. Subcutaneous layer
3. Superficial musculoaponeurotic system (SMAS) layer
4. Loose areolar tissue
5. Periosteum and deep fascia, or buccal mucosa

• BOX 28.2 Retaining Ligaments of the Cheek

- Tear trough ligament
- Orbicularis retaining ligament
- Zygomatic cutaneous ligaments (McGregor's patch)
- Masseteric cutaneous ligaments
- Mandibular cutaneous ligament
- Platysma auricular ligament

order to gain sufficient mobilization of flaps, or to recreate the effect of the retaining ligaments using deep sutures. They are discussed in greater detail in other chapters.

Muscles

The majority of the muscles of the cheek are muscles of facial expression (Box 28.3). They are embryologically derived from the second branchial arch and are supplied by the nerve of that arch: the facial nerve. The exception is masseter. As a muscle of mastication it is derived from the first branchial arch, and is supplied by the mandibular division of the trigeminal nerve.[6,10]

• BOX 28.3 Muscles of the Cheek

- Orbicularis oculi
- Levator labii superioris
- Levator labii superioris alaeque nasi
- Depressor anguli oris
- Risorius
- Zygomaticus major
- Zygomaticus minor
- Platysma
- Levator anguli oris
- Buccinator
- Masseter

Arteries

Branches of the external carotid artery supply all the tissues of the cheek. The facial artery (once known as the external maxillary) arises from the external carotid artery in the region of the carotid triangle, crosses the margin of the mandible

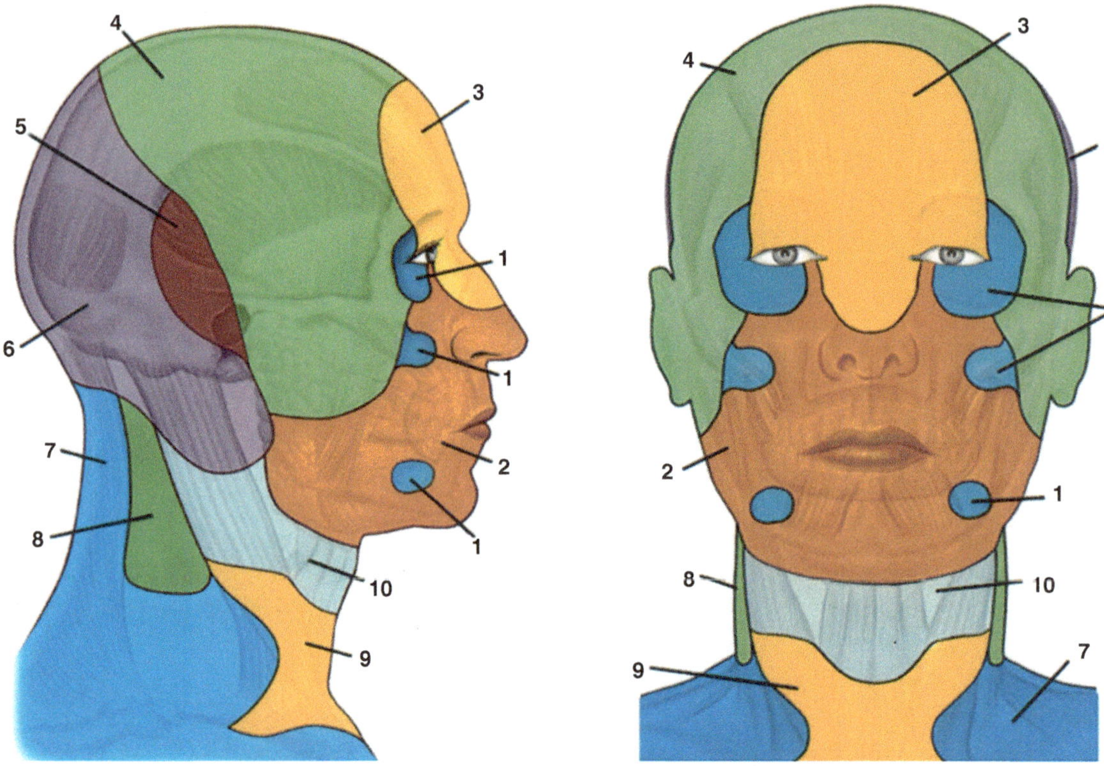

• **Fig. 28.2** Angiosomes of the face: *1*, maxillary; *2*, facial; *3*, ophthalmic; *4*, superficial temporal; *5*, posterior auricular; *6*, occipital; *7*, transverse cervical; *8*, deep cervical; *9*, inferior thyroid; *10*, superior thyroid. (From Houseman ND, Taylor GI, Pan W-R. The angiosomes of the head and neck: anatomic study and clinical applications. *Plast Reconstr Surg*. 2000;105(7):2287–313.)

anterior to the insertion of masseter where it may be palpated, then runs convex anteriorly across the cheek deep to the zygomaticus muscles and becomes the angular artery at the medial canthus. Its named branches are the ascending palatine, tonsillar, submental, glandular, inferior labial, superior labial, and lateral nasal.[6,10] The angiosome of the facial artery includes the majority of the cheek (Fig. 28.2).[11]

Three branches of the maxillary artery supply areas on the cheek, one from each of its parts. The inferior alveolar artery branches from the first part of the maxillary artery in the infratemporal fossa, running along the medial surface of the ramus of the mandible to the mandibular foramen. It emerges via the mental foramen and supplies the skin of the chin and inferomedial cheek. The buccal artery branches from the second part of the maxillary artery, then runs anteriorly on lateral pterygoid to supply buccinator and a small area of skin on the medial cheek. The infraorbital artery branches from the third and final part of the maxillary artery in the pterygopalatine fossa, then runs through the infraorbital canal to emerge on the face from the infraorbital foramen. There are extensive anastomoses between all three and branches of the facial artery.

The superficial temporal artery runs upward within the substance of the parotid gland between the TMJ and the external acoustic meatus over the posterior zygomatic arch. It gives off two branches in the cheek: the transverse facial artery, and the zygomatico-orbital artery. The parotid duct of Stensen and the buccal branches of the facial nerve accompany the transverse facial artery, which supplies the skin overlying the parotid gland and lateral cheek. The zygomatico-orbital artery runs superior to the zygomatic arch in parallel with the transverse facial artery as far as the orbicularis oculi muscle.

Veins

The facial vein accompanies the facial artery, running immediately lateral to it, but follows a less tortuous course. The infraorbital vein accompanies the artery in its course and is a tributary of the facial vein. The retromandibular vein is formed by the union of the superficial temporal and maxillary veins from the pterygoid plexus and may be found accompanying the superficial temporal artery. It divides into anterior and posterior branches, the former joining the facial vein before emptying into the internal jugular vein, the latter forming the external jugular vein with the posterior auricular vein.[6]

Lymphatics

The pattern of lymphatic drainage of the cheek roughly mirrors the venous system, and is chiefly to the submental, submandibular, and periauricular nodes.[6,12]

Nerves

The anatomic structure of chief importance in the cheek is the facial nerve. As the sole motor supply to the muscles of facial expression, any facial nerve injury can have significant and lasting effects on patients' quality of life. After emerging from the stylomastoid foramen the facial nerve enters the parotid gland. From this point on the ramification pattern of the facial nerve is highly variable.[13] In general, upon emerging from the parotid it has frontal, temporal, buccal, mandibular, and cervical branches, and various landmarks have been described for locating individual branches.[14] Depth of facial nerve branches also varies according to the area of the cheek being examined and the presence of tissue spaces, though in general they are deep to the SMAS laterally before becoming more superficial to supply muscles of facial expression medially.

The skin of the cheek, and of the face in general, is supplied almost exclusively by branches of the Vth cranial nerve: the trigeminal. The sole exception is an area of skin overlying the parotid gland and the angle of the mandible, which is supplied by the great auricular nerve, a branch of the cervical plexus. The remainder of the cheek is supplied by branches of the lower two divisions of the trigeminal nerve. The maxillary division provides two branches to the skin of the cheek. The infraorbital nerve supplies the cheek immediately beneath the eyelid, while the zygomaticofacial nerve supplies an area over the zygoma just lateral to the eye. The infraorbital nerve may be blocked by infiltration of local anesthetic around where it exits the infraorbital foramen, which is located below the medial third of the infraorbital margin. The mandibular division also provides two branches. The buccal nerve supplies an area beneath the zygoma, between the distribution of the infraorbital and great auricular nerves. The mental nerve emerges from the mental foramen in line with the second premolar tooth and supplies the lower lip and surrounding skin.[10]

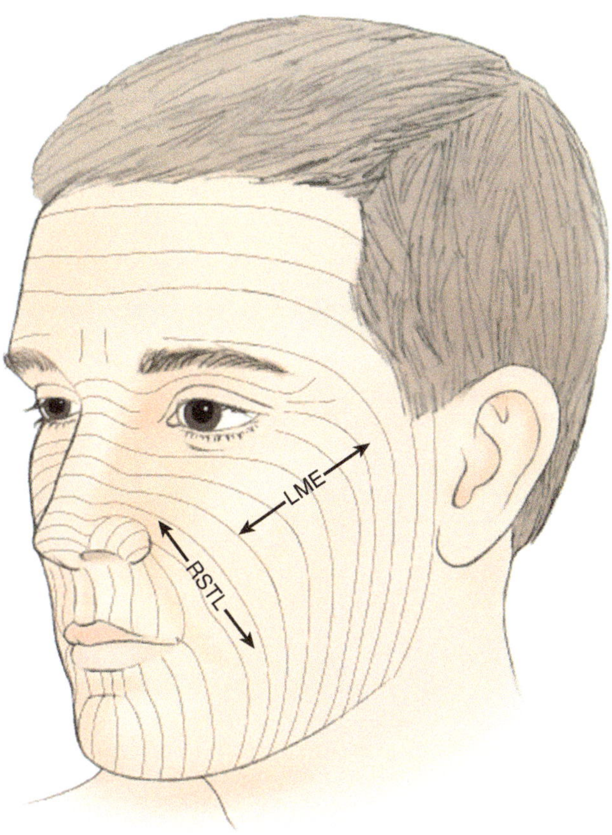

• **Fig. 28.3** Relaxed skin tension lines (RSTLs) of the face. *LME*, Line of maximum extensibility. (From Bhrany AD, Bradley DT, Murakami CS. Reconstruction of the cheek. In: Baker SR, ed. *Local Flaps in Facial Reconstruction* [electronic resource]. 3rd edn. Philadelphia: Elsevier Saunders; 2014:530–562.)

Management

As is the case throughout reconstructive plastic surgery, the approach to reconstructing a cheek defect should be individualized for the patient, considering their overall health, prognosis, and functional status. The defect should be examined and characterized, noting such features as defect site, size, shape, and depth, in addition to wound condition and etiology, and any associated injury, where relevant. Clinical photography may be helpful as a record.

General principles are helpful to bear in mind while planning and executing the reconstruction, and Menick has provided some useful guidelines for reconstruction of facial units, which may be applied to cheek reconstruction.[15] It should be borne in mind that in the cheek the crucial element for a good esthetic result is uniformity of skin color and texture, rather than contour or outline. For this reason, local and regional flaps from adjacent units are generally preferred over grafting. Exceptions to this rule are in cases requiring total facial resurfacing, in which case a complete skin graft or complete flap are preferred to a combination of other techniques.

Distant skin is a poor match for facial skin, but for some wounds (large, contaminated, irradiated) transfer of distant tissue using microvascular techniques is the only solution. In these situations a free flap may be used to provide mucosal lining and tissue build, with local and regional flaps mobilized secondarily to provide permanent external skin. For smaller defects which may be amenable to direct closure, scars should be placed either in the borders of esthetic units or in parallel with relaxed skin tension lines (RSTLs), which are perpendicular to lines of maximum skin extensibility (Fig. 28.3).[12]

All of the techniques on the reconstructive ladder are useful in the management of defects of the cheek (Box 28.4). However, as discussed above, nearby tissues provide the best color and texture match for cheek skin, and as such local and cervicofacial flaps are generally preferred where the lesion is not amenable to direct closure. Use of each of these techniques in reconstruction of the cheek is discussed below.

Secondary Intention

Wounds able to form granulation tissue may be allowed to heal by secondary intention following resection of tumor, or debridement of devitalized tissue following trauma. Defects less than 1 cm may produce an acceptable

• BOX 28.4 General Principles for Reconstruction of Facial Units

1. Characterize the defect both aesthetically and functionally, ensure that it is ready for reconstruction prior to planning.
2. Aim to rebuild or resurface entire aesthetic units.
3. If necessary, excise tissue to alter the defect to aid reconstruction.
4. For unilateral defects, use the contralateral for comparison.
5. Match donor tissue to the recipient site in colour, texture, thickness, and hair-bearing.
6. Facial skin is preferred for resurfacing, though other donors may provide bulk.
7. Bone or cartilage grafts should be used to recreate underlying architecture.
8. More than one reconstructive technique (local flaps, non-vascularized grafting, and free vascularized tissue transfer) may be required for the best result.
9. Defects that involve multiple facial units, especially when including the nose, may need to be staged due to the unpredictable outcome of contracture and distortion during healing.

result when left to heal by secondary intention, however the esthetic appearance is generally inferior to other approaches due to scar contraction.[12] It is therefore generally not appropriate for defects close to the eyelid, nose, and lip due to the potential for distortion. It may be employed with acceptable results in the lateral cheek, in particular in the periauricular area.[3]

Direct Closure

The simplest means of reconstructing a cheek defect is direct closure. It has been suggested that defects of up to 4 cm in size are amenable to direct closure, and that this should be the technique of choice where scars may be concealed in borders of esthetic units or in parallel with RSTLs. Prior to attempting direct closure, it is important to check that there is sufficient skin laxity to allow tension-free closure. Preoperative examination and intraoperative tailor-tacking may be of assistance in assessing this.[12,16]

Undermining of wound edges may allow further mobilization of wound edges to directly close defects that would otherwise be under excessive tension.[12] Standing cones should be excised at the time of initial closure, as the cheek is an area in which they are unlikely to settle. M-plasty may be employed where excision of a standing cone would intrude on critical areas.[3,12]

The perialar and preauricular areas are particularly amenable to direct closure with their abundance of tissue laxity and proximity to the border of the cheek, allowing large defects to be closed with a well-concealed scar.[16]

Tissue Expansion

Tissue expansion is a useful adjunct for managing a defect in the cheek. Internal or external tissue expanders may be used to increase available skin to enable a repair that would otherwise result in excessive wound tension.[17] Caution should be exercised to avoid injury or compression of branches of the facial or trigeminal nerves. Furthermore, since weeks are required for useful tissue expansion, the need for immediate reconstruction prevents its use in many cases.

Local Flaps

The most robust and esthetic means of reconstructing cheek defects not amenable to direct closure are local flaps. The use of skin from the same esthetic unit provides a good tissue match with little wound contraction. Local flaps are particularly useful for closure of defects in the midcheek, where scars may be concealed along the natural creases of the face.

A selection of flaps that may be used for defects of the cheek are shown (Fig. 28.4). Deep anchoring sutures to take tension off the leading edge of flaps, especially in areas of fixation such as the periorbital region.[12] V–Y advancement and nasolabial island flaps are particularly useful for medial defects, due to the relative mobility and elasticity of tissues.[16,18] These flaps are useful in the lateral cheek due to the relative paucity of subcutaneous fat and denser connections to the underlying fascia via retaining ligaments. Other flaps such as transposition flaps, rotation-advancement flaps, and geometric flaps including rhomboid, bilobed, and Dufourmental flaps, are of use in cheek reconstruction but are described in greater detail in other chapters.

Cheek Rotation-Advancement and Cervicofacial Flaps

Cheek rotation-advancement flaps were originally designed by Mustardé,[19] who described their use for closure of eyelid defects. The technique was further developed and found its full expression in the cervicofacial flaps of Juri and Juri.[20] By wide undermining of tissue throughout the cheek and extended into the neck where necessary, this is a versatile technique that is used to close wounds that are too large for direct closure or other local flaps, providing a good match for facial skin color, texture, and thickness.[16] They have become the method of choice to reconstruct cheek defects that are too large for a local flap, and are the preferred method for even medium-sized defects (larger than 2 cm) for some authors, who find that local flaps may result in an esthetically unpleasing scar.[16] They are useful for large defects of both the lateral cheek, where there is relatively less skin laxity, and the medial cheek, where the scar may be concealed along the borders of the cheek. Cervicofacial flaps may be anteriorly or posteriorly based depending on the position of the defect and the direction of advancement of the flap. Posteriorly-based cervicofacial flaps have a more robust blood supply than anteriorly-based flaps due

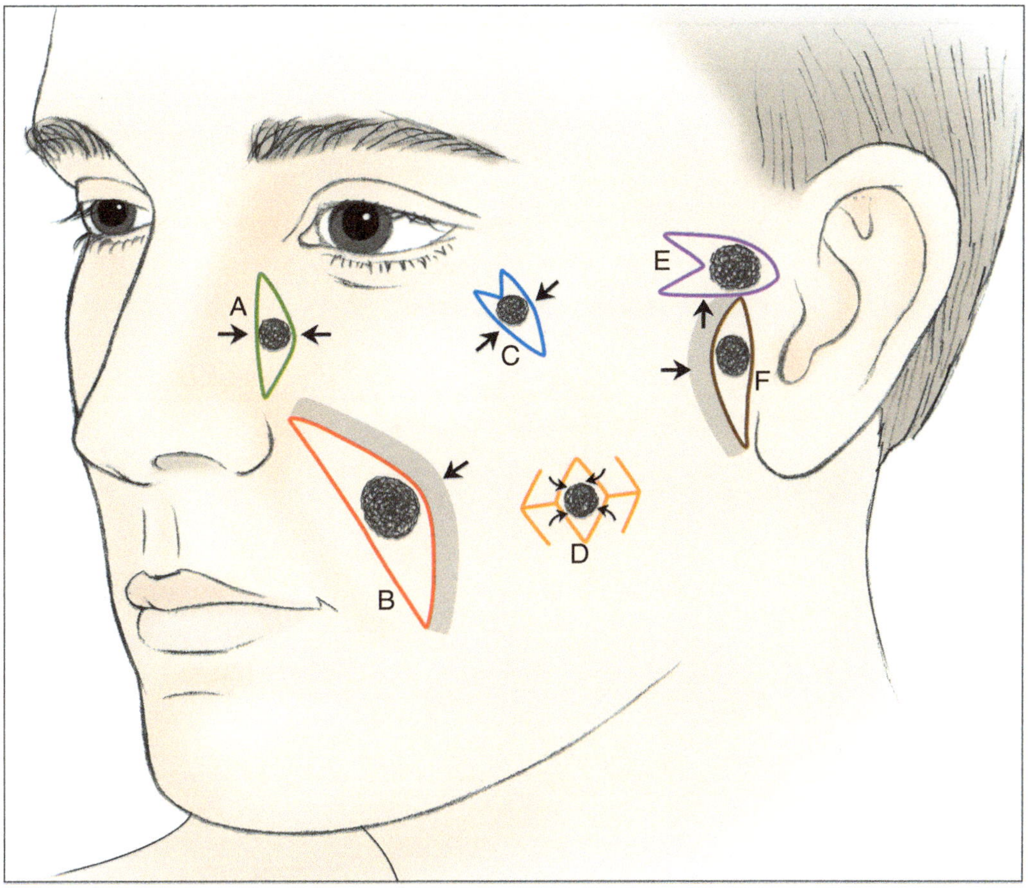

• **Fig. 28.4** Local flaps in the cheek: *A*, primary closure; *B*, primary closure with asymmetric undermining; *C*, elliptical closure with M-plasty; *D*, rhombic flaps; *E*, advancement with M-plasty; *F*, primary closure with asymmetric undermining. (From Bhrany AD, Bradley DT, Murakami CS. Reconstruction of the cheek. In: Baker SR, ed. *Local Flaps in Facial Reconstruction* [electronic resource]. 3rd edn. Philadelphia: Elsevier Saunders; 2014:530–562.)

to preservation of the transverse branches of the facial and superficial temporal arteries.

Technique

The incision follows the borders of the cheek and is extended down the neck. In anteriorly-based flaps, the incision follows the superior border of the cheek, the preauricular crease, around the ear toward the occipital hairline, before being extended inferiorly for as far as is necessary to mobilize sufficient tissue prior to back-cutting, where possible following a variation of a facelift type incision.[2] For larger defects or those extending into the neck, the incision may be extended further inferiorly, creating a cervicothoracic flap. For a posteriorly based flap, the incision follows the nasolabial crease and extended onto the upper neck. Flaps extending to the posterior neck should be kept posterior to the anterior border of trapezius to avoid webbing of the scar.

Following the incision, the flap must be dissected in order to mobilize it into position. The dissection may be either subcutaneous or sub-SMAS (Fig. 28.5). The deep plane cervicofacial flap is based on the technique of the sub-SMAS facelift and incorporates the SMAS in the flap (Fig. 28.6).[21] It is designed to include branches of the facial artery in the case of anteriorly-based flaps, or of the superficial temporal artery in posteriorly based flaps. Advocates of the deep plane approach emphasize its more robust blood supply, enhanced mobility of the flap, and greater thickness providing a more aesthetically pleasing contour.[22] Opponents of this approach argue that deep plane dissections are more difficult with a greater risk of facial nerve injury and a greater risk of ectropion due to the increased weight of the flap.[16,23] The deep plane approach may be preferred in patients in whom blood supply to the flap is a significant concern, such as diabetics, smokers, or those who have undergone radiotherapy to the area.

The senior author's preference is to dissect in the subcutaneous layer above the zygoma and overlying the parotid only, and in the sub-SMAS plane elsewhere. Regardless of which plane is chosen, the dissection should be extended into the temporal region to create sufficient laxity to prevent tension from the weight of the flap, which may result in ectropion (Figs. 28.7 and 28.8).[16] Periosteal suspension sutures should be used to anchor the leading edge of the flap at the cheek/eyelid junction.[2,24] Care should be taken during dissection to avoid injury to the branches

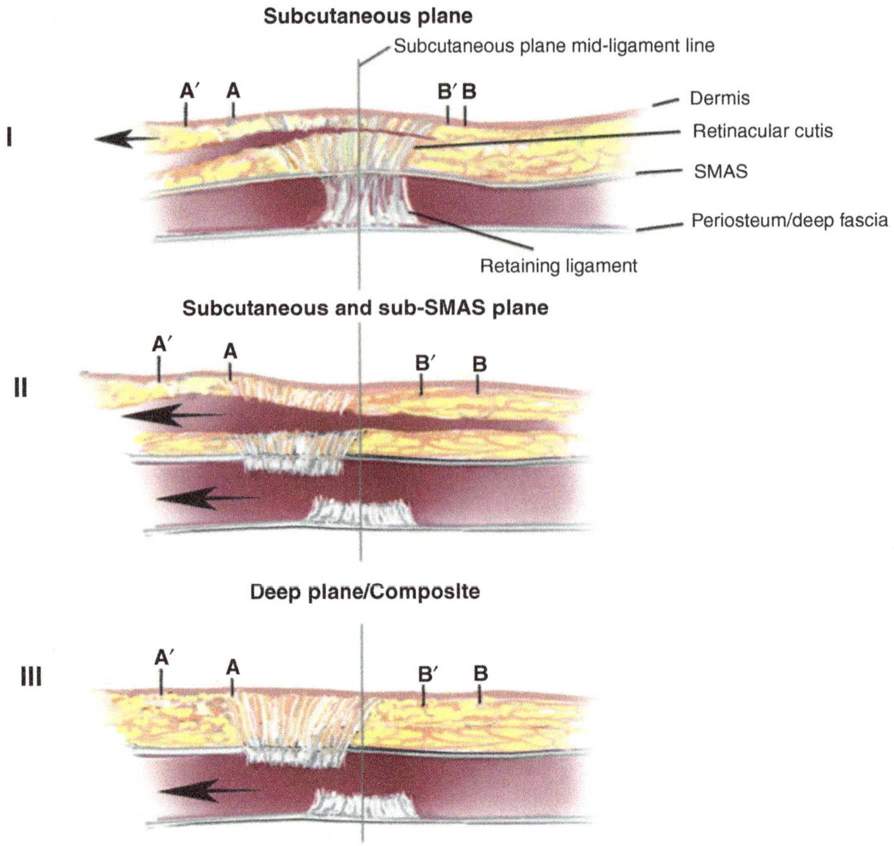

• **Fig. 28.5** Subcutaneous and deep plane facelift techniques demonstrating plane of dissection and release of retaining ligaments. Points A and B are advanced to A′ and B′, respectively, demonstrating the greater mobilization permitted by the deep plane technique. (From Alghoul M, Codner MA. Retaining ligaments of the face: review of anatomy and clinical applications. *Aesthet Surg J*. 2013;33(6):769–782.)

of the facial nerve, particularly immediately anterior to the parotid where the branches are no longer protected by intervening parotid tissue.[22] The cutaneous branches of the cervical plexus and mandibular division of the trigeminal nerve should also be protected. Following dissection, the flap is advanced into the defect and sutured into place.

Regional Flaps

For patients with large defects of the cheek in whom cervicofacial flaps are not viable, regional pedicle flaps are a useful option. Commonly used flaps include the supraclavicular and deltopectoral flaps. The supraclavicular flap is an axial pattern flap based on the supraclavicular artery, which originates from the transverse cervical. After raising the flap, it may be tunneled subcutaneously to reach the cheek, though care should be taken to avoid pressure on the pedicle. The deltopectoral is supplied by perforators from the internal mammary artery, though the distal part is supplied by branches of the thoracoacromial trunk which are cut during raising of the flap. For this reason a delay prior to transfer of the flap is required to ensure adequate vascularization of the distal part of the flap.

For full-thickness defects of the cheek, musculocutaneous flaps such as the pectoralis major flap are a useful option (Fig. 28.9). Originally described by Hueston and McConchie[25] and first used for head and neck reconstruction by Ariyan,[26] this is a versatile flap which may be harvested with either single or multiple skin paddles for reconstructing multiple surfaces. In addition, bone from the fifth rib may be harvested if required for bony reconstruction.

Skin Grafts

Skin grafts are not ideal for reconstruction of cheek defects as they generally provide a poor match for facial skin. Furthermore, secondary contracture may result in distortion which may not be desired, especially in proximity to eyelid, nose, and lip.[2] Nevertheless, there is a place for skin grafting for patients with large defects not amenable to direct closure or a local flap, and in whom a more complex reconstruction may not be practical, such as the elderly or those with significant comorbidities. Full-thickness skin grafts are generally preferred as they are less likely to contract and have a better match for color, texture, and thickness. Common donor sites for facial defects are the preauricular and supraclavicular areas, and the nasolabial fold.[27] Due to their disadvantages, split-thickness skin grafts are generally used

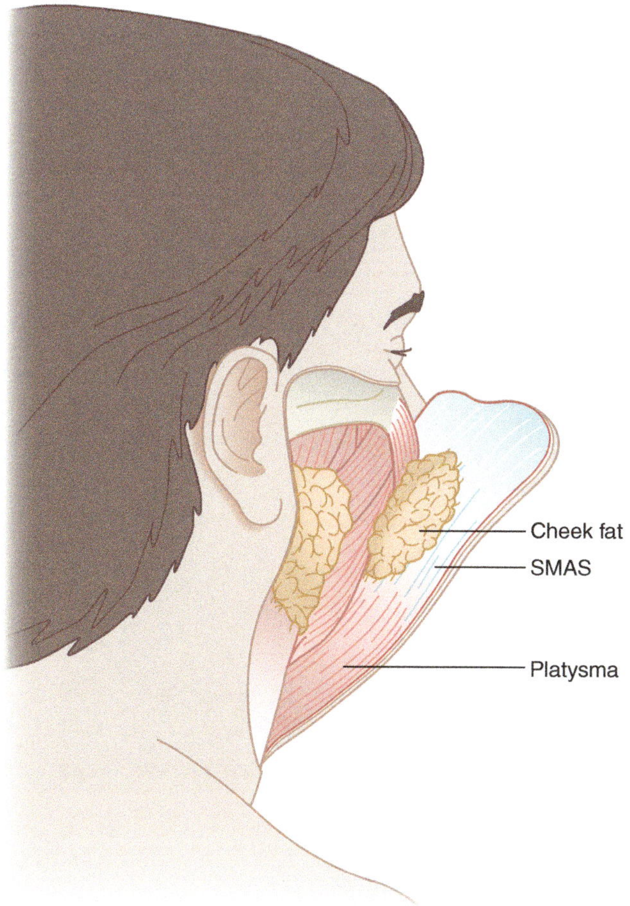

• **Fig. 28.6** Deep plane cervicofacial flap incorporating cheek fat, superficial musculoaponeurotic system (SMAS), and platysma. (From Kroll SS, Reece GP, Robb G, Black J. Deep-plane cervicofacial rotation-advancement flap for reconstruction of large cheek defects. *Plast Reconstr Surg*. 1994;94(1):88–93.)

only for temporary coverage while a definitive reconstruction is planned, or when incomplete excision is suspected.

Free Flaps

The most advanced option for reconstruction of very large defects, or in patients in whom other reconstructive options are not viable, is free tissue transfer. Fasciocutaneous flaps are preferred as they provide a thin, pliable flap that may be molded to restore the contour of the cheek. Suitable flaps include the subscapular and parascapular, radial forearm, and anterolateral thigh flap. For patients requiring a bony element to their reconstruction, the osteocutaneous free fibular flap is particularly useful for reconstructing mandible. Musculocutaneous flaps based on rectus abdominis or latissimus dorsi may also be useful, though their use usually results in a bulky reconstruction requiring substantial revision.

Prefabrication and Allotransplantation

Prefabricated and prelaminated flaps were devised by Pribaz for reconstruction of complex defects in the head and neck.[28] He defined prefabrication as the "pre-transfer implantation of a non-native vascular pedicle into tissue desired for reconstruction," while prelamination describes the "pre-transfer implantation of anything else."[29] Thus while prefabrication is a technique allowing the transfer of otherwise nontransferable tissue, prelamination allows the assembly of tissue to reconstruct a composite defect prior to transfer. One disadvantage of these techniques is that they require at least two and perhaps several staged procedures. However, they may be useful where simpler alternatives are not viable, as in extensive burns or trauma.

The first facial allograft signaled the dawn of an era of vascularized composite allotransplantation (VCA).[30] Though the significant morbidity associated with lifelong immunosuppression currently prohibits widespread use of these techniques, anatomical proof of concept studies have been performed.[31] Currently, allotransplantation is considered a "last resort," to be considered only when less morbid reconstructive techniques are considered inadequate.

Complications

Complications of cheek reconstruction may be divided into surgical, functional, and esthetic complications (Box 28.5). Surgical complications include wound complications such as breakdown and infection and flap necrosis, which may be subdivided into superficial, partial, and total necrosis according to the area of tissue involved. It is generally acknowledged that the rate of surgical complications is vastly increased in smokers or those with vascular disease.[16] Functional complications, such as oral incompetence and lower eyelid ectropion, result from displacement of the angle of the mouth or the lateral canthus due to excessive flap tension, swelling, or weight. These complications may be avoided by careful flap design and the use of strategically placed deep sutures to fix the flap to underlying structures.[1] Finally, esthetic complications such as loss of symmetry, loss of skin quality, and abnormal hair distribution generally result from inappropriate selection of tissue used for the reconstruction. Revisional procedures may be required to improve the final result.

• BOX 28.5 Complications of Cheek Reconstruction

- Surgical
- Wound complications
- Flap necrosis
- Functional
- Oral incompetence
- Eyelid ectropion
- Esthetic
- Loss of symmetry
- Loss of skin quality
- Abnormal hair distribution

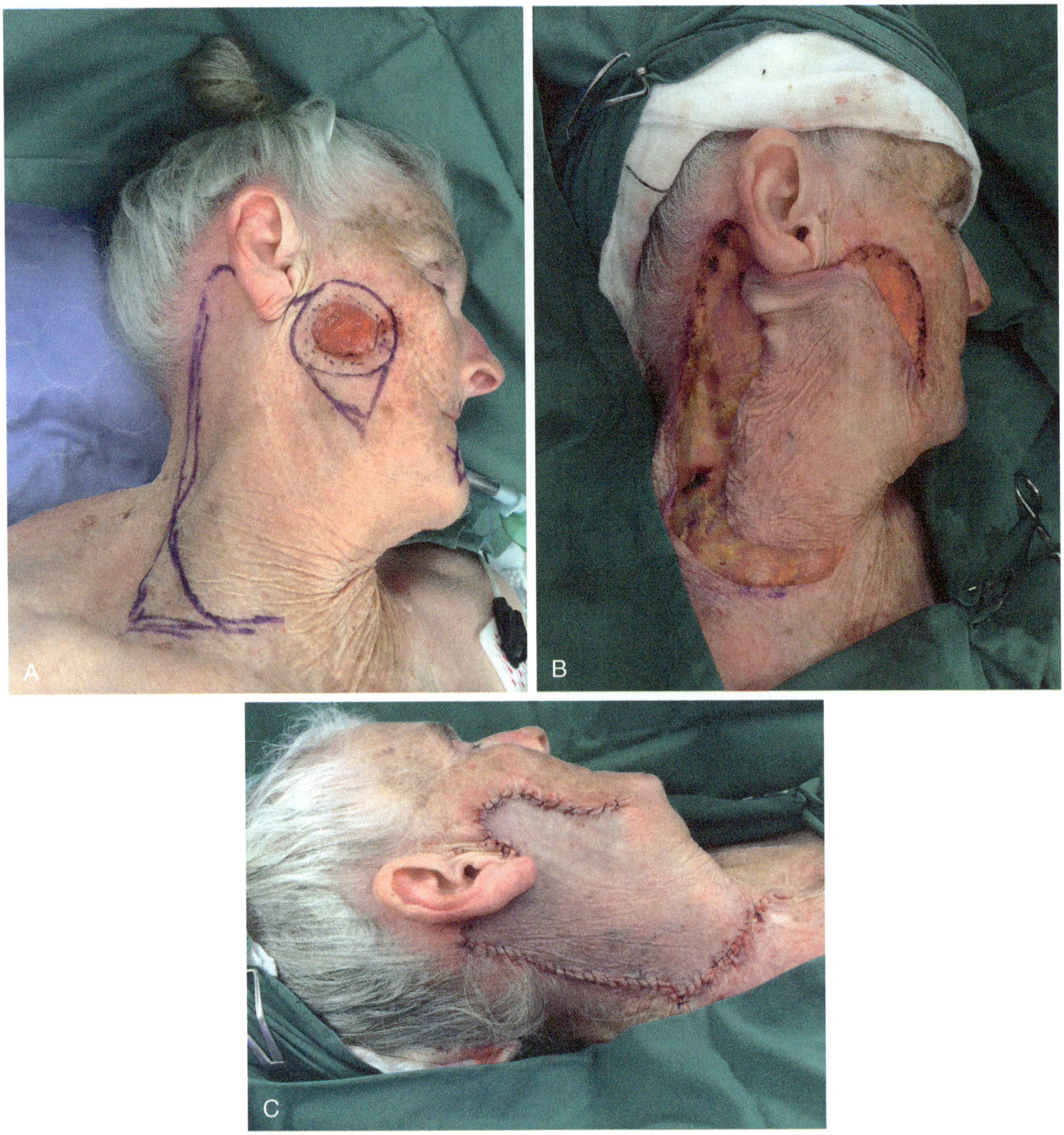

• **Fig. 28.7** (A) Cervicofacial flap, preoperative marking. (B) Intraoperative appearance following raising of the flap. (C) Intraoperative appearance following flap inset.

Contour Defects

Some patients may present with a complex deformity resulting from a condition causing widespread facial atrophy. Since the predominant contour of the cheek is that of a smooth convex surface, this has a significant effect on facial appearance, producing obvious asymmetry when unilateral, or a "starved" appearance when bilateral. The etiology of the progressive syndrome is unknown. The eponymous names for the unilateral and bilateral types are Parry–Romberg and Barraquer–Simons, respectively. In addition, there are a wide range of other known causes of facial atrophy, including scleroderma, trauma, tumor, radiation injury, and HIV infection.

A number of techniques may be used in the treatment of facial atrophy. These include the use of autologous tissue, as in fat grafting or free flap surgery, or synthetic material. Synthetic fillers that have been used for facial atrophy include biodegradable materials such as hyaluronic acid gel, and nonbiodegradable materials such as silicon.[32] However, due to concern regarding long-term complications, these materials have fallen out of favor.[33] The mainstay of treatment of contour defects thus comprises autologous tissue. Detailed study of the role and technique of fat grafting has seen a surge in its use in reconstructive

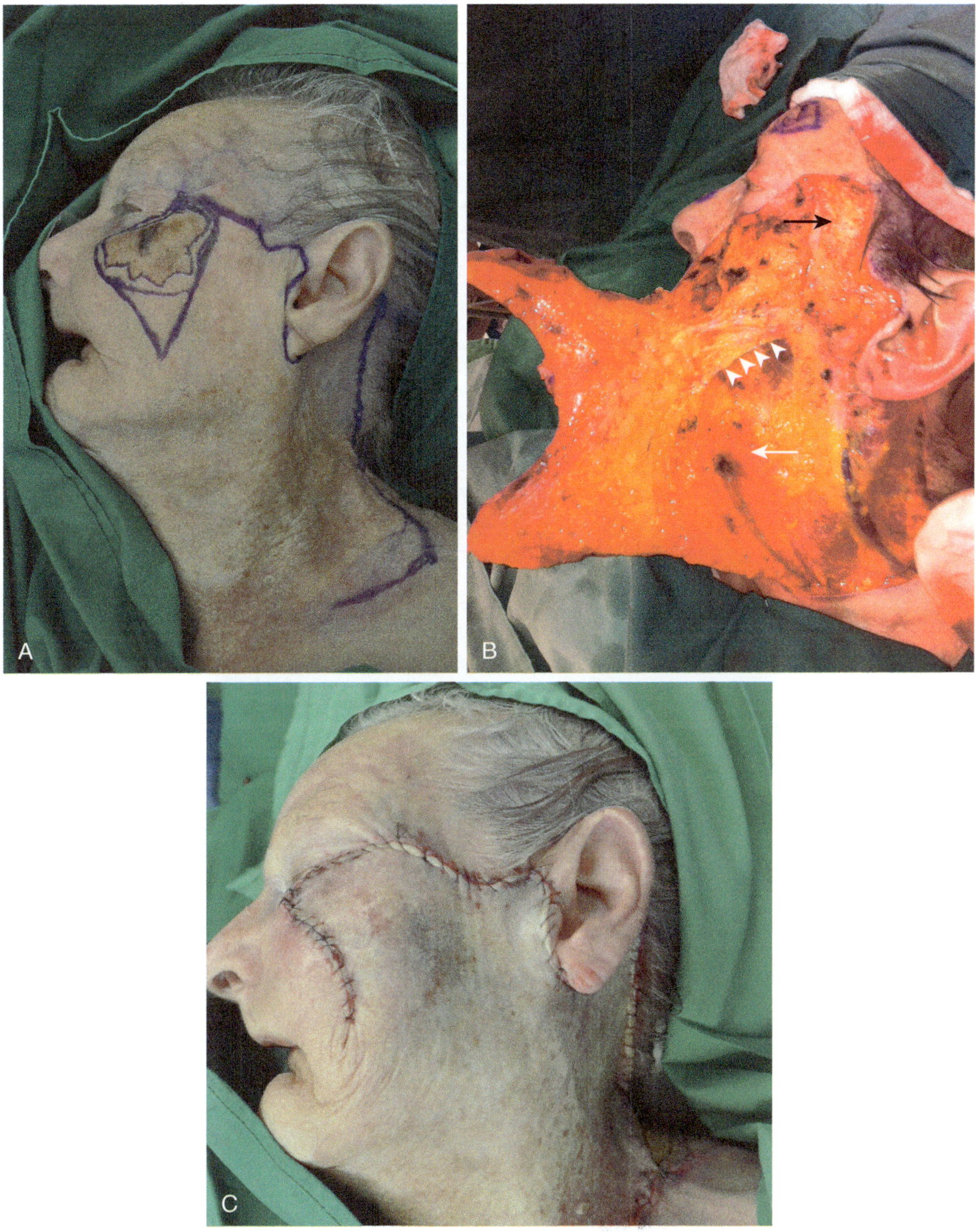

• **Fig. 28.8** (A) Cervicofacial flap, preoperative marking. (B) Flap raised, demonstrating subplatysmal plane in neck, facial nerve branches emerging from parotid, and subcutaneous dissection into temple (note that this image is taken from a different procedure to the other images in this series). *Black arrow*, subcutaneous dissection into temple; *white arrow*, subplatysmal dissection into neck; *white arrowheads*, facial nerve branches emerging from parotid. (C) Intraoperative appearance following flap inset.

surgery, and the restoration of the cheek contour is a place where it finds a natural home. In addition, the action of adipose-derived stem cells contained within fat graft may modify the underlying pathology, particularly in the case of radiation damage.[34] A variety of free flaps have been used for soft tissue restoration in facial atrophy, including omentum, TRAM, scapular and parascapular, and groin flaps.[33,35] Ultimately, the choice of technique will be determined by the degree of atrophy and the volume of tissue required, and risk of morbidity associated with the chosen reconstruction compared with the effect of the deformity on the patient's quality of life.

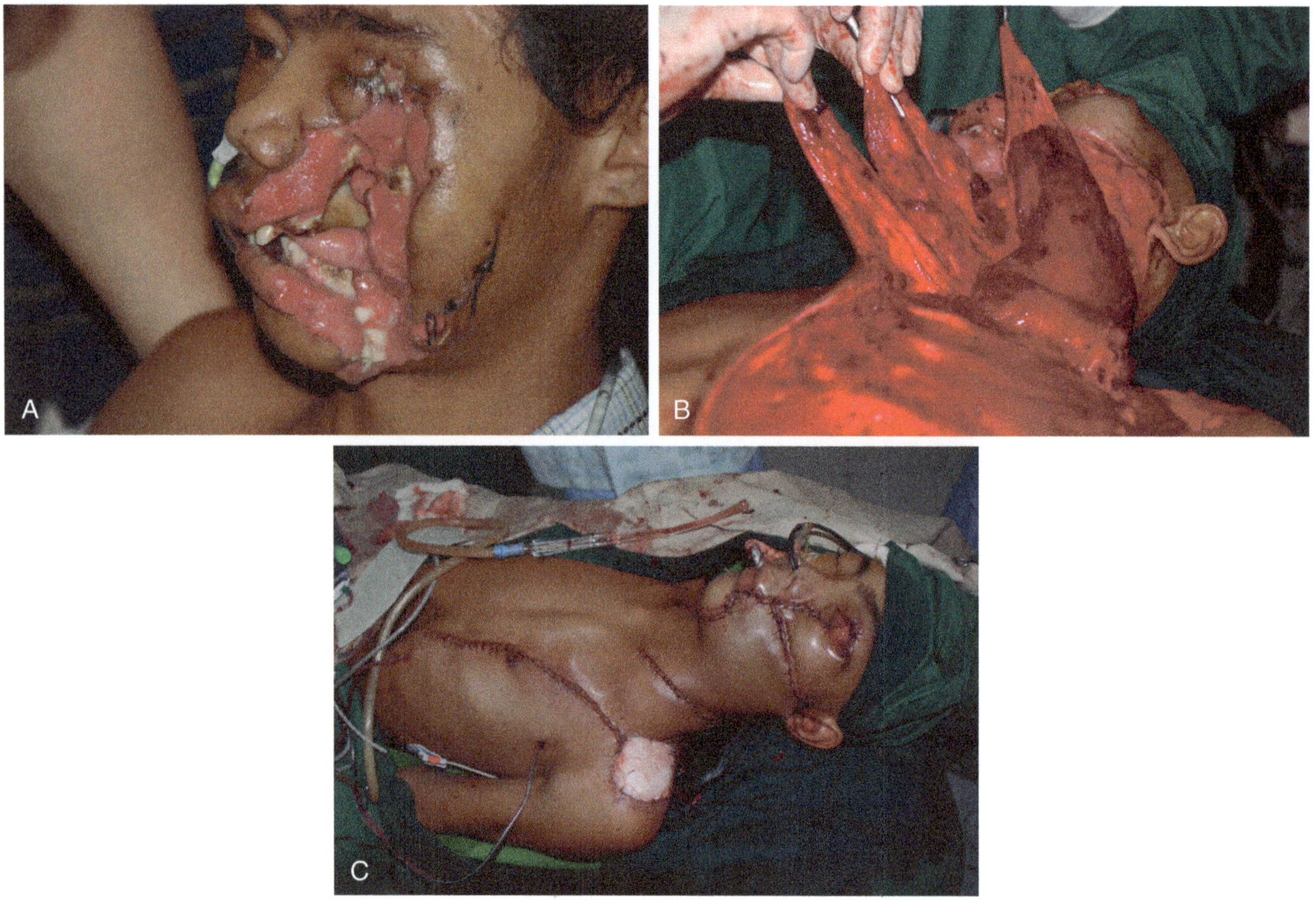

• **Fig. 28.9** (A) Full-thickness cheek defect secondary to gunshot wound. (B) Pectoralis major flap raised, demonstrating multiple skin paddles for reconstruction of the intraoral defect, a deltopectoral flap for the neck donor site and a cervicofacial flap for the cheek defect, incorporating muscle for vascularity and contour restoration. (C) Postoperative appearance. (Photos courtesy Associate Professor Michael Leung.)

Conclusion

The approach to reconstructing a cheek defect should be tailored to the individual patient. Assessment of the patient's overall health, in addition to the characteristics of the defect, is essential in order to select an appropriate reconstructive technique. Detailed understanding of the facial anatomy and esthetics are vital to the creation and execution of a sound plan. Taking these basic principles into consideration allows the surgeon to achieve harmonious esthetic and functional results in reconstructing the full range of cheek defects.

Acknowledgments

The authors would like to thank Associate Professor Michael Leung in the preparation of this chapter.

References

1. Menick FJ. Reconstruction of the cheek. *Plast Reconstr Surg.* 2001;108(2):496–505.
2. Jowett N, Mlynarek AM. Reconstruction of cheek defects: a review of current techniques. *Curr Opin Otolaryngol Head Neck Surg.* 2010;18(4):244–254.
3. Cass ND, Terella AM. Reconstruction of the cheek. *Facial Plast Surg Clin North Am.* 2019;27(1):55–66.
4. Pepper J-P, Baker SR. Local flaps: cheek and lip reconstruction. *JAMA Facial Plast Surg.* 2013;15(5):374–382.
5. Mendelson BC, Jacobson SR. Surgical anatomy of the midcheek: facial layers, spaces, and the midcheek segments. *Clin Plast Surg.* 2008;35(3):395–404.
6. Larabee WF, Makielski KH, Henderson JL. *Surgical Anatomy of the Face.* 2nd edn. Philadephia, PA: Lippincott Williams & Wilkins; 2004.
7. Mitz V, Peyronie M. The superficial musculo-aponeurotic system (SMAS) in the parotid and cheek area. *Plast Reconstr Surg.* 1976;58(1):80–88.
8. Mendelson B. Facelift anatomy, SMAS, retaining ligaments and facial spaces. In: Aston SJ, Steinbrech DS, Walden JL, eds. *Aesthetic Plastic Surgery.* Elsevier Health Sciences; 2012:53–71.
9. Furnas DW. The retaining ligaments of the cheek. *Plast Reconstr Surg.* 1989;83(1):11–16.
10. McMinn RMH. *Last's Anatomy.* 9th edn. Sydney: Elsevier Churchill Livingstone; 2019.
11. Houseman ND, Taylor GI, Pan W-R. The angiosomes of the head and neck: anatomic study and clinical applications. *Plast Reconstr Surg.* 2000;105(7):2287–2313.
12. Bradley DT, Murakami CS. Reconstruction of the cheek. In: Baker SR, ed. *Local Flaps in Facial Reconstruction [electronic resource].* 2nd ed. Philadelphia: Saunders; 2007:525–556.

13. O'Brien JX, Ashton MW. Relationship of the temporofrontal rami of the facial nerve to the fascial layers of the temporal region. *Ann Plast Surg.* 2012;68(6):547–548.
14. Davis RA, Anson BJ, Budinger JM, Kurth LR. Surgical anatomy of the facial nerve and parotid gland based upon a study of 350 cervicofacial halves. *Surg Gynecol Obstet.* 1956;102(4):385–412.
15. Menick FJ. Defects of the nose, lip, and cheek: rebuilding the composite defect. *Plast Reconstr Surg.* 2007;120(4):887–898.
16. Rapstine ED, Knaus II WJ, Thornton JF. Simplifying cheek reconstruction. *Plast Reconstr Surg.* 2012;129(6):1291–1299.
17. Radovan C. Tissue expansion in soft-tissue reconstruction. *Plast Reconstr Surg.* 1984;74(4):482–492.
18. Baker SR. Advancement flaps. In: Baker SR, ed. *Local Flaps in Facial Reconstruction [electronic Resource].* 2nd edn. Philadelphia: Saunders; 2007:157–187.
19. Mustardé JC. The use of flaps in the orbital region. *Plast Reconstr Surg.* 1970;45(2):146–150.
20. Juri J, Juri C. Advancement and rotation of a large cervicofacial flap for cheek repairs. *Plast Reconstr Surg.* 1979;64(5):692–696.
21. Alghoul M, Codner MA. Retaining ligaments of the face: review of anatomy and clinical applications. *Aesthet Surg J.* 2013;33(6):769–782.
22. Kroll SS, Reece GP, Robb G, Black J. Deep-plane cervicofacial rotation-advancement flap for reconstruction of large cheek defects. *Plast Reconstr Surg.* 1994;94(1):88–93.
23. Austen Jr WG, Parrett BM, Taghinia A, Wolfort SF, Upton J. The subcutaneous cervicofacial flap revisited. *Ann Plast Surg.* 2009;62(2):149–153.
24. Robinson JK. Suspension sutures in facial reconstruction. *Dermatol Surg.* 2003;29(4):386–393.
25. Hueston JT, McConchie IH. A compound pectoral flap. *Aust N Z J Surg.* 1968;38(1):61–63.
26. Ariyan S. The pectoralis major myocutaneous flap: a versatile flap for reconstruction in the head and neck. *Plast Reconstr Surg.* 1979;63(1):73–81.
27. Jewett BS. Skin and composite grafts. In: Baker SR, ed. *Local Flaps in Facial Reconstruction [electronic resource].* 2nd ed. 2007:337–365.
28. Pribaz JJ, Fine N, Orgill DP. Flap prefabrication in the head and neck: a 10-year experience. *Plast Reconstr Surg.* 1999;103(3):808–820.
29. Mathy JA, Pribaz JJ. Prefabrication and prelamination applications in current aesthetic facial reconstruction. *Clin Plast Surg.* 2009;36(3):493–505.
30. Devauchelle B, Badet L, Lengele B, et al. First human face allograft: early report. *Lancet.* 2006;368(9531):203–209.
31. Pomahac B, Lengele B, Ridgway EB, et al. Vascular considerations in composite midfacial allotransplantation. *Plast Reconstr Surg.* 2010;125(2):517–522.
32. Rees TD, Ashley FL, Delgado JP. Silicone fluid injections for facial atrophy: a ten-year study. *Plast Reconstr Surg.* 1973;52(2):118–127.
33. Jurkiewicz MJ, Nahai F. The use of free revascularized grafts in the amelioration of hemifacial atrophy. *Plast Reconstr Surg.* 1985;76(1):44–55.
34. Coleman SR. Structural fat grafting: more than a permanent filler. *Plast Reconstr Surg.* 2006;118(Suppl):108S–120S.
35. Longaker MT, Siebert JW. Microvascular free-flap correction of severe hemifacial atrophy. *Plast Reconstr Surg.* 1995;96(4):800–809.

29 Lip Reconstruction

MARLENE SEE, ANDREW MORRITT, AND NAVID JALLALI

Introduction

The lips constitute the main feature of the lower third of the face, and have been a focus of interest by reconstructive, cleft, and esthetic surgeons. Functionally, the lips play many important roles articulation and enunciation in speech; maintenance of oral competence during eating, drinking, and forceful blowing; and expression of emotion and kissing. These roles are possible because, unlike the other elements of the face, the lips are dynamic and mobile. Esthetically, the vermilion is the hallmark; discrepancies of 1 mm are noted by the naked eye across the room. Reconstruction of the lips, therefore, aims to maintain these characteristics both for function and appearance.

This chapter reviews the anatomy of the lips and presents an algorithm for reconstruction.

Anatomy

Embryology

The upper lip is derived from two distinct structures, namely the paired maxillary and nasomedial processes. Fusion of these processes gives rise to the characteristic features of the upper lip, such as the philtral columns, philtral dimple, Cupid's bow and white roll. The lower lip is formed from fusion of the paired mandibular processes, which result in a less defined lower lip. The topographical landmarks of the lip are illustrated in Fig. 29.1.

Musculature

The muscles that animate the lips are illustrated in Fig. 29.2. The principle muscle is the orbicularis oris, which forms a complex sphincter muscle. This muscle arises both from intrinsic fibers of the lip as well as from other muscles which insert into the lip. The deep and oblique fibers of orbicularis oris approximate the lips to the alveolar arch, while the superficial fibers purse and protrude the lips. The orbicularis oris can be dissected from its supportive muscles while preserving its viability, sensation, and motor function, an important consideration in the choice of reconstruction.[1]

Levator labii superioris elevate the upper lip, levator anguli oris and zygomaticus major draw the lateral upper lip up and back, while buccinator and risorius clear the gingival sulcus. The lower lip is depressed and retracted by the platysma, depressor anguli oris, and depressor labii inferioris. The mentalis muscles cause elevation and protrusion of the central aspect of the lower lip. Loss of these muscles leads to lip incompetence and incisor show.

Vasculature

The blood supply to the upper and lower lips is the superior and inferior labial arteries, respectively. These originate from the facial artery from either side of the face. The average distance of the superior labial artery from the oral commissure (as it branches off the facial artery) is 12 mm, and can be found along its course within 10 mm from the inferior border of the lips. However, the anatomy of the labial arteries can be variable. Magden et al reported that 29% of superior labial arteries have a unilateral origin.[2] This finding has important implications when raising pedicled flaps, such as the Abbe or Estlander flaps. The superior labial artery has a mean diameter of between 1 and 2 mm at its origin, and is therefore large enough for microsurgical anastomosis.[3,4] There are numerous reports and case series of lip replantation in the literature, and problems attributed to replantation are mainly related to the venous drainage of the replanted tissue.

The origin of the inferior labial artery varies between the lower margin of the mandible and the oral commissure.

Lymphatic Drainage

The lymphatic drainage of the lips is ipsilaterally into the submental, submandibular, and parotid nodes. Tissues in the midline drain bilaterally. Submental lymph nodes then drain into ipsilateral submandibular nodes. Submandibular and parotid nodes secondarily drain into the ipsilateral jugulodigastric lymph nodes.

Innervation

The facial nerve (VIIth cranial nerve) provides the motor innervation to the perioral musculature via its buccal and marginal mandibular branches. There are interconnections between both branches of the facial nerve distal to the parotid gland. The motor nerves are located on the

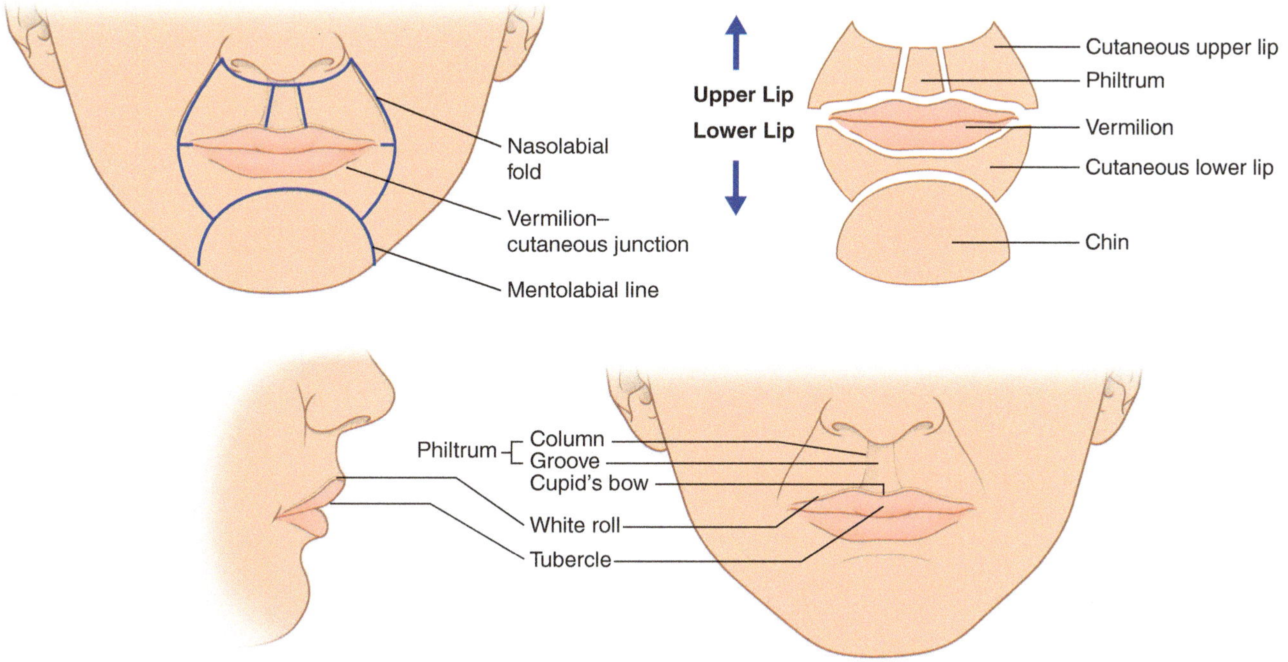

• **Fig. 29.1** Topographical anatomy of the lips. (From Robinson JK. Anatomy for procedural dermatology. In: Robinson JK, Siegel DM, Fratila A, Bhatia AC, Rohrer T, eds. *Surgery of the Skin*. 3rd edn. London: Elsevier; 2015.)

undersurface of all the perioral musculature except for buccinator, levator anguli oris, and mentalis, where the nerve lies on the superficial surface of these muscles.

The maxillary and mandibular branches of the trigeminal nerve (Vth cranial nerve) provide sensory innervation to the perioral region. Specifically, the infraorbital nerve, which is a terminal branch of the maxillary nerve, innervates the upper lip. The infraorbital foramen faces downward and medial and lies 4–7 mm below the infraorbital rim, on a vertical line that descends from the medial limbus of the iris. The nerve runs beneath the levator labii superioris and superficial to the levator anguli oris to supply the lateral nasal sidewall, ala, columella, medial cheek, and upper lip. The lower lip, down to the labiomental fold, is innervated by the mental nerve, which originates from the inferior alveolar nerve, a branch of the mandibular nerve. The mental foramen is located below the apex of the second mandibular bicuspid with 6–10 mm of lateral variability.

Etiology of Lip Defects

The commonest indication for lip reconstruction is following tumor extirpation. The lower lip is much more frequently affected by neoplasia compared to the upper lip, presumably due to greater actinic exposure. The vast majority of skin cancers are squamous cell carcinoma in origin and are more frequently encountered in males (2.4 times) as a result of greater sun exposure, alcohol, and tobacco.[5] Fortunately, these lesions often involve the area between the midline and the oral commissure, avoiding the need for commissural reconstruction. Other causes of lip defects include trauma, infection (e.g., noma), vasculitis, and congenital causes such as vascular malformation or clefts.

Reconstruction: General Principles

Goals

The three main goals of lip reconstruction are:

1. Preservation of oral continence – this requires a muscular integrity, normal sensation and an adequate oral aperture.
2. Preservation of function for speech and ingestion of food.
3. Cosmesis.

Anesthesia

Surgical procedures to the perioral region should be preceded by a regional block, followed by local infiltration to the affected area for the adrenaline-facilitated vasoconstriction. Prior to local infiltration of the lip tissue, it is important to mark or tattoo the white roll of the lip either side of the planned resection in order to match this up afterwards. Any local infiltration, particularly with adrenaline, will obliterate the white roll. A 1-mm discrepancy between the vermilion and skin is noticeable at conversational distance.

The entire upper lip can be anesthetized by bilateral infraorbital nerve block. This can be carried out either

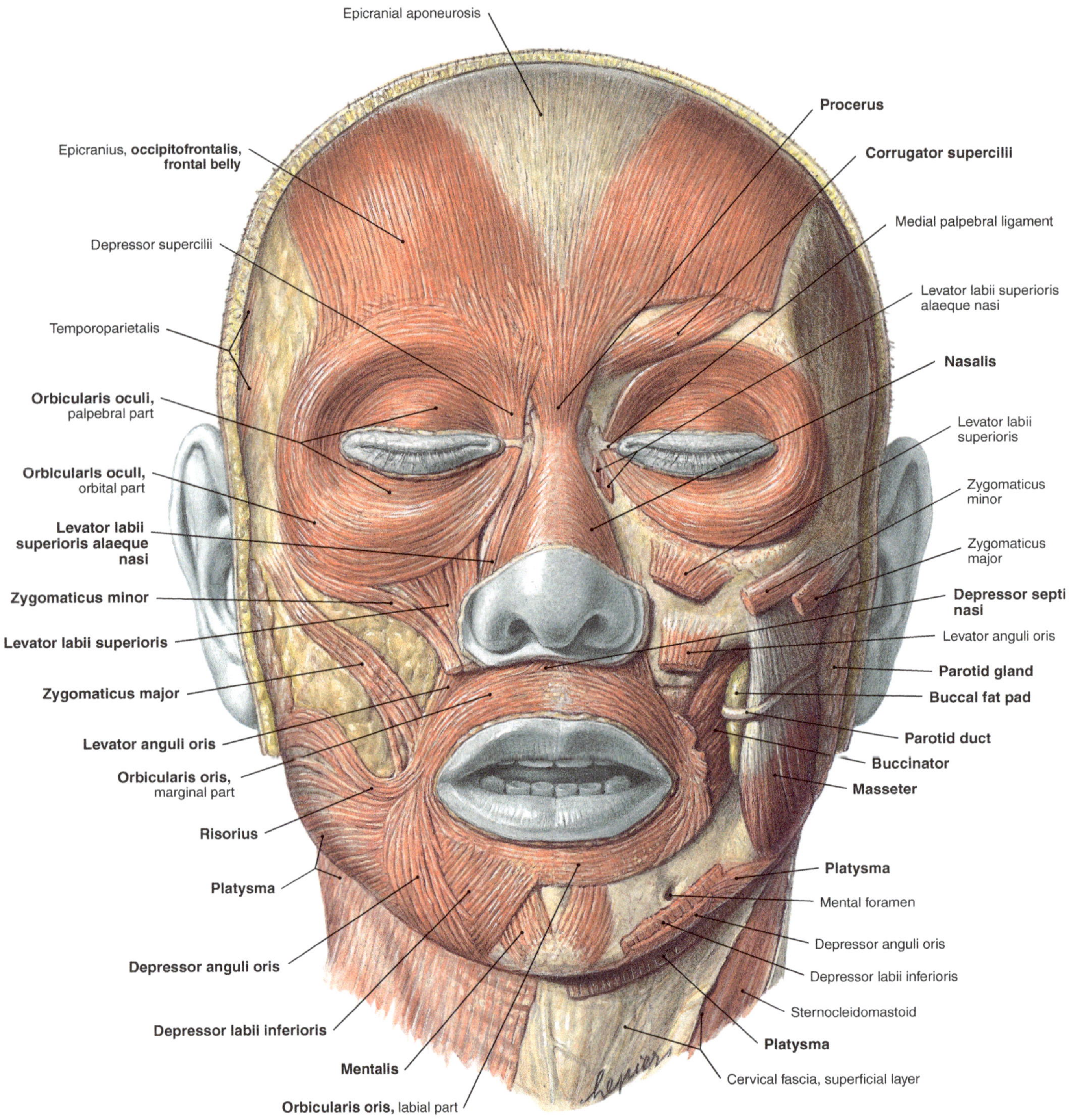

• **Fig. 29.2** Facial musculature. (From Paulsen F. Head. In: Paulsen F, Waschke J., eds. *Sobotta Atlas of Human Anatomy*. 15th edn. Vol. 3: *Head, Neck, and Neuroanatomy*. Munich: Elsevier GmbH; 2013.)

percutaneously or transorally.[6] A 25–27G needle is used and does not need to pass into the foramen to desensitize the lip. For the percutaneous route, the needle is placed medial to the nasolabial fold but lateral to the alar base. For the transoral route, the needle is passed transmucosally above the canine eminence.

The lower lip is anesthetized by bilateral mental nerve blockade. This is performed intraorally by rolling the lower lip outward and stretching the mucosa to visualize the mental nerve just below the mucosa at the canine root. If the nerve is not readily visible, the surgeon should infiltrate local anesthetic into the submucosa at the apices of the canines into the lower lateral buccal sulcus.

Analysis of the Defect

Before embarking on lip reconstruction, the following factors need to be contemplated.

Site

The upper lip has more topographical landmarks compared to the lower lip. The lower lip, lacking in features, is theoretically more expendable as donor tissue for reconstruction. However, functionally and socially, the lower lip deserves more consideration. The lower lip serves to maintain oral competence by containing solids and liquids within the oral cavity. Therefore, any reduction in sulcus depth, compounded by loss of sensation and poor muscle function, will result in liquids leaking out of the mouth. The lower lip can be thought of as one subunit and the upper lip can be thought of either as two subunits (left and right) or as three (two laterals and a central).

Hence, the surgeon needs to deliberate carefully in the following situations: using lower lip tissue to reconstruct the upper lip, denervating the lower lip during the raising of local flaps, or the use of insensate and nonfunctional tissue such as the nasolabial or cheek tissue to reconstruct the lower lip.

Size

Whilst the absolute size of the tumor and excision margins is important, the percentage of the lip which has been ablated is crucial in deciding the reconstructive option. As previously mentioned the lower lip is more expendable, especially in elderly patients with more laxity in the tissues, thereby permitting transposition, advancement or rotation flaps more readily. However, it is vital not to leave the patient with a microstomia. Although amenable to stretching, microstomia does result in imminent problems with dental care, insertion and removal of dentures.

Depth

The four layers of the lip from the oral cavity outwards are mucosa, muscle, vermilion, and skin. With regards to the depth of the defect, the surgeon should "replace like with like" and consider the reconstructive options accordingly.

Involvement of Commissure

If the lip defect involves the oral commissure, then effort must be made to reconstruct the commissure as this is an important esthetic landmark of the lips and face.

Algorithm for Reconstruction

Vermilion Defects

The vermilion is a unique feature of the lip. The vermilion is the transition zone between the stratified keratinized squamous epithelium of the skin and the nonkeratinized squamous epithelium of the oral mucosa. This exists only in humans, and is the partially keratinized layer, which is red due to the reflection of the underlying blood vessels. The wet and dry vermilions are distinct, and in women, the dry vermilion tends to take on lipstick more readily.

For small lesions confined within the vermilion, the lesion should be excised as a vertical ellipse and sutured directly avoiding extension of the incision onto the skin. This technique can also be employed for notch or whistle deformities of the lip, with the addition of a *Z*-plasty to avoid recurrence.

Large superficial defects confined to the vermilion can be left to heal by secondary intention, and tend to heal within 3–4 weeks with a good cosmetic result.

For full-thickness defects resulting in a deficiency of less than 50% of the total vermilion, the options include the axial musculovermilion advancement flap described by Goldstein[7] or a musculomucosal V–Y advancement flaps.[8] For the axial musculovermilion advancement flap, the position of the labial artery is identified from the resection of the lesion and the flap is elevated deep to the labial artery, and then advanced into the defect (Fig. 29.3). Although cross-lip flaps for vermilion reconstruction have been widely reported in the literature,[9–11] it is our opinion that they should be avoided. Cross-lip flaps should not be undertaken lightly as they not only compromise the other intact lip, but also are difficult to tolerate as they are executed as a staged procedure with an intervening period of lip adhesion, i.e., the pedicle of the flap attached.

The facial artery myomucosal flap (FAMM) described by Pribaz in 1992[12] is a good option for vermilion defects of more than 50%.This flap can also be used for total vermilion reconstruction by raising bilateral flaps. The FAMM flap is a composite flap, which is raised from the lateral cheek, based

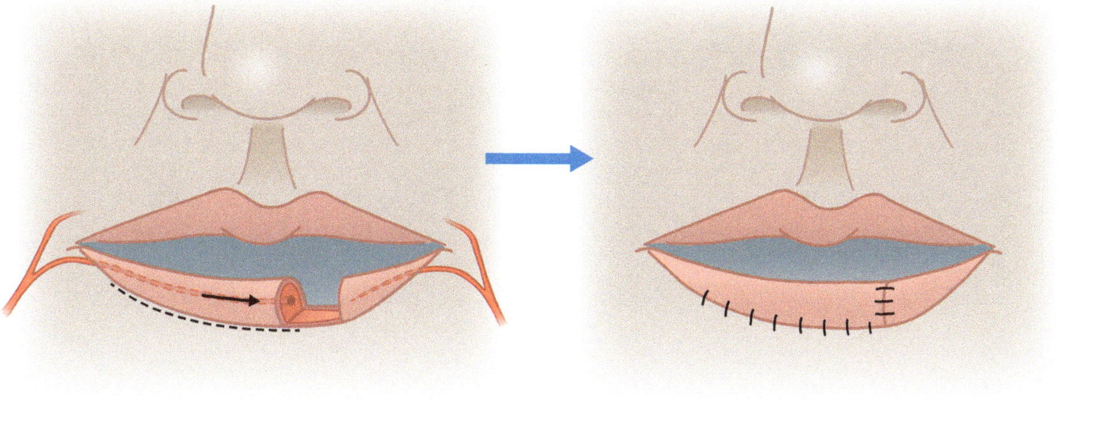

• **Fig. 29.3** The axial musculovermilion flap for full-thickness vermilion defects less than 50% of the total vermilion. The flap is elevated deep to the labial artery.

on the facial artery as it courses though the cheek lateral to the buccinator muscle. It consists of mucosa, submucosa, a small amount of buccinator, a segment of the facial artery and venous plexus. It may be used as a superiorly based flap, which has retrograde perfusion via the angular artery, for the upper lip. Alternatively, the inferiorly based flap based on the facial artery is used for the lower lip. Wide flaps, up to the entire width of the cheek, and up to 7–8 cm in length, can be raised safely but the authors advocate thin flaps to reduce donor site morbidity (Fig. 29.4).

Some patients undergo total vermilionectomy for severe actinic damage or unstable residual epithelium adjacent to a malignant lesion. In these cases of total vermilion deficiency, buccal mucosal advancement as a bipedicled flap described by Lustig et al[13] can be raised to resurface the defect. An incision is made in the buccal sulcus, and the bipedicled flap is advanced as a myomucosal flap including the labial artery. The donor site is left to heal by secondary intention (Fig. 29.5).

Full-Thickness Lower Lip Defect

In addressing full-thickness defects of the lower lip, the rule of thirds provides an effective algorithm for reconstruction (Fig. 29.6).

Defects Less than One-Third Width

For defects up to a third of the total width of the lower lip, the edges of the defect can be approximated directly. It is important to carry out primary closure according to the layers, i.e., the lining (buccal mucosa), the muscle, and the cover (vermilion and skin). The buccal mucosa is sutured using an absorbable suture (e.g., polyglactin/Vicryl or Vicryl Rapide (Ethicon Inc., Cornelia, GA, USA)). The orbicularis oris muscle is also approximated with an absorbable suture (e.g. Vicryl, Monocryl (Ethicon Inc.) or polydiaxonone (PDS, Ethicon Inc.). The vermilion is sutured using an absorbable suture such as Vicryl Rapide.

As previously mentioned, prior to infiltration of any local anesthetic agent, the vermilion junction and/or the white roll must be carefully marked to facilitate accurate approximation of the edges. Techniques for marking the vermilion junction or the white roll include tattooing or placing a single suture at the corresponding points either side of the defect. In some elderly patients, defects between a third to half of the width of the lower lip can be approximated primarily due to increased laxity and redundancy of the tissues with age (Fig. 29.7), however, for the majority of patients, defects greater than a third in width require flap reconstruction to avoid microstomia.

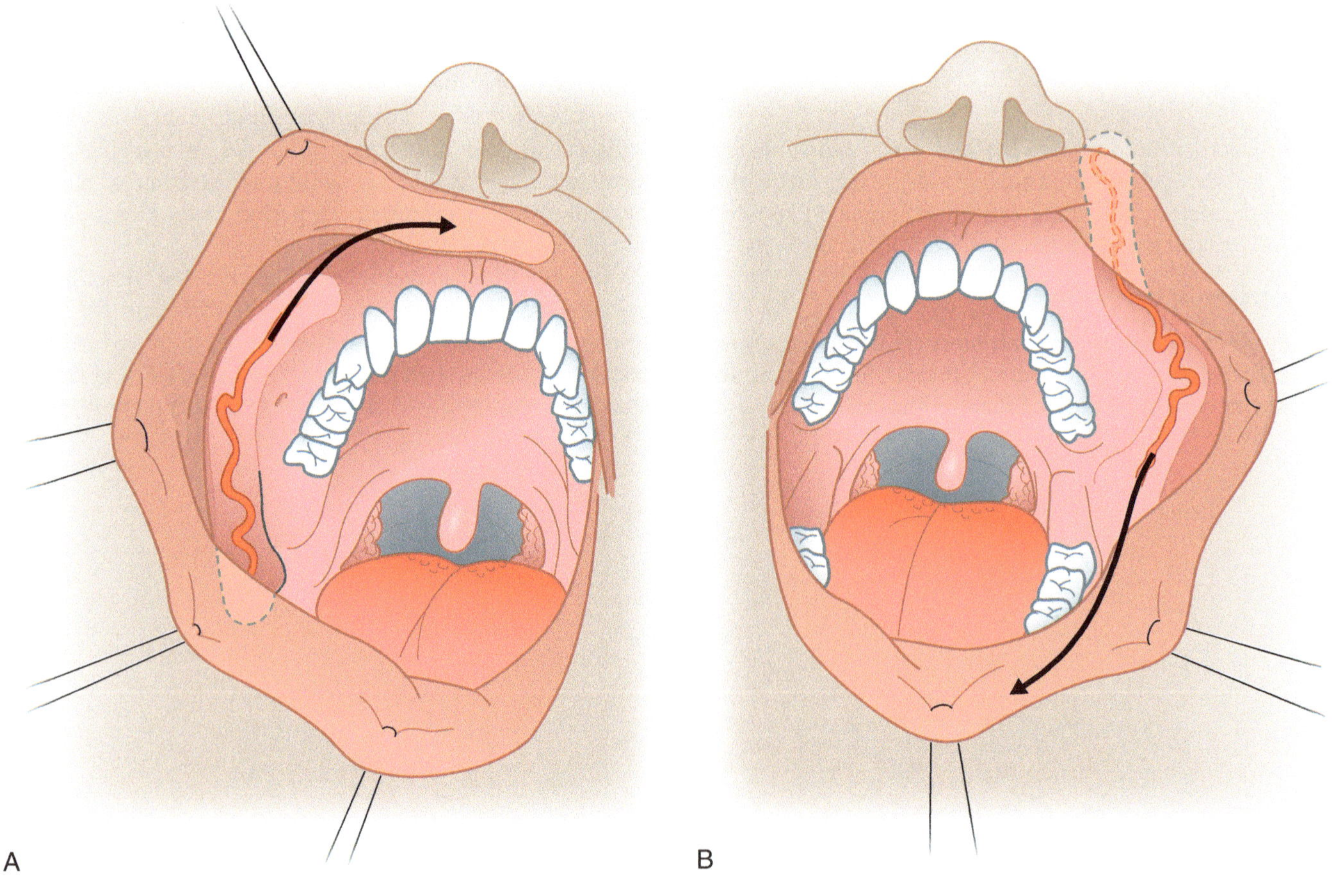

• **Fig. 29.4** Illustrations of the (A) superiorly based and (B) inferiorly based facial artery myomucosal flaps (FAMM flaps) described by Professor Julian Pribaz.[12]

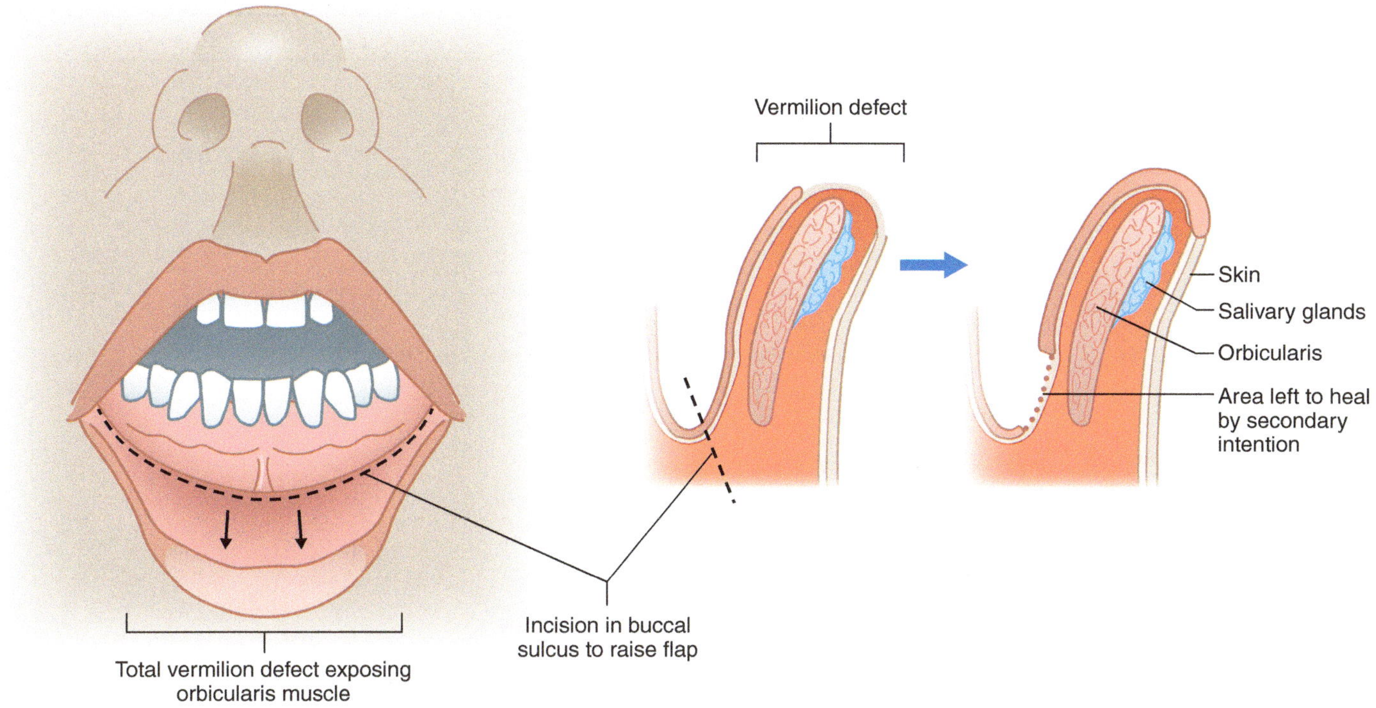

• **Fig. 29.5** A schematic diagram of the bipedicled myomucosal advancement flaps described by Converse for total vermilion reconstruction. The donor defect is left to heal by secondary intention.

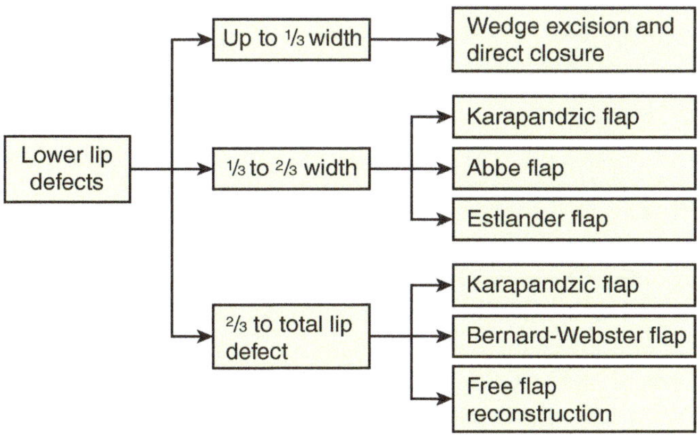

• **Fig. 29.6** The rule of thirds as an algorithm for reconstruction of full-thickness lower lip defects.

Defects between One- and Two-Thirds Width

Defects between a third and two-thirds of the width of the lower lip will require reconstruction with a flap. For these defects, local flaps offer the best option. The three main choices are the Karapandzic flap, Abbe flap, and Estlander flap.

The Karapandzic flap, first described in 1974,[14] is a rotation-advancement flap, which reestablishes the circumoral sphincter. The Karapandzic flap contains skin, innervated orbicularis oris, and mucosa, and can be used to reconstruct both upper and lower lip defects (Fig. 29.8). The key element in raising this flap is to translate the vertical height of the lip defect to the width of the flap. Curvilinear incisions are made through skin, and muscle, releasing the muscle fibers and suspensory ligaments but preserving the superior and inferior labial arteries and buccal branches of the facial nerve. The mucosal incisions are more limited, placed in the buccal sulcus long enough simply to enable advancement of the musculocutaneous component of the flaps. In the superiorly based Karapandzic flaps for lower lip defects, the mucosal incisions should only extend up to the mental nerve at the canine root in order to preserve sensation to any residual lower lip tissue. Limited mucosal incisions also prevent effacement of the buccal sulcus, which can lead to salivary incompetence.

The Karapandzic flap should be the first choice of reconstruction for moderate sized defects as it is innervated, dynamic, and therefore functional. The main disadvantage of the Karapandzic flap is the potential risk of microstomia, and the need for surgical revision to deepen the buccal sulcus if it is effaced.

The Abbe flap, described in 1898,[15] is a staged lip-switch flap that provides effective reconstruction of defects of up to two-thirds of the width of the lip not involving the oral commissure. The Abbe flap is raised from the junction of the middle and lateral thirds of the opposite lip, with a flap of approximately half the width of the defect but equal in height. Prior to raising the flap, the vermilion border on either side of the incisions, i.e., four points, is carefully marked to enable accurate closure of the donor site and inset of the flap. The flap is pedicled on the corresponding labial artery, its location identified on the free edge of the flap as the artery can be palpated. The pedicle is divided 14–21 days later (Fig. 29.9).

The main advantage of the Abbe flap is the ability to replace the vertical height of the defect and import

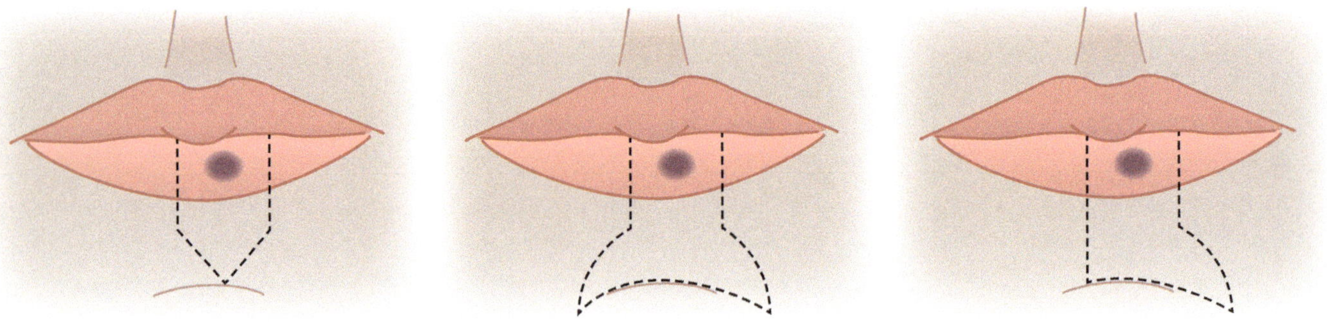

• **Fig. 29.7** Variation in wedge excision and primary closure of lower lip defects.

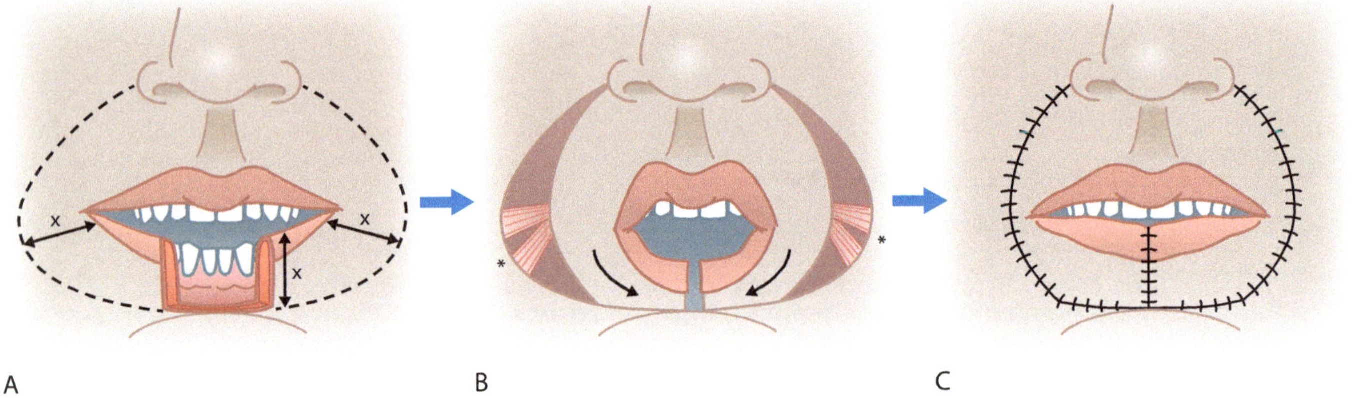

• **Fig. 29.8** Schematic diagram of the Karapandzic flap. (A) The defect following tumor extirpation. Note the height of the defect, *x*, is equivalent to the width of each flap. The mucosal incisions are more limited. (B) The flap raised, preserving the neurovascular bundles (*) to each flap. (C) The final appearance of the lips, with a smaller oral aperture.

vermilion tissue into the defect. However, the disadvantages include a period of lip adhesion, imbalance of the white roll and vermilion and the insensate segment of imported tissue. Furthermore, as previously mentioned, around a third of the population have a unilateral origin of the superior labial artery, which has implications on the pivot point of the flap, i.e., the pivot point should be more proximal whereby the caliber of the artery is larger.

The Estlander flap, described in 1872,[16] is a single-stage lip-switch flap for defects involving the oral commissure (Fig. 29.10). The flap is based medially, and is rotated into the defect to reconstruct the commissure and lip. Similar to the Abbe flap, the flap is designed to be equal in height but half the width of the defect. The reconstructed oral commissure usually has an obtuse or blunted angle, and frequently requires revision by means of a commissuroplasty. This is described further in the chapter.

Defects More than Two-Thirds Width or Total Lip Defect

Lower lip defects greater than two-thirds of the total width can be addressed with local flaps in selected cases. The Karapandzic flap previously described can be used for defects up to 80% of the total width. The main advantage of this flap is that it is innervated and therefore dynamic. However, the disadvantage of the Karapandzic flaps is the resulting microstomia. Other local flaps, such as the Gillies fan, McGregor and Nakajima flaps, have been described for large defects of the lower lip but these flaps are largely obsolete in our practice. The Gillies fan flap distorts the oral commissure, the McGregor and Nakajima flaps reconstruct the lip but the muscle fiber direction is changed and a new vermilion is required.

The Bernard flap (described in 1853)[17] with the Webster modification provides the best reconstructive local option for total lip defects. The original Bernard operation involves a triangular wedge excision of the whole lower lip. The incision is extended laterally from both oral commissures with full-thickness triangular excision at the nasolabial area to enable direct closure of the lower lip wedge (Fig. 29.11). The Webster modification, described in 1960,[18] employs the principles of:

- Quadrilateral or rectangular resection
- Medial advancement of one or two cheek-lip flaps
- Excision of skin and subcutaneous tissue only for removal of tissue excess
- Minimal incisions through the muscle laterally
- Buccal mucosa flaps for vermilion replacement
- *Z*-plasties on all vertical suture lines.[19]

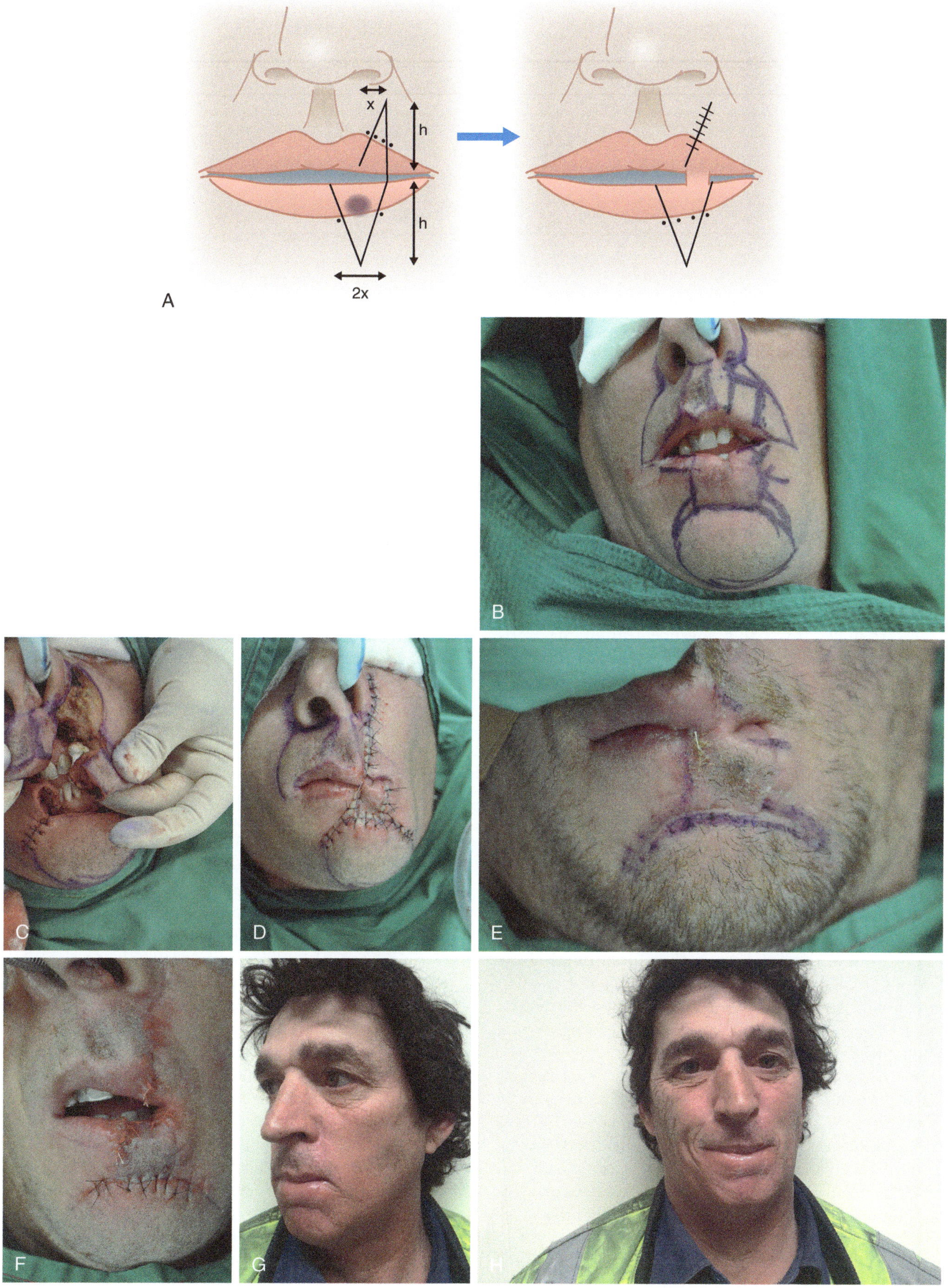

• **Fig. 29.9** (A) Schematic diagram of the Abbe flap. The flap is raised at the junction of the middle and lateral thirds of the contralateral lip. The four points denoting the vermilion border either side of the incisions for the flap are marked. The width of the flap (*x*) is half that of the defect (2*x*), but the height of the flap (*h*) is equivalent to that of the defect. The flap pedicle containing the labial artery is left attached for 2–3 weeks before division. (B) Design of upper lip Abbe flap for recurrent squamous cell carcinoma following previous wedge resection. (C) Raised flap and nasolabial excisions at donor site. (D) Inset of the first-stage Abbe flap. (E, F) Division and inset during second stage at 21 days. (G, H) Postoperative result. (B–H, Photos courtesy Dr. Rostam D. Farhadieh.)

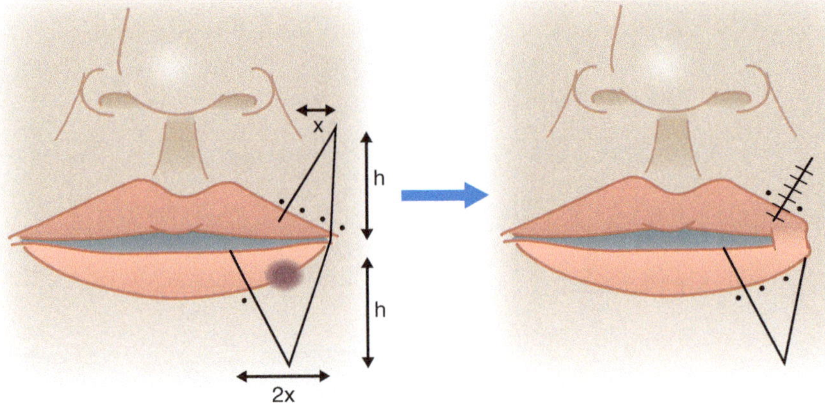

• **Fig. 29.10** Schematic diagram illustrating the Estlander flap to reconstruct defects involving the oral commissure. The four points denoting the vermilion border either side of the incisions for the flap are marked. The width of the flap (*x*) is half that of the defect (2*x*), but the height of the flap (*h*) is equivalent to that of the defect. Note the blunted neocommissure, which is a common sequelae of this flap. This may require a commissuroplasty at a later stage.

Hence, the planning of the Bernard–Webster flap begins with the cheek advancement flaps. The length of each advancement flap is equivalent to half the length of the horizontal lip defect. Then, superior curvilinear incisions are made along the nasolabial fold, integrated into Burrow's triangles, to enable advancement of the horizontal cheek advancement flaps. Inferiorly, incisions are made along the labiomental fold, also incorporated into Burrow's triangles. These incisions are deepened through skin, subcutaneous tissue, and muscle to the level of the mucosa. The mucosa is only incised medially to allow advancement of the cheek tissue, preserving as much of the intraoral lining as possible. These medial incisions are also placed superior to the skin flap design to allow mucosa to be delivered anteriorly and everted to create the vermilion of the reconstructed lip. Finally, the medial edges of each flap are inset with a three-layer closure. There is a relative contraindication for this flap in patients who have had previous facial surgery, or neck dissections resulting in ligation of the facial artery, thus compromising the cutaneous circulation. The other disadvantages of this flap are the potential for microstomia, notching of the central lip and effacement of the buccal sulcus, leading to oral incompetence.

The other less favored option for total lip reconstruction is free tissue transfer. Whenever possible, local tissue must be used to reconstruct the lips. However, this may not be possible due to the need to reconstruct composite defects involving the whole lip and adjacent regions such as the chin and cheeks, the lack of suitable local tissue as the result of previous surgery or radiotherapy, and finally the increasing proficiency of plastic surgeons in performing microsurgical reconstruction. Care and attention should be paid when deciding on the choice of free flap reconstruction. Factors to take into consideration include skin color match, the volume required to fill the defect, the ability to contour the flap to fit the defect, and the feasibility of suspending the flap to prevent ptosis. Surgeons have proposed a multitude of flaps for lower lip reconstruction. The list includes radial forearm, anterolateral thigh, parascapular, rectus abdominis,[20] and lateral arm flaps. These flaps can either be used in isolation, in combination with another flap, either locally based or free tissue transfer, or prelamination of a free flap. The radial forearm free flap is the most popular choice because it provides a good color match, thin and therefore can be easily folded, has a long pedicle, can be harvested simultaneously during the oncological resection of the lower lip or preparation of neck recipient vessels, and can be harvested with the palmaris longus tendon as a static sling to suspend the lower lip reconstruction (Fig. 29.12).

When undertaking free flap reconstruction, the first step involves obtaining a template of the defect. The surgeon needs to be aware that the defect usually appears larger than the actual size of the tissue lost. This is due to the pull of the perioral and facial mimetic muscles, which retract the edge of the defect laterally. Thus, it is important to place tension on the edges of the defect medially before obtaining the template. Once the free flap has been raised, insetting the flap is another crucial process. The tension of the flap needs to be taut enough to prevent ptosis leading to salivary incompetence, but not too tight resulting in compromise to flap perfusion. Attention must also be directed towards the depth of the gingivobuccal sulcus, ensuring adequate depth to prevent drooling. If a static sling is placed simultaneously to suspend the flap, the sling is attached to a relatively stable structure, and the senior author prefers the periosteum of the zygomatic arch. Some authors advocate attaching the sling to remnants of zygomaticus major muscle to obtain a measure of dynamic movement.

The disadvantage of free flap reconstruction is that both the tissue and sling can relax with time, leading to ptosis, and oral incompetence. Furthermore, the results are esthetically inferior to local flaps.

Full-Thickness Upper Lip Defect

We previously alluded to the topographical difference between the upper and lower lips, and due consideration has to be given to the philtral columns and Cupid's bow

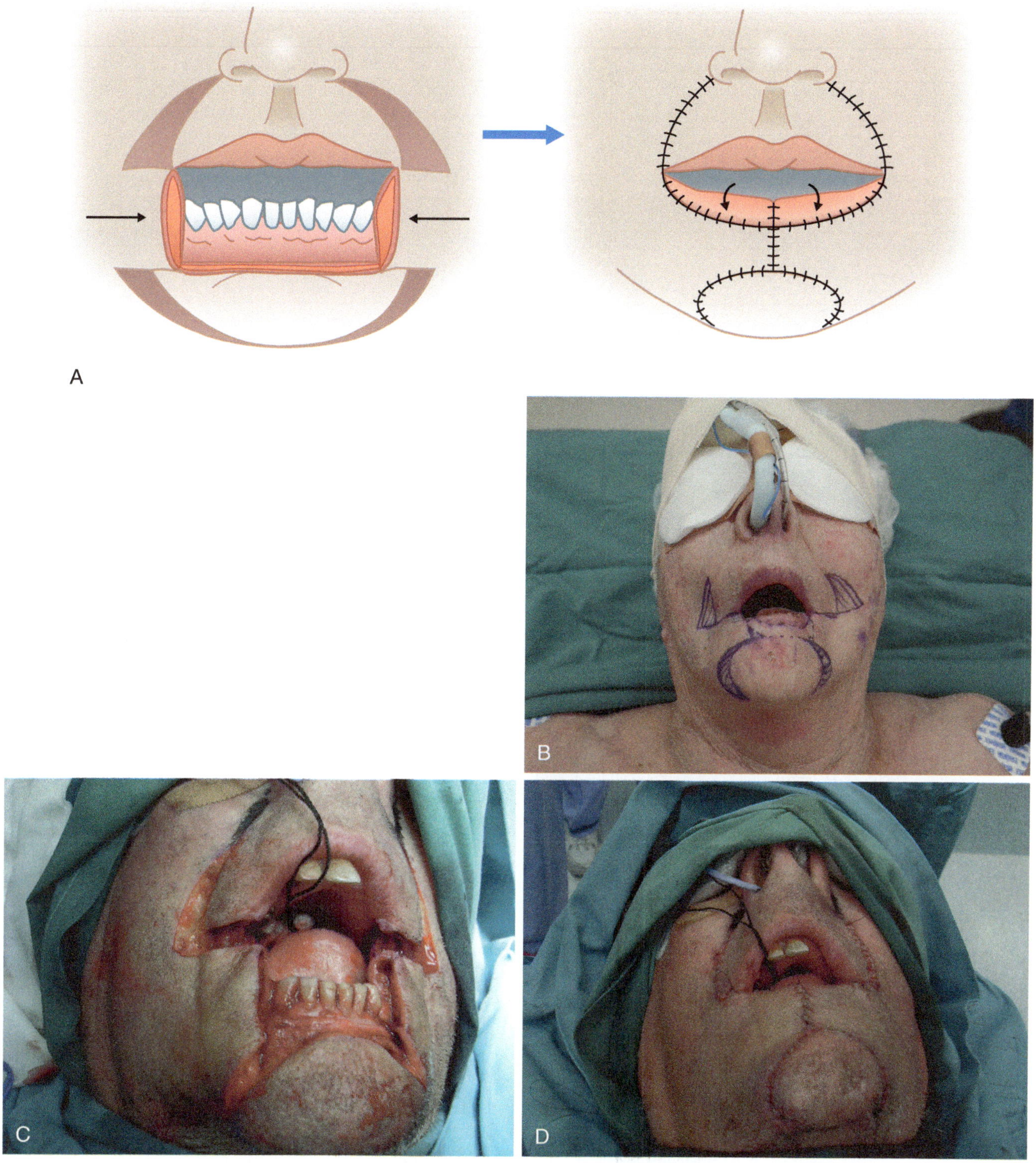

• **Fig. 29.11** The Bernard–Webster flap: (A) Illustration demonstrating the quadrilateral or rectangular defect following tumor extirpation, medial advancement of the two cheek–lip flaps, excision of skin and subcutaneous tissue only for removal of tissue excess (hashed area), minimal incisions through the muscle laterally and buccal mucosa flaps for vermilion replacement. (B–D) Clinical photographs of a modified Bernard–Webster flap for a total lower lip reconstruction following excision of a recurrent squamous cell carcinoma. (B–D, photos courtesy Dr. Rostam D. Farhadieh.)

when planning the reconstruction. In men, the hair-bearing area of the upper lip is a further confounding factor in choice of reconstruction.

Similar to the lower lip, the rules of thirds are also used for the upper lip. Fig. 29.13 illustrates a useful algorithm for upper lip defects.

Defects Less than One-Third Width

Upper lip defects that do not involve the vermilion can be reconstructed with a full-thickness skin graft or local flaps such as the nasolabial flap. In men, hair-bearing tissue from the temporal scalp[21–23] provides a reconstructive option that restores the moustache.

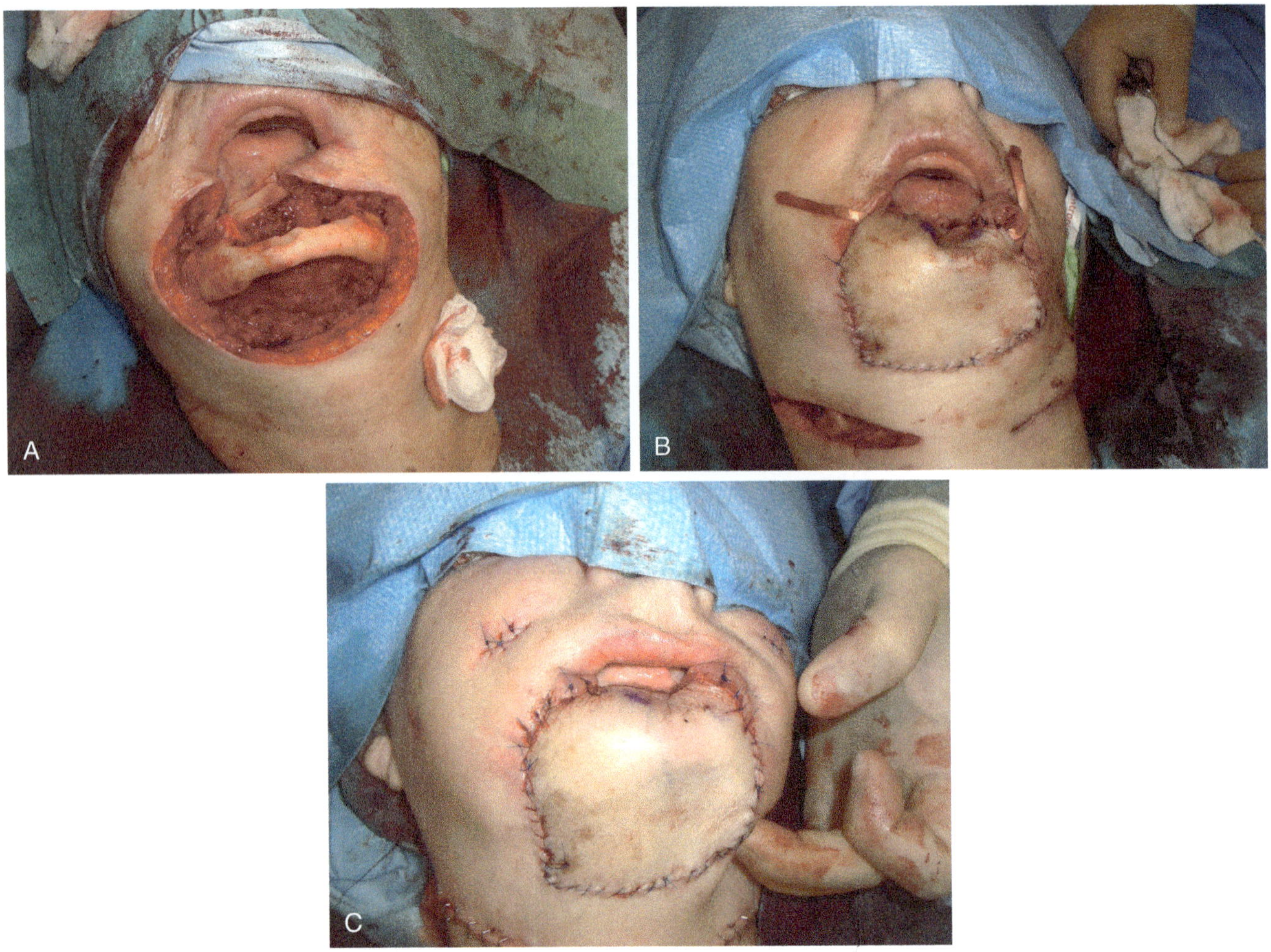

• **Fig. 29.12** (A–C) Total lower lip reconstruction with radial forearm free flap. The flap has been suspended over a palmaris longus graft which was secured to the zygomatic arches.

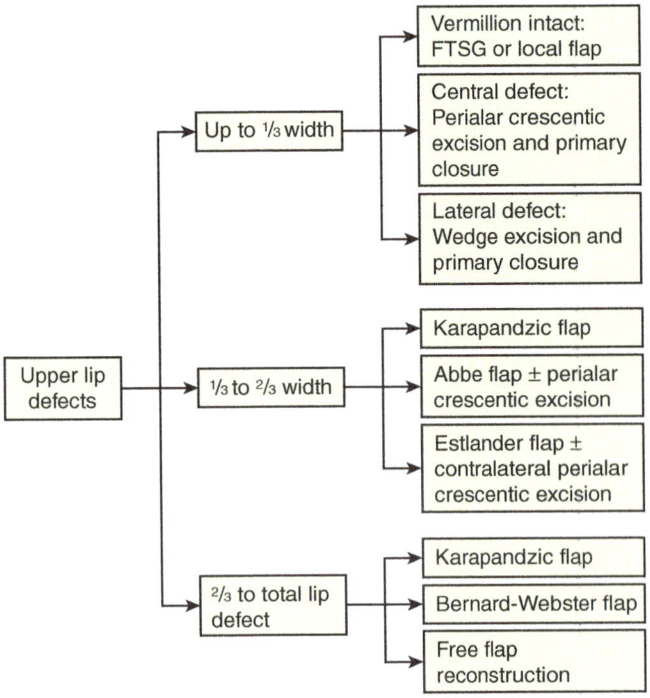

• **Fig. 29.13** The rule of thirds is a useful algorithm for reconstruction of full-thickness defects of the upper lip. FTSG, full-thickness skin graft.

Lateral defects located between the philtral columns and the oral commissures are closed directly as for the lower lip, ensuring accurate approximation of the white roll and vermilion border. Central defects involving the philtral columns and Cupid's bow are also closed directly, but a useful adjunct is Webster's perialar crescentic excision and bilateral cheek advancement flaps (Fig. 29.14).

Defects between One-Third and Two-Thirds Width

As for the lower lip, the Karapandzic flap remains the first choice for local flap reconstruction of the upper lip, as it is dynamic and innervated, thereby providing a functional reconstruction. The alternatives are the Abbe and Estlander flaps. The former is employed for central defects, and the latter for defects involving the oral commissure. The perialar crescentic excision is a useful adjunct for the Abbe flap in reconstructing central defects, and can also aid in closure of lateral defects together with the Estlander flap (by means of a contralateral perialar crescentic excision).

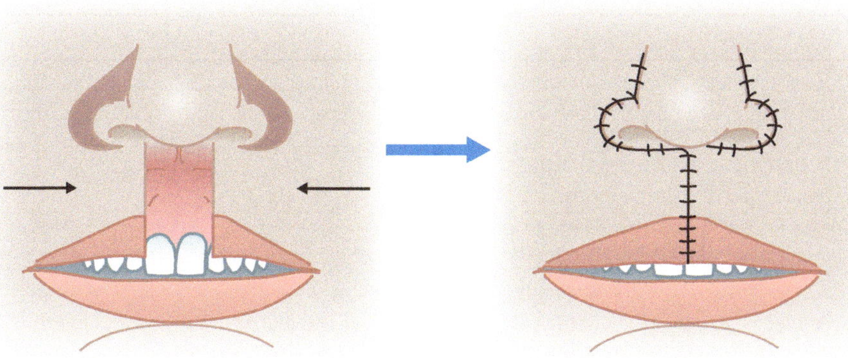

• **Fig. 29.14** Schematic diagram illustrating the Webster's perialar crescentic advancement flaps. The hashed area denotes skin excision only.

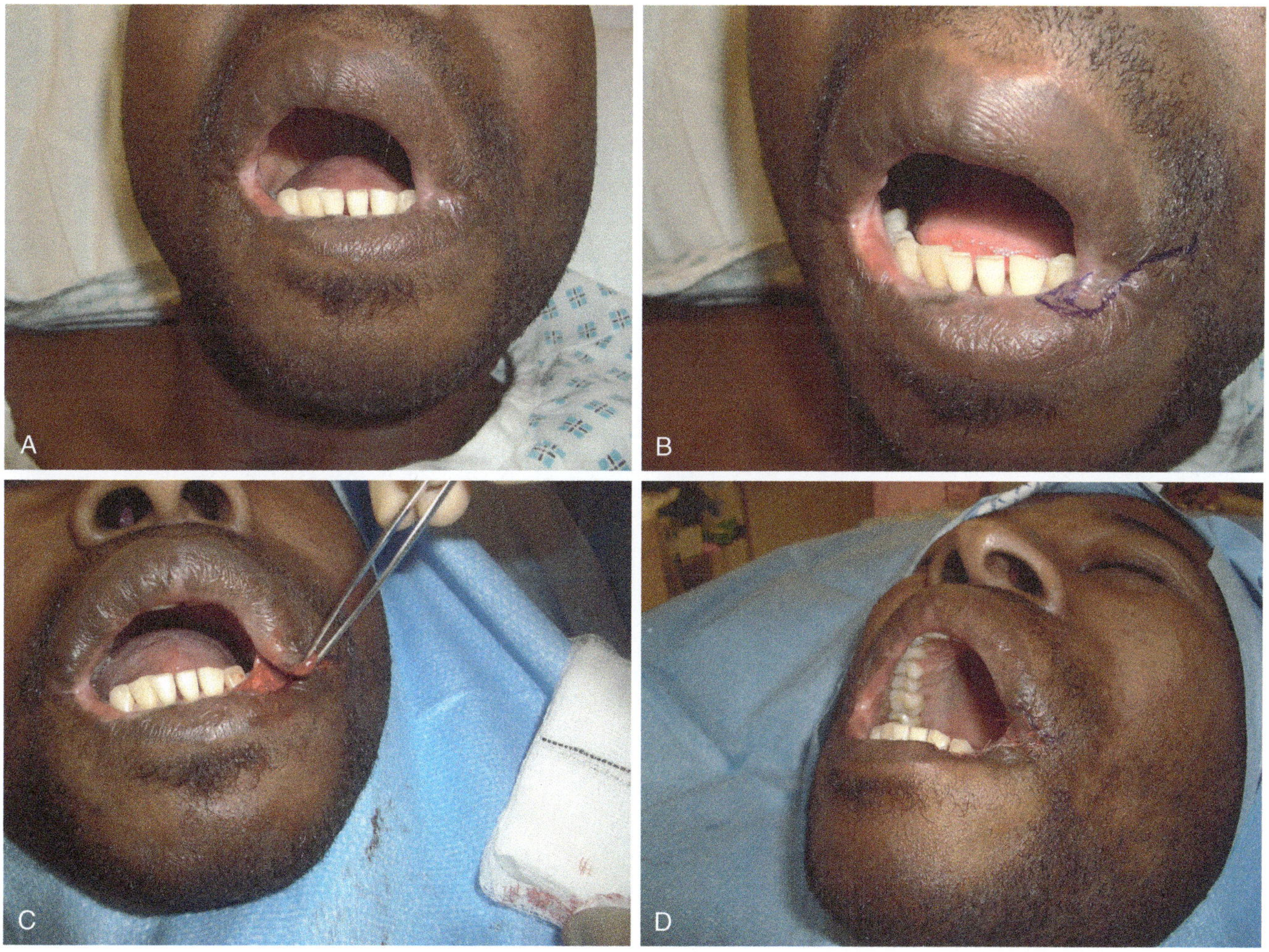

• **Fig. 29.15** (A–D) Left commissuroplasty following an acid burn. The right had been previously released.

Defects More than Two-Thirds Width or Total Lip Defect

The same algorithm as for the lower lip applies for the upper lip, i.e., the Karapandzic flap, Bernard–Webster flap or free tissue transfer.

Commissuroplasty

Commissuroplasty is indicated in patients with microstomia, or a blunted oral commissure following lip reconstruction with local flaps such as the Estlander or Karapandzic flaps.

In these patients, wherever possible, the vermilion is utilized either as advancement or transposition flaps. If the vermilion is too small or inadequate, then the buccal mucosa is used instead or in combination. Several methods have been modified from Dieffenbach's approach in 1831,[24] whereby a triangular wedge of scar tissue is excised and superior, lateral and inferior mucosal flaps are advanced to resurface the corner of the mouth.

A popular contemporary method is Converse's commissuroplasty, described in 1959 (Fig. 29.15).[25] A triangular area of skin is excised to accommodate the elongated commissure.

The buccal mucosal flaps are designed as shown in Fig. 29.15, incised, and advanced to form the neovermilion.

Conclusion

Lip defects can be approached with a step-wise algorithm ranging from primary closure to free tissue transfer. This chapter has by no means provided a comprehensive catalog of the reconstructive options available. We have not explored here the surgical techniques for congenital lip defects, such as cleft lips (see Chapter 16), craniofacial clefts (see Chapter 19), macrostomia or microstomia; nor have we elaborated on the indications and techniques of face transplantation (see Chapter 11). However, as surgeons, it is imperative we adhere to the basic principles of replacing like with like, and focus on both function and form for lip reconstruction.

References

1. Jabaley ME, Orcutt TW, Clement RL. Applications of the Karapandzic principle of lip reconstruction after excision of lip cancer. *Am J Surg*. 1976;132(4):529–532.
2. Magden O, Edizer M, Tayfur V, Atabey A. Anatomic study of the vasculature of the submental artery flap. *Plast Reconstr Surg*. 2004;114(7):1719–1723.
3. Pinar YA, Bilge O, Govsa F. Anatomic study of the blood supply of perioral region. *Clin Anat*. 2005;18(5):330–339.
4. Magden O, Edizer M, Atabey A, Tayfur V, Ergür I. Cadaveric study of the arterial anatomy of the upper lip. *Plast Reconstr Surg*. 2004;114(2):355–359.
5. Abreu LP, Kruger E, Tennant M. Oral cancer in Western Australia, 1982–2006: a retrospective epidemiological study. *J Oral Pathol Med*. 2010;39(5):376–381.
6. Zide BM, Swift R. How to block and tackle the face. *Plast Reconstr Surg*. 1998;101(3):840–851.
7. Goldstein MH. "Orbiting the orbicularis:" restoration of muscle-ring continuity with myocutaneous flaps. *Plast Reconstr Surg*. 1983;72(3):294–301.
8. Kolhe PS, Leonard AG. Reconstruction of the vermilion after "lip-shave." *Br J Plast Surg*. 1988;41(1):68–73.
9. Mazzola RF, Lupo G. Evolving concepts in lip reconstruction. *Clin Plast Surg*. 1984;11(4):583–617.
10. Standoli L. Cross lip flap in vermilion reconstruction. *Ann Plast Surg*. 1994;32(2):214–217.
11. Kawamoto HK. Correction of major defects of the vermilion with a cross-lip vermilion flap. *Plast Reconstr Surg*. 1979;64(3):315–318.
12. Pribaz J, Stephens W, Crespo L, Gifford G. A new intraoral flap: facial artery musculomucosal (FAMM) flap. *Plast Reconstr Surg*. 1992;90(3):421–429.
13. Lustig J, Librus H, Neder A. Bipedicled myomucosal flap for reconstruction of the lip after vermillionectomy. *Oral Surg Oral Med Oral Pathol*. 1994;77(6):594–597.
14. Karapandzic M. Reconstruction of lip defects by local arterial flaps. *Br J Plast Surg*. 1974;27(1):93–97.
15. Abbe R. A new plastic operation for the relief of deformity due to double harelip. *Plast Reconstr Surg*. 1968;42(5):481–483.
16. Estlander JA, Estlander A. A method of reconstructing loss of substance in one lip from the other lip. *Plast Reconstr Surg*. 1968;42:361–366.
17. Bernard C. Cancer de la lèvre inférieure: restauration à l'aide de deux lambeaux lateraux quadrilatère. *Bull Mem Soc Chir Paris*. 1853;3:357.
18. Webster RC, Coffey RJ, Kelleher RE. Total and partial reconstruction of the lower lip with innervated muscle-bearing flaps. *Plast Reconstr Surg Transplant Bull*. 1960;25:360–371.
19. Zide BM. Deformities of the lips and cheeks. In: McCarthy JG, ed. *Plastic Surgery*. Vol. 3. Philadelphia, PA: W.B. Saunders; 1990:2009–2056.
20. Jallali N, Malata CM. Reconstruction of concomitant total loss of the upper and lower lips with a free vertical rectus abdominis flap. *Microsurgery*. 2005;25(2):118–120.
21. Hyakusoku H, Okubo M, Umeda T, Fumiiri M. A prefabricated hair-bearing island flap for lip reconstruction. *Br J Plast Surg*. 1987;40(1):37–39.
22. Lyons GB, Milroy BC, Lendvay PG, Teston LM. Upper lip reconstruction: use of the free superficial temporal artery hair-bearing flap. *Br J Plast Surg*. 1989;42(3):333–336.
23. Wilson JS, Galvao MS, Brough MD. The application of hair-bearing flaps in head and neck surgery. *Head Neck Surg*. 1980;2(5):386–409.
24. Dieffenbach JF. Chirurgische Erfahrungen, besonders über die Wiederherstellung zerstörter Theile des menschlichen. *Körpers nach neuen Methoden*. 1829.
25. Kazanjian VH, Converse JM. *Kazanjian and Converse's Surgical Treatment of Facial Injuries*. Vol. 1. Baltimore: Williams & Wilkins; 1974:795.

30

Nasal Reconstruction

DAVID W. MATHES, ALINE RAU, AND RYAN CONSTANTINE

Introduction

The nose maintains the central position on the face and often can be a challenging structure to successfully reconstruct, both its form and the function. The fundamental techniques of reconstruction emerged early in history as a response to the use of nasal rhinokopia (nasal amputation) as a punishment.[1,2] Sushruta Samitha (600 BC) described both the use of pedicled cheek flaps and the paramedian forehead flap for nasal reconstruction.[2,3] In 15th-century Italy, Antonio Branca first described the use of a pedicled flap from the arm for nasal reconstruction (often known in Europe as the Italian technique). This technique was further popularized by Gaspare Tagliocozzi with his version of this flap (Tagliocozzi flap). Later, a series of surgeons in France further refined the use of the pedicled cheek flap.

In the modern era, nasal defects are commonly encountered after cancer resection and trauma. While there are multiple options available for reconstruction of the nose, the surgeon's challenge is to select the most appropriate option for the defect. There has been a continuous process of improvement of results as the plastic surgeon now pays closer attention to reconstructing the details of the nose (including color and texture match) while minimizing the donor site morbidity.

Surgical Anatomy

The nose is a composite structure composed of three layers: the nasal skeleton, the nasal lining, and the external cover.

Nasal Skeleton

The nasal skeleton is the supporting structure of the nose. It consists of the nasal bones and ascending processes of the maxilla in the upper third, the paired upper lateral cartilages in the middle third, and the lateral paired alae in the lower third.

The upper lateral cartilages are attached lightly to the caudal edge of the nasal bones and the dorsal border of the nasal septum, the "keystone area," allowing them to remain suspended above the nasal cavity. At the junction of septum and upper lateral cartilages, the dorsal border of the septum widens to form a "T." This broadening is crucial, as it maintains the aperture of the internal valve during nasal inspiration.

The paired alae support the lower third of the nose by uniting to form a tripod configuration with the nasal tip, as first described by Anderson.[4] The paired medial crura form the central leg of the tripod and are attached to the anterior nasal spine and septum in the midline. The lateral crura compose the two lateral legs of this tripod, and they are attached to the pyriform aperture. Between the lateral and medial crura, the dome defines the apex of the alar cartilage. It supports the nasal tip and is responsible for the light reflex of the tip. The region of fibrous connection of the ala with the upper lateral cartilages is known as the "scroll" area. The normal ala does not contain cartilage but a compact stiff fibrofatty tissue. Alar reconstruction has to include cartilage, however, to prevent collapse and retraction.

Nasal Lining

The nasal lining consists of a thin layer of vascular mucosa. The nasal vestibule is lined by stratified squamous epithelium, while internally it is lined by mucosa. The lining tightly adheres to the deep surface of the nasal skeleton. The mobility of the mucosa is limited by this dense adherence. Consequently, only the smallest of mucosal defects (<5 mm) can be closed primarily. The anterior septal branch of the labial artery and medial internal nasal branch of the anterior ethmoid artery may be used for lining flaps as described below.

Nasal Cover

From deep to superficial, the nasal skeleton is covered by perichondrium/periosteum, an areolar tissue plane, a musculoaponeurotic plane, a subcutaneous layer (a few millimeters of fat), dermis, and epidermis. In the upper two-thirds of the nose, the skin is thin, loose, and mobile, with a slight excess. It contains few sebaceous glands. Proceeding inferiorly from the glabella, skin thickness decreases over the cartilaginous dorsum and upper lateral cartilages. Conversely, as it reaches the tip and ala, the skin becomes thick, sebaceous, and tightly adherent to the ala, which limits mobility.

Thus, regardless of design, local flaps will generally mobilize the upper thirds of skin excess to resurface inferior defects.

Blood Supply

Nasal vasculature runs in the subcutaneous layer. On each side of the nose, the blood supply is derived from the dorsal nasal branch of the ophthalmic artery, which creates an axial network for the dorsal and lateral nasal skin. The angular artery, a branch of the facial artery, passes medially along the cephalic margin of the lateral crura, just above the alar groove, supplying the lateral surface of the caudal nose. The columellar artery, a branch of the superior labial artery, supplies the nasal sill, septum, and base of the columella. Finally, the infraorbital branch of the internal maxillary artery supplies the dorsum and lateral sidewalls of the nose. Venous drainage parallels the arterial system.

The anterior septal branch of the superior labial artery, medial internal nasal branch of the anterior ethmoid artery, septal branch of posterior ethmoid artery, posterior septal branch of sphenopalatine artery, and greater palatine artery supply nasal mucosa (Fig. 30.1).

Innervation

Sensation of the nose is provided by two divisions of the trigeminal nerve. The ophthalmic division (V_1) innervates the radix, rhinion, and cephalic portion of the nasal sidewalls, as well as the skin from dorsum to tip. The maxillary division (V_2) innervates the lateral tissue on the lower half of the nose as well as the lateral vestibule. The facial nerve supplies

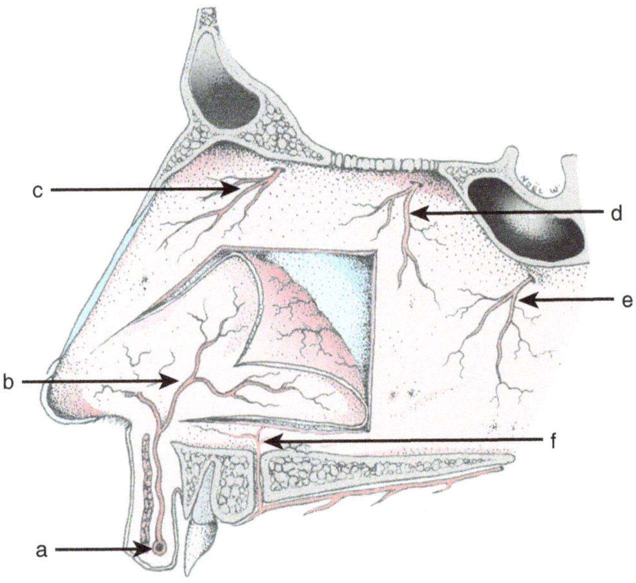

• **Fig. 30.1** Demonstration of the vascular supply of the nose: *a*, superior labial artery; *b*, anterior septal branch of superior labial artery; *c*, medical internal nasal branch of anterior ethmoid artery; *d*, septal branch of posterior ethmoid artery; *e*, posterior septal branch of sphenopalatine artery; *f*, branch of the greater palatine artery.

the muscles of the nose, specifically the nasalis, procerus, and depressor septi nasi.

Principles of Reconstruction

The goals of nasal reconstruction are to optimize nasal esthetics while maintaining nasal function and airway patency. After a thorough presurgical evaluation of the patient, the extent of the nasal defect is defined by what tissue is missing. The reconstruction is then designed based on addressing all three layers to obtain a satisfactory outcome. In addition, the defect location will often dictate the best reconstructive option to achieve a satisfactory reconstruction.

Presurgical Evaluation

To ensure a satisfactory reconstruction, complete patient evaluation must be undertaken. The general health of the patient must be considered, specifically the comorbidities that may limit the reconstructive options available to the surgeon. Health issues may limit the amount of surgical stages the patient can undertake, the type and duration of the anesthesia, materials that can be harvested from the patient, and techniques that can be applied to the problem.

The nasal wound is next examined with a focus on what is missing anatomically (e.g., cover, lining, or support). To obtain a complete understanding of the defect, it is beneficial to review the patient's old photographs, take normative measurements, and in complex defects consider creating a facial moulage or model. The local and donor tissue are assessed for skin irregularities, overall skin quality, and any existing asymmetries.

When the reconstruction follows the oncologic resection, it is mandatory to confirm negative margins prior to undertaking a reconstruction. Frozen sections obtained at the time of resection risk may not identify residual tumor that will be detected on permanent pathology. If there is any question of the pathology the reconstruction should be delayed with dressing changes or allograft until final pathology results are available.

Defect Analysis

A functionally patent nasal airway and a good esthetic outcome are the basic reconstructive aims. These goals can be met by careful analysis of the defect and meticulous design of the flaps to reconstruct the defect. Often, the contralateral side of the nose is an ideal guide for planning reconstruction.[5] Defect analysis determines the size, location, and thickness of the defect, as well as the quality and laxity of the remnant skin and lining. It is important to note that wound retraction, when present, will give the illusion of a smaller defect.

Nasal defects are categorized by their size, location, and depth. When a defect is less than 5 mm, it can often be closed primarily. Superficial defects with intact support structure and less than 1.5 cm in size can be reconstructed with skin grafts or local flaps. Larger defects, or defects involving the underlying cartilage, usually require reconstruction with interpolated flaps.[6]

Three-Layered Reconstruction

A three-layered reconstruction is often essential to successful reconstruction. The surgeon must consider the lining, support, and cover when planning nasal reconstruction. Each component must be repaired individually if involved in the defect. Overlooking a lining or cartilage loss because it is hidden by skin covering will lead to retraction, collapse that will result in distortion. The surgeon must also assess surrounding structures such as the cheek and lip. These must be reconstructed first, because aberrant surrounding structures will lead to an abnormal-appearing nose, even if the nose itself has a satisfactory reconstruction.

Subunit Principle

As described by Millard[7] and modified by Burget and Menick,[8,9] the naturally lit ridges and shadowed valleys of the nose divide its surface into nine esthetic subunits (dorsum, sidewalls, alar lobules, soft triangles, columella, and tip that can be divided into two hemi–tips) (Fig. 30.2). Using the esthetic subunits during surgical planning allows for a logical approach to reconstruction that achieves a satisfactory esthetic result. The contralateral subunit may be used as a guide for reconstruction, and if the defect is large, it may be divided into multiple subunits using this principle. When reconstructing an esthetic subunit, the defect should be reconstructed with tissue of similar quantity and quality of the missing tissue.[6] The subunit principle also endorses that when more than 50% of a unit is involved in the defect, the entire subunit is excised and reconstructed. This will position the scars between subunits, camouflaging them and minimizing contour distortion such as pincushioning or trapdoor contraction.[5,6]

However, the subunit principle should not been seen as an absolute rule and even Menick,[10] does not apply the subunit rule when reconstructing dorsal or sidewall defects. These areas have indistinct border outlines and are relatively flat surfaces, and as such the reconstructions can be limited to the defect alone. It has also been reported that in these areas skin grafts do not undergo trapdoor contraction. Other authors use the subunit principle as a guideline and often use defect-only reconstruction. In defect-only reconstruction, as described by Rohrich et al,[11] the defect is reconstructed without excising healthy tissue in the subunit. These authors use adjunct procedures, such as dermabrasion, to improve the esthetic result and decrease the need for additional revisions.

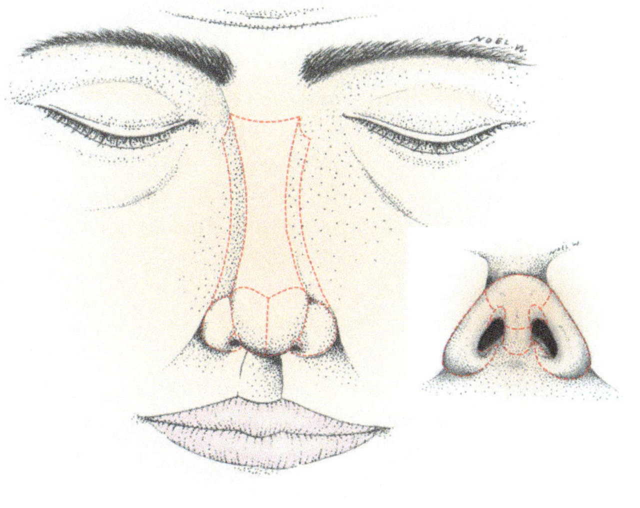

• **Fig. 30.2** Esthetic subunits of the nose: 1 dorsum, 2 sidewalls, 1 tip (divided into two hemi–tips), 2 alar lobules, 2 soft triangles, 1 columella.

Small and Superficial Defects

Nasal defects can be classified into two groups: small superficial defects and large and/or full-thickness defects. The first group typically only requires skin replacement whereas the second will often necessitate a three-layered reconstruction consisting of inner lining, cartilage, and skin. Small and superficial defects entail the loss of skin and underlying subcutaneous fat or muscle that can be left to heal by secondary intention or repaired by direct closure, full-thickness grafts, or local skin flaps. These small and superficial defects can generally be repaired with a single-stage procedure.

Secondary Intention Healing

All superficial defects on the nose, provided that they are well vascularized, will heal over time. For example, after rhinophyma excision, it is recommended to let the entire nose surface heal by secondary intention. Granulation tissue, epithelialization, and wound contracture will lead to a flat, thin, shiny, and atrophic scar initially. Thus, secondary intention is best suited to thin skin areas and flat or concave surfaces (upper two-thirds of the nose). Conversely, healing by secondary intention for defects encompassing adjacent landmarks or the alar rim would result in distortion of the shape and normal appearance of the nose.

Healing by secondary intention is best indicated on sidewalls (especially near the internal canthus) and dorsum defects. This method can also provide good results on the tip and in alar regions when the defect is small (less than 5 mm) and more than 8–10 mm away from the alar rim. The postoperative care is typically simple for the patient, and involves daily cleansing of the wound and moist dressing changes. Antibiotics or local antiseptic is rarely necessary.

Direct Closure

Direct closure is often the best technique when certain that it will not distort the nasal landmarks or result in nostril margin retraction. Primary closure will generally leave an acceptable scar, especially when its axis is longitudinal and in the midline, or the defect is less than 5 mm. Undermining is often necessary in order to decrease tension.

Generally, direct closure is possible in wounds in the upper two-thirds of the nose where there is a slight excess of skin. Conversely, direct closure is not recommended on the ala, tip or columella, which are areas of poor skin laxity, as it would distort landmarks and retract the nostril.

Full-Thickness Graft

Despite their often unpredictable final outcome, full-thickness skin grafts (FTSG) can be a useful tool in many cases, provided that the recipient bed is well vascularized. Avascular surfaces such as cartilage and bone cannot support a skin graft. Skin grafts can be considered in patients who have superficial defects less than 1 cm in size. Ideally, candidates for skin grafting would be nonsmokers in order to optimize the chances of graft take.[12]

Immobility and direct contact with the recipient bed is vital. Quilting sutures and a tie-over bolster dressing using a petroleum gauze can aid in immobilizing skin grafts. Generally, the bolster is removed within 4–7 days, earlier if any signs of infection are noted. Depending on the wound's depth, it can be employed as a full-thickness skin graft or as a composite graft if underlying soft tissue is carried with the skin. Skin grafts can provide good results in thin skin and flat areas such as dorsum, sidewall, and columella. Skin grafts are a poor match for defects in thick and sebaceous skin zones such as ala, tip, and supratip; however, when circumstances necessitate utilizing an FTSG to reconstruct these thick, sebaceous areas, McCluskey et al advocate using forehead skin, as this area has similar sun exposure and character to these sites.[10,12] If the inferior border of the defect involves the alar rim, an FTSG should be avoided, as alar notching can result.[13]

Skin graft color match is one of the most challenging aspects of this type of reconstruction.[13] The use of FTSGs often result in a patchwork appearance secondary to color mismatch and contour irregularities. This seems to be less prominent when it is performed in individuals with fair skin tone and with superficial defects involving the upper third of the nose.[6] Preauricular, retroauricular, supraclavicular, and forehead skin are often the preferred donor sites. In order to optimize final contour and color match, dermabrasion can be utilized starting 6 weeks postoperatively.

Local Skin Flaps

Local skin flaps mobilize the slight excess of skin within the upper two-thirds of the nose and glabellar zone. Unlike skin grafts, the final color and texture of such flaps are predictable since the intrinsic blood supply of the raised skin is preserved. As they are also thicker than grafts, they can better supply missing subcutaneous tissue, but local skin flaps should be avoided when significant cartilaginous support is missing. In such cases, the reconstructed cartilage framework would most likely not resist the skin tension of a local flap and would risk losing its resistance and shape, leading to collapse and landmark distortion.

The dorsal nasal flap and bilobed flap, described below, should be used with caution during alar reconstruction, as they can have limited reach. If placed under tension, these local flaps can result in alar notching and blunting of the alar groove.

Dorsal Nasal Flap (Rieger's Flap)

Described by Rieger in 1967, the dorsal nasal flap is vascularized by vessels of the sidewall and medial canthus.[14] The skin, subcutaneous tissue and muscles of the upper two-thirds of the nose and glabellar area are elevated just above perichondrium and periosteum and mobilized toward the lower third of the nose. A dog-ear is excised inferiorly and the glabellar donor site is then closed with a V–Y closure (Fig. 30.3). Mobilization of this flap can be increased by Marchac's modification, which narrows the pedicle around the medial canthus zone with a counter-incision at the junction between cheek and sidewall.[15]

The dorsal nasal flap is particularly suitable for nasal tip defects that are less than 2.5 cm, and where a forehead flap may be unsuitable or undesirable for the patient. When utilizing the dorsal nasal flap, the defect should be at least 1 cm away from the alar rim, as it tends to retract causing nasal tip and nostril margin displacement. It is also useful for upper third nasal defect (Fig. 30.4). Additionally, this flap approximates the eyebrows and creates a radix fullness that often necessitates a revision.

Bilobed Flap

Zitelli's bilobed flap is a double transposition flap widely used for defects up to 1.5 cm in diameter located within the lower third of the nose (Fig. 30.5).[16] This flap provides excellent skin and texture match, and is particularly suited for defects involving the ala with an intact alar rim, lateral tip, or supratip. In patients with nasal valve collapse secondary to loss of alar support, this flap can accommodate the use of a cartilage graft.[6]

The first lobe is designed adjacent to the defect with the same diameter. The slightly smaller second lobe is designed adjacent to the first one, and has to lie in an area of laxity to allow its direct closure (upper two-thirds). The angle of transposition is approximately 45° for each lobe. In general, the flap is based laterally for tip and supratip defects and medially for alar defects. After resection of the inferior dog-ear between pivot point and defect, the flap is incised and elevated. Wide undermining of the defect borders, flap base, and donor site just above the perichondrium and periosteum facilitates transposition and minimizes distortion. The first lobe is then mobilized to cover the defect and the second lobe shifts to repair the defect created by the first lobe. This final defect is closed directly.

Though a useful single-stage local flap, the bilobed flap does have the disadvantage that it has a complex design,

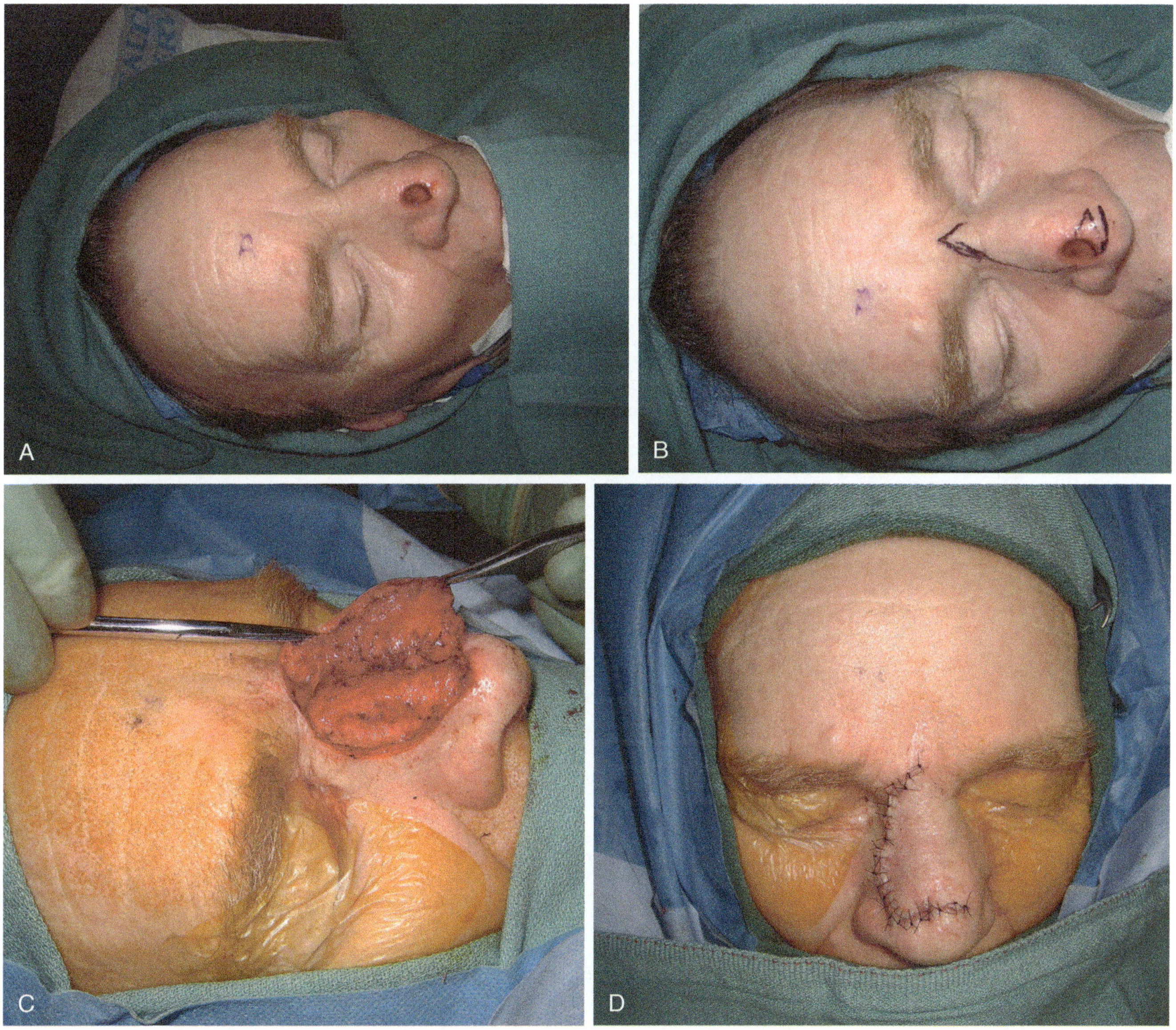

• **Fig. 30.3** Dorsal nasal flap lower third of the nose (classic indication): (A) distal nasal defect; (B) flap design; (C) flap elevated to periosteum; (D) flap final inset.

violates the esthetic subunit principle, and can potentially greatly distort the nasal tip and ala if not planned precisely.[6] In addition, the flap often require a revision to treat pincushioning or irregular scars.

V–Y Flap Based on Perforators from the Facial Artery

This flap can be designed in the nasal-alar groove and is often the first choice for reconstruction of the soft triangle and lateral portion of the nose. It does not lead to pincushioning or have the issues associated with a patterned flap. The defect is measured and a flap designed that has enough tissue to fill the defect and allow the closure of the V to a Y (Fig. 30.6). Once designed, the flap is elevated down to the perforators (these can be identified with a hand-held Doppler). The perforators do not need to be skeletonized as this puts the flap at risk. It is then closed with deep dermal sutures and external nylon sutures.

Single-Stage Regional Skin Flaps

Regional skin flaps mobilize skin of nearby units of the face from the glabellar and nasolabial area.

Glabellar Flap

Like the Rieger's flap, the laxity in the glabellar area affords the glabellar flap the utility to cover defects of dorsum, medial canthus, or lateral wall. It can accommodate defects up to 2 cm in diameter. This flap is based on the medial canthus, and it can be mobilized using advancement, rotation or transposition. The glabellar flap technique is simple, and

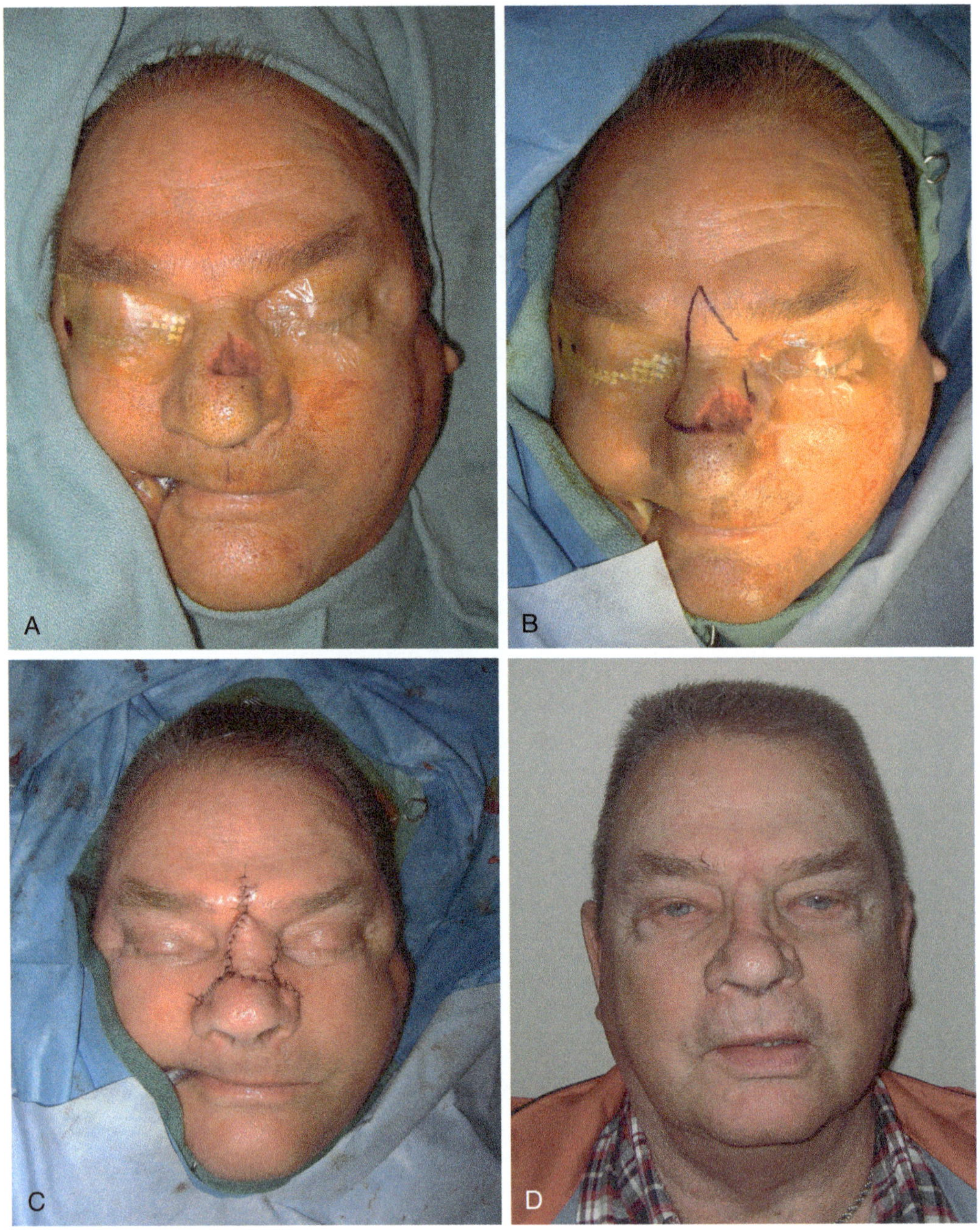

• **Fig. 30.4** Dorsal nasal flap for upper third defect: (A) initial defect; (B) flap design; (C) flap inset; (D) final result.

has low morbidity for the patient and can be rotated into the defect (Fig. 30.7). The donor site can usually be closed primarily with a V–Y closure.[6] While the scars are well hidden, the flap can lead to eyebrow approximation. It is an excellent reconstruction option for frail and elderly patients who need a simple and single-staged reconstruction.

Single-Stage Nasolabial Flap

Directly adjacent to the nasolabial fold, the excess skin of the medial cheek can provide skin for lateral defects of the nose. The color and texture of the single-stage nasolabial flap are similar to those of the alar and sidewall subunits. The nasolabial flap is generally indicated for defects up to 2 cm in diameter (Fig. 30.8). This size corresponds to the maximum width of skin that can be harvested from the medial cheek without leading to unacceptable distortions of the nasolabial fold or asymmetry of the oral commissure due to excessive tension during donor site closure.

In contrast to the two-stage flap, the single-stage nasolabial flap mobilizes the excess skin of the medial cheek as a random pattern flap. As such, the blood supply is not via arterial perforators of the facial artery, but rather from subcutaneous and dermal vessels of the cheek.

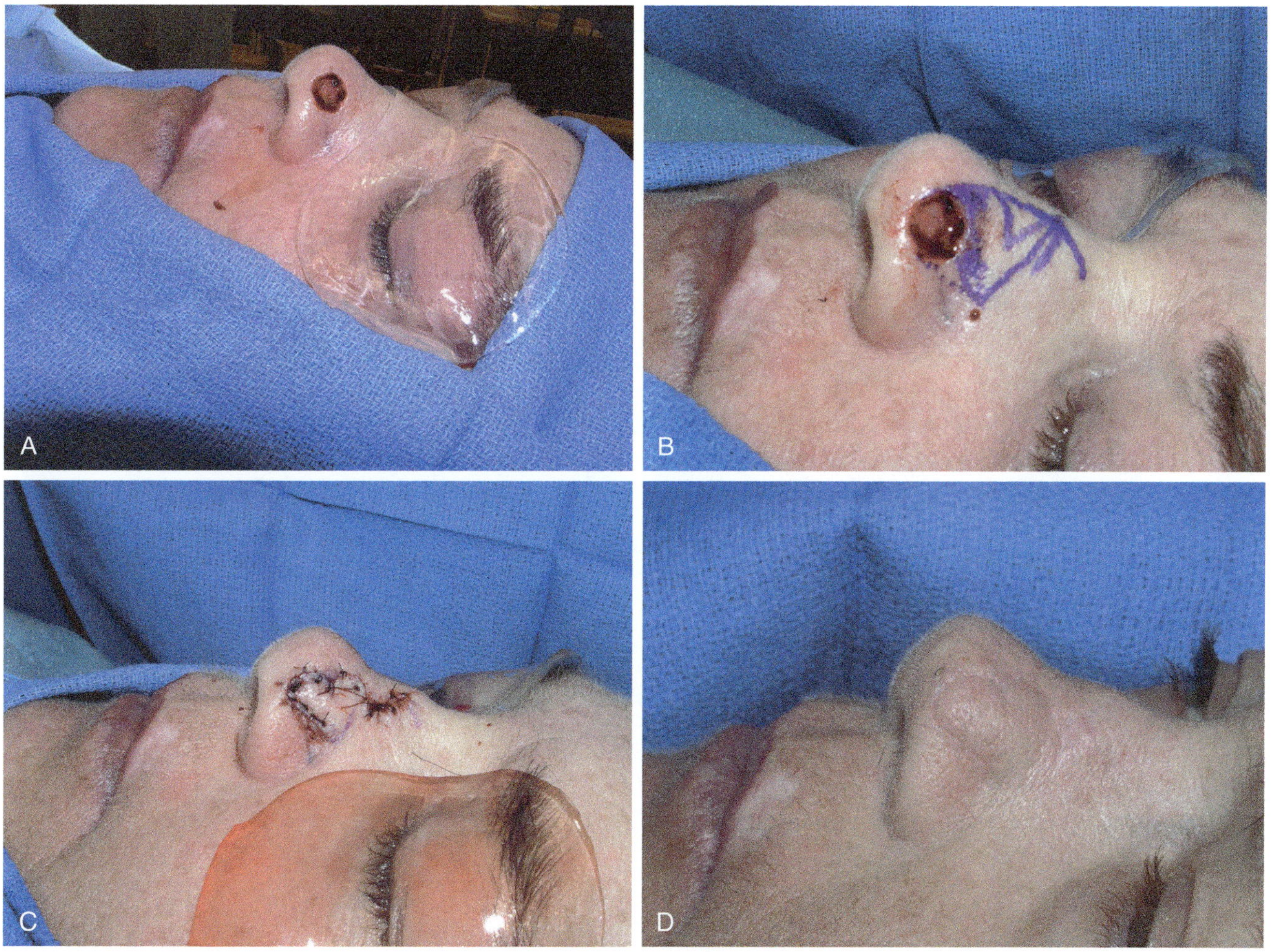

• **Fig. 30.5** Bilobed flap: (A) initial defect; (B) flap design; (C) flap inset; (D) final result. (Case courtesy James Thornton, MD.)

The nasolabial fold has to be outlined on an awake patient, especially in young people, as the crease can be indistinct and only a wide smile can precisely locate it. Prior to skin replacement, an extra-anatomical cartilage graft should brace the lining to prevent collapse and nostril margin retraction. This graft should be quilted to the lining and be of good shape and size.

The flap is designed immediately adjacent to the nasolabial crease. The distal margin of the flap lies within the dog-ear and may be trimmed at closure. The nasolabial flap and its distal dog-ear are incised and raised in continuity with 2 or 3 mm of subcutaneous fat. The lateral incision should not extend higher than the top of the nasolabial fold, as this may compromise the blood supply. The cheek is then elevated just above the superficial musculoaponeurotic system (SMAS). The wider the nasolabial flap, the more extensive undermining of the cheek is required in order to decrease tension at closure. The cheek flap is advanced and attached to deep tissues with solid underlying absorbable sutures along the groove between nose and cheek. This fixation is of vital importance as it will recreate this groove, close the nasolabial incision, and eliminate tension on the nasolabial extension flap. A dog-ear appears on the sidewall, just above the defect, and should be trimmed. Ideally, the alar crease may be recreated with quilting sutures between the flap and lining, at the superior border of the cartilage graft. Attention should be directed at the blood supply and viability of the flap after the quilting sutures are placed, and if there is suspicion of flap ischemia they should be removed. Finally, the flap is thinned again (if necessary), precisely trimmed on its distal margin to fit perfectly, and all incisions are closed.

A disadvantage of the nasolabial flap is that it is prone to pincushioning secondary to contraction. The nasolabial flap will also not reach the dorsum or tip.[5] If more than 2 cm of width is needed for a significant alar defect, the pattern will have to lay parallel to the nasolabial fold, therefore a two-stage flap will be necessary. Often the V–Y perforator flap is a better option for these reconstructions.

Large and/or Deep Defects

While many cases are amenable to a single-stage technique for defect closure, other defects necessitate a multistaged

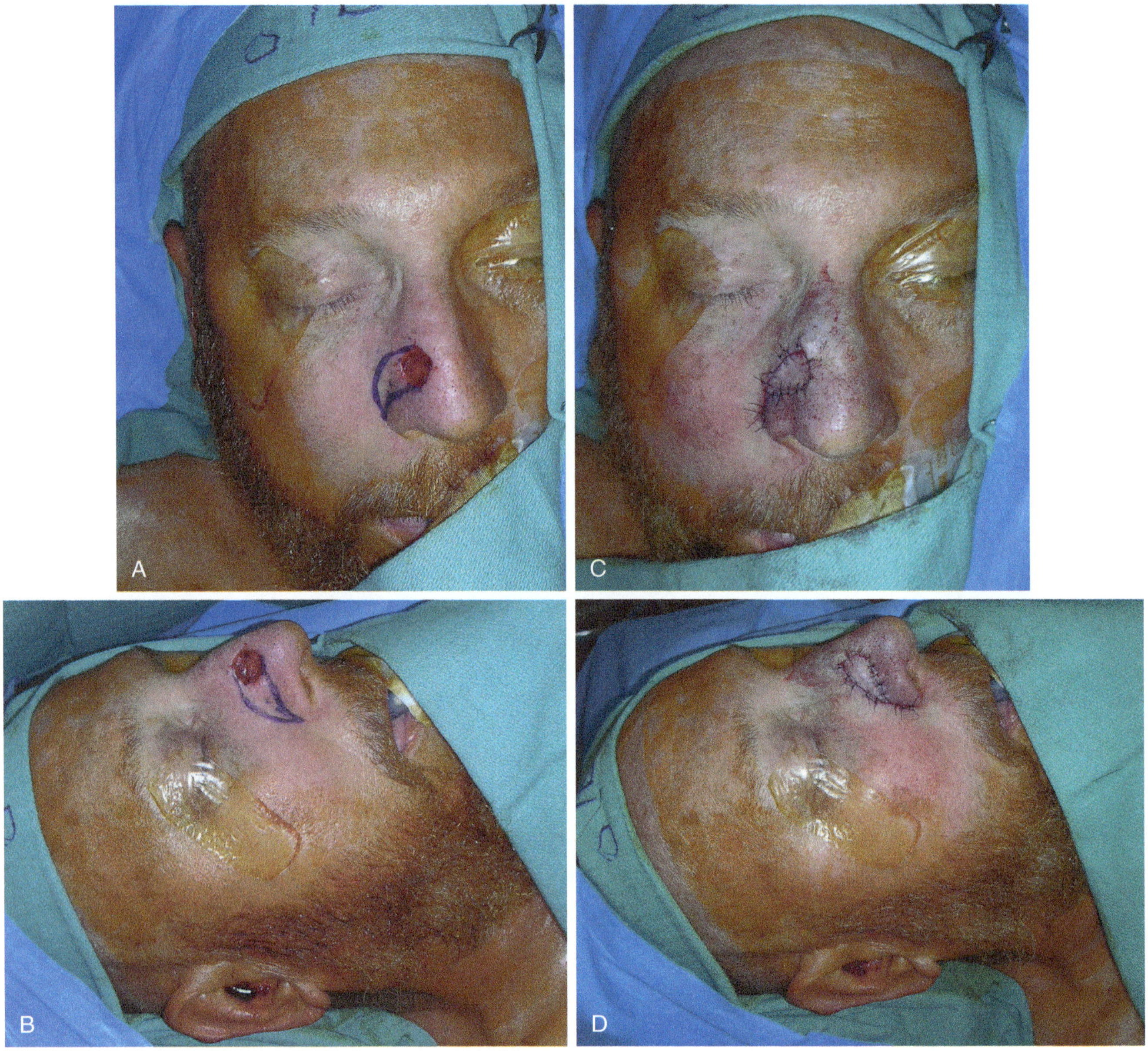

• **Fig. 30.6** V–Y nasal flap: (A) flap design frontal view; (B) flap design lateral view; (C) flap inset frontal view; (D) flap inset lateral view.

approach in order to improve cosmetic and functional outcomes. In such cases, the different possibilities have to be discussed with the patient in terms of result, total recovery time, and number of operations.

Even in larger defects, greater than 1.5–2 cm, remnant skin of the nose may be sufficient to close the defect but insufficient to resurface nasal skin without any distortion of the landmarks and rim or cause columellar retraction. A large skin graft is always an option, but color, thickness, and texture are unpredictable and may not be satisfactory, especially in the lower part of the nose. In such cases, additional skin mobilized from the cheek or forehead should be used, which necessitates at least two stages.

Concerning the depth of the nasal defect, as soon as it involves cartilage, the reconstruction needs cartilage replacement. If support is not restored, it will lead to cosmetic failure (landmark deformities, nostril and columellar retractions) as well as functional problems (nasal airway collapse). A cartilage graft precludes the use of a skin graft. The columella, infratip lobule, and defects very close to the nostril rim will generally need additional skin in order to avoid distortion in these delicate areas.

Skin Replacement

Large and/or deep defects need additional skin, occasionally necessitating harvest from a distant location (Washio flap or distal free flap). Scarred external skin must also be discarded, which will increase the size of the defect.[17]

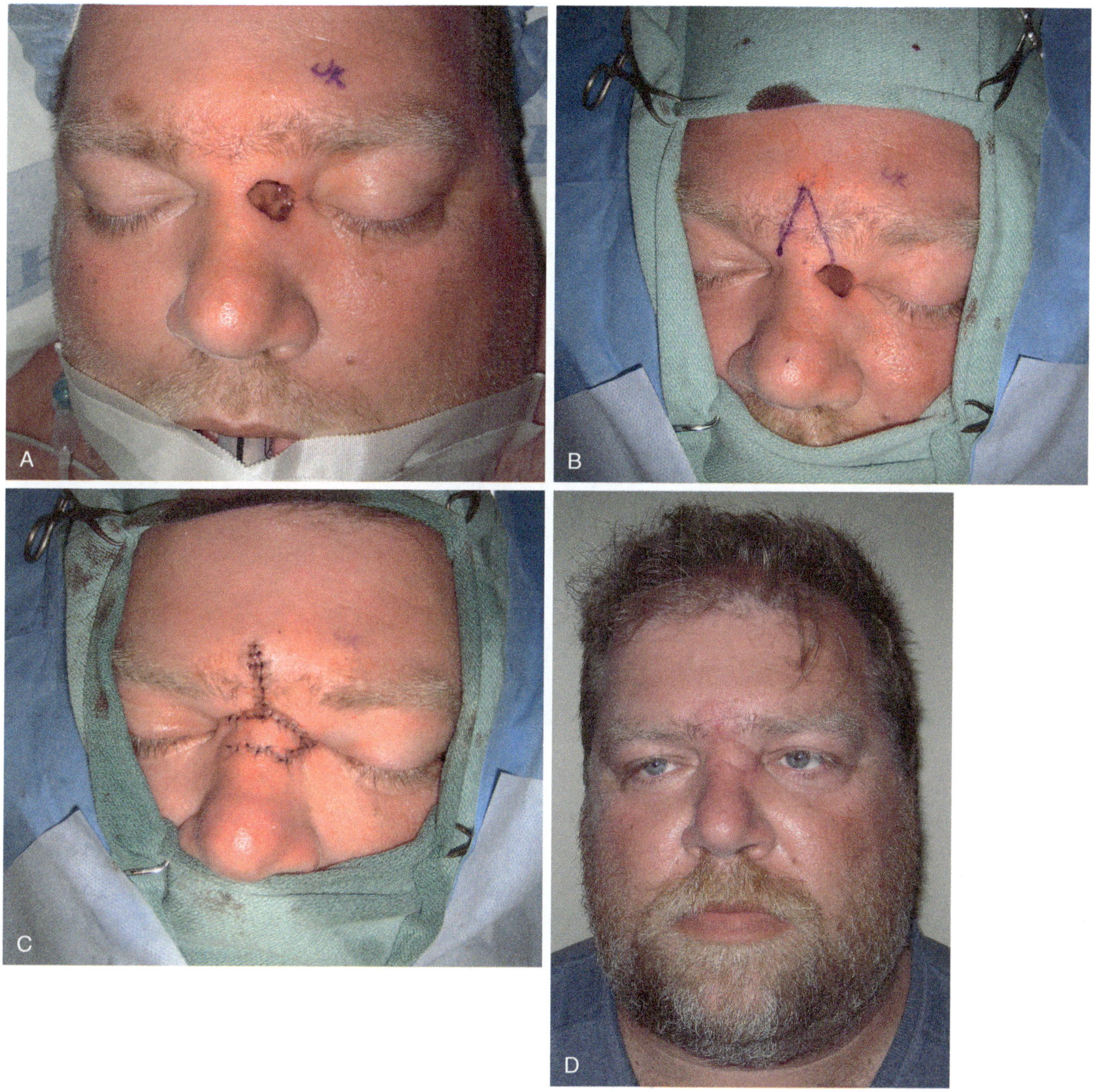

• **Fig. 30.7** Glabellar flap: (A) initial defect; (B) flap design; (C) flap inset; (D) final result.

The best skin match is the skin closest to the defect, and therefore the best donor sites are most often the medial cheek and forehead. As mentioned previously, FTSGs can be used to reconstruct large defects. Often, this technique is utilized in patients who are high risk and cannot tolerate general anesthesia, as well as those patients who need surveillance for recurrence of malignancy.[6]

Two-Stage Nasolabial Flap

This flap is well-suited for reconstruction of alar defects between 1.5 and 2 cm in diameter. It can also be used to replace lining defects when mucosal flaps are insufficient. The flap transfers excess skin from the medial cheek to the lateral part of the lower nose, directly adjacent to the nasolabial fold. When harvested in two stages, the nasolabial flap is vascularized by perforating vessels coming from the facial artery and crossing the muscular plane below, through and above levator labii muscle. Therefore, this flap is a transposition island flap, with the pivot point located at the junction between cheek, alar groove, and lip.

First Stage

The nasolabial fold must be outlined on an awake patient. A very precise template of the contralateral alar

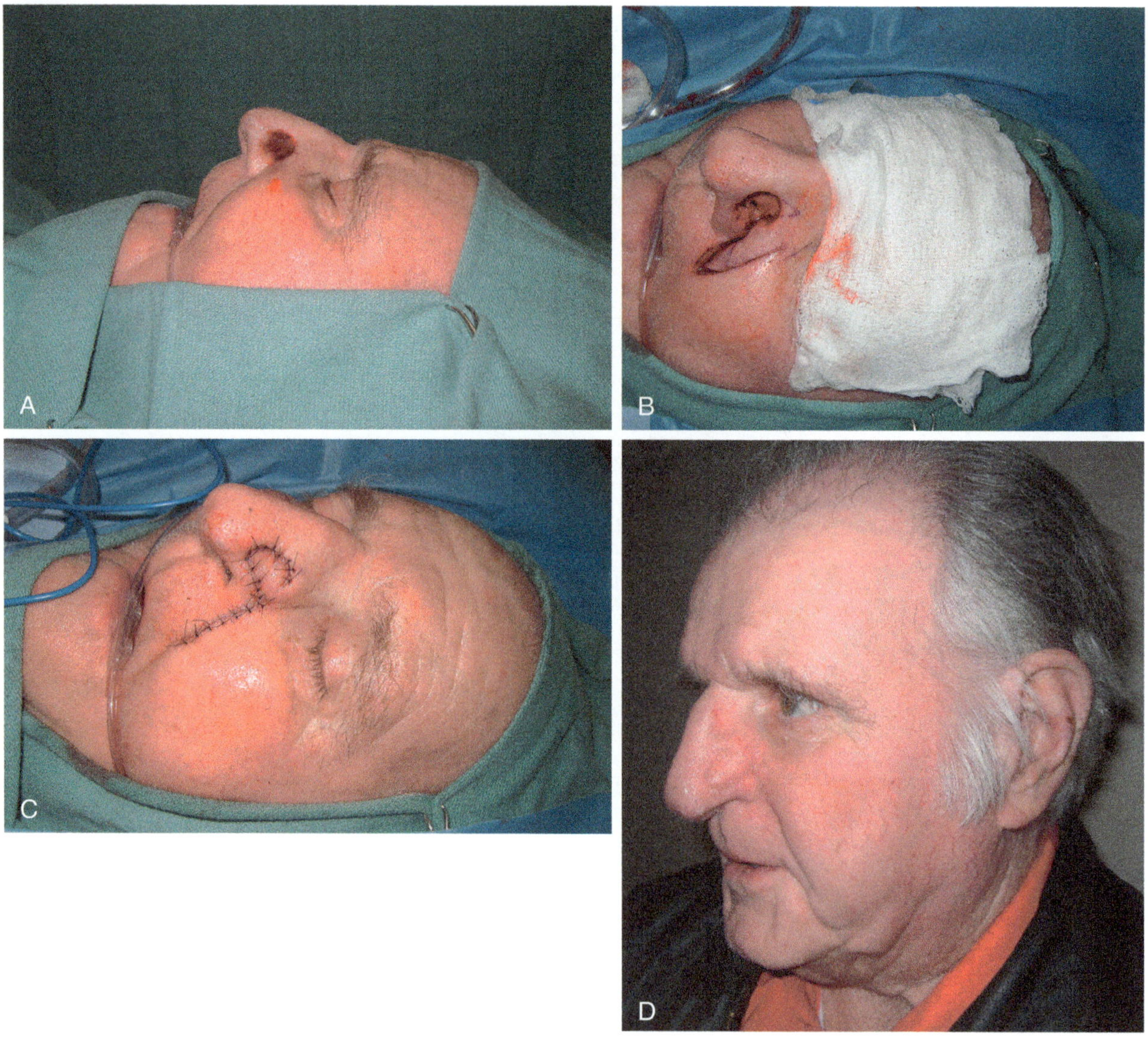

• **Fig. 30.8** Single-stage nasolabial flap: (A) initial defect; (B) flap design; (C) flap inset; (D) final result.

subunit is then transposed adjacent to the nasolabial fold (Fig. 30.9). The flap is designed at least 1–2 mm larger than the defect to allow for contraction postoperatively.[6] As the flap will be transposed with an angle of about 110 degrees, the medial portion of the template should be placed distally in the flap. Positioning of the template has to be calculated to reach the ala without any tension. Usually, this is achieved by positioning the flap just above the oral commissure.

Before harvesting the flap, it is strongly recommended to brace the lining (reconstructed or not) with a cartilage graft to avoid collapse and alar rim retraction. Despite lack of cartilaginous support in the normal ala, the fibrofatty middle layer is normally able to act against collapse during nasal inspiration. With a significant amount of alar skin loss, however, this counteracting force decreases and collapse is more likely to occur. Furthermore, this cartilage graft will help to recreate the round shape of the ala, and its upper and external border will help reconstruct the alar groove. In this location, conchal cartilage can be used because of its natural round shape. This graft is designed a few millimeters smaller than the skin template.

The flap is elevated where possible. Dissection is performed from distal to proximal. The distal part of the flap is elevated with 2 or 3 mm of fat to avoid secondary thinning of this region, but dissection becomes deeper proximally as it nears the perforators. Medially, the subcutaneous base is protected and dissection must be deliberate in order to preserve the perforators. The muscles should be spared. Once the flap reaches the defect without any tension, undermining is stopped and the medial part of the flap is precisely sutured to the defect. The surgeon should be aware that, although reliable, blood supply is more tenuous than that in the forehead flap, and distal necrosis may occur when there is tension or extensive dissection of the pedicle.

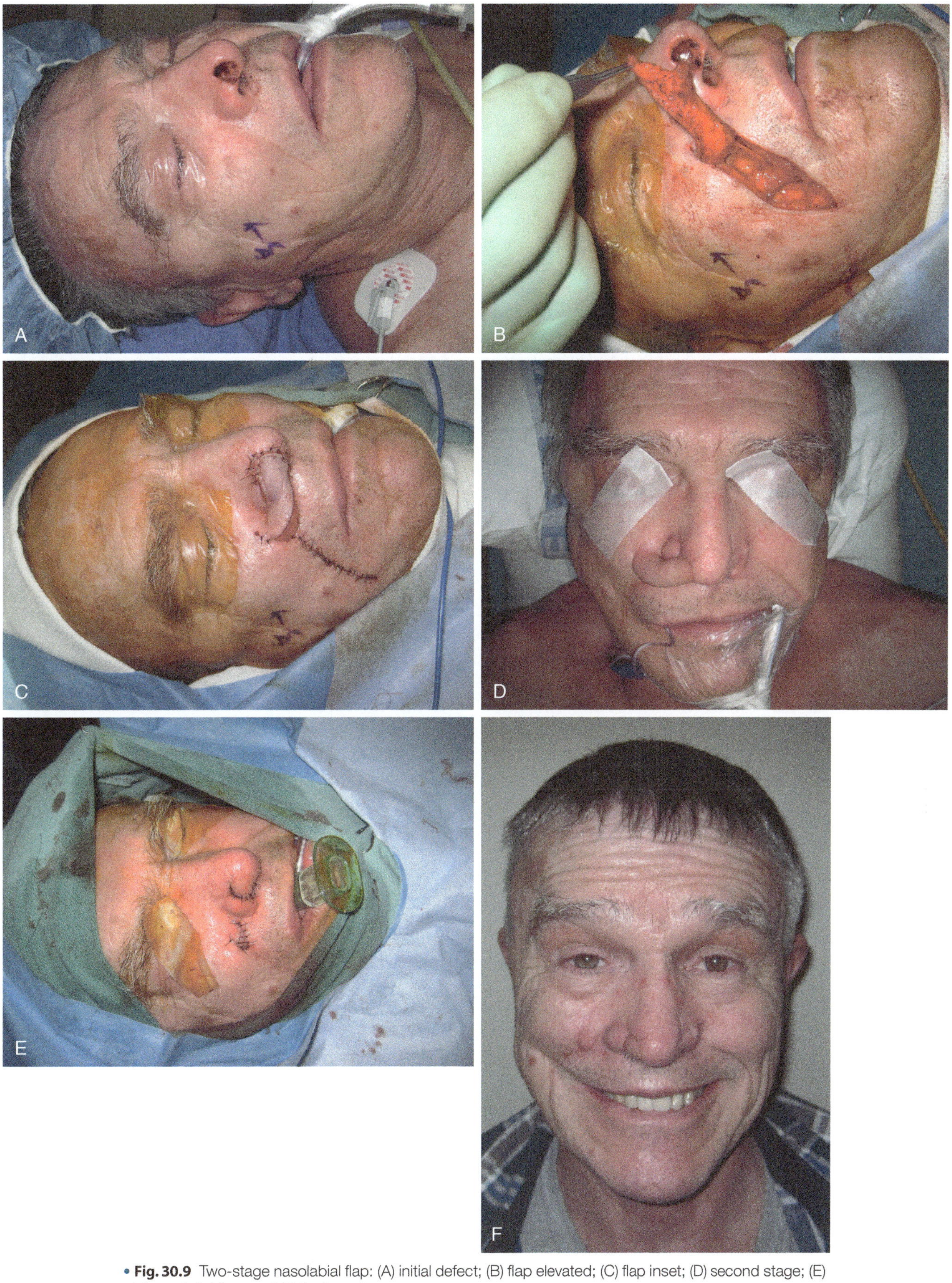

• **Fig. 30.9** Two-stage nasolabial flap: (A) initial defect; (B) flap elevated; (C) flap inset; (D) second stage; (E) at time of division; and (F) final result.

Second Stage

After approximately 3 weeks, the pedicle may be divided. As it was already thinned during elevation, the medial part of the flap does not need additional work. Conversely, as dissection was deep laterally during the first stage, this area is often thicker than needed. Therefore, after division, the external skin flap is re-elevated and thinned, keeping just 2–3 mm of underlying fat. The tail is then sutured and the superior dog-ear (the flap's pivot point) is excised (see Fig. 30.9).

In general, the skin color matches well with the remnant nasal skin and the trapdoor effect will contract the flap into a spherical shape, which will often improve the result with time. A well-planned design and location of the donor site makes the final scar well hidden. Nevertheless, in some cases the cheek may be flattened and necessitate a contralateral excision of nasolabial fold to reestablish symmetry.

This technique usually provides good cosmetic results and a suitable choice for reconstruction of the entire alar subunit. Once the defect involves part of the tip or sidewall, however, a forehead flap would be a more appropriate reconstruction technique.

The Two-Stage Paramedian Forehead Flap

The paramedian forehead flap is indicated for defects of the ala greater than 2 cm, defects of the nasal tip and ala, or large nasal defects. Its color, texture, thickness, and amount of available tissue make it an excellent choice for large and/or deep defects.[3] Considered a workhorse flap for nasal reconstruction, this flap can be used for resurfacing the entire nose.[5,6] A width of up to 3 cm can be harvested from the forehead while still being able to close the donor site primarily.

Forehead flaps have been described and used in numerous fashions and designs, depending on the flap's blood supply (one or two supratrochlear arteries, supraorbital artery, superficial temporal artery), its localization on the forehead (median, paramedian, lateral), and its axis (vertical or oblique). Median forehead flaps, which are based on paired supratrochlear vessels, are pivoted on high and wide pedicles, which limits the reach of the flap. The Converse scalping flap is based on the contralateral superficial temporal vessels. This flap is a high-morbidity procedure for the patient as it will temporarily blind one of the patient's eyes with a large, heavy, hairy, and uncomfortable pedicle, and necessitates the use of an evident and unsightly skin graft to resurface the lower forehead, just above the eyebrow.[5,18] Finally, the oblique forehead flap is designed in such a way to increase the flap's reach. This design, however, leads to increased donor site scarring and prohibits a second flap harvest from the contralateral forehead due to compromise of the axial vessels supplying that area.[5] The standard paramedian forehead flap is very reliable and can provide enough skin to resurface the entire nose. The lower part of the scar is generally camouflaged, and, if designed narrow enough, the eyebrow approximation is very acceptable. Furthermore, if the upper part of the donor site is too wide to close, it can be left to heal by secondary intention.

Vascular Supply of the Forehead Flap

The forehead flap is well perfused on one supratrochlear pedicle. This artery is a branch of the ophthalmic artery, which originates from the internal carotid artery. The supratrochlear artery leaves the orbit at its medial angle, crosses the orbital rim, between corrugator and frontalis muscles, before coursing vertically upwards. The artery is initially subperiosteal, but as it passes over the brow the supratrochlear artery courses above the periosteum, protected by the corrugator first and then by the frontalis. This means that above the orbital rim the flap can be safely elevated over the periosteum. Under the orbital rim, dissection must be beneath the periosteum. At about the mid-forehead level, the artery will course through the frontalis muscle to lie in the subcutaneous plane, increasingly becoming superficial as it reaches the hairline.

First-Stage

When the nasal defect is lateral, the flap is harvested on the ipsilateral side. When it is median, the paramedian forehead flap can be elevated from either side. The glabellar rhytid should be outlined on an awake patient, especially for young people. We favor localization of the supratrochlear artery preoperatively with a hand-held Doppler. If a significant amount of cartilage is missing, the lining should be supported with a cartilage graft to avoid collapse, and retraction. This can be completed before harvesting the flap.

A precise template of the defect (respecting the subunit principles and, when intact, derived from the contralateral side) is designed and transposed to the paramedian forehead, just off the midline. This is positioned as high as possible, but below the hairline if possible to avoid hair transfer to the nose. The pedicle of the flap is then marked out, narrowed from the pattern to the glabellar rhytid. The base pedicle width can be 1.2–1.5 cm in width. A narrow pedicle will augment the arc of rotation, decrease closure tension and limit approximation of the brow.

The flap is elevated vertically downwards. As a two–stage flap, the distal part of the flap is thinned directly at this first stage. This means that it is elevated with a few millimeters of fat (trying to obtain the same thickness as the remnant skin of the nose), but respecting the frontalis muscle. This decreases blood supply and may lead to local necrosis in smokers or in very large flaps. In such cases, it may be safer to elevate the flap with muscle and plan an intermediate stage for thinning (Fig. 30.10).

About 1 cm above the mid-forehead level, dissection proceeds under the frontalis muscle, but over the periosteum, to protect the artery. Dissection can stay in this plane until the brow, after which dissection should continue under the periosteum. The flap is then rotated medially and when the paddle reaches the defect it can be closed precisely without tension in a single layer.

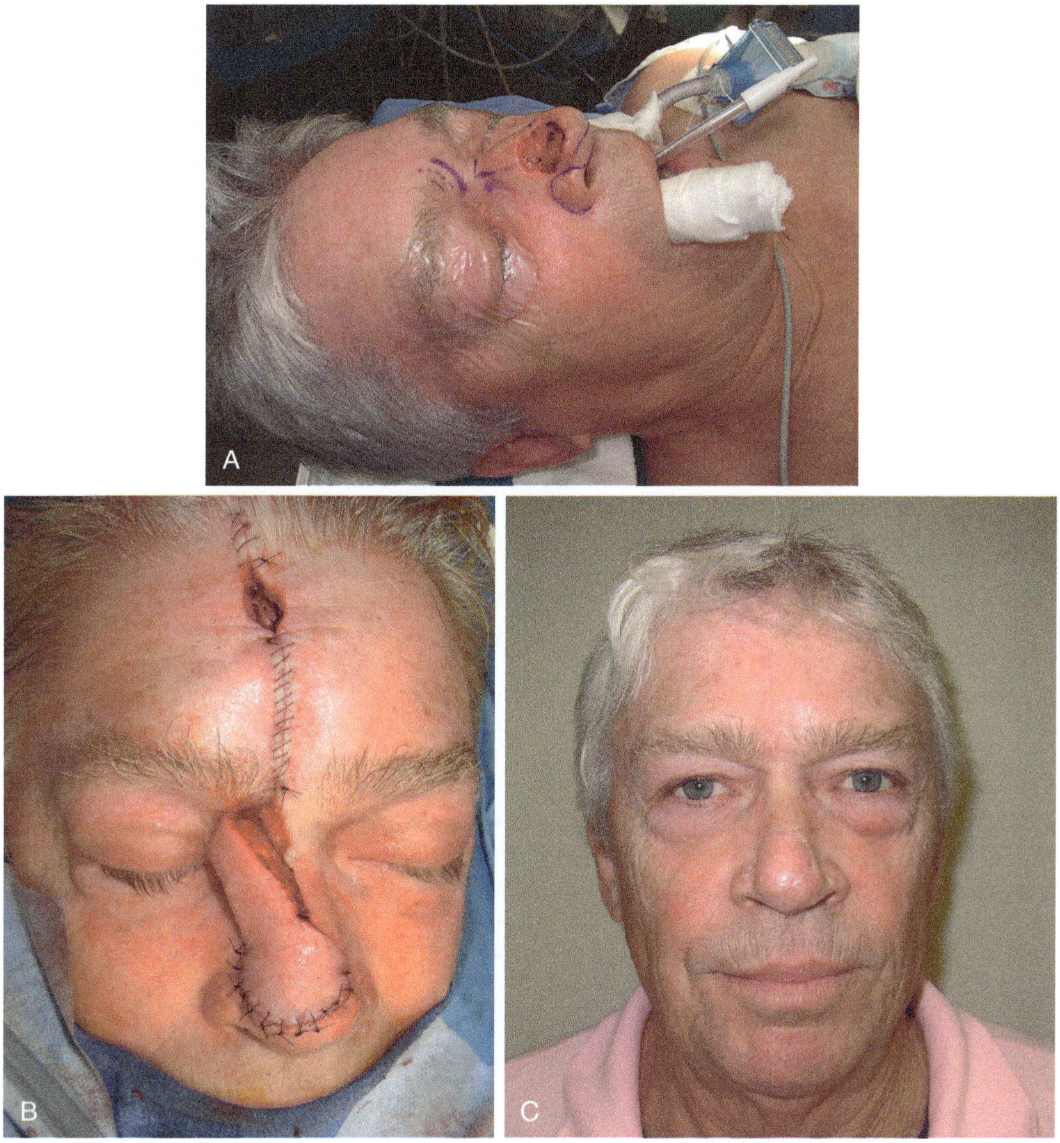

• **Fig. 30.10** Two-stage forehead flap: (A) initial defect; (B) flap inset; (C) final result.

The forehead is then undermined on both sides in the subgaleal plane to decrease tension and precisely sutured in layers. Special care is given to maintaining eyebrow level during closure. If the upper part is too wide to be closed, it can heal by secondary intention. With secondary intention healing, the brow will not distort and the final result is generally better than with a skin graft.

Finally, the pedicle can be dressed with bacitracin and diced Surgicell. This significantly decreases bleeding, which generally completely stops after 2 days. Obviously, this dressing should not compress the artery. In rare cases one can skin graft the pedicle.

Second Stage

After approximately 3 weeks, the second stage can be performed. Before division, the viability of the flap should be checked with compression of the pedicle. If flap perfusion is maintained, the pedicle can be divided.

After transection, the superior part of the flap is re-elevated, and excess subcutaneous tissue is excised to recreate the natural convexities and creases of the nose. Elevation further than 1.5 cm of distal flap margin risks devascularization of the flap. When the desired shape and thickness is obtained, the superior flap margin is trimmed to fit the defect precisely and is sutured (see Fig. 30.10).

Finally, the inferior forehead scar is reopened and the proximal pedicle is returned to the donor site and sutured in a small inverted "V" with quilting sutures to avoid hematoma. The proximal pedicle can also be completely excised, leaving a barely visible scar on the eyelid; however, this will likely bring the eyebrows closer together.

The Three-Stage Paramedian Forehead Flap

Thinning the flap at the first stage could compromise blood supply in smokers or when a large flap is needed. In such cases, the paramedian forehead flap can be constructed over three stages for greater safety and improved results. Adding an intermediate stage supports increased vascularity, avoids piecemeal thinning, allows more intensive soft tissue sculpting, and allows structural support placement.[5]

Millard first introduced an intermediate stage that was later modified by Burget.[12] During the intermediate stage, the pedicle is left intact and the distal inset is left attached up to 1.5 cm from its distal margin. This effectively creates a bipedicled flap, allowing the middle part of the flap to be thinned safely; however, there are difficulties due to poor visibility, and the distal part of the flap could not be addressed at this stage.

Menick describes the full-thickness three-stage forehead flap.[10] During the first stage, except if a skin graft or a folded forehead flap is used for lining replacement, primary cartilage grafts are placed. Then, a full-thickness forehead flap, including frontalis muscle, is elevated and sutured to the recipient bed. In the second stage, 3 or more weeks later, the flap can be completely re-elevated safely in the subcutaneous plane due to the delay phenomenon. The most proximal part of the flap can be thinned during the final stage. The underlying recipient bed, comprised of fat, frontalis muscle, scar, and cartilage, is then sculpted precisely to recreate landmarks and creases. If needed, additional grafts can be used. The thinned flap is then repositioned. Finally, division is performed 3–4 weeks later (Fig. 30.11). This technique has produced improved results as well as decreased the need for revisions.[5]

Lining Restoration

Many surgeons feel that restoring the nasal lining is the most important aspect of nasal reconstruction.[17] Even the smallest of defects can result in cicatricial contraction resulting in distortion of the nasal framework. Unrepaired lining defects also expose the underlying structures, which can potentially lead to infection of the soft tissue and underlying cartilage as well as bone necrosis.[17,19] nasal lining defects often lead to nasal shortening and loss of projection with retraction of the nostril margins. When the lining of the nasal floor is also involved, the scarring becomes circumferential, and can affect the upper lip, which leads to lip shortening and retrusion.[17] Several options are available to restore nasal lining. The ideal reconstruction should be well vascularized in order to support bone and cartilage grafts, restore nasal airway, and decrease donor site morbidity.[2]

Full-Thickness Skin Graft

The main indication for an FTSG is to reconstruct the donor site for the bi-pedicled vestibular advancement flap discussed below. Full-thickness grafts are otherwise not often used, as they have a tendency to undergo contraction. They are also unable to support underlying cartilage grafts, unless multiple stages of reconstruction are performed.[2,19] Examples of this would be with the prefabricated forehead flap and the "classical" skin graft as described by Menick.

Prefabricated Forehead Flap

The prelaminated forehead flap was first described by Konig. Later, it was popularized by Gillies and then modified by Converse.[20,21] In this technique, the flap lining and cartilage framework are first built on the forehead and then transferred onto the nose. The first stage consists of designing a precise template of the skin defect and another template for the lining defect. The template of missing skin is transferred to the forehead, exactly like a traditional forehead flap. In this technique, only the distal part of the flap is incised and undermined between frontalis and periosteum.

An FTSG is then harvested with the template of the missing lining. This skin graft is sutured with fine absorbable sutures to the underside of the frontalis muscle.

Finally, cartilage grafts are inserted in a tunnel between skin and frontalis muscle. In order to maintain maximum connection between the skin and muscle, when possible, it is better to introduce the cartilage grafts through an incision on the lateral border of the flap. Four weeks later, the flap is completely elevated, positioned and sutured into the defect. Before division, an intermediate stage can be added.

Though effectively able to replace intranasal lining, this flap is not ideal. The number of stages is not reduced and it is difficult to obtain optimal results because precise positioning of the cartilage framework is difficult to achieve given that the three-dimensional shape is difficult to predict when the flap is still flat on the forehead.

"Classical" Skin Graft

Although frequently described, the classical skin graft has given poor results for the restoration of nasal lining. Menick recently modified the technique.[10] An FTSG can be sutured to the borders of the lining defect. Then a full-thickness forehead flap is elevated and positioned on the nose. Quilted absorbable sutures fix the graft to the flap. A skin graft naturally precludes the use of a cartilage graft.

Four weeks later, during an intermediate stage, the flap is re-elevated with 2–3 mm of subcutaneous fat. Excess scar, subcutaneous tissue, and frontalis muscle are excised from the recipient bed. The graft is normally well vascularized and the cartilage framework can be placed without compromising the graft vascularization during this stage. The flap is replaced and sutured to the nose. Finally, after an additional 4 weeks, the final stage is completed as the pedicle is divided.

With this technique, skin graft take is often unpredictable and for this reason the patient is checked regularly. If the skin graft fails, it can be replaced with another, delaying the intermediate stage.

Hingeover Flaps

After a full-thickness amputation, sutured together or not, remnant skin and lining will join by scar. After several weeks (6–8 depending on the author), neighboring

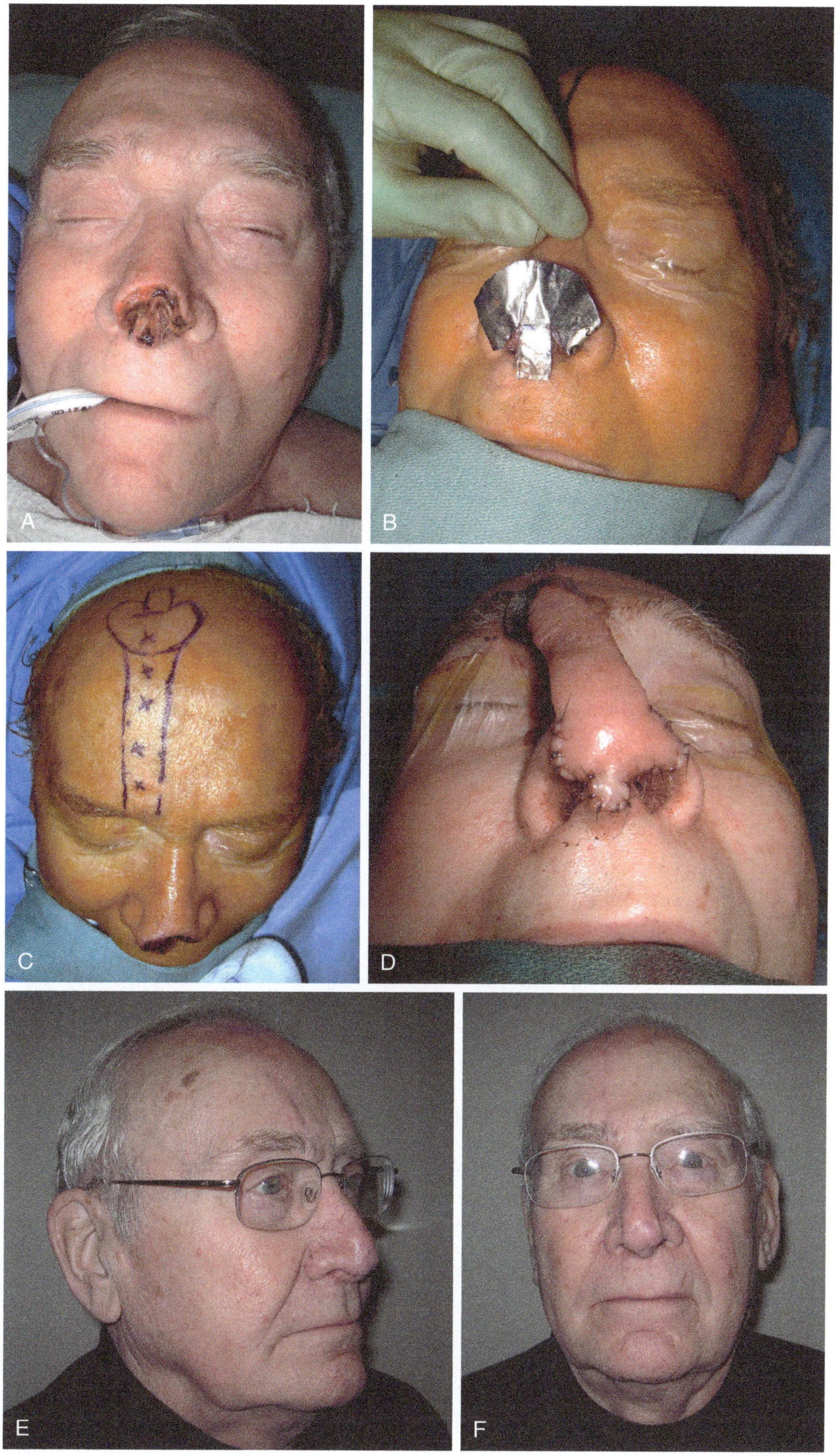

• **Fig. 30.11** Three-stage forehead flap: (A) initial defect; (B) making a template; (C) flap design; (D) flap inset with special attention to insetting the columella; (E) lateral view after three-stage reconstruction; (F) frontal view after three-stage reconstruction.

skin vascularized across the scar can be elevated and hinged over to replace lining. Most commonly, the medial cheek, nasal sidewall, and cephalic edge of an alar defect are used as donor sites. The flap is based on a subcutaneous pedicle composed of scar tissue adjacent to the defect margin.[19] This limits the vascularity and functionality of the flap. Its length is typically limited to 1.5 cm and often these flaps are thick and not conducive to shaping with a cartilage graft as they contain scar tissue.[5] Nevertheless, they can be very useful for small defects or in association with intranasal lining flaps when only a few millimeters of lining are required.

Intranasal Lining Flaps

Intranasal flaps are typically the preferred method of reconstructing lining defects, because they replace missing tissue with similar tissue. The following lining flaps can be used alone or in conjunction with one another. Although these flaps are well-vascularized, caution is necessary in smokers. These flaps are generally used with primary cartilage grafts and should be used if necrosis of the lining leads to cartilage graft exposure, resulting in probable infection and graft resorption.

These flaps can be technically difficult to perform, especially when the full-thickness defect is small, owing to poor visibility. Even when strongly fixed with cartilage graft, such flaps will often tend to retract toward their pivot point, which means inside the nose. For this reason, stenosis regularly occurs and may necessitate a revision. Additionally, intranasal lining flaps will often lead to bleeding and crusting that can obstruct airway and compromise patient comfort. Nevertheless, they are often very useful for lining restoration and reconstruction.

Residual Nasal Lining Advancement

When the lining defect is less than 4 mm along the nostril rim, the remnant vestibular lining can be separated from the ala to be pulled downward. To avoid secondary retraction, this lining advancement should be braced in position with a primary cartilage graft.

Bipedicle Flap

Defects up to 1 cm within the ala or hemi-tip can be lined by a bipedicled vestibular skin advancement flap. This flap is based medially at the junction of the anterior vestibular lining with the septum and laterally at the nasal floor. An incision is made at the vestibular lining, and the flap is elevated and rotated inferiorly to the level of the nostril margin. Structural support is provided by a cartilage graft. The donor site may require a full-thickness skin graft to prevent scar contracture and subsequent alar notching.[13,19]

Ipsilateral Septal Flap

Described by Burget and Menick, this flap is vascularized by the septal branch of the superior labial artery (Fig. 30.12).[2,15] This artery comes from the facial artery and passes medially through the orbicularis oris muscle, at the junction between skin and vermilion. Just lateral to the philtrum, it gives rise to the septal branch that goes vertically upward from lip to septum, passing laterally to the nasal spine.

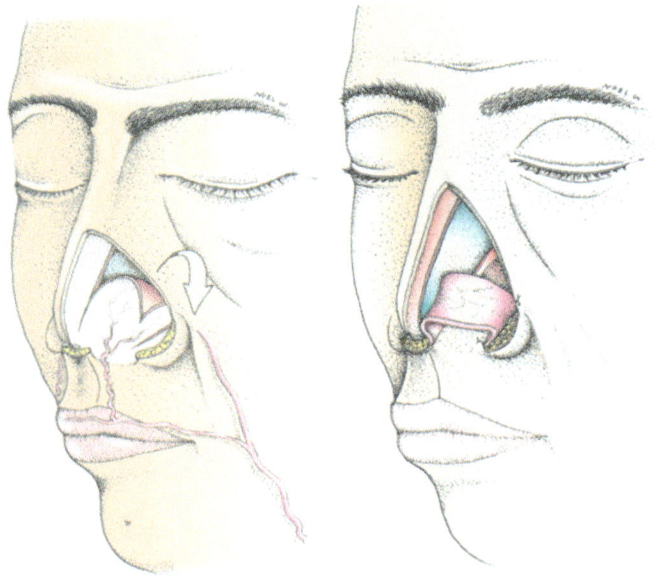

• **Fig. 30.12** Ipsilateral septal flap: elevation of the ipsilateral mucosal flap based on the anterior branch of the superior labial artery and then rotated into a position to be sutured to the ala. (Courtesy Dr. Warren Noel.)

This branch is theoretically able to vascularize the entire ipsilateral septal lining. Thus, an ipsilateral septal mucoperichondrial flap can be elevated from posterior to anterior and can restore lining losses of the lower third of the nose. A disadvantage of this flap is that it extends across the vestibule to cover a lateral defect, resulting in obstruction of the nasal airway. The pedicle is divided after 3 weeks.[13,19] Additionally, when the defect is small this flap can be challenging to harvest because of poor visibility.

Contralateral Septal Flap

This flap is vascularized by the medial branch of the anterior ethmoidal artery that runs parallel to the dorsum. After elevation of the ipsilateral mucosa (used as a flap too or replaced after contralateral flap elevation, depending on lining loss), the septal cartilage is removed, preserving a septal L strut for nasal support. Then, a dorsally based flap of contralateral septal mucosa is incised, maintaining at least 1 cm of its dorsal blood supply. This flap is then swung laterally in order to line the mid-vault. Finally, if the ipsilateral mucosa is not used to line the lower part, it is replaced in order to repair the fistula. Ipsilateral and contralateral flaps are frequently used for large defects of the hemi–nose (Fig. 30.13). Repair of such a large defect will result in a large septal fistula. This defect, however, is largely asymptomatic due to its width.[19,22]

Septal Pivot Composite Flaps

This flap, described by Burget and Menick, is useful for central full-thickness defects of the lower half of the nose (Fig. 30.14).[8] This flap provides the dorsal support and restores the lining of the mid-vault, but it is not able to

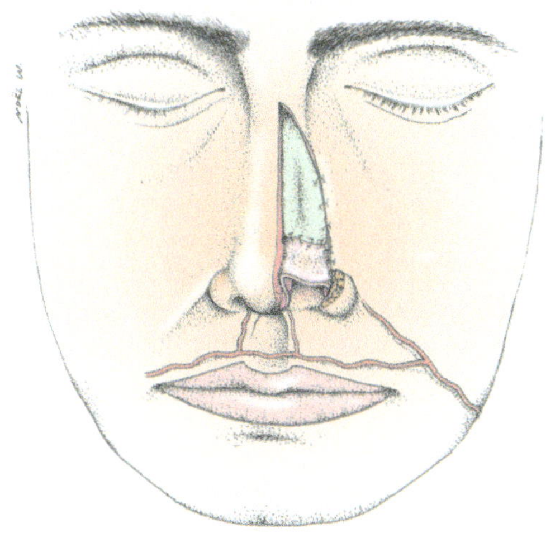

• **Fig. 30.13** Ipsilateral and contralateral flaps are frequently used for large defects of the hemi–nose. (Courtesy Dr. Warren Noel.)

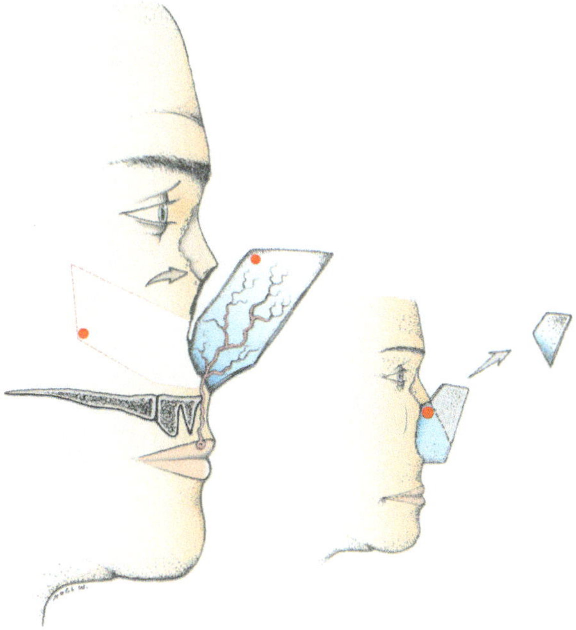

• **Fig. 30.14** Septal pivot composite flaps. (Courtesy Dr. Warren Noel.)

restore lining of the entire lower third of the nose. The septal pivot composite flap can be used when an amputation leaves the posterior part of the septum intact, which is normally the case. The minimum requirement to perform this flap is that the remaining septum is flush with the face. If the resection involves more of the septum, the septal branches of the superior labial arteries are likely compromised and flap survival is poor.

The full-thickness septum is cut superiorly, posteriorly, and inferiorly until 1.2 cm from the nasal spine. In the region of the nasal spine, the mucosa is preserved as it contains the two septal branches. The flap is now only retained by attachments between cartilage and nasal spine. Therefore, mucoperichondrium has to be very cautiously separated from each side in this region in order to release the septal cartilage attachments without compromising vascularization. The composite flap is then rotated forward, out of the nose, and fixed superiorly to the nasal bones and/or upper lateral cartilages. This recreates the midline support of the nose. The caudal aspect of the flap becomes the support and lining for the columella.

Alloplast

If the patient has no history of nasal radiation exposure, intranasal lining defects, particularly in the upper two-thirds of the nose, may be repaired with titanium mesh. Titanium mesh is useful in that it resists cicatricial contracture, while mucosalization can still occur through the mesh.[13]

Regional Flaps

The use of a nasolabial flap for lining was popularized by Millard.[7] Vascularized by perforators from the facial artery, it can restore the lining of alar bases and vestibule. Nevertheless, the risk of necrosis with proximal dissection and of not being able to thin the flap adequately, an alternative flap may be better suited for lining replacement to prevent the risk of airway obstruction and lateral displacement of the alar base.

A second paramedian forehead flap can be used to resurface a hemi-nose lining defect. If the cause of amputation was a skin malignancy; however, the risk of recurrence must be considered when utilizing this flap given that another forehead flap cannot be utilized.

Three-Stage Folded Forehead Flap

Until recently, folding the end of a forehead flap for lining reconstruction was a part of the traditional two-stage method. Adding an intermediate stage, Menick modified this technique and it has become a preferred technique for the reconstruction of unilateral and bilateral defects of up to 3.5 cm in the lining.[23] Preserving septal lining minimizes bleeding, permanent crusting, and intranasal retraction of lining flaps.

During the first stage, a precise template of the defect is created using the contralateral subunits when possible. It is turned 180 degrees to account for the pivotal movement of the forehead flap, and then transferred to the forehead as an extension of the forehead flap. If required, this pattern can lie in the hair line as it will replace lining. A few millimeters of extra skin are added between the two patterns in order to fold the flap more easily during its inset. After elevation of the full-thickness forehead flap, the distal lining extension is folded inward and sutured to the residual mucosal lining. No cartilage graft is added at this stage. The donor site is closed primarily, or allowed to heal by secondary intention if under too much tension, and a full-thickness skin graft is placed upon the raw surface of the pedicle.

Three to four weeks later, the second stage of the procedure is performed. A marginal incision is made, and the proximal portion of the flap is completely re-elevated, leaving the reconstructed lining on the nose. Each side of the flap is sculpted before the cartilage framework is precisely reconstructed. The flap is then sutured back onto the nose.

At the third stage, again 3–4 weeks later, the surgeon undertakes division and inset. The pedicle is divided and any residual thickness to the proximal portion of the tissue to be inset is thinned (see Fig. 30.14)

Unfortunately, this technique is not without complications. Folding of the forehead flap at the new nostril margin can result in a thickened ala, minimal skin rim support, and external nasal valve obstruction. Also, the folding of the flap on itself may compromise its vascularity. Commonly, three months after division of the pedicle a fourth procedure that debulks the nostril is necessary for adequate cosmesis and function.[5,19]

Distant Free Flaps

When the lining loss is too great, possibly involving the adjacent check and lip, microvascular distant tissue transfer must be considered. The radial forearm free flap is the most commonly used for inner lining reconstruction due to its thinness, reliability, and long pedicle. As mentioned previously, the surgeon must also ensure that the nasal platform is restored prior to nasal reconstruction. Often, the septum is not reconstructed to ensure patency of the airway.[5] The radial forearm free flap is harvested suprafascially and is anastomosed to the facial or neck vessels. Unfortunately, this distant skin does not match the recipient site, so a forehead flap is required to resurface the nasal skin at a later date. At that time, cartilage grafts can be added as well (Fig. 30.15).[24,25]

Structural Support

The nasal bones, upper lateral cartilages, septum, and fibrofatty ala support the normal nose structure. These structures are not only critical to allow nasal air passage, but are

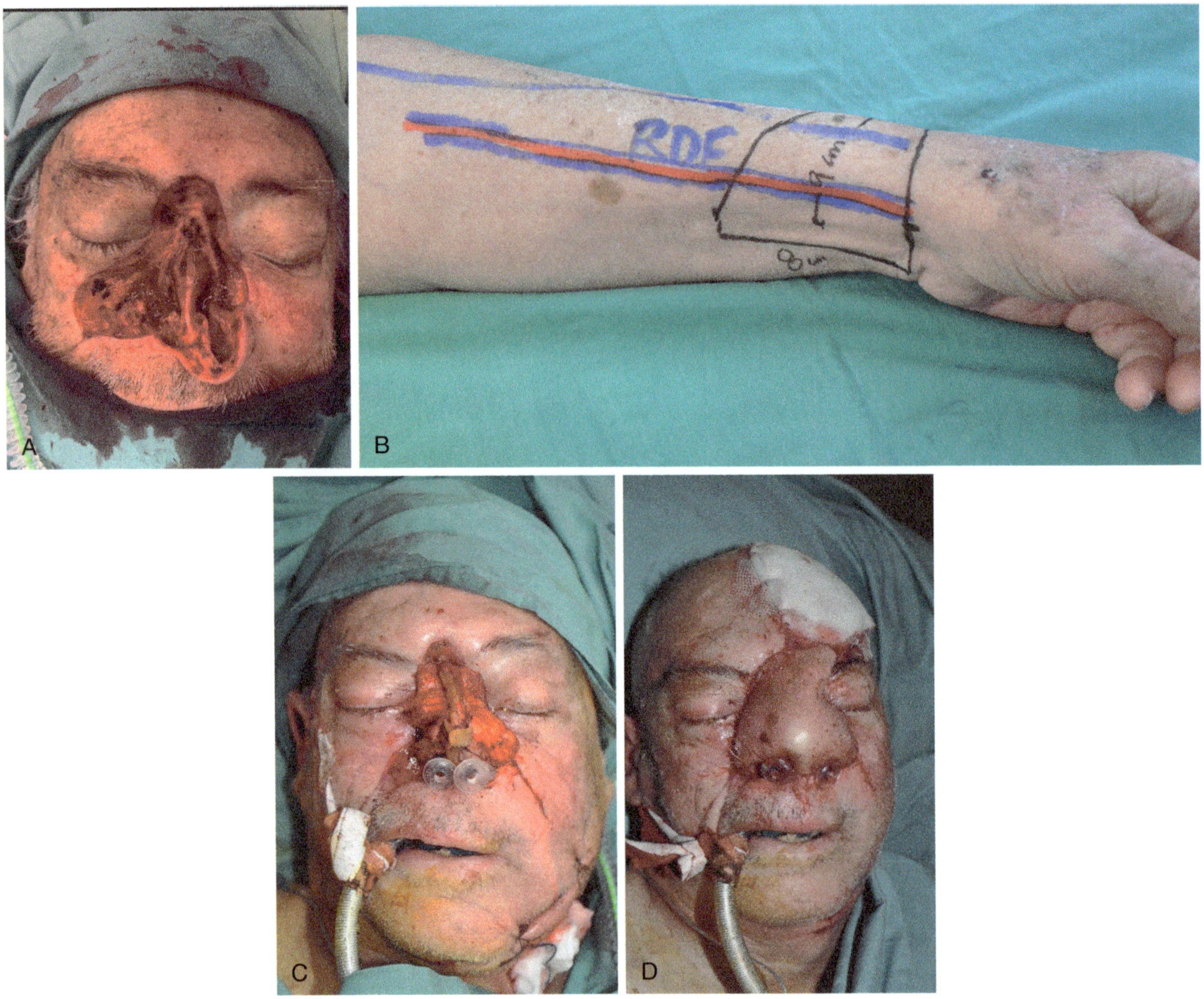

• **Fig. 30.15** (A) Defect shows total rhinectomy and cheek defect following locally invasive squamous cell carcinoma, excised with negative margins. (B) Radial forearm flap designed for lining and dissected in suprafascial plane. (C) Osteochondral septal graft secured into the frontal bone, cartilage grafts for columellar, alar, and tip reconstruction. (D) Forehead flap for cover. (Courtesy Dr. Rostam D. Farhadieh.)

also critical for an esthetic reconstruction. If not precisely replaced, in spite of reconstructive technique, the result will be poor in terms of esthetic and functional outcome. The structural defect determines the type of material necessary for reconstruction. Septal, ear, rib bone or cartilage, or cranial bone are all options for reconstruction depending on the shape, strength, and malleability required to replace the defect.[2,5]

The ideal time for the reconstruction of the structural support is during the primary or intermediate stages rather than secondarily. Although possible to perform small augmentations and refinements with grafts, the skin is more difficult to mold and a complete framework will be difficult to recreate at that time.

Midline Support

L-Strut Technique

Described by Gillies, the L-strut consists of a longitudinal piece of cartilage that is seated on the nasal radix and extended along the dorsum to the tip. The caudal part of the L is strongly sutured to the anterior nasal spine with figure-of-eight sutures.[26]

Hinged Septal Flap

Described by Millard, this L–shaped flap is carved from the remaining septum and hinged on the caudal end of the septal bones. As it pivots upward, the flap augments the nasal angle and recreates the dorsal support. The caudal part of the L is strongly sutured to the anterior nasal spine.[27]

Septal Pivot Flap

As described above, this flap can provide dorsal support as well as restoring lining of the mid-vault. In this flap, the entire septum is rotated forward out of the nasal cavity, and maintained by the superior labial artery.[10]

Cantilever Rib Graft

Described by Converse and Millard, this graft consists of a longitudinal graft extending from the dorsum down to the tip, which does not require fixation support of the distal tip. Proximally it can be embedded in the frontal bone, screwed to the nasal bone, or both. In order to keep the same dorsal projection, it is often necessary to lower the nasal bone before fixing the cantilever graft (see Fig. 30.15).[28,29]

The best material for cantilever graft is the ninth and tenth ribs. Designed at the osteocartilaginous junction, the bony portion of the graft is in contact with the nasal bones while the distal cartilaginous portion keeps the nasal tip pliable and resists resorption.

Lateral Support

The paired nasal ala are essential for providing nasal symmetry and the functionality of the external nasal valve. They also are an important esthetic structure, providing the natural creases with the cheek, nasal sidewall, and nasal tip. Defects in this area often do not lend themselves to healing by secondary intention, and are not amenable to being closed primarily. The ala are unique in that their structural support is provided by fibrofatty tissue. This tissue cannot be replaced with like tissue, and thus often requires reconstruction with cartilage grafts. If they are not braced, contraction during healing will tend to collapse and retract the soft triangle, alar rim, and ala. Isolated alar defects are best treated with grafts that are positioned and buried in adjacent subcutaneous pockets and secured with temporary percutaneous sutures. This nonanatomical grafting will aid in preventing alar notching and external nasal valve collapse.

Free Cartilage Graft

The nasal septum and auricle most commonly provide cartilage for free grafts. Auricular cartilage is often preferred, as the contour of the conchal cartilage is similar to the natural convexity of the ala. The surgical technique for harvest is associated with minimal donor site morbidity, and can easily be performed through either anterior or posterior skin incisions. After harvest, the cartilage can be thinned to 1 mm thick and still maintain its curvature.

Grafts can either be placed in anatomical or nonanatomical position to provide lateral nasal support. Anatomical grafts are shaped to resemble normal lateral crura and are anchored to the remaining medial crura and columella. Nonanatomical grafts are used to support the nasal ala without obstructing the nasal airway.

Composite Cartilage Graft

Composite cartilage grafts are indicated for repair of intermediate and full-thickness defects. Auricular composite grafts most often consist of conchal cartilage and its overlying skin. For intermediate defects that have intact internal lining, the posterior concha is harvested so as to provide both cartilage and external skin coverage. If the defect is full-thickness, the anterior choncha and skin can be harvested to provide internal lining and structural support under a regional flap. Additionally, both anterior and posterior chonchal skin can be harvested and transplanted as a three-layered graft for full-thickness defects.[13] These grafts are limited to 1.5-cm defects. The microvascular free flap variation of this was first described by Parkhouse and Evans in 1985.[30] It remains an elegant and reliable solution for alar defects >10 mm (Fig. 30.16).

Alloplasts

When alloplasts are used to provide a structural framework for the nose, they are used in combination with autogenous tissue. The dorsal support of the nose can be provided by titanium mesh. While titanium mesh is easily malleable and can be stabilized against the dorsal and lateral nasal walls without difficulty, it is susceptible to exposure and infection. When creating a strut or a large sheet of framework, porous polyethylene can be utilized.

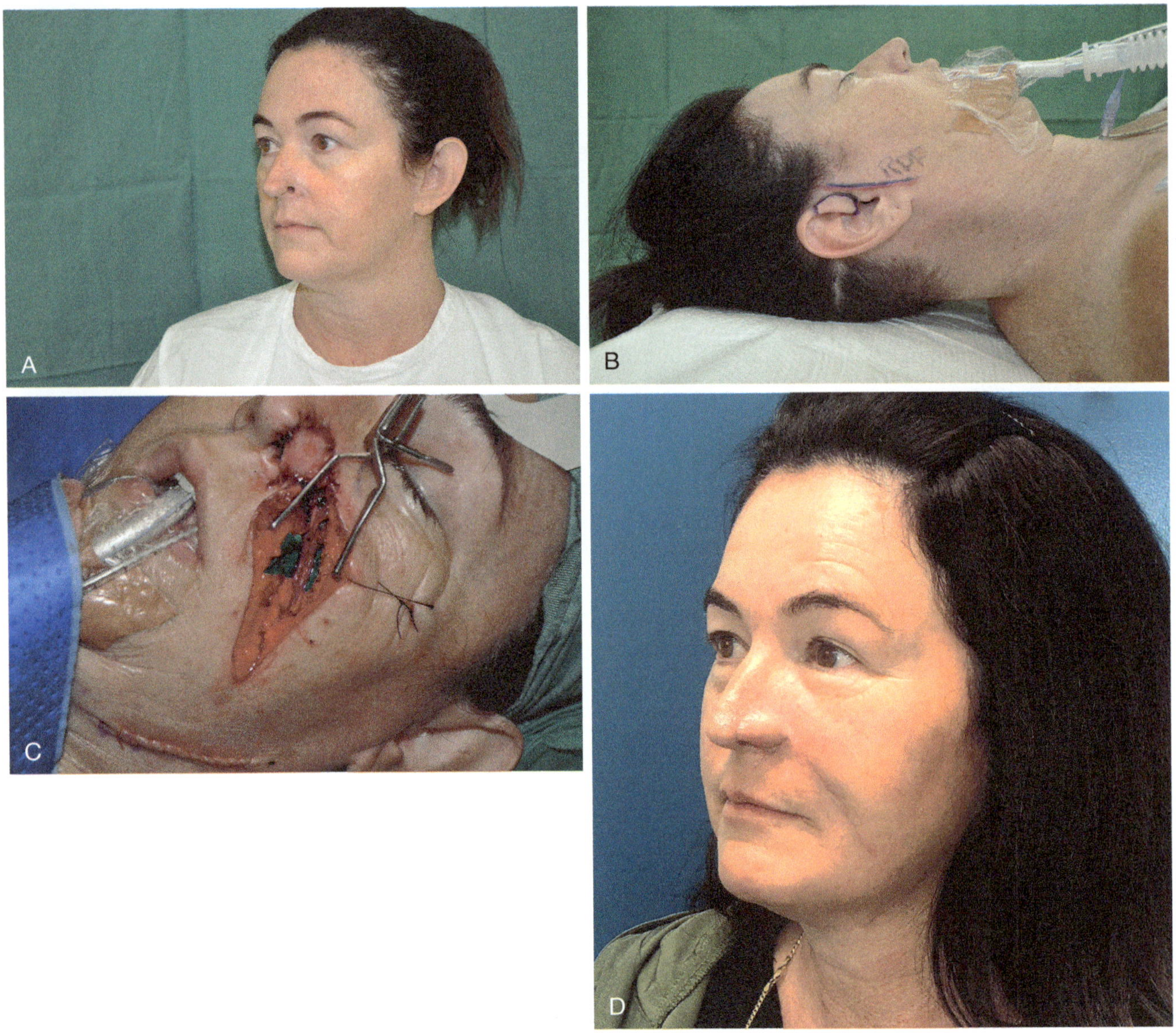

• **Fig. 30.16** A 44-year-old woman with a previous basal cell carcinoma excision elsewhere presented for reconstruction options. (A) The left alar defect. (B) Outline of the ascending helical rim (Evans' flap). (C) Flap inset and microsurgery: previous excision resulted in no local recipient artery; distal superficial temporal artery from the flap was used as an arterial graft to the left superior labial artery, identified and dissected with protection of the marginal mandibular nerve through a submandibular incision. (D) Results at 3 months postoperatively. (Courtesy Dr. Rostam D. Farhadieh.)

This material becomes incorporated into the tissue with time, but like titanium, is susceptible to implant exposure and infection.[13]

Composite and Extended Defects

Frequently the defect may encompass several adjacent facial subunits, including the lip and the cheek. Each cosmetic area should be treated individually as each facial subunit has different reconstructive requirements that could not be recreated with a single flap. Several flaps with multiple stages will be required to recreate the features of the normal face.

As discussed previously, the ideal nose has its foundations on a solid and symmetrical platform which should be reconstructed first, and for this reason it is advised to start with maxillary, cheek, and lip reconstruction followed by nasal reconstruction.

Use of an Algorithm for Flap Selection for Nasal Reconstruction

Flap section in nasal reconstruction should be based on defect location and orientation (Table 30.1), with the nose

TABLE 30.1 **Guide to Flap Selection for Nasal Reconstruction Based on Location**

Proximal Third of the Nose	
Central	
Horizontal defect	Dorsal nasal flap
Round defect	Glabella flap
Vertical defect	V–Y flap
Lateral	
Horizontal defect	Glabella flap, first choice Dorsal nasal flap, second choice
Vertical defect	V–Y flap
Combined defect	Forehead flap
Middle Third of the Nose	
Central	
Horizontal and round defect	Dorsal nasal flap
Vertical defect	V–Y flap
Lateral	
Horizontal defect	Dorsal nasal flap
Vertical defect	V–Y flap, first choice Nasolabial flap, second choice
Combined defect	Forehead flap
Distal Third of the Nose	
Alar defect	Nasolabial flap, first choice V–Y flap, second choice Ascending free helical rim flap
Domal-alar groove defect	Nasolabial flap, first choice V–Y flap, second choice
Dome defect	Bilobed flap
Central tip defect	Bilobed flap
Columella defect	Composite graft, skin graft, ascending helical free flap
Nasal sill defect	Nasolabial flap
Combined defect	Forehead flap, first choice Nasolabial or extended V–Y flap, second choice
Rhinectomy	Lining: free radial forearm flap Support: fee rib cartilage (osteochondral) Cover: extended forehead flap

divided transversely into three zones (proximal third, middle third, and distal third). Most of these reconstructions can be performed under local anesthesia in an outpatient setting. However, when defects exceed 2 cm in size, it can become difficult to rotate local tissue and often the use of a forehead flap is the best option.

Proximal Third

Defects most often encountered in the proximal third of the nose can be centrally located on the dorsum or radix area or laterally on the upper sidewalls. These defects often have exposed periosteum or bone but rarely require bony reconstruction.

Defects in the upper third are often reconstructed with a glabella flap transposed from the midforehead or glabella region. If the lesion is centrally located it can often be reconstructed with a dorsal nasal advancement flap. Lateral defects that are horizontally orientated can be reconstructed with the glabellar flap whereas those defects that are vertically orientated can be treated with a V–Y flap from the dorsum of the nose. Larger combined defects are best treated with a forehead flap but can be amenable to an extended glabella flap or modified glabella-bilobed flap.

Medial Third

The middle third of the nose is divided into central and lateral zones, and includes the nasal bones and upper lateral cartilages. The medial third is an excellent place to apply the dorsal nasal flap. The lateral defects encountered in the medial third can be closed with a V–Y flap, nasolabial flap, bilobed flap or a dorsal nasal flap. A very useful flap is a V–Y flap based on perforators from the facial artery. Larger defects will most often require a forehead flap.

Distal Third

The distal third zone of the nose is the most common location for nasal defects after cancer excision. Alar defects can be reconstructed with a staged nasolabial flap. However, for alar defects sparing the rim, a V–Y advancement flap may used. Any remaining alar rim will need a cartilage graft for support to prevent collapse of the rim. Small alar rim defects (up to 8 mm) can be reconstructed with a composite graft of skin and cartilage from the root of the ear helix. If the defect is full-thickness then lining can be provided by turnover flaps or skin graft, cartilage from the nasal septum or ear concha (placed along the alar edge), and skin from a nasolabial flap or forehead flap.

Defects located in the domal-alar groove can be reconstructed with a nasolabial flap but more recently these defects are often reconstructed with the V–Y flap advanced laterally to cover the defect in a single stage. Those defects confined to the dome of the nose are usually best reconstructed with a forehead flap. Alternative options include the use of the dorsal nasal flap or the use of a bilobed flap. Cartilage tip grafts may need to be placed if there is deficient or weakened cartilage. Lining can be reconstructed with a mucoperichondrial flap or FTSG.

If the defect involves only the columella and is small then a composite graft from the antihelix of the ear can be used. If no cartilage is deficient and there is intact periosteum, an FTSG may be placed. If the columella defect is large or encompasses the entire columella, a multistaged nasolabial flap may be required. When a more complex reconstruction is required (e.g., bilateral alar rims and columella), the total central forehead flap should be used. The best approach to the more complex lower third defects is to use the three-stage technique described by Menick.[23]

The key to complete survival of the flap is the position of its base; this should be at the medial canthal level or below. In this way, the vascular anastomosis on the side of the nose between the cheek and forehead vessels can provide a satisfactory flap to close the defect. With the base correctly positioned, the midline flap will comfortably reconstruct the nasal tip and the columella without tension. The forehead is closed directly, but if there is tension in the area just anterior to the hairline, it should be left to close spontaneously. The scar resulting from this rarely, if ever, requires any reconstruction. The pedicle is divided at 3 weeks, depending on the inset, and the nasal tip is fashioned. Apart from thinning, it is unusual to require further adjustments. If there is any concern about vascularity, the flap base is delayed.

If a total nasal reconstruction is required, a larger amount of forehead skin is harvested in the transverse dimension, but again, the base should be positioned at or below the medial canthal ligament. The septal mucosa is used for lining. For closure of the midline forehead defect, the skin can frequently be mobilized extensively and advanced. If there is concern, a tissue expander can be inserted to expand the whole forehead.

This gives a large amount of skin with a good blood supply. If nasal support is needed, a cranial bone graft from the outer table of the skull is taken from an area where the curvature is similar to that required for the defect reconstruction, the shape can be chosen to some extent. This may be done at the same time with secure screw stabilization of the bone graft in the forehead/nose junction. It may be safer to delay grafting to the time of flap division or to a third procedure. Noses may be prefabricated elsewhere (e.g., on the forearm using a radial flap) and subsequently transferred by microvascular techniques.

References

1. Yong JS, Christophel JJ, Park SS. Repair of intermediate-size nasal defects: a working algorithm. *JAMA Otolaryngol Head Neck Surg*. 2014;140(11):1027–1033.
2. Seth R, Revenaugh PC, Scharpf J, et al. Free anterolateral thigh fascia lata flap for complex nasal lining defects. *JAMA Facial Plast Surg*. 2013;15(1):21–28.
3. Bhishagratna KKL, ed. *Sushruta Samitha*. Calcutta: Bose; 1907–1916.
4. Anderson JR. In: *The Dynamics of Rhinoplasty*. Presented at *Proceedings of the 9th International Congress of Otorhinolaryngology*. Excerpta Medica; 1969.
5. Menick FJ. Nasal reconstruction. *Plast Reconstr Surg*. 2010;125(4):138e–150e.
6. Konofaos P, Alvarez S, McKinnie JE, Wallace RD. Nasal reconstruction: a simplified approach based on 419 operated cases. *Aesthetic Plast Surg*. 2015;39(1):91–99.
7. Millard Jr DR. Aesthetic reconstructive rhinoplasty. *Clin Plast Surg*. 1981;8(2):169–175.
8. Burget GC. Aesthetic restoration of the nose. *Clin Plast Surg*. 1985;12(3):463–480.
9. Burget GC, Menick FJ. The subunit principle in nasal reconstruction. *Plast Reconstr Surg*. 1985;76:239–247.
10. Menick FJ. *Nasal Reconstruction: Art and Practice*. Philadelphia: Saunders; 2009.
11. Rohrich RJ, Griffin JR, Ansari M, et al. Nasal reconstruction – beyond aesthetic subunits: a 15-year review of 1334 cases. *Plast Reconstr Surg*. 2004;114:1405.
12. McCluskey PD, Constantine FC, Thornton JF. Lower third nasal reconstruction: when is skin grafting an appropriate option? *Plast Reconstr Surg*. 2009;124:826.
13. Chen C, Patel R, Chi J. Comprehensive algorithm for nasal ala reconstruction: utility of the auricular composite graft. *Surg J*. 2018;4(2):e55–e61.

14. Rieger RA. A local flap for repair of the nasal tip. *Plast Reconstr Surg*. 1967;40:147–149.
15. Marchac D. Lambeau de rotation fronto-nasal. *Ann Chirurg Plast*. 1970;15:44–49.
16. Zitelli JA. The bilobed flap for nasal reconstruction. *Arch Dermatol*. 1989;125:957–959.
17. Menik FJ, Salibian A. Primary intranasal lining injury: cause, deformities, and treatment plan. *Plast Reconstr Surg*. 2014;134(5):1045–1056.
18. Converse JM. Reconstruction of the nose by the scalping flap technique. *Surg Clin North Am*. 1959;39:259–335.
19. Weber SM, Wang TD. Options for internal lining in nasal reconstruction. *Facial Plast Surg Clin North Am*. 2011;19(1):163–173.
20. Gillies HD. A new free graft applied to the reconstruction of the nostril. *Br J Surg*. 1943;30:305.
21. Converse JM. Composite graft from the septum in nasal reconstruction. *Transact Latin Am Congress Plast Surg*. 1956;8:281.
22. Burget GC, Menick FJ. Nasal support and lining: the marriage of beauty and blood supply. *Plast Reconstr Surg*. 1989;84:189.
23. Menick FJ. A new modified method for nasal lining: the Menick technique for folded lining. *J Surg Oncol*. 2006;94:509–514.
24. Burget GC, Walton R. Optimal use of microvascular free flaps, cartilage grafts and a paramedian forehead flap for aesthetic reconstruction of the nose and adjacent facial units. *Plast Reconstr Surg*. 2007;120:1171–1207.
25. Menick FJ, Salibian A. Microvascular repair of heminasal, subtotal, and total nasal defects with a folded radial forearm flap and a full–thickness forehead flap. *Plast Reconstr Surg*. 2011;127:1–15.
26. Gillies HD, ed. *Plastic Surgery of the Face*. London: Oxford University Press; 1920.
27. Millard Jr DR. Hemirhinoplasty. *Plast Reconstr Surg*. 1967;40:440.
28. Converse JM, ed. *Reconstr Plast Surg*. 2nd edn. Vol 2. Philadelphia: WB Saunders; 1977.
29. Millard Jr DR. Total reconstructive rhinoplasty and a missing link. *Plast Reconstr Surg*. 1966;37:167.
30. Parkhouse N, Evans D. Reconstruction of the ala of the nose using a composite free flap from the pinna. *Br J Plast Surg*. 1985;38:306–313.

31 Eyelid Reconstruction

EBBY ELAHI AND IRINA BELINSKY

Introduction

Reconstructive surgery of the face and eyelids has undergone significant changes in the past half century. The increased specialization and advanced understanding of anatomy and physiology of the periocular region has coincided with an increased number of reconstructive options available to the surgeon. With this widened armamentarium and a changing expectation of patients, aesthetic awareness is now a significant part of reconstructive surgery even if the primary goal is protecting the eye and restoring or preserving function (Fig. 31.1).

One of the most significant advances in the past several decades is the awareness of the role of volume in functional and esthetic restoration. Patients with protuberant eyes (negative vector orbit) resulting from exophthalmos or hypoplastic orbit and midface encounter significantly more challenges in reconstruction than those with relative enophthalmos.[1] Similarly, procedures outside the immediate periocular region (e.g., microvascular free flap reconstruction of the midface) can cause significant distortions to the eyelid and secondary functional deficits. The patient's age is an important factor in the decision to pursue a particular reconstructive option. Older patients with more tissue laxity have generally better options with local tissue rearrangements than younger patients in whom free flaps may be superior.

Finally, an important, but often overlooked element in periocular reconstruction is the dynamic physiology of the periocular region. A number of neurological reflex pathways govern the position and function of the eyelids. Hering's law of equal innervation refers to the shared efferent pathway of the third cranial nerve to both levator palpebrae superioris (LPS) muscles.[2] A patient with unilateral ptosis will often have retraction of the contralateral eyelid and vice versa. Furthermore, in a majority of patients elevation of the eyebrow occurs on the ipsilateral side (Sherrington's reflex).[3] These combined reflexes often result in retraction of the orbital fat and deepening of the superior sulcus on the ipsilateral side. Matsuo et al have also shown that ipsilateral ptosis can result in increased scleral show by causing a reflex contraction of the inferior rectus muscle in response to the contraction of the levator palpebrae superioris and superior rectus muscles.[4] Rootman et al have demonstrated a 15% change in brow height in patients undergoing ptosis repair[5] (Fig. 31.2). Ignoring such dynamic shifts in reconstructive surgery can lead to functional deficits and aesthetic dissatisfaction with the final outcome (Fig. 31.3).

Periocular Physiology

The eyelids are a dynamic structure and their function is to protect the ocular surface, simultaneously maintaining corneal wetting and normal tear outflow. Normal horizontal eyelid tension created by the medial and lateral suspensory ligaments maintains the eyelids snug against the eye. The vertical balance of eyelid protractor and retractor muscles ensures complete closure of the eyelids with passive blinking and adequate opening of the eyelids to clear the pupil and visual axis. Contraction of the orbicularis oculi muscle during blinking pumps tears into the lacrimal outflow tract. A complex neural pathway involving cranial nerves V and VII regulates the balance between tear production and outflow. Excessive tearing, or epiphora, from overproduction is most commonly a result of reflex tearing from corneal irritation, such as aberrant lashes or corneal exposure. Exposure keratopathy caused by eyelid malposition can lead to corneal dryness, chronic pain, scarring, infection, loss of vision, and even loss of eye. Epiphora from insufficient drainage can

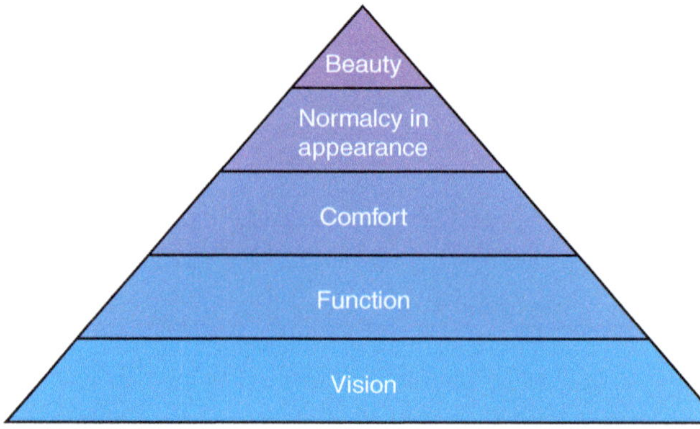

• **Fig. 31.1** Pyramid of goals in periorbital reconstruction.

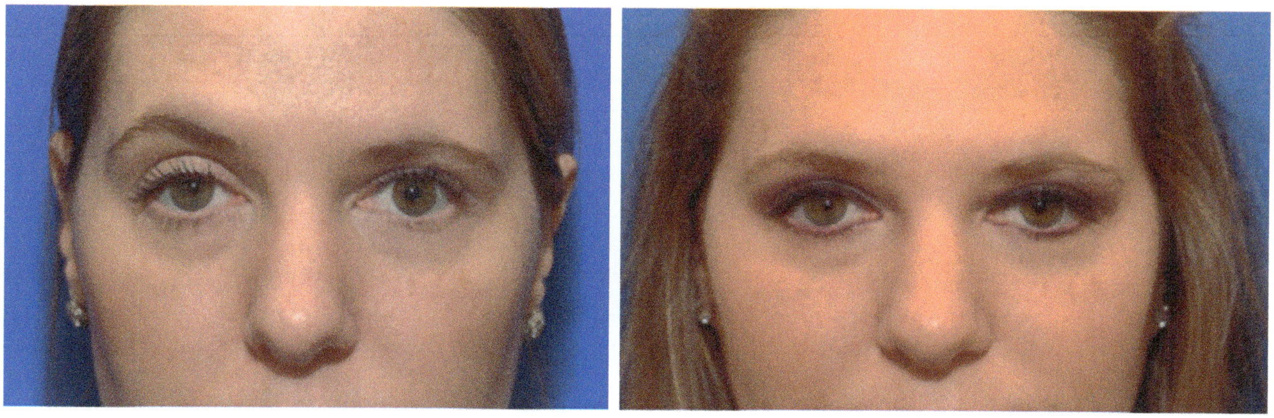

• **Fig. 31.2** Sherrington's reflex as demonstrated by ipsilateral brow elevation on the side of eyelid ptosis. Note change in brow position following ptosis repair.

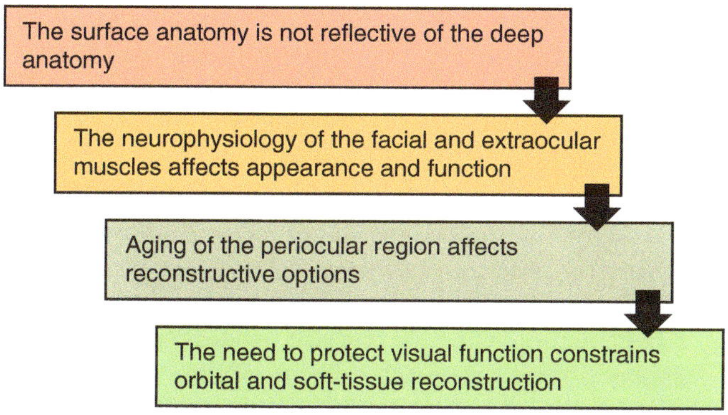

• **Fig. 31.3** Challenges in periorbital reconstruction.

occur when any part of the lacrimal outflow system is interrupted, so special attention is paid to this during medial eyelid surgery.

Periocular Anatomy: Fundamentals of Eyelid Anatomy

The eyelid subunits include the upper and lower lids as well as the lateral and medial canthi. The eyelids can generally be considered a bilaminar structure enveloping the orbital septum and fat (aka the middle lamella).

The anatomical features of the eyelid vary with the distance from the eyelid margin. The vertical height of the central upper eyelid tarsus is 10–12 mm and in the central lower eyelid it is 4–5 mm with some variation between sexes and ethnicities. In most instances the levator aponeurosis is bifurcated in its aponeurotic layer. The eyelid crease is defined by the anterior extensions of the aponeurosis onto the pretarsal skin.[6] Superior to this eyelid crease, the layers include skin, orbicularis oculi muscle, septum, preaponeurotic fat, levator aponeurosis, Müller's muscle, and conjunctiva. The lower eyelid has a similar multilayer, with the capsulopalpebral fascia analogous to the levator muscle and the inferior tarsal muscle analogous to Müller's muscle. The eyelid margin from posterior to anterior includes: the mucocutaneous junction, the meibomian gland orifices, the gray line (formed by the marginal portion of the palpebral orbicularis muscle), and the eyelash line.

The levator palpebrae superioris (LPS) and Müller's muscles in the upper eyelid are the main retractors. The levator muscle originates from the lesser wing of the sphenoid bone and inserts on the anterior surface of the tarsus as a broad aponeurosis and is innervated by the superior division of cranial nerve III (oculomotor nerve). The Müller's muscle, which is sympathetically innervated, originates from the posterior surface of the levator and inserts onto the superior border of tarsus. The orbicularis oculi muscle is the main protractor of the eyelids and receives its innervation from cranial nerve VII (facial nerve). The superficial musculoaponeurotic system (SMAS) of the cheek interdigitates with the orbicularis oculi muscle in the lower eyelid. Posterior to the orbicularis oculi muscle is the orbital septum. It is an avascular fascial extension of the arcus marginalis of the orbital rim and separates the superficial eyelid adnexa from the orbit, making it an important surgical landmark. Incision of the orbital septum allows access to the various extraconal orbital fat compartments.

The lateral canthal tendon inserts posteriorly and superolaterally onto Whitnall's tubercle on the inner aspect of the lateral orbital rim. The medial canthal tendon is anatomically more complex because it includes the lacrimal system. The anterior and posterior limbs surround the lacrimal sac. The posterior limb acts as the horizontal supporting band of the lower eyelid, directing the medial eyelid posteriorly to follow the curvature of the globe. Reconstruction at either canthus is aimed at recreating the deep attachments of the canthal tendons inside the orbit to avoid problematic eyelid malpositions.

The conjunctiva is a mucous membrane that forms a single continuous lining over the anterior surface of the eye and posterior eyelids. In reconstructive eyelid surgery, conjunctiva can be rotated or advanced as a flap, grafted from the ipsilateral or contralateral eye, or replaced with analogous nonkeratinizing mucosal epithelium.

A rich vascular supply to the eyelids comes from branches of both the internal and external carotid arteries. These branches form a highly vascularized anastomotic network of vessels that contribute to the high survival rate of grafts and flaps in periocular reconstruction. In general this obviates the need to design flaps based upon specific vessels. As in any surgery, attention to careful hemostasis is important, especially in the periocular region where a retrobulbar hemorrhage resulting in an orbital compartment syndrome can lead to vision loss.

General Principles of Reconstruction

The goal of periocular reconstruction is the restoration of eyelid function, appearance, and maintenance of visual function. Because myriad choices are available to the surgeon (e.g., graft vs. flap), it is valuable to review some general principles that can underlie these choices.

- *Protection*: Since the eyelid's function is primarily to protect the sight organ, reconstruction should be directed to protect vision. The role of the upper lid is critical in humans. The eyelid must be able to cover the majority of the cornea with a blink and during sleep. Small degrees of opening (lagophthalmos) can be tolerated by many patients during sleep as a result of Bell's phenomenon whereby the eye is in an upgaze position during most sleep hours. The cornea cannot tolerate significant exposure for long periods of time and must be protected by other means if a staged operation is planned. A number of methods have been employed such as placement of temporary gold weight on the upper lid, tarsorrhaphy, or injection of botulinum toxin to the levator muscle.
- *Mobility*: The eyelid position under normal circumstances is defined by the static anatomy of the periocular structures and the neurophysiology of the protractor and retractor muscles. In reconstructing the eyelid, special attention must be paid to avoid cicatricial changes resulting in inadvertently connecting these separate layers. Patients with scarring between the LPS and orbicularis oculi muscle or orbital septum may have the inability to open and close the eyelids resulting from significantly diminished levator function.
- *Esthetics*: It is critical for the reconstructive surgeon to be familiar with the esthetic principles underlying oculoplastic surgery. For optimal functional and cosmetic outcomes, the surgeon must consider the anatomical relationship of the eyelids to neighboring regions of the face. The face is divided into several esthetic units. Most relevant to periocular reconstruction are its neighboring esthetic regions: the forehead, the cheek, and the nose. Taking into account the unique topography of these borders will aid in incision design, scar camouflage, construction of flaps and grafts, and volumetric balance. It is also helpful to think of normative features that are universal regardless of ethnic origin. Useful examples include the following:
  - The outer canthus should be approximately 5–10 degrees (or 2 mm) above the medical canthus.
  - The upper lid generally covers the upper border of the iris on primary gaze.
  - The lower lid is generally at or within 1 mm of the lower iris border. Any further scleral show is generally considered displeasing.
  - The upper eyelid peaks nasally to the pupil. Lateralization of this peak can alter a person's esthetic identity.

A number of technical principles should also be considered in guiding the reconstructive surgeon.

- *Maintain vascularity.* Although recently challenged by some researchers, it is generally accepted that continuous vascularity is necessary in at least one layer of the eyelid if the other layer is to be grafted. A bilaminar grafting of the eyelid can result in necrosis and subsequent tissue loss. Several classically described procedures such as the Hughes or Cutler–Beard procedure (described below) take advantage of these principles.
- Diminish excess tension, especially as it applies to the lower lid. Due to the weak support of the eyelid at the canthus, any excess tension especially on the midface will result in an ectropion of the eyelid. For this reason, no downward pull must be felt by the eyelid during reconstruction. In cases where canthal laxity is present, a canthal tightening procedure (canthopexy, canthoplasty or tarsal strip procedure) can be performed. However, the inferior vector pull of the midface must be addressed separately by supporting the midface. Under certain circumstances, a staged approach may provide the ideal esthetic and functional outcome while minimizing scar size (Fig. 31.4).
- Choose ideal skin match. Generally, the best match for a defect is the local surrounding tissue that retains the esthetic characteristics of the missing tissue. Thus, whenever possible, a local flap would be preferable. This principle must be weighed against the overall size of the incision necessary to mobilize tissue to cover the defect. If distal tissue is used, the ideal donor size is in descending order: eyelid skin, retroauricular skin or other sources of thin, non-hair-bearing regions such as the supraclavicular skin.
- Minimize incision size. It is sometimes said that with a sufficiently long scar most facial defects can be primarily closed. The goal of every reconstructive surgery is therefore not only to repair the existing defect, but minimize the length of incisions and potentially resultant scarring. In addition to gaining familiarity with specific techniques, it is helpful to consider these principles in the perioperative decision planning:
  - Whenever possible, incisions should follow Langer's relaxed skin tension lines (RSTLs) of the face that result in more inconspicuous scarring.
  - Delaying the repair often results in a smaller defect, allowing for a smaller incision.
  - With cautious and judicious exercise in clinical judgment, both the anterior and posterior lamella of the ipsilateral or contralateral eyelid can be very useful sources of tissue. In patients with upper lid dermatochalasis, the use of upper lid skin can not only provide

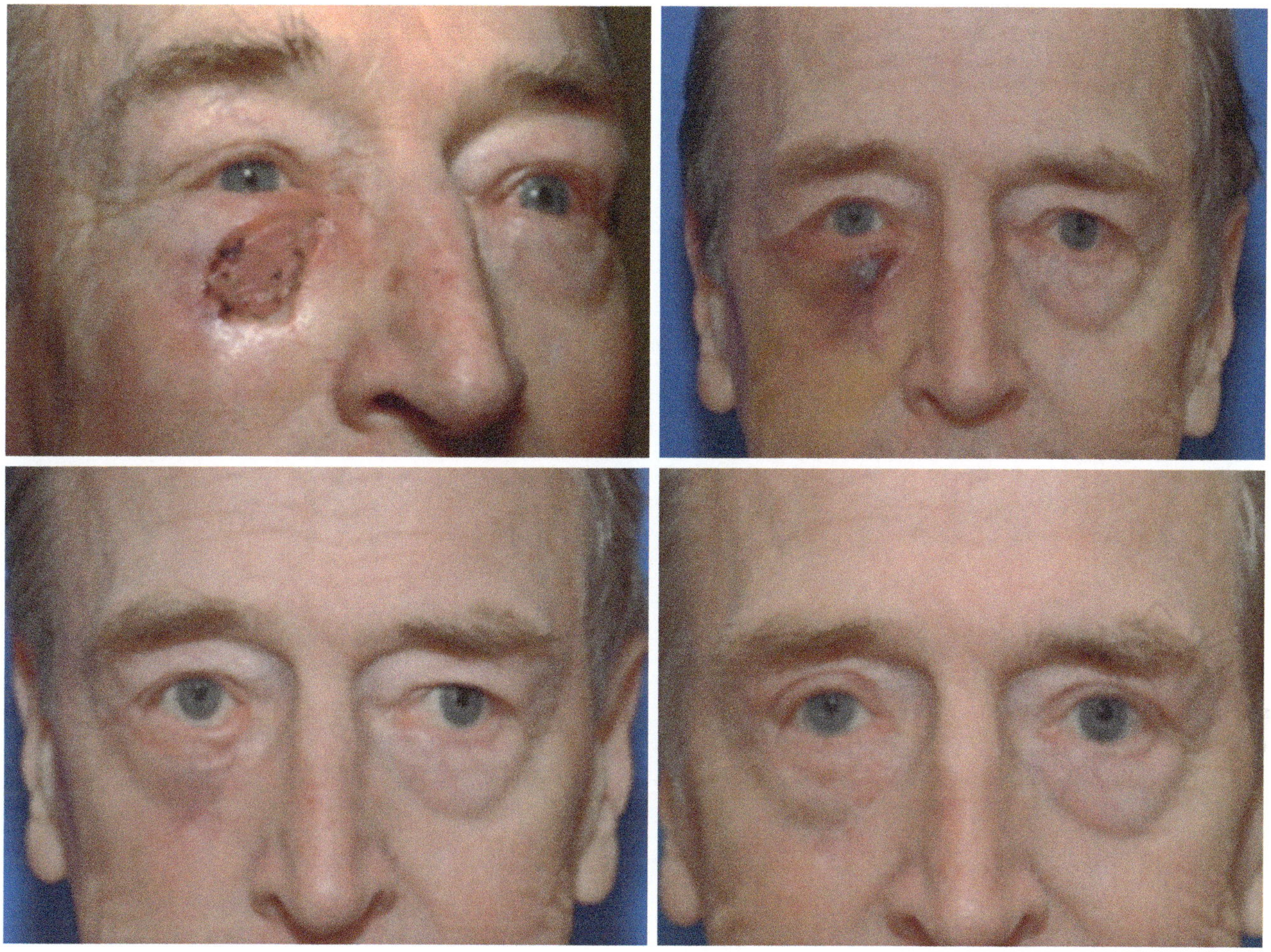

• **Fig. 31.4** Staged approach to lower eyelid reconstruction. First, the lower eyelid defect is closed with a local advancement flap. Two months later, cicatricial ectropion is noted, which is sometimes unavoidable in older individuals with lower eyelid laxity. This is repaired with a free skin graft from the upper eyelid, paired with a contralateral blepharoplasty for optimal cosmesis.

an ideal coverage of a defect but result in an overall improved facial appearance. Due to the surgeon and patient bias alike, cosmetic enhancement is often not thought of as a goal of reconstructive surgery, often to the detriment of the patient (Fig. 31.5).

- Similarly with a conservative approach, another very useful source of posterior lamellar reconstruction is the upper tarsus. As long as 4 mm of vertical upper tarsus is preserved, the remainder can be used to reconstruct a posterior lamellar defect, often obviating the need for more invasive procedures that would require stages.

Anesthesia and Perioperative Tips

Many extensive procedures require the use of general anesthesia, the risk of which must be weighed against the use of local anesthetic in an outpatient setting. This is especially true for patients who are anticoagulated and the elderly. Thus, the appropriate use of local anesthesia can be immensely helpful in reducing perioperative risk. In our practices, we generally use a 50:50 mix of lidocaine 1% with 1:100,000 epinephrine and bupivacaine 0.75% combined with 8.4% sodium bicarbonate in a 1:9 dilution. Occasional hyaluronidase is added to help local anesthetic diffusion. Whenever possible, we inject our local anesthetic with a cannula to minimize ecchymosis. In addition, the use of oral medications containing benzodiazepines, inhaled nitrogen oxide, or combined preparations such as sublingual MKO (midazolam 3 mg, ketamine HCl 25 mg, ondansetron 2 mg – Imprimis, New Jersey, USA) can provide safe and effective means of controlling patient anxiety in an outpatient setting.

Topical proparacaine 0.5% or tetracaine 1% is used before preparation to anesthetize the ocular surface. Corneal shields lubricated with ophthalmic ointment are used to protect the eye during eyelid surgery. When a corneal shield is not used or otherwise temporarily removed intraoperatively, frequent rewetting with ophthalmic petrolatum ointment is done to prevent corneal dryness and abrasions. Surgical marking is done before infiltration with local anesthetic because fine eyelid creases and RSTLs are easily lost

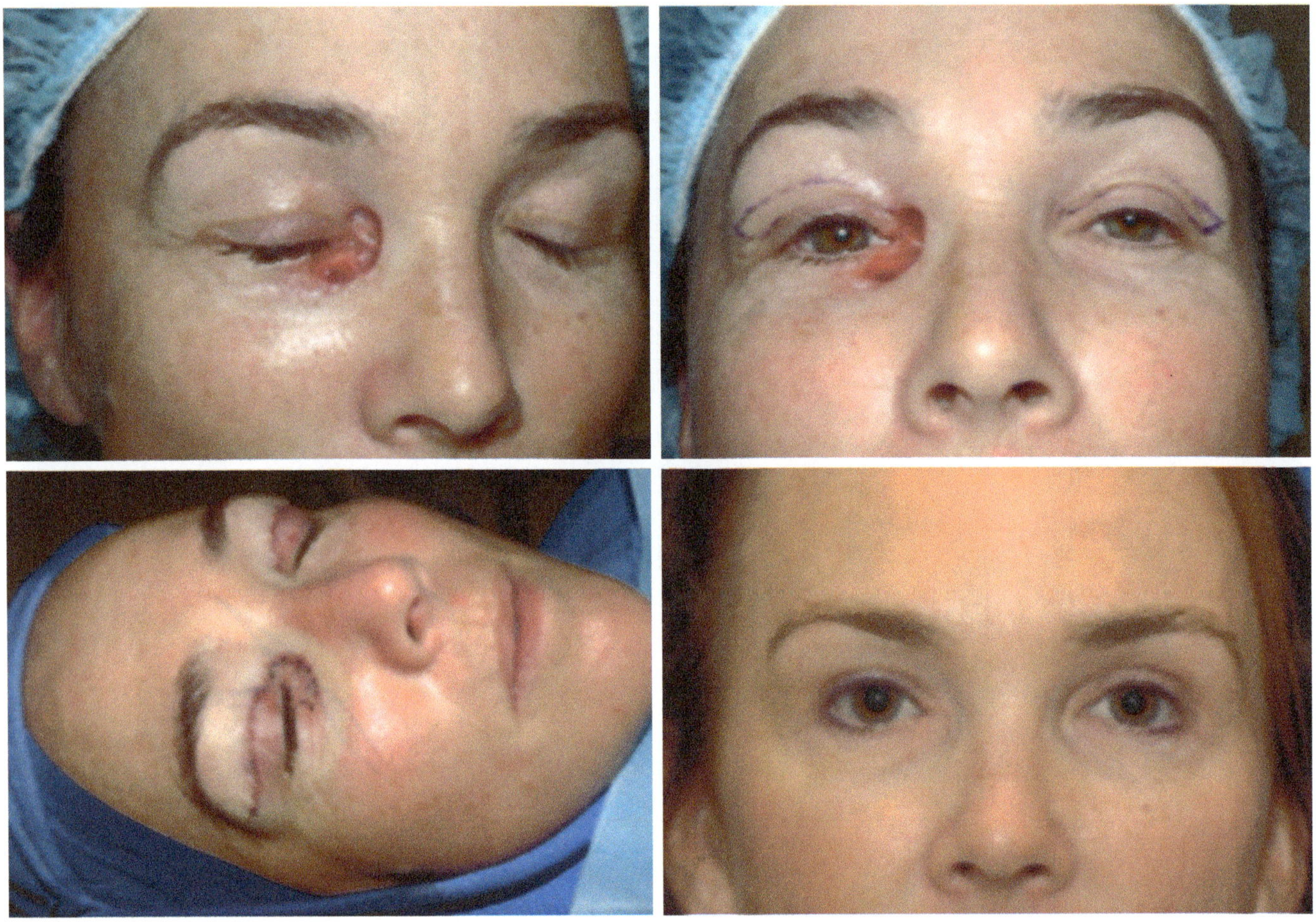

• **Fig. 31.5** Free skin graft from the ipsilateral upper eyelid was used to reconstruct a medial canthal defect. This was paired with a contralateral blepharoplasty for optimal esthetic result.

when volume is added. Local anesthetic is delivered slowly, making sure to direct the needle in such a way that patient movement does not result in globe penetration. It is useful to slightly bend the needle at 30 degrees and direct it away from the globe while pulling the eyelid away from the globe during injection. In this manner any penetration of the eyelid is immediately observed, and the needle redirected. Depending on the case, a 27G, 30G, or 33G needle can be useful. Transconjunctival injection is less painful than skin injection and is especially useful to anesthetize a lower eyelid full-thickness defect. The needle should penetrate conjunctiva in the fornix (below the inferior edge of tarsus, not into tarsus). In the lateral canthus, additional anesthesia is administered over the orbital rim. In the medial canthus, direct injection into the puncta or canaliculus is avoided.

Techniques

No two defects will be the same. Defects can be described as primarily anterior lamellar, posterior lamellar, or full thickness. A full-thickness eyelid defect involving one-third of the eyelid may be repaired with simple direct closure in an elderly patient with significant eyelid laxity, but in a young patient would require lateral canthal release to achieve closure. In many cases there is more than one design that works and selection is based on surgeon experience and preference. The following provides a list of reliable and predictable reconstructive techniques that, when guided by the principles previously described, will help achieve successful eyelid reconstruction.

Anterior Lamellar Defects

Primary Closure

Healing by granulation or secondary intention may be appropriate for small wounds away from the mobile eyelids, such as in the medial canthal region. Conjunctival incisions in the inferior cul-de-sac can heal nicely without closure. However, in most other periocular areas, scar contracture can cause eyelid malposition.

The simple ellipse may be used to remove most superficial periocular skin lesions and it can be closed primarily. The ellipse should be oriented vertical to eyelid RSTLs to avoid vertical cicatricial tension. Since the ellipse sacrifices normal tissue in addition to the surface area of the original defect, modifications of the ellipse such as the double-S ellipse and O-to-Z-plasty can be used to conserve more normal tissue.[7] Closure is typically performed using interrupted sutures with slight eversion of the wound edges, skin-to-skin, using 6-0 dissolvable material (such gut,

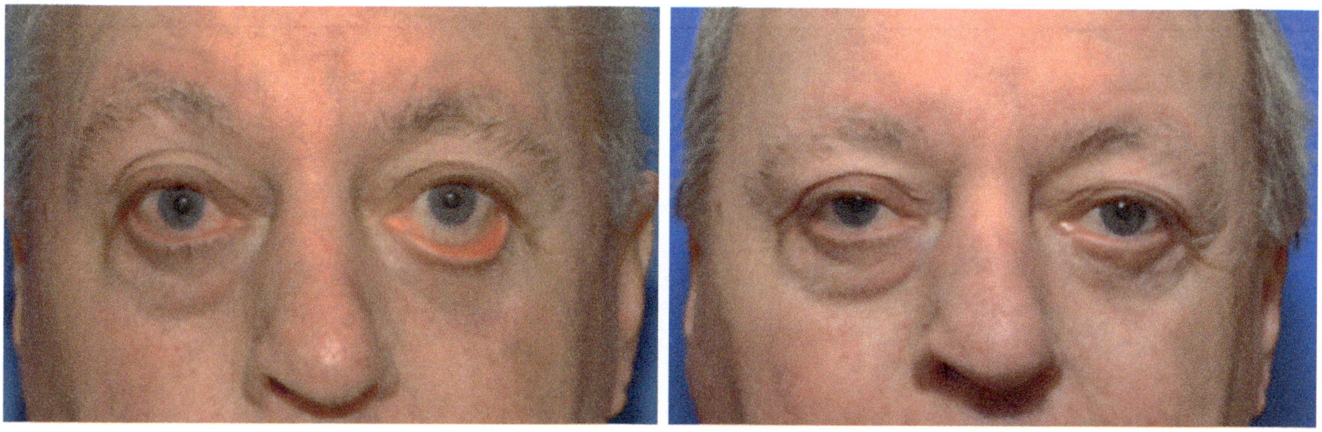

• **Fig. 31.6** Left lower eyelid cicatricial ectropion repaired with a retroauricular free skin graft.

polyglactin or poliglecaprone 25) or nondissolvable material (such as nylon or polypropylene, to be removed in 5–7 days).

Local Flaps

For larger anterior lamellar defects, where there is adequate skin elasticity, tissue can be mobilized in the form of advancement or rotational flaps.

Advantages of flaps over free skin grafts are better skin color and texture match, they undergo less contraction, they can support free grafts for posterior lamellar reconstruction, following healing there is near normal innervation of the skin, and they require shorter surgical time (locally available tissue means less injecting, prepping, and draping of a different body site). They also carry a native blood supply, so they are a good choice in smokers and patients with irradiated tissues where vascular supply is already compromised.

Advancement Flaps

The standard unipedicle or bipedicle advancement flaps can be used to repair lower eyelid, upper eyelid, and eyebrow defects. Parallel incisions are designed beginning at one edge of the defect, which becomes the leading edge of the rectangular-shaped flap. The resulting scars fall parallel or into the eyelid creases and any resulting dog-ears are excised.

Transposition Flaps

Hemi-Tripier Flap.[8] A bipedicled flap designed to reconstruct a lower eyelid defect using upper eyelid tissue in patients who have adequate upper dermatochalasis. It can be transferred as a cutaneous or musculocutaneous flap. The vascular pedicle and pivot point is usually at the lateral canthus and can extend to cover a lower eyelid defect from the lateral to the medial canthus.

Technique

1. The upper eyelid skin crease is marked like for a blepharoplasty. At least 20 mm of eyelid skin should be preserved.
2. A template of the lower eyelid defect is made.
3. The template is transferred to the upper eyelid, with the inferior margin of the lower lid defect aligned with the upper eyelid crease incision.
4. More skin is taken from the upper lid than is required to cover the defect, to allow room for graft contracture.
5. The upper eyelid flap is dissected in the suborbicularis plane.
6. The flap is sutured into the defect using interrupted 6-0 nonabsorbable monofilament suture.

Postoperative Management. Topical ophthalmic ointment and ice packs are applied three times daily. Sutures are removed in 5–7 days.

Fricke Flap. The Fricke flap is a similar, though less frequently utilized, transposition cutaneous flap from the supraorbital area for both upper and lower eyelid anterior lamellar defects.[9] In the first stage, the length of the flap is marked out just above the brow, with the lateral aspect of the flap kept wide. In the second stage the flap is transposed to either an upper or a lower eyelid defect, followed by wound closure.

Rhomboid Flap

These are versatile flaps, especially useful in the periocular region for reconstruction in the medial canthus. Glabellar and median forehead flaps are also used in this anatomical space, but are not discussed in this chapter.

The median forehead flap, not discussed in detail here, is commonly used to repair larger anterior lamellar defects involving the medial eyelid, medial canthus, and/or bridge of the nose especially when down to bare bone. It can be combined with other procedures such as the Mustardé cheek rotation for large combination defects. The flap is constructed along the axis of the contralateral supraorbital and supratrochlear neurovascular bundle and, by necessity, leaves a vertical scar in the forehead. It is debulked during a second stage procedure approximately 6 weeks later.

Full-Thickness Skin Grafts (Fig. 31.6)

There are several donor sites ideal for replacing eyelid anterior lamella, which have thin, hairless skin with a close

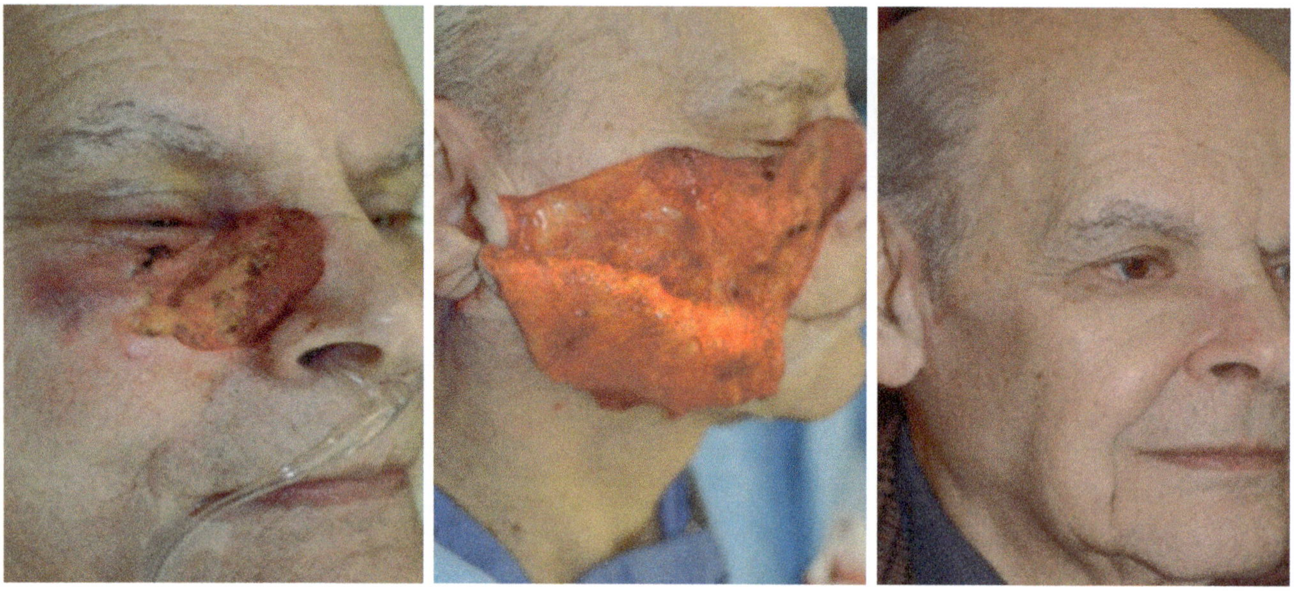

• **Fig. 31.7** Large anterior lamellar defect involving the lower eyelid, cheek, and bridge of nose repaired with a Mustardé cheek flap.

match in color and texture. The graft should be placed on a well-vascularized bed of tissue.[10] Full-thickness skin grafts do not take well on bare bone.

- *Upper eyelid*: Ideal for patients with dermatochalasis, this site has the best color and texture match. A contralateral blepharoplasty can be done at time of reconstruction to achieve aesthetic balance.
- *Pre- and post-auricular region*: Results in inconspicuous donor site scars. The skin color, especially post-auricular, is somewhat lighter and thicker. Availability is also limited by variation in patient's hairline.
- *Supraclavicular*: Larger surface area available for harvesting. In some patients this area has a similar sun-exposed color match.
- *Inner upper arm*: Large surface area available of thicker and generally lighter skin.

Technique

1. The margins of the defect are cleaned.
2. Perform any appropriate direct closure of the defect prior to sizing a graft.
3. A template is made of the defect using sterile paper dressing, such as Telfa, which can then be cut along its outline.
4. The template is transferred to the donor site and traced with a surgical marking pen.
5. The skin graft is harvested using a No. 15 blade, toothed forceps, and scissors.
6. The graft is thinned to the level of the Rete pegs using curved Stevens scissors. Cautery to the graft should not be done.
7. The base of the donor site is cauterized for hemostasis and sutured closed.
8. The graft is sutured within the defect using the surgeon's suture of choice, usually 6-0 nonabsorbable monofilament.
9. A No. 11 blade or sharp-tipped scissors are then used to create small full-thickness stab incisions within the graft. This facilitates egress of blood should a hemorrhage occur beneath the graft (which could risk graft necrosis). These stab incisions will heal by secondary intention without scarring.
10. A pressure bolster is applied over the graft and if it is located in the inferior eyelid, a Frost suture is placed.

Postoperative Management. The pressure dressing and the sutures can be removed in 5 days. Topical ophthalmic ointment is applied three times daily. The graft will usually look dark at week 1. Normal color and texture will return several weeks postoperatively. A small amount of shrinkage of the graft is expected.

Mustardé Cheek Rotation Flap[11] (Fig. 31.7)

Used for reconstruction of a total lower eyelid anterior lamellar defect. There must be an intact posterior lamella, or otherwise reconstructed separately. This is a single-stage procedure. Note that the donor flap tissue lacks protractor muscles.

Technique

1. The flap is marked by starting upwards at the lateral canthus aiming toward the hairline, then extending inferiorly anterior to the tragus.
2. The skin is cut with a No. 15 blade and dissection is carried out in the subcutaneous plane along the temple and cheek.
3. Care is taken in the region of the zygomatic arch to avoid the zygomatic branch of the facial nerve, again remaining in the subcutaneous/fat plane.
4. Once sufficient dissection is completed, the flap is rotated into place.
5. Dog-ear deformities may need to be excised both in the preauricular region and the cheek.

6. The highest point of the flap is anchored a few millimeters superior to the intended position of the lateral canthus at the inner lateral orbital rim with a 5–0 braided, absorbable suture.
7. Skin is closed with 6–0 nonabsorbable monofilament.

Postoperative Management. A firm dressing is applied for 3–5 days to reduce the risk of hematoma formation. A topical antibiotic ointment can be applied three times a day to both the eye and wound for up to 2 weeks. All sutures can be removed at 10 days.

Full-Thickness Eyelid Defects

Primary Eyelid Margin Closure

Whether performing an eyelid wedge biopsy, fixing a congenital coloboma, or repairing a tumor excision or traumatic laceration, primary eyelid margin repair is an essential technique to master. Generally, defects involving 30% of the eyelid width or less will have enough horizontal laxity to permit direct closure. In some cases, even larger defects of up to 50% can be closed primarily if the eyelid is sufficiently lax, as in much older individuals. An extra 3–5 mm can be gained by performing a lateral canthotomy and cantholysis. The goal is to realign: (1) tarsus, (2) eyelid margin, and (3) skin.

Technique (***Fig. 31.8***)

1. The margins of the defect are cleaned. Conversion to a pentagonal defect using a No. 15 blade and making clean tarsal edges will optimize alignment.
2. The eyelid margins are grasped with toothed 0.5 forceps and approximated to each other. If there is too much tension, do a canthotomy and cantholysis (see 3, otherwise skip to 4).
3. A lateral canthotomy incision is made using a blade. Next the inferior eyelid margin is grasped with toothed Adson forceps or a 0.5 mm Castroviejo forceps and then scissors or a protected electrosurgical tip (Colorado needle) are used to cut the inferior crus of the lateral canthal tendon. Once fully released, tactile feedback from the forceps will offer free movement of the lower eyelid.
4. For eyelid margin repair, the first suture must establish perfect alignment. A 7-0 absorbable braided suture (such as Vicryl Rapide) is passed through the gray line in a vertical mattress fashion and tied. The tails are left long. The wound edges should be slightly everted to minimize notching. 6-0 silk sutures can also be used for eyelid margin alignment.
5. Next, close the tarsus using 5-0 Vicryl passed partial thickness through the tarsal plate (2 bites in the lower eyelid, 3 bites in the upper eyelid). Make sure the suture knot is buried.
6. A second vertical mattress suture is passed through the eyelash line and also left long. Any aberrantly directed lashes are epilated intraoperatively.
7. The orbicularis oculi muscle is closed with buried interrupted 5-0 or 6-0 dissolvable sutures.
8. The skin is closed in an interrupted fashion using a 6-0 suture material of the surgeon's choice. The long tails of the margin sutures are incorporated. In children or patients in whom suture removal will not be possible in the office setting, dissolvable material is a better choice.
9. The lateral canthal angle can be recreated into a sharp "V" shape by placing a buried mattress suture through the most lateral edges of the superior and inferior eyelid margins. This minimizes risk of lateral canthal rounding.
10. The canthotomy skin incision can be closed with the same 6-0 suture material.
11. Inspect that none of the sutures are in touch with the corneal surface.

Postoperative Management. Topical ophthalmic ointment and ice compresses are applied three times daily. While the skin sutures can be removed in 5–7 days, the vertical mattress margin sutures are removed later at 10–14 days. Complications may include notching, trichiasis, lower eyelid retraction, upper eyelid ptosis, and corneal abrasion.

The Tenzel Semicircular Advancement Flap[12–14]

This technique is used when a full-thickness eyelid defect cannot be closed primarily or after a lateral canthotomy and cantholysis, typically for defects of 50%–75%.

Technique (***Fig. 31.9***)

1. Beginning at the lateral canthal angle, draw an arched line extending superiorly with a relatively steep angle and a diameter of approximately 20 mm. For upper eyelid reconstruction, create a mirror marking.
2. Perform a lateral canthotomy to be incorporated in the incision of the flap followed by inferior cantholysis to fully free the lower eyelid.
3. As usual, clean the defect and freshen the tarsal edges of the wound.
4. Make the skin incision along the marking using a No. 15 blade. Dissect the musculocutaneous flap in the preseptal plane, undermining thoroughly until the flap can be adequately advanced medially. The edges of the defect should align without undue tension.
5. The flap can now be anchored medially by suturing it to the lateral canthal rim periosteum using one or two 4-0 PDS sutures. One bite should be into the inner aspect of the rim, with the sutures placed such that the lateral canthus is overcorrected superiorly and snug against the globe. This prevents lateral sagging of the eyelid.
6. Repair the eyelid margin as previously described.
7. The lateral incision site is closed with 6-0 nonabsorbable, monofilament suture.

The Tarsoconjunctival Advancement Flap: Hughes[15–17]

This procedure is used to reconstruct the posterior lamella of a full-thickness lower eyelid defect, usually encompassing the majority of the lower eyelid 50%–100%. It offers a rectangular pedicle of tarsus and conjunctiva from the upper eyelid and is sutured into the lower eyelid defect. The

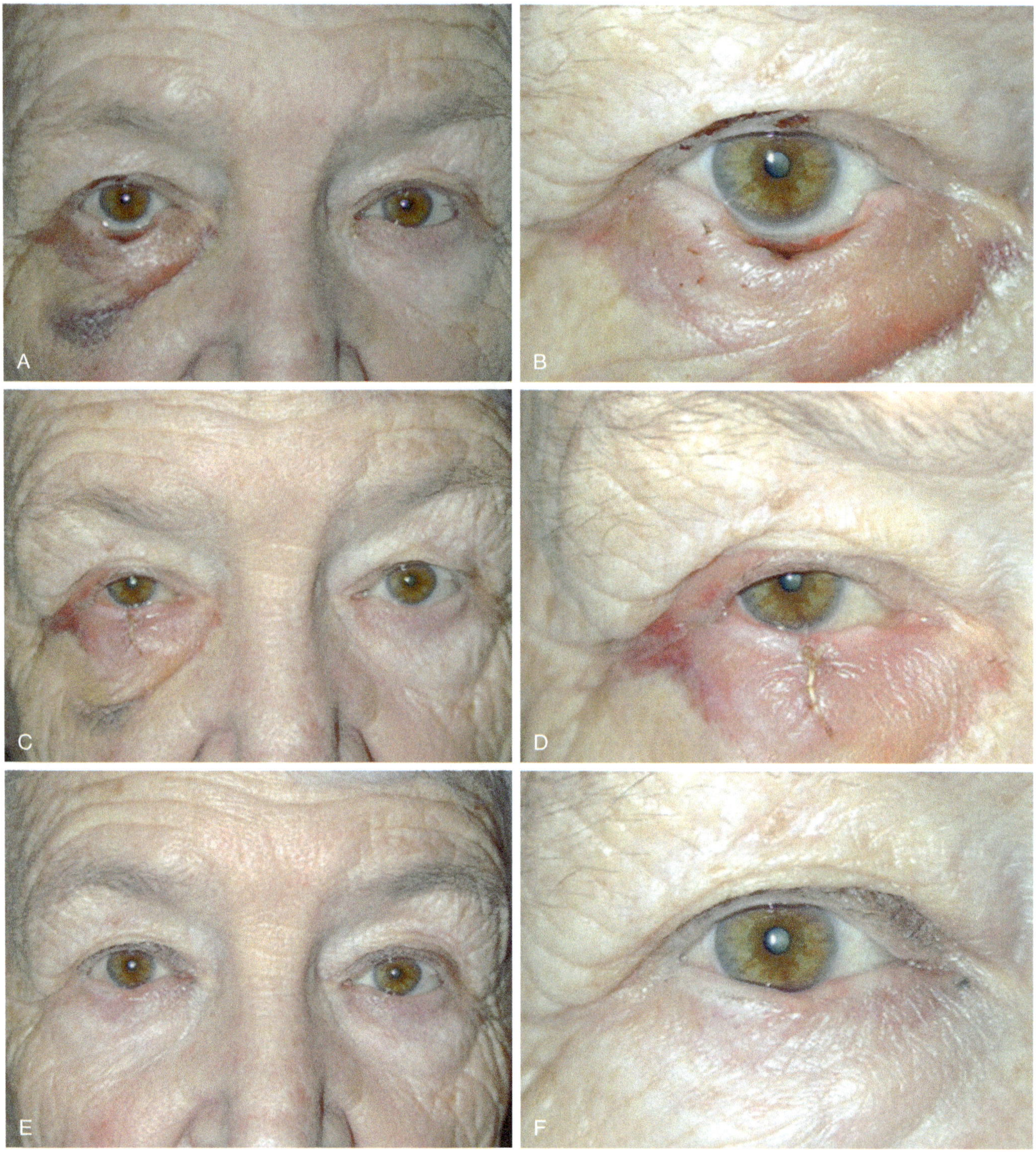

• **Fig. 31.8** Primary closure of full-thickness defect. (A,B) Approximately 50% full-thickness defect of the right lower eyelid with baseline eyelid laxity. (C,D) Primary closure of full-thickness after wedge excision. (E,F) 6-month postoperative appearance. (From Guanning NL, Pelton RW, Humphrey CD, Kriet JD. Defect of the eyelids. *Facial Plast Surg Clini North Am*. 25(3):377–392. Copyright © 2017 Elsevier Inc. Figure 8.)

blood supply to the tarsal graft comes from the conjunctiva, which remains attached to the superior fornix. It is divided 2–6 weeks later, so during this time the patient's vision is obstructed by the flap. This procedure is usually combined with a myocutaneous flap or full-thickness free skin graft to repair the anterior lamella.

Technique

1. Local anesthesia is administered in the region of the lower eyelid defect and in the ipsilateral upper eyelid subcutaneously. In addition, the upper eyelid is everted and anesthetic is delivered subconjunctivally above the superior tarsal border using a 30-gauge needle.

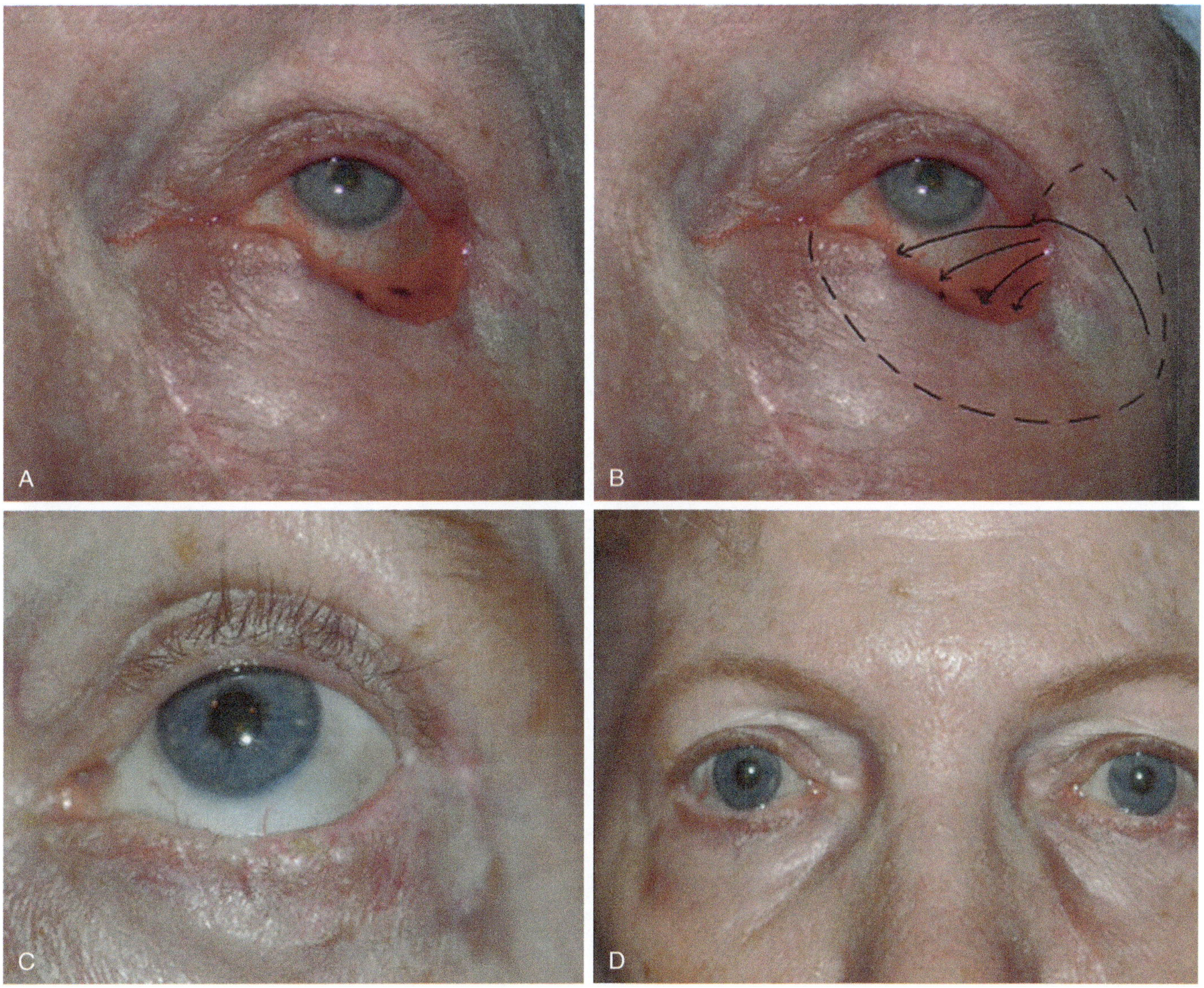

• **Fig. 31.9** Tenzel flap repair. (A) Defect involving approximately two-thirds of the left lower eyelid. (B) Dotted line represents area of undermining in the suborbicularis plane. Solid black line represents extension of incision into lateral canthal skin. *Arrows* represent advancement of Tenzel flap to close defect. (C) Postoperative close-up view. (D) Satisfactory symmetry to right eye achieved postoperatively. (From Guanning NL, Pelton RW, Humphrey CD, Kriet JD. Defect of the eyelids. *Facial Plast Surg Clin North Am.* 25(3):377–392. Copyright © 2017 Elsevier Inc. Figure 9.)

2. The lower eyelid defect margins are freshened, defect size is assessed by grasping both ends with forceps and bringing them together, and subsequently measured with a ruler.
3. The upper tarsal graft should be sized such that it is slightly smaller than the defect, to restore adequate horizontal tension and avoid eyelid malposition due to laxity post operatively.
4. In cases involving the entire width of the lower eyelid, the medial and lateral support for the tarsoconjunctival graft can be provided with periosteal flaps.
5. A 4-0 silk traction suture is placed through the grey line of the upper eyelid and the eyelid is everted over a Desmarres retractor.
6. The upper tarsus is marked using calipers and a surgical marking pen. A line is made parallel to and 4 mm away from the eyelid margin, to preserve this 4 mm of upper eyelid tarsus for future stability. The width then corresponds to the size of the lower eyelid defect and the height extends to and includes the superior edge of tarsus.
7. A No. 15 scalpel or No. 69 Beaver blade is used to make the incisions full thickness through tarsus only. The graft is dissected off the orbicularis (and levator aponeurosis) base using 0.5 forceps and blunt-tipped Wescott scissors.
8. At the superior tarsal border, dissection is carried out in the subconjunctival plane taking care to avoid Muller's muscle, the associated vascular arcade, and conjunctival buttonholes.
9. The donor tarsus can now be flipped down on its broad conjunctival pedicle and secured to the lower eyelid

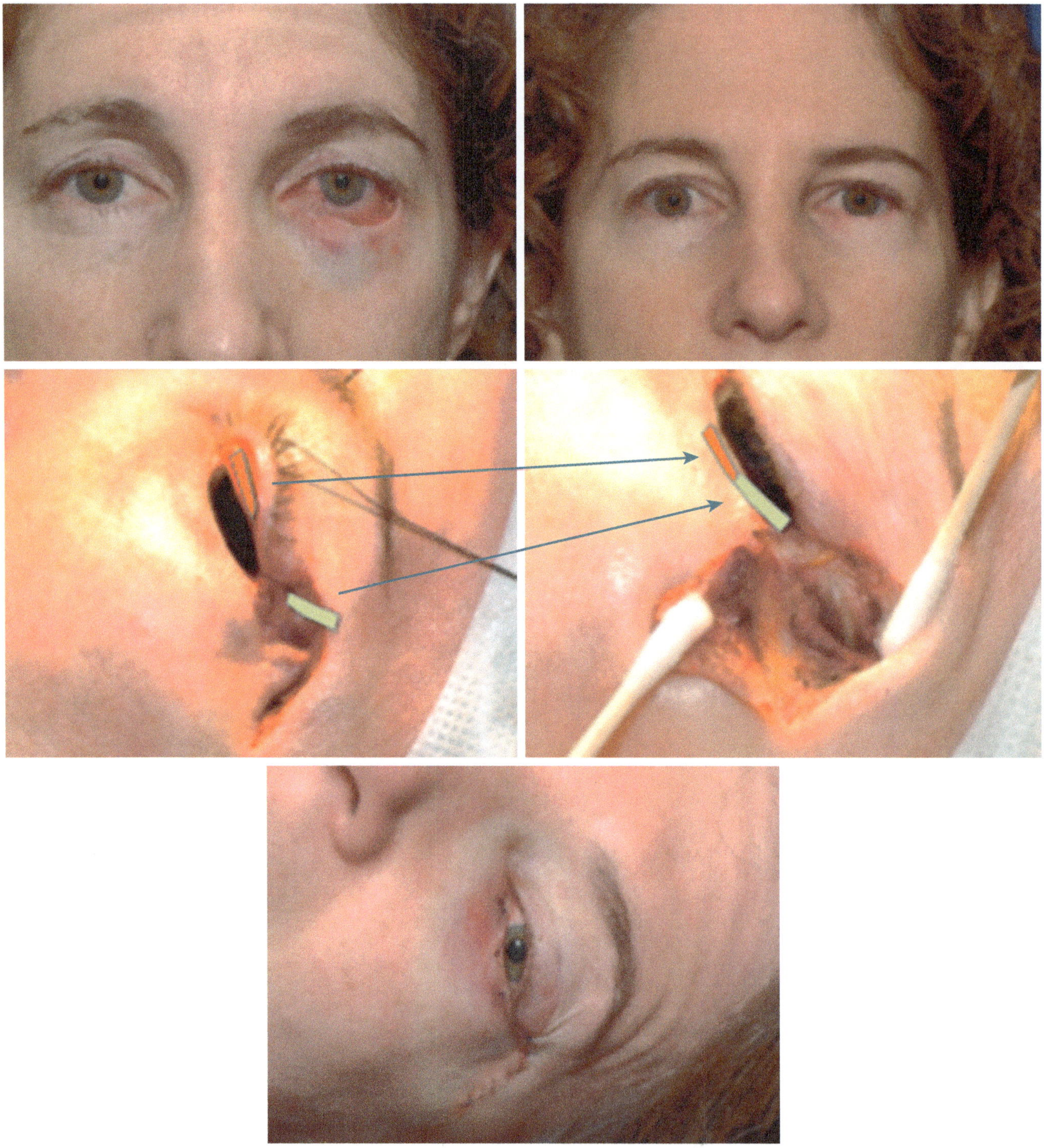

• **Fig. 31.10** Large inferior full-thickness defect repaired in a single-staged procedure with a free tarsal graft from the superior eyelid and an attached periosteal flap for posterior lamellar support. The anterior lamella is achieved via a myocutaneous advancement flap anchored on the periosteum.

defect using 5-0 polyglactin suture on a S-14 spatula needle. Anchor sutures can be placed first, ensuring there is no excessive tension, followed by running sutures along the borders.

Postoperative Management. Topical ophthalmic ointment is applied three times daily. The conjunctival flap is divided in 2–6 weeks under local anesthesia. Whenever possible, extra conjunctiva should be draped over the new lower eyelid margin, to maintain a mucocutaneous junction at the cornea.

It is valuable to note that in many instances the authors believe this two-staged procedure may be avoided by using a combination of a free tarsal graft,[18] a periosteal flap,[19] and a cheek advancement (Fig. 31.10). This can result in a more comfortable patient experience and potentially a superior esthetic outcome.

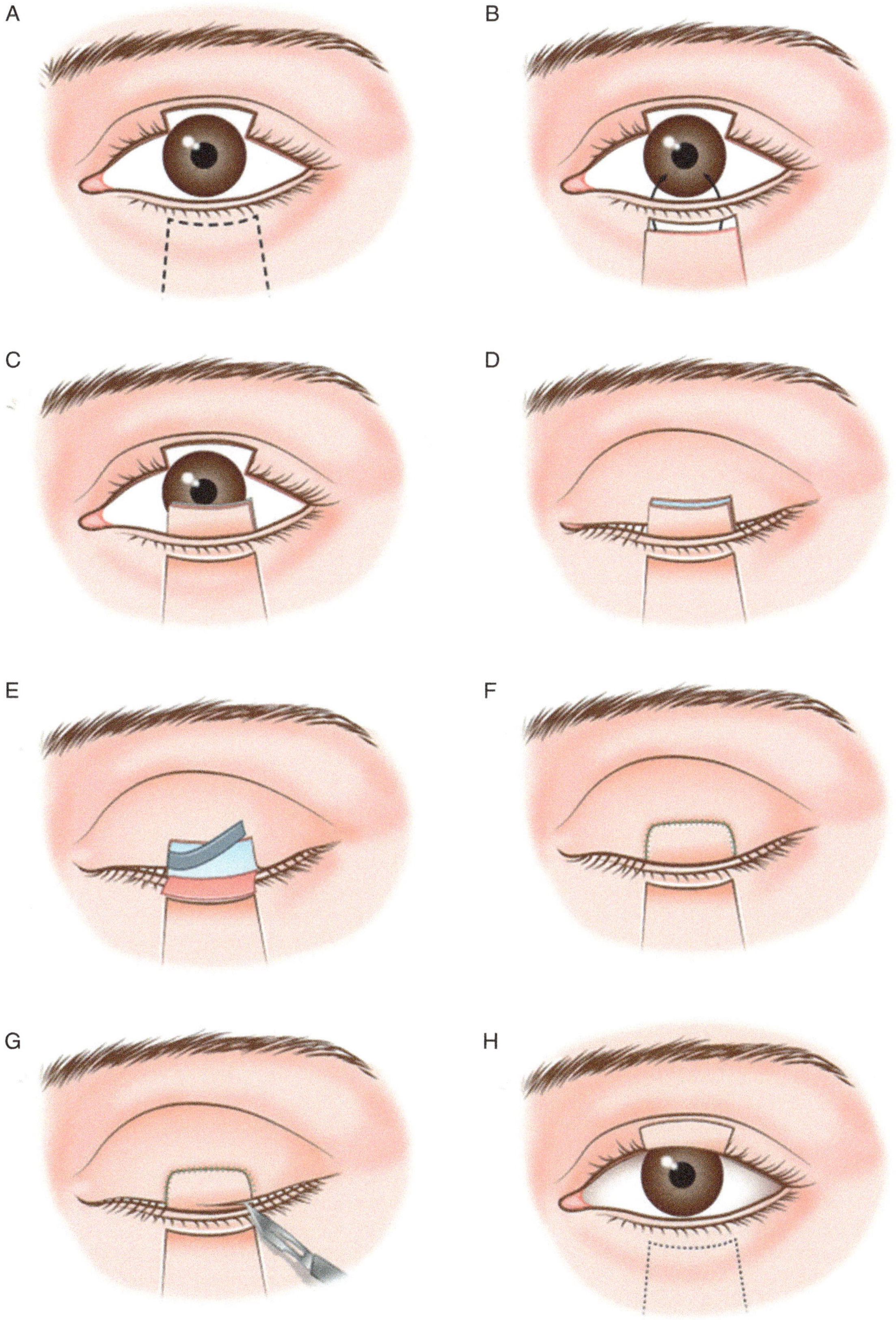

• **Fig. 31.11** Cutler–Beard flap. (A) Upper eyelid full-thickness defect and planned incisions along lower lid (*dotted line*). (B,C) Skin–muscle–conjunctiva flap raised from lower lid and tunneled underneath intact lower eyelid tarsus. (D) Conjunctiva separated from lower lid flap and secured along defect to replace posterior lamella. (E) Additional grafting (e.g., contralateral tarsus, cartilage, perichondrium) may be placed between the reconstructed posterior and anterior lamellae. (F) Skin and orbicularis is secured to the upper eyelid and left attached for 2–4 weeks. (G,H) Pedicle is divided and remaining flap replaced along the lower lid. (From Guanning NL, Pelton RW, Humphrey CD, et al. Defect of the eyelids. *Facial Plast Surg Clin North Am*. 25(3):377–392. Copyright © 2017 Elsevier Inc. Figure 12.)

Technique

1. The periosteum of the superior lateral orbital rim is access and marked with a marking pen. A 5x12 mm band of periosteum is then elevated and kept attached to the superior lateral orbital rim
2. A free tarsal graft is harvested from the left upper lid and attached to the remaining stump of the tarsus medially and to the periosteal flap laterally
3. A myocutaneous cheek flap is then elevated and secured to the periosteum of the lateral orbital rim, thus providing anterior lamellar coverage. It is important to provide a superior lateral vector of elevation in order to avoid scleral show postoperatively
4. The "new" posterior lamella is then secured to the anterior lamella via polypropylene mattress sutures.

The Tarsoconjunctival Advancement Flap: Cutler–Beard[20]

This is a two-stage, lid-sharing procedure for the reconstruction of large full-thickness upper eyelid defects that cannot be closed with a Tenzel flap. It involves a skin-muscle-conjunctival flap advanced from the lower eyelid to the upper eyelid, with temporary closure of the eye for 4–6 weeks, as in the Hughes procedure.

Technique (***Fig. 31.11***)

1. The edges of the upper eyelid defect are freshened and the upper eyelid defect is measured.
2. A horizontal incision line is marked on the skin of the lower eyelid 5 mm below the eyelid margin followed by vertical lines extending 15–20 mm inferiorly on either end.
3. Two 4-0 silk traction sutures are placed through the gray line of the inferior lower eyelid.
4. A wide malleable is placed between the globe and inferior eyelid, which is stretched superiorly over the malleable.
5. A No. 15 blade is used to make a full-thickness blepharotomy along the horizontal line followed by skin incisions along the vertical lines.
6. Straight scissors are used to complete the vertical incisions to the level of the inferior fornix.
7. The flap is brought up and under the inferior eyelid bridge. The anterior and posterior lamella of the flap are separated using Wescott scissors.
8. The conjunctival flap is sutured to the conjunctival edges of the wound, incorporating if possible the cut edge of the levator muscle, using 6-0 polyglactin.
9. The anterior lamella of the flap is sutured to the upper eyelid defect using 6-0 polyglactin or silk.
10. The inferior eyelid blepharotomy is not sutured closed. Ophthalmic ointment is applied to the site three times daily and the eyelids are separated 6–8 weeks later.
11. Second stage: The inferior eyelid margin is retracted inferiorly with a Desmarres. A horizontal mark is made 2 mm inferior to the expected upper eyelid margin. The flap is then separated by layer such that the skin edge is kept shorter than the conjunctival edge.
12. After initial hemostasis, the conjunctival edge is rolled over the eyelid margin anteriorly and sutured to the skin edge with 7-0 Vicryl sutures. Alternatively, it can be anteriorized with Tisseel glue. It is important that the final upper eyelid edge is mucosalized, not keratinized.
13. The inferior edge of the lower eyelid bridge is freshened with scissors and sutured to the base of the lower eyelid flap in a layered fashion.

Posterior Lamellar Grafting

Several options exist for replacing the structural element of the eyelids. The Hughes flap, previously discussed, is not appropriate for every case. Free grafts are more often used. Where canthal support is missing medially or laterally, a periosteal flap can be fashioned.

- Contralateral upper eyelid: The upper part of the tarsus of the upper eyelid can be harvested for use as a graft. At least 4 mm height of tarsal plate should be left behind to avoid destabilizing the donor eyelid. The advantage of this graft is that it is identical tissue and has a conjunctival covering. Disadvantages include possible upper eyelid entropion and a limited size graft.
- Hard palate[21]: This has the advantage of being readily harvested and has superior structural rigidity. Disadvantages include discomfort associated with oral mucosal recovery and the potential to cause corneal abrasion as the mucosal surface is rougher than conjunctiva. Therefore it is generally avoided in the central upper eyelid.
- Auricular cartilage: Disadvantages include a lack of mucosal covering and too much rigidity. Vertical partial-thickness cuts are made across the graft to improve its bend. It is most useful in the inferior eyelid as a vertical spacer graft.Despite shaping, the graft often returns to its original shape that can distort the eyelid.
- Nasal septal cartilage: Similar to auricular cartilage, it has no mucosal covering. An advantage is its relatively flat shape, but disadvantages include possible donor site comorbidity (e.g. nasal strut collapse and septal perforation).
- Other options for tarsal replacement or spacer grafting include acellular dermal allograft, AlloDerm (Lifecell, Branchburg, NJ, USA), which is a collagen framework from donated cadaveric skin.[22] ENDURAGen (Stryker Corp., Kalamazoo, Michigan, USA) and TarSys (IOP Ophthalmics, Costa Mesa, CA, USA) are xenografts from porcine dermal collagen and are not lined with a mucous membrane so should be used medially or temporally away from the cornea (otherwise need to be lined with mucous or amniotic membrane graft).[23] AmnioGuard (Bio-Tissue, Inc., Miami, FL, USA) is a more rigid form of Amniograft and has a mucous lining safe for central lower and upper eyelid.

By being aware of the vector forces that are applied to the mobilized tissue, the surgeon can create opposing flaps that result in smaller relaxing incisions and tissue undermining. A thoughtful approach in determining the techniques best suited to the patient, and ultimate esthetic and functional outcomes, yield the best results. Ultimately, the eyelid reconstruction remains highly dependent on individual skill and creativity (Figs. 31.12 and 31.13).

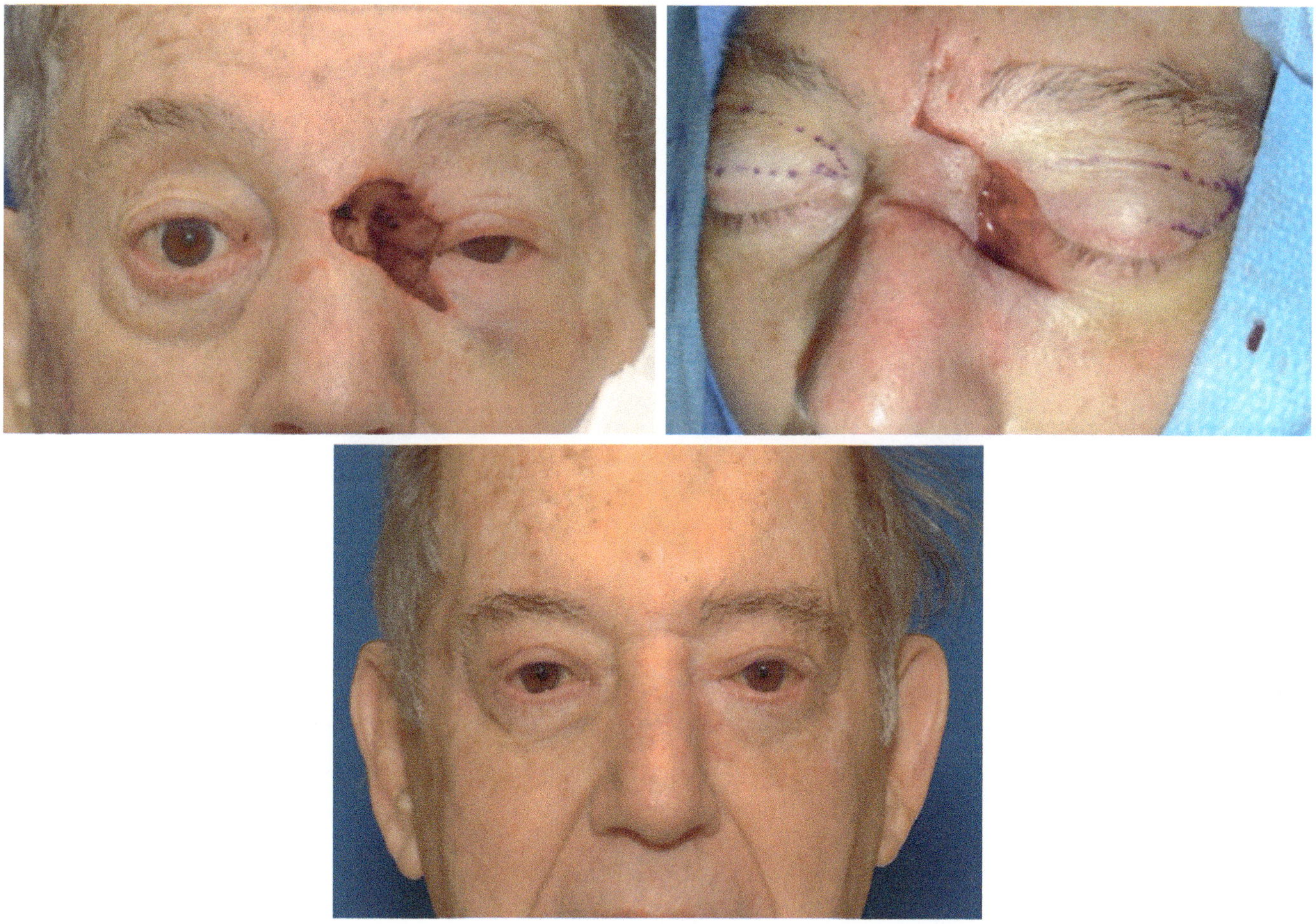

• **Fig. 31.12** Complex reconstruction of the medial canthus with multiple flaps and grafts. The use of combined reconstructive options can minimize ultimate scar length and resultant deformity.

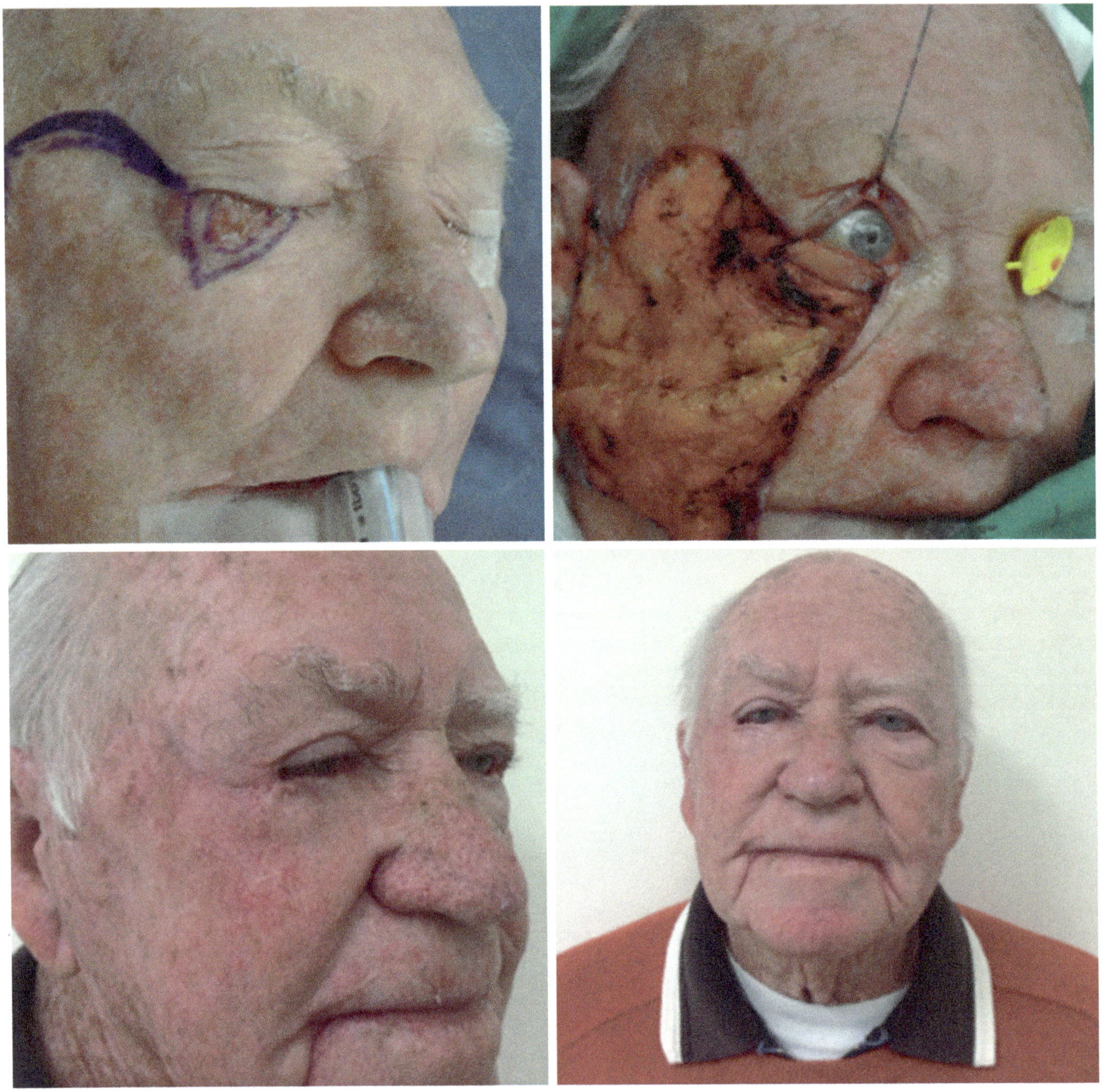

• **Fig. 31.13** Total right lower eyelid reconstruction, mucochondral nasal septum graft, and Mustardé cheek rotation flap. (Courtesy Dr. Rostam D. Farhadieh.)

References

1. Jelks GW, Glat PM, Jelks EB, et al. The inferior retinacular lateral canthoplasty: a new technique. *Plast Reconstr Surg.* 1997;100(5):1262–1270.
2. Hering E. *Die Lehre Om Binokularem Sehen*. Leipzig: Engelmann; 1868.
3. Sherrington CS. Reciprocal innervation of antagonistic muscles. Fourteenth note. On double reciprocal innervation. *Proc R Soc London Set B*. 1909;81:249–268.
4. Matsuo K, Kondoh S, Kitazawa T, et al. Pathogenesis and surgical correction of dynamic lower scleral show as a sign of disinsertion of the levator aponeurosis from the tarsus. *Br J Plast Surg.* 2005;58(5):668–675.
5. Rootman DB, Karlin J, Moore G, et al. The effect of ptosis surgery on brow position and the utility of preoperative phenylephrine testing. *Ophthalmic Plast Reconstr Surg.* 2016;32(3):195–198.
6. Ng SK, Chan W, Marcet MM, et al. Levator palpebrae superioris: an anatomical update. *Orbit.* 2013;32(1):76–84.
7. Patrinely JR, Marines HM, Anderson RL. Skin flaps in periorbital reconstruction. *Surv Ophthalmol.* 1987;31:249.
8. Elliot D, Britto JA. Tripier's innervated myocutaneous flap 1889. *Br J Plast Surg.* 2004;57(6):543–549.
9. Fricke JCG. *Die Bildung neuer Augenlider (Blepharoplastik) nach Zerstorungen und dadurch hervorgebrachten Auswartswendungen derselben*. Hamburg: Perthes and Bessler; 1929.

10. Putterman AM. Viable composite grafting in eyelid reconstruction. *Am J Ophthalmol.* 1978;85:237–241.
11. Mustardé JC. *Repair and Reconstruction in the Orbital Region.* New York: Churchill Livingstone; 1971.
12. Tenzel RR, Stewart WB. Eyelid reconstruction by the semicircle flap technique. *Ophthalmology.* 1978;85:1164.
13. Tenzel RR. Reconstruction of the central one half of an eyelid. *Arch Ophthalmol.* 1975;93:125–126.
14. Jordan DR, Anderson RL, Holds JB. Modifications to the semicircular flap technique in eyelid reconstruction. *Can J Ophthalmol.* 1992;27:130–136.
15. Hughes WL. Total lower eyelid reconstruction: technical details. *Transact Am Ophthalmol Soc.* 1976;74:321–329.
16. McNab AA. Early division of the conjunctival pedicle in modified Hughes repair of the lower eyelid. *Ophthalmic Surg Lasers.* 1996;27:422–424.
17. McNab AA, Martin P, Benger R. A prospective randomized study comparing division of the pedicle of modified Hughes flaps at two or four weeks. *Ophthalmic Plast Reconstr Surg.* 2001; 17:317–319.
18. Hawes MJ. Free autogenous grafts in eyelid tarsoconjunctival reconstruction. *Ophthalmic Surg.* 1987;18:37–41.
19. Weinstein GS, Anderson RL, Tse DT, et al. The use of a periosteal strip for eyelid reconstruction. *Arch Ophthalmol.* 1985;103:357.
20. Cutler NL, Beard C. A method for partial and total upper eyelid reconstruction. *Am J Ophthalmol.* 1955;39:1.
21. Siegel RJ. Palatal grafts for eyelid reconstruction. *Plast Reconstr Surg.* 1985;76:411.
22. Taban M, Douglas R, Li T, et al. Efficacy of "thick" acellular human derived (AlloDerm) for lower eyelid reconstruction: comparison with hard palate and thin AlloDerm grafts. *Arch Facial Plast Surg.* 2005;7(1):38–44.
23. Symbas J, McCord C, Nahai F. Acellular dermal matrix in eyelid surgery. *Aesthet Surg J.* 2011;31:101–107.

32 Ear Reconstruction

FRANÇOISE FIRMIN AND NEIL W. BULSTRODE

Introduction

A variety of traumatic ear defects are observed after amputation, be they partial, subtotal or total, all of which require complex contour reconstruction.

There are multiple causes of ear amputations and this summary chapter aims to define some principles and guidelines that permit a precise surgical management plan.

Initial Assessment Concerning a Posttraumatic Amputation

Mechanism of Ear Amputation

Clean Amputations

These are usually secondary to trauma involving a knife, surgical resection or sharp bites (animals or human). Primary treatment consists of debridement and suturing of the edges of the wound.

If we exclude surgical amputation for cutaneous malignancy, it is tempting to replant the amputated segment of ear. Many different techniques have been proposed to ensure success of such replantation (burying, fibrocartilage fenestration, cartilage storage, and secondary replantation). Whatever the degree of success of such a surgical approach, the final result will be disappointing. Even though it may be difficult to make the decision not to attempt replantation and sacrifice the amputated ear segment, this will preserve the skin potential for a superior secondary reconstruction.

Replantation should only be considered when vascular anastomosis is possible and reliable.

Crush Injury

These injuries occur after a fall, road traffic accident, blunt trauma ,and violent compression. In such circumstances the ear defect is generally only part of complex injury involving the surrounding soft tissue.

Burn Injury

Thermal, chemical or electrical injury are frequent causes of traumatic ear defects. Both ears are frequently affected and the burn area extends around the auricular area. Besides the zone directly injured by the burn, a secondary chondritis often results in severe resorption of the fibrocartilage.[1] When limited to the ear, the defect usually affects the scapha and helix, but often retroauricular skin and the scalp is affected with scars and alopecia.

Burn patients are generally managed in a burns unit where initial stabilization and grafting is performed. Reconstruction of the ear is a last step of management. These patients, who have undergone multiple surgical procedures, may opt not to have an ear reconstruction. In some cases, an ear prosthesis is indicated.

Analysis of the Defect

A precise analysis of the defect is critical in all reconstructive efforts. The missing contours must be appreciated and reconstructed in all dimensions.

To correctly appreciate the defect it is essential to draw the normal ear on a transparent template and place it on the injured ear to appreciate the missing contours needing reconstruction. Skin alone is not adequate to reconstruct the contours of the ear and depending upon the size of the defect either fibrocartilage or rib cartilage is required as part of the reconstruction.

Analysis of the Skin Potential

The specific problem encountered in cases of posttraumatic amputation is the presence of scars. It is essential to analyse their location and the skin availability to cover the reconstructed cartilage construct. The following three factors need consideration:

1. The quality and quantity of skin in the auricular area must be appreciated. The presence of lax and scarless retroauricular skin provides the best conditions for coverage of the cartilage framework.
2. Scars. After inspection of scars, a surgical approach is chosen to minimize the use of new scars and ensure vascularity of the skin to cover the cartilage construct.
3. Deficit of skin. In cases where there is no skin available in the auricular area, surrounding fascia (temporoparietal

or occipital) or the use of skin expansion will have to be considered to cover the cartilage framework.

Reconstruction in Partial Amputations

Partial traumatic defects of the ear are always located along the free border of the ear.

In this discussion we will exclude defects of the helix that can be closed directly or using skin flaps or chondrocutaneous flaps. The Antia–Buch flap[2] can be used for small defects but its principle of moving the helix after a scaphoid resection always reduces the size of the ear.

In partial amputation skin availability is usually adequate and the main concern is to choose the best support to reproduce the missing cartilage contours. Either fibrocartilage or rib cartilage may be used. It is essential to draw the normal ear on a template, and then transpose the template on the affected ear to work out what is missing and what contours need reconstructing.

The rule is that fibrocartilage can only be used to reconstruct a partial defect after trauma if it is no more than a quarter of the border of the ear and includes no more than two adjacent planes. Harvesting all of the concha can only reproduce two adjacent planes and just a quarter of the ear. If the defect is less than a quarter but includes three planes, then rib cartilage should be harvested to correctly reproduce the missing contours (Fig. 32.1).

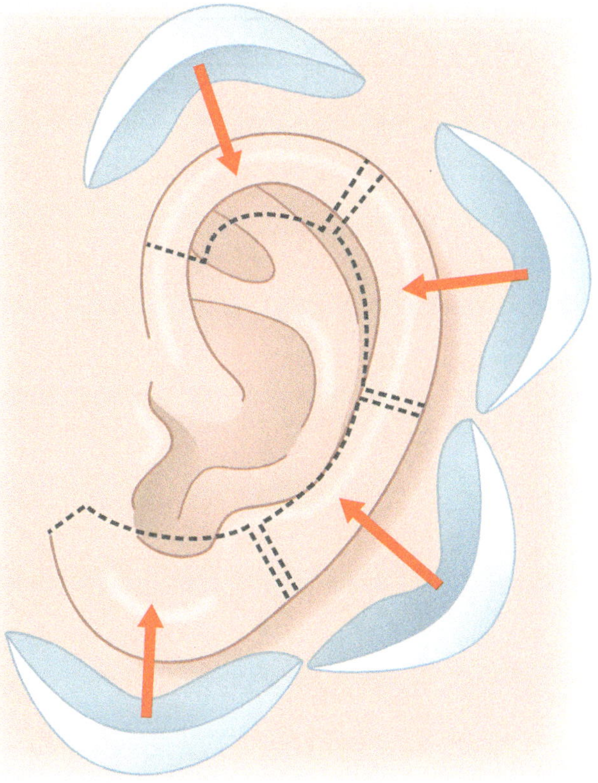

• **Fig. 32.1** Fibrocartilaginous conchal graft can only be used when the defect is no more than a quarter of the ear and no more than two adjacent planes.

Reconstruction Using Fibrocartilage

Harvesting the Fibrocartilage Graft

The concha is the best donor site considering its size and the fact that it will not be visible if harvested correctly. The entire concha has to be harvested taking care to preserve the root of the helix and enough posterior wall of the concha.

Depending on the case, it can be harvested through an anterior or posterior approach from the ipsi- or contralateral ear.

The choice concerning the skin approach (anterior or posterior) depends on the defect and the skin vascularity. The choice concerning the harvesting on the ipsi- or contralateral side may be discussed with the patient, who sometimes is reluctant to have surgery performed on the normal ear.

Depending on the location of the defect and the skin potential, the reconstruction will be performed in one or two stages.

Case 1 **(*Fig. 32.2*).** Reconstruction in one stage using ipsilateral conchal graft. The defect is secondary to chondritis after trauma. It is a quarter of the contour of the ear and no more than two adjacent planes.

Case 2 **(*Fig. 32.3*).** The defect being a quarter and no more than two planes, the reconstruction was performed using a contralateral conchal graft covered with retroauricular skin. Creation of the retroauricular sulcus behind the reconstructed part of the ear will be performed in a second stage. Elevation of the ear is performed respecting the soft tissues behind the ear, to cover the area with a small full-thickness skin graft harvested from the opposite retroauricular sulcus.

Reconstruction Using Costal Cartilage

There is an abundant amount of cartilage when harvesting from the thorax but when harvesting for reconstruction of partial defects, only one segment of cartilage is required. In such situations the scar on the thorax will be short.

Harvesting cartilage is a routine procedure with minimal risk. Pain is avoided by injecting local anesthetic into the muscles.

Using only a skin flap to reconstruct a partial amputation located on the periphery of the ear cannot reproduce complex contours and will give a poor result.

It is important to differentiate cases were the entire antihelix has been preserved from cases where part of it is missing, particularly the posterior wall of the concha. If part of the antihelix is missing it has to be reconstructed respecting the anatomical unit of the antihelix and the base that supports it.

Cases with Normal Antihelix

Case 3 **(*Fig. 32.4*).** Clean amputation with a defect that is no more than two adjacent planes but more than a quarter of the ear or the border of the ear requiring the use of rib cartilage support. The reconstruction will be performed in one stage as there is enough retroauricular skin to cover the narrow cartilaginous graft.

Case 4 **(*Fig. 32.5*).** The amputation is secondary to a human bite. An unsuccessful replantation has left a defect involving half of the inferior border of the ear, including the lobule. The reconstruction was performed

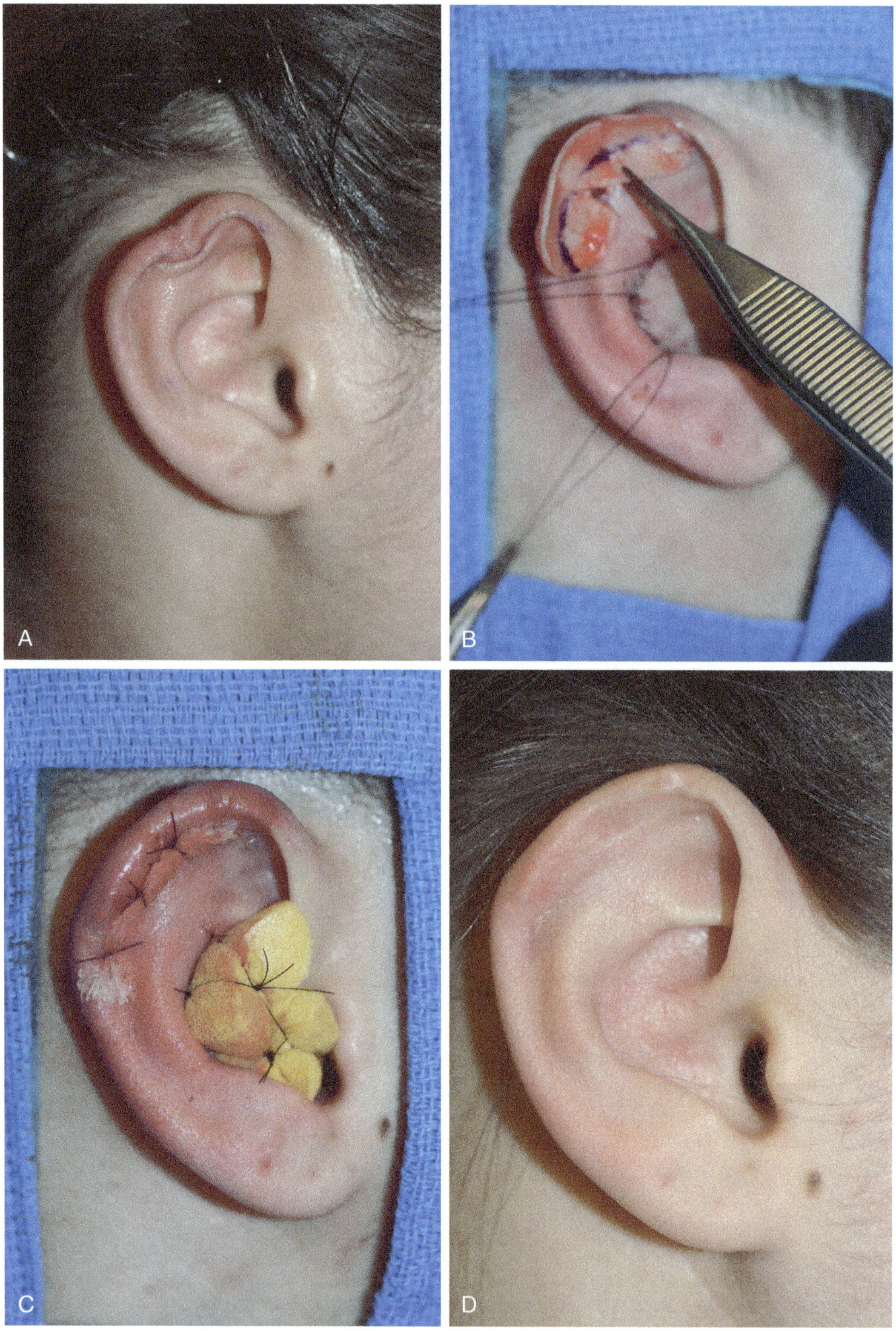

• **Fig. 32.2** Case 1. (A) The defect is a quarter of the ear and no more than two planes. (B) The conchal graft harvested on the same ear by an anterior approach will be reduced to reproduce the missing contours. (C) Bolster sutures apply the skin to the underlying contours. (D) Result.

in two stages with a very good result. The former scar was used to prepare the flap to cover the cartilage framework during the first stage. Advancement of the retroauricular skin and grafting the posterior surface of the reconstructed ear was done 4 months later during the second stage.

***Case 5* (*Fig. 32.6*).** Using a rib cartilage graft on a 60-year-old patient is possible as there is no correlation between the age and ossification. Texture and color of the cartilage will just be different. The rib segments are thicker so the scapha and helix can be sculpted in one segment. Elevation of the reconstructed upper third of the ear will be performed 4 months later.

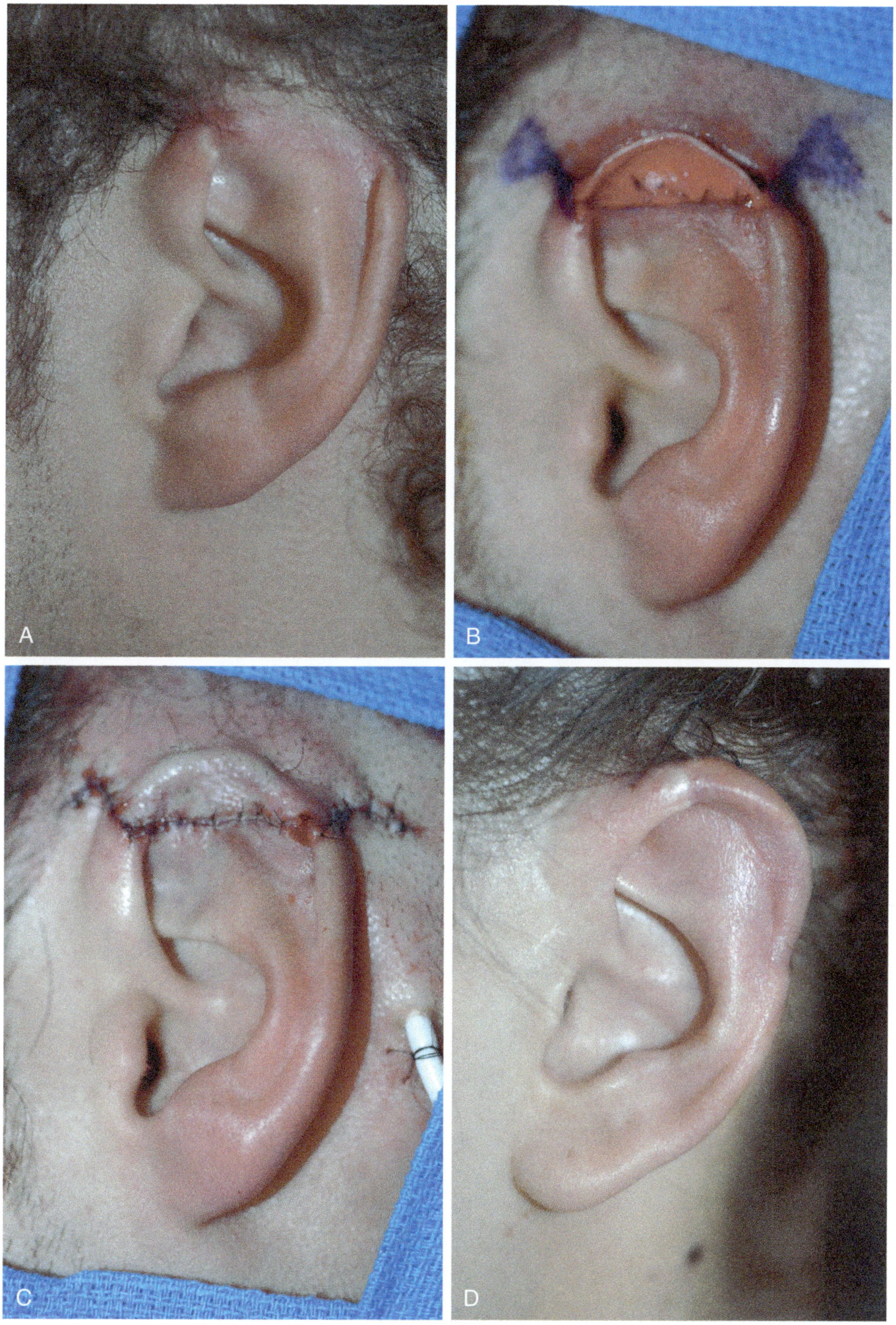

• **Fig. 32.3** Case 2. (A) The defect is a quarter and no more than two adjacent planes. (B) The conchal graft harvested on the contralateral ear is sutured to the fibrocartilage and the retroauricular skin will cover it. (C) Appearance after the first stage. (D) Result after elevation of the reconstructed contours using a full-thickness skin graft harvested from the contralateral retroauricular sulcus.

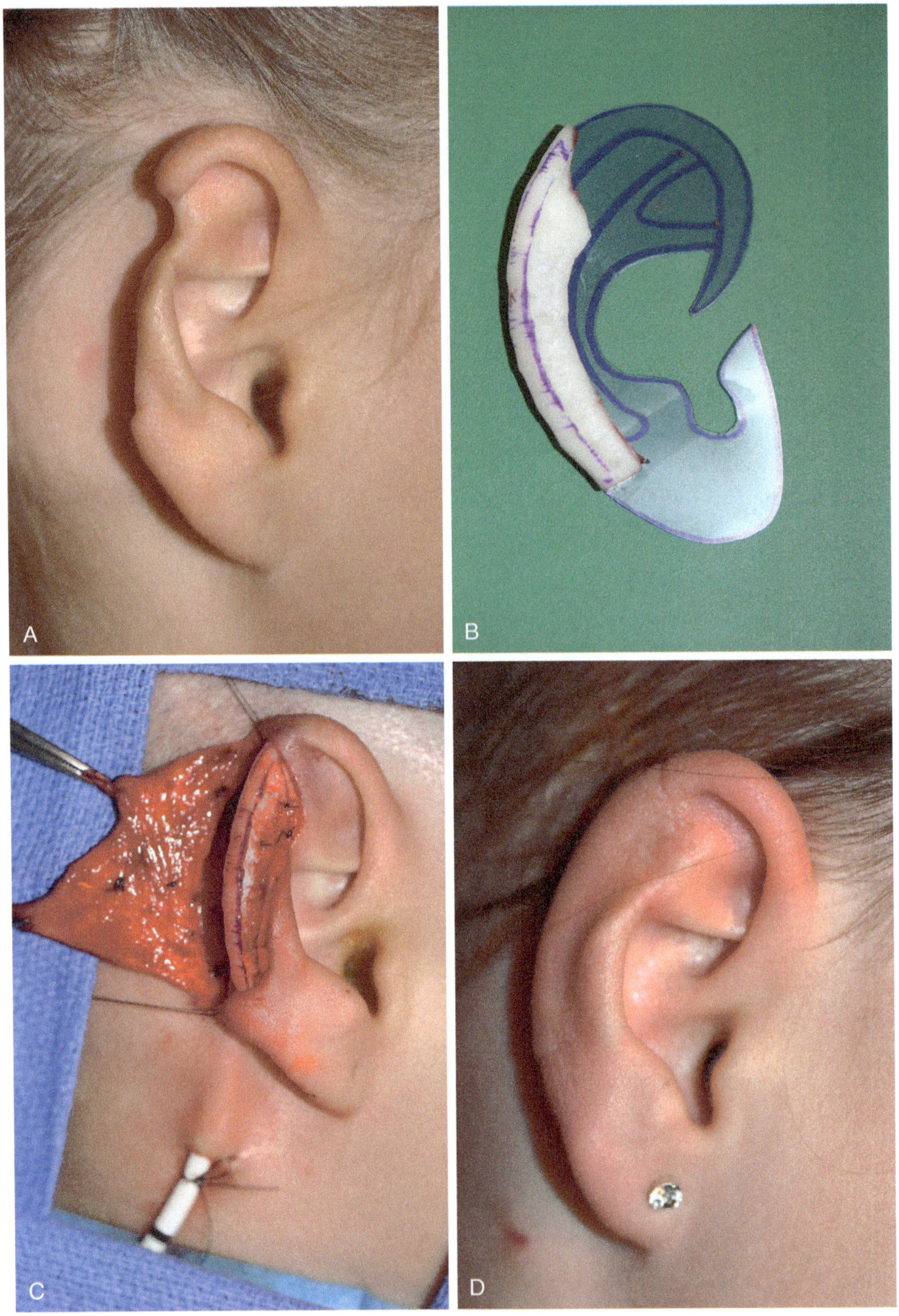

• **Fig. 32.4** Case 3. (A) Even though the defect is no more than two adjacent planes, it is more than a quarter of the border of the ear. (B) Perfect adaptation of the sculpted rib cartilaginous graft to the contours of the other ear drawn on a template. (C) Coverage of the reproduced contours by an advanced retroauricular skin flap. (D) Result obtained in one stage.

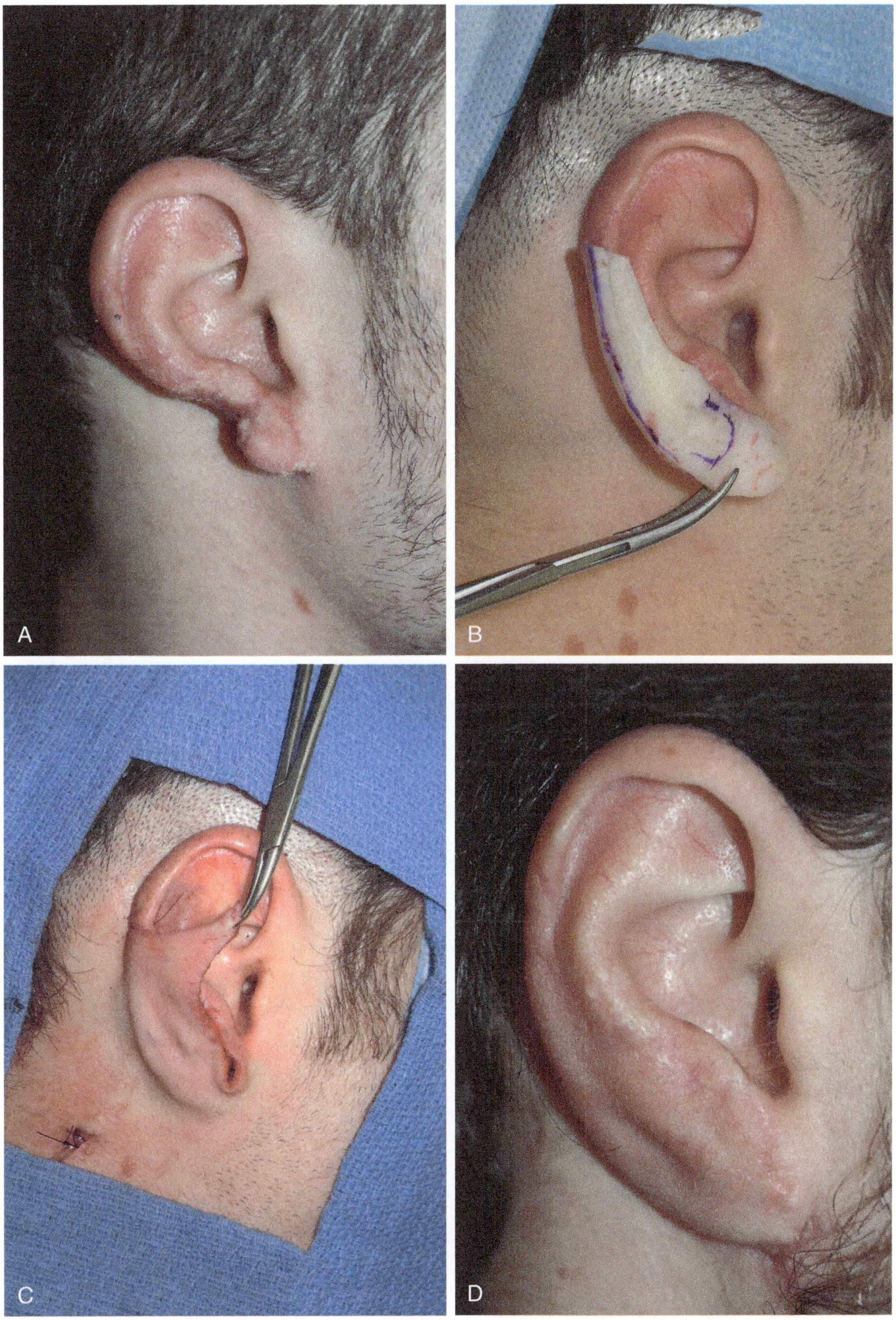

• **Fig. 32.5** Case 4. (A) Defect after unsuccessful replantation. (B) Rib cartilaginous graft reproducing the missing contours. (C) Skin flap covering the reconstructed contours. (D) Final result after elevation using a split-thickness skin graft harvested from the scalp.

Cases with an Injured Antihelix

In cases where the antihelix has been destroyed, a framework including a base must be fabricated to be able to fix the antihelix to obtain correct projection of the antihelix and middle part of the ear.

Case 6 (***Fig. 32.7***). The amputation is secondary to a dog bite. It is clear that part of the antihelix is missing and that the entire antihelix anatomical unit has to be reconstructed.

Even though this patient is 52, her cartilage is not ossified but presents with the usual yellow discoloration and is particularly dense.

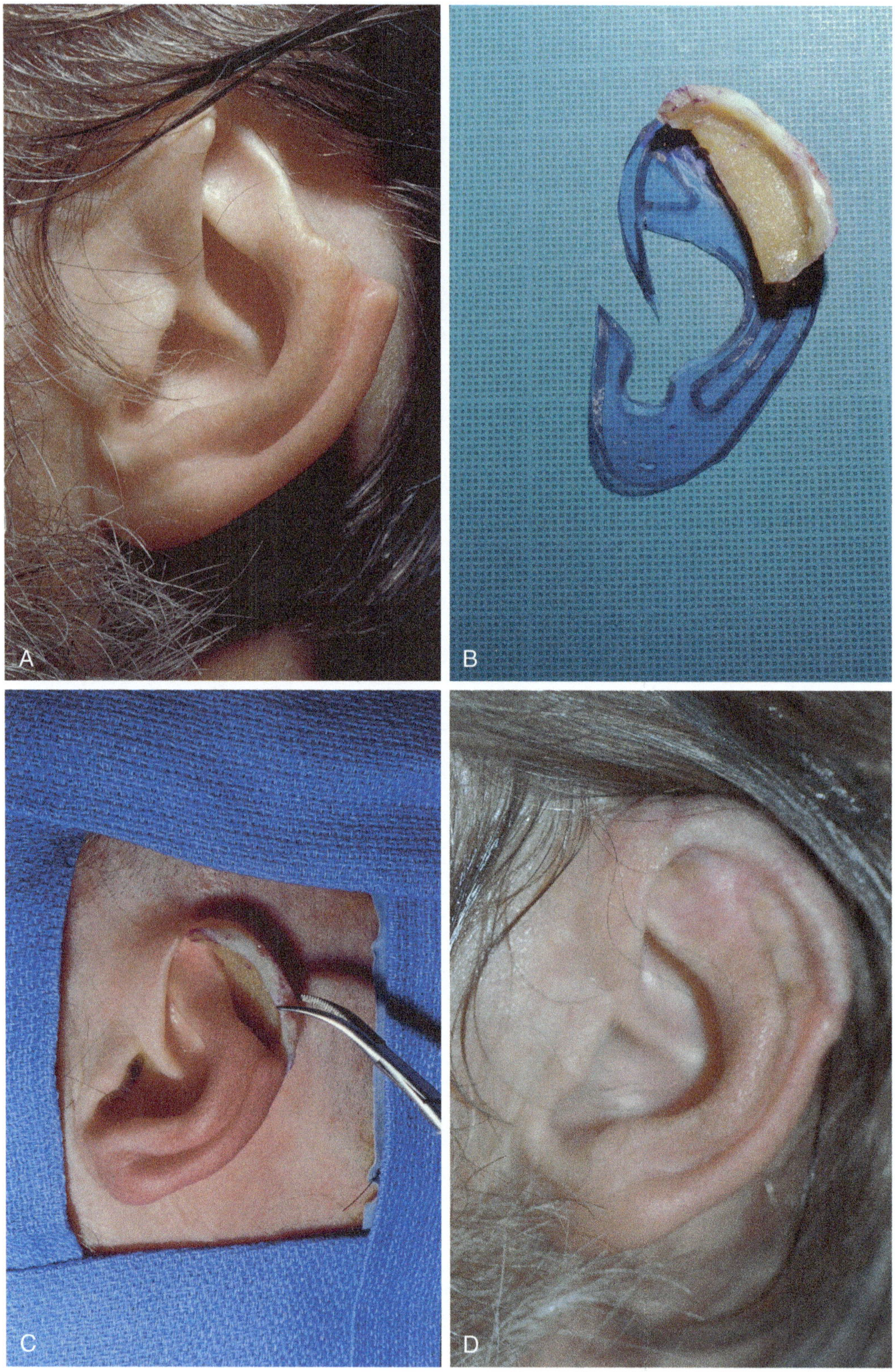

• **Fig. 32.6** Case 5. (A) The defect is more than a quarter and only two planes (helix and scapha). (B) Cartilaginous rib graft sculpted after appreciation of the missing contours using a transparent template. (C) Good match of the graft with the contours of the ear. (D) Result after elevation of the upper part of the ear using a skin graft.

Total and Subtotal Amputation

Total amputation does not always imply that there are no auricular remnants. Total or subtotal amputation implies that most of the contours are missing and that the reconstruction has to be done with a cartilage framework reproducing all of the ear's contours with rib cartilage.

A framework will be carved from several segments of ribs. Even though many synthetic materials have been proposed to avoid rib cartilage, autologous rib cartilage remains the best material.

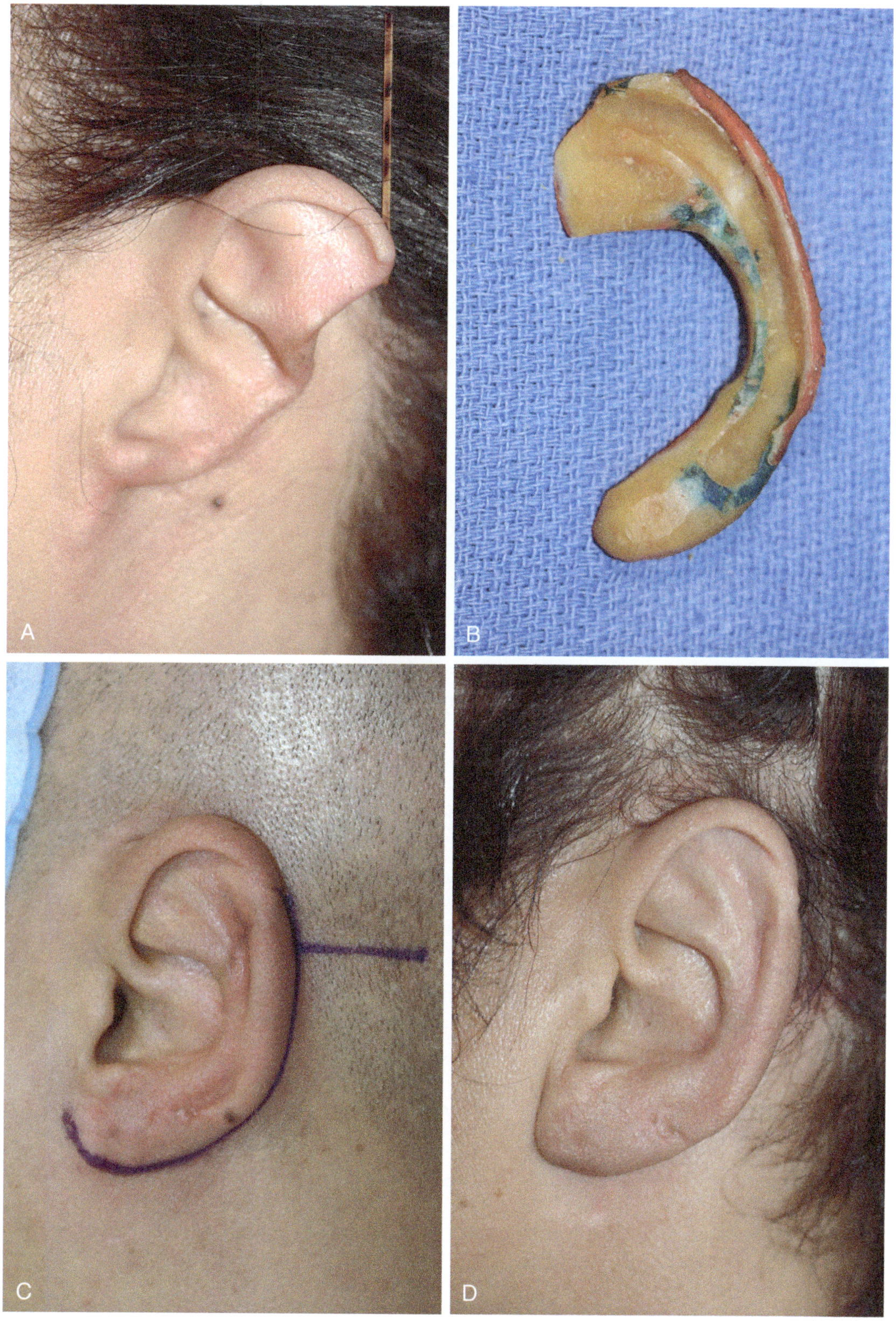

• **Fig. 32.7** Case 6. (A) The roots of the antihelix have been preserved but not the posterior wall of the concha and the inferior part of the antihelix. This case must be considered like a subtotal amputation. (B) Antihelix with its two roots is carved in one segment of cartilage and just the missing part of the helix is added on the base. This is the typical color of a nonossified cartilage of a 52-year-old patient. (C) Reconstruction of the retroauricular sulcus 6 months later by retroauricular skin advancement and skin graft of the posterior surface of the ear elevated with soft tissues. (D) Result after 1 year.

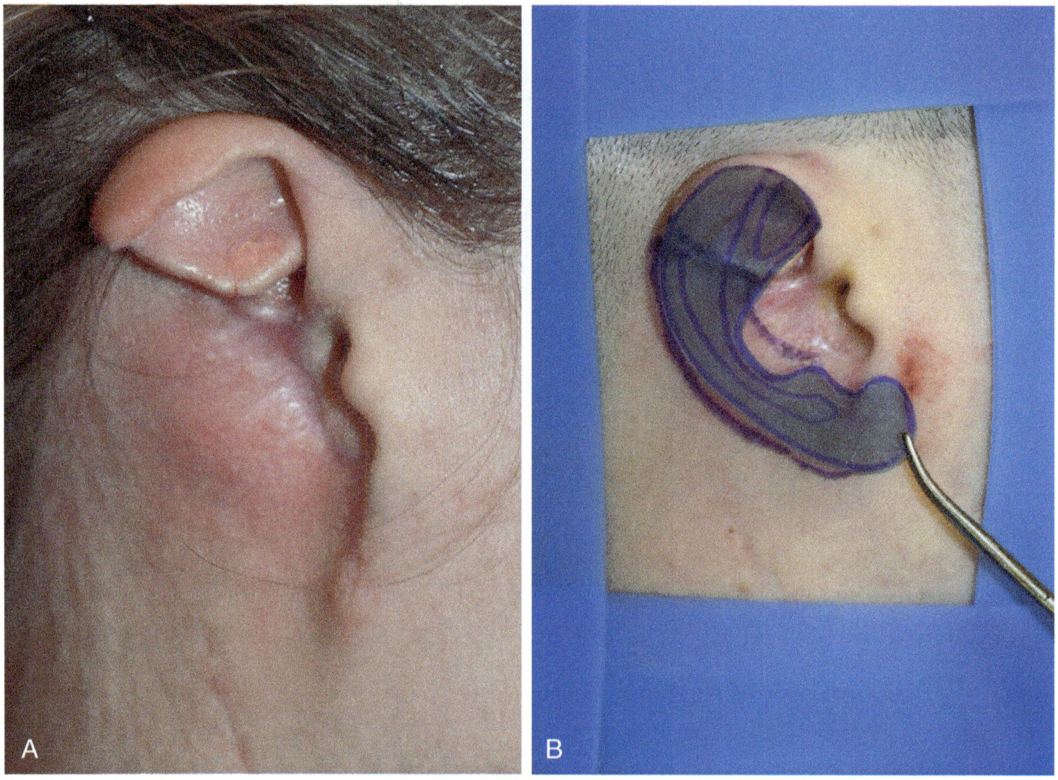

• **Fig. 32.8** (A) Only the upper part of the helix and the tragus have been preserved. (B) After drawing a template of the other ear, the missing contours to be reproduced are drawn on another transparent template.

In these cases, two stages are required for ear reconstruction. The first stage involves creation of the cartilage construct with all the contours, followed by the second stage of elevation and creation of a postauricular sulcus, performed 4–6 months later.

Technique

First Stage: Reconstruction of the Ear Contours

The contours of the normal ear are drawn on a transparent template. Under general anesthesia the operative field is prepared and the head is placed in a lateral position. The template is then transposed on the affected ear to correctly analyse the missing contours and to appreciate the symmetry at the end of the operation. Landmarks are taken on the normal side and then transposed on the affected side to reconstruct the ear in an ideal position and axis (Fig. 32.8).

The first stage includes three steps: harvesting of the rib cartilage, carving the cartilagenous framework, and preparation of the skin in the auricular area to insert the framework.[3]

Harvesting Rib Cartilage

Three or four segments of rib cartilage are harvested on the same side of the injured ear. The skin approach on the thorax is oblique and located close to the inferior border of the thoracic wall. This gives access to the anterior surface of the 6th, 7th, 8th, and 9th rib segments.

A template of the other ear having been sterilized is used to select the adequate segments of cartilage. Once selected these segments will be harvested preserving the posterior perichondrium. When the framework includes the helix, the 7th or the 8th segment is chosen to obtain no less than 7 cm in length. The template is also used to select the two adjacent segments united by their synchondrosis which are the most appropriate for the base. Preservation of the posterior perichondrium reduces the risk of injury to the pleura. Before closing the different planes, local anesthetic is injected into the muscles to minimize postoperative pain. The muscles' edges are approximated by interrupted sutures, including the edges of the anterior and posterior of the aponeurosis. Care must be taken to reduce the prominent residual cartilage to avoid visible thoracic irregularities. There are no functional sequelae after harvesting these segments of cartilage.

Carving the Framework

With experience, this is the most routine step of the reconstruction. A specific set of instruments (Storz, Germany) and double-ended wire sutures are used to construct the framework. Using a silicone board for stabilization is very helpful.

The posterior surface of the segments, free of perichondrium, becomes the anterior surface of the base and the segments of cartilage are cleaned, removing any perichondrial remnants. The template of the other ear is drawn on a clotting paper which is dipped into ink and applied on the cartilage. The base is placed on two adjacent ribs.

The 8th rib is prepared to reproduce the helix and will be lengthened with an additional piece if needed. It is then carved with a gouge to increase pliability. The lobule is lowered and shaped as well as the area of the intertragal notch and antitragus. The posterior edge of the base is cut obliquely to look thinner from behind.

The base is carved and a segment reproducing the antihelix with its two crura is added to give more projection to the antihelix. The antihelix is fixed on the base using double-ended wire sutures. The antihelix once added to the base is reshaped. The helix is then added. Its root is fixed onto an extra piece of cartilage to give more projection and stability. The overall size and shape of the framework is checked with the template.

All the double wire sutures used to fix the construct are tightened, cut short and buried in the cartilage. In cases of trauma there is usually no need to reconstruct the tragus.

The final touch accentuates the curve of the junction between the antihelix and the antitragus. An additional piece is sometimes added behind the base to deepen the concha and increase projection.

Framework Classification. We have established a classification for the different types of cartilaginous frameworks[3]:

- Type I is a complete framework including the tragus and the antitragus
- Type II is including the antitragus but not the tragus
- Type III does not include the tragus and the antitragus.

In cases of traumatic amputation the tragus is often preserved and the most frequent frameworks used are type II and type III (Fig. 32.9).

Insertion of the Framework Under the Auricular Skin

A correct analysis of the skin potential in the auricular area is essential to choose the best skin coverage for the framework. When the retroauricular skin has been preserved it represents an ideal coverage and the retroauricular sulcus will be reconstructed during a second stage. When it has been damaged it is necessary to use temporoparietal fascia and a skin graft. If the skin is too tense to cover the tridimensional framework it is possible to use indirect expansion.

The following scenarios represent different skin conditions.

Good Skin Availability in the Auricular Area. If the retroauricular skin has not been damaged and has not been sutured under tension it can be used to cover the framework. The skin approach to prepare the skin pocket and to insert the framework must be through a previous scar. Dissection will be performed respecting the subdermal plexus.

Case 7 **(*Fig. 32.10*).** Total amputation preserving the tragus on an adult patient 55 years old. A preoperative computed tomography (CT) scan with 3D colored printing is very useful to appreciate the degree of ossification of the cartilage at that age. The nonossified segments of cartilage being larger and thicker, it is sometimes possible to carve the base of the framework and the antihelix in one piece and just add the helix generally carved from the eighth costal cartilage segment. There is just enough skin to cover the 3D framework. Six months later elevation of the reconstructed ear was performed taking into account the projection of the other ear. Here a temporoparietal fascia flap was used to cover the posterior surface of the framework after adding a crescent-shape piece of cartilage behind the antihelix stored since the first stage under the thoracic skin.

Good Scarless Skin but Under Tension. It is very important to appreciate the elasticity of the retroauricular skin to decide if it can adapt to a 3D framework without too much tension, particularly on the helix. If not, an expander may be placed under the adjacent scalp prior to the formal first stage. This expansion is indirect expansion because it will not expand the non-hair-bearing skin in the auricular area but will increase the skin potential, which will be redistributed during placement of the framework, reducing the skin tension and avoiding the risk of skin necrosis and cartilage exposure.

Crescent-shape expanders are used (150 cm^3) and filled over a period of 6–8 weeks.[4]

Case 8 **(*Fig. 32.11*).** In this case a type III framework was carved as tragus and antitragus have been preserved. To avoid excessive tension and allow good adaptation of the skin to the contours, indirect expansion is used. Reconstruction of the retroauricular sulcus will be performed 6 months later.

No Available Skin. When there are scars in the retroauricular area that impair skin vascularity making it impossible to cover the framework without a high risk of skin necrosis, other options are needed. A temporoparietal fascia flap based on the superficial temporal artery, if not damaged, is planned to cover the framework. This is then covered with a scalp split-skin graft. When the superficial temporal artery has been damaged it is still possible to use a random pattern fascial flap.

After shaving of the temporal area, the course of the superficial temporal artery is mapped with Doppler. A zigzag incision is then performed on the scalp to expose the fascia. To facilitate the rotation of the fascial flap a narrow pedicle including the artery is designed and raised. Once inset the fascial flap is covered with a scalp split-thickness skin graft, which is a superior donor site for color match and donor site visibility.

Two to three suction Blake drains are placed during the first stage. The aims of the drains are to minimize hematoma formation and apply the skin on to the underlying cartilage contours. Drains are removed after 3 days during the first dressing change.

Definition of the contours and quality of the result can only be judged after 1 year to allow the scarring to have minimized. When elevation of the ear, to create the retroauricular sulcus, is indicated, it is usually performed after 1 year.

Case 9 **(*Fig. 32.12*).** After a road traffic accident, the auricular region had been grafted. A temporoparietal fascia is indicated. The temporoparietal fascia is covered with a scalp split-thickness skin graft placed on the upper two-thirds of the framework. Elevation of the upper part of the ear was performed 1 year later.

Second Stage: Reconstruction of the Retroauricular Sulcus

There are different techniques to elevate the reconstructed ear:

- Elevation of the ear preserving soft tissues on the posterior surface of the framework. A split-thickness skin graft is used to cover the posterior surface of the ear. The posterior

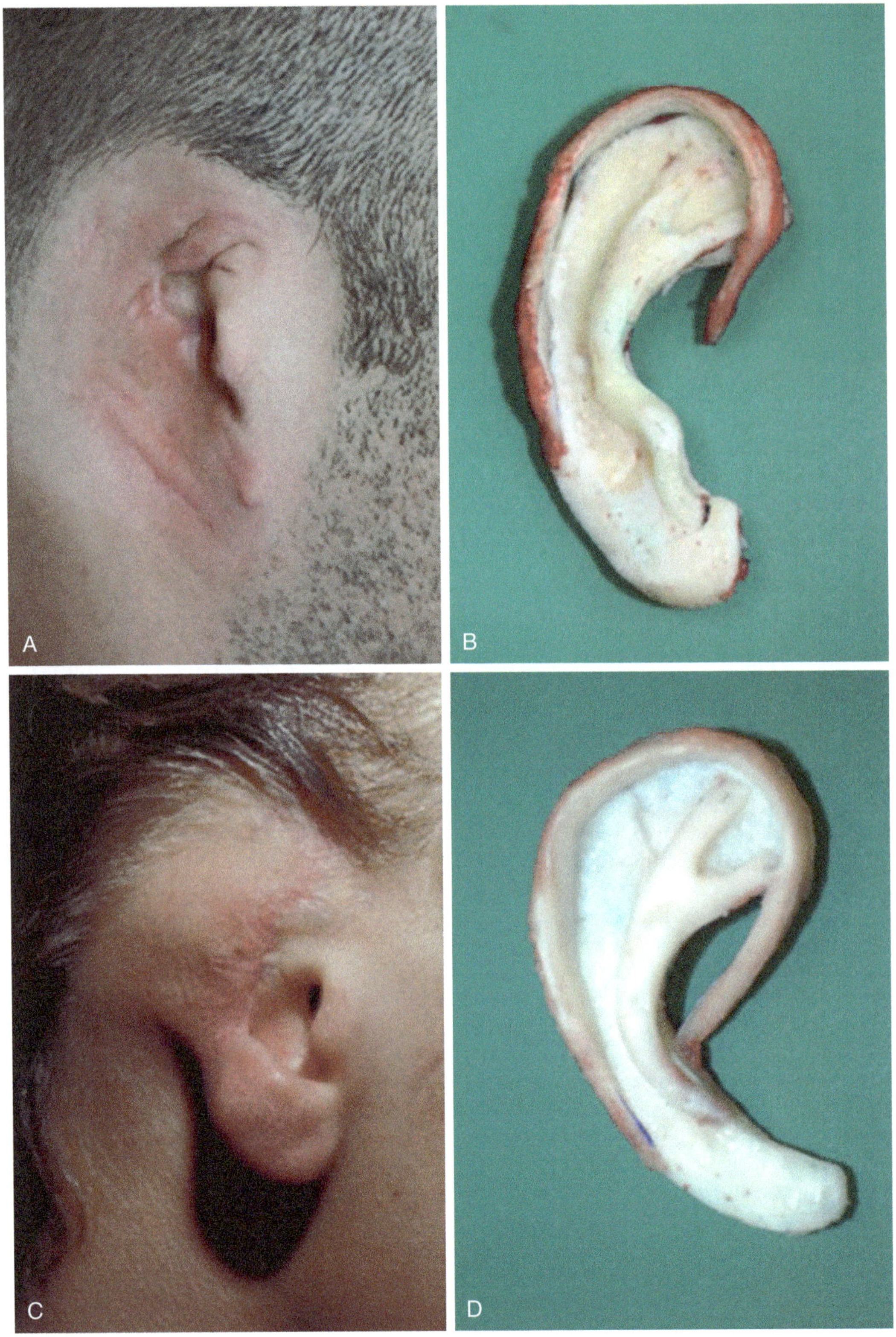

• **Fig. 32.9** The most frequent types of cartilage in cases of total amputation. (A,B) All the contours except tragus must be reconstructed: type II cartilage. (C,D) All the contours except tragus and antitragus must be reconstructed: type III cartilage.

edge of the incision around the ear is brought forward after undermining the skin. This is the technique advocated by Brent except that he was not using a split-thickness skin graft harvested from the calvarium[5] (see Fig. 32.6C).

- Use of a temporoparietal fascia covering a piece of cartilage placed behind the antihelix to deepen the concha and give more projection to the ear. This procedure was advocated by Nagata in cases of microtia[6] (see Fig. 32.10D).
- Improving the projection of the ear after its elevation by inserting a piece of cartilage behind the framework, into a tunnel, which will be placed behind the anterior root of the anthelix or the antihelix or the antitragus.[3]

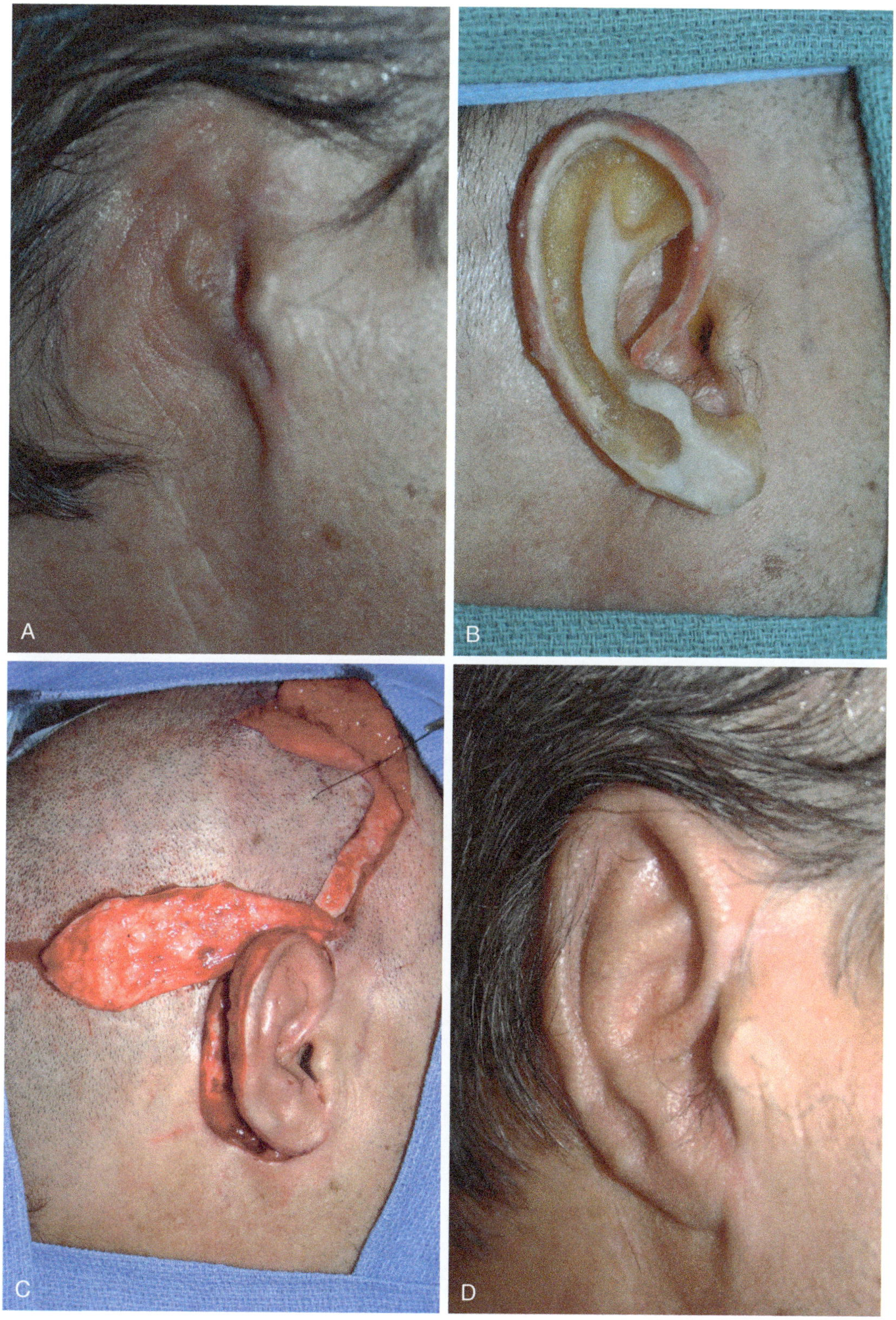

• **Fig. 32.10** Case 7. (A) Only the tragus has been preserved. (B) Framework type II, reproducing all the contours except the tragus. Only two segments of ribs (7th and 6th) have been harvested. The antihelix has been carved in the base. (C) After the first stage all the contours are present but there is no retroauricular sulcus. (D) Elevation of the ear is performed using a temporal fascia which covers the posterior surface of the ear and an additional cartilage graft placed behind the antihelix to give projection to the ear and deepen the concha. Some hair-bearing skin on the helix can also be excised.

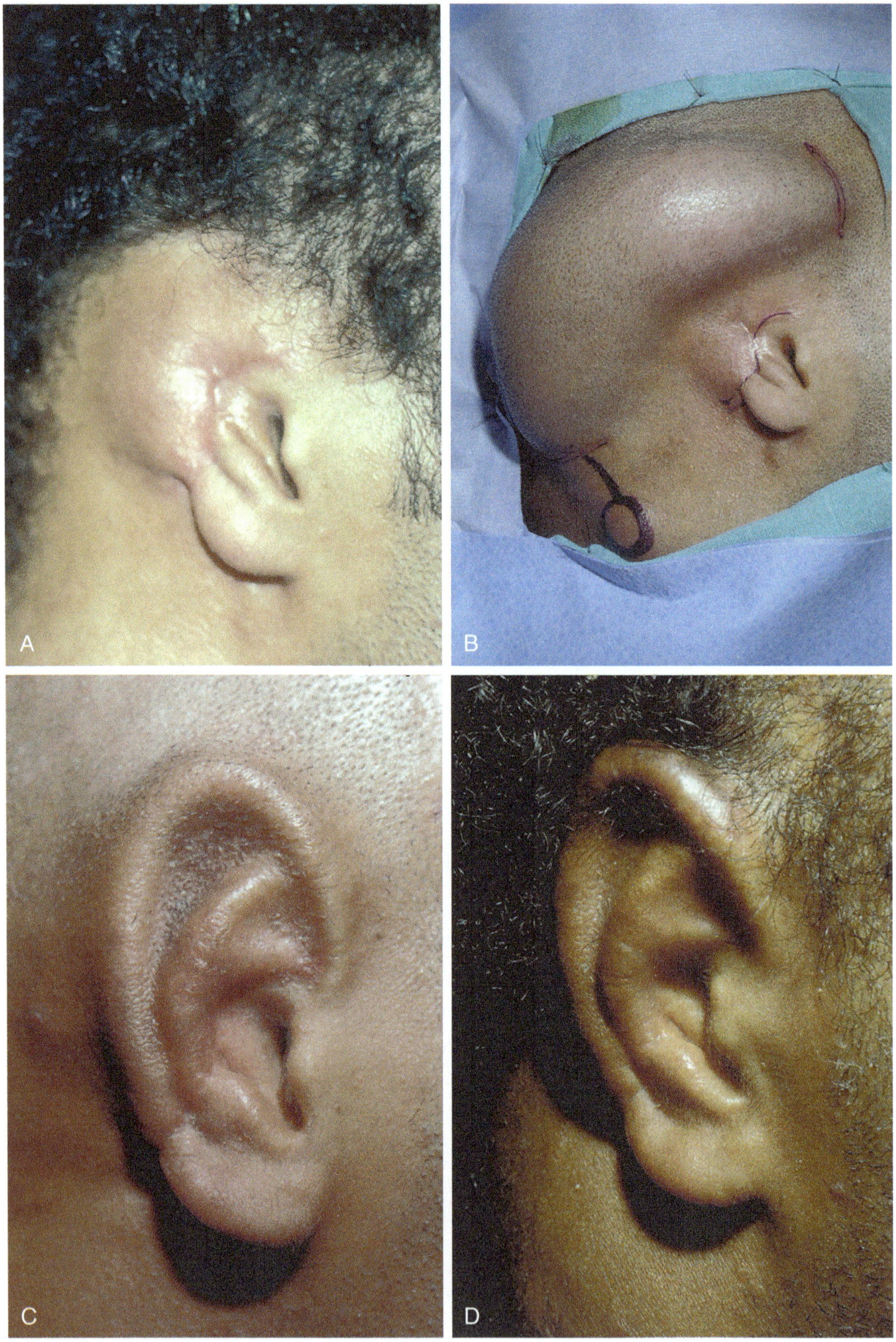

• **Fig. 32.11** Case 8. Indirect skin expansion. (A) Primary closure has been performed under some tension. (B) A crescent-shape expander (150 cm^3) has been placed under the skin behind the hair-bearing skin superior and posterior to the auricular area, and filled. (C) The tridimensional framework has been inserted without excessive tension. (D) Result after elevation of the ear.

The criterion to select the most appropriate procedure is the need to obtain symmetry concerning the projection of the ears, taking into account the local conditions. Analysing the projection of the contralateral ear is essential before performing the second stage.

Prosthesis

In cases of poor local conditions, including severed superficial temporal and occipital arteries, the prosthetic solution should be considered. It may be indicated for older patients when

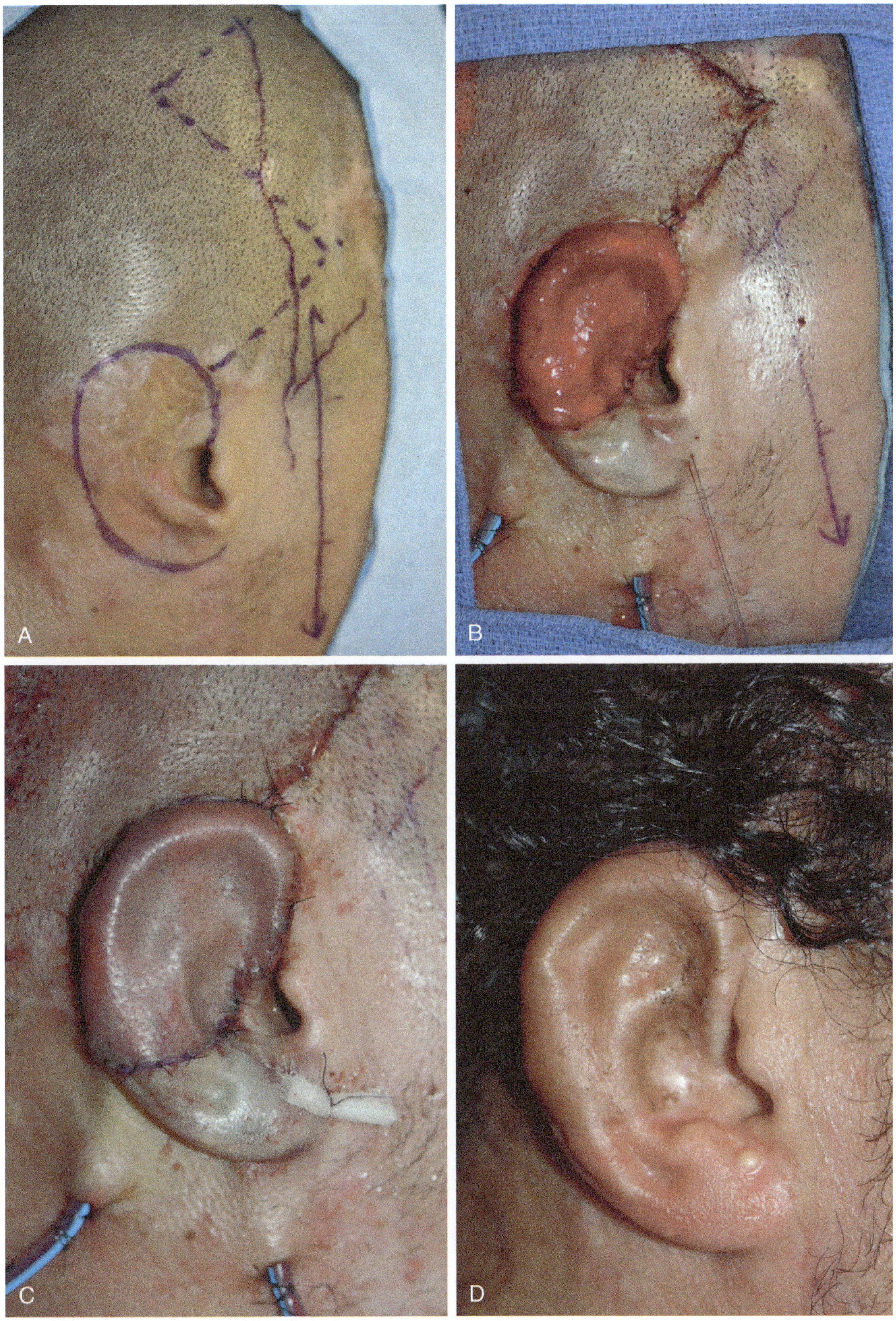

• **Fig 32.12** Case 9. (A) The skin of the auricular area cannot be used. The route of the superficial temporal artery has been drawn using a Doppler. A zig-zag incision will allow good exposure of the fascia and reduce the risk of a noticeable scar. (B) The well-vascularized fascia flap covers the framework. (C) A split-thickness skin graft taken on the scalp with a dermatome covers the fascia. Suction drainage will avoid hematoma. (D) Result after 1 year and before elevation.

rib cartilage may be ossified or when a patient has undergone multiple surgical procedures and opts for this solution.

Placement of Brånemark implants is performed in one or two stages depending on local condition and auricular remnants. The result of course relies on the quality of the prosthesis and the good adaptation of the patient to the management of the prosthesis and the percutaneous abutments.

Case 10 **(*Fig. 32.13*).** Patient with total amputation of the ear after an automobile accident who needed primary coverage of the temporal bone by a scalp flap. The temporal artery

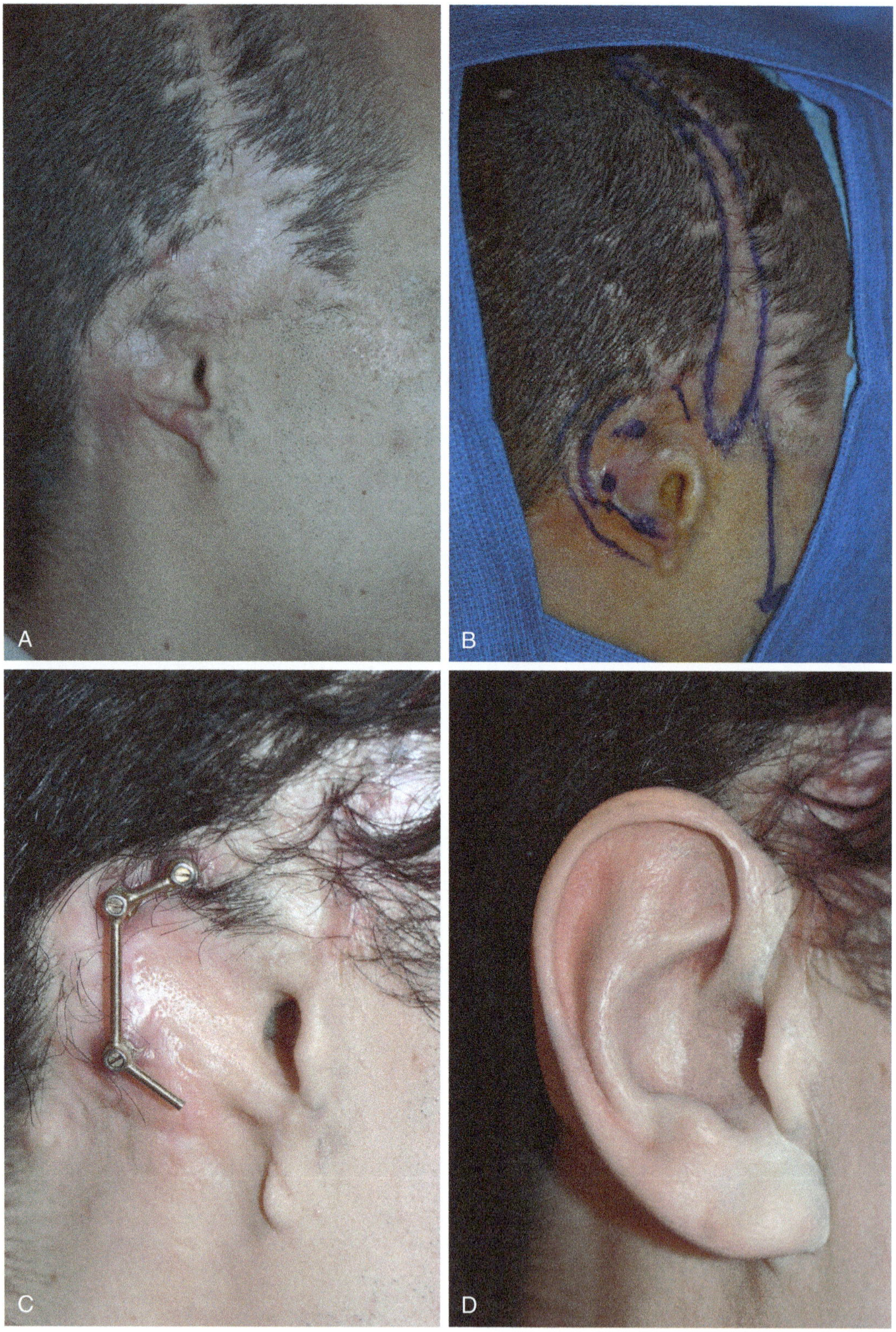

• **Fig. 32.13** Case 10. Prosthesis. (A) Temporal fascia cannot be used and there is no skin available in the auricular area. (B) Revision of the temporal scar and correct location of the implants. (C) Brånemark implants. (D) Prosthesis.

and fascia have been damaged and there is no skin available in the scarred auricular area. Three Brånemark implants are placed in one stage and a prosthesis by an experienced anaplastologist (Dr Pillet) give the patient great satisfaction.

Complications

The use of suction drains correctly located and removed after 3 days helps to avoid hematomas. Unsatisfactory results may result from inappropriate planning in carving the framework or selecting the wrong skin approach. Extrusion of wire sutures, retraction of the sulcus, and hypertrophic scarring may occur.

Infection and skin necrosis with exposure of the cartilaginous framework are the most serious complications.

Infection

Infection is the most severe complication as it will be responsible for cartilage resorption. It has to be prevented by a very vigorous preparation of the operating field (shaving around the ear, cleaning the skin invaginations, cleaning of the auditory canal and exposed face and scalp).

Cleaning the auditory canal and prescription of antibiotic drops some days before surgery is helpful. Antibiotics during the operation and postoperatively is essential.

Infection when diagnosed must be treated by repeated drainage and appropriate antibiotic therapy. If the infection is serious enough it is usually responsible for resorption of the cartilage, which may in some cases necessitate the carving of another framework.

Skin Necrosis

Necrosis occurs secondary to a poor blood supply of the skin flaps or excess skin tension over the contours of the cartilaginous framework and is generally due to poor surgical planning. A small exposure less than 2 mm may close by spontaneous healing from the skin edges which must be cleaned to induce granulation and epithelialization over the exposed cartilage. A larger exposure needs to be covered. Random fascial flaps all around the ear are available as well as temporal fascia when possible and needed.

Case 11 (***Fig. 32.14***)**.** A small exposure can be managed with correct local treatment inducing spontaneous healing.

Case 12 (***Fig. 32.15***)**.** When skin necrosis is responsible for a large exposure of the framework, a fascial flap can save the situation and must be performed once the necrosis is confirmed, which means some days after the first dressing. Antibiotics must be prescribed after a bacteriological exam. A random flap of fascia covered with a skin graft harvested on the scalp will save the situation with a good color match.

Case 13 (***Fig. 32.16***)**.** Too much tension of the skin over the framework can lead to skin necrosis on the antihelix. The situation cannot be solved by trying to approximate the skin edges with sutures. Only a short temporal fascia with axial vascularization (ATS) can solve the problem and avoid secondary infection and resorption of the cartilage.

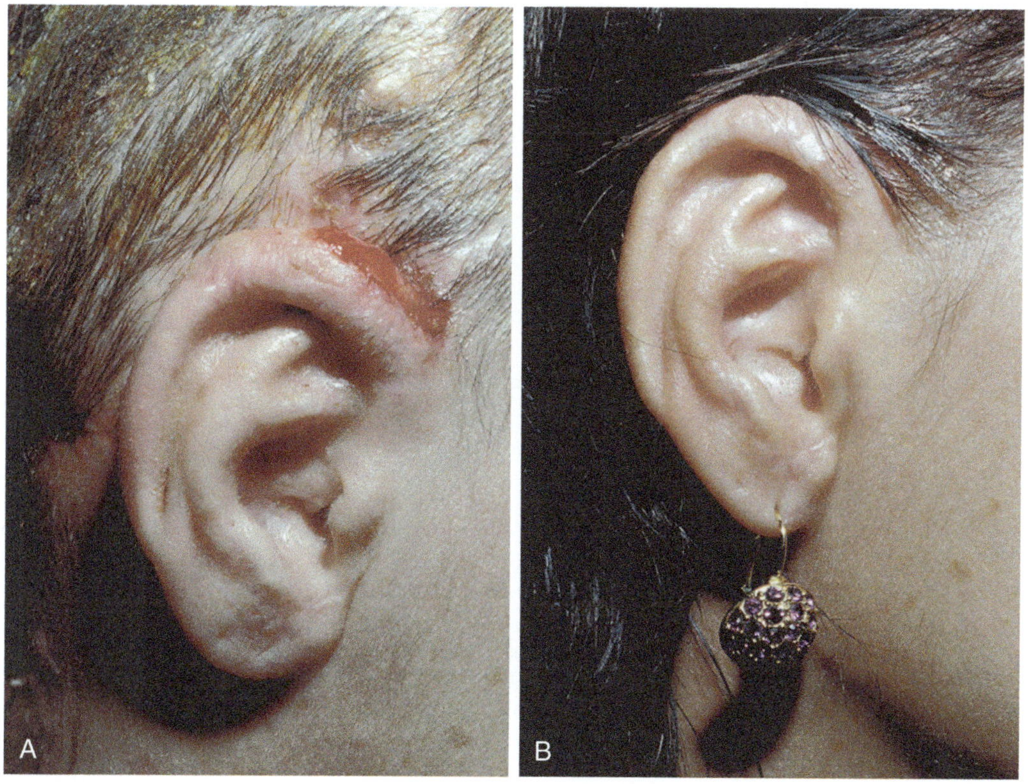

• **Fig. 32.14** Case 11. Exposure treated by spontaneous healing. (A) Exposure of the root of the helix after elevation of the reconstructed ear. (B) Granulation of the skin edges will cover the exposed cartilage followed by epithelialization.

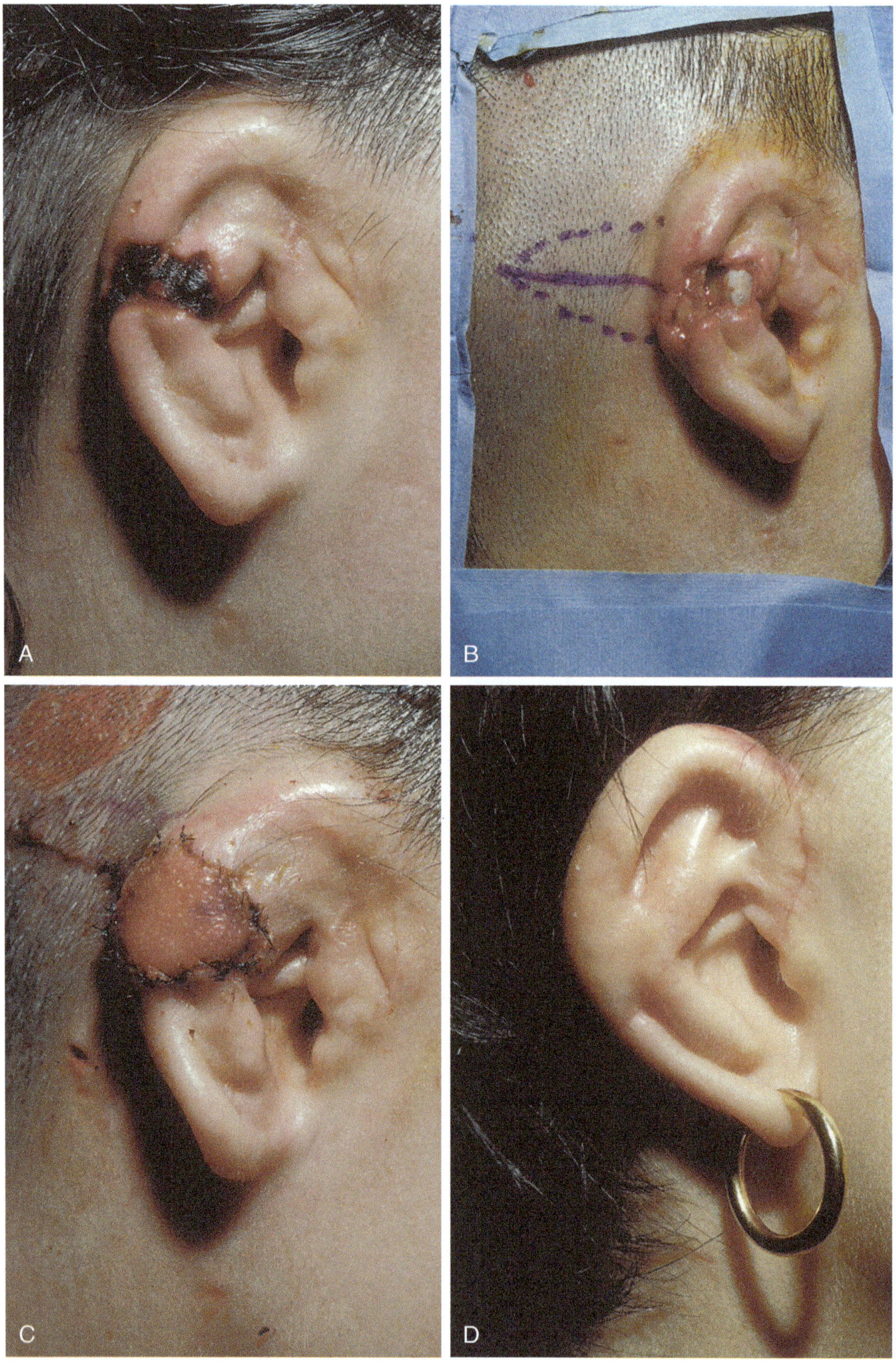

• **Fig. 32.15** Case 12. (A) Large skin necrosis at the level of the previous sutures. (B) Clean exposure of the cartilage framework and drawing of the skin approach to dissect a random fascial flap (dotted line). (C) Fascial flap covered with a split-skin graft taken from the scalp. (D) Final result with good color match of the skin graft.

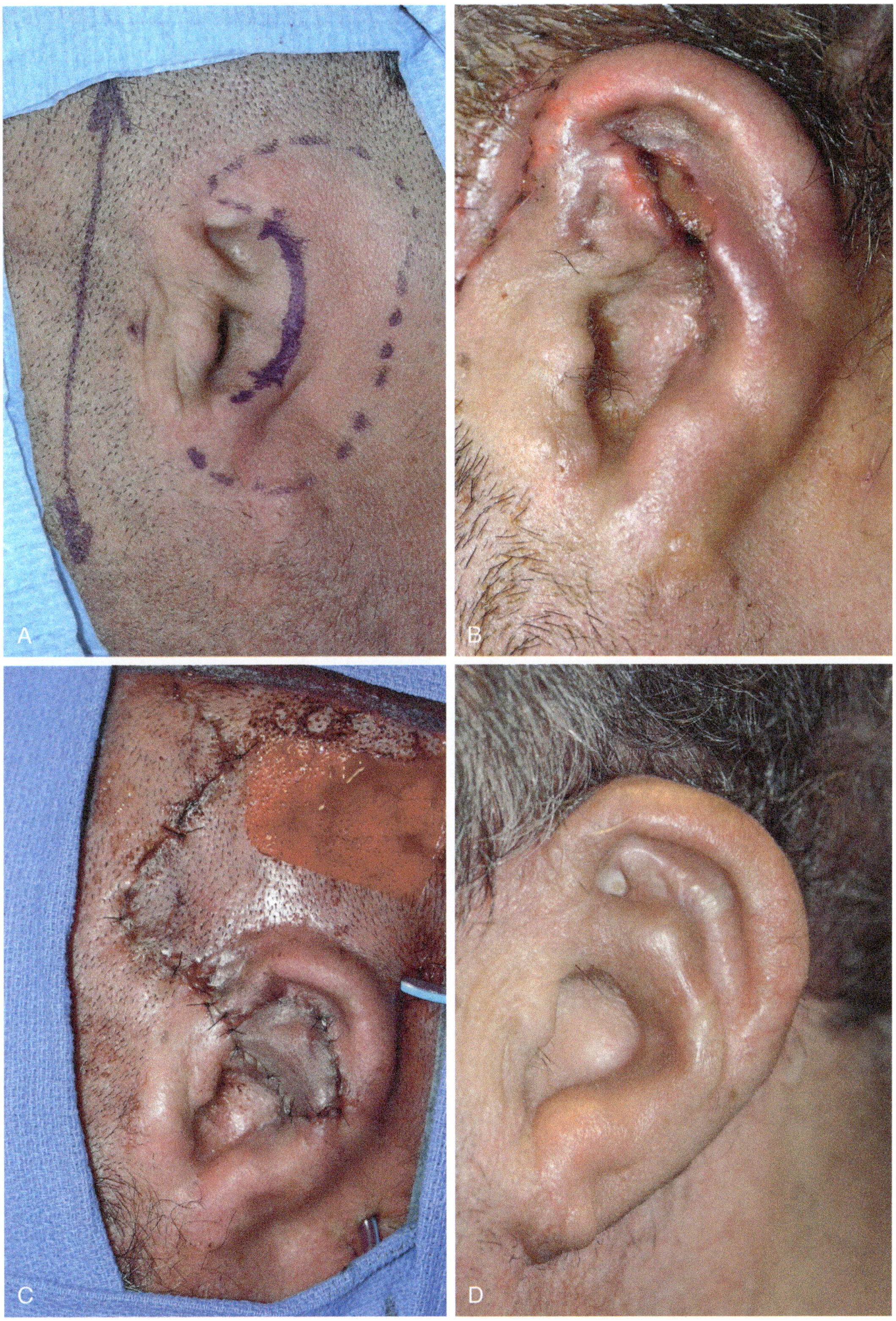

• **Fig. 32.16** Case 13. (A) Total amputation after human bite. The former scar in the concha is used as the skin approach to prepare the skin pocket. (B) Skin necrosis and exposure of the cartilage. (C) The temporal fascia flap has been placed in front of the exposed cartilage avoiding any tension of the skin, and is covered with split-thickness skin from the scalp. (D) Final result.

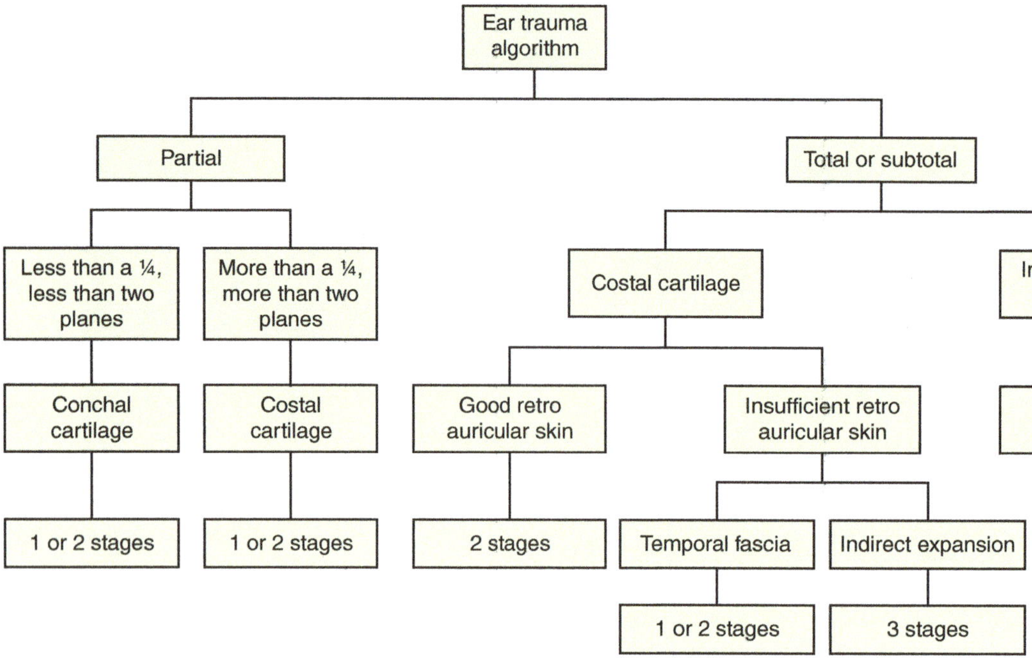

• **Fig. 32.17** Ear trauma algorithm.

Algorithm

It is essential when reconstructing an ear after trauma to have in mind the principle and guidelines of this surgery. It can be useful to follow a precise algorithm, such as that offered here which has been established by the senior author after three decades of experience in ear reconstruction, including 654 reconstructions after traumatic amputation (Fig. 32.17).

References

1. Brent B, Byrd HS. Secondary ear reconstruction with cartilage grafts covered by axial, random and free flaps of temporoparietal fascia. *Plast Reconstr Surg*. 1983;72(2):141–152.
2. Antia NH, Buch VI. Chondrocutaneous advancement flap for the marginal defect of the ear. *Plast Reconstr Surg*. 1967;39(5):472–477.
3. Firmin F, Marchac A. A novel algorithm for autologous ear reconstruction. *Semin Plast Surg*. 2011;25(4):257–264.
4. Firmin F. Value of tissue expansion in total reconstruction of the external ear. *Ann Chir Plast Esthet*. 1996;41(5):495–502.
5. Brent B. Technical advances in ear reconstruction with autogenous rib cartilage grafts: personal experience with 1200 cases. *Plast Reconstr Surg*. 1999;104(2):319–334.
6. Nagata S. A new method for total reconstruction of the auricle for microtia. *Plast Reconstr Surg*. 1993;92(2):187–201.

33 Scalp and Calvarial Reconstruction

YUN-HUAN (BARRY) HSIEH AND FU-CHAN WEI

Introduction

Scalp comprises the forehead and the hair-bearing regions. It extends from the supraorbital ridge anteriorly to the highest nuchal line posteriorly, while ears and zygomatic arches define its lateral borders.[1] In surgical practice, the scalp refers to the hair-bearing region exclusively, separating forehead from the frontal hairline. Hair-bearing scalp represents an irreplaceable tissue unit with esthetic importance. Its reconstructive approach should adhere to the basic principle of the reconstructive ladder, while providing durable coverage to protect intracranial contents with esthetically pleasing contour. The reconstruction also needs to preserve hair-bearing patterns and avoid neighboring structure distortions. Hair restoration should be considered to refine postreconstruction esthetics.

Anatomy of the Scalp

Anatomical Layers

The acronym of scalp compositions is represented by its own capital letters, SCALP, representing Skin, Connective tissue (subcutaneous tissue), Aponeurosis (galea aponeurotica), Loss of connective tissue, and Pericranium. The skin of the scalp is the thickest in the body (3–7 mm), and the occipital region is its thickest portion.[1] The scalp has the highest hair follicle density and is highly sebaceous. Connective tissue consists of adipose tissue and fibrous septa, allowing skin anchorage to galea aponeurotica. The aponeurosis layer is a broad and thin layer of tendinous sheet that unites the paired frontalis and occipitalis muscles. It extends bilaterally and fuses with the external auricular muscles. Its continuance forms temporoparietal fascia bilaterally, and the superficial musculoaponeurotic system (SMAS) of the face anteriorly.[2] The tight and inelastic nature of the galeal layer provides the explanation of "tight" and "loose" portions of the scalp. The "loose" portion refers to the region where the galeal edges blend with the temporoparietal fascia and scalp musculatures, whereas the "tight" portion extends from the same edges towards the scalp vertex.[2] Recognizing the tight and loose portion of the scalp facilitates the design of local flaps and placement of tissue expanders. Loose connective tissue (areolar tissue) connects the galeal layer to the pericranium while permitting union gliding of the galeal layer and above, allowing contraction movements of occipitofrontalis.[1] Emissary veins (posterior condyloid, mastoid, occipital, and parietal emissary vein) penetrate through this layer, connecting the superficial venous system of the scalp to cranial diploic veins and intracranial venous sinuses. Pericranium is the periosteum of the cranial bones; it fuses bilaterally with the deep temporal fascia at the superior temporal crest, and extends interiorly as endosteum at the cranial sutures.

Arterial Supply

The rich arterial plexus supply to the scalp is formed by extensive arterial anastomoses from terminal branches of both internal and external carotid arteries. Posterolaterally, the arterial supply of the scalp derives from branches of the external carotid arteries, including a pair of occipital, posterior auricular, and superficial temporal arteries. Anteriorly, its blood supply derives from the internal carotid arteries, including a pair of supratrochlear and supraorbital arteries. The arteries are located at the deepest layer of the dermis in the connective tissue layer.

Venous Drainage

The veins of the scalp are located in the connective tissue layer accompanying their corresponding arteries. They form a complex venous network, anastomosing with each other and via emissary veins. The occipital vein drains into the suboccipital venous plexus around the semispinalis capitis muscle and continued into vertebral veins, or less commonly into the internal jugular vein. The posterior auricular vein drains the post-auricular region as well as receiving the mastoid emissary vein from the sigmoid sinus. It joins the retromandibular vein at its exit from the parotid gland, forming the external jugular vein. The superficial temporal vein courses with its artery until its union with the maxillary vein in the parotid gland, forming the retromandibular vein. Anteriorly, the supraorbital and supratrochlear veins accompany their respective arteries before uniting medial to the orbit. They are drained by the angular vein into the facial vein.[1]

Lymphatic Drainage

The lymphatic system is located within the subdermal and subcutaneous level. There are no lymph nodes in the scalp. Posteriorly, the lymphatic channels drain into occipital and postauricular nodes. Anteriorly, it drains to the parotid gland, preauricular, submandibular, and upper cervical lymph nodes. The lymph eventually reaches the nodes of the deep cervical chain.

Nerve Supply

Motor Nerves

Anteriorly, frontalis is supplied by the ipsilateral frontal branch of the facial nerve. The frontal nerve exits the parotid gland approximately 2.5 cm anterior to the tragus, ascends on the periosteum of the zygomatic arch, then continues adherent to the deep surface of, and eventually within, the temporoparietal fascia towards a point approximately 1.5 cm lateral to the orbital rim. Pitanguy's line is the most widely used landmark to estimate the course of the frontal nerve, and is defined by a line drawn from 0.5 cm inferior to the tragus to 1.5 cm superior and lateral the eyebrow.[3] Posteriorly, the posterior auricular branch of the facial nerve supplies both occipitalis and extrinsic auricular muscles, which leaves the facial nerve before it enters the parotid.

Sensory Nerves

Sensory innervation of the scalp is provided by the trigeminal nerve, cervical spine nerves, and branches from the cervical plexus.[1] Anteriorly, the scalp is supplied by the paired supratrochlear and supraorbital nerves; both arise from the ophthalmic division of the trigeminal nerve. The supratrochlear nerve courses with its artery and provides sensation to the conjunctiva, upper eyelid, nasal sidewall, medial forehead, frontal scalp, and its vertex. The supraorbital nerve travels with its artery, and divides into superficial and deep branches to provide sensation to the forehead and frontoparietal scalp. Laterally, the scalp is supplied by the zygomaticotemporal nerve and auriculotemporal nerve. They arise from maxillary and mandibular branches of the trigeminal nerve respectively.[1] Posteriorly, the sensation of the scalp is supplied by the greater occipital nerve (posterior ramus of C2), lesser occipital nerve (anterior ramus of C2), and third occipital nerve (posterior ramus of C3).[1]

Reconstructive Principles

Patient Evaluation and Examination

Holistic evaluation of the intrinsic and extrinsic patient factors is an integral part of surgical assessment. Multidisciplinary unit assessments for oncological resection and reconstruction are essential for patient outcome maximization. Collaboration with neurosurgeons may be necessary if further calvarial reconstruction is required. Patients' baseline functions, medical comorbidities, history of cigarette smoking, immunocompetence status, histological and clinical staging of the malignant neoplasm, as well as history and planned chemoradiotherapy are to be explored in detail. Surgically, knowledge of previous incision, hair status, and the patient's expectation are important factors of reconstruction design. Comprehensive understanding of the defect size, location, and nature of the defect (simple versus composite defect) facilitates surgical planning and choice of surgical technique.

Reconstruction Goals

The goals of scalp reconstruction are both functional and esthetic. The functional goal is to provide a durable, in some cases, sensate coverage for the protection of calvarium or alloplastic cranioplasty prosthesis in prevention of desiccation and infection. Esthetic goals include an esthetically placed incision, replacing "like with like," adequate contouring, preservation of hairlines and their growth patterns, limits to postoperative alopecia, avoidance of neighboring structure distortion (anterior hairline, sideburns, eyebrow, upper eyelids, and auricles), and if appropriate, utilizing adjuvant hair transplantation to restore trauma and reconstruction-induced hair loss.

Reconstruction Options

Healing by Secondary Intention

The rich vascular network plexus of the scalp and its high-density skin appendages permit superior healing potential by secondary intention. This approach is most suitable for small wounds in patients who are intolerant of anesthesia or related donor site morbidity.[4] Superficial partial-thickness wounds from abrasions or burns, after minimal debridement, can expect to heal adequately with simple but frequent dressing regimens. Deep partial-thickness wounds may heal sufficiently with dressing only, however, they may result in sparse hair growth and scar contracture. In small defects with an exposed outer table of the calvarium, granulation tissue can form secondarily if a moist environment is provided through adequate dressings. Becker et al[4] presented their series of 205 patients with secondary intention healing of exposed scalp following Mohs surgery. The mean healing time in exposed calvarium with intact pericranium was 7 weeks, and the average time for bare calvarium to heal was 13 weeks.

Vacuum-assisted closure (VAC) dressing should be considered in large and complex scalp wounds in patients who are unsuitable for complex reconstruction.[5] VAC therapy is believed to promote wound healing in the negative-pressure environment by increasing blood flow and stimulating granulation tissue formation, thus enhancing its healing by secondary intention. Marathe and Sniezek[6] reported their experience in VAC dressing for scalp and calvarial defects with exposed dura. They achieved 25% reduction of defect size while gaining a granulation wound bed, successfully simplifying the complexity of scalp reconstruction options.

Primary Closure

The applicability of primary closure of scalp is tightly associated with defect size and location. Primary closure is generally attainable in most acute scalp defects up to 10 cm^2 in size.[6] Primary closure of larger defects is possible in the "loose" area of the scalp where underlying muscles are located. Primary closure limits alopecia, provides good contouring, and allows monitor of tumor recurrence. In traumatic cases, limited debridement of hair-bearing scalp is advisable. Dual-layer closure allows the galeal layer to endure wound closure tension, allowing tension-free skin closure.[2] Tension-free closure reduces scar widening and its associated alopecia.[7] Surgical techniques commonly employed to facilitate primary closure in larger defects or tight areas of the scalp include undermining, galeal scoring, induction of mechanical creep, and stress relaxation of the skin. These techniques are also applicable during advancement and inset of local flaps.

Skin Grafts, Adjuvant Techniques, Dermal Matrix and Dermal Substitutes

In the presence of a noninfected vascularized wound bed with intact pericranium, skin graft is an easy and quick solution for scalp defect reconstruction. It is a reliable technique and able to reconstruct medium to large defects. It shortens healing time and allows oncological surveillance. The major disadvantages of skin grafts are alopecia, contouring deficiency, and hypopigmentation. Split-thickness skin graft (STSG) is more commonly used than its full-thickness variant. In contrast to full-thickness skin graft (FTSG), STSG is suitable for medium to large defects, but creates greater contour deficiency and wound contracture. Donor site morbidity is considerably more significant in STSG than FTSG.

If bare calvarium is exposed, several adjuvant techniques can be utilized to convert a non-skin-graftable wound bed to a graftable defect. A large subgaleal, periosteal, and temporoparietal fascia flap can be raised, to either rotate or advance into the defect. These flaps enhance vascularity of the wound bed, allowing immediate skin grafting. Decortication of cranial outer table also coverts cranium into a graftable wound bed.[8] These reconstructions, however, commonly result in unstable wounds and are subject to recurrent breakdowns and risk of subsequent infection. VAC dressing converts bare calvarium into a graftable wound bed by promoting granulation. Second-stage skin graft is thus achievable with prolonged VAC dressing application. Dermal matrix and dermal substitute simplified the complexity of scalp wound by its adherence to non-graftable structures such as calvarium. Onlay skin grafting to dermal matrix or dermal substitutes enhances the durability and pliability of the reconstruction, and lessens contour deformity when compared with skin grafting alone.[9] They are, however, expensive and frequently require delayed skin grafting up to 3 weeks. Careful patient selection is thus imperative.

Skin graft is also used for secondary defect reconstruction after transposition or bipedicled flaps. In addition, skin graft can be utilized as temporary biological dressing prior to the definitive reconstruction. This concept is valuable in oncological cases when staged operation is planned and clearance of resection margin is being assessed.

Locoregional Flaps

Locoregional flaps are indicated when recruitment and advancement of neighboring tissue is inadequate for tension-free closure. Locoregional flaps are applicable to wide ranges of defect sizes, and are important options for complex scalp wound reconstructions, principally for those with exposed calvarium and alloplastic cranioplasty prosthesis. Utilizing local flaps adheres to the "replace like with like" principle of plastic surgery. Advantages are hair bearing, superior contouring, and color matching, and thus they are more esthetically pleasing. Successful local flap reconstruction requires familiarity with regional vascular anatomy, flap designs, judicious assessments of regional tissue pliability, and avoidance of neighboring tissue distortions. Based on the concepts of "tight" and "loose" portion of the scalp, the feasibility of using local flap is greater in the frontal, temporoparietal, and occipital region, in contrast to vertex of the scalp. General surgical pearls for successful local flap reconstruction include designing a large flap with a wide base, minimizing the number of flaps, and avoiding suture lines in critical areas. If skin grafting is planned, it should be designed to locate inconspicuously so it can be camouflaged with hairstyling. Importantly, resist the temptation of trimming the dog-ears as they will invariably settle. Revising the dog-ear on the scalp narrows the skin pedicle and reduces vascular supply and drainage.

Although a surfeit of locoregional techniques were described for scalp reconstruction, the workhorse options are variations of rotation and transposition flaps. In contrast, an advancement flap shares less success due to the innate inelasticity of the scalp. In a smaller defect, a random pattern fasciocutaneous flap can be reliably raised, and serves as an alternative option to skin graft. For medium and large scalp defects, designing a local flap based on the named vascular pedicles is preferred. A pinwheel flap consists of four small rotation flaps bordering the defect that are 90 degrees apart from each other. It is used for small circular defects of the scalp. Recent modification by Simsek and Eroglu[10] extended its application to scalp defects up to 50 mm in size. It is an alternative choice if a large rotation flap is to be avoided.

A rotation flap is the classical solution for a scalp defect of up to 50 mm diameter (Fig. 33.1). The flap is based on

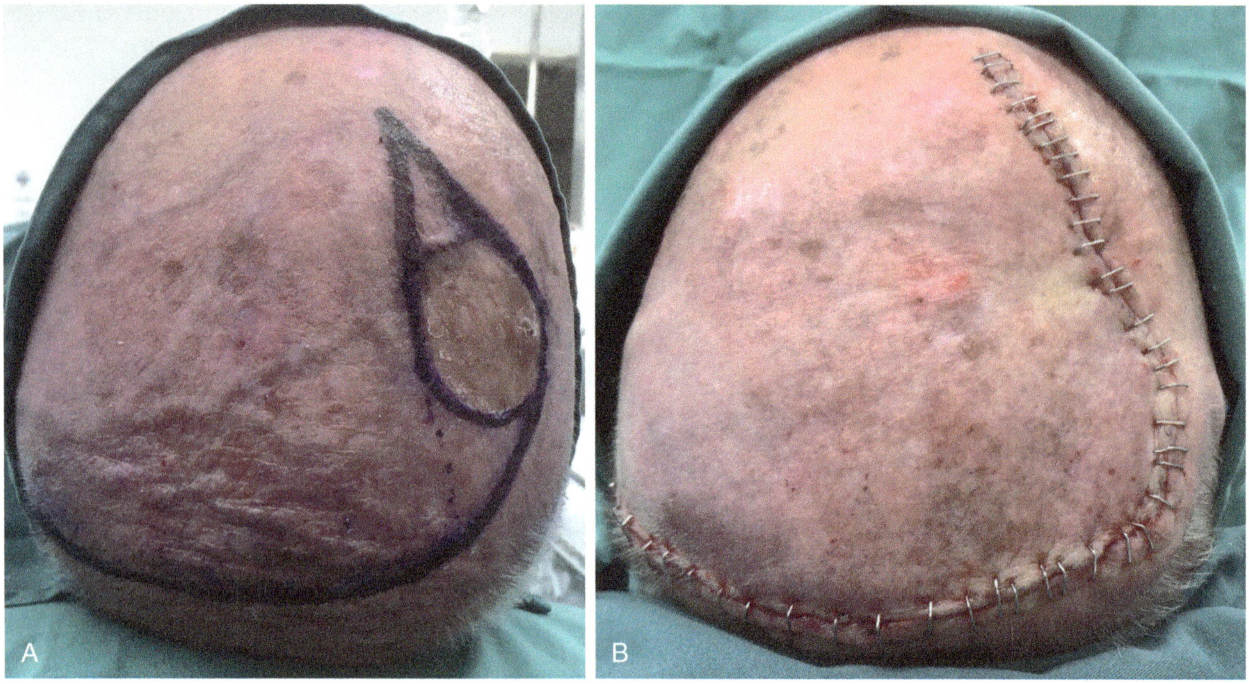

• **Fig. 33.1** (A) Preoperative marking of rotation flap of the scalp. (B) Immediate postoperative appearance. (Courtesy Dr. Cameron Keating.)

an axial pattern blood supply, incorporating at least one of the named arteries. Although the ideal flap circumference and defect width ratio is inconsistently described, an experimental study by Lo and Kimble[11] demonstrated that the effect in decreasing tension becomes minimal once the flap circumference exceeds approximately 5 times. Meticulous reverse planning with careful attention to pivot point, blood supply, sensory supply, and defect/flap dimensions are critical. A transposition flap is used in medium to large scalp defect. As a transposition flap creates a secondary defect and requires skin grafting, it is typically reserved for large scalp defect reconstruction (Fig. 33.2). Similar to the design of a rotation flap, it should be raised based on an axial pedicle with a wide skin paddle.

A bipedicled flap is an uncommonly described, yet a useful local flap for scalp reconstruction. It is raised like a bucket handle based on two opposing axial arteries, and is useful for large scalp defect reconstruction (Fig. 33.3). Analogous to a transposition flap, it creates a secondary defect requiring skin graft reconstruction. Orticochea flap, initially described by Miguel Orticohea in 1967 as a local advancement and rotation flap, consists of 3-flap and 4-flap variants.[12] The flap design represents the greater understanding and utilization of regional vascular anatomy, and is used for large scalp defects with an attempt to preserve hairlines. Despite the best intention of hairline preservation, the Orticochea flap is known to be associated with high risks of postoperative alopecia, unnatural direction of hair growth, wound healing problems, and potential requirement for skin grafting. With advances in flap diversity, the introduction of tissue expanders, and microvascular reconstruction, the Orticochea flap is now less commonly used.

Numerous regional flaps were described for scalp constructions, however, microsurgical reconstruction has replaced many of the regional options. Regional flap reconstructions are now reserved for unsuitable microsurgical reconstruction candidates, or as a second-line option. Commonly described regional flaps for scalp reconstruction are the pedicled trapezius myocutaneous, pedicled latissimus dorsi, temporoparietal fascia fasciocutaneous, and spenius capitis muscle/myocutaneous flaps. The trapezius flap is classically described as upper and lower trapezius myocutaneous flap. The complexity of the vascular anatomy of the region gives rise to further classification of the flap into four types: (1) type 1, based on the occipital artery; (2) type 2, based on the superficial branch of the transverse cervical artery (SCA); (3) type 3, based on the dorsal scapula artery (DSA); (4) type 4, based on the intercostal artery. Scalp reconstruction with a pedicled trapezius myocutaneous flap commonly uses either type 2 and type 3 flaps. The DSA-based flap provides a greater arch of rotation and greater pedicle length in comparison to the SCA-based trapezius flap. DSA-based flaps can safely reach the neck and lower face, whereas SCA-based flaps can safely reach the neck and lower face.[13] The trapezius myocutaneous flap provides pliable yet durable reconstruction to the scalp and is currently underused in surgical practice (Fig. 33.4).

Tissue Expander

Tissue expansion is indicated when local flap coverage is inadequate due to defect size, regional traumatized tissue, unacceptable postreconstruction hair pattern or distortion of the hairline. In contrast to one-stage reconstruction, tissue

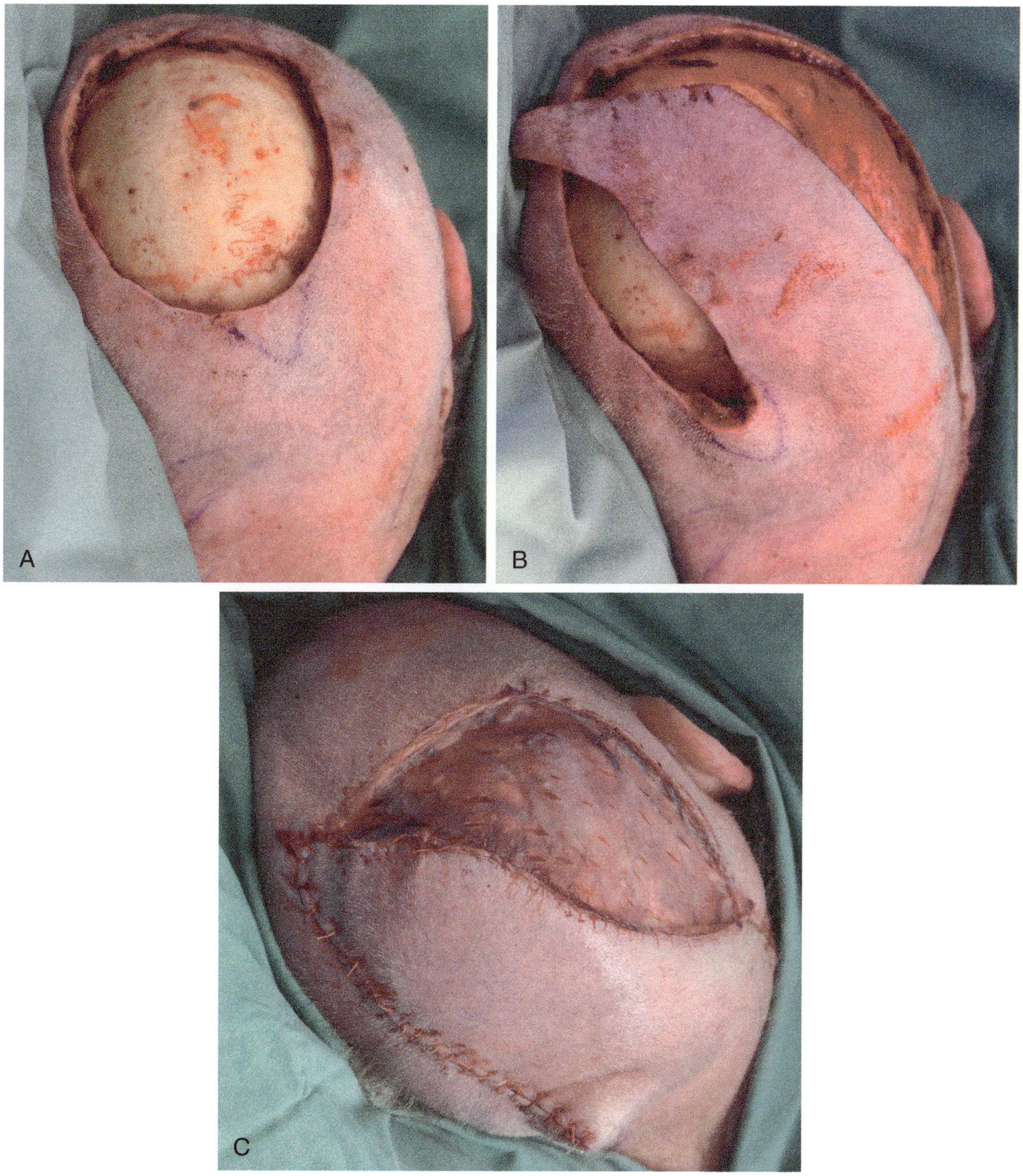

• **Fig. 33.2** (A) Large vertex defect post wide local excision of squamous cell carcinoma exposing calvarium. (B) Raising transposition flap for exposed calvarium reconstruction. (C) Final inset of transposition flap and STSG to secondary defect. (Courtesy Dr. Rostam D. Farhadieh.)

expansion enhances the reconstructive area and facilitates the reach of the rotation-advancement flap, thus avoiding the need for a skin graft to the secondary defect and allowing primary closure. A tissue expander, however, requires staged operations and a lengthy expansion period. Patient collaboration, etiology of the defect, psychological suitability, and tissue expander-associated complications should be considered and weighed against esthetically inferior reconstruction options. Stable scalp coverage must be achieved prior to the expansion to prevent unnecessary calvarial desiccation and osteomyelitis. Tissue expander is the combined clinical application of three concepts that include stress relaxation, mechanical and biological creeping of the skin. Approximately 50% of the scalp can be resurfaced with tissue expanders.[14] The shape of the expander generally correlates with the shape of the intended flap design. A single large expander is preferred, allowing greatest gain in tissue per volume of expansion, and minimizes tissue expander-associated complications. However, multiple expanders are frequently needed for sizable defect reconstruction of the scalp.

Judicious planning with a particular focus on placement of expander pockets, ports, and incisions is the key to reduce morbidity. General guidelines for tissue expansion in the scalp region include the following:

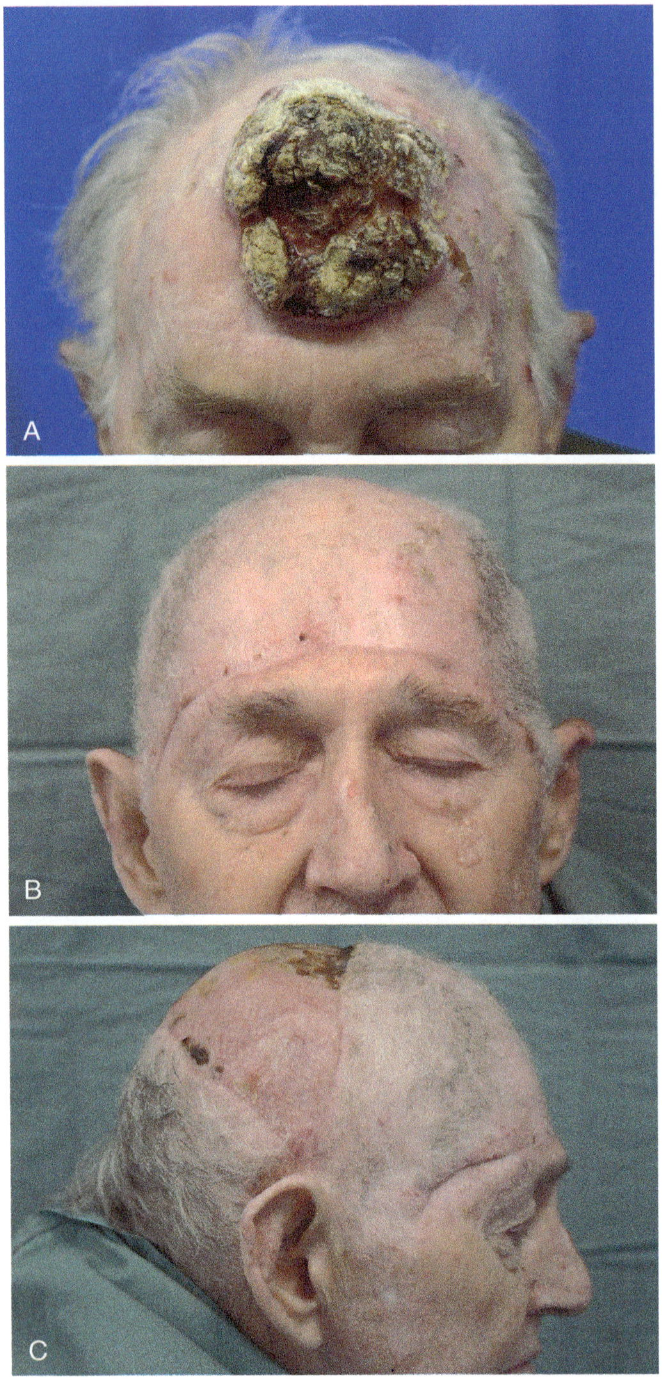

• **Fig. 33.3** (A) Large rapid growing frontal squamous cell carcinoma. (B) Frontal and (C) lateral views, 1 month post bipedicled flap reconstruction with STSG to secondary defect. (Courtesy Dr. Rostam D. Farhadieh.)

- The expander should be placed in the subgaleal plane.
- The expander base area should be 2.5 to 3 times the defect area.
- Design the incision perpendicular to the direction of intended expansion. The incision should be located away from the defect and flap incision sites, and should be made as small as possible.
- The expander valve is placed in a healthy area above and/or lateral to the expander, at least 7 cm away.

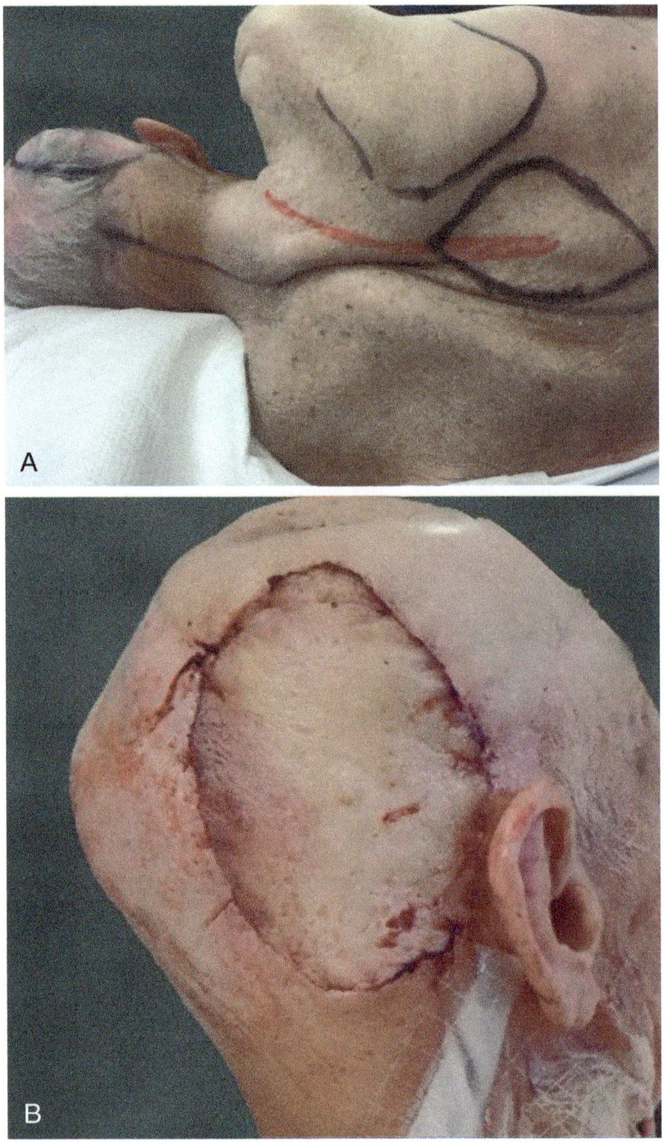

• **Fig. 33.4** (A) Design of trapezius flap for posterolateral scalp defect reconstruction. (B) Postoperative appearance of the trapezius flap. (Courtesy Dr. Rostam D. Farhadieh.)

- Fill the expander at the conclusion of the operation to reduce seroma/hematoma and the need for drains.
- Allow 2 weeks for healing before expansion, and continue weekly thereafter. The capsule can be incised to increase stretch, but avoid a full capsulectomy.
- Elasticity and contractility of the expanded flap depend on individual factors, but an estimation of gained flap length is the distance over the dome of the expander minus the corresponding measurement of its base.
- The estimated flap advancement for an expanded flap in scalp region is about 8 cm; the expected expanded flap width is between 12 cm and 16 cm.
- Overexpansion by 30%–50% is suggested to account for flap contraction, as the theoretical flap gain is rarely, if ever, yielded in vivo.[15]

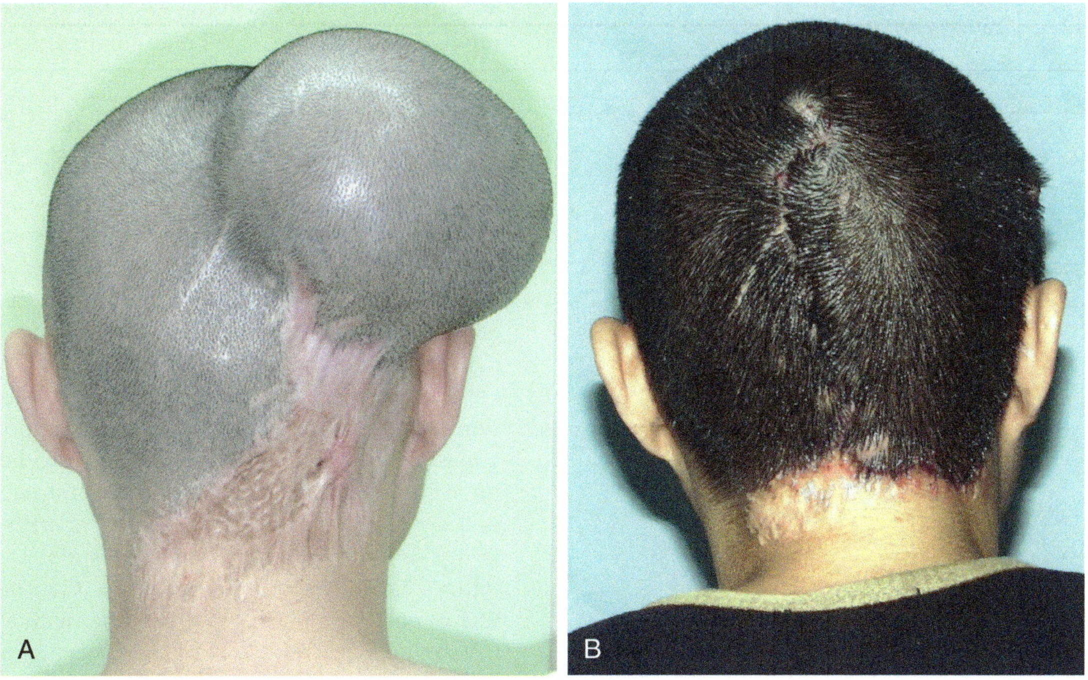

• **Fig. 33.5** (A) Alopecia in the occipital region treated with a tissue expander. (B) Postoperative appearance at 2 months. (Courtesy Dr. Shiow Shuh Chuang.)

Meticulous alignment of hair growth direction should be attempted, especially when multiple tissue expanders are used for multiple local flap expansions (Fig. 33.5).

Microsurgical Free Tissue Transfer

Free flap, the highest order in the reconstructive ladder, is indicated in large to extensive scalp defects, composite defects, CSF leak, and insufficient healthy local tissues due to trauma, irradiation, infection, or repetitive history of surgery. A free flap can also be used for postcranioplasty implant exposure salvage.[16] Free flap reconstruction offers a one-stage operation, and transfers fresh healthy tissue from a distant site that is unaffected by regional pathology. It imports robust vascular supply to the wound bed, enhances wound healing in the heavily irradiated defect, and facilitates antibiotic delivery to previously infected wound. Diversity of free flap harvesting techniques permits reconstruction targets beyond resurfacing of the scalp. With suitable flap choices, each component of a composite defect (bone, muscle, fascia, and skin) can be reconstructed individually with "like" tissues. Oversize design of the free flap allows dead space obliteration and provides a resilient tissue reconstruction if further radiotherapy is needed. Similarly, utilizing myocutaneous flaps with either chimeric or composite free flap design can also obliterate dead space successfully. The principle drawbacks of free flap reconstructions to scalp are contour disparity and the inability to provide hair restoration. Free flaps are generally thicker than scalp, and do not adhere to skull as tightly as native skin. If a muscle component is incorporated, an acceptable scalp contour may result as the muscle atrophies. Similarly, radiotherapy potently reduces flap volume once commenced, therefore, an oversize flap is frequently necessary to prevent postradiation hollowing.

Primary or secondary debulking of cutaneous or fasciocutaneous flaps can be offered, if necessary, to reduce contour disparity. Occasionally, an ablative composite defect spares the hair-bearing skin. In these instances a de-epithelialized fasciocutaneous or adipofascial free flap with or without muscle can be used for dead space obliteration and contour restoration, leaving a small monitoring paddle. The monitoring paddle can be strategically hidden in the nonvisible region and removed under local anesthetic once its purpose has been fulfilled. Wide ranges of free flap donor sites have been proposed in the literature for scalp and calvarium reconstruction. They include fasciocutaneous flaps (anterolateral thigh, parascapular, scapular, and radial forearm free flaps), muscle free flaps (latissimus dorsi, rectus abdominis, and gracilis), as well as omentum flap. The anterolateral thigh (ALT) flap may be the most versatile donor site for a composite scalp defect. It allows harvesting of vascularized fascia lata for dura replacement, vastus lateralis muscle for volume replacement and dead space obliteration, and fasciocutaneous tissue for scalp resurfacing. It has consistently lengthy vascular pedicles with dependable caliber, allowing ipsilateral, in some cases, contralateral microvascular anastomoses with superficial temporal vessels (Fig. 33.6). In addition, eccentric flap design at the vascular hilum can further lengthen the vascular pedicle for alternative recipient vessels in the neck. However, if the defect is located at the vertex, vein grafts may still be needed. As a distant flap, away from the head and neck region, a simultaneous two-team approach

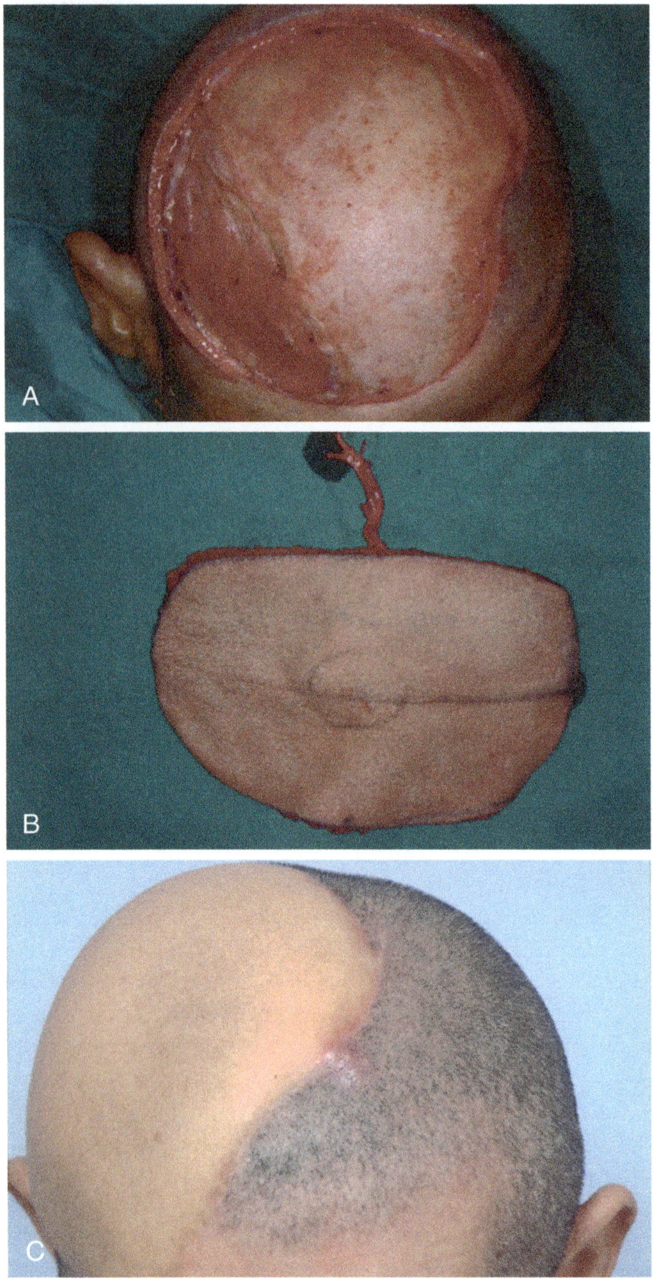

• **Fig. 33.6** (A) Scalp defect after skin cancer excision. (B) Harvested anterolateral thigh flap ready for inset and revascularization at the defect. (C) Postoperative appearance of the ALT flap.

smooths surgical logistics, shortens surgical time, and facilitates patient anesthetic recovery.

In the case of subtotal or total scalp resurfacing, the latissimus dorsi muscle flap and omentum flap may provide greater defect coverage. The latissimus dorsi muscle flap is preferred as the donor site can be closed directly without breaching into the abdominal cavity. An intraabdominal donor site may have a negative impact on a potentially ill patient. Abdominal discomfort limits inspiration effort, worsens lung atelectasis, impairs respiratory function, and increases the risk of pneumonia and sepsis. A large fasciocutaneous flap can also be used for subtotal or total scalp reconstruction. However, the need for extensive skin grafting to the donor site makes it an unattractive approach.

Scalp Replantation

Scalp avulsion is a devastating injury and potentially life-threatening. The classical mechanism is avulsion injury from entanglement of loose long hair into rotary machinery. Other common causes of scalp avulsion include animal bite and "scalping" assaults. Owing to the rich vascular network of the scalp, catastrophic hemorrhage can occur. An early management of severe trauma (EMST) protocol should be adhered to for early hemorrhage control, followed by initiation of aggressive fluid and blood resuscitation. If required, a massive transfusion protocol should also be activated. Be mindful of associated head and neck injuries; up to 9.4%[17] of scalp avulsion injuries are associated with cervical spine injury, and 4%–8% of patients will suffer concurrent head injury that is clinically significant.[18] Contraindications of scalp replantation are multitrauma with hemodynamic instability, a severely crushed or macerated amputate, and fragmented injuries.

All the avulsed parts of the scalp should be rescued from the scene, wrapped in saline wet gauze/cloth, placed in the sealed plastic bag, and preserved in a bag of ice. As a non-replaceable tissue, scalp replantation should be attempted whenever possible, as no other reconstructive alternative provides superior results. Scalp avulsions typically tear through loose areolar tissue separating galea aponeurotica and pericranium. As scalp vasculature resides in the connective tissue layer, the vascular network supplying the scalp is likely preserved, allowing replantation. Extensive vascular intercommunication permits successful replantation of the scalp based on one set of microvascular anastomoses. All major pieces of avulsed scalp should be revascularized unless tissue damage is beyond salvage. Intraoperatively, the entire scalp and amputate should be shaved to approximately 1 mm in length. This allows better visualization of tissue damage, wound edge, and patterns of hair growth. The wound and amputate should be judiciously debrided and washed-out, avoiding damage to hair follicle by iatrogenic means. Vascular anatomy should be accurately evaluated and identified. Traumatized vasculature should be replaced with vein graft, especially if the corkscrew sign is observed. Superficial temporal vessels are the principle recipients for revascularization. In the scalp avulsion scenario, they are likely to be found proximally in the parotid gland. It is, however, possible to utilize other scalp vessels for anastomoses including supraorbital, occipital, and posterior auricular vasculatures. To reduced overall ischemia time, arterial anastomoses should be performed first, followed by at least two sets of venous anastomoses. The scalp flap should be inspected carefully for both perfusion and drainage to ensure adequate circulation is restored, and reassess the need for additional vascular anastomoses. Leeching therapy with ciprofloxacin (for *Aeromonas* cover), mechanical (VAC dressing),[19,20] or chemical leeching (subdermal clexane or heparin injection)[20]

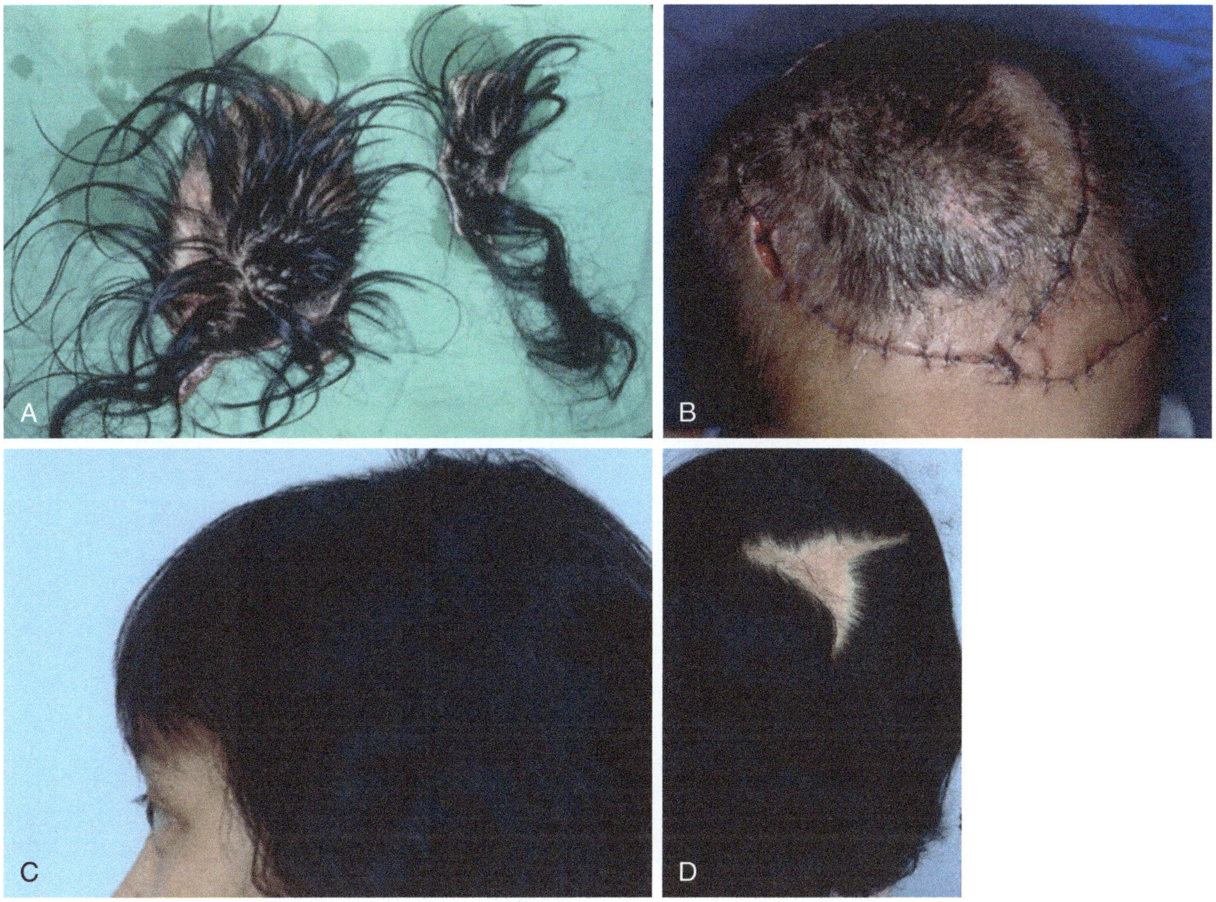

• **Fig. 33.7** (A) Avulsed scalp. (B) Appearance 3 months after microsurgical replantation. (C,D) Appearance 1 year after replantation.

may be necessary postoperatively if venous drainage remains insufficient.

Several salvage procedures are available for failed scalp replantation. Depending on the residual scalp defect, a reconstructive strategy ranging from VAC dressing-assisted closure to free flap reconstruction can be employed. The surgical outcome of these options, however, is less esthetically sound (Fig. 33.7).

Minimization of Iatrogenic Alopecia

Minimization of iatrogenic alopecia is essential in scalp reconstruction surgery, as preservation of hair follicles enhances overall esthetic outcomes. Principles of tension free closure, sparing use of electrocautery for hemostasis, and prevention of crushing injury at the wound edge by instruments should be followed strictly.

Incorporating meticulous trichophytic closure technique used by hair transplantation surgeons may further enhance hair follicle preservation and patient satisfaction. Major concepts of trichophytic closure are: (1) scalp laxity assessment; (2) incision at the side in line with the direction of hair growth; (3) parallel incision to hair follicles to avoid follicular injury; (4) trichotomy performed on one or both wound edges. Trichotomy is aimed at changing the direction of the hair follicle, encouraging hair growth through the scar, and camouflaging the presence of the scar.[21]

Hair Restoration

The nonsurgical options are more suitable for nontraumatic induced alopecia. Minoxidil and finasteride are the only FDA-approved agents for hair restoration. The discovery of platelet-rich plasma creates a new frontier in regeneration medicine; its application in hair restoration needs further evaluation to establish its use.[22] Surgical procedures remain the gold standard for hair restoration post reconstruction, as the hair follicles are largely damaged or absent due to initial trauma and subsequent resurfacing procedures. The common surgical techniques include tissue expansion, scalp reduction, and hair transplantation. A recently described vascularized island hair-bearing flap[23] based on temporal vascular pedicles may be used to restore patients' former esthetics in selective cases. Hair transplantation provides target-specific refinement of hair restoration and has become the surgical treatment of choice.

The goal of hair transplantation is to mimic the natural hair pattern in the area of alopecia that aligns and blends into its surroundings. Careful inspection and analysis of native hair, including its color, density, and direction of growth, facilitates surgical planning, execution, and esthetic success.

The hair follicle harvesting techniques that are commonly used include follicular unit transplantation (FUT) and follicular unit extraction (FUE). In FUT an occipital strip was taken in elliptical fashion followed by microdissection of follicular units. The donor site strip is designed horizontally between the occipital protuberance and 1 cm above the top of the auricles. Generally, each follicle unit contains 1–4 hair follicles. The normal hair density is around 100 units/cm^2, and the density achieved with hair transplantation is approximately 30–40 units/cm^2.[23] Conversely, FUE extracts multiple follicular units, performed manually or, more recently, robotically. The follicular grafts are prepared under loupe or microscopic magnification. Surrounding epithelium and connective tissue of the hair root are removed prior to their transplantation. The grafts should be kept viable in cool saline-soaked gauze throughout the procedure. Hypodermic needles, mini-knives, or micropunches can be used to create recipient ports at the recipient site for graft insertion. Careful positioning of the grafts in the intended direction and depth enhances the graft survival and hair esthetics. In hairline restoration, it is advisable to place the graft in an irregularly irregular stepping manner and plant them in triangular instead of linear fashion. Gentle transition is required from hair-bearing to non-hair-bearing regions to recreate a natural appearances. The result of transplantation can be evaluated after 8 months, allowing hair follicles to be appropriately cycled through the expected telogenic and anogenic phases (Fig. 33.8).

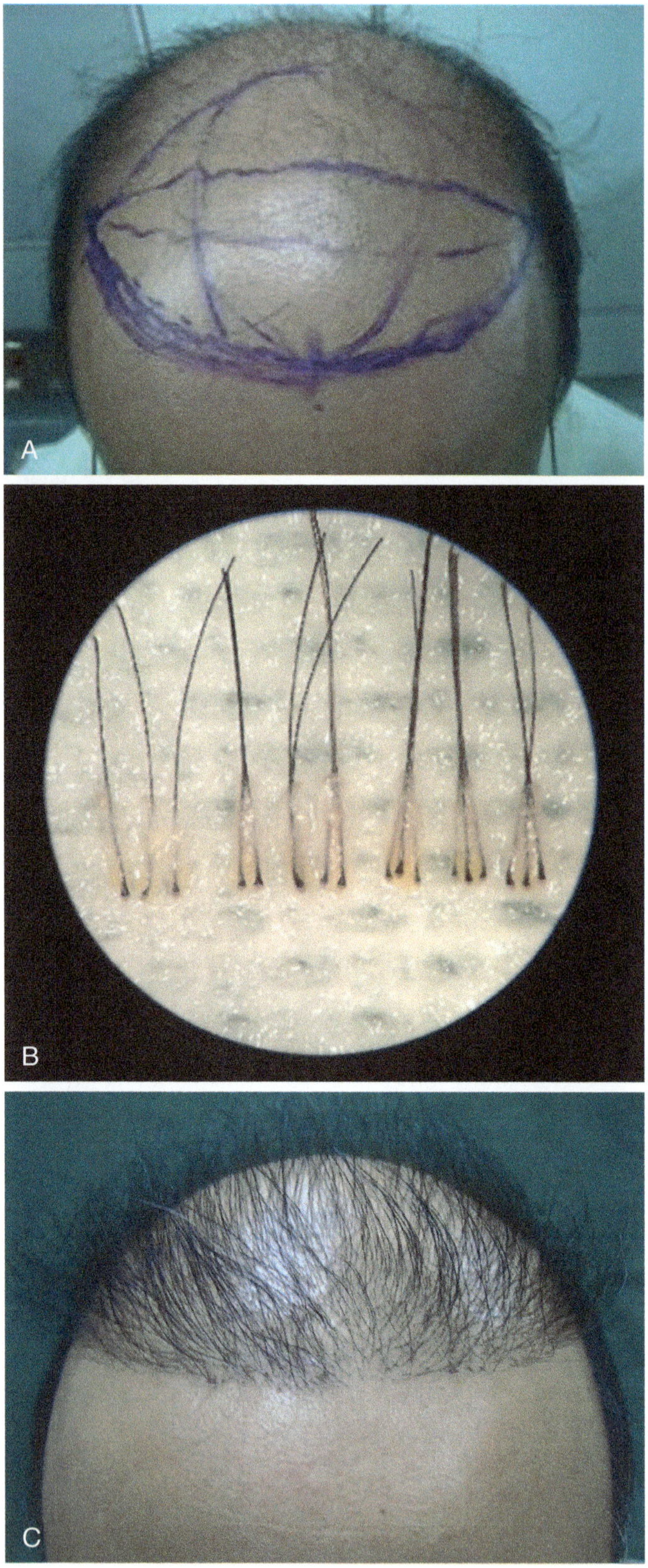

• **Fig. 33.8** (A) A 45-year-old male with frontal alopecia. (B) Follicular hair unit preparation. (C) Appearance 1 year after 2049 follicular hair transplantation. (Courtesy Dr. Yau-Li Huang.)

Allotransplantation

In extensive scalp injuries, on the scale of subtotal or total scalp defects, the esthetic results from limited reconstruction options are invariably displeasing. The lack of donor site for hair restoration in extensive defects inspires surgeons to seek new frontiers. As tissue engineering and cloning of the hair remain experimental, vascularized composite allotransplantations (VCA) seems to be the most feasible solution for extensive scalp defects. Bastidas et al[24] demonstrated the probable surgical approach for total facial and scalp allotransplantation through their anatomical studies. Since 2013, three reported cases of scalp allotransplantation have been performed, and all were part of more extensive head and neck allotransplantations.[25–27] The targeted need for scalp allotransplantation is less apparent when compared with facial allotransplantation. However, the regional data from Choi et al[28] revealed an increased public acceptance of scalp specific allotransplantation. Given the risk of lifelong immunosuppression, scalp allotransplantation should be reserved for patients with a combined extensive defect in the head and neck region.

Conclusion

Hair-bearing scalp is an integral unit of overall head and neck esthetics. Suboptimal reconstruction gravely impacts on patients' biopsychosocial wellbeing. The surgical techniques presented here offer sturdy autologous reconstructions, and esthetics can be greatly enhanced with subsequent hair restoration. VCA offers superior functional and esthetic outcome, yet is accompanied by risks associated with lifelong immunosuppression. VCA of the scalp should, therefore, be performed only as part of extensive facial allotransplantation.

References

1. Last RJ, McMinn RMH. *Last's Anatomy, Regional and Applied.* Edinburgh: Churchill Livingstone; 1994.
2. Desai SC, Sand PJ, Sharon JD, et al. Scalp reconstruction: an algorithmic approach and systematic review. *JAMA Facial Plast Surg.* 2015;17(1):56–66.
3. Pitanguy I, Ramos AS. The frontal branch of the facial nerve: the importance of its variations in face lifting. *Plast Reconstr Surg.* 1966;38(4):352–356.
4. Becker GD, Adams LA, Levin BC. Secondary intention healing of exposed scalp and forehead bone after Mohs surgery. *Otolaryngol Head Neck Surg.* 1999;121:751–754.
5. Dedhia R, Luu Q. Scalp reconstruction. *Curr Opin Otolaryngol Head Neck Surg.* 2015;23(5):407–414.
6. Marathe US, Sniezek JC. Use of the vacuum-assisted closure device in enhancing closure of a massive skull defect. *Laryngoscope.* 2004;114:961–964.
7. Hoffmann JF. Reconstruction of the scalp. In: Baker SR, ed. *Local Flaps in Facial Reconstruction.* St. Louis, MO: Mosby; 2007:638.
8. Lin SJ, Hanasono MM, Skoracki RJ. Scalp and calvarial reconstruction. *Semin Plast Surg.* 2008;22(4):281–293.
9. Khan MA, Ali SN, Farid M, Pancholi M, Rayatt S, Yap LH. Use of dermal regeneration template (Integra) for reconstruction of full-thickness complex oncologic scalp defects. *J Craniofac Surg.* 2010;21(3):905–909.
10. Simsek T, Eroglu L. Versatility of the pinwheel flap to reconstruct circular defects in the temporal and scalp region. *J Plast Surg Hand Surg.* 2013;47(2):97–101.
11. Lo CH, Kimble FW. The ideal rotation flap: an experimental study. *J Plast Reconstr Aesthet Surg.* 2008;61(7):754–759.
12. Badhey A, Kadakia S, Abraham MT, Rasamny JK, Moscatello A. Multiflap closure of scalp defects: revisiting the orticochea flap for scalp reconstruction. *Am J Otolaryngol.* 2016;37(5):466–469.
13. Wei FC, Mardini S. *Flaps and Reconstructive Surgery.* Amsterdam: Elsevier; 2016.
14. Manders ER, Schenden MJ, Furrey JA, et al. Skin expansion to eliminate large scalp defects. *Plast Reconstr Surg.* 1984;74:493.
15. Wieslander JB. Tissue expansion in the head and neck. A 6-year review. *Scand J Plast Reconstr Surg Hand Surg.* 1991;25:47–56.
16. Chou P-Y, Lin C-H, Hsu C-C, Yang W-H, Kane AA, Lin C-H. Salvage of postcranioplasty implant exposure using free tissue transfer. *Head Neck.* 2017;39(8):1655–1661.
17. Zhang Y, Cheng K, Dong J, et al. Incidence and features of vertebral fractures after scalp avulsion injuries. *J Craniofac Surg.* 2015;26:2217–2220.
18. Hills MW, Deane SA. Head injury and facial injury: is there an increased risk of cervical spine injury? *J Trauma.* 1993;34:549–553.
19. Qiu SS, Hsu C-C, Hanna S, et al. Negative pressure wound therapy for the management of flaps with venous congestion. *Microsurgery.* 2016;36:467–473.
20. Azzopardi EA, Whitaker IS, Rozen WM, Naderi N, Kon M. Chemical and mechanical alternatives to leech therapy: a systematic review and critical appraisal. *J Reconstr Microsurg.* 2011;27:481–486.
21. Yamamoto K. Double trichophytic closure with wavy two-layered closure for optimal hair transplantation scar. *Dermatol Surg.* 2012;38:664–669.
22. Kayiran O, Cihandide E. Evolution of hair transplantation. *Plast Aesthet Res.* 2018;5:9.
23. Tellioglu AT, Çimen K, Açar HI, Karaeminogullar G, Tekdemir I. Scalp reconstruction with island hair-bearing flaps. *Plast Reconstr Surg.* 2005;115(5):1366–1371.
24. Bastidas N, Runyan CM, Jones DC, et al. Anatomic study of full facial and scalp allografts without cutaneous facial scars. *J Plast Surg Hand Surg.* 2013;47:528–531.
25. Jiang HQ, Wang Y, Hu XB, et al. Composite tissue allograft transplantation of cephalocervical skin flap and two ears. *Plast Reconstr Surg.* 2005;115:31e–35e; discussion 36e–37e.
26. Sosin M, Ceradini DJ, Levine JP, et al. Total face, eyelids, ears, scalp, and skeletal subunit transplant: a reconstructive solution for the full face and total scalp burn. *Plast Reconstr Surg.* 2016;138(1):205–219.
27. Selber JC, Chang EI, Clemens MW, et al. Simultaneous scalp, skull, kidney, and pancreas transplant from a single donor. *Plast Reconstr Surg.* 2016;137(6):1851–1861.
28. Choi JH, Kim KS, Shin JH, Hwang JH, Lee SY. Risk acceptance and expectations of scalp allotransplantation. *Arch Craniofacial Surg.* 2016;17(2):68–76.

34 Facial Trauma

DAVID J. DAVID

Introduction

The modern management of facial trauma had its origins in the trenches of World War I, when disciplines united to deal with the devastating results of missiles. Plastic surgeons, neurosurgeons, dentists, and anesthetists worked together in a structured environment to deal with this complex situation. A great boost to the management of facial trauma occurred when Paul Tessier successfully advocated the extended multidisciplinary care of the craniofacially deformed.

This chapter deals with trauma to the naso-fronto-orbital region, the middle third of the face, encompassing the upper jaw and zygomas, the mandible, and panfacial fractures.

The principles of treatment are set out for each fracture type and from them flow the descriptions of operative management, conservative management, and long-term care.

Frontal Bone and Naso-orbital Fractures

The frontal bone and naso-orbital region constitute the upper third of the face. Trauma to this region of the face is often accompanied by brain injury and damage to the cranial nerves. The impacting forces may be transmitted to the base of the skull, producing a range of effects from transient loss of consciousness to loss of life. The injuring force may impact directly on the frontal bone, causing blunt or penetrating brain injury. With this in mind, it becomes obvious that the treating surgeon should be part of a team capable of assessing and treating such injuries.[1] The injuries therefore fall into three categories: injuries to the bone without cerebral involvement, externally compound fractures or penetrating wounds with underlying dural and cerebral injury, and internally compound fractures often of the cribriform plate region resulting in a cranionasal fistula with or without cerebrospinal fluid (CSF) leak.

Some of the causes of craniofacial trauma include falls, assaults, sporting injuries, industrial accidents, and missile injuries. The epidemiology varies with the community, so when organizing multidisciplinary care and planning preventative strategies, an understanding of the causes and incidences in a particular community is essential.[2]

Anatomy

The anterior cranial fossa is formed in the front and at the sides by the *frontal bones*, and they are attached to the facial skeleton at the front nasal, frontomaxillary, and frontozygomatic sutures (Fig. 34.1). The frontal bone also articulates with the ethmoid bone in the anterior cranial fossa, which bone forms part of the orbit and its vertical plate forms part of the nasal septum and indeed is said to play a part in facial development. Laterally, the anterior fossa forms the thin superior orbital plates; they dip down medially to articulate with the cribriform plate of the ethmoid, the posterior articulation of which is the body of the sphenoid bone. The lesser wings of the sphenoid bone form the crescentic posterior borders of the anterior fossa. The optic canal is formed by the two roots of the lesser wing of the sphenoid and runs forward and laterally in the superolateral wall of the sphenoid sinus to the orbital apex.

The complex sphenoid bone is the keystone of the craniofacial skeleton; it forms part of the anterior cranial fossa, the middle cranial fossa, the lateral orbital wall, where its articulation with the zygoma is an important landmark in the reduction of orbitozygomatic fractures, and the infratemporal fossa.

The rest of the facial skeleton is composed of the lacrimal bones, the nasal bones, the ethmoids, the zygomas, the maxillae, and the mandible. It is customary to describe the face as being divided into three thirds. The upper third is formed mostly by the frontal bone, which forms the orbital rooves. The middle third contains the maxillae, zygomas, and the nasoseptal complex with a contribution from the lacrimal bone and the ethmoid. These elements articulate laterally with the zygomatic processes of the temporal bones, and serve as a good measure of the anterior projection of the face. Posteriorly they articulate with the sphenoid to form the orbit and centrally and laterally with the frontal bone. The lower third is said to be formed by the mandible, however this is somewhat of a convention as the body only is in the lower third, the ramus in the middle third, and the temporomandibular joint has a major component formed by the base of skull.

The midfacial skeleton is designed to transmit the powerful forces of mastication to the base of skull. The horizontal

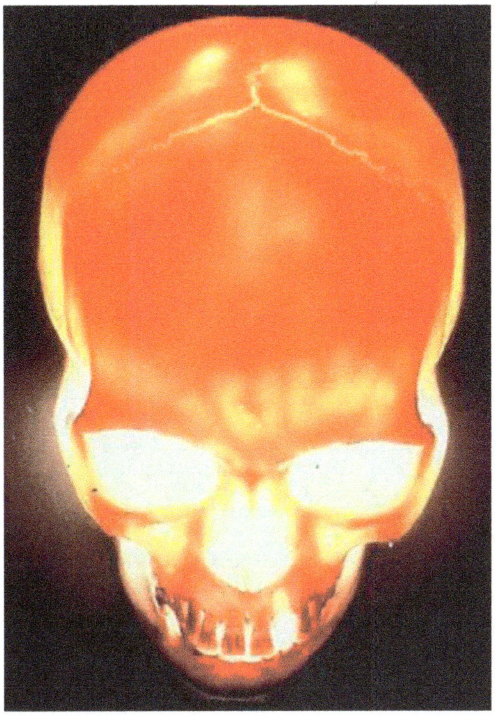

• **Fig. 34.1** A transilluminated adult skull demonstrates the paranasal sinuses and the supporting buttresses of the face.

elements in the maxilla, the alveolus, and hard palate support three paired vertical buttresses, at the pyriform margins, at the zygomatico-maxillary junction, and more posteriorly at the pterygo-maxillary junction. The two pairs of anterior buttresses provide the best places for internal fixation with plates and screws.

The *orbital cavity* is formed of seven bones in the shape of a four-sided pyramid. There is a relatively strong rim anteriorly, four more flimsy walls, and a thick apex. The zygoma contributes to the lateral and inferior orbital margins, the lateral orbital wall, and the orbital floor. The maxillary component of the orbital floor medial to the zygoma is thin and delicate (lamina paparycea).

The anterior orbital floor medial to the infraorbital canal is concave downwards, but posterior to the globe it becomes convex upward. A point to be noted for successful restoration of the orbital floor after injury: the medial wall is composed of the lacrimal bone anteriorly and the thin lateral plate of the ethmoid posteriorly.

The *paranasal air sinuses* are rudimentary at birth and do not reach adult proportions until puberty. The degree of pneumatization varies, particularly that of the *frontal sinus.* They range from being barely pneumatized to extending superiorly in the frontal bone for a variable distance; laterally they can go as far as the lateral margins of the orbit and also extend into the orbital roof.

The frontonasal ducts open inferomedially and drain into the frontal recess of the nasal cavity.

The *ethmoid sinuses* constitute an interconnected series of thin-walled cells that lie between the upper lateral nasal cavity and the orbit, and are separated from the orbit by the thin lateral wall. Their roof forms part of the anterior fossa lateral to the cribriform plate. The ethmoid sinuses are related to the maxillary sinuses inferiorly, the frontal sinuses superiorly, and the sphenoid sinuses posteriorly.

The *sphenoid sinuses* are within the body of the sphenoid and may sometimes spread into the lesser wing of the bone; they are divided by a septum and may be asymmetrical. They lie under the central part of the floor of the anterior fossa and are closely related to the internal carotid artery, the pituitary gland, and the optic nerve. They connect through their anterior wall with the upper nasal cavity.

The *maxillary sinuses* usually fill the entire body of the maxilla and may extend into the zygoma and below the floor of the nose; their walls are fragile and easily broken. They also are rudimentary at birth.

Management Principles

Management involves investigation and treatment, and should be based on a thorough knowledge of the *pathophysiology.*

With respect to the *cranial cavity*, the dura is firmly attached around the cribriform plate through which the filaments of the olfactory nerve pass sheathed by arachnoid. A dural arachnoid tear with a fracture communicating with the nose or paranasal sinuses will lead to CSF leak.

The frontal lobes of the *brain* are particularly vulnerable to the effects of frontal impact, and by anterior fossa fractures, when the orbital rooves are shattered or buckled. Bilateral frontal lobe injury can result in long-term neuropsychological problems.

The *olfactory nerve* filaments may be damaged by fractures crossing the cribriform plates resulting in anosmia as well as CSF leak.

The *optic nerve* may be compressed by a displaced fracture through the optic canal, by shearing forces that devascularize the nerve, by contusion or hematoma within the canal without a fracture, or by direct injury to the orbit.

The *orbit* itself may be fractured directly or indirectly as part of frontal, nasoethmoid, and midface or zygomatic fractures.

In addition to the pathophysiology, it is essential to have knowledge of the effects resulting from the various *mechanisms of injury.*

Frontal impact is the most common mechanism of craniofacial injury; it may result in linear fractures or depressed fractures, and the forces may be transmitted to the cranial base and cause fracturing there.

Fractures of the skull base are rarely significant in themselves, however the force required in producing such a fracture is considerable and is often associated with injuries of the soft tissues, brain, cranial nerves, major vessels, etc.

The pattern of fracture lines resulting from blunt trauma follows the points of weakness and in the frontal bone is influenced by the extent of the frontal sinuses and the particular honeycomb structure of the particular sinus (Fig. 34.2). The age of the patient is a significant influence, younger bones being more pliant and less brittle.

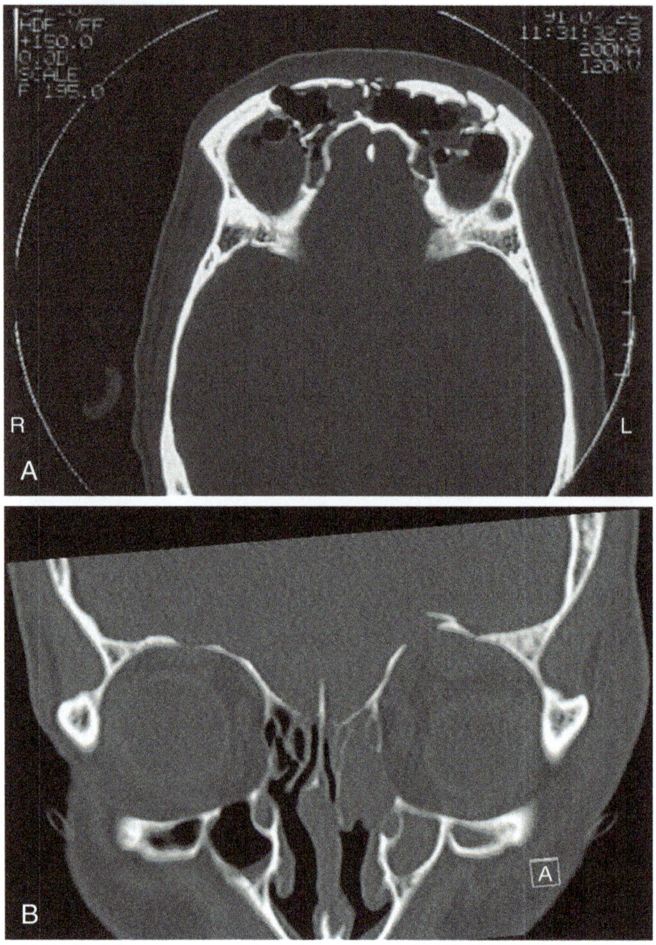

• **Fig. 34.2** (A) CT scan showing a depressed comminuted fracture of the frontal sinus affecting both inner and outer tables resulting from blunt trauma. (B) A fracture of the orbital roof resulting from a billiard cue entering the orbit, sparing the globe, and penetrating the orbital part of the frontal bone and brain.

Fracture patterns, however, rarely conform to a predictable formula.

Penetrating and missile wounds have no particular pattern. The tissue damage resulting from low-velocity penetration is confined to the pathway of the penetrating agent.[3]

Gunshot wounds may be penetrating, perforating or ablative, depending on the velocity and nature of the projectile: the higher the velocity, the greater the damage. High-velocity missiles cause massive avulsion with loss of bone and soft tissue, which is often more extensive than immediately apparent because tissues may be devitalized or injured by the traction of avulsion. The eyes and brain may be injured directly or by vascular injury, which can be delayed.[1] *Crushing injuries* may result in severe fracturing of the frontal bone and skull base; however, in infants and children the pliability of the bones means that the pattern of fracture is different, with greenstick fractures.

Initial Management

Remember to save the patient! Fractures of the frontal bone and nasoethmoid complex can occur in isolation but more commonly are associated with other facial and systemic trauma. Severe craniofacial injuries often pose an immediate threat to life. Airway obstruction, displaced dentures, and collapse of the mandibular arch with retrodisplacement of the tongue may cause severe hypoxia. Particular care should be taken with cases of frontofacial fractures, where the possibility of a breach in the anterior cranial fossa exists, not to forcibly insufflate the patient or to pass tubes via the nose.

Emergency Assessment and Resuscitation

The primary survey, setting the priorities for management, follows resuscitation, secondary survey, and stabilization, and in the craniofacial region these are: airway, breathing, and circulation.

Airway

The following is a list of problems that may be encountered when trying to secure the airway in severe frontofacial fractures. These same problems also potentially occur in fractures of other regions of the face.

- Distortion of the bony facial skeleton
- Swelling of the lips, tongue, and floor of mouth
- Broken teeth and dentures
- Multiple fractures of the mandible with loss of tongue support
- Hemorrhage into the soft tissues of the neck hindering cannulation of the airway
- Disruption of the anterior cranial fossa
- Trismus
- Blood and vomit in the airway
- Fracture of the larynx

Breathing

Associated chest injuries must be excluded. A brain injury may cause central problems with breathing, as can the overzealous or inappropriate use of pain relief. It therefore behooves the treating team to assess and secure the airway safely and soon. This may be difficult and intubation requires a skilled and experienced anesthetist. Nasal intubation in patients with fractures potentially involving the anterior base of skull should be undertaken with great care. There are various anesthetic strategies to minimize the risks.

Tracheostomy in an awake patient under local anesthesia may be considered, however if the neck tissues are suffused, cricothyroidotomy can be used.

Circulation

Craniofacial injuries, especially those of the midface, can involve severe bleeding from the branches of the external carotid artery that supply the region. Superficial arterial bleeding may be controlled by pressure or by wound exploration and ligation of the bleeding vessel. Packing may control bleeding from the nasal cavity or oropharynx. In the rare case when this cannot be achieved, arterial ligation may be considered, the maxillary artery via a transantral approach and/or ligation of the anterior ethmoidal artery, which is a branch of the internal carotid system and enters the orbit through the medial orbital wall. Interventional radiological techniques are emerging as useful tools in controlling deep bleeding in this area.

Clinical Assessment

This assessment applies to all fractures of the craniofacial skeleton and precedes the special investigations.

The *neurological state* should be determined early using the Glasgow Coma Scale to record consciousness. It is necessary to examine the cranial nerves, and careful ophthalmological assessment may lead to urgent consultation with an ophthalmologist. Testing for light touch in the various zones identifies facial sensory nerve function. The facial nerve is tested by observation and by response to painful stimuli.

The *face* should be examined for lacerations and contour deformities. Bruising around the orbits may indicate an anterior fossa fracture, and bruising around the mastoid process indicates a temporal bone fracture. CSF leakage should be suspected, but in the presence of blood and mucus it is very hard to identify with certainty at this early stage.

Jaw movements and the muscles of facial expression are tested; the cervical spine is palpated for tenderness or deformity and the scalp for lacerations and hematomas.

Each facial region should be palpated systematically from the frontal bone to the mandible, looking for evidence of deformity or abnormal movement. Cooter[4] has described a systematic sequence of examination by palpation.[2] Palpation of the inferior orbital margin may help differentiate isolated fractures of the zygoma, where the lateral rim is depressed, from nasomaxillary fractures, where the medial rim is depressed.

The mandible is examined with the patient's mouth slightly open; the margins of the bones are palpated externally. Intraorally, with a gloved finger the alveolar ridges and the hard palate are palpated. Grasping the maxillary alveolar ridge or pressing on the anterior hard palate behind the teeth and applying a rocking movement while palpating the face with the other hand can elicit abnormal movements of the midface.

Imaging

Early Imaging

- *Computed tomography (CT)*: A cranial CT is performed after the initial resuscitation to assess for possible brain injury. It may be extended to include other areas of suspected injury. Fractures of the anterior fossa may warrant fine-cut bone windows at this stage, but it is the later investigations that will give the definitive information.
- *Angiography*: At this stage, angiography is indicated for penetrating injuries in the region of major vessels or blunt injuries where there is suspicion of vascular damage.

Later Imaging

The detailed diagnostic imaging is usually planned after full clinical investigation is complete. It has become regular practice for the first and principal investigation to be a CT scan, however some of the standard radiographic projections can be most useful and in some circumstances essential (e.g., the panoramic radiograph (orthopantomogram, OPG) that shows the mandible, temporomandibular joints, and teeth).

Axial CT scanning is vital in managing severe craniofacial trauma of the frontal and nasoethmoid region. Fine-cut two-dimensional CT is the best method for assessing craniofacial fractures around the fronto-orbito-ethmoid region and the fractures are seen most clearly on the scan at right angles to the bone that is fractured. The acquired CT slices, usually axial, can be used to produce a three-dimensional image of the skeleton and/or soft tissues. These images can be rotated and viewed from all angles and are indispensable for surgical planning.

These data can be used to create solid nylon models of the injured skull, which can be sterilized and used for reference at surgery or for mock surgical planning.[5]

Magnetic resonance imaging (MRI) is often useful later in tracking the origins of CSF leakage. It is used to assess ocular injuries and also to identify nonmetallic foreign material, especially wood.

Definitive Management

Having resuscitated the patient, established the presence of brain injury, established an infection control regimen, and made a clinical and radiological diagnosis, the next step is to establish the priorities in managing the craniofacial injury, in this case the frontal and naso-orbital fractures. Urgent surgical intervention within hours is indicated by the presence of acute neurosurgical problems of intracranial bleeding, penetrating brain injuries or externally compound fractures. Otherwise, delayed treatment is preferred, by an appropriate team after full investigation and planning in the "cold light of day."

Urgent operative intervention may be necessary for injuries to other body systems, and appropriate discussions will determine what parts of the management can be done simultaneously.

Operative Surgical Principles

Modern craniofacial surgical technique is based on wide exposure of the craniofacial skeleton, the capacity to reduced bony fragments precisely and implement rigid interfragmentary fixation with titanium mini- and microplates. Where there is absence of bone from the trauma, primary bone grafting of defects is undertaken at this stage.

The most effective and commonly used approach to the naso-orbito-frontal region is the *coronal scalp flap* (Fig. 34.3). The incision is placed well behind the hairline and is made in a wavy or zigzag fashion to better disguise the

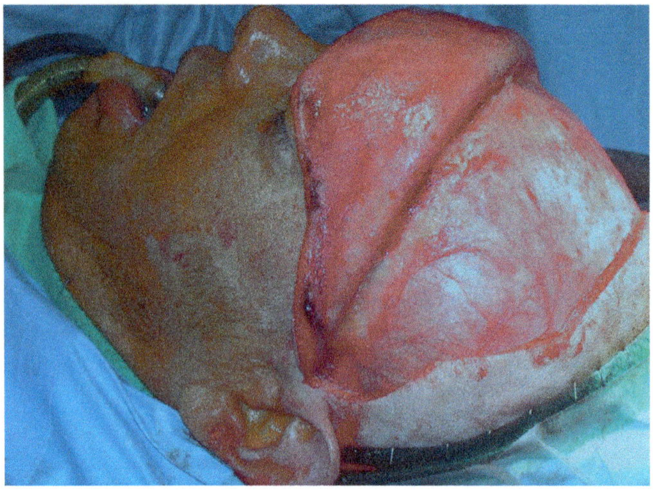

• **Fig. 34.3** A zigzag or wavy coronal incision gives a better final scar. The flap is raised over the pericranium and superficial temporal fascia. The pericranium is incised 1 cm superficial to the superior orbital margin and the dissection continued subperiosteally into the orbit. Staying deep to the fat pad over the superficial temporal fascia will protect the frontalis branch of the facial nerve.

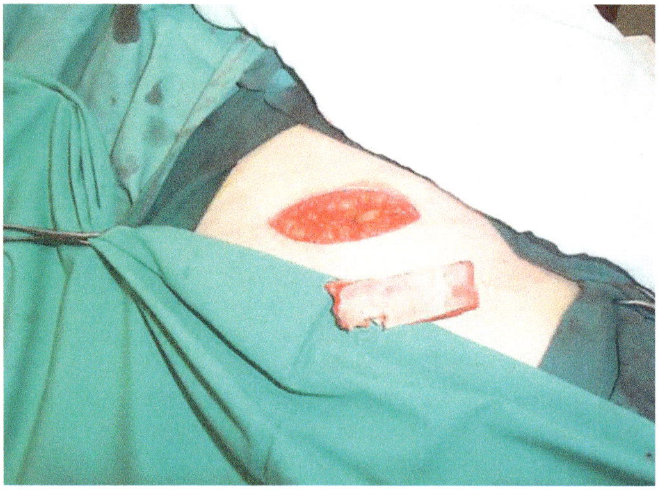

• **Fig. 34.4** A graft taken from the inner table of the right hip.

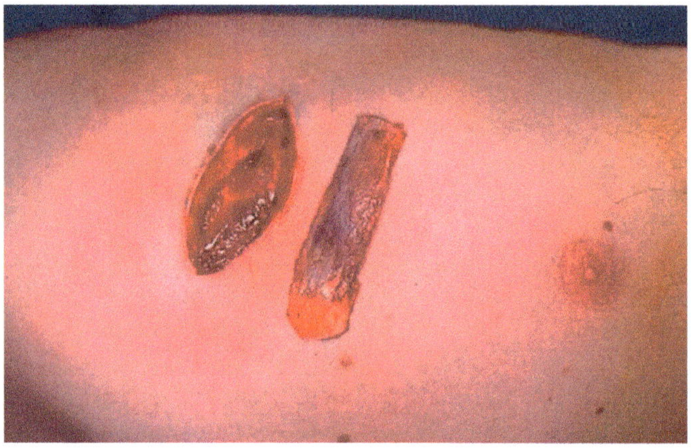

• **Fig. 34.5** Rib with attached costal cartilage can be used to support the crushed nasal dorsum.

scar. The flap is raised in the subgaleal plane down to a level about 2 cm above the orbital margins or the site of any fractures of the frontal bones. The dissection then proceeds subpericranially, scraping the bone, and extends over the orbital rim into the orbit. The supraorbital neurovascular bundle is preserved and, if necessary, chiseled out of its canal. More medially, the dissection disconnects the trochlea without obvious deleterious effect.

Laterally, it is important to dissect strictly against the temporal fascia beneath the fatty layer directly superficial to it in order to preserve the frontalis branch of the facial nerve. Within the orbit the periorbita may be safely dissected to within 1 cm of the apex, however in traumatic cases the walls may be breached, the periorbita torn and orbital fat trapped in fracture lines, making dissection more difficult.

Medially, in the region of the glabella, the dissection can be taken down over the nose, anteriorly and posteriorly to the canthal ligaments and nasolacrimal ducts. These structures, so often injured, must be identified and preserved.

Access to the anterior part of the medial orbital wall can be obtained via a transcaruncular approach. The floor is exposed by subciliary eyelid incisions or best by transconjunctival incisions with or without lateral canthotomy.

Bone Grafting

Bone loss demanding early replacement can occur over the frontal sinus, in the orbital walls, especially medial, and the floor, and after comminuted depressed fractures of the nasal pyramid. In the middle third of the face the vertical bony pillars may need to be grafted to secure midfacial height.[2]

The common donor sites for harvesting bone are the iliac crest and medial surface of the ilium, the ribs (both bone and cartilage), and the calvaria. The most important factors for the survival of bone grafts are: rigid fixation, good soft tissue coverage, a well-vascularized bed, and absence of hematoma.

There is a wide selection of all plastic materials to reconstruct the midface and orbits, none of which are favored by this author. In particular, their use in relation to open sinuses should be avoided.

Donor Sites

Hip grafts provide strong malleable bone (Fig. 34.4). The inner table can be harvested, and additional cancellous bone scooped out for packing (e.g., the nasofrontal duct). The full thickness of the ilium can be used but it is important to preserve the crest in both adults and children.

Rib grafts are harvested through a submammary incision, cartilage can be taken in the form of the costochondral junction for use in the nose and the temporomandibular joint. Ribs can be used whole or more usually split for calvarial or orbital reconstruction (Fig. 34.5).

Calvarial grafts have the disadvantage of being less malleable than hip or rib grafts. Small portions can be taken from the outer table where the skull is thick enough, obviating a need for extra visible scars, however contour defects of the skull are often a problem as are complications arising from damage to the underlying dura and brain arising from

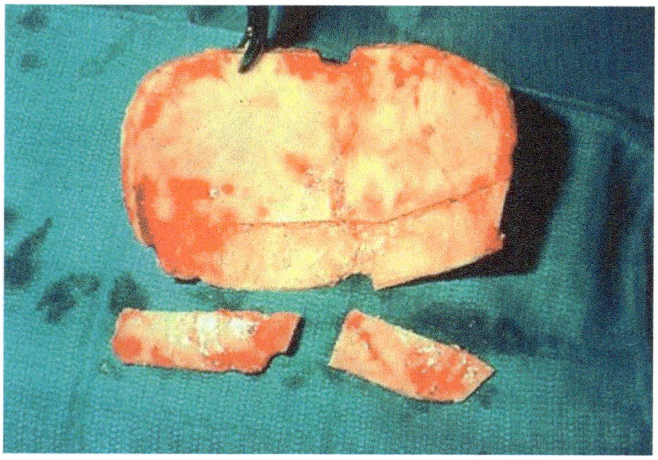

• **Fig. 34.6** Bone can be taken from the inner table of the craniotomy bone flap if the skull is thick enough.

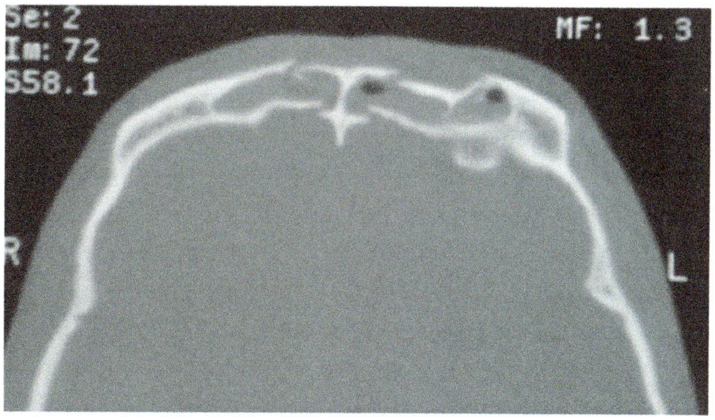

• **Fig. 34.7** CT scan showing fractures of the anterior and posterior walls of the frontal sinus.

inexperienced operators. The inner table can be harvested when a craniotomy is being performed and the bone is thick enough. Good quantities of high-quality bone can be obtained in this fashion (Fig. 34.6).

Operative Management

This depends on the nature of the fracture pattern. Each case must be managed on its merits but there are a number of consistent and significant variations, such as:

- A fracture or the outer table of the frontal sinus with skin intact and a contour defect of the forehead
- A compound fracture with the outer table involvement as above
- A compound depressed fracture involving the anterior and posterior walls with suspected involvement of dura and brain
- Depressed fractures of the frontal bone lateral to the sinus with or without involvement of the orbital roof.

Penetrating wounds need separate consideration due to the extreme risk of contamination.

The *simple depressed fracture* with a contour defect can be approached via a coronal flap; the fragments can be repositioned and secured with microplates or fine wires. If there is an overlaying or adjacent wound this can be debrided and the same procedure undertaken.

A *compound depressed fracture* involving both walls is also approached through a coronal scalp flap (Fig. 34.7). A small frontal craniotomy is made above the sinus area to expose the posterior wall, the depressed fracture being approached extradurally. If the dura is torn, the posterior wall of the sinus is nibbled and drilled away (cranialized) and the sinus mucosa meticulously stripped. The dura is repaired in a watertight manner by primary suture and may be augmented by a graft of temporalis fascia or pericranium (Figs. 34.8–34.10).

The *frontonasal duct* can be plugged with muscle and/or bone chips. A pericranial flap pedicled inferiorly is turned in and sutured to the dura in order to seal the frontal sinus. The anterior wall of the sinus is preserved and, if fragmented, treated as in the case of a simple depressed fracture.

Closed anterior and posterior wall fractures associated with CSF leakage are treated expectantly and if the leak persists for more than a week dural repair is performed.

Depressed fractures lateral to the sinuses are usually managed by the neurosurgical team by elevation and if necessary repair of any underlying dural or cerebral damage; however, if the orbital rim and roof is involved, a combined craniofacial approach is often used to reposition the orbital margins and graft the roof.

Penetrating injuries are likely to be associated with contamination along the wound track and consideration must be given to opening the wound track and removing foreign material. Remember that wood is often best visualized by an MRI scan. A frontal craniotomy is performed and if the wound is orbitocranial, the frontal crown can be removed for greater access and replaced. Where there is dural repair under an orbital roof defect, a bone graft will add additional security.

Central depressed fractures of the frontal region may be associated with naso-orbito-ethmoid fractures that extend to the floor of the anterior cranial fossa, hence often complicated by CSF rhinorrhea. A combined neurosurgical/craniofacial approach is needed to deal with this situation. The anterior fossa is explored and the fistula repaired intradurally and the naso-orbito-ethmoid fractures are repaired in sequence from posteriorly to anteriorly with grafts, fixation plates and canthopexies (Fig. 34.11).

Naso-orbito-ethmoid Fractures

These fractures occur as a result of direct trauma to the midface and, although they can occur in isolation, are frequently associated with other craniofacial fractures. Management is challenging because of the intricate and complex skeletal anatomy in close juxtaposition with the canthal ligaments, the nasolacrimal apparatus, and the cribriform plate and brain above. Exposure, reduction and maintaining fixation have always been and still remain difficult.

Classification

These fractures may be unilateral or bilateral, simple or comminuted, closed or compound; they may occur in isolation

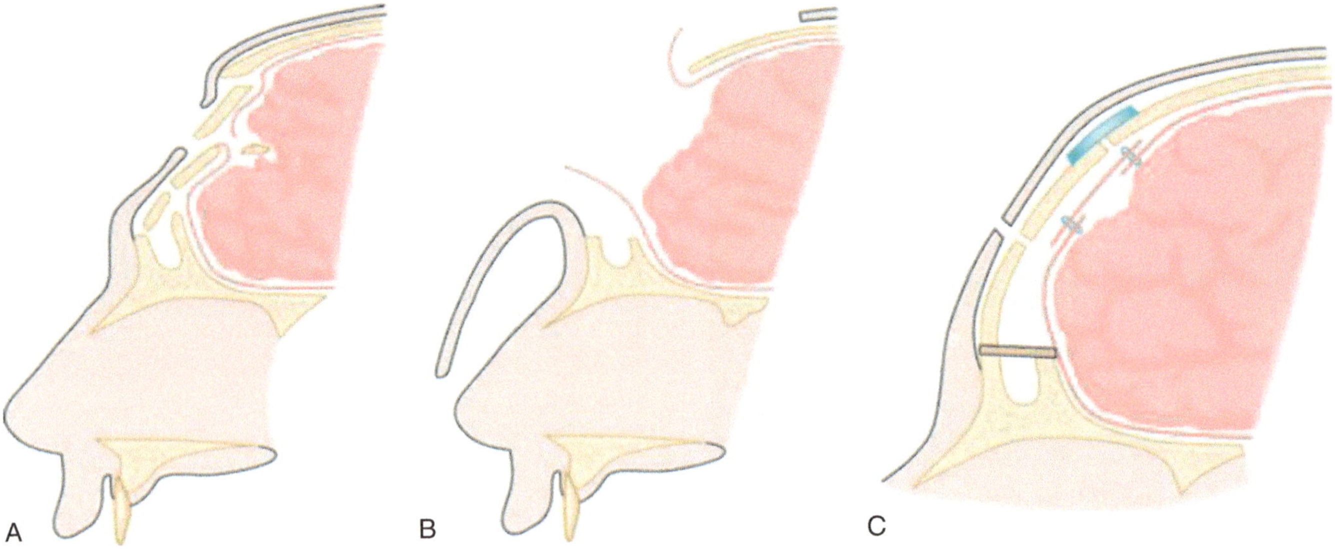

• **Fig. 34.8** (A) When there is a compound comminuted depression of the frontal bone involving both tables of the sinus and tearing dura and/or brain, (B) the coronal flap exposes the area, the depressed fragments are removed, the area is gently cleansed, (C) the dura repaired, the posterior sinus wall removed, the sinus ostia blocked, and the frontal bone reconstructed with microplates or fine wires.

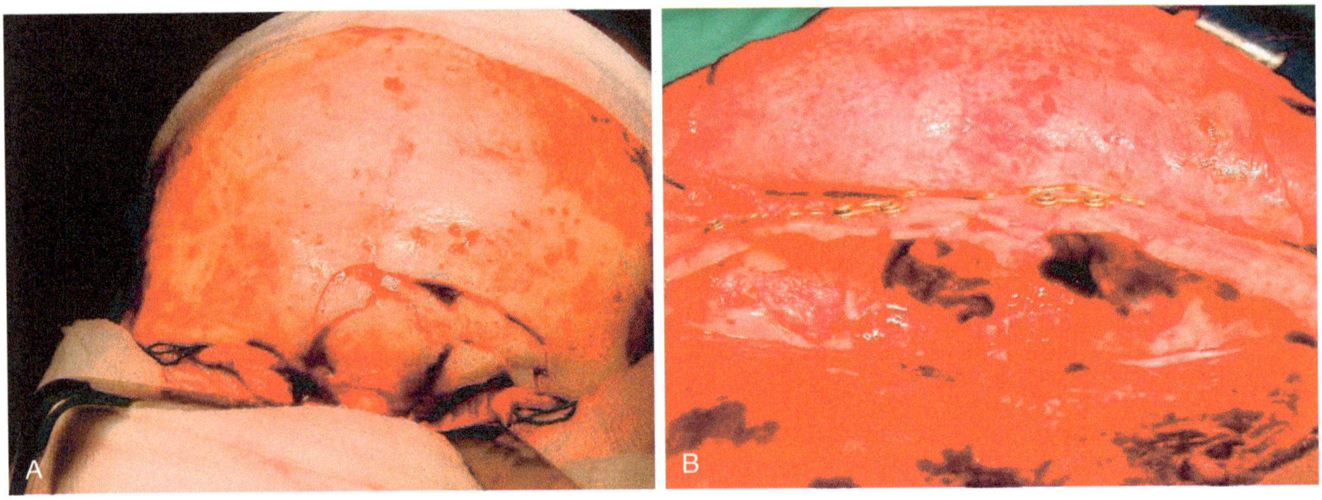

• **Fig. 34.9** (A) The fracture exposed via the coronal flap. (B) The sinus has been cranialized, the dura repaired, and the outer table fragments plated.

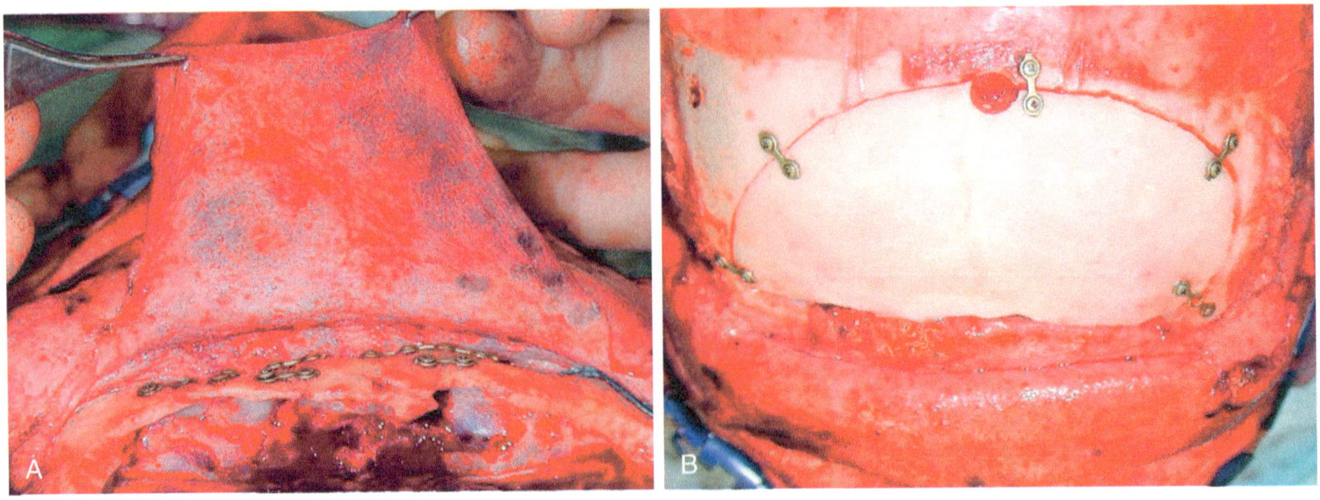

• **Fig. 34.10** (A) An anteriorly based galeal or pericranial flap can be raised, and used to help obliterate the sinus and close off the ducts. (B) The flap is attached to the dura and coats the floor and walls of the anterior fossa; it is seen here "posted" between the frontal bone flap and the reconstructed frontal crown.

or in association with more extensive damage to the craniofacial skeleton.

Multiple classifications have been proposed. Markowitz et al[6] proposed Types I–III with increasing measure of complexity in each group. Gruss[7] attempts to relate to the fractures in adjacent bones. The problem with classifications in this area is the complexity and the difficulty of finding a language that reflects the reality of each clinical situation.[8] The author's view is that the closest method that is useful for measurement and comparison is one of alphanumeric scoring, which quantifies the extent and pattern of bony damage in a global fashion.[9]

Principles of Treatment

Historically, these fractures were treated by closed reduction and external splintage; the results were not only poor but rendered the secondary corrective surgery very difficult. Credit must be given to Mustardé,[10] Dingman and Natvig,[11] and Stranc[12] for identifying the need for open reduction and internal fixation, at the time, with wire. However restricted access and limited radiological assistance with diagnosis meant that the results remained suboptimal.

The modern approach is much aided by CT scanning, involves wide exposure using the coronal approach, accurate anatomical reduction becomes possible and fixation with micro- and miniplates and screws ensures stability. In addition, primary bone grafting to delicate medial walls and graft support for the depressed comminuted nasal pyramid has vastly improved patient outcomes (Fig. 34.12).

Operative Management

The coronal scalp flap extended to the supraorbital margin then subperiosteally into the orbit will give tension-free exposure of the medial orbital walls, nasal bones, and frontal processes of the maxillae as well as the orbitofrontal region.

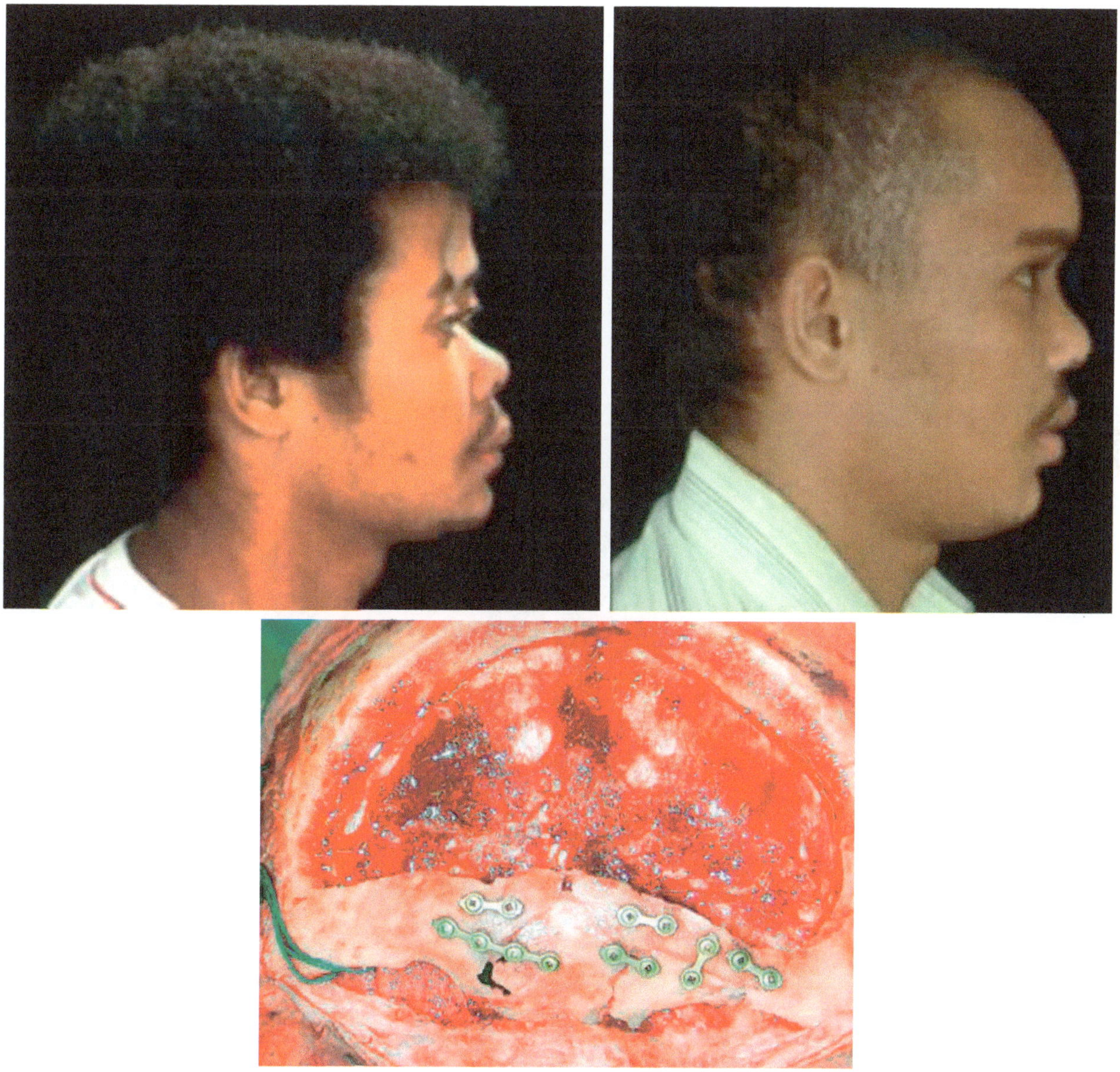

• **Fig. 34.11** A completed frontal reconstruction after a severe frontal crush.

Care must be taken to preserve whatever bony attachment there is of the medial canthal ligament.

Transconjunctival incisions or subciliary lower eyelid incisions are used to expose the inferomedial orbital wall and orbital floor. An upper buccal sulcus incision exposes the nasomaxillary buttress and the margins of the pyriform aperture. In the case of compound fractures, local lacerations may be useful for access.

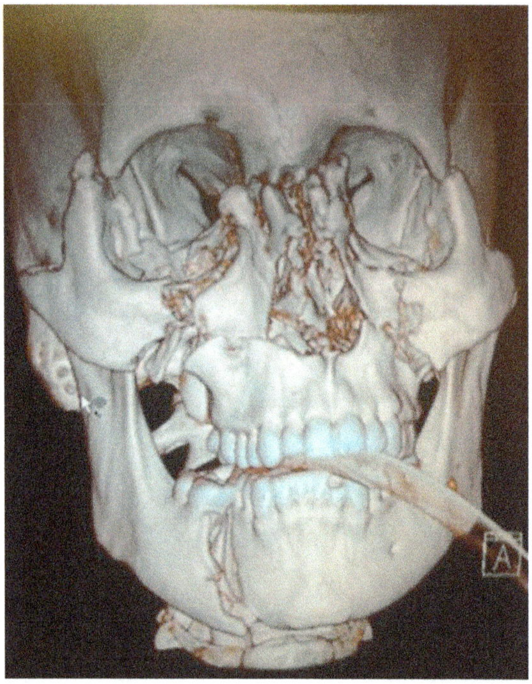

• **Fig. 34.12** 3D CT scan showing panfacial fractures.

When the naso-orbito-ethmoid complex is fractured and displaced en bloc the fragments can be reduced and controlled by plate and screw fixation to the adjacent stable skeleton. In these cases the canthal attachments in continuity with the major bony fragment and its correct position is restored. In the more severe comminuted cases it is necessary to determine if the canthal ligament is attached to a fragment of bone. If this is so, this attachment is preserved and may be used to maintain the correct intercanthal distance. Transnasal wiring of the canthi is achieved by placing the wires posterior and superior to the lacrimal fossa. The wires are tightened; if there is much loss of bone the wire that is attached to the ligament can be passed through a small bone graft on one or both sides. Reconstruction of the medial walls is usually necessary; the author prefers thinned out inner table of ilium for this purpose. It is important to remember to reconstruct this area before tightening the intercanthal wires thus denying you access! The repair proceeds from back to front (Figs. 34.13 and 34.14).

In the comminuted cases, use of a costochondral graft fixed as a cantilever restores the nasal bridge projection and maintains the soft tissue expansion, which aids and minimizes secondary reconstruction, which is so often necessary in this condition.

With respect to the nasal septum, primary open reduction is not attempted beyond centralization by closed manipulation.

The associated frontal sinus and cranial fractures are repaired at the same time. This implies a team working in harmony. It is the author's experience that a written preoperative plan setting out the sequence of events from beginning to end of the procedure facilitates harmony.

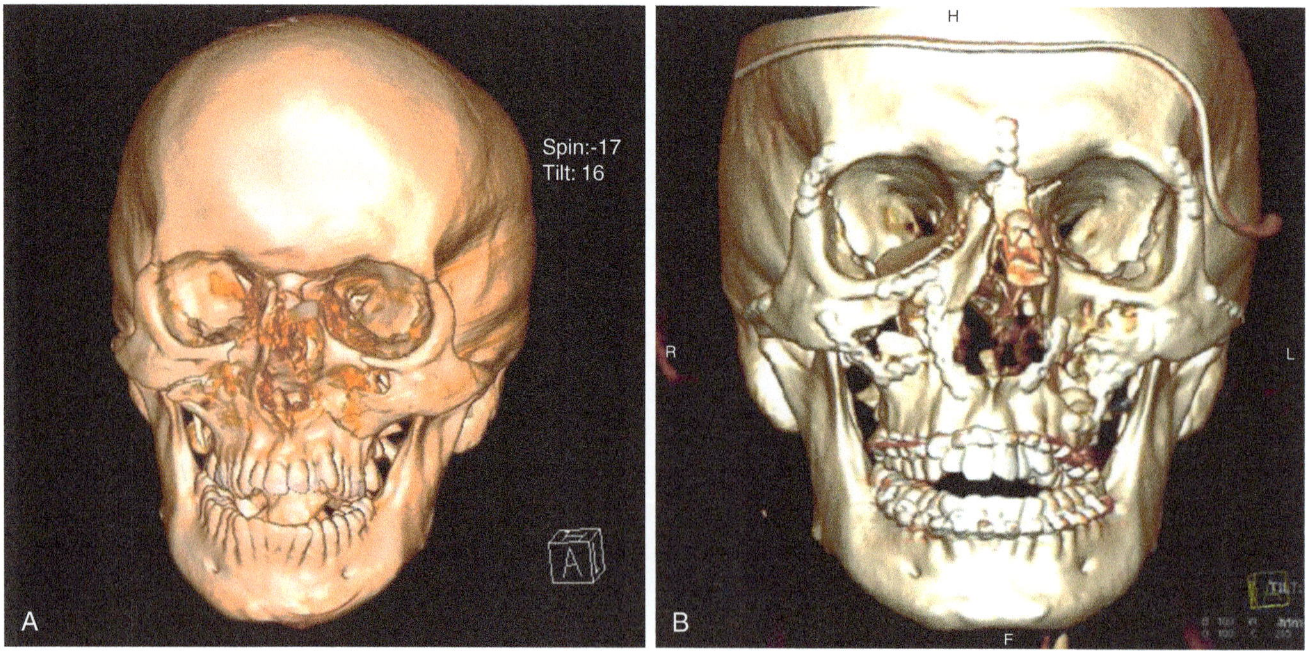

• **Fig. 34.13** (A,B) A panfacial fracture where the naso-orbito-ethmoid complex has been repaired from posterior to anterior: the medial orbital walls grafted, the nasomaxillary processes plated, hence restoring the canthal ligaments, and a cantilever bone graft to the dorsum of nose to support the integument against collapse and contracture.

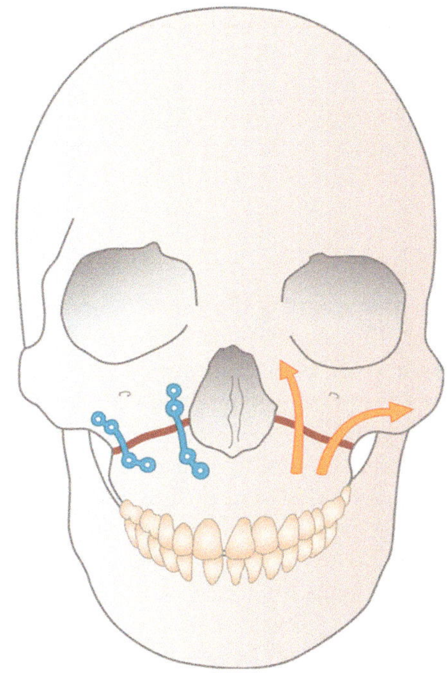

• **Fig. 34.14** This shows the load-bearing direction of the buttresses, and on the right how plates are positioned on these lines.

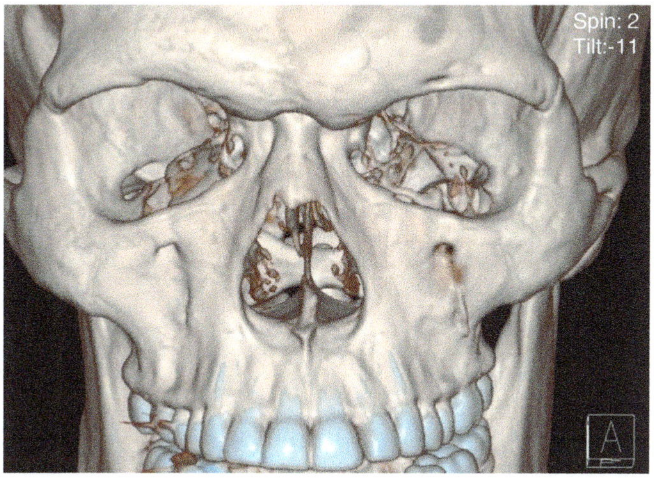

• **Fig. 34.15** This 3D image of the skull shows a fractured zygoma on the left and a normal bone on the right. The articulation with the sphenoid bone forms the lateral orbital wall, with the frontal bone at the frontozygomatic suture, with the temporal bone to form the zygomatic arch (visibly deformed in this image), with the maxilla in two places to form the inferior orbital rim and the zygomatico-maxillary buttress.

Management of nasolacrimal injuries does not usually involve early exploration, except where there is an obvious lacrimal system transection in an external laceration. Repairing this over a silicone tube is the preferred option. Despite its intimate proximity to the fractures, the nasolacrimal system is not often damaged, even with severe injuries. When late obstruction does occur, it is usually in the bony nasolacrimal canal. The more accurate the initial reduction, the less need for later dacryocystorhinostomy (see Fig. 34.14).

Zygomatico-maxillary Fractures

The face is generally described as having an upper, middle, and lower third. The middle third is formed mostly by the maxillae, zygomatic bones, and the nasoseptal complex. This section deals with fractures of the zygoma and maxilla. As these bones articulate with each other, form part of the orbit, and the tooth-bearing maxillae form the upper jaw which articulates with the base of skull and occludes with the mandible, fractures of this complex may not be simple. Trauma to the middle third of the face has the potential for severe functional, psychosocial, and esthetic consequences. Whereas fractures of the mandible remain the most common form of single facial fracture, the zygoma is the commonest when multiple facial fractures occur. The ratio of males to females remains high, 3–4:1.[13]

Anatomy

The zygoma and maxillae are part of the face between the lower jaw and the base of skull that, together with the nasoethmoid complex, compose the majority of the bones generally described as the middle third. It is important to understand the blood and nerve supply to the maxilla and upper dental arch. This assists with planning, safe incisions, and for understanding the patterns of numbness of the skin and palate associated with maxillary fractures. The greater palatine canal transmits the greater palatine artery and nerve, which supplies all of the bone and mucosa of the hard palate. Branches of the maxillary artery and maxillary nerve pass into the posterior maxilla through small foramina to become the posterior superior alveolar artery and nerve. This nerve supplies the molar teeth with a dental plexus. Branches from the infraorbital artery and nerve enter the anterior maxillary bone from the orbital floor and supply the anterior teeth. Fractures of the orbital floor and the anterior maxilla may result in numbness of the anterior teeth, whereas fractures extending low in the maxilla posterior to the first molar region may result in numbness of the posterior teeth. It is important to know that the maxilla gains blood supply from the gingival attachments to the alveolar bone and through its attachments to the soft palate from the pharyngeal palatine branches of the facial artery and the ascending pharyngeal branches of the external carotid artery. Both the trauma and the surgical exposure may significantly compromise the blood supply to fracture fragments.

There are strong horizontal elements in the maxillae, alveoli, and hard palate which make up a foundation to support the three paired vertical bony condensations or buttresses (Fig. 34.15). The most anterior of these extends from the dentoalveolar arch in the region of the lateral incisor/canine region superiorly along the pyriform margin to the medial orbital rim and frontomaxillary suture. The middle buttress extends from the first molar tooth to the body of the zygoma and through this bone as the lateral orbital wall to the frontozygomatic suture. The posterior buttress is represented by the attachment of the maxillary tuberosity to the pterygoid plates and hence to the sphenoid bone.

The biomechanical stresses in the midface have been harder to assess than those in the mandible; however, the load paths for distribution of force appear to be the buttresses described above.[2]

The zygoma makes a key contribution to the orbital contour, facial width, and projection. Comprising as it does the inferolateral orbital rim, the zygoma articulates with the frontal bone superiorly, the maxilla inferiorly and medially and with both sphenoid and temporal bones posteriorly and laterally.

Four bony processes radiate from the zygomatic bone, providing strong articulations with the frontal, maxillary, and temporal bones as well as the greater wing of the sphenoid bone. The bony junction between the temporal process of the zygoma and the zygomatic process of the temporal bone constitutes the zygomatic arch. The temporal fascia and masseter muscle are attached to the arch. These muscles are usually considered to be the major deforming force in maintaining displacement of a depressed zygomatic fracture. The superficial temporal vessels and frontal branch of the facial nerve lie immediately superficial to the arch. Deep to it pass the internal maxillary vessels, temporalis muscle and coronoid process. It is important to understand the value of maintaining the zygomatic arch when locating the zygoma appropriately in relation to the skull base in an anteroposterior, vertica, and transverse dimension.[14]

Classification

In classifying occlusal fractures of the maxilla we seem to be stuck with Le Fort's original description. The Le Fort I pattern is a low horizontal fracture through the pyriform aperture and the zygomatic buttresses and pterygoid plate. The Le Fort II fracture has the upper detachment at a fracture line running across the nasal bones, through the inferior orbital rims and through the zygomatic buttresses and pterygoid plates. The Le Fort III pattern has the upper jaw detached from the base of skull at a fracture line running through the nasofrontal suture, ethmoid bone, frontozygomatic suture and arches of the zygomas, and the pterygoid plates.

The language associated with this form of description is now so embedded that it ceases to be scientifically meaningful; it does not take into account the degrees of comminution and displacement of fragments, nor does it mention the parasagittal fractures of the hard palate and the smaller dentoalveolar segment fractures of the upper jaw. It certainly does not relate the severity of the maxillary fracture to other areas of the craniofacial skeleton. It is the author's belief that alphanumeric classifications are superior in this respect.[14]

Classifications of zygomatic fractures are many and varied. With the advent of CT scanning together with improved methods of operative exposure and fixation of the orbital zygomatic region, the extent rather than the pattern of fracturing was seen to be of greater significance. Gruss[14] recognized the role of the zygomatic arch in accurate reduction and classified these injuries according to the level of bony damage to the zygomatic body and zygomatic arches. Cooter and David[9] quantify the degree of bony comminution of each element of the zygoma as well as the level of displacement of the skeletal articulations.

Clinical Assessment

With respect to fractures of the *maxilla*, the signs depend on the degree of displacement and comminution and indeed whether the fracture extends into the orbits and skull base, and whether the zygomas are involved as well. Intraoral examination may show the upper dental arch to be intact or it may be fragmented. There may be mobile dental alveolar segments as well. Malocclusion may be evident: the patient may notice it or it may be obvious on inspection. It is important to be mindful of preexisting occlusal disharmony. In the typical fracture of the upper jaw with an intact alveolar arch, posterior and inferior displacement the occlusal surface will result in an open bite.

The external examination shows cheeks that are typically swollen, and there may be bleeding from the nose and bruising. There may also be emphysema from the air forced out of the paranasal sinuses. If the fracture extends into the orbit, swelling and bruising of the eyelids may be a dominant feature. A gloved figure on the hard palate exerting an upward and rocking force may elicit pain, crepitus, and abnormal mobility. Diastases at the fracture sites may be felt at the nasofrontal and frontal zygomatic sutures.

When managing fractures of the zygoma, it is important to record the mechanism, direction, and particularly the force of the impact, as this will assist in understanding the pattern of fracture. These observations may be very important in later medicolegal proceedings, particularly in cases of interpersonal violence. The association of zygomatic fractures with other midface injuries, in particular fractures of the maxilla, has been noted above (see Fig. 34.15).

The symptomatology typically relates to the effect of the displaced zygomatic bone on the surrounding soft tissues. The orbital soft tissues manifest swelling, ecchymosed and subconjunctival hemorrhages, particularly laterally. Double vision or blurred vision may be complained of due to orbital soft tissue swelling, ocular dystopia or primary ocular injury. Numbness or altered sensation in the distribution of the infraorbital nerve indicates a fracture in the region of the orbital rim. If the zygoma is medially displaced, trismus and complaints of malocclusion are noted when the arch fractures impinge on the underlying temporalis muscle. Patients sometimes complain of altered occlusion and in this situation occlusal disturbance by extension of the zygomatic fracture into the maxillary alveolar process must be excluded by careful intraoral examination.

Physical examination and especially palpation will readily identify displacement. Observation from above the patient provides an impression of loss of the zygomatic prominence.

The examining fingers are placed on the prominent part of the zygomatic body and will give a comparison with the noninjured side. When there is displacement of the inferior rim, there may be a palpable step at the infraorbital margin and this is usually painful. In isolated fractures of the zygomatic arch there may be a depression which is palpable. When the zygomatic fractures are part of extensive midface fracturing, for example in conjunction with maxillary fractures, the zygomatic arches bow outwards and the anteroposterior projection of the zygomatic prominence is diminished.

Intraoral examination shows bruising in the upper buccal sulcus. Alveolar extensions of the fracture or malocclusion caused by trismus or associated with midfacial and mandibular fractures can be noted at this time.

It is important to have a detailed ophthalmological examination similar to that necessary in isolated fractures of the orbital walls.

Imaging

Fractures of the middle third of the face were once investigated by plain radiology. This has almost completely disappeared and the most useful radiological investigation has become the CT scan with axial, coronal, and three-dimensional reformatting. This is the standard radiological examination for fractures of the upper jaw and orbit and all but the most simple fractures of the zygoma.

Axial cuts show fractures of the posterior wall of the maxillary antrum and of the pterygoid plates. It is possible to identify midline fractures of the hard palate as well as dentoalveolar segmental fractures. Coronal CT scans of the midface give detailed information of the anterior maxilla and the relationships with nasoethmoid and orbitozygomatic fractures. When the fractures are primarily of the orbitozygomatic region, then the radiological analysis is similar to that described in the section on orbital fractures.

Principles of Management

The mainstay of surgical treatment for zygomatic fractures was for many years the Gillies technique of elevating by leverage from an incision in the hair-bearing scalp of the temple.[15] The Dingman and Natvig variation[11] or elevation from a lateral eyebrow incision is a more useful and elegant method as it also affords access to the lateral orbital wall and allows for frontozygomatic interfragment fixation.

An intraoral upper buccal sulcus approach gives access to the arch and body of the bone which can be elevated and fixation can be made at the zygomatico-maxillary buttress. Because of the pull of the masseter muscle, it became common practice, in order to prevent relapse, to add fixation using a wire at the frontozygomatic suture. It is now standard practice to employ miniplate fixation. Miniplate or microplate fixation together with wide operative exposure of the orbitozygomatic skeleton allows anatomical restoration of the zygomatic prominence with fewer positional disturbances of the globe, such as enophthalmos and vertical global dystopia.

Following clinical examination and CT confirmation of the fracture pattern, it becomes important to identify fracturing and comminution in and around the zygomatico-maxillary buttress and the inferior orbital rim, disruptions of the arch and at the zygomatico-frontal suture. Because of the deforming and displacing effects of the masseter muscle, the placement of adequate mini- or microplate fixation is necessary. The techniques of exposure, reduction, and fixation are now well described. It becomes logical to subdivide fractures of the zygoma to those where there is no orbital wall involvement (the isolated zygomatic arch fracture) and the more common orbitozygomatic fracture and also those associated with other midfacial fractures, or the panfacial fracture.

Isolated Zygomatic Arch Fractures

These result in the main from low-velocity injuries and the characteristic symptoms are those of trismus and a depression at the site of impact. This injury is usually best treated by the Gillies technique of closed reduction. A short oblique incision in the hair-bearing temple allows passage of an elevator deep to the temporalis fascia behind the depressed arch. This technique produces a stable reduction in the majority of cases. If the arch fracture is not corrected, the cosmetic deformity remains and in extreme cases there is some long-term disturbance of jaw opening.

Orbitozygomatic Fractures

An undisplaced fracture does not need operative intervention. Displaced orbitozygomatic fractures require careful open reduction and internal fixation on an individualized basis. Exposure via an eyebrow incision, a lower eyelid subciliary skin muscle flap or transconjunctival incision reveals the zygomatico-frontal suture, lateral orbital wall inferior orbital rim, orbital floor, and interior zygomatic arch. An upper buccal vestibular incision permits exposure of the zygomatico-maxillary articulation and anterior attachment of the masseter muscle to the zygoma. Following fracture mobilization and elevation, either by the intraoral approach or by using the elevator through the eyebrow approach, an anatomical restoration is achieved by visualizing the zygomatic articulations and checking the alignment of the zygoma with the greater wing of sphenoid. Miniplate fixation in the zygomatico-maxillary buttress is effective, however there may be comminution in this area and sometimes the bony attachments of the plate are thin. The zygomatico-frontal suture on its own is often not enough but it does provide the strongest bone for miniplate fixation. Two-site fixation will provide sufficient stability in the majority of fractures. When the orbital floor needs exploring then the orbital rim can be plated as well through the lower lid or transconjunctival incision.

Comminuted and grossly displaced orbitozygomatic fractures seldom occur in isolation and are almost always the result of high-velocity impacts producing major midface fractures involving the maxillae. In those cases, recognizing the disruption and restoring the arch is key to restoration of zygomatic projection and hence a very good marker for fixation of adjacent fractured bones. In these cases a coronal scalp flap facilitates exposure, mobilization, and reduction of the arch fractures.

Comminution and loss of bone at the major articulations, the anterior maxillary wall, the orbital floor, and the lateral orbital wall demands careful operative exposure, reduction, and reconstruction by primary bone grafting to avoid enophthalmos and orbito-ocular dystopia.

When dealing with *maxillary fractures*, it is important to have a preoperative dental assessment. Impressions of the dental arches and teeth can be used to cast a plaster model which is then cut through the site of the fractures. Restoration of the premorbid occlusion can be planned and an acrylic bite wafer constructed, which can be used intraoperatively and postoperatively to maintain correct occlusal relationships.

There is some discussion in the literature about the timing of definitive treatment of maxillary fractures. The desirability of performing surgical correction of midface fracture as early as possible after injuring has been championed by Gruss and Mackinnon[16] and Manson et al,[17] their argument being that early accurate bony reconstruction will prevent the development of soft tissue contractures and hence post-traumatic deformity.

It is the author's belief that there are other factors that must be considered when deciding on the correct timing of surgery.

The foremost of these is consideration of the priorities of management of other injuries, such as associated brain injuries and other associated limb and intraabdominal problems. It is also useful to have time to properly plan and assemble an operative team to be able to give the appropriate time and expertise to the restoration of the facial injury.[2]

Airway management may be compromised with other jaw fractures and great care needs to be taken when considering placement of endotracheal tubes at the time of surgery. Particular care should be taken with panfacial fractures, which may extend through the cranial base. Where there is massive craniofacial disruption with hemorrhage then there is a role for tracheotomy.

Fracture reduction by disimpaction used to be carried out using somewhat brutal forceps inserted with one prong in the nasal cavity, the other in the oral cavity so as to grip the palate bilaterally. It is possible to inflict further damage with this instrument. With the advent of wider exposure through coronal, buccal, and conjunctival approaches, more delicate instrumentation can be used to disimpact the fracture sites.

Stabilization of fractures is of course now achieved with miniplate fixation and when there is comminution and loss of bone at the buttresses, primary bone grafting is performed.

Once the impacted displaced maxilla has been reduced, the upper and lower jaws are stabilized in the pretraumatic occlusion using arch bars, the wafer, and intermaxillary wiring. Where the zygomas are also fractured, these should be reduced as described above. They then provide a reference point for reestablishing the vertical buttresses.

In the case of an uncomplicated Le Fort I fracture, the vertical height can be determined easily by opposing the vertical buttresses at the pyriform margin and zygomaticomaxillary region, which can then be plated. Even when there are other fractures of the midface, at least one of the four anterior vertical midface buttresses will usually not be severely comminuted and so provide a guide for the correct vertical relationship. Once this has been established, miniplates are used to stabilize the reduced fracture using at least two screws on either side of the fracture. If there is loss of bone then bone grafting may be needed in one or more of these vertical buttresses. Once the vertical height has been established and stabilized, with or without bone graft, the maxillary fixation can be released, the surgical fields irrigated, and the wounds closed. The jaw opening is controlled with light elastics and the wafer removed after several days when the patient is able to bite in the correct position (Figs. 34.16–34.18).

Management of complex midfacial fractures when the zygomas, maxillae, and indeed nasal ethmoid fractures are involved (that is, fractures above the Le Fort I level) need different treatment sequences. The occlusal complex (i.e., mandible and maxilla) is stabilized and bought together in occlusion with the help of a preplanned occlusal wafer. The zygomatic orbital complexes are stabilized usually via a coronal scalp flap to give the forward projection offered by accurate reduction of the zygomatic arch. The occlusal complex can then be united with the orbital complex via the four vertical buttresses. Fixation of the buttresses can be with miniplates and/or bone grafting if necessary. Finally, the nasal ethmoid complex can be reconstructed by meticulous interfragmentary miniplate fixation and the nasoethmoid area as described earlier.

Complications

Zygoma

These include:

- Deformity
- Prominent plates
- Disturbance of globe position
- Ocular injury
- Nerve injury.

Deformity was more common with older techniques of management where there was inadequate exposure and fixation. Soft tissue deformities, including sagging of the eyelid and cheek, after zygomatic dissections require meticulous repositioning of soft tissues (Figs. 34.19–34.22).

Prominent plates are a common complication that may require plate removal on a subsequent occasion.

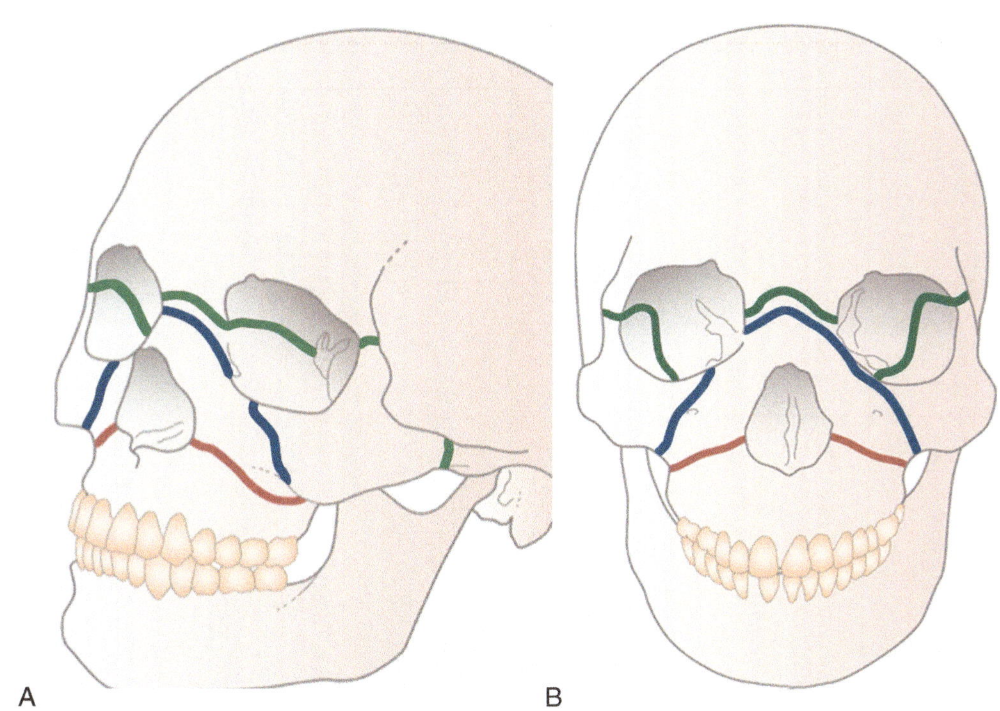

• **Fig. 34.16** (A,B) Maxillary fracture classification of Le Fort. The classical fracture lines – horizontal (I, *red*), pyramidal (II, *blue*), total disjunction (III, *green*).

Disturbance of globe position in both the anteroposterior and vertical dimensions remains a major long-term complication. Enophthalmos and vertical global dystopia are cosmetically and functionally disturbing. They are very hard to correct and in some cases may require osteotomies of the orbit to reposition part or the entire orbital box.

With regard to ocular injury, direct globe injuries are common in association with these fractures. The fracture of the lateral wall of the zygoma that produces the "cigar cutter technique" can injure the optic nerve. Ophthalmological investigation will determine whether or not there are any retinal injuries as a result of the trauma.

Nerve injuries most commonly involved are those of the infraorbital nerve, causing persistent numbness, paresthesia or hyperesthesia in the distribution of this nerve. Most patients experience significant recovery of function early but occasional patients experience progressive improvement over a longer period of time, up to 18 months or more. A very small number go on to have dysesthesia, which can be distressing.

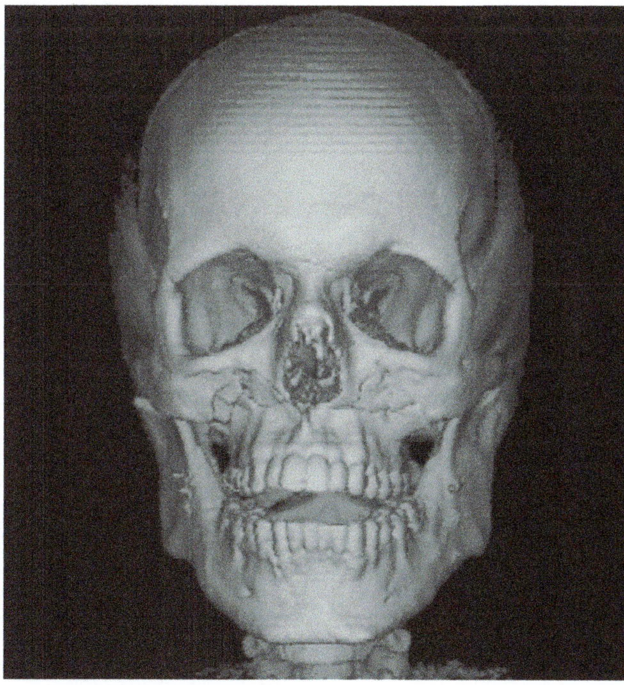

• **Fig. 34.17** A typical Le Fort I fracture of the upper jaw – the fracture line is horizontal; there is an intact alveolar arch. The posterior and inferior displacement of the arch and palate result in the open bite seen clearly on this 3D image.

The Maxillae

These include:

- Malunion and malocclusion
- Non-union
- Facial deformity
- Infection
- Nasal obstruction
- Lacrimal obstruction.

Malunion with associated malocclusion and loss of normal facial form are most significant complications of upper jaw fractures, particularly where there has been severe comminution in and around the midfacial buttresses. Deformity may require early intervention if there has been some relapse; however, long-term assessment leading to osteotomies and onlay bone grafts may be the answer in complex cases.

Facial deformity can also result from an alteration to the facial contour, for example where the anterior wall of the

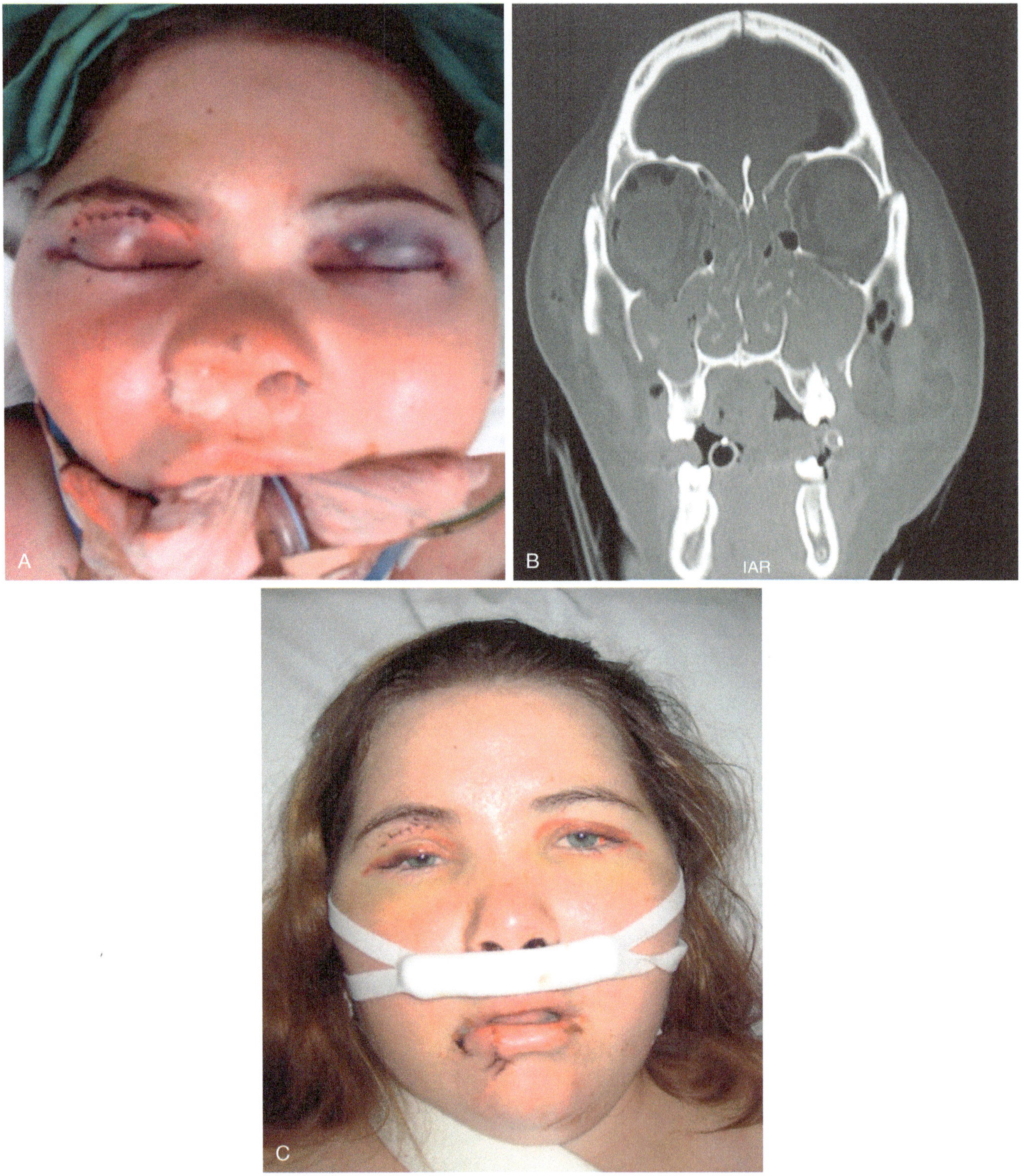

• **Fig. 34.18** A patient with fractures at all three Le Fort levels. (A) Swollen, bruised, nasal and oral packing to control hemorrhage, and intubated to protect her airway. (B) The coronal CT slice shows the endotracheal tube, the oral packing, and the fractures. (C) After 7 days, extubated, lacerations sutured, swelling abating, clinically there is right enophthalmos, flattening of the cheeks, flattening and widening of the nasoethmoid region, and an anterior open bite.

maxilla has been fragmented and there is scarring between the maxillary fragment and the overlying integument. The wide dissection necessary to secure adequate reduction is itself a cause of scarring at the periosteal level, which produces an aging effect.

Infection tends to occur in and around plates and screws but, in the long term, patients can come back possibly many years later with sinusitis resulting from obstruction to the sinus drainage or indeed screws that have eroded into the sinus cavities.

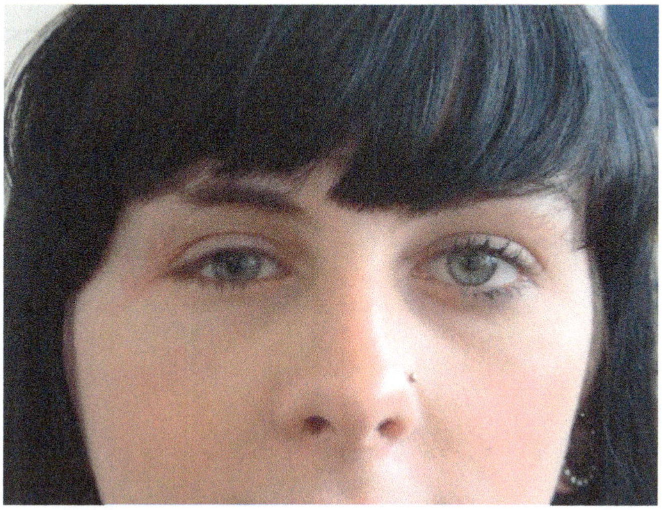

• **Fig. 34.19** Flattened right zygoma, the arch is bowed out, and the palpebral fissure is narrowed due to the enophthalmos.

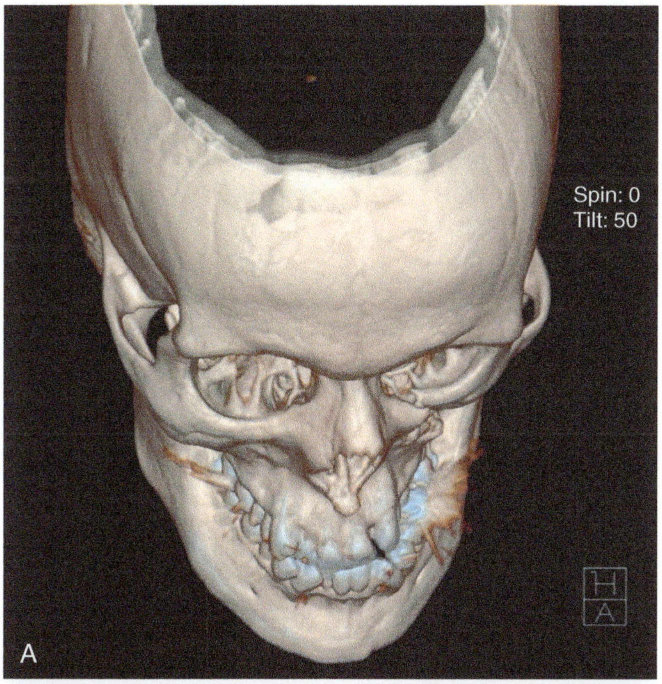

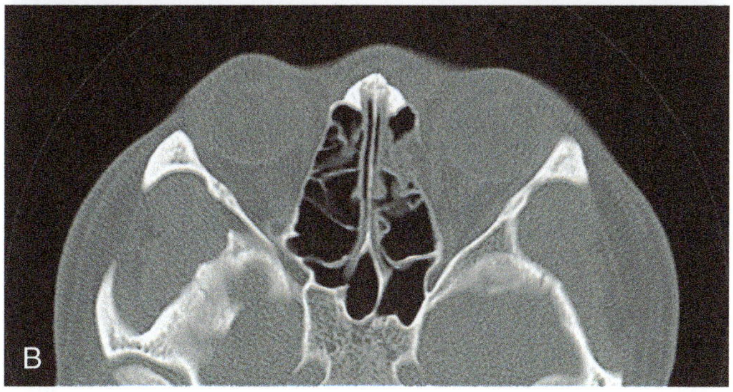

• **Fig. 34.20** (A,B) Depression of the zygoma, which is both visible and palpable.

Nasal obstructive symptoms may follow upper jaw fractures through fracture dislocations of the nasal central cartilage bone. Correction is usually performed once the mucosa has soundly healed, at which time a septorhinoplasty may be performed.

Lacrimal obstruction is common in those fractures that involve the nasal ethmoid complex (Figs. 34.23–34.29).

Orbital Fractures

Because the orbit is situated between the cranium above and the midface below, it is frequently involved in the other fractures described in this chapter, that is, the zygoma and midface, the naso-orbito-ethmoid, frontal, and orbito-zygomatic fractures. Advances in imaging have led to a greater understanding of the anatomy of fractures; this in turn has led to more meaningful correlation between observed pathology and symptoms. A good example of this is the ability to image the medial orbital wall and understand the relationship between these fractures and persisting enophthalmos when they go uncorrected (Fig. 34.30).[2]

Advances in imaging permit preoperative planning; the possibility of wide exposure enables reconstruction of both skeletal and soft tissues; techniques of grafting and rigid fixation give rise to a high level of predictable skeletal anatomical restoration. The team approach is vital in managing orbital injuries; especially important is the relationship between the craniofacial surgeon and the ophthalmologist.

Anatomy

The orbit is composed of seven bones and shaped like a quadrilateral pyramid; it has a strong anterior rim and four thin walls that converge on a strong bony apex (Fig. 34.31). The thick protective outer rim is formed by the frontal, zygomatic, and maxillary bones. At the rim the orbit is ovoid in coronal section, becoming more rectangular towards the apex which is almost triangular. The roof, medial, lateral, and inferior (floor) are thin and respond to trauma each in their own way. The portion of the orbit in front of the transverse axis of the globe has little effect on the orbital volume, and hence the projection of the globe of the eye, but more influence on its vertical and transverse position. Alterations to the size and shape of the part of the orbit behind the axis of the globe determine the meaningful skeletal volume and therefore influence the projection of the globe.

Lang, citing Oehmann,[18] gives the mean lengths of the adult orbit as: roof – 50.5 mm; floor – 48.4 mm; lateral wall – 47.2 mm; medial wall – 40.5 mm.

The eye is protected from blunt trauma by the orbital rim, this being least effective in the inferolateral area. The optic canal enters the orbit at the apex of the pyramid. The canal is on average 9.8 mm long and 4.6 mm wide at its narrowest point. The optic nerve may be injured within the canal, either by forces transmitted through the intact bony canal or the orbital contents, or when a fracture enters the

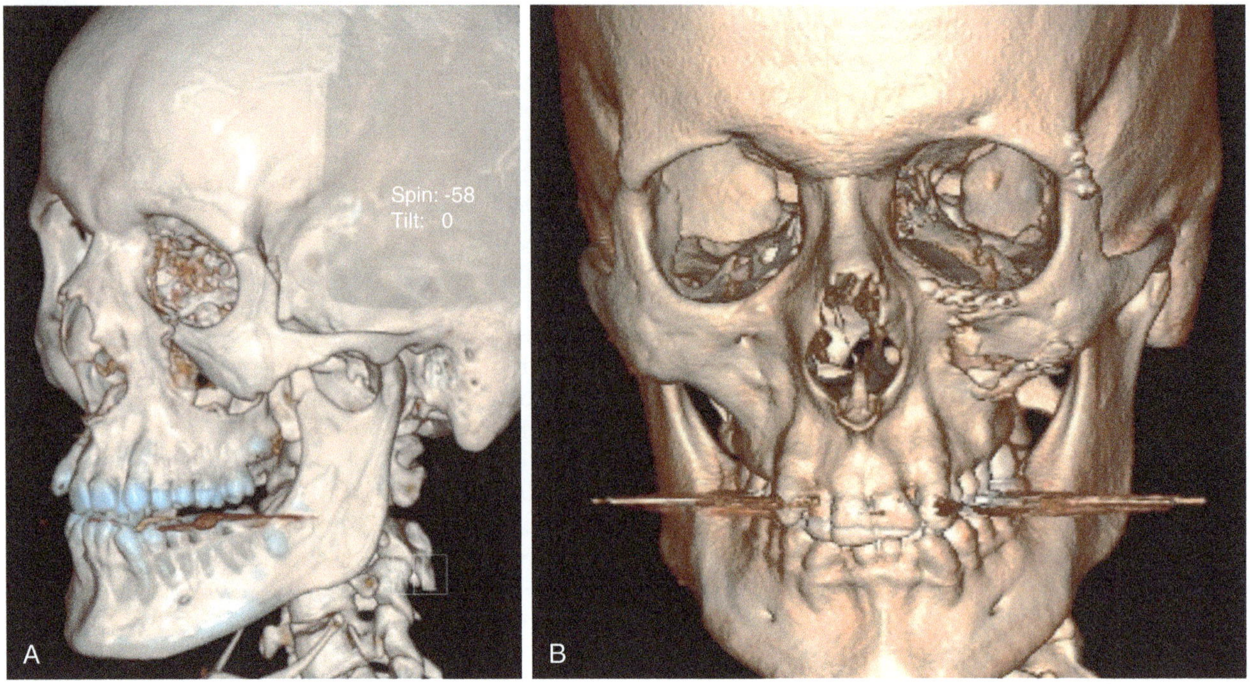

• **Fig. 34.21** (A,B) Open reduction and internal fixation of a fracture of the left zygoma. Access was gained via a buccal sulcus incision, an eyebrow incision, and a transconjunctival incision. Plates are seen at the frontozygomatic suture, the inferior orbital rim and the zygomatico-maxillary buttress. The orbital floor has been reconstructed with iliac bone.

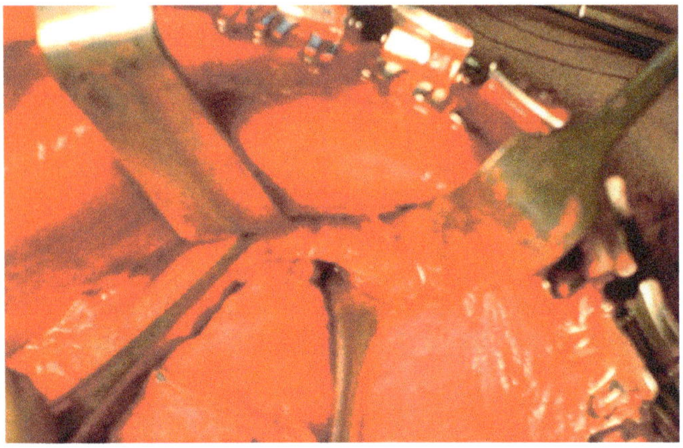

• **Fig. 34.22** Right zygomatic arch fracture exposed via a coronal scalp flap.

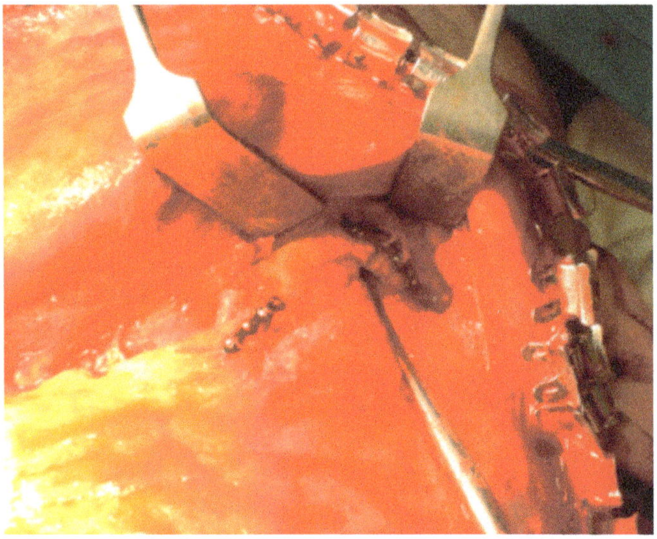

• **Fig. 34.23** The forward projection of the zygoma is assured by accurate reduction and plating of the zygomatic arch. Access is via the coronal flap and the fronto-zygomatic diastasis has been reduced and plated.

canal. The nerve is further protected from impact by the orbital fat and from stretching by its tortuosity.

Surgical Pathology and Pathogenesis

Disruption of the orbit may result from fracture of the orbital rim and walls by extension of extrinsic fractures, that is, those arising external to the orbit which are classified according to their major anatomical component (Table 34.1). Intrinsic fractures arise from indirect forces transmitted via the globe and periorbital soft tissues, which produce "blow-out" fractures of the orbital floor and medial orbital wall (Fig. 34.32).

The *orbital roof* is formed by the frontal bone, which is thick at the rim and the roof is arched in both the anteroposterior and transverse dimensions. It is relatively resistant to fracturing. Inferior displacement of the roof is the most frequent fracture in this area and in most cases is associated with disruption of the orbital rim. Roof fractures resulting from high-impact injuries to the frontal bone and extensions into the face are more frequently seen in children (Fig. 34.33).

The *orbital floor* is the site of the classic blow-out fracture. The anterior part of the orbital floor medial to the

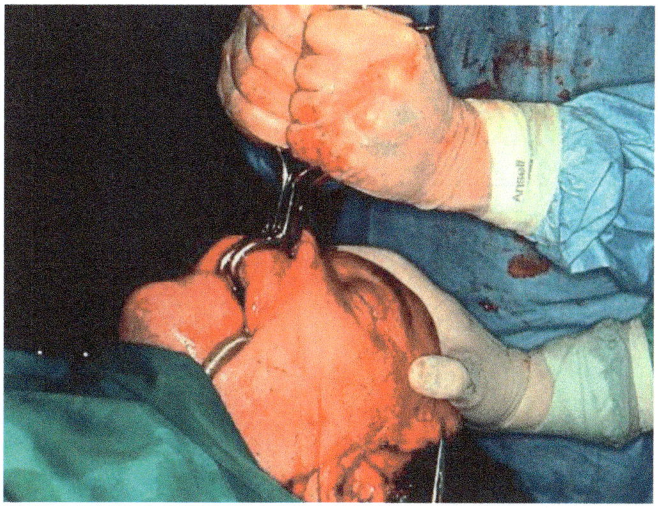

• **Fig. 34.24** Row's disimpaction forceps can cause further damage to already compromised tissue.

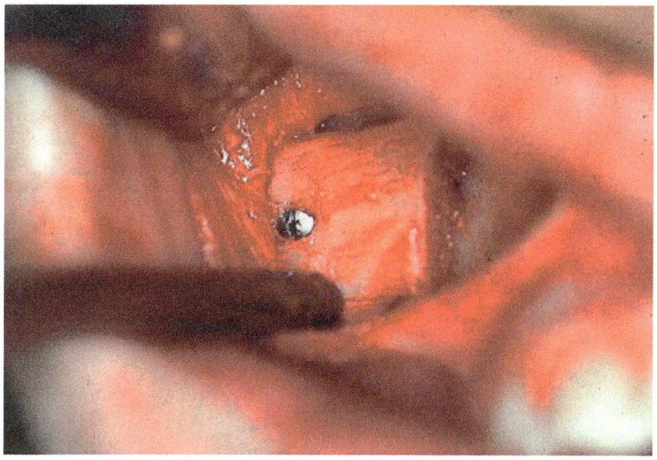

• **Fig. 34.25** A graft across the absent buttress.

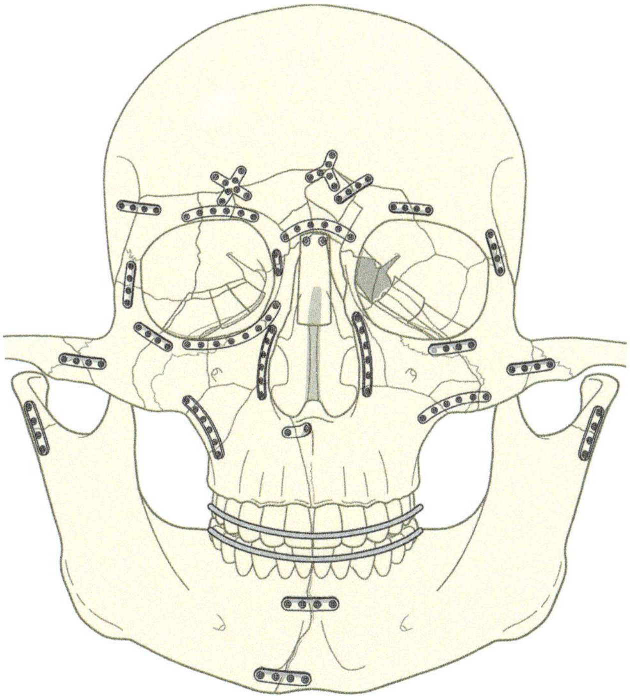

• **Fig. 34.26** Schematic of final panfacial fracture fixation with orbital volume and nasal projection restored with grafts. (From Holland IS, McMahon JD, Koppel DA, et al. Maxillary and panfacial fractures. In: Booth PW, Eppley BL, Schmelzeisen R, eds. *Maxillofacial Trauma and Esthetic Facial Reconstruction*. Philadelphia: Saunders; 2012:239, with permission from Elsevier.)

infraorbital nerve canal is concave from front to back, posterior to the axis of the globe it becomes convex upwards because the maxillary antrum bulges superiorly and obliterates the angle between the floor and the medial wall. When reconstructing the floor it is important to restore this posterior convexity in order to prevent enophthalmos (Fig. 34.34).

The *medial walls* are almost vertical and have a slight three-dimensional wave formation. The lacrimal bone and the lamina papyracea of the ethmoid bone form the thin, vulnerable portion of the medial wall that is subject to blow-out and "blow-in" fractures. Isolated medial wall defects in the middle and posterior third of the orbit increase the orbital volume and may cause enophthalmos. Until the advent of CT scanning these injuries were difficult to diagnose and often went undetected. The lacrimal drainage system lies at the anterior aspect of the medial orbital wall and is intimately associated with the medial canthal ligament. Injuries of these structures are most frequently seen with naso-orbito-ethmoid fractures (Fig. 34.35).

The *lateral orbital wall* is formed by the greater wing of sphenoid and the orbital process of the zygoma, it lies entirely posterior to the transverse axis of the globe. Isolated fractures are rare; fracturing usually being part of a zygomatic injury (Fig. 34.36).

The *orbital apex* is formed by thicker bone which surrounds the inferior and superior orbital fissures and the optic foramen. The extraocular muscles are separated from the bony walls of the orbit in its anterior half by fat pads. In the posterior orbit they are close to the bony walls and more vulnerable to trauma from fracture of orbital dissection.

Fractures of the orbit may be classified as being intrinsic to the orbital walls and those fractures of the walls that are associated with fractures of the bones that form the orbital rim. Intrinsic fractures of the orbital walls are characterized as blow-out or blow-in fractures. When there is extension of the fracture to involve the orbital rim these fractures are often referred to as "impure!"

The application of sudden blunt trauma to the periorbital soft tissues is transmitted as a hydraulic pressure wave to the orbital walls resulting in the fracture.[19] The orbital floor medial to the infraorbital nerve is thin and unsupported and breaks easily, as does the fragile lateral plate of the ethmoid bone. The sequelae of this disturbance include enophthalmos from the expanded volume of the orbital box combined with prolapse of orbital contents into the adjacent sinus, possible muscle involvement in the fracture, damage to the infraorbital nerve, and diplopia. These fractures usually

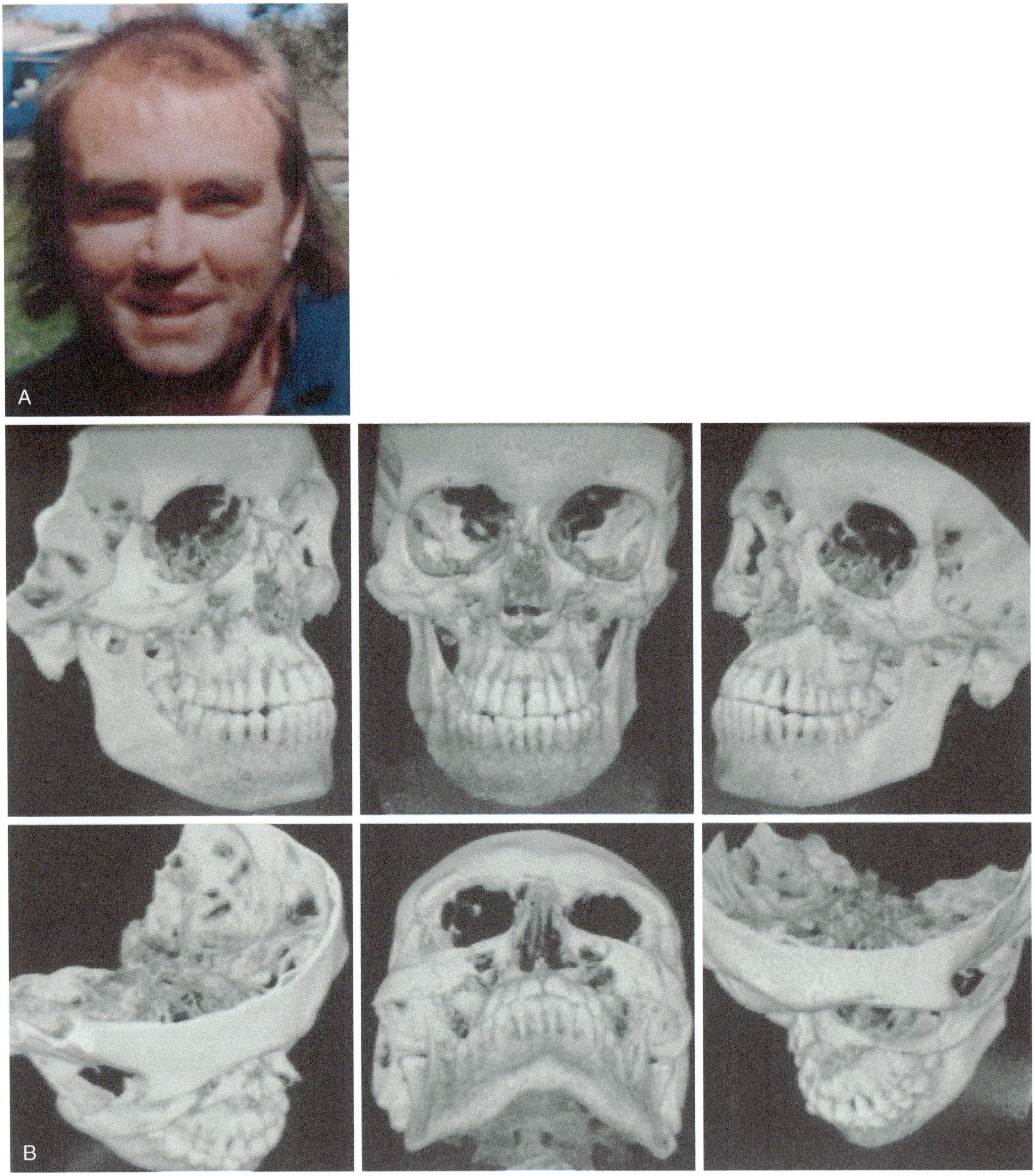

• **Fig. 34.27** A case study of the sequence of events in repairing this panfacial fracture. (A) Knowledge of the patient's premorbid appearance. (B) Detailed study of the fracture pattern.

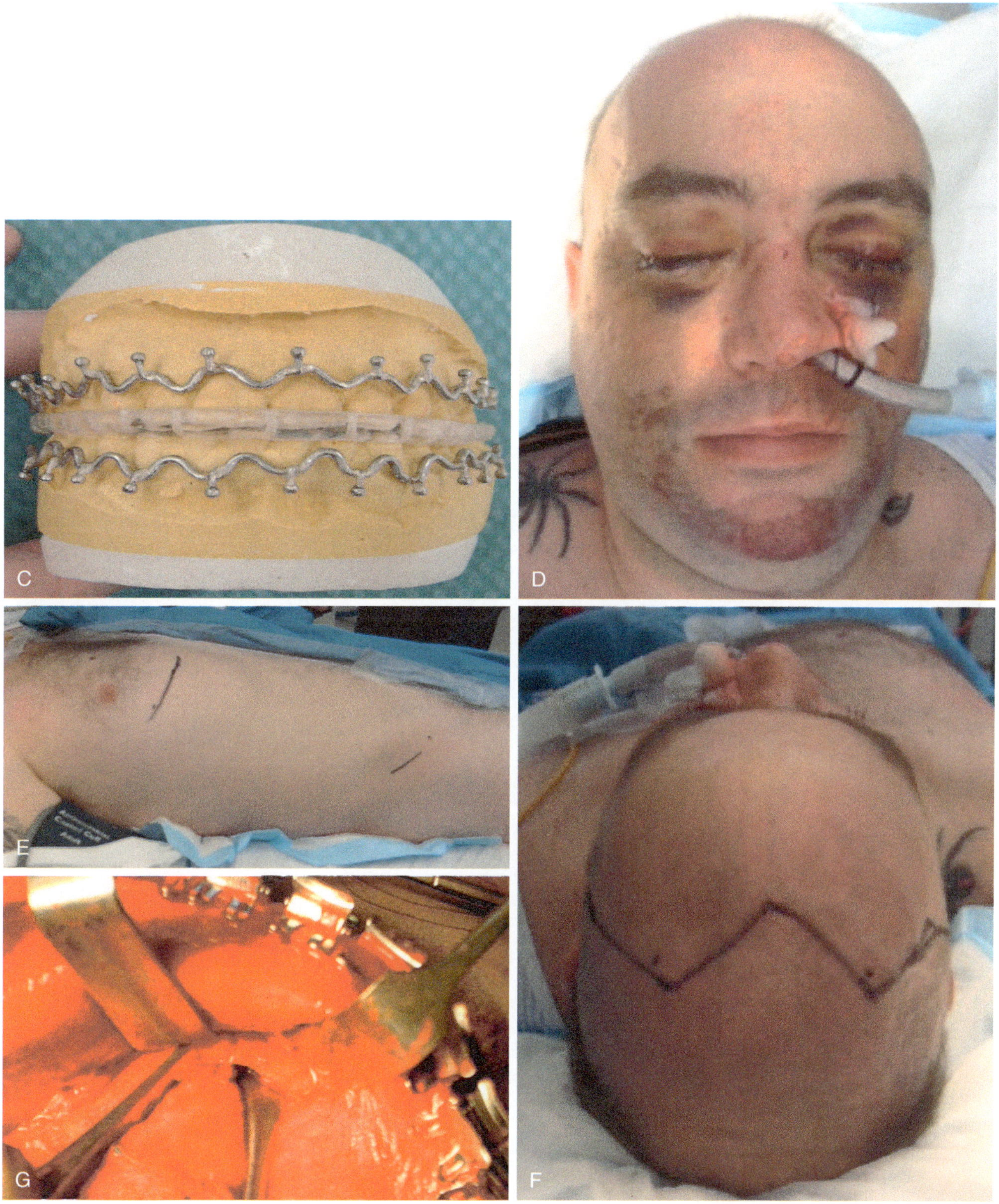

• **Fig. 34.27 cont'd** (C) Planned occlusal restoration with a wafer and preformed arch bars. (D) The nasal intubation. (E) The bone graft sites. (F) The coronal scalp flap. (G) Exposure of the zygomatic arch.

Continued

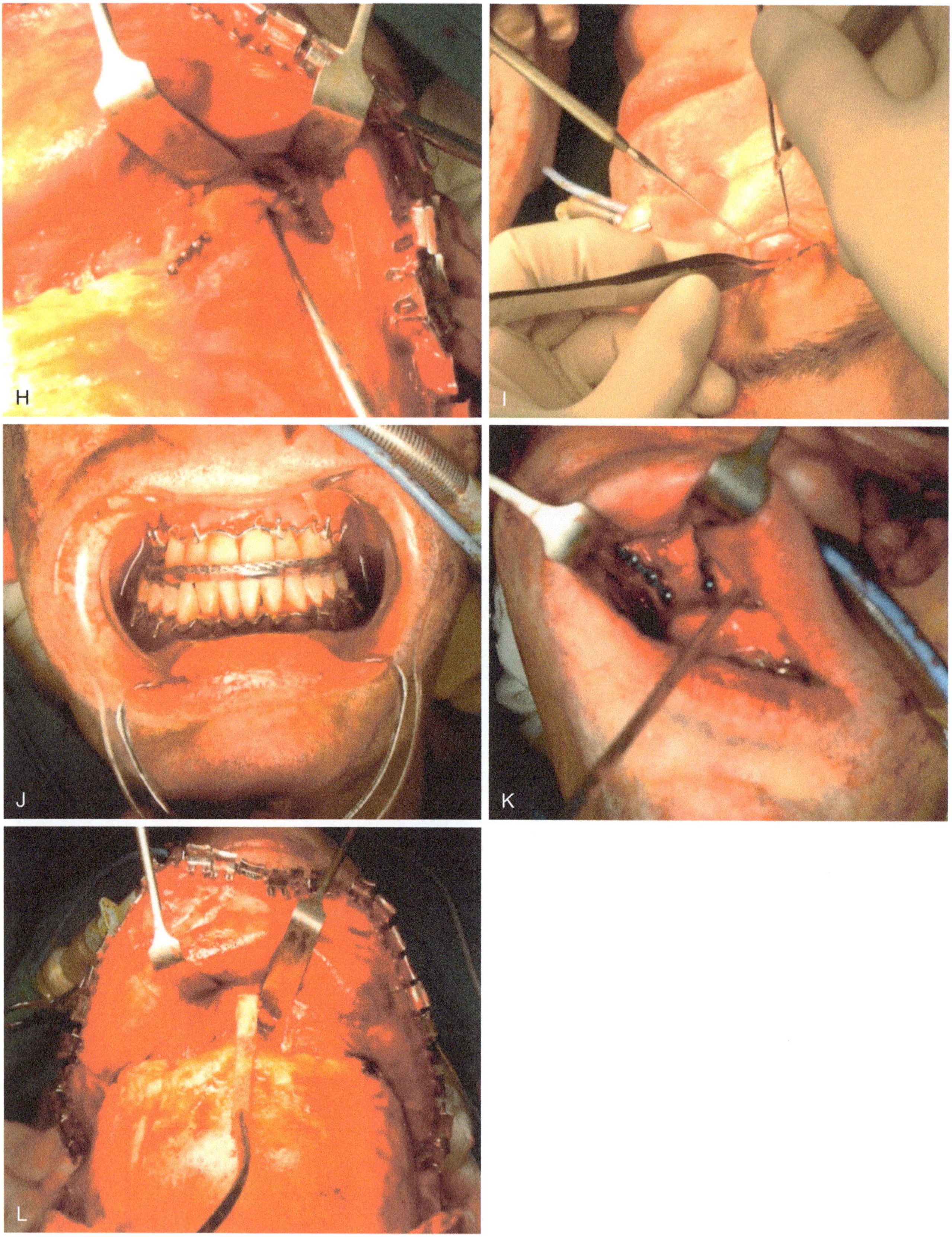

• **Fig. 34.27 cont'd** (H) Plating of the frontozygomatic suture and arch. (I) The transconjunctival incision to expose the orbit. (J) The occlusion restored using the wafer, and intermaxillary fixation. (K) The buttresses plated. (L) The nasoethmoid region reconstructed and the dorsum of the nose grafted with a split costochondral graft.

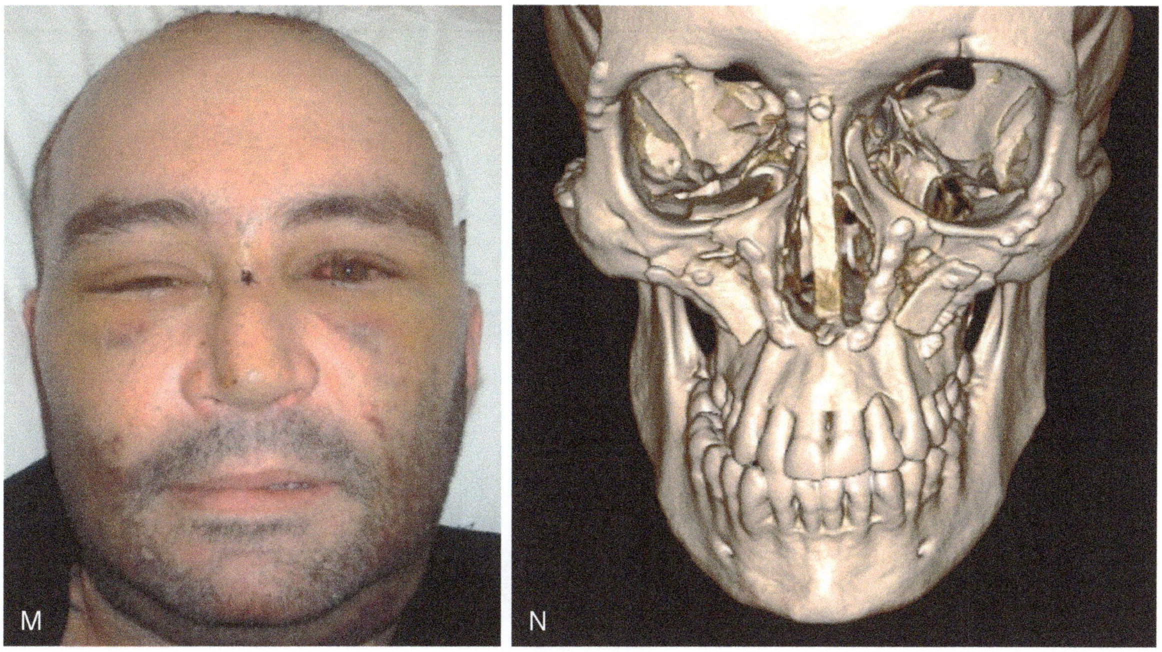

• **Fig. 34.27 cont'd** (M) Seven days post surgery. (N) Postoperative 3D CT.

result from a low-energy impact (e.g., a champagne cork in the eye!). The blow-in fracture[20] is characterized by inward displacement of bony fragments of the walls and/or margins which results in decreased orbital volume and proptosis (Fig. 34.37).

Low-velocity impacts from assaults or falls tend to produce simple linear or blow-out types of fracture involving one or two orbital walls. Medium-velocity injuries have a similar pattern of wall disruption but may be associated with disruption of the orbital rim. The orbital fractures that extend to the orbit from fractures of adjacent bones invariably result from medium- to high-velocity impacts.

The multiple wall fractures resulting from high-velocity impacts that are part of a panfacial fracture exhibit less well-defined patterns and have more comminution and bone loss.

Clinical Assessment

Ophthalmological examination is an essential part of the clinical assessment of a patient with orbital trauma, the ophthalmologist being an essential member of the craniofacial team. In addition to the routine examination for fractures such as those of the zygoma, the orbital contents need to be examined by everting the lids with appropriate retractors lest globe destruction be missed. Visual disturbance must be investigated further. The clinician must test for altered sensation in the distribution of the nerves passing through the orbit. Enophthalmos is difficult to determine in the presence of swelling but becomes obvious as the swelling abates. Early marked exophthalmos is indicative of reduction of the orbital volume and requires urgent ophthalmological and radiological examination to determine if there is impingement of bone on the orbital contents or damage at the orbital apex. It is important to test ocular motility. In children, the rare damage to the muscle early intervention is recommended. These patients are often very distressed by attempted eye movements (Fig. 34.38).

Imaging

CT examination is the diagnostic investigation of choice in orbital trauma; this form of imaging is mandatory for accurate diagnosis and when planning surgical reconstruction.

High-resolution axial CT examination with films of both bone and soft tissue windows show damage to the medial and lateral walls and extensions of fractures beyond the orbit into the adjacent bones. Direct coronal views show the orbital roof, medial orbital wall, and orbital floor. When a pure blow-out fracture is suspected, direct coronal scans of the orbit will identify both the extent of the floor and the medial wall involvement and the nature of the soft tissue abnormality. Modern programs have the tools to define and measure the area of bone destroyed and give a guide to the amount of reconstructive material that may be used at operation. Careful studies will identify the prolapsed fat and the relationship of the orbital muscles to the fracture. Submucosal hematomas or mucosal polyps of the maxillary sinus can be differentiated from herniated soft tissues. Sagittal images viewed in the line of the inferior rectus muscle will show the relationship to the bony damage and also demonstrate the nerves as they pass through the orbital floor.

Comparison with the contralateral orbit provides a qualitative assessment of the degree of enophthalmos.

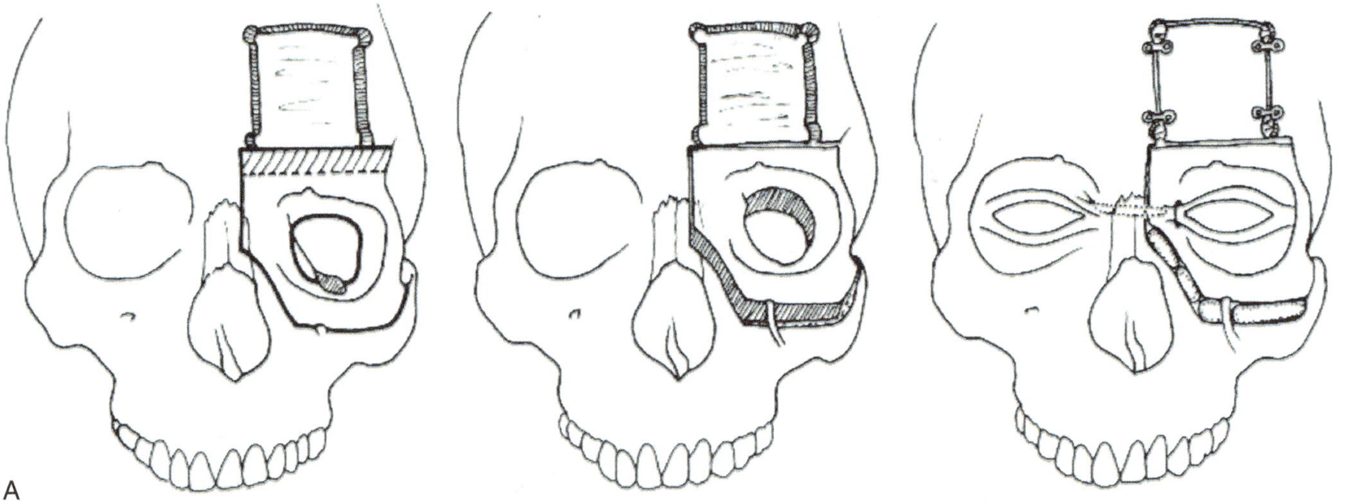

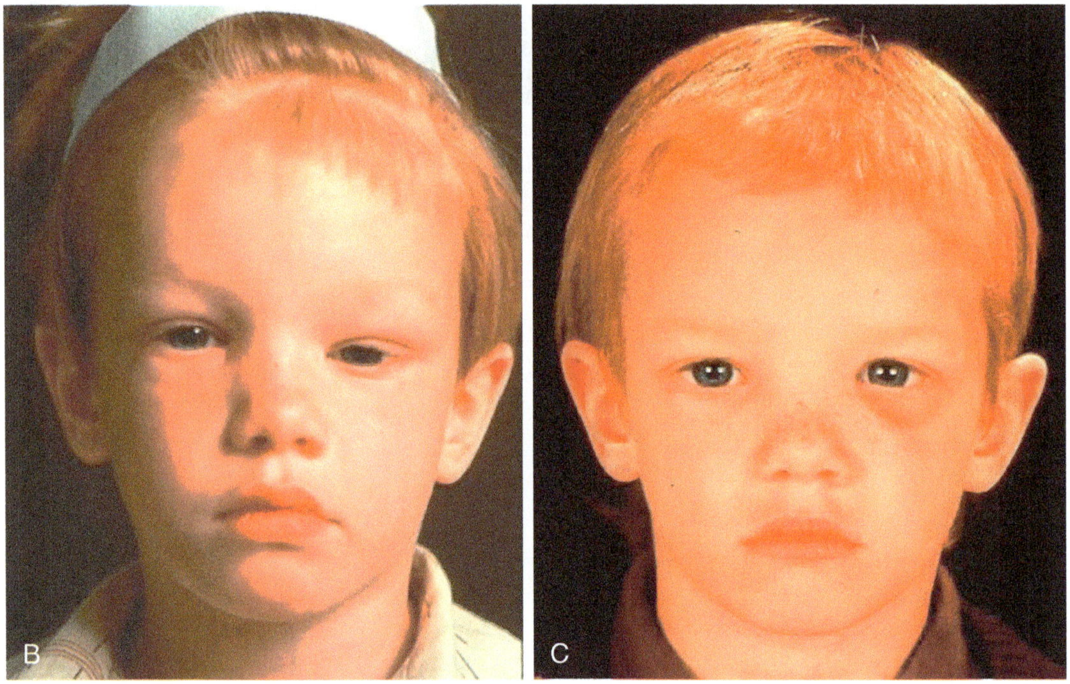

• **Fig. 34.28** (A–C) Old orbital trauma requiring a box osteotomy to correct the vertical dystopia.

Postoperative CT scanning reveals the results of surgery (Fig. 34.39).

Management

As always with craniofacial trauma, the management of orbital fractures is multidisciplinary, the craniofacial surgeon relying heavily on the relationship with the ophthalmologist. Minor disruptions that do not exhibit clinical signs or cause symptoms are managed conservatively, but followed for some weeks to ensure that late problems such as developing enophthalmos do not occur.

The aim of surgical treatment is accurate restoration of the orbital rim, followed by reconstruction of the orbital walls. The orbital rim is reduced and fixed with miniplates or microplates. The orbital walls are usually reconstructed with bone graft (the author's preference) or alloplastic material. It is important to perform the operative repair as early as possible to minimize the development of soft tissue fibrotic changes. Early swelling and insufficient multidisciplinary work-up usually prevent immediate intervention, however there are exceptional circumstances such as bony fragments impinging on the globe or optic nerve, as can occur in some lateral wall fractures and blow-in fractures.

Surgical exposures to the orbit are described elsewhere. The coronal scalp flap giving the widest access to the medial wall in its middle and posterior third. It also gives good access to the lateral orbital wall, roof and, in the experienced craniofacial surgeon's hands, the orbital floor.

The latter can be approached via a subconjunctival route with or without lateral canthotomy, a subciliary approach, or via a lower lid crease incision. More recently

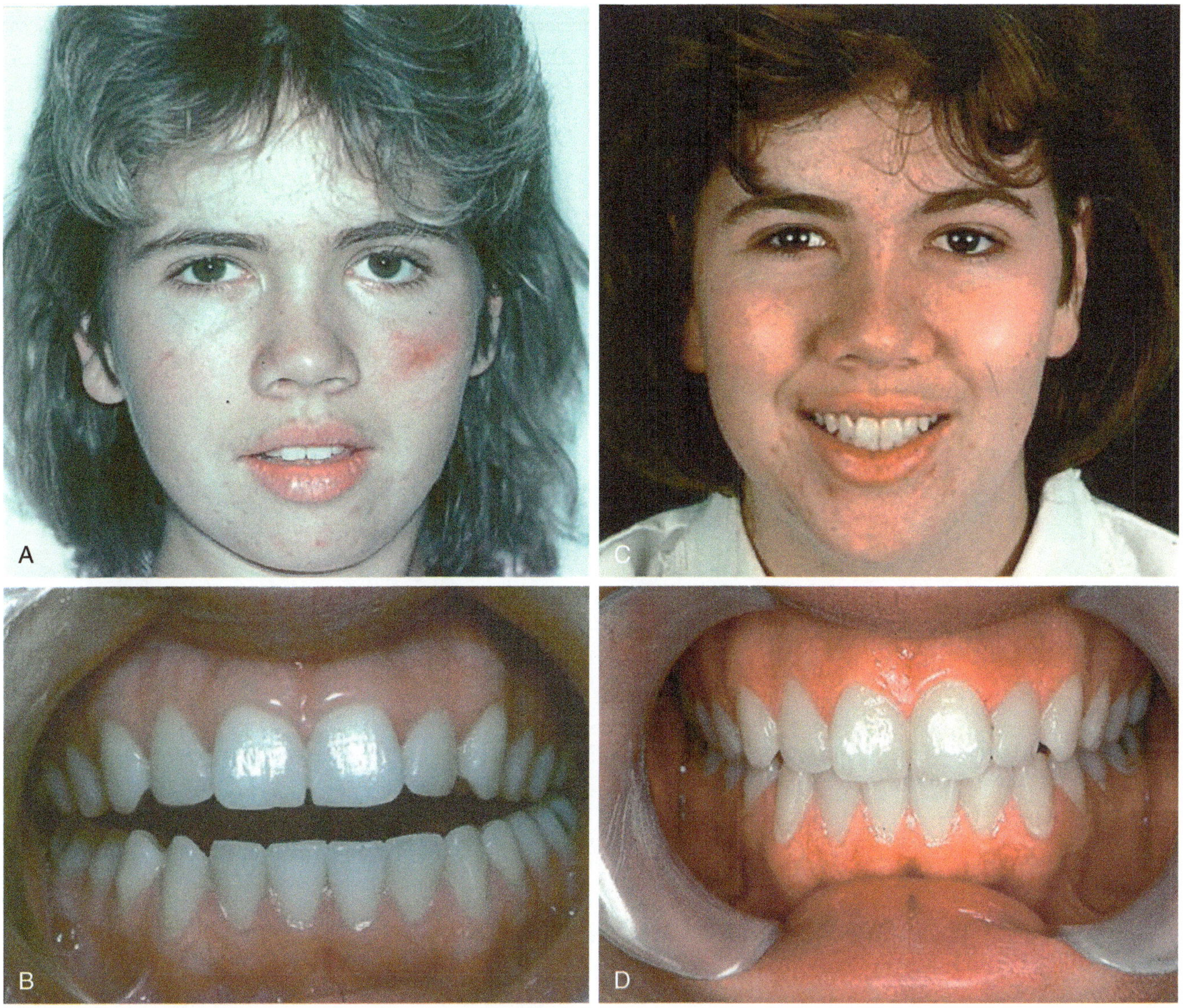

• **Fig. 34.29** (A,B) An uncorrected Le Fort I fracture with malunion and an anterior open bite (C,D) corrected by an osteotomy. (From Winn HR. *Youmans Neurological Surgery.* 6th edn. Philadelphia: Saunders; 2011, with permission from Elsevier.)

there have been advocates of a medial wall repair via a transcaruncular approach to the medial orbital wall (Figs. 34.40 and 34.41).[21,22] The endoscope has been employed by some surgeons to enhance access to fractures near the orbital apex.[23]

Proper reconstruction of the orbital "box" returns the globe to its preinjury position with full maintenance of ocular mobility. Subperiosteal dissection of the orbital walls delineates the fracture and dissection continues so as to expose the surrounding stable bony margins. The herniated soft tissue must be retrieved from the defect in order to restore intraorbital volume and prevent fibrosis.

If the blow-out fracture of the orbital floor is small and isolated, it may be possible to elevate and manipulate the fragment to override the solid margins of the defect. For most defects this is inadequate, and the introduction of an orbital wall graft is required.

The choice of materials for orbital wall reconstruction lies between autogenous bone or cartilage and various forms of alloplastic implants. Historically, there are many materials used; at one time Silastic sheeting was popular, but its tendency to extrude has led to other materials being preferred. Titanium mesh is well tolerated, but with the ingrowth of fibrous tissue it makes reoperation difficult and it is hard to remove. Porous polyethylene (Medpore) has become popular for reconstruction. It does not show on postoperative radiology. The author believes that autogenous bone remains the best material for orbital repair. It has minimal tendency to extrude or become infected and it readily remolds and shapes to the normal orbital contour. The disadvantage is donor site morbidity, which becomes minimal with operator experience.

Calvarial bone enjoyed widespread popularity and is best used when a craniotomy is part of the treatment regimen,

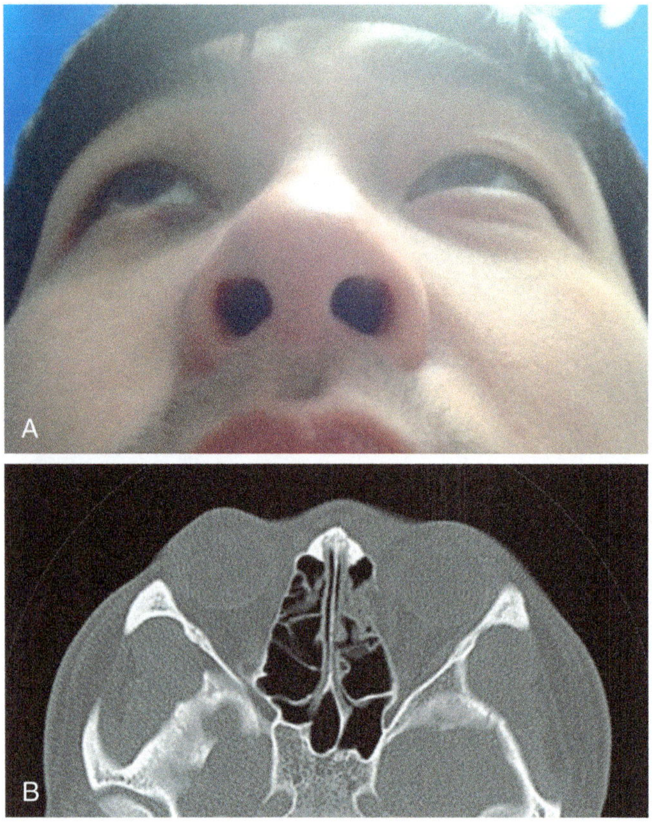

• **Fig. 34.30** A blow-out fracture of the left medial orbital wall produces enophthalmos seen (A) clinically and (B) radiologically.

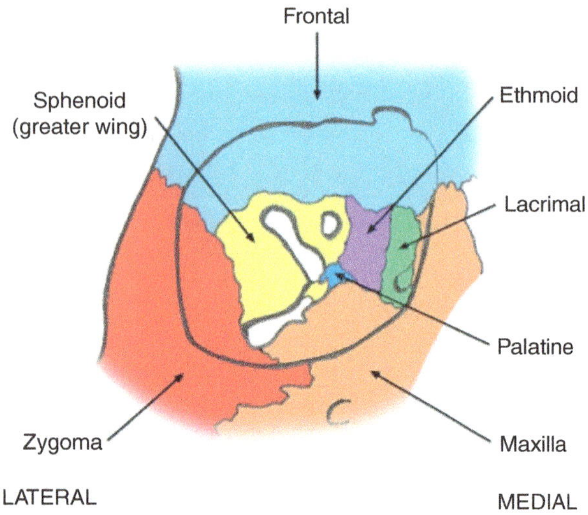

• **Fig. 34.31** Osteology of the orbit showing the contributing bones.

TABLE 34.1 Classification of Orbital Fractures

1. Intrinsic – orbital rim intact	(a) Blow-out (b) Blow-in
2. Extrinsic – orbital rim fractured	(a) Blow-out (b) Blow-in

From David DJ, Simpson DA, eds. *Craniomaxillofacial Trauma*. Edinburgh: Churchill Livingstone; 1995, with permission from Elsevier.

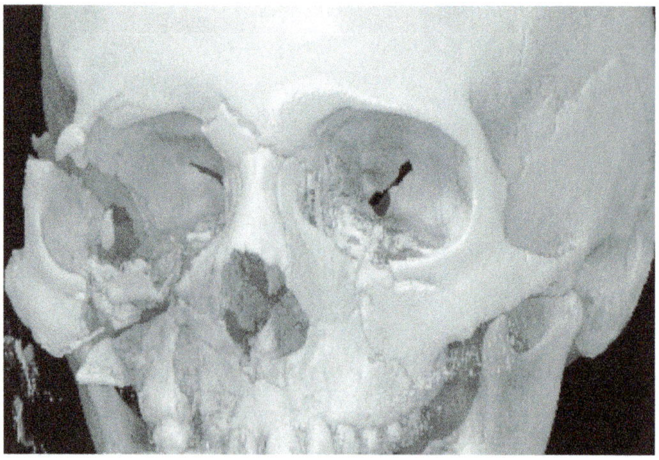

• **Fig. 34.32** Fracture of the zygoma extending into the lateral orbital wall and floor which is so disrupted as to require reconstruction.

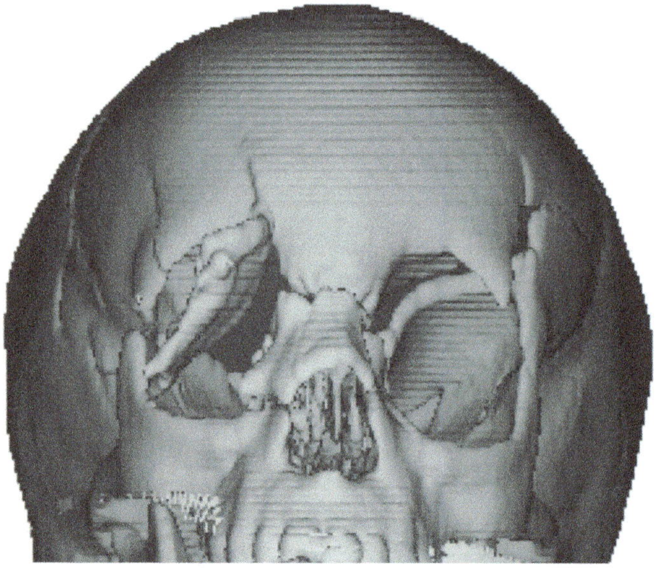

• **Fig. 34.33** High-impact injury in a child producing a blow-in fracture of the orbital roof.

and it can be harvested from the inner table of the calvarial bone flap. Splitting off a layer of the outer table risks damage to the brain or at least an unsightly contour defect of the skull. The bone thus harvested is often rigid and difficult to shape.

Split-rib graft is available in large quantities; however the author's preferred option is the smooth inner surface of the blade of the ilium approached via an iliac crest incision which can be minimal in length. The quantity and quality of the bone is most suitable for the task of orbital wall reconstruction (Fig. 34.42).

In uncomplicated blow-out fractures, after anatomical restoration of the orbital bony anatomy, with or without a graft, the orbital soft tissues are allowed to redrape.

A forced duction test is performed by grasping the rectus muscle insertions with forceps and moving the globe to demonstrate that muscle entrapment has been relieved. The lid and conjunctival incisions can be closed in a single layer.

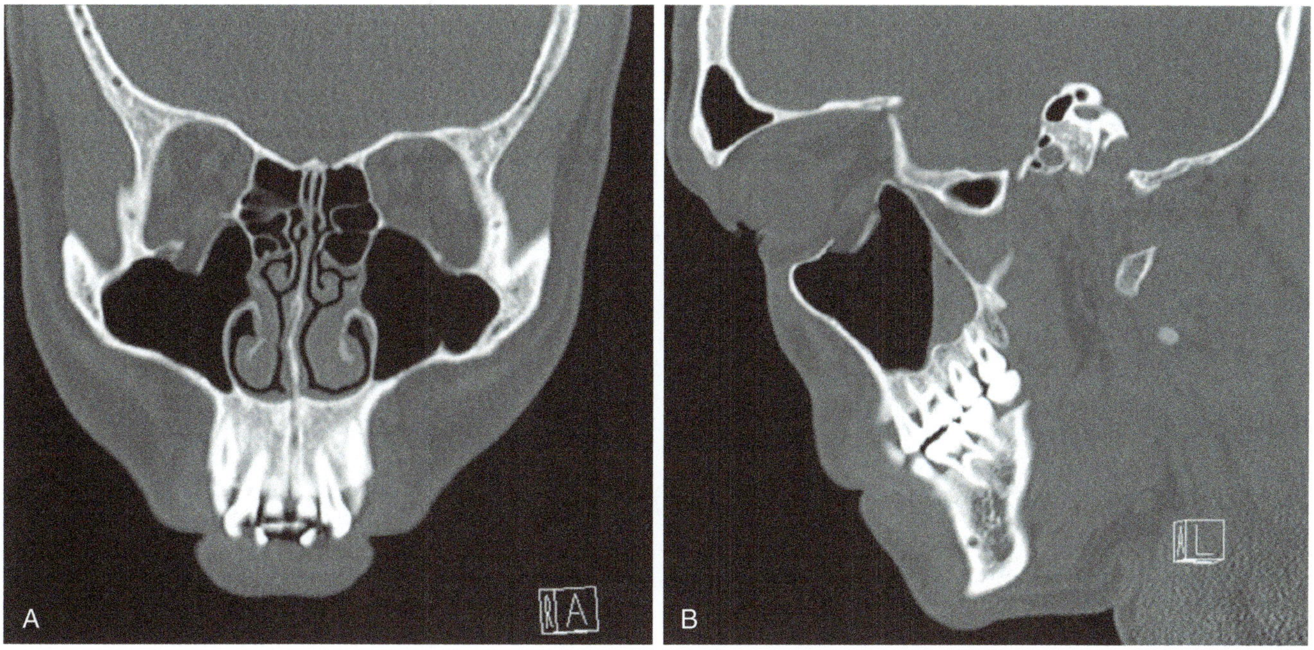

• **Fig. 34.34** A blow-out fracture of the orbital floor. (A) Shows the fragment hinged medially. (B) Shows the same fracture in the sagittal view and also shows the upward bulge of the posterior floor.

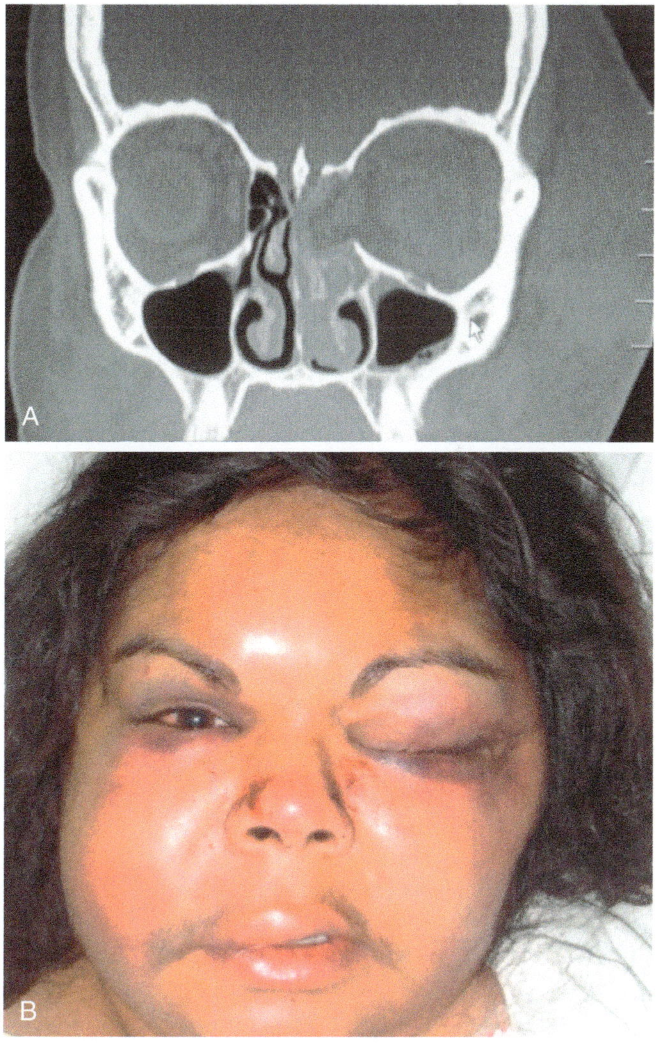

• **Fig. 34.35** A massive medial wall blow-out fracture; the swelling and hematoma hide the inevitable severe enophthalmos.

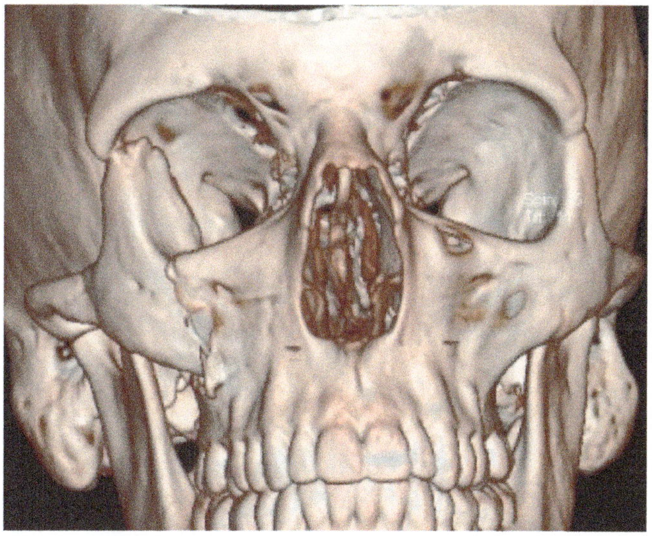

• **Fig. 34.36** The fractured zygoma is displaced posteromedially, overlapping the sphenoid and decreasing the orbital volume.

In the case of a very extensive defect when the posterior margins may be difficult to reach and define, Tessier suggested removal of the orbital rim, placing microplates on the fragment, thus obtaining a much better exposure. Once the repair is completed, the plated rim is replaced (Fig. 34.43).

Complications of Orbital Fractures

Complications are still seen in spite of the use of modern treatment modalities. Residual problems may stem from the initial injurious process, from incomplete surgical restoration, or from the operative exposure itself.[23]

Ocular problems usually relate to the initial injury and are not affected by the bony reconstruction. Persistent diplopia

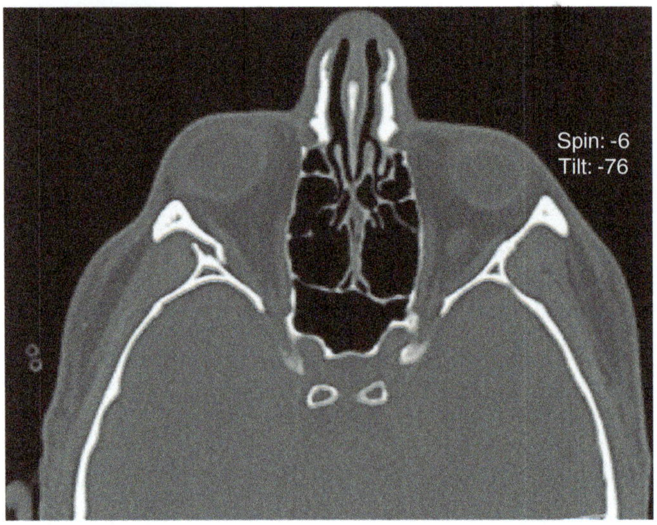

• **Fig. 34.37** The displaced zygoma decreases the orbital volume and causes proptosis.

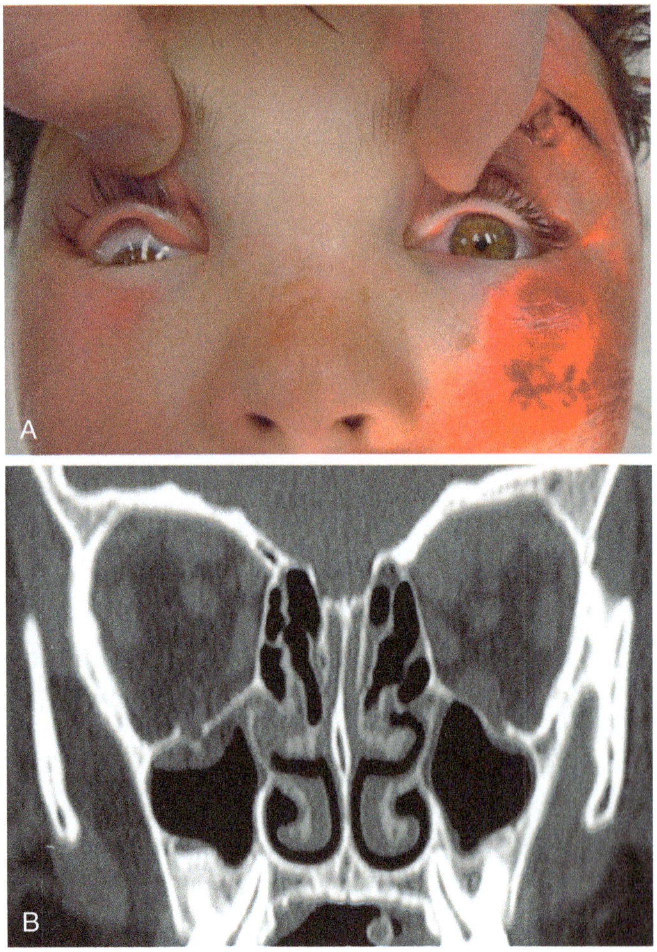

• **Fig. 34.38** The cause of (A) the restriction of upward gaze can be seen in (B) the coronal CT scan: the belly of the inferior rectus muscle is pinched in a small orbital floor fracture. Early release is indicated.

in the initial postoperative period is not uncommon but is seldom noted in long-term follow-up. Careful ophthalmological assessment will detect any muscle weakness or restriction of gaze and some of these patients may need ocular muscle surgery.

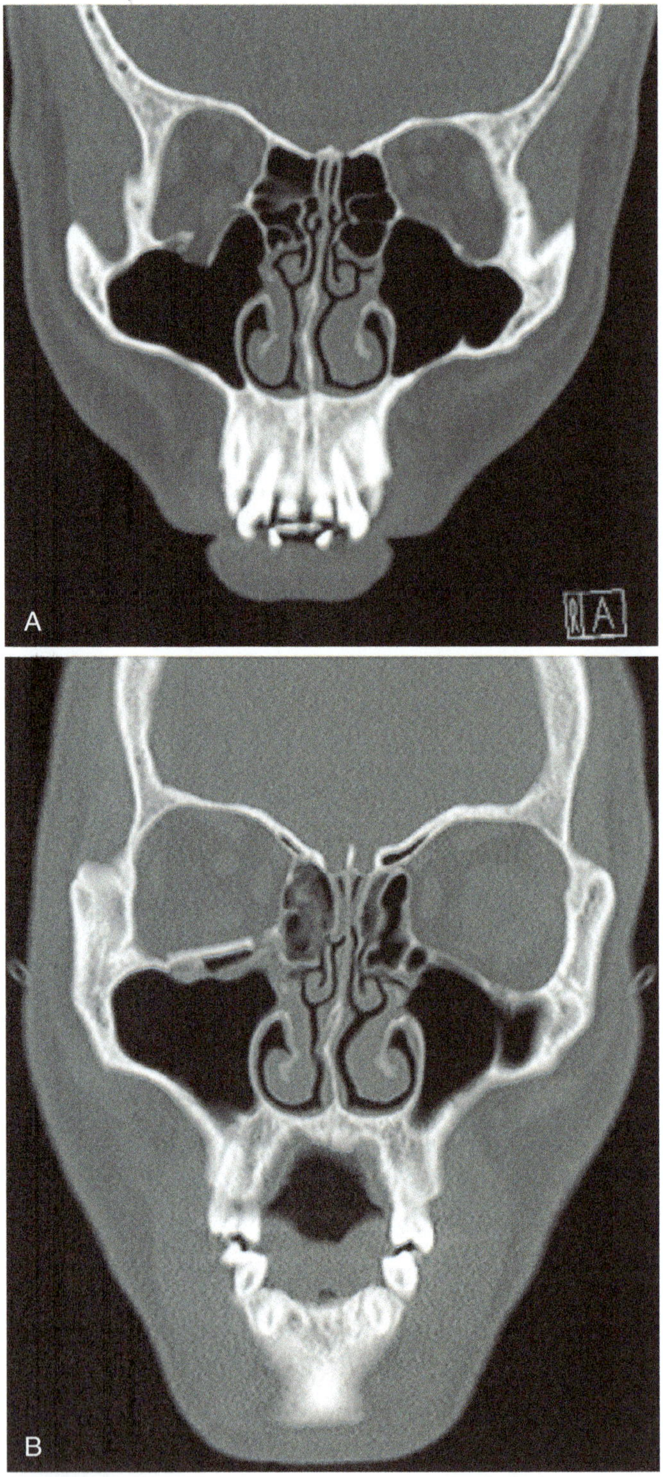

• **Fig. 34.39** (A) Before and (B) after coronal CT showing the repair of a severe blow-out fracture of the orbital floor with a bone graft taken from the blade of the ilium.

With significant bony displacement at the orbital apex and superior orbital fissure, optic nerve damage and/or ophthalmoplegia can occur.

Enophthalmos is the commonest complication; this has become less since the recognition of and the ability to treat medial wall fractures. It remains hard for the treating surgeon to judge the volume of orbital contents lost or

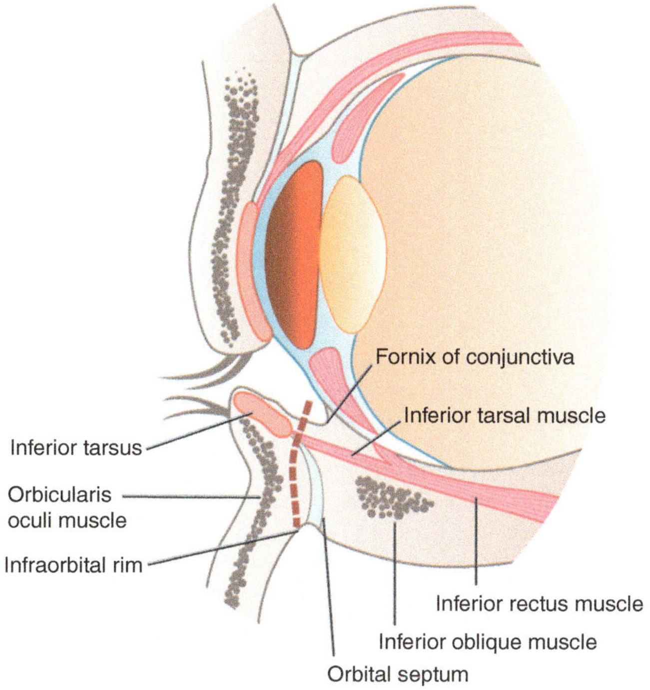

• **Fig. 34.40** A sagittal illustration of the transconjunctival approach to the orbital floor. The approach to the orbital floor begins inferior to the tarsal plate of the lower eyelid. The incision is made in front of the orbital septum down to the maxilla just inferior to the orbital rim. The periosteum is then elevated over the rim to expose the floor.

damaged by the trauma and hence if and by how much to overcorrect the orbital wall defect.

Global dystopia may occur with poorly reduced fractures of the bones constituting the orbit, as well as under- or overcorrection of the walls. In a very few cases this may need secondary orbital osteotomy to correct the deformity.

Canthal dystopia occurs medially when the ligament has been disrupted and not correctly reattached, and laterally, most commonly when a lateral canthotomy has been performed and inaccurately repaired.[24]

Mandible Fractures

Fractures of the mandible are common; in a report from a major Australian trauma center these fractures were the most common requiring surgery, although orbital fractures, many of which did not require surgery, were the most common in the series.[25] The incidence of mandibular fracture is higher in males than in females with a peak incidence in the third decade of life. Interpersonal violence accounts for the majority of fractures in males, whereas falls account for the majority of fractures in females. With the aging population in Western society, the incidence of mandibular fractures in the elderly resulting from falls is increasing.

The mandible is a very strong bone, designed to withstand forces applied in mastication, however it has areas of weakness that include the condylar processes, the angle, and the anterior body in relation to the deep root of the canine tooth. The fact that it has an articulation with the base of the skull at the temporomandibular joint complicates the management of fractures of the mandible. The joint's integrity needs to be restored and its position and function respected in the management of fractures of this bone.

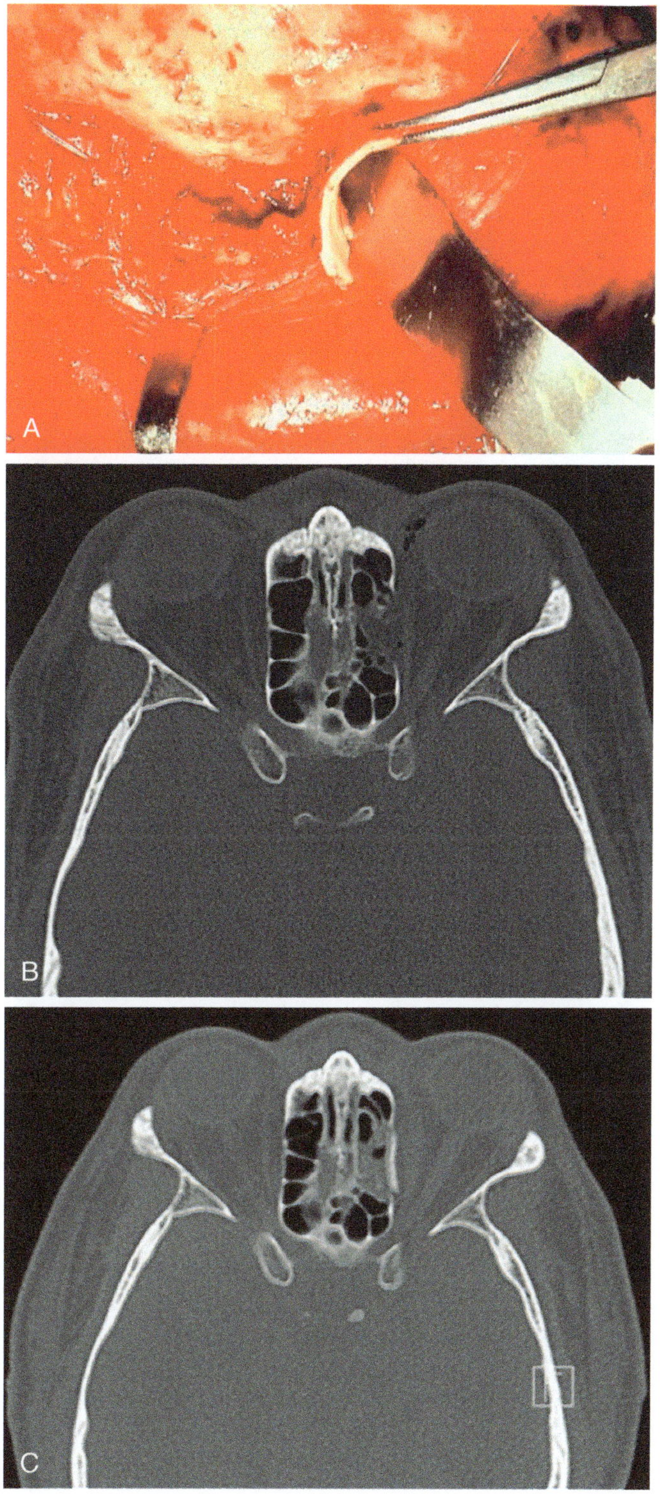

• **Fig. 34.41** (A) Bone being inserted into the medial orbital wall via a coronal flap. (B) A medial wall blow-out fracture. (C) Postoperative scan showing the bone graft in situ.

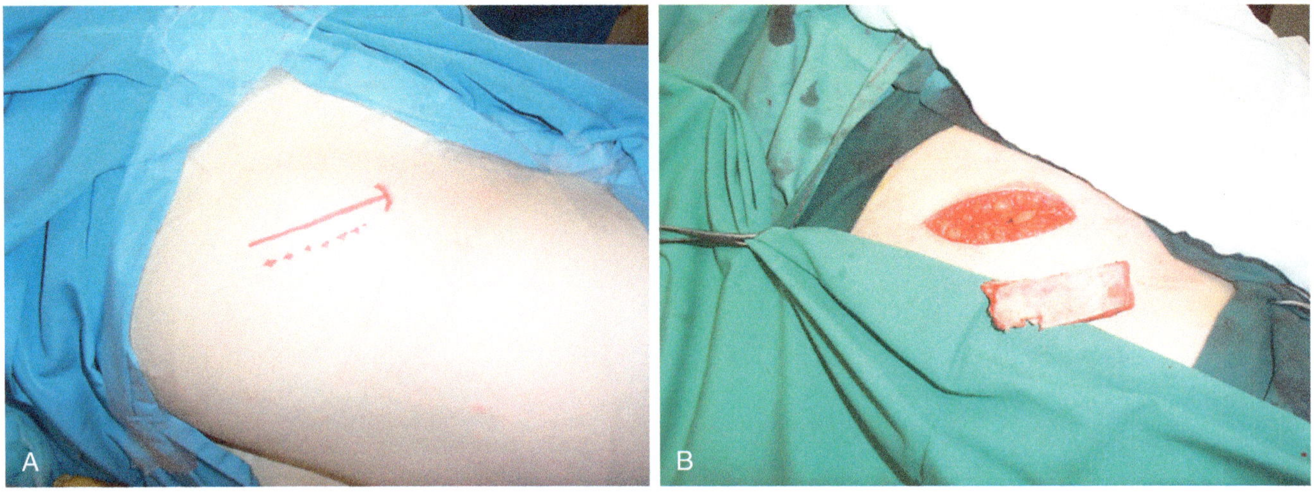

• **Fig. 34.42** Bone harvested from the inner side of the ilium is smooth, and can be easily contoured for orbital reconstruction.

Anatomy

This robust bone occupies a prominent exposed position in the facial skeleton. It articulates with the cranial base through its condyles, which lie in the glenoid fossae. The joint is divided into two cavities by a disc of fibrocartilage. The joint acts as a hinge but also allows a sliding movement in the anteroposterior plane. The mandible comprises a number of components: the condyles, the coronoid processes, the rami, the angles, and the two halves of the body joined arterially at the symphysis. Viewed from the lateral aspect, the ramus forms an angle of about 120 degrees with the body of the bone in the adult, slightly more than the very young and elderly. When viewed from the superior aspect there is a slight divergence of the rami. The alveolar portion of the bone supporting the molar teeth does not follow the same line as that formed by the lower border of the mandible.

Functionally, the mandible can be regarded as two conjoined L-shaped cantilevers, acting under the influence of the masticatory muscles. The temporalis muscle inserts predominantly into the medial surface of the coronoid processes, the masseter into the lateral surface of the angle of the ramus. The medial pterygoid muscle inserts on the medial surface of the angle and lower ramus; together with the masseter, it forms a powerful sling acting on the ramus. The two heads of the lateral pterygoid muscles unite to insert into the anterior part of the capsule of the temporomandibular joint and the pterygoid plate. The action of this muscle is important in functional recovery after intracapsule fractures of the condyle and its insertion must be preserved.

In cross-section, the body of the mandible is seen as being composed of strong inner and outer cortical plates of bone between which are inserted the teeth and their roots which are imbedded in cancellous bone. Between the two plates of cortical bone runs the inferior dental canal, which contains the inferior dental nerve, entering the bone at the mandibular foramen and exiting at the mental foramen.

Mandibular fractures may be classified simply on the anatomical site of the fracture (Fig. 34.44). They may be linear or comminuted, and the fragment size may be displaced or undisplaced. The distinction between compound and non-compound mandibular fractures is important, as any displaced fracture through a tooth root is inevitably compound and fractures of the ramus and condylar region are not compound unless caused by an entering agent, such as a gunshot. The presence or absence of teeth on either side of the fracture line is also important from the viewpoint of treatment by intermaxillary fixation or interfragment fixation, and this justifies the classification (Fig. 34.45):

- Class I – teeth on either side of the fracture
- Class II – teeth on the one side only
- Class III – edentulous.

Clinical Assessment

The clinical assessment is based on a thorough history and complete examination, the history being very important because many cases of fractured mandible are due to assault and vehicle accidents which may involve subsequent litigation. The history should establish whether dentures were worn at the time of the accident and whether there had been any previous disease. The fractured mandible may be a part of multiple traumas and resuscitation is the first priority; nevertheless, it is important even in cases with life-threatening injuries to make a thorough preliminary assessment by palpation of the facial skeleton and examination of the oral cavity, including the dentition.

Where possible, get the patient to point out the areas of pain or tenderness and ask the patient to feel the teeth with the tongue tip to detect dental irregularities, chipping, and loss of dental restoration. The patient is asked to map out any areas of numbness on the face and an accurate record of bruising is made.

External and internal lacerations may give a clue to the mechanism of fracture and external chin lacerations may point to a condylar fracture. Steps in the dental arch are noted as they indicate a fracture, as may local swelling and bruising of the gingival tissues or lacerations of the oral mucosa. When the patient is asked to bite the teeth together, they can determine whether the occlusion feels normal and the nature of the occlusion is noted. If the patient is edentulous, the dentures are inspected for signs of injury. The assessor then proceeds to palpate the mandible through the overlying soft tissues from behind and from in front, and notes tenderness and deformity. Compression of the angles will usually cause pain in an otherwise occult fracture. Examination of the

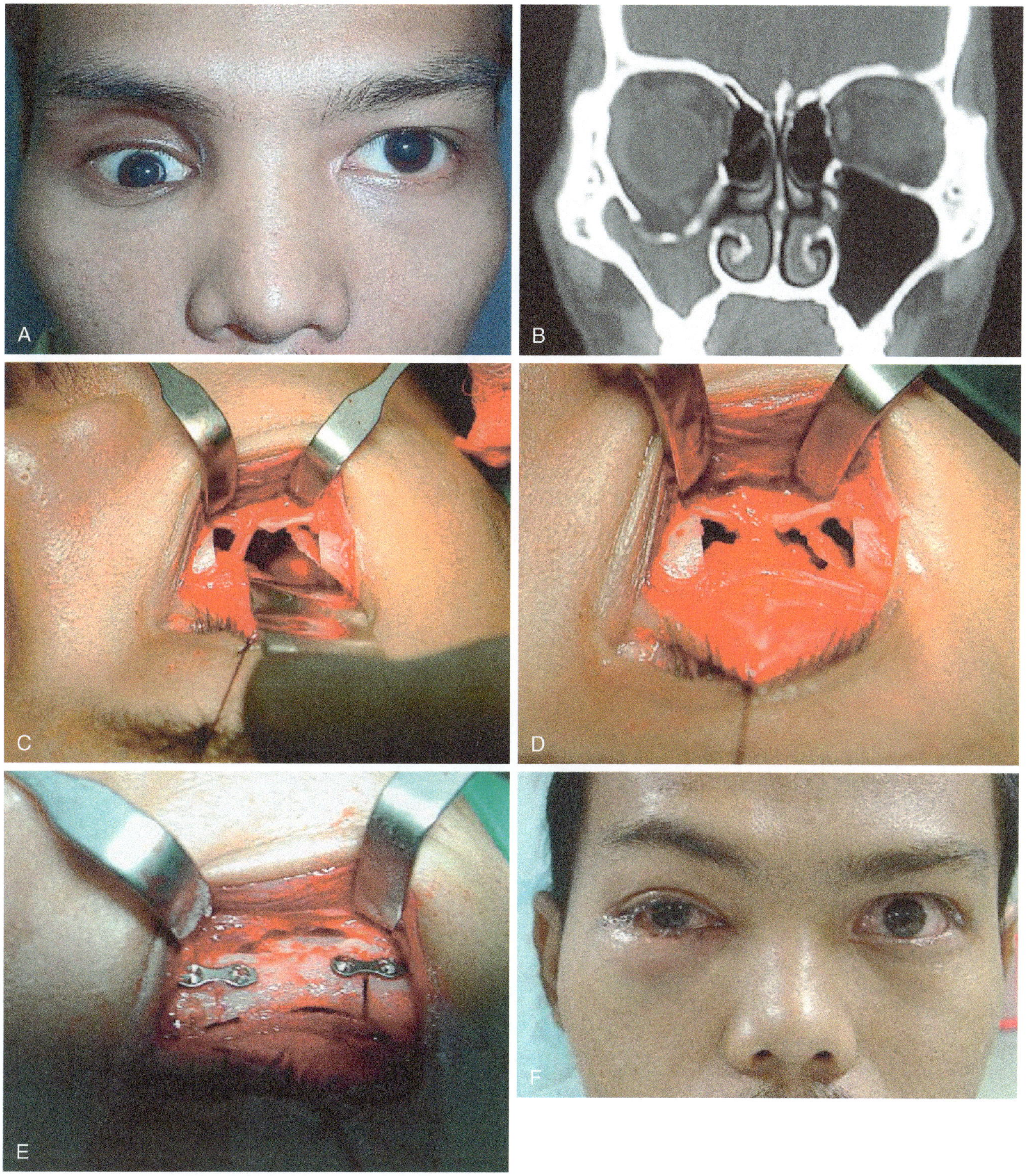

• **Fig. 34.43** (A,B) Patient with a massive orbital floor fracture and global dystopia. (C,D) Removal of a segment of orbital rim exposes the orbital floor which is reconstructed with bone graft. (E) The rim replaced and fixed with microplates (after Tessier). (F) Postoperative correction. (From Winn HR. *Youmans Neurological Surgery*. 6th edn. Philadelphia: Saunders; 2011, with permission from Elsevier.)

temporomandibular joint for pain, swelling, loss of mobility and abnormal movement or crepitus is important.[10] Neurological examination may show sensory loss in the lower lip from damage to the inferior dental nerve.

Imaging

Radiological assessment classically involved the OPG and the Towne's anteroposterior view. The OPG allowed inspection of the entire mandible and mandibular dentition on a single film, being a composite of the two lateral views. However, the tomographic process results in blurring in the symphyseal region and fractures here may be missed. Moreover, the patient needs to sit and this may be impossible in severely injured or uncooperative patients. This technique remains the mainstay of assessment and follow-up radiology for mandibular fractures. CT images give the most useful information on the integrity of the buccal and lingual plates and modern CT scanning can also give good views of the temporomandibular joints when they are involved in the fracture pathology (Fig. 34.46).

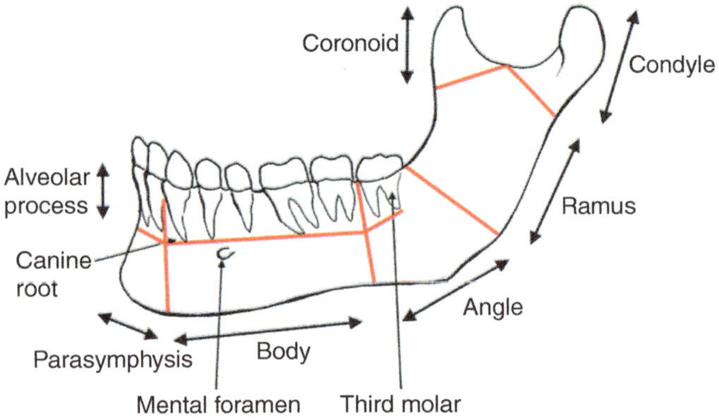

• **Fig. 34.44** Common fracture sites of the mandible. The commonly used descriptive terms for the anatomy of the mandible.

Early Management

Patients with compound mandibular fractures need to be admitted to hospital, treated with intravenous antibiotics, given appropriate pain management and prescribed an adequate fluid intake, and instructed in maintaining oral hygiene. In dentate patients with a displaced fracture, dental impressions are taken to provide a plaster cast of the occlusion in the position resulting from injury; these casts are then cut at the fracture site and mounted on an articulator in a predicted pretraumatic position so that they can be used as models in planning how to restore

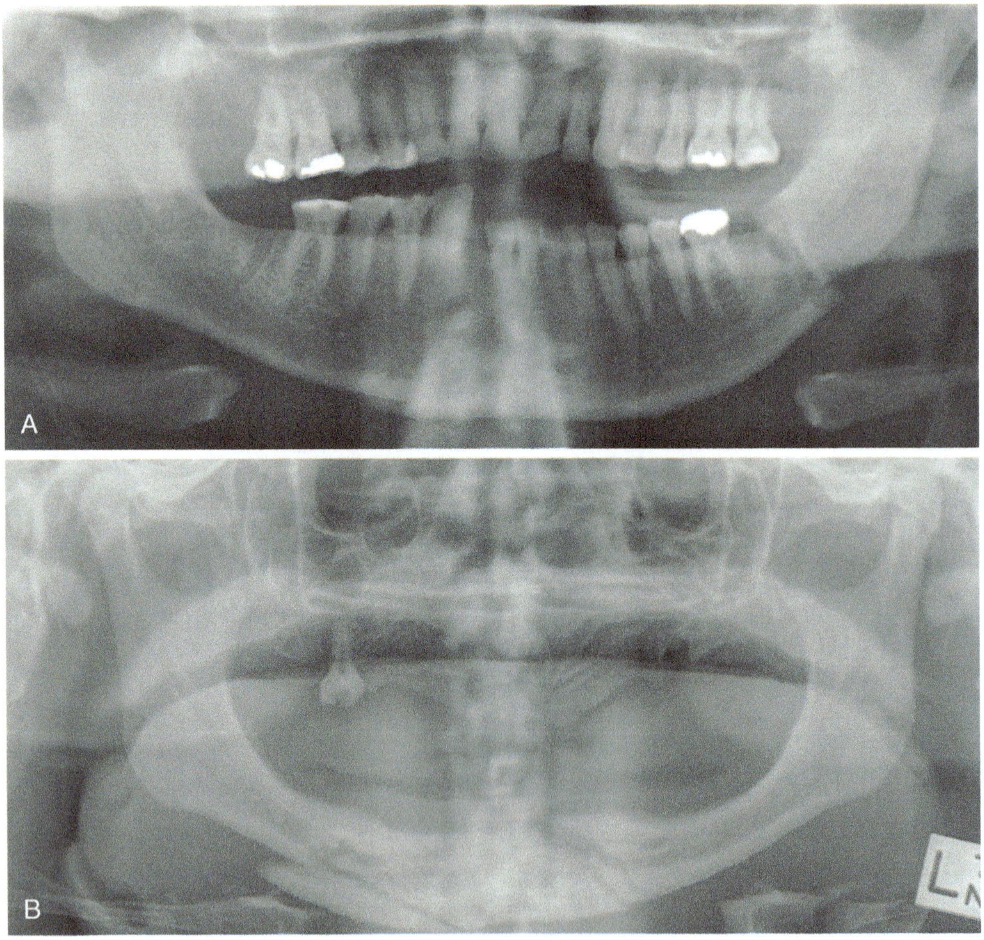

• **Fig. 34.45** (A) A parasymphyseal fracture with teeth on both fragments – Class I. A left angle fracture with a tooth on one fragment – Class II. (B) Fractures in an edentulous mandible – Class III.

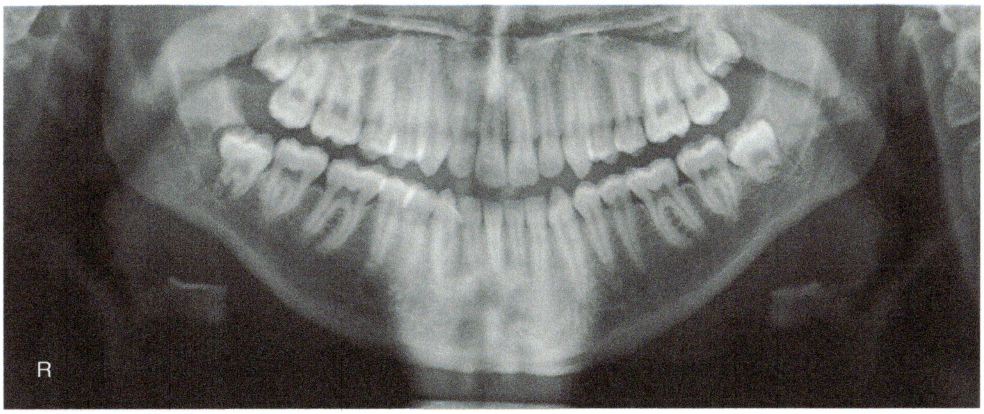

• **Fig. 34.46** An orthopantomogram showing a fracture of the right angle of mandible involving the partially erupted wisdom tooth. Note the clarity of the image laterally compared with the relative lack of definition at the symphysis.

the pretraumatic occlusion as accurately as possible. From this structure an acrylic wafer can be made for use in the surgical reduction and fixation of the fracture.

Timing of Definitive Treatment

Often the clinical priorities of other injuries have to be taken into account. Soft tissue lacerations should be debrided and sutured within 12 hours of the injury. Some authorities favor early reduction and immobilization of compound fractures of the mandible.[26]

Others[27] believe that the best results occur if operations are done with good instrumentation with experienced staff after thorough assessment and work-up, and this may extend the period of time between trauma and definitive treatment if an increased infection rate was not noticed under these circumstances.

Conservative Management

Stable fractures without displacement are best treated conservatively by a liquid nonchewed diet and analgesics. Sometimes a soft padded neck collar may be worn to support the chin. This regimen can be used for unilateral fractures of the angle and body of the mandible in elderly edentulous patients and in greenstick fractures of children. Some ramus fractures are splinted by the masseter muscle laterally and the medical pterygoid muscle medially and lend themselves to conservative management. Undisplaced hairline fractures of the body or angle which extend infection o a dental root may cause more of a problem with respect to affecting the viability of the tooth, so long-term dental follow-up is mandatory. In a sensible patient who is likely to comply with good follow-up and dental management, conservative treatment would have a good chance of success.

Principles of Operative Fixation

Historically, mandibular fractures were fixed by external intermaxillary fixation, but this method has faded into antiquity. More recently, closed reduction and intermaxillary fixation, where the jaws were fixed together in occlusion for a prolonged period of time, has been used, aided in class II fractures by interfragmentary wiring. However, these methods are rarely practised today, or even thought of since the advent of internal osteosynthesis with miniplates. Although there is still much debate about the number, siting, and composition of the plates, this mode of treatment is widely preferred and allows early release of intermaxillary fixation, followed by support of the mandible with light elastics, which entails minimal time in hospital, ability to feed and facilitation of oral hygiene. It also avoids the risks associated with prolonged intermaxillary fixation and the presence of the devices that are used to secure it.

When a fracture extends into a dental root, it is arguable as to whether it is necessary to extract the tooth or not in order to lessen the risk of subsequent infection. The consequence of removing such teeth and converting a potentially stable fracture into an unstable fracture is less of an issue with miniplate fixation used as the primary treatment. The author's rational has been to retain teeth in the fracture line where these teeth have potential function, either in establishing the occlusion or as a fixation post for subsequent prosthodontic work, assuming that the teeth have a chance of survival. When there is severe fracturing of the tooth with comminution of the surrounding alveolar bone, infection is almost certain and the tooth should be extracted. When an impacted third molar is involved in an angle fracture it is customary to extract it as the tooth rarely has a function part in the occlusion, and retention of such a tooth may lead to future infection. Rubin et al[28] have shown that completely erupted molars may be left in a fracture line without increasing risk of complications.

Miniplate Osteosynthesis

Miniplate fixation in the modern context goes back to 1958, when the Association for Osteosynthesis/Association for the Study of Internal Fixation (AO/ASIF) system was introduced and showed the value of rigid mobilization and coaption of bone ends and securing bone union. Initially the plates were made of stainless steel before Hans Luhr developed a system in Würzburg using vitallium and producing compression with bicortical screws. More recently, titanium plates have been preferred because they are malleable, radiolucent, and have high biocompatibility. The search continues for suitable resorbable implants for mandibular fixation.

Success in plating fractures of the mandible depends on an understanding of the mechanical forces acting through the mandible during mastication. The mandible is normally subjected to tension forces of its upper border and to compression forces at the lower border unless the fracture is inherently self-stabilizing. There will therefore be distraction of the upper or alveoli end of the fracture and the plating system must counteract this distraction. Champy et al[29] described an ideal line for the siting of the plate, as shown in Fig. 34.47. They demonstrated the presence of rotational torsion forces in the anterior mandible, which is a three-dimensional structure upon which bilateral muscular groups act. They also recommended a lower border plate as well as an upper border plate to give better control of these torsional forces. In the tooth-bearing alveolar area the thickness of the bone is variable and unsuitable for screw fixation; the upper boarder of the mandible is therefore the ideal site.

Champy et al showed that the average thickness of the outer cortex of the mandible is 5 mm but in some areas the cortex is less than 3 mm thick. There is therefore some danger of injuring the inferior dental nerve. Care should therefor be taken to drill only through the outer cortex and use the smallest possible screws.

In certain situations the usual tension/compression relation-ships can be reversed. This may be the case when a bite load is placed just anterior to an angle fracture and the contralateral muscle sling is functioning normally but the ipsilateral sling is ineffective from posttraumatic oedema and bruising. In addition to this theoretical concept of intermittent reversal of the normal tension–compression zones, there is also some clinical evidence of unfavorable results with angle fractures treated with only a single plate as Champy suggests. Levey et al[30] had a significantly higher complication rate with using one plate rather than two. It has been the author's experience that the Champy principle with a single upper border plate for angle fractures has been more than satisfactory. It has emerged, however, that in noncompliant patients firmer bracket fixation by applying a second plate may be needed.

The Champy technique of upper border single-plate osteosynthesis is mostly successful for angle fractures providing the patient is compliant and does not chew and the reduction is accurate.

Compression Plates

Because the mandible is an asymmetrical structure, bicortical screws and compression plates are required. The compression plating systems have a consistent potential drawback. Because the compression is applied across the buccal plate

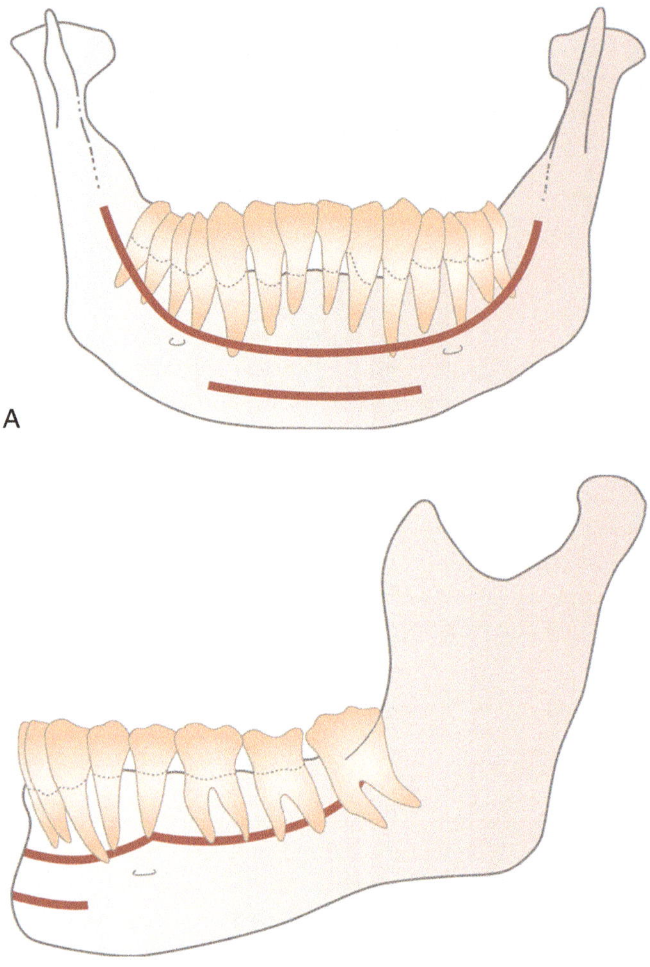

A

B

• **Fig. 34.47** (A) The mandibular tension line is at the junction of the dentoalveolar bone and the mandibular base bone (Champy). (B) The anterior body reverse tension line. The anterior lower borderline is the site for lower border plates in conjunction with upper border plates when fractures cross this area (Champy).

of bone there is the possibility that the fracture line may be opened on the lingual side and this can lead to a significant cross bite. Efforts have been made to contour the plates extremely accurately so that this does not occur. In practice, it does not appear that the healing claimed by compression systems is any more advanced than that of noncompression systems.

Operative Management According to Champy

The patient is prepared in the usual fashion using an acrylic wafer to register the occlusion and the application of arch bars or intermaxillary fixation screws. A nasoendotracheal tube is usually necessary. The incision to explore an angle fracture is placed just lateral to the anterior boarder of the ramus and runs down beyond the third molar just lateral to the inferior buccal sulcus. The incision is deep into the bone and the fracture line exposed by subperiosteal dissection down to the inferior border of the mandible. A posterior border retractor combined with a notched anterior border retractor will give good exposure. When the third molar is to be extracted, care is taken not to fracture the external oblique ridge of the bone as this is important for the fixation.

After removal of the tooth, the socket is cleaned and irrigated; care is taken not to injure the inferior dental nerve, which is sometimes exposed by the fracture. It is important to spend some time cleaning the edges of the fracture of granulation tissue and irrigating the area thoroughly in order to wash away debris. The fracture is reduced manually into its correct anatomical position. The occlusion is established and intermaxillary fixation is applied. The pretraumatic position of the occlusion is established by the use of the dental wafer. Once the jaw is secured with the intermaxillary wiring and the fracture reduced anatomically, it is relatively easy to apply the miniplate according to Champy's principles. A four-hole titanium miniplate with two monocortical 5 mm screws on either side of the fracture line is adequate (Fig. 34.48).

The incision to explore a fracture of the body is placed to the labial side of the inferior sulcus. In order to preserve the mental nerve, the scalpel is angled back sharply under the sulcus down to the bone, the periosteum is incised and the fracture exposed by subperiosteal dissection in the usual manner. If the fracture is laterally placed, the mental nerve in its foramen must also be exposed and preserved. In both the angle and body fractures, care must be taken to drill only the outer cortex and the plates are bent as accurately as possible to conform to the contours of the mandible. Some plating systems use malleable titanium with no memory and these can be contoured very accurately with the screw pressure.

Sometimes it is warranted to modify the standard method in fractures in the angle area on the external oblique ridge, some operators preferring the six-hole plate and longer screws and, where there is some doubt about the reduction of the fracture at the lower order of the mandible, some operators prefer to place the second plate in this region, still using an intraoral approach but combined with percutaneous drilling and screwing through a cannula.

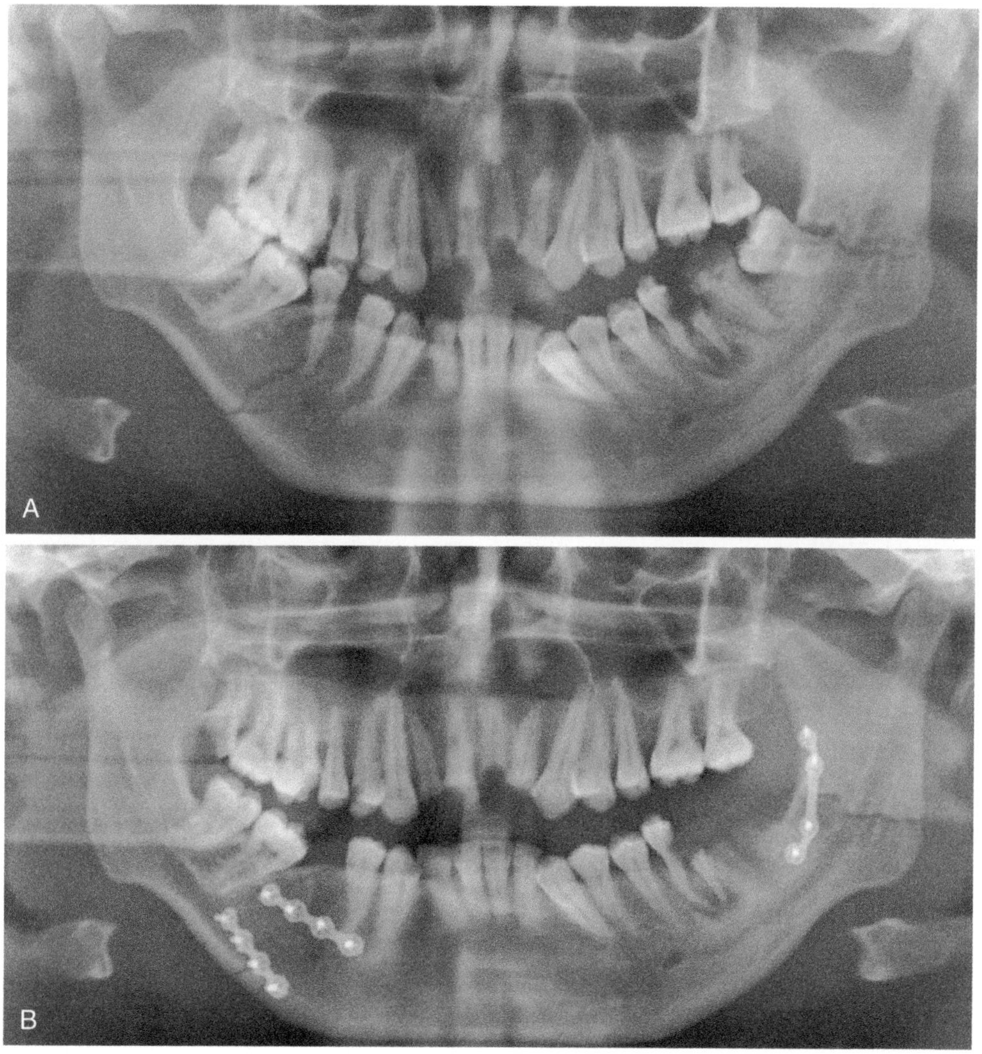

• **Fig. 34.48** A left angle and right body fracture in a jaw with carious teeth and teeth involved in both fractures. The monocortical plates have been used according to Champy after removal of the teeth in the fractures.

With body fractures, it is usual to apply the four-hole plate to the upper border of the body with two monocortical screws on either side of the fracture line and a similar plate applied to the lower border, avoiding the nerve. Intraoral wounds are usually closed with an absorbable suture. The temporary intermaxillary fixation is removed and the excursions of the mandible are checked with special attention to the ability to bite into occlusion. The arch bars or fixation screws are left in situ and the jaws are supported by light elastic rubber traction to overcome any imbalance in the masticatory muscles caused by injury and swelling. The elastic traction may be maintained for a number of days, being removed once the patient settles into their normal occlusion.

The postoperative management includes a dose of intravenous antibiotics at the time of surgery, clear fluids, soft diet, and mouth toilet. Postoperative radiology is important to check the reduction of the fracture. This regime facilitates early discharge from hospital and encourages self-care. Follow-up at regular intervals including a postoperative dental assessment is important and long-term follow-up is routine for 12 months. If there are clinical reasons, the patient may be seen beyond that in order to check the healing of scars, the recovery of any areas of sensory loss, and the return of normal mastication.

Complications of Fractures of the Body and Angle of the Mandible

Complications include:
- Infection
- Nonunion
- Malocclusion and malunion
- Plate exposure
- Nerve injury and/or dental injury due to drilling the body of the mandible.

Infection

The instance varies in different reports and the causes are disputed. The argument that early surgery on the mandible prevents infection[26] has been made; others[30] reported a high incidence of infection when plates were used. Anderson and Alpert[31] gave special attention to fractures of the mandibular angle when only one miniplate was used without intermaxillary fixation, giving it an infection rate of 22%. Once infection is diagnosed and a wound culture is taken, intravenous antibiotics are started. If radiology reveals a fracture displacement or bone sequestrum or any complication relating to a plate, the fracture is explored and the foreign and necrotic material removed. Teeth in the fracture line need to be extracted. The occlusion can be reestablished and where there is bone contact with the fracture, replating can be undertaken. If there is discontinuity of the bone, a bone graft may be inserted with rigid fixation and adequate drainage.

Nonunion

This is clinically indistinguishable from infection and in principle the treatment is the same.

Malocclusion and Malunion

Some malocclusion can result from inadequate or inappropriate reduction of the fracture but may also be a consequence of orthodontic movement of teeth that have been wired to arch bars or the result of imbalanced masticatory muscles and the management can be relatively conservative. If the cause of malocclusion is shown by X-ray to be due to inadequate reduction of the fracture, it may have been due to the operative procedure and reoperation is necessary to reduce the fracture again and fix it more strongly in its correct position. If there is true malunion and the bone is united and there is a malocclusion then an osteotomy will be required.

Plate Exposure

Miniplate exposure may be due to poor operative technique and suturing mucosa or due to postoperative trauma. It is usually safe to leave the plate exposed until healing is complete in 6 weeks, in which case the plate can be removed without compromising the result.

Nerve Injury

Injury to the inferior dental nerve is usually the result of the trauma but may occur with poor operative technique and radiology will show whether a screw is impinging on the inferior dental nerve canal. Sensory recovery or failure of recovery to the inferior dental nerve should be watched for over 12–18 months. Some operators would uncover the canal and attempt to anastomose the nerve or indeed graft it.[32]

Fractures and Fracture Dislocations of the Condyle

Surgical Pathology

The condyle is the part of the mandible that passes vertically up from the posterior border above the sigmoid notch to the glenoid fossa of the temporal bone. Fractures may occur at any level in the sigmoid notch, thereby including a variable amount of the ramus in the condylar fragment (Fig. 34.49).

Sagittal fractures of the condylar head are rare; however, there may be dislocation of the fractured condyle in a posterior, anterior, medial or lateral position, and very rarely vertical dislocation into the cranial fossa.

Attempts at Classification

The classification devised by Lund[33] has the merit of being very simple:
- Type I: enlocated head with or without displacement at the fracture site with no more than 60 degrees angulation
- Type II: a dislocated head with 90 degrees or more angulations.

Lund also described this fracture as either high, involving the head or neck, or low, at the base of the condylar process.[33]

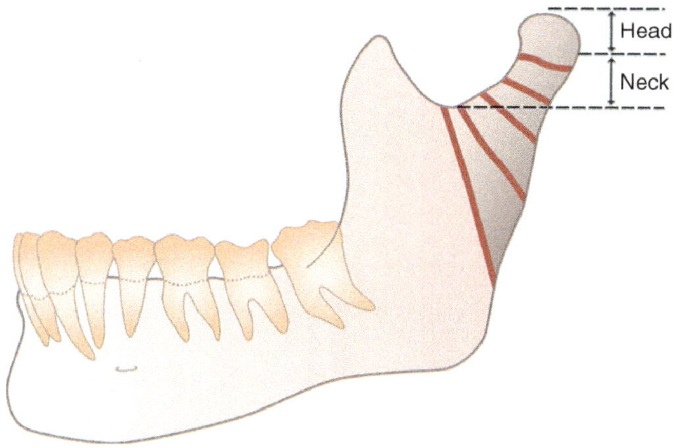

• **Fig. 34.49** Anatomy of condylar fractures. A condylar fracture is one that separates the condylar head from the corpus of the mandible, but excludes the coronoid. These fractures all pass through the sigmoid notch and are deemed high or low.

Clinical Assessment

A proper clinical assessment commences with a thorough history as well as a complete examination, and a history of the causation of the fracture will often point in the direction of the temporomandibular joint. Pain in the region, together with trismus, is a common combination in these circumstances. Attempting to open the mouth will be painful and the movement restricted, and this may be bilateral. When the fracture is unilateral, any attempt at opening of the mouth will cause deviation of the chin point towards the affected side.

Bleeding from the external auditory canal may indicate a compound fracture into the external ear canal and otoscopic examination of the meatus may show a tear in the lining of the canal. Bimanual palpation of the condyles during movement may detect swelling, tenderness, and the absence of a normal condylar head. With respect to occlusion, typically bilateral condylar fractures cause an anterior open bite not present before injury, whereas a unilateral fracture causes lateral cross bite. The clinician should always keep in mind the possible presence of multiple facial fractures.

Radiological Assessment

The standard OPG and Towne's views have mostly now been replaced by CT scanning, and the modern fine-cut CT scan can be reproduced as a solid image and even converted to nylon models which may, in complicated cases, be of great help in surgical planning (Fig. 34.50).

Principles of Treatment

The management of these injuries is controversial. In children, there may be restitution of the fractured condylar head and remodeling of the displaced fracture and associated compensatory growth which would support a conservative plan of management in the young. This is not repeated, however, as growth nears completion.[34] When the fractures are intracapsular and unable to be successfully reduced in an open fashion then the management is conservative, relying on reduction of pain, supporting the occlusion and early mobilization with the application of dental arch bars and elastic traction.

In the mature patient, when there is a fracture that can be fixed by open reduction and internal fixation with plates or other devices, this can be undertaken when the fragment is dislocated or when fixation of other fractures in the face require an intact mandible. Because the surgical approach to the temporomandibular joint is not an easy one and may be associated with complications such as facial nerve damage, there are several criteria that should be fulfilled for operative procedures to be acceptable.[35]

- The operative procedure must provide full restoration of normal function and occlusion within 6–12 weeks.
- The fracture must be reduced so that the muscles that act on the condyle regain normal tension and position.
- The displaced fragment must be large enough to be reduced and stabilized in three dimensions.
- The stabilization must be able to maintained until bone union occurs.
- The operation must not damage the attachments of the lateral pterygoid muscle for the condylar head.
- There must be no operative morbidity from injury to the nerves and other important structures or to mandibular growth.

Operative Management

Zide and Kent[35] produced a list of absolute indications for open reduction and internal fixation of fractures of the condyle. Other authors have slight variation on this list but the principles are essentially the same:

- Fracture dislocation of the head into the middle cranial fossa or into the temporal fossa if associated with clinical disability
- Intra-articular foreign body
- Lateral extracapsular dislocation of the condyle
- Inability to open the mouth or to bring the mandible into occlusion after a week with evidence of bony block
- Compound injuries (e.g., gunshot wounds)
- Displaced condylar fracture where the fracture line is near the lower border of the sigmoid notch and the head is dislocated from the glenoid fossa
- Condylar fracture where the vertical displacement is associated with displaced fracture of the upper jaw.

The ideal situation is where there is enough bone substance to hold two plates, giving rigid fixation and a capacity for immediate mobilization. The condyle may be approached through an intraoral incision and various skin incisions. Lately, some authors have used endoscopic assistance in this surgery. The author has found the most acceptable approach in his practice is through a coronal scalp flap, but extended in front of the ear to the level of the tragus. It is often unnecessary to make the full coronal incision. Once the zygomatic arch has been exposed, the masseter muscle is

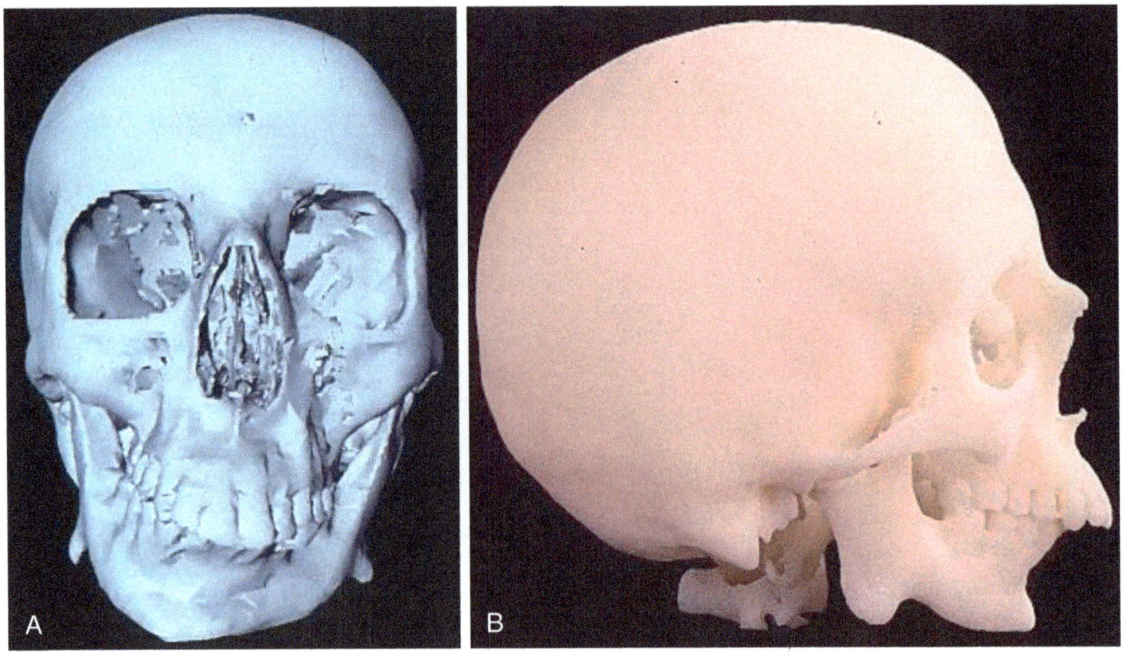

• **Fig. 34.50** (A) A 3D CT image of a patient injured in infancy; there is left temporomandibular joint ankylosis and a typical growth deformity. (B) A nylon model showing the pathology can be useful when planning reconstructive surgery.

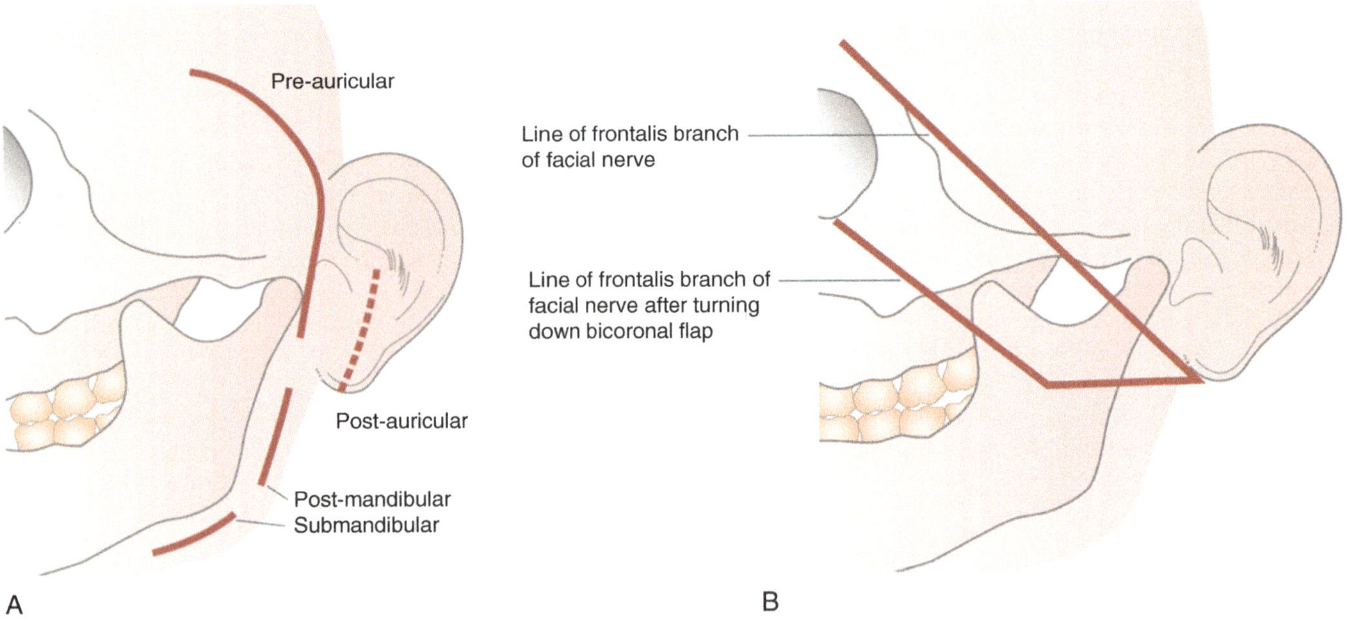

• **Fig. 34.51** (A,B) External incisions for exposure of the condyle. The coronal flap "relocates" the frontalis nerve: the act of turning down the flap relocates the nerve to a level below the sigmoid notch.

exposed and may be transacted giving a very good exposure to the condyle, upper part of the mandible, and hence the fragments (Figs. 34.51 and 34.52).

Various methods of fracture stabilization have been used once it has been exposed and reduced. Surgeons have used various types of interosseous wiring, Steinmann pins with or without wiring and external fixators and miniplates; the latter have the great advantage of giving three-dimensional stabilization while allowing early return to normal function.

The recent trend for endoscopic-assisted surgery shows promising results, however there is a steep learning curve with increased surgical time.

Complications of Condylar Fractures

These include:

- Growth disturbance
- Avascular necrosis

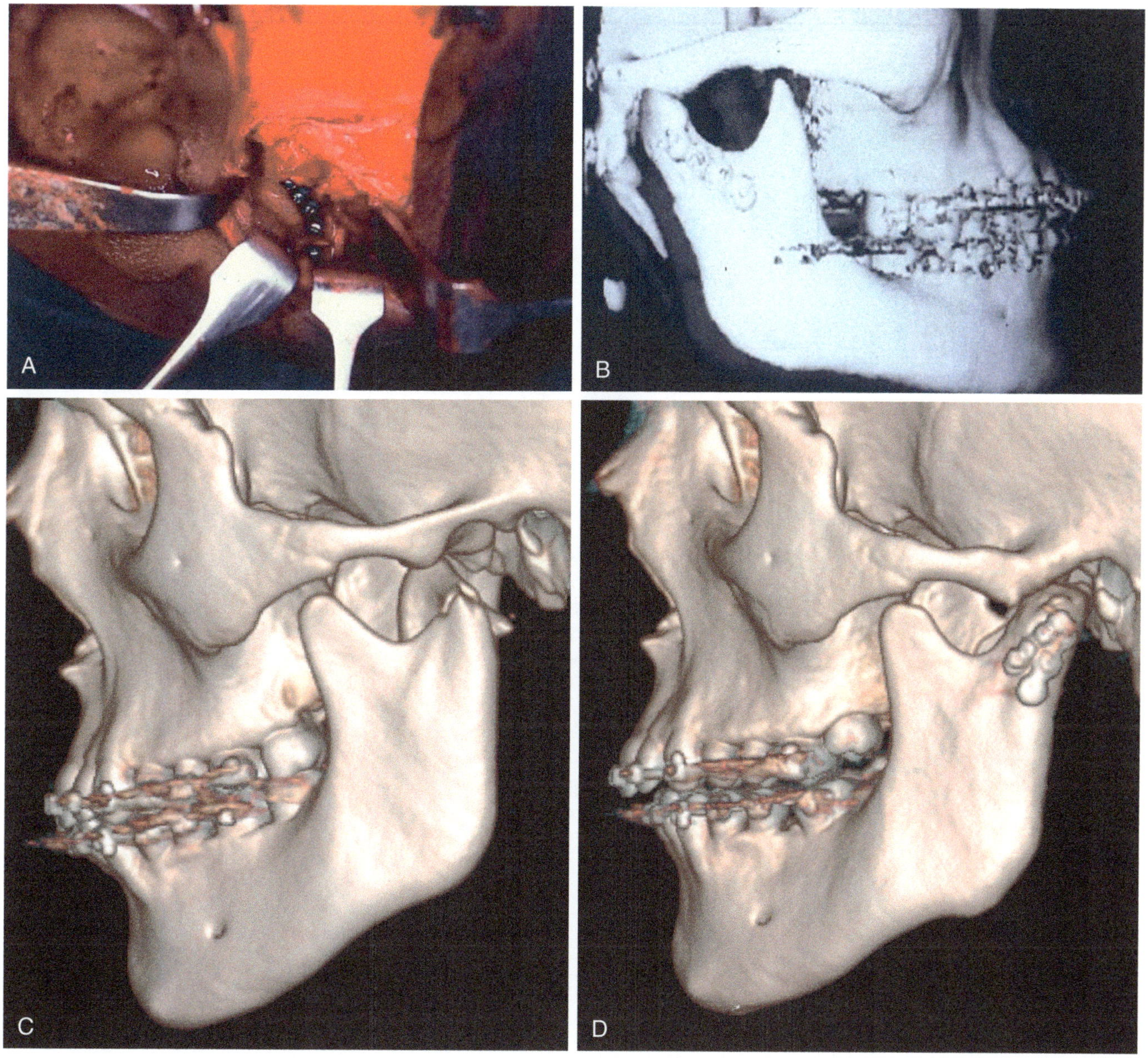

• **Fig. 34.52** (A) The fracture has been exposed via a coronal scalp flap reduced and plated. (B) The postoperative position is shown, with a single plate. (C) A similar severe fracture dislocation on the left. (D) Fixed with two plates, which is the ideal.

- Ankylosis of the temporomandibular junction
- Malunion and other temporomandibular junction dysfunctions.

Growth Disturbance

The problem is peculiar to childhood, of course, and may give rise to considerable facial asymmetry. Where the fracture is associated with infection, then severe growth disturbance may occur. This is often seen in developing countries, where malnutrition may play a part (Fig. 34.53).

Avascular Necrosis

This can be seen when an intracapsular fracture detaches a fragment of the head of the condyle which is denuded of its bloody supply. It may lead to pain and temporomandibular joint dysfunction. The avoidance of a vascular necrosis is assisted by maintaining all residual capsule attachments of the proximal fragment.

Ankyloses of the Temporomandibular Joint

This complication may develop when there has been tearing or disruption of the articular disc associated with comminution of the condylar articular surface as an intracapsular fracture. Its occurrence is minimized by early mobilization of the jaw and by careful follow-up. The patients at risk are those who have, for other reasons, a long period of intermaxillary fixation or where they have disturbed consciousness from head injuries and the problem has not been one of the first priorities in management. The long-term management of such problems can be extremely difficult.

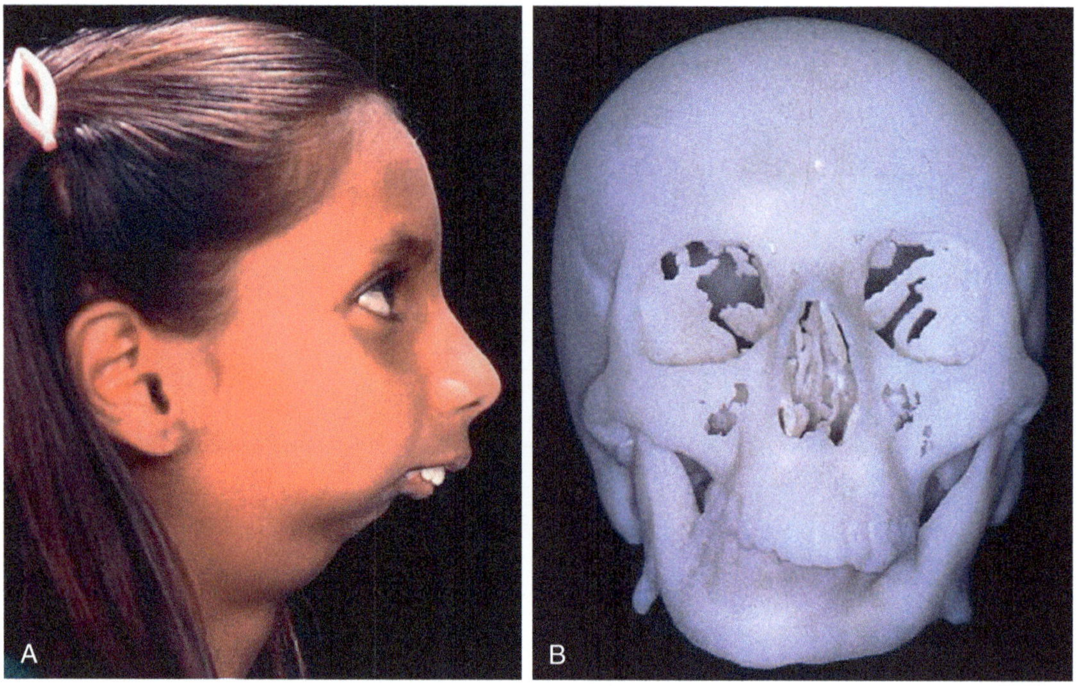

• **Fig. 34.53** (A) The result of bilateral intracapsular fractures of the mandibular condyles in childhood. The severe growth disturbance is accompanied by ankylosis of the joints. (B) A nylon model of a patient at maturity who suffered a high condylar fracture without treatment. Note the facial asymmetry, malocclusion, and fused joint.

Malunion and Other Temporomandibular Joint Dysfunctions

Standard osteotomies may restore any occlusal discrepancy due to the malunion; however, the temporomandibular joint dysfunctions that produce pain and trismus may in some patients result in crippling and chronic disruptions to their lives in spite of intensive physiotherapy and long-term pain relief.

References

1. Reilly PL, David DJ. Craniofacial injuries. In: Winn HR, ed. *Neurological Surgery*. 6th edn. Philadelphia, PA: Elsevier; 2011:3479–3496.
2. David DJ, Simpson DA, eds. *Craniomaxillofacial Trauma*. Edinburgh: Churchill Livingstone; 1995:263–342.
3. Balasubramanian C, Kaliaperumal C, Jadun CK, et al. Transorbital intracranial penetrating injury – an anatomical classification. *Surg Neurol*. 2009;71:238–240.
4. Cooter RD. *Craniofacial Fracture Patterns*. MD Thesis. University of Adelaide: Department of Surgery; 1990.
5. Hemmy DC, David DJ, Herman GT. Three-dimensional reconstruction of craniofacial deformity using computed tomography. *Neurosurgery*. 1983;13:534.
6. Markowitz BL, Mansom PN, Sargent L, et al. Management of the medial canthal tendon in nasoethmoid orbital fractures: The importance of the central fragment in classification and treatment. *Plast Reconstr Surg*. 1991;87:843–853.
7. Gruss JS. Fronto-naso-orbital trauma. *Clin Plast Surg*. 1982;9:577.
8. David DJ. Invited editorial: facial fracture classification: current thoughts and applications. *J Cranio-Maxillofac Trauma*. 1999;5:31–36.
9. Cooter RD, David DJ. Computer-based coding of fractures in the craniofacial region. *Br J Plast Surg*. 1989;42:17–26.
10. Mustardé JC. Epicanthus and telecanthus. *Br J Plast Surg*. 1963;16:346–356.
11. Dingman RO, Natvig P. *Surgery of Facial Fractures*. Philadelphia, PA: Saunders; 1964.
12. Stranc MF. Primary management of naso-ethmoid injuries with increased intercanthal distance. *Br J Plast Surg*. 1970;23:8–25.
13. Kim K, Ibrahim AM, Koolen PG, et al. Trends in facial fracture treatment using the ACS-NSQIP database. *Plast Reconstr Surg*. 2014;133(3):627–638.
14. Gruss JS, Van Wyck I, Phillips JH, et al. The importance of the zygomatic arch in complex midfacial fracture repair and correction of post traumatic orbitozygomatic deformities. *Plast Reconstr Surg*. 1990;85:875–890.
15. Gillies HD, Kilner TP, Stone D. Fractures of the malar-zygomatic compound, with description of a new X-ray position. *Br J Surg*. 1927;14:651–656.
16. Gruss JS, Mackinnon SE. Complex maxillary fractures: role of buttress reconstruction and immediate bone grafts. *Plast Reconstr Surg*. 1986;78:9–24.
17. Manson PN, Crawley WA, Yaremchuk MJ, et al. Midface fractures: advantages of immediate extended open reduction and bone grafting. *Plast Reconstr Surg*. 1985;76:1–12.
18. Lang J. *Clinical Anatomy of the Head, Neurocranium, Orbit, Craniocervical Regions*. Berlin: Springer; 1983.
19. Ahmad F, Kirkpatrick WN, Lyne J, et al. Strain gauge biomechanical evaluation of forces in orbital floor fractures. *Br J Plast Surg*. 2003;56(1):3–9.
20. Antonyshyn O, Gruss JS, Kassell EE. Blow-in fractures of the orbit. *Plast Reconstr Surg*. 1989;84:10–20.
21. Choi M, Flores RL. Medial wall fractures and the transcaruncular approach. *J Craniofac Surg*. 2012;23(3):696–701.

22. David DJ. Exploration of the orbital floor through a transconjunctival approach. *Aust N Z J Surg.* 1974;44(1):25–27.
23. Wencan W, Wentao J, Selva D, et al. Endoscopic transcaruncular repair of large medial orbital wall fractures near the orbital apex. *Ophthalmology.* 2013;120(2):404–409.
24. Mackinnon CA, David DJ, Cooter RD. Blindness and severe visual impairment in facial fractures: And 11 year review. *Br J Plast Surg.* 2002;55:1–7.
25. Cabalag MS, Wasiak J, Andrew NE, et al. Epidemiology and management of maxillofacial fractures in an Australian trauma centre. *J Plast Reconstr Aesthet Surg.* 2014;67(2):183–189.
26. Maloney PL, Welch TB, Doku HC. Early mobilisation of mandi ular fractures: a retrospective study. *J Oral Maxillofac Surg.* 1991;49:698–702.
27. Moore MH, Abbott JR, Abbott AH, et al. Monocortical noncompression miniplate osteosynthysis of mandibular angle fractures. *Aust N Z J Surg.* 1990;60:805–809.
28. Rubin MM, Koll TJ, Sadoff RS. Morbidity associated with incompletely erupted third molars in the line of mandibular fractures. *J Oral Maxillofac Surg.* 1990;48:1045–1047.
29. Champy M, Pape HD, Gerlach KL, et al. Mandibular fractures. The Strasbourg miniplate osteosynthesis. In: Kruger E, Schilli W, eds. *Oral and Maxillofacial Traumatology.* Vol. 2. Chicago, IL: Quintessence Publishing; 1986.
30. Levy FE, Smith RW, Odland RM, et al. Monocortical miniplate fixation of angle fractures. *Arch Otorhinolaryngol Head Neck Surg.* 1991;117:149–154.
31. Anderson T, Alpert B. Experience with rigid fixation of mandibular fractures and immediate function. *J Oral Maxillofac Surg.* 1992;50:555–560.
32. Jones RHB. Repair of the trigeminal nerve: A review. *Aust Dental J.* 2010;55:112–119.
33. Lund K. Mandibular growth and remodelling processes after condylar fracture. A longitudinal roentgencephalometric study. *Acta Odontol Scand Suppl.* 1974;32(64):3–117.
34. Brukmoser E, Undt E. Management and outcome of condylar fractures in children and adolescents: A review of the literature. *Oral Surg Oral Med Oral Pathol Oral Radiol.* 2012;114:86–106.
35. Zide JE, Kent JN. Indications for open reduction of mandibular condyle fractures. *J Oral Maxillofac Surg.* 1983;41:89–98.

35 Breast Augmentation

BENJAMIN H.L. HOWES AND ROSTAM D. FARHADIEH

For video accompanying this chapter see ExpertConsult.com. See inside cover for access details.

Introduction

Breast augmentation is the most popular esthetic surgery procedure.[1] In the United States 450,000 implants are placed for reconstructive surgery purposes and 5,083,717 for breast augmentation annually.[2] Given its history, there is a vast amount of literature devoted to differing opinions, philosophies,[3] and controversy regarding its safety.[4] Many injectable and implantable materials have also been used over the years, including shellac, beeswax, epoxy resin, petroleum jelly, Teflon, polyurethane and polyvinyl alcohol.[3] In recent times, controversy again has surrounded silicone implants, with an increased association with breast implant-associated anaplastic large cell lymphoma (BIA-ALCL).[5] The popularity of this procedure would behoove all plastic surgeons to remain abreast of the science and the clinical literature in this rapidly evolving field.

Implant Evolution

Silicone (dimethylpolysiloxane) was first developed during World War II as part of aircraft engineering. Its soft, inert nature made it a perfect prosthetic substrate for medicine.[3] Silicone breast implants can be divided into five generations based on shell thickness, texture, and implant fill (Table 35.1). Current implants are divided by gel fill into saline or silicone.[3] The silicone fill is further subdivided into stable and soft, based on level of molecular cross-linkage. By shell, they are divided into textured and smooth, all made of silicone polymers, and finally, by shape, into round and anatomical.

First-generation implants manufactured by Dow Corning in 1962 were composed of viscous silicone gel containing a thick teardrop shell.[1] In the 1970s, high capsular contracture rates led to an evolutionary step towards a second generation of softer implants; these were smooth, round, seamless, and contained less viscous silicone.[3] Although reducing capsular contracture rates, they were associated with "gel bleed" from small molecular weight particles of silicone diffusing across the thin silicone elastomer shells, which has also been implicated in capsular contractures.[6] This led to third-generation implants which had a strengthened silicone shell, two layers of high performance elastomer with a fluorosilicone barrier between layers. The fourth generation of textured implants were made in part to emulate polyurethane foam's natural pores. Foam delamination resulted in a noncontractile capsule, yielding immobile implants that had a soft feel. They were, however, withdrawn in 1990 after animal studies showed the carcinogenic nature of the polyurethane byproducts. Kirkpatrick et al implanted 1266 polyurethane implants in 490 animals (3 implants each) which caused the formation of 340 tumors over a 2-year period.[7] The study concentration, however, was 3000 times that used in humans.

Biocell, developed by McGhan Medical (owned by Allergan), is composed of an irregular open pore textured surface with an average density of 3.1 pores/mm^2 and an average pore size of 289 μm. These pores, created by a lost salt technique, are developed through an adhesive effect. This is similar to polyurethane except for delamination. This shell characteristic has been used for both saline- as well as silicone-filled implants, resulting in immobile yet soft feel implants and lower contracture rates.[1] Biocell was withdrawn from the European markets in December 2018, followed by the Canadian and Australian regulators, the latter banning a large number of textured implants and tissue expanders. In July 2019 Allergan issued a worldwide recall of their textured implants and breast expanders after the US Food and Drug Administration (FDA) notified the company of the increased risk associated with their textured implants. Eighty percent of the reported 573 cases were Allergan textured implants. Of these, there have been 33 deaths. Given the rarity of BIA-ALCL the FDA have not recommended removal from women with implants currently in situ. The FDA conducted their own analysis and concluded that the use of Biocell textured implants from Allergan was associated with a sixfold risk of BIA-ALCL compared with textured implants from other companies. It is clearly evident that research into the appropriate implant materials is an evolving field and will require greater understanding of biocompatibility.

Siltex, developed by Mentor (owned by Johnson & Johnson), has a textured surface characterized by a pattern of nodules ranging in height of from 65 μm to 150 μm and in width from 60 μm to 275 μm. These do not adhere to the surrounding tissues, meaning they are mobile in the pocket

TABLE 35.1 Alloplastic Material Evolution Over Time

Implant Generation	Production Period	Shell Characteristics	Silicone Gel Characteristics	Shape
First	1962–1970	Thick shell (average 0.25 mm), Dacron patch	Thick viscous	Anatomical
Second	1970–1982	Thin shells (average 0.13 mm), no patch, smooth surface	Less viscous softer gel	Round
Third	1982–1992	Thick low bleed shells, smooth surface	More viscous than second generation	Round
Fourth	1993–present	Thick, strong, low bleed shell, smooth and textured surfaces	More viscous cohesive gel	Round and anatomical
Fifth	1993–present	Thick, strong, low bleed shell, smooth and textured surfaces	Cohesive and form stable gel	Round and large array of anatomical

resulting in lower contracture rates (saline- or silicone-filled). Fifth-generation silicone implants are textured with form stable silicone achieved by increasing the cross linkage of the silicone gel, which assists in maintaining their shape (Table 35.1).[3]

Saline implants were first reported by the French in 1965, aiming for a less invasive and smaller scar surgery.[3] The main disadvantage of these devices is their deflation rate and feel. The deflation rates in the initial offerings were as high as 75% at 3 years. The shells were thickened by a room temperature vulcanized process which reduced their deflation rates. However, they contained surface wrinkles and a round-ball appearance when overfilled. The current accepted rate of deflation is approximately 1–4% for the first 10 years.[3]

Indications

Glandular hypomastia may occur as a developmental or involutional process and affects a significant number of women. Developmental hypomastia is seen as primary mammary hypoplasia, or as a sequela of thoracic hypoplasia (Poland's syndrome). Involutional hypomastia may develop in the postpartum setting and be exacerbated by breastfeeding or significant weight loss. Inadequate breast volume may lead to a negative self-body image, feelings of inadequacy, and low self-esteem. Such disturbances may adversely affect a patient's interpersonal relationships, sexual fulfillment, and quality of life.

Initial consultation for augmentation should begin with open-ended questions about the patient's goals and expectations. Patients today have often invested time researching the internet, Facebook forums, chat rooms and learning from friends who have had the procedure. The surgeon should be able to form an impression of the patient. Any concerns about the patient's level of understanding, unrealistic expectations, or self-esteem issues should be explored prior to proceeding with surgery. A medical history and physical examination is essential for assessment of risk factors and candidacy for breast augmentation.

The *ideal* size and shape of the female breast is subjective and relates to both personal preference and cultural norms. However, most surgeons agree there are certain shared characteristics representing the esthetic ideal. These include a profile with a sloping or full upper pole and a gently curved lower pole with the nipple–areola complex at the point of maximal projection. The breast structure itself contains breast parenchyma, skin, and subcutaneous fat. The resulting form of the breast after augmentation will be determined by the dynamic interaction of the breast implant, parenchyma, and soft tissue envelope.

Assessment and Implant Selection

Physical examination begins with observation of signs of chest wall deformity or spinal curvature. It is imperative to document and draw attention to any asymmetry of breast size, nipple position, or inframammary fold (IMF) position. Palpation of all quadrants of breasts and axillae is required to rule out masses or suspicious lymph nodes. The surgeon should carefully assess the quantity and compliance of the parenchyma and soft tissue envelope. The soft tissue pinch test involves gathering the superior pole of the breast between the examiner's thumb and index finger, measuring the thickness of the intervening tissue. A pinch test result of <2 cm indicates a need for subpectoral placement of the implant. It is also important to characterize the amount, quality and distribution of the breast parenchyma as it may be necessary to reshape or redistribute tissues to achieve the desired shape of the breast mound. The elasticity of the skin should also be characterized by observing its resistance to deflection and noting any signs of skin redundancy or stretch marks. Most manufacturers have developed a preoperative planning system to facilitate patient assessment and implant selection. Standard discussion centers around information about implant shapes (anatomical vs. round) or projection levels. The patient's perception of the desired look is simulated utilizing different size and style implants and sizers or with computer simulation. Interestingly, Hidalgo and Weinstein's level 1 study did not demonstrate a statistically significant difference between anatomical or round implants.[8]

Operative Techniques

Preoperative Markings

Preoperative markings are a useful reference point during the procedure and are made with the patient in the upright position. The surgeon should mark the chest midline in the frontal view from the suprasternal notch to the xiphoid process, the existing IMFs, and the likely position of the new IMFs as the proposed limits of the dissection. The senior surgeon's approach is dynamic, using the intrinsic mobility, movement and excursion of the patient's tissues, as well as implant measurements and dimensions. The central sternum is used as a static reference point to the more laterally placed breast and nipple areolar complex (NAC) during standard arm excursion. In the seated position, a line from the center of the nipple is marked with the arms in both the resting position and with the hands behind the head to the sternal point. The lower pole of breast skin and glandular elasticity is assessed by simulating expansion with an implant. This allows the surgeon to assess how much skin may be recruited from below the native IMF and optimal placement of the incision. The dimensions of the implant in relation to the breast mound footprint is used as another measure for establishing the new IMF position. The ideal natural appearance of the NAC is at mid-height of an anatomical form stable implant. The NAC is elevated with augmentation. Based on these markings the mid-height of the implant is determined on the chest wall. This translates to approximately 1.0 cm for small breasts, 1.0–1.5 cm for moderately sized breasts, and 1.5–2.0 cm for larger breasts.

Access Incisions

Inframammary

This is the most common and versatile access incision. It allows for clear dissection and subsequent visualization of the implant pocket. The technique may reduce the rate of capsular contracture through clear visualization and "dry" technique. This allows good hemostasis and reduced risk of bacterial contamination through the incision and operative field. Its direct access to the glandular–muscular interface and overlap allows manipulation for the best symmetrical and esthetically pleasing outcome. The drawback of this incision is the relative visibility of the scar. The incision should be placed in the predicted location of the new IMF, which has been determined and marked preoperatively. An incision length of up to 5.0–7.5 cm (depending on shape and size of the implant) is required, especially for anatomical implants. The incision should be designed lateral to the breast midline, this will place the resulting scar in the deepest portion of the new IMF.

Periareolar

The principle advantage of this incision is the resulting scar, which is usually considered well camouflaged and inconspicuous. The periareolar approach allows easy adjustment of the IMF and direct access to the parenchyma for scoring and release when the lower pole of the breast is constricted. Whether this is a transparenchymal approach, or periparenchymal via dissection to the inferior pole, the incision allows for access and creation of subglandular, and submuscular pockets. In addition to the higher risk of contamination and capsular contracture rates, it is associated with reduced sensitivity of the NAC as well as increased rates of periareolar pain.[9] It is also more likely to interfere with lactation and breastfeeding.

In pigmented skin the risk of keloid and/or depigmentation remains high. It is also exceedingly difficult to place many cohesive or anatomically shaped implants through this incision. Despite the evidence, this access is used by many surgeons who appreciate the "direct" access, "remote" control of the IMF and "invisible" incision. In the opinion of the authors, the basic science and clinical series evidence suggests there is no justification for using the periareolar incision.

Transaxillary

This was first developed in the 1970s as an open technique, before being adapted to a minimally invasive approach. Although this technique theoretically offers access and creation of all three implant pockets, the traditional open technique involved blunt dissection of the inferior origins of the pectoralis major muscle, for creation of the submuscular pocket. The open blunt technique led to a series of suboptimal esthetic outcomes, due in part to uneven coverage of the implant and its malposition owing to a lack of controlled dissection of the vascular inferomedial aspect of pectoralis major. In this space lie the major intercostal vessels, which increases the risk of hematoma. As saline implants became popular, especially in the United States, proponents of this technique increased. Introduction of endoscopic assistance allowed the insertion of saline implants through a 2–3 cm incision, enabling precision view, thus becoming a new standard. Currently, the technique is performed with a slightly longer incision of 4–5 cm. Although textured implants can be placed via the incision, anatomical-shaped implants cannot. The IMF is lowered 1–2 cm depending on size and asymmetry. Proponents of this technique support its safety, small incision hidden in the axilla, remote access, and better control of the IMF. Despite evidence suggesting this incision increases capsular contractures, the authors believe that this technique is more anatomically and surgically sound than the periareolar technique, but less versatile than the inframammary incision. However, the purported control over the IMF is offset by the fact that there is little or no possibility for a nuanced manipulation of the gland–muscle interface or position at the IMF. This is imperative in the view of the authors, as it gives a more direct control of the NAC to IMF distance as well as the shape of the lower pole. However, Tebbetts reports excellent equivalent outcomes with dual plane and transaxillary approaches at long-term follow-up.[10]

Transumbilical

This technique was developed in the 1990s, and the first large series reported by Dowden argued for its use based on its versatility (access to both subpectoral, as well as subglandular pockets), minimal scarring with no implant tension on the wound, reduced loss of nipple sensation, elimination of dead space, and good control of the implant pocket.[11] This technique has limited application and is only suited for inflatable saline implants. It involves blunt dissection over the rectus sheath toward the breast. Creation of the subglandular or subpectoral pockets is achieved by avulsion of the tissues, including the inferior pectoralis major (for the subpectoral pocket). Although good results have been reported by Dowden and other surgeons, the authors feel this is not a surgically sound technique. It has poor visibility of the operative field. Its safety, based on basic surgical principles, cannot be recommended in comparison to the other incisions.

Pocket Creation

Subglandular

The original implant pockets were dissected in a subglandular plane. Where the soft tissue envelope is considered thick enough, many surgeons continue to use the subglandular pocket for implant placement.

Submuscular

This approach was first developed to reduce the risk of capsular contractures, the theory and clinical supportive evidence being that increased movement over the implants disrupt capsular contracture formation. However, these are associated with implant animation superiorly on pectoralis major contraction independent of the overlying breast tissues.

Dual Plane

This approach is developed in either a complete or partial submuscular pocket. The lower edge of the pectoralis major is dissected off the chest wall and lower sternum. For a total submuscular pocket it may be necessary to also dissect serratus anterior and the external oblique from the chest wéll. The issues of animation of the implants with contraction, the implants riding too high, and the wide cleavage are well-known drawbacks of the submuscular plane. By definition, with this technique, it can sometimes be difficult to place the NAC on the most projected part of the breast tissue.[10]

Tebbetts described the dual-plane technique as a means of addressing the various shortcomings of each technique and allowing a nuanced approach to implant placement and pocket dissection.[10] He described dissection of tissue in both submuscular and subglandular planes. The lower edge of the pectoralis major is dissected, followed by dissection of the breast tissue from the underlying pectoralis major. He described three different levels of dissection of the breast tissue–muscle interface and redraping of the pectoralis major muscle on the implant as the projected NAC level (Fig. 35.1):

- Type I: No dissection, the inferior border of the muscle covers the implant and entire NAC level.
- Type II: The inferior border of the muscle drapes over the implant to the level of the NAC.
- Type III: The inferior border of the muscle retracts to the superior margin of the NAC.

Utilization of dual-plane technique provides the most flexible and nuanced approach for implant positioning and placement. It mostly alleviates implant animation problems due to muscle contraction by allowing good soft tissue coverage of the upper pole. Dual-plane technique also facilitates expansion of the lower pole and eases adjustment of the IMF should it be necessary. In addition, this technique has been shown to reduce capsular contracture rates.[10]

Subfascial

Subfascial plane is a more recent technique. Here the implant is placed under the pectoralis major fascia which results in very low or no capsular contracture. The authors have little experience with this technique, however the senior author has extensive experience with pectoralis major in reconstructive settings and we contend that the pectoralis major fascia is rather thin and would not alleviate the issues of implant animation or optimal NAC position on the breast mound.

Sterile Technique, Betadine, and Adams' Solution

Authors' Preference

The general principles of surgery need to be observed even more stringently with the use of prosthetic material. Once informed consent has been obtained by the surgeon, decisions relate to access incision and pocket creation, use of sterile technique, no touch approach, and perioperative antibiotics.

The patient is then placed in the supine position, centered on the operating table with the pelvis directly over the flexion point of the bed. The arms are tucked in with adequate ulnar nerve protection. This way the patient may be placed in the upright seated position as needed during the procedure. Sterile preparation and draping of the anterior chest must provide visualization of the patient's shoulders as an important anatomical reference point. Triple antibiotic solution irrigation is used for all implant cases regardless of the incision type.

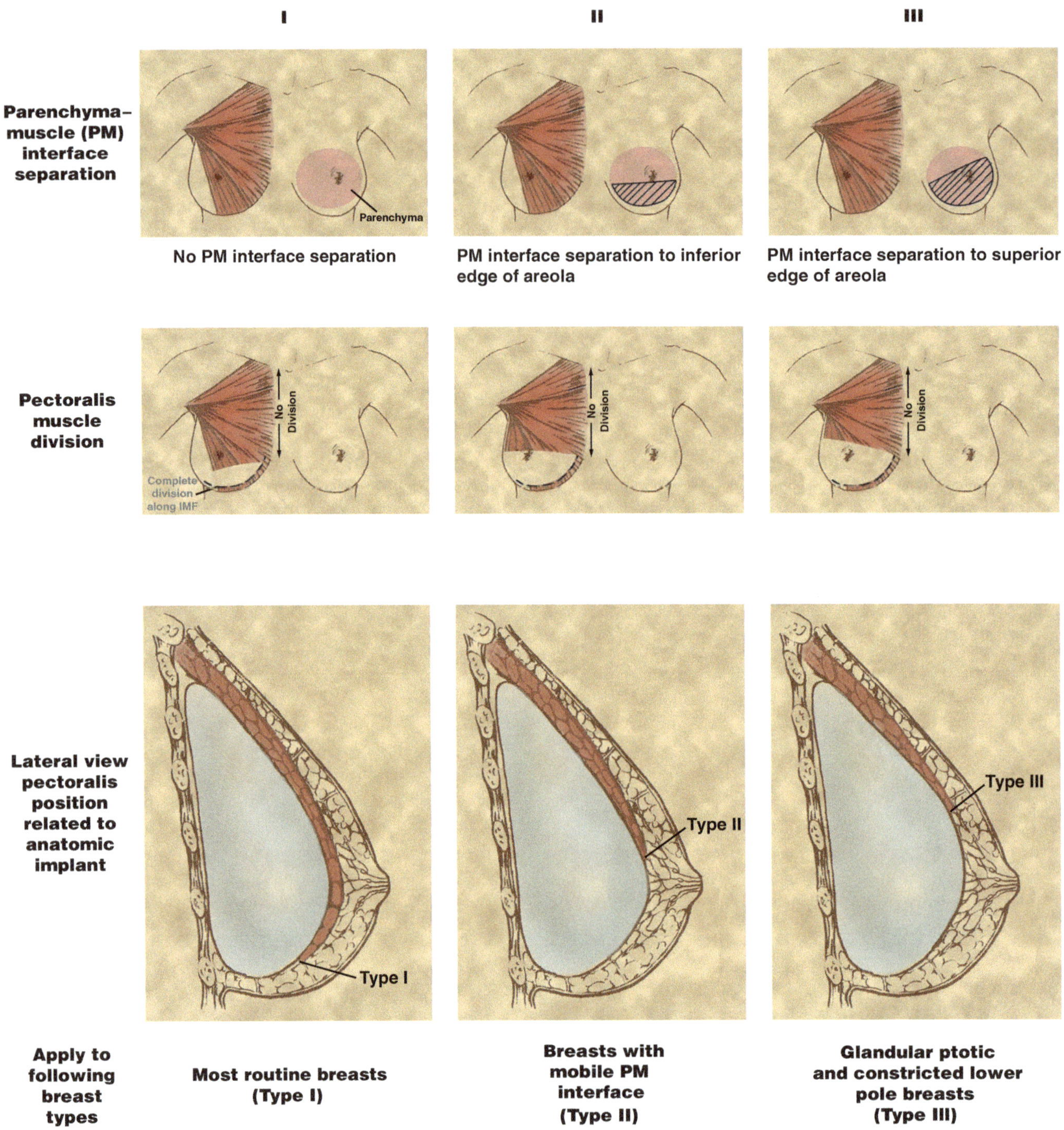

• **Fig. 35.1** Schematic diagram representing the extent of dissection of breast parenchyma off the pectoralis major and subsequent pectoral release in dual-plane breast augmentation. (Reproduced with permission from Tebbetts JB. Dual plane breast augmentation: optimizing implant-soft-tissue relationships in a wide range of breast types. *Plast Reconstr Surg*. 2006;118(7 Suppl):81S–98S; discussion 99S–102S.)

The authors use the IMF incision approach in all procedures. The senior author in most cases creates a dual-plane II–III pocket with silicone implants. The pocket is precisely dissected to snugly accommodate the implant. After creation of the subglandular plane, the lateral border of the pectoralis major muscle is identified. The muscle edge can be lifted by forceps to allow easy entry into the submusculofascial plane. This plane is readily identified by the loose areolar connective tissue and ease of dissection. An extended electrocautery instrument is used to complete the dissection. The inferior origin of the pectoralis major is released from lateral to medial at the level of the IMF. Division of the pectoralis continues medially to the sternal border. The internal mammary vessels in the subpectoral dissection pocket are visualized and cauterized as the dissection is extended medially maintaining a "dry" dissection field. Partial deep division may selectively be carried out 1–3 cm above the xiphoid, depending on implant shape and size. Lateral dissection is avoided in order to let the implant push the pocket out itself and to reduce the risk of injury to the lateral neurovascular bundles. The nerves can be stretched to accommodate the implant but should be preserved to minimize postoperative sensory changes. When the pectoralis major muscle is elevated, care must be taken to leave the pectoralis minor down on the chest wall. This will minimize bleeding and allow correct placement of the implant. Once adequate hemostasis is obtained and pocket dimensions are finalized, the pocket is irrigated with betadine first and then antibiotic-containing solution, and the implants are carefully placed by a minimal-touch technique and change of glove. Repeated use of implant "sizers" is avoided to reduce unnecessary pocket manipulations and possible contamination. A multilayer closure is performed with absorbable suture. It is important to close off the implant pocket with a separate layer of suture before closing the skin prior to application of skin glue. No drains are placed, the NAC is covered with film and chloramphenicol antibiotic ointment (Figs. 35.2 and 35.3).

In order to reduce the incidence of bacterial biofilm production, and subsequent capsular contracture, a variation Adams' solution is employed (1 g cephazolin, 160 mg gentamicin, and 500 mL saline for each pocket). This triple antibiotic irrigation has conflicting reports regarding its efficacy (See section on Capsular contracture, below.).

Complications and Treatment

There are inherent risks involved with all surgical procedures, especially when they involve a prosthetic device. Such risks are significant and have to be considered over longer follow-up time periods. While some risks may be minimal, others are potentially devastating for both patient and surgeon. Regardless of estimated likelihood, these all should be discussed in detail with patients undergoing esthetic surgery. They generally pertain to surgical complications and esthetic outcomes.

Surgical Complications

Hematoma

This is uncommon, with a range of 0–6.7% risk,[1] but must be evacuated. Many authors have noted persistent hematoma or significant seromas lead to capsular contractures.[1]

Device Failure

More recent generations of implants have proved to be more reliable; as noted previously, saline implants undergo approximately 4% deflation over the first 10 years.[12] The Inamed 6-year follow-up study of silicone implants reports a 3.5% device failure.[13] These are consistent across all recent studies, with the largest study, by Coroneos et al, reporting rupture rates at 2 years of 2.5% for saline implants versus 0.5% for silicone ($P<0.001$).[4]

Infection and Exposure

This is a dreaded complication for both patient and surgeon. The reported rates of proven infection are between 0 and 2.6%.[1] The clinical picture presents along a spectrum. Traditionally, the implants were removed and the patient was prescribed antibiotics. Recently, however, salvage procedures have become more common. These range from closed system antibiotics irrigation, to conservative wound care and passive drainage in addition to systemic antibiotics. The more aggressive end of the spectrum involves exchange of the implant and provision of coverage with muscle or using posterior capsule. Bachour et al report a very good salvage rate of infected or exposed implants with seemingly good medium-term follow-ups.[1] However, as discussed later, capsular contracture and presence of biofilms inevitably leads to the development of capsular contracture. Except in the mildest cases the authors advocate capsulectomy and exchange of implant after the initial infection has been treated and the tissues have regained some of their suppleness.

Late Seromas

Appearance of a late seroma in an augmented breast is a source of concern for both patient and surgeon alike. Its management hinges on surgical principles and judgment. This relates to the three principle causes: idiopathic, infective, and neoplastic. A 20-mL estimated volume on ultrasound remains the threshold for seroma diagnosis. If a patient presents with a new onset late seroma an ultrasound-guided diagnostic aspiration is mandatory.

Esthetic Outcomes Complications

These include: capsular contractures; malposition of implant; implant visibility/palpability/rippling; sensory and asymmetrical position changes to the NAC; breast size asymmetry; contour deformities; galactorrhea; skin stretch deformities; glandular atrophy over time; and need for device change with passage of time. All are salient in the discussion with the patient.

Rotation

This is not a problem with traditional implants. The anatomical implants have the advantage of filling the lower pole and are especially useful with patients with mild ptosis (grade II with good skin envelope), but not suitable if preferring augmentation mastopexy. However, up to 1% of anatomical implants undergo rotation in their pockets, which requires secondary corrective surgery.[12]

Malposition

This is the second most common problem associated with breast augmentation and one of the most common reasons for revisional surgery. This occurs in about 1.2%–1.6% of cases.[14] Malpositioned implants can be difficult to treat. The implant

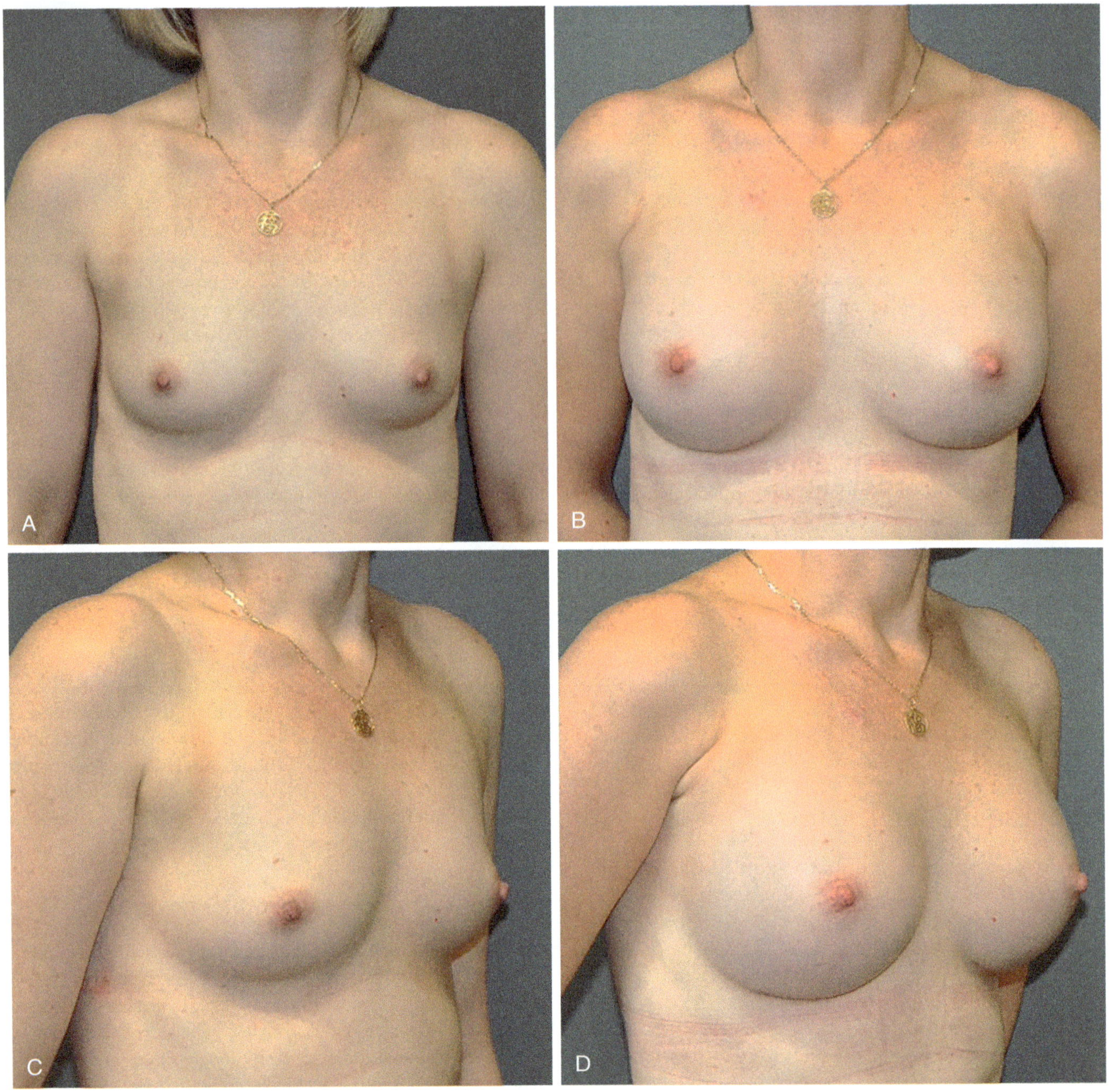

• **Fig. 35.2** (A–D) A 41-year-old woman 3 months postoperatively following dual-plane II primary breast augmentation with 330-mL moderate profile, moderate height, moderate projection, anatomical textured implants.

may be displaced in any direction – medially, laterally, superiorly or inferiorly. Synmastia occurs when medial displacement of the breast is bilateral, centralizing the breast mounds. Conversely, when both implants move laterally, into the axilla, this can cause a double-bubble deformity. Double-bubble deformity is defined in two types. Type I, dubbed "waterfall deformity," occurs when the breast and skin envelope slip over the implant with ptosis, placing the implant in a superior position. This type is seen when complete submuscular pockets are used or when the breast has significant ptosis (grade III) prior to augmentation (rather than augmentation-mastopexy). Type II deformity is related to incorrect lowering of the IMF during surgery when the implant sits below the well-formed IMF and breast tissue. Lateral implant displacements are most commonly due to over-dissection of the implant pocket or contraction of the pectoralis major muscle. The lateral part of the pocket can be excised and closed; or simply closed to tighten the pocket displacing the implants medially. Use of acellular dermal matrix (ADM) in all malposition revisional surgery has been described and must be considered in the planning stage. Synmastia is notoriously difficult to treat, it is the result of over-dissection of the medial pocket and the sternal origins of the pectoralis major muscle in the submuscular planes. Here ADM can be useful as the capsule can be used to augment the medial border of the pocket in

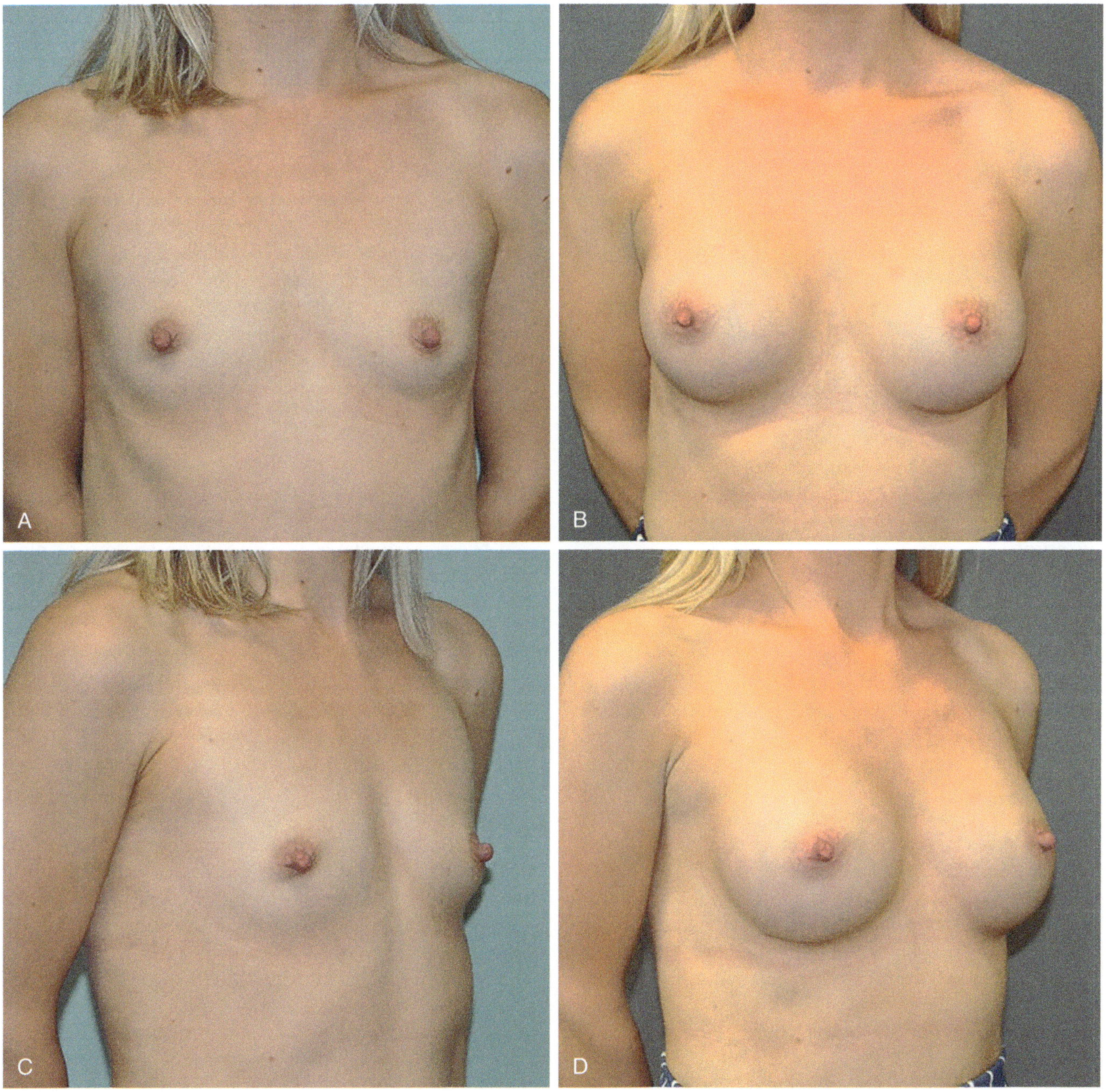

• **Fig. 35.3** (A–D) A 43-year-old woman, 3 months postoperative after dual-plane II primary breast augmentation with 350-mL moderate profile round smooth implants.

addition to a layer of ADM placed medially.[15] A reduction in implant size where possible is helpful.[15]

Wrinkling/Rippling

This is most commonly reported with saline implants, particularly in textured subtypes. It was not related to whether the implant was underfilled, recommended fill or overfilled. It is also more common when implant to parenchymal ratio is greater than 50%.[1]

Asymmetries

All breasts are asymmetrical, therefore, preoperative observation and documentation is good practice. The patient is made aware of these differences preoperatively making asymmetries as a result of augmentation more acceptable.

NAC Sensory Changes

These are more common in periareolar approaches. In the normal course of an inframammary or transaxillary approach, transient altered sensation may occur. Generally it is considered that permanent changes are more common when implants larger than 350 mL are used.[1]

Scar Formation

Keloid and hypertrophic scar formation need to be discussed with the patient preoperatively. Their treatment is part of the standard algorithm discussed elsewhere in this book (see Chapter 1).

Capsular Contracture

Pathophysiology and Study Outcomes

Capsular contracture remains the most significant drawback of breast implants. Contracture can cause deformation of the implant resulting in altered esthetics, and women may complain of discomfort or pain, making it the most common reason for reoperation.

They are clinically classified by the degree of contracture, which has previously been described by Baker:[16]

- Grade I: breast is soft to palpate whilst implant is either not visible or palpable, or visible
- Grade I: breast firm and/or palpable implant but the implant is not visible
- Grade III: moderate breast firmness with palpable implant and visible breast deformity
- Grade IV: severe contracture with breast firmness and distortion.

The rates of capsular contracture based on multiple studies vary. A recent systematic review by Bachour et al comprehensively reviewed studies addressing capsular contracture following breast augmentation.[1] The follow-up of 5373 women within a Danish registry indicated that 4% of women, over a mean follow-up period of 3.8 years, underwent secondary surgery. Coroneos et al, in the largest study of its kind, reported that the capsular contracture rate was higher for silicone at 5% versus 2.8% for saline ($P<0.001$) with incidence of capsular contracture ranging from 7.2% to 18.3% over a 7-year period.[4] Short-term reoperation necessitating implant removal was higher for silicone (6.5% and 3.4% at 2 years, $P<0.001$). At follow-up of 7 years the most common reason for reoperation was capsular contracture post primary augmentation, with a rate of 11.7%.[4] A limitation of this study may be the perceived inherent bias of outcomes data collection by companies with vested interest, with differing protocols for collection.

A plethora of clinical studies have been produced to implicate material- and surgical-related factors that may cause contracture: the device fill and shell; surgical access incision and pocket; use of antiseptics and antibiotics; and use of drains.[1,16] Calobrace et al conducted a study spanning 10 years identifying 2277 women which demonstrated that implants of sizes >350 mL were associated with higher capsular contracture rates.[17] This may relate to a tighter skin envelope which impedes implant mobility causing an increased likelihood of contracture. Calobrace also outlined timing towards capsular contracture of 41% in the first 2 years and 80% within 5 years.[17] This outdates older information which suggested that most capsular contractures occur within 12–18 months.[17]

Headon et al compared single study results of six authors involving 3716 patients with an average follow-up of 1.24–8 years and a capsular contracture rate of 10.6%.[16] One of these studies was a long-term multicenter study assessing highly cohesive silicone. At 6 years there was a 4.6% capsular contracture rate.[16] Another of the studies on Mentor round silicone in 1007 women at 3 years follow-up noted a 8.1% rate of Baker's grade III/IV capsular contracture.[16]

Two theories have emerged for the pathogenesis of capsular contracture: the scar formation and infective theories. Histologically, these capsules are made of an inner layer of cellular elements, synovial type metaplasia, fibrocytes, and multinucleated giant cells, with a middle layer of vascular networks and an outer layer of collagen bundles.[18] In order to reduce scar formation, subpectoral pockets were designed to afford more protection, coverage, and regular contraction of the muscle hindering the formation of periprosthetic capsule. The fact that no definitive study exists controlling for all variables indicates that capsular contractures are most likely multifactorial.[1,16]

The second theory, periprosthetic subclinical infection theory, is well documented.[1,16,19] However, what is less clear is how this process causes capsular contracture. It has been shown that up to 80% of female breast capsule samples contain bacteria.[1] Bacterial presence in up to 83% of nipple secretions is considered a cautionary tale for the use of periareolar incisions. The most commonly implicated organism is a coagulase-negative *Staphylococcus epidermidis*, although other organisms have been isolated.[1] Basic science evidence of an accelerated capsular contracture following *Staphylococcus aureus* contamination has also been demonstrated.[1,9]

In general, the considerations for reducing likelihood of capsular contracture are as follows.

Access Incision

The most commonly used access incisions available for primary breast augmentation are transaxillary, inframammary, and periareolar. Umbilical incision remains in the realms of surgical possibilities with little reasonable surgical philosophical justification in the opinion of the authors. The ferocious debate regarding the merit of each access site is ongoing. There is compelling evidence that periareolar and transaxillary incisions, in addition to reduced access, expose the implant to potentially higher risks of bacterial contamination increasing capsular contracture rates[1,9,14] These all lend support to use of inframammary incisions as the safest choice.

Implant Type

Originally, one of the major advantages of saline implants was thought to be their lower rate of capsular contracture. Histologically, macrophages were shown to have engulfed silicone from silicone implants after inflammatory reaction. This was suggested to be an indicator of saline implant superiority. However, a recent systematic analysis of randomized controlled trials failed to demonstrate a clear reduction of the capsular contractures with the use of saline implants.[20]

Surgical Pockets

These studies are divided into implant type (textured vs. smooth) and surgical pockets used.

Subglandular. A systemic review published in 2018 reviewed the results of various trials comparing polyurethane, textured, and smooth implants in subglandular breast augmentation which totaled 48 studies.[1] There were 16 studies which directly reviewed capsular contracture rates between textured and smooth. Three studies demonstrated textured having higher capsular contracture rates but these finding were not statistically significant. There were 13 studies demonstrating higher contracture rates for smooth implants. Ten of these studies made significant findings[1].

Subpectoral. A study of 55 breasts, the only randomized trial of this kind, compared silicone implants placed in the submuscular pocket. The final outcome trended towards less capsular contracture rates in the textured group but it was not statistically significant (15% textured vs. 8.6% controlled).[6]

Finally, a more recent meta-analysis using the majority of the above studies demonstrated a fivefold increased incidence of capsular contracture with smooth implants.[6] This is consistent with previously reported papers.[9,14,16]

Periprosthetic Drains

There is some evidence that periprosthetic drains are associated with a higher risk of infection and capsular contractures.[1] Many surgeons advocate not using drains in primary breast augmentation.

Perioperative Antibiotics and Pocket Irrigation

Antibiotic and betadine irrigation have previously been shown to reduce the rates of capsular contracture, but results are contradictory. Betadine irrigation of the implant pocket was first championed by Burkhardt and colleagues as a means of reducing bacterial biofilm. Adams and colleagues used a triple antibiotic solution, the Adams' solution, consisting of: 1 g cephazolin, 80 mg gentamycin and 50,000 IU bacitracin, replaced 50mL povidone-iodine from 2000 onwards mixed with 500 mL normal saline.[1] They managed to show a reduction of capsular contracture (Baker III/IV) rates to 1.8%. This is far lower than the documented 7.2%–18.3% by Coroneos et al for primary augmentation.[4] A recent systematic review and meta-analysis by Yalanis et al reviewed the safety and efficacy of povidone-iodine irrigation on reducing capsular contracture rates.[19] There were nine studies totaling 5153 patients who had esthetic augmentation. The meta-analysis concluded that the use of povidone-iodine solution reduced the rate of capsular contracture (2.7% vs. 8.9%) with less than 1% implant failure rate.[19]

An interesting meta-analysis by Drinane et al reviewed eight studies examining the role of antimicrobial irrigation and outlines the contradictory information amongst studies.[21] Seven studies were included. Paradoxically, they found that patients who received either iodine, antibiotic or a combination of the two for irrigation demonstrated an increased likelihood of developing capsular contracture. They argue that in order for the antimicrobial therapies to be efficacious the contact time for topical use may be too brief and may only treat nonresistant bacteria. However, the studies used were retrospective and heterogenous.[21]

Treatment of Capsular Contracture

Treatment of capsular contractures of Baker's grade III–IV requires surgery. This can take the form of: capsulotomy, scoring, and device exchange; capsulectomy and device exchange; or neo-pocket creation and device exchange. Considering the discussion in the previous sections about the cause of capsular contractures and the roles of biofilms, bacterial inoculation, and contamination of the capsule, the authors feel it is a good surgical principle to excise the capsule, create a new implant pocket, and exchange the device.

More recently, the use of ADM has found a place in the debate on capsular contracture.[15] Much like the concept of a "fire break" skin graft in Dupuytren's disease, ADM has been found to prevent incorporation into the forming capsule. Histological, basic science and clinical evidence indicate that placement of ADM yields an abrupt disruption of the capsule formation thereby alleviating capsular contractures. The authors favor the use of ADM in revisional augmentation surgery.

Breast Implant-Associated Illnesses

Breast implant illness-type symptoms were increasingly reported by patients as far back as the 1980s/early 1990s along with a series of autoimmune disorder that were linked with women who had breast implants. This resulted in temporary withdrawal from the US market by the FDA between 1992 and 2006.[22] These were replaced by saline-filled, single lumen implants. In the event of rupture, extravasation of saline solution was thought preferable to leakage of silicone. Breast implant-associated illness remains a controversial topic and in the only study of its kind, in 1997, Peters et al reported the effects of explantation in 100 women compared with a control group of 100 women.[22] Subgroup analysis of the women who had explantation was as follows:

- Group 1: In this group of women the symptoms experienced were pain, breast firmness, fatigue, joint pain, GI symptoms, rashes, memory loss, and sleep disturbance. They experienced the most positive effects of implant explantation without evidence into rheumatic or autoimmune disease.
- Group 2: This group had proven rheumatic disease and complaints similar to group one. The majority of patients who had improved symptoms post explantation had these return within 12 months, with six patients having ongoing severe symptoms.
- Group 3: Proven autoimmune disease (rheumatoid arthritis, systemic lupus erythematosus, Raynaud's, multiple sclerosis). None of these patients had improvement post explantation.

Autoantibody titer analysis for autoimmune diseases did not show a statistically significant difference between groups. The authors admitted a limitation of the study was an inherent bias as all patients had been referred by their rheumatologists for negative symptoms.

Recently, a controversial cohort study by Coroneos et al addressed safety and efficacy of implants in 99,993 patients. This is the largest multicenter implant outcomes study and the first with significant power to identify risks of acquiring connective tissue disorders.[4] They highlighted the potential problems in relation to breast implants. They found that there was an increased risk of developing Sjögren syndrome, scleroderma, rheumatoid arthritis, stillbirth, and one recorded case of melanoma.

The study highlights the low potential overall risk of developing any of the published illnesses for multiple reasons:

1. Data show a combination of increased and decreased illness risk with breast implants.
2. Reported risk rates are extremely low when looking at the data, ranging from 0.004% to 0.6%.
3. Most data rely on self-reporting by patients and is related to the single manufacturer "Mentor" implants only. Allergan self-reported data are confirmed by a physician with "true" diagnoses (but has shorter follow-up of only 2 years).

Breast implant patients are grouped together, but cosmetic and reconstructive groups are very different (e.g., melanoma risk may be significantly increased in cosmetic patients, who are more likely to sunbathe after their augments). General population figures for comparison are taken from heterogenous studies that include significantly older data with a broad spectrum of different cases. Significant attrition rate is demonstrated during follow-up in these studies, with retrospective analysis and no control group comparison. This suggests unreliable conclusions despite high numbers in the study. Table 35.2 highlights the combination of increased and decreased illness risk.

The study by Coroneos et al shows illness risk increase, but also a "protective" nature of breast implants and in all cases the percentage of risk protection is extremely small. However, patient-reported symptoms are real and must be taken seriously. Properly designed, prospectively enrolled, controlled, diagnosis-confirmed, long-term follow-up studies are required to present the data accurately.

Autoimmune disease was identified as a potentially related factor, however Shon and Schubert's 1992 study did not support this, with only 28 cases being reported from 1 million to 2 million women in the United States who had implants.[23] A small study of 38 implant cases by Rohrich et al, retrospectively matched for implant removal, found temporary improvement in breast implant-related illness-type symptoms.[24] Fryzek et al's study in 2500 patients randomly selected from the Swedish breast implant registry, when compared to 3500 breast reduction patients, found that although breast augmentation patients were more likely to report illness-type symptoms, the lack of specificity and absence of a dose–response relationship suggests no causal association.[25]

In an attempt to offer a pathological basis for these symptoms De Jong et al's study of 42 silicone breast implant patients self-reported illness-type symptoms in a questionnaire.[26] They found 12/48 had increased polymer binding immunoglobulins and none of these patients were categorized as being "severe" in their symptoms and clinical examination reports. Furthermore, the 17 years (average) silicone exposure in the "minimal symptoms group" did not result in induction of polymer binding Ig. The only conclusion here is that there is no strong association between silicone exposure and detectable immunoglobulins levels in the blood.

There have been a variety of generalized symptoms reported making it difficult to ascertain "true" related illness features. There have been no biochemical associations demonstrated. There may also be a psychological predisposition for developing symptoms, such as in the case of 100 capsulectomy patients who had improved symptoms from implant illness post explantation.[4,26]

Breast Implant-Associated Anaplastic Large Cell Lymphoma

Incidence

The first reported case of a patient with anaplastic T-cell lymphoma was by Keech in 1997. The Food and Drug Administration (FDA) has been notified by the American Society of Plastic Surgeons (ASPS) of 414 cases of BIA-ALCL.[27] The current risk based on cited cases of BIA-ALCL with textured implants is a range of 1:3817 to 1:30,000, therefore, the FDA does not recommend any changes in medical care and follow-up in asymptomatic patients.[27] The systematic review by Leberfinger et al identified 115 articles on BIA-ALCL involving 93 reported cases.[28] Initially, in Australia, spanning a 5-year period, there were 55 recorded cases of BIA-ALCL involving textured implants.[27] There have been four related cases of death. Eleven patients had complications of either rupture, contracture or infection. All patients underwent total capsulectomy and resection of capsule. Histologically, the sample analyzed were CD30-positive and ALK-negative. The incidence in reported cases has recently risen to 81, with the majority of cases being related to grade 4 implants (polyurethane, rough).[5]

More recent studies suggest a BIA-ALCL incidence of 1 in 6920 women who have breast augmentation.[2] The recent patient registry and outcomes for breast implants and anaplastic large cell lymphoma etiology and epidemiology (PROFILE) study noted a median time frame of implantation to diagnosis of 11 years.[29] Almost all implants implicated in BIA-ALCL formation are textured. Only four patients had smooth implants at the time of diagnosis but they had previously had textured permanent implants and in one case textured tissue expander.[29]

Pathophysiology

The pathophysiology includes an admix of genetic predisposition, textured type implants creating an immune reaction,

TABLE 35.2 Main Findings from Study by Coroneos et al[4] on Breast Implant-Associated Illness

	Mentor	Allergan
SLE	0.65% risk = 1.11× increased risk vs. general population	0.006% risk = 9× protective vs. general population
RA	0.35% risk = 5.96× increased risk vs. general population	0.008% risk = 7× protective vs. general population
Scleroderma	0.04% risk (but reported as 7× more likely vs. general population)	No reports
Sjögren syndrome	0.06% risk (but reported as 8× more likely vs. general population)	No reports
Breast cancer	No difference in general population	No reports
Lung cancer	9× protective vs. general population	No reports
Melanoma	0.08% risk (but reported as 3.71× more likely vs. general population – increased sunbathing in breast augment patients?)	No reports

RA, Rheumatoid arthritis; SLE, systemic lupus erythematosus.

and biofilm growth. Chen et al purported that the main pathway in enhancing tumor growth activity is Janus kinase/signal transducer and activator of transcription mutations (JAK/STAT), which transmits cell surface signals from cytokines to increase phosphorylation of proteins.[30] Similarly, anaplastic lymphoma kinase (ALK) is oncogenic through transcription mutations. Janus kinase inhibitor therapy may be useful to treat various ALK-ALCL malignancies in the presence of JAK/STAT mutations. Another target for therapy was due to the finding that the majority of ALCL cases carry TRG or TRB arrangements, and in vitro studies reveal a genetic cytokine profile. Aggressive cases of BIA-ALCL express Notch 1, which is strongly pronounced by phosphorylated STAT3 pathways.[2] Interleukin-17 T-cells are the predominant driver of inflammation in the tissue-specific response.[2] Doren et al calculated a lifetime prevalence of 33 per 1 million persons with textured implants based on 100 pathological confirmed cases of BIA-ALCL.[31] This was 67.6 times higher than that of primary ALCL of the breast in the general population. Textured implants have been implicated as a causal factor in several manuscripts to date. Loch-Wilkinson et al, who investigated the surface area of textured implants, found a higher surface area leads to more bacterial biofilm infection.[27] Chronic inflammation recruits T-cells during a premalignant lymphoproliferative phase (lymphomatoid papulosis) which potentiates CD30+ clonal expansion. Clinically this presents with a late benign seroma. The genetic markers that may be implicated in the development of T cell diseases may be able to be tested via identification of point mutations, deletions, and insertions. Low mutant T-cell populations differ from the wider range of malignant wild-type cells. This would assist in differentiating between a benign T-cell lymphocytosis and identify high CD30+ with morphology. Further in vitro and in vivo studies are being conducted on bacterial antigenic interaction mechanisms and interaction with cancer cells.[5]

Management

Patients may present with asymmetry secondary to effusion or masses, capsular contracture or lymphadenopathy.[27] Lymphadenopathy has been reported in 35% of cases.[2] Seroma fluid and the capsule around the implant must be sent for analysis, which includes microscopy, culture, and cytology. Wright Giesma stained smears, positive immunohistochemistry of CD30+ cells, anaplastic lymphoma kinase protein, translocation studies are indicated in consultation with a hematology/oncology team. Sterile fluid of idiopathic seroma may be an indication of subclinical infection in the biofilm, which may not be picked up by microscopy or culture. In these cases of persistent and unresolved seroma with a course of antibiotics, the authors advocate a capsulectomy and device exchange.

Those with proven lymphoma should undergo removal of implants and capsulectomy in both disease-affected and normal sides. Cases of confirmed disease with lymphocytic hyperplasia in the capsule, CD 30-positive and ALK-negative status should then be discussed at a multidisciplinary meeting for consideration of postoperative chemoradiotherapy. There may also be a role for preoperative neoadjuvant chemoradiotherapy or bone marrow transplant in advanced disease. Leberfinger et al saw 84% of their patients have capsulectomy. Sixty-one percent had chemotherapy (cyclophosphamide, hydroxydaunorubicin, vincristine, and prednisolone, CHOP) and 30% received radiotherapy.[28] The ability to perform capsulectomy for a lymphoma is beneficial for disease control, owing to the fact that BIA-ALCL behaves more like a solitary tumor.[28] Targeted immunotherapies for suppression of IL-4/IL-13/

IL-6, and JAK/STAT may be shown to suppress growth of BIA-ALCL and research is underway to determine their role as adjuvant therapies.[28,30] The margin recommendations of normal breast cancer surgery are not indicated in these cases. Standard follow-up should include appropriate surveillance every 3–6 months with interval imaging with CT staging and PET every 6 months for 2 years.[28]

Prognosis

There is insufficient data to establish a time course for morbidity and mortality of BIA-ALCL. Presumably early intervention and treatment alters the time course of the disease favorably. There have been recorded deaths from metastatic disease, sepsis, complications post bone marrow transplantation and obstructive respiratory failure.[28]

Patient Counseling

Currently, BIA-ALCL remains a rare disease but the risks should be discussed nonetheless. Clinicians should give patients the breast implant manufacturer's labeling and educational material prior to implantation. The risks associated with textured implants should be outlined.

The Plastic Surgery Foundation or National Comprehensive Cancer Network can aid in developing individualized treatment plans. Currently Wang et al are exploring whether there is a difference in lymphoma rates between smooth versus textured implants.[32]

Autologous Fat Grafting

Fat grafts have become a popular means of soft tissue augmentation and breast reconstruction in recent years.[33] Capitalizing on the benefits of pluripotent STEM cells from adipose tissue remains the holy grail of tissue engineering and regeneration.[33] Initially, Coleman et al injected fat into the face and then used the same technique to inject into the breast.[33] Bircoll was first to note calcifications in the breast post fat grafting.[33] That same year, these concerns prompted the American Society of Plastic Surgery to ban its use. Fat necrosis microcalcification could mimic calcifications associated with breast cancer. This could result in patient distress and high false-positive reporting of breast cancer on mammography. As imaging modalities improved in the 21st century this concern was soon dispelled with the appearance of breast cancer calcification noted to be spiculated compared with the benign eggshell-shaped appearance of fat necrosis.[33] The American Society of Plastic Surgeons has since overturned their previous decision and the number of procedure has increased internationally.

The benefits of fat grafting are diverse, ranging in the reversal of the effects of radiotherapy post breast cancer surgery and scar contracture from burns, to an adjustment for minor defect correction in breast augmentation.[33] Its use has also been described for women who have undergone breast conserving surgery and total mastectomy.[33] There have been many changes in recent years with better understanding of fat and stem cells as well as better techniques for harvesting and engrafting.[33] However, following recent concerns regarding BIA-ALCL in women who have breast implants there is an unknown risk regarding the introduction of stem cells from adipocytes and lymphoma proliferation.[33] Seth et al led a comparative study of women who had prostheses combined with autologous fat grafting as an adjunct, versus women who had implants only. He did not find an increase in the recurrence risk of breast cancer.[33]

Basic Sciences and Oncogenesis

Preadipocytes begin differentiation during embryonic stages of development with cross-talk induced by type IV collagen, LPL release which activates c-jun, jun-B, c-myc and c-fos.[33] The promotion of insulin sensitivity, lipogenesis, and lipolysis is by means of four proto-oncogenes regulating CAAT/enhancer-binding proteins (C/EBPβ and C/EBPδ), and subsequent activation of proliferator–activator receptor gamma (PPARϒ).[33] Other governing regulators that assist with adipocyte formation include: WNT inhibition, hedgehog (HH) signaling pathway, ribosomal protein S6 kinase 1 (S6K1), gluthione, transforming growth factor β, and activin.[33] When adipocytes are transferred as a graft, without an associated blood supply, the following has been observed to occur: degenerative changes associated with apoptosis, macrophage-induced phagocytosis, elevated expression of hypoxia-inducible factor 1α, which assists in homeostasis and angiogenesis.[33] For this reason, autologous fat grafting to the breast continues to attract controversy regarding oncogenesis. There are conflicting reports from in vitro and in vivo studies compared with clinical studies as to whether or not fat potentiates quiescent breast cancer cell proliferation.[33]

Efficacy

In regard to meaningful breast augmentation, fat-based autologous augmentation remains a goal rather than an attainable outcome. Due to fat graft loss from reabsorption, fat necrosis, and cyst formation, its efficacy remains to be seen.[33] Rohrich et al explored the efficacy of centrifugation to improve the quality of graft and determined that centrifugation did not improve viability.[34] Cell enrichment techniques involve the separation of fat into two distinct layers prior to injection: mature adipocytes and preadipocytes,[33] the latter having been yielded by placing adipocytes in stroma with collagenase during a period of centrifugation. The premise is that by placing an admix of mature adipocytes with preadipocytes (increased concentration cellularity) this will enhance graft take.[33] Other methods include gravity separation, washing, gauze rolling, and filtration.[33] Washing and gauze rolling may result in a loss of stromal vascular fraction, which may contain growth factors that allow differentiation of preadipocytes to adipocytes.[33]

Imaging studies that have explored fat graft retention rates over time have noted graft retention volumes of 0–43%.[33] Rates may be lower post breast cancer surgery with radiotherapy and higher in cases of breast augmentation where women have native breast tissue.[33] The improved vascularity of the recipient bed and ability for nutrient tissue from the surrounding area to supply the graft, would be greater than in areas of radiotherapy damage.[33]

Smaller amounts of fat grafting volumes (10–100 mL) can be a useful adjunct to improve the transition from chest wall to implant and to conceal rippling.[33] In this manner, fat can be grafted into the decolleté and cleavage area, lateral hollows behind the midaxillary line and implant fold.[33] Cohort studies have shown a decrease of capsular contracture (Baker grade from IV to I) using a single fat grafting session.[33] Results were recorded at 20.3 months' follow-up. The same paper noted avoidance of implant exposure in four patients by using fat grafting compared to a control group who had not had fat grafting.

The BRAVA external expander device was on the market for 10 years, has been theorised to exert an isotropic distraction force on the breast resulting in an expanded fibrovascular scaffold, which is fertile ground for fat engraftment. A multicenter study of 488 patients who used the device showed promising results visually as well as through the clinically reported data[35]. A mean augmentation volume of 233 ml is reported at 12 months based on 3D calculations. The patients had a baseline MRI preoperatively, a 3-month and a second follow up MRI at least 6 months postoperatively. The key findings were a stable volume between the first and second postoperative MRI, indicating permanency of fat graft. The fat graft retention rate was not explored as percentage augmentation was deemed to be a more suitable measure of assessment. Percentage augmentation is only a meaningful measure in women who have native breast tissue and are undoing augmentation for additional volume. It is likely to be an inaccurate measure in women who have had a total mastectomy and radiotherapy who are not being augmented, but are undergoing breast reconstruction. The BRAVA device has since been removed from the market.

When measuring breast volume, there is equivalence between 3D laser scanning and MRI for volume measurement[33] and these modalities have also been shown to be useful when planning complex reconstruction to establish breast volume asymmetry, volume necessary to inject for correction and to monitor fat graft retention rates over time.[33]

The usefulness of external expansion devices (e.g., BRAVA device) appears to be in cases where women have native breast tissue that is more responsive to the negative pressure. In case where women have undergone breast conserving surgery, or total mastectomy and adjuvant radiotherapy, it appears to be less efficacious.[33] However, autologous fat grafting appears to reverse the deleterious effects of the radiotherapy, making the skin supple and pliable.[33]

When used for breast reconstruction, autologous fat grafting can assist with volume correction for minor defects in lumpectomy sites, post sector resection in breast conserving surgery, and for reconstruction post total mastectomy.[33]

Larger controlled augmentation volumes remain in the realm of promising trials. Breast augmentation surgery remains the most popular cosmetic plastic surgery procedure. Since its inception it has endured controversies. The future shows hope for autologous options along with a need for a good understanding of the esthetics, techniques as well as potential complications facing this patient population which underpins good and safe surgical practice.

References

1. Bachour Y, Bargon CA, de Blok CJM, et al. Risk factors for developing capsular contracture in women after breast implant surgery: a systematic review of the literature. *J Plast Reconstr Aesthet Surg.* 2018;71(9):e29–e48.
2. Quesada AE, Medeiros LJ, Clemens MW, et al. Breast implant-associated anaplastic large cell lymphoma: a review. *Mod Pathol.* 2019;32(2):166–188.
3. Spear S. The breast implant story. *Ann Plast Surg.* 2006;56(5):573–583.
4. Coroneos CJ, Selber JC, Offodile AC 2nd, Butler CE, Clemens MW. US FDA breast implant postapproval studies: long-term outcomes in 99,993 patients. *Ann Surg.* 2019;269(1):30–36.
5. Magnusson M, Beath K, Cooter R, et al. Special Update: the epidemiology of breast implant associated large cell lymphoma in Australia and New Zealand confirms the highest risk for grade 4 surface breast implants. *Plast Reconstr Surg.* 2019;143(5):1285–1292.
6. Wong C, Samuel M, Tan BK, Song C. Capsular contracture in subglandular breast augmentation with textured versus smooth breast implants: a systematic review. *Plast Reconstr Surg.* 2006;118(5):1224–1236.
7. Kirkpatrick CJ, Alves A, Kohler H, et al. Biomaterial-induced sarcoma: a novel model to study preneoplastic change. *Am J Pathol.* 2000;156(4):1455–1467.
8. Hidalgo DA, Weinstein AL. Intraoperative comparison of anatomical versus round implants in breast augmentation: a randomized controlled trial. *Plast Reconstr Surg.* 2017;139(3):587–596.
9. Li S, Chen L, Liu W, Mu D, Luan J. Capsular contracture rate after breast augmentation with periareolar versus other two (inframammary and transaxillary) incisions: a meta-analysis. *Aesthet Plast Surg.* 2018;42(1):32–37.
10. Tebbetts JB. Dual plane breast augmentation: optimizing implant-soft-tissue relationships in a wide range of breast types. *Plast Reconstr Surg.* 2006;118(suppl 7):81S–98S; discussion 99S–102S.
11. Dowden RV. Dispelling the myths and misconceptions about transumbilical breast augmentation. *Plast Reconstr Surg.* 2000;106(1):190–194.
12. Young VL, Watson ME. Breast implant research: where we have been, where we are, where we need to go. *Clin Plast Surg.* 2001;28(3).
13. Spear S, Murphy D, Slicton A. Inamed silicone breast implant core study results at 6 years. *Plast Reconstr Surg.* 2007;120(suppl 7): 8S–16S.
14. Henriksen TF, Fryzek JP, Hölmich LR, et al. Surgical intervention and capsular contracture after breast augmentation: a prospective study of risk factors. *Ann Plast Surg.* 2005;54(4):343–351.
15. Vardanian AJ, Clayton JL, Roostaeian J, et al. Comparison of implant-based immediate breast reconstruction with and without acellular dermal matrix. *Plast Reconstr Surg.* 2011;128(5):403e–10e.

16. Headon H, Kasem A, Mokbel K. Capsular contracture after breast augmentation: an update for clinical practice. *Arch Plast Surg*. 2015;42(5):532–543.
17. Calobrace MB, Stevens WG, Capizzi PJ, et al. Risk factor analysis for capsular contracture: a 10-year Sientra study using round, smooth, and textured implants for breast augmentation. *Plast Reconstr Surg*. 2018;141(4S Sientra Shaped and Round Cohesive Gel Implants):20S–28S.
18. Maxwell GP, Gabriel A. The evolution of breast implants. *Clin Plast Surg*. 2009;36:1–13.
19. Yalanis GC, Liu EW, Cheng HT. Efficacy and safety of povidone-iodine irrigation in reducing the risk of capsular contracture in aesthetic breast augmentation: a systematic review and meta-analysis. *Plast Reconstr Surg*. 2015;136(4):687–698.
20. Schaub TA, Ahmad J, Rohrich RJ. Capsular contracture with breast implants in the cosmetic patient: saline versus silicone – a systematic review of the literature. *Plast Reconstr Surg*. 2010;126(6):2140–2149.
21. Drinane JJ, Chowdhry T, Pham TH, et al. Examining the role of antimicrobial irrigation and capsular contracture: a systematic review and meta-analysis. *Ann Plast Surg*. 2017;79(1):107–114.
22. Peters W, Smith D, Fornasier V, et al. An outcome analysis of 100 women after explantation of silicone gel breast implants. *Ann Plast Surg*. 1997;39(1):9–19.
23. Shons AR, Schubert W. Silicone breast implants and immune disease. *Ann Plast Surg*. 1992;28(5):491–499; discussion 499–501.
24. Rohrich RJ. The FDA approves saline-filled breast implants: what does this mean for our patients? *Plast Reconstr Surg*. 2000;106(4):903–905.
25. Fryzek JP, Signorello LB, Hakelius L, et al. Self-reported symptoms among women after cosmetic breast implant and breast reduction surgery. *Plast Reconstr Surg*. 2001;107(1):206–213.
26. De Jong WH, Goldhoorn CA, Kallewaard M, et al. Study to determine the presence of antipolymer antibodies in a group of Dutch women with a silicone breast implant. *Clin Exp Rheumatol*. 2002;20(2):151–160.
27. Loch-Wilkinson A, Beath KJ, Knight RJW, et al. Breast implant-associated anaplastic large cell lymphoma in Australia and New Zealand: high-surface-area textured implants are associated with increased risk. *Plast Reconstr Surg*. 2017;140(4):645–654.
28. Leberfinger AN, Behar BJ, Williams NC, et al. Breast implant-associated anaplastic large cell lymphoma: a systematic review. *JAMA Surg*. 2017;152(12):1161–1168.
29. McCarthy CM, Loyo-Berrios N, Qureshi AA, et al. Patient registry and outcomes for breast implants and anaplastic large cell lymphoma etiology and epidemiology (PROFILE): initial report of findings, 2012–2018. *Plast Reconstr Surg*. 2019;143(3S A review of breast implant-associated anaplastic large cell lymphoma):65S–73S.
30. Chen J, Zhang Y, Petrus MN, et al. Cytokine receptor signaling is required for the survival of ALK- anaplastic large cell lymphoma, even in the presence of JAK1/STAT3 mutations. *Proc Natl Acad Sci U S A*. 2017;114(15):3975–3980.
31. Doren EL, Miranda RN, Selber JC, et al. U.S. epidemiology of breast implant-associated anaplastic large cell lymphoma. *Plast Reconstr Surg*. 2017;139(5):1042–1050.
32. Wang C, Luan J, Panayi AC, Orgill DP, Xin M. Complications in breast augmentation with textured versus smooth breast implants: a systematic review protocol. *BMJ Open*. 2018;8(4):e020671.
33. Howes B. *The Role of Autologous Fat Grafting for Breast Reconstruction* [DPhil]. Adelaide, South Australia: Flinders University; 2018.
34. Rohrich RJ, Sorokin ES, Brown SA. In search of improved fat transfer viability: a quantitative analysis of the role of centrifugation and harvest site. *Plast Reconstr Surg*. 2004;113(1):391–395; discussion 396–397.
35. Khouri RK, Rigotti G, Khouri Jr RK, et al. Tissue-engineered breast reconstruction with Brava-assisted fat grafting: a 7-year, 488-patient, multicenter experience. *Plast Reconstr Surg*. 2015;135(3):643–658.

36

Breast Reconstruction

ROBERT J. ALLEN Jr AND BABAK J. MEHRARA

Introduction

The female breast is a defining characteristic of femininity, and its distortion or absence may result in significant quality of life impairment and psychological distress. As a result, a variety of surgical techniques have been developed for reconstruction of congenital, traumatic, or oncological defects of the breast. These procedures have naturally and iteratively evolved over time, resulting in better cosmetic results and decreased surgical morbidity. Improvements in reconstructive outcomes increase overall satisfaction, self-esteem, body image, quality of life, and psychological well-being.[1] In a testament to the benefits of breast reconstruction, the Women's Health and Cancer Rights Act was enacted in 1998, mandating insurance coverage for breast reconstructive procedures in the United States. These advances are important because nearly 1 in 9 women will develop breast cancer in their lifetime. In the United States alone, nearly 250,000 new cases are detected annually, accounting for nearly 33% of all new cancer diagnoses per year.

This chapter is an overview of current practices in breast reconstruction and aims to cover the general principles of these procedures. It is not the intent of the authors to provide an encyclopedic discussion of this topic as entire textbooks have been written on portions of this chapter. As a result, the interested reader is guided to several excellent texts and landmark papers and manuscripts through this review.

Reconstructive Goals

The goals of breast reconstruction are to recreate a natura-appearing breast in clothing and, ideally, also when undressed, while limiting surgical morbidity. This process is individualized to best fit the reconstructive needs for volume and skin while taking oncological, social, and other concerns into consideration. As a result, a detailed history and physical examination paying close attention to social history, oncological history (when applicable), personal preferences of the patient, and availability of donor sites for reconstruction is necessary. This is a complicated process and requires practice and sensitivity. Nevertheless, successful completion of breast reconstruction is highly gratifying and personally rewarding.

Despite the nuances in anatomy, the breast can be defined by its fixed anatomical boundaries or "footprint" on the chest wall. Specifically, these boundaries include the inframammary fold (IMF) inferiorly; the second rib superiorly, the lateral border of the sternum medially; and an area located 1–2 cm posterior to the anterior axillary line laterally. Several authors have even attempted to quantify the ideal characteristics of an esthetic breast. However, while these measurements may represent the "ideal" breast shape, the reconstructive surgeon should aim for symmetry and pay attention to the patient's desire which, in some cases, may differ substantially from these ideals. With this as a background, the reconstructive surgeon can begin to analyze surgical options for reconstruction of the complex three-dimensional shape of the breast. As the breast is naturally made up of skin, fat, and glandular tissues, a patient's own skin and fat provide the most analogous tissue for a natural-appearing reconstruction. Shaping this tissue into an esthetically pleasing breast, however, can be a challenging task. Implants are also useful in many patients and can provide a pleasing reconstructive outcome.

Mastectomy Incisions

Mastectomy can be performed with a variety of incisions, including nipple sparing, skin sparing, Wise pattern, among others. The selection of the mastectomy incision should be made in conjunction with the breast surgeon and depends on oncological and esthetic factors. Esthetic factors include the size and shape of the breast, the degree of ptosis and the patient's desires. This last point is very important. A large-breasted patient who desires a reduction and lift following their mastectomy is not served well with a nipple-sparing mastectomy since failure to fill the breast envelope will result in contour deformities that are difficult to manage. One option in these cases is to proceed initially with a breast reduction and lift, wait until the skin has fully healed and the blood supply to the nipple–areola complex (NAC) is restored through the periareolar scar, and then proceed with mastectomy. This option is not always possible or advisable

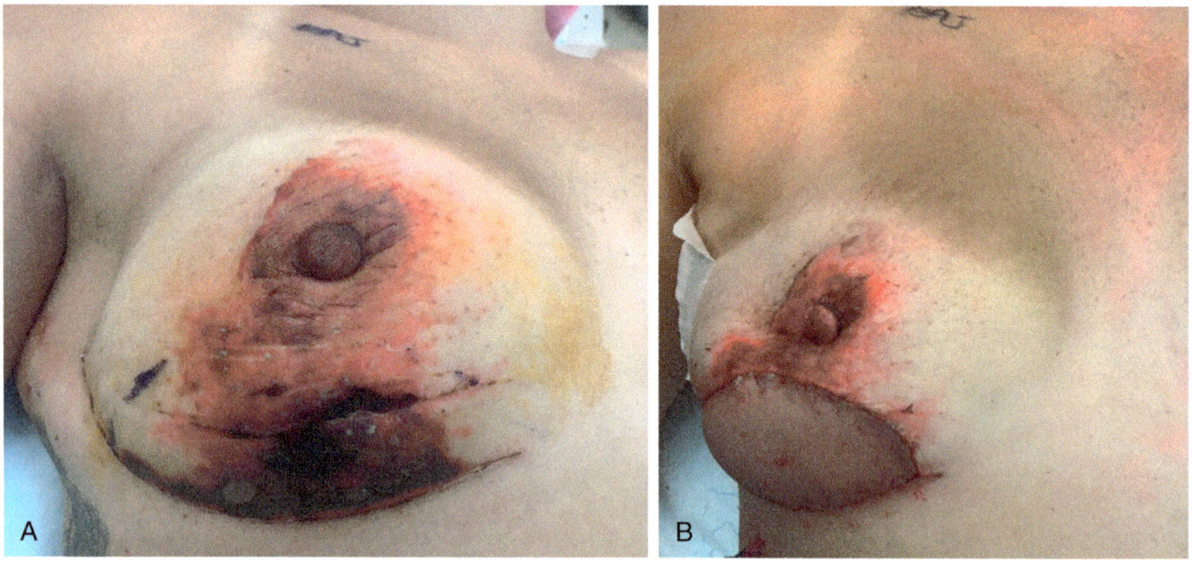

• **Fig. 36.1** (A) Photograph of a patient 2 weeks after nipple-sparing mastectomy through an IMF incision. Note ischemia of the triangle below the nipple. (B) Immediate postoperative photograph after salvage with thoracodorsal artery perforator flap.

in women who have active breast cancer. In most cases, an excellent outcome is achievable with virtually any breast incision if a reasonable mastectomy that does not overly thin the breast skin or violate the borders of the breast is performed.

Nipple-Sparing Mastectomy

Nipple-sparing mastectomy is an excellent option for most women. However, this approach may not be feasible in cases where the breast tumor is close to or involves the NAC. Nipple-sparing mastectomy is also not a good option in women with significant ptosis or those with very large breasts. The skin tone and thickness, as well as a sound approach to mastectomy taking care to preserve the blood supply of the skin and avoiding undue tension with retraction, are vitally important.

Nipple-sparing mastectomies can be performed with an incision in the inframammary fold, lateral breast incision with or without a periareolar extension, or a vertical incision. These incisions all have advantages and disadvantages. For example, a lateral incision decreases the length of the mastectomy skin flap and allow excellent exposure of the upper/outer part of the breast. In addition, if mastectomy or skin flap or nipple–areola necrosis occurs following surgery with this incision, the skin can simply be excised and re-expanded with an expander converting the procedure to skin-sparing mastectomy. However, the lateral breast nipple-sparing mastectomy incision has a higher rate of nipple–areola necrosis (particularly if the incision is extended around the NAC). This incision is also more likely to result in outward malposition of the nipple–areola by decreasing the relative potential of expansion of the lateral breast skin as compared to the medial breast skin. As a result, the medial breast area may be overexpanded, thus shifting the position of the nipple laterally.

The inframammary incision avoids all incisions on the breast and can hide the mastectomy incision in the fold. This incision also avoids cicatricial distortion of skin expansion and is less likely to cause nipple malposition. However, the inframammary incision is more technically challenging, particularly in patients with large or more ptotic breasts. This incision also limits exposure of the upper part of the breast and may complicate resection of upper–outer or upper–medial breast tumors. Excess tension on the skin with retraction or disturbance of skin perfusion may result in skin necrosis that is difficult to deal with in patients treated with inframammary mastectomy since there is little excess skin laxity in this area and excision of necrotic skin will almost certainly result in distortion of the reconstructed breast. In severe cases, mastectomy skin ischemia may involve a triangular-shaped area that includes the NAC and the skin incision (Fig. 36.1). Full-thickness necrosis in these cases necessitates reconstruction with a flap to replace the skin and restore the normal shape of the breast. Finally, the inframammary skin incision may make it difficult to expose recipient vessels for free flap breast reconstruction. Nevertheless, in experienced hands, the inframammary incision results in excellent esthetic outcomes (Fig. 36.2).

The vertical nipple-sparing mastectomy incision is an excellent choice in cases where autologous reconstruction is planned. This incision facilitates excellent exposure of the breast for mastectomy and dissection of the internal mammary artery/vein for microvascular anastomosis. Likewise, the vertical incision is less likely than the lateral breast incision to cause nipple–areola malposition. However, in our experience, this incision has a higher rate of nipple–areola ischemia than the inframammary incision, particularly when an extensive mastectomy is performed. Nevertheless, in cases where perfusion of the mastectomy skin is damaged, these areas can simply be excised and expanded or replaced by skin from the free flap.

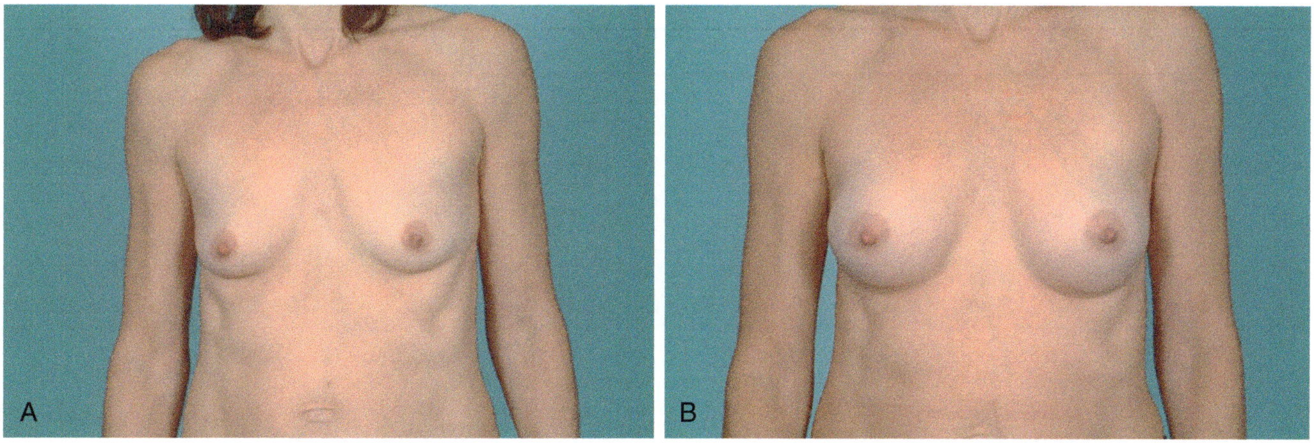

• **Fig. 36.2** (A) Preoperative and (B) 1-year postoperative photographs of a patient following bilateral nipple-sparing mastectomy via an IMF incision and reconstruction with implants.

Skin-Sparing Mastectomy

Skin sparing mastectomy is a good option in most cases and provides flexibility for reconstruction and excellent exposure for mastectomy. Skin-sparing mastectomy is safe and does not increase the risk of local recurrence or distant metastasis.[2] The most aggressive skin-sparing mastectomy is an areola-sparing mastectomy in which the nipple but not the areola is resected along with the breast. This is an excellent option in women who wish to maximally minimize their risk of breast cancer by removing as much breast tissue as possible since the areola, unlike the nipple, does not contain breast ducts. The areola-sparing mastectomy can also help hide the scar from the procedure within the areola or just outside it thus decreasing the final length of the mastectomy incision because a large elliptical excision of the NAC is avoided. Finally, the preserved areola skin is thicker than the surrounding breast skin and regains muscular activity following mastectomy. These features preserve the ability of the areola skin to respond to cold or touch thereby permitting reconstruction of a highly esthetic nipple. This incision is not ideal, however, for patients with excess ptosis or those in whom the breast tumor extends close to or involves the NAC.

Skin-sparing mastectomy can also be performed by simply excising the NAC with a circular incision and replacing this area with skin from a flap. A vertical or medial extension of this incision can greatly increase the exposure of recipient vessels while preserving the overall esthetics of the breast. This incision has also been reported for use with tissue expander/implants closing the mastectomy skin in a "cross-shaped" fashion. However, in our experience, we have found that this approach limits expansion of the central breast area and decreases projection where it is most needed. In most cases, an elliptical incision removing the NAC and skin lateral/medial to this area is the best option for skin-sparing mastectomy when tissue expander/implant reconstruction is planned. This approach allows excision of all excess skin and redraping to avoid medial/lateral breast dog ears. Wider elliptical excisions also allow lifting the breast and repositioning the reconstruction higher up on the chest; however, this approach can result in long, unsightly incisions that are difficult to hide.

Non-Skin-Sparing Mastectomy or Delayed Reconstruction

In some cases, skin-sparing mastectomy is not possible. This is an issue, for example, in patients who have been previously treated with radiation and have unfavorable prior partial mastectomy scars (i.e., incisions that are not in-line with the NAC or located in anatomically unfavorable areas of the breast). These patients are at high risk of developing mastectomy skin flap necrosis if a standard skin-sparing mastectomy is performed. In other patients, the skin may be involved with tumor and may require wide resection, or the skin may be previously damaged by radiation and thereby not suitable for reconstruction. In these cases, it is often better to remove the damaged skin and replace it with healthy flap skin thus, at the minimum, restoring the natural shape of the breast but at the cost of larger breast incisions.

Wise Pattern Mastectomy

Wise pattern mastectomy is an excellent option for patients with breast ptosis or macromastia. This incision enables reduction of the skin envelope and simultaneous narrowing of the breast width. In addition, preservation of the lower mastectomy skin flap increases lower pole projection and covers the T-point, thus providing an extra layer of protection in case of skin breakdown or mastectomy skin flap necrosis. The Wise pattern mastectomy is designed as would be performed for a standard breast reduction. In our experience, it has been helpful to make the vertical limbs of the pattern slightly longer than usual (8–10 cm rather than the typical 7 cm used for Wise pattern breast reduction). The mastectomy is done using the vertical and upper

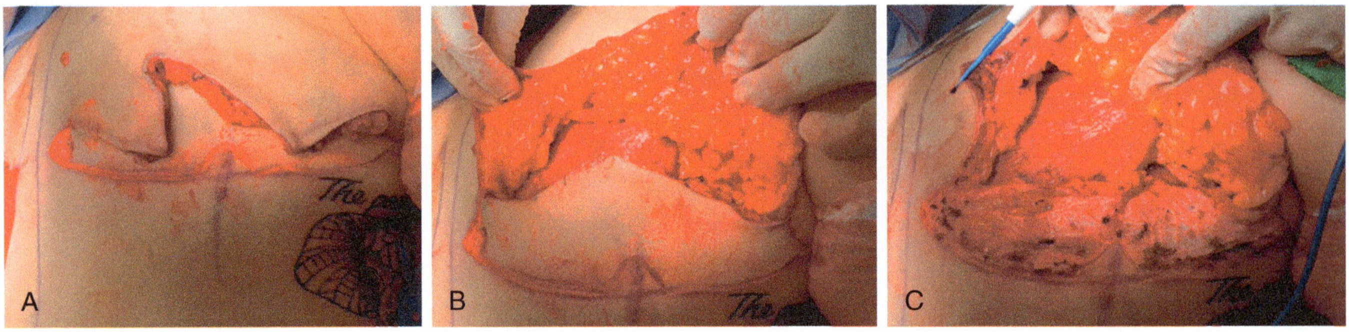

• **Fig. 36.3** Technique for Wise pattern mastectomy and implant reconstruction. (A,B) The lower skin flap that is ordinarily discarded with a Wise pattern breast reduction is preserved and de-epithelialized. (C) The resulting flap is then sutured to the inferior border of the pectoralis major flap to cover the lower pole of the reconstruction.

flap incisions, and the breast is dissected from the lower skin flap that would ordinarily be removed following breast reduction. This skin flap is then de-epithelialized and used to cover the lower portion of the reconstruction (either a tissue expander or autologous breast reconstruction) to improve projection and contour of the lower breast pole. The Wise pattern mastectomy can be technically challenging for breast surgeons, particularly in women with severe macromastia. Aggressive mastectomy with violation of the later breast fold or dissection above the level of the second rib greatly increase the risk of mastectomy skin flap necrosis. In these situations, the lower mastectomy skin flap can be used to replace the ischemic breast skin, and indocyanine green angiography (ICGA) is helpful to assess the degree of skin resection necessary. This results in the placement of a triangle of skin in the inferior portion of the breast; however, the long-term results can still be excellent (Fig. 36.3).

Autologous Tissue Breast Reconstruction

Autologous tissue breast reconstruction, in the appropriately selected patient, offers several advantages over implant-based techniques. This approach usually results in a more natural-appearing and more natural-feeling reconstructed breast and avoids the long-term complications of breast implants such as capsular contracture, implant rupture, and asymmetry due to weight gain or aging (Fig. 36.4). Autologous breast reconstruction is, however, more technically challenging and demands a thorough understanding of anatomy and tissue perfusion. As a result, progress in surgical techniques together with advanced knowledge of anatomy have led to continuous improvement and evolution of autologous breast reconstruction resulting in better esthetic outcomes and decreased donor site morbidity.

In 1965, the microsurgery pioneers Tamai and Komatsu successfully replanted an amputated thumb at the metacarpophalangeal joint, marking the beginning of the microsurgical renaissance in plastic and hand surgery.[3] This was followed in 1973 by Taylor and Daniel's report of a successful free microvascular skin flap and then in 1975 by Toyomi Fujino, who performed the first microvascular reconstruction of a congenital breast aplasia defect with a free myocutaneous flap from the buttocks anastomosed to the thoracoacromial vessels. These technical advances facilitated transplantation of tissues from one part of the body to another and increased the number of options available for reconstruction.

Ground-breaking anatomical dissections by Taylor and Palmer in the late 1980s described the concept of skin angiosomes, identifying source vessels for various regions of the body. This was an important discovery and suggested that large areas of skin could survive based simply on a single artery and vein (i.e., a perforator), leading the way for the development of a variety of flaps. The angiosomes concept has thus served as a basis for rational, anatomically-based flap design and has greatly advanced autologous tissue breast reconstruction using donor sites that include the abdomen, the inner/outer thighs, the back, and the gluteal areas.

Abdominally-Based Flaps

Pedicled Transverse Abdominis Myocutaneous Flap (pTRAM)

History

The abdomen is the ideal donor site for autologous breast reconstruction because this area can provide ample tissue, and the donor site scar can be placed in a favorable position. The abdomen also enables harvesting of a large skin paddle that is suitable for reconstruction of large chest wall defects. The use of abdominal tissues for reconstruction can be traced back to Sir Harold Gillies, who first described the use of tubed abdominal flaps for breast reconstruction in 1942. These operations required multiple delay procedures and often resulted in flap failure. This history is nicely reviewed by Uroskie and Colen.[4] In 1977, Drever described the use of the epigastric island flap, now commonly referred to as the vertical rectus abdominis myocutaneous flap (VRAM), for breast reconstruction.[5] This flap had an excellent blood supply and, unlike the previously

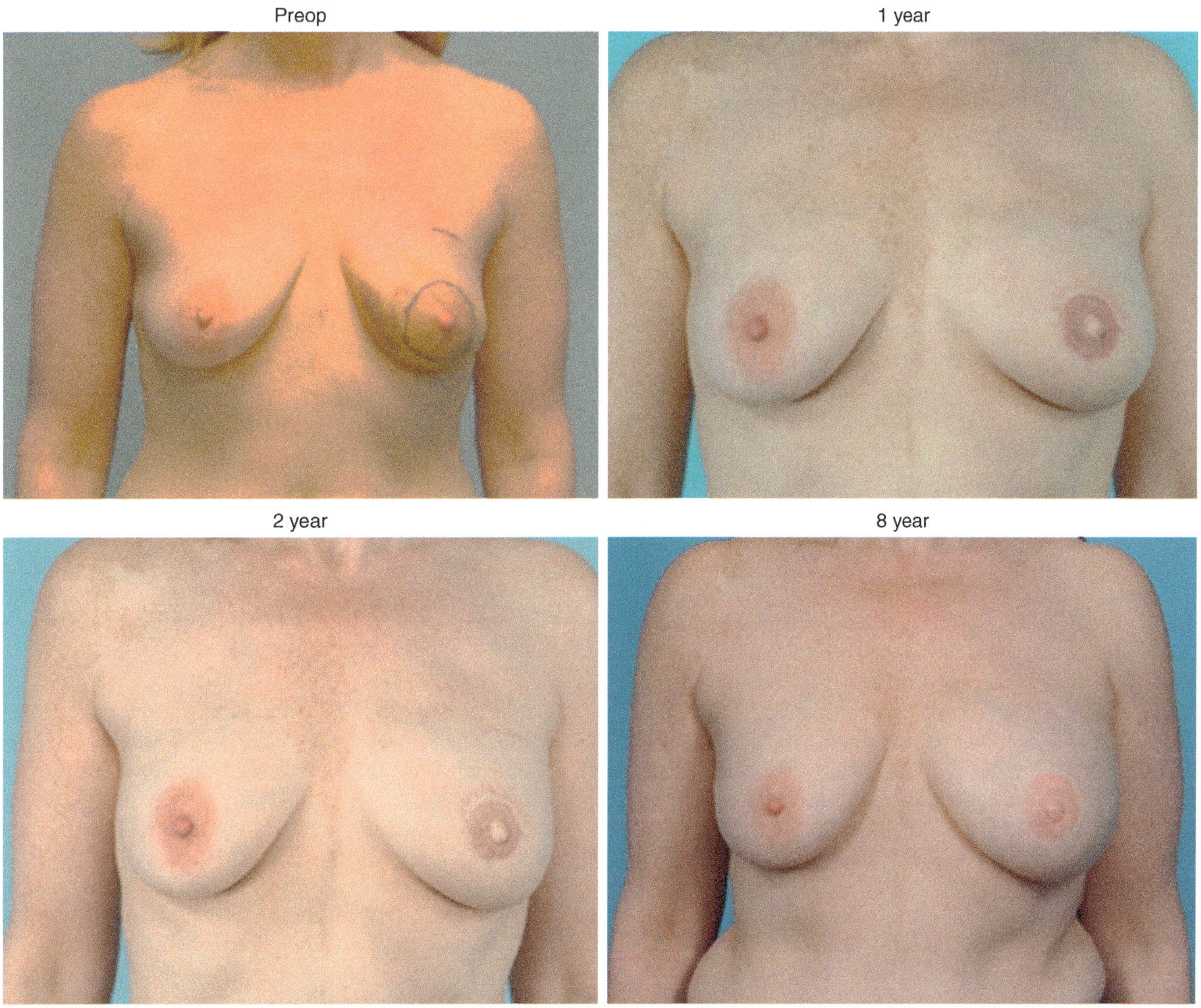

• **Fig. 36.4** One-year postoperative and long-term photographs of the same patient after left breast reconstruction with a DIEP flap. Note how the flap changes over time with weight gain, maintaining a good symmetry with the right breast over time

reported tubed flaps, could be transferred in a single operation. A few years after this initial report, Robbins described the use of the VRAM flap for breast reconstruction.[6] The abdominal donor site rapidly gained popularity and became the workhorse for reconstruction following the description of the pedicled transverse rectus abdominis myocutaneous flap (pTRAM) flap by Hartrampf et al, in 1982.[7] This flap is based on skin perforators arising from the deep superior epigastric artery and vein, and enabled surgeons to place the abdominal scar in the lower abdomen. The ability to improve the contour of the abdomen while reconstructing the breast was intuitively appealing to both patients and plastic surgeons. In addition, unlike the latissimus flap (the other commonly used autologous option at the time), the pTRAM flap provides a large amount of skin and soft tissues that could be used to replace the missing skin/volume of the breast without an implant. This was particularly important in the early 1980s since at that time, immediate breast reconstruction was rarely performed, and most women who presented for breast reconstruction had large skin and soft tissue deficits.

Patient Selection

The pTRAM can be performed in patients who have a suitable body habitus and sufficient lower abdominal skin and fat to restore the volume of the breast. Obesity, active smoking, significant co-morbid conditions, and history of prior abdominal surgery are relative contraindications. Obesity and smoking significantly increase the risk of complications, including partial flap loss, fat necrosis, and abdominal wall complications. Patients with a history of open cholecystectomy are at high risk of abdominal skin necrosis and hernia. The right upper rectus muscle is also transected in this operation, thereby precluding harvest of a right-sided flap. A prior history of abdominoplasty is a contraindication for pTRAM flap breast reconstruction. Other abdominal operations such as cesarean section, midline laparotomy, laparoscopy and appendectomy, increase the risk of abdominal complications but may be feasible if the rectus muscle has not been injured. Prior chest wall surgery, including medial sternotomy or procedures in which the internal mammary artery/vein have been damaged or resected, usually preclude the use of a pTRAM flap for breast reconstruction.

Surgical Technique

The pTRAM is still commonly performed in many areas of the United States and Europe. This procedure is relatively simple to perform, does not require microsurgical skills and, in experienced hands, can provide excellent outcomes. The flap is marked in the lower abdomen with the upper skin incision line usually drawn 1–2 cm above the umbilicus. This upper incision placement does place the lower abdominal incision higher than a typical abdominoplasty or free TRAM flap (see below), however, capturing the periumbilical perforators greatly improves the blood supply of the flap and decreases complications such as fat necrosis or partial flap loss. The upper skin incision is performed, and the upper skin flap is elevated to the level of the xyphoid centrally and the costal margin laterally. The lower incision is then performed, and the flap is carefully elevated from lateral to medial taking care to preserve the cutaneous perforators arising from the rectus muscle in these areas. The flap dissection is continued to expose the medial and lateral row perforators arising from the rectus muscle and supplying the overlying skin. The anterior abdominal wall fascia is then incised, and the intercostal branches to the rectus muscle are ligated. The inferior epigastric artery and vein are identified and dissected distally for 5–8 cm and ligated. The inferior epigastric pedicle can be used as a fallback and anastomosed to recipient vessels in the chest in case the perfusion from the superior epigastric artery/vein is inadequate. The rectus muscle is then dissected from inferior to superior taking care to avoid injury to the pedicle vessels that run on the deep surface of the muscle. The flap may be transferred to the breast from the ipsilateral or contralateral abdominal area. In the authors' experience, we have found that an ipsilateral flap has a longer reach and results in less significant disruption of the inframammary fold. Once the flap is dissected, a tunnel is made connecting the abdominal site to the breast, and the flap is carefully pulled through to avoid avulsion of the cutaneous perforators of the flap. The perfusion of the flap is then assessed, and the flap is inset into the defect to reconstruct the breast.

Hartrampf divided the abdominal tissues into four zones: zones 1 and 2 are ipsilateral to the harvested muscle while zones 3 and 4 cross the midline to the other side (Fig. 36.5). Zones 1 and 2 can be consistently transferred with a pTRAM. However, extended flaps with large segments of zone 3 are less reliable and susceptible to distal necrosis. Zone 4 is not well perfused and should not be used with a pTRAM. Perfusion across the midline of the abdomen can be improved by anastomosing the deep inferior epigastric vein to a recipient vein in the axilla, a process known as supercharging a flap. Less commonly, the deep inferior epigastric artery may also require anastomosis. Another

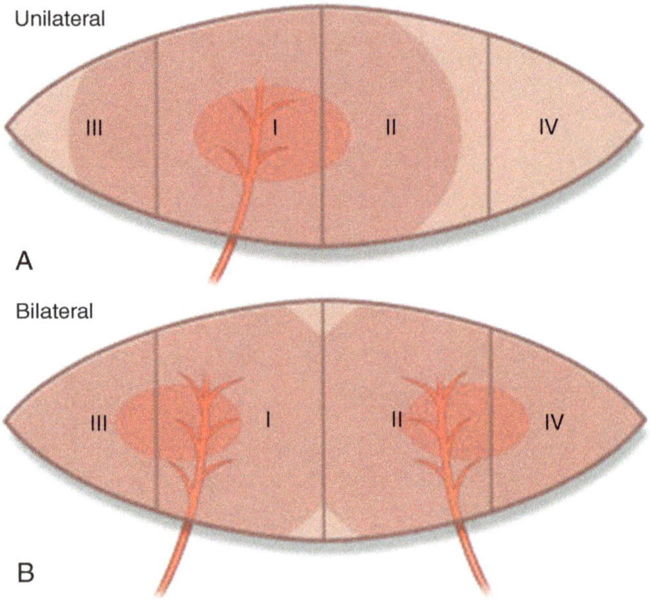

• **Fig. 36.5** The blood supply zones of a TRAM flap based on the right rectus abdominis muscle perforators. (A) Unilateral; (B) bilateral. (From Nahabedian MY. The free TRAM flap. In: Nahabedian MY, Neligan PC, eds. *Plastic Surgery*, Vol. 5: *Breast*. Elsevier; 2018.)

option is to delay the flap by incising the skin and ligating the deep inferior epigastric vessels 2–4 weeks prior to flap transfer. Other authors have described the use of bipedicle TRAM flaps in which both rectus muscles are harvested, thus providing a dual blood supply to the skin. This surgical approach enables transfer of virtually all of the lower abdominal skin/fat and greatly increases the perfusion of the flap even in patients with comorbid conditions such as obesity; however, removal of both rectus muscles can be quite morbid, decreasing abdominal/core strength and resulting in higher rates of hernia formation as compared to a unilateral pTRAM or other abdominally-based flaps.

The abdominal fascia is closed either primarily, or more commonly, using permanent mesh that is placed as an inlay between the edges of the fascia. The contralateral fascia is often plicated to bring the umbilicus back to the midline. The patient is brought into a slightly flexed position, and the abdominal skin is closed over drains. Progressive tension sutures repairing the skin to the abdominal fascia are helpful to avoid excess tension on the abdominal skin incision and decrease the rates of abdominal seromas. These sutures usually enable the surgeon to remove the abdominal drains in a week or less following surgery.

Outcomes

The pTRAM flap is safe, with very low reported rates of complete flap loss. However, the rate of partial flap loss is significant (2%–10%) and can result in delayed healing, distortion of the reconstructed breast, and poor esthetic outcomes. The reported rates of fat necrosis with pTRAM flap reconstruction are also highly variable, ranging from 2%–3% to as high as 20% and depend largely on the surgical technique, the surgeon experience, and the definition of a clinically significant area of fat necrosis. These ischemic flap complications occur because the superior epigastric artery and vein are not the dominant blood supply of the lower abdominal skin and because there is considerable variability in the number/size of connections between the superior and inferior deep epigastric vessels. Thus, placing the flap higher up on the abdomen improves the blood supply by increasing the likelihood of capturing perforators that arise from the deep superior epigastric vessels. However, this flap design decreases the arc of rotation of the flap and results in a higher/less aesthetic lower abdominal donor scar.

The pTRAM also can be associated with high rates of abdominal wall complications such as abdominal wall laxity or hernia. These complications can occur in as many as 10%–12% of patients, although very low hernia rates have been reported by some authors.[8] Nevertheless, the closure of the abdominal wall is crucially important since the long fascial incision, together with the removal of the entire muscle clearly disrupts the abdominal wall and can result in significant morbidity.

Free TRAM (fTRAM) and Muscle-Sparing TRAM (msTRAM)

History

With time comes experience, and the high rate of fat necrosis and abdominal wall complications of the pTRAM led surgeons to experiment with other techniques aiming to decrease the incidence of these problems. In 1979, Holmström reported the use of the free TRAM flap in a series of experiments conducted on discarded abdominoplasty tissues.[9] Using angiography studies and a clinical series, he showed that the blood supply to the lower abdominal skin was reliable and that the procedure was technically feasible. The msTRAM was an evolution of the fTRAM and aimed to further decrease the morbidity of a fTRAM by decreasing the amount of muscle and fascia harvested with the flap.

Patient Selection

The fTRAM and msTRAM have the same indications and relative contraindications as the pTRAM. However, because of the improved perfusion of the free flap options, these procedures are usually well tolerated, with low rates of complications even in obese patients. Active smokers have higher rates of wound healing complications; however, free flap breast reconstruction is an option if the patient understands the risk. These complications are generally self-limited and usually resolve without the need for additional surgical intervention. Similarly, prior abdominal surgery or a history of prior abdominal liposuction do not preclude fTRAM or msTRAM breast reconstruction; however, it may be necessary to confirm the continuity of the pedicle vessels with imaging studies. A history of clotting abnormalities is a relative contraindication to these procedures as the risk of vascular complications is significantly increased in these patients. However, this risk may be mitigated by judicious use of anticoagulation.

Surgical Technique

To perform an fTRAM, the lateral and medial edges of the rectus muscle are identified, and the abdominal fascia is incised. The rectus muscle is transected superiorly and inferiorly, and the inferior portion of the muscle together with the deep inferior epigastric artery and vein are harvested. The flap is then transferred to the chest and perfusion is restored with microvascular anastomosis to the thoracodorsal artery/vein or the internal mammary artery/vein.

In the msTRAM, the lateral and medial borders of the rectus muscle are identified, and the dissection continues with exposure of the lateral and medial row perforators. The flap is elevated to spare as much of the fascia as possible. The fascia is incised, and the perforating vessels are harvested together with a portion of the rectus muscle. Usually, the central portion of the rectus muscle is harvested leaving the medial and lateral borders of the muscle intact and in continuity with the upper portion of the muscle. This is important since the neurovascular supply to the rectus muscle is derived from the lateral intercostal nerve branches leaving at least some of the muscle innervated. This procedure also decreases the amount of fascia that is removed, thus decreasing the need for mesh reconstruction.

A two-team approach is usually used for flap harvest and preparation of recipient vessels. The internal mammary vessels are the recipient vessels of choice for most surgeons, as they are of similar caliber to the deep inferior epigastric vessels and can be exposed widely for ease of microsurgical anastomosis. In most instances, the 3rd rib cartilage is removed in part or in whole to provide access to the underlying internal mammary artery/vein; however, a rib-sparing approach can be used. Alternately, the thoracodorsal vessels can be used as recipient vessels.

Once the flap dissection is completed, and recipient vessels have been prepared, the anterior surface of pedicle vessels is marked with methylene blue or a marking pen, and the vessels are divided. Marking the anterior surface of the pedicle helps to avoid twisting of the pedicle during microvascular anastomosis. The microsurgical anastomosis is performed, and the flap is inset. The abdominal wall is repaired, and mesh is used as necessary to reinforce the abdominal fascia repair. Transversus abdominis plane blocks are used at our center for postoperative pain control in the abdomen. The patient is brought into a slightly flexed position, and the abdominal skin is closed as discussed for the pTRAM.

Outcomes

Several groups have compared outcomes between the fTRAM flap with the pTRAM and demonstrated decreased rates of partial flap loss, fat necrosis, abdominal wall laxity, and hernias. The use of the fTRAM also avoids the unsightly bulge in the epigastrium that can occur with the tunneling of the pTRAM into the breast area. The improved blood supply of the fTRAM enables the safe transfer of larger amounts of abdominal tissues, facilitates inset of the flap, and improves esthetic outcomes in the breast and the abdomen.

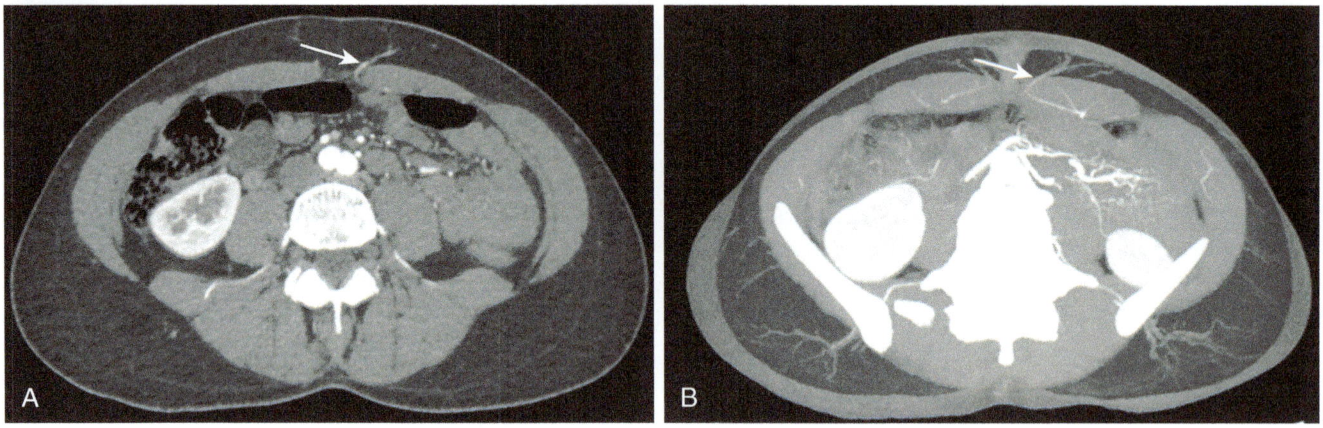

• **Fig. 36.6** (A) Preoperative MRA of abdomen showing a paramuscular perforator from the deep inferior epigastric vessels. (B) Delayed imaging showing course of perforator around rectus abdominis muscle before joining the deep inferior epigastric pedicle.

The msTRAM and the fTRAM have an excellent blood supply and tissue perfusion that routinely enable the transfer of tissues across the midline, including most or all of zone 3 and, occasionally, even zone 4. In experienced hands, these flap options have excellent outcomes with low rates of total flap loss (<1%) and fat necrosis (5%–8%).[10] A recent meta-analysis of 11 studies comparing outcomes following 1891 pTRAM vs. 866 fTRAM flaps found a significantly lower risk of fat necrosis and partial flap loss with microvascular techniques.[11] Another meta-analysis of outcomes following msTRAM and fTRAM reported a pooled rate of 4.9% for fat necrosis, 1.8% partial flap loss, and 1% total flap loss.[12] The msTRAM and fTRAM also have lower rates of abdominal wall complications and decreased abdominal weakness as compared to the pTRAM. The pooled rates of abdominal wall bulge/laxity/weakness in a meta-analysis of 14 studies was 5.9% while the rate of abdominal hernia was 3.9%.

Deep Inferior Epigastric Artery Perforator (DIEP) and Muscle-Sparing TRAM Flaps

History

In 1989, Koshima and Soeda first described the concept of the "inferior epigastric artery skin flaps without rectus abdominis muscle" for the reconstruction of a groin defect and a defect of the oral cavity.[13] A few years later, Robert Allen Sr reported the use of the deep inferior epigastric artery (DIEP) flap for breast reconstruction.[14] Since its original description, numerous authors have published favorable outcomes with the DIEP flap, and its use has become routine in centers that specialize in microvascular autologous tissue breast reconstruction.

Patient Selection

The DIEP flap is usually the first choice for microsurgical autologous reconstruction because of its long pedicle length, the caliber, and ease of dissection of the inferior epigastric artery and vein, the large amount of skin and fat that can be harvested, and the inconspicuous donor site scar. The ability to simultaneously reconstruct a bilateral mastectomy with one donor site scar is also a major advantage of the DIEP flap. The DIEP flap has the same indications and relative contraindications as the fTRAM/msTRAM.

Surgical Technique

The DIEP flap is the natural evolution of the muscle-sparing flap. In this procedure, the perforating vessels that perfuse the skin are dissected free from the rectus muscle, and the innervation of the muscle is largely maintained. The size and location of the abdominal wall perforators can be assessed preoperatively using computed tomographic angiography (CTA) or magnetic resonance angiography (MRA) (Fig. 36.6). This information may enable the surgeon to assess the feasibility of performing a DIEP, decrease operative time, and provides an estimate of the amount of tissues available for breast reconstruction. The position of the perforators is usually marked in relation to the umbilicus, and the flap is designed to capture the largest perforators. In some cases, however, preoperative imaging may not be available, and the procedure can simply be performed by surgically exposing the perforators and selecting the best option for reconstruction. The use of a handheld Doppler may help identify perforators preoperatively in these cases; however, in general, this is not necessary.

Flap dissection is begun as with the msTRAM to elevate the upper abdominal flap and to identify the perforating vessels to the skin. The superficial inferior epigastric vein (SIEV), if present, should be identified and dissected for several centimeters. This vessel may be useful as an additional venous outflow option if the flap is congested following the completion of perforator dissection. If a preoperative MRA or CTA was performed, this is used to guide the surgeon to the "ideal" perforator. Without imaging, the surgeon should choose the largest perforator encountered. This can be judged based on size, visible pulsation, or handheld Doppler ultrasound. Once a perforator(s) is chosen, the anterior abdominal wall fascia is incised, taking care to avoid

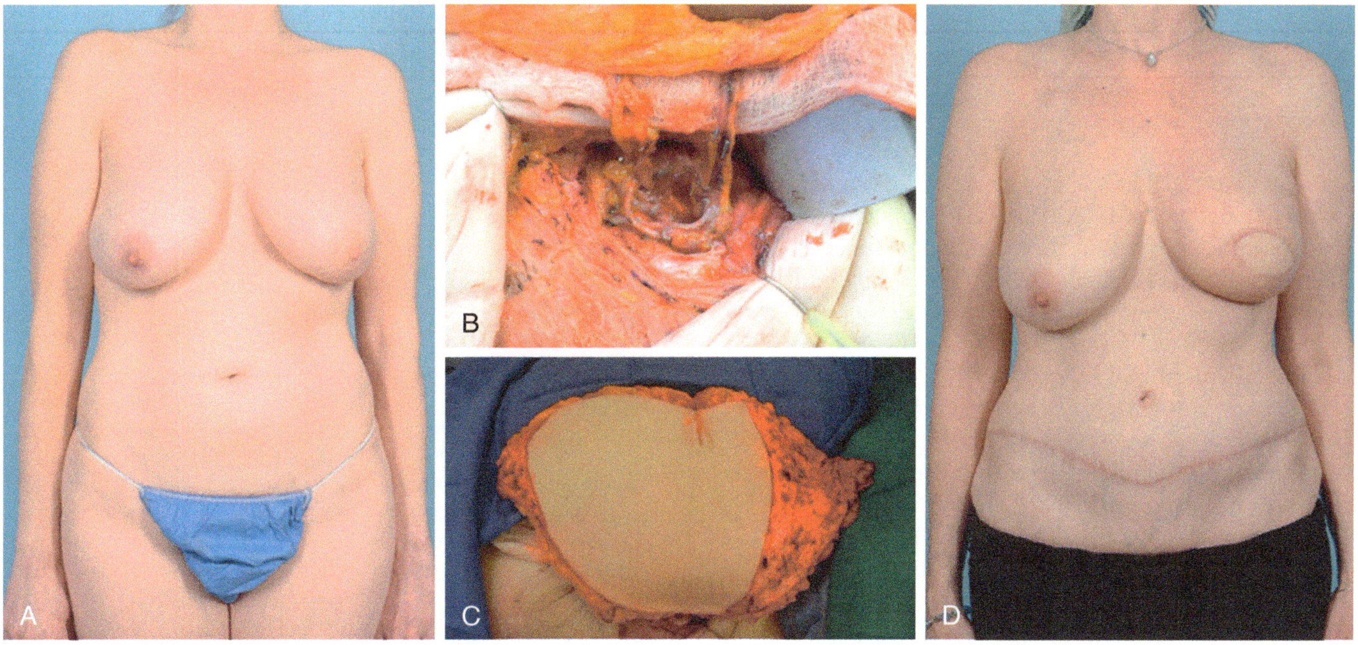

• **Fig. 36.7** Example of stacked or conjoined DIEP flaps for unilateral breast reconstruction. (A) Preoperative photo. (B) Anastomosis of both pedicles in an antegrade and retrograde fashion to the internal mammary vessels. (C) Perfusion of entire abdomen following anastomoses. (D) Postoperative result at 5 months with no revisions.

injury to the vessel. The perforator is then carefully dissected through the rectus muscle back to the main pedicle. The length of the pedicle dissection is guided by the size of the recipient vessels and the surgeon's preference. In cases where multiple perforators are harvested, it may be necessary to divide motor branches that travel between the perforators. These motor nerve branches can usually be microsurgically repaired.

Prior to division of the pedicle, it is prudent to assess the perfusion of the flap by checking capillary refill and bleeding from the edges of the flap. These clinical signs can alert the surgeon to areas of the flap that are not well perfused. This assessment can be confirmed using ICGA. This technology can also be used to assess perfusion of mastectomy skin flaps, thereby possibly decreasing the risk of postoperative complications.

The DIEP flap can reliably transfer tissues across the abdominal midline in most patients. In some cases, perfusion is inadequate, most commonly manifesting as venous congestion. In these cases, the SIEV contralateral to the pedicle vessels can be anastomosed either to a branch of the DIEV or, more commonly, to the internal mammary vein. This may necessitate a vein graft. In other cases when the entire lower abdominal flap is needed for reconstruction, perforating vessels on both sides of the abdomen can be dissected, and both pedicles anastomosed to the internal mammary artery/vein in an anterograde/retrograde fashion. These so-called "stacked flaps" have excellent perfusion and facilitate the shaping of the breast to create ptosis or reconstruct large volume defects (Fig. 36.7).

Once the flap has been harvested, it is weighed and transferred up to the chest for microvascular anastomosis. In most cases, a flap harvested from the contralateral abdominal wall is used since this orientation allows the pedicle vessels to run along the medial border of the chest and place the SIEV in close proximity to the internal mammary vessels, giving the surgeon the option of additional venous outflow or supercharging of the flap. However, an ipsilateral flap is also commonly performed if the perforating vessels in this area are superior in size/caliber as compared with the contralateral flap. In this case, the SIEV can easily be anastomosed to the axillary vessels if necessary. Following microvascular anastomosis, the flap is shaped and secured to the chest wall. Any twisting, kinking, or tension on the pedicle should be avoided. A skin paddle is usually left visible for postoperative flap monitoring, and the remainder of the flap is de-epithelialized. The skin is closed in layered fashion after placement of a closed suction drain.

The abdominal donor site is closed as outlined for the msTRAM. Mesh may be used as necessary if the fascia is attenuated or in patients with a prior history of abdominal operations. The abdominal wall may be plicated to improve the contour of the abdominal wall.

Postoperatively, patients are treated with an enhanced recovery after surgery (ERAS) protocol in which they are monitored for 4–6 hours in the recovery room and then transferred to a regular room. "Flap checks" are performed every 15 minutes for 1 hour, every 30 minutes for 2 hours and then every 1 hour for the next 24 hours. Patients are treated with subcutaneous heparin or Enoxaparin just prior to surgery and then daily for up to 1 month based on their risk of deep venous thrombosis as assessed by the Caprini Score.[15] After discharge from the hospital, patients are asked to avoid strenuous activity, and lifting objects greater than 10 pounds for 6 weeks to prevent abdominal wall dehiscence.

Outcomes

Although some older studies had suggested that the DIEP flap may have a higher risk of partial flap loss and fat necrosis as compared with fTRAM/msTRAM, more recent studies suggest that the risk of these complications is similar in experienced hands and in properly selected patients.[12] DIEP flaps also have lower rates of abdominal wall laxity and hernia as compared with fTRAM and pTRAM flaps. The pooled abdominal wall bulge/laxity/weakness rate reported in 11 studies with 930 DIEP flaps was 3.1%. This rate compares favorably with the pooled rate of 5.9% reported in 14 studies with 2015 fTRAM flaps. Similarly, the pooled rate of abdominal wall hernia in 10 studies reporting on 1529 DIEP flaps was 0.8% as compared to a rate of 3.9% in 18 studies reporting on 2609 msTRAM flaps.[12]

Superficial Inferior Epigastric Artery (SIEA) Flap

History

The SIEA flap is an axial adipocutaneous flap based on the superficial inferior epigastric vessels and was first described in 1971 by Antia and Buch for the repair of a soft tissue defect of the face.[16] Robert Allen Sr reported the first use of the SIEA flap for partial and total breast reconstruction.

Patient Selection

The SIEA flap has the same indications and contraindications as the DIEP flap. However, the use of this flap option may be limited by the caliber of the pedicle vessels, which are variable among individuals. These vessels can be analyzed preoperatively using imaging with CTA or MRA or with a handheld Doppler. In practice, the major indication for this flap is whether the superficial inferior epigastric artery is present, has a suitable size, and a palpable/visible pulse. The superficial inferior epigastric artery branches off of the common femoral or the superficial circumflex femoral artery and, when present, has a diameter of 1.1–1.9 mm.[17] However, the artery has considerable anatomical variability and is absent in as many as 57% of individuals and, by some estimates, only adequate in diameter for microvascular anastomosis in fewer than 25% of cases.[18]

Surgical Technique

The flap markings and patient setup are the same as for the DIEP flap. The procedure begins with the inferior skin incision just through the dermis, followed by careful dissection through the subcutaneous tissues to identify the SIEV. Deeper dissection, usually lateral to the SIEV and 4–7 cm from the midline, is performed through Scarpa's fascia to identify the SIEA. If the SIEA is present and suitable for microsurgical anastomosis, the dissection is continued to the origin of the vessels, and the flap dissection is completed by ligating the DIEP perforators. Flap perfusion can be

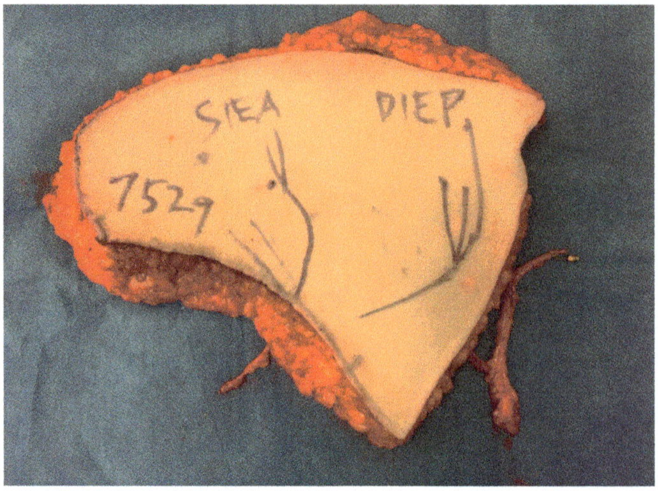

• **Fig. 36.8** An example of a hemiabdominal flap raised on both the superficial inferior epigastric and deep inferior epigastric vessels. Note the more superficial location of the superficial vessels compared to the deep vessels.

assessed prior to ligation of the DIEP perforators to ensure that adequate blood supply is present. If not, the SIEA is aborted, and a DIEP flap is elevated instead. The flap is then ligated, and microsurgical anastomosis is performed to the internal mammary vessels. The contralateral flap is preferred since this orientation places the pedicle vessels at the medial border of the flap, decreasing the risk of tension or kinking on the anastomosis. If an ipsilateral flap is chosen for the reconstruction, the flap is rotated 180 degrees to line up the SIEA/SIEV with the internal mammary vessels.

Great care is taken during insetting of an SIEA flap to avoid kinking of the pedicle vessels since these vessels are relatively short and exit the tissues more superficially than the pedicle for the DIEP flap (Fig. 36.8). This anatomical orientation, particularly in obese patients with thick flaps, can result in a sharp turn of the pedicle vessels through the pectoralis muscle to reach the internal mammary vessels, making it more likely to kink or place the anastomosis under tension. The superficial nature of the pedicle in the SIEA flap also increases the possibility of compression by the mastectomy skin flaps as may occur in patients with a history of radiation. The breast and abdominal incisions are closed as described for the DIEP flap. The abdominal fascia may be plicated as necessary to improve the contour of the lower abdomen.

Outcomes

The primary advantage of the SIEA flap as compared to other abdominally based tissue options is lack of injury to the abdominal wall fascia or musculature. Patients treated with SIEA flaps have essentially no risk of abdominal wall hernia and retain abdominal core strength. However, this advantage is balanced by an increased risk of microvascular complications because the SIEA is usually smaller in diameter as compared to the DIEA and because the pedicle for the SIEA flap is relatively short. As a result, even experienced surgeons reporting large series of cases have reported total flap loss rates of 3%–5%; a number that is considerably higher than msTRAM or DIEP flaps. The rate of fat necrosis following SIEA flaps is also higher than other abdominally-based options due to the anatomical variability of the vascular supply of this flap.

Thigh-Based Flaps

While the abdominal donor site is an excellent option in many patients, this area may not be suitable in some individuals due to paucity of abdominal tissue, a history of previous abdominal surgery, or an aversion to abdominal scars. In these cases, tissues harvested from the medial or lateral thighs may be a good option.

Gracilis Flaps

Transverse Upper Gracilis (TUG)/Transverse Myocutaneous Gracilis (TMG) Flap

History

The transverse myocutaneous gracilis (TMG) or transverse upper gracilis (TUG) flap is the most commonly cited thigh-based flap used for breast reconstruction since its first description by Yousif et al in 1992.[19] This flap is oriented transversely, extending anteriorly along the groin crease to the posterior midline of the thigh along the gluteal crease. This orientation is analogous to a medial thigh lift, and the blood supply to the flap is the gracilis pedicle, which is a branch of the profunda femoris artery. The pedicle for the flap is reliably found deep to the adductor longus muscle approximately 6–8 cm distal to the groin crease. Musculocutaneous perforators from the gracilis pedicle and septocutaneous perforators around the gracilis muscle provide perfusion to the skin and soft tissues of this flap.

Patient Selection

Gracilis-based flaps are good options for patients who are not candidates for abdominally-based flaps or would like to avoid the abdominal scar and have sufficient tissue of the medial and posterior thigh for breast reconstruction (i.e., patients with a pear-shaped body habitus). Poor candidates for the thigh donor site include those with peripheral vascular disease, severe venous insufficiency or history of deep vein thrombosis, and any unexplained swelling suspicious for primary lymphedema. Morbidly obese patients or those with large amounts of adipose tissues in the medial thigh areas are also poor candidates for gracilis-based flaps.

Surgical Technique

The groin crease and inferior gluteal fold are marked with the patient in the standing position. The superior border of the flap will be 1–2 cm below this line and should not extend beyond the posterior midline of the thigh. Anteriorly, the tip of the flap is located 2–5 cm anterior to the adductor longus muscle, which is easily marked with the patient in the frog-legged position. An ellipse is drawn to connect the anterior- and posterior-most portions of the flap after pinch test confirms the amount of tissue that can be harvested (reliably 6–8 cm). A conservative approach to flap width is essential, as this transversely oriented flap results in the greatest tension lines on closure. Excess tension can result in labial spreading and/or flattening of the inferior gluteal crease.

The patient is prepped and positioned in the frog-legged (or less commonly, lithotomy position). A two-team approach can be used for flap harvest, while the recipient vessels are being prepared or the mastectomies performed. The anterior portion of the flap is incised, and a superficial dissection proceeds posteriorly to avoid skeletonizing the greater saphenous vein and reduce the risk of lower extremity lymphedema. The adductor longus muscle is identified, and this fascia is incised throughout the width of the flap over the muscle, ensuring capture of septocutaneous perforators between the adductor longus and gracilis muscles. The adductor longus muscle is then retracted anteriorly revealing the gracilis pedicle. At this point, the pedicle can be easily dissected to its takeoff (6–8 cm). It is isolated circumferentially before the final skin incisions are made and the entire gracilis muscle is harvested. Care should be taken to avoid beveling to include greater volumes of the flap to improve the contour of the final donor site.

The ipsilateral flap is used for breast reconstruction with anastomosis to the internal mammary vessels. The flap is inset to the chest wall following microvascular anastomosis, leaving a skin paddle for postoperative monitoring. Patients are monitored postoperatively as noted above. Compressive garments are routinely applied over the donor site. There are no specific precautions besides avoiding trauma to the incision and strenuous activity until the donor site is well healed.

Outcomes

Excellent results and high patient satisfaction have been reported following TUG flap breast reconstruction; however, this flap does have limitations. These include a short pedicle, smaller flap size, limited skin available for reconstruction and muscle sacrifice. Aggressive harvest of this tissue is associated with wound dehiscence, labial spreading, poor cosmesis, and lymphedema with complication rates of up to 60% demonstrated in the literature.[20] With this flap, the resulting incision on closure lies in the lines of greatest tension of the thigh. Thus, a conservative approach to tissue harvest is essential. Donor-site wound complications have been reported to be as high as 27%, with rates of labial spreading and a visible scar being 11% and 78%, respectively.

One devastating complication that can result following TUG flap harvest is lymphedema of the lower extremity. This can result from skeletonization of the proximal femoral vein in the anterior portion of the flap, where the major lymphatic drainage of the lower extremity is found. Lakhiani et al report limiting the anterior dissection in this area to avoid lymphedema and to prevent visibility of the incision from the frontal view.[21] Despite these potential complications, up to 83% of patients report satisfaction following use of this flap for breast reconstruction.[22]

Diagonal Upper Gracilis (DUG) Flap

History

To account for some of the limitations experienced with the TUG flap (see above), Dayan et al modified the orientation of the flap along Langer's lines, calling it the diagonal upper gracilis (DUG) flap.[23] The benefits of the orientation are an increased flap width along the lines of least tension, low risk of wound healing issues, and avoidance of the femoral triangle and the lymphatics vessels. Like the TUG flap, the DUG flap is based on the gracilis pedicle (medial circumflex femoral vessels). Patient selection is also similar to the TUG flap, with ideal patients being those with excess skin laxity and tissue of the proximal posteromedial thigh that are not candidates for, or prefer to avoid abdominally-based flaps.

Surgical Technique

The flap is a diagonally-oriented ellipse over the gracilis muscle in the proximal thigh. This orientation not only results in less tension on the incision but also captures the angiosome of the flap. The DUG flap is marked with the patient in the frog-legged position on the operating room table by first palpating the adductor longus (AL) prominence. The anterior incision is placed vertically along the posterior border of the AL muscle for approximately 10 cm, keeping the anterior border of the flap away from the draining lymphatics of the lower extremity. From here, the incision line is drawn posteriorly in a curvilinear fashion over the gracilis muscle. A pinch test determines the width of the flap, which is reliably 10–12 cm depending on patient body habitus and the posterior incision is marked connecting the proximal and distal aspects of the flap.

The proximal 10 cm of the anterior incision is made first with dissection proceeding down and through the AL fascia. The AL muscle is then distracted anteriorly revealing the gracilis pedicle. Pedicle dissection is quick, and the remainder of the incisions are performed following its isolation. The entire gracilis muscle is harvested with this flap. A straight-lined closure is performed over a closed suction drain. The closure is oriented in the resting skin tension lines and thus results in no postoperative mobility restrictions. Additionally, the area supplied by the obturator nerve is largely removed with harvest of the flap, resulting in little to no sensory loss to the patient.

Outcomes

Given the novelty of this flap, there is little data available on complication profile and long-term outcomes; however, Dayan and Allen Jr report a 6-year experience with over 60 DUG flaps, showing an excellent complication profile.[24] In this series, flaps averaged 10.3 cm in width, ranging from 8 to 13 cm. One patient experienced 20% flap necrosis, and the overall incidence of donor-site complications was 10%.

The main disadvantages of the DUG flap include a visible posterior scar, short pedicle (6–8 cm), muscle sacrifice and a smaller flap to use for breast reconstruction. Atrophy of the gracilis muscle with time can also result in shrinking of the flap, though this can be minimized with primary fat grafting of the gracilis during breast reconstruction or stacking the flaps for a unilateral reconstruction (Fig. 36.9). Overall, this flap is technically easy to perform, provides a reliable blood supply and can result in excellent satisfaction in the appropriately selected patient.

Profunda Artery Perforator (PAP) Flap

History

Robert Allen Sr described the PAP flap for breast reconstruction in 2010 during the XIIth International Course on Perforator Flaps in Mexico City.[25] This flap is based on perforating vessels off the profunda artery that course through the adductor magnus and supply the posterior thigh skin and fat.[26] The profunda femoris artery originates from the common femoral artery 3–4 cm distal to the inguinal ligament coursing posterior to the femur from lateral to medial, where it then gives off several perforators to supply the posterior and medial thigh. Key perforators are located within 7 cm of the inferior gluteal crease (IGC) and within 4 cm of the posterior border of the gracilis muscle. Unlike gracilis muscle-based flaps (see above), the PAP flap does not sacrifice any thigh muscles.

Patient selection

The PAP flap is a good option in patients who are not candidates for abdominal tissue harvest or who wish to avoid

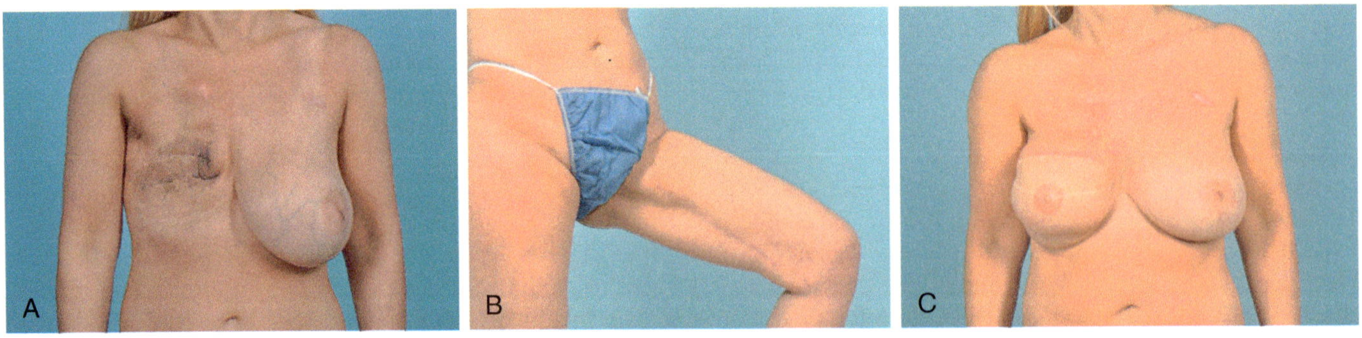

• **Fig. 36.9** (A) Preoperative and (B,C) 1-year postoperative photographs of a patient after right stacked DUG flap reconstruction. This patient also had an implant placed at a later time below the DUG flaps for additional projection.

abdominal scars. Tissue harvested from one or both thighs (i.e., stacked PAP flaps), ideally should also have sufficient volume and skin for reconstruction. This is not, however, a contraindication to surgery since volume may be augmented during revision surgery with fat grafts or even a small implant. A recent study reporting surgical outcomes in 101 consecutive PAP flaps reported an average flap weight of 425 grams with a range of 170–815 grams.[27] A larger study on 164 PAP flaps reported an average flap weight of 367 grams, suggesting that this flap option is best used for relatively small breast reconstructions unless a stacked procedure is performed.[28]

Surgical Technique

Preoperative imaging with MRA or CTA is useful for identifying the main perforators of the PAP flap that usually arise 5–7 cm below the IGC (Fig. 36.10). In most cases, the PAP flap is oriented transversely and measures 5–7 cm wide and 20–28 cm long. The flap width is determined by the pinch test, and the flap is drawn with an elliptical shape with the anterior most portion located over the middle/posterior border of the adductor longus muscle (Fig. 36.11). The planned incision site is hidden in/just below the IGC, and as a result, it is helpful to mark the patient in the standing position. It is important to remember that the main perforators for the PAP flap are located in the midline of the thigh deep to the posterior border of the gracilis muscle.

Intraoperatively, the patient is placed in the supine position, and the dissection can be performed with the patient in the frog-legged, split-legged, or lithotomy position. The frog-leg dissection, however, does place considerable strain on the surgeon's neck/back and, as a result, we prefer the lithotomy or split-legged position. The lithotomy position enables dissection of the flap with the surgeon in a sitting position and improves the ergonomics of the procedure.

Flap harvest is usually performed while the mastectomy is performed and/or the recipient vessels are prepared. The procedure starts with the incision of the anterior half of the flap to expose the perforating vessels. Typically, one or sometimes two perforators are selected. The perforators are dissected down to the fascia overlying the adductor magnus or gracilis muscles. Here, the surgeon may encounter the transverse branch of the greater saphenous vein that can be dissected and preserved with the flap for additional venous drainage. The gracilis muscle is identified, and the fascia overlying it is incised with electrocautery along the entire width of the flap. The gracilis muscle is then retracted

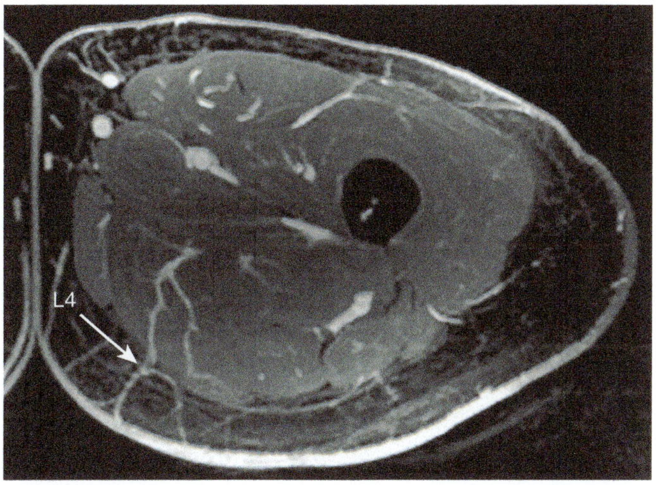

• **Fig. 36.10** Preoperative MRA showing a profunda artery perforator (*arrow*) supplying the posteromedial thigh skin and fat and coursing through the adductor magnus muscle to the profunda femoris artery.

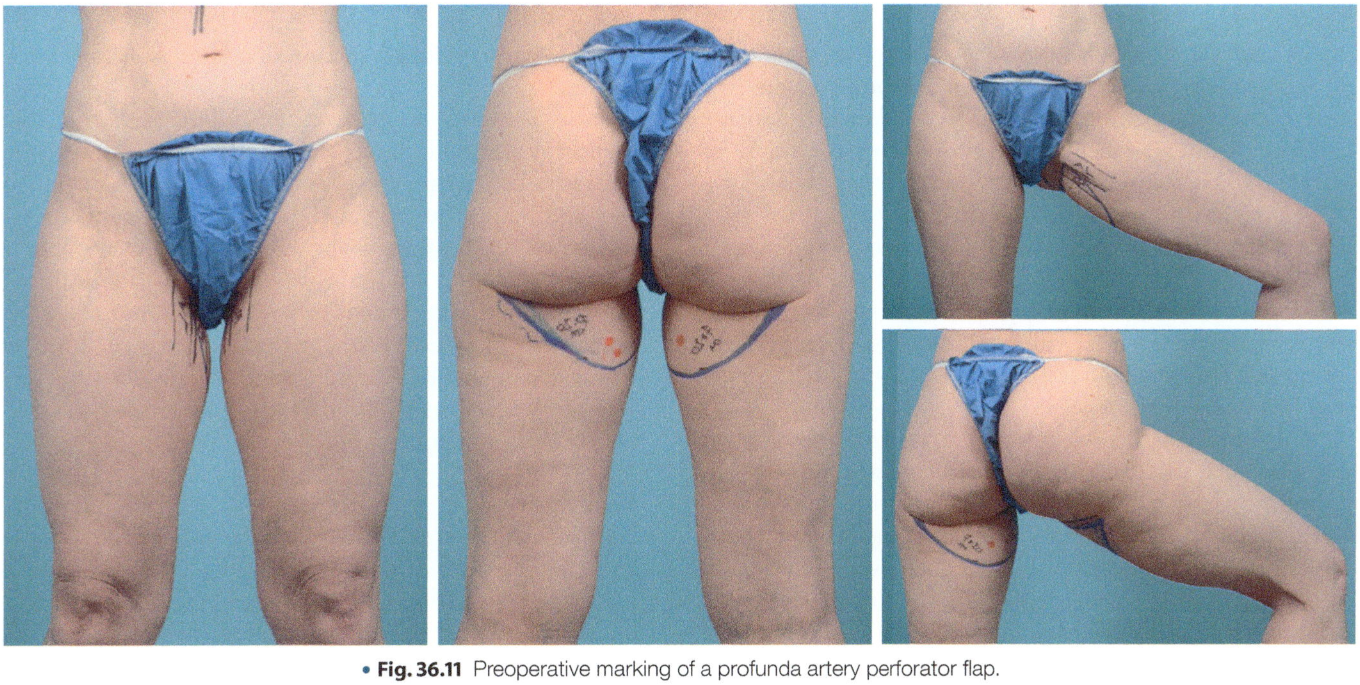

• **Fig. 36.11** Preoperative marking of a profunda artery perforator flap.

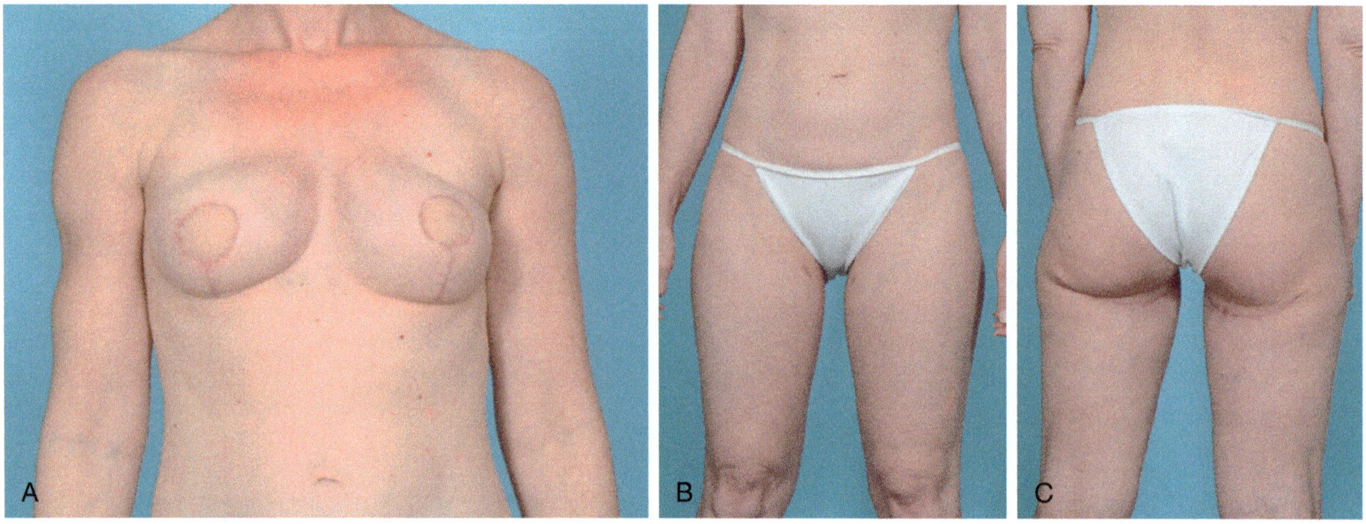

• **Fig. 36.12** Three-month postoperative photographs of the (A) recipient site and (B,C) donor sites following bilateral breast reconstruction with profunda artery perforator flaps. Note the superior pole insufficiency that can result given the smaller flap size obtained. This can be addressed with fat grafting during the second stage.

anteriorly to visualize adductor magnus muscle. The anterior fascia of the adductor magnus muscle is then incised along the width of the flap and subfascial dissection over the muscle to expose the perforating vessels. The muscular septum is then incised, and the perforators are dissected through the adductor magnus muscle to their origin from the profunda femoris. A vascular pedicle length of 8–15 cm can be obtained quite easily in this fashion. One common mistake is to ligate the pedicle before dissecting it completely through the adductor magnus muscle. This is problematic because while the veins at this level are quite large, the artery can be small, thereby complicating microvascular anastomosis. At the profunda vessels, the artery and vena comitantes are isolated and divided. Because it is difficult to regain exposure to this area while waiting for the mastectomy or recipient vessel exposure to be completed, it is possible to ligate the vessels at this point as the flap remains perfused through its posterior skin attachments and the musculocutaneous perforators that have yet to be divided. Once the surgeon is ready to harvest the flap, the remainder of the incisions are performed, and the dissection is completed expeditiously. It is important to note that the incisions through the thigh fat should not be beveled and should be performed perpendicular to the skin incision. Beveling of the thigh fat will result in contour deformities of the posterior thigh after flap closure and may increase the risk of wound dehiscence.

The ipsilateral flap is transferred up to the chest for microvascular anastomosis, where the flap is oriented in a horizontal or oblique fashion. While some reports suggest coning of the flap, this frequently results in a breast mound that is too narrow for the chest wall. Ideally, the flap should provide good medial and inferior pole fullness, as these areas are the hardest to correct for during revision procedures. The microvascular anastomosis is performed in the standard fashion to the internal mammary vessels, and the flap is inset with absorbable sutures to the chest wall. The flap is selectively de-epithelialized, leaving a skin paddle for monitoring and/or subsequent nipple reconstruction. Closed suction drains are placed in the pocket, and the skin is closed.

The donor site closure is performed by elevating the inferior thigh skin/subcutaneous fat off of the thigh fascia to enable a tension-free closure. This should be done carefully to prevent injury and avoid devascularizing the skin. The superior border of the defect should not be elevated as this will cause distortion of the IGC. The inferior thigh tissue can be advanced and secured with quilting sutures to the deep thigh fascia to decrease tension on the incision. The superficial fascia is then reapproximated, and the skin is repaired over a closed-suction drain in a standard layered fashion.

Postoperatively, the patient is placed in compression garments for the thigh donor site. Patients are asked to avoid strenuous activity for 6 weeks but encouraged to ambulate and climb stairs as tolerated. Compression garments aid in decreasing the time that donor-site drains are needed. Without them, drains can be expected to stay in for up to 3 weeks, given the dependent nature of this donor site. Additionally, many patients benefit from an elevated toilet seat to use in the first 4 weeks after surgery. This takes the pressure off the donor site, limiting pain in the area, which is a frequent but temporary complaint.

Outcomes

The PAP flap offers reliable, pliable tissue for breast reconstruction that has a long pedicle, adequately sized donor vessels for microvascular anastomosis, and an inconspicuous donor site scar (Fig. 36.12). Patient positioning also allows for a two-team approach to reconstruction, thereby decreasing surgical time. The flap limitations include the width of the flap (limited to 5–8 cm), superior pole insufficiency given small flap dimensions, postoperative pain with sitting, and a cumbersome donor site to close because of positioning. One option that can be used to decrease these limitations is to design the flap in a vertical or diagonal fashion. The diagonally oriented flap lies along Langer's lines and enables harvesting of a wider flap (up to 11–12 cm). The tradeoff for this flap orientation, however, is a more visible scar on the medial/posterior thigh. Alternately, PAP flaps from both thighs can be stacked together to create one breast, thus increasing the volume of the reconstruction and decreasing the likelihood of superior-pole insufficiency. This approach may also allow for a more conservative flap marking, thus improving donor site closure and contour. Whichever orientation is chosen, it is important to note that the ideal fat to be used for breast reconstruction is in the proximal part of the thigh. The thickness and quality of the fat diminish as you travel distally on the thigh.

The reported rate of donor site complications is variable, with one study of 164 flaps reporting a low rate of 1.9% while another study of 101 consecutive flaps reporting a higher rate of donor site complications with wound dehiscence in 11% and donor site cellulitis in 5.9%.[27,28] The total flap loss rate, however, is low, occurring in only 1–2% and fat necrosis in 7%.

Lateral Thigh Perforator (LTP) and Septocutaneous Tensor Fascia Lata (scTFL) Flap

History

The lateral thigh perforator (LTP), or septocutaneous tensor fascia lata (scTFL), flap is based on the ascending branch of the lateral circumflex femoral (LCF) vessels which supply the proximal lateral thigh or "saddle bag" region. This flap was first described for breast reconstruction in 1998 by Robert Allen Sr.

Patient Selection

The LTP or TFL flaps are less commonly used than abdominal or medial thigh autologous tissues. This is because the flap donor site scar is more conspicuous, and the flap pedicle is shorter and more tedious to dissect. The ideal patient for the LTP/TFL flap has sufficient skin laxity and subcutaneous fat in the lateral thigh area to enable a tension-free closure while simultaneously providing enough skin/fat for breast reconstruction. Lateral thigh skin harvest in patients who have minimal skin laxity can result in a significant contour deformity that is nearly impossible to revise. This flap, like other thigh-based flap options, usually provides less skin and adipose tissue for reconstruction and is, therefore, less useful for reconstruction of large, ptotic breasts. The median flap weight reported in a prospective series of 138 flaps was 348 grams (range 175–814 g).[29]

Surgical Technique

Preoperative imaging is helpful for LTP/TFL flap planning and can help delineate the length of the pedicle available for harvest (Fig. 36.13). This is important because the pedicle is ordinarily short in length and somewhat variable. Thus, use of this flap in patients with shorter pedicle lengths may be more difficult, and other options may be more favorable. Key landmarks to localize the perforator on preoperative imaging include the anterior superior iliac spine (ASIS), pubic symphysis, and greater trochanter.[30]

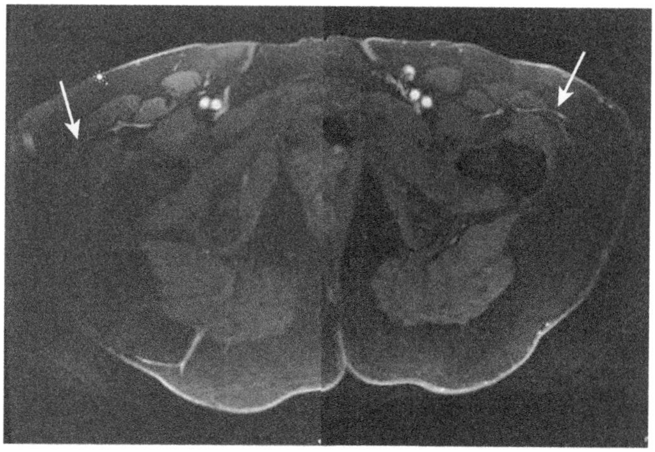

• **Fig. 36.13** Preoperative MRA of lateral thigh or septocutaneous tensor fascia lata perforators.

The perforators for the LTP/TFL flap arise from the ascending branch of the lateral femoral circumflex artery, which in turn is a branch of the common femoral, profunda femoral or external iliac arteries. The perforators for the LTP/TFL flap have a variable anatomy and can arise as septocutaneous vessels traveling through the anterior septum between the TFL and rectus femoris/vastus lateralis muscles (Type 1), musculocutaneous through the TFL muscle (Type 2), or septocutaneous traveling through the posterior septum between the TFL and gluteus medius/minimus muscles (Type 3). While any of these perforators can be chosen for basis of the LTP flap, Type 3 perforators are preferred because they are generally larger and less eccentrically placed on the flap. Type 3 perforators are nearly always present and simplify dissection because of their septocutaneous course, obviating the need for muscle disruption during harvest.

It is usually preferable to mark the patient in the standing position by outlining the saddle bag deformity such that the flap can capture this excess tissue. Next, the patient is placed in the supine position, and a line connecting the ASIS and the lateral border of the patella is marked. This marks the anterior border of the TFL muscle or the anterior intermuscular septum. Next, the pubic symphysis is marked, extending laterally and beyond the line connecting the ASIS and patella. Finally, the greater trochanter can be marked for reference. A handheld Doppler is then used to identify the septocutaneous perforators located in the inferolateral quadrant of these intersecting lines. The flap can be designed around the key perforator(s) in a transverse, oblique or S-shaped pattern, but the design should stay within the marked saddle bag deformity to avoid a major contour deformity of the lateral thigh. The flap dimensions

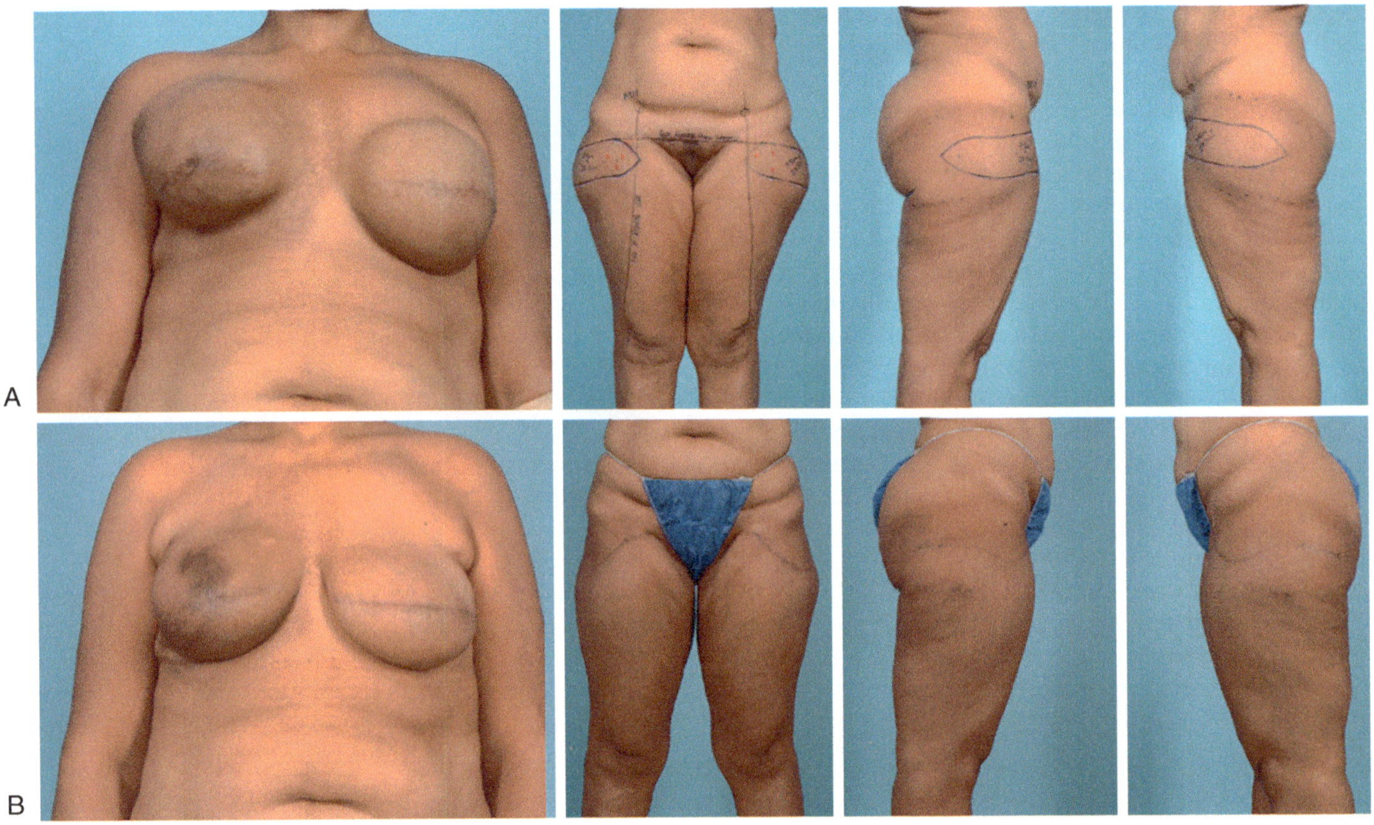

• **Fig. 36.14** (A) Preoperative and (B) 1-year postoperative photographs of a 36-year-old female who underwent delayed bilateral breast reconstruction with lateral thigh perforator flaps.

are based on patient habitus and skin laxity of the lateral thigh, averaging 5–9 cm in width by 18–28 cm in length (Fig. 36.14).

The flap is harvested with the patient in the supine position with a small bump placed under the hip to aid in the dissection of the posterior-most portion of the flap. The ipsilateral arm is usually prepped in the field and placed on the belly to avoid excessive arm abduction during flap harvest. Flap dissection is started by incising the anterior overlying the TFL muscle. The lateral femoral cutaneous nerve may be present in this area depending on the flap marking and should be preserved unless the plan is for a sensate flap reconstruction. Dissection proceeds straight down to the fascia of the thigh and beveling to include additional volume in the flap should be avoided since this would result in an unacceptable contour deformity following closure. The first key step is to identify the posterior intermuscular septum between the TFL and gluteus medius muscles on both the superior and inferior borders of the flap. This alerts the surgeon to the course of the septum through the flap and to the location of the perforators that the flap will be based upon. The septum is easily identified based on the appearance of the fascia of the TFL and gluteus medius muscles. While the TFL fascia is thin with visible muscle fibers underneath, the gluteus fascia is thick and white with no visible underlying muscle fibers. Once this is identified, the flap is elevated in the suprafascial plane from anterior to posterior. Musculocutaneous perforators can be ligated. The septocutaneous perforators are approached with caution and then surrounded once identified. The posterior intermuscular septum is then widely opened throughout the width of the flap to allow for placement of non-penetrating retractors and dissection of the pedicle. The pedicle is dissected to its origin from the lateral circumflex femoral vessels and then divided. The flap then maintains perfusion from gluteal perforators posteriorly. Once the recipient vessels and breast pocket have been prepared, the remainder of the flap can be harvested. One mistake is not to include all the gluteal fat in the posterior portion of the flap by beveling anteriorly. This will decrease the volume of the flap and is unnecessary. Gluteal perforators through the gluteus medius should be identified and ligated when raising the remainder of the flap in the suprafascial plane.

An ipsilateral flap is used for anastomosis to the internal mammary vessels, where the pedicle artery and vein calibers are similar to the recipient vessels. Given the short pedicle length, it is important to pay close attention when orienting the flap during inset. Any tension or kinking of the pedicle should be avoided by meticulously securing the anterior border of the flap to the chest wall. The flap provides for excellent reconstruction of the medial and inferior portions of the breast when used alone. Patients with a significant saddle bag deformity can also obtain excellent total breast reconstruction with this flap.

The donor site is closed primarily over a closed suction drain. All efforts should be towards providing for a tension-free closure, and this is best achieved by mobilizing the inferior thigh skin and subcutaneous tissues widely for advancement and quilting to the underlying fascia on advancement superiorly. When done properly, this will avoid a major contour deformity of the lateral thigh.

Postoperative flap monitoring is similar to the other flaps already mentioned. We recommend that all thigh-based flaps are placed in compression garments for the first 3 months postoperatively. This decreases the time that the drains are needed and decreases the chances of postoperative seroma formation. Drains in the donor area typically stay in for 2 weeks. Patients are mobilized from bed on postoperative day 1. There are no restrictions with ambulation, but patients are encouraged to avoid strenuous activity for a total of 4–6 weeks postoperatively.

Outcomes

The LTP flap is a useful flap for autologous breast reconstruction in the appropriately selected patient and has the lowest risk of donor site lymphedema of the thigh-based flaps (see Fig. 36.14). The blood supply for this flap is most commonly septocutaneous, thus requiring no muscle dissection. The pedicle vessels are also of suitable caliber for microvascular anastomosis to the internal mammary artery/vein. A review of 138 LTP for breast reconstruction revealed a total flap loss rate of 1.4% while 8% of patients required operative re-exploration.[29] Donor site complications were common in the initial experience occurring in as many as 40% of patients but decreased to 6.3% with refinements in surgical techniques.

However, the LTP flap is relatively difficult to shape due to the quality of the fat in the lateral thigh area as well as the short pedicle length making inset more difficult. The limited amount of skin that can be harvested with the flap together with the short pedicle length also makes this flap less useful for delayed mastectomy reconstruction, particularly in patients previously treated with radiation. In these cases, the LTP flap may need to be combined with autologous tissues harvested from other areas and inset as a stacked flap. In this scenario, the LTP flap is used to reconstruct the inferior portion of the breast, with the DIEP used to reconstruct the superior portion of the breast. Finally, the donor site is unforgiving, and the scar may be conspicuous. Donor site contour deformities, particularly in patients who undergo unilateral flap harvest, may be difficult to manage and may necessitate contralateral liposuction and skin excision for symmetry.

Gluteal Flaps

History

In 1983, William Shaw described the use of the superior gluteal myocutaneous flap for breast reconstruction.[31] The inferior gluteal myocutaneous flap was subsequently described in 1989 by Paletta et al.[32] Robert Allen Sr later described the superior and inferior gluteal artery flaps (SGAP and IGAP, respectively).[33,34] These perforator flap options represented a significant advance since they decreased donor site morbidity while simultaneously increasing the pedicle length and technical ease of the procedure. Later refinements of the IGAP were reported with the positioning of the scar in the gluteal crease and decreasing donor site contour deformities. Nevertheless, the SGAP and IGAP are used less commonly than abdominal or thigh-based flaps due to the fact that reposition of the patient is usually necessary for flap harvest and because these flaps are more technically demanding.

Patient Selection

The SGAP and IGAP flaps are useful options in patients who do not have sufficient tissues in the abdominal or thigh donor sites or wish to avoid scars in these areas. The ideal candidate has a moderate amount of soft adipose tissue in the buttock area and has sufficient skin laxity to allow a tension-free closure. We avoid these flaps in obese patients or those with very thick or hard fatty tissues. In these patients, flap dissection and shaping of the flap is difficult and may be associated with increased rates of vascular compromise. The SGAP flap has a relatively short pedicle (depending on where the perforator enters the skin). This may complicate reconstruction of delayed mastectomy defects in patients with a high mastectomy scar since the short pedicle precludes placement of the flap at the lower breast border.

Surgical Technique

As with most perforator flaps, the use of preoperative imaging is helpful (but not essential) in surgical planning of SGAP or IGAP flaps. The position of the perforator is marked based on anatomical landmarks (e.g., posterior superior iliac spine) and confirmed using a handheld Doppler. The flap is marked with the patient in the standing position, and the patient is prepped in the lateral decubitus or corkscrew position. Patients can be positioned in a prone position when harvesting bilateral gluteal flaps. In bilateral cases, we usually prepare the internal mammary vessels and the breast donor site first, position the patient in the prone position, harvest both flaps, close the gluteal donor sites, repositioning the supine position, and complete the microsurgical anastomosis. In these cases, it is often helpful to have a co-surgeon to facilitate simultaneous flap dissection and minimize prone positioning.

Selection of perforators that are lateral in the muscle, particularly when harvesting an SGAP flap, is helpful as this will increase the length of the pedicle and facilitate perforator dissection. More medial perforators tend to have a short run to the main pedicle and are, in our experience, more difficult to dissect. Usually, only one perforator is selected for dissection since dissection of multiple perforators is difficult and requires muscle transection. The perforator of choice is dissected by splitting the gluteus maximus muscle in the direction of its fibers and continued below the gluteus medius. The pedicle continues below the piriformis muscle until the

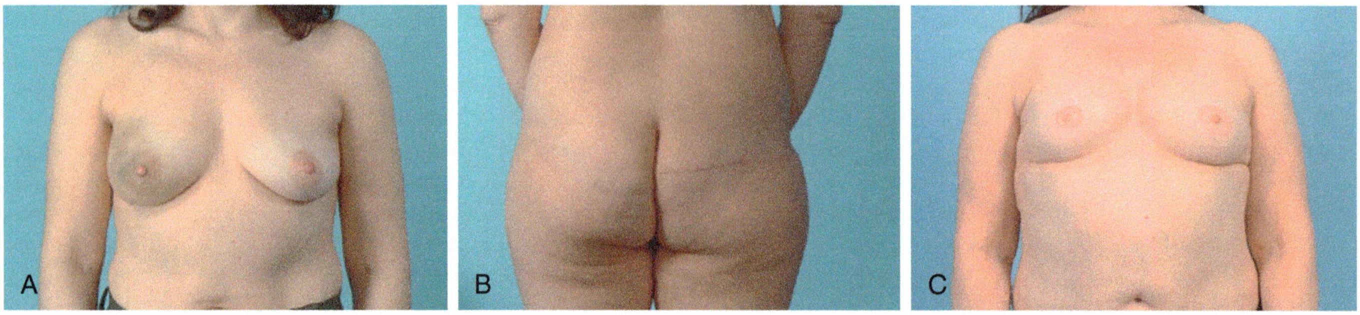

• **Fig. 36.15** (A) Preoperative and (B,C) 1-year postoperative photographs of a patient after right breast reconstruction with an SGAP flap and left breast mastopexy.

artery is a suitable diameter. This can be tricky because the vein is often very large, but the artery is small. In fact, in some patients, the vein becomes quite large at a level when the artery is suitable for microvascular anastomosis. In these cases, we often perform the anastomosis in a staggered manner cutting the vein more proximally and avoiding the dilated area of the vein and leaving the superior gluteal artery longer (and cutting the internal mammary artery) to obtain a better size match for the anastomosis. This makes it easier also to separate the vessels since, at the level below the piriformis, the gluteal artery and vein give off many large branches.

Dissection of the IGAP, or in the crease IGAP, is very similar and technically easier. This is because the diameter of the inferior gluteal artery perforator tends to be larger and proximal dissection where the vein becomes quite large is rarely necessary. Care should be taken with this flap, however, to avoid beveling of the flap edges as this will result in a contour deformity that is difficult to manage.

The gluteal area is closed over drains with care taken to avoid dog ears and to obtain an excellent approximation of the fascia to avoid late contour deformities. Liposuction of the ipsilateral and/or contralateral buttock, and more rarely, fat grafting of the gluteal flap donor site, may be necessary to improve the contour of this donor site.

The microsurgical anastomosis is performed to the internal mammary artery and vein. Anastomosis at the level of the 4th rib on the right side may enable positioning of the flap lower on the breast in patients who undergo delayed mastectomy reconstruction. In the left chest, this is rarely possible as the internal mammary vein tends to be smaller, creating an unacceptable size mismatch with the gluteal vein.

The flap is inset horizontally across the breast and can be coned somewhat to create a more pleasing lateral contour (Fig. 36.15). Ideally, the flap should be used to reconstruct the medial and inferior border of the breast. Because gluteal flap tends to be relatively narrow, insetting of the flap in this manner may result in an upper breast hollow that may require fat grafting to correct. Fat grafting can be performed either at the same time or at a later date (or often, both).

Outcomes

Historically, gluteal flaps have had a higher rate of microvascular complications as compared with abdominally-based flaps. This is due to the fact that the myocutaneous flaps (particularly the superior gluteal) have short pedicle lengths and very large veins resulting in size mismatch with recipient vessels in the breast. However, the advent of perforator flaps greatly simplified flap harvest providing a longer pedicle and greater opportunities to manage the vein size. This is reflected by the fact that several groups have published excellent outcomes with low rates of flap loss (ranging between 0% and 3%). Nevertheless, SGAP, and to a lesser extent, IGAP flap harvest is still more challenging than DIEP or other perforator flap harvest. Other complications of gluteal flap harvest include seroma (10%), fat necrosis (10%), and donor site contour deformities.

Implant Breast Reconstruction

History

The history of implant breast reconstruction can be traced to Cronin and Gerow, who first reported the use of the silicone gel implant in 1962 (refer to Chapter 35, Breast Augmentation for more detail). Although silicone gel implants were initially used for breast augmentation, reconstructive surgeons soon reported delayed postmastectomy breast reconstruction by elevating breast skin flaps from the chest wall and inserting an implant. This delayed approach was based on hypothetical concerns that immediate breast reconstruction would increase the risk of cancer recurrence or metastasis. As a result, the first case of immediate breast implant reconstruction was not reported until nearly a decade later when, in 1971, Snyderman and Guthrie reported their experience with placement of a silicone gel implant subcutaneously at the time of radical mastectomy.[35]

Although immediate reconstruction gained some popularity over the next decade, the vast majority of procedures were still performed in a delayed fashion which limited the size and esthetics of the reconstruction due to a relative paucity of skin. This changed in 1982 when Radovan described his experience with breast tissue expanders in 68 women.[36] The average size of the implant in this series was 300–400 cm^3 enabling the surgeon to consider contralateral symmetry procedures, thereby improving esthetic outcomes. Today, implants are the most common method of breast reconstruction, and refinements in surgical technique, and

TABLE 36.1 A Timeline Showing the History of Breast Implants

Year	Event
1962	Thomas Cronin and Frank Gerow introduce the silicone breast implant
1976	The United States Food and Drug Administration (FDA) develops controls and performance standards for silicone breast implants
1982	The FDA requires reports of adverse events from silicone implant manufacturers
1991	First successful lawsuit against silicone implant manufacturer Dow Corning
1992	FDA and European agencies announce voluntary moratorium for the use of silicone gel breast implants. Silicone gel implants could only be used for breast reconstruction
1995	Dow Corning Company files for bankruptcy
2000	Ban on silicone implants in France is lifted
2006	FDA lifts ban on silicone gel implants

implant design has significantly improved long-term outcomes. Nevertheless, implant-based breast reconstruction has been the focus of controversy through the years as a result of safety concerns for silicone implants and, more recently, the development of anaplastic large cell lymphoma around the implant capsule in some patients. These concerns are, however, balanced by excellent outcomes in a large number of women necessitating additional research and improvements in implant technology.

Types of Implants

Implants can be broadly categorized as saline-filled or silicone-filled devices. Importantly, all implants have a silicone shell. Saline implants have the advantage that, in the event that they leak, the saline fluid is simply absorbed by the body. In this manner, it is easy to tell if the implant has leaked and, more importantly, there is no exposure to liquid silicone in the event of a leak. On the other hand, saline implants tend to come in fewer shapes and sizes, are more prone to rippling, and do not feel as soft or natural as silicone-filled implants. Structured saline implants are a new type of saline implant and are designed to have a more natural feel than standard saline devices. These implants gained FDA approval for breast augmentation in 2014 and have an internal structure that controls fluid movement and is thought to improve fluid movement when the device is upright. Importantly, these implants are not currently FDA approved for breast reconstruction. Nevertheless, the initial experience with these implants has been positive, with high rates of satisfaction.[37]

Silicone gel implants were originally filled with liquid silicone and the history of these implants is summarized in Table 36.1. Silicone gel implants are very soft and natural; however, liquid silicone implants tend to ripple, and in the event of a break in the implant shell, the liquid silicone can leak into the breast capsule, and occasionally, into the tissues. This leakage can cause inflammation, lymph node enlargement, and the development of granulomas. In response to these issues, implant manufacturers developed semi-solid or cohesive silicone gel implants. There are implants with varying degrees of cohesivity. The most cohesive silicone gel implants have the lowest rippling and, although these implants can break, they, in theory, do no leak liquid silicone. However, some patients do not like the feel of highly cohesive implants and complain that the implant feels hard or uncomfortable. Less cohesive implants are a middle ground between highly cohesive and liquid silicone gel implants and have some of the advantages of the former (i.e., less rippling, decreased possibility of a leak) but may feel softer and natural in some patients.

Silicone gel implants have been a source of significant controversy over the years and were even taken off the market by the FDA in 1992 over concerns that leaky silicone implants may increase the risk of rheumatological or other diseases. However, a 1999 review of the literature by a committee appointed by the National Academy of Science Institute of Medicine concluded that there was no identifiable association between silicone gel implants and immunological disorders, connective tissue disease, or neurological conditions.[38] This report, along with other reviews, lifted the voluntary moratorium on the use of silicone gel implants in 2006. Since then, other comprehensive reviews of the literature have found no significant association between silicone gel implants and a variety of adverse events including cancer, rheumatologic/autoimmune/connective tissues diseases, reproductive issues, and mental health problems.[39,40] However, it should be noted that these studies have significant limitations and that studies to date have rarely controlled for potential confounding variables. As a result, the FDA, the American Society of Plastic Surgery, and patient advocacy groups continue to develop and conduct studies that will answer these questions more definitively in the future.

Implants are marketed as either round or anatomic/"tear drop"-shaped implants. Round implants have been available for decades and are simple to use since the rotation of the implant or shifting of its position will not make a difference in the breast shape. Round implants, however, do have a front and back directionality and flipping of the implant within the breast pocket can occur. This results in a flattened-appearing breast with minimal projection at the anatomical midpoint of the device. The main disadvantage of round implants is that they have a uniform projection in the anterior–posterior dimension and may result in unwanted/unnatural upper pole fullness.

Anatomically-shaped implants were designed to have a more natural shape and decreased upper pole fullness. These implants come in a variety of shapes and sizes and are more likely to match a contralateral breast. Anatomical implants also have more projection in the lower pole of the breast and help create a more natural breast shape. These implants may be used to improve nipple position

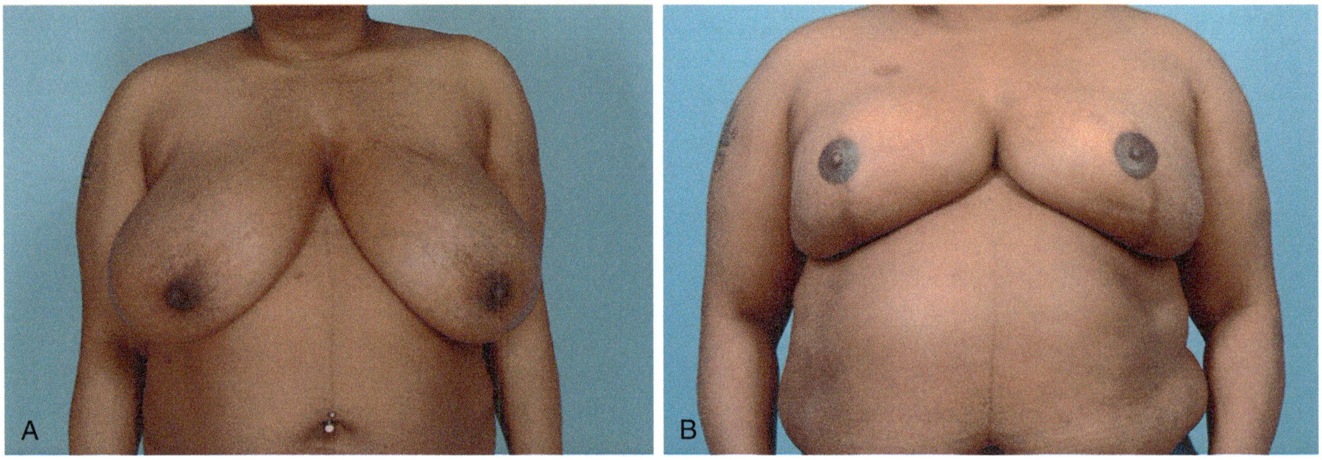

• **Fig. 36.16** (A) Preoperative and (B) 1-year postoperative photographs of a patient with bilateral breast reconstruction with implants, using a Wise pattern mastectomy scar.

during breast augmentation thereby potentially avoiding a mastopexy in some patients. Unfortunately, these implants are prone to malposition/rotation resulting in an obvious breast deformity. This malposition almost always required surgical intervention. Anatomical implants also always have a textured surface that is designed to adhere to the implant capsule and prevent implant rotation.

The texturing of the implant surface has recently been linked with breast implant-associated anaplastic large cell lymphoma (BIA-ALCL), a low-grade tumor of lymphocytes that grows around textured implant capsules (refer to Chapter 35 for more detail).[41] Importantly, although BIA-ALCL has developed in patients with smooth devices, all reported cases have had a history of textured implant use. As a result, it is thought that textured devices have the highest risk for developing this disease, and this observation has led to a significant decrease in the use of anatomic breast implants. In fact, some countries have removed textured implants from the market.

BIA-ALCL tumors tend to present with acute swelling of the breast, fluid accumulation around the implant, palpable mass in the breast or the skin, or axillary/cervical lymphadenopathy. The diagnosis of BIA-ALCL requires a high level of suspicion and histological or cytological testing for lymphoma cells which express CD30, a cell surface antigen, among other markers. Although the risk of ALCL remains unknown, recent studies have suggested that the disease develops in as many as 1 in 2832 women.[41] However, estimating the risk of this disease has been complicated by implant usage records and lack of uniform follow-up. It is possible, therefore, that the actual risk of the disease is lower or higher. In addition, the rate of disease development appears to be influenced by the length of time the implant has been in place with most patients presenting 8–10 years after surgery. To date, nearly 700 cases of BIA-ALCL have been reported to the FDA. In the majority of these women, the disease was treated effectively with a complete capsulectomy. However, some patients do develop metastatic disease and require treatment with chemotherapy or radiation. Sadly, the disease has been fatal in a small minority of women in whom the diagnosis was delayed.

Patient Selection

The ideal patient for implant-based breast reconstruction has relatively small breasts (<800 g) with well-defined breast contours and minimal ptosis. However, implant reconstruction is feasible in most patients, particularly if care is taken to select the best incision given anatomical considerations. Thus, patients with small to medium-sized breasts with minimal ptosis have excellent outcomes following nipple-sparing or skin-sparing mastectomy. Women with large breasts or significant ptosis may benefit from skin reduction techniques such as Wise pattern breast reduction (Fig. 36.16). The Wise pattern approach has the added benefit of preserving the lower breast skin and dermis. This flap is deepithelialized and used to cover the lower pole of the breast. Not only does this skin flap decrease the rate of complications, but it also increases lower pole projection and lateral breast contours, thereby improving outcomes. Implants are also useful as a temporary reconstruction, preserving the breast skin following mastectomy to enable eventual autologous breast reconstruction. This approach preserves the contours of the breast and the breast pocket; thus, reconstruction simply requires replacement of the volume of the breast.

Obesity, smoking history, uncontrolled diabetes, and high blood pressure have all independent predictors of complications following mastectomy and implant or tissue expander breast reconstruction.[42] Even patients who had previously smoked but are not current smokers have an increased risk of implant loss and infection. As a result, these factors should be optimized as much as possible. In most cases, however, patients with a diagnosis of breast cancer require surgery in a timely manner and, as a result, this information is important only for informed consent. Other contraindications to implant reconstruction include a history of mastectomy and radiation and extensive skin involvement with the tumor. Radiation damage usually results in the development of tough, nonpliable mastectomy skin flaps that are not amenable to implant reconstruction and increase the risk of complications. Patients who have previously been treated with partial mastectomy and radiation and those

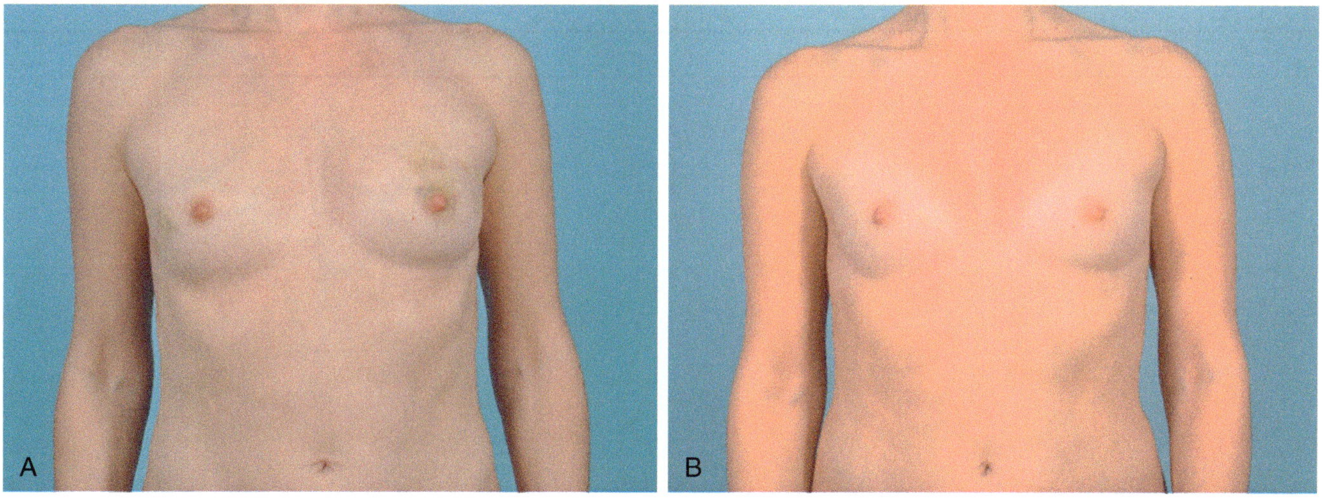

• **Fig. 36.17** (A) Preoperative and (B) 1-year postoperative photographs of a patient after right-sided DTI breast reconstruction.

with a history of mantle radiation may have less significant radiation-induced skin injury. These patients may, therefore still be candidates for implant reconstruction, albeit at a higher rate of complications.[43] Patients with extensive skin resection may not be candidates for implant reconstruction as the skin has only a finite amount of stretch and over-resection of the skin may prevent adequate expansion. Finally, patients with very large breasts or those with very small breasts may be difficult to reconstruct with implants due to the availability of implants at the extremes of sizes. However, these patients may be candidates for contralateral procedures (e.g., reduction or augmentation) that may help with symmetry.

Implant Reconstruction Surgical Technique

Implant reconstruction can be performed in a variety of ways. For example, a permanent implant may simply be placed immediately after mastectomy (i.e., direct-to-implant or DTI reconstruction). More commonly, tissue expanders are placed followed by conversion of the tissue expander to a permanent implant once the expansion has been completed. Tissue expanders may be placed completely under the pectoralis and serratus muscles (subpectoral), partially under the pectoralis muscle with coverage of the inferolateral portion of the expander using acellular dermis or other material (partial subpectoral), or under the skin, usually covered by acellular dermis (prepectoral). These surgical options all have advantages and disadvantages that must be carefully considered.

Direct to Implant (DTI) Reconstruction

Excellent outcomes with DTI reconstruction have been published by a number of groups (nicely reviewed by Bertozzi et al) (Fig. 36.17).[44] In most cases, the pectoralis muscle is elevated, and the implant is placed in the subpectoral position. The inferior portion of the pectoralis muscle is usually sutured to the acellular dermis or other material (Vicryl mesh, bovine collagen matrix, etc.) which is, in turn, sutured to the inframammary fold inferiorly and the chest wall laterally to keep the implant in the correct anatomical position. Some authors have also recently described good results following the prepectoral placement of the implant with coverage of the device with acellular dermis. For example, in a review of 134 cases of DTI breast reconstruction, Antony and colleagues compared reconstructive outcomes following DTI with the implant in the subpectoral (n = 57) or prepectoral (n =77) position and found no significant difference in the rate of complications (although esthetic outcomes were not reported).[45] Other groups, however, have reported higher rates of implant loss following prepectoral versus subpectoral DTI reconstruction.[46]

DTI is only possible in patients with healthy mastectomy skin flaps since the placement of a full-size implant in patients with borderline skin perfusion may result in mastectomy skin flap necrosis and implant removal. In addition, in most cases, this option is best in patients with minimal ptosis, good skin tone, and relatively small breasts who are being treated with nipple-sparing mastectomy. In a review of 160 DTI reconstructions following nipple-sparing mastectomy, the average implant size was only 376.2 cm^3, and the reconstructive failure rate was 5.6%.[47] Implant size greater than 400 cm^3 was a significant predictor of overall complications and implant loss, as was age over 50. Another report of a multicenter randomized trial with 59 patients (91 breasts) found that mastectomy weight was a significant predictor of complications (odds ratio (OR) 1.94, 95% confidence interval (CI) 1.33–2.83).[48]

The advantages of DTI include a single-stage approach to breast reconstruction and return to full recovery. The disadvantages of this technique include higher complication rates, particularly if the patients are not carefully selected, although this point is debated. Nevertheless, a systematic review of 16 studies comparing 561 reconstructions, found a pooled complication rate of 30% for DTI versus 20.3% for patients treated with tissue expanders and implants.[49]

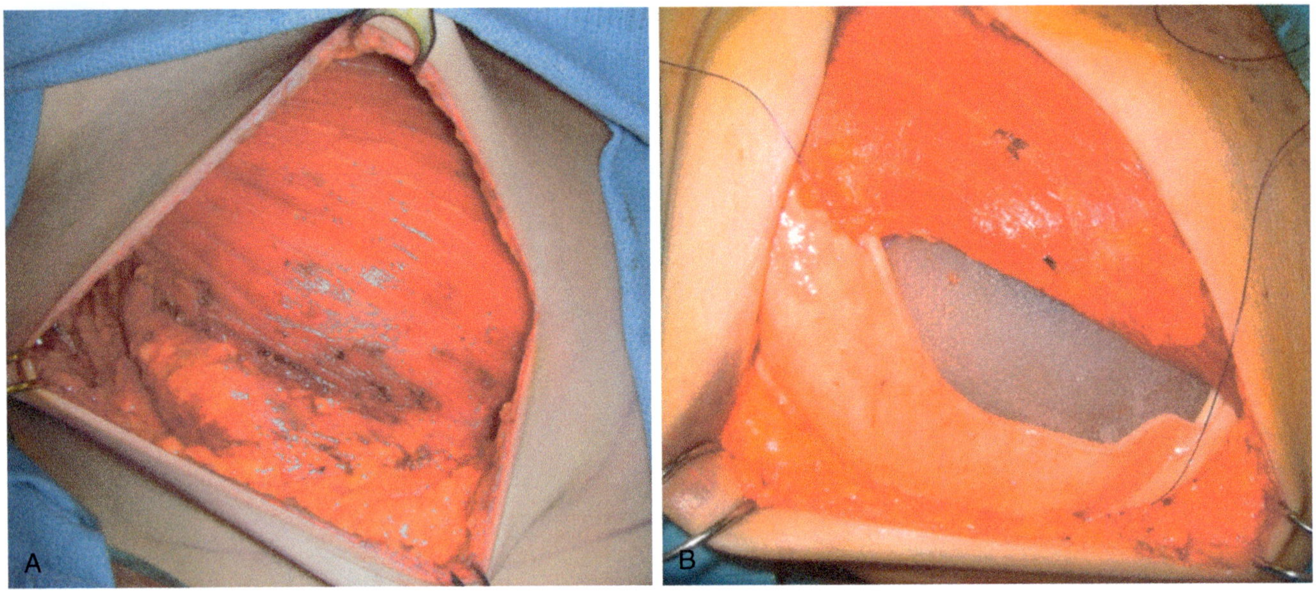

• **Fig. 36.18** (A) Total submuscular and (B) partial submuscular placement of a tissue expander. Note inferolateral placement of acellular dermis in the partial submuscular (dual plane) reconstruction.

Patients who underwent DTI were more likely to have mastectomy skin flap necrosis, wound healing complications, infection, seroma, and hematoma. DTI, in carefully selected patients, does not increase the need for revision surgery.[50]

Tissue Expander/Implant (TE-I) Reconstruction

Tissue expanders can be placed in the subpectoral or prepectoral position. In patients treated with subpectoral expander placement, the device may be either completely (total subpectoral) or partially covered with the muscle (dual plane) (Fig. 36.18). In dual plane reconstructions, the inferior/inferolateral portion of the expander is covered with acellular dermal matrix or other similar material. The acellular dermal matrix in these cases connects the inferior portion of the pectoralis muscle to the inframammary fold and prevents window-shading of the muscle superiorly after disruption of its inferior attachments. In some cases, the inferior insertion of the pectoralis muscle may be disrupted, and the lower pole of the expander placed in the subcutaneous position. This is most commonly done in delayed reconstruction when the skin is not elevated off of the pectoralis muscle and, as a result, this new anatomical orientation prevents window-shading of the muscle back to its origin.

Prepectoral Tissue Expander Technique

A variety of surgical techniques have been described for prepectoral expander reconstruction.[51] In most cases, the expander is covered either partially or completely on the back table with acellular dermis or other biologic materials and placed in the subcutaneous pocket. The expander is then secured using suture tabs on the device. Additional sutures may be placed to secure the acellular dermis to the chest wall laterally to prevent lateral migration of the device and to promote rapid incorporation of the material with the native tissues. Other biologic materials have also been used for coverage of the expander, including decellularized bovine collagen and porcine dermis, among others. In all cases, the use of perforated acellular matrix is encouraged since seroma formation is a common problem. The thickness of the biologic material has been debated, with some groups preferring thick material while others have advocated the use of thin acellular matrices. Which material has lower rates of complications and is better tolerated is still largely unresolved in the literature, although a number of studies have compared biologic material derived from various donor tissues and manufacturers.

Proponents of prepectoral breast expander placement cite the lack of pectoralis muscle animation deformity and decreased postsurgical pain. Some have even suggested that prepectoral reconstruction may have lower rates of capsular contracture, although these reports remain anecdotal and require validation.[52] Other purported advantages of prepectoral reconstruction include a more natural shape, increased projection, improved medial fullness, and avoidance of changes in pectoralis muscle strength. The disadvantages of prepectoral reconstruction are debated but primarily include increased costs due to the use of larger portions of acellular dermis to cover the entire expander. Prepectoral reconstruction also increases the risk of rippling, upper pole contour deformities, and routine need for fat grafting.[52] Whether or not prepectoral expander reconstruction increases the risk of implant exposure or infection is highly debated. However, several groups have reported retrospective reviews with encouraging results. For example, Sbitany et al compared 175 breasts reconstructed with immediate prepectoral tissue expanders with 236 reconstructions using expanders in the submuscular plane and found no difference in the overall rate of complications in all patients as well as those treated with postmastectomy radiation.[51] Similarly, Manrique and colleagues reported results comparing 187 prepectoral with

124 subpectoral breast reconstructions. With a median follow-up of nearly 1.5 years, the authors found no difference in the rate of total complications, breast infections, wound dehiscence, or device loss between the groups.[53] However, the rate of device loss in both groups (5.4% and 6.5%, respectively) is higher than the rates reported for other large series of total subpectoral breast reconstructions.[54] Nevertheless, prepectoral breast reconstruction is an interesting technique with promising early results in a variety of settings. Longer-term studies are needed to assess complication rates, esthetic rates, the patient-reported outcomes and resource utilization costs.

Subpectoral Tissue Expander Technique

Subpectoral expander placement is started by elevating the pectoralis muscle laterally from the chest wall and creating a pocket for the expander. Medial dissection is important to avoid excessive distance between the implants and may require ligation of internal mammary perforators between the 3rd and 4th intercostal spaces. Rarely, the pectoralis muscle may need to be partially disinserted to allow proper positioning of the expander. However, this should be done with care to avoid synmastia.

The dissection of the inferior border of the pectoralis muscle is extremely important as this area determines the position and shape of the inframammary fold (IMF). If the inferior border of the pectoralis muscle is at or just above the IMF, then the muscle may be elevated, and its insertion into the rectus sheath can be divided just at or slightly below the IMF. In this manner, the expander is completely covered by muscle. Some surgeons advocate placement of the expander below the IMF at a variable distance as this will preferentially expand the lower mastectomy skin flap and create a more natural ptotic breast. This is useful for symmetry in women who have a contralateral ptotic breast. However, the preferential expansion of the lower skin flap displaces the mastectomy scar superiorly, necessitating an additional scar for nipple reconstruction in most cases, and in some patients, the resultant high mastectomy scar may be visible in bathing suits or a low-cut dress. In addition, placement of the expander below the IMF effectively ablates this natural structure and requires resuturing of the fold at the time of implant exchange. This increases the complexity of the exchange procedure and the risk of implant malposition if the sutures are misplaced or disrupted.

If the inferior border of the pectoralis muscle is far from the IMF (i.e., >2–3 cm) or if a significant amount of intraoperative expansion is needed to fill the breast envelope (for example, in patients treated with nipple-sparing mastectomy), then acellular dermis or collagen matrix may be used. In these cases, the inferior insertion of the pectoralis muscle is disinserted, and the biologic material is then used to bridge the distance between the lower border of the muscle and the IMF. This will allow preservation of the IMF and facilitates expansion. Alternatively, the pectoralis muscle may be elevated in continuity with the rectus sheath inferiorly to a point just below the IMF. The rectus sheath is then transected horizontally to allow lower pole expansion. This approach is useful if acellular dermis is not available, or total submuscular coverage is desired either due to technical concerns (e.g., mastectomy skin flap ischemia) or patient wishes.

Laterally, the serratus fascia or a strip of the serratus muscle is elevated carefully while avoiding injury to the long-thoracic nerve. The lateral dissection should continue to a line drawn inferiorly from the anterior axillary line. More lateral dissection should be avoided since this may result in lateral malposition of the expander. In patients who have undergone nipple sparing mastectomy, the expander should be centered on the nipple areola complex. The advantages of subpectoral or partial subpectoral breast expander reconstruction are the fact that these procedures have been used for many years and several large studies have reported long-term outcomes evaluating the rate of complications, the patient-reported outcomes, the effects of postmastectomy radiation, and esthetic outcomes. However, it is noteworthy that the rate of complications among groups is somewhat variable with some groups reporting larger rates of revision or implant loss. Nevertheless, subpectoral two-stage implant reconstruction in experienced hands and in appropriately selected patients is a safe procedure with predictable outcomes. Patients treated with this approach have high rates of satisfaction and low rates of surgical morbidity.

Outcomes

Overall Complications

Implant breast reconstruction is safe and effective in most patients with low rates of reconstructive failure, and acceptable esthetic/patient-reported outcomes. A multicenter, prospective study of 11 centers in the United States and Canada reporting on complications occurring 1 year after surgery in 1615 patients (the Mastectomy Reconstruction Outcomes Consortium (MROC)) found that the overall complication rate of implant reconstruction was 24% and that major complications occurred in 18% of patients.[55] These rates compared favorably with patients who underwent free flap breast reconstruction (34% any complication and 24% major complication for DIEP flaps). Major complications that occurred in patients who underwent implant reconstruction included hematoma (3.5%), wound dehiscence (1.6%), wound infection (10.0%), mastectomy skin flap necrosis (6.6%), seroma (2.9%), capsular contracture (0.8%), and implant malposition/leakage/rupture (1.6%). Overall, implants had a low reconstructive failure rate of 5.9% at 1 year. This rate likely will increase in the years to come due to late effects of implant reconstruction (e.g., capsular contracture or asymmetry due to weight gain). Nevertheless, it is clear that at least in the short-term, implant reconstruction is successful for most patients.

The independent predictors of major complications with implant reconstruction in the MROC study were older age (particularly with patients over 65; odds ratio (OR) = 2.3 vs. women age <35), BMI >30.0 (OR 1.5), bilateral reconstruction (OR = 1.5), immediate

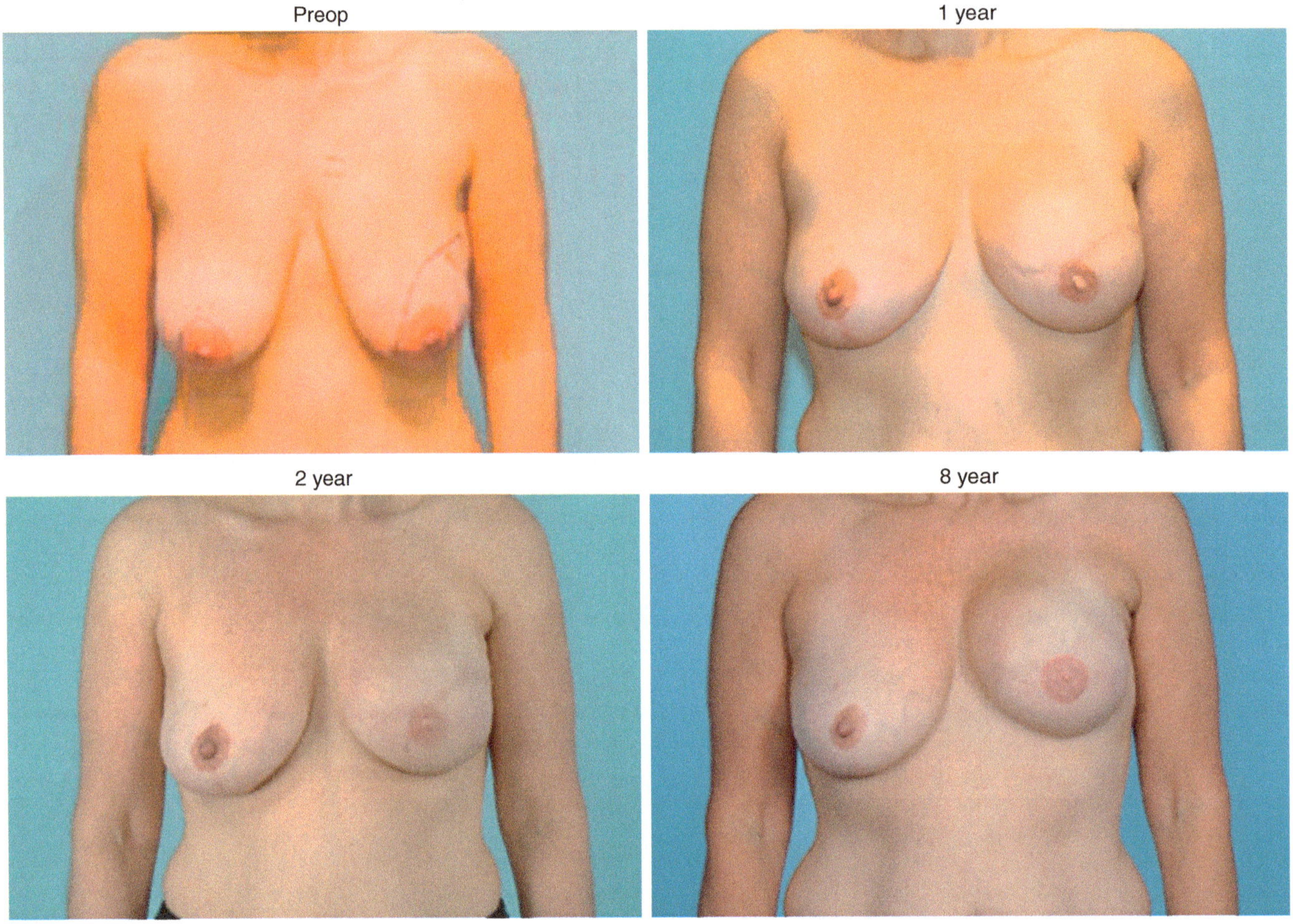

• **Fig. 36.19** One year postoperative and long-term photographs of the same patient after left breast reconstruction with an implant and right breast mastopexy. Note how capsular contracture of the implant has caused significant asymmetry in the long-term follow-up photograph.

reconstruction (OR = 1.8), radiation therapy (OR = 1.5), morbidity score (Charlson score above 1; OR = 1.6), and chemotherapy during or after reconstruction (OR = 1.35). The effect of radiation in this study is likely an underestimate since the follow-up was limited to 1 year from surgery. In addition, the study did not assess the incidence of asymmetry. As a result of these issues, long-term satisfaction and esthetic outcomes with implant-based breast reconstruction tend to decrease over time necessitating additional procedures and "maintenance" (Fig. 36.19).[56] A study of 360 patients followed prospectively over a 9-year period revealed that cosmetic outcomes following implant breast reconstruction deteriorated linearly over the course of the study. While 86% of patients had a cosmetically acceptable result at 2 years, this number decreased to only 54% by 5 years.

Animation of the pectoralis muscle in patients with subpectoral breast implants is usually not problematic; however, in some patients, this can result in significant distortion of the reconstruction. This outcome is not necessarily a complication since the contraction of the muscle is normal. However, the so-called animation deformity can be a source of dissatisfaction in some patients. This outcome may be treated, to a certain extent, with fat grafting to improve coverage of the implant. In severe cases, the implant may be repositioned in the prepectoral position or, less frequently, by ligating the pectoral nerves to decrease pectoral muscle movement.

Implant Leak and Capsular Contracture

Implant leak and long-term maintenance is an important aspect of implant breast reconstruction.[57] It has, however, been difficult to accurately document implant leak rates because of a lack of standardized methods for documentation and verification. Nevertheless, this data was reported in some form by the major implant manufacturers in their application for FDA approval (core studies). At 6 years follow-up, Mentor MemoryGel implants had an overall rupture rate of 1.1% for primary augmentation, 11.6% for revision augmentation, 3.8% for primary reconstruction, and 5.9% for revision reconstruction.[58] The clinically significant capsular contracture rates (Baker III/IV) for these implants was 9.8% for primary augmentation and 13.7% for primary reconstruction. This study was conducted on 1008 patients with 1898 implants enrolled at 48 sites (refer to Chapter 35 for more detail).

The 10-year leak rate (assessed by MRI in 264 patients) of Allergan Naturelle round silicone gel implants was 9.3% for primary augmentation, 5.3% for revision augmentation, and 35.4% for primary reconstruction. The overall patient reported rupture rate was 13%. The 10-year clinically significant capsular contracture rate in 715 patients was 18.9% for augmentation, 28.7% for revision augmentation, and 24.6% for reconstruction.[59]

The core study from Sientra had 1788 patients, with MRI follow-up in 571. The 8-year MRI documented rupture rates for these cohesive silicone gel implants was 6.4% for primary augmentation, 5.2% for revision augmentation, and 2.8% for primary reconstruction. The overall capsular contracture rate was 12.6%.[60]

Implants and Radiation

Postmastectomy radiation therapy (PMRT) is an adjuvant therapy that is increasingly used in patients with breast cancer. This treatment improves local control and decreases the incidence of local recurrence. However, PMRT has significant effects on breast reconstruction outcomes, particularly in patients who undergo implant breast reconstruction. Patients treated with PMRT have significantly increased risk of implant loss, infection, capsular contracture, and the need for revision surgery. A meta-analysis of seven studies with 2921 patients (520 treated with PMRT and 2401 who were not treated with PMRT) revealed that radiation therapy increased the risk of revision surgery by 2.2-fold, reconstructive failure by 2.5-fold, and capsular contracture by more than 10-fold.[61] In addition, PMRT significantly decreased patient satisfaction and cosmetic outcomes. Nevertheless, implant reconstruction is indicated in some women, even if PMRT is needed. This is based on the fact that in some cases, other reconstructive options are either not available or not suitable due to patient-specific, medical, or oncological concerns. In addition, implants may serve as a good option to bridge patients to autologous reconstruction after PMRT. This is important because PMRT can also have significant negative effects on autologous reconstruction, particularly when insufficient tissues are available for reconstruction.

The timing of implant exchange relative to PMRT has been a topic of debate in the literature. Most authors have advocated for changing the expander to the permanent implant after PMRT has completed. The rationale for this approach is that there is no delay of radiation following completion of chemotherapy or mastectomy and, if PMRT-induced capsular contracture occurs, then it can be addressed at the time of exchange. Other investigators have proposed the exchange procedure to be done following completion of chemotherapy but prior to radiation. The rationale for this approach is to decrease wound healing complications that may occur when the procedure is performed on radiated tissues. Both approaches have merit. A meta-analysis of 20 studies revealed that PMRT of tissue expanders followed by implant exchange had a 2.3-fold higher rate (20% vs. 13.4%) of reconstructive failure as compared with the exchange of the expanders to implants followed by PMRT. However, the exchange of the expander to permanent implant prior to PMRT increased the rate of capsular contracture by nearly 2-fold (49.4% vs. 24.5%).[62] Ultimately, the results are likely dependent on a number of variables, including the thickness of the mastectomy flaps, the size of the implant, the reconstructive techniques, radiation technique/delivery, and the response of the patient to radiation. Unfortunately, PMRT use will likely increase until long-term studies of its efficacy in various clinical scenarios are completed, and more rational guidelines are developed. This will be a challenge for plastic surgeons for years to come.

Latissimus Dorsi Flap

History

Schneider and colleagues described the use of the latissimus flap for breast reconstruction in 1977.[63] These techniques were refined by McCraw et al, and later by Bostwick and associates who published on the use of the latissimus flap for immediate breast reconstruction.[64,65] The limited volume of tissues available for breast reconstruction with the latissimus flap was an issue in many patients and led some groups to describe extended latissimus flaps. However, the use of extended latissimus flaps fell largely out of favor due to donor site complications and partial flap loss. Nowadays, the latissimus flap is usually used in combination with tissue expanders or implants to increase the volume and projection of the reconstruction. More recently, immediate fat grafting of the latissimus has been proposed as a means of increasing the volume of reconstruction.

Patient Selection

The latissimus flap is useful in patients who have previously been treated with radiation and do not have adequate tissues in other donor sites for autologous reconstruction or those who wish to avoid other donor site scars. The latissimus is also useful in obese patients who have unfavorable abdominal donor sites and, in these situations, can provide a large amount of tissues for reconstruction (Fig. 36.20). Some surgeons use the latissimus flap as a first-line option for breast reconstruction. In these cases, the latissimus flap skin paddle can replace the NAC and provide an esthetically pleasing reconstruction (Fig. 36.21). The diagnosis of ipsilateral arm lymphedema is considered a relative contraindication to the use of the latissimus flap by some groups since harvesting additional axillary tissues may increase the severity of lymphedema. Interestingly, however, other groups have reported improvements in lymphedema following latissimus flap transfer.[66] The latissimus flap is also most likely not a good option in patients who are highly physically active as the harvest of this muscle may cause muscular weakness and decreased range of motion. However, in most cases the use of this flap for breast reconstruction is well tolerated. A prospective patient-reported outcome study of 1096 patients treated in 270 centers in the United Kingdom revealed that 78% of patients reported no problems with

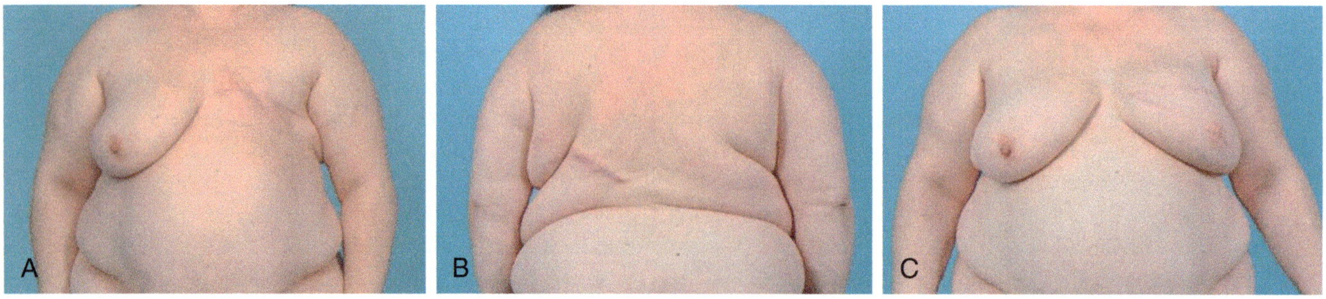

• **Fig. 36.20** Morbidly obese patient shown (A) preoperative and (B,C) 1-year postoperative after delayed latissimus flap and implant reconstruction.

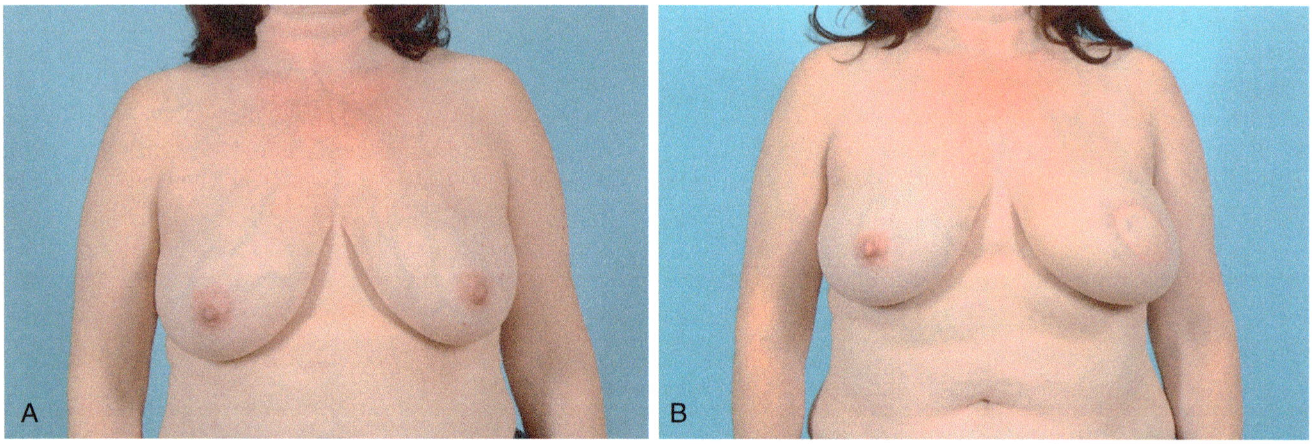

• **Fig. 36.21** (A) Preoperative and (B) postoperative photographs of a patient following immediate left breast reconstruction with a latissimus flap.

the appearance of the back-donor site; however, 40% of patients did report some degree of functional morbidity.[67] Concerns regarding functional problems in the latissimus donor site has led some investigators to advocate the use of segmental latissimus flaps to preserve muscle function.[68]

Surgical Technique

The patient is usually marked in the standing position, and the scar is usually placed along the orientation of Langer's lines and centered on the latissimus muscle. The arc of rotation of the muscle is assessed to ensure proper placement of the flap on the breast. Alternatively, the flap scar may also be positioned in the bra line if a limited amount of skin is needed for the reconstruction. Orienting the flap in this manner places the skin paddle in the middle of the breast and is ideal for replacing the skin deficit following mastectomy and nipple–areola resection. A typical skin paddle measures 6–12 cm in width by 15–25 cm in length. These measurements depend on the degree of skin laxity and reconstructive needs.

The patient is placed in the lateral position and padded appropriately. It is also possible to harvest the flap with the patient in a modified lateral position with a few bumps placed under the patient to elevate the ipsilateral arm/back (so called "sloppy lateral" position). It is very helpful to prep the arm into the field as this will allow intraoperative movement of the arm during flap dissection. The skin incisions are made, and skin flaps are elevated to expose the latissimus muscle. Leaving a small amount of fat below the Scarpa's fascia is helpful to increase the volume of the reconstruction and to prevent abnormal adherence of breast skin flaps to the latissimus dorsi flap. However, this should be done with care as over-resection of the fat in this area can result in noticeable contour deformities. In a standard muscle flap harvest, the latissimus muscle is exposed circumferentially, and the dissection is started from distal to proximal separating the flap from the paraspinous, serratus, oblique, teres major, and trapezius muscles. The pedicle vessels are identified and preserved. The serratus branch of the thoracodorsal artery/vein may be ligated if the proximal pedicle is intact. This will increase the arc of rotation of the flap. However, in patients previously treated with axillary lymph node dissection or extensive sentinel lymph node resection, it may be more prudent to preserve the serratus branch since the flap can be perfused in a retrograde manner if the primary pedicle has been injured.

The decision to either disinsert the muscle or not is made based on the arc of rotation of the flap and esthetic requirements. It is usually helpful to disinsert the latissimus muscle in thin patients because otherwise the bulk of the muscle in the axilla may be noticeable. This is difficult to treat postoperatively. In these cases, the disinserted head of the latissimus muscle is transposed anteriorly and used to reconstruct the defect resulting from resection of the tail of the breast. It is helpful to fully dissect the pedicle vessels in these patients to avoid kinking or twisting of the vein. In heavier patients or in those with extensive scarring that precludes dissection of the thoracodorsal artery and vein, disinserting the muscle is usually not necessary and may increase the risk of pedicle injury. However, even in this scenario, the flap should be completely mobilized to allow transposition into the breast defect and avoid axillary/lateral breast fullness as much as possible.

In cases where latissimus muscle function is important or preferable, then a partial latissimus muscle harvest can be performed. In some cases, it is possible to harvest the skin paddle based on a perforator (thoracodorsal artery perforator flap), in which case the latissimus muscle function is completely preserved. Partial harvest of the latissimus muscle can be performed by harvesting either the lateral or medial portion of the muscle and preserving the thoracodorsal nerve to the remaining segment of the latissimus. The lateral (descending) branch of the thoracodorsal artery is slightly longer than the medial (transverse) branch. The flap, together with the overlying skin, is harvested, and the pedicle dissection is completed to allow transposition of the flap into the breast defect. This flap is particularly useful for reconstruction of partial mastectomy defects. The thoracodorsal artery flap is harvested in a similar manner. In this case, the flap is marked 8–10 cm below the axillary crease, and a Doppler is used to identify cutaneous perforators that arise from the lateral border of the latissimus muscle. The superior (upper) skin incision is performed, and the flap is elevated carefully using blunt dissection to expose the perforator. The perforator is then dissected through the muscle to expose the thoracodorsal artery/vein. In some cases, the descending branch of the thoracodorsal nerve runs over or between the flap vessels and must be divided to transfer the flap. In these cases, the nerve is sharply divided and sutured using standard microsurgical techniques. Once the perforator dissection is completed, the remainder of the flap dissection is performed rapidly to completely mobilize the flap.

The back-donor site is closed over drains. Quilting sutures in the skin are extremely helpful to decrease the risk of seroma formation. The combination of fibrin sealant and quilting sutures is even more effective, decreasing the incidence of seromas by more than 70%. Injection of bupivacaine or liposomal bupivacaine is also helpful for decreasing postoperative pain.

The patient is brought back to the supine position, and the latissimus flap is transposed into the breast defect. The flap is medialized as much as possible to avoid axillary fullness. The medial border of the breast is repaired by suturing the flap in place. The latissimus flap is then sutured to the inframammary fold. The lateral border of the breast is similarly formed by suturing the latissimus muscle to the lateral chest wall at a line drawn just anterior to the anterior axillary line. If an implant or tissue expander is required, the device is placed below the latissimus muscle, and the remainder of the muscle is sutured to the pectoralis muscle. In some cases, the pectoralis muscle may be elevated to increase the size of the pocket for the tissue expander. This is particularly helpful for patients with a ptotic contralateral breast. The breast incisions are then closed over drains. A loose postoperative bra may be used for keeping the drains in place; however, compression of the flap pedicle should be avoided.

Outcomes

The most common complication of latissimus dorsi flap harvest is seroma formation in the donor site occurring in as many as 60% of patients.[69] As previously noted, quilting sutures with or without fibrin glue markedly decrease the incidence of this complication. Other minor complications include hematoma (5%) and wound infection (2%). Flap ischemia and total flap loss are rare and occur most commonly due to undiagnosed pedicle injury that had occurred during axillary lymph node dissection. Preoperative evaluation of latissimus dorsi muscle function is helpful as a quick test of possible pedicle injury (if the muscle is active and the thoracodorsal nerve is intact, then the rest of the pedicle was likely preserved). An angiogram can also be helpful to identify pedicle injury prior to flap harvest. Other causes of flap ischemia include twisting or kinking of the pedicle with flap transfer. Prepping the arm in the field is helpful to avoid this complication since the position of the pedicle with arm movement can easily be assessed intraoperatively after flap inset.

The latissimus dorsi flap has a reliable and robust blood supply. As a result, partial flap loss is also relatively uncommon, occurring in approximately 7% of cases.[70] Even in smokers, diabetics, and obese patients, the latissimus flap has low rates of ischemic complications.

Functional morbidity resulting from latissimus muscle harvest is a significant concern. A systematic review of 13 studies showed that 30%–50% of patients experience prolonged tightness, numbness, and impairment of range of motion following the latissimus dorsi flap harvest.[71] However, in most cases, these symptoms improve with time and, in most cases, resolve. For example, a prospective study of 22 patients who underwent latissimus flap harvest demonstrated significant impairment in strength, disability scores, pain, and range of motion 6 months following surgery.[72] However, by 1 year post operation, these abnormalities normalized and there were no significant changes in strength or function at this time. Patients who underwent extended latissimus flap harvest tended to have more complaints and slower recovery as compared with women treated with latissimus flap and implants. These findings were supported by a prospective study of 47 immediate latissimus dorsi flaps, demonstrating a decreased range of motion in the early recovery period and gradual resolution over time (1 year). Patients in this study had minor deficiencies in abduction and flexion capacities (5%–10% decrease) from the baseline that did not resolve; however, these patients did not have restriction of flexion or abduction. Injury to the long thoracic nerve may cause winging of the scapula and result in permanent morbidity.

Animation deformity with the latissimus flap is occasionally symptomatic in cases where the thoracodorsal nerve is not divided at the time of flap transfer. This can be addressed at a later date with exposure and division of the nerve. As a result of this issue, some surgeons advocate ligation of the thoracodorsal nerve in all patients who undergo latissimus dorsi flap breast reconstruction. The advantage of this approach is it avoids animation deformity. The disadvantage is late fibrosis and shrinkage of the muscle that may result in asymmetry. In general, it is our preference to not divide the nerve at the initial operation as in our experience this complication is rare and easily treated.

Conclusions

The techniques available for breast reconstruction have improved significantly over the past 50 years. The evolution of these procedures has improved outcomes and made reconstruction more widely available. Development of perforator flaps has decreased donor site morbidity and greatly improved the patient experience. The surgical myths that reconstruction changes the biology of breast cancer or makes recurrences more difficult to diagnose have been debunked, and immediate reconstruction is routinely performed. Nevertheless, plastic surgeons and breast cancer survivors face new and complex challenges. The timing and indications for postmastectomy radiation continue to evolve and expose more women to the deleterious effects of these treatments on their reconstruction. Controversies with implants such as implant-related illness or ALCL still exist even though implants have been in use since the early 1960s. Recent studies have shown that even modern breast reconstruction techniques have relatively high rates of complications with significant room for improvement. Thus, the quest for the ideal breast reconstruction technique continues and will be the challenge for the next generation of plastic surgeons.

References

1. Wilkins EG, Cederna PS, Lowery JC, et al. Prospective analysis of psychosocial outcomes in breast reconstruction: one-year postoperative results from the Michigan Breast Reconstruction Outcome Study. *Plast Reconstr Surg.* 2000;106(5):1014–1025; discussion 1026–1027.
2. Kroll SS, Khoo A, Singletary SE, et al. Local recurrence risk after skin-sparing and conventional mastectomy: A 6-year follow-up. *Plast Reconstr Surg.* 1999;104(2):421–425.
3. Tamai S. Digit replantation. Analysis of 163 replantations in an 11 year period. *Clin Plast Surg.* 1978;5(2):195–209.
4. Uroskie TW, Colen LB. History of breast reconstruction. *Semin Plast Surg.* 2004;18(2):65–69.
5. Drever JM. The epigastric island flap. *Plast Reconstr Surg.* 1977;59(3):343–346.
6. Robbins TH. Rectus abdominis myocutaneous flap for breast reconstruction. *Aust N Z J Surg.* 1979;49(5):527–530.
7. Hartrampf CR, Scheflan M, Black PW. Breast reconstruction with a transverse abdominal island flap. *Plast Reconstr Surg.* 1982;69(2):216–225.
8. Ireton JE, Kluft JA, Ascherman JA. Unilateral and bilateral breast reconstruction with pedicled TRAM flaps: An outcomes analysis of 188 consecutive patients. *Plast Reconstr Surg Glob Open.* 2013;1(2):1–7.
9. Holmström H. The free abdominoplasty flap and its use in breast reconstruction. An experimental study and clinical case report. *Scand J Plast Reconstr Surg.* 1979;13(3):423–427.
10. Mehrara BJ, Santoro TD, Arcilla E, et al. Complications after microvascular breast reconstruction: experience with 1195 flaps. *Plast Reconstr Surg.* 2006;118(5):1100–1109; discussion 1110–1111.
11. Jeong W, Lee S, Kim J. Meta-analysis of flap perfusion and donor site complications for breast reconstruction using pedicled versus free TRAM and DIEP flaps. *Breast.* 2018;38:45–51.
12. Man LX, Selber JC, Serletti JM. Abdominal wall following free TRAM or DIEP flap reconstruction: A meta-analysis and critical review. *Plast Reconstr Surg.* 2009;124(3):752–764.
13. Koshima I, Soeda S. Inferior epigastric artery skin flaps without rectus abdominis muscle. *Br J Plast Surg.* 1989;42(6):645–648.
14. Allen RJ, Treece P. Deep inferior epigastric perforator flap for breast reconstruction. *Ann Plast Surg.* 1994;32(1):32–38.
15. Pannucci CJ, Bailey SH, Dreszer G, et al. Validation of the Caprini risk assessment model in plastic and reconstructive surgery patients. *J Am Coll Surg.* 2011;212(1):105–112.
16. Antia NH, Buch VI. Transfer of an abdominal dermo-fat graft by direct anastomosis of blood vessels. *Br J Plast Surg.* 1971;24(1):15–19.
17. Arnez ZM, Khan U, Pogorelec D, et al. Breast reconstruction using the free superficial inferior epigastric artery (SIEA) flap. *Br J Plast Surg.* 1999;52(4):276–279.
18. Piorkowski JR, DeRosier LC, Nickerson P, et al. Preoperative computed tomography angiogram to predict patients with favorable anatomy for superficial inferior epigastric artery flap breast reconstruction. *Ann Plast Surg.* 2011;66(5):534–536.
19. Yousif NJ, Matloub HS, Kolachalam R, et al. The transverse gracilis musculocutaneous flap. *Ann Plast Surg.* 1992;29(6):482–490.
20. Pulzl P, Schoeller T, Kleewein K, et al. Donor-site morbidity of the transverse musculocutaneous gracilis flap in autologous breast reconstruction: short-term and long-term results. *Plast Reconstr Surg.* 2011;128(4):233e–242e.
21. Lakhiani C, Lee MR, Saint-Cyr M. Vascular anatomy of the anterolateral thigh flap: A systematic review. *Plast Reconstr Surg.* 2012;130(6):1254–1268.
22. Fansa H, Schirmer S, Warnecke IC, et al. The transverse myocutaneous gracilis muscle flap: A fast and reliable method for breast reconstruction. *Plast Reconstr Surg.* 2008;122(5):1326–1333.
23. Dayan E, Smith ML, Samson W, et al. The diagonal upper gracilis (DUG) flap: A safe and improved alternative to the TUG flap. *Plast Reconstr Surg. Global Open.* 2013;132(4S-1):33–34.
24. Dayan JH, Allen Jr RJ. Lower extremity free flaps for breast reconstruction. *Plast Reconstr Surg.* 2017;140:77S–86S. 5S Advances in Breast Reconstruction.
25. Allen RJ, Haddock NT, Ahn CY, et al. Breast reconstruction with the profunda artery perforator flap. *Plast Reconstr Surg.* 2012;129(1):16e–23e.
26. Saad A, Sadeghi A, Allen RJ. The anatomic basis of the profunda femoris artery perforator flap: A new option for autologous breast reconstruction – a cadaveric and computer tomography angiogram study. *J Reconstr Microsurg.* 2012;28(6):381–386.
27. Haddock NT, Gassman A, Cho M-J, et al. 101 Consecutive profunda artery perforator flaps in breast reconstruction: Lessons

learned with our early experience. *Plast Reconstr Surg.* 2017;140(2):229–239.
28. Allen Jr RJ, Lee Z-H, Mayo JL, et al. The profunda artery perforator flap experience for breast reconstruction. *Plast Reconstr Surg.* 2016;138(5):968–975.
29. Tuinder SMH, Beugels J, Lataster A, et al. The lateral thigh perforator flap for autologous breast reconstruction: A prospective analysis of 138 flaps. *Plast Reconstr Surg.* 2018;141(2):257–268.
30. Tuinder S, Baetens T, De Haan MW, et al. Septocutaneous tensor fasciae latae perforator flap for breast reconstruction: radiological considerations and clinical cases. *J Plast Reconstr Aesthet Surg.* 2014;67(9):1248–1256.
31. Shaw WW. Breast reconstruction by superior gluteal microvascular free flaps without silicone implants. *Plast Reconstr Surg.* 1983;72(4):490–501.
32. Paletta CE, Bostwick J 3rd, Nahai F. The inferior gluteal free flap in breast reconstruction. *Plast Reconstr Surg.* 1989;84(6):875–883; discussion 884–885.
33. Allen RJ, Tucker Jr C. Superior gluteal artery perforator free flap for breast reconstruction. *Plast Reconstr Surg.* 1995;95(7):1207–1212.
34. Allen R, Guarda H, Wall F, et al. Free flap breast reconstruction: the LSU experience (1984–1996). *J La State Med Soc.* 1997;149(10):388–392.
35. Snyderman RK, Guthrie RH. Reconstruction of the female breast following radical mastectomy. *Plast Reconstr Surg.* 1971;47(6):565–567.
36. Radovan C. Breast reconstruction after mastectomy using the temporary expander. *Plast Reconstr Surg.* 1982;69(2):195–208.
37. Nichter LS, Hardesty RA, Anigian GM. IDEAL IMPLANT structured breast implants: Core study results at 6 years. *Plast Reconstr Surg.* 2018;142(1):66–75.
38. Bondurant S, Enster V, Herdman R. *Safety of Silicone Breast Implants.* National Academy Press; 1999.
39. McLaughlin JK, Lipworth L, Murphy DK, et al. The safety of silicone gel-filled breast implants: A review of the epidemiologic evidence. *Ann Plast Surg.* 2007;59(5):569–580.
40. Balk EM, Earley A, Avendano EA, et al. Long-term health outcomes in women with silicone gel breast implants: A systematic review. *Ann Intern Med.* 2016;164(3):164–175.
41. Collett DJ, Rakhorst H, Lennox P, et al. Current risk estimate of breast implant-associated anaplastic large cell lymphoma in textured breast implants. *Plast Reconstr Surg.* 2019;143:30S–40S. 3S A Review of Breast Implant-Associated Anaplastic Large Cell Lymphoma.
42. McCarthy CM, Mehrara BJ, Riedel E, et al. Predicting complications following expander/implant breast reconstruction: an outcomes analysis based on preoperative clinical risk. *Plast Reconstr Surg.* 2008;121(6):1886–1892.
43. Bacilious N, Cordeiro PG, Disa JJ, et al. Breast reconstruction using tissue expanders and implants in Hodgkin's patients with prior mantle irradiation. *Plast Reconstr Surg.* 2002;109(1):102–107.
44. Bertozzi N, Pesce M, Santi P, et al. One-stage immediate breast reconstruction: A concise review. *BioMed Res Int.* 2017;2017:6486859.
45. Han HH, Kim HB, Kim EK, et al. Direct-to-implant as a frontline option for immediate breast reconstruction: A comparative study with 2-stage reconstruction. *Ann Plast Surg.* 2018;81(3):274–279.
46. Bernini M, Calabrese C, Cecconi L, et al. Subcutaneous direct-to-implant breast reconstruction: surgical, functional, and aesthetic results after long-term follow-up. *Plast Reconstr Surg. Global Open.* 2015;3(12):e574.
47. Choi M, Frey JD, Alperovich M, et al. Breast in a Day": examining single-stage immediate, permanent implant reconstruction in nipple-sparing mastectomy. *Plast Reconstr Surg.* 2016;138(2):184e–91e.
48. Negenborn VL, Dikmans REG, Bouman MB, et al. Predictors of complications after direct-to-implant breast reconstruction with an acellular dermal matrix from a multicentre randomized clinical trial. *Br J Surg.* 2018;105(10):1305–1312.
49. Corban J, Shash H, Safran T, et al. A systematic review of complications associated with direct implants vs. tissue expanders following Wise pattern skin-sparing mastectomy. *J Plast Reconstr Aesthet Surg.* 2017;70(9):1191–1199.
50. Clarke-Pearson EM, Lin AM, Hertl C, et al. Revisions in implant-based breast reconstruction: how does direct-to-implant measure up? *Plast Reconstr Surg.* 2016;137(6):1690–1699.
51. Sbitany H, Gomez-Sanchez C, Piper M, et al. Prepectoral breast reconstruction in the setting of postmastectomy radiation therapy: An assessment of clinical outcomes and benefits. *Plast Reconstr Surg.* 2019;143(1):10–20.
52. Sbitany H. Important considerations for performing prepectoral breast reconstruction. *Plast Reconstr Surg.* 2017;140:7S–13S. 6S Prepectoral Breast Reconstruction.
53. Manrique OJ, Banuelos J, Abu-Ghname A, et al. Surgical outcomes of prepectoral versus subpectoral implant-based breast reconstruction in young women. *Plast Reconstr Surg. Global Open.* 2019;7(3):e2119.
54. Antony AK, McCarthy CM, Cordeiro PG, et al. Acellular human dermis implantation in 153 immediate two-stage tissue expander breast reconstructions: Determining the incidence and significant predictors of complications. *Plast Reconstr Surg.* 2010;125(6):1606–1614.
55. Wilkins EG, Hamill JB, Kim HM, et al. Complications in postmastectomy breast reconstruction: one-year outcomes of the mastectomy reconstruction outcomes Consortium (MROC) study. *Ann Surg.* 2018;267(1):164–170.
56. Clough KB, O'Donoghue JM, Fitoussi AD, et al. Prospective evaluation of late cosmetic results following breast reconstruction: I. Implant reconstruction. *Plast Reconstr Surg.* 2001;107(7):1702–1709.
57. Hillard C, Fowler JD, Barta R, et al. Silicone breast implant rupture: a review. *Gland Surg.* 2017;6(2):163–168.
58. Cunningham B, McCue J. Safety and effectiveness of Mentor's MemoryGel implants at 6 years. *Aesthet Plast Surg.* 2009;33(3):440–444.
59. Spear SL, Murphy DK. USCCSG. Allergan Silicone Breast Implant, Natrelle round silicone breast implants: Core study results at 10 years. *Plast Reconstr Surg.* 2014;133(6):1354–1361.
60. Stevens WG, Calobreace MB, Harrington J, et al. Nine-year core study data for Sientra's FDA-approved round and shaped implants with high-strength cohesive silicone gel. *Aesthet Surg J.* 2016;36(4):404–416.
61. Magill LJ, Robertson FP, Jell G, et al. Determining the outcomes of post-mastectomy radiation therapy delivered to the definitive implant in patients undergoing one- and two-stage implant-based breast reconstruction: A systematic review and meta-analysis. *J Plast Reconstr Aesthet Surg.* 2017;70(10):1329–1335.
62. Ricci JA, Epstein S, Momoh AO, et al. A meta-analysis of implant-based breast reconstruction and timing of adjuvant radiation therapy. *J Surg Res.* 2017;218:108–116.

63. Schneider WJ, Hill Jr HL, Brown RG. Latissimus dorsi myocutaneous flap for breast reconstruction. *Br J Plast Surg.* 1977;30(4):277–281.
64. Bostwick 3rd J, Scheflan M. The latissimus dorsi musculocutaneous flap: A one-stage breast reconstruction. *Clin Plast Surg.* 1980;7(1):71–78.
65. McCraw JB, Dibbell DG, Carraway JH. Clinical definition of independent myocutaneous vascular territories. *Plast Reconstr Surg.* 1977;60(3):341–352.
66. Abbas Khan MA, Mohan A, Hardwicke J. Objective improvement in upper limb lymphoedema following ipsilateral latissimus dorsi pedicled flap breast reconstruction – a case series and review of literature. *J Plast Reconstr Aesthet Surg.* 2011;64(5):680–684.
67. Browne JP, Jeevan R, Pusic AL, et al. Measuring the patient perspective on latissimus dorsi donor site outcomes following breast reconstruction. *J Plast Reconstr Aesthet Surg.* 2018;71(3):336–343.
68. Ding Y, Cao DS, Huang XY, et al. Segmental latissimus dorsi free flap attempting to preserve function at the donor site: Anatomical and clinical experiences. *J Reconstr Microsurg.* 2017;33(4):268–274.
69. Menke H, Erkens M, Olbrisch RR. Evolving concepts in breast reconstruction with latissimus dorsi flaps: results and follow-up of 121 consecutive patients. *Ann Plast Surg.* 2001;47(2):107–114.
70. Hokin JA, Silfverskiold KL. Breast reconstruction without an implant: results and complications using an extended latissimus dorsi flap. *Plast Reconstr Surg.* 1987;79(1):58–66.
71. Smith SL. Functional morbidity following latissimus dorsi flap breast reconstruction. *J Adv Pract Oncol.* 2014;5(3):181–187.
72. Glassey N, Perks GB, McCulley SJ. A prospective assessment of shoulder morbidity and recovery time scales following latissimus dorsi breast reconstruction. *Plast Reconstr Surg.* 2008;122(5):1334–1340.

37 Congenital Breast Anomalies

SABRINA CUGNO AND ALAIN J. AZZI

Embryology

Breast development begins at approximately the 5th to 6th embryonic week. It proceeds from a single ectodermal bud and begins developing along the ventral side of the embryo as paired longitudinal bands of thickened ectoderm called *milk lines* (mammary ridges). The latter extend from axilla to groin. The majority of the mammary ridge involutes by the 9th week of gestation except for a focus of epithelial cells at the fourth intercostal space that subsequently form a single pair of mammary buds.[1] Failure of complete involution results in polythelia/polymastia along the mammary ridge. The primary buds form the secondary buds as ectodermal cells begin to invade the underlying mesenchyme by the 12th week of gestation.[2] While the epithelial cells grow downward as mammary ducts, terminating in lobular buds, the mesenchymal cells differentiate into smooth muscle of the nipple and areola. This specialized epithelium differentiates into 15–20 branches that first consist of solid epithelial columns and then, by the 20–24th week of gestation, develop inner lumens and eventually canalize to form the lactiferous ducts and their branches.[3] These branched epithelial tissues are stimulated to canalize by the placental hormones that enter the fetal circulation during the third trimester. The ends of these branches differentiate into lobulo–alveolar structures that contain *colostrum*, which is a yellow, sticky, and serous fluid. This colostral milk, stimulated by the placental hormones, can be expressed for 4–7 days after birth in both male and female newborns ("witch's milk"). Sebaceous glands, sweat glands, and specialized apocrine glands (Montgomery glands) develop in the second trimester. During the final weeks of gestation, the mass of the mammary gland increases consistently and the nipple–areola complex (NAC) develops and becomes pigmented. With the withdrawal of placental hormones after birth, the secretion of colostrum stops and the breast begins to involute. The supporting structure of the breast, composed of connective tissue and fat, originates from the mesenchyme that invades and surrounds the epithelial system. Failure of some of these stages in breast development to take place can result in congenital abnormalities of the breast.

After birth, circulating maternal estrogens may cause breast enlargement. Thereafter, maternal estrogens are metabolized resulting in involution of breast tissue and a period of quiescence during childhood. At puberty, hormonal flux results in breast growth or *thelarche*, with estrogens affecting ductal and stromal tissue proliferation and progesterone causing alveolar budding and lobular growth. Thelarche occurs at an average of 11 years of age (range, 8–15). The Tanner Scale describes breast development as proceeding through five stages, with growth generally reaching completion at 16–18 years of age.

Polythelia and Polymastia

Polythelia or presence of supernumerary nipples or nipple–areola complexes are often noted at birth, with the majority located along the embryonic milk line (Fig. 37.1). These form due to failure of regression of the mammary ridge. However, uncommon locations include the back, thigh, neck, and face.[4] The condition usually occurs sporadically, but may be familial, and has a reported incidence as high as 5.6%.[5,6] The supernumerary nipple is most commonly located in the inframammary region. There is little evidence to support an association with other congenital anomalies or syndromes nor is there any correlation with gender or predilection for the right or left side, however, it has been suggested that the prevalence is higher on the left side and in males.[5–7] The clinical significance of supernumerary nipples is the possibility of growth and development of similar pathologies as a normal breast, including breast neoplasia. Traditionally, the management of polythelia has been observation. However, pigmented lesions along the embryonic lines are routinely excised before puberty in order to avoid wider tissue excision secondary to glandular growth, which may be necessary after the onset of puberty in girls.[8,9] If multiple nipple–areola complexes are present on the breast proper, magnetic resonance imaging may be required to determine the complex associated with glandular/ductal tissue.[9] Changes to the pigmented lesion should be treated as for any melanocytic nevus, with early excision and histopathological assessment.

An oncologist should evaluate nipple growth that occurs at a time other than childhood, puberty, or pregnancy.

Polymastia occurs due to failure of the mammary ridge to completely regress in utero, leading to the development of breast tissue following hormonal stimulation. Ectopic breast tissue may or may not have an overlying NAC, but it is not uncommon for the nipple and areola to be absent or rudimentary. Polymastia has an even lower incidence than polythelia (1–2%), and also occurs along the embryonic milk line.[10] Unlike polythelia, polymastia may only be noticed during puberty, pregnancy or lactation. A common location is the axilla and unusual locations include the vulva, lower extremities and dorsal trunk.[10] Like polythelia, it is usually sporadic, but can have familial inheritance. Unlike polythelia, polymastia can be associated with other congenital anomalies, particularly congenital renal anomalies.[11] Treatment of polymastia is variable and depends on the size and location of the supernumerary breast gland and nipple.

In view of the fact that ectopic breast tissue is subject to the same pathology as normal breast parenchyma, complete resection is recommended. Simple mastectomy is the option of choice in patients who present with a third distinct breast mound; however, disruption of the inframammary fold and soft tissue envelope of the remaining breast should be prevented when possible. In cases where the accessory breast is adjoined to the native breast, tissue-sparing techniques with skin de-epithelialization and accessory nipple excision can usually restore the mound to a normal appearance and location. Corrective surgery for polymastia should be performed when breast development is complete and final breast tissue volumes have been achieved. It is often difficult to predict the form and position of the accessory breast mound or nipple and early excision may ultimately compromise the eventual outcome. Delaying excision until the final shape and position of the native breast tissue is complete will prevent eventual deformities from inadvertent iatrogenic insult to the developing breast.

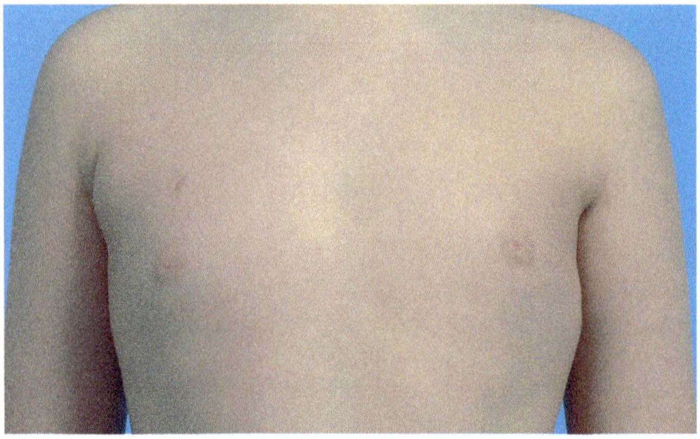

• **Fig. 37.1** A 10-year-old male with polythelia seen along the right mammary ridge superior to the true nipple–areola complex.

Gynecomastia

Gynecomastia, or abnormal benign proliferation of the male breast tissue, affects up to 65% of boys, peaking between the ages of 13 and 14 years (Fig. 37.2).[12,13] Physiological pubertal gynecomastia is attributed to a disruption of balance between testosterone and estrogen, where there is a lag between rising testosterone and estradiol levels through puberty.[14] This transient period of excess estradiol promotes glandular proliferation of the breast. Gynecomastia should not be confused with pseudogynecomastia, defined as adipose tissue giving the appearance of a female breast, without the presence of glandular tissue. Only 5–10% of gynecomastia persists beyond one year and spontaneous resolution occurs in the majority of patients.[13] If the condition persists beyond one year, fibrosis and hyalinization occur, with regression of epithelial proliferation. These changes render the condition less amenable to medical therapy and increase the necessity for surgical intervention. Timing of surgical correction is based on the absence of a secondary cause for gynecomastia (e.g., endocrine), persistence of breast enlargement for greater than one year, as well as psychosocial impact on the patient. Simon proposed a classification

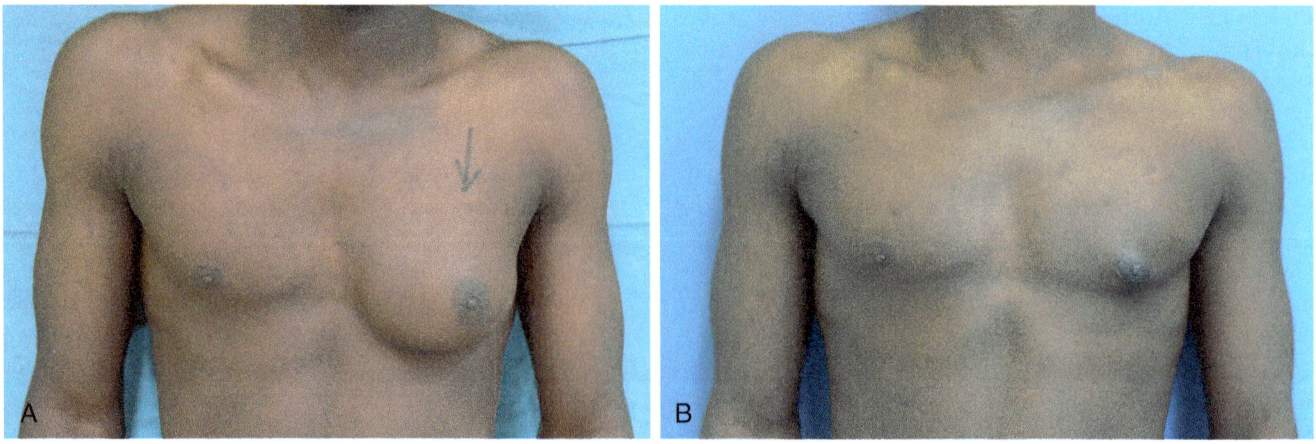

• **Fig. 37.2** A 21-year-old male with (A) left gynecomastia, who underwent (B) correction with liposuction and periareolar gland excision. (Courtesy Dr. Rostam D. Farhadieh.)

system for gynecomastia, with *grade 1* characterized by slight breast enlargement without skin redundancy, *grade 2a* moderate breast enlargement without skin redundancy, *grade 2b* moderate breast enlargement with marked skin redundancy, and *grade 3* both marked breast enlargement and skin redundancy.[15] Albeit physiological in the majority of cases, secondary gynecomastia must be ruled out by performing a thorough physical exam and history. Drug-induced gynecomastia is the most common secondary cause. A breast and testicular exam is recommended to rule out any rare secondary causes such as testicular malignancies. Other secondary causes include tuberous sclerosis, adrenal malignancies, and steroid hormone synthesis abnormalities.[10] Preoperative evaluation by endocrinology should be considered if endocrinopathy is suspected on history or physical examination (such as galactorrhea, abnormal testicular examination, features of Klinefelter syndrome, abnormal visual field or funduscopic testing, rapid progression). Routine workup by an endocrinologist in patients with suspected physiological gynecomastia lasting less than a year with no suspicious findings is likely not necessary. Some authors suggest a more selective evaluation, recommending referral to endocrinology if gynecomastia persists beyond 16 years of age.[13]

Management consists of excising the breast tissue and removing excess skin, if present. A semicircular periareolar incision is commonly used for breast tissue excision. Liposuction (traditional suction-assisted or ultrasonic-assisted) is used to remove the surrounding stromal hypertrophy or fibrofatty accumulation around the breast. The breast bud is often too firm and liposuction alone is difficult, however it could be used to fragment the breast tissue, facilitating subsequent excision through a limited excision (pull-through technique).[16,] Arthroscopic shavers have been used to remove the firm fibrous breast tissue, obviating the need for a periareolar incision in certain cases. Mild skin excess may resolve after gland excision due to skin contraction. In view of the capacity for contraction of the skin envelope with the exception of dramatic skin excess, a staged approach may be considered with volume reduction as an initial treatment, followed by revision surgery if necessary 6–12 months later.[16] When skin resection is necessary, an algorithm similar to that implemented for mastopexy may be applied. In cases of significant skin excess, a circumareolar, circumvertical, or wise-pattern skin resection can be considered depending on the severity.

Virginal Hypertrophy

Virginal hypertrophy or gigantomastia is defined as massive enlargement of the breast, usually defined as a breast volume requiring a reduction of at least 1800 g per side.[8] The condition is usually bilateral and is associated with rapid and disproportionate growth of the breast, which typically commences shortly after puberty. The growth is so rapid that it often outgrows the existing blood supply. There is no association with endocrine abnormalities. Gigantomastia is generally sporadic and secondary to abnormally sensitive glandular tissue to normal levels of pubertal hormones. The standard treatment is breast reduction. Continued growth following breast reduction of the hypertrophied breast is frequent and also reported to occur years later during pregnancy. Some authors have recommended skin and nipple-sparing mastectomy in order to control an aggressive process in patients who demonstrated continued regrowth following a reduction.[10] Pharmacological treatment with tamoxifen (antiestrogen medication) has been reported to control breast growth and/or ablate recurrence but its use is still controversial considering the significant side effects. Clinically, unilateral virginal hypertrophy should be distinguished from excessive breast growth secondary to a mass such as phyllodes tumor or fibroadenoma.

Athelia and Amastia

The absence of nipple (athelia) and/or glandular breast tissue (amastia/amazia, respectively) is a rare occurrence. According to Lin and Nguyen, there are different presentations of amastia and each can be attributed to different underlying pathologies: (1) ectodermal defects may cause bilateral absence of breasts in males and females and is related to failure of development of the ectodermal layer and its appendages (abnormalities of the skin, teeth and nails); (2) bilateral amastia may be an isolated occurrence or be associated with other anomalies of the palate and upper extremities; (3) unilateral amastia may be a variant of Poland syndrome and should be treated accordingly (Fig. 37.3).[17] Treatment of amastia and athelia may follow the principles of post-oncologic breast reconstruction with special attention paid to the placement of the inframammary fold and nipple. However, reconstruction in patients with amastia should be performed keeping in mind potential aberrations of the blood supply to the skin.[9] Very often, reconstruction for amastia is initiated prior to physical maturity with placement of a tissue expander, which is inflated commensurate with the growth of the normal contralateral breast or in bilateral cases, initiated at thelarche and continued proportionate with body habitus.

Tuberous Breast

Rees and Aston first described the *tuberous breast deformity* in 1976, after its resemblance in shape to a tuberous plant root.[18] This deformity is characterized by constriction of the breast base, parenchymal hypoplasia, pseudoherniation of the breast tissue through the areolar region, skin deficiency in the subareolar region and superior malposition of the inframammary fold.[19] Since their initial description, many similar breast deformities have been described, including *herniated areolar complex*, *snoopy deformity*, *tubular breast*, *constricted breast*, *lower pole hypoplasia*, and *narrow-based breast*.[20] Indeed, most consider these deformities to be various degrees of the same pathology, with the commonality being breast base anomaly. Tuberous breast remains the most widely used nomenclature to describe the pathological

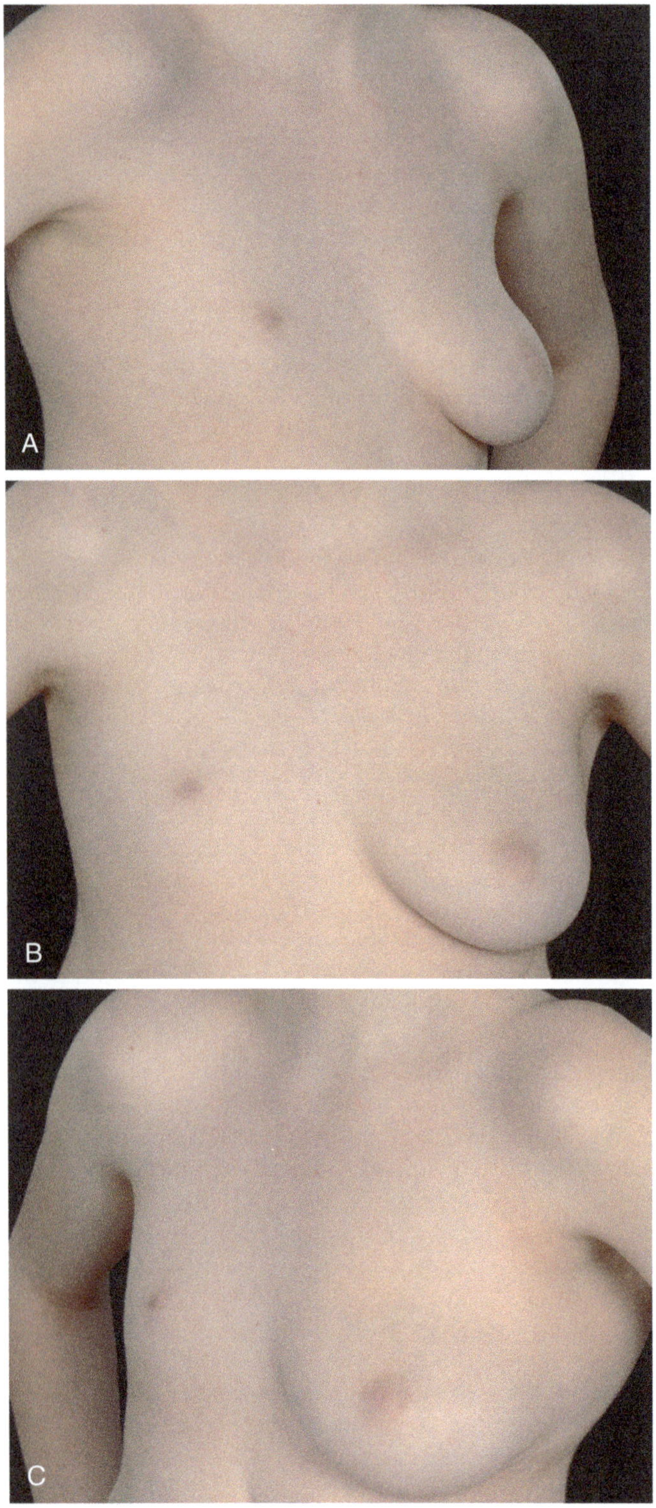

• **Fig. 37.3** (A–C) A 17-year-old female with right-sided amazia.

condition of glandular hypoplasia with a deficiency in the circumferential skin envelope of the breast base. The incidence remains unknown and there is no evidence to suggest a familial association. The deformity can be unilateral or bilateral, and usually asymmetric.

The etiology remains unclear, although several authors have proposed developmental sequences to account for the deformity. Grolleau et al attribute the deformity to an anomaly of the superficial muscular fascia in the lower pole of breast, such that the superficial fascia is aberrantly adherent to the dermis and muscular plane.[21] This restricts peripheral expansion, exaggerating forward growth resulting in a tubular breast shape and enlarged areola. Additionally, the deformity may arise secondary to involution of the mammary ridge, in light of the fact that the inferior portion of the deformed breast possesses a deficiency of milk ducts. Alternatively, Mandrekas and Zambacos proposed that the deformity is a result of a constricting ring at the base of the breast.[22] The authors propose that this pathological process begins in puberty explaining why no anomaly is discernible prior to the onset of breast development. As a result of the ectodermal origin of the breast and its invagination into the underlying mesenchyme, the breast parenchyma is contained within a fascial envelope, the superficial fascia. This fascia consists of a superficial layer, which covers the breast parenchyma and a deep layer, which forms the posterior boundary of the parenchyma and lies on the muscular fascia of the pectoralis major and serratus muscles. The two layers of superficial fascia are joined by fibrous attachments (suspensory ligaments of Cooper) extending from the dermis to the pectoralis fascia. The region beneath the NAC is devoid of superficial fascia. Thus, the pathological constricting ring at the periphery of the NAC in the tuberous breast deformity is thought to represent a thickening of the superficial fascia, which coupled with the absence of superficial fascia beneath the areola inhibits inferior expansion of the breast and leads to herniation of the breast parenchyma through the areola. As a result, the authors proposed complete vertical transection along the inferior portion of the breast parenchyma. In 1996, von Heimburg et al proposed a classification system for the tuberous breast deformity, based primarily on the degree of breast hypoplasia and deficiency of skin in the lower pole, including *Type I*, hypoplasia of the lower medial quadrant, *Type II*, hypoplasia of the lower medial and lateral quadrants, with sufficient skin in the subareolar region, *Type III*, hypoplasia of the lower medial and lateral quadrants, with a deficiency of skin in the subareolar region, and *Type IV*, severe breast constriction with minimal breast base.[23] Grolleau et al proposed a more simplified classification system, which is more commonly adopted. In *type I* deformity, only the lower medial quadrant is deficient.[21] Both lower medial and lateral quadrants are deficient in a *type II* anomaly (Fig. 37.4), and in type III deformity all four quadrants are deficient and the breast base is constricted both horizontally and vertically (Fig. 37.5). Meara et al[19] expanded on the latter classification system to aid in development of a specific treatment strategy.

The surgical management of the tuberous breast deformity varies as widely as the nomenclature. Rees and Aston first described the principles of correction and recognized an implant alone was insufficient to adequately correct the areolar herniation and proposed release or scoring to expand the breast base, with lowering of the inframammary fold.[18] The principles of treatment were further expanded in more

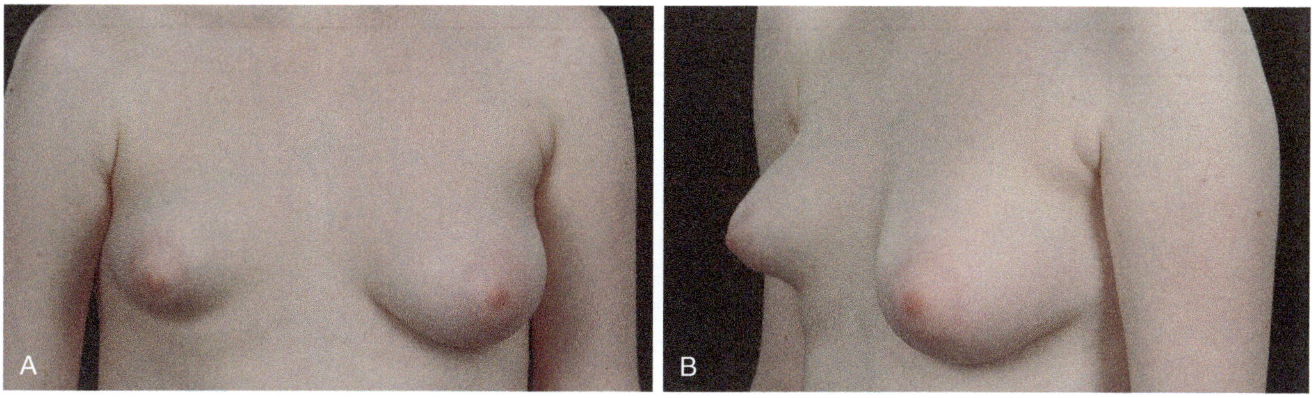

• **Fig. 37.4** (A,B) A 16-year-old female with type 2 tuberous breast deformity (Grolleau). The inferior medial and lateral quadrants are deficient, without constriction of the upper pole when compared to the contralateral breast. Superior malposition of the inframammary fold is also noted.

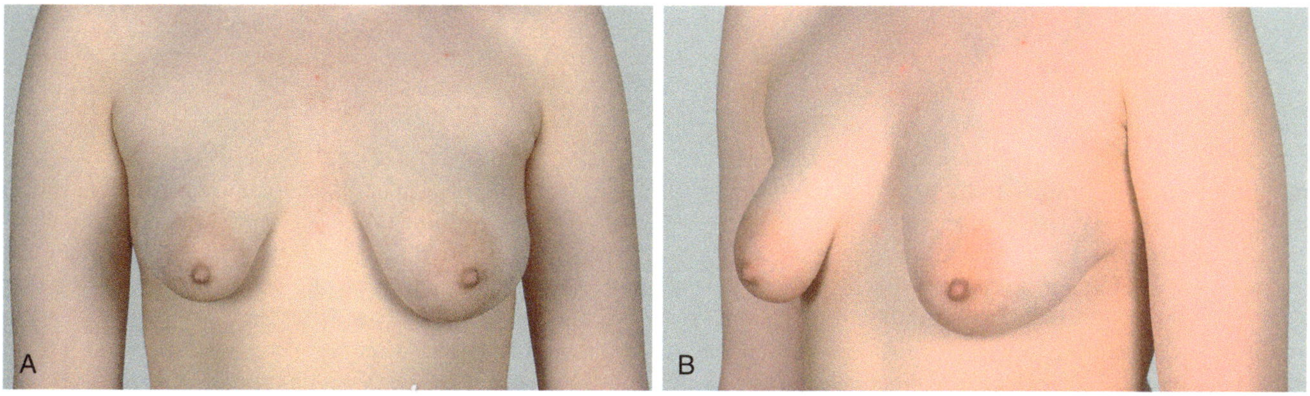

• **Fig. 37.5** (A,B) A 16-year-old female with type 3 tuberous breast deformity (Grolleau). The breast is constricted in all four quadrants. The deformity is more advanced and the upper pole is more constricted than the patient in Fig. 37.4.

recent literature and include expansion of the constricted base, lowering of the inframammary fold, increasing the skin envelope when required, augmentation of breast volume, reduction of breast tissue herniation through the areola and correction of areola size when necessary. In type I breasts, the lower lateral quadrant is distended, ptotic, and has excess skin. As such, the lateral cutaneous and glandular excess are used to fill the cavity created by undermining of the lower lateral quadrant, using a mammaplasty technique with a superior glandular pedicle and a triangular dermoglandular flap with a lower lateral pedicle.

In type II breasts, correction is achieved with placement of an implant and releasing the constricted base. As simple insertion of an implant creates a *double-crease deformity* in the lower quadrant, accentuating the tuberous deformity, Rees and Aston were the first to advise using radial incisions at the base of the gland.[18] Through an inframammary incision, the posterior surface of the breast is exposed to effect radial parenchymal incisions. Dinner and Downden, attributed the constriction in the inferior pole of the breast to the *skin envelope* and thus advocated full-thickness incision through the skin.[24] The role of the skin in breast base constriction is not supported by all authors. Others advocated transecting the breast parenchyma horizontally and then unfolding the flap. Puckett and Concannon, and Ribeiro et al performed periareolar de-epithelialization and undermined the lower pole to the position of the new inframammary fold.[20,25] Ribeiro et al maintained that the primary goal of correction of this deformity is to *transect the constricting ring*.[25] The authors described the use of an inferiorly based glandular adipose flap. The areola is drawn with a diameter of 4 cm and the exceeding halo is marked, as well as the position of the corrected inframammary fold. The circumareolar region is de-epithelialized and an inferiorly based parenchymal flap is made by dividing the breast horizontally down to the muscular plane below the NAC. Following parenchymal division, the inferior pole is freed from the skin envelope and lateral and medial prolongations of the inferior flap are resected. The creation of this flap results in disruption of the constriction ring, which is responsible for the herniation. The inferior flap is then fixed to the pectoral fascia by folding it over itself to project the lower pole of the breast. The superior pedicle (with the overlying NAC) then drapes over the inferior flap and is rearranged so that the mammary base is enlarged. In cases of severe hypoplasia, augmentation with a prosthesis is added. After parenchymal rearrangement, a periareolar Benelli-type purse-string suture is done. Unlike Ribeiro et al,[25] Puckett and Concannon[20] divided the parenchyma from the posterior aspect of the gland, allowing an "unfurling" of the lower pole downward. The inferior flap is then used to enhance the projection of the hypoplastic breast, thereby negating the use of implants. While Ribeiro's technique allows greater ease of dissection, the vascularization of the glandular flap is less reliable if significant undermining is required for implant placement, even in the retropectoral position.[21] Mandrekas et al also emphasized the importance to adequately release the constricting ring within the breast parenchyma.[22,26] Similar in principle to the Ribeiro technique, the breast is divided but in a *vertical* rather than horizontal plane creating two inferior pillars that are then reapproximated and folded over each other to fill the inferior pole of the breast, with the option of adding an implant to correct any deficiency in breast volume.

The type III deformity is characterized by areolar herniation and inadequate skin envelope. Correction of the type III breast usually requires a two-stage approach with tissue expander or definitive implant placement concomitantly with the release of the constricted base, followed by periareolar skin excision. Kolker and Collins[27] proposed correction through a periareolar incision, with dissection in a perpendicular fashion through the gland directly to the prepectoral fascia. Prefascial dissection is then extended to the new inframammary fold. The inferior dermoglandular flap is scored in a radial fashion to expand and release the lower pole constriction. The pectoralis major is then horizontally incised across its inferior margin, retropectoral dissection is completed, and an implant (one-stage) or tissue expander (two-stage) in placed. The gland is then reapproximated and circumareolar mastopexy is performed.

Poland Syndrome

In 1841, Alfred Poland, a medical student, described the syndrome which bears his name.[28] The latter is the combination of chest wall and upper limb anomalies, and is more commonly unilateral on the right and in males.[29] The prevalence of 1 in 20,000–30,000 births is likely underestimated.[30] Most cases are sporadic, although there are some linked to a genetic transmission. While its cause remains to be definitively elucidated, most authorities contend that an abnormal development of the fetal vasculature in the area is responsible. One theory suggests interruption of the subclavian artery during the 6th to 7th week of gestation.[31] An alternate hypothesis stipulates a developmental failure of the embryonic mesodermal plate that gives rise to the pectoralis muscle.[29] There is an association with other syndromes, including Möbius, Klippel–Feil, and Sprengel deformity. Severity ranges from severe deformity with absence of ribs to minor and subtle asymmetry. Complete absence of the pectoralis major muscle presents as an absence of the anterior axillary fold (Fig. 37.6). Occasionally, an anomalous fibrous band extending from the thorax to the humerus may result in webbing of the axilla. Hypoplasia or aplasia of the breast, NAC, and subcutaneous tissue is also observed. Neighboring muscles may likewise be diminutive or absent, including the serratus and latissimus dorsi muscles, and there may be asymmetry or elevation of the shoulder and scapula, as well as narrowed hemithorax. The ipsilateral upper limb is often shorter with brachysyndactyly of the hand. Alopecia in the axillary or mammary regions, aplasia/deformity of the costal cartilages or ribs, and absence of the pectoralis minor are also possible findings.[10] An entity distinct from Poland anomaly, referred to as *anterior thoracic hypoplasia*, is also characterized by unilateral depressed chest wall, hypoplasia of the breast, superiorly displaced NAC.[32] However, in the latter, there is a normal pectoralis muscle, whereas absence of the sternal head of the pectoralis major muscle is a pathognomonic finding in Poland syndrome.

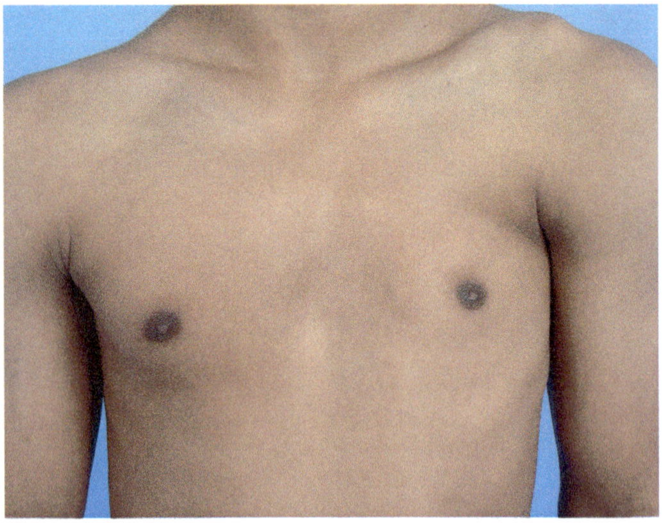

• **Fig. 37.6** A 15-year-old male with unilateral left-sided Poland syndrome. Partial absence of the pectoralis major muscle is noted. The superior portion of the anterior axillary line is present, representing the clavicular portion of the pectoralis muscle. Hypoplasia of the subcutaneous tissue can also be noted.

Reconstruction is dictated by the affected components. The most frequently affected ribs are the second to fourth, or third to fifth, which may result in lung herniation and chest wall instability.[29] Re-establishment of thoracic wall integrity is often accomplished with split rib grafts. The sternum may be rotated and rib cartilages more prominent on the affected side, requiring correction in selected cases. Beyond the chest wall, surgical management is influenced by the sex of the patient. In males, a custom-made prosthesis may serve to camouflage the flattened appearance. This is recommended in cases where a muscle transfer is needed to recreate the anterior axillary fold. Insertion of a prosthesis under a skin flap with minimal subcutaneous tissue has an unnatural appearance and a higher complication rate.[33] In cases where the anterior axillary fold is present, consideration of de-epithelialized dermal-adipose flaps or fat grafting without muscle transfer can reliably provide satisfactory contour restoration. With regards to reconstruction of the pectoralis muscle, functional muscle transfer depends on the presence or absence of the anterior axillary fold. When the superior portion of the pectoralis muscle and axillary fold are present, soft tissue augmentation alone is sufficient. In the absence of the anterior axillary fold, a dynamic muscle transfer is considered. Classically, the ipsilateral latissimus dorsi muscle is preferred. The muscle is usually harvested through a midlateral thoracic incision, which allows for both muscle harvest and elevation of anterior skin flap for muscle insertion. The tendon is also reinserted on the humerus through a short incision. The latissimus muscle is larger and thinner than the pectoralis muscle so it is folded on itself to provide more bulk, particularly in the subclavicular area and laterally at the level of the axillary fold. In cases of severe depression in the subclavicular area, a de-epithelialized skin paddle can be transferred with the muscle to increase the thickness. The arm is kept adducted for 6 weeks postoperatively. The donor site deformity is minimal as the posterior axillary fold is preserved with the tendon of the teres major, and the resultant scar well tolerated as it is hidden under the resting arm. Free innervated muscle transfers are needed in cases where the ipsilateral latissimus muscle is absent. Alternatives are the contralateral latissimus or free transverse myocutaneous gracilis flap.

In general, reconstruction of the female breast is performed once growth of the contralateral normal breast is complete. Augmentation with prosthesis is preferred in cases where there is some breast tissue on the affected side and the normal contralateral breast is small and nonptotic. Alloplastic augmentation alone in minor cases may be satisfactory but accentuation of the subclavicular hollowing and potential migration of the implant into this space can occur.[33] The prosthesis can be placed over or under the latissimus muscle at the time of muscle transposition depending on the amount of overlying soft tissue. Indeed, if a small contralateral breast is present, latissimus muscle transfer without concomitant implant placement is considered. If the location of the nipple-areolar complex (NAC) is acceptable, the prosthesis can be inserted at the time of muscle transfer. When the location of the NAC is relatively high, preliminary tissue expansion is performed to lower it to an appropriate level. When growth of the contralateral breast is incomplete, a permanent expander/implant can be used for volume adjustment during continued breast development. A modest-size autologous breast augmentation can also be obtained with a buried latissimus dorsi myocutaneous flap, a buried free transverse myocutaneous gracilis flap or fat grafting. Autologous augmentation is considered in cases of complete absence of the breast, and when the normal contralateral breast is relatively large, to obtain better symmetry and progressive ptosis with aging. A tissue expander is inserted at the time of muscle transposition and overexpansion is achieved prior to autologous tissue transfer. Options include pedicled or free transverse rectus abdominis myocutaneous flap, deep inferior epigastric perforator flap, free inferior or superior gluteus myocutaneous or perforator flap.[34] In teenagers, the relative lack of abdominal fat is such that free inferior or superior gluteus musculocutaneous or perforator flap options are favored. Of note, anomalies of the vascular anatomy may complicate the use of the ipsilateral latissimus dorsi as the donor site and may render thoracodorsal vessels inadequate donors in free tissue transfers.[10] When the thoracodorsal vessels provide the blood supply to a transferred latissimus dorsi muscle, the internal mammary vessels are the preferred recipient vessels. The same midlateral thoracic incision is used for muscle transposition, expander insertion, or definitive breast augmentation with a prosthesis or free flap unless microvascular anastomosis requires exposure of the internal mammary vessels.

Breast Hypoplasia

Breast asymmetry more commonly occurs in isolation, secondary to a disparate response of each individual breast to hormones during development. Unilateral hypoplasia is present when a significant discrepancy in breast size exists, without evidence of macromastia of the contralateral breast (Fig. 37.7). Bilateral hypoplasia may be symmetric or asymmetric. Hypoplasia may be isolated or associated with chest wall deformities or syndromes (see "Tuberous Breast" and "Poland Syndrome"). The isolated pathology may be congenital or acquired. Secondary causes include chest wall deformities, Becker's nevus (unilateral cutaneous hamartoma), burn scar, vascular anomalies, radiation therapy and trauma to the developing breast from surgical intervention (Fig. 37.8). Treatment of the breast asymmetry should consider both developmental abnormality of the breasts and skeleton. Scoliosis and chest wall deformity need to be assessed before definitive treatment can be undertaken. Traditionally, reconstruction is deferred to completion of breast development, where breast volume has been stable for one year and the patient has maintained a stable adult weight.[35] More recently, some authors have advocated for earlier correction, typically with progressive tissue expansion through the stages of breast maturation. Otherwise, following completion of breast maturation, management of breast asymmetry may be undertaken using appropriate procedure(s) for each individual breast. Advantages of implant-based reconstruction include an easier initial operation without precluding the ability to perform autologous tissue transfer at a later date. Thus, it may be used as a bridge to allow maturation of the patient while concurrently correcting the deformity. However, the difficulty in achieving symmetry with a natural contralateral breast remains an important disadvantage, as is the possibility of capsular contracture and implant rupture, and the eventual need for reoperation should be considered in the adolescent population.

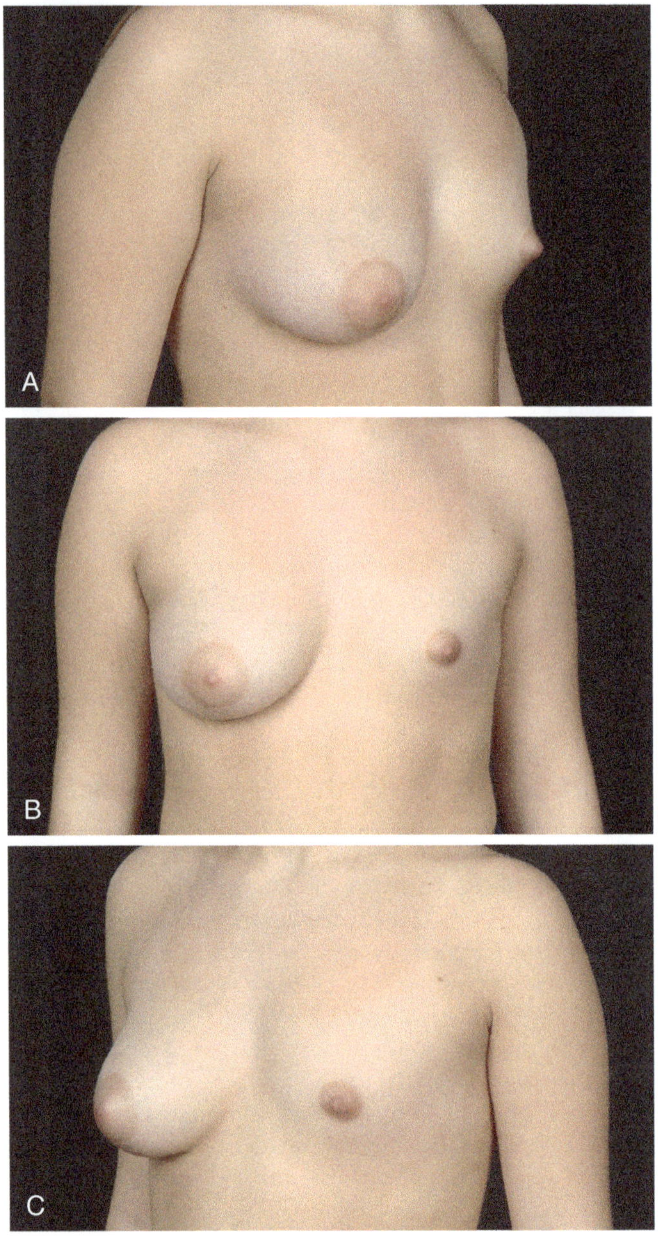

• **Fig. 37.7** (A–C) A 15-year-old female who presents with left unilateral breast hypoplasia, without evidence of chest wall involvement (Poland syndrome or anterior thoracic hypoplasia).

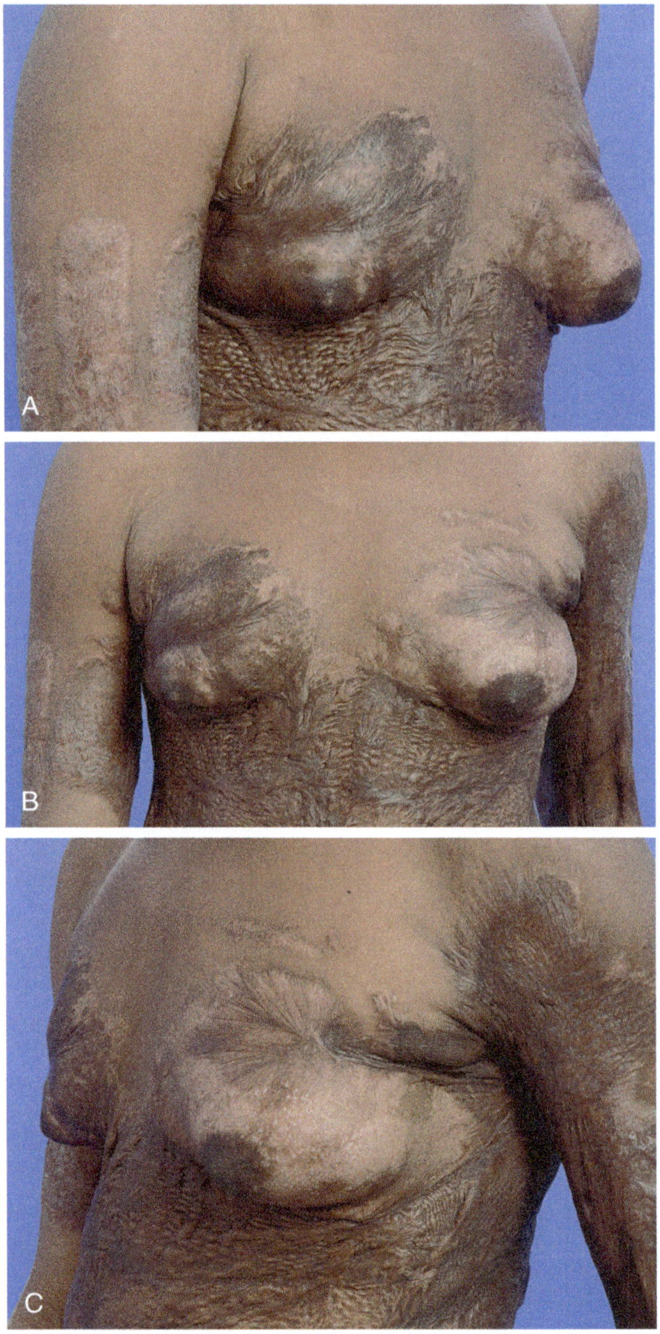

• **Fig. 37.8** (A–C) A 14-year-old female with bilateral constrictive breast hypoplasia (more severe involvement on the right) following severe burn and skin grating to her chest at 9 years of age.

References

1. Hassiotou F, Geddes D. Anatomy of the human mammary gland: current status of knowledge. *Clin Anat.* 2013;26(1):29–48.
2. Russo J, Russo IH. Development of the human breast. *Maturitas.* 2004;49(1):2–15.
3. Lemaine V, Simmons PS. The adolescent breast. *Semin Plast Surg.* 2013;27(1):3–4.
4. Velanovich V. Ectopic breast tissue, supernumerary breasts, and supernumerary nipples. *South Med J.* 1995;88(9):903–906.
5. Mimouni F, Merlob P, Reisner SH. Occurrence of supernumerary nipples in newborns. *Am J Dis Child.* 1983;137(10):952–953.
6. Schmidt H. Supernumerary nipples: prevalence, size, sex and side predilection – a prospective clinical study. *Eur J Pediatr.* 1998;157(10):821–823.
7. Casey HD, Chasan PE, Chick LR. Familial polythelia without associated anomalies. *Ann Plast Surg.* 1996;36(1):101–104.
8. Pryor LS, Lehman Jr JA, Workman MC. Disorders of the female breast in the pediatric age group. *Plast Reconstr Surg.* 2009;124(suppl 1):50e–60e.
9. Sadove AM, van Aalst JA. Congenital and acquired pediatric breast anomalies: a review of 20 years' experience. *Plast Reconstr Surg.* 2005;115(4):1039–1050.

10. Latham K, Fernandez S, Iteld L, et al. Pediatric breast deformity. *J Craniofac Surg*. 2006;17(3):454–467.
11. Grossl NA. Supernumerary breast tissue: historical perspectives and clinical features. *South Med J*. 2000;93(1):29–32.
12. Braunstein GD. Gynecomastia. *N Engl J Med*. 1993;328(7):490–495.
13. Malhotra AK, Amed S, Bucevska M, et al. Do adolescents with gynecomastia require routine evaluation by endocrinology? *Plast Reconstr Surg*. 2018;142(1):9e–16e.
14. Johnson RE, Murad MH. Gynecomastia: pathophysiology, evaluation, and management. *Mayo Clin Proc*. 2009;84(11):1010–1015.
15. Simon BE, Kahn S. Classification and surgical correction of gynecomastia. *Plast Reconstr Surg*. 1973;51:48–52.
16. Hammond DC. Surgical correction of gynecomastia. *Plast Reconstr Surg*. 2009;124(suppl 1):61e–68e.
17. Lin KY, Nguyen DB, Williams RM. Complete breast absence revisited. *Plast Reconstr Surg*. 2000;106(1):98–101.
18. Rees TD, Aston S. The tuberous breast. *Clin Plast Surg*. 1976;3(2):339–347.
19. Meara JG, Kolker A, Bartlett G, et al. Tuberous breast deformity: principles and practice. *Ann Plast Surg*. 2000;45(6):607–611.
20. Puckett CL, Concannon MJ. Augmenting the narrow-based breast: the unfurling technique to prevent the double-bubble deformity. *Aesthet Plast Surg*. 1990;14(1):15–19.
21. Grolleau JL, Lanfrey E, Lavigne B, et al. Breast base anomalies: treatment strategy for tuberous breasts, minor deformities, and asymmetry. *Plast Reconstr Surg*. 1999;104(7):2040–2048.
22. Mandrekas AD, Zambacos GJ. Aesthetic reconstruction of the tuberous breast deformity: a 10-year experience. *Aesthet Surg J*. 2010;30(5):680–692.
23. von Heimburg D, Exner K, Kruft S, et al. The tuberous breast deformity: classification and treatment. *Br J Plast Surg*. 1996;49(6):339–345.
24. Dinner MI, Dowden RV. The tubular/tuberous breast syndrome. *Ann Plast Surg*. 1987;19(5):414–420.
25. Ribeiro L, Canzi W, Buss Jr A, et al. Tuberous breast: a new approach. *Plast Reconstr Surg*. 1998;101(1):42–50; discussion 51–52.
26. Mandrekas AD, Zambacos GJ, Anastasopoulos A, et al. Aesthetic reconstruction of the tuberous breast deformity. *Plast Reconstr Surg*. 2003;112(4):1099–1108; discussion 1109.
27. Kolker AR, Collins MS. Tuberous breast deformity: classification and treatment strategy for improving consistency in aesthetic correction. *Plast Reconstr Surg*. 2015;135(1):73–86.
28. Poland A. Deficiency of the pectoral muscles. *Guy's Hosp Rep*. 1841;6:191.
29. Fokin AA, Robicsek F. Poland's syndrome revisited. *Ann Thorac Surg*. 2002;74(6):2218–2225.
30. Baban A, Torre M, Bianca S, et al. Poland syndrome with bilateral features: case description with review of the literature. *Am J Med Genet*. 2009;149A(7):1597–1602.
31. Bavinck JN, Weaver DD. Subclavian artery supply disruption sequence: hypothesis of a vascular etiology for Poland, Klippel–Feil, and Möbius anomalies. *Am J Med Genet*. 1986;23(4):903–918.
32. Spear SL, Pelletiere CV, Lee ES, et al. Anterior thoracic hypoplasia: a separate entity from Poland syndrome. *Plast Reconstr Surg*. 2004;113(1):69–77; discussion 78–79.
33. Seyfer AE, Fox JP, Hamilton CG. Poland syndrome: evaluation and treatment of the chest wall in 63 patients. *Plast Reconstr Surg*. 2010;126(3):902–911.
34. Caouette-Laberge L, Borsuk D. Congenital anomalies of the breast. *Semin Plast Surg*. 2013;27(1):36–41.
35. Caouette-Laberge L, Bortoluzzi P. Correction of breast asymmetry in teenagers. In: Hall Findley E, Evans GRD, eds. *Aesthetic and Reconstructive Surgery of the Breast*. Philadelphia, PA: Saunders Elsevier; 2010:601–629.

38 Mastopexy and Breast Reduction

ELIZABETH J. HALL-FINDLAY

For videos accompanying this chapter see ExpertConsult.com. See inside cover for access details.

Introduction

The best way to approach esthetic breast surgery is to work with gravity – not against it. Remove tissue where it is in excess and add tissue where it is deficient. Although this sounds simplistic, it forms the basis of the principles of esthetic breast surgery.[1] Although in some cases the skin brassiere can be used to shape the breast, it is better to rely on parenchymal reshaping for a consistent, long-lasting result. The parenchyma can be reshaped most easily by following this "excess/deficiency" principle.

The surgeon needs to understand what various surgical maneuvers can achieve and what our limitations are as surgeons. With that knowledge, we can then manage surgical results (and therefore patient expectations) more appropriately.

Because the upper breast border will not change with either a breast reduction or mastopexy, the result can be predictable (but not always what either the surgeon or the patient desires).[2] Some patients are high-breasted and some are low-breasted. The breast is lifted – not at the upper breast border – but by controlling the glandular ptosis. Once the patient (and the surgeon) understands this concept, it becomes clear what can be "removed" in a breast reduction or "moved" in a mastopexy.

Patients and surgeons often think that the breast can be pushed up the chest wall, but the upper breast border will only be elevated if something is added (an implant raises the upper breast border on average 2 cm and fat grafting far less).

The surgeon can transpose drawings onto the patient's photographs (Fig. 38.1) and the decision-making process becomes simplified. Remove (or move) any ptotic gland below the ideal breast shape. Determining the ideal nipple position then becomes simple once the shape is outlined.

This involves an understanding of the inferior wedge principle.[3,4] The inferior ptotic gland needs to be "removed" in a breast reduction. It is best "moved" in a mastopexy using Liacyr Ribeiro's method[5,6] where it can be separated and moved up to the center of the breast (not the upper pole). Filling the upper pole usually requires either an implant or the addition of tissue (e.g., fat grafting). The inferior wedge is that tissue below the Wise pattern.

When Robert Wise[7] deconstructed a brassiere and developed the "Wise pattern," it was designed to be used for the skin to shape and hold up the breast (Fig. 38.2). Unfortunately, skin is often not a good brassiere and it stretches with tension (as it does with skin expansion procedures). If the surgeon, on the other hand, uses the Wise pattern for the parenchyma – and leaves behind a Wise pattern (with no tension on either the parenchyma or the skin), the result will be predictable and long-lasting. The Wise pattern shown below starts flat but then develops a nice conical shape when put together with the inferior wedge removed.

Because the upper breast border is the more stable (and predictable) landmark, the inframammary fold (IMF) becomes less important. In the past, I marked the new nipple position at the level of the IMF until I realized how variable the fold can be. Some patients not only have a variable footprint location on the chest wall, the distance between the upper breast border and the lower breast border (inframammary fold) can vary from a few centimeters to well over 15 cm.

Because of the variability of the IMF, the Regnault classification of ptosis can be misleading. Paule Regnault[8] classified breast ptosis based on the relationship of the nipple to the IMF. If the nipple was well below the level of the fold, then a mastopexy would be required. Unfortunately, sometimes the nipple is in a good position on the breast mound, but the fold is abnormally high (especially in tuberous

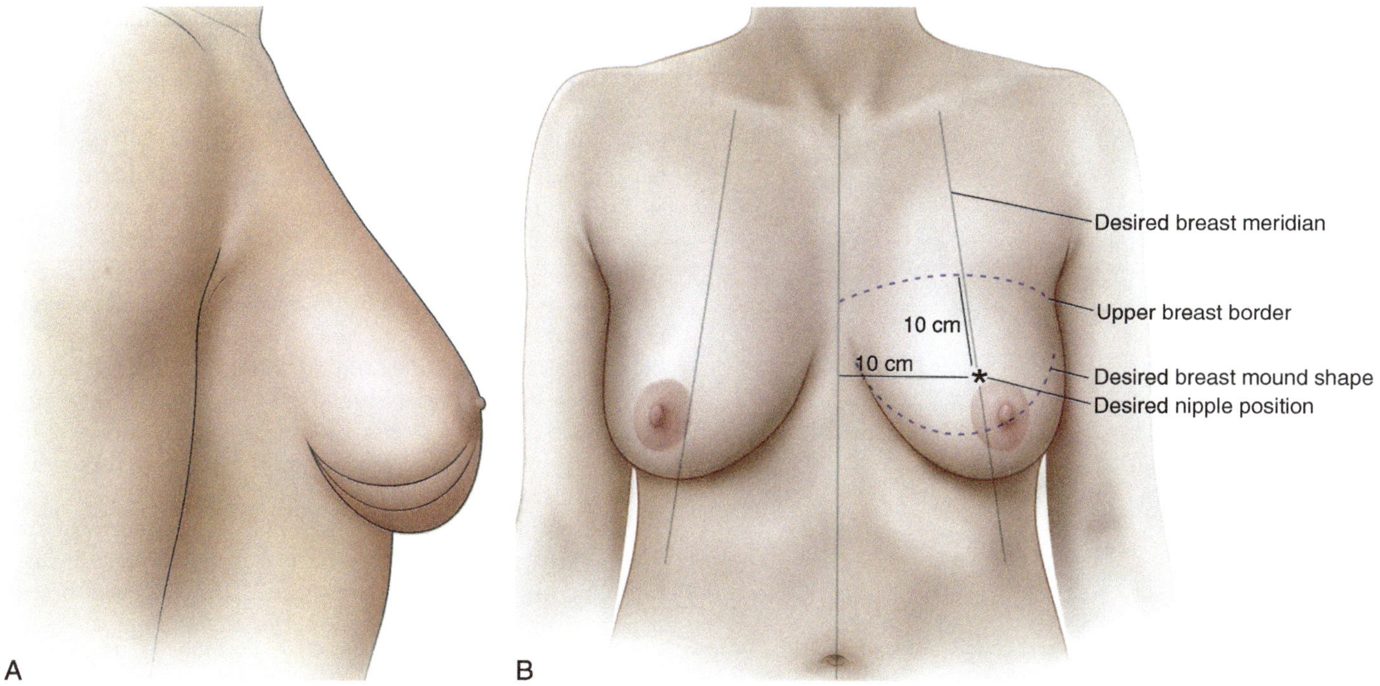

• **Fig. 38.1** Principles. (A) The upper breast border does not change in a breast reduction or mastopexy. The key to a good result is for the surgeon to understand that the excess in the lower pole needs to be "removed" in a breast reduction or "moved" in a mastopexy. (B) The surgeon can visualize the shape of the final result by marking what is desired. The excess beyond that shape needs to be removed in a breast reduction. The ideal nipple position should be determined at about 10 cm below the upper breast border (since this remains unchanged) in an average "C" cup breast. The new breast meridian should be drawn where it "should" be, not where it exists and the ideal breast meridian is about 10 cm from the chest midline (straight, not around the curve of the breast) in the "average" patient. (© Elizabeth J. Hall-Findlay.)

breasts) and the approach should instead be to fill the lower pole of the breast and give a better breast shape by centralizing an implant behind the existing nipple position. If the breast is large and the nipple is high then the best approach would be to remove some of the ptotic gland. The nipple should be moved only if it is too low on what will be the final breast mound.

We should instead look at the amount of glandular ptosis or nipple ptosis in relation to the upper breast border and upper pole of the breast. Once the inferior wedge of glandular ptosis is removed, the new nipple position can be easily determined. The ideal nipple position on an average "C" cup breast is about 10 cm down from the upper breast border and about 10 cm from the chest midline (drawn straight – not around the breast).

The upper breast border remains at the preoperative level with a breast reduction or mastopexy but it can be elevated on average 2 cm with an augmentation or mastopexy-augmentation.[2]

It is easier to plan surgery if the surgeon first assesses glandular ptosis and then nipple ptosis. The level of the IMF is the least important landmark. Sometimes it is better to fill the lower pole of the breast (and lower the IMF) with an implant to centralize the breast mound behind the existing nipple position than it is to move the nipple.

Macromastia

Assessment

History

It is important for the surgeon to first assess patient desires in terms of size. Any previous biopsies, mammogram results, and personal and family breast history should be outlined. The patient should be asked about past experience and wishes related to pregnancy and breastfeeding.

Then details of other patient requests, such as shape and upper pole fullness, should be determined.

Examination and Photographs

The consultation is far easier if photographs are taken and used for the discussion. The surgeon can then mark on the photos to illustrate what kind of result can be achieved (Fig. 38.3). The upper breast border is marked (here with a dotted line). The distance of "flat" chest wall is marked with the vertical arrow on both the frontal and the lateral views. Note that the drawing shows removal of the glandular ptosis – removal of both inferior and lateral breast tissue where it is in excess. Once the desired inferior border of the breast is determined, the new nipple is placed about one-third up the breast mound. Note that the IMF is not marked – and not needed.

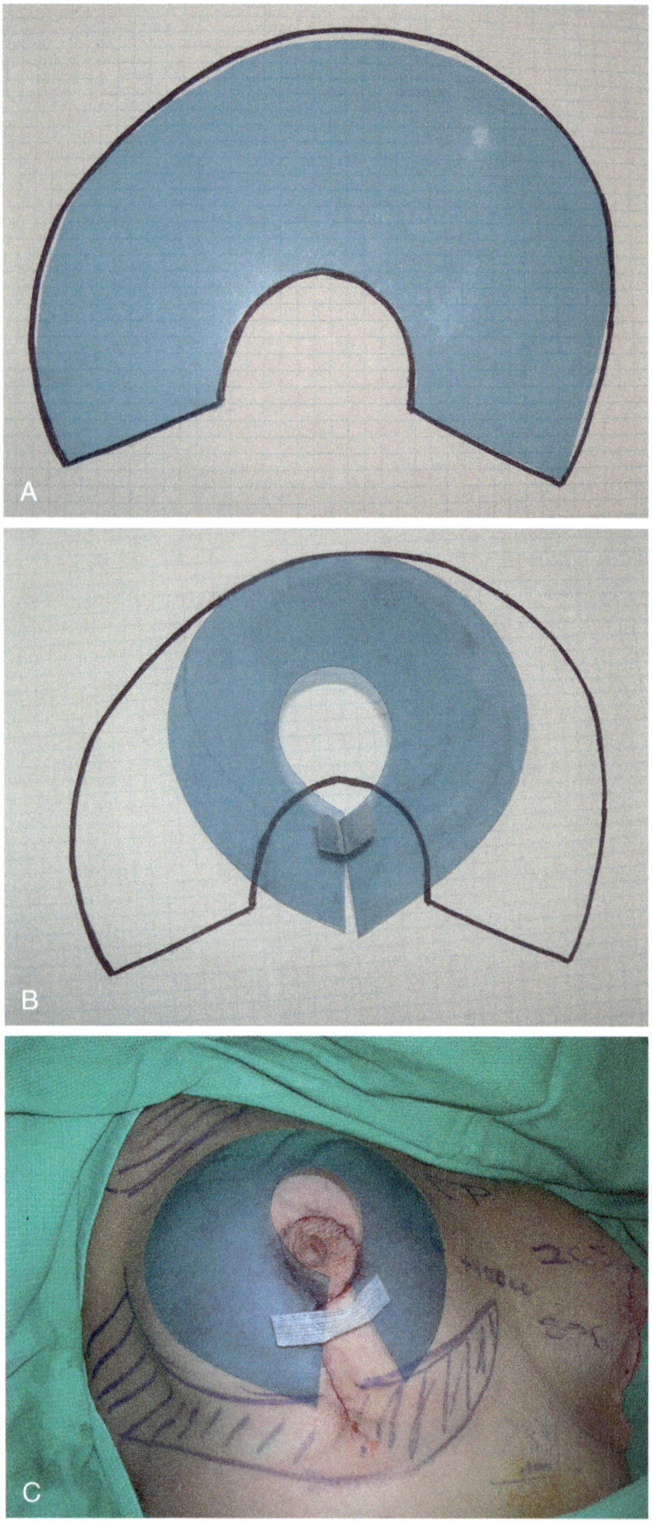

• **Fig. 38.2** The "Wise" pattern. The Wise pattern was adapted from a deconstructed brassiere by Dr Robert Wise[5] and it forms the basis of an ideal breast shape. Once the flat pattern is coned (by removing or moving the inferior wedge) a good shape with good projection is achieved. (A) The Wise pattern. (B) The Wise pattern coned. (C) The Wise pattern is an excellent design for what should be left behind to achieve a good breast shape rather than using it as a skin brassiere pattern. (© Elizabeth J. Hall-Findlay.)

There is still a bit of overhang in the final result because it is difficult to lift the breast completely up onto the footprint without some overhang. Having the breast shape completely confined to the breast footprint is difficult unless the footprint is long vertically or without lowering the IMF (as often happens with an inverted T inferior pedicle breast reduction).

Patients need to be warned that they will not achieve the "double push up brassiere effect" without clothes. There is normally a vertical distance of flat chest wall (this can vary from about 9 cm to 16 cm in an average height patient) between the clavicles and the upper breast border. The breasts do not normally come up close to the clavicle and the upper breast border should never be higher than the preaxillary crease. This has become an important part of managing patient expectations over the past few years with the new fashions in brassieres.

If a patient has very poor upper pole fullness, some of the inferior wedge can be moved up[5,6] (separated from all surrounding breast tissue but left attached as a chest wall-based flap) to provide better projection, but any attempt to try to fill the upper pole is usually doomed to failure. The tissue that is mistakenly pushed up will inevitably fall down resulting in unattractive glandular ptosis.

Patients often see more in the photographs than they do in the mirror and by showing patients their photographs, they can better understand the limitations of the procedure. Patients need to understand that they cannot achieve either a higher footprint or more upper pole fullness. They can, however, achieve better projection.

Management Principles and Operative Options

Reduction/Mastopexy

There are numerous designs and labels for various breast reduction and mastopexy techniques. The design should be divided into two categories:

1. pedicle design, and
2. skin resection pattern.

Pedicle Design

The breast is a superficial structure attached to the skin at the nipple. Most of the blood supply to the breast is superficial. It starts out in a deep location around the periphery of the breast and then both the arteries and veins travel around the breast in the subcutaneous tissue.

Most of the blood supply to the breast comes from the internal mammary system (Fig. 38.4). The inferior or central pedicle is supplied by the deep artery and vein that penetrates through the intercostal muscles and the pectoralis muscle from the fourth interspace. That this artery (and venae comitantes) comes from the fourth interspace makes sense because the breast is a fourth interspace structure.[1]

There is also some blood supply from the superficial branch of the lateral thoracic system and this artery supplies a lateral pedicle.

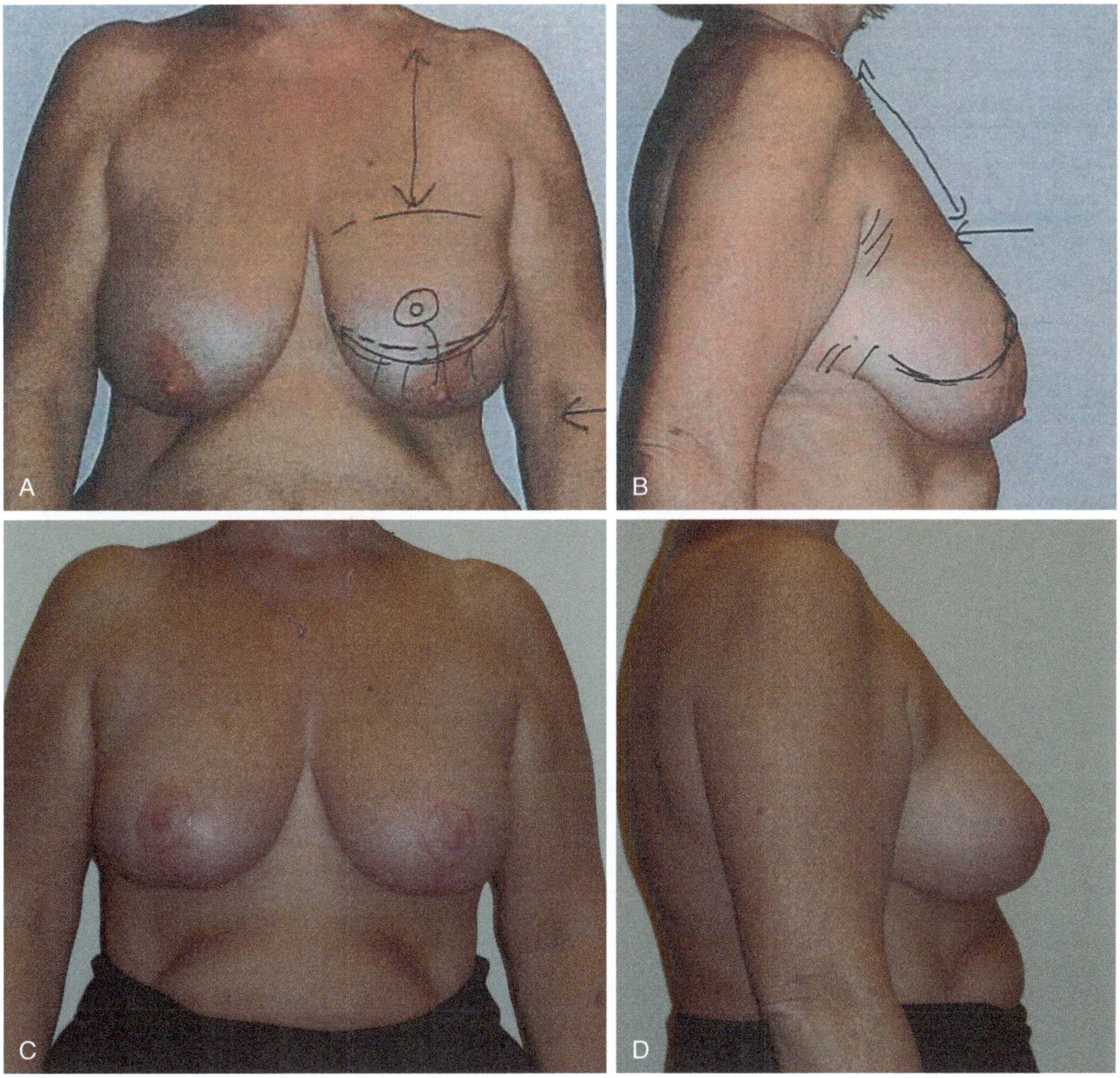

• **Fig. 38.3** Managing patient expectations through consultation photographs. Patient photographs taken at consultation can be used to manage patient expectations. Once the surgeon understands that the upper breast border will not change, the expected result can be drawn on the preoperative photograph. More projection can be achieved by coning the breast tissue after the inferior wedge is removed. The breast cannot be elevated on the chest wall and the upper pole cannot be filled, but the angle (projection) can be increased. The surgeon will also know if tissue needs to be removed in the upper pole in the occasional patient where reduced projection is desired. (A) Preoperative frontal breast reduction candidate showing the desired final breast shape with inferior and lateral tissue removed. (B) Preoperative lateral of same breast reduction candidate showing the patient that the upper breast does not change but the lower pole is removed. (C) Postoperative view of same patient showing the postoperative result. The frontal view matches the preoperative drawing. (D) Postoperative view of same patient showing the postoperative result. The lateral view matches the preoperative drawing. The breast footprint remains unchanged but the glandular ptosis is corrected and the nipple repositioned to the most projecting part of the breast. (© Elizabeth J. Hall-Findlay.)

Most of the arteries are within the first centimeter deep to the skin surface at the level of the areola. The veins travel separately from the arteries and they are more superficial – just under the dermis. They can often be seen through the skin when examining the patient and they can be seen to drain mainly superomedially.

Because the blood supply to an inferior or central pedicle comes up through the chest wall, the pedicle must be full thickness. Because the blood supply to the superior, lateral, and medial pedicles is in the subcutaneous tissue the pedicles can be created as dermal-subcutaneous pedicles. The pedicle should be thick where the vessels are deep at the breast periphery and then can be thinned out closer to the areola where the vessels are found usually within the first centimeter of tissue depth beneath the skin.

Pedicle design is based on blood supply. If the surgeon does not believe that there is a safe pedicle available, then a free nipple graft may be an option. Usually, however, there

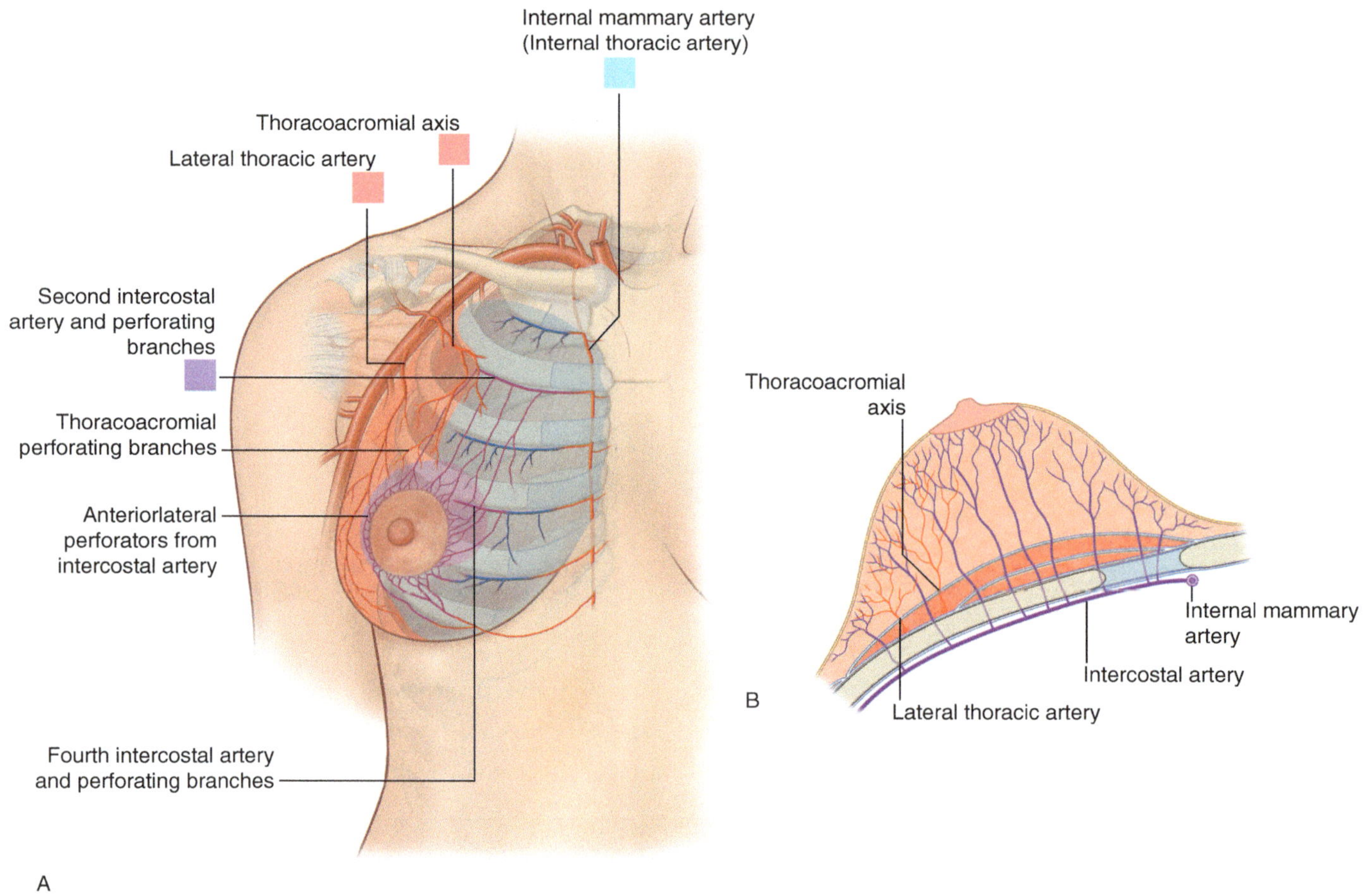

• **Fig. 38.4** Blood supply. The major blood supply to the breast comes from the internal mammary (thoracic) system. There is also some contribution from the superficial branch of the lateral thoracic artery. (A,B) The arteries penetrate up from the chest wall around the periphery of the breast and then they pass around the breast parenchyma itself, up in the subcutaneous tissue. The arteries are superficial as they course toward the areola. The veins are even more superficial as they course just under the dermis (and are often visible through pale skin) with the majority draining superomedially. The branch of the internal mammary artery from the fourth interspace actually penetrates directly up into the breast parenchyma just medial to the breast meridian just above the fifth rib. This artery has accompanying venae comitantes. This makes sense because the breast is a fourth interspace structure attached to the skin at the nipple and sliding loosely over the pectoralis fascia. The breast is held in place by skin–fascial structures at the IMF and over the sternum. The superior and lateral aspects of the breast slide freely over the underlying tissues. (From Harmann EC, Spring MA, Stevens WG. One- and two-stage considerations for augmentation mastopexy. In: Nahabedian MY, Neligan PC, eds. *Plastic Surgery.* Vol. 5: *Breast*. London: Elsevier; 2018.)

are good pedicle designs that can be used. The main choices are inferior (and central), superior, medial, lateral, or a combination (Fig. 38.5).[9,10]

The superior pedicle is supplied by the internal mammary system by the descending branch of the artery from the second interspace and the medial pedicle is supplied by the third interspace. There is clearly some variability but a true superomedial pedicle can be designed to include these two axial arteries.

Fig. 38.6 shows the artery and vein to the inferior wedge that is about to be removed in a vertical breast reduction using a true superomedial pedicle.

Innervation to the nipple comes from various sources.[11] There are nerves that come from all directions but they are mainly medial and lateral. There are several medial branches but also a major nerve from the lateral fourth intercostal nerve. This nerve splits with a superficial branch that courses up in the subcutaneous tissue and a deep branch that travels along the pectoralis fascia. The deep nerve branch then turns upward at the breast meridian and can be included in a full-thickness pedicle. Evaluation of my patients has shown that the medial pedicle actually has better return of sensation than either the lateral or superior pedicles.[1] Other studies have shown that there is not much difference in sensation recovery among the various pedicles.

Skin Resection Pattern

The pedicle design determines the design of the parenchymal resection pattern, but the skin pattern can vary. The classic inverted T (Wise pattern) skin resection pattern[12,13] was designed to use the skin brassiere to hold up the remaining breast parenchyma. In those cases where the skin has good elasticity, it can be used to shape the breast.

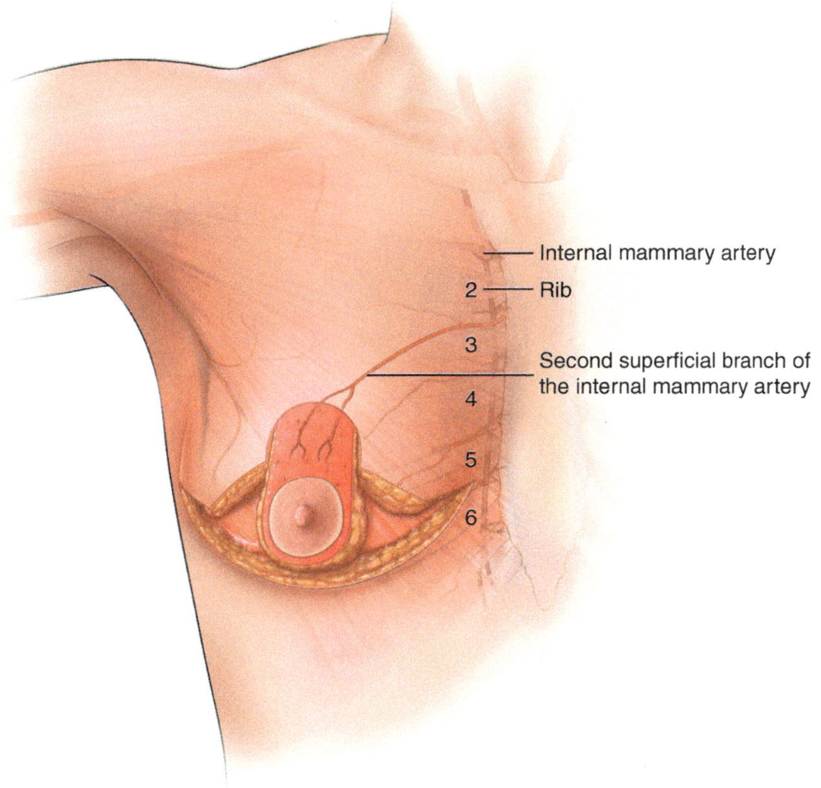

A

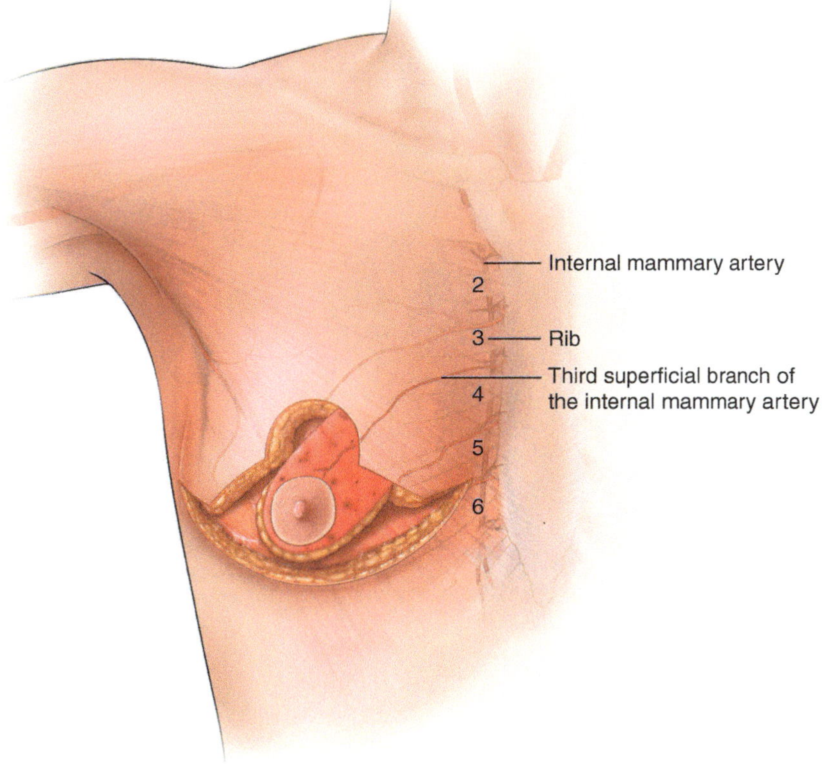

B

• **Fig. 38.5** The various pedicle designs for the nipple and areolar complex. The four classic pedicle designs. (A) Superior pedicle: The blood supply comes from the descending branch of the internal mammary (thoracic) system at the second interspace. (B) Medial pedicle: The blood supply comes from the third interspace branch of the internal mammary system.

Continued

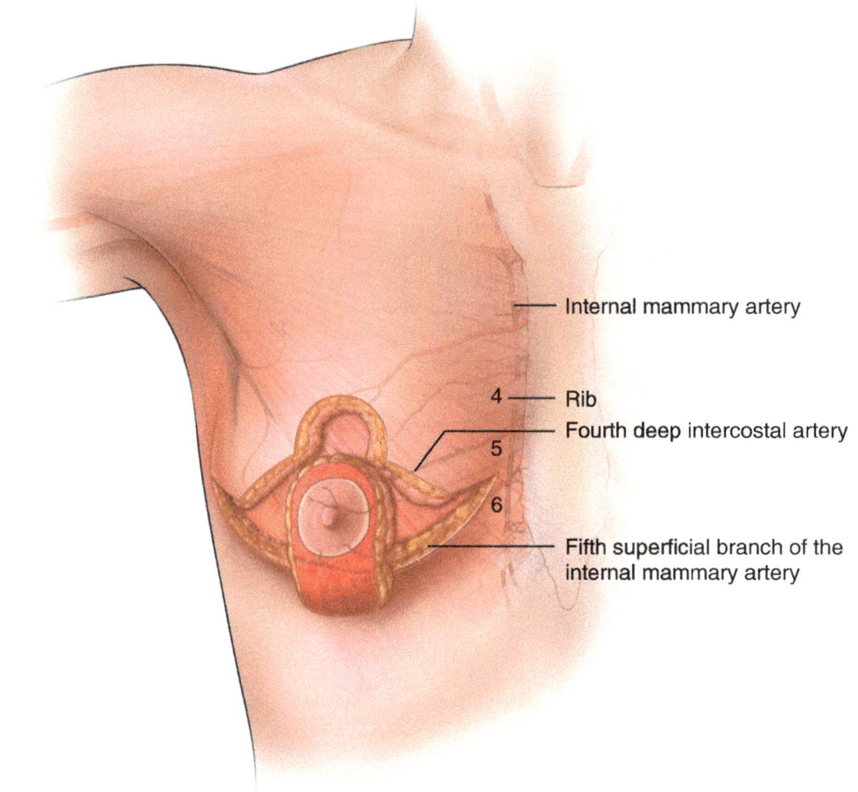

C

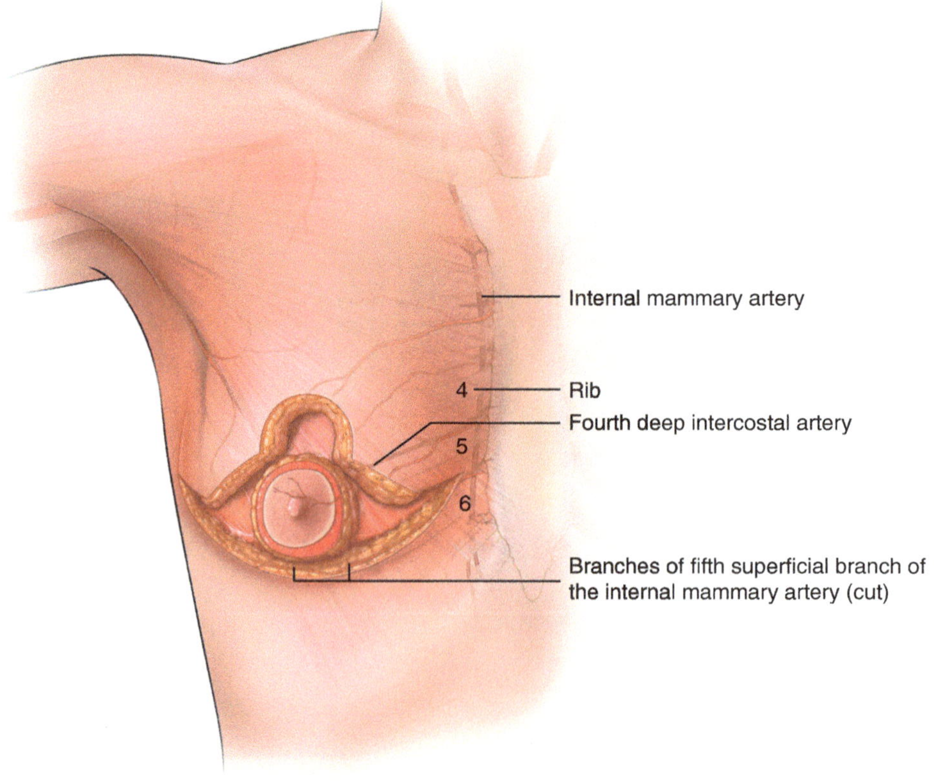

D

Fig. 38.5 cont'd (C) Inferior pedicle: The blood supply comes from the perforator that comes up at the fourth interspace, along with its venae comitantes. This deep branch also comes from the internal mammary system. There are also blood vessels that come up through the IMF. (D) Central pedicle: The central pedicle has a more restricted blood supply than an inferior pedicle because it does not have the vessels coming through the IMF.

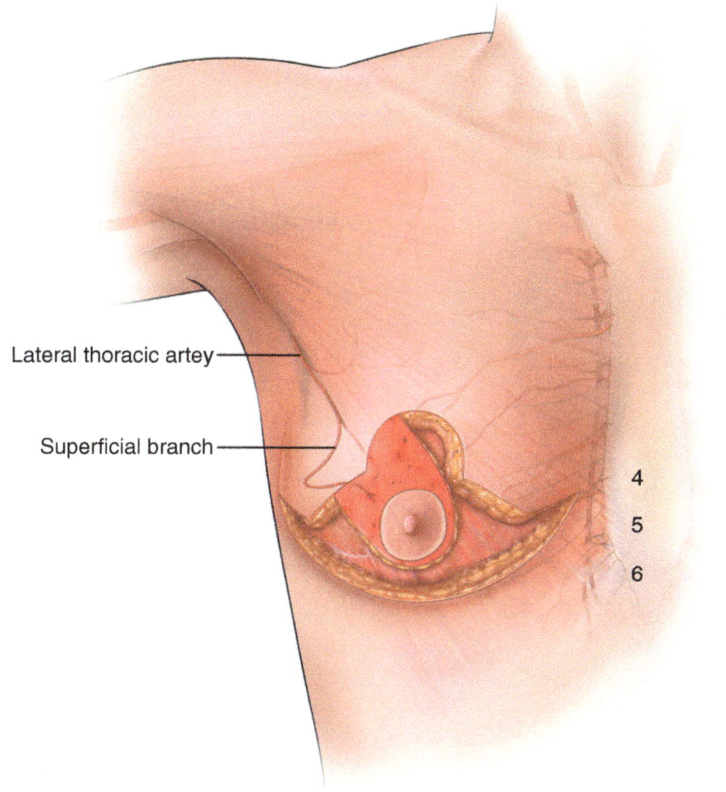

E

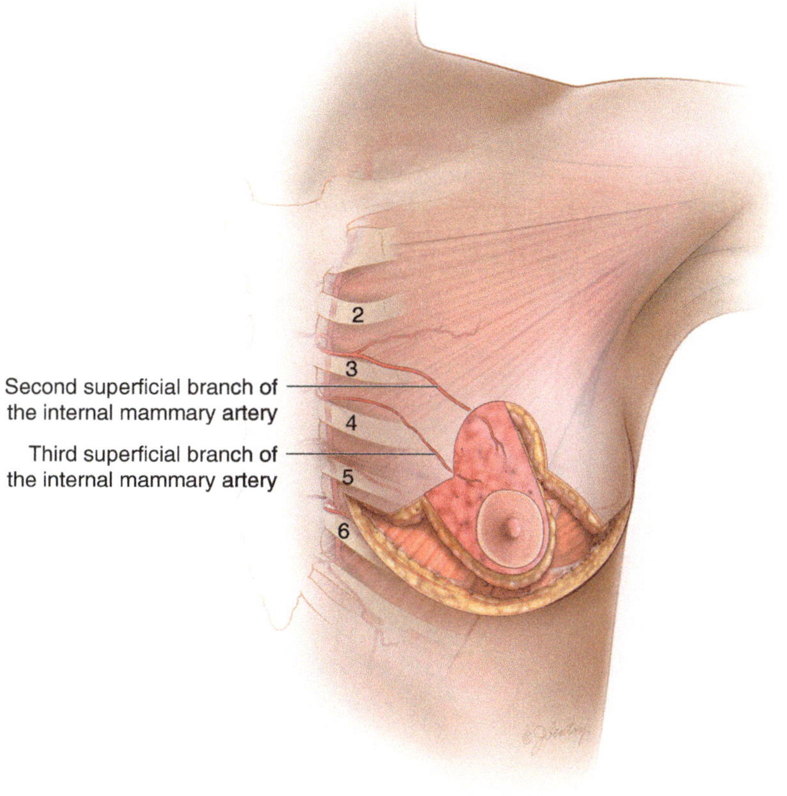

F

Fig. 38.5 cont'd (E) Lateral pedicle: The blood supply comes from the superficial branch of the lateral thoracic artery. (F) A true superomedial pedicle combines both superior and medial pedicles to include two axial arteries. The majority of the venous drainage is superomedial. (From Mackinnon S. *Nerve Surgery*. New York: Thieme. 2015.)

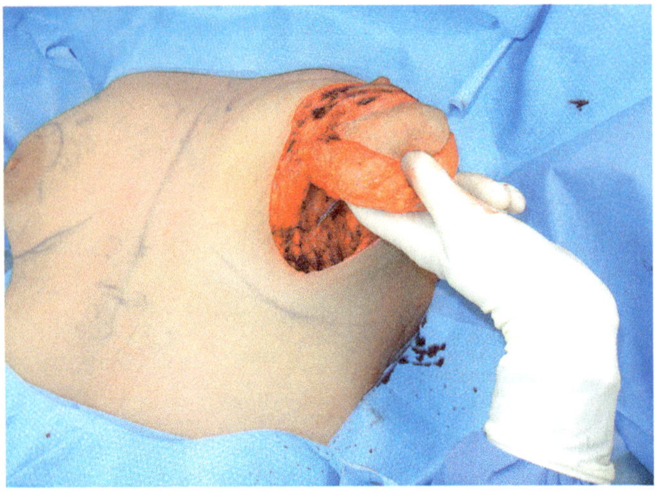

• **Fig. 38.6** This photo shows the artery and vein to the inferior wedge that is about to be removed in a vertical breast reduction using a superomedial pedicle. (© Copyright Elizabeth J. Hall-Findlay.)

Unfortunately, skin tends to stretch under tension and many surgeons are now using the inferior wedge resection principle to remove the heavy inferior breast tissue, then closing the pillars together following the Wise pattern[7] for the parenchymal resection and closure instead of using the Wise pattern for the skin resection pattern. The skin resection pattern will then depend on how much skin redundancy there is because it is used to redrape around the breast parenchyma instead of being used as a handle or support.

Not all "vertical" (or "inverted T") breast reductions are the same. They can be designed with various pedicles. Usually, however, the term "vertical" is associated with the superiorly (superior, medial or lateral)-based pedicles and the term "inverted T" is associated with inferior or central pedicles.[14–26] The excess breast tissue is removed inferiorly (and laterally) with the superiorly-based pedicles and the excess breast tissue is removed superiorly (and laterally and medially) with the inferiorly-based pedicles.

It makes more sense to work with gravity rather than against it. The inferior pedicle tends to bottom out with time, pushing the IMF down. Over time, the IMF can end up several centimeters below the horizontal scar.[27]

Periareolar skin resection patterns (where the outer doughnut skin edge is sutured to the inner doughnut hole skin edge) are used only rarely because not much skin can be resected. If the patient has a significant amount of redundant skin, then more skin needs to be resected, using either a vertical or inverted T pattern. The breast is not well reshaped when the skin alone is tightened – surgeons need to be aware that Benelli's description[28] of a periareolar mastopexy did not just tighten the skin; he reshaped the underlying breast parenchyma as well. Failure to follow this advice has resulted in unsatisfactory results.

Indications

Some surgeons believe that the inferior pedicle is a safer pedicle for the very large breast reduction. I believe that the true superomedial pedicle has the best blood supply because it includes two axial arteries. I have pencil-Dopplered more than 85 patients[1] and the descending artery from the second interspace is usually just medial and occasionally just lateral to the breast meridian.

When the breast enlarges, the blood vessels also enlarge and travel down with the nipple. The risk in a longer pedicle is not that the blood vessels do not travel to the nipple but that creation of the pedicle might not actually include those particular vessels.

An inferior pedicle (using the inverted T skin resection technique) is the easiest to inset but the weight of the breast is left inferiorly. The medial and lateral pedicles are easy to inset because they rotate into position. The superior pedicle can be harder to inset because it needs to be folded or forced up. Superior pedicles often need to be thinned in order to allow an easier inset without compression and this leaves an empty concave lower pole.

The true superomedial pedicle (with the main base medial but extending upward and across just lateral to the breast meridian) can be harder to inset than a true medial pedicle. But if the surgeon understands that the blood supply is superficial, debulking deep tissue which is causing the restriction can be performed safely. This not only provides a good reliable blood supply but it also gives a nice elegant curve to the lower pole of the breast on the table because the inferior border of the medial pedicle becomes the medial pillar.

The lateral pedicle can be used, but it is often difficult to remove some of the lateral bulk in a breast reduction because the tissue that is in excess (laterally) forms the base of the lateral pedicle. Although there are some veins that drain superolaterally, the majority of the venous drainage is superomedial.

With a mastopexy, breast tissue needs to be rearranged because tightening the skin brassiere alone is not very effective. Patients who have developed ptosis have already demonstrated that their skin envelope cannot hold up the breast parenchyma. A small breast reduction is the easiest mastopexy, especially when an inferior wedge of breast tissue is removed. When the patient wants to maintain their volume, then an inferior flap (described by Liacyr Ribeiro) can be created, moved up, and the pillars closed around caudal to the flap.[5,6] When this method of a mastopexy is used, the pedicle is therefore based superiorly (superior, superomedial or superolateral). This method of "moving" breast tissue (that is "removed" in a breast reduction) is a good way of reshaping the breast when the skin brassiere has lost elasticity.

Operative Technique for Superomedial Vertical Breast Reduction

Assessment

The surgeon needs to assess the footprint – whether the patient is high- or low-breasted. Then he or she needs to visualize what needs to be removed – usually inferiorly and laterally. The patient needs to be consulted on her preferred breast size (and of course warned that an exact size and shape cannot be achieved). It is always a balance between size and shape to achieve a good result.

The superomedial pedicle can be used with either the vertical or inverted T skin resection pattern[29] – this will depend on the desired final size of the breast and the elasticity and amount of excess skin. The vertical distance from the lower border of the areola to the IMF is usually about 7 cm in a "B" cup breast, 9 cm in a "C" cup breast and 11 cm in a "D" cup breast. Surgeons are often warned to keep the vertical scar length at 5–7 cm in an inferior pedicle inverted T breast reduction because the weight of the breast stretches out the skin. In a vertical type of breast reduction, however, the extra vertical length is needed to accommodate projection and weight is not an issue.

Markings

First the surgeon should mark the ***upper breast border*** because this is a landmark that does not change. This is best determined by finding the pre-axillary indentation laterally and marking the upper breast border medial to that indentation. The breast can be folded (not pushed up) to see where the fold between the breast and the chest wall occurs.

Next, the surgeon should draw the ***chest midline*** and ***breast meridian***. The "ideal" breast meridian should be marked and not the "existing" breast meridian. The surgeon can then draw what the resultant breast shape would be (Fig. 38.7A, B). This can help to mark the new nipple position.

The *ideal nipple position* on an average "C" cup breast on an average patient should be about 10 cm below the upper breast border and 10 cm from the chest midline (not drawn around the curve of the breast but with a straight ruler on a line parallel to the chest wall). If a surgeon places the new nipple (for example) at 24 cm from the suprasternal notch, that distance will not change postoperatively. It will remain at 24 cm. An arbitrary SSN-N distance can be misleading, leading to a nipple placement which is too high. The surgeon needs to understand that the footprint cannot be changed; a low-breasted patient will remain low-breasted.

Because the vertical approach leads to increased breast projection, it is important for the surgeon to place the new nipple lower than they are used to doing with an inverted T, inferior pedicle, because, although the SSN-N distance will stay where marked, the nipple will be elevated vertically with the increased projection that results.

It is always better to err on the side of leaving a nipple slightly lower because it is almost impossible to lower a nipple that is too high. I believe that the idea that the nipple should be 45% down and 55% from the bottom of the breast[30] will lead to many patients who have nipples that slip up over the edge of clothing. I believe that the ideal nipple is slightly lower than the horizontal midline and slightly lateral to the breast meridian.

The *new areolar opening* should be marked about 2 cm above the new nipple position. The opening can be drawn freehand to be about 14–16 cm in length. A 14 cm circumference matches a 4.5-cm diameter areola and a 16-cm circumference matches a 5-cm diameter areola. A large paperclip is 16 cm long and can serve as a good template when unfolded. There is no need to draw out the opening laterally in a mosque-type shape. It is in fact better to take out length vertically rather than horizontally.

It is important to mark the medial part of the areolar opening where desired and allow the lateral part to be variable. The medial marking should fit the desired Wise pattern. The lateral side is more mobile and can be moved medially to fit the desired shape and positioning.

In order to mark the *skin resection pattern*, the breast can then be rotated laterally and the vertical meridian marked to match the breast and chest wall meridians. The breast is then rotated medially and the lateral meridian marked. The breast can be held up with the surgeon's thumb of the opposite hand and the two lines can be joined in a "U" or "V" shape but the bottom of the design should remain at least 2–4 cm above the IMF. The surgeon can then test the skin resection pattern by pinching the skin.

A vertical breast reduction using the superomedial pedicle does not rely on the skin brassiere so there is no need to design a wide skin resection pattern. There should be no tension on the vertical skin closure. If an inverted T design is needed, the medial and lateral extensions are drawn about 7 cm down the vertical limbs because the ideal vertical parenchymal distance is about 7 cm. These extensions are then drawn to meet the IMF both medially and laterally. The skin resection pattern should not result in a tight closure in any direction – it is used only to allow the skin to redrape loosely.

A pure *medial pedicle* is designed with the base about 4 cm below the areolar opening along the vertical skin resection pattern and 4 cm above into the areolar opening. A true *superomedial pedicle* takes the medial pedicle base and extends it up and across the breast meridian. This allows it to include two axial arteries (as opposed to one artery in a medial pedicle) but it does make it a bit harder to inset occasionally. If it does prove to be too stiff to inset easily then excess tissue can be safely debulked deep to the pedicle because the blood supply is superficial.

Finally, the areas that may need to be liposuctioned (preaxillary fullness and lateral chest wall areas) are marked (Fig. 38.7C, D).

Positioning

The patient is supine on the operating table with the arms outstretched to the sides.

Infiltration

It is not a good idea to infiltrate along the incisions because the veins can be damaged. Lidocaine with epinephrine is used in the areas to be suctioned. If the patient has a higher body mass index, then tumescent type of infiltration may be indicated for the lateral chest wall in particular – in the areas where liposuction will be performed.

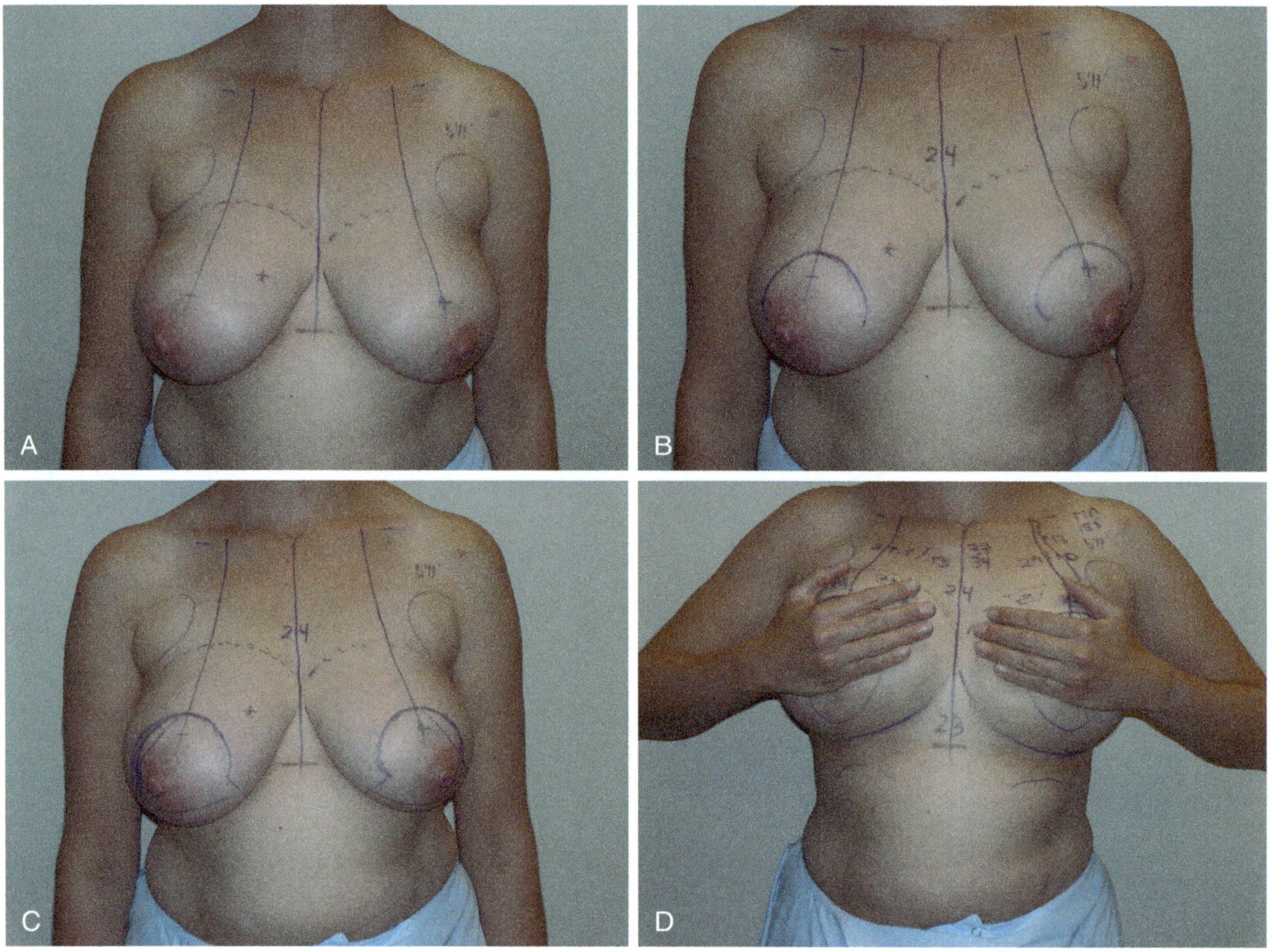

• **Fig. 38.7** Markings for a vertical breast reduction using a superomedial pedicle. (A) The upper breast border and desired breast meridian are marked. The new nipple position is marked about 10 cm below the upper breast border. The IMF is marked at the chest midline (it is often different from one side to the other) but it is not used to determine the new nipple position because it is often too high or too low. Because the upper breast border remains unchanged from the preoperative position to the postoperative result, it is the better landmark to use to determine the new nipple position. (B) The areolar opening is drawn freehand about 2 cm above the new nipple position. The drawing should be performed so that the final result is a circle. A large paperclip is 16 cm long and it can be folded out and used as a template if desired. The skin opening will determine the new areolar diameter because the areolar skin is so elastic that it will stretch to fit the skin pattern. A 16-cm circumference matches a 5-cm diameter areola and a 14-cm circumference matches a 4.5-cm diameter areola. (C) A true superomedial pedicle is drawn. A pure medial pedicle has a base that is about 4 cm up into the areolar opening and about 4 cm below along the vertical limb. A true superomedial pedicle has an extension of the base up and slightly across the breast meridian to capture the descending artery from the second interspace. A true superomedial pedicle contains the arteries from both the second and third interspaces and still allows the lower border of the pedicle to become the medial pillar (giving an elegant shape to the lower pole) while avoiding some of the difficulties inherent in insetting a superior pedicle. (D) The lower skin resection pattern is drawn while rotating the breast medially and then laterally to match the desired breast meridian drawn on the breast and continued down onto the chest wall. The pattern should be joined usually about 4 cm above the IMF to take into account the fact that the fold often rises but also to avoid the scar extending onto the chest wall. Closure of an ellipse ends up with a longer scar at each end. The pattern should be designed only to remove the excess, not to use the skin as a handle or brassiere. The key is to reshape the parenchyma (by removing the inferior wedge) and then allowing the skin to redrape. (© Elizabeth J. Hall-Findlay.)

Technique (Fig. 38.8)[31]

De-epithelialization

The incision lines are incised around the areola and vertically making sure that the vertical skin resection pattern remains about 4 cm above the IMF. A lap pad is then placed around the base of the breast and held with a Kocher clamp to tighten the breast skin and facilitate de-epithelialization.

The veins are just deep to the dermis, so whatever method is used, the surgeon should keep the dermis intact during de-epithelialization. The skin is easier to remove in a superomedial pedicle than in an inferior pedicle.

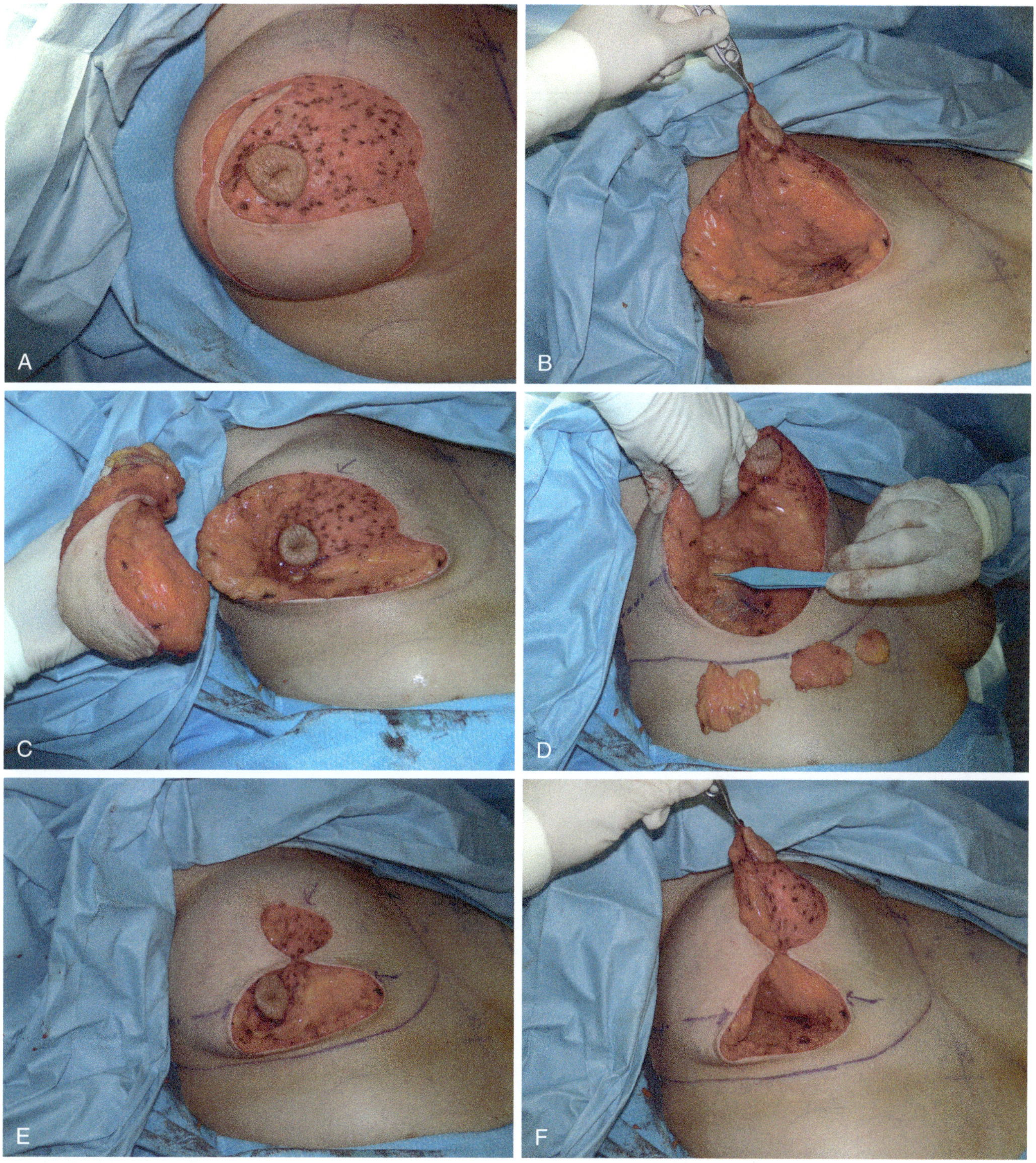

• **Fig. 38.8** Operative technique for superomedial vertical breast reduction. (A) De-epithelialization of a superomedial pedicle. Note that the base of the pedicle extends along the vertical limb but that the upper base extends across to just lateral to the breast meridian. This allows the pedicle to include two axial arteries (from the second and third interspaces). (B) The superomedial pedicle is created as a full-thickness pedicle to include the ascending branch of the fourth intercostal nerve that travels above the pectoralis fascia and then turns upward toward the areola at the breast meridian.[11] (C) Resection of the parenchyma is performed initially around the pedicle but mainly as an inferior wedge resection. An initial inferior vertical wedge resection is performed while leaving a 2-cm thick lateral pillar (about 7 cm long). The medial pillar will be formed by the inferior border of the medial pedicle. Extra parenchyma is removed from under the lateral flap – where there is excess. (D) Extra breast tissue is removed inferiorly above the IMF and below the Wise pattern (which is marked in blue on the skin). This is performed to prevent bottoming out and to prevent an inferior pucker (which is usually a problem of lack of subcutaneous tissue excision rather than a skin redundancy problem). Aggressively removing this tissue will result in a higher IMF level. The blue forceps are pointing to the excess parenchyma that needs to be removed under the lateral flap. In a very glandular breast (young women) this tissue needs to be carved out under the flap but also to remove any tissue lateral to the desired Wise pattern. In older patients, this excess can be liposuctioned but it must be completely removed or else the breast will end up too wide and full laterally. Tissue needs to be removed where it is in excess. (E) The lower border of the areola is closed first to allow the surgeon to assess the extent of resection. No dermal undermining is needed for this closure. (F) The superomedial pedicle is easily rotated up into position. This maneuvre of pulling the areola cephalad allows the medial and lateral pillars to fall together. The arrows marked on the skin show the lower edges of the pillars. This is usually about half-way up the vertical skin resection with tissue removed inferiorly. The pillars do not extend as far down as the skin opening or as far down as the IMF. The pillars are closed with a few relatively superficial sutures with no tension. The pillars should be sutured only enough to allow them to stay together during the postoperative period so that they can heal together. Deep bites are not necessary and may lead to tissue necrosis. Tension should not be relied upon to shape the breast because it will inevitably fail over time. The key is to remove all tissue where it is in excess.

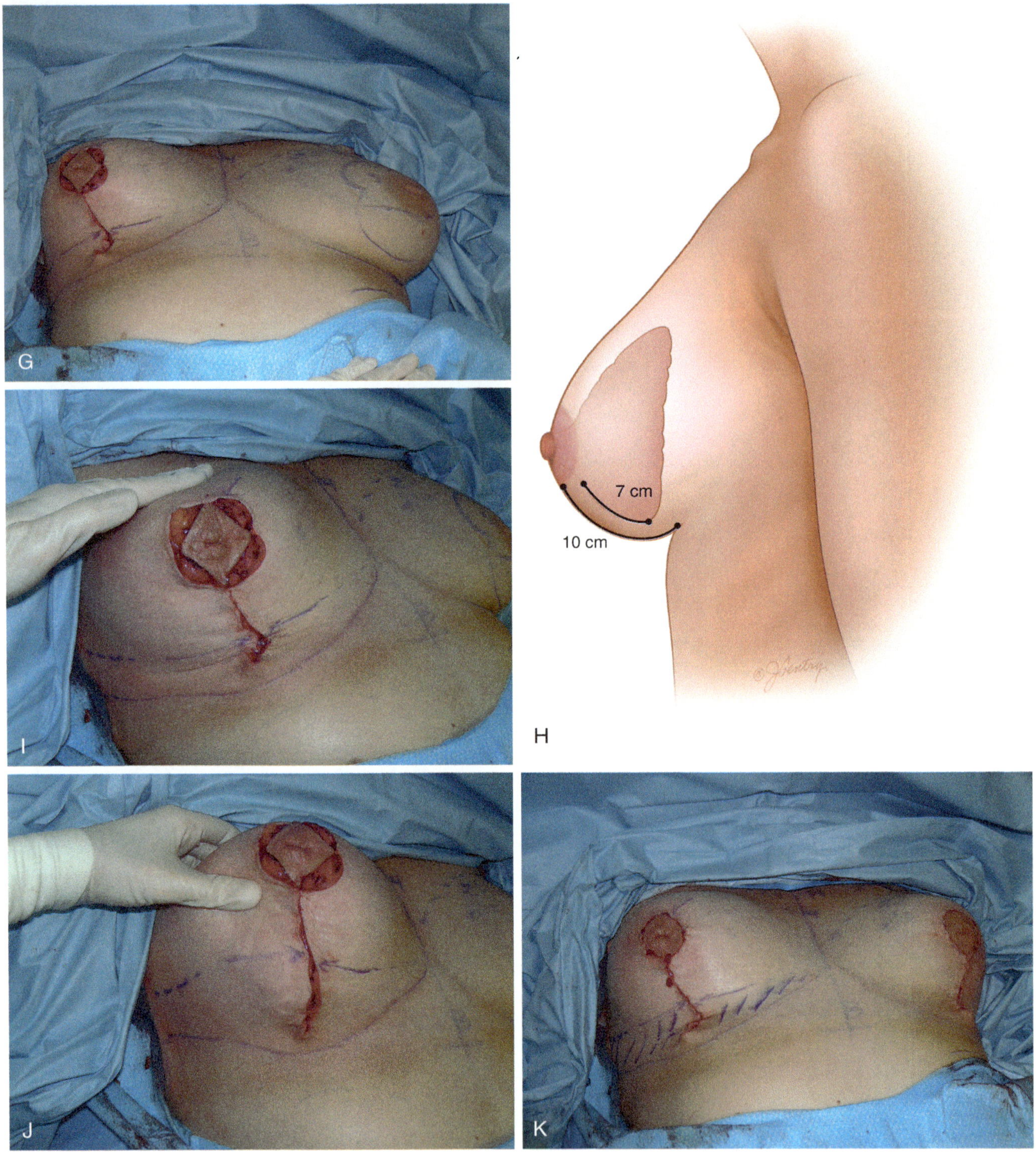

Fig. 38.8 cont'd (G) The dermis is closed loosely both vertically and around the areola. Note the shape of the right breast. Good projection is achieved along with narrowing of the breast base as compared with the unoperated left breast. (H) Although the pillars are often about 7 cm long, the skin can be much longer because it tucks up under and behind the pillars. (I) The photograph shows that the breast does not settle by dropping as shown. In order to determine whether a horizontal scar needs to be added, it is better to lift up the breast and then push down. Pushing it down like this will make the surgeon think that a horizontal scar is needed. (J) The final breast shape and extent of excess skin can be shown by using this maneuver where the breast is elevated and pushed down so that it slides down the chest wall to its original position. This allows the surgeon to determine if any more subcutaneous tissue or parenchyma needs to be removed but also to assess whether a horizontal skin excision needs to be added. The excess inferior skin in this example will just curve up under the parenchyma around the pillars and does not need to be modified. (K) Final closure. The cross-hatched area shows where the liposuction has been performed (usually after deep dermal closure before subcuticular closure). Liposuction is also performed along the lateral chest wall and (not to excess) in the preaxillary areas.

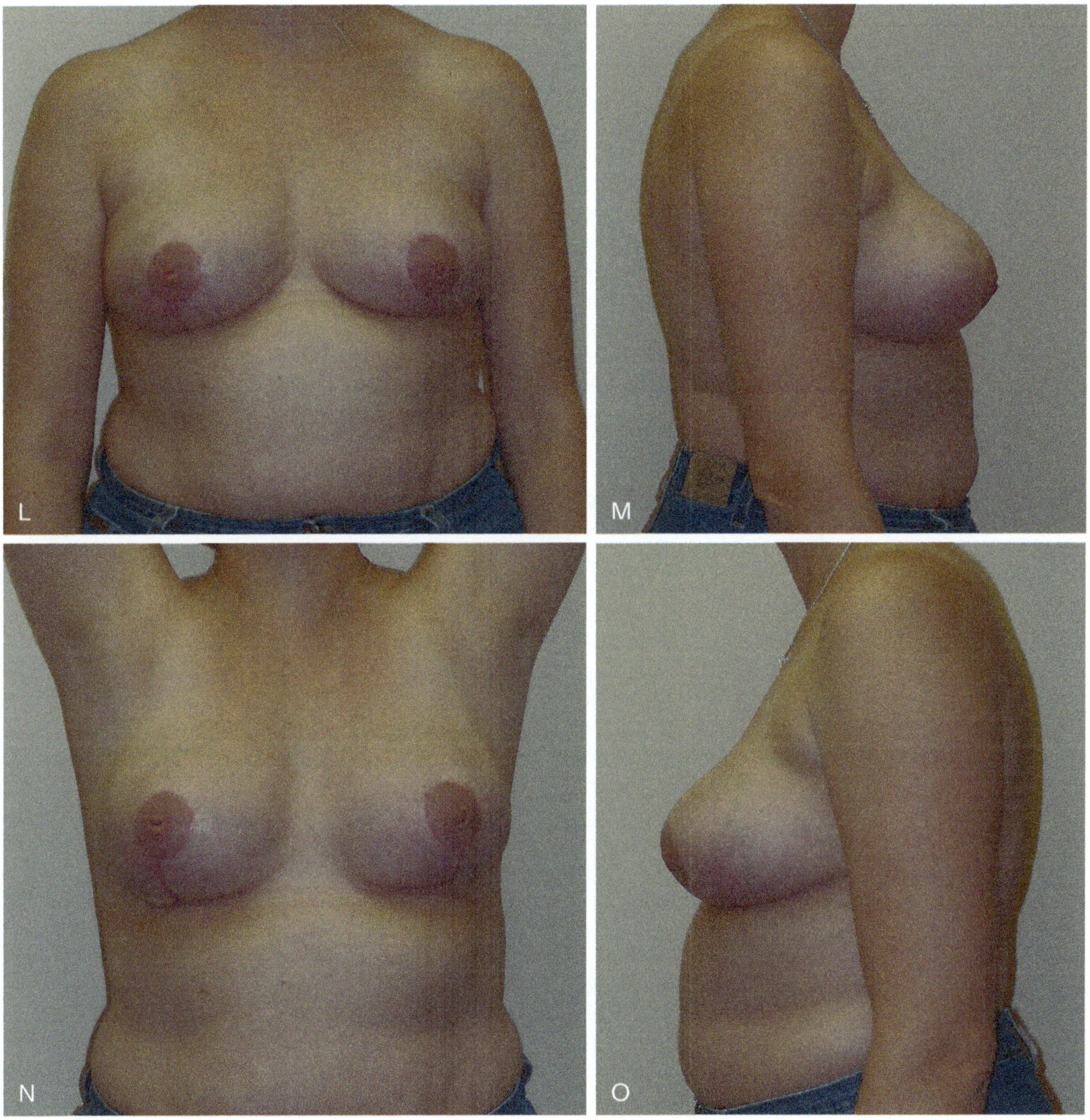

Fig. 38.8 cont'd (L–O) Postoperative photographs at 5 months. The patient was 41 years old, 5'11" tall, weighed 82 kg and wore a 34G brassiere. She had 346 g removed from the right breast and 325 g from the left breast. She had 400 ml of fat suctioned from the inferior breast along the IMF as well as along the lateral chest wall and in the preaxillary areas. (© Elizabeth J. Hall-Findlay.)

Pedicle Creation

The pedicle is created initially as a full-thickness pedicle cutting straight down toward the chest wall. Most of the bleeding occurs in the first few centimeters as initially the veins are encountered just under the dermis and then the arteries are severed in the subcutaneous tissue. There is not much bleeding from the breast parenchyma itself. The only artery and vein (and lateral branches) that course through the parenchyma to the nipple penetrate through the intercostals (and pectoralis muscle) at the fourth interspace. This is the artery and vein that supply an inferior and central pedicle. Of course there are vessels that supply the parenchyma, but no other vessels that course through the parenchyma to supply the nipple. All the other pedicles are supplied by superficial vessels in the subcutaneous tissue.

No alteration is made at this stage for insetting the pedicle. If the pedicle is stiff then deep tissue can be debulked later to allow for an easier inset.

Parenchymal Resection

The inferior wedge of parenchyma is then removed cutting straight down to the chest wall. A 2-cm thick lateral pillar should be created before undermining the lateral flap. It is important to remove tissue down toward the pectoralis fasbia but there will be less bleeding if the fascia itself is left undisturbed. The surgeon will encounter the deep perforators coming just up above the fifth rib (fourth interspace) just medial to breast meridian. There are some branches that perforate more laterally as well but all from the internal mammary system.

The excess parenchyma in a breast reduction is inferior and lateral. Once the inferior wedge of breast tissue is removed, then more tissue can be beveled out under the lateral flap. The lateral parenchymal pillar should be about 2 cm thick and about 7 cm in length. If the tissue is thick glandular tissue (as in a teenager) the surgeon needs to carefully carve out all tissue until a good Wise pattern of parenchyma is left behind. If the lateral excess tissue is comprised mainly of fat, it can be removed later with liposuction, but any "white" glandular tissue needs to be directly excised.

Rarely does any parenchyma need to be removed medially except just above the IMF. It is good to leave behind some parenchyma in the lateral aspect of the areolar opening to serve as a platform so that the areola does not retract once it is inset. Even a full-thickness pedicle will appear to be undermined once it is created.

The surgeon should consciously leave behind a Wise pattern of parenchyma. This will mean not only removing the inferior wedge of tissue and tissue under the lateral flap but also tissue caudal to the Wise pattern above the IMF. This will result in some elevation of the IMF – another reason to keep the lower border of the vertical skin resection pattern about 4 cm above the original IMF.

The surgeon who is less familiar with the vertical approach will initially remove less parenchyma than required – the breast looks smaller on the table than it is when sitting.

Pillar Closure

It is best to close the areolar opening first to best assess the shape and to effectively close the pillars. The dermis does not need to be undermined or released for this suture (usually a 3-0 Monocryl). Once the areola is closed, the pedicle can be easily rotated up into the opening. If there is any resistance, the deep tissue of the pedicle can be debulked because the blood supply is superficial.

If the pedicle is pulled up in a cephalad direction using forceps, the pillars will automatically fall together. The inferior border of the medial pedicle becomes the medial pillar and the first suture should be placed at the caudal end of the lateral pillar (about 7 cm down from the areolar opening as shown by the arrows on the photograph) and where the inferior border of the medial pedicle meets the skin (i.e., at the caudal end of what is now the medial pillar).

Deep bites are not necessary (and can actually lead to tissue necrosis). It is only necessary to make sure that parenchyma (not fat) is apposed on each side so that healing can occur. I usually use only 3–4 sutures of 3-0 Monocryl to hold the pillars in contact with each other. Any tension on parenchyma (which I mistakenly tried with lateral pedicles in a vain attempt to pull lateral tissue inward) will eventually release and the tissue will return toward its original position.

Skin Closure

The deep dermis is then closed with interrupted 3-0 Monocryl sutures, again with the goal of achieving only dermis-to-dermis contact so that the circulation to the skin edges is not compromised. The vertical skin is then closed with a subcuticular 3-0 or 4-0 Monocryl but it is important not to "cinch" or "gather" the vertical incision. It was initially thought that it was important to shorten the vertical incision because of the fear of bottoming-out that occurred when the skin stretched with the inferior pedicle, inverted T breast reduction.

Not only does the gathering compromise blood supply to the skin edges, but it is ineffective in shortening the vertical skin length.[32] It is important for surgeons to change their thinking and realize that a longer vertical length is actually needed to accommodate the increased projection that occurs with the vertical approach. Bottoming out occurs with the inferior pedicle procedures because the weight of the tissue is left in the lower pole and the skin brassiere stretches; bottoming-out occurs with vertical procedures with inadequate resection of the lower pole (inferior wedge). The skin is allowed to redrape with a vertical approach as it is not used as a handle to hold the breast up. Any procedures that use skin (or dermis) as slings tend to fail over time because skin (and dermis) stretches.

There is some tissue overhang in a vertical breast reduction and the vertical length from the lower border of the areola to the IMF is usually about 7 cm in a "B" cup breast, about 9 cm in a "C" cup breast and about 11 cm in a "D" cup breast. It is important to warn patients that they will still be able to "hold a pencil" underneath their breasts. Although the pillars are about 7 cm, the skin is longer and it tucks up underneath the breast.

The decision to add a "T", a "J" or an "L" can be a difficult one. It will depend on the quality and amount of excess skin. As a guideline, a vertical incision length of up to 12 cm can be tolerated in patients with poor quality skin and up to 15 cm with good quality skin for an average "C" to "D" cup breast. The way to test to see if the inferior end of the incision will tuck up underneath the breast is to hold the breast up and push it down by lifting and sliding (see Fig. 3.8J), and if the end of the incision tucks up under the pillars, no further correction is necessary.

Areolar Closure

The pedicle is allowed to sit comfortably in the areolar opening and it is usually rotated slightly to fit. Debulking of deep tissue in the superomedial pedicle to allow unrestricted inset can be performed at any time during the procedure.

Four deep 3-0 Monocryl sutures are used to close the dermis and the skin is closed with a subcuticular 3-0 or 4-0 Monocryl. If the skin opening is not completely circular, the skin can be trimmed prior to closure.

The areola will eventually stretch out to match the skin opening circumference. A 16-cm circumference (of the skin opening, not the areola) will match a 5-cm diameter areola. A 14-cm circumference matches a 4.5-cm diameter areola. Areolar skin is quite elastic and will stretch to fit the skin opening. A permanent Gore-Tex type of suture can be used in a circumvertical type of breast reduction (which is used to shorten the vertical length) but at the expense of some stretching that can occur beyond the Gore-Tex pursestring.

Liposuction for Tailoring

After the deep dermis is closed, liposuction is easier to perform because there is some resistance to the tissues and because it is easier to visualize the final Wise pattern. Liposuction is performed beyond the Wise pattern to remove any excess tissue (this must be carved out and excised directly in young patients who have more parenchyma and less fat) (Fig. 38.9). Liposuction can also be used to reduce fat in the lateral chest wall and preaxillary areas.

Drains

Drains can be used if desired. If a patient has a large lateral dead space or had an unusual amount of bleeding during surgery then drains might be indicated. Seromas do occur and drains would need to be left in for a long time to treat seroma formation. The advantage of the vertical approach is that seroma fluid can easily work its way through the tissues with gravity without being blocked by an inframammary incision.

Antibiotics

The breast is often considered "clean" surgery, but it is well known that breast ducts contain bacteria and it may be best to give a prophylactic dose of antibiotics before surgery (usually a cephalosporin). In my experience, when patients are given a full week of postoperative antibiotics, almost all problems with suture spitting disappear. Some of those problems recurred

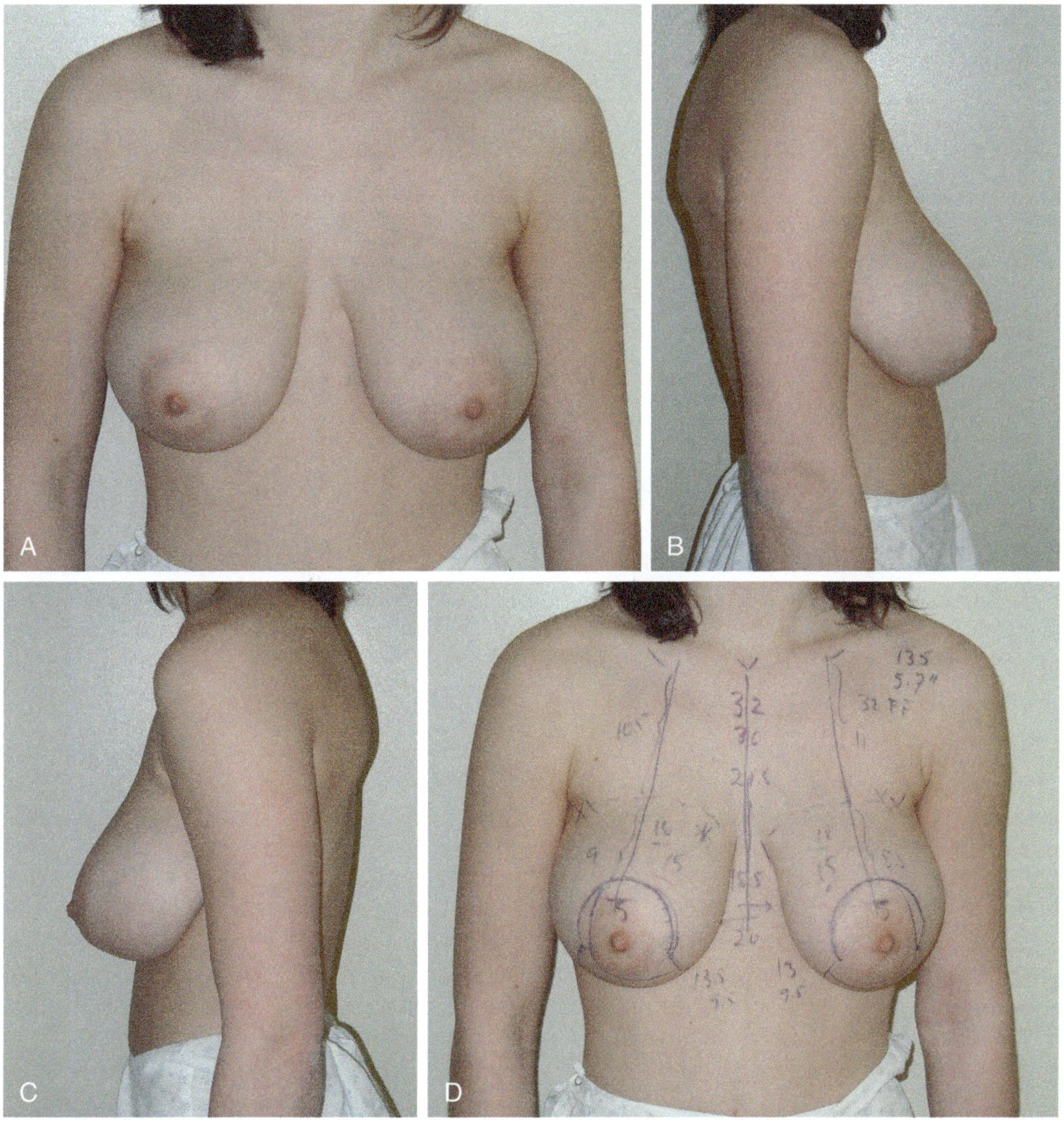

• **Fig. 38.9** Vertical breast reduction. (A–D) A 16-year-old patient who was 5′7″ tall, weighed 61 kg and wore a 32FF brassiere.

Continued

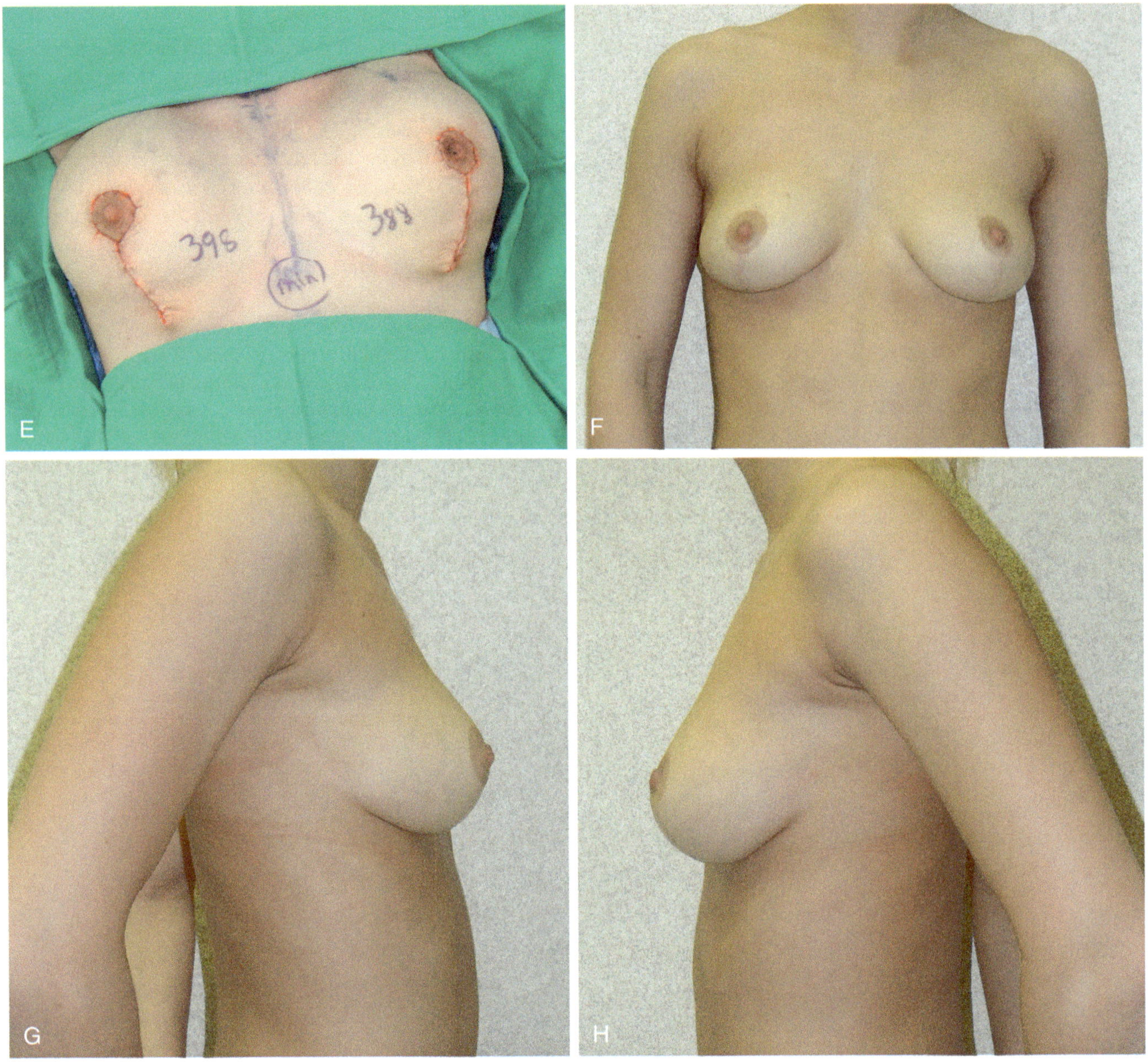

Fig. 38.9 cont'd (E) She had a true superomedial pedicle vertical breast reduction with 398 g removed from the right breast and 388 g removed from the left breast. She only had a minimal amount of fat removed with liposuction. (F–H) Postoperative photographs at just over one year. (© Elizabeth J. Hall-Findlay.)

when only a single prophylactic dose was given, but the use of triclosan (an antibacterial, not an antibiotic) impregnated sutures helped reduce the incidence of suture spitting.

Taping and Garments

The incisions are best managed by covering them with paper tape. Steristrips can be used, but if they are placed across the incision, blisters can occur from the shear forces as the breast swells. Tape should be placed along the incision and glue is not necessary. The incisions are then covered with gauze and the patient is placed in a non-compressive surgical brassiere. It is unnecessary (and ineffective) to tape all the breast skin in an attempt to shape the breast.

Patients are allowed to shower the next day. The paper tape will stay in place (without being changed) for 3–4 weeks.

The pucker at the lower end of the vertical incision may swell and protrude for a few weeks and then it will tuck in under the pillars. Some patients may need a revision but this should not be performed for at least 6 months. Because the parenchyma (and skin) is removed as a vertical ellipse, there is a dog-ear that disappears into the areola and one that can be a nuisance inferiorly. The inverted T, inferior pedicle type of breast reduction results in a horizontal type of excision of skin and parenchyma with a medial and lateral dog-ear – both of which can be a nuisance.

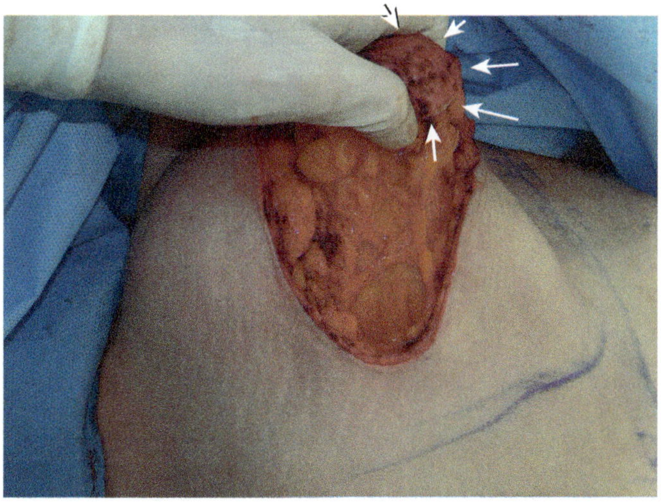

• **Fig. 38.10** The inferior wedge that is normally removed in a breast reduction is shown as an inferior flap left attached to its chest wall-based blood supply but separated from breast and skin on all four sides to allow good mobilization.

Operative Technique for Vertical Mastopexy

It is important to understand that the skin will not act as a good brassiere in a patient who has already developed breast ptosis. An inferior wedge of breast needs to be removed in a breast reduction or small mastopexy. If a patient likes her breast size, then the inferior wedge of breast tissue needs to "moved" rather than "removed". Any attempt to push and hold up the parenchyma with the skin will be doomed to failure.

Liacyr Ribeiro[6,7,8] describes an inferior flap along with a superior pedicle. The flap needs to be separated on all four sides and left as a chest wall-based flap (Fig. 38.10). The flap can be easily mobilized and moved up the chest wall and the medial and lateral pillars can then be closed caudal to the flap to hold it up. The flap is sutured up to the chest wall long enough that breast tissue will heal to breast tissue. The flap does not heal to pectoralis fascia even when sutured up but it will heal to the overlying breast tissue. The arrows in Fig. 38.10 outline the dermis: it can be seen how much mobility this flap has because the dermis originated just above the IMF.

Any attempt to suture breast tissue to pectoralis fascia will either fail or result in scar contracture that will cause the breast to move unnaturally every time the muscle is contracted. In normal circumstances, this flap can provide extra breast projection and can prevent recurrent glandular ptosis but it will not result in increased upper pole fullness (Fig. 38.11).[1]

The blood supply to this inferior flap is the deep artery and vein from the internal mammary system at the fourth interspace. It is important to create the flap while being careful to preserve the attachments to the chest wall just above the fifth rib and just medial to the breast meridian. The flap is de-epithelialized not to maintain blood supply but to serve as something somewhat substantial to help suture the flap upwards. Either a superior or superomedial pedicle can be used with this inferior flap.

A superior pedicle is often used because a concave inferior aspect to the breast will not occur because the central aspect of the breast is filled with the flap. A superomedial pedicle can be used if the nipple and areola have a long distance to travel – where rotation is better than folding.

Ruth Graf[33] has described a similar mastopexy but using a strip of pectoralis muscle to act as a handle to hold the flap up higher on the chest wall. This does attach the flap to the chest wall but the remaining breast will still tend to drop down around the flap, back into its original position. This flap can improve upper pole fullness to some degree but it can cause a problem in weight loss patients when the flap stays up and the breast drops down below the flap. Some surgeons complain that this procedure puts breast tissue behind the pectoralis muscle, but in reality all that happens is that a strip of muscle acts as a handle over the breast tissue.

Operative Technique for Vertical Augmentation-Mastopexy

The problem with the inferior flap in a mastopexy-augmentation is that the blood supply to the inferior flap is damaged when the implant is placed in either a subglandular or subpectoral location. The artery and vein to this flap come up through the intercostal muscles just above the fifth rib and they are cauterized with insertion of the implant. The procedure can be performed while preserving the flap but it is difficult and skin closure can be a problem.

It is best to perform a "reduction-augmentation" or "plus-minus" procedure[34,35] when both a mastopexy and an augmentation are desired (Fig. 38.12). Some surgeons believe that the mastopexy and the augmentation involve opposing forces, but that is not really the best way to approach the problem.[36–38] The implant is used to add volume to the upper and central poles of the breast and the inferior wedge resection is used to take care of the glandular ptosis.

A superior pedicle is often used because a concave inferior aspect to the breast will not occur because the central aspect of the breast is filled with the implant. A superomedial pedicle can be used if the nipple and areola have a long distance to travel – where rotation is better than folding.

Closing the skin under tension is not only unnecessary but can lead to wound healing problems. The skin will not act as a good brassiere and skin tension should not be relied upon to hold the implant up. Even a subfascial inferior sling fails to hold up the implant in the long term.[1] The ptotic gland needs to be removed and patients need to understand that a large implant will be subject to gravity.

Some surgeons will insert an implant into the subpectoral pocket, first keeping inferior muscle and fascia intact to close up the pocket completely. They then perform the mastopexy so that there is no contact between the implant and the bacteria present in the breast ducts.

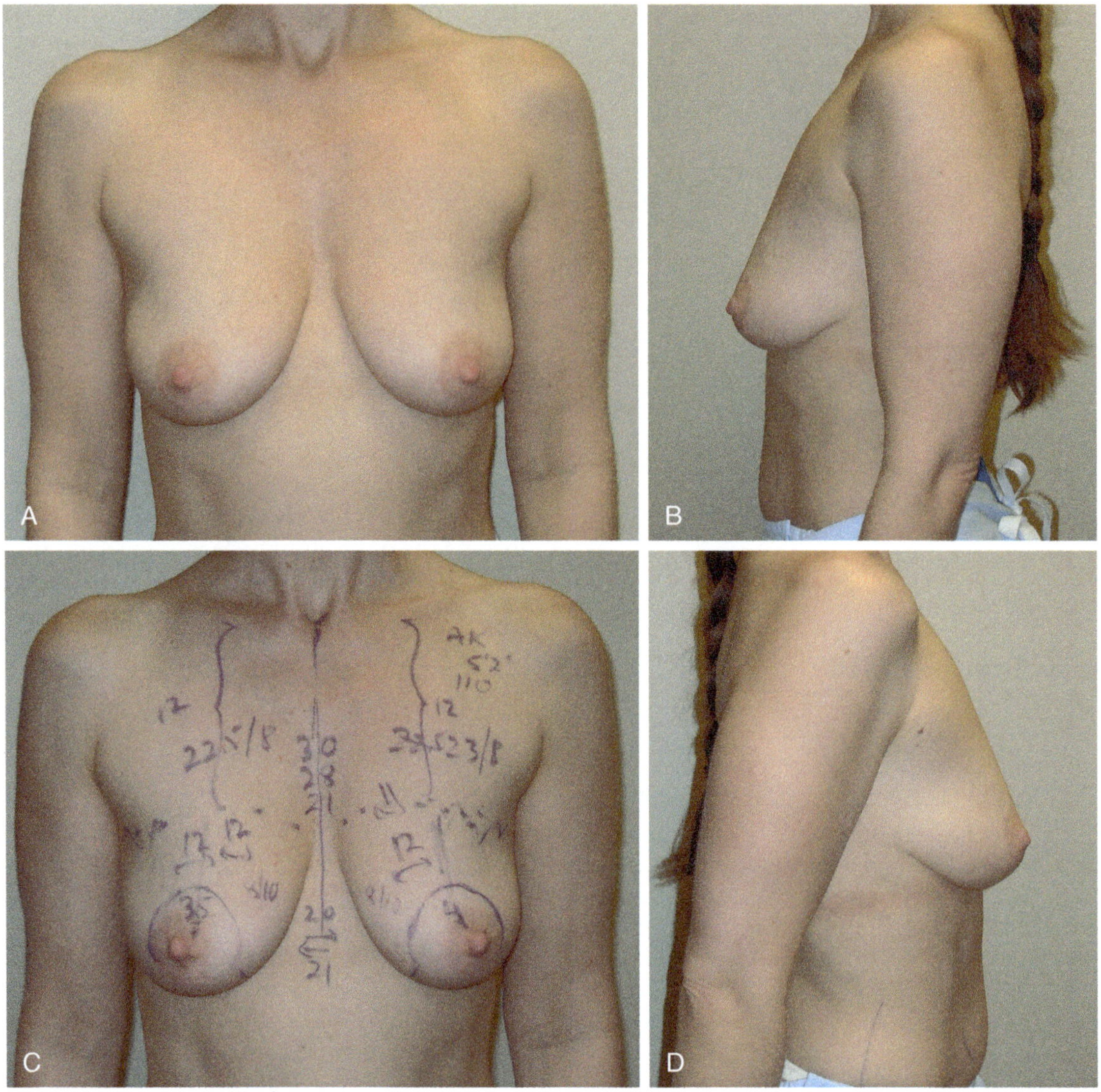

• **Fig. 38.11** Vertical mastopexy. (A–D) Patient who had a mastopexy using an inferior flap and a superior pedicle to rearrange (rather than remove) the inferior glandular ptosis.

Complications

The potential complications are basically the same for all breast procedures: blood loss, infection, necrosis, hematoma, seroma, dehiscence, and unsatisfactory esthetic results.

Blood loss: It is unusual to need a transfusion or even an autologous transfusion for most esthetic breast surgery. Blood loss is higher for the inverted T inferior pedicle breast reductions (about 300–400 ml) than a vertical reduction (about 100–200 ml). A vertical mastopexy as described here has a blood loss of about 100 ml and a vertical mastopexy-augmentation rarely exceeds 100 ml.

Infection: The breast ducts contain bacteria and breast surgery should not be considered completely "clean". A single dose of prophylactic antibiotics is indicated but postoperative antibiotics should probably only be considered when an implant is used. Even this is controversial. In my experience, suture spitting (festering) is a low-grade infection and it can be prevented to some degree by using antibacterial impregnated sutures such as Monocryl Plus. It appears that larger breast reductions and a higher BMI may lead to a higher infection rate.

Necrosis: Nipple necrosis is a definite risk inherent in all breast procedures that involve a transposition of the nipple and areola complex (Fig. 38.13). The rate is usually less than 1%. A good understanding of the blood supply to the breast will help minimize the risk but the occurrence of nipple necrosis is probably inevitable in any large volume practice. Although there are many recommendations on what to do with incipient necrosis, it is probably best only to intervene if it is possible that there is compression causing obstruction on either arterial inflow or venous outflow. The latter may develop obvious venous congestion. Once it is clear that some necrosis is likely, it is best to leave things alone and let the extent of necrosis declare itself. The nipple areolar complex seems to be a "privileged" construct and it often recovers far better than expected with no intervention.[1]

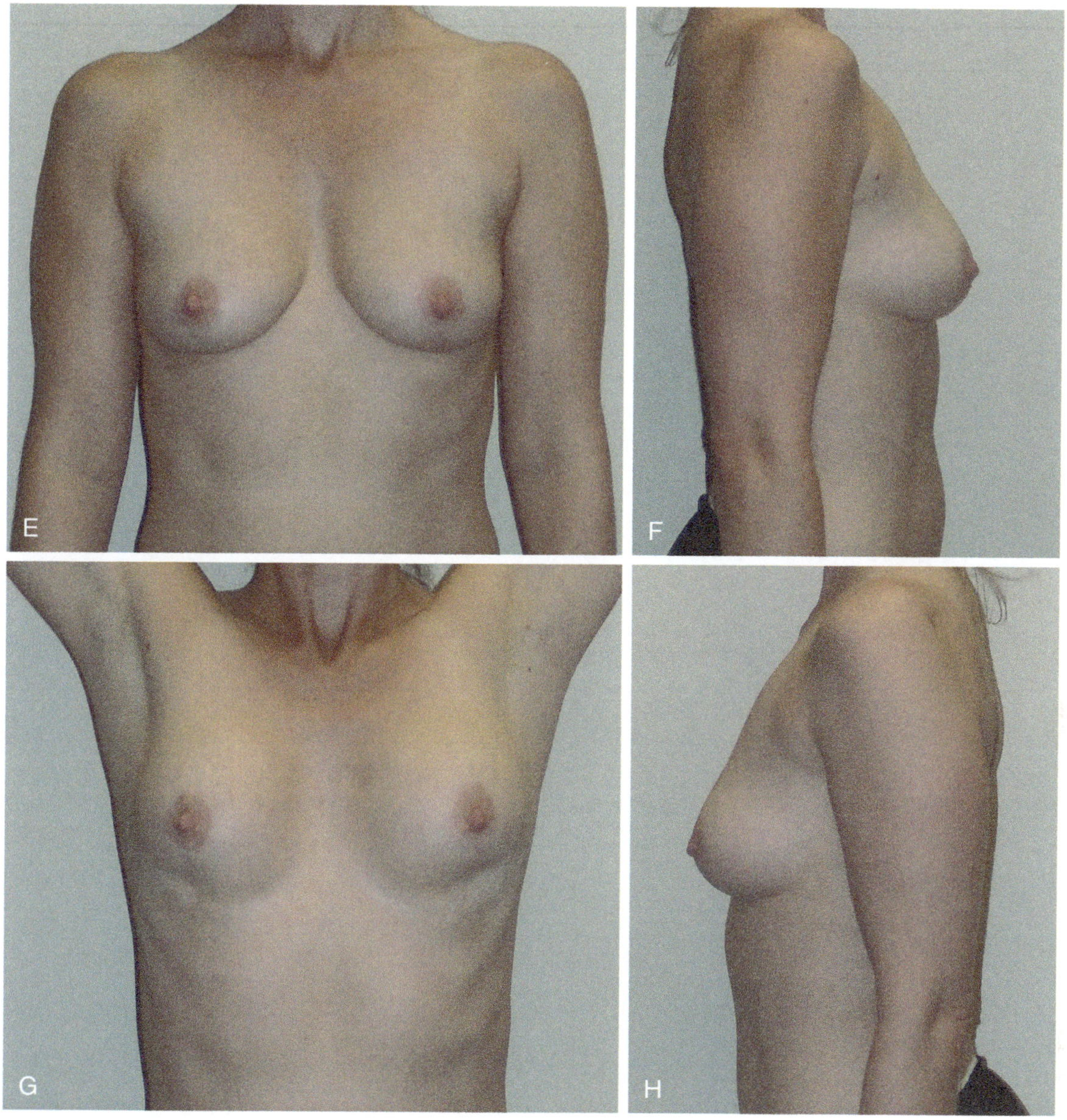

Fig. 38.11 cont'd (E–H) She is shown just over a year after her surgery with better projection and a long-lasting shape. (© Elizabeth J. Hall-Findlay.)

There are recommendations to remove the nipple–areola and apply it as a free nipple graft but this is probably not indicated in most cases. Removing sutures or taking the patient back to the operating room to inspect the pedicle for compression may be indicated but the surgeon needs to weigh the potential consequences of action versus inaction. Inaction is often a good choice.

Hematoma: All plastic surgery procedures have a risk of hematoma. The rate is probably close to 1% of cases. The best way to prevent a hematoma is to understand the main arterial supply and to check those areas for secure hemostasis before closure. There is an artery that comes up at the fourth interspace just medial to the breast meridian along with some branches appearing laterally as well at the fourth interspace. There are some vessels coming up in the subcutaneous tissue at the level of the IMF and there is the superficial branch of the lateral thoracic artery that enters the breast laterally and courses up into the breast initially deep peripherally and then in the subcutaneous tissue. The veins are even more superficial and usually lie just beneath the dermis. Drains do not prevent or treat hematomas but they may be indicated if there is an unusual amount of "ooze" that is evident during surgery.

Seroma: Seromas occur where there is a lot of dead space and where there is some friction between the overlying flap and underlying chest wall. Drains are needed for as long as shearing movement allows friction to occur. This can range from several days to weeks. Quilting sutures are very effective in the abdomen but somewhat harder to use along the lateral chest wall.

Dehiscence: This can occur when sutures fail to hold. More frequently the problem is excess tension on the closure which leads to constriction of blood supply to the skin edges (Fig. 38.14).

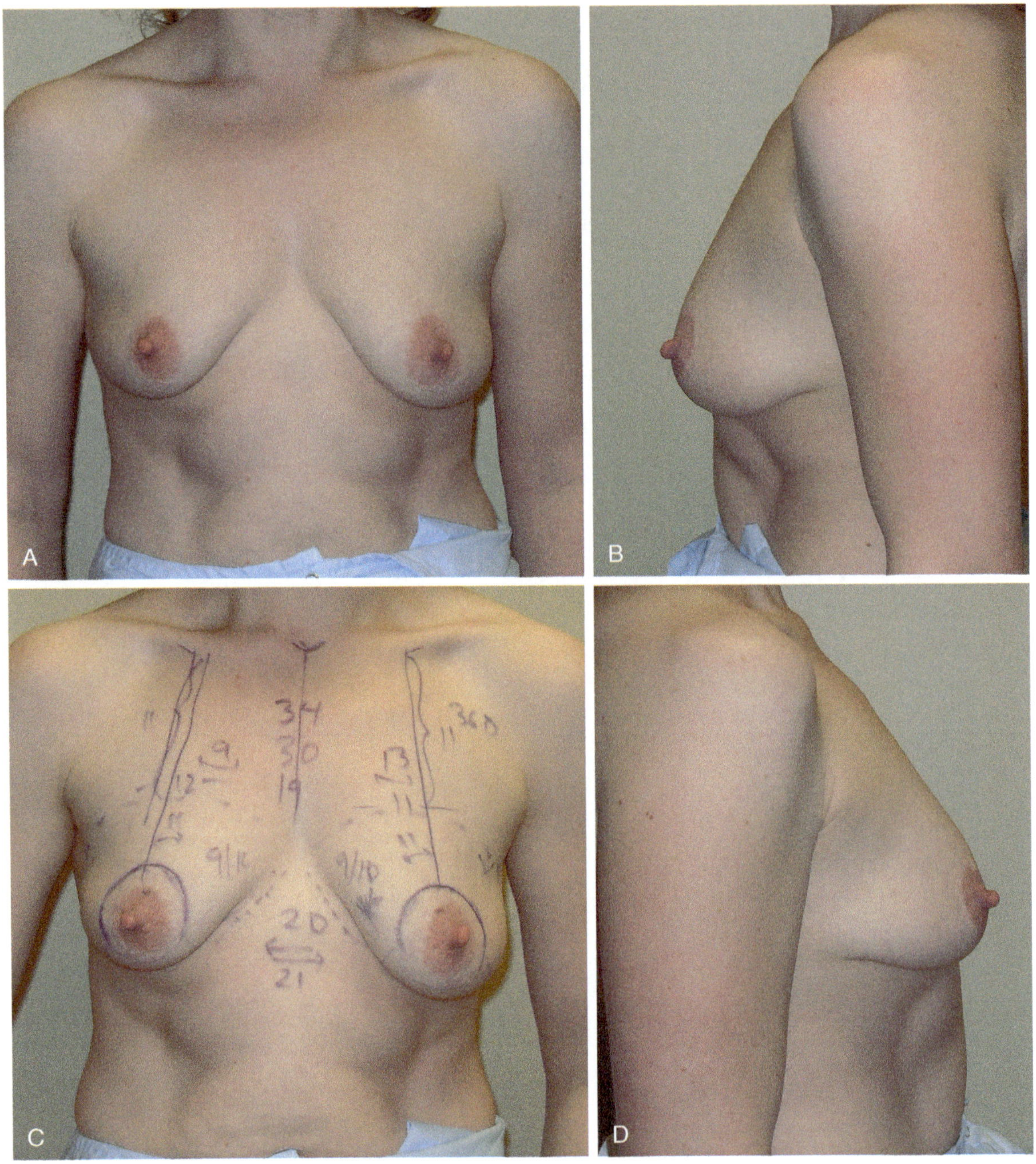

• **Fig. 38.12** Vertical mastopexy-augmentation. (A–D) Patient shown with a superior pedicle vertical mastopexy-augmentation with the implant (Allergan Style 15, each 339 ml) placed in a subglandular pocket. She did not have much glandular ptosis and only 15 g was removed from the right breast and 25 g from the left breast.

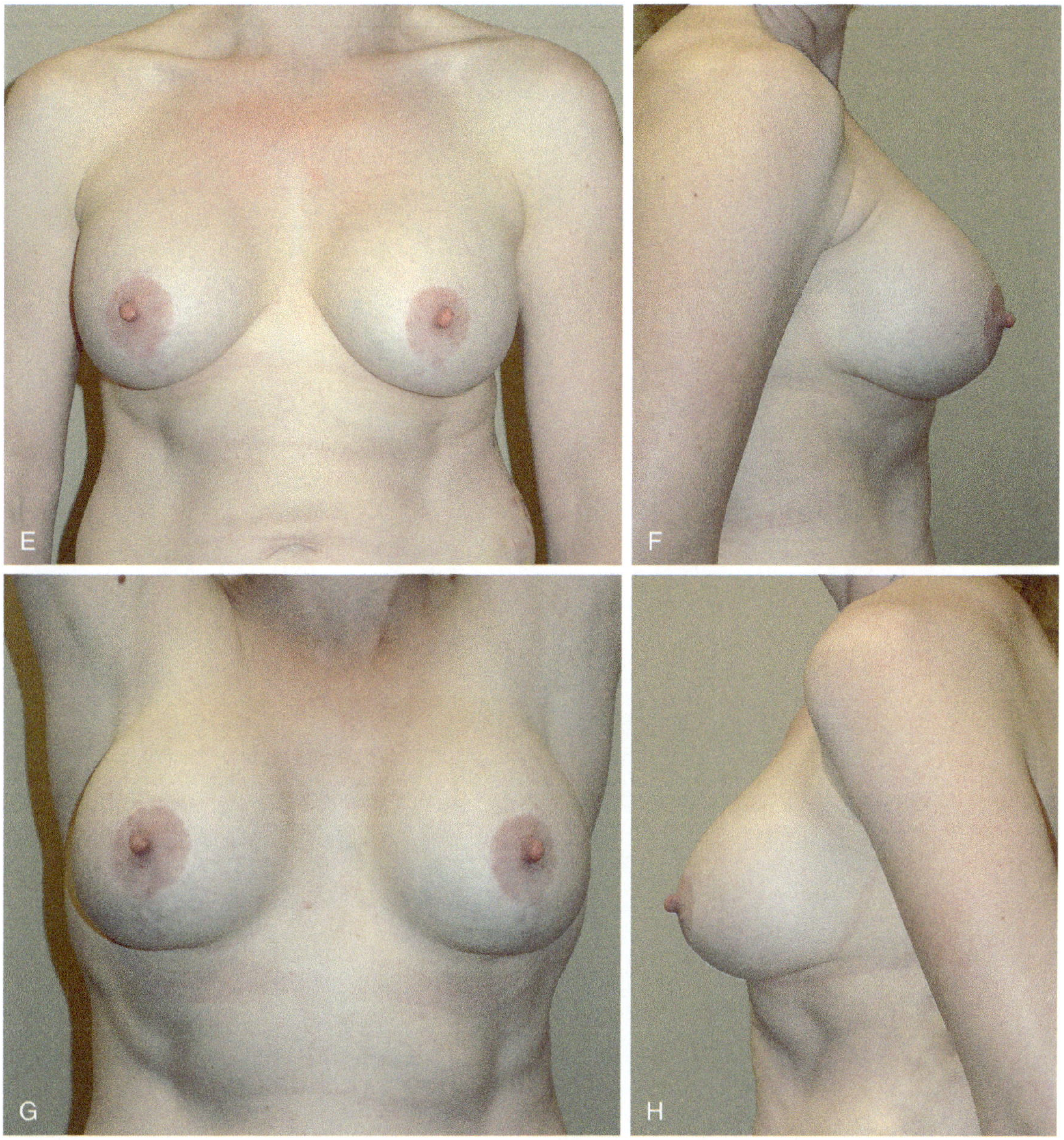

Fig. 38.12 cont'd (E–H) 3 years after her surgery. (© Elizabeth J. Hall-Findlay.)

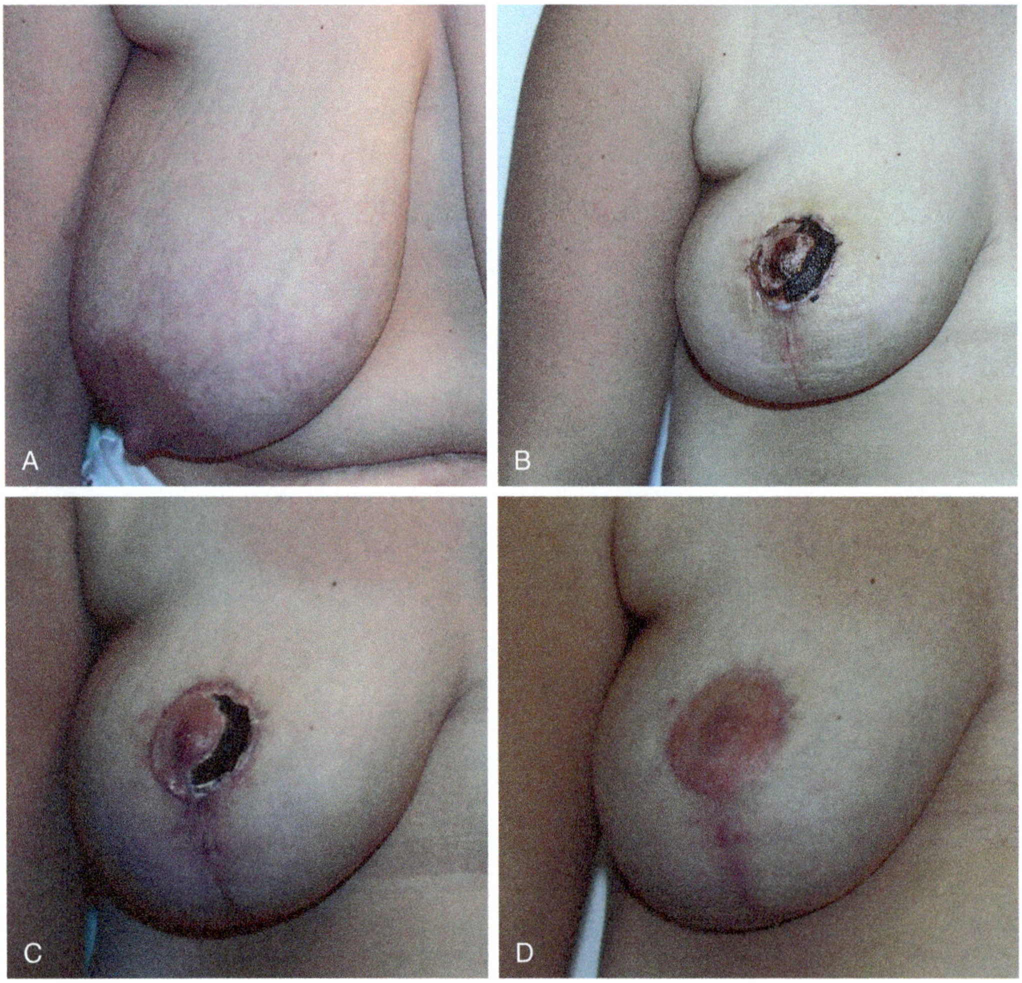

• **Fig. 38.13** Nipple necrosis. (A–D) Once established, sometimes nipple and areolar necrosis heals surprisingly well without intervention. The photos were taken at 2 weeks, 6 weeks, and 3 months postoperatively. (© Elizabeth J. Hall-Findlay.)

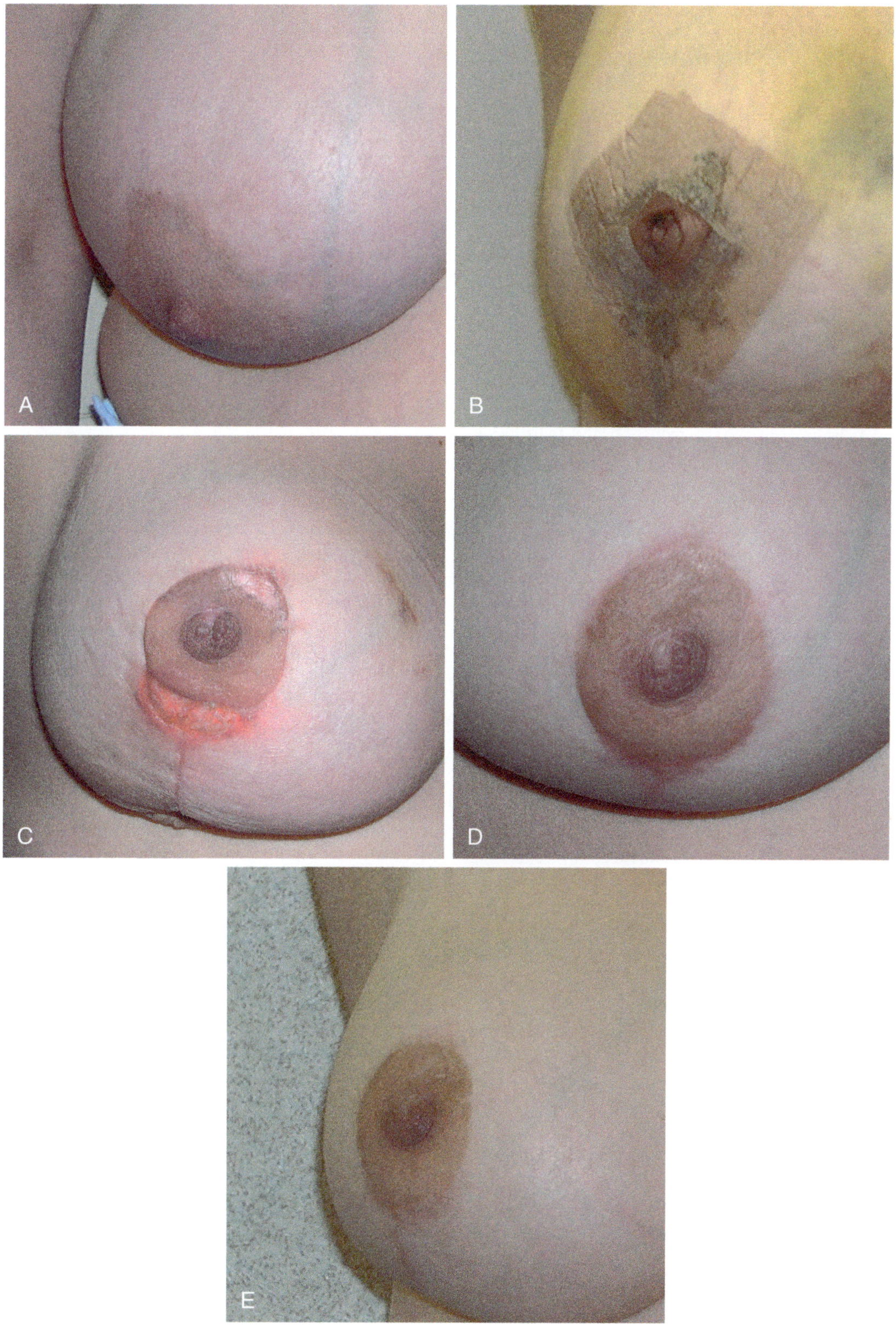

• **Fig. 38.14** Dehiscence. Sometimes a dehiscence is best left alone for healing by secondary intention. (© Elizabeth J. Hall-Findlay.)

References

1. Hall-Findlay EJ. *Aesthetic Breast Surgery, Principles and Techniques*. St Louis: Quality Medical Publishing; 2010.
2. Hall-Findlay EJ. The three breast dimensions: analysis and effecting change. *Plast Reconstr Surg*. 2010;125:1632.
3. McKissock PK, Discussion of Mathes SJ, Nahai F, Hester TR. Avoiding the flat breast in reduction mammaplasty. *Plast Reconstr Surg*. 1980;66:63–70.
4. McKissock PK. Reduction mammaplasty with a vertical dermal flap. *Plast Reconstr Surg*. 1972;49:245–252.
5. Ribeiro L. A new technique for reduction mammaplasty. *Plast Reconstr Surg*. 1975;55:330.
6. Ribeiro L. Creation and evolution of 30 years of the inferior pedicle in reduction mammaplasties. *Plast Reconstr Surg*. 2002;110(3):960–970.
7. Wise RJ. A preliminary report on a method of planning the mammaplasty. *Plast Reconstr Surg*. 1956;17:367.
8. Regnault P. Breast ptosis, definition and treatment. *Clin Plast Surg*. 1976;3:193–203.
9. Hall-Findlay EJ. Pedicles in vertical reduction and mastopexy. *Clin Plast Surg*. 20:379–391.
10. Hamdi M, Hall-Findlay EJ. Pedicle choices in breast reduction. In: Hamdi M, Hammond D, Nahai F, eds. *Vertical Scar Mammaplasty*. Berlin: Springer-Verlag; 2005.
11. Schlenz I, Kuzbari R, Gruber H, et al. The sensitivity of the nipple–areola complex: an anatomic study. *Plast Reconstr Surg*. 2000;105:905–909.
12. Robbins TH. A reduction mammaplasty with the areola-nipple based on an inferior pedicle. *Plast Reconstr Surg*. 1977;59:64–67.
13. Courtiss EH, Goldwyn RM. Reduction mammaplasty by the inferior pedicle technique. An alternative to free nipple and areola grafting for severe macromastia or extreme ptosis. *Plast Reconstr Surg*. 1977;59:500.
14. Skoog T. A technique of breast reduction. *Acta Chir Scand*. 1963;126:453.
15. Wiener DL, Aiache AE, Silver L, et al. A single dermal pedicle for nipple transposition in subcutaneous mastectomy, reduction mammaplasty or mastopexy. *Plast Reconstr Surg*. 1973;51:115.
16. Finger RE, Vasquez B, Drew GS, et al. Superomedial pedicle technique of reduction mammaplasty. *Plast Reconstr Surg*. 1989;83:471.
17. Strombeck JO. Reduction mammaplasty with horizontal pedicle technique. In: Noone RB, ed. *Plastic and Reconstructive Surgery of the Breast*. Philadelphia: BC Decker; 1991:195–206.
18. Robbins LB, Hoffman DK. The superior dermoglandular pedicle approach to breast reduction. *Ann Plast Surg*. 1992;29:211–216.
19. Asplund O, Davies DM. Vertical scar breast reduction with medial flap or glandular transposition of the nipple–areola. *Br J Plast Surg*. 1996;49:507–514.
20. Marchac D, de Olarte G. Reduction mammaplasty and correction of ptosis with a short inframammary scar. *Plast Reconstr Surg*. 1982;69:45–55.
21. Lassus C. Breast reduction: evolution of a technique. A single vertical scar. *Aesthet Plast Surg*. 1987;11:107–112.
22. Lejour M, Abboud M, Declety A, et al. Reduction des cicatrices de plastie mammaire: de l'ancre courte à la verticale. *Ann Chir Plast Esthet*. 1990;35:369.
23. Hall-Findlay EJ. A simplified vertical reduction mammaplasty: shortening the learning curve. *Plast Reconstr Surg*. 1999;104:748.
24. Hammond DC. Short scar periareolar inferior pedicle reduction (SPAIR) mammaplasty. *Plast Reconstr Surg*. 1999;103:890.
25. Cardenas-Camerena L, Vergara R. Reduction mammaplasty with superior-lateral dermoglandular pedicle: another alternative. *Plast Reconstr Surg*. 2001;107:693–699.
26. Blondeel PN, Hamdi M, Van de Sijpe KA, et al. The latero-central glandular pedicle technique for breast reduction. *Br J Plast Surg*. 2003;56:348.
27. Mistry RM, MacLennan SE, Hall-Findlay EJ. Principles of breast re-reduction: a reappraisal. *Plast Reconstr Surg*. 2017;139(6):1313–1322.
28. Benelli L. A new periareolar mammaplasty: the "round block" technique. *Aesthet Plast Surg*. 1990;14:93.
29. Davison SP, Mesbahi AN, Ducic I, et al. The versatility of the superomedial pedicle with various skin patterns. *Plast Reconstr Surg*. 2007;120:1466.
30. Mallucci P, Branford OA. Population analysis of the perfect breast: a morphometric analysis. *Plast Reconstr Surg*. 2014;134(3):436–447.
31. Hall-Findlay EJ. Vertical breast reduction with a medially based pedicle. Operative strategies. *Aesthet Surg J*. 2002;22(2):185–195.
32. Matthews JLK, Oddone-Paolucci E, Lawson DM, et al. Vertical scar breast reduction: does gathering the incision matter? *Ann Plast Surg*. 2016;77(1):25–31.
33. Graf R, Auersvald A, Bernardes A, et al. Reduction mammaplasty and mastopexy with shorter scar and better shape. *Aesthet Surg J*. 2000;20:99–106.
34. Baroudi R, Lewis JR. The augmentation-reduction mammaplasty. *Clin Plast Surg*. 1976;3:301–308.
35. Regnault P, Daniel RK, Tirkanits B. The minus-plus mastopexy. *Clin Plast Surg*. 1988;15(4):595–600.
36. Brink RR. Evaluating breast parenchymal maldistribution with regard to mastopexy and augmentation mammaplasty. *Plast Reconstr Surg*. 2000;106:491–496.
37. Spear SL, Boehmler JH, Clemens MW. Augmentation/mastopexy: a 3-year review of a single surgeon's practice. *Plast Reconstr Surg*. 2006;118:136S–147S.
38. Stevens WG, Freeman ME, Stoker DA, et al. One-stage mastopexy with breast augmentation: a review of 321 patients. *Plast Reconstr Surg*. 2007;120:1674–1679.

39 Chest Wall Reconstruction

NAGARAJAN MUTHIALU, MAZYAR KANANI, OLIVER J. SMITH, ROBERT PEARL, AND SIMON WITHEY

Overview of the Thoracic Cage

The thoracic cage serves two principal functions: to protect the thorax and upper abdomen and their associated viscera, and to allow movement for ventilation. It consists of 12 pairs of ribs and their respective costal cartilages; the manubrium and sternum anteriorly, and the thoracic vertebrae posteriorly. The costal cartilages of the true ribs (1–7) articulate directly to the manubrium/sternum. The costal cartilages of the false ribs (8–10) unite as a single synchondrosis and join the costal cartilage of the 7th rib. The floating ribs (11 and 12) have no anterior articulation. Three layers of intercostal muscles exist between each rib (external, internal, and innermost) and a neurovascular bundle (artery, vein, nerve) runs in a groove below each rib between the internal and innermost layers of muscle. The thorax is defined inferiorly by the diaphragm and superiorly by the clavicles.

CONGENITAL DEFECTS

Nagarajan Muthialu and Mazyar Kanani

Congenital chest wall anomalies may present at any age up to adolescence and may occur in isolation, or represent one marker in a spectrum of defects.

Pectus Deformities

In this spectrum of malformations, there is an abnormal contour of the anterior chest wall. It is thought the underlying problem lies with the relative rate of growth of the costal cartilages in relation to the growth of the ribs and sternum. If the elongated cartilages cause the anterior chest wall to buckle inwards, pectus excavatum results. If there is buckling outwards, the result is pectus carinatum.[1] However, some have proposed that the defects arise from abnormal growth of the diaphragm.[2]

Both conditions may be symmetric or asymmetric in nature, with a varying composite of anomalies, such as sternal angulation, tilt, and rotation about the long axis – all of which need to be taken into account during cosmetic correction. Within the broad spectrum, some patients may even have a mixed defect.

Pectus Excavatum

In this condition, there is a depression in the anterior of the chest wall of varying shape and severity (Fig. 39.1).

Morphologic Varieties

In most cases, the depression is symmetrical on either side of the midline and limited to the lower half of the sternum. More severe forms are deeper and extend further upwards toward the manubrium. At the more severe end of the scale is the so-called "Grand Canyon" variety where there is a deep and long depression. It can be a challenge to treat successfully, particularly since many of these are asymmetrical. In about 5% of cases, there is a combined excavatum/carinatum deformity.

Epidemiology

The incidence of the defect is 1 in 150–1000 live births.[1] Although the defect may be present anytime after birth, most patients present around the time of puberty during their phase of rapid body growth. There is also an association with connective tissue disorders such as Marfan's and Ehlers–Danlos syndromes where scoliosis is also more frequent.[3]

Clinical Evaluation

Prior to surgical correction, we undertake a number of investigations to determine the severity and extent of morphology, as well as impact on physiology.

Imaging

We routinely perform a plain chest radiograph that demonstrates the overall shape of the thoracic cavity. A plain chest

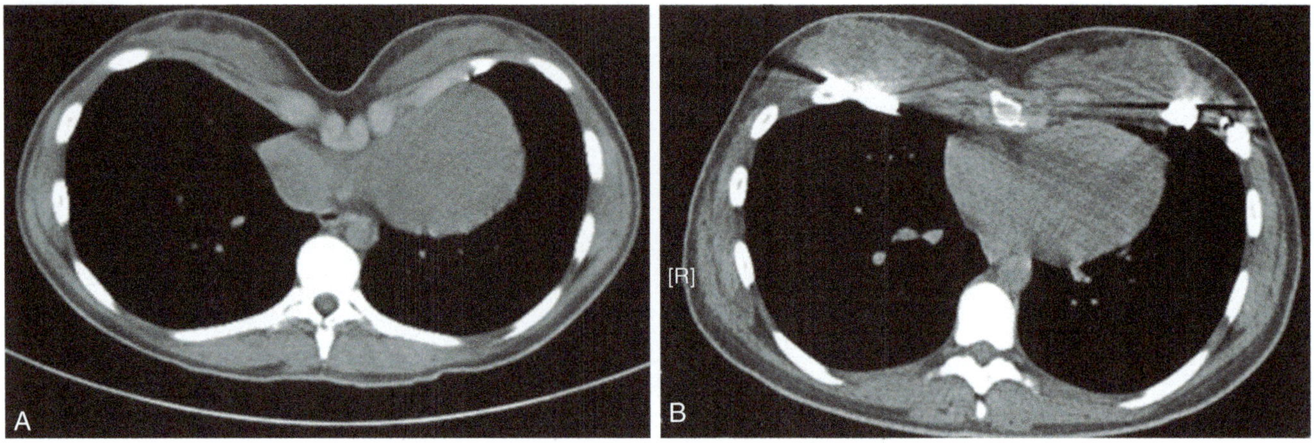

• **Fig. 39.1** Transverse section of a computerized tomography (CT) scan of a patient with pectus excavatum, (A) before and (B) after Nuss correction. Note the cardiac compression seen before correction.

radiograph is also a very useful screening tool to assess the spinal curvature initially.

This is followed by computerized tomography (CT scan) imaging, which can be used to construct the 3D anatomy of the thoracic cavity.[4] The Haller index of severity can be calculated from this. This is the ratio of the transverse diameter and the anteroposterior diameter of the rib cage. A normal ratio is 2.5. Of special importance is the shape and axis of the body of the sternum. Sternal torsion and asymmetry have an impact on the type of surgery. CT scan can also show associated anomalies including spinal deformities and also the extent of cardiac compression.

We also routinely perform transthoracic echocardiography to assess overall ventricular function. There is an association with mitral valve prolapse, which may be seen with connective tissue disorders.[3]

Functional Assessment

As part of our initial evaluation, we also perform exercise testing of the patient. This is following some reports of a modestly reduced functional capacity arising from the combination of right ventricular compression and reduced pulmonary capacity in some patients.[5]

Lung function testing including spirometry becomes useful whenever a restrictive lung capacity is suspected. In combination with exercise testing, this offers a very useful physiological way to assess functional implication of the pectus deformities, and also serves as a prognostic index for postoperative recovery.

Surgery for Pectus Excavatum

Timing

There are advantages and disadvantages to both early and late repair.[6–8] Each case is considered individually. Important factors to consider include the age at presentation, symptoms, severity of the deformity, and type of surgical approach. As a general rule, younger patients have a more malleable chest, which will make the minimally-invasive Nuss procedure an attractive option here. However, it has to be tempered with the fact that some of these children will outgrow their bar and need further bar insertion. Also, early bar removal in younger patients may result in recurrence as the chest continues to remodel with age. Nevertheless, the severity will reduce the age at intervention.

In the literature, surgery has been performed successfully from the ages of 1 year to 50.[7,8] In our experience, for the reasons noted above, the ideal is around the age of puberty.

Influence of Morphology

We reserve the minimally-invasive Nuss procedure for symmetric cases.[9] If the symmetry extends to a so-called Grand Canyon-type deformity, we may either use two Nuss bars, or elect to perform an open sternochondroplasty.[10] If it is likely that any second bar needs to be inserted high up, we favor an open approach due to the risk of placement over the great arteries in the mediastinum. In some cases with mild asymmetry, the Nuss bar can be molded appropriately.

Nuss Procedure

The patient is usually positioned supine on the operating table with the arms abducted following induction of anesthesia and epidural catheter placement.

Once positioned, necessary landmarks are drawn on the chest – the deepest part of the chest that indicates the level where the bar will lie, the point beneath the nipples at the level of where the bar will lie, and the two lateral points where the vertical skin incisions are made for the introduction of the bar and stabilizers.

The two lateral skin incisions are made, and the subcutaneous plane is developed to the marked point beneath the nipples at the level of where the bar will lie. These will be the points at which the bar will exit the chest wall on either side. Then, the thoracoscope is introduced into the right pleura through a port placed either just beneath or into the lateral skin incision. Carbon dioxide insufflation permits exposure. Next, the bar introducer creates a subcutaneous tunnel from the skin incision to the point of entry into the chest. Entry through the chest wall is observed via

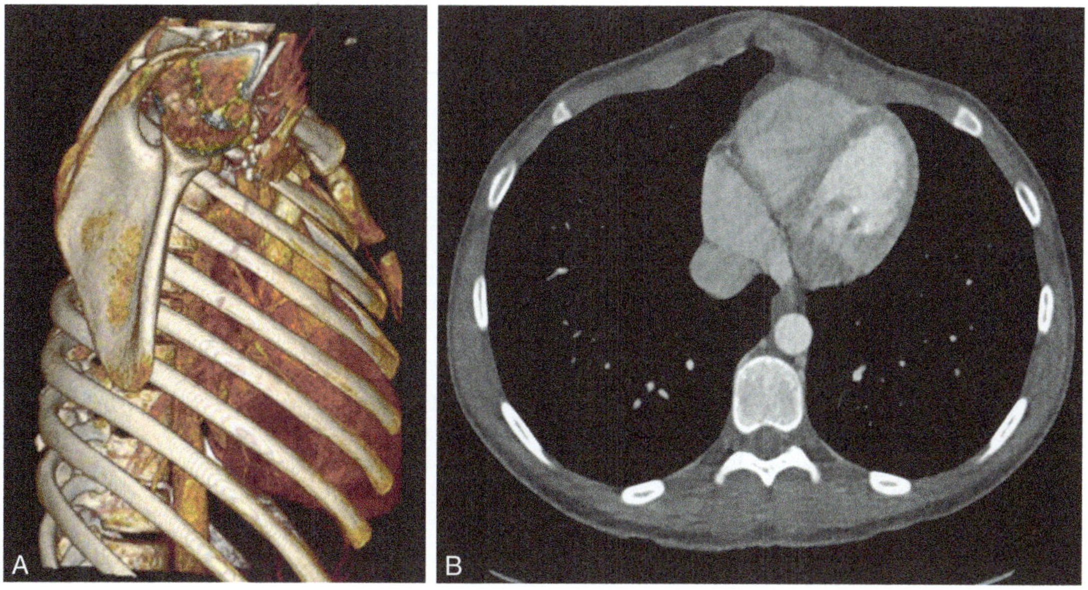

• **Fig. 39.2** Pectus carinatum as seen on (A) 3D CT reconstruction and (B) transverse CT scan. Note the 90 degree angulation between the body of the sternum and xiphisternum.

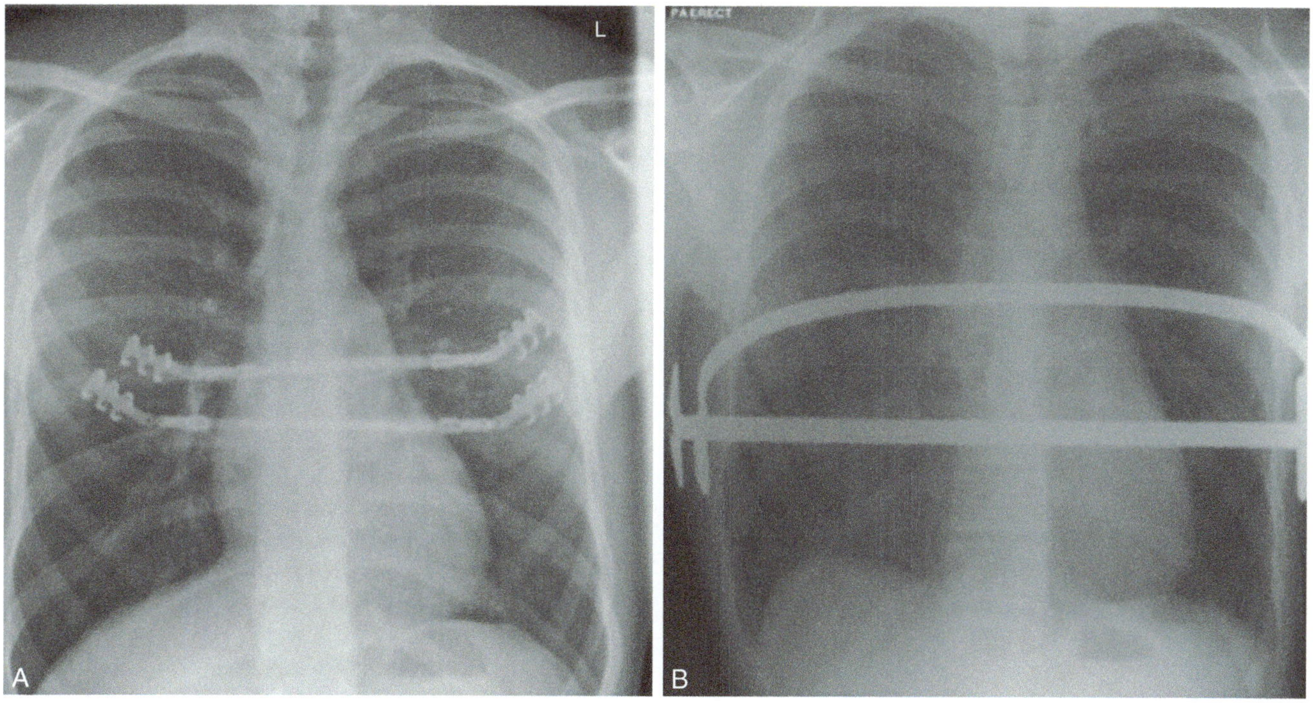

• **Fig. 39.3** (A) STRATOS bars in place for stability following repair of pectus carinatum. (B) Two Nuss bars in situ following repair of pectus excavatum.

thoracoscopy. The introducer is passed to the pleural cavity on the other side, anterior to the pericardium under direct vision. It is guided through the chest wall. Once safely out of the skin, it is tied by umbilical tape to a molded Nuss bar of appropriate size. As the introducer is removed, the bar is carried with it into the chest. The bar is then finally flipped with a specially-designed flipper and secured to the chest wall by bilateral stabilizers secured to it by steel wire (see Fig. 39.3B).

Following the procedure, the patient is extubated on table and a chest radiograph is taken immediately to check for pneumothoraces and bar position.

Once on the ward, the patient is observed in the high dependency unit for the duration of the epidural catheter – usually 4–5 days. Adequate analgesia is very important here once the epidural is removed. Mobilization aided by physiotherapy is the final step before discharge. A final posteroanterior and lateral chest radiograph check the bar position.

Bar Removal. We elect to remove the bar anywhere between 2 and 3 years. Although the bar can be left in for 4 years without problems, the longer it is left, the greater the degree of calcification around the bar, which can make removal more challenging. Removal is performed as a day-case procedure under general anesthesia. The greatest risk comes from pneumothorax, and there are also isolated reports of injury to great vessels.[11]

Pectus Carinatum

This is also known as "pigeon" or "keel" chest. In this condition, there is variable protrusion of the chest.[12] It is less common than pectus excavatum, being seen in about 0.06 of all live births (Fig. 39.2).

Morphologic Varieties

Depending on the exact extent of the protrusion, there are a number of variations.

- *Symmetrical*: The sternum is arched forwards. If there is some depression of the costal cartilages, the sternal prominence is exaggerated. In some cases, the body of the sternum fuses with the xiphoid at a 90-degree angle.
- *Symmetrical deformity with a normal sternum*: here, the anterior prominence comes from protrusion of the costal cartilages with a relatively normal sternal contour.
- *Asymmetry with combined carinatum and excavatum*: protrusion of costal cartilages on one side only causes rotation of the sternum about its long axis, causing a relative excavatum on the contralateral side.
- *Pouter pigeon chest*: there is prominence of a thickened manubrium so that the deformity is limited to the upper sternum only.

Surgery for Pectus Carinatum

Timing of Operations

This deformity becomes most apparent during adolescence when the infantile potbelly recedes to make the anterior chest more prominent during the period of rapid body growth. Although we do not have a distinct cut-off age, surgery is mainly reserved after this final adolescent growth-spurt has begun and chest wall natural chest wall modeling is complete.[12]

Reconstructive Aims

The main aim of surgery is to remodel the anterior chest wall to the normal contour – through trimming the elongated costal cartilages and returning the sternum to its natural alignment. Surgery will provide an immediate result, but in order for the remodeling to be complete, we encourage physiotherapy and muscle-building exercises to enhance the muscular contribution to chest wall shape.

Technique of Repair

Our method of repair is based on that of Ravitch,[10] but with the addition of any of the metal implants that we may have to consider, if needed for further stability. Chest wall stabilization using the Strasbourg Thorax Osteosyntheses System (STRATOS, MedXpertGmbH, Heitersheim, Germany) of costal bars[13] (Fig. 39.3A) was considered very effective, till we recently reported on a high fracture rate of these bars.[14]

The patient is positioned supine, with the arms by the side. We prefer to mark the skin first – indicating both the line of incision, and the most prominent areas of cartilage/sternum. The incision is horizontal at the level of the xiphisternal junction, being some 10 cm with a gentle upwards curve. The subcutaneous plane is developed, at first, superiorly to the highest cartilage involved then inferiorly to the xiphisternum. This is seldom above the 3rd rib. Then the pectoralis major muscles are detached, sparing their clavicular origins. Care must be taken not to enter the intercostal spaces, especially in thin patients. Next, the plane inferior to the incision is developed. The uppermost origins of the rectus abdominis muscles may have to be detached if the underlying cartilages are involved. At this point, the xiphisternum is also detached from the body of the sternum with diathermy.

Once the underlying involved costal cartilages and ribs are exposed, resection can begin. The cartilages are initially detached at the sternocostal joints through a combination of diathermy and sharp dissection. Care must be taken not to damage the underlying internal thoracic vessels, or parietal pleura. In order to preserve growth potential in the juvenile sternum, we try to preserve the underlying perichondrium when shelling out the exuberant cartilage. Generally, the lower the cartilage level, the greater the lateral extent of resection. The lateral extent of resection will be determined by the final position of the sternum.

A sternal osteotomy is performed at a level determined by the angle and position of protrusion. This allows the sternum not only to be straightened, but also rotated appropriately to the normal anatomical plane. The sternum is fixed in the correct position using absorbable suture, or stainless steel wires depending on the size of the patient.

Next, the free ends of the ribs are fixed to the lateral edge of the sternum with a figure-of-eight absorbable sutures, making sure that they lie flat without protrusion. The xiphisternum is also reattached to the body of the sternum with absorbable sutures.

If there has been multilevel involvement with the risk of chest wall instability, we add STRATOS titanium rib bridges to provide final stability.

The muscles are reapproximated, ensuring that the two pectoralis major muscles on either side are brought together in the midline. This will help determine the final contour of the chest, and allow better healing of the bone beneath. Two drains are inserted and placed in the subcutaneous plane. If the pleural cavity has been entered, a suction catheter is placed at the end of the case to evacuate air. The rest of the tissues are closed in layers and dressing applied. Once the patient is in the recovery room, a chest radiograph is taken to ensure there is no pneumo- or hemothorax.

Poland Syndrome

Poland syndrome is a rare congenital anomaly characterized by hypoplasia of the breast and nipple, absence of the costosternal portion of the pectoralis major muscle, absent pectoralis minor, aplasia or deformity of the costal cartilages and ribs 2–4 or 3–5, alopecia of the axillary and mammary region, and unilateral brachysyndactyly.[15]

Epidemiology and Etiology

The incidence of Poland syndrome ranges from 1 in 7000 to 1 in 100,000 live births. Males are affected more frequently, with a 2:1 to 3:1 ratio. The right side of the body is involved in 60%–75% of patients.[15]

There are a number of theories as to why it develops. One suggests that there is hypoplasia and interruption of the subclavian artery during the 6th week of development. Another theory suggests a disruption of the lateral plate mesoderm affecting the development of the upper limb girdle.[16] There is an association with Klippel–Feil syndrome and Möbius syndrome, with bilateral congenital facial nerve palsy and paralysis of the eye abductors.

Clinical Manifestations

Although there is some variation upon the theme, the most consistent feature is the absence of the sternocostal head of the pectoralis major muscle. The underlying pectoralis minor may be absent altogether. Other chest wall muscles, such as the latissimus dorsi and serratus anterior, may also be absent – which is important when considering surgical soft tissue coverage. In up to a third of females, there is absence of breast development.

Absence of underlying ribs and costal cartilages causes the ipsilateral chest to be sunken. The most frequently absent or hypoplastic ribs are 2–4, or 3–5. As a result, upwards of 10% of patients may also have lung herniation and chest wall instability leading to paradoxical movements during respiration.[15] Hand abnormalities in Poland syndrome include shortness of the middle phalanges with cutaneous webbing (or even full syndactyly), to complete absence of the hand (ectrodactyly). These tend to be ipsilateral to the chest wall anomalies.

Reconstructive Aims and Indications for Surgery

Surgical intervention may be indicated for the following reasons:[15]

- Unilateral depression of the chest wall with cosmetic implications
- Lack of adequate protection of the heart and lung with lung herniation
- Chest wall instability with resulting paradoxical chest movement
- Hypoplasia or aplasia of the female breast.

Surgical Management

This will be influenced by the age and sex of the patient, as well as pattern of involvement. Both the chest wall contiguity and muscular coverage need to be addressed. Many have advocated a two-stage approach in children – first repairing the chest wall defect, followed by a second procedure, which provides chest wall soft tissue coverage and sculpting of the absent anterior axillary fold. A single-stage approach may be reserved for older children and adolescents.

The approach is via a transverse incision – which will provide excellent access not only to the rib defects, but also to the sternum, which may be rotated as part of the constellation of defects.[15] A subperichondral resection of the costal cartilages is performed of the affected rib ends. A sternal osteotomy is performed to allow it to be rotated to the corrected plane. Where there is rib aplasia, rib grafts may be used to bridge the defect. Synthetic mesh has also been used to provide a wider coverage. We have, however, in more recent cases been using artificial bone or STRATOS bars to bridge the defect and provide chest wall stability.[13]

A musculocutaneous flap of the latissimus dorsi can be used for coverage and provide reconstruction of the absent axillary fold. In our center, such cases are performed as a joint procedure between the thoracic and plastic surgeons.

Sternal Cleft

This is a rare malformation characterized by failure of fusion of the sternum in the midline. It may be partial, where there is a U-shaped dip at the upper end of the manubrium, to a more extensive defect extending all the way to the xiphisternum, where there are two bars of bone to which attach the costal cartilages.[17]

This defect in the sternum may occur in isolation, but it may also herald associated anomalies, such as cardiac malformations.[17]

Surgical Approach and Timing

Our preference is to repair this defect in the neonatal period or at least as early as possible, as the more pliable tissues allow for a better chance for primary repair with autologous tissues.

The repair is traditionally carried out via a midline vertical incision and the subcutaneous plane developed over the sternum and adjoining costal cartilages. A wedge osteotomy is performed of the bony bridge between the two sternal bars. This will allow better mobilization when bringing the two sides together without tension.

If the two sides of bone can be brought together, they may be sutured together with either stainless steel wire, or else a heavy absorbable suture. In neonates or early infancy we use heavy absorbable suture. We have recently developed a primary repair with a periosteal flap and sliding osteochondroplasty, thereby avoiding the use of metal implants.[18]

If there is tension laterally, the sternocostal joints may have to be released and resutured or bridged with STRATOS bars.

We close the soft tissues over the bone by suturing the pectoralis major, rectus abdominis, and sternocleidomastoids to their counterparts in the midline. The subcutaneous tissues and skin are then closed primarily to complete the operation.

Jeune Syndrome: Asphyxiating Thoracic Dystrophy

This autosomal recessive condition leads to characteristic skeletal abnormalities in the form of generalized chondrodysplasia, limb defects, mild dwarfism, and importantly, a constricted chest. This latter feature makes the resulting physiological problems particularly difficult to manage.[19]

Epidemiology and Clinical Features

The incidence is 1:100,000 to 1:130,000 live births. Since 2006, this has been classified under the umbrella of *short rib skeletal dysplasias with or without polydactyly.* The natural history of the condition is that the majority of patients do not live beyond the age of 10, mainly from the complications of respiratory or renal failure, which are some of the extraskeletal manifestations of the disease.

Chest Wall Morphology

Failure of normal costal cartilaginous growth leads to cessation of normal chest wall expansion and a persistently narrowed, bell-shaped rib cage. The result of the defect is that the ribs and costal cartilages are shortened, with a fixed horizontal orientation. This results in failure of normal lung development with resulting respiratory failure and pulmonary hypertension, recurrent chest infections and restrictive lung disease.

Chest Wall Surgery

There is no easy surgical solution to the chest wall defects seen in this condition. A number of approaches have been attempted, often through staged interventions.

Lateral thoracic expansion was first outlined in 1995 by Davis et al[20] as a staged approach for patients who are older than 12 months. Dissection is carried down to the beds of the 4th to 9th ribs. Those ribs are divided along their shaft, and their adjoining intercostal muscle released. This will permit the rib to be connected to the rib below by a titanium plate in order to expand the chest. Additional chest wall support is obtained by uniting the supperiosteal tissue of rib bed to its counterpart below. In those where this technique has been used, new bone formation has been demonstrated.[21]

While staged approach seems to contribute to better perioperative management in the past, we demonstrated that single stage bilateral repair offers overall improvement in respiratory dynamics in such a way that the ventilatory as well hemodynamic managements become simpler when bilateral surgery is performed at the same time.[22] The operative time is shortened overall, as well as the length of intensive care time, thereby potentially limiting the risk of overall morbidity and burden of care.

Less frequently, there are reports of the modified Nuss technique being used to provide expansion. In the former technique, two bars are implanted bilaterally to provide expansion in the lateral plate. It has been reserved for older children and is limited by the need for a bar change.

More recently, thoracoplasty using the vertical expandable titanium rib technique, has been described.[23] A vertical titanium device is anchored bilaterally to ribs 2 and 10. Ribs 3–8 are then transected and pulled laterally, and finally connected to the titanium device. Growth is allowed by progressively adjusting the device.

ACQUIRED DEFECTS

Oliver J. Smith, Robert Pearl, and Simon Withey

In adult patients the acquisition of chest wall defects almost always occurs due to one of four etiologies: midline sternal wound dehiscence following cardiothoracic surgery; trauma; neoplasms; tissue damage secondary to radiotherapy. Each of these pathologies presents different reconstructive challenges in relation to patient factors such as overall health and adjuvant therapy, and local factors such as tissue quality, infection, and excision margins.

Sternal Wound Dehiscence

The midline sternotomy incision was introduced into cardiac surgery in the 1950s. Early management of sternal wound dehiscence involved debridement and packing of the wound, leaving it to heal by secondary intention. This led to high mortality rates with surviving patients often requiring prolonged hospitalization. In the 1970s the technique of early debridement and introduction of fresh, well-vascularized omental flaps into the wound defect was pioneered by Lee et al.[24] The use of muscle flaps to reconstruct the sternal dehiscence was developed from this,[25] and has become the gold standard treatment leading to a significant reduction in mortality rates.[26]

Etiology

Wound dehiscence is reported in 0.5%–5% of midline sternotomies and is a serious complication which can lead to potentially fatal mediastinitis.[27] The primary underlying causative factor in dehiscence in most patients is partial or complete devascularization of the hemisternum after harvest of the internal mammary artery (IMA) for cardiac bypass. When both IMAs are harvested the risk of wound complications increases dramatically.[28] Risk is increased in patients who are already suffering with underlying vascular disease and are therefore less able to perfuse the sternum through collateral circulation, such as those with poorly controlled diabetes or heavy smokers. Other generalized factors such as obesity, cardiac or respiratory failure, or immunosuppression also increase the risk, as well as local factors such as previous chest wall irradiation.

Infection is often not the causative factor of wound dehiscence and is usually a secondary complication. A wide range

TABLE 39.1 **Pairolero's Classification and Starzynski's Classification of Sternal Defects**

Pairolero	Presentation	Timing
Type I	Serosanguinous discharge only	0–3 days
Type II	Cellulitis and purulent mediastinitis	3 days to 3 weeks
Type III	Chronic sinus and osteomyelitis	Months to years
Starzynski	**Anatomical Involvement**	**Physiological Deficit**
1	Upper sternal body and adjacent ribs (2–5)	Mild
2	Entire sternal body and adjacent ribs (2–7)	Moderate
3	Manubrium, upper sternal body and ribs (1–5)	Severe

of Gram-positive and negative organisms can be detected from wound cultures, with the commonest being *Staphylococcus aureus* and *Pseudomonas aeruginosa.*[29] However, organisms cultured may not be pathologically active and may be commensal to the wound surface. Antibiotic resistance in organisms that are active in causing infection is becoming a serious problem and treatment will be based on local guidelines.

Pairolero and Arnold[30] proposed a classification system of sternal wound infections as outlined in Table 39.1. However, this is limited by the fact that it fails to categorize the degree of vascularity in these wounds and is focused mainly on the secondary complication of infection. Starzynski[31] categorizes sternal defects based on the degree of anatomical involvement following operative debridement. This can help to predict the degree of physiological compromise, however as all patients react differently, its use clinically can be limited.

Preoperative Management

Preoperative planning is key to ensuring successful management of wound dehiscence and a multidisciplinary team approach is essential. A full history should be taken, paying particular attention to any previous cardiothoracic or abdominal surgeries which may affect the reconstructive options. The patient should be optimized medically prior to any major reconstructive procedures and they should be seen regularly by a dietitian to improve their nutritional status. Early involvement of the microbiology team is important to ensure the correct antibiotics are prescribed and wound swabs or tissue samples from the wound should be sent early and at each stage of debridement. Imaging is of limited use, although in selected chronic cases a CT scan may provide information on the extent of bone necrosis or osteomyelitis. Prior to surgery, a full anesthetic assessment should be undertaken. If a patient is too unwell for reconstruction or radical debridement then a limited debridement and washout followed by medical optimization may buy some time.

Debridement

The wound should be irrigated extensively and all non-viable tissue removed; multiple tissue and bone samples should be sent for microbiological culture. The bone of the devascularized hemisternum will be soft and there is often purulent fluid in the bone and tissues. Any bone that does not feel firm in the teeth of a bone nibbler should be removed along with any affected costal cartilages. When undertaking this debridement great care should be taken when mobilizing the sternum so as not to damage the underlying pericardium, myocardium or vasculature. Any sharp bony edges should be removed before finishing the debridement to ensure that these do not penetrate deeply and cause damage. The risk of damage from sharp bony edges is increased when negative-pressure therapy is used.

In some cases, immediate reconstructive surgery following debridement is appropriate, however this depends on the health of the patient and whether the surgeon is confident that the debridement is complete. In patients who are on large doses of inotropic or vasopressive support, the process of devsacularization of the sternum may continue. In cases where the patient is not fit or ready for reconstruction then careful use of negative-pressure therapy may be appropriate.

Negative-Pressure Therapy

Vacuum therapy, in the form of a sponge dressing and negative-pressure pump, can assist in reducing wound oedema and bacterial load. It is a very useful temporizing therapy in sternal wound dehiscence as it can buy time in the unstable patient. It also helps in restoring a degree of thoracic integrity by splinting the sternal defect, encouraging wound contracture and a fibrous union. This can help the patient to mobilise earlier and reduce the time they are dependent on ventilatory support.

Neoplasms

Chest wall tumors, if large enough, can cause significant chest wall defects requiring reconstructive surgery to fill skin defects or provide stability to the thorax. Their etiology can be split into: primary chest wall lesions (e.g., sarcoma); invading adjacent malignancies (e.g., breast, lung); and metastases.

Management

Multidisciplinary management of patients with complex chest wall tumors is essential and a close relationship should be developed between the surgical and oncological teams to ensure the best treatment outcome. Prior to reconstructive surgery, patient factors such as expectation the surgery will be curative, prognosis and adjuvant therapy should be considered. Local factors, such as size of the defect, and previous surgery or irradiation, also affect reconstructive options. Planning of the likely reconstructive flap should be done before resection of the primary lesion is undertaken so that the flap and its vascular supply are preserved.

Chest Wall Radiation

A relatively large proportion of patients with breast cancer, and other malignancies, will undergo radiotherapy treatment of the chest wall. This can lead to tissue and bone damage through cell death and a compromise in blood supply. Osteoradionecrosis is a rare side effect that can occur years after treatment and may present with chest pain due to pathological fractures or chronic non-healing wounds. Reconstruction of defects associated with radiation damage is complicated by poor vascularity and fibrosis of local tissues. Local flaps are often limited by both of these factors and the quality of recipient blood vessels may limit the use of free tissue transfer. All of these factors must be considered before embarking on resection of nonviable tissue in order to minimize the reconstructive requirements.

Chest Wall Trauma

It is rare that trauma to the chest requires reconstructive surgery, however it can be required in some cases of high-energy injury. In these patients the priority is always immediate management of life-threatening injuries by a multi-disciplinary team and stabilization of the patient. Once a patient is well enough, reconstruction can be planned, but there may be limitations on the types of flaps that can be offered as these are dependent on the degree of tissue loss or damage.

Reconstruction of Chest Wall Defects

Two factors are crucial to ensuring adequate reconstruction of the chest wall:

1. Does the thoracic cage require supporting to ensure its stability?
2. Which type of tissue reconstruction is best suited to a particular patient? Here the surgeon must bear in mind systemic and local factors whilst also choosing the best flap that will obliterate any dead space and provide strong soft tissue coverage.

Restoring Stability of the Thoracic Cage

When a chest wall defect involves loss of a significant part of the underlying bony thoracic cage (more than four ribs or an area >5 cm), structural reconstruction is often required to maintain mechanical integrity, preserve pulmonary compliance, and to ensure protection of the thoracic viscera.[32] However, larger defects in the upper posterior chest wall can usually be tolerated without structural support due to the stability provided by the scapula. Similarly, structural stabilization can be avoided in the anterior chest wall due to the splinting effects of the sternum, clavicles, and large muscles. Even when part or all of the sternum is lost due to debridement, the loss of mechanical stability rarely occurs due to the development of a fibrous union. The opportunity to use structural support in the form of metalwork or prothesis is contraindicated in cases of infection.

Choice of Structural Support

Prostheses are an excellent choice for structural support of the thoracic cage, as they avoid donor site morbidity and they allow the reconstruction of much larger defects than autologous tissue alone could achieve. The types of prostheses available can be split into synthetic/composite meshes (e.g., prolene, Gore-Tex) and allograft (e.g., Alloderm) or xenograft (e.g., Strattice, Permacol, Surgimend) biomaterials. Use of an individual type of prothesis often comes down to surgeon preference and availability.

Synthetic/composite meshes can be contoured well to the chest wall, however their use can be complicated by infection and seromas. If infection occurs then the entire prosthesis will need removal. Stronger structural support, such as titanium plates, may be required for additional stability and these are usually combined with a synthetic or biomaterial prosthesis.

The use of biomaterials in the form of acellular dermal matrices (ADM) is becoming commonplace in chest wall reconstruction, particularly after oncological resection. These come in the form of allografts or xenografts. The basic principle of these biomaterials is that the cellular components have been removed, preventing an immune response, whilst also allowing vascularization and tissue integration at the recipient bed. They are not rigid materials but they do help in stabilizing tissues and reducing paradoxical movement. ADMs can be used in combination with pedicled or free tissue flaps to good effect,[33] however there is little evidence to support one type of biomaterial prosthesis over another. Risks include infection, which may be increased when they are used in high-risk areas such as irradiated beds or sites of fungating tumors.[34]

Soft Tissue Coverage

As with all aspects of plastic surgery, there are a myriad of options for chest wall reconstruction and each defect must be treated individually. In some cases of very large defects, a combination of flaps may be required or free tissue transfer may be the best option. However, the majority of chest wall defects can be treated with the following four pedicled flaps:

- Pectoralis major

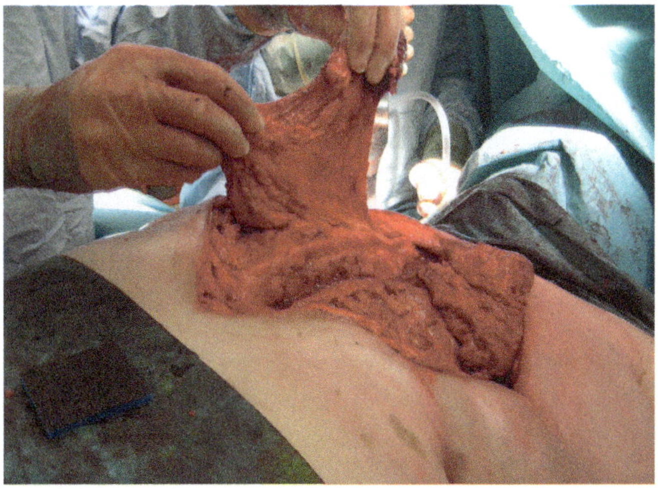

• **Fig. 39.4** Pectoralis major raised as a turnover flap based on the IMA perforators.

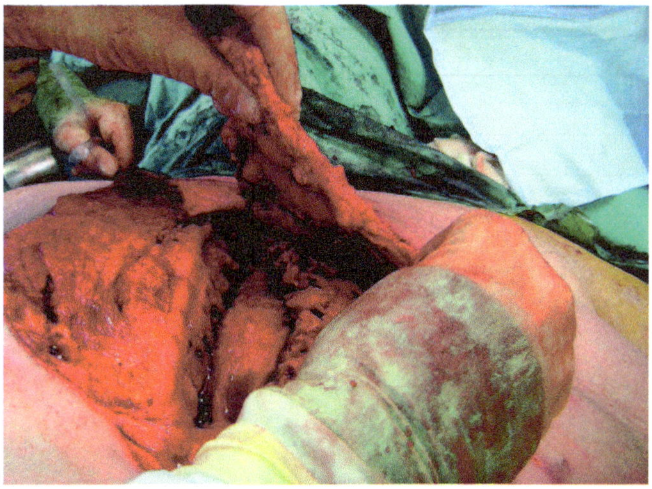

• **Fig. 39.5** Pectoralis major raised as an advancement flap based on the thoracoacromial vessels.

- Omentum
- Latissimus dorsi
- Rectus abdominis

Pectoralis Major Flap

The pectoralis major muscle flap is supplied by a single dominant vessel from the thoracoacromial axis as well as multiple small perforators medially from the IMA (Type V blood supply). It can therefore be advanced on its lateral supply from its dominant pedicle after division of the tendinous insertion, or used as a turnover flap on the medial vessels (provided the IMA on this side has not been previously harvested). A combination of both a turnover flap from one side (Fig. 39.4) and an advancement from the other (Fig. 39.5) is a highly effective method of filling the dead space and providing soft tissue coverage to the sternum. The pectoralis flap is therefore a highly versatile workhorse for reconstruction of sternal wound dehiscence or for central defects left following tumor resection. However care should be taken when using this flap in female patients with large breast volume, as harvesting both the IMA perforators and thoracoacromial supply may devascularize the breast tissue leading to significant fat necrosis, particularly when perfusion pressures are low in an unwell patient.

Prior to utilizing this flap for reconstruction it is important that a full surgical history is obtained, particularly as the left IMA is typically harvested for cardiac bypass surgery and therefore could not be used as a turnover flap on this side. Bilateral IMA harvest is rare and therefore the right pectoralis major can often be mobilized on its IMA perforators. The use of this flap in cases of osteoradionecrosis is often limited as it is likely to be within the previously irradiated field.

Omental Flap

The greater omentum is a large fold of visceral peritoneum which extends from the greater curvature of the stomach and hangs over the intestines. It has two individual dominant vascular pedicles (left and right gastroepiploic arteries), meaning it is a richly vascularized piece of tissue which has sufficient bulk to reconstruct large chest wall defects. In those patients with large defects it is very effective in forming tissue fibrosis, which improves the structural integrity of the chest and assists in respiratory rehabilitation. It is particularly useful in cases of osteoradionecrosis, as it provides large volume vascularized tissue which is well away from the irradiated area. Previous abdominal surgery and episodes of peritonitis may prevent its use and a full history should be taken.

The omentum can be harvested either laparoscopically or via an upper midline laparotomy incision. The larger right gastroepiploic vessel is the preferred pedicle to harvest the flap on, and this can be identified by transilluminating the omentum near the greater curvature of the stomach. To deliver the flap to the chest, it can either be tunneled subcutaneously over the costal margin or via a window in the anterior diaphragmatic tendon. A large tunnel is often required due to the size and bulk of the flap and therefore there is a risk of herniation of abdominal viscera. Our preferred technique involves the creation of a generous transdiaphragmatic window to allow passage of the flap and to prevent compression of the pedicle. A second omental flap is then created and is wrapped around the pedicle and sutured to the diaphragmatic defect on the abdominal side (Figs. 39.6 and 39.7). This obliterates the defect and helps to prevent herniation of abdominal contents into the chest.[35]

Latissimus Dorsi (LD) Flap

The LD flap is a common workhorse flap that is simple to harvest and provides reliable coverage to most anterolateral chest defects with minimal donor site morbidity. It can be raised as a muscle-only flap or with an attached skin paddle. As with the pectoralis major, the LD has a type V blood supply, with the thoracodorsal pedicle being its dominant supply and the tendinous insertion into the humerus can be divided to allow greater mobilization. The LD can also be advanced or transposed to cover defects on the back, or it

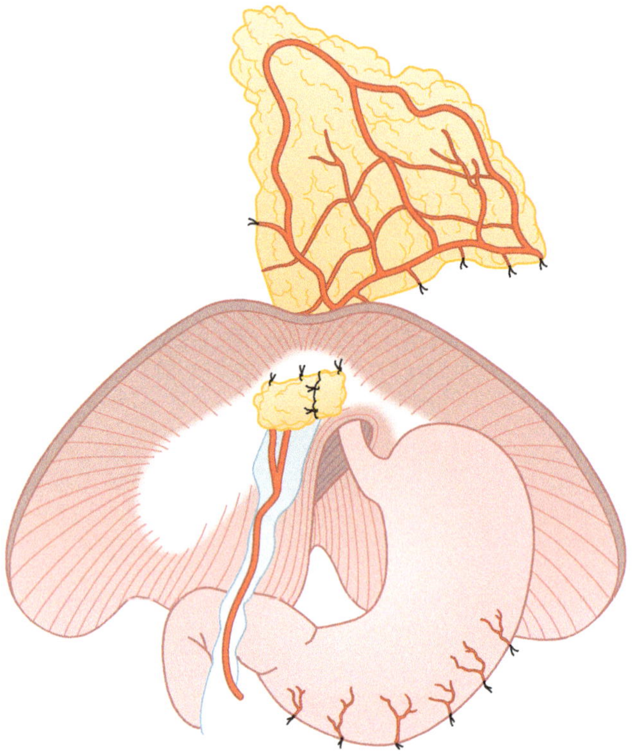

• **Fig. 39.6** The "omental wrap." (From Tansley P, Kakar S and Withey S. A novel modification of omental transposition to reduce the risk of gastrointestinal herniation into the chest. *Plast Reconstr Surg*. 2006;118(3):676–680. Reproduced with permission from Lippincott Williams & Wilkins.)

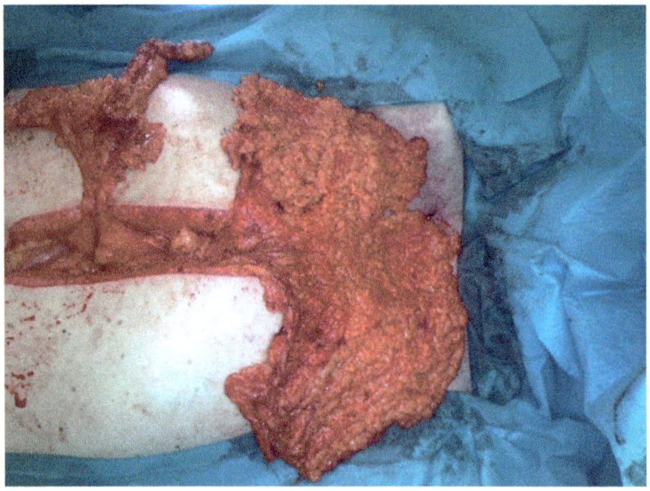

• **Fig. 39.7** The omental flap raised with secondary flap isolated.

can be raised on its secondary lumbar perforators and used as a turnover flap.

Rectus Abdominis

As with the greater omentum, the rectus abdominis has two dominant vascular pedicles (inferior and superficial epigastric arteries), and it is therefore a type III muscle flap. When reconstructing lower chest wall defects it is raised on its superior pedicle and transposed into the defect with the pivot point at the costal margin. It can be used as a muscle-only flap, or with an attached vertical (VRAM) or transverse (TRAM) skin paddle. The superior epigastric vessel is supplied from the IMA and therefore in instances where this has been harvested flap reliability is unpredictable, although it may remain perfused through communication with intercostal vessels. A good tip is to preserve a length of the deep inferior epigastric artery and vein when harvesting the flap, as this allows supercharging if perfusion is inadequate.

Congenital Chest Wall Defects in the Adult Patient

Although the management of congenital chest wall defects has been covered in the previous section, patients with congenital defects can also present in adulthood. These patients are often asymptomatic and their concerns are usually esthetic. A full history should bc taken in order to identify the patient's goals with regards to the surgery.

With regards to pectus carinatum and excavatum, the treatment offered in adult patients is much the same as described in the previous section.

In adult cases of Poland syndrome, these patients are often treated with custom-made pectoral silicon implants in order to camouflage the defect. Although these are modelled to the patient's anatomy, they are often mobile, leading to positional changes of the implants known as "ghosting." This is particularly noticed by patients on standing where the lower pole of the implant often rides too inferiorly and the border can be palpable beneath the anatomical confines of the chest. To prevent this phenomenon, an indent can be created in the inferior aspect of the prosthesis which allows it to straddle the linea alba, preventing movement inferiorly.

References

1. Fokin AA, Steuerwald NM, Ahrens WA, et al. Anatomical, histologic and genetic characteristics of congenital chest wall deformities. *Semin Thorac Cardiovasc Surg*. 2009;21:44–57.
2. Harcke HT, Grissom LE, Lee MS, et al. Common congenital skeletal anomalies of the thorax. *J Thorac Imaging*. 1986;1:1–6.
3. Tocchioni F, Ghionzoli M, Messineo A, et al. Pectus excavatum and heritable disorders of the connective tissue. *Pediatr Rep*. 2013;5:15.
4. Swanson JW, Avansino JR, Phillips GS, et al. Correlating Haller Index and cardiopulmonary disease in pectus excavatum. *Am J Surg*. 2012;203:660–664.
5. Malek MH, Berger DE, HoushTJ, et al. Cardiovascular function following surgical repair of pectus excavatum: a meta-analysis. *Chest*. 2006;130:506–516.
6. Kim DH, Hwang JJ, Lee MK, et al. Analysis of the Nuss procedure for pectus excavatum in different age groups. *Ann Thorac Surg*. 2005;80:1073–1077.
7. Nuss D. Minimally invasive surgical repair of pectus excavatum. *Semin Pediatr Surg*. 2008;17:209–217.
8. Schalamon J, Pokall S, Windhaber J, et al. Minimally invasive correction of pectus excavatum in adult patients. *J Thorac Cardiovasc Surg*. 2006;132:524–529.

9. Dzielicki J, Korlacki W, Janicka I, et al. Difficulties and limitations in minimally invasive repair of pectus excavatum-6 years experience with Nuss technique. *Eur J Cardio Thorac Surg.* 2006;30:801–804.
10. Ravitch MM. Unusual sternal deformity with cardiac symptoms: operative correction. *J Thorac Surg.* 1952;23:138.
11. Leonhardt J, Kubler J, Feiter J, et al. Complications of the minimally invasive repair of pectus excavatum. *J Pediatr Surg.* 2005;40:e7-e9.
12. Lester CW. Pigeon breast (pectus carinatum) and other protrusion deformities of the chest of developmental origin. *Ann Surg.* 1953;137:482–489.
13. Brichon PY, Wihlm JM. Correction of a severe pouter pigeon breast by triple sternal osteotomy with a novel titanium rib bridge fixation. *Ann Thorac Surg.* 2010;90(6):e97–e99.
14. Muthialu N, McIntyre D, McIntosh N, et al. Disturbingly high fracture rate of STRATOS bars in pectus corrections. *Eur J Cardio Thorac Surg.* 2019;55(2):300–303.
15. Ravitch MM. Poland's syndrome. In: Ravitch MM, ed. *Congenital Deformities of the Chest Wall and Their Operative Correction.* Philadelphia: WB Saunders; 1977:233–271.
16. Bavinck JNB, Weaver DD. Subclavian artery supply disruption sequence: hypothesis of a vascular etiology for Poland, Klippel–Feil, and Möbius anomalies. *Am J Med Genet.* 1986;23:903–918.
17. Biswas G, Khandelwal NK, Venkatramu NK, et al. Congenital sternal cleft. *Br J Plast Surg.* 2001;54:259–261.
18. Muthialu N. Primary repair of sternal cleft in infancy using combined periosteal flap and sliding osteochondroplasty. *Interact Cardiovasc Thorac Surg.* 2013;16(6):923–925.
19. Phillips JD, van Aalst JA. Jeune's syndrome (asphyxiating thoracic dystrophy): congenital and acquired. *Semin Pediatr Surg.* 2008;17(3):167–172.
20. Davis JT, Ruberg RL, Lippink DM, et al. Lateral thoracic expansion for Jeune's asphyxiating dystrophy: a new approach. *Ann Thorac Surg.* 1995;60:694–696.
21. Davis JT, Long FR, Adler BH, et al. Lateral thoracic expansion for Jeune syndrome: evidence of rib healing and new bone formation. *Ann Thorac Surg.* 2004;77:445–448.
22. Muthialu N, Mussa S, Owens CM, et al. One-stage sequential bilateral thoracic expansion for asphyxiating thoracic dystrophy (Jeune syndrome). *Eur J Cardio Thorac Surg.* 2014;46(4):643–647.
23. Waldhausen JHT, Redding GJ, Song KM. Vertical expandable prosthetic titanium rib for thoracic insufficiency syndrome: a new method to treat an old problem. *J Pediatr Surg.* 2007;42(1):76–80.
24. Lee AB, Schimert G, Shatkin S, et al. Total excision of the sternum and thoracic pedicle transposition of the greater omentum. *Surgery.* 1976;80:433.
25. Jurkiewicz MJ, Bostwick J, Hester TR, et al. Infected median sternotomy wound: successful treatment by muscle flaps. *Ann Surg.* 1980;191:738.
26. Lazar HL, Salm TV, Engelman R, et al. Prevention and management of sternal wound infections. *J Thorac Cardiovasc Surg.* 2016;152:962.
27. Olbrecht VA, Barreiro CJ, Bonde PN, et al. Clinical outcomes of noninfectious sternal dehiscence after median sternotomy. *Ann Thorac Surg.* 2006;82:902.
28. Kouchoukos NT, Wareing TH, Murphy SF, et al. Risks of bilateral internal mammary artery bypass grafting. *Ann Thorac Surg.* 1990;49:210–219.
29. Ma JG, An JX. Deep sternal wound infection after cardiac surgery: a comparison of three different wound infection types and an analysis of antibiotic resistance. *J Thorac Dis.* 2018;10(1):377–387.
30. Pairolero PC, Arnold PG. Management of infected median sternotomy wounds. *Ann Thorac Surg.* 1986;42:1e2.
31. Starzynski TE, Snyderman RK, Beattie EJ. Problems of major chest wall reconstruction. *Plast Reconstr Surg.* 1969;44(6):525–535.
32. Chang RR, Mehrara BJ, Hu Qun-Ying, et al. Reconstruction of complex oncologic defect: a 10 year experience. *Ann Plast Surg.* 2004;52(5):471–478; discussion 479.
33. Catherine CC, Gallego K, Anderson ED, et al. Chest wall reconstruction with acellular dermal matrix (AlloDerm) and a latissimus muscle flap. *Plast Reconstr Surg.* 2004;114(4): 1015–1017.
34. Weyant MJ, Bains MS, Venkatraman E, et al. Results of chest wall resection and reconstruction with and without rigid prosthesis. *Ann Thorac Surg.* 2006;81:279–285.
35. Tansley P, Kakar S, Withey S. A novel modification of omental transposition to reduce the risk of gastrointestinal herniation into the chest. *Plast Reconstr Surg.* 2006;118(3):676–680.

40 Abdominal Wall Reconstruction

ANNE C. O'NEILL, WILLIAM A. TOWNLEY, AND STEFAN O.P. HOFER

Anatomy

The abdominal wall is a multilayered structure that wraps around and protects the abdominal viscera. In addition, it is involved in numerous other functions including trunk movement, respiratory effort (active expiration), and an adjunctive force in micturition and defecation. Anatomically, it is bound by the xiphoid process and costal margin superiorly and the iliac crests and pubis inferiorly.

The abdominal wall consists of skin, superficial fat, muscles, transversalis fascia, and parietal peritoneum.

Skin, Subcutaneous Fat, and Fascia

The skin envelope of the abdomen is compliant and of intermediate thickness. Traditionally, two distinct layers of fascia are recognized – Camper's fascia and Scarpa's fascia. Camper's fascia represents the superficial layer, which contains variable amounts of fat. In males it is continuous with dartos fascia in the penis. Scarpa's fascia is deeper and more fibrous. Scarpa's fascia merges with the deep thigh fascia and superficial perineal fascia to contribute to fascia lata and Colles' fascia, respectively. In reality, it is more practical to think of three layers between the skin and abdominal musculature – superficial fat, membranous fascial layer (Scarpa's), and deep fat. The superficial fat layer is evenly distributed throughout the abdomen and is more vascular. The deeper fat layer is of variable thickness, being thicker in the upper abdomen compared with the lower abdomen.[1]

Muscles

The central abdominal wall is formed by the two paired rectus abdominis muscles and pyrimidalis muscles inferiorly.

The paired rectus abdominis muscles are long and flat muscles involved in trunk flexion, forced expiration, and in creating increased abdominal pressure such as in coughing. They originate from the pubic symphysis and pubic crest and insert into the xyphoid process and costal cartilages 5–7, interdigitating with the inferior fibers of pectoralis major. The two paired muscles are enclosed within the rectus sheath and separated from each other by a midline band of connective tissue, the linea alba. The vertical muscle fibers are separated by three or four tendinous interconnections, which are horizontal bands of connective tissue. It is a type III muscle with a dual co-dominant blood supply (deep inferior and superior epigastric arteries). It is segmentally innervated from the 7th to 11th intercostal nerves.

The pyrimidalis muscles originate from the pubis and insert into the linea alba.

The lateral abdominal wall muscles include three sets of paired muscles — external oblique, internal oblique, and transversus abdominis, which all contribute to the rectus sheath medially (Fig. 40.1).

The external oblique is the most superficial and largest of the three lateral muscles. It originates from ribs 5–12 and runs in an inferiomedial direction to insert into the linea semilunaris, where it contributes to the anterior rectus sheath, and iliac crest. The aponeurosis of external oblique forms the inguinal ligament inferiorly. It is innervated and nourished by the intercostal neurovascular bundles (intercostal nerves 5–12).

The internal oblique originates from the thoracolumbar fascia and iliac crest and runs in a superomedial direction, perpendicular to the external oblique fibers. It becomes aponeurotic medially contributing to both anterior and posterior rectus sheath before inserting into the linea alba and ribs 10–12. It is innervated by the lower intercostal nerves and the first lumbar spinal nerve. There are multiple source vessels feeding the muscle, including the deep circumflex iliac artery, deep inferior epigastric artery and lower intercostal vessels.

The transversus abdominis is the deepest of the three lateral muscles and runs transversely towards the midline from the iliac crest and thoracolumbar fascia. The transversalis fascia is a continuous fascial sheet that lies on the deep surface of transversus abdominis.

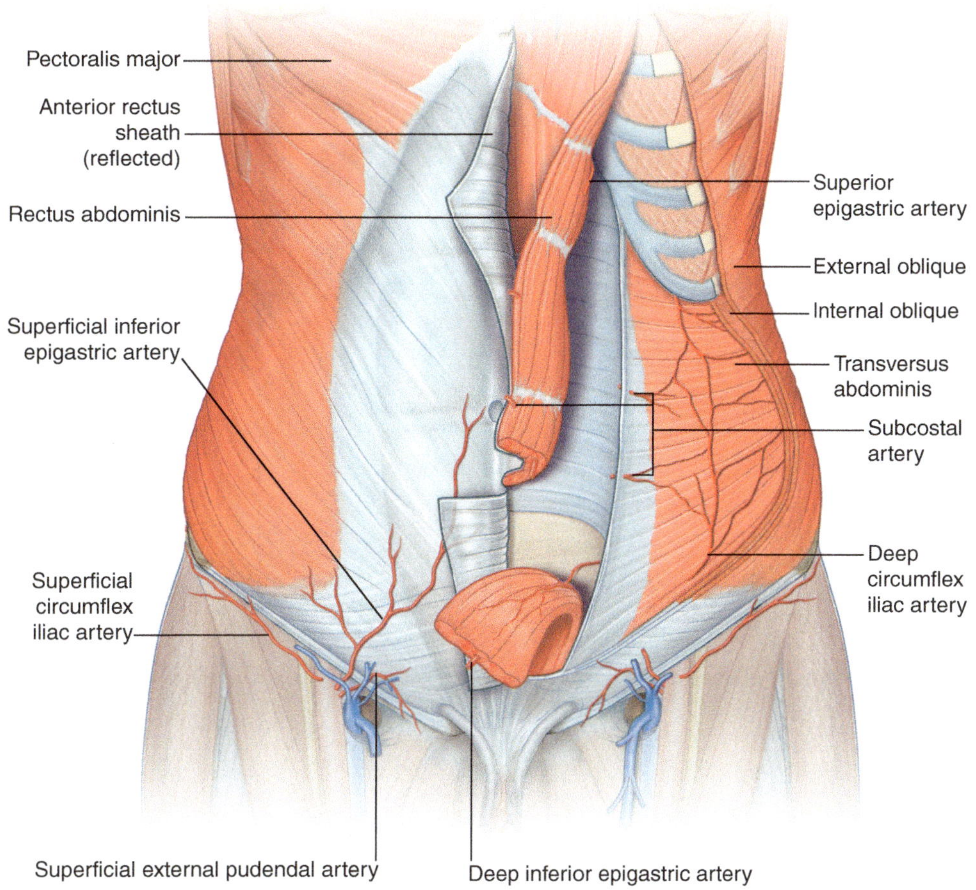

• **Fig. 40.1** Anteroposterior view of abdominal wall muscles (lateral and central components). (From Richter DF, Schwaiger N. Abdominoplasty procedures. In: Rubin JP, Neligan PC, eds. *Plastic Surgery*. Volume 2: *Aesthetic Surgery* 4th edn. Philadelphia: Elsevier; 2018: Fig. 23.2A.)

Blood Supply

The blood supply of the abdominal wall is robust, with multiple independent sources and extensive collateralization. Huger considered the skin and subcutaneous components of the abdominal wall in terms of three zones of perfusion, as illustrated in Fig. 40.2.[2]

Zone I encompasses the central abdominal tissue overlying the paired rectus abdominis muscles. It is bound by the xyphoid process, pubic symphysis, and lateral edges of the rectus sheath. The skin and subcutaneous tissue of Zone I is perfused by musculocutaneous perforators from the deep inferior epigastric (branch of external iliac artery) and to a lesser extent the superior epigastric arteries (branch of internal mammary artery). The perforators are predominantly arranged in two rows – medial and lateral. The highest concentration of perforators is within 3 cm of the umbilicus. The medial row perforators provide greater perfusion across the midline than their lateral counterparts.[3]

Zone II refers to the lower abdominal wall, below the line of the anterior superior iliac spines. Zone II is perfused by three separate branches of the common femoral artery – the superficial circumflex femoral artery, the superficial inferior epigastric artery, and the external pudendal artery. Zone III refers to the flank and abdominal wall lateral to the rectus muscles. It is supplied by the lower intercostal arteries and first lumbar artery – a robust blood supply that can perfuse the entire abdominal wall after division of Huger's Zone 1 and II as demonstrated after an abdominoplasty.

Innervation

The motor and sensory innervation of the anterior abdominal wall is derived from the anterior rami of the 7th to 12th intercostals and first lumbar root. The intercostal neurovascular abdominal bundles pierce the transversus abdominis and travel in a plane deep to internal oblique. Preservation of the motor supply is essential for maintaining the integrity of the abdominal wall to prevent hernia formation or bulging.

Fascia

A detailed understanding of the fascia of the abdominal wall muscles is essential in abdominal wall surgery

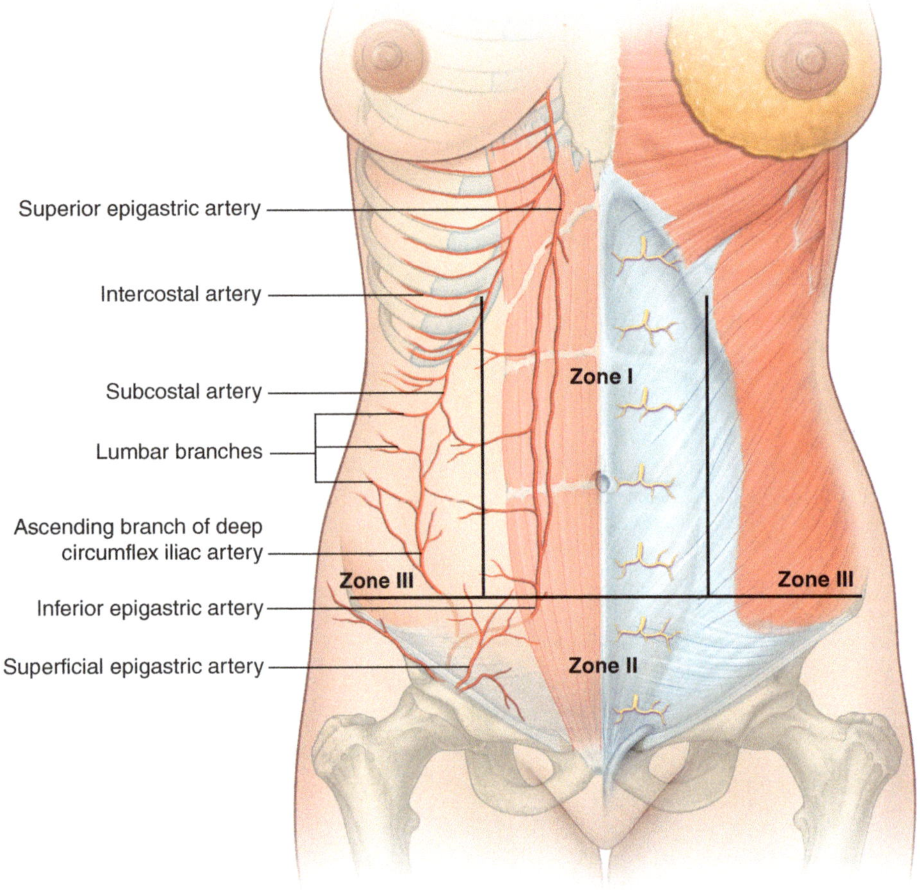

• **Fig. 40.2** Huger's abdominal skin perfusion zones. (From Richter DF, Schwaiger N. Abdominoplasty procedures. In: Rubin JP, Neligan PC, eds. *Plastic Surgery*. Volume 2: *Aesthetic Surgery*. 4th edn. Philadelphia: Elsevier; 2018: Fig. 23.4.)

(Fig. 40.3). The rectus sheath is formed laterally at the linea semilunaris by the condensation of the aponeuroses of external oblique, internal oblique, and transversus abdominis. The anterior rectus abdominis is covered by sheath throughout its course. Posteriorly, the rectus is covered by sheath only above the arcuate line, a transverse line at the level of the anterior superior iliac spine. Below the arcuate line, only transversalis fascia and parietal peritoneum lie deep to the rectus.

Above the arcuate line, the anterior rectus sheath is composed of external oblique and the superficial leaf of the internal oblique fascia, whereas the posterior rectus sheath is formed by the condensation of deep leaf of internal oblique and transversus abdominis fascia. Below the arcuate line, the transversus abdominis fascia and deep leaf of the internal oblique fascia also contribute to the anterior rectus sheath, whereas the posterior rectus sheath is devoid of muscular aponeurosis. The rectus abdominis muscle is tightly adherent to the sheath at the tendinous intersections.

Etiology and Classification of Abdominal Wall Hernia Defects

Abdominal wall hernias can be congenital or acquired. Congenital hernias include umbilical hernias, periumbilical hernias, Spigelian hernias (between rectus and linea semilunaris), lumbar hernais, and epigastric hernias. Gastroschisis and omphalocele represent two severe types of congenital abdominal wall defects that are commonly associated with other developmental anomalies. An omphalocele is a large defect where the abdominal contents protrude through the umbilicus and are maintained in a peritoneal sac. A gastroschisis is a smaller defect where the abdominal contents protrude freely without coverage from the peritoneum. Both conditions occur infrequently (1 in 5000 births) but are often detected antenatally by ultrasound.[4]

Most acquired hernias are iatrogenic and arise in a previous surgical incision. Other acquired causes include infection, trauma, and tumors. There are a number of known risk factors for incisional hernias. Systemic factors include poor

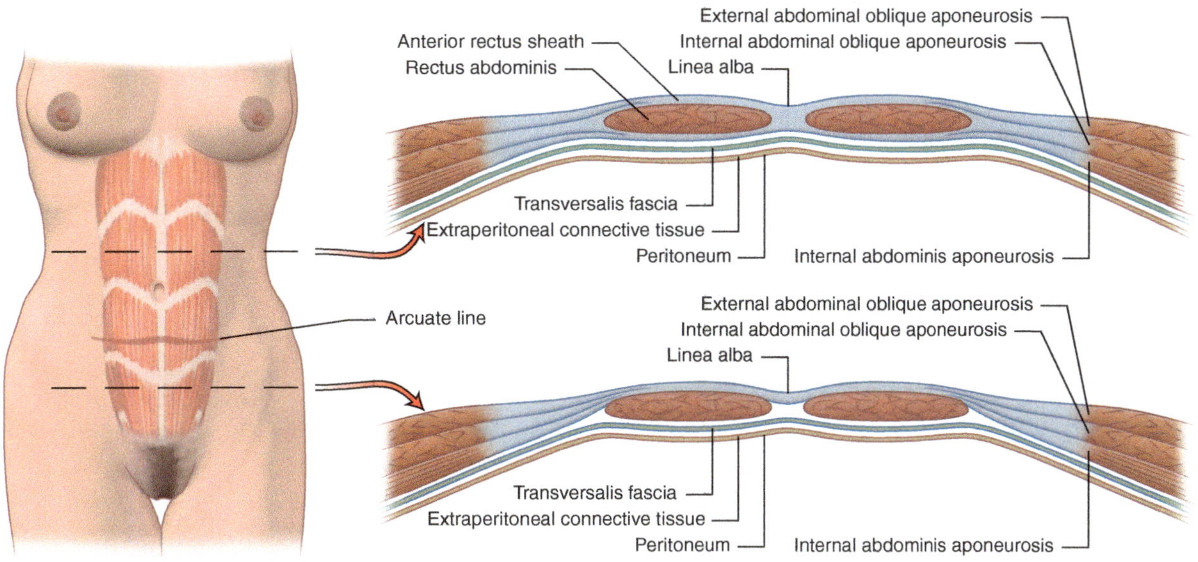

• **Fig. 40.3** Formation of rectus sheath above and below the arcuate line. (From Hunstad JP, Repta R. *Atlas of Abdominoplasty*. Philadelphia: Elsevier; 2009: Fig. 2.4DEF)

intrinsic wound healing, obesity, older age, comorbidities, and malignancy. Local factors include suboptimal wound closure, infection, ischemia, prior radiation, increased intraabdominal pressure and prolonged ventilation. Initial surgical technique plays an important role in the prevention of hernias with evidence suggesting that low dehiscence rates are best achieved by taking wide tissue bites (>1 cm from the fascia margin) with short stitch intervals (1 cm) and avoiding strangulating tension on the suture. However, even in the absence of identified risk factors, incisional hernias develop in 11% of primary laparotomies and may be as high as 33% in obese patients.[5] Recurrent incisional hernias are especially challenging and the incidence of recurrent herniation after repair increases with each subsequent hernia repair operation.[6]

The European Hernia Society has proposed a classification system of abdominal hernias to deliver conformity and allow ease of comparison in published clinical studies.[7] This classification system distinguishes between primary and incisional ventral hernias. For primary ventral hernias, the two parameters are location and size (hernia diameter), as illustrated in Table 40.1. The location is subdivided into midline defects (epigastric, umbilical) and lateral defects (Spigelian, lumbar). For incisional hernias, there are additional criteria, including whether the hernia is recurrent or not.

TABLE 40.1 European Hernia Society Classification of Primary Ventral Hernias

Location		Diameter		
		Small <2 cm	Medium ≥2–4 cm	Large ≥4 cm
Midline	Epigastric			
	Umbilical			
Lateral	Spigelian			
	Lumbar			

ASSESSMENT OF THE ABDOMINAL WOUND

Clinical

Initial assessment must start with an appropriately directed clinical history and physical examination. Local and systemic risk factors for impaired wound healing should be identified. A clear history and timeline of the wound must be elucidated to determine whether it is acute or chronic in nature. Any prior surgical interventions and their effects should be noted.

The examination should evaluate both the wound itself and the quality of the surrounding tissues. The abdomen should be inspected for scars, fistulas, sinuses, radiation injury or evidence active infection. The wound should be characterized in detail and include evaluation and documentation of the components that are absent. In chronic wounds the potential for malignant change should be considered and ruled-out with tissue biopsy where indicated.

Imaging

Preoperative imaging is very helpful in defining the pathology and in preoperative planning. Both abdominal computed tomography (CT) and magnetic resonance imaging (MRI) can successfully identify the extent of the abdominal wall defect and the integrity of adjacent musculofascial structures. However, CT angiography (i.e., with intravenous contrast) is superior at delineating the vascular anatomy, especially when planning pedicled flaps or free tissue transfer (Fig. 40.4). An abdominal and pelvic CT scan with

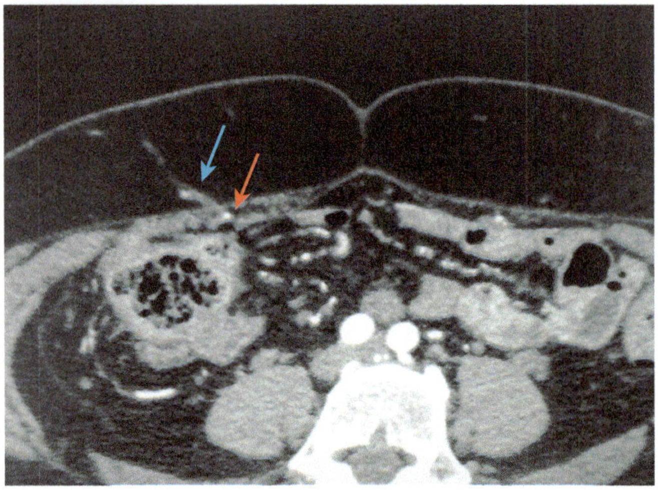

• **Fig. 40.4** CT image demonstrating a musculocutaneous perforator (*blue arrow*) traversing the rectus abdominis muscle from the right deep inferior epigastric artery (*red arrow*) at the level of the umbilicus.

oral contrast enables detailed understanding of the wound and intraabdominal contents.

Goals of Reconstruction

The goal of abdominal wall reconstruction is twofold. The first goal is to restore function and integrity of the musculofascial abdominal wall to prevent visceral exposure and provide dynamic muscle support. The second is to provide skin resurfacing.

Management of Abdominal Wounds

Acute Wounds

Acute abdominal wounds may be the result of dehiscence post laparotomy, infection, trauma or neoplasms.

Most acute abdominal wounds following laparotomy can be managed with local wound care, including bedside debridement of necrotic tissue and daily dressing changes or application of negative-pressure wound therapy (NPWT). In select cases, secondary closure following wound excision may be feasible and has been shown to be superior to healing by secondary intention.[8] Fascial dehiscence post laparotomy may occur in the acute setting without a skin defect. The typical history involves persistent drainage of serous fluid through the wound after 1 week. Fluid cultures are often positive. Fascial reclosure has a high chance of failure. Ideally, tension-free fascial closure is achieved and this may require use of a biologic or synthetic mesh with skin closure or NPWT.

In the acute trauma setting an abdominal wound may be left open because visceral edema makes it impossible to close, to facilitate further exploratory surgery or to prevent intraabdominal hypertension and compartment syndrome. In most cases NPWT is used as a temporizing measure.[9] Although this approach may have benefits in selected cases, it may be associated with high rates of complications such as entero-atmospheric fistula or frozen abdomen.[10] Early definitive closure should be performed as soon as possible, preferably within 7 days of the index surgery.[11] In cases where this cannot be achieved, a "planned ventral hernia" procedure may be performed where the skin is closed or skin-grafted but the fascial defect is not addressed in the acute setting. Skin graft excision and formal hernia repair can be performed at a later date.

Chronic Wounds

Chronic uncomplicated wounds without fistula can be managed in a number of ways. Small wounds may be managed with simple dressings and closed directly at the time of hernia repair. Moderate to large wounds are probably best skin-grafted initially to allow a temporizing wound closure. The skin graft can be excised at the time of definitive hernia repair. In cases where there is exposed mesh, the mesh should be removed if grossly contaminated. However, exposed mesh can be readily salvaged with application of NPWT and subsequent split-thickness skin grafting once sufficient granulation tissue has developed.

Small sinuses with retained foreign material but no fistula (e.g., stitch abscess) should be managed by removal of the foreign body. Healing by secondary intention usually follows.

The presence of an enterocutaneous fistula, defined as an epithelial-lined connection between the skin and internal organ, poses an immense clinical challenge. Treatment must be individualized and despite involvement of experienced multidisciplinary teams, outcomes are often poor with a high morbidity, mortality and psychosocial dysfunction.[12]

Prevention is key. Enterocutaneous fistulas most commonly develop in patients who have suffered a postoperative anastomotic leak. In wounds with exposed abdominal viscera, wet-to-dry dressings should be avoided as they can cause mechanical debridement of friable bowel mucosa and subsequent fistula development. Instead, the bowel should be covered with omentum where possible or absorbable mesh if omentum is unavailable.

Once a fistula is established, initial therapy should be directed at systemic measures to facilitate wound healing and maintain bowel function. These include aggressive treatment of sepsis, nutritional supplementation, and attention to fluid and electrolyte disturbances. Patients have high caloric and metabolic needs. In addition, vitamins and trace elements such as copper and zinc can be rapidly depleted through fistula-related losses. Total parenteral nutrition (TPN) can reduce enteric losses by as much as 50%, although enteral may also be used to provide trickle feeds.[13] Reduction of fistula output may increase the chance of spontaneous closure.

Once systemic factors have been addressed adequately, a surgical closure should be carefully planned. Imaging is critical to determine the anatomy of the fistula. This may include CT, MRI, fistulograms, and small bowel imaging.

In the early stages, the wound may be skin-grafted to convert the fistula into an ostomy, which can be managed more easily with a pouch system. Other techniques have been used to divert the fistula effluent from the wound bed in the early stages, such as NPWT and bridging dressings, which isolate the fistula. In either case, the periwound skin should be adequately protected with topical barrier ointments (containing zinc oxide, petrolatum, dimethicone or a combination) to prevent chemical denudation. A pouch system is used to collect the effluent and in addition may suppress odour.

The fistula can then be allowed to close spontaneously or be closed secondarily. Secondary fistula closure is best achieved by bowel resection and reanastomosis with abdominal wall reconstruction using acellular dermal matrices or components separation.

Management of Fascial Defects

Mesh reinforcement has been widely reported to improve outcomes following ventral hernia repair, with reduced recurrence rates compared to primary fascial closure.[14,15]Although an increasing number of synthetic and biological products are now available, none meets all the requirements of an ideal mesh and so the relevant risks and benefits must be considered in each individual clinical case. The ideal mesh would not adhere to the underlying bowel, would allow tissue ingrowth without shrinkage, prevent recurrence and fistula formation, and would not cause additional pain.[16] The material should be inert, non-carcinogenic, sterile, resistant to infection and capable of withstanding significant changes in intraabdominal pressure that range from 1.55 mmHg in patients lying supine up to 150 mmHg maximum peak pressure in coughing patients.[17]

Synthetic Mesh

Among the commonest meshes are permanent synthetic meshes that can be made from a variety of polymers, including polypropylene, polyester, and polytetrafluoroethylene (PTFE). Polypropylene is the most commonly used mesh due to its proven efficacy and relatively low cost. Individual filaments are knit together to form a flat sheet and the density of the filaments and the intervening pore size influence the clinical behavior of the material. Lighter weight meshes contain a lower density of polypropylene and are believed to be more favorable as they are associated with less foreign body response, superior compliance, increased tissue ingrowth, and less shrinkage of the material. The increased pore size is also believed to be beneficial in cases where bacterial contamination occurs, with salvage rates of up to 100% reported.[18] Conversely, materials such as PTFE have very small pores, in the order of microns, that prevent macrophage penetration and make salvage very difficult in cases of infection. However, decreased pore size is associated with reduced adhesion formation and may therefore be preferable in some cases where the mesh is placed in the peritoneum.[19] Meshes that combine PTFE and other non-adherent materials with other polymers such as polypropylene have been developed for use when mesh is in contact with bowel.

A range of resorbable meshes are also available and commonly comprise a formulation of polyglycolic acid (PGA), polylactic acid (PLA), trimethyl carbonate (TMC), or poly-4-hydroxybuturate (P4HB). These components are frequently combined to exploit their respective properties. These meshes aim to support the abdominal wall repair temporarily while wound healing occurs and then degrade completely leaving no permanent foreign material. Composite meshes have also been developed that combine permanent and resorbable polymers. These products offer some long-term tensile strength while reducing the amount of permanent foreign materials and its associated complications.

Biologic Mesh

A wide range of biologic meshes is now available, originating from different species (human, porcine, bovine) and anatomical locations (skin, intestine, pericardium). Tissues are processed and sterilized using a variety of techniques that remove the cellular component while preserving the extracellular matrix. The method of decellularization and sterilization may affect the efficacy of the mesh as any injury to the material may result in increased host inflammatory response and resorption.[20] The mesh may also be crosslinked to varying degrees to strengthen and stabilize the collagen network but excessive crosslinking will impede recellularization and neovascularization.

Biologic meshes are far more expensive than synthetic products but may have advantages in certain clinical scenarios as they have the potential for revascularization and superior integration.[21] They are more resistant to infection and can therefore be used in contaminated fields.[22] In addition, biologic meshes can be placed directly on the abdominal viscera as they have a low rate of adhesion formation.

Although biologic meshes have a number of theoretical advantages they are not without associated complications. Among the most significant concerns is hernia recurrence, with rates as high as 80% frequently reported.[23] Although the source and composition of the mesh is likely to influence recurrence rates there is a lack of well-designed studies that directly compare products. Some studies suggest that porcine products may have lower recurrence rates.[24] The method of mesh inset is also important, with interpositional placement associated with higher recurrence rates.[25] Repairs are more successful in cases where fascial approximation can be achieved.

Other complications included infection, seroma, and skin necrosis. Although relatively common, infection rarely leads to matrix extrusion and can often be managed with targeted antibiotics as early capillary ingrowth allows effective delivery of antimicrobial agents and innate host defenses. Even when implanted in a contaminated field, infection has been demonstrated to be as low as 16%.[26] Seromas are common

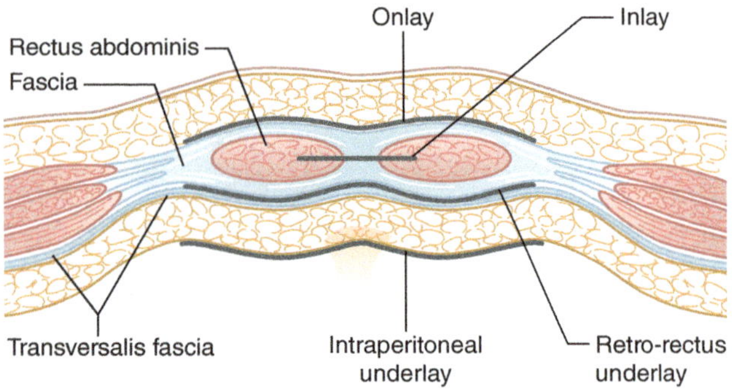

• **Fig. 40.5** Cross-sectional image of abdominal wall above arcuate line demonstrating different positions of mesh placement – onlay, inlay, underlay. (From Jamadar DA, Jacobson JA, Girish G, et al. Abdominal wall hernia mesh repair: sonography of mesh and common complications. *J Ultrasound Med: Official Journal of the American Institute of Ultrasound in Medicine*. 2008;27(6):907–917.)

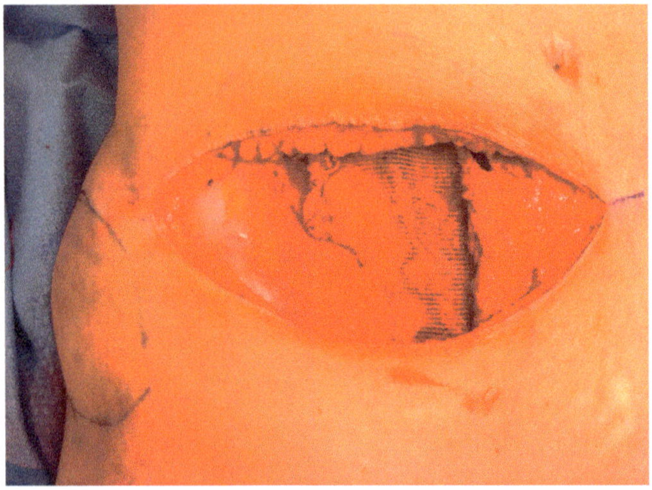

• **Fig. 40.6** Inlay mesh technique for repair of DIEP donor site hernia.

but rarely affect outcome. Strategies to reduce seroma formation include avoiding wide undermining of abdominal skin over fascia, preservation of suprafascial fat, use of quilting sutures, and abdominal binders.[27]

Surgical Techniques for Mesh Placement

The general principles of a successful mesh repair technique involve wide coverage with adequate overlap and secure suture fixation to the fascia. The mesh may be inserted above the fascia (onlay or overlay), underneath the fascia (inlay) or deep to the rectus (underlay, Fig. 40.5).[28]

Mesh can be used to reinforce a fascial repair or as an interpositional strut where a fascial defect exists. Fig. 40.6 demonstrates an inlay mesh placement of a donor site hernia post DIEP flap breast reconstruction.

Both inlay and only mesh repair techniques are popular methods of bridging fascial defects and seem to be equally effective.[29] However, with inlay mesh placement, the mesh is in direct contact with the abdominal viscera over a greater surface area than onlay placement, increasing the theoretical risk of erosion into the bowel and fistula formation. The key component is ensuring there is sufficient overlap between the margins of the fascia and the mesh.

Components Separation

Ramirez and colleagues described the technique of components separation to reconstruct midline defects although the use of external oblique fascial relaxing incisions had previously been described for epigastric hernia repairs.[30,31] The technique involves medial advancement of innervated musculofascial flaps involving a complex of rectus abdominis, internal oblique and transversus abdominis. Preoperative CT imaging is critical in determining the presence or absence of the rectus muscle complex, particularly in massive midline defects where the rectus muscles have been widely displaced laterally.

The procedure commences with elevation of the skin flaps off the underlying abdominal musculature. This can be continued to the anterior axillary line as required. Subsequently, the linea semilunaris is identified (condensation of internal and external oblique fascia into rectus sheath). A vertical incision is made through the external oblique fascia 2 cm lateral and parallel to the linea semilunaris. It should be just medial to the myofascial junction of the external oblique muscle itself. This is continued from the level of the costal margin superiorly to the arcuate line inferiorly. The plane between external oblique and internal oblique is developed, being careful to avoid damage to the internal oblique fascia or segmental intercostal neurovascular bundles supplying rectus. The dissection is continued lateral to the level of the mid-axillary line. At this point, the mobility of the rectus abdominis/internal oblique/transversus musculofascial complex is assessed. If further advancement is required, the dissection can be continued to the posterior axillary line.

Each hemicomplex can deliver 4 cm of advancement in the upper abdomen, 8 cm in the mid-abdomen, and about 3 cm in the lower abdomen (Fig. 40.7). Release of the posterior rectus sheath from the under surface of the muscle can increase medial translocation further by 2 cm at each point, making the total movement 6 cm, 10 cm, and 5 cm, respectively. Therefore, components separation can reconstruct defects of 20 cm or more in the midline. The fascia is closed and the skin is advanced to the midline and closed in a layered fashion over suction drains.[32]

Components separation has allowed the reconstruction of large midline and paramedian abdominal wall defects with well-vascularized innervated tissue and acceptable donor site morbidity compared with other autologous techniques. In addition, it frequently obviates the need for mesh and its associated complications, such as infection, extrusion, and enterocuatneous fistula development.

The hernia recurrence rates in published series ranges from 0% to 32%, suggesting that it can be a very effective technique.[33] Recurrence rates are reduced further by additional use of onlay synthetic meshes. In most cases, the strength of the abdominal wall is increased but does

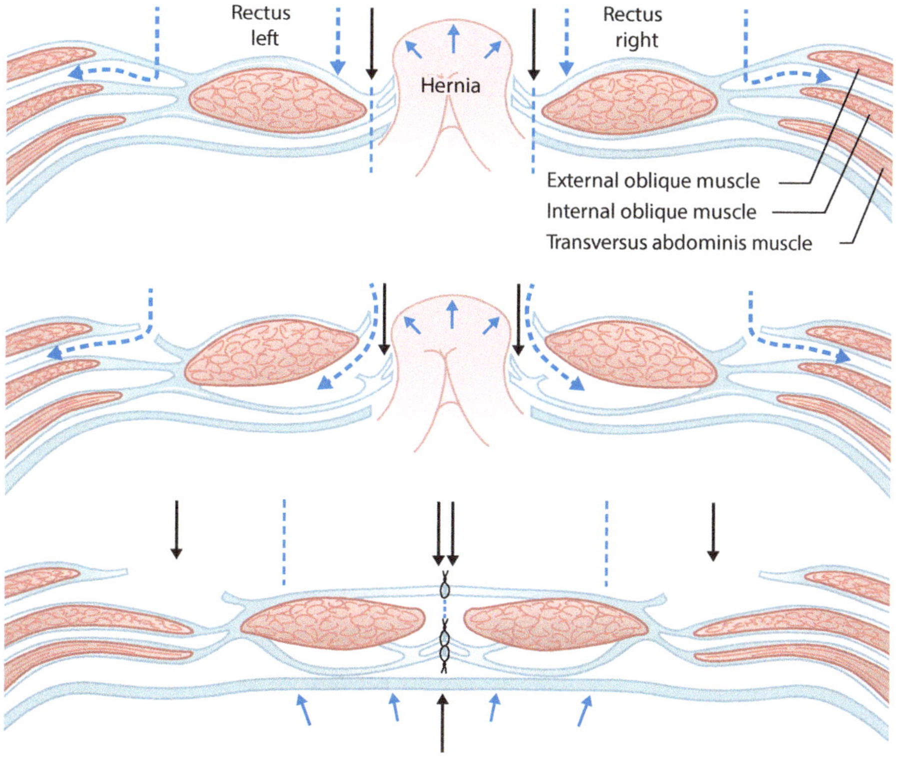

• **Fig. 40.7** Cross-sectional view illustrating components separation technique. (From addendum to Dragu A, Klein P, Unglaub F, et al. Tensiometry as a decision tool for abdominal wall reconstruction with component separation. *World J Surg*. 2009;33(6):1174–1180.)

not return to premorbid levels. Although commonly used in adults, the components separation technique has also been applied successfully to closure of congenital abdominal wall defects in neonates, including gastroschisis and omphaloceles.[34]

One of the potential pitfalls of the components separation technique is ischemia of the medial skin edges and ensuing necrosis, infection, or dehiscence. Compromise of the medial margin occurs due to the extensive undermining of the skin flaps required to allow sufficient exposure for division of the external oblique muscles. Modifications to the original procedure that reduce midline wound healing complications include endoscopic-assisted components separation and techniques that preserve periumbilical perforators.[35,36] Posterior component separation techniques have also been described in an effort to eliminate the need for extensive subcutaneous dissection and the associated complications.[37] The posterior approach creates a retromuscular space for mesh placement while allowing myofascial advancement of the external and internal oblique to achieve midline fascial closure. This technique divides the neurovascular bundles of the rectus abdominis muscle, which may predispose to bulge formation or hernia recurrence. Further modifications, including the transversus abdominis release, have been more recently described to avoid these sequelae.[38] A chemical component separation technique which uses botulinum toxin to weaken abdominal musculature and allow myofascial advancement has also been described.[39]

Soft Tissue Reconstruction in Abdominal Wall Reconstruction

Following oncological resection there is frequently a composite defect of the abdominal wall that requires both reconstitution of the myofascial integrity and replacement of the skin and subcutaneous tissues. A classification system (MD Anderson) has been proposed for these defects based on the anatomical location and the tissues that are absent.[40] The reconstructive algorithm for soft tissue reconstruction includes local skin advancement, local flaps, regional pedicled flaps, and free tissue transfer.[41]

Skin Advancement and Direct Closure

Due to the laxity of the abdominal wall skin envelope, direct closure is often feasible. If required, wide undermining in the prefascial plane can be performed to deliver additional advancement of the skin flap edges, such as in an abdominoplasty or components separation.

Flap Reconstruction

Soft tissue flaps can be used to reconstruct both skin and fascial components of abdominal wall defects, delivering robust well-vascularized tissue to aid primary wound healing and maintain abdominal wall integrity. Flaps are often used to repair fascial defects in contaminated wounds, where

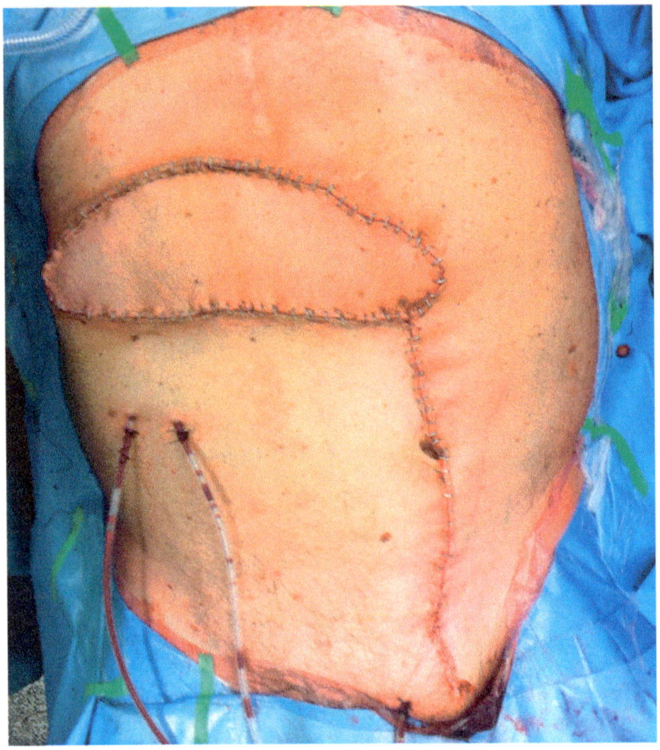

• **Fig. 40.8** VRAM reconstruction of a full-thickness right upper quadrant abdominal wall defect following excision of a liposarcoma in a 59-year-old man.

synthetic mesh is best avoided. Another common indication for flaps is to provide soft tissue cover of mesh or acellular dermal matrices in clean wounds following tumor extirpation. Flaps provide an alternative autologous reconstruction in situations where components separation is not feasible.

The pedicled rectus abdominis flap is the workhorse flap in abdominal wall reconstruction (Fig. 40.8). It can be taken with or without a skin paddle and a variety of orientations of the skin paddle are possible providing flexibility in design. Based superiorly, the flap is perfused by the superior epigastric artery or inferiorly on the deep inferior epigastric system.

The anterolateral thigh flap (ALT) can be used to reconstruct large composite abdominal wall defects providing both fascial and skin components. A very large area of fascia lata can be harvested from the thigh with the flap to reinforce or reconstruct large fascial defects. As a pedicled flap, it can easily reach above the umbilicus. Once elevated on the lateral circumflex femoral artery, the flap is passed deep to the rectus femoris and sartorius muscles to be delivered to the abdomen. The fascia lata is sutured to the fascial margins of the defect and the skin is closed in a layered fashion over suction drains. In upper abdominal wall defects and in cases where the flap does not reach the defect adequately, a pedicled ALT can be converted into a free ALT with similar outcomes.[42] Where a free ALT is performed, the deep inferior epigastric vessels are first choice recipient vessels due to their accessibility and size. If unavailable, the gastroepiploic vessels provide a reliable alternative.

The tensor fascia latae (TFL) flap can also be used to reconstruct composite defects of the lower abdominal wall but is inferior to the ALT flap, which has a larger, more reliable skin territory and longer vascular pedicle. Fig. 40.9 demonstrates an example of a TFL flap. In particular, tip necrosis is common in both free and pedicled TFL flaps, being reported to occur in up to 43% of flaps used in abdominal wall reconstruction.[43]

The pedicled rectus femoris muscle has also been described for use in reconstruction of lower abdominal wall defects. In contrast to TFL flaps, it provides considerable muscle bulk, which is useful for dead-space filling. It has the same pedicle as the ALT flap (descending branch of the lateral circumflex artery), although the pedicle length is shorter than the ALT flap as the rectus branch typically comes off higher up than the ALT perforators.

Other flaps used in abdominal wall reconstruction include vastus lateralis, gracilis, internal oblique, external oblique, and in cases where large skin defects exist, free latissimus dorsi flaps.

Abdominal Wall Transplantation

Abdominal wall transplantation is an evolving technique used to facilitate abdominal wall closure in patients undergoing intestinal or multivisceral transplantation.[44] In this group of patients, abdominal closure can be very difficult due to loss of domain and swelling after organ transplantation. In addition, they have a high mortality and morbidity. The abdominal wall graft is a vascularized composite allograft composed of skin, subcutaneous tissue, and the rectus abdominis myofascial complex. The flap is vascularized through anastomosis of donor and recipient inferior epigastric vessels or from an iliac vessel anastomosis in continuity with the femoral vessels. The muscle is not innervated and although muscle hypotrophy develops, significant hernia formation does not seem to be a problem.[45] Models for composite flaps innervated by the intercostal nerves have also been proposed and may permit functional muscle transfer and enhanced abdominal wall integrity.[46,47]

Management of the Postoperative Bulge

Abdominal wall complications after primary abdominal surgery or flap harvest can manifest as either an abdominal wall hernia or myofascial laxity (bulge). It can be difficult to distinguish clinically between a hernia and a bulge. A bulge is a contour abnormality of the abdominal wall with underlying myofascial continuity that is the result of global weakness. In contrast, a hernia is associated with a discrete myofascial defect. Bowel entrapment and obstruction are therefore a less common sequela of bulges compared with hernias.

Predisposing factors to development of bulges include muscle denervation (abdominal flap harvest), inadequate mesh tension, native myofascial laxity, and increased intraabdominal pressure. In a recent systematic review, the

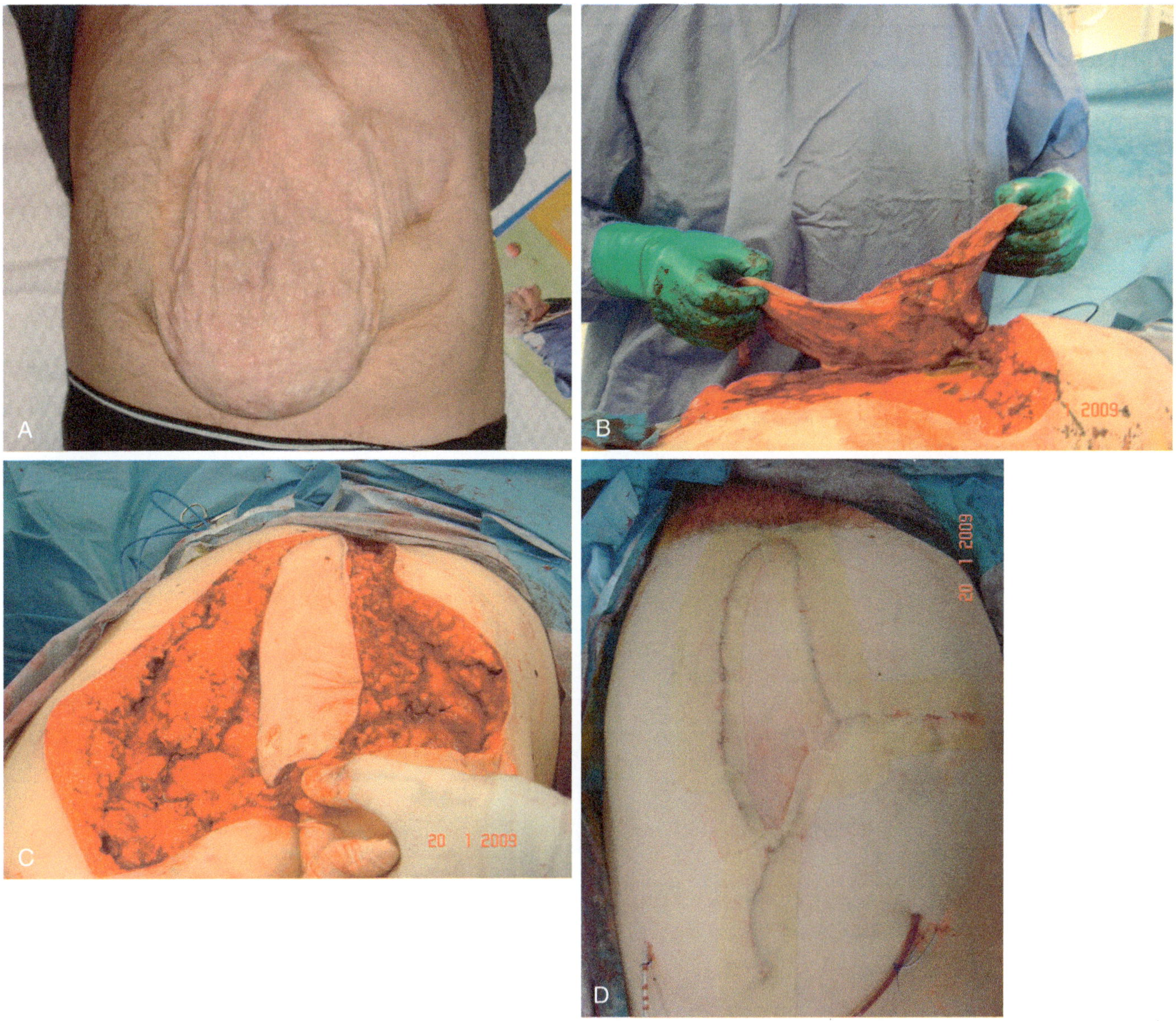

• **Fig. 40.9** Elderly man with ventral hernia following previous laparotomy wound treated definitively by extended TFL flap composite reconstruction. (A) Skin graft on laparostomy wound. (B) TFL flap raised with fascial extension. (C,D) Flap inset. (Courtesy Professor Wayne Morrison and Dr. Rostam D. Farhadieh.)

risk of bulging associated with DIEP flap harvest was one-third of muscle-sparing TRAMs.[48] Most frequently, a bulge presents as a contour abnormality that changes with posture and activity and can be associated with a dull ache. In severe cases, it can significantly interfere with daily activities and cause progressive skin attenuation with ulceration and infection. Diagnosis can be made by clinical examination and imaging, including contrast-enhanced CT scan and dynamic ultrasound assessment, which looks at the effect of posture and intraabdominal pressure on abdominal wall integrity.

Indications for operative repair include massive bulges with loss of function due to truncal instability, progressive skin changes or significant esthetic concerns. Pain relief is not a guaranteed outcome following repair. The principles of surgical correction include: (1) resect or plicate the area of myofascial laxity; (2) reapproximate intact dynamic fascial tissue under physiological tension; (3) reinforce the repair with adjunctive procedures such as mesh or components separation.[36] It is important to appreciate that bulges are associated with a global central or lateral fascial attenuation, often due to muscle denervation. Therefore, simple patching of the defect often results in recurrent bulges in adjacent areas. This is best achieved by use of inlay mesh across the entire central or lateral bulge with fixation of mesh to stable points beyond the bordering oblique muscle complexes, ideally to innervated myofascia or bone. Postoperatively, patients can ambulate on day 1 but should avoid heavy physical activity and sports for 6 weeks.

Conclusion

Defects of the abdominal wall can arise in a number of settings and present a difficult clinical challenge. A wide range of reconstructive options are available. Careful evaluation of the defect and prioritization of the requirements in each individual case is necessary so that an optimal management strategy can be formulated and long-term abdominal wall integrity can be restored.

References

1. Harley OJ, Pickford MA. CT analysis of fat distribution superficial and deep to the Scarpa's fascial layer in the mid and lower abdomen. *J Plast Reconstr Aesthet Surg*. 2013;66(4):525–530.
2. Huger Jr WE. The anatomic rationale for abdominal lipectomy. *Am Surg*. 1979;45(9):612–617.
3. Wong C, Saint-Cyr M, Mojallal A, et al. Perforasomes of the DIEP flap: vascular anatomy of the lateral versus medial row perforators and clinical implications. *Plast Reconstr Surg*. 2010;125(3):772–782.
4. Stoll C, Alembik Y, Dott B, et al. Associated malformations in cases with congenital diaphragmatic hernia. *Genet Counsel*. 2008;19(3):331–339.
5. Diener MK, Voss S, Jensen K, et al. Elective midline laparotomy closure: the INLINE systematic review and meta-analysis. *Ann Surg*. 2010;251(5):843–856.
6. Flum DR, Horvath K, Koepsell T. Have outcomes of incisional hernia repair improved with time? A population-based analysis. *Ann Surg*. 2003;237(1):129–135.
7. Muysoms FE, Miserez M, Berrevoet F, et al. Classification of primary and incisional abdominal wall hernias. *Hernia*. 2009;13(4):407–414.
8. Dodson MK, Magann EF, Meeks GR. A randomized comparison of secondary closure and secondary intention in patients with superficial wound dehiscence. *Obstet Gynecol*. 1992;80(3 Pt 1):321–324.
9. Cirocchi R, Birindelli A, Biffl WL, et al. What is the effectiveness of the negative pressure wound therapy (NPWT) in patients treated with open abdomen technique? A systematic review and meta-analysis. *J Trauma Acute Care Surg*. 2016;81(3):575–584.
10. Chiara O, Cimbanassi S, Biffl W, et al. International consensus conference on open abdomen in trauma. *J Trauma Acute Care Surg*. 2016;80(1):173–183.
11. Coccolini F, Roberts D, Ansaloni L, et al. The open abdomen in trauma and non-trauma patients: WSES guidelines. *World J Emerg Surg*. 2018;13:7.
12. Draus Jr JM, Huss SA, Harty NJ, et al. Enterocutaneous fistula: are treatments improving? *Surgery*. 2006;140(4):570–576; discussion 576–578.
13. Gardiner KR. Management of acute intestinal failure. *Proc Nutr Soc*. 2011;70(3):321–328.
14. Burger JW, Luijendijk RW, Hop WC, et al. Long-term follow-up of a randomized controlled trial of suture versus mesh repair of incisional hernia. *Ann Surg*. 2004;240(4):578–583; discussion 583–585.
15. Luijendijk RW, Hop WC, van den Tol MP, et al. A comparison of suture repair with mesh repair for incisional hernia. *N Engl J Med*. 2000;343(6):392–398.
16. Raptis DA, Vichova B, Breza J, et al. A comparison of woven versus nonwoven polypropylene (PP) and expanded versus condensed polytetrafluoroethylene (PTFE) on their intraperitoneal incorporation and adhesion formation. *J Surg Res*. 2011;169(1):1–6.
17. Doctor HG. Evaluation of various prosthetic materials and newer meshes for hernia repairs. *J Minim Access Surg*. 2006;2(3):110–116.
18. Petersen S, Henke G, Freitag M, et al. Deep prosthesis infection in incisional hernia repair: predictive factors and clinical outcome. *Eur J Surg Acta Chir*. 2001;167(6):453–457.
19. Jenkins ED, Yom V, Melman L, et al. Prospective evaluation of adhesion characteristics to intraperitoneal mesh and adhesiolysis-related complications during laparoscopic re-exploration after prior ventral hernia repair. *Surg Endosc*. 2010;24(12):3002–3007.
20. Nahabedian MY, Sosin M, Bhanot P. A current review of biologic meshes in abdominal wall reconstruction. *Plast Reconstr Surg*. 2018;142(3 suppl):74S–81S.
21. Blatnik J, Jin J, Rosen M. Abdominal hernia repair with bridging acellular dermal matrix – an expensive hernia sac. *Am J Surg*. 2008;196(1):47–50.
22. Itani KM, Rosen M, Vargo D, et al. Prospective study of single-stage repair of contaminated hernias using a biologic porcine tissue matrix: the RICH Study. *Surgery*. 2012;152(3):498–505.
23. Janis JE, O'Neill AC, Ahmad J, et al. Acellular dermal matrices in abdominal wall reconstruction: a systematic review of the current evidence. *Plast Reconstr Surg*. 2012;130(5 suppl 2):183S–93S.
24. Huntington CR, Cox TC, Blair LJ, et al. Biologic mesh in ventral hernia repair: outcomes, recurrence, and charge analysis. *Surgery*. 2016;160(6):1517–1527.
25. Jin J, Rosen MJ, Blatnik J, et al. Use of acellular dermal matrix for complicated ventral hernia repair: does technique affect outcomes? *J Am Coll Surg*. 2007;205(5):654–660.
26. Patton JH Jr, Berry S, Kralovich KA. Use of human acellular dermal matrix in complex and contaminated abdominal wall reconstructions. *Am J Surg*. 2007;193(3):360–363; discussion 363.
27. Patel KM, Bhanot P. Complications of acellular dermal matrices in abdominal wall reconstruction. *Plast Reconstr Surg*. 2012;130(5 suppl 2):216S–224S.
28. Jamadar DA, Jacobson JA, Girish G, et al. Abdominal wall hernia mesh repair: sonography of mesh and common complications. *J Ultrasound Med*. 2008;27(6):907–917.
29. Hawn MT, Snyder CW, Graham LA, et al. Long-term follow-up of technical outcomes for incisional hernia repair. *J Am Coll Surg*. 2010;210(5):648–657.
30. Ramirez OM, Ruas E, Dellon AL. "Components separation" method for closure of abdominal-wall defects: an anatomic and clinical study. *Plast Reconstr Surg*. 1990;86(3):519–526.
31. Young D. Repair of epigastric incisional hernia. *Br J Surg*. 1961;48:514–516.
32. Dragu A, Klein P, Unglaub F, et al. Tensiometry as a decision tool for abdominal wall reconstruction with component separation. *World J Surg*. 2009;33(6):1174–1180.
33. Heller L, Chike-Obi C, Xue AS. Abdominal wall reconstruction with mesh and components separation. *Semin Plast Surg*. 2012;26(1):29–35.
34. Levy S, Tsao K, Cox Jr CS, et al. Component separation for complex congenital abdominal wall defects: not just for adults anymore. *J Pediatr Surg*. 2013;48(12):2525–2529.
35. Albright E, Diaz D, Davenport D, et al. The component separation technique for hernia repair: a comparison of open and endoscopic techniques. *Am Surg*. 2011;77(7):839–843.
36. Saulis AS, Dumanian GA. Periumbilical rectus abdominis perforator preservation significantly reduces superficial wound complications in "separation of parts" hernia repairs. *Plast Reconstr Surg*. 2002;109(7):2275–2280; discussion 2281– 2282.

37. Carbonell AM, Cobb WS, Chen SM. Posterior components separation during retromuscular hernia repair. *Hernia.* 2008;12(4):359–362.
38. Novitsky YW, Elliott HL, Orenstein SB, et al. Transversus abdominis muscle release: a novel approach to posterior component separation during complex abdominal wall reconstruction. *Am J Surg.* 2012;204(5):709–716.
39. Motz BM, Schlosser KA, Heniford BT. Chemical components separation: concepts, evidence, and outcomes. *Plast Reconstr Surg.* 2018;142(3 suppl):58S–63S.
40. Mericli AF, Baumann DP, Butler CE. Reconstruction of the abdominal wall after oncologic resection: defect classification and management strategies. *Plast Reconstr Surg.* 2018;142(3 suppl):187S.
41. Rohrich RJ, Lowe JB, Hackney FL, et al. An algorithm for abdominal wall reconstruction. *Plast Reconstr Surg.* 2000;105(1):202–216; quiz 217.
42. Kayano S, Sakuraba M, Miyamoto S, et al. Comparison of pedicled and free anterolateral thigh flaps for reconstruction of complex defects of the abdominal wall: review of 20 consecutive cases. *J Plast Reconstr Aesthet Surg.* 2012;65(11):1525–1529.
43. Williams JK, Carlson GW, Howell RL, et al. The tensor fascia lata free flap in abdominal-wall reconstruction. *J Reconstr Microsurg.* 1997;13(2):83–90; discussion 91.
44. Levi DM, Tzakis AG, Kato T, et al. Transplantation of the abdominal wall. *Lancet.* 2003;361(9376):2173–2176.
45. Selvaggi G, Levi DM, Cipriani R, et al. Abdominal wall transplantation: surgical and immunologic aspects. *Transplant Proc.* 2009;41(2):521–522.
46. Broyles JM, Berli J, Tuffaha SH, et al. Functional abdominal wall reconstruction using an innervated abdominal wall vascularized composite tissue allograft: a cadaveric study and review of the literature. *J Reconstr Microsurg.* 2015;31(1):39–44.
47. Broyles JM, Sarhane KA, Tuffaha SH, et al. Reconstruction of large abdominal wall defects using neurotized vascular composite allografts. *Plast Reconstr Surg.* 2015;136(4):728–737.
48. Egeberg A, Rasmussen MK, Sorensen JA. Comparing the donor-site morbidity using DIEP, SIEA or MS-TRAM flaps for breast reconstructive surgery: a meta-analysis. *J Plast Reconstr Aesthet Surg.* 2012;65(11):1474–1480.

41

Genitourinary and Perineal Reconstruction

NIRI S. NIRANJAN, CHARLES Y.Y. LOH, ADEYEMI A. OGUNLEYE, GORDON K. LEE, KATHRYN EVANS, AND IMRAN MUSHTAQ

PERINEAL RECONSTRUCTION

Niri S. Niranjan and Charles Y.Y. Loh

Perineal reconstruction is a challenging feat and there are multiple considerations for the surgeon. Discussed here are the relevant anatomy, common workhorse flaps for perineal reconstructions, our tips and tricks from experience, especially – from its conception – with the lotus petal flap, and the importance of reconstructing the perineal body.

Introduction

The management of advanced pelvic malignancy is challenging and requires a multidisciplinary approach. The potential method of resection and reconstruction for total perineal defects should be discussed by a multidisciplinary team (MDT), which should consist of a colorectal surgeon, urologist, gynecologist, oncologist, radiologist, plastic surgeon, specialist nurse practitioner, physiotherapist, and psychologist. Factors that dictate the choice of method are the patient's general condition and habits (age, sex, diabetes, atherosclerosis, obesity, smoking, and nutritional state) and the defect created (skin, pelvic viscera, pelvic muscles). Some of the patients would have already undergone surgery and radiotherapy. In these patients, the local option would have either already been used or not be possible because of radiotherapy. The patient should be fully informed of the surgical treatment, the outcome, and possible major life adjustment postoperatively (e.g., colostomy and urinary conduit). An anesthetist who is regularly involved in this type of procedure should assess the patient.

Total perineal reconstruction, including skin and pelvic viscera, may be indicated for advanced cancer and post-irradiated cancer recurrence, total perineal skin loss in extensive debilitating infection or following full-thickness burn or trauma.

The "clockface" assessment of the defect is a very useful method of considering anatomically sound options available. There are numerous perforator-based or myocutaneous flaps available beyond the clockface territory of the lotus petal flaps[1] and extended lotus petal flaps, which serve this purpose.[2,3] These flaps are away from disease and irradiated areas of the perineum and hence will provide well-vascularized tissue for primary healing. The aim is to achieve wound closure with primary healing. Sexual function has to be sacrificed and excretory function is diverted. One should consider using a larger flap either on its own or in combination with local flaps if available. The preferred large flaps are the vertical rectus abdominis myocutaneous (VRAM) or deep inferior epigastric perforator (DIEP) flaps at 12 o' clock; the anterolateral thigh (ALT) or transverse myocutaneous gracilis (TMG) flaps at 9 and 3 o' clock; and the superior/inferior gluteal artery perforator (SGAP/IGAP) or posterior thigh flaps at 7 and 5 o' clock. If and when there is a defect beyond the perineum, a larger flap like an extended VRAM, DIEP or bilateral ALTs may be considered. The bilateral TMG flap, either with a transverse or longitudinally-oriented skin paddle, is a secondary option.

The perineal region has two important components, one excretory and one sexual. Malfunction or dysfunction of either of these can affect the whole body. The perineum has a very rich blood supply, fed by both the femoral and the iliac arteries (similar to the face by external and internal carotid vessels). Branches from these vessels anastomose with each other around the urogenital and anal orifices and this enables reconstructing surgeons to use skin flaps based on the perforators from these vessels.

The soft tissue reconstruction is challenging both in terms of functional and esthetic outcomes. Local flaps based on perforators are the ideal as they replace like tissues. Regional myocutaneous flaps continue to have their place in reconstruction of the region.

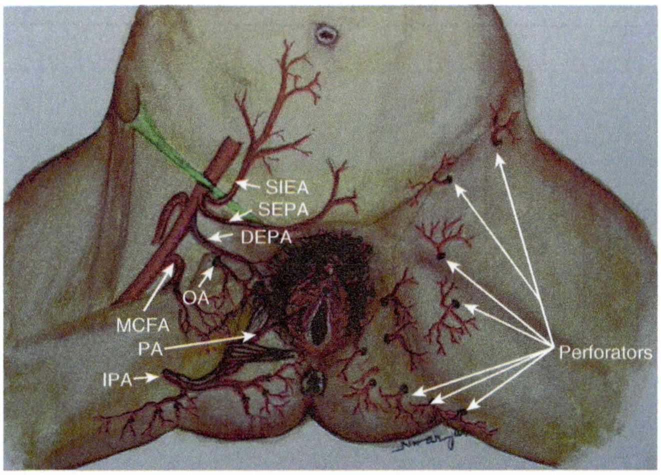

• **Fig. 41.1** Blood supply of the perineum. SIEA, superficial inferior epigastric artery; SEPA, superficial external pudendal artery; DEPA, deep external pudendal artery; OA, obturator artery; MCFA, medial circumflex femoral artery; PA, perineal artery; IPA, internal pudendal artery

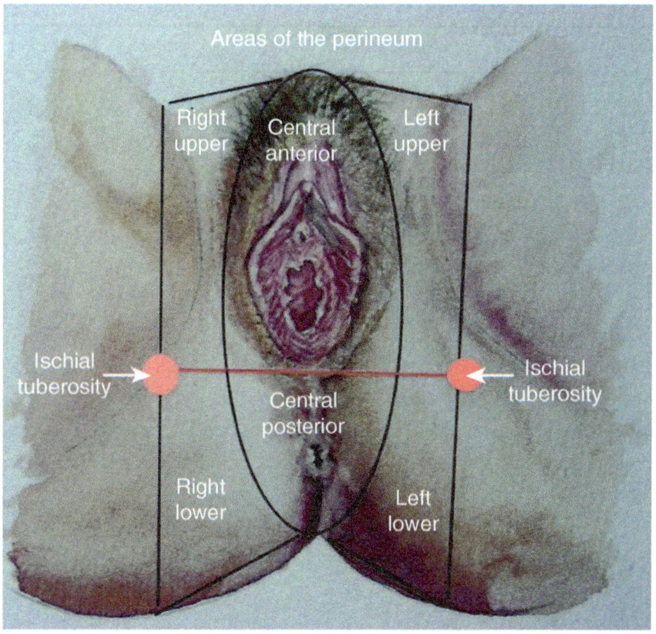

• **Fig. 41.2** Schematic division of the perineum.

Anatomy of the Blood Supply of the Perineum

In 1889 Carl Manchot[4] divided the cutaneous area of the perineum into anterior and posterior regions. He also described the blood supply of the perineum in great detail. Branches of the femoral and internal iliac arteries form the rich vascular network of the perineum. The anterior region is supplied by the superficial external pudendal artery and deep external pudendal artery. The obturator artery, internal pudendal artery, and branches of the inferior gluteal artery supply the posterior half of the perineum.

The internal pudendal artery gives out two terminal branches: the penile/clitoral branch and the perineal artery. The perineal artery supplies the labial/scrotal part of the perineum via its terminal branches, which anastomose with their contralateral counterpart. The perineal artery also gives off medial and the lateral branches. The medial branch supplies the perianal region and the lateral branch supplies an area of posterior surface of the upper thigh. All these branches anastomose with their counterpart from the opposite side and hence form a rich circle of vascular anastomoses around the orifice. This vascular network provides the basis of the perforator flaps (Fig. 41.1).

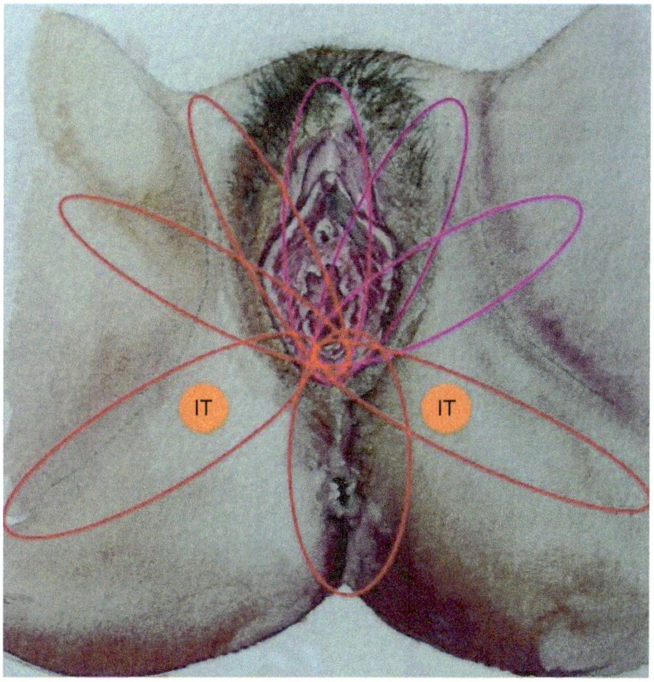

• **Fig. 41.3** Lotus flap schema based on local perforators. IT, ischial tuberosity.

Reconstruction of the Perineum

The ideal flap for any perineal defect should use reliable and robust like tissue, not be too bulky, and should have protective sensation to maintain normal function and appearance. There should also be minimal donor site morbidity. For practical purposes the perineum can be divided into right, left, and central areas. A line drawn between the ischial tuberosity divide these areas into anterior and posterior halves (Fig. 41.2). The central area contains the urogenital orifice in the anterior half and the anal orifice in posterior half. In the majority of the cases the defect to be reconstructed is created in the central area, for example due to vulvar/vaginal or anal neoplasia. Other situations where flap reconstruction is used are congenital malformations and severe debilitating infections (like hidradenitis suppurativa). Traumatic defects requiring local flaps are uncommon. For defects in the upper quadrant, donor skin flaps could come from the groin and/or mons pubis area,[5] whilst for the lower quadrant the donor site may be from the gluteal fold and/or gluteal area.[6,7] The mid-thigh can also provide a flap for these situations. For the central area of the perineum the donor could be selected from any of the above sites. The selection depends on the site and size of the defect. There are three ways of moving local perforator flaps, namely rotation (lotus petal flaps, Fig. 41.3), V–Y advancement flaps (Fig. 41.4), and transposition (pudendal, mons pubis flaps, Fig. 41.5).

Horton et al in 1973 reported local random pattern flaps designed around the genital area. Other types of skin flaps used during the 1970s and 1980s were mostly myocutaneous flaps. Among these are, the gracillis (reported by McCrow et al in 1976), tensor fascia lata (Nahai et al in 1979 and Chafe et al in 1983) and rectus abdominus (Tobin and Day in 1988[8]). These flaps were obviously bulky and accompanied by considerable donor site morbidity. The fasciocutaneous flap emerged in the early 1980s and in 1987 Wang et al advocated medial thigh fasciocutaneous flaps, whilst Wee and Joseph in 1989[9] described a pudendal thigh flap with an intact nerve supply for vaginal reconstruction. Woods et al modified the same flap in 1992. Where possible, the senior author attempts reconstruction using local perforator fasciocutaneous flaps, which schematically form the petals of a lotus.

Surgery may be performed either under general or regional anesthesia. The patient is placed in the Lloyd Davies position. A urinary catheter is inserted. Prophylactic antibiotics should be given at induction and for 48 hours postoperatively. The defect is created during the resection for either cancer or infection or the debridement of traumatized tissue. Once the dimension of the defect is studied and assessed, the required flap is planned over the donor area. The flap is planned in a reverse manner by using a swab or a pattern of the defect turned towards the selected donor site in reverse. The success of perforator flap reconstruction depends on the selection of the perforator vessel at or around the base of the selected flap. Before the operation, perforator vessels are mapped using a hand-held Doppler ultrasound probe at the base of the skin flap. An exploring incision is made along one edge of this flap down to the muscle. The flap is elevated with the deep fascia and the perforating vessel is reassessed. In rotation or transposition flaps, perforators should be selected closer to the defect. However, for V–Y advancement flaps, perforators can be anywhere in and around the mid-axis of the V–Y flap.

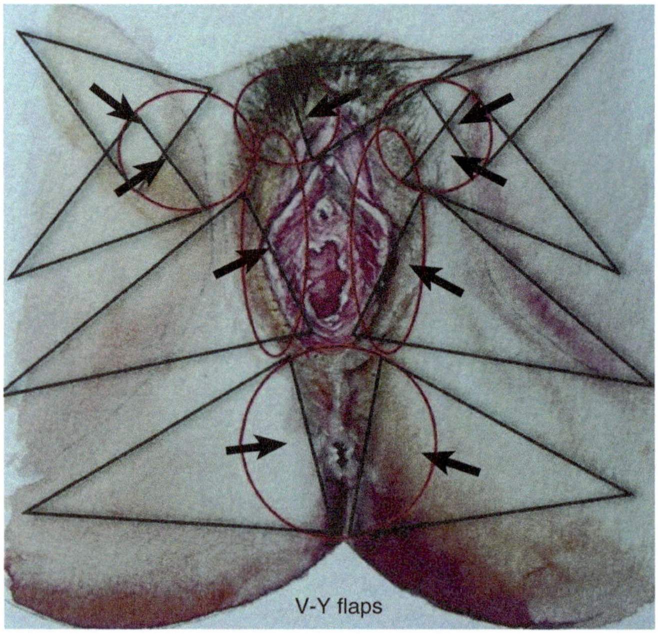

• **Fig. 41.4** V–Y advancement flap.

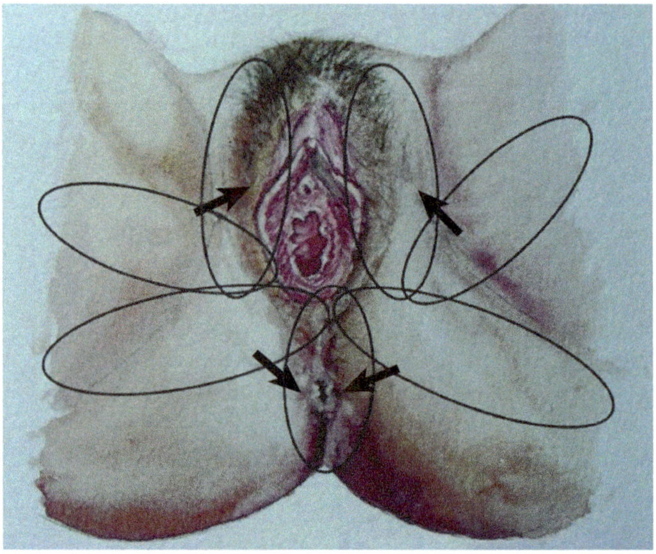

• **Fig. 41.5** Transposition of pudendal and mons pubis flaps.

Reconstructing the Perineal Body

In 1989, MacAlister introduced the term *perineal body* to describe the site that separates the cloacal sphincter into anal and urogenital portions.[10] The perineal body is a complex fibromuscular mass into which many structures insert. It is bordered cephalad by the rectovaginal septum (Denonvilliers' fascia), caudad by perineal skin, anteriorly by the posterior wall of the vagina, posteriorly by the anterior wall of the anorectum and laterally by the ischial rami. The perineal body has been compared to that of a red pine cone, with each "petal" representing insertion of the fascia or muscles of the perineum.

The perineal body is an important part of the perineum. It provides a physical barrier between the vagina and the rectum, both of which it anchors, maintaining urinary and fecal continence. When the perineal body is damaged following, for example, gynecological surgery or obstetric perineal trauma, the patient may suffer from pain, dyspareunia, aerovagina, and fecal and/or urinary urgency or incontinence. The perineal body is also an important part of the "orgasmic platform," which can be damaged when the perineal body is damaged by an injury or disease.

Optimal primary repair followed by training of the perineal body can reduce most distressing physical and psychosexual consequences. However, if a patient requires subsequent surgery, it would be advisable to have a multidisciplinary perineal team approach (gynecologist, colorectal surgeon, urologist, and plastic surgeon). The team should also involve expertise in dealing with psychosexual problems.

The plastic surgeon's role is usually focused on scar revision and reconstruction following tissue loss over the perineal body. This can be achieved using local perforator flaps to build a tissue bridge between the vagina and the anorectum.

Regional Flaps

Deep Inferior Epigastric Artery-Based Flaps

The VRAM flap should be considered as first choice for patients who are undergoing abdominoperineal resection. This is an ideal flap in total perineal resection, i.e., pelvic exenteration. The perforators of the deep inferior epigastric artery are marked over the abdomen using ultrasound Doppler and/or CT angiogram. Following completion of resection, the perineal defect is re-assessed in terms of the size of skin defect and the volume of pelvic cavity. The deep inferior epigastric vessels can be inspected through the abdominal wound and the required skin paddle is re-marked working out the required length of the pedicle (Figs. 41.6–41.8).

The midline incision is extended superiorly and the lateral incision of the skin paddle is incised down to the rectus sheath. The rectus sheath is incised just laterally to the lateral row of perforators and a strip of the fascia is kept intact all along the rectus muscle. The flap, consisting of muscle, a strip of fascia, and an island of skin, is elevated. The deep inferior vessel is identified and carefully dissected right down to its origin. The lower attachment of the muscle is also divided, which helps in orienting the flap in the pelvic cavity and in delivering the skin paddle through the perineal wound.

The muscle is sutured to the pelvic floor. The skin paddle is usually larger than the defect hence it is de-epithelialized, leaving the exact amount of skin required. The skin paddle is inset keeping two drains, and the abdominal wound is also closed in layers. Postoperatively, the patient is mobilized as soon as possible.

Lateral Circumflex Femoral Profunda Artery-Based Flaps

The ALT flap is now a workhorse in reconstructive surgery, first described by Song et al in 1984[11] as a septocutaneous flap. The major advantages of this flap are that it provides a large amount of skin for harvest and that the pedicle is close enough to reach the perineum, but far enough to be away from diseased and irradiated areas of the perineum.

The blood supply of the ALT flap is dependent upon the perforators of the descending branch of the lateral circumflex profunda femoral artery. In general, a large skin flap can be raised but a width of up to 8 cm can be closed directly and any wider skin flap requires a skin graft. The perforators are assessed for a visible pulsation and for venae comitantes. Where of septocutaneous type, the vessels traverse the septum between rectus femoris and vastus lateralis muscles. If the perforators are of a muscular type, which usually comes from the vastus lateralis, that part of the muscle may also be included to add bulk to the flap. The flap is passed under the rectus femoris muscle and through the subcutaneous tunnel to reach the perineum, making sure that there is no tension on the pedicle. The perineal wound is closed in layers with a drain and the donor area is either closed directly, or with a skin graft.

Postoperatively, the patient may be nursed in slight flexion and also abduction of the thighs to prevent any compression on the pedicle, although this is rarely necessary. The patient is mobilised after 48 hours.

Gluteal Artery-Based Flaps

The gluteus maximus muscle is a large muscle of the buttock area. It has two dominant blood supplies as a type III muscle flap. The superior and inferior gluteal arteries arise from the internal iliac artery and they emerge on either side of the pyriform muscles. The superior gluteal artery supplies the upper part of the gluteus maximus and the inferior gluteal supplies the lower half. The inferior gluteal artery is a direct continuation of the internal iliac artery emerging below the pyrifomis muscle, accompanying the sciatic nerve, inferior gluteal nerve, the internal pudendal vessel, and posterior femoral cutaneous nerves. The cutaneous perforators of the inferior gluteal artery, about 8 ± 4, are concentrated in the middle third of the gluteal region, parallel to the gluteal crease. The SGAP or myocutaneous flaps would be suitable for the sacral part of the defect whilst the IGAP or myocutaneous flaps would be suitable for a large part of the perineum and also in pelvic exenteration (Figs. 41.9–41.11).

These flaps are considered when VRAM or ALT flaps are not possible for reconstruction. When chosen for abdominoperineal reconstruction, the surgery requires two different positions of the patient. Initially, the resecting surgeon will carry out the abdominal part of the operation, including colostomy and urinary conduit, and the abdominal wound is closed. The patient is then positioned in the prone, jackknife position. Using ultrasound Doppler, the lateral groups of perforators of the IGA are selected in the ellipse of the skin so that the pedicle is long enough to reach without tension. The skin flap is elevated from the lateral aspect and a small portion of the gluteus maximus muscle may be included, which not only adds to the bulk but also includes a number of perforators for the flap. Once the flap is islanded, the pedicle is dissected, ligating all other branches of the IGA. When the flap is transposed over the perineum, the deep layer is sutured with the pelvic floor and the skin is sutured in two layers of the perineum, with two drains.

Posterior Thigh Flap

The blood supply of this flap arises from the descending branch of the IGA. This flap contains the posterior cutaneous nerve of the thigh, which makes it a sensate flap. The course of the artery and the perforators can be mapped out by using ultrasound Doppler or by CT angiography. This helps in planning the required flap. A line is drawn from the ischial tuberosity to the lateral epicondyle of the femur. The

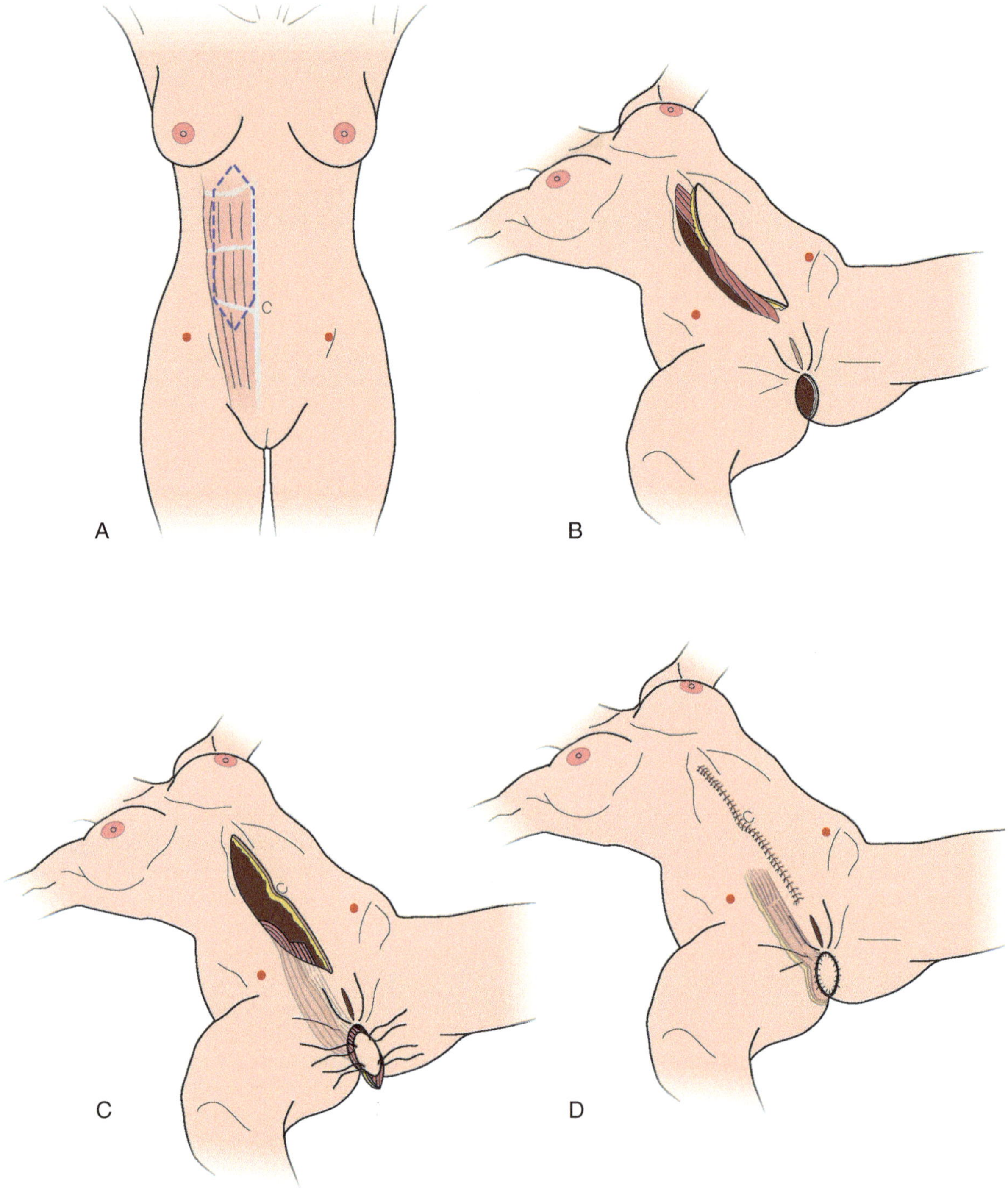

• **Fig. 41.6** Vertical rectus abdominis myocutaneous (VRAM) flap. (A) Skin paddles. (B) VRAM flap. (C) VRAM to perineal defect. (D) Wound closed.

skin paddle is centered at the midpoint of this line, with the width of the skin paddle being either the amount that can be closed directly or more if skin grafting is required. It is also possible to take two flaps or to use this in combination with other flaps. The flap is elevated by incising its lateral border and extending it towards the gluteal crease to expose the pedicle and following it up to its origin. Extra length can be obtained by dissecting the IGA. The flap may then be tunneled under the skin to the perineal defect and inset.

The postoperative regime is as described before. The donor scar of the IGAP flap does cause some discomfort for the patient during sitting for about 4–6 weeks postoperatively.

Medial Circumflex Femoral Profunda Artery-Based Flaps

Orticohea in 1972 and McCraw et al in 1976 described the gracilis myocutaneous flap. The gracilis myocutaneous

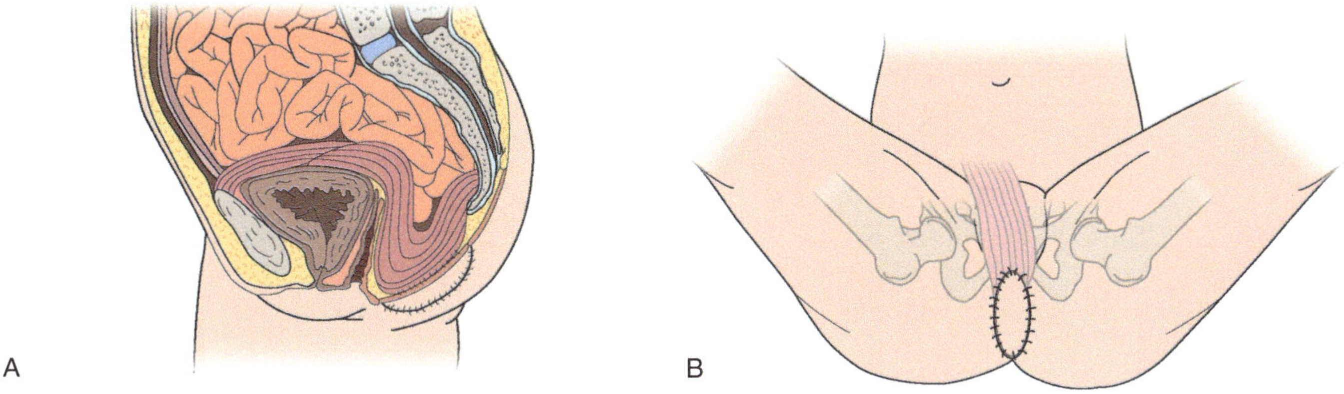

• **Fig. 41.7** (A) Rectus muscle sutured to the pelvic floor. (B) Inset VRAM flap.

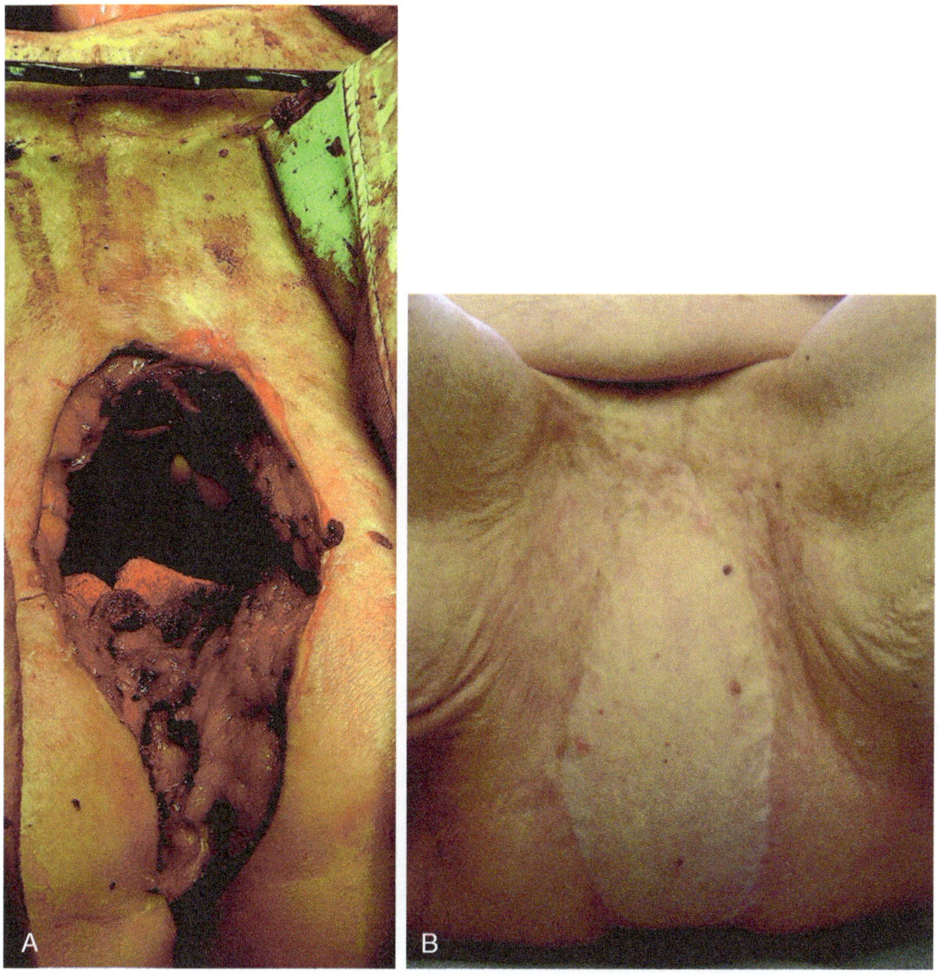

• **Fig. 41.8** VRAM flap. (A) Defect following total perineal resection. (B) Five-year follow-up. (From Blondeel PN, Morris SF, Hallock GG, eds. *Perforator Flaps: Anatomy, Technique, and Clinical Applications*, 2nd edn. Boca Raton, FL: CRC Press; 2013: Fig. 64.15.)

flap is a type II muscle flap, the blood supply of which is from the ascending branch of the medial circumflex femoral artery. The skin flap paddle orientation is usually in the line of the gracilis muscle, but in recent years, following the paper from Yousif et al[12] in 1992, a transverse orientation of the cutaneous paddle has been shown to be more reliable (Fig. 41.12). This is now called a TMG or TUG flap. The muscular artery for the gracilis enters the muscle at about 8–10 cm from the pubic tubercle. The gracilis muscle can be used as a myocutaneous flap, or a muscle flap in combination with other skin flaps.

The gracilis myocutaneous flap is indicated for abdominoperineal resection with surgery carried out in the Lloyd Davies position. A skin paddle is drawn about 1–2 cm

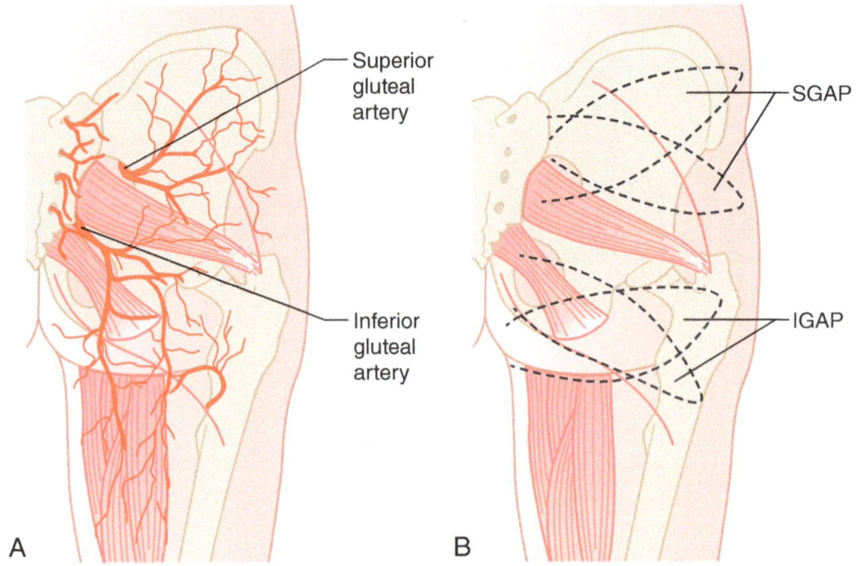

• **Fig. 41.9** Superior (SGAP) and inferior (IGAP) gluteal artery perforator-based flaps. (A) Anatomy. (B) Skin paddle of SGA and IGA.

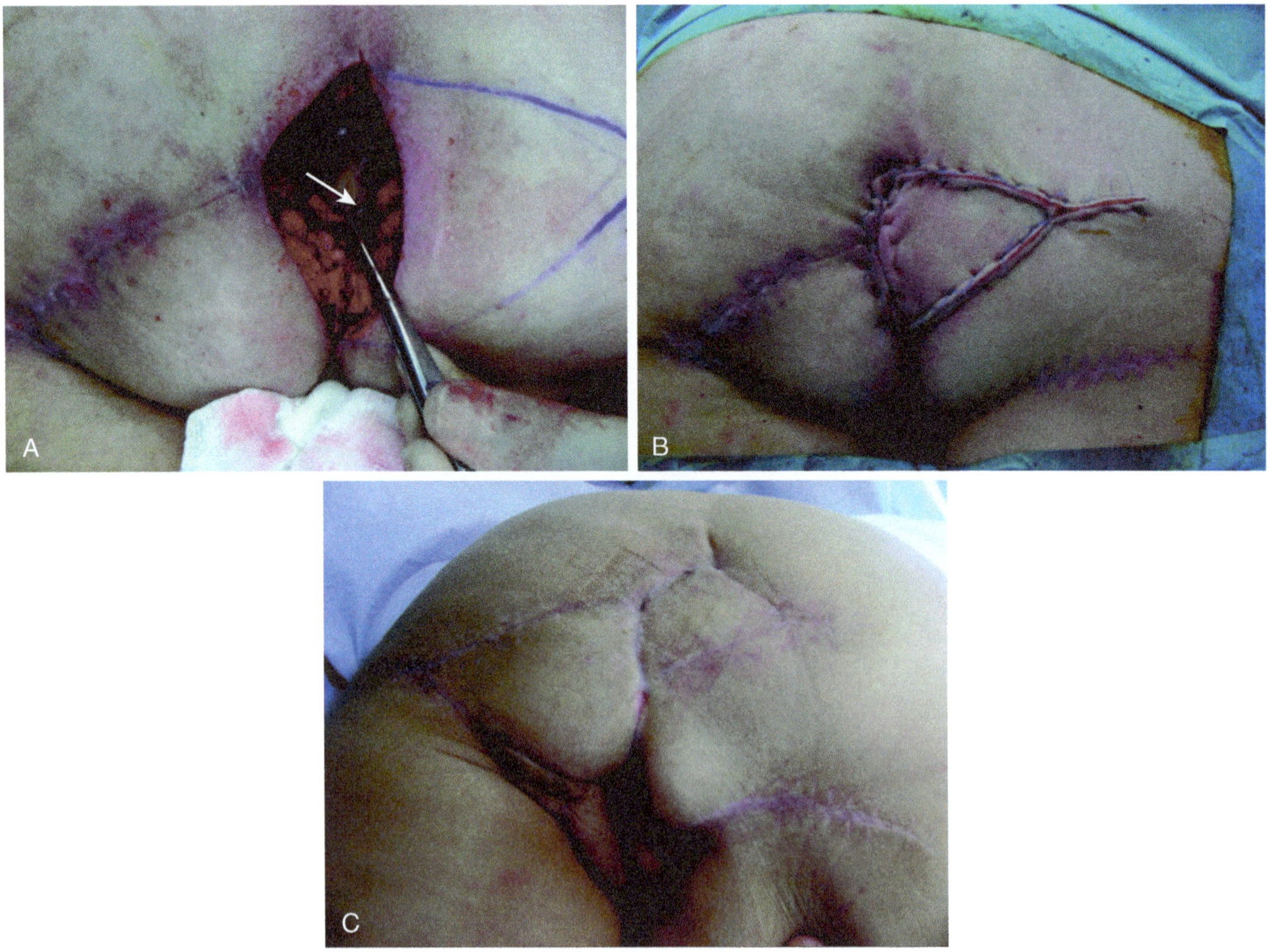

• **Fig. 41.10** Inferior gluteal artery flap, island flap V–Y advancement. (A) Postperineal reconstruction wound showing intact gluteal fold flap. (B) Immediate postoperative result. (C) Three months postoperative result.

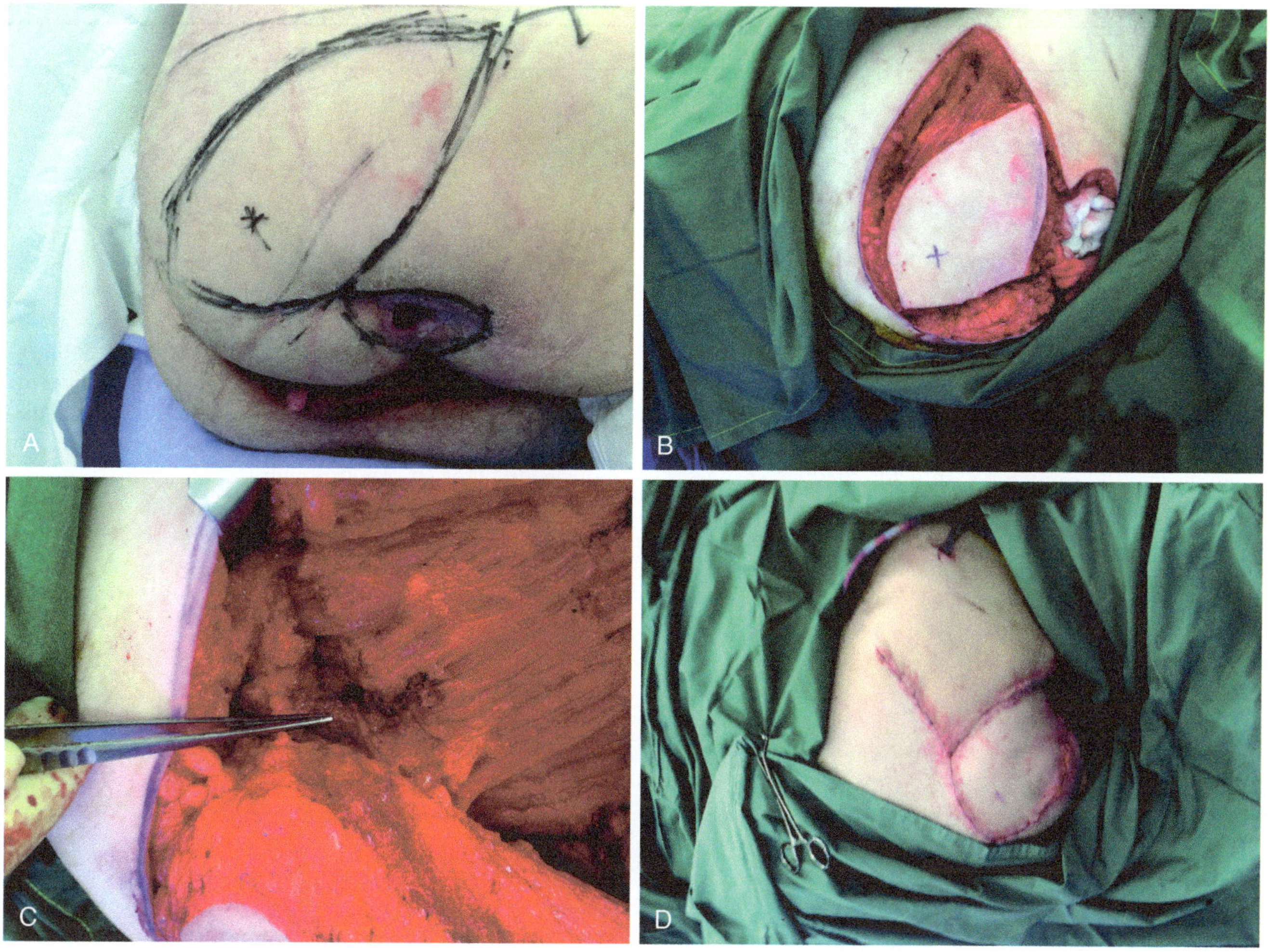

• **Fig. 41.11** Superior gluteal artery flap, islanded transposition flap. (A) Reverse flap design around the perforator. (B) Islanded flap. (C) Perforator isolation and dissection through the muscle towards the pelvis. (D) Transposition, inset, and closure of donor site. (Photographs courtesy Dr. Rostam D. Farhadieh.)

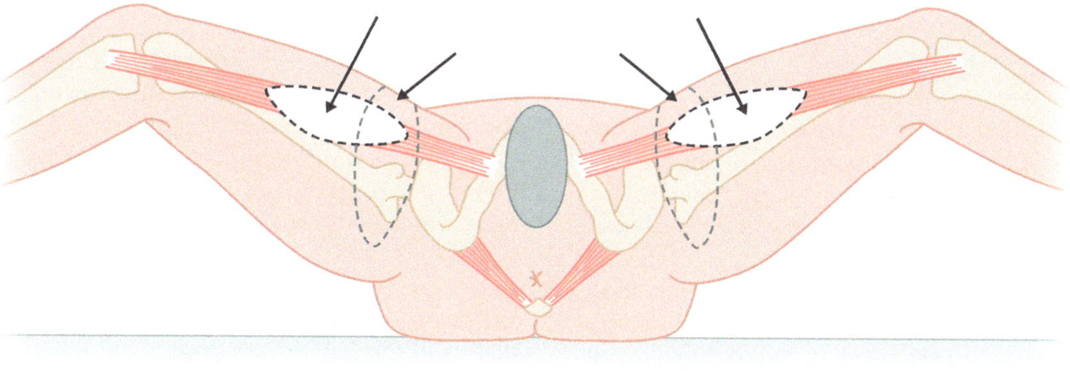

• **Fig. 41.12** Bilateral transverse myocutaneous gracilis (TMG) design.

below and parallel to the groin crease and the inferior line is drawn depending on the amount of skin available for direct closure. This gives an ellipse measuring 18–20 cm in the anterior posterior direction.

The flap is elevated from anterior to posterior in the subfascial plane until the intramuscular septum between adductor longus and gracilis is encountered. The great saphenous vein is protected and preserved (i.e., not included in the flap). The adductor longus muscle can be identified easily and the fascia over the adductor longus muscle is included with the flap. The gracilis muscle is below adductor longus and the septum between the two can be easily separated by finger dissection, exposing the distal part of gracilis. The pedicle of gracilis, ascending branch of the medial circumflex profunda femoris artery, and the vein can easily be seen under the fascia.

Postoperatively, the patient is kept in a supine position with the legs slightly abducted, with a pillow under the knees to keep them flexed. After 24–48 hours, the drains are removed and the patient is mobilized.

The gracilis muscle may also be considered for functional transposition for perineal reconstruction by preserving the nerve to the muscle.

Discussion

Perineal reconstruction is complex and involves a multidisciplinary approach. The ablative surgery often leaves the patients with significant and sometimes difficult lifestyle changes. Adherence to basic reconstructive surgery principles with provisions of a watertight, and reliable reconstruction offer patients the best chance of meaningful recovery and quality of life. The lotus petal flap and the V–Y perforator fasciocutaneous flaps have become workhorses in perineal reconstruction. The perineum is basically divided into an anterior and posterior half by a line joining the ischial tuberosities. When one-half of the perineum requires reconstruction, any one of the petals of a lotus petal flap would be sufficient. When both halves or the whole of the perineum require reconstruction, an extended petal of the lotus petal is selected according to the required size and volume. Generally, one needs three structures to reconstruct when the whole of the perineum is resected: pelvic floor, dead space, and skin cover. The first can be reconstructed either by acellular dermal matrix or de-epithelialized skin flaps. The second needs bulky but vascularized muscle or a de-epithelialized myocutaneous or fasciocutaneous flap, and the last, a skin flap.

GENITAL RECONSTRUCTION

Adeyemi A. Ogunleye and Gordon K. Lee

Introduction

Congenital anomalies of the genitalia result from a variety of genetic and prenatal causes. Abnormal genitalia are seen in patients with 46,XX chromosomes, 46,XY chromosomes, and mixed sex chromosomes. The expressions of these chromosomal abnormalities are the results of complex biological interplay. The manifestations range broadly and can affect multiple areas of human anatomy and physiology. In males, testosterone promotes development of the epididymis, vas deferens, and seminal vesicle; and Müllerian-inhibiting substance (MIS) prevents the maturation of the uterus, cervix, and upper vagina. In females, the absence of MIS allows maturation of the uterus, cervix, and upper vagina. At approximately the 9th week of gestation, normal males have produced enough testosterone to allow synthesis of DHT (dihydrotestosterone). DHT then induces fusion of the genital folds and promotes growth of the genital tubercle.[13]

A defect in any of the genes or environmental milieu that affect this developmental process can result in abnormal genitalia. Certain developmental problems, such as bladder exstrophy, can simply disrupt normally developing anatomy. Other developmental problems, specifically those disrupting gender-specific development, result in anatomy that lies on a spectrum between normal female and male external genitalia. The Prader scale, originally described by Andrea Prader in 1954, is often used to describe this anatomy. It is a 5-level scale where 1 represents normal female external genitalia with clitoromegaly and 5 represents normal male external genitalia.[14]

The type of reconstruction required for each patient varies depending on the cause of ambiguous genitalia and the resulting appearance. The most common causes of anomalous genitalia in those patients undergoing feminization procedures are congenital adrenal hyperplasia and mixed gonadal dysgenesis. Gender assignment in those with anomalous genitalia is crucial although the timing of surgery is a controversial issue. Some have suggested that the birth of ambiguous genitalia is a neonatal emergency and requires immediate intervention. Others have advocated delaying surgery until the patient can give informed consent. Most physicians, however, suggest performing surgery prior to the age of 3. Performing surgery during this earlier time increases compliance with dilatations and decreases parental concern about their child's gender. The goals in vaginal reconstruction of ambiguous genitalia include preserving fertility, adequate sexual function, and eliminating the risk of malignancy in the intraabdominal gonads.[15]

Vaginal Reconstruction

Acquired vaginal defects are commonly due to oncological resections, although other causes include trauma and infection. Rectal adenocarcinoma frequently is cited as the most common indication for vaginal resections, accounting for approximately half of all reconstructions. Other causes include anal squamous cell cancer, cervical carcinoma, bladder or urethral transitional cell, bladder or urethral squamous cell cancer, vaginal or vulvar squamous cell cancer, endometrial adenocarcinoma, and trauma.[16,17] According to Crosby et al, the most common surgical procedures resulting in vaginal defects are abdominoperineal resections and pelvic exenterations.[17]

In 2002, Cordeiro and colleagues published a classification system to define full-thickness vaginal defects.[16] Type I defects include those involving the anterior, lateral, or posterior walls of the vagina. Type IA defects involve the anterior or lateral vaginal wall, whereas type IB defects involve the posterior wall. Type II refers to circumferential vaginal defects. Type IIA defects encompass up to two-thirds of the upper portion of the vagina while type IIB defects are the result of circumferential total vaginectomies. The most common vaginal defect is a Cordeiro type IB or full-thickness posterior wall defect.[16,17]

Vaginal reconstruction has positive effects on the psyche and has been shown to improve wound healing. Placing healthy, well-vascularized tissue in a previously radiated area prevents enteroperineal fistulas and limits dead space, thereby reducing pelvic fluid collections and risk of postoperative abscess and infection.

Nonsurgical Options

In cases of vaginal agenesis where a dimple of vaginal mucosa is present, often nonsurgical techniques are preferred to surgical creation of a neovagina. The Frank procedure involves the use of serial vaginal dilators. Using the dilator, pressure is placed on the vaginal dimple for 30 minutes to 2 hours per day. Over time the width and length of the dilator are increased to allow for a neovagina that is appropriately sized for sexual activity. Some discomfort is expected during dilatations, but after dilatations are complete, only intermittent dilatation is required if sexual activity is frequent enough to maintain patency. Edmonds et al document a 94.9% success rate with dilatation treatment in patients with Mayer–Rokitansky–Küster–Hauser syndrome.[18] Ingram described a modification of the Frank procedure in which the serial dilators are attached to a bicycle seat upon which the patient sits.[19] The modified positioning allows for improved patient comfort during serial dilatations.

Surgical Options

The reconstructive surgeon must consider multiple factors when planning the surgical creation of a neovagina. The location and size of the defect is the most important factor. However, it is also valuable to consider the patient's position on the operating room table. The oncological surgeon may have completed the procedure with the patient in the prone or supine position. This may influence the options that are available without repositioning the patient. The type of incision, particularly whether a laparotomy incision was performed, and whether the initial incision remains open or has been closed, can alter the operative plan. The desired neovagina length and width should be based on the patient's postoperative goals for sexual activity. The need for a connection between the neovagina and the uterus, when present, must be considered in congenital reconstruction.

Small defects of the vagina are amenable to *primary closure* if they do not significantly alter the length or width of the vagina. For larger defects, which are superficial or partial thickness, a *skin graft* can be considered. A vaginal conformer is often used to help promote take of the skin graft, which provides compression and immobilization of the graft to the underlying wound bed. In the pediatric gynecology literature, the preferred method for surgical creation of a neovagina in patients with vaginal agenesis is the Abbé–McIndoe procedure. First documented in 1938, this involves creating a space between with rectum and bladder and inserting a skin graft-lined mold to create the neovagina. This procedure requires the use of a mold or vaginal conformer for 6–12 months postoperatively and dilatations to maintain a vagina that can be used for sexual activity. Fussey et al. have also described the use of continuous negative pressure therapy to aid in skin graft take during vaginoplasty.[20]

The *pedicled rectus abdominis myocutaneous flap* is the workhorse of vaginal reconstruction. Cordeiro described the use of the rectus flap for both partial posterior vaginal defects and circumferential upper two-thirds defects.[16] The myocutaneous flap can be designed and harvested with a vertical or transverse skin paddle. The senior author (G.K.L.) prefers the vertical rectus abdominis myocutaneous (VRAM) flap as it is aligned with the midline incision that is most often used for a laparotomy incision, and, therefore, provides the greatest length of flap and greatest reach for the vaginal and perineal defect. The flap is based upon the deep inferior epigastric artery and can be passed directly into the pelvis/vaginal defect. Authors have recently described the harvest of the flap as a perforator flap for vaginal reconstructions noting decreased donor site morbidity.[21] However, incorporation of the rectus muscle provides additional bulk and blood supply, which can be helpful in eliminating pelvic dead space and facilitating healing.

The *pedicled gracilis myocutaneous flap*, based on the medial femoral circumflex vessels, is another versatile option for vaginal and perineal reconstruction. The flap can be harvested with a transverse or longitudinal skin paddle. Cordeiro favored the longitudinal skin paddle for total circumferential vaginal defects while the transverse skin paddle can be used for labial reconstruction (Fig. 41.13). It is important to note past reports of necrosis of the gracilis skin paddle when designed

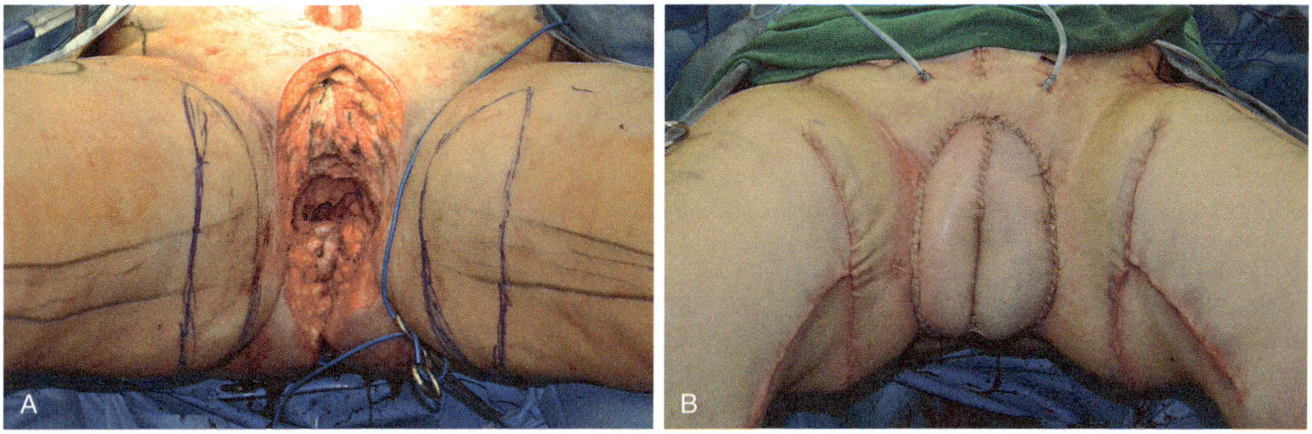

• **Fig. 41.13** Transverse upper gracilis (TUG) flap for total vaginal reconstruction. (A) Defect after oncological resection and flap design. (B) Final flap inset with donor site closed.

distally on the muscle down the thigh. Surgeons should note that the gracilis muscle tapers distally and becomes more tendinous, and that the blood supply of an overlying skin paddle at this level becomes less reliable. Hence, a skin paddle that incorporates the proximal major skin perforator, which enters at approximately 8–10 cm below the pubic ramus, is important for maintaining maximal perfusion.

The *pudendal thigh flap* was first published by Wee and Joseph in 1989, and is often referred to as the "Singapore flap."[22] The flap is an innervated fasciocutanous flap based off perforators from the internal pudendal artery, which travel from posterior to anterior. The skin flaps are designed over the proximal medial thigh and harvested deep to the fascia of the adductor muscles. Proponents of this flap cite the benefit of an inconspicuous donor site and more reliable blood supply than the gracilis myocutaneous flap. This technique has been used in the reconstruction of both congenital and acquired defects. This flap is of limited bulk, and should be considered for defects that do not require a large amount of dead space obliteration.

Intestinal conduits, including the colon and jejunum, have also been utilized for vaginal reconstruction. This type of reconstruction is more widely documented for congenital defects. Erman Akar et al described their experience with vaginal reconstruction for congenital defects (33 of 34 patients) using a free vascularized jejunal flap.[23] At a mean follow-up of 50 months, the authors noted satisfactory vaginal depth and diameter. However, six patients noted jejunal hypersecretion post-reconstruction and 10 patients required two lengths of jejunum opened along its antimesenteric border in order to increase luminal diameter. In contrast, the benefit of the colon in vaginal reconstruction is its larger diameter in comparison to the jejunum. Lima et al reviewed their 34-year experience treating 46 cases of vaginal agenesis with sigmoid colon interposition.[24] While they noted no cases of excessive mucus production, eight patients had stenosis, six of whom required operative intervention. Of note, 34% of the group was sexually active at a mean follow-up of 12 years. Anecdotally, some patients may report a foul odor with the use of intestinal conduits as a result of mucus secretions.

Omental flaps, which have been used to treat rectovaginal and vesicovaginal fistulas as well as to close off the pelvic inlet after pelvic exenteration, can be modified for vaginal reconstruction. Authors have documented the use of a cylindricized omental flap based off the left gastroepiploic artery with a skin graft for neovaginal creation.[25] The minimal donor site morbidity and ease of flap harvest are among the benefits of this flap. However, like other skin graft-based reconstructions, stenting is necessary for up to 6 months postoperatively to maintain adequate vaginal depth and to prevent strictures and stenoses.

The *anterolateral thigh (ALT) flap* has emerged as another option for vaginal and perineal reconstruction. Based on the descending branch of the lateral femoral circumflex artery, the ALT flap is a versatile flap for reconstruction. The flap can be harvested as a fasciocutaneous, an adipofascial, or a musculocutaneous flap. This versatility is beneficial for reconstruction in the perineum where dead space obliteration may be required or thinner pliable tissue may be ideal. The flap is tunneled beneath the rectus femoris and sartorius to improve pedicle length.

Complications

The most common complication after vaginal reconstruction is delayed wound healing or dehiscence. Other more devastating complications include: flap necrosis, fistula formation, and pelvic abscesses. Strictures may develop that require dilatations or revision surgery. Donor site infections may also be seen, as vaginal reconstruction is not a clean procedure. It is advised to use a separate clean set of instruments for flap harvest outside of the abdominal cavity if practical. After vaginal reconstruction with a rectus abdominis myocutaneous flap or an intestinal conduit, neovagina prolapse can occur which becomes bothersome to the patient. This may require secondary correction with sacral suspension.

Penile Reconstruction

Aphallia (complete absence of the penis) is a severe congenital anomaly estimated to occur in 1 in 30 million live births and may be associated with other malformations of the perineal area such as urogenital septum malformation sequence.[26] Options for reconstruction include a single-stage random pattern midline pubic flap with mucosal flap for urethral reconstruction,[26] or a two-stage random pattern parascrotal skin flap for the shaft and midline perineal skin flap for the urethra at the second stage. The absence of erectile tissue will require separate management at adulthood, which typically involves the use of a prosthetic implant.

Acquired penile defects may be secondary to trauma, infection, or oncological resections. Penile trauma is rather uncommon since the penis has a relatively protected position between the thighs and pubic bone, but can occur particularly in military injuries where the trunk is often protected but the lower extremities and pelvis are not and vulnerable to explosive devices. Penile skin loss occurs from necrotizing infections, burns, constrictive bands, degloving injuries as well as dog and human bites. Avulsions are most often caused by power tool injuries or motor vehicle accidents. They have also occurred from self-inflicted causes such as insertion of the penis into vacuum cleaners or other suction devices. Penetrating penile trauma is usually secondary to stab or gunshot wounds.

The most common cause of penile carcinoma requiring major resection is squamous cell cancer. Approximately 1500 new cases are diagnosed each year in the USA, accounting for less than 1% of all malignancies in men. The tumor is age-related, with a peak incidence in the fifth and sixth decades. In addition to squamous cell carcinoma, almost all tumors that involve the skin, subcutaneous tissue, and smooth muscle have been found in the penis. Resection can include circumcision for foreskin lesions, Mohs micrographic surgical resections, glansectomy, wide local excision, partial penectomy, and total penectomy.

Surgical Options

Preoperatively, the surgeon should discuss with the patient his sexual history as well as his goals for reconstruction. The need for multiple procedures in order to fully restore sexual function should be discussed in detail with the patient. If the defect is self-inflicted, a psychiatric evaluation is necessary prior to reconstruction. Akin to vaginal reconstruction, the reconstructive surgeon must consider the size and location of the defect.

Subtotal Reconstruction

Subtotal injuries to the penis may involve the shaft and/or glans. For injuries involving the skin only, such as those due to avulsion or infection, a skin graft is the best option for reconstruction. A full-thickness skin graft is preferred for shaft resurfacing due to decreased contracture during the healing process. Injuries to the glans only can be reconstructed using a split-thickness skin graft or a urethral flap. A urethral flap involves dissection of the penile urethra from the corpora cavernosa. The distal end of the urethra is then spatulated and folded ventral to create a pseudoglans.

Total Reconstruction

Total penile reconstruction may be based on the tube within a tube concept to create the shaft and glans as well as the penile urethra. Gillies was among the first to describe a technique for total penile reconstruction.[27] Because of the unique anatomy of the erectile tissue of the penis, urologists recommend maintaining penile length whenever possible and then utilizing secondary procedures, such as excision of the suprapubic fat pad or division of the suspensory ligament, to increase penis length. However, if the trauma, tumor or infection is so severe that total penile reconstruction is required, local/regional flaps as well as free tissue transfer techniques are available.

Local and regional flaps available for phallus reconstruction include the pedicled rectus abdominis, groin, and tensor fascia lata flaps. Recently, the ALT flap has been described for total penile reconstruction.[28] The available width and length of skin and soft tissue which can be harvested and tailored as well as the favorable donor site make the ALT flap the favored option for many reconstructive surgeons (Fig. 41.14). A neurorrhaphy between the lateral femoral cutaneous nerve harvested with the ALT flap and the dorsal pudendal nerve gives sensation to the neophallus. Insertion of a prosthetic stiffener can allow the patient to have an erect reconstruction.

Free tissue transfer techniques have allowed the use of the radial forearm free flap (RFFF), based on the radial artery, and the free fibula, based on the peroneal vessels, for penile reconstruction. The use of bone within the flap avoids a second-stage surgery for implantation of penile prosthesis, which is required in soft tissue only reconstructions if erectile function is desired. However, this creates a permanently erect penile reconstruction, which can potentially be problematic. With regards to the RFFF, the conspicuous donor site involving the majority of the skin on the forearm can leave an unsightly scar.

Penile transplantation is a novel option that was first successfully performed in 2014, with achievement of urinary, erectile and sexual function.[29] Transplantation allows replacement of the unique erectile tissue of the penis and eliminates donor site morbidity, but must be balanced against the risks of long-term immunosuppression. Psychological considerations must be considered during patient selection and a multidisciplinary team of plastic surgeons, urologists, and transplant physicians is essential for success.

Gender-Affirming Surgery

Gender affirming surgery can be performed in patients with gender identity disorder to help alleviate gender dysphoria. Gender identity disorder is defined as the disturbance from a strong and persistent cross-gender identification and it cannot be concurrent with a physical intersex condition. A variety of treatments exist, ranging from medical and hormonal therapy to gender-affirming surgery. Similar to gender-assignment surgery for ambiguous genitalia, gender-affirming surgery aims to create an outcome that optimizes appearance, urinary function, and sexual function.

The timing of gender-affirming surgery is important for developing a lasting benefit. Studies of prepubertal children who were referred to clinics for gender dysphoria have suggested that less than 30% of those patients had persistence of this dsyphoria into adulthood.[30] The percentage of lasting gender dysphoria increases with increasing age of initial presentation.

Upon embarking on gender-affirming procedures, a number of steps should be taken prior to surgery. These include social changes and reversible hormonal treatments.[30] The World Professional Association for Transgender Health (WPATH) recommends carrying out genital surgery only when the patient has reached a legal age to give informed consent and after the patient has lived for at least 12 continuous months in the gender role that is congruent with their gender identity. A multidisciplinary approach with psychiatrists, endocrinologists, speech, and language therapists, breast surgeons, plastic surgeons, gynecologists, or urologists is often employed.

Conclusion

Successful genital reconstruction requires open communication between the surgeon, the patient, and other medical personnel. The reconstructive surgeon must have a comprehensive picture of the patient's postoperative goals. In cases of tumor resection, the oncological and reconstructive surgeons should develop a team approach. For congenital reconstructions or gender dysphoria cases, a psychologist or psychiatrist should be involved to help the patient navigate

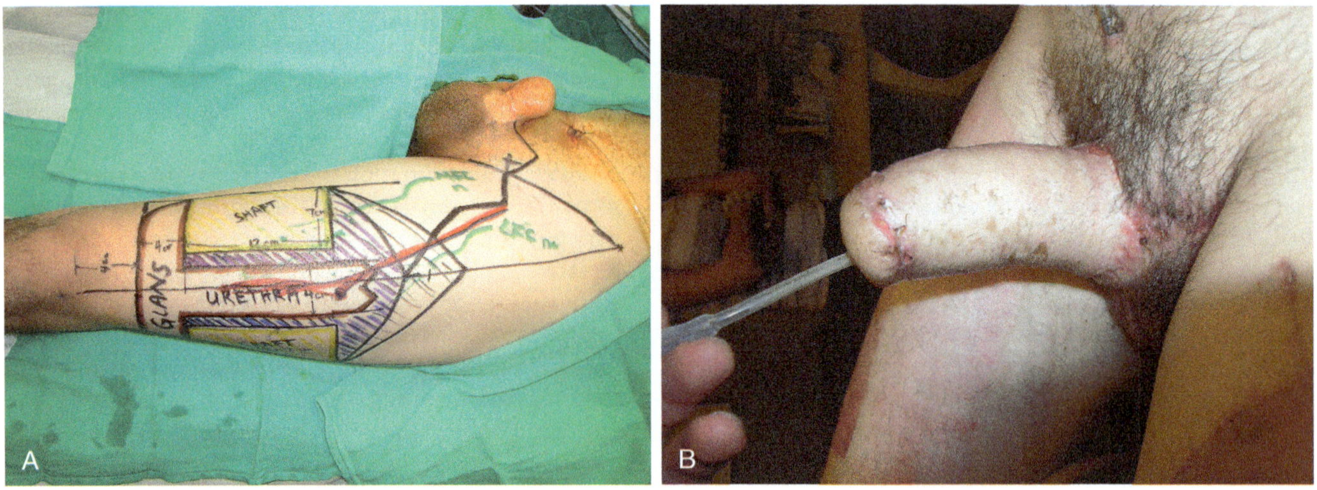

• **Fig. 41.14** Anterolateral thigh flap for penis reconstruction. (A) Flap design prior to reconstruction. (B) Completed reconstruction 1 month postoperatively.

the complex and diverse psychosocial issues involved in gender assignment and affirmation. The reconstructive surgeon has a variety of options available to achieve functional and satisfying results in vaginal and penile reconstruction.

HYPOSPADIAS

Kathryn Evans and Imran Mushtaq

Introduction

Hypospadias is the most common congenital abnormality of the penis. It is characterized by the association of three anatomical abnormalities that are present in a variable manner:

- A proximally located urethral meatus on the ventral aspect of the penis
- A ventral curvature of the shaft of the penis (chordee)
- A dorsally hooded prepuce that is deficient and incomplete ventrally.

Hypospadias results from the deficiency of the tissues forming the ventral aspect of the penis beyond the division of the corpus spongiosum, most likely due to incomplete virilization of the genital tubercle. As a consequence, there is a ventral triangular defect with the apex located at the division of the corpus spongiosus, the sides formed by the two pillars of the atretic spongiosum, and the base by the glans. The typical hypospadiac penis has the glans open ventrally, with an absent segment of the urethra of variable length. In place of the normal tubular urethra is the urethral plate, which extends from the ectopic meatus up onto the glans. The urethral plate is often hypoplastic or dysplastic, and may be partially responsible for the chordee. For this reason the fibrotic tissue that forms a part of the urethral plate is referred to as the "chordee tissue." The corpus spongiosum, which would normally encircle the urethra, is either absent or displaced laterally in the region of the urethral plate. More proximal to the ectopic urethral meatus, the structures forming the ventral aspect of the penis are mostly normal.

The diagnosis of hypospadias is usually made at birth, but occasionally when the child is brought for cultural or religious circumcision. In both instances, the parents should be advised not to have the child circumcised as the foreskin may be required for surgical reconstruction.

Classification

Hypospadias is most commonly classified anatomically according to the position of the urethral meatus (Fig. 41.15), with 70% of cases being located at the glanular, coronal, and subcoronal level (distal hypospadias). The remaining 30% are described as midshaft, penoscrotal, midscrotal, and perineal (proximal hypospadias). Mouriquand et al[31] have proposed that a more accurate means of classification would be according to the level of the division of the corpus spongiosum, as the urethra can be hypoplastic and adherent to the ventral skin distal to the division of the spongiosum.

Incidence and Etiology

Hypospadias occurs in around 1 in every 250 male births, with a degree of geographical variation. In Western countries the incidence of hypospadias has been noted to increase over the past 15 years.[32] Some of the differences in prevalence reported between countries and over time are artefacts of study methodology. However, there appears to be a genuine increase in the incidence of related abnormalities such as cryptorchidism and testicular cancer, as well as a fall in male fertility. The precise cause is unknown but likely to be multifactorial. The main etiological factor is believed to be exposure to endocrine-disrupting chemicals. These are exogenous substances that interfere with endocrine pathways. Examples would include dietary phytoestrogens, pesticides (e.g., dichlorodiphenyltrichloroethane (DDT)) and other toxins that are known to disrupt reproduction. There is also a genetic component, as the incidence is higher if there is a positive family history (1 in 100 to 1 in 80 male

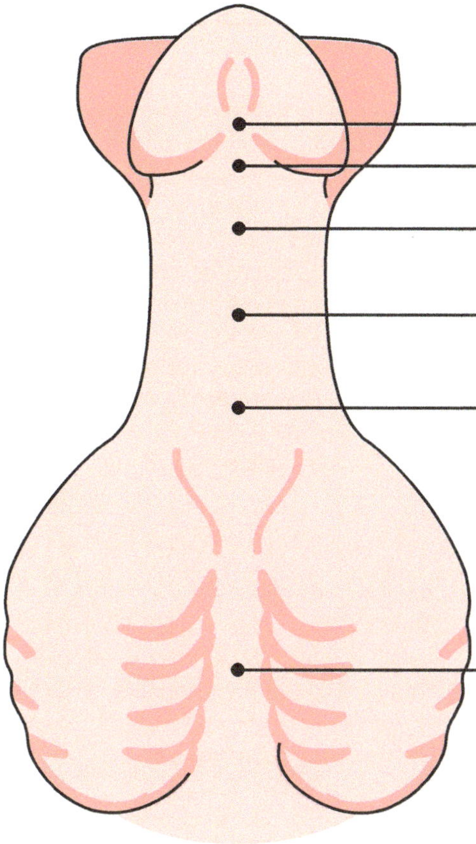

• **Fig. 41.15** Classification of hypospadias according to the position of the urethral meatus.

births). For example, brothers of affected individuals have a 6%–17% chance of also being affected. In a series of 205 hypospadias patients compared to 205 controls, the risk of having another child with hypospadias was increased 17-fold. In a Swedish series of 2500 patients, 7% reported one additional family member with hypospadias.[33]

Associated Anomalies

Although hypospadias is mostly an isolated anomaly, 10%–15% of patients have additional congenital malformations, primarily affecting the urogenital system. Some of these will have a pattern of malformations suggestive of recognizable chromosomal abnormalities, as summarized in Table 41.1. Boys with hypospadias and an undescended testis should be investigated for the possibility of an underlying disorder of sex development. Karyotyping should therefore be performed in children who have hypospadias in association with other anomalies.

Management

Nonoperative Management

In cases of distal hypospadias (especially glanular and coronal) the option of nonoperative management should be discussed with the parents. The potential minimal benefit of advancing the meatus with a urethroplasty should be weighed up against the potential high risk of complications. They may be offered a circumcision or a foreskin reconstruction for cosmesis.

TABLE 41.1 Syndromic Gene Mutations Associated with Hypospadias

Gene	Disorder
SF1	No adrenal glands
WT1	Wilms' tumor Denyus–Drash syndrome (Wilms' tumor and renal failure) Frasier syndrome
SOX9	
HOXA13	Hand–foot–genital syndrome

Surgical Principles

The main aims of surgery are to straighten the penis, to reconstruct the urethral defect, to create a slit-like meatus in a near terminal position on the glans and finally to reconstruct the penile shaft skin, either with or without circumcision. A successful surgical reconstruction should allow the individual to micturate standing up with a single, straight urinary stream and to allow for sexual intercourse with a straight erection. At the same time, the cosmetic result must be acceptable to the parents and the individual. This is a formidable challenge, which is perhaps why more than 300 different operations have been described for hypospadias repair.

Correction of Chordee

The first step in hypospadias surgery is the correction of chordee. This begins with fully degloving the penis all the way down to the base of the penis, and sometimes beyond the penoscrotal junction. In the majority of cases (87%) this maneuver alone will straighten the penis as the chordee commonly results from an abnormal attachment of the ventral skin to the penile shaft. If the chordee persists after degloving then some surgeons would advocate mobilizing the urethral plate off the ventral surface of the corpora cavernosa. This can jeopardize the blood supply to the urethral plate and is thus not a popular technique.

Most surgeons in Europe would perform a dorsal plication in the corpora cavernosa to correct the residual chordee. The two most common techniques for this are the Nesbit procedure and the Baskin modification. The Nesbit procedure was initially described in 1965 and modified in 1994. It is performed by plicating the tunica albuginea by suturing two parallel incisions with a 6-0 monofilament suture. The Baskin modification[34] is performed in the midline to avoid injury to the neurovascular bundles. The correction of the chordee can be confirmed by means of manual pressure on the bulbospongiosus, without the need for a formal artificial erection test. The potential disadvantage of a dorsal plication is that it may cause shortening of the penis. For this reason some surgeons, particularly those in North America, would favor ventral lengthening. There are essentially two ways to achieve ventral lengthening. The first involves multiple superficial transverse incisions along the corpora cavernosa and the second involves a single incision through the tunica albuginea at the point of maximal curvature and the placement of a graft into the resulting defect, using dermis,[35] tunica vaginalis[36] or small intestinal mucosa.[37]

Reconstruction of the Urethra

When the urethral defect is relatively short and the urethral plate is wide, the urethra can be reconstructed by simple tubularization of the lateral edges (Thiersch–Duplay technique). If the urethral plate is narrow then a midline longitudinal incision may provide further width to allow tubularization (Snodgrass technique). The other option would be to suture a pedicalized rectangular flap of penile or preputial skin to the lateral edges (onlay island flap procedure). With a lengthier urethral defect, there are essentially two options. The first would be to perform the surgery in a staged manner, with the first stage involving placing a free or pedicalized graft (inner prepuce, penile skin, postauricular skin or buccal mucosa) on the ventral aspect of the corpora and glans. Once the graft is mature (after 6 months) this can be used to fashion the urethra by tubularization in the second stage. This two-stage technique is has gained significant popularity worldwide. The alternative would be to substitute the urethra with a tubularized flap of pedicalized inner prepuce (Duckett procedure) or buccal mucosa. The Duckett procedure, once very popular in the 1980s, has lost favor due to high reoperation rates.

Reconstruction of the Penile Shaft Skin

Once reconstruction of the urethra has been completed, it is customary to cover the urethroplasty with a "waterproofing" layer, which is harvested from the adjacent dartos tissue or a dorsal pedicle of dartos tissue which is brought ventrally to cover the urethra. Finally, the penile skin is reconstructed with or without a circumcision.

Surgical Techniques

The main challenge of hypospadias surgery is whether the desired outcome can be achieved in a single operation or will require a staged procedure. In some cases this cannot be determined until during the actual surgery. Most surgeons focus on two or three preferred techniques and at the present time the Snodgrass technique or tubularized incised plate (TIP) repair is the favored technique for distal hypospadias. For the more proximal repairs, most surgeons use a two-stage repair. The remainder of this section will focus on these two most common techniques for hypospadias repair.

The surgery is ideally performed between 6 and 18 months age. If a two-stage procedure is anticipated, then the aim should be to complete both stages by the age of 2 years. This is based on emotional, cognitive, and psychosexual factors as well as improved tissue healing in the younger patient. Some surgeons prefer to do the surgery around the age of 5 years due to anesthetic limitations. Another advantage of performing surgery at an older age is that the tissues may be more robust, making the repair somewhat easier. There is considerable debate regarding preoperative penile hormonal stimulation when the penile size is very small. It can be administered systemically as beta-human chorionic gonadotrophin (beta-HCG) or testosterone or topically in the form of dihydrotestosterone gel. There is emerging evidence, however, that their use can lead to delays in healing.[38]

Tubularised Incised Plate (Snodgrass) Repair

Warren Snodgrass described the technique in 1994.[39] It is versatile, easily performed, has fewer complications and results in a cosmetically acceptable slit-like meatus. Relative contraindications include proximal hypospadias, a distal hypospadias with significant chordee or a poor glans groove, which would be too narrow for tubularization.

Operative Technique

Degloving the Penis and Chordee Correction

A polypropylene traction suture is placed in the glans just beyond the anticipated dorsal lip of the neomeatus. The urethra and overlying skin are assessed with a urethral sound or the tip of the forceps. The distal portion of the urethra may be quite thin and adherent to the skin. Usually, a circumscribing skin incision is made 1–2 mm proximal to the meatus and the shaft skin is degloved to the penoscrotal junction. If the urethra is excessively thin, a U-shaped incision is made extending to more healthy tissues. At this stage the penis is assessed for any chordee and this can be corrected (as described above) (Fig. 41.16).

Urethroplasty

The urethral plate is separated from the glans wings by parallel longitudinal incisions. The glans wings are mobilized laterally, taking care to avoid damage to the margins of the urethral plate. In most cases the urethral plate is not sufficiently wide at this point to tubularize into a functional urethra. Therefore a relaxing incision is made in the midline from within the meatus to the end of the urethral plate. This incision should extend through the epithelium to near the underlying corpora cavernosa. An 8Fr stent is passed into the bladder. The urethral plate is then tubularized over this stent using a fine monofilament suture. The neomeatus should be generously sized. Adjacent dartos layer is then used to cover this suture line; alternatively a dartos pedicle is developed from the dorsal shaft skin and transposed to the ventral surface. Following this the glans wings are mobilized and then closed in two layers using a fine monofilament suture.

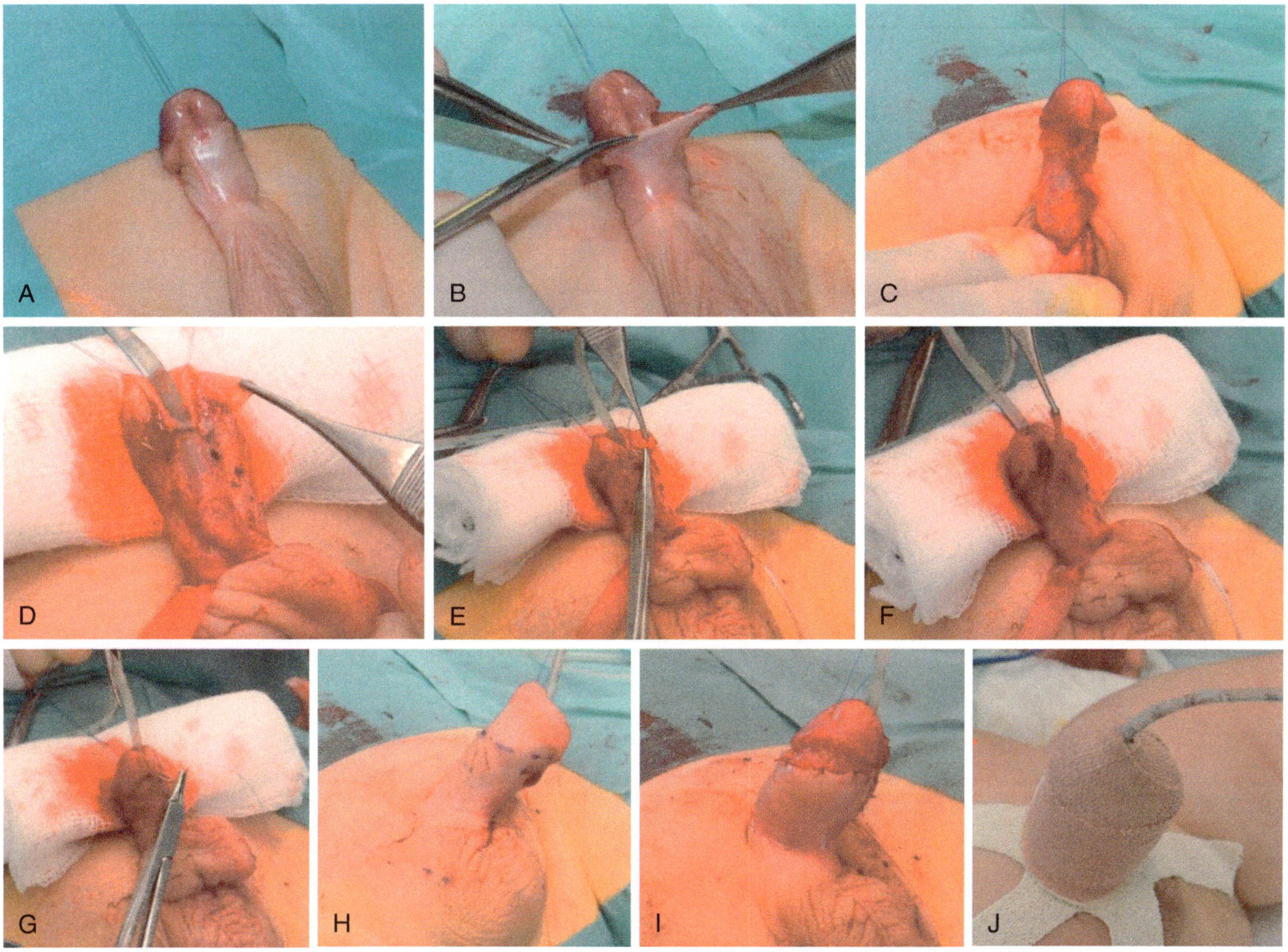

• **Fig. 41.16** (A) Placement of the glans stitch. (B) Degloving of the penis. (C) Assessment of chordee once fully degloved. (D) Glans wings are formed. (E) The urethroplasty is performed. (F) Dartos waterproofing layer is secured over the completed urethroplasty. (G) The glans wings are closed in one or two layers. (H) The excess dorsal skin is excised. (I) The excess skin is reconfigured to complete circumcision. (J) Cavicare and Elastoplast dressing are applied.

Skin Closure and Dressing

The skin is then reconfigured, ensuring that there is enough skin to cover the deficiency of skin on the ventral surface. The excess dorsal skin is excised to complete the circumcision. The stent is secured in place using the traction suture and a pressure dressing (e.g., MepilexXT or Allevyn Gentle) is applied and this is then covered with Elastoplast. This remains in situ for 7 days with a one-week course of antibiotics and anticholinergics to prevent bladder spasms.

Outcomes

With careful patient selection, the results of the TIP repair are very favourable and reproducible. Snodgrass et al reported a multicenter experience using the TIP urethroplasty.[40] The study included 148 boys operated on by six pediatric urologists. All patients had a vertically-orientated and normally-placed meatus. The cosmetic appearance was considered superior to that obtained by standard flap techniques, with a 7% complication rate. Five boys developed a fistula, two of these closed spontaneously, three boys developed meatal stenosis,and three had a partial glans dehiscence.

The two-stage technique described by Bracka[41] is indicated when the meatus is located at the midshaft or more proximally, in the presence of severe chordee and in those with an inadequate urethral plate. This technique is also excellent for failed hypospadias repairs.[42] The main aim of the first stage is to lay the foundation for the construction of a straight, esthetic, and normally-functioning penis in the second stage. The first stage comprises correction of the chordee, circumcision, and grafting the ventrum of the penile shaft and glans. The ideal material for the graft should be non-hair-bearing, robust, and supple. It should be able to be harvested without leaving a cosmetic defect. The inner preputial skin is most commonly used for the graft, as it is readily available. In its absence posterior auricular skin is a good alternative as it is relatively thin, pliable, and essentially non-hair-bearing. It also leaves an inconspicuous scar. Some surgeons would prefer to use buccal mucosa, as it is abundant and particularly useful when balanitis xerotica obliterans is a complication of previous repairs with skin grafts. Buccal mucosa can be harvested from the inner cheek or a combination of inner cheek and inner lip. The parotid duct located near the upper second molar should be identified and carefully preserved.

First-Stage Operative Technique

Degloving and Chordee Correction

The penis is fully degloved down to the penoscrotal junction following a circumscribing incision. Dorsally the dissection continues superficial to Buck's fascia and on the ventral aspect the urethral plate, Buck's fascia, and the corpus spongiosum are mobilized from the corpus cavernosa and excised. The meatus moves to a more proximal position and this should be opened ventrally to ensure it is of adequate size. The glans is incised in the midline, deep enough to clearly visualize the corpora cavernosa. The dorsal limit of this incision will correspond to the dorsal margin of the future external urethral meatus. At this stage if there is still residual chordee then one of the techniques described previously can be utilized (Fig. 41.17).

Harvesting the Graft

The size of the graft needs to be adequate to fully cover the ventral defect without tension. The graft is usually harvested from the inner and/or outer aspect of the prepuce, or alternatively the posterior auricular skin or buccal mucosa. On occasions, composite grafts may be required if the defect is large. The graft is tacked down to a silicone board to facilitate removal of the surplus subcutaneous fat and alveolar tissue. This process should result in a translucent membrane.

Securing and Immobilizing the Graft

The graft is placed onto the defect, trimmed to size, and secured with fine monofilament sutures. Fenestrations may be made in the graft to allow any hematoma to escape. A few midline quilting sutures are recommended to secure the graft in place. A roll of petroleum jelly gauze dressing

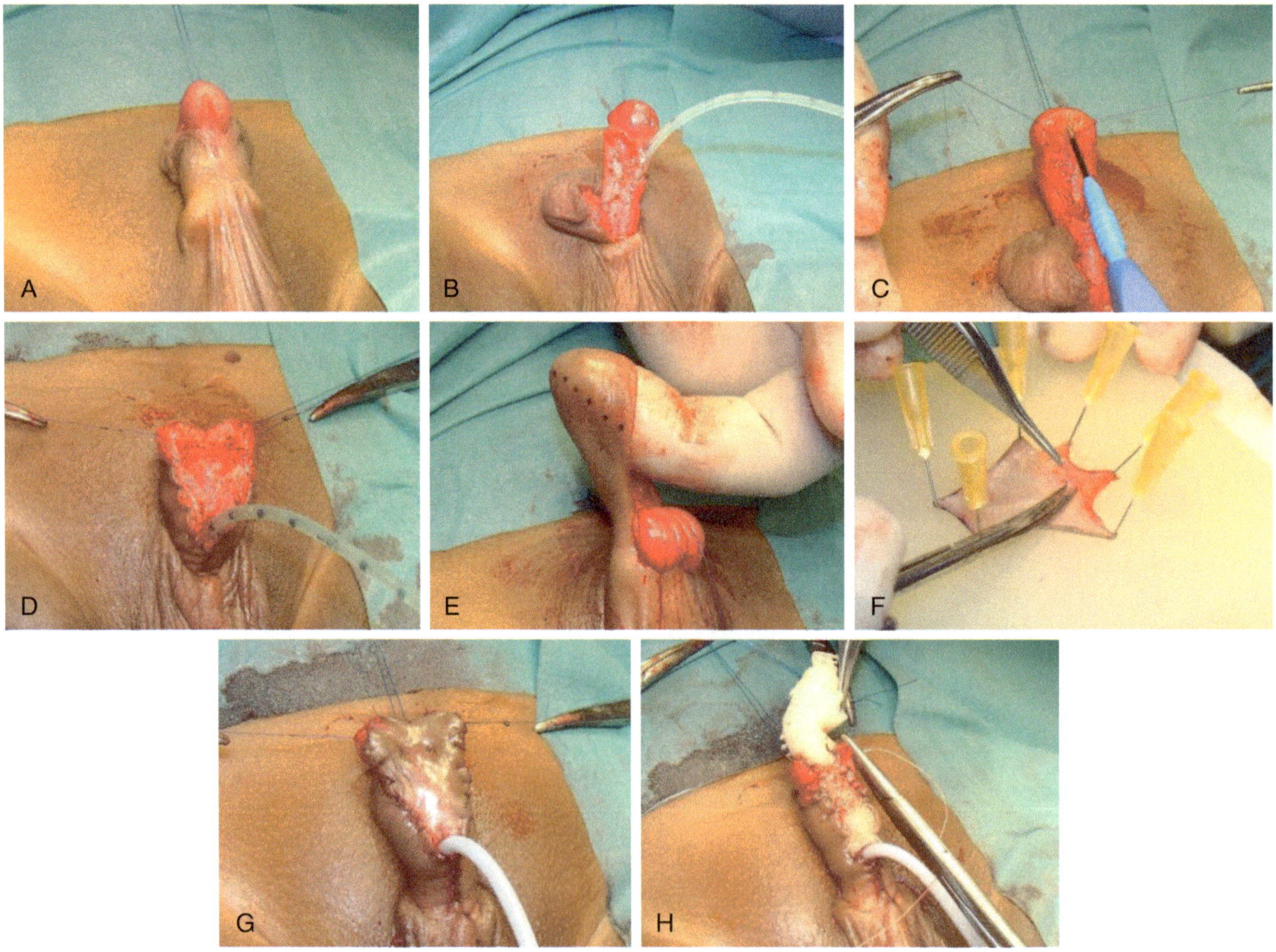

• **Fig. 41.17** (A) Midshaft hypospadias suitable for a two-stage procedure. (B) Penis is fully degloved and any chordee is corrected. (C) The glans is split in the midline. (D) The penis is split in the midline to allow placement of the graft. (E) The graft is harvested from the dorsal prepuce. (F) The graft is prepared on a silicone block. (G) The graft is secured in place. (H) The Vaseline gauze dressing is secured in place.

is secured onto the graft with sutures. This will minimize shearing forces on the graft and is supplemented with a pressure dressing and Elastoplast. The dressing is left in situ with a dripping stent for 7 days.

Postoperative Care

The dressing should be removed under general anesthetic, at which stage the graft can be inspected. The parents should be instructed to apply an antibiotic ointment (chloramphenicol) three times daily to the graft for a period of 2 weeks. After a further 4 weeks the graft should be moisturized daily with a simple emollient cream.

Second-Stage Operative Technique

The second stage is usually performed after a minimum period of 6 months. The graft should be smooth, well vascularized, and the glans cleft sharply delineated. A U-shaped incision on the grafted skin is marked from the ventral limit of the neourethral meatus with the lower limits skirting closely around the margin of the proximal urethral meatus (Fig. 41.18). The marked ventral strip is incised and mobilized to allow tubularization of the neourethra over an 8Fr stent. A layer of adventitia should be used to cover the urethroplasty. The glans wings are mobilized and closed in one or two layers, although this may not be possible in all cases. The skin is approximated and the stent is secured using the glans traction suture. A pressure dressing is applied and secured with Elastoplast. The dressing and stent are then removed after 7 days in the outpatient setting.

Outcomes

A study on the outcome of the two-stage repair in 62 boys was performed in 2006.[43] Indications for a two-stage repair included proximal meatus (midshaft, penoscrotal or perineal), poor glans groove, and lichen sclerosis with a median age at surgery of 27.6 months. Inner preputial skin was the graft of choice and was successful in all the patients. One patient developed a hematoma. Overall cosmetic results were subjectively excellent. Complications included partial glans dehiscence (three patients), residual mild curvature (three patients), and meatal stenosis (three patients).

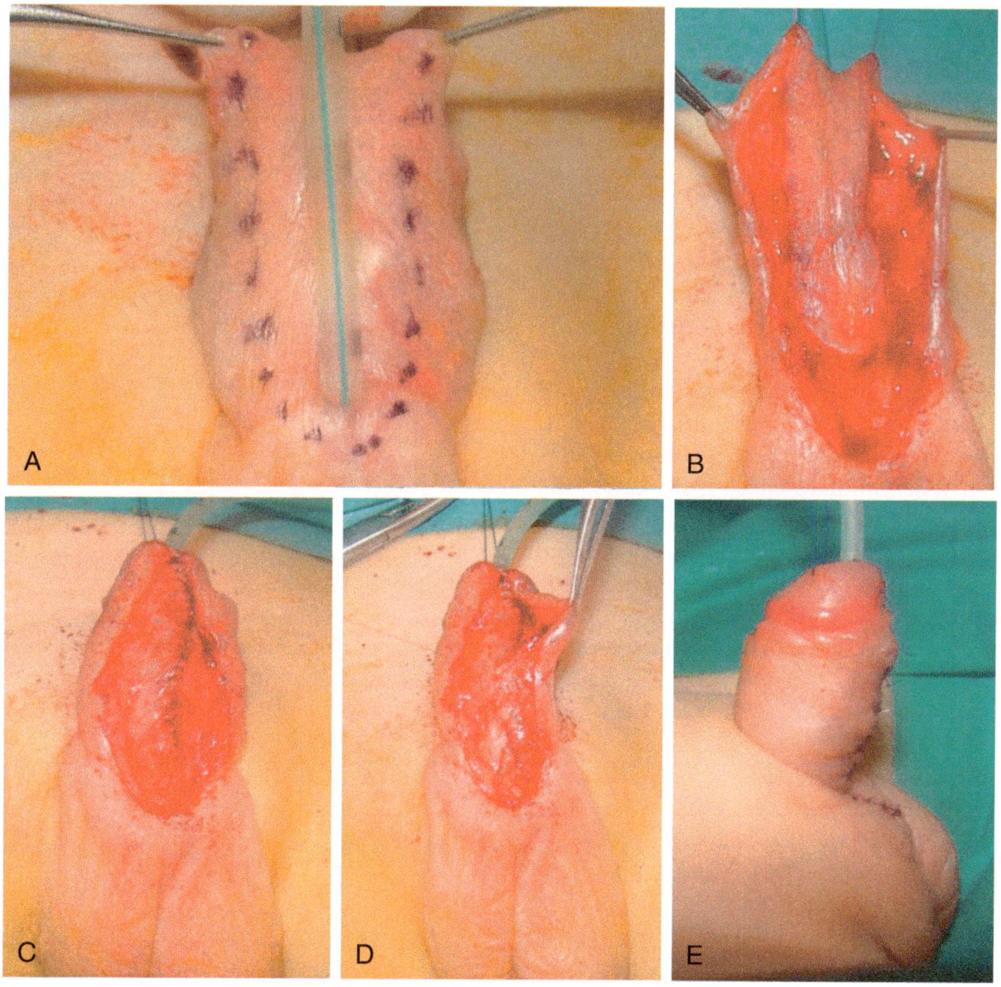

• **Fig. 41.18** (A) The location of the incision is marked. (B) The incision is made with a scalpel and/or monopolar diathermy. (C) Urethroplasty is performed in one or two layers. (D) Waterproofing layer is secured over the urethroplasty. (E) Skin closure.

A study from the same institution in 2017[44] reported a single surgeon's experience using a free graft. This study included 301 boys (208 primary, 93 revision). Overall reoperation rate was 6.3% which is considerably lower than previous studies.

Complications

Complications include bleeding, infection, meatal stenosis, urethrocutaneous fistula, and urethral stricture.

Bleeding

The most common early complication is bleeding but it is rarely significant. Bipolar diathermy is used during the surgery for precise pinpoint cauterization. Excessive cauterization should be avoided to avoid tissue ischemia. The risk of bleeding is minimized by using the supportive pressure dressing and applying the compressive Elastoplast. Early hematoma formation can lead to infection, fistula formation, and breakdown of the repair. It is rare for a patient to return to theater for bleeding, and if required the hematoma should be evacuated, the bleeding controlled, and the dressing reapplied.

Infection

Skin infections following hypospadias repair are uncommon as the patients are maintained on a 7-day course of oral antibiotics. If following dressing removal an infection is evident, the antibiotic treatment should be broadened and continued for a further 7–10 days.

Meatal Stenosis

Ensuring a wide distal anastomosis while preserving good blood supply can minimize the incidence of meatal stenosis. It may result from ischemia of the glans wings or an overzealous attempt to terminalize the urethral meatus in the setting of an inadequate glans. In such cases it may be pertinent to leave the meatus in a coronal location. The child may present with straining to void, a fine urinary stream, spraying, or urinary tract infections due to incomplete emptying of the bladder. When meatal stenosis is suspected, the child should be evaluated with an assessment of the urinary flow rate and a careful external inspection. If confirmed, the patient will require a meatal calibration and meatoplasty. Meatal stenosis can occur many years following the hypospadias repair and in these delayed cases balanitis xerotica obliterans should be suspected.

Urethrocutaneous Fistula

Fistulas are the most common significant complication following hypospadias repair. A fistula may be seen at the time of dressing removal and some of these may heal spontaneously. The patient may present with a history of passing urine with two streams or dripping from the ventral surface of the penis. Usually a dimple can be seen on the ventral surface proximal to the neomeatus. It is always important to exclude a distal obstruction at the time of fistula repair.

The reported fistula rate for a single stage repair is 10%–15%. This may be lower than the actual incidence as small fistulas may not become apparent until years after the procedure. Success rates for fistula repair are in the region of 90%.[45]

Urethral Stricture

Urethral strictures are less common with modern techniques. They may respond to urethral dilatation but more often require a two-stage redo urethroplasty.

References

1. Yii NW, Niranjan NS. Lotus petal flaps in vulvo-vaginal reconstruction. *Br J Plast Surg*. 1996;49:547–554.
2. Taylor GI, Palmer JH. The vascular territories (angiosomes) of the body experimental study and clinical application. *Br J Plast Surg*. 1987;40:113–141.
3. Salmon M. Arteries of the skin. In: Taylor GI, Tempest M, eds. Edinburgh: Churchill Livingstone; 1998.
4. Manchot C. The Cutaneous Arteries of the Human Body. Trans Ristic J, Morain WD. New York: Springer-Verlag 1983.
5. Spear S, Pellegrino CJ, Attinger CE, et al. Vulvar reconstruction using a mons pubis flap. *Am Plast Surg*. 1994;32:602–605.
6. Ragoowansi R, Yii N, Niranjan W. Immediate vulvar and vaginal reconstruction using the gluteal fold flap: long term results. *Br J Plast Surg*. 2004;57:406–410.
7. Hashimoto I, Nakarishi H, Nagae H, et al. The gluteal fold flap for vulvar and buttock reconstruction: anatomic study and adjustment of flap volume. *Plast Reconstr Surg*. 2001;108(9):1998–2005.
8. Tobin GR, Day TG. Vaginal and pelvic reconstruction with distally based rectus abdominis myocutaneous flaps. *Plast Reconstr Surg*. 1988;81:62–70.
9. Wee JT, Joseph VT. A new technique of vaginal reconstruction using neurovascular pudendal thigh flaps: a preliminary report. *Plast Reconstr Surg*. 1989:701–709.
10. Woodman PJ, Graney DO. Anatomy and physiology of the female perineal body with relevance to obstetrical injury and repair. *Clin Anat*. 2002;15:321–334.
11. Song YG, Chen GZ, Song YL. The free thigh flap: a new free flap concept based on the septocutaneous artery. *Br J Plast Surg*. 1984;37(149).
12. Yousif NJ, Matloub HS, Kolachalam R, et al. The transverse gracilis musculocutaneous flap. *Ann Plast Surg*. 1992;29(6):482–490.
13. Hutson JM, Warne GL, Grover SR. *Disorders of Sex Development*. New York: Springer; 2012:311.
14. Rink RC, Adams MC, Misseri R. A new classification for genital ambiguity and urogenital sinus anomalies. *Br J Urol Int*. 2005;95(4):638–642.
15. Graziano K, Teitelbaum DH, Hirschl RB, et al. Vaginal reconstruction for ambiguous genitalia and congenital absence of the vagina: a 27-year experience. *J Pediatr Surg*. 2002;37(7):955–960.
16. Cordeiro PG, Pusic AL, Disa JJ. A classification system and reconstructive algorithm for acquired vaginal defects. *Plast Reconstr Surg*. 2002;110(4):1058–1065.
17. Crosby MA, Hanasono MM, Feng L, et al. Outcomes of partial vaginal reconstruction with pedicled flaps following oncologic resection. *Plast Reconstr Surg*. 2011;127(2):663–669.
18. Edmonds DK, Rose GL, Lipton MG, et al. Mayer–Rokitansky–Kuster–Hauser syndrome: a review of 245 consecutive cases managed by a multidisciplinary approach with vaginal dilators. *Fertil Steril*. 2012;97(3):686–690.
19. Ingram JM. The bicycle seat stool in the treatment of vaginal agenesis and stenosis: a preliminary report. *Am J Obstet Gynecol*. 1981;140(8):867–873.

20. Fussey JM, Luesley DM, Sterne GD. Vaginoplasty: a modern approach: a report of 2 cases. *J Reprod Med.* 2013;58(9–10):441–444.
21. Qiu SS, Jurado M, Hontanilla B. Comparison of TRAM versus DIEP flap in total vaginal reconstruction after pelvic exenteration. *Plast Reconstr Surg.* 2013;132(6):1020e–1027e.
22. Wee JT, Joseph VT. A new technique of vaginal reconstruction using neurovascular pudendal-thigh flaps: a preliminary report. *Plast Reconstr Surg.* 1989;83(4):701–709.
23. Erman Akar M, Ozkan O, Ozkan O, et al. Sexual function and long-term results following vaginal reconstruction with free vascular jejunal flap. *J Sex Med.* 2013;10(11):2849–2854.
24. Lima M, Ruggeri G, Randi B, et al. Vaginal replacement in the pediatric age group: a 34-year experience of intestinal vaginoplasty in children and young girls. *J Pediatr Surg.* 2010;45(10):2087–2091.
25. Kusiak JF, Rosenblum NG. Neovaginal reconstruction after exenteration using an omental flap and split-thickness skin graft. *Plast Reconstr Surg.* 1996;97(4):775–781; discussion 783.
26. Goyal A, Bianchi A. The parascrotal flap phallo-urethroplasty for aphallia reconstruction in childhood: report of a new technique. *J Pediatr Urol.* 2014;10:769–772.
27. Gillies H, Millard R. *The Principles and Art of Plastic Surgery.* Vol II. London: Little Brown & Company; 1957:369–388.
28. Lee GK, Lim AF, Bird ET. A novel single-flap technique for total penile reconstruction: the pedicled anterolateral thigh flap. *Plast Reconstr Surg.* 2009;124(1):163–166.
29. Bateman C. World's first successful penis transplant at Tygerberg Hospital. *S Afr Med J.* 2015;105:25.
30. Coleman E, Bockting W, Botzer M, et al. Standards of care for the health of transsexual, transgender, and gender-nonconforming people, version 7. *Int J Transgend.* 2012;13(4):165–232.
31. Mouriquand PDE. Hypospadias. In: Atwell JD, ed. *Paediatr Surg.* London: Arnold; 1998:603–616.
32. Paulozzi LJ, Erickson JD, Jackson RJ. Hypospadias trends in two US surveillance systems. *Pediatrics.* 1997;100:831–834.
33. Morera AM, Valmalle AF, Asensio MJ, et al. A study of risk factors for hypospadias in the Rhhone–Alpes region (France). *J Pediatr Urol.* 2006;2:169–177.
34. Baskin LS, Erol A, Li YW, et al. Anatomical studies of hypospadias. *J Urol.* 1998;160:1108.
35. Caesar RE, Caldamone AA. The use of free grafts for correcting penile chordee. *J Urol.* 2000;165:1691.
36. Perlmutter AD, Montgomery BT, Steinhardt GF. Tunica vaginalis free graft for correction of chordee. *J Urol.* 1985;134:311.
37. Weiser AC, Franco I, Herz DB, et al. Single layered small intestinal submucosa for corporal body grafting in cases of severe penile curvature. *J Urol.* 2003;170:1593.
38. Gilliver SC, Ashworth JJ, Ashcroft GS. The hormonal regulation of cutaneous wound healing. *Clin Dermatol.* 2007;25:56–62.
39. Snodgrass WT. Tubularised incised plate urethroplasty for distal hypospadias. *J Urol.* 1994;151:464.
40. Snodgrass W, Koyle M, Manzoni G, et al. Tubularized incised plate hypospadias repair: results of a multicenter experience. *J Urol.* 1996;156:839–841.
41. Bracka A. A versatile two-stage hypospadias repair. *Br J Plast Surg.* 1995;48:345.
42. Nitkunan T, Johal N, O'Malley K, et al. Secondary hypospadias repair in two stages. *J Pediatr Urol.* 2006;2(6):559–563.
43. Johal NS, Nitkunan T, O'Malley K, et al. The two-stage repair for severe primary hypospadias. *Eur Urol.* 2006;50(2):366–371.
44. Pfistermuller KLM, et al. Two-stage hypospadias repair with a free graft for severe primary and revision hypospadias: a single surgeon's experience with long-term follow-up. *J Pediatr Urol.* 2017;13:35.e1–35.e7.
45. Hayashi Y, Mogami M, Kojima Y, et al. Results of closure of urethrocutaneous fistulas after hypospadias repair. *Int J Urol.* 1998;5:167–169.

42 Pressure Injuries

ADAM C. GASCOIGNE AND STEPHEN FLOOD

Introduction

Pressure sores, also known as pressure injuries, pressure ulcers, decubitus ulcers, and bedsores, are a common problem. A pressure sore comprises a "localized injury to the skin and/or underlying tissue usually over a bony prominence, as a result of pressure, or pressure in combination with shear and/or friction."[1] The development of a pressure sore has significant implications for patients and healthcare providers, increasing length of admission and requiring increased utilization of healthcare resources. A US study published in 2019 estimated that hospital-acquired pressure injuries (HAPI) resulted in US$ 26.8 billion in additional healthcare costs annually, the majority due to treatment of higher grade (stage 3 or greater) injuries.[2] With an aging population and rising prevalence of chronic conditions predisposing to pressure injuries, the incidence of pressure sores and their associated costs are likely to increase. This necessitates the development of specialist multidisciplinary teams for the care of patients with pressure injuries, including reconstructive surgeons for the management of advanced, complex, or refractory pressure sores.

Epidemiology

Pressure sore incidence and prevalence are determined by the characteristics of the population studied. Specific patient populations are particularly at risk of developing a pressure sore. The normal response to injury, such as the prolonged application of pressure, is withdrawal from the noxious source. However, in some individuals this does not occur, either because the pain stimulus is not present, as in sensory impairment, or because of an inability to reposition the body in order to redistribute pressure. Such patients include the elderly, the acutely unwell, patients who are immobilized as a result of spinal cord injury or following surgery, and patients with sensory impairment due to diabetes or chronic neurological conditions. Other risk factors include a past history of pressure sores, obesity, smoking, and peripheral vascular disease, among others (Box 42.1).

The prevalence of pressure sores in the general population is low. An early study of the general population of a county in Denmark found a prevalence of 0.04%,[3] and a study of elderly patients seen in general practice found a prevalence of 0.31–0.7%.[4] However, the epidemiology of pressure sores among hospitalized patients is of greater interest, both due to the increased risk of pressure sores while admitted to a hospital or institution, and also because nosocomial pressure sore incidence is increasingly used as an indicator of healthcare quality and safety. A number of studies have examined the epidemiology of pressure sores among hospital inpatients, resulting in prevalence ranging from 10.2% to 19.7%, and incidence from 0 to 7.3%.[5] Such wide variation partly results from differences in study design. However, there are two further major difficulties that prohibit study comparison.

The first is the variable nature of the population studied. As noted above, it has long been recognized that pressure sores are more common among certain patient populations, such as the elderly, among patients with spinal cord injuries, and among patients with sensory impairment.[3] As such, the prevalence of pressure sores in a given hospital or institution more likely represents the patient population serviced by that facility than any difference in quality of care or pressure injury prevention strategies. As an example, a centre which specialises in the care of patients with spinal cord injuries is likely to have a much higher incidence of pressure sores than other institutions which many be identical in every other regard. The second difficulty is how the study defines a pressure sore. Though most studies now use the International classification system (see Table 42.1), they may differ on whether or not the milder forms are included, and frequently exclude grade 1 pressure injury which comprises only non-blanching erythema (see below, under Patient Assessment). The EPUAP collected detailed data in 2001 and 2002 and found an overall prevalence of pressure sores in five European hospitals of 18.1%.[6] However, the majority of these consisted of only a grade 1 pressure injury, with a minority (2.5% of the total) suffering the most severe, a grade 4 pressure injury. For these reasons it is important to carefully review the methodology when interpreting a given study of the epidemiology of pressure sores, and it should be interpreted warily if used as an indicator of healthcare quality and safety.

Pathophysiology

Pathologically, pressure sores are areas of localized tissue necrosis resulting from external forces. As the name suggests, external pressure is the key causative element in their

• BOX 42.1 Risk Factors for Development of Pressure Sores

- Past history of pressure sores
- Immobility (spinal cord injury, post-surgery/injury, critical illness)
- Neuropathy (spinal cord injury, diabetic neuropathy, other neurological causes)
- Abnormal posture (musculoskeletal abnormalities, spastic contractures)
- Anemia
- Poor nutrition
- Diabetes
- Peripheral vascular disease
- Obesity
- Poor skin quality (age, endocrine disorders)
- Smoking

pathogenesis. In experimental studies of the effect of pressure on limb vascular volume using human volunteers in the 1940s, Landis established a threshold pressure of 35 mmHg, noting that external pressures above this figure resulted in reduced vascular volume, likely reflecting capillary occlusion.[7] This process, if repeated or sustained, ultimately results in ischemic necrosis of skin, subcutaneous tissue, and deeper tissues. Further studies by Kosiak demonstrated irreversible changes in muscle of rats subjected to 70 mmHg of constant pressure for a period of 2 hours or more. Such changes were also seen in rats exposed to pressure which was applied and removed at 5-minute intervals, but only at much higher pressures (155 mmHg). Importantly, it was also established that denervated muscle required the same magnitude and duration of pressure in order to demonstrate signs of injury and that normal and denervated muscle had the same susceptibility to pressure injury. This was contrary to prior thinking which supposed that the absence of neurotrophic factors secreted by functional nerves was causative in pressure sore pathogenesis.[8]

Studies in animal models have demonstrated pressure sore formation and progression resulting from repeated and sustained application of pressure, the extent of injury varying according to these two factors. In combination with external pressure, shear stress and the presence of moisture may contribute to the extent of injury.[9] Shear stress is a mechanical force acting in parallel to the surface under compressive pressure. In the presence of a significant degree of shear stress, the magnitude of external pressure required to cause a pressure injury is significantly reduced.[10] This is hypothesized to occur due to the deforming effect of shear stress on tissues deep to the skin resulting in direct injury through sustained deformation of cells and worsening of ischemia by microcirculatory injury.[11] Recent research has also identified reperfusion injury as an important factor in the pathogenesis of pressure sores, with greater tissue necrosis and reduction in functional capillary density following repeated compression and release of tissues by comparison with compression alone.[12] The interaction of these

TABLE 42.1 International Pressure Injuries Classification System

Stage	Features
Stage I	Non-blanching erythema of intact skin. Area may also be painful, firm, soft, warmer, or cooler by comparison to adjacent tissue
Stage II	Partial-thickness skin loss involving epidermis and/or dermis presenting as a shallow open ulcer with a pink wound bed without slough/eschar. May also present as open/ruptured fluid-filled blister
Stage III	Full-thickness skin loss with subcutaneous fat visible but without exposure of deeper structures such as bone, tendon, or muscle
Stage IV	Full-thickness tissue loss with extensive tissue necrosis and exposure and/or involvement of deeper structures such as bone, tendon, or muscle. Slough or eschar may be present
Suspected deep tissue injury	Area of discolored intact skin or blood-filled blister. Skin integrity maintained with suspected damage to deeper tissues
Unstageable	Full-thickness tissue loss in which actual depth of ulcer is obscured by slough and/or eschar in the wound bed

Modified with permission from European Pressure Ulcer Advisory Panel, National Pressure Injury Advisory Panel and Pan Pacific Pressure Injury Alliance. *Prevention and Treatment of Pressure Ulcers/Injuries: Quick Reference Guide*. Emily Haesler (ed.). EPUAP/NPIAP/PPPIA; 2019.

biomechanical factors in the pathogenesis of a pressure sore is complex, and research into their relative contributions is ongoing. However, it is clear that the key pathological insult in the formation of a pressure sore is repeated compression of tissues by external pressure over a prolonged period, which may be exacerbated by contributory factors including shear forces, moisture, and reperfusion injury (Fig. 42.1).

Pressure sores have been described as occurring in many locations, though the vast majority occur over bony prominences in the lower limb. The aforementioned EPUAP study found the following to be the commonest sites of pressure injury of any severity, in descending order (percentages stated according to data collected in the United Kingdom): sacrum (37.5%), heel (26.2%), ischium (13.7%), elbow

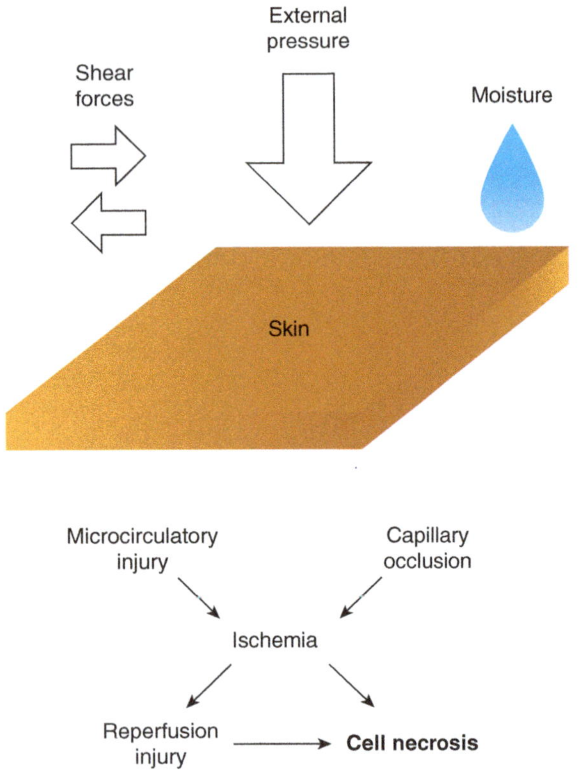

• **Fig. 42.1** Pressure injury pathogenesis.

(10.3%), ankle (6.4%), and hip (5.8%).[6] The reason for pressure injuries occurring most frequently over bony prominences may seem intuitively obvious, nevertheless the physiological explanation follows. Sangeorzan et al compared the effects of applied external pressure to skin overlying the subcutaneous surface of the tibia with that over tibialis anterior. The researchers established that much greater external pressure was required to reduce capillary perfusion in skin over muscle than in skin over bone.[13] Crucial to this is the realization that the subcutaneous (interstitial) tissue pressure is of much greater significance than the external pressure, and the interstitial pressure resulting from a given external pressure is determined by the nature of those tissues and whether they overlie bone. As such, over bony prominences where there is a thinner layer of soft tissue between skin and bone, a relatively minor external pressure may result in significant, ischemia-inducing interstitial pressure.

Prevention

Effective pressure sore prevention requires ongoing assessment of patients for risk factors together with appropriate interventions to minimize risk to vulnerable patients. Pressure sore risk factors are common in the hospitalized population (see Epidemiology, above).

Assessment of Risk

Pressure sore risk assessment should be performed for all patients on admission and repeated regularly in order to identify at-risk patients and track response to interventions. A number of structured risk assessment tools have been developed to identify patients at risk of developing a pressure sore. The Norton scale was developed in 1962, from which were developed the Waterlow and Braden scales in 1985 and 1987, respectively. The latter two are in widespread use today and have been demonstrated to have a high sensitivity in predicting patients likely to develop a pressure sore. There is, however, no good-quality evidence to suggest that the use of these tools results in a decreased incidence of pressure sores.[14] Regardless of whether or not a scale is used, assessment of patients for pressure sore risk allows identification of patients likely to benefit from prevention strategies.

Prevention Strategies

Interventions for the prevention of pressure sores are of two general types. First, the extrinsic causes of pressure sores (see Pathophysiology, above) should be minimized. The effect of external pressure may be ameliorated using pressure redistribution strategies, such as manual repositioning and the use of appropriate lifting devices for patient transfers. There is no good evidence to recommend any particular manual positioning regimen over any other.[15] Use of pressure-relieving support surfaces such as gel-filled overlays during surgery and air mattresses or cushions on the ward are also beneficial, though again there is nothing to suggest the superiority of any particular surface type, except over basic mattresses.[16,17] Medical-grade sheepskins are also of benefit in reducing pressure sore risk, which may be particularly relevant in the nursing home environment.[18]

However, if achievable, early mobilization is the best strategy for external pressure reduction. Daily skin care, including moisturization of dry skin in areas prone to pressure sore development, and prompt cleaning and changing following episodes of incontinence reduces the effect of moisture and may allow the identification of early stage pressure injuries. Secondly, modifiable risk factors should be managed. The management of any medical comorbidities should be reviewed and the patient's nutritional state assessed and managed if necessary. Patients should be discouraged from smoking, and obese patients should be counseled regarding the benefits of weight reduction. These strategies are summarized in the Institute for Healthcare Improvement (IHI)'s recommendations for pressure sore prevention (Box 42.2).

Assessment of the Patient with a Pressure Sore

The aims of assessment are: to establish the severity of the pressure sore; to evaluate treatment options and their appropriateness and acceptability for the individual patient; and to assess risk of complications and recurrence of pressure sores.

• BOX 42.2 Institute for Healthcare Improvement Recommendations for Pressure Sore Prevention

1. Conduct a pressure sore admission assessment for all patients
2. Reassess risk for all patients daily
3. Inspect skin daily
4. Manage moisture
5. Optimize nutrition and hydration
6. Minimize pressure

Patient Assessment

If the patient has a past history of pressure sores, a complete history of their prior management should be taken. Their medical history should be reviewed, in particular to identify comorbidities such as diabetes mellitus, peripheral vascular disease, and sensory impairment, which may increase their risk of complications such as recurrence or the development of further pressure sores. In particular, diabetic control should be assessed through regular blood sugar level checks and testing of HbA_{1c} levels, and referral to a specialist endocrinologist considered if control is poor. A complete functional assessment should be completed in order to determine the patient's cognitive state and capacity for ambulation. A full nutritional assessment should be performed, including testing of serum albumin. Where there are concerns regarding the patient's mood or mental state, formal psychological assessment is recommended. The patient's social situation and support network including the availability and appropriateness of caregivers should be examined, and the goals of care should be discussed with the patient and their family, especially in cases where overall prognosis is poor. In palliative patients, or if the patient's medical or nutritional status indicate that a poor outcome following surgery would be likely, conservative management of the pressure sore is indicated.

Wound Assessment

Features of the pressure sore should be ascertained by taking a history from the patient regarding symptoms, including pain and associated features to indicate infection, such as fever and localized swelling. Relevant characteristics to note are summarized in Box 42.3. The familiar four-stage grading system for pressure sores was devised by Shea in 1975.[19] This system was subsequently revised to include two new categories: suspected deep tissue injury and unstageable (Table 42.1). The addition represents the recognition that pressure sores may develop from bottom-to-top rather than progressing through the classic four stages, resulting in rapid development of an advanced pressure sore. Comprehensive assessment and staging of the pressure sore is important in order to accurately estimate severity and to determine management. This may necessitate debridement to ascertain depth of tissue loss. It is important to note that in the special situation of a pressure sore on the heel, the eschar layer is an important part of the wound healing process and it is recommended that it not be removed.[20] If osteomyelitis is suspected, appropriate imaging with scintigraphy or magnetic resonance imaging is indicated.

• BOX 42.3 Pressure Sore Features

- Size of pressure sore
- Location of pressure sore
- Stage of pressure sore
- Presence of eschar or exudate
- Signs of local infection and collections
- Evidence of osteomyelitis

Initial Management

Management of the patient with a pressure sore should involve a multidisciplinary team to allow collaboration between reconstructive surgeons, rehabilitation medicine physicians, specialist wound care nurses, and members of Allied Health disciplines including occupational therapists, physiotherapists, dietitians, and social workers if required.

Wound Care

Cleansing the wound with an antiseptic solution, packing any cavities, and covering it with a nonadherent dressing (such as hydrocolloids, hydrogels, hydrofibers, foams, films, alginates, and soft silicones) provide an optimum wound healing environment. There is little evidence to recommend a particular type of dressing or antiseptic over any other, though some trials have found a benefit for hydrocolloid dressings over saline gauze.[21] Negative-pressure wound therapy (NPWT) is frequently used in management of chronic ulcers, including pressure sores.[22] It has advantages in reducing frequency of dressing changes and may have a beneficial effect on wound healing.[23] Some new devices provide wound instillation in addition to negative pressure, which may have particular utility in infected wounds.[24]

Constant assessment for signs of infection allow early diagnosis and treatment. Tissue obtained during debridement and any swabs taken of fluid exudate should be sent for microbiological examination to allow tailoring of antimicrobial agents to the pathogenic organism and its sensitivities.

Pain Control

Patients with pressure sores frequently have multiple sources of pain. The pressure sore itself causes pain, the patient may have chronic pain issues related to musculoskeletal abnormalities or neuropathy, and healthcare interventions may also cause pain. Wound debridement is a particular cause of pain that may require additional analgesia, sedation, or even

• BOX 42.4 Surgical Debridement

- Drainage of all collections
- Adequate debridement of necrotic, infected, and scarred tissue
- Excision of pseudobursa
- Removal of infected bone
- Hemostasis, drainage
- Closure if possible

general anesthesia. Strategies to reduce pain include regular repositioning, regular and adequate analgesia, coordination of interventions such as dressing changes, debridement, and wound examination with analgesia administration, prescription of breakthrough analgesia as required, use of low adherence dressings, and adjuvant analgesia for neuropathic pain.

Nutrition

It is important to ensure the patient with a pressure sore is adequately nourished and to give nutritional supplementation for wound healing. Enteral feeding by nasogastric tube may be necessary in patients unable to tolerate oral feeding. Mixed nutritional supplementation with protein, arginine, zinc, and vitamin C has been demonstrated to be effective in clinical trials. Suggested daily intakes for patients with pressure sores are: energy: 30–35 kcal/kg, protein: 1.2–1.5 g/kg.[25]

Adjunctive Treatments

Many experimental treatments have been trialled in the treatment of pressure sores. These include therapies such as electrical stimulation, pulsed electromagnetic field treatment, ultraviolet light C, ultrasound, and hyperbaric oxygen. Currently there is little good quality evidence to recommend their routine use in the management of pressure sores.

Surgical Debridement

The pressure sore and its sequelae must be resected in order to provide an adequate environment for any subsequent reconstruction (Box 42.4). Debridement of necrotic and infected tissue is an essential part of the care of any wound. Devitalized tissue provides a focus for infection, prevents healing by stimulating a persistent inflammatory response, and prevents wound contraction.[20] Pressure sores are commonly associated with pseudobursae, collections of fluid surrounded by a wall of scar tissue. These and any other serous or infected collections should be excised or drained. Nonviable or infected bone should also be resected, though bone excision should be minimized if possible, as removal of bone results in alteration of pressure distribution patterns and the potential for development of new pressure sores in novel areas. If it is then possible to close the wound directly without tension, this should be done with drain tubes left in situ. If not, then an appropriate dressing regimen should be used while planning reconstruction (see above).

Reconstruction

Careful patient selection is vital in order to ensure that surgical reconstruction is the appropriate course for the individual patient. Factors that may increase the risk of failure of a surgical reconstruction or recurrence of a pressure sore postoperatively include any of the risk factors listed (Table 42.2) and poor compliance with previous treatment. Patients in whom these risk factors are present should only be considered for reconstructive surgery if there is a clear plan in place to ameliorate or reduce the effect of the risk factor, as a poor outcome is otherwise highly likely. In addition, patients with a poor overall prognosis are generally unsuitable for reconstructive surgery for pressure sores.

Preoperative Management

Prior to embarking on surgical reconstruction of a defect resulting from a pressure sore, all of the initial management strategies should be instituted to minimize the need for surgery and to improve the chance of success of any reconstruction. The physiological stress resulting from a prolonged operation such as is generally required for the reconstruction of a pressure sore would have a dire effect on any patient who is acutely unwell. The management of any medical conditions should therefore be optimized and any nutritional deficiencies remedied preoperatively. The preoperative period is also a good time in which to educate patients and caregivers regarding the operation and strategies for prevention of further pressure sores.

Reconstructive Ladder

The reconstructive ladder is a concept every plastic and reconstructive surgeon should be familiar with. It arranges options for surgical reconstruction in order of increasing complexity, from basic healing by secondary intention to the technically and physically demanding free vascularized tissue transfer. It is important to note that this does not necessarily mean that the simplest reconstructive option is the most appropriate for the individual patient; there are often situations where a more advanced procedure will have benefits over a simpler procedure. This is particularly true in the management of the patient with a pressure injury, in whom reconstructive options that do not provide tissue bulk, such as healing by secondary intention, primary closure, and skin grafting, are likely to result in recurrence. For this reason musculocutaneous or fasciocutaneous flaps are usually the treatment of choice, as they provide vascularized tissue bulk to fill dead space and allow wider distribution of pressure over bony prominences. Local or regional flaps are most commonly used, though free flaps may be a viable

TABLE 42.2 Indications and Contraindications for Reconstruction of Pressure Sores

Indications	Contraindications
Stage 3/4 pressure sore	Poor overall prognosis
Unlikely to/has not responded to more conservative management	Poor compliance
	Acutely unwell
	Malnourished/cachectic

alternative where all other options have been exhausted. In general, procedures should be planned so as to preserve other options, as pressure sore recurrence is common and another flap may be required in future.

Reconstructive Techniques by Location

Sacral

The area overlying the sacrum and coccyx is very commonly affected by pressure sores, usually occurring in bedridden patients who remain in the supine position for prolonged periods. Local musculocutaneous flaps based on the gluteus maximus muscle, or fasciocutaneous flaps based on the overlying fascia, are versatile and effective methods for reconstructing these defects.[26] Techniques include V–Y advancement flaps, rotation flaps, and split flaps. Note that musculocutaneous flaps based on the gluteus maximus muscle are not generally recommended for ambulatory patients due to the resultant functional deficit. Other techniques include the superior gluteal artery perforator flap and the transverse back flap. In particular, the perforator-sparing rotation technique allows rerotation in patients likely to experience recurrence of a pressure injury.[27]

Ischial

Pressure sores overlying the ischial tuberosities are common in wheelchair-bound patients, such as patients with spinal cord injuries. Similarly techniques to those used for sacral pressure sores may be effective in the reconstruction of defects caused by ischial pressure sores, such as musculocutaneous flaps based on the gluteus maximus muscle, or fasciocutaneous flaps based on inferior gluteal perforators. The posterior thigh flap is another useful option, its advantages including a reliable blood supply, good long-term outcomes, no functional deficit, and the preservation of other options for repeat flap repair in cases of recurrence (Fig. 42.2). It is a fasciocutaneous flap composed of posterior thigh skin and subcutaneous tissue, based on perforators from either the first and second perforating arteries of the profunda femoris or the inferior gluteal artery.[28] Other options include flaps based on the hamstring muscles, such as the V–Y advancement biceps femoris musculocutaneous flap, or the gracilis flap.

Trochanteric

Patients spending a prolonged period in the lateral recumbent position are at risk of developing pressure sores overlying the greater trochanter of the femur. A common option for reconstruction of these defects are flaps based on the tensor fascia lata (TFL) muscle.[29] This flap is based on a branch of the lateral circumflex femoral artery and may be composed of muscle and skin or muscle alone. It may also be used for reconstruction of ischial pressure sores, and is particularly useful in situations where both trochanteric and ischial sores are present. Other options include the anterolateral thigh flap, which may provide additional tissue bulk where the size of the TFL may be insufficient. Another option is the groin flap, based on the superficial circumflex iliac artery, which may be useful if the TFL has already been used as a local or free flap for reconstruction of pressure sores elsewhere.

Heel and Lateral Malleolus

Pressure sores on the posterior aspect of the heel and overlying the lateral malleolus are common in neuropathic or insensate patients. They pose a challenge to the reconstructive surgeon due to the scarcity of local tissue for coverage. Options for reconstruction of a pressure sore on the heel or elsewhere in the foot include the lateral calcaneal and medial plantar artery flaps.[30,31] The lateral supramalleolar flap (Fig. 42.3), based on a distal perforator of the peroneal artery,[32] is a rotation flap which provides coverage of a lateral malleolar defect, while the donor region can be safely covered with a split-thickness skin graft.[33] For recurrent or refractory pressure sores, the distally based superficial sural artery flap is a versatile option which may be rotated to cover either of the malleoli or the heel.[34]

Last Resort

If the above strategies fail, or if they have been used in prior reconstructions, then the situation is a difficult one. The management of a patient suffering from recurrent pressure sores is complex, and requires the involvement of all members of the multidisciplinary team to evaluate the causes of recurrence. If all potential causes of recurrence have been addressed, then further reconstruction may be considered. Further procedures should be tailored to the patient, and may require some creativity. Free flaps from distant sites, or tubed pedicle flaps from the contralateral side are options, and choice of one over another is reserved for the surgeon's clinical judgment.

Postoperative Care

Excellent postoperative care and follow-up following surgical reconstruction of a pressure sore is essential if complications and a poor outcome are to be avoided. Potential complications to be vigilant for include: sepsis, wound dehiscence (superficial and deep), hematoma, seroma, partial or total flap loss, and pressure injury recurrence. Good operative technique with low tension skin closure and use of drains reduces the risks of hematoma, seroma, and wound dehiscence. Rates of partial or total flap loss may be reduced by attentive nursing care, and early return to

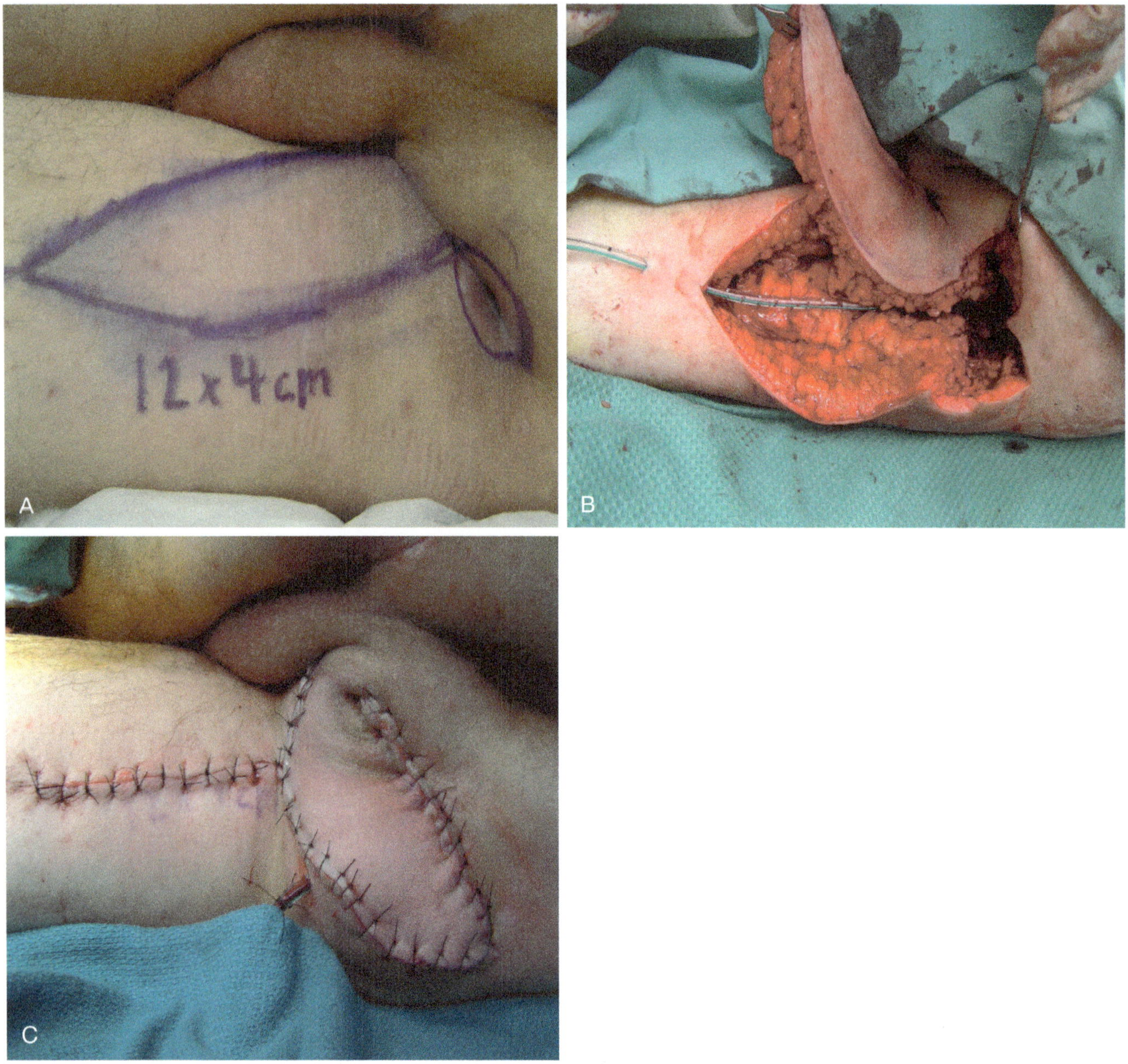

• **Fig. 42.2** Posterior thigh flap for reconstruction of an ischial pressure sore. (A) Preoperative markings. (B) Raising of flap based on medial perforator. (C) Flap sutured into defect, donor site closed primarily.

theater to revise flaps that appear to be failing. Recurrence or the development of a new pressure sore is unfortunately very common. Following reconstruction, it is crucial to continue prevention strategies for pressure sores. As stated above, in patients with recurrent or refractory pressure sores, the causes for recurrence should be addressed. Pressure sores provide a focus of necrotic tissue which acts as a nidus for bacterial growth, increasing the risk of postoperative wound infection. For this reason broad-spectrum antibiotics are frequently continued for extended periods, though this should be discussed with antimicrobial stewardship services. Other potential complications following pressure sore reconstruction are corollaries of immobility. Loss of muscle and bone mass results from prolonged bed rest, and immobilization of joints may result in the development of contractures. It is also important to be aware of the risk of deep venous thrombosis and pulmonary embolism, and staff should be especially vigilant for the signs of these conditions in the postoperative period.

A general protocol followed by the senior author is for surgical sutures and drains to be left in situ for 2–3 weeks to minimize the risk of complications such as seroma, hematoma, and wound dehiscence, all of which may compromise flap viability. Appropriate broad-spectrum antibiotics, administered orally or intravenously, should be continued for up to 6 weeks, with a low threshold for referral to specialist infectious diseases physicians if there is uncertainty regarding choice of agent, especially if there is suspicion of osteomyelitis or if multiresistant organisms are present. In the absence of major bleeding, prophylactic doses

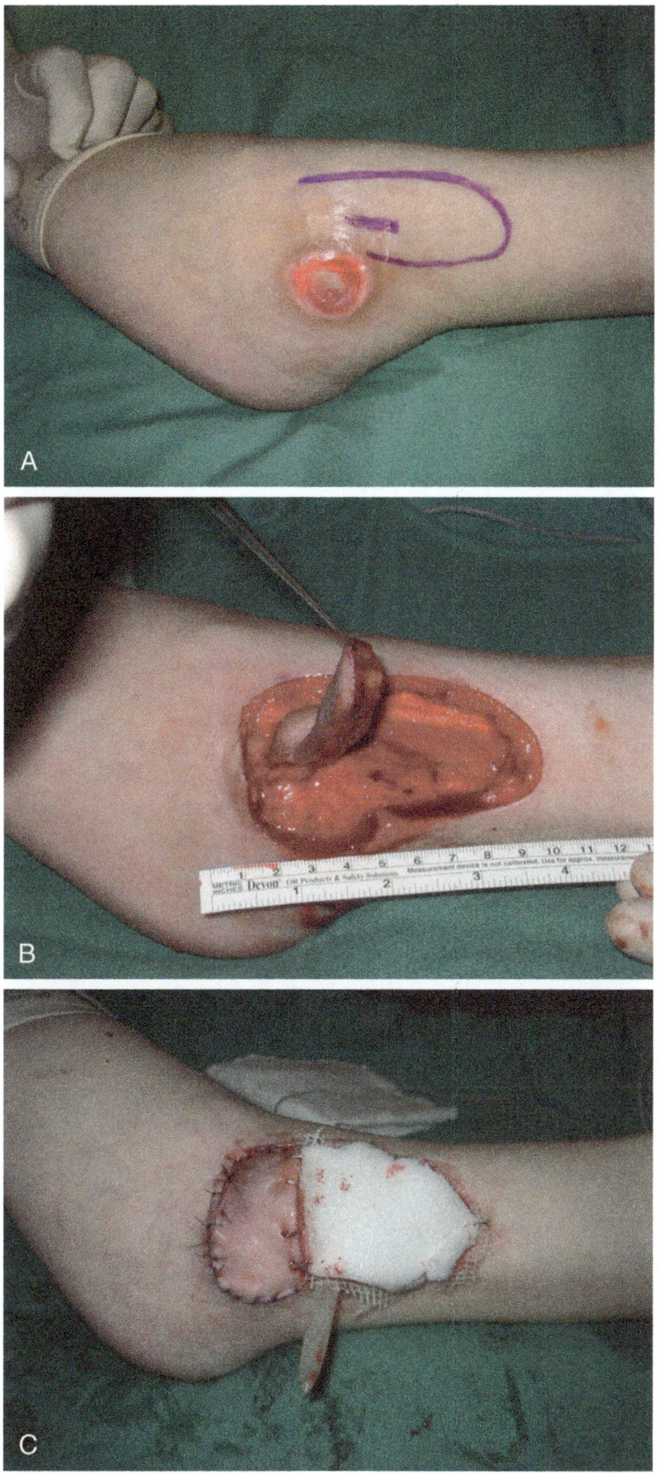

• **Fig. 42.3** Lateral supramalleolar perforator flap reconstruction of a lateral malleolar pressure sore. (A) Preoperative markings. (B) Flap raised on peroneal artery perforator. (C) Flap sutured into defect, donor site closed with split-thickness skin graft.

of anticoagulation should be administered from the first postoperative day for prophylaxis of deep venous thrombosis and embolic events. The strategies outlined in the prevention and general management sections above should be continued to prevent recurrence or the development of a new pressure sore, including repositioning and use of pressure-relieving support surfaces. Minimizing shear and pressure on the operative site is especially important in the postoperative period. Protection of the flap pedicle should be a priority, and intensive monitoring of flap viability using clinical examination including bedside Doppler ultrasound by resident medical staff and specialist nurses is essential. Once the immediate postoperative period has passed, the patient is likely to require a period of rehabilitation with graduated increase in pressure on the operative site. During this period any required devices, such as wheelchairs, should be evaluated and customized for the patient.

Conclusion

Pressure sores are a common problem in the inpatient population, particularly among patients with sensory impairment or reduced mobility. The development of a pressure sore has implications for patient length of stay and increased use of healthcare resources. Through a sound knowledge of the pathophysiology of pressure sores, and using the prevention strategies outlined in this chapter, occurrence of pressure injuries and their attendant costs may be reduced. The patient with a pressure sore is best managed with a multidisciplinary team approach, incorporating physicians and allied health practitioners. Their general medical condition and nutrition should be optimized and any management of modifiable risk factors reviewed. Following initial surgical debridement and treatment of any infection, further reconstructive procedures may be considered if indicated. Careful patient selection is necessary prior to embarking on any advanced reconstructive procedure to avoid a poor outcome. Ideally, a local fascio- or musculocutaneous flap should be chosen to provide well-vascularized tissue bulk. Following the procedure, attentive postoperative care will reduce the risk of complications and pressure sore recurrence.

References

1. Black J, Baharestani MM, Cuddigan J, et al. National Pressure Ulcer Advisory Panel's updated pressure ulcer staging system. *Adv Skin Wound Care*. 2007;20(5):269.
2. Padula WV, Delarmente BA. The national cost of hospital-acquired pressure injuries in the United States. *Int Wound J*. 2019;16(3):634–640.
3. Petersen NC, Bittmann S. The epidemiology of pressure sores. *Scand J Plast Reconstr Surg*. 1971;5(1):62–66.
4. Margolis DJ, Bilker W, Knauss J, Baumgarten M, Strom BL. The incidence and prevalence of pressure ulcers among elderly patients in general medical practice. *Ann Epidemiol*. 2002;12(5):321–325.
5. Vandenkerkhof EG, Friedberg E, Harrison MB. Prevalence and risk of pressure ulcers in acute care following implementation of practice guidelines: annual pressure ulcer prevalence census 1994–2008. *J Healthc Qual*. 2011;33(5):58–67.
6. Clark M, Bours G, Defloor T. Summary report on the prevalence of pressure ulcers. *EPUAP Review*. 2002;4(2):49–56.
7. McLennan CE, McLennan MT, Landis EM. The effect of external pressure on the vascular volume of the forearm and its relation to capillary blood pressure and venous pressure. *J Clin Invest*. 1942;21(3):319–338.

8. Kosiak M. Etiology of decubitus ulcers. *Arch Phys Med Rehabil.* 1961;42:19–29.
9. Reuler JB, Cooney TG. The pressure sore: pathophysiology and principles of management. *Ann Intern Med.* 1981;94(5):661–666.
10. Bennett L, Kavner D, Lee BK, Trainor FA. Shear vs pressure as causative factors in skin blood flow occlusion. *Arch Phys Med Rehabil.* 1979;60(7):309–314.
11. Stekelenburg A, Strijkers GJ, Parusel H, et al. Role of ischemia and deformation in the onset of compression-induced deep tissue injury: MRI-based studies in a rat model. *J App Physiol.* 2007;102(5):2002–2011.
12. Tsuji S, Ichioka S, Sekiya N, Nakatsuka T. Analysis of ischemia-reperfusion injury in a microcirculatory model of pressure ulcers. *Wound Repair Regen.* 2005;13(2):209–215.
13. Sangeorzan BJ, Harrington RM, Wyss CR, et al. Circulatory and mechanical response of skin to loading. *J Orthop Res.* 1989;7(3):425–431.
14. Moore ZEH, Cowman S. Risk assessment tools for the prevention of pressure ulcers. *Cochrane Database Syst Rev.* 2008;(3):CD006471.
15. Moore ZE, Cowman S. Repositioning for treating pressure ulcers. *Cochrane Database Syst Rev.* Wiley Online Library. 2009(2):CD006898.
16. Reddy M, Gill SS, Rochon PA. Preventing pressure ulcers: a systematic review. *J Am Med Assoc.* 2006;296(8):974–984.
17. McInnes E, Jammali-Blasi A, Bell-Syer SE, et al. Support surfaces for pressure ulcer prevention. *Cochrane Database Syst Rev.* Wiley Online Library. 2011(4):CD001735.
18. Mistiaen P, Achterberg W, Ament A, et al. The effectiveness of the Australian Medical Sheepskin for the prevention of pressure ulcers in somatic nursing home patients: a prospective multicenter randomized-controlled trial (ISRCTN17553857). *Wound Repair Regen.* 2010;18(6):572–579.
19. Shea JD. Pressure sores: classification and management. *Clin Orthop Relat Res.* 1975;112:89–100.
20. Bellingeri A, Hofman D. Debridement of pressure ulcers. In: Romanelli M, Clark M, Colin D, eds. *Science and Practice of Pressure Ulcer Management.* London: Springer Verlag; 2006:129–137.
21. Moore ZE, Cowman S. Wound cleansing for pressure ulcers (Review). *Cochrane Database Syst Rev.* 2005(4):CD004983.
22. Argenta LC, Morykwas MJ. Vacuum-assisted closure: a new method for wound control and treatment: clinical experience. *Ann Plast Surg.* 1997;38(6):563–576; discussion 577.
23. Wanner MB, Schwarzl F, Strub B, Zaech GA, Pierer G. Vacuum-assisted wound closure for cheaper and more comfortable healing of pressure sores: a prospective study. *Scand J Plast Reconstr Surg Hand Surg.* 2003;37(1):28–33.
24. Kim PJ, Attinger CE, Steinberg JS, et al. The impact of negative-pressure wound therapy with instillation compared with standard negative-pressure wound therapy. *Plast Reconstr Surg.* 2014;133(3):709–716.
25. Thomas DR. Clinical management of pressure ulcers. *Clin Geriatr Med.* 2013;29(2):397–413.
26. Becker H. The distally-based gluteus maximus muscle flap. *Plast Reconstr Surg.* 1979;63(5):653–656.
27. Wong C-H, Tan B-K, Song C. The perforator-sparing buttock rotation flap for coverage of pressure sores. *Plast Reconstr Surg.* 2007;119(4):1259–1266.
28. Rubin JA, Whetzel TP, Stevenson TR. The posterior thigh fasciocutaneous flap: vascular anatomy and clinical application. *Plast Reconstr Surg.* 1995;95(7):1228–1239.
29. Erçöçen AR, Apaydin I, Emiroğlu M, et al. Island V–Y tensor fasciae latae fasciocutaneous flap for coverage of trochanteric pressure sores. *Plast Reconstr Surg.* 1998;102(5):1524–1531.
30. Holmes J, Rayner CR. Lateral calcaneal artery island flaps. *Br J Plast Surg.* 1984;37(3):402–405.
31. Roblin P, Healy CMJ. Heel reconstruction with a medial plantar V–Y flap. *Plast Reconstr Surg.* 2007;119(3):927–932.
32. Masquelet AC, Beveridge J, Romana C, Gerber C. The lateral supramalleolar flap. *Plast Reconstr Surg.* 1988;81(1):74–84.
33. Sham E, Choi W-T, Flood SJ. Lateral supramalleolar flap in reconstruction of pressure ulcers in patients with spinal cord injury. *ANZ J Surg.* 2008;78(3):167–171.
34. Hasegawa M, Torii S, Katoh H, Esaki S. The distally based superficial sural artery flap. *Plast Reconstr Surg.* 1994;93(5):1012–1020.

43

Lower Limb Reconstruction

MICHEL SAINT-CYR, ABIGAIL M. RODRIGUEZ, AND STACY WONG

Introduction

Worldwide, lower extremity trauma is associated with significant cost, as well as considerable morbidity and even mortality. In the United States, open tibial shaft fractures are most common in young adult males and typically result from motor vehicle collisions (MVCs).[1] Quantifying the cost of such injuries is challenging. To improve understanding of the financial and medical implications of limb-threatening lower extremity trauma and its management, the Lower Extremity Assessment Project (LEAP) was of paramount importance.[2] For both limb salvage and amputation patients, total lifetime costs were found to be remarkably high, though salvage was shown to offer higher utility and to cost less compared to amputation (by at least 93,606–154,636 USD for a 40-year-old patient).[2] Lower extremity trauma is both common and costly, and an ongoing evolution in management has been instrumental to improving outcomes. It has become increasingly evident that a multidisciplinary approach is critical. Care by emergency medicine, general surgery, and vascular surgery teams is acutely required, followed by careful planning and coordinated efforts from the orthopedic surgery and plastic surgery teams. This "orthoplastic approach" can provide optimal and definitive care of limb-threatening lower extremity trauma.[3] Importantly, the role of the plastic surgeon in the "orthoplastic approach" can involve reconstructive efforts for both limb salvage and limb amputation.

This chapter aims to review the history of lower extremity reconstruction, injury classification, early assessment and initial management, patient selection for limb salvage versus amputation, principles of skeletal fixation, principles of soft tissue reconstruction, and postoperative considerations.

History

Lower extremity trauma management has undergone significant progress over many centuries, periodically catapulted forward around times of war.

Amputation of the lower extremity is thought to have occurred as a form a punishment or in religious ceremony as far back as Neolithic times, based on archeological evidence.[4] As a form of medical practice, however, amputation is first mentioned in the Hippocratic treatise *On Joints* (460–370 BC).[5] The amputation of gangrenous extremities was described with surgical intent, recommending amputation be done distal to the "boundary of blackening," thus limiting pain and blood loss.[5] Later, around 25 BC–AD 50, Celsus promoted the concept of thorough debridement to healthy tissue followed by bone shortening with very deliberate management of the soft tissue at the stump.[5] He described that "the face of the bone ... is smoothed down, and the skin drawn over it: this must be sufficiently loosened in an operation of this sort to cover the bone all over as completely as possible."[5]

Further developments were described by Archigenes and Heliodorus (AD 100), who designed flaps for complete soft tissue closure after amputation of digits, though not specifically for the lower extremity.[5]

The introduction of gunpowder to warfare in 1338 resulted in a drastic shift in injury patterns, greatly increasing the number of amputation cases that presented to military surgeons.[4]

A paramount figure in surgical advancement, Ambroise Paré (1509–1590) rejected the widely held notion that gunpowder was poisonous and thus discouraged the common practice of dressing the wounds with caustic hot oil.[5] Paré also refined the amputation technique by using vessel ligation rather than nonspecific cauterization.[5] Introducing a pivotal concept, Paré was the first to consider amputation in a reconstructive manner.[4] For instance, he considered the functional implications of the amputation location, recommending amputation five fingerbreadths below the knee to accommodate a wooden leg prosthesis, and he fashioned the first artificial limbs.[5]

Acute management of lower extremity trauma shifted dramatically in the early 1800s. Through extensive experience managing combat injuries, Larrey of France and Guthrie of Great Britain noted that early or primary amputation (within the first 24 hours) of the lower extremity reduced mortality, hastened stump healing, and reduced infection and overall blood loss.[4,5] Indications for primary amputation of the lower extremity included compound fractures resulting from gunshot wounds, all fractures of joints, all gunshot wounds of joints, significant soft tissue loss (especially with critical nerve injury), and loss of major blood supply of an extremity.[5]

The advent of ether and chloroform anesthesia in the 1840s permitted surgeons to prioritize technique over speed.[4] Surgical hygiene also saw a significant advancement with Joseph Lister in 1867. Lister drew from Louis Pasteur's research and posited that, in order to prevent infection, "septic organisms" must be eliminated from the wound and from anything coming into contact with the wound.[4] His method of antisepsis involved spraying carbolic acid in the air overlying the surgical field and applying a carbolic acid-soaked dressing to the wound.[4] Carl Thiersch and Richard von Volkmann of Germany adopted these antisepsis methods and, with them, demonstrated lower mortality rates, faster healing, and fewer complications.[4] This contributed to the gradual acceptance of later developments, such as the use of steam sterilization technique, sterile gowns, and face masks.[4]

At the time of the First World War (1914–1918), more powerful and accurate weapons were employed which caused significant mutilation and resulted in half a million amputations.[4] High concentrations of bacteria in the battlefield soil resulted in frequent infections.[4] Works from Ollier and Orr were integrated by Carrel into his practice of thorough debridement, plaster immobilization, antisepsis with 0.5% sodium hypochlorite (Dakin's) solution, and delayed wound closure.[4]

Subsequently, during the Spanish Civil War (1936–1939), Trueta synthesized the recommendations of preceding surgeons by treating open fractures with wound debridement, fracture reduction, packing the wound with sterile gauze, plaster cast application, and tetanus prophylaxis administration.[4]

Through the Second World War (1939–1945) and the Korean conflict (1950–1953), indications for amputation remained largely unchanged from the time of Larrey and Guthrie. Improvements implemented over that period of time notably improved outcomes, with the mortality from lower extremity trauma dropping from 8% during the First World War to 4.5% in the Second World War.[4] By the time of the Vietnam War, through the 1960s and early 1970s, compound fractures and gunshot injuries of the joints were no longer considered indications for amputation.[4] Without many options for large soft tissue transfer, extensive soft tissue injury remained an indication for amputation, along with extensive bone trauma and nerve injury.

In 1975, Taylor harnessed the developing fields of bone reconstruction, vascular surgery, and microsurgery to perform a free vascularized bone graft. Distraction osteogenesis, pioneered by Codivilla and Ilizarov in the 20th century, was a means to provide stable fixation and bone stock without the donor site morbidity of a bone graft.

Soft tissue reconstruction progressed dramatically following the arrival of anesthesia in the 1840s. A surgical innovator, Hamilton performed the first cross-leg flap for lower extremity reconstruction in 1854 and is also credited with furthering the basic understanding of skin grafts that arose centuries prior. Daniel and Taylor applied emerging microsurgical techniques and performed the first free soft tissue transfer in 1973, using a free groin flap to the lower leg. Free tissue transfer for lower extremity reconstruction was a critical addition to the reconstructive armamentarium and has bourgeoned into a reliable method for limb salvage and outcome optimization.

Initial Management

Out of necessity, lessons learned during wartimes of the 19th and 20th centuries helped develop efficient methods of evacuation, stabilization, and early critical treatments of injuries in the military. An orthopedic surgeon, Jim Styner, helped to bridge this concept to the civilian world by devising a methodical, concise approach to trauma patient care with the Advanced Trauma Life Support (ATLS) program. The first ATLS course, held in 1978, championed the multidisciplinary approach, and encouraged process standardization to improve outcomes. Today, initial management of the lower extremity trauma patient should adhere to the ATLS protocol, focusing on respiratory and cardiovascular stabilization and neurological evaluation before specifically addressing the lower extremities. A stable airway should be ensured and breathing assessed. A circulatory exam should be performed, examining peripheral perfusion and acutely managing hemorrhage with pressure, splint application, or pelvic binders. Ideally, a neurological exam is performed prior to analgesia or sedation, with particular focus on peripheral motor and sensory nerve function of the lower extremity. Complete exposure of the patient with removal of clothing and dressings is critical and may reveal unexpected soft tissue injury. Any indicated imaging and laboratory tests should be ordered, and adequate intravenous access and a Foley catheter placed.

On secondary survey, a focused exam of the lower extremity is performed to consider the following:

- *Skin*: The area, size, and degree of soft tissue damage should be documented. The degree of contamination of an open fracture will guide administration of prophylactic antibiotics and tetanus immunization[6] (Table 43.1).
- *Nerve function*: Motor and sensory function should be examined thoroughly throughout both lower extremities. Special attention should be given to the tibial nerve, where trauma can cause loss of plantarflexion and sensory loss to the plantar foot. The finding of an insensate plantar surface has historically been a key reason to selecting amputation rather than limb salvage. However, in a LEAP study, 55% of patients presenting with an insensate foot who underwent limb reconstruction ultimately regained sensation at 2 years after injury, indicating that an insensate foot is not an accurate indicator of the need for amputation.[7]
- *Vascular status*: Peripheral pulses should be palpated and evaluated with Doppler. CT angiography is the imaging

TABLE 43.1 **Tetanus Prophylaxis Immunization Schedule**

Tetanus Immunization History	Clean, Minor Wounds		Contaminated, Complex Wounds	
	Td or Tdap	TIG	Td or Tdap	TIG
Unknown or <3 doses	Yes	No	Yes	Yes
≥3 doses	No[a]	No	No[b]	No

Td, Tetanus–diphtheria vaccine; Tdap, tetanus–diphtheria and acellular pertussis vaccine; TIG, tetanus immune globulin.
[a]Yes, if >10 years since the last tetanus booster.
[b]Yes, if >5 years since the last tetanus booster.
From Valenziano CP, Chattar-Cora D, O'Neill A, Hubli EH, Cudjoe EA. Efficacy of primary wound cultures in long bone open extremity fractures: are they of any value? *Arch Orthop Trauma Surg*. 2002;122(5):259–261.

of choice to diagnose vascular injury, as they have been shown to have both high sensitivity and specificity in detecting traumatic arterial injury.[8]

- *Musculoskeletal*: Muscle functions and musculotendinous integrity should be assessed. Compartments should be palpated and, in conjunction with the neurovascular exam, a determination should be made if compartment syndrome is suspected. Standard radiographs should be obtained to include a joint above and below the injury site.

Injury Classification

After the secondary trauma survey and review of the lower extremity imaging results, an assessment of the injury pattern can be described and classified according to various systems. The Gustilo[9] and the Byrd[10] classifications are used most commonly (Table 43.2). Other systems include the Mangled Extremity Severity Score (MESS), which aims to predict which limbs should be salvaged rather than amputated.[11] The MESS and other lower extremity injury-severity scores have failed to demonstrate clinical utility and should be used cautiously in determining if a lower extremity trauma patient is best served with an amputation or limb salvage.[11]

Orthoplastic Approach

For patients with moderate-severe trauma injury, the transfer to a trauma center is warranted, with in-hospital mortality rate being significantly lower at trauma centers compared to non-trauma centers (7.6% vs. 9.5%), as well as a lower one-year mortality rate (10.4% vs. 13.8%).[12] While the specific reason for the improved outcome of lower extremity trauma patients at trauma centers is uncertain, the availability of the multidisciplinary team is likely a significant factor.

To further optimize care and outcomes for lower extremity trauma patients, a combined approach by orthopedic and plastic surgery teams is preferred.[3] Success in limb reconstruction requires the surgeon to abandon the tissue-specific perspective and to adopt a holistic approach, considering the extremity in totality. Indeed, decreased rates of complications and revision surgery were noted in patients with Gustilo grade IIIB open tibial fractures when treated at trauma centers with an orthoplastic team instead of a tertiary center without an orthoplastic team.[13]

Compartment Syndrome

The five "Ps" (pain, pallor, paralysis, paresthesia, poikilothermy) suggest compartment syndrome, with paresthesia and disproportionate pain on passive stretch being the earlier signs. Traditionally, intracompartmental pressure (ICP) of 30 mmHg or less was an indication for fasciotomy. Newer evidence suggests that the differential pressure (diastolic minus compartment pressure) over 30 mmHg is a more sensitive indicator of compartment syndrome requiring fasciotomy.[14] Fasciotomy incisions should be placed precisely to avoid compromising perforators for possible local fasciocutaneous flap and to avoid undue tibial exposure (Figs. 43.1 and 43.2).

Vascular Injury

Evidence of arterial injury on CT angiography can include sudden narrowing of an artery, loss of arterial opacification, pseudoaneurysm formation, active contrast material extravasation, and arteriovenous fistula formation.[8] An ischemic limb should have circulation restored ideally within 3–4 hours of injury to avoid irreversible muscle damage. Preoperative angiography should not delay revascularization attempts. When vascular disruption is present in combination with bone injury, the order of repair is debatable. On one hand, fracture reduction and skeletal fixation will require manipulation that can potentially jeopardize an adjacent, delicate vascular repair. On the other hand, prompt reversal of ischemia is critical to avoid muscle damage and to ensure limb salvage. No definitive evidence exists to indicate that surgical sequence has any impact on the rate of subsequent lower extremity amputation.

TABLE 43.2 **Classification of Lower Extremity Injury**

System	Grade	Soft Tissue	Bone
Gustilo[25]	I	Wound <1 cm	Simple fracture No comminution
	II	Wound >1 cm Minimal soft tissue damage	Moderate comminution
	III	Extensive soft tissue damage (ex: degloving, contusion, flaps)	Comminuted fracture
	IIIA	III with adequate soft tissue coverage	Comminuted fracture
	IIIB	III with extensive soft tissue loss Inadequate soft tissue coverage	Periosteal stripping Exposed bone
	IIIC	III with arterial injury requiring repair	Any open fracture pattern
Byrd[26]	I	Wound <2 cm Clean	Low energy Spiral or oblique fracture
	II	Wound >2 cm Moderate adjacent skin/ muscle contusion No devitalized muscle	Moderate energy Comminuted or displaced fracture
	III	Extensive skin loss Devitalized muscle	High energy Significantly displaced fracture Severe comminution Segmental fracture or bone defect
	IV	Crush, degloving, or associated vascular injury requiring repair	As III but extremely high energy

Free flap reconstructive options can be limited by the availability of native recipient arteries and veins in the traumatized lower extremity. To circumvent the shortage of peripheral recipient vessels, a temporary arteriovenous (AV) fistula can be created. The fistula is designed with a long, reversed vein graft anastomosed to a large artery at one end and a large vein at the other end. The vein graft is preferably harvested from the ipsilateral limb to minimize donor site morbidity.[15] Alternatively, the Corlett loop technique, originally described by Mulholland et al in the neck,[16] can be applied to the lower extremity. The ipsilateral lesser saphenous vein can be utilized "in situ" to create the fistula by preserving the proximal end where it merges into the popliteal vein, thereby avoiding a second microvascular anastomosis.[15] The distal end of the vein is transposed to be anastomosed to an artery. Anastomosis of the vein can be performed to a major artery such as the popliteal artery in an "end-to-side" fashion or to a sural artery branch in an "end-to-end" fashion.[15] The fistula loop should be positioned adjacent to the defect to be reconstructed (Fig. 43.3).[15] Ideally, the fistula location permits the microvascular anastomosis to be performed outside the zone of injury. Division of the fistula loop and anastomosis to the flap vessels can be performed as a single-stage surgery or in a delayed fashion. If this is done as a single stage, it is recommended to perfuse the AV fistula for one hour intraoperatively prior to division of the loop and anastomosis to the flap.[15] A single-stage technique is beneficial as early thrombotic occlusion of the fistula can theoretically be identified immediately and anastomotic revision performed.

Antibiotics

Open tibial fractures are particularly susceptible to infection given the low vascularization compared to other long bones. The relatively poor blood supply confers a suboptimal resistance to bacterial invasion, further increasing the likelihood of infection. Antibiotic prophylaxis is widely recommended for these patients, though no definitive international consensus exists with regard to antibiotic choice or duration of coverage.

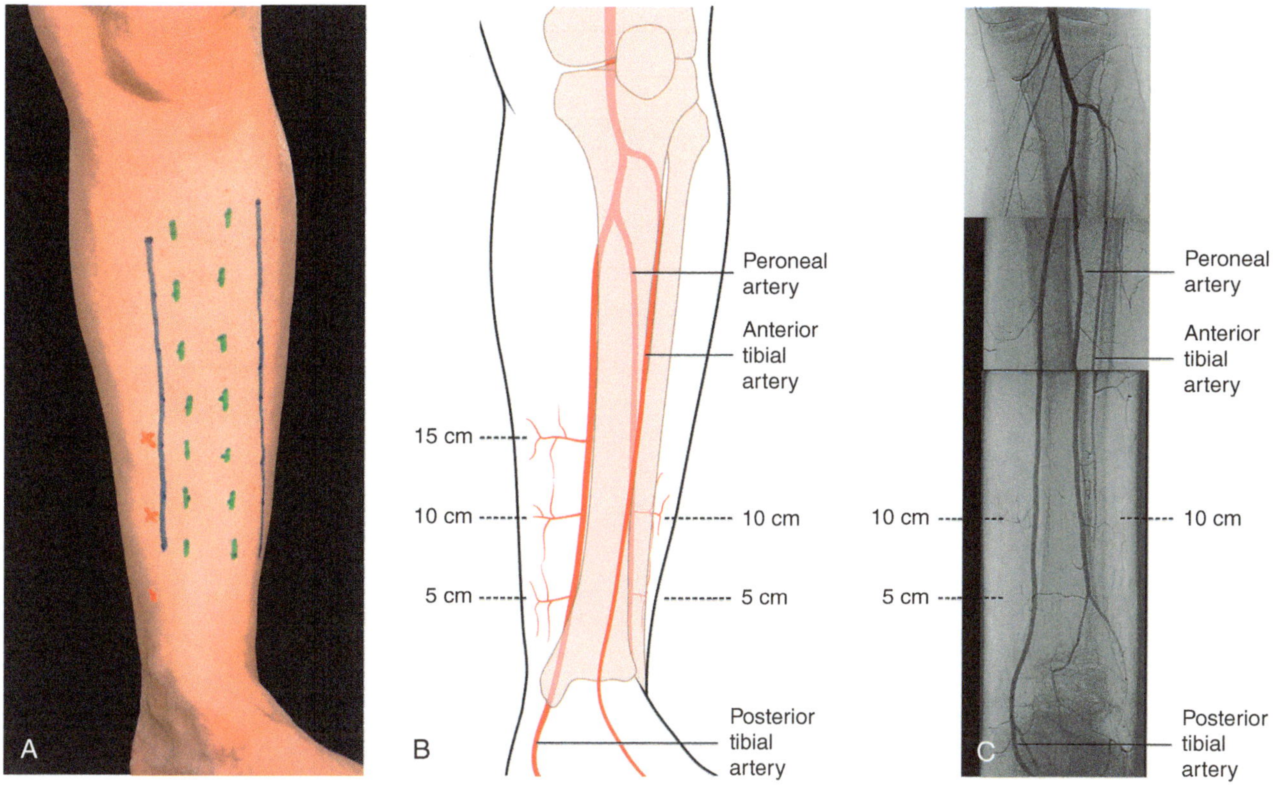

• **Fig. 43.1** Recommended incisions for fasciotomy and wound extensions. (A) Margins of subcutaneous border of tibia marked in green, fasciotomy incisions in blue, and the perforators on the medial side arising from posterior tibial vessels in red. (B) Line drawing depicting the location of the perforators. (C) Arteriogram demonstrating perforators. The 10 cm perforator on the medial side is typically the largest and most reliable for distally-based fasciocutaneous flaps. In this patient, the anterior tibial artery had been disrupted following an open dislocation of the ankle; hence the poor flow evident in this vessel in the distal one-third of the leg. The distances of the perforators from the tip of the malleolus are approximate and can vary between patients.

Common organisms that cause open fracture infection include Gram-negative rods or Gram-positive cocci, primarily *Staphylococcus aureus.*[17] Rather than contaminating organisms from the time of initial injury, it appears that nosocomial organisms tend to cause infection of open fractures.[18] As such, antibiotic regimens have been tailored to address the potential nosocomial infection arising after presentation. In addition, there is limited utility in obtaining initial wound cultures in open long bone fractures, as the cases that develop infection from the organism noted on initial wound culture are rare.[19] Post-debridement cultures are slightly more predictive, as the organism noted on culture causes infection about 42% of the time.[19]

Antibiotics are recommended to be administered ideally within 1 hour of injury and no later than 3 hours after injury.[18] Early initiation of antibiotic prophylaxis within 3 hours of injury has been shown to lower infection rates.

The duration of antibiotics is determined by the severity of injury. For Gustilo I and II injuries, antibiotics can be discontinued 24–48 hours following wound closure.[18] For Gustilo III injuries, antibiotics are continued for 48–72 hours after the initial injury or until 24 hours after definitive soft tissue coverage, whichever comes first.[17,18]

In general, a first- or second-generation cephalosporin is recommended, such as cefazolin 1–2 g load then 1 g IV q8 hours or cefuroxime 1.5 g IV q8 hours.[17,18] For patients with penicillin allergy, clindamycin is an acceptable alternative.[17,18] Particularly for Gustilo III injuries, additional coverage should be added at the time of first surgical debridement with gentamicin 1–2 mg/kg IV, either one dose or q8 hours for 48 hours.[17,18] Also, at the time of skeletal stabilization and definitive soft tissue coverage, an additional one-time dose of gentamicin plus vancomycin 1 g IV can be considered.[18]

Wound Debridement

For many years following Gustilo and Anderson's landmark study, the standard of care for patients with open tibial fractures involved early debridement (within 6–8 hours of the time of injury) and copious irrigation.[20] Some studies of open lower extremity fractures have corroborated this practice. Malhotra et al demonstrated an 18% infection rate when wound debridement and irrigation was delayed over 8 hours, compared to an 11% infection rate when debridement and irrigation was completed within 8 hours.[21] On the other hand, a LEAP study demonstrated that a longer

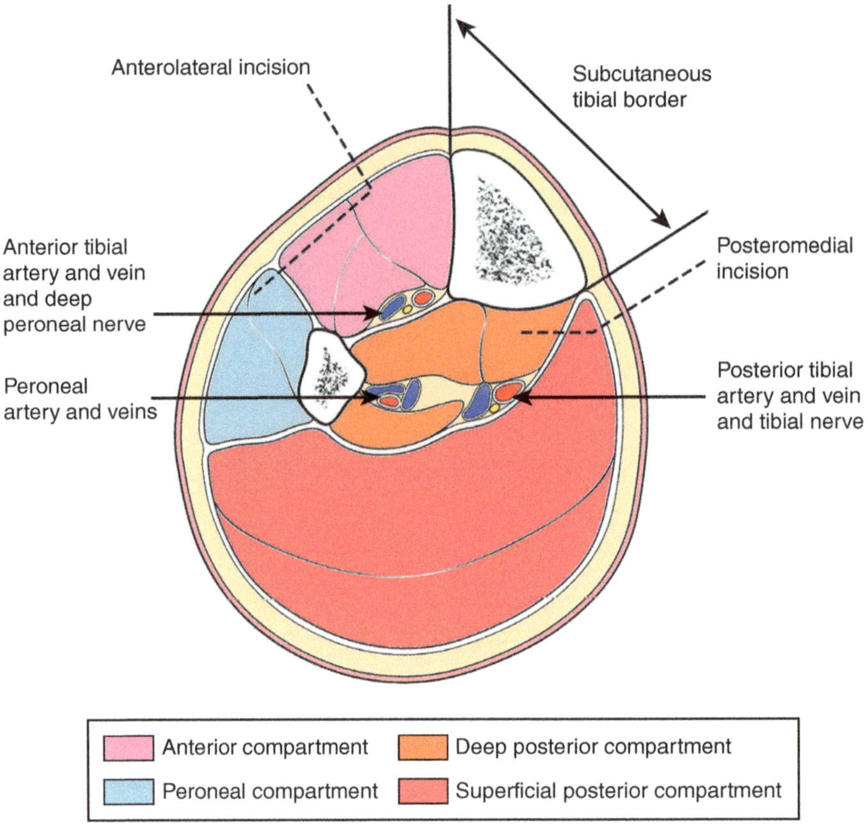

• **Fig. 43.2** Cross-section through the leg showing incisions to decompress all four compartments. The medial incision is situated 1.5 cm from the medial subcutaneous border of the tibia. The lateral incision is placed 2 cm lateral to the lateral subcutaneous tibial border. The lateral dissection continues subfascially until the peroneal septum, which must then be divided.

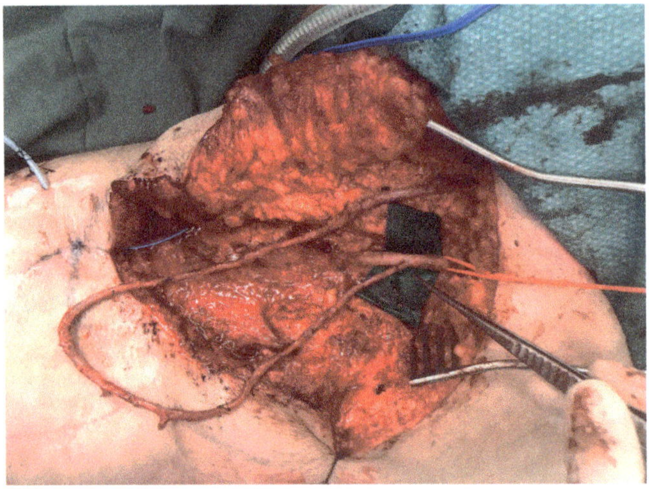

• **Fig. 43.3** Temporary arteriovenous fistula of the lower extremity with a long, reversed vein graft anastomosed to an artery at one end and a vein at the other. Note the positioning of the fistula with the apex towards the defect, which will permit facile anastomosis to the free flap vessels. (Courtesy Dr. Rostam D. Farhadieh.)

time from injury to debridement (approximately 11–13 hours) was not a significant independent predictor of the risk of infection.[22] Given the lack of consistent evidence to support early debridement, it has become accepted practice to defer debridement until the next operating day.

Debridement should be performed by the orthoplastic team. Careful debridement of devitalized tissues and identification of all structures should be performed, starting at the peripheral uninvolved tissue and progressing from "known to unknown" into the wound bed. The end-point of debridement can be guided by bleeding at the cut edges. Degloved skin may require debridement but should not be thoughtlessly discarded. An avulsed skin flap, if notably devascularized, can be used as a donor site for a skin graft.

Copious irrigation should be performed but high-pressure pulsatile lavage should be avoided as this may further propagate bacteria into soft tissue. A sterile dressing should be applied, and a splint placed for immobilization. After thorough debridement of the wound, negative pressure wound therapy can be applied. This can be used to bridge the wound between debridements and the final reconstruction, while encouraging rapid granulation of the wound bed.

Principles of Skeletal Fixation

Early fracture reduction and stabilization is of utmost importance and is preferably performed at the time of initial wound debridement. Fracture stabilization can reduce the propensity for bacterial spread and can improve blood flow and venous return. Current fixation techniques include external fixators, plates and screws, and either reamed or unreamed locking nails. The injury pattern will principally guide selection of a skeletal stabilization method. External fixation is typically reserved for complex fractures, whereas internal fixation methods are used for less severe fractures.

External Fixation

Tibia fractures can be treated with a variety of types of external fixation devices. In the past, pin-to-bar external fixation was used regularly for definitive treatment of open tibial shaft fracture. However, pin-tract infections, higher rates of malunion, patient dissatisfaction, and the need for prolonged application (upwards of 3–4 months) have caused pin-to-bar external fixation popularity to wane.[23] Pin-to-bar external fixation remains quite helpful as a temporizing method of fracture stabilization if the wound will require repeat debridement or if the patient is too ill for definitive fixation and coverage.[23]

Definitive external fixation can be performed with a monotube unilateral fixator or circular external fixator. The circular external fixator can be helpful for periarticular fractures and allow for earlier mobilization.[23] In general, definitive external fixation has been found to have a much higher rate of reoperation (68.5%) and malunion (20%) compared to unreamed intramedullary nailing and other skeletal fixation techniques.[23]

The orthoplastic team should confer prior to placing pins and bars/frames. Haphazard selection of pin sites can potentially compromise or complicate microvascular anastomosis. Bar and frame positioning should be planned to accommodate postoperative edema. An elevation frame can be applied to suspend the extremity in elevation, thereby facilitating edema resolution and eliminating pressure on the flap, pedicle, and wound.

Plates and Screws

Conventionally, internal fixation with plate and screws was unpopular for open tibia fractures. Application of the plate requires additional soft tissue elevation which can potentially exacerbate devitalization of injured tissues. Modern designs of plates that minimize the disruption of periosteal blood supply have gained some popularity. Gopal et al demonstrated the safety of the "fix and flap" method of immediate internal fixation with plate and screws with free flap soft tissue coverage.[24] The limb salvage rate was 95% and the majority of fractures progressed to primary bony union with this technique alone.[24] When compared to the external fixator, the low profile nature of the plate understandably causes fewer practical difficulties for subsequent procedures, including free flap coverage.[24]

Intramedullary Nailing

Intramedullary nailing for tibia fractures is accepted as an effective treatment for both open and closed types. Reamed intramedullary nails offer greater biomechanical stability when compared to unreamed nails. However, the reaming of the intramedullary canal can disrupt endosteal blood flow and can thereby contribute to bone necrosis and infection.

A 2008 randomized SPRINT trial found that there was no significant difference in reoperation rates between the reamed and unreamed intramedullary nailing groups, with rates being 29% in the reamed group and 24% in the unreamed group.[25] Rates of bone grafting, implant exchange or removal, and implant breakage were comparable, without a statistically significant difference.[25] Yet, other studies have noted improved outcomes with reamed intramedullary nailing. Debate regarding the superiority of reamed over unreamed nails is ongoing.

Principles of Soft Tissue Reconstruction

Timing

Most believe that early definitive soft tissue coverage of open fractures leads to better outcomes. This is supported by the study by Godina et al in which the timing of microsurgical reconstruction was analyzed with respect to flap failure, infection, bone-healing time, length of stay, and number of operations.[26] Those reconstructed by 72 hours had the best outcomes, and those between 72 hours and 3 months had the highest rates of flap failure and infection. Recent guidelines advocate definitive coverage ideally within 72 hours and no later than 7 days after the injury.[18] Although early coverage is preferable, immediate reconstruction is not an option for every patient.

Interestingly, there is a documented trend towards later soft-tissue coverage. Sheckter et al demonstrated that, over 10 years, there was a significant trend in the mean hospital day of soft-tissue coverage from 6.12 days in 2002 to 12.50 days in 2011.[27] This is theorized to be partly due to increased utilization of negative-pressure wound therapy as a bridge to definitive soft tissue coverage.[27] The outcomes of delayed reconstruction, in light of current management options, are not yet fully understood.

Reconstructive Ladder versus Reconstructive Elevator

In lower extremity trauma, numerous reconstructive options should be considered to provide the patient with a reliable, functional outcome. The reconstructive ladder traditionally guides the orthoplastic team to select oftentimes the simplest reconstruction possible for the patient. With the refinement of fixation techniques and locoregional and free flap options, as well as improvements in perioperative care to improve flap survivability and general outcomes, the algorithmic approach may be more aptly named the reconstructive elevator. In present times, greater gain may be obtained with a more complex procedure, such as a free flap, compared to gain obtained in the past. This may validate saltatory movement along the reconstructive ladder (i.e., the reconstructive elevator). Major lower extremity trauma may have extensive soft tissue injury and a wide zone of injury which preclude local options, and free flap reconstruction may be required. Consideration is given to defect size and location, functional needs, zone of injury, recipient vessels for free flap reconstruction, and need for future operative interventions.

Rule of Thirds

Location of the soft tissue defect is often a major factor in the reconstructive choice. Defects of the proximal third of the leg include the pedicled gastrocnemius muscle flap. Middle third defects favor the proximally-based soleus muscle flap. Distal third reconstructive choices include perforator flaps, propeller flaps, reverse sural artery flap, but frequently require free flap reconstruction. Certainly, other factors including depth and type of tissue missing (i.e., skin, subcutaneous tissue, fascia, muscle, periosteum, etc.), size, and donor site availability/morbidity are other important considerations when planning soft tissue coverage.

Locoregional Flaps

Local Muscle Flaps

There are a limited number of muscles available for reconstructive options; however, they are important workhorses for many proximal and middle third defects.

Gastrocnemius Flap

The gastrocnemius muscle is a bipennate muscle, and its medial or lateral heads may be used for proximal third defects. It is useful for coverage of the knee but may not reach as far as the proximal aspect of the patella in some patients (Fig. 43.4). It is a Mathes and Nahai type I flap, and its dominant blood supply consists of the sural artery with clear separation between the two heads. The gastrocnemius muscle is the most superficial of the calf muscles, superficial to the underlying plantaris and soleus. Approach to the muscle may be performed through a posterior or medial longitudinal incision. Dissection is carried proximally to the muscular origin at the medial or lateral femoral condyle for the medial or lateral heads, respectively. Division of the origin of the muscle may increase the reach of the flap but may place greater tension on the vascular pedicle. Dissection continues distally to the common insertion of the gastrocnemius muscle and soleus muscle at the Achilles tendon. Harvest of a small cuff of Achilles tendon while maintaining its integrity facilitates inset. Increased reach and greater surface area may be covered with fascial scoring. The muscle is then tunneled through a subcutaneous window or the skin bridge opened to allow inset, and finally covered with a split-thickness skin graft. Harvest of a single head is associated with little to no functional loss.

Soleus Flap

A proximally-based soleus muscle flap is typically favored for middle third defects. A Mathes and Nahai type II muscle flap, its vascular supply consists of branches from the popliteal artery, posterior tibial artery, and peroneal artery. The soleus muscle lies deep to the gastrocnemius and the plantaris, and distally fuses with the gastrocnemius to form the Achilles tendon. Depending on defect location, elevation of the flap may be approached through a medial longitudinal incision or midlateral incision.

Other Muscle Flaps

Other local muscles may be used for reconstruction, including tibialis anterior, flexor digitorum longus, extensor digitorum longus, flexor hallucis longus, and extensor digitorum hallucis; however, the utility of these flaps is limited as they typically cover fairly small defects and/or are associated with some degree of function loss.

Local Fasciocutaneous Flap

The lower extremity is an anatomical region rich with perforators for flap design. Local fasciocutaneous flaps may be advantageous by providing replacement of "like with like," and may have shorter operative times and decreased complexity. A greater understanding of angiosomes has allowed these flaps to be safely performed when based on known perforators. Perforator flaps can be particularly useful in select distal third defects when the alternative would require free tissue transfer.

Perforator Flaps

Surrounding the knee there are perforators from the femoral artery, and septocutaneous branches from the descending genicular artery, medial and lateral superior genicular arteries, medial and lateral inferior genicular arteries, anterior tibial recurrent artery, and popliteal artery cutaneous branch. There is a rich density of perforators of the leg for flap design and harvest (Fig. 43.5).

Posteriorly, the sural artery flap is based on perforators of the medial or lateral sural artery and the venae comitantes that run with the sural nerve, with perforators from the medial head of the gastrocnemius muscle tend to be more reliable. Although the medial sural artery perforator flap has gained popularity, especially for head and neck reconstruction as it provides thin and pliable soft tissue, a relatively long pedicle, and minimal donor site morbidity, its pedicled use for lower extremity reconstruction is more limited. A review of 70 flaps found that up to 36% developed necrosis, particularly in the presence of comorbidities such as diabetes, venous insufficiency, and peripheral arterial disease.[28]

The distally-based (reverse) sural artery flap is often considered a neurofasciocutaneous flap, as the sural nerve runs with the median superficial sural artery. Its retrograde arterial supply is classically described as septocutaneous perforators from the peroneal artery to the superficial sural artery; however, there is also some contribution from

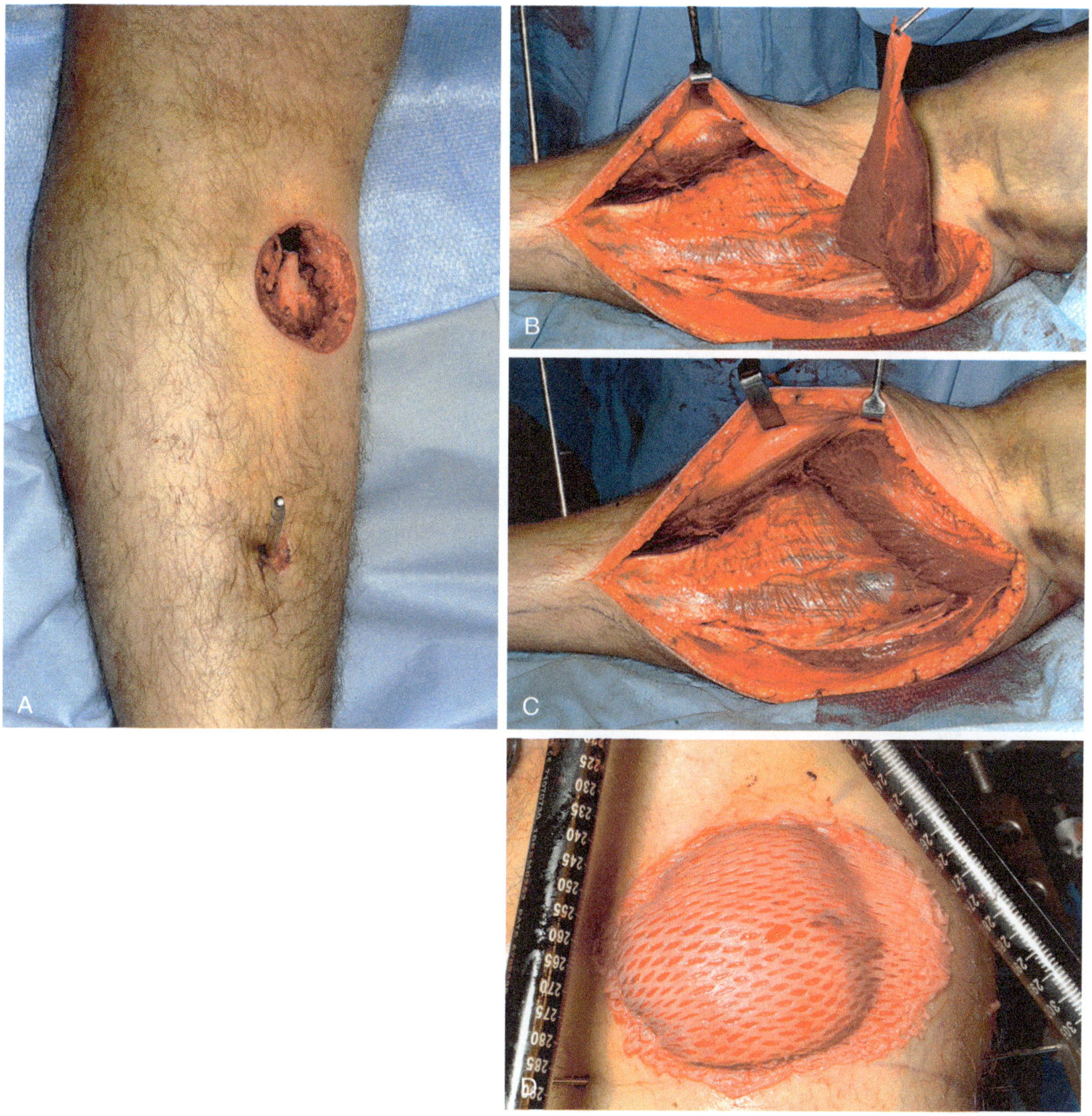

• **Fig. 43.4** Gastrocnemius local muscle flap. (A) A proximal open tibial fracture with a small anteromedial soft tissue defect. Half pins used for the preliminary bridging external fixation (BEF) were retained for the circular external fixation (CEF). (B) The medial head of gastrocnemius, with a portion of Achilles tendon, was raised via a posterior incision. (C) The muscle was tunneled beneath intact medial tissues and (D) covered with a split-thickness skin graft. (Case courtesy Mr. Jon Simmons.)

septocutaneous perforators from the posterior tibial artery, as well as from small arteries accompanying the sural nerve and lesser saphenous vein. It is critical to include the sural nerve and lesser saphenous vein during dissection of this flap. Despite multiple sources of vascularity, it is not particularly robust. Incidence of partial flap necrosis has been described as from 11% to 36% (Fig. 43.6).[28]

In the leg, perforators can arise from the anterior tibial artery, posterior tibial artery, and peroneal artery. Anterior tibial artery-based perforators emerge either from the tibialis anterior muscle or between the tibialis anterior and extensor hallucis longus, or from the anteromedial septum between the peroneus tertius and peroneus brevis muscles. The posterior tibial perforator flap utilizes perforators from the intermuscular septum between the soleus and flexor digitorum longus. Peroneal artery perforators arise from the posterolateral septum between the peroneus longus and soleus muscles.

Free Flaps

With the advancement of microsurgery, use of free tissue transfer has progressed the treatment paradigm of lower extremity defects and contributed to the shift from the reconstructive ladder to the reconstructive elevator. A multitude of defects can be reconstructed using free transfer of fasciocutaneous tissue, muscle, bone, and a combination of these tissues via chimeric flaps. Recipient vessels, in particular the venae comitantes, can be injured at the level of the fracture and intimal injuries may not be outwardly apparent. It is critical to trace recipient vessels for anastomosis outside the zone of injury, with preference to vasculature proximal to the defect when possible.

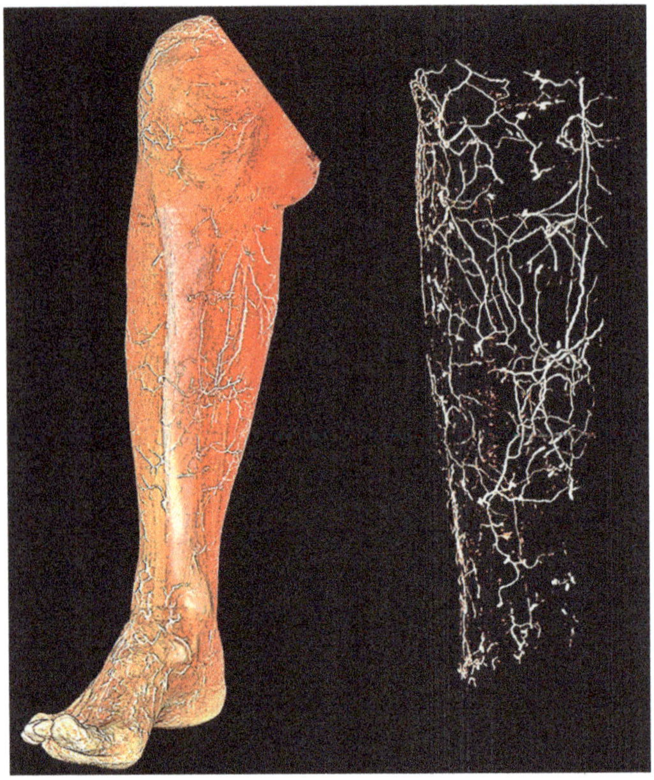

• **Fig. 43.5** Computed tomography angiography of perforators of the leg.

The posterior tibial vessels are less likely to have been injured during the initial trauma and are more reliable. The posterior tibial vessels can be identified just deep to the fascia covering the flexor hallucis longus distally, and proximally the vessels lie deep to soleus. Vein grafting or temporary arteriovenous fistulas, as previously described, may be required to avoid anastomosis within the zone of injury and to improve recipient vessel options.

Muscle flaps are versatile to fill various defects, especially to obliterate dead space. Latissimus dorsi muscle is especially useful in resurfacing broad, large surface area defects; positioning and trunk/upper extremity strength and stability are considerations. Smaller defects may be filled with free gracilis muscle. Vastus lateralis muscle can also be harvested with little donor site morbidity. Rectus abdominis has waned in popularity due to potential abdominal wall weakness and bulge. To limit donor site morbidity in smaller size defects, muscle-sparing flaps can be raised with the latissimus dorsi flap and vastus lateralis. Although initially bulky, the denervated muscle atrophies and has better contour with time. Disadvantages include need for split-thickness skin grafting over the muscle flap and difficulty raising the flap should the underlying bony trauma require reoperation.

Fasciocutaneous free flaps provide reconstruction with minimal donor site morbidity and can potentially be sensate. One of the most common choices is the anterolateral

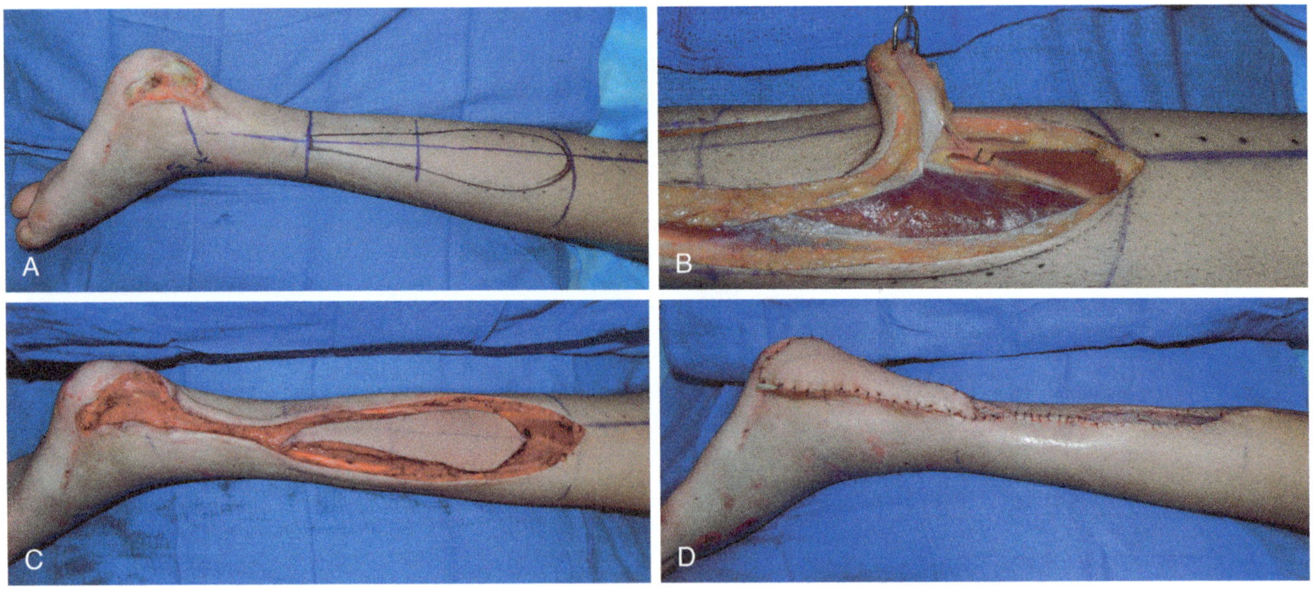

• **Fig. 43.6** (A) Exposed Achilles tendon and calcaneus. A reverse sural artery flap is designed along a vertical axis centered from the midpoint between the lateral malleolus and the Achilles tendon and the midpoint of the popliteal fossa. Maximal peroneal perforator density can be found within 8 cm of the lower transverse line, which is the proximal extent of flap. (B) Subfascial elevation of the sural artery flap from proximal to distal with early identification of the sural nerve and artery. (C) Reverse sural artery flap in situ following elevation and recipient site debridement. (D) Final flap inset. Donor site is closed primarily and with split-thickness skin graft as needed.

thigh fasciocutaneous flap, based off the descending branch of the lateral femoral circumflex artery. The pedicle is long and large areas can be reconstructed. The flap can be made into a sensate flap with incorporation of the lateral femoral cutaneous nerve (Fig. 43.7). Other free flap options include the scapular or parascapular flaps, radial forearm flap, and anteromedial thigh flap.

Choice of Muscle versus Fasciocutaneous Flaps

The optimal reconstructive flap helps restore form and function, promotes osseous union, and minimizes donor-site morbidity. A recent multicenter retrospective study analyzed 518 lower extremity free flaps and determined that muscle and fasciocutaneous flaps achieved similar limb salvage rates in acute and chronic trauma subgroups. There was no significant difference in the rates of flap thrombosis, flap salvage, flap loss, or tibial nonunion requiring bone grafting. The fasciocutaneous flap group were more commonly re-elevated for subsequent orthopedic procedures compared to the muscle flap group and required fewer secondary skin-grafts.[29] Although this review did not demonstrate a clinical difference on bony union, other studies have suggested superior fracture healing with muscle flaps. In order to utilize the benefits of both muscle and fasciocutaneous free flaps, an anterolateral thigh flap harvested with some vastus lateralis would provide the benefits of a fasciocutaneous flap with muscle for dead-space obliteration and hematoma prevention.

Skeletal Reconstruction

Bone defects of the lower extremity can be reconstructed by bone graft (both nonvascularized and vascularized) or distraction osteogenesis. Small defects under 5 cm can be successfully treated with autogenous cancellous bone graft, whereas significant graft resorption will occur when applied to defects over 5 cm. The Masquelet technique utilizes nonvascularized bone graft for slightly larger defects.[30] This two-stage technique starts with bone debridement and polymethylmethacrylate antibiotic spacer application into the defect.[30] An "induction membrane" with a rich vascular network is formed over the course of 6–8 weeks.[30] At the second stage of surgery, the spacer is removed from under the membrane and cancellous bone graft, typically harvested from the iliac crest, is packed into this space. Disadvantages of the Masquelet technique include donor site morbidity and limited graft availability.

Defects over 5 cm can also be reconstructed with a free vascularized bone graft. This is most commonly harvested from the fibula, though skeletal reconstruction with vascularized bone flaps from the iliac crest and scapula are also possible.[30] The free fibula bone graft requires a lengthy surgery with added donor site morbidity. An ispilateral island fibula transfer, or pedicled fibula bone flap, is also an option for reconstruction of segmental tibial defects in patients that are not candidates for microsurgical procedures. Fracture of the bone graft can pose a threat to the reconstruction viability. To improve long-term stability and shorten the time of osseous consolidation, a double-barrel fibula flap can also be considered.

Defects over 10 cm and up to 15 cm can be reconstructed at a rate of about 1 mm per day with the Ilizarov distraction osteogenesis technique.[30] A corticotomy is made adjacent to the fracture site and the fracture ends are gradually separated. The Ilizarov method allows for immediate weight bearing and permits dynamic adjustment of the limb alignment. Potential disadvantages include pin site infection, stress fracture, and significant psychological stress due to the protracted treatment course.[30]

Amputation

Indications for primary amputation include incomplete traumatic amputation, devascularization with warm ischemia time greater than 4–6 hours, severe foot crush injury, and severe lower extremity trauma in the setting of an unstable polytrauma. Amputation should be considered when there is loss of two or more fascial compartments, two or more vessels injured, severe muscle loss, and older age/poor functional status of the patient (Fig. 43.8). Although classically loss of plantar sensation was an indication for amputation, the LEAP study found otherwise. In patients who underwent limb salvage, those who did not have plantar sensation initially had outcomes similar to those of patients who did have plantar sensation, and half regained sensation in 2 years.[7]

Many studies have evaluated the injury severity to determine whether a patient should receive an amputation; however, an independent, prospective evaluation of five scoring systems (Mangled Extremity Severity Score; the Predictive Salvage Index; the Limb Salvage Index; the Nerve Injury, Ischemia, Soft Tissue Injury, Skeletal Injury, Shock, and Age of Patient Score; and the Hanover Fracture Scale-97) demonstrated they have limited utility.[11] A staged orthoplastic approach and early education for the patient and their family is imperative to reach the appropriate decision.

Outcomes, Patient Satisfaction, Cost–Utility

Limb salvage and reconstructive efforts must be compared to functional outcomes of transtibial amputation, and the choice must be tailored to each patient and his/her individual circumstances. In severely injured lower extremities (Gustilo type IIIB and IIIC fractures), functional outcomes of limb salvage and successful primary transtibial amputation are similar. Amputation has been associated with shorter hospital stay, fewer surgeries, and more rapid return to ambulation.[31]

The Lower Extremity Assessment Project (LEAP) study analyzed surgeon and patient satisfaction with outcome at 24 months and found discordance between overall outcome and cosmesis. Patients were particularly

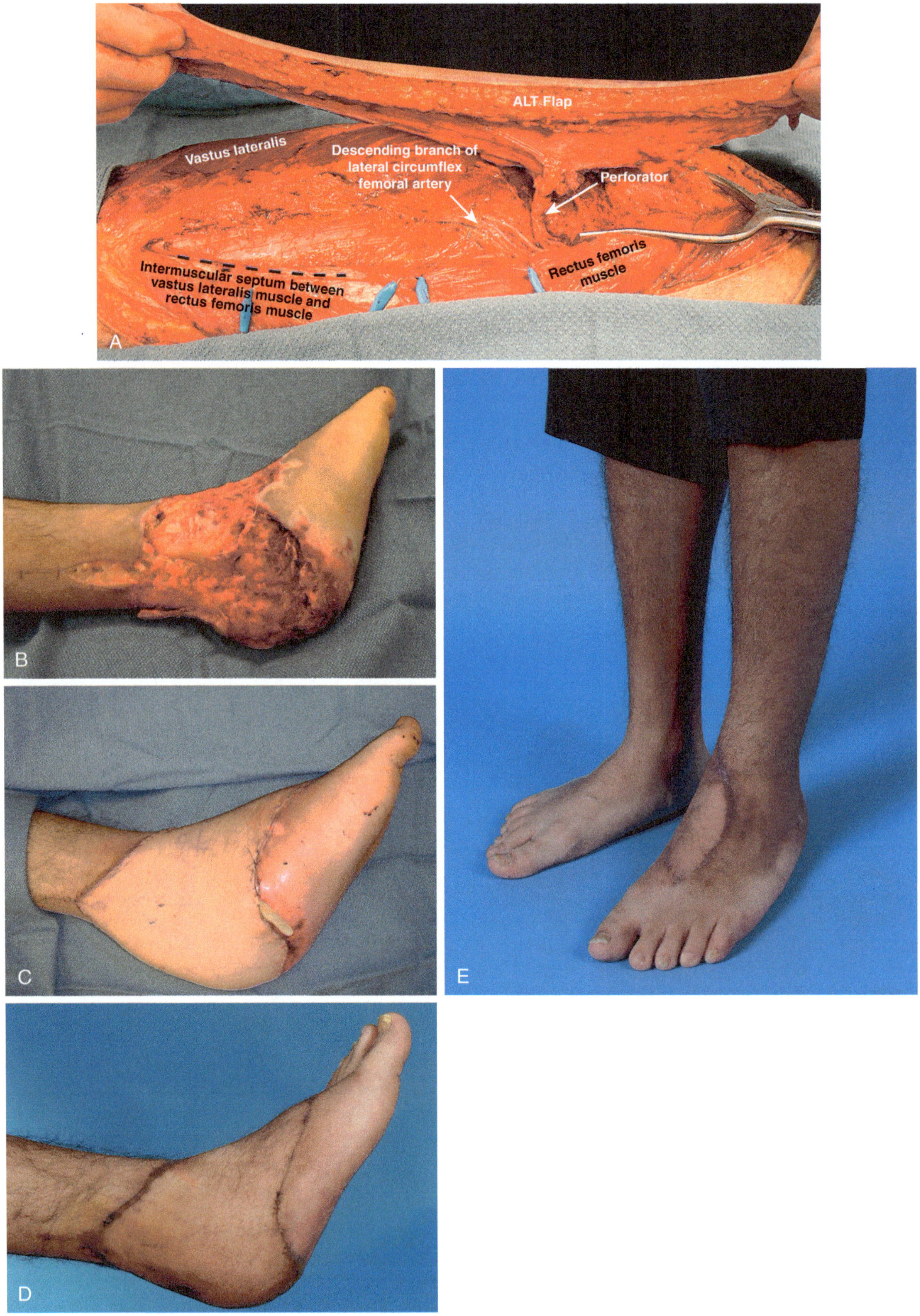

• **Fig. 43.7** (A) In situ elevation and labeled anterolateral thigh (ALT) flap. (B) Large degloving injury of the left lower extremity with exposure of the medial malleolus, Achilles tendon, calcaneus, and extensor tendons. (C) Following radical debridement, anterolateral thigh free fasciocutaneous flap was used for reconstruction. (D) It was later liposuctioned for improved contour. (E) The patient was able to wear his normal footwear and ambulate at his preinjury level.

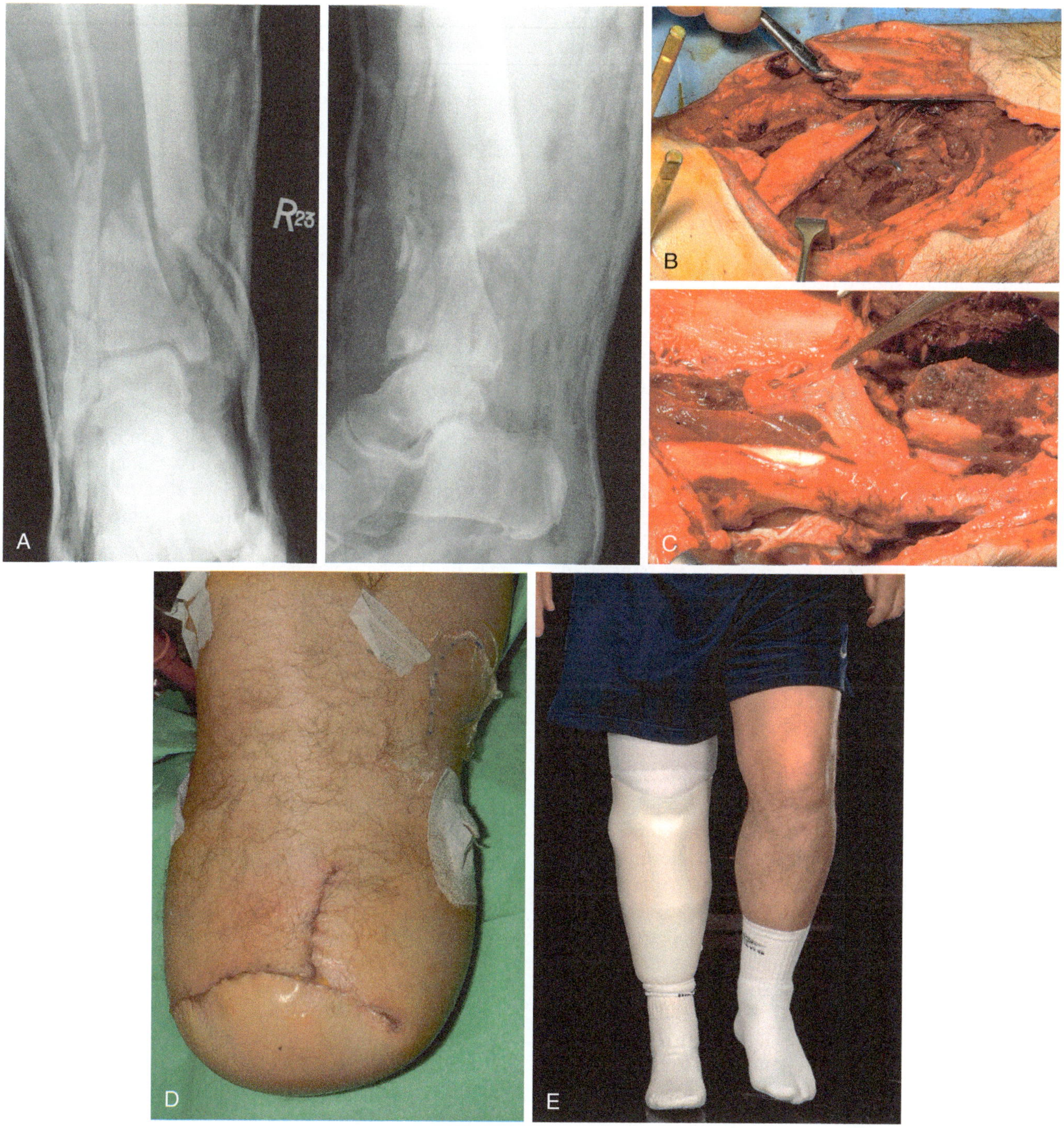

• **Fig. 43.8** Transtibial amputation. A 62-year-old man fell from a roof sustaining a grade IIIB open tibial fracture that was unsalvageable. (A) Initial radiographs show a displaced fracture of the distal tibial shaft with a significant intraarticular component. There were also segmental comminuted fractures of the fibula. (B) There was periosteal stripping of the exposed bone ends and approximately 4 cm bone loss following debridement. (C) The tibial nerve, held in the forceps, was partially divided and severely contused. (D) Postamputation appearance highlighting a cylindrical-shaped residual limb with normal skin where possible and tension-free wound closure avoiding end-bearing wounds. (E) Progress at 3 months showing successful limb fitting and unaided walking.

less satisfied on cosmetic outcome compared to their surgeons.[32] Overall, 66% of patients were satisfied and 34% were not. No preexisting patient factors were identified as predictive of their satisfaction. The only factors that correlated with satisfaction were measures of physical function, psychological distress, clinical recovery, and return to work.[33]

When outcomes are similar, cost–utility must also be studied and considered. When costs associated with rehospitalization and postacute care were factored in, the overall cost at 2 years was similar between salvage and amputation. When factoring in costs relating to prostheses, which require maintenance and replacement, projected lifetime cost was significantly greater for amputees.[2]

Amputation Surgery

The goal of amputation is the creation of a residual limb that can fit a prosthesis, a functioning myodesis, no end neuroma, and sensate skin throughout. Ideally, 12–15 cm of residual tibial length should be preserved. Transtibial amputation with a prosthesis results in 10%–30% increase in ambulation energy expenditure compared to 40%–70% for transfemoral amputation.[34] In cases where there is inadequate soft-tissue coverage for coverage of a bony stump, it is possible to use free flaps to maintain length or use of "spare parts" surgery, where portions of the amputated extremity can be used to reconstruct the remaining stump.

Targeted muscle reinnervation has been utilized for improved control of myoelectric prosthetics but has also shown promise for treating end neuromas. Transected peripheral nerves in the amputated extremity are transferred to recipient motor nerves of residual muscle with the goal of reestablishing muscle innervation, preventing muscle atrophy, and diminishing symptomatic neuroma and phantom limb pain.

Complications

Wound Complications

The goal of lower extremity reconstruction is to provide stable, durable, and healed soft tissue coverage and prevent secondary complications of the injury such as nonunion and infection. The LEAP study analyzed wound complications according to type of reconstruction. Although more severe injuries were often treated with free flaps, there was no significant difference in wound complication rates. When regression analysis was used to stratify according to osseous injury, rotational flap patients were more likely to have wound complications requiring a return to the operating room when compared to free flaps.[31]

Infection/Osteomyelitis

Severe lower extremity trauma is at high risk for wound infection, especially with a contaminated wound bed, potential underlying hardware and biofilm formation, devitalized tissue, and stagnant hematoma which is a nutrient-rich environment for pathogens with limited penetration by the immune system and antibiotics. Agricultural injuries, delayed presentation/debridement, extensive zone of injury, vascular injury, and bone loss are at particularly high risk. Adequate debridement prior to reconstruction is paramount.

Acute infection is typically classified as occurring within 4 weeks of injury. Erythema, drainage, and fluid collection under the flap are signs that warrant prompt surgical exploration to prevent deep infection. The most common organisms include *Staphylococcus aureus*, *Enterococcus*, *Enterobacter*, and *Pseudomonas*.[17] Debridement of any devitalized tissue should be aggressive and contaminated internal fixation converted to external fixators.

The tibia is known to be a common site of infected nonunion and chronic posttraumatic osteomyelitis. The LEAP study had demonstrated an incidence of 7.7% developing osteomyelitis, and 84% required further operative intervention.[35] There are four types of osteomyelitis as it pertains to the anatomic location on the bone: medullary, superficial (bone surface), localized (full-thickness cortex extending to medullary canal), and diffuse. The patient is also classified according to immune status: type A – normal immune response; type B – some immune compromise (i.e., smoking); and type C – severe immune compromise (i.e., diabetes).

Treatment of osteomyelitis involves removal of hardware, debridement until viable bone with punctate red bleeding occurs, possible local antibiotic therapy in the form of antibiotic-impregnated beads/spacers, and temporary external fixator placement until the infection is eradicated. Flaps may need to be readvanced, or Gustilo grade I/II fractures may convert to large soft tissue defects after debridement requiring flap coverage. Bone grafting, if needed, can be performed once the soft tissue envelope has healed and infection is under control, typically 6–8 weeks after soft tissue coverage. In some instances, amputation may be required.

Key Points

- A combined orthoplastic approach optimizes care and outcomes for lower extremity patients.
- Evaluation begins with the Advanced Trauma Life Support protocol.
- Identification of injuries to critical structures, like vessels and nerves, is imperative.
- Initial management includes early irrigation and debridement.
- Reconstruction is tailored to the patient's defect, available donor sites, and overall health status, and may include local muscle/fasciocutaneous flaps, bony reconstruction, and/or free flaps.
- The choice between amputation and limb salvage in the severely traumatized lower extremity is balanced between the patient's goals and anticipated functional outcome.

References

1. Anandasivam NS, Russo GS, Swallow MS, et al. Tibial shaft fracture: a large-scale study defining the injured population and associated injuries. *J Clin Orthop Trauma*. 2017;8(3):225–231.
2. Chung KC, Saddawi-Konefka D, Haase SC, et al. A cost-utility analysis of amputation versus salvage for Gustilo type IIIB and IIIC open tibial fractures. *Plast Reconstr Surg*. 2009;124(6):1965–1973.
3. Levins LS. The reconstructive ladder. An orthoplastic approach. *Orthop Clin North Am*. 1993;24(3):393–409.

4. Aldea PA, Shaw WW. The evolution of the surgical management of severe lower extremity trauma. *Clin Plast Surg.* 1986;13(4):549–569.
5. Kirk NT. The development of amputation. *Bull Med Libr Assoc.* 1944;32(2):132–163.
6. Center for Disease Control. Tetanus. [Online] Available at: https://www.cdc.gov/vaccines/pubs/pinkbook/downloads/tetanus.pdf.
7. Bosse MJ, McCarthy ML, Jones AL, et al. The insensate foot following severe lower extremity trauma: an indication for amputation? *J Bone Joint Surg.* 2005;87(12):2601–2608.
8. Miller-Thomas MM, West OC, Cohen AM. Diagnosing traumatic arterial injury in the extremities with CT angiography: pearls and pitfalls. *Radiographics.* 2005;25(suppl 1):S133–S142.
9. Gustilo RB, Mendoza RM, Williams DN. Problems in the management of type III (severe) open fractures: a new classification of type III open fractures. *J Trauma.* 1984;24(8):742–746.
10. Byrd HS, Spicer TE, Cierney G 3rd. Management of open tibial fractures. *Plast Reconstr Surg.* 1985;76(5):719–730.
11. Bosse MJ, Mackenzie EJ, Kellam JF, et al. A prospective evaluation of the clinical utility of the lower-extremity injury-severity scores. *J Bone Joint Surg Am.* 2001;83:3–14.
12. MacKenzie EJ, Rivara FP, Jurkovich GJ, et al. A national evaluation on the effect of trauma-center care on mortality. *N Engl J Med.* 2006;354:366–378.
13. Naique SB, Pearse M, Nanchahal J. Management of severe open tibial fractures: the need for combined orthopaedic and plastic surgical treatment in specialist centres. *J Bone Joint Surg Br.* 2006;88-B:351–357.
14. McQueen MM, Court-Brown CM. Compartment monitoring in tibial fractures: the pressure threshold for decompression. *J Bone Joint Surg Br.* 1996;78(1):99–104.
15. Demiri EC, Hatzokos H, Dionyssiou D, Megalopoulos A, Pitoulias G, Papadimitriou D. Single stage arteriovenous short saphenous loops in microsurgical reconstruction of the lower extremity. *Arch Orthop Trauma Surg.* 2009;129:521–524.
16. Mulholland S, Boyd JB, McCabe S, et al. Recipient vessels in head and neck microsurgery: radiation effect and vessel access. *Plast Reconstr Surg.* 1993;92(4):628–632.
17. Glass GE, Barrett SP, Sanderson F, Pearse MF, Nanchahal J. The microbiological basis for a revised antibiotic regimen in high energy tibial fractures: preventing deep infections by nosocomial organisms. *J Plast Reconstr Aesthet Surg.* 2011;64(3):375–380.
18. Nanchahal J, Nayagam S, Khan U, et al. Standards for the Management of Open Fractures of the Lower Limb. [Online] Available at: http://www.bapras.org.uk/docs/default-source/commissioning-and-policy/standards-for-lower-limb.pdf?sfvrsn=0.
19. Valenziano CP, Chattar-Cora D, O'Neill A, Hubli EH, Cudjoe EA. Efficacy of primary wound cultures in long bone open extremity fractures: are they of any value? *Arch Orthop Trauma Surg.* 2002;122(5):259–261.
20. Gustilo RB, Anderson JT. Prevention of infection in the treatment of one thousand and twenty-five open fractures of long bones. *J Bone Joint Surg Am.* 1976;58(4):453–458.
21. Malhotra AK, Goldberg S, Graham J, et al. Open extremity fractures: impact of delay in operative debridement and irrigation. *J Trauma Acute Care Surg.* 2014;76:1201–1207.
22. Pollak AN, Jones AL, Castillo RC, LEAP Study Group, et al. The relationship between time to surgical debridement and incidence of infection after open high-energy lower extremity trauma. *J Bone Joint Surg Am.* 2010;92(1):7–15.
23. Tejwani N, Polonet D, Wolinsky PR. External fixation of tibial fractures. *J Am Acad Orthoped Surg.* 2015;23(2):126–130.
24. Gopal S, Majumder S, Batchelor AGB, Knight SL, DeBoer P, Smith RM. Fix and flap: the radical orthopaedic and plastic treatment of severe open fractures of the tibia. *J Bone Joint Surg Br.* 200;82(7):959–966.
25. Bhandari M, Guyatt G, Tornetta P, et al. Randomized trial of reamed and unreamed intramedullary nailing of tibial shaft fractures. *J Bone Joint Surg Am.* 2008;90(12):2567–2578.
26. Godina M. Early microsurgical reconstruction of complex trauma of the extremities. *Plast Reconstr Surg.* 1986;78(3):285–292.
27. Sheckter C, Pridgen B, Li A, Curtin C, Momeni A. Regional variation and trends in the timing of lower extremity reconstruction: a 10-year review of the nationwide inpatient sample. *Plast Reconstr Surg.* 2018;142(5):1337–1347.
28. Baumeister SP, Spierer R, Erdmann D, Sweis R, Levin LS, Germann GK. A realistic complication analysis of 70 sural artery flaps in a multimorbid patient group. *Plast Reconstr Surg.* 2003;112(1):129–140; discussion 141–142.
29. Cho EH, Shammas RL, Carney MJ, et al. Muscle versus fasciocutaneous free flaps in lower extremity traumatic reconstruction: a multicenter outcomes analysis. *Plast Reconstr Surg.* 2018;141(1):191–199.
30. Kovach SJ, Levin LS. Skeletal reconstruction. In: Neligan P, ed. *Plastic Surgery: Lower Extremity, Trunk, and Burns.* 3rd edn. Edinburgh: Elsevier Saunders; 2013:174–188.
31. Saddawi–Konefka D, Kim HM, Chung KC. A systematic review of outcomes and complications of reconstruction and amputation for type IIIB and IIIC fractures of the tibia. *Plast Reconstr Surg.* 2008;122(6):1796–1805.
32. Bosse MJ, MacKenzie EJ, Kellam JF, et al. An analysis of outcomes of reconstruction or amputation after leg–threatening injuries. *N Engl J Med.* 2002;347(24):1924–1931.
33. O'Toole RV, Castillo RC, Pollak AN, et al. Surgeons and their patients disagree regarding cosmetic and overall outcomes after surgery for high-energy lower extremity trauma. *J Orthop Trauma.* 2009;23(10):716–723.
34. Mattes SJ, Martin PE, Royer TD. Walking symmetry and energy cost in persons with unilateral transtibial amputations: matching prosthetic and intact limb inertial properties. *Arch Physical Med Rehabil.* 2000;81(5):561–568.
35. Harris AM, Althausen PL, Kellam J, et al. Complications following limb-threatening lower extremity trauma. *J Orthop Trauma.* 2009;23(1):1–6.

44

Lymphedema: Anatomy, Pathophysiology, Evaluation, and Treatment

BABAK J. MEHRARA, MICHELLE CORIDDI, JOSEPH DAYAN, AND RAGHU KATARU

Introduction

Lymphedema is a chronic, debilitating disease resulting from infections, obesity, congenital abnormalities, or traumatic injuries. Congenital abnormalities of the lymphatic system resulting in lymphedema are referred to as primary lymphedema. In contrast, lymphedema resulting from trauma, injury, infections, or other external factors is known as secondary lymphedema. Regardless of the type, patients who have lymphedema experience swelling, pain, recurrent infections, and have impaired quality of life.

In the Western world, the most common cause of lymphedema is cancer treatment and iatrogenic lymphatic injury (i.e., secondary lymphedema). Breast cancer, due to its high incidence, is the most common cause of secondary lymphedema afflicting as many as 50% of patients who undergo axillary lymph node dissection. The advent of sentinel lymph node biopsy has decreased the need for lymph node dissection in many patients, and as a result, has decreased the risk of lymphedema. However, it is important to note that lymphedema can still develop in 5%–7% of patients who undergo sentinel lymph node biopsy.[1] In addition, lymphedema is not a disease that is restricted to breast cancer survivors, developing in nearly 1 in 6 patients who undergo surgical management of gynecological/urological tumors, sarcoma, or melanomas. As a result, lymphedema is prevalent, affecting nearly 6 million Americans. However, this number pales in comparison to worldwide figures, with an estimated 200 million individuals who suffer from lymphedema as a result of chronic parasitic infections. Because the mainstay of current treatment is palliative measures such as compression garments and physical therapy, it is incumbent on the medical community to develop effective medical and surgical treatment options for this disease. This chapter will review the anatomy and physiology of the lymphatic system and outline current advances in the surgical management of lymphedema.

Anatomy of the Lymphatic System

Lymphatic Capillaries and Collectors

The lymphatic system has several functions, including absorption of interstitial fluid and macromolecules, migration of immune cells and regulation of inflammation, initiation of adaptive and innate immune responses, intestinal fat absorption, and cholesterol metabolism among others. Interstitial proteins, immune cells, and particulate matter that are too large to enter the capillary venous system are passively and, in some cases, actively absorbed by initial lymphatics. The initial lymphatics drain into successively larger collecting lymphatics that then actively transport these substances via coordinated pumping of smooth muscle cells that cover the collectors and one-way valves that prevent backflow of lymph (Fig. 44.1). Lymphatic fluid is eventually returned to the blood circulatory system via connections of the thoracic duct to the internal jugular vein.

The capillary lymphatics, located in the dermis, have a single layer of lymphatic endothelia cells connected by overlapping or intercalating button-like junctions. These cells are tethered to the surrounding tissue by anchoring filaments, which pull open the button-like junctions between individual cells and widen the lymphatic vessel lumen as interstitial volume increases. This allows fluid and molecules to enter the lymphatic system. Once in the system, fluid and particulate matter reach the collecting lymphatics. These collecting lymphatics are comprised of continuous or zipper-like endothelial cell junctions that prevent fluid leak, a surrounding basement membrane and smooth muscle cells that coordinately contract to propel fluid forward, and bicuspid valves that ensure one-way flow. Passive forces such as muscle contractions, respiration, regional arterial pulsation, and gravity also assist in moving lymphatic fluid within collecting vessels.

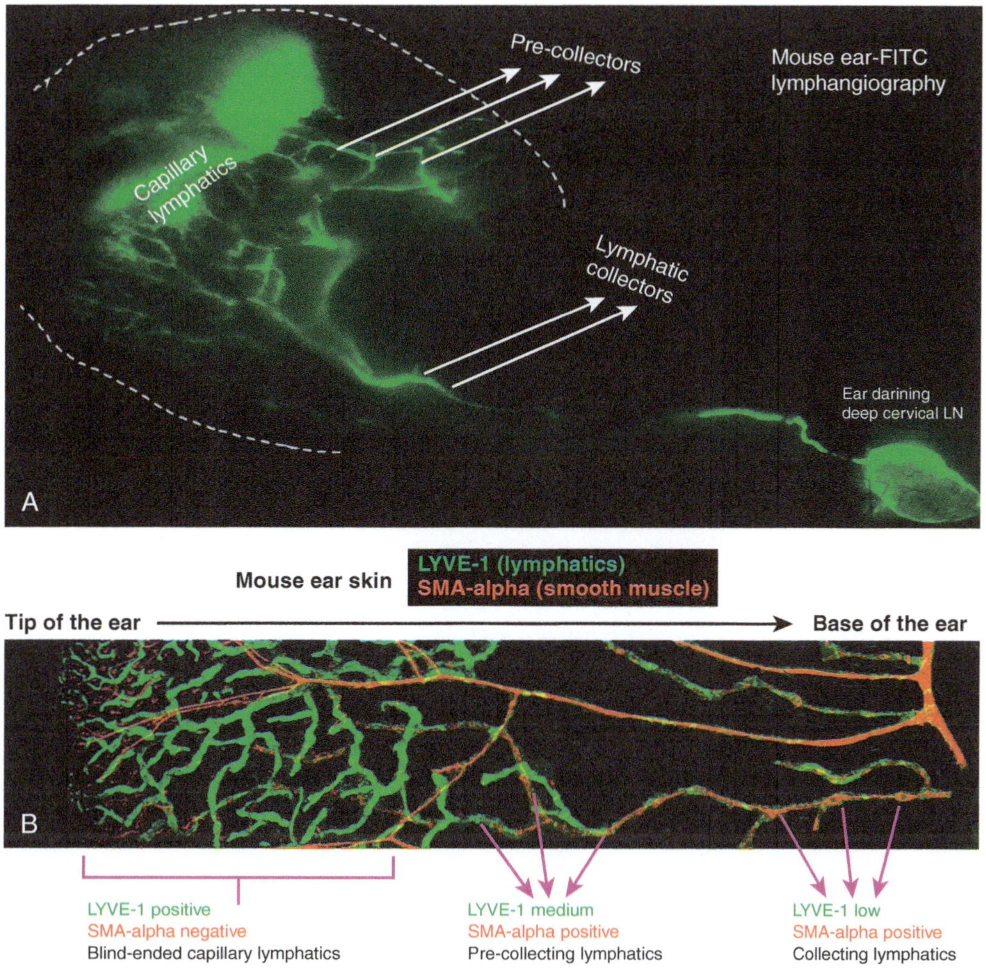

• **Fig. 44.1** Microscopic anatomy of lymphatic drainage system in a mouse ear model. (A) Drainage from capillary lymphatics to pre-collectors to collectors to lymph node on fluorescein isothiocyanate (FITC) lymphangiography. (B) Staining of mouse ear skin with lymphatic vessel endothelial hyaluronan receptor 1 (LYVE-1) and smooth muscle actin, alpha (SMA-alpha) showing a progressively increasing number of smooth muscle cells along the drainage pathway from capillary lymphatics to pre-collecting lymphatics to collecting lymphatics.

The lymphatic system is composed of superficial and deep collecting lymphatic vessels, divided by the deep fascia. The superficial and deep systems have no direct connections between them, although lymphatic vessels do diverge and converge within each system. The lymphatic drainage of the skin can be divided into lymphatic territories called lymphosomes. Anatomical dissections in canine specimens by Suami and colleagues, and more recently indocyanine green lymphography in the clinical setting, have revealed multiple lymphosomes draining the skin. In addition, these studies have shown that collateral lymphatics may develop following injury bypassing the area of lymphatic obstruction. This observation is important and may provide an anatomical rationale for the finding that lymph node dissection does not result in the development of lymphedema in all patients.

In the upper extremity, lymphatic collectors emerging from the fingers and palm run axially in the dorsal hand and divide into radial and ulnar bundles. These collecting lymphatic vessels travel up the forearm, converging towards each other, and gradually changing course at the elbow to the anteromedial aspect of the limb. The primary drainage pathway of the upper extremity drains along the medial aspect of the upper extremity, within the bicipital groove, eventually draining into the axillary region (Fig. 44.2). An alternate pathway in some individuals extends from the dorsal surface of the lateral upper arm and drains into the supraclavicular lymph nodes, bypassing the axillary lymph nodes. This pathway can develop as a collateral drainage route in some patients who undergo axillary lymph node dissection.

In the lower extremity, lymphatics emerging from the toes and soles of the feet travel from the medial and anterior foot, ascending axially along the medial border of the leg (see Fig. 44.2). The vessels in the lower extremity range in size from 0.2 mm to 2.2mm in diameter and travel in the subcutaneous tissues. These lymphatic channels have a tortuous course and drain along the lesser saphenous vein, draining into the popliteal lymph nodes. Other collectors bypass the popliteal region and drain along the medial

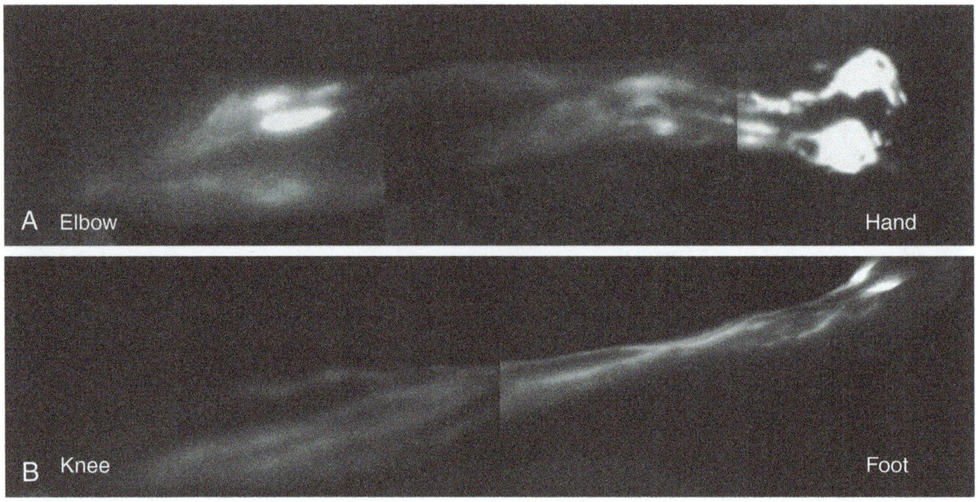

• **Fig. 44.2** (A) ICG anatomy of a healthy upper limb (volar view). Note dual drainage from the hand along radial and ulnar bundles of lymphatic channels and convergence of these pathways at the elbow. (B) ICG anatomy of a healthy lower limb (anteromedial view). Note drainage along the medial border of the leg.

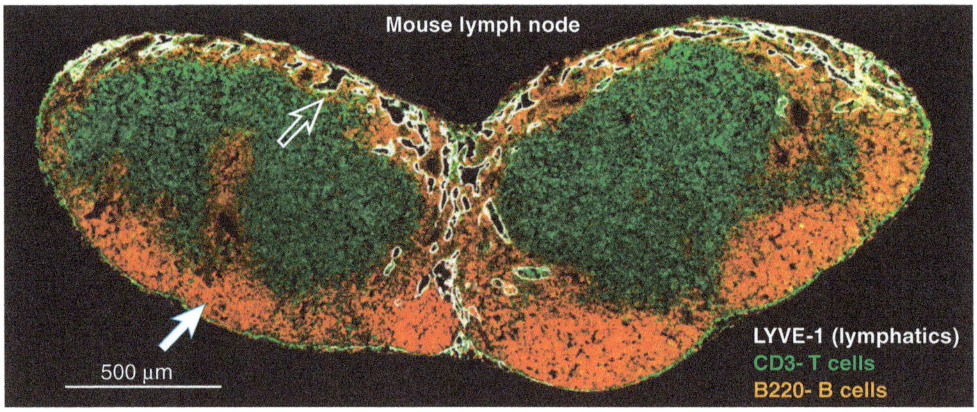

• **Fig. 44.3** Anatomy of a mouse lymph node. Open arrow shows subcapsular sinus. Closed arrow shows medulla of lymph node.

aspect of the thigh along the greater saphenous vein, draining into the inguinal lymph nodes.

Lymph Nodes

Lymphatic fluid is filtered by lymph nodes to allow sampling of bacterial antigens, removal of particulate matter, and transport of antigen-presenting cells to areas where T and B cell activation can occur. Lymph nodes are localized in the abdominal cavity as well as at the junction of the extremities and the head with the trunk. Interstitial fluid in the afferent lymphatics drains into the subcapsular sinus of the lymph node and through lymphatic sinuses surrounding B cell follicles (Fig. 44.3). Lymphatic sinuses are lined by reticular endothelial cells and dendritic cells that are activated by antigens within the lymphatic fluid. Particulate matter and bacteria are phagocytosed by lymph node-resident macrophages that process the antigens and promote activation of immune responses. Immune cells from the systemic circulation enter and leave the lymph node through high endothelial venules that border lymphatic sinuses, thus enabling the exchange of cells, and to a lesser extent, interstitial fluid with the systemic circulation. The lymphatic fluid continues to drain to the medulla (central portion) of the lymph node and exits the node via efferent lymphatics that continue to drain into the remaining lymph node chains and eventually into the thoracic duct to empty into the venous system.

Etiology of Lymphedema

Primary Lymphedema

Recent advances in DNA sequencing have identified a variety of genetic abnormalities that are associated with the development of primary lymphedema. These abnormalities involve a broad spectrum of pathologic changes, including abnormal lymphangiogenic growth factor signaling, lymphatic valve defects, leaky tight junctions, smooth muscle cells coverage, and alterations in lymphatic contractility.

The most common cause of primary lymphedema is an insufficient number of collecting lymphatics. These genetic defects may be familial or may develop spontaneously as a result of germline or somatic mutations.

In most cases of primary lymphedema, the genetic defects that underly the development of the disease remain unknown. Nevertheless, it is generally thought that lymphatic abnormalities in these cases are present at birth and gradually worsen with time.

The presentation of familial forms of lymphedema is highly variable both in terms of timing and severity of symptoms. These differences may be related, at least in part, to the penetrance of the genetic abnormalities. Other causes of differences in severity or timing of lymphedema presentation include interaction with environmental factors (e.g., obesity) or hormonal fluctuations. As a result, some cases of primary lymphedema referred to as *congenital lymphedema*, present early in life or shortly after birth. More commonly, primary lymphedema becomes manifest later in life, a condition termed *lymphedema praecox* or *lymphedema tarda.*

Congenital lymphedemas account for 10%–25% of all cases of primary lymphedema and occur most commonly in the lower extremity of females. The severity of this disease is highly variable, ranging from mild to severe swelling. In addition, congenital lymphedema may occur unilaterally or differentially between limbs. Milroy's disease is a classic form of congenital lymphedema and accounts for 2%–3% of all patients with this form of lymphedema. Patients with this familial, sex-linked disease have heterozygous inactivating mutations of vascular endothelial growth factor 3 (VEGFR3) and usually, present shortly after birth, with limb swelling and/or chylothorax. Abnormalities in VEGFR3 signaling are important because activation of this receptor by its ligands, vascular endothelial growth factor C (VEGF-C) and the closely related VEGF-D, is necessary for lymphatic endothelial cell development, proliferation, differentiation, and migration. As a result, patients with Milroy's disease have hypoplastic lymphatic vessels. Interestingly, however, the severity of lymphatic vessel abnormalities can vary between the upper and lower extremities (lower extremities are more severely affected) and abnormalities are often absent in intestinal lymphatics.

Patients diagnosed with *lymphedema praecox* present with lymphedema before the age of 35. Most patients diagnosed with lymphedema praecox are female (ratio of 4:1 with males) and develop unilateral lower extremity lymphedema at or around the time of puberty, suggesting that sex hormones may contribute to the development of this disease. Although pathological changes in the lymphatic system in patients with lymphedema praecox are highly variable, most patients display decreased numbers of initial lymphatics and hypoplastic collecting vessels.

Patients who develop primary lymphedema after the age of 35 have *lymphedema tarda* (Fig. 44.4). This is a diagnosis of exclusion and other causes of lymphedema or diseases that may cause swelling must be ruled out. This presentation of primary lymphedema is also infrequent and, like other forms of primary lymphedema, occurs most commonly in the lower extremity of women. Recent genetic studies have suggested that some patients with lymphedema tarda have mutations in *FOXC2*, a gene that regulates lymphatic valve development and function.

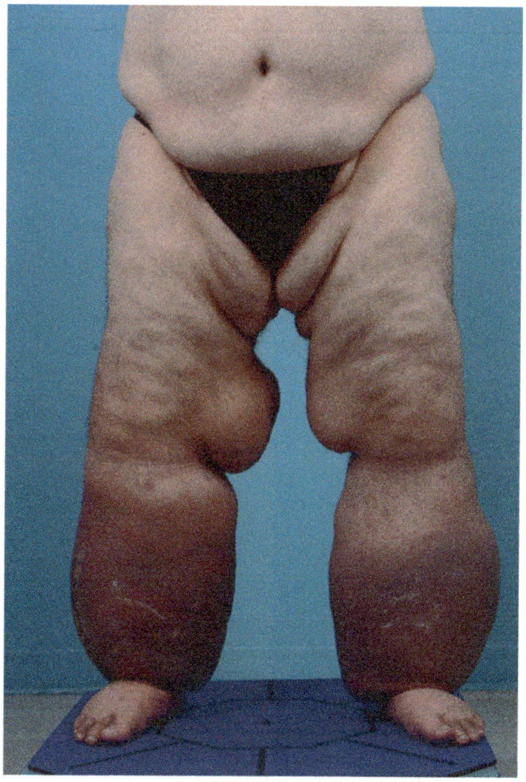

• **Fig. 44.4** Example of a patient with severe congenital lymphedema tarda.

An arbitrary classification of primary lymphedema based on the age at which symptoms present is an oversimplification and most likely not helpful when evaluating individual patients. These schemes do not, for example, provide any basic knowledge of the pathophysiology of the disease and, as a result, do not help in devising logical treatment options. More recent studies have developed classification schemes that combine presentation of the disease and genetic mutations. This approach categorizes congenital lymphedemas into five main groups: syndromic, systemic or visceral, disturbed growth, congenital onset, and late onset. This classification is more precise and may be more useful than the timing of presentation alone in developing diagnostic or therapeutic interventions.

Secondary Lymphedema

Secondary lymphedema results from obstruction or injury to the lymphatic system. Worldwide, the most common cause of lymphedema is infection by roundworms (*Wuchereria bancrofti*, *Brugia malayi*, and *Brugia timori*). The roundworms, commonly transmitted by mosquitos, grow in the tissues and release larvae that occlude lymphatic channels. This occlusion, and the resultant severe inflammatory response, cause progressive and often devastating limb swelling. Treatment for filariasis is symptomatic and primarily limited to antiparasitic medications that kill the developing larvae rather than the adult worm residing in the tissues. Patients with severe filariasis-induced lymphedema often require disfiguring reductive surgery.

In the developed world, the most common cause of secondary lymphedema is iatrogenic injury to the lymphatic system in the course of cancer treatment. Lymphedema can occur from the treatment of all solid tumors, including breast, gynecological tumors, melanoma, sarcoma, pelvic tumors, and even head and neck tumors. Although the rates of and severity of the disease vary depending on the extent of the surgery and adjuvant therapies (e.g., radiation), most patients who undergo lymph node dissection or even wide skin excision are at risk for developing lymphedema.

The development of lymphedema after surgery is usually delayed and occurs 3–12 months postoperatively. Thus, while most patients have transient postoperative swelling immediately after surgery, these changes typically resolve only to recur in a progressive manner in a subset of patients who go on to develop lymphedema. Lymphedema tends to develop more rapidly in the lower extremities as compared with the upper extremities. Thus, patients who undergo pelvic surgery and develop lymphedema typically do so within a few months of surgery. In contrast, patients treated for breast cancer usually develop lymphedema 8–10 months following surgery. Nearly 75% of patients who develop lymphedema after axillary lymph node dissection for breast cancer do so within the first 3 years following surgery. However, lymphedema develop even 30 years after the initial surgical insult has been reported.

Progression of lymphedema, once it develops, is highly variable with some patients displaying slowly progressive disease, even without compression, while others exhibit a more fulminant form of the disease with rapidly progressive symptoms despite aggressive therapy. Nevertheless, early diagnosis and aggressive physical therapy/compression is helpful in most patients and should be instituted as soon as possible as early intervention has been shown to improve long-term outcomes. Other nonsurgical interventions, for example, exercise or weight loss programs, can also be helpful in preventing the development of disease or decreasing the rate of progression once it has developed. The concept that exercise or weight lifting can increase "lymphatic load" has been disproven by several level 1 randomized prospective control studies demonstrating the efficacy of these interventions for the treatment of lymphedema. Thus, patients who are at risk for developing lymphedema, as well as those who have developed lymphedema, should be encouraged to maintain a healthy weight and participate in aerobic and resistance exercise.

Risk Factors for Lymphedema

There are many known risk factors for the development of lymphedema, including obesity, radiation, infection, advanced age, and genetic factors. *Obesity* has long been recognized as an important risk factor for the development of lymphedema following cancer surgery. For example, Helyer et al found that patients with a body mass index (BMI) of greater than 30 had a more than threefold increase in the risk of developing lymphedema following breast cancer treatment as compared with patients with a BMI less than 25.[2] McLaughlin et al examined breast cancer patients treated with either sentinel lymph node biopsy or axillary lymph node dissection and found those with a higher baseline BMI had a significantly higher incidence of lymphedema.[1] Interestingly, these authors found that even postoperative weight gain (independent of the presurgical weight) significantly increased the risk of lymphedema development. Importantly, a randomized, controlled, prospective trial showed that patients who had nutritional counseling and lost weight over a 12-week period of time had significant reductions in their upper extremity limb volumes as compared to a control group that did not receive nutritional counseling and did not lose weight.[3] Other studies have shown that exercise programs improve lymphedema symptoms at least in part by promoting weight loss. These findings are supported by prospective longitudinal studies demonstrating that the incidence of lymphedema is increased nearly twofold in patients with a sedentary lifestyle.

Several lines of evidence support the idea that obesity may increase the risk of lymphedema by decreasing lymphatic function. For example, macromolecule transport in obese patients is significantly decreased as compared with healthy volunteers.[4] Other studies have shown that obese patients (BMI >59) spontaneously develop lower extremity lymphedema even without surgery or other injuries.[5] Preclinical studies have shown that increasing obesity is linearly correlated with impaired lymphatic pumping capacity, lymphatic vessel number, and lymphatic vessel leakiness.[6] These changes are partially reversible with exercise or weight loss. Taken together, these findings suggest that weight loss and exercise programs may be beneficial in patients who are considered for lymphatic surgery since these behavioral modifications improve lymphatic function and regeneration.

Radiation therapy, mainly when used as adjuvant therapy in conjunction with surgical extirpation, is also a significant risk factor for the development of lymphedema increasing the relative risk of disease two- to fivefold. Radiation in isolation rarely (<7%) results in lymphedema development.[7] However, radiation and obesity appear to increase the risk of lymphedema in an additive manner since the risk of disease development is significantly higher in obese patients treated with adjuvant radiotherapy. Some researchers have questioned the link between radiation and development of breast cancer-related lymphedema, having failed to show a significant increase in risk in some studies. However, it is likely that these studies are confounded by the fields used for radiation and heterogeneous populations of patients that had radiation treatment to the chest wall rather than regional lymph node basins.

Postoperative infections and cellulitis have also been linked to the development of lymphedema following lymph node dissection for a variety of cancers. This clinical finding is supported by recent studies demonstrating that bacterial toxins and inflammatory responses can permanently injure lymphatic endothelial cells and lymphatic smooth muscle cells. Other studies have shown that lymphatic injury can result in impaired innate and adaptive immune responses, thereby increasing the risk of infections.[8] Thus, patients with lymphatic injury are at high risk for developing infections and when these infections develop, they may cause additional injury to the lymphatic system, thereby setting up a vicious cycle that leads to rapid progression of the disease.

Advanced age also infers increased risk of developing lymphedema in some series. One study of 287 Australian breast cancer survivors showed that women who were more than 50 years old were 3.1 times more likely to develop lymphedema following axillary lymph node dissection as compared with those who were less than 50 years old at the time of surgery.[9] However, the importance of age as a predictive factor for lymphedema development is debated, as other studies have failed to show a significant correlation. Nevertheless, recent preclinical studies have shown that aging decreases lymphatic pumping capacity, lymphatic permeability, and lymphatic endothelial cell proliferation potential with resultant decreased lymphatic function. It is therefore conceivable that these physiological changes may infer a higher risk of developing lymphedema after surgery.

Recent studies have identified *genetic mutations* and alternative coding regions that increase the risk of secondary lymphedema development. For example, Finegold et al showed that mutations in the connexin 47 or hepatocyte growth factor genes significantly increased the risk of breast cancer-related lymphedema.[10] Other studies have shown that normal variants of four genes, so-called single-nucleotide polymorphisms (SNPs), confer a significant risk for the development of secondary lymphedema following axillary lymph node dissection for breast cancer treatment. A recent meta-analysis reviewed reports of the association of secondary lymphedema and genetic variations in coding sequences of 18 genes, including *HGF*, *MET*, *GJC2*, *IL1A*, *IL4*, *IL6*, *IL10*, *IL13*, *VEGF-C*, *NFKB2*, *LCP-2*, *NRP-2*, *SYK*, *VCAM1*, *FOXC2*, *VEGFR2*, *VEGFR3*, and *RORC*.[11] Taken together, these studies demonstrate that lymphedema is a complex disease and that the risk of this disease can be modified by intrinsic and extrinsic risk factors. It is also clear that these independent variables interact with each other, further modulating the risk of disease development.

Pathophysiology of Secondary Lymphedema

Recent studies have helped elucidate the pathophysiology of secondary lymphedema and provided some answers to vexing questions about this disease. To understand these discoveries, it is essential to have a historical perspective of clinical and experimental studies aiming to understand this disease.

For many years, it was assumed that the pathophysiology of secondary lymphedema is related to lymphatic injury and the failure of lymphatics to regenerate or form collateral pathways that bypass the zone of injury. This failure of regeneration resulted in a mismatch between lymphatic transport capacity and interstitial fluid production, leading to the development of lymphedema. Indeed, this hypothesis was supported by laboratory studies demonstrating that delivery of lymphangiogenic growth factors such as VEGF-C improved lymphatic regeneration and resulted in resolution of lymphedema in animal models. The discovery of associations between coding variants or mutations in genes regulating lymphatic vessel development or differentiation in a small subset of patients who developed secondary lymphedema also supported this hypothesis.[11] However, more recent studies demonstrated that the delivery of lymphangiogenic growth factors does not improve lymphedema, and in some circumstances, the expression of these factors (including VEGF-C) is paradoxically *increased* in lymphedematous tissues harvested from clinical biopsy specimens.[12] More importantly, the lymphatic injury hypothesis failed to provide a rationale for the clinical characteristics of the disease. For example, lymphatic injury alone does not explain why lymphedema develops in a delayed manner, usually months and sometimes years after the initial surgical insult. If lymphatic damage is the cause of lymphedema, then why do some patients develop the disease while others do not? Why do some patients with seemingly minor lymphatic injury (e.g., sentinel lymph node biopsy) develop lymphedema? Why is lymphedema progressive, and why is the rate of progression so highly variable? These characteristics of secondary lymphedema suggested that lymphatic injury is an initiating event and that in some patients additional pathways are activated, leading to disease development and progression.

Lymphedema is a progressive disease of the entire lymphatic vascular tree rather than an isolated injury at the site of lymph node dissection. This concept is supported by progressive changes noted in indocyanine green (ICG) lymphography demonstrating incremental increases in lymphatic vascular leakiness (as evidenced by dermal backflow), loss of collecting lymphatics, and formation of aberrant lymphatic channels to bypass lymphatic obstruction at multiple levels of the limb. The end-stage of the disease is characterized by loss of all functional lymphatics and pooling of lymphatic-specific dyes in the skin. These changes have led to the development of ICG lymphedema classification systems (see below).

Histologically, lymphedema is characterized by progressive accumulation of fibroadipose tissues in the skin. This fibrotic process also involves the lymphatic vessels encasing the initial and collecting vessels in thick collagen bundles. As lymphedema progresses, collecting lymphatics become progressively sclerosed with the proliferation of lymphatic smooth muscle cells and obliteration of the vessel lumen and resultant lymphatic dysfunction. Although the mechanisms that regulate the proliferation of smooth muscle cells remain unknown, it is hypothesized that increased afterload resulting from the initial surgical insult (and tissue fibrosis) may, in a fashion like hypertensive cardiomyopathy, lead to a compensatory increase in the number of smooth muscle cells. Progressive fibrosis and lymphatic vessel obliteration provide a rationale for the finding that lymphedema develops in a delayed fashion after surgery since these changes take time to happen. In this manner, lymphedema may simply be fibrotic organ failure of the lymphatic system. This hypothesis is supported by the fact that fibrosis is a common end-pathway for organ failure in all other organ systems. In these diseases, similar to lymphedema, the progression of the disease is often highly variable and influenced by genetic or environmental factors. For example, obesity, recurrent infections, and radiation (i.e., important risk factors for lymphedema) are also essential regulators of fibrosis in a variety of other fibroproliferative disorders. Thus, it is possible that surgical injury to the lymphatic system in some patients initiates progressive changes in the tissues/lymphatics of the limb that then lead to the development of lymphedema in some individuals if a critical threshold of decreased lymphatic function is reached. Patients with risk factors for fibrosis such as obesity, infections, radiation, genetic abnormalities, advanced age, etc. are more likely to reach this threshold because these risk factors independently increase the risk of fibrosis.

Fibrosis in lymphedema is regulated by chronic inflammatory responses that involve T-helper cells. These cells produce profibrotic growth factors such as interleukin 4 (IL4), IL13, and transforming growth factor beta-1 (TGF-β1) that promote collagen deposition, decrease matrix breakdown, and regulate fibroblast differentiation.[8] These T cell inflammatory reactions also regulate lymphatic pumping, leakiness, and formation of collateral pathways suggesting that T cells play a key role in the pathophysiology of lymphedema.

The discovery that inflammation is a crucial regulator of lymphedema development led to studies aiming to determine the efficacy of antiinflammatory drugs in lymphedema treatment. An early preclinical study in this area showed that ketoprofen, a nonsteroidal antiinflammatory drug, was effective in decreasing the severity of lymphedema in mouse models.[13] This finding led to a clinical trial of ketoprofen with 55 patients.[14] Interestingly, although the authors failed to show significant improvements in limb volumes (the primary endpoint of the study), they did note significant improvements in skin fibrosis and thickness.[14] Subsequent studies have shown that the beneficial effects of ketoprofen are primarily related to activation of leukotriene B4 and have led to the initiation of new clinical trials using more targeted approaches.

Other studies have more directly targeted T cells for the treatment of lymphedema. For example, a recent study by our lab showed that topical application of tacrolimus, a drug that decreases T cell proliferation and differentiation, could prevent the development of lymphedema in a mouse model of the disease.[15] This treatment was also highly effective in this mouse model for treating established lymphedema. These findings suggest that inflammatory pathways activated by lymphatic injury play a key role in the development of lymphedema. More importantly, these studies continue to identify novel means of treating lymphedema. These treatments may be even more effective when combined with surgery to prevent the development of lymphedema or treat it once it has developed. This is an exciting new area in lymphedema research.

Lymphedema Diagnosis

Lymphedema is diagnosed by history, physical exam, and objective measures. Symptoms of lymphedema include gross or perceived swelling of the limb, pain, decreased range of motion, subjective sensation of heaviness, and tightness. These symptoms can significantly impair quality of life and limit the ability of affected individuals to participate in activities of daily living. Some patients also have a history of recurrent infections that often require intravenous antibiotic treatment. A history of trauma, surgery, or radiation as well as family history, should also be elicited. The history should also include a detailed analysis of the onset and course of lymphedema and the treatments that the patient has had for the condition, including physical therapy, compression, and manual lymphatic massage.

Physical Examination

Physical exam findings in patients with lymphedema are variable and can range from a healthy limb to an enlarged limb with pitting edema, to an enlarged limb with thickened, fibrotic, and nonpitting skin. Swelling can be diffuse or focused in some regions of the limb. The dorsal aspect of the arm just distal to the elbow and the lateral/dorsal aspect of the upper arm are frequently involved (Fig. 44.5). Less common, though more problematic, is hand or finger swelling. The differential diagnosis of lymphedema includes infection, venous insufficiency, recurrent malignancy with resultant venous or lymphatic obstruction, and, less frequently, heart failure.

Quantification of Swelling and Diagnosis of Lymphedema

Swelling is an important clinical feature of lymphedema and, as a result, a variety of techniques to quantify limb swelling have been reported. These efforts can be broadly categorized as techniques that estimate limb volume or those that measure limb circumference at defined intervals. Water displacement is a highly accurate method that has been used for millennia to calculate volumes. However, this approach is rarely used clinically due to practical considerations such as sterility and space requirements. The perometer is an automated machine that scans the limb using light-emitting diodes and photosensors. These measurements are then used

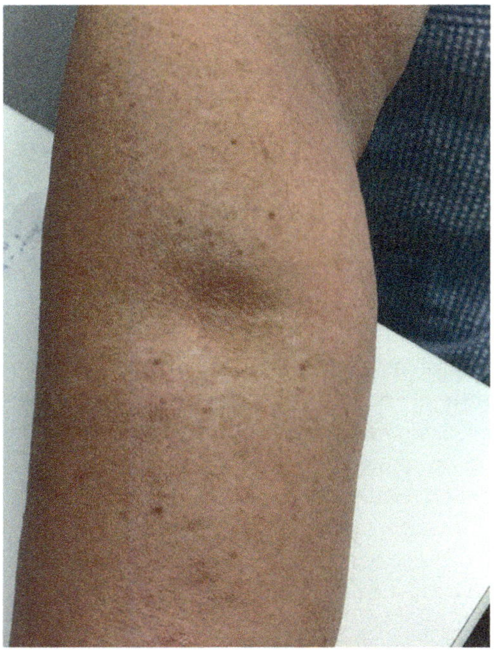

• **Fig. 44.5** Pitting edema of the dorsum of the arm just distal to the elbow in a patient with breast cancer-related lymphedema.

in a truncated cone formula to calculate limb volumes. The perometer is simple to use and can reproducibly estimate limb volumes. However, the use of the perometer for longitudinal measurements requires some training since even minor changes in the areas where the measurements are performed can produce significant changes in limb volumes. Manual circumference measurements of the limb at defined intervals (e.g., 5 cm above and below the olecranon) have been used in many studies. However, there is methodologic heterogeneity in the literature in the areas that are measured, and although this technique is simple to perform, the validity of this method for quantification of the swelling has been questioned due to high inter- and intraoperator variability. In addition, even minor errors in measurement can have significant effects when longitudinal studies are performed since most authors report changes in limb circumference as compared with the normal contralateral limb rather than absolute changes in circumference measurements. Brorson described a simple method to improve the validity of circumferential measurements and estimating upper and lower extremity limb volumes by measuring limb circumference at 4-cm intervals and using these values in the truncated cone formula.[16] This technique is highly accurate with low inter- and intra-user variability and enables comparison of absolute volume changes from baseline measurements.

Limb swelling can be used to diagnose lymphedema if other causes of this symptom are excluded. Most studies consider an absolute difference of more than 2 cm in circumference measurements between the affected and normal limb (or as compared from preoperative measures) as consistent with lymphedema. Differences greater than 5 cm are considered by most groups to represent severe lymphedema. However, this is somewhat arbitrary and potentially misleading since baseline differences in limb circumference exist and because absolute differences in patients with different body habitus may be less meaningful. Thus, a 2-cm difference in a thin patient may be consistent with severe swelling, whereas this difference may be barely noticeable in an overweight individual. Volume differences of greater than 200 mL or 10% increase as compared to the contralateral limb or preoperative measures are also consistent with the diagnosis of lymphedema. In some series, even a 5% increase or a volume increase of 100 mL has been used to diagnose lymphedema. However, this can be tricky if the comparison is made between limbs rather than compared with preoperative values since this small change may simply be related to baseline differences in limb volumes.

Bioimpedance and Estimation of Fluid Content

Bioimpedance is a test that can be used to estimate the fluid content of the lymphedematous and contralateral healthy limb by measuring the rate of electrical current transmission through tissues. This approach is based on the fact that electrical currents transmit more quickly through fluid as compared with fat or muscle. The ImpeiMed L-Dex machine has been used in several studies and calculates a proprietary measure termed the lymphedema index (L-Dex), ranging from −10 to +10 in healthy individuals. An L-Dex score higher than +10 or a change of 10 points from baseline is diagnostic of lymphedema. Other studies have suggested that a cut of +7.1 is diagnostic of lymphedema.[17] This technique has excellent sensitivity and specificity (80% and 90%, respectively) for the diagnosis of breast cancer-related lymphedema and has been used as a method for early diagnosis of the disease.

Imaging

Lymphoscintigraphy

Lymphoscintigraphy is a nuclear medicine test in which radiolabeled technetium sulfur colloid is injected into the dermis of the distal extremity, and the radioactive uptake is analyzed in the draining lymph node basins. Although some investigators have attempted to quantify lymphatic function by calculating the rate of radiotracer clearance from the injection site (a measure termed the lymphatic transport index), most radiologists report changes in lymphoscintigraphy using qualitative language to report the presence or absence of dermal backflow and evaluate lymph node uptake after a defined period of time (e.g., 3 hours). As a result, lymphoscintigraphy findings can be variable, and some authors have reported low sensitivity and specificity for this test, particularly when performed in patients with early-stage disease.[18] Other authors have reported high sensitivity and specificity for this test for the diagnosis of lymphedema.[19]

Magnetic Resonance Imaging/Angiography

Magnetic resonance angiography (MRA) has also been used to visualize lymphatic vessels, and the pathological changes that occur with lymphedema. This imaging modality is particularly useful as it can examine both superficial and deep lymphatics, as well as the venous and arterial systems. Therefore, contributing factors such as venous obstruction and malignancy can be detected. Additionally, with the progression of lymphedema, the proportion of fluid and adipose tissue in the affected extremity can be estimated using MRA.[18] This analysis may help differentiate between early and later stage disease. Unfortunately, however, the technique requires optimization and close collaboration with radiologists.

Indocyanine Green Lymphography

Indocyanine green (ICG) lymphography is a safe and minimally invasive test that can be used to evaluate lymphatic vessel anatomy and function in patients with limb swelling. ICG is a large molecule that when injected into the dermis is picked up selectively by the lymphatics because its molecular size excludes absorption by the venous capillary system. It is important to note that the use of ICG is FDA approved only for intravenous injection. Therefore, intradermal injection is an off-label use. However, this test has been used extensively in the lymphatic literature over the past decade with no reported adverse effects. Stimulation of ICG in the tissues with laser light following intradermal injection causes near infrared light emission that can be visualized using specialized cameras. This technique can visualize lymphatic collectors and pre-collectors 5–10 mm below the skin. Using this approach, lymphatic pumping and leakage (as evidenced by dermal backflow of dye) can be visualized leading some authors to conclude that ICG lymphography is more sensitive than lymphoscintigraphy in patients with early stage lymphedema.[20]

Lymphedema Classification

International Society of Lymphology (ISL) Staging

The most widely used lymphedema classification is the International Society of Lymphology (ISL) staging system (Table 44.1). Stage 0 lymphedema in the ISL staging scheme is also known as latent lymphedema and is used to refer to patients who have had lymphatic injury (e.g., lymph node dissection) but have no swelling or clinical manifestations of lymphedema. Stage 1 lymphedema, also known as spontaneously reversible lymphedema, is diagnosed in patients who meet volume requirements for the diagnosis of lymphedema and in whom pitting edema and swelling is completely resolved with elevation and compression garment use. Patients with stage 2 lymphedema (termed spontaneously irreversible lymphedema) have persistent swelling, pitting edema, and tissue fibrosis that does not resolve with compression. Stage 3 lymphedema (also known as lymphostatic elephantiasis) is characterized by extensive fibrosis, adipose deposition, skin thickening, and severe irreversible swelling of the limb.

NECST Classification System

ISL staging of lymphedema relies almost entirely on physical examination and is less useful for surgical classification of patients with lymphedema. These deficiencies have led some researchers to develop other classification schemes that may be more reflective of the physiology of the disease. For example, Koshima and colleagues have used intraoperative photography and histological analysis of samples obtained at the time of lymphovenous bypass procedures to develop a 4 stage classification system that represents progression of pathological changes in the lymphatic vasculature.[21] This scheme is referred to as the NECST system (an acronym for Normal, Ectasis, Contraction, Sclerosis Type). In the initial stage of the disease, encountered in patients with early-stage lymphedema or minimal swelling, the lymphatic collectors appear normal with a thin layer of surrounding smooth muscle cells. Patients with ectatic lymphatics had dilated lymphatic vessels with flattened lymphatic endothelial cells. In contrast, patients with more severe lymphedema display a contraction pattern with loss of intraluminal diameter and thickening of the smooth muscle cell coverage. Patients with end-stage disease displayed the sclerosis type in which the entire lumen of the collecting lymphatic is obliterated with proliferative smooth muscle cells. This staging system is interesting and pathologically sound; however, it is invasive (requiring a biopsy of a lymphatic collector) and therefore is not useful for preoperative staging or longitudinal analysis. In addition, it is likely that at any given time in the same patient, there will be varying stages of pathological changes in the lymphatic vasculature since these changes do not occur simultaneously throughout the entire limb.

Koshima ICG Classification System

Other investigators have proposed staging systems based on physiological changes noted on ICG lymphography. In a follow-up paper to their NECST staging system, Koshima and colleagues evaluated ICG patterns that purportedly correlated with the histological changes in the NECST staging system.[18] They proposed an ICG classification system that had four stages: linear, splash, stardust, and diffuse (Fig. 44.6). This classification system was primarily used for the lower extremity but could be used for the upper extremity as well. *Linear* patterns display the normal anatomy of the lymphatic collectors with longitudinal arrangement of the lymphatic collectors and no dermal backflow. The *splash* pattern is characterized by primarily a linear pattern of drainage but with isolated areas of dermal backflow resulting from leaky lymphatics. Often, these changes are also accompanied by the formation of abnormal appearing, hyperplastic lymphatic vessels. The *stardust* pattern has more diffuse areas of dermal backflow even though linear lymphatics can still be seen in some regions of the limb. Finally, the *diffuse*

TABLE 44.1 **Classification Systems Commonly Used for Lymphedema Including the International Society of Lymphology (ISL) Classification, the NECST Classification, the Koshima ICG Classification, and the MD Anderson ICG Classification**

Stage	ISL	NECST	Koshima	MD Anderson
0	Latent phase with no clinically evident swelling	Normal and fully functional lymphatic vessels	Normal superficial lymphatic vessels appear as a "linear" pattern with no dermal backflow	n/a
1	Swelling that is reversible with elevation and compression	Ectatic and dilated lymphatic vessels with flattened endothelial cells	Lymphatic vessels appear dilated and torturous with areas of ICG accumulation as a "splash" pattern	Normal appearing, patent lymphatics with minimal to no dermal backflow
2	Swelling that is not reversible with elevation or compression	Contracted lymphatic vessels with loss of intraluminal diameter and thickening of the smooth muscle cell coverage	Lymphatic vessels are disrupted causing increased areas of ICG accumulation as "stardust" pattern	Moderate number of normal lymphatics with segmental dermal back
3	Lymphostatic elephantiasis	Sclerotic lymphatic vessels with obliteration of the lumen and proliferation of smooth muscle cells	No lymphatic vessels can be seen and there is ICG accumulation as a "diffuse" pattern	Few normal lymphatics with dermal backflow throughout the limb
4	n/a	n/a	n/a	Normal lymphatics absent with diffuse dermal backflow throughout the entire limb

ICG, Indocyanine green; n/a, not applicable; NECST, Normal, Ectasis, Contraction, Sclerosis Type.

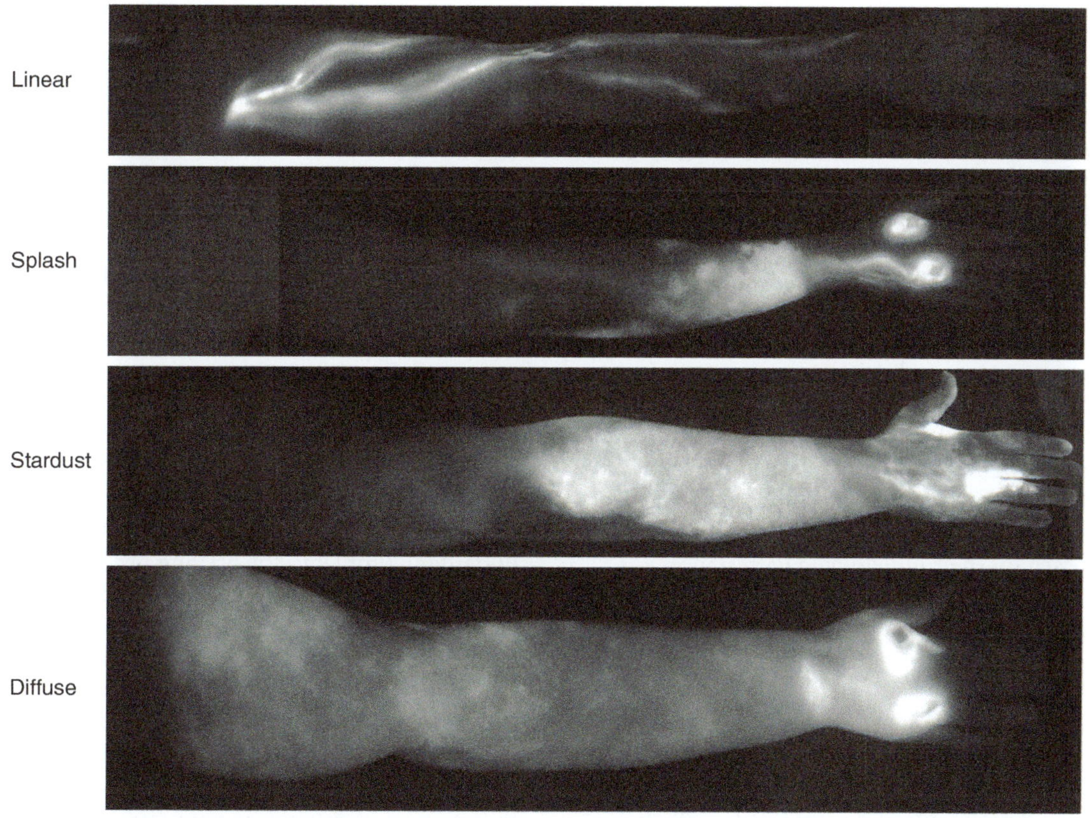

• **Fig. 44.6** Koshima ICG lymphedema classification system. Stage 1 (top): normal superficial lymphatic vessels appear as a "linear" pattern with no dermal backflow. Stage 2 (second from top): lymphatic vessels appear dilated and torturous with areas of ICG accumulation as a "splash" pattern. Stage 3 (second from bottom): lymphatic vessels are disrupted causing increased areas of ICG accumulation as "stardust" pattern. Stage 4 (bottom): no lymphatic vessels can be seen and there is ICG accumulation as a "diffuse" pattern.

pattern is characterized by dermal backflow involving the entire limb and no evidence of functional lymphatic vessels. This classification scheme is helpful, although it remains quite subjective, and differentiation between splash and stardust is often difficult. Nevertheless, in our opinion, this approach is helpful for preoperative evaluation of patients seeking surgical intervention for lymphedema.

MD Anderson ICG Classification System

The MD Anderson classification scheme is similar to the Koshima classification and has four stages based on ICG findings and analysis of dermal backflow.[22] This classification scheme was developed for patients with upper extremity lymphedema resulting from breast cancer treatment and used for patient selection for lymphovenous bypass. Patients classified as stage I disease have normal appearing, patent lymphatic vessels with minimal to no dermal backflow. Patients who have progressed to stage 2 have a moderate number of normal lymphatic vessels with segmental dermal backflow. Stage 3 patients have very few patent lymphatics and dermal backflow throughout the entire limb. Stage 4 disease is characterized by no patent lymphatics and diffuse dermal backflow throughout the entire arm. This classification scheme, like the Koshima ICG classification system, is subjective rather than quantitative. Nevertheless, the authors reported improved outcomes in patients who had early-stage disease as compared with stage 3 or stage 4 disease following lymphovenous bypass.

Lymphedema Treatment

Lymphedema can be treated either medically, surgically, or using a combination of both methods. Medical treatments consist primarily of behavioral modification (e.g., weight loss, exercise), physical therapy, and compression garments. However, recent studies have proposed additional options such as laser treatment, stem cells, growth factor therapy, and antiinflammatory medications. Surgical treatments can be broadly categorized as reductive procedures aiming to remove excess fibroadipose tissue deposited by the disease process or physiological procedures that attempt to reconstruct the damaged lymphatic system. The complex pathophysiology of the disease requires a deep understanding of all options available for treatment and tailoring of the approach for a patient based on their individual circumstances.

Medical Treatments

Weight Loss and Exercise

Obesity or postoperative weight gain significantly increase the risk of developing lymphedema, and numerous randomized clinical trials have shown that weight loss can significantly decrease the severity of secondary lymphedema.[3] For example, one study found that patients with breast cancer-related lymphedema who participated in a medically directed diet plan for 12 weeks not only lost weight but also had significant decreases in their arm volumes as compared with women who were given nutritional advice only.[3] Other studies have shown that aerobic and resistance training exercises result in changes in overall body composition and decrease the severity of lymphedema. This concept is supported by experimental studies demonstrating that even mild aerobic exercise that does not produce weight loss does increase lymphatic function by improving collecting lymphatic vessel pumping and decreasing lymphatic vessel leakiness. Thus, it is reasonable to hypothesize that the combination of weight loss and exercise may be even more effective, and that nutritional counseling is an important aspect of lymphedema therapy.

Decongestive Therapy, Compression, Intermittent Pneumatic Pumps

The mainstay of therapy for patients with lymphedema is complete decongestive therapy (CDT), an intensive combination of manual lymphatic massage (MLD), bandaging, light exercises, skin care, and compression garments aiming to decrease fluid accumulation in the lymphedematous tissues. MLD is a soft-tissue massage that gently stretches the skin and the initial lymphatics using light strokes moving lymphatic fluid in a directional manner away from the zone of injury towards alternate drainage pathways. Although MLD alone is not sufficient for the treatment of lymphedema, there is some evidence that MLD in combination with compression garments is more effective than compression alone in decreasing the symptoms of lymphedema. MLD is commonly used in conjunction with short-stretch bandages during the intensive phase of CDT. These bandages have a more rigid structure for skeletal muscles to press against, thereby increasing lymphatic pumping through the exogenous pump mechanism, and are less likely to impinge on skin folds when compared with more widely available long-stretch bandages. Short-stretch bandages are also used in combination with foam or other padding material to form a multilayer compression garment. This combination is much more effective in decreasing limb volumes as compared with compression garments. However, multilayer bandages are bulky, cumbersome, and hot and therefore are a significant source of patient discontent. In addition, although CDT is helpful in most patients, it is important to note that this treatment is palliative in nature and designed to decrease the symptoms of the disease rather than cure the underlying problem. The lifelong need for intensive therapy in combination with the expense of this treatment is a major cause of noncompliance.

Intermittent pneumatic compression (IPC) devices are also commonly used for the treatment of lymphedema and are designed to automate MLD and compression. These pumps vary in design, but in general, have one or more pneumatic cuffs that sequentially inflate and mimic the pump effect of muscular contraction to increase lymphatic flow. There are currently many different devices on the market, each with varying pressures, cycle times, and pump design. In addition, there is some debate regarding the efficacy of this treatment. However, recent meta-analyses and systematic reviews have shown that IPC is effective for volume reduction in patients with secondary lymphedema either when used alone or in combination with other treatments.[23] Unfortunately, these treatments are expensive and, in some cases, not covered by commercial insurance carriers.

Low-Level Laser Therapy

Low-level laser therapy (LLLT), or so-called cold lasers, are low-power lasers that stimulate tissue changes via nonthermal mechanisms and have been used for a variety of inflammatory disorders, including tendinitis and arthritis. Experimental studies in mouse models have shown that LLLT has antifibrotic, lymphangiogenic, and antiinflammatory effects suggesting that treatment may also be effective for the treatment of lymphedema. This hypothesis has been tested in a few recent studies demonstrating that LLLT is moderately effective in treating patients with secondary lymphedema. A systematic review and meta-analysis of nine smaller studies found that LLLT either alone or in combination with other lymphedema treatments significantly decreased swelling and pain.[24] Patients treated in this manner had an average volume reduction of 90 mL and the treatment was well tolerated, with only 1 patient experiencing an episode of cellulitis. Additional studies with larger patient populations and longer follow-up are needed to evaluate this therapeutic modality fully.

Stem Cells

Several studies have attempted to use bone marrow or adipose tissue-derived mesenchymal stem cells (MSCs) for the treatment of secondary lymphedema. Hou and colleagues tested the hypothesis that autologous bone-marrow-derived MSCs can decrease limb volumes in patients with breast cancer-related lymphedema (BCRL) by injecting MSCs intramuscularly in the affected extremity of 10 patients and comparing these patients with a control group of 35 patients with BCRL treated with CDT.[25] Patients treated with stem cells were not treated with compression or CDT. The authors showed that both groups had significant reductions in arm volumes 1, 3, and 12 months after initiation of the trial as compared to pretreatment figures. At 1-year follow-up, patients treated with MSCs had significantly improved arm volumes (81% decrease vs. 55% decrease in patients treated with CDT; P <0.001) and decreased pain/symptoms of lymphedema. However, it is intriguing why the authors have not provided additional follow-up or larger trials since their initial report over a decade ago.

Maldonado and colleagues used a similar approach in 20 patients with BCRL divided equally between bone marrow-derived stem cell therapy (without compression) or CDT alone and followed for 12 weeks.[26] Similar to Hou et al, this study also noted significant, though modest, reductions in arm volumes in both groups. However, unlike Hou et al, stem cell therapy was not more effective as compared to CDT. In addition, two patients in the MSC treatment group developed recurrent cellulitis after treatment necessitating hospitalization and antibiotic treatment. In another study, Toyserkani and colleagues documented a case report in which freshly isolated adipose-derived stem cells were injected in the axilla of a single patient with BCRL. The authors noted improvements in arm volume and lymphedema symptoms 4 months after treatment.[27]

Although additional work is necessary to study the efficacy of stem cells in the treatment of lymphedema, preclinical studies have provided some mechanistic rationale for the observation that MSCs may be beneficial in this disease process. For example, in vitro and studies in mouse models of lymphedema have suggested that MSCs can differentiate into lymphatic endothelial-like cells in specialized conditions and can increase lymphatic function in vivo.

Lymphangiogenic Growth Factors

Since the discovery of vascular endothelial growth factor-C (VEGF-C) in the late 1990s, several other growth factors that increased lymphatic sprouting and growth, a process termed lymphangiogenesis, have been discovered. These discoveries led to numerous preclinical studies in a variety of animal models which, by and large, demonstrated that local delivery of lymphangiogenic growth factors significantly increases collateral lymphatic formation and is effective in decreasing the severity of lymphedema.[28] Other studies have shown that VEGF-C gene therapy significantly increases lymphatic regeneration following lymph node transplantation in a porcine model of lymphadenectomy. These findings have led to clinical trials combining VEGF-C gene therapy (Lymfactin, Herantis Pharma, Inc.) with vascularized lymph node transplantation for the treatment of BCRL. The results of this phase II clinical trial have not yet been reported. Nevertheless, clinical translation of VEGF-C gene therapy in cancer patients may be complicated by the fact that this growth factor is also a key regulator of breast cancer growth and metastasis.

Antiinflammatory Treatments

Chronic inflammation is a critical histological feature of lymphedema and has, more recently, been shown to contribute to the pathology of the disease. As a result, recent studies have evaluated the efficacy of antiinflammatory therapies for the treatment of this disease. Rockson and colleagues reported on the effectiveness of ketoprofen (75 mg p.o., t.i.d. for 4 months), a nonsteroidal antiinflammatory drug (NSAID), for the treatment of primary or secondary lymphedema in an open-label and a placebo-controlled trial.[14] Twenty-one patients were treated in the open-label trial and treatment was found to significantly improve skin histopathology and decrease skin thickness at the conclusion of the trial. In the follow-up randomized trial, 16 patients were treated with ketoprofen, while 18 patients were treated with placebo. This trial, like the open-label study, reported significantly improved skin histopathology scores, decreased plasma granulocyte CSF (G-CSF) expression, and reduced the infiltration of neutrophils and macrophages. There were no major adverse effects reported in this study. A follow-up study demonstrated that ketoprofen blockade of leukotriene-B4 is responsible for its beneficial effects in lymphedema, and these drugs are currently being tested in a new clinical trial.

Surgical Treatments

Early stages of lymphedema are characterized by fluid accumulation in the interstitial tissues and are amenable to decongestive therapy and surgical procedures that aim to restore lymphatic function, so-called physiological procedures. Late stages of lymphedema result in progressive fibroadipose tissue deposition and are, as a result, less amenable to treatment with compression. In general, these pathological changes are also less responsive to physiological procedures and are more effectively treated by reductive techniques aiming to remove the excess fibrofatty tissues surgically. In some cases, physiological and reductive procedures can be combined to improve lymphatic fluid transport and remove fibroadipose tissues. Thus, both surgical approaches are useful and have a role in the treatment of lymphedema. Selection of the procedure depends on accurate preoperative assessment and realistic goals.

Reductive Methods

Reductive techniques, including direct excision and liposuction, are appropriate in patients who have a predominantly fibrofatty component to their lymphedema (i.e., later stages of disease). Direct excision techniques such as the Charles or Sistrunk procedures have been described for the treatment of end-stage upper and lower extremity or genital lymphedema. In these procedures, skin and subcutaneous tissue are excised down to the level of investing fascia and covered with skin grafts or local flaps. These procedures are still used, often as a last resort, in cases of severe lymphedema with a massive localized accumulation of fibrofatty tissues and fibrotic changes of the skin. However, these operations are extremely invasive and can result in a large amount of blood loss and physical deformity. Consequently, these operations can result in significant morbidity, infections, and delayed healing.

Hakan Brorson pioneered the use of liposuction for the treatment of lymphedema and has published excellent long-term outcomes in elegant, well-designed studies.[29] In these procedures, like cosmetic liposuction, fat is aspirated circumferentially using epinephrine containing tumescent to decrease blood loss. Liposuction is most effective in patients with nonpitting lymphedema who have significant adipose deposition (>600 mL volume differential). These treatments are highly effective for the treatment of late-stage BCRL and can, on average, decrease arm volume excess by 50%–100%. The volume reduction is maintained long term (even years later) if compression garments are worn continuously. In addition, skin resection is seldom necessary with the natural tightening of the skin over time and with compression use. Patients treated with liposuction also had decreased rates of cellulitis. Liposuction is well tolerated and can be performed as an outpatient procedure. Reported complications are relatively minor and self-limited, including paresthesia, cellulitis, and minor wound healing complications.

Hoffner et al reported their findings in a recent long-term study of 105 patients with upper extremity lymphedema with an average preoperative volume excess of 1573 ± 645 mL and followed for a minimum of 5 years following liposuction.[30] Liposuction was used to remove an average of 1831 ± 599 mL and resulted in an average volume reduction of 117%. These findings are consistent with a recent systematic review of four high-quality studies reporting an average excess volume reduction of 97% (95% CI = 86.2–107%; $I^2 = 0.0\%$).[31] It is important to note that the majority of studies that have evaluated liposuction as a treatment modality for lymphedema have been performed in patients with upper extremity lymphedema. More recently, several investigators have reported the efficacy of this approach for the treatment of lower extremity lymphedema.[32] In one study, 69 patients (72 legs) with lower extremity lymphedema were treated with liposuction.[32] These patients had a mean preoperative volume excess of 4372 mL and underwent an average resection of 4550 mL of lipoaspirate. The average volume reduction at 1 year was 88%. Longer follow-up of a smaller group of patients at 2 years and 5 years demonstrated that these volume reductions were maintained. Patients with secondary lymphedema had the best outcomes, while men with primary lymphedema responded more poorly. Importantly, these authors reported no major complications in their series.

Physiological Methods

Physiological procedures can be divided into two categories, including lymphatic bypass procedures that surgically re-route lymphatic drainage and lymph node transplants that transfer lymph nodes from an unaffected region of the body to the lymphedematous limb. These techniques are commonly performed, and each has its own advantages and disadvantages. In some instances, lymphovenous bypass and lymph node transplants (and in some cases, liposuction) are combined to treat an individual depending on the pathological changes that are present. Advances in microsurgical techniques and imaging technologies have led to rapid advances in the surgical management of lymphedema with improved outcomes and a deeper understanding of the pathology of lymphedema.

Lymphovenous Bypass

Lymphovenous bypass (LVB) was first described in the 1970s, and detailed anastomosis of lymphatic collectors to large superficial veins. This technique had mixed results due, at least in part, to the fact that pressures in the larger veins in some cases exceeded the low pressures in the lymphatic system. Improvements in microsurgical techniques and equipment enabled surgeons to repair smaller vessels (usually less than 0.5 mm in diameter), and the focus shifted to bypass of smaller lymphatics to smaller venules using supermicrosurgery (Fig. 44.7). Identification and analysis

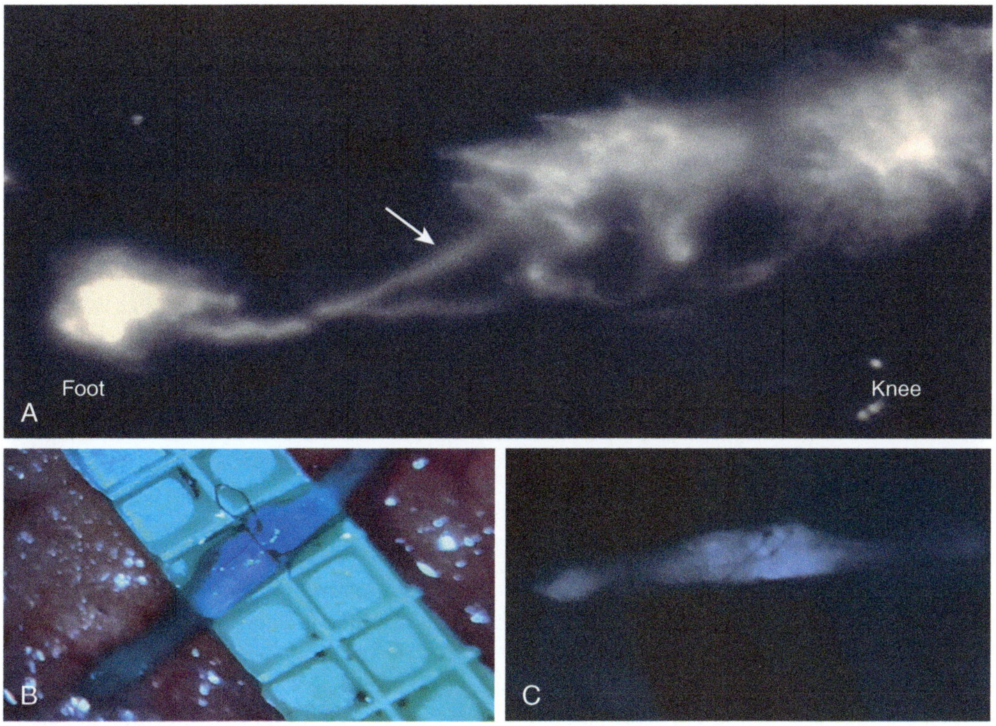

• **Fig. 44.7** (A) ICG lymphography showing functional lymphatic ending in dermal backflow, allowing for precise identification of lymphovenous bypass target site (arrow). (B) Lymphovenous bypass of lymphatic (left) to vein (right). Note flow of blue dye from lymphatic, through anastomosis, into vein. (C) ICG of lymphovenous bypass. Note flow of ICG from lymphatic, through anastomosis, into vein.

of lymphatic drainage patterns with ICG lymphography have also been a significant advance in this technique as this approach enables precise identification of leaky and functional lymphatics (see Fig. 44.7). Since then, several authors have shown that LVB can be effective in patients with early-stage lymphedema, reducing the excess volume, and improving the symptoms of the disease. For example, Chang and colleagues followed 100 patients treated with LVB and noted that 96% of patients with breast cancer-related upper extremity lymphedema had symptomatic improvement (lighter, softer, less painful arms) and 74% had a quantitative reduction in excess volume.[22] Patients with early-stage disease (MD Anderson stage I or II ICG disease) upper extremity lymphedema experienced significantly better outcomes as compared with women with late-stage (MD Anderson stage III/IV) or lower extremity lymphedema. One year following surgery, patients with stage I/II disease had an average decrease of 61% in excess volume. In contrast, patients with stage III/IV disease experienced much more modest improvements (average =17%). Nevertheless, these procedures were safe and well tolerated with few reported complications. While the benefits of LVB continue to be clarified, these procedures appear to be safe and well tolerated. The findings reported by Chang and colleagues are consistent with a recent systematic review of 18 studies with 939 patients. In this review, all analyzed studies reported objective improvements in lymphedema measures, subjective improvement in 50%–100% of patients, and a reduction in the number of cellulitis episodes.[33]

Chang and colleagues found that only 57% of the patients treated for lower extremity lymphedema with LVB reported symptomatic improvement, leading these authors to conclude that this procedure is less helpful for this patient population. In contrast, Campisi et al found that LVB was equally effective for the treatment of both upper and lower extremity lymphedema.[34] These authors reported their outcomes with over 2600 patients treated over 40 years and found that 84% of their patients had a long-term improvement in excess limb volumes, and more than 86% of those with early-stage lymphedema stopped using compression garments. They also found that more than 90% of their patients had a decreased incidence of cellulitis. However, these conclusions require additional study since the authors used a variety of techniques and follow-up was variable. In addition, changes in patient satisfaction were assessed with nonvalidated methods, and the report was retrospective in nature. Thus, future prospective studies using standardized techniques, follow-up times, and validated lymphedema questionnaires are needed to assess the efficacy of LVB for the treatment of lower extremity lymphedema.

Recent studies have reported outcomes of LVB performed at the time of lymph node dissection to prevent the development of lymphedema. Although the available published data are limited, the results from these studies are generally promising. For example, in the largest published series to date, Boccardo and colleagues reported their 4-year outcomes in 74 patients treated with prophylactic LVB, a procedure they termed LYMPHA ("lymphatic microsurgical preventing healing approach") for the treatment of patients who underwent axillary lymph node dissection.[35] Their technique involves intussusception of multiple lymphatics into one vein, as opposed to an end-to-end anastomosis commonly performed in LVB for the treatment of existing lymphedema. Using outcomes that included volumetric analysis and lymphoscintigraphy, the authors found that only 4% (3 patients) treated with LYMPHA as compared with 30% of patients who underwent axillary lymph node dissection alone developed lymphedema at 4 years follow-up. In a smaller, though methodologically similar study, Feldman et al followed 27 patients treated with axillary lymph node dissection and LYMPHA and compared them to 10 patients who underwent axillary lymph node dissection in whom LYMPHA could not be performed for technical reasons.[36] At a mean follow-up of 6 months (a relatively short period for secondary lymphedema studies), the authors noted lymphedema in 12.5% of patients treated with LYMPHA versus 50% of those in whom bypass could not be performed. This study is somewhat problematic since it can be argued that the groups are not comparable, and the rate of lymphedema at 6 months even in the LYMPHA group is quite high as compared to historical reports. Nevertheless, if one projects the findings of LVB for early-stage disease as compared with late-stage lymphedema, then it makes sense that the prevention of lymphedema should be even more successful.

More recent publications have reported outcomes following LYMPHA for the prevention of lower extremity lymphedema in patients who underwent inguinofemoral lymphadenectomy.[37] Although these reports are still preliminary with short follow-up times and small numbers of patients (27 in the largest series), the early results are promising, with documented lymphedema development in only 1 patient (3%). Future studies using a randomized approach and prospective follow-up with more advanced imaging techniques (e.g., ICG lymphography) and validated lymphedema outcomes questionnaires are needed.

Vascularized Lymph Node Transplantation (VLNT)

VLNT is a procedure popularized by Corrin Becker in which lymph nodes and soft tissues are harvested from an unaffected region and transferred to the lymphedematous area using microsurgical techniques to restore the arterial and venous blood supply of the transplanted tissues. Importantly, the afferent and efferent lymphatic channels are not repaired. Therefore, the lymphatic circulation to the lymph node is restored by lymphangiogenesis and spontaneous reconnection of transected lymphatics.

Lymph nodes may be transplanted to the area where lymph node dissection was performed (orthotopic transplantation) or to a region distal to the zone of injury (heterotopic transplantation). Some authors have reported simultaneous orthotopic and heterotopic transplantation. Although the cellular mechanisms by which VLNT may aid in the treatment of lymphedema remain unknown, emerging experimental and clinical studies suggest that transplanted lymph nodes spontaneously reestablish connections to regional lymphatic vessels and that shunting of interstitial fluid to the venous system occurs in the lymph node high endothelial venules.

Many donor areas for donor lymph nodes used in VLNT have been described, including the inguinal area, axilla, lateral thoracic area, cervical area, submental area, omentum, and mesenteric (Fig. 44.8). A systematic review of 24 studies reporting on 271 VLNTs, reported that the inguinal region was the most common donor site reported in the literature (68%).[38] However, this trend is likely to change due to relatively high rates of donor site complications with this area including seroma (7.6%), chronic pain (1.6%), and worryingly, donor site lymphedema (1.6%). The rate of donor site lymphedema, particularly in the inguinal region, is likely even higher than the reported rates since it has been shown that 5%–7% of patients who undergo sentinel lymph node biopsy develop lymphedema. The technique of reverse lymphatic mapping in which a radioactive tracer is injected in the distal limb enabling surgeons to identify and avoid lymphatic pathways that drain the extremity and instead harvest lymph nodes that drain the trunk is helpful and may decrease the incidence of donor site lymphedema.[39]

Concerns about donor site lymphedema have led some investigators to harvest lymph nodes from the omentum and, less commonly, from the mesentery. The omentum is easy to harvest and has a long pedicle with large and reliable vascular anatomy (Fig. 44.9). This donor site eliminates the risk of donor site lymphedema completely, and lymph nodes can be harvested using minimally invasive techniques. In addition, the omentum can easily be split into two flaps enabling simultaneous orthotopic and heterotopic lymph node transplantation. Nevertheless, intraabdominal surgery has potential risks such as hernia, small bowel obstruction, and pancreatitis. Thus, the risks and benefits of donor site complications for VLNT should be carefully considered and discussed with patients.

Analysis of outcomes following VLNT has been difficult due to heterogeneity in surgical techniques, patient selection criteria, and clinical outcome measures. Many investigators report outcomes of circumference measurements or change in circumference while others have reported volumetric changes. There is also significant variability in patient selection criteria with some investigators offering VLNT to all patients regardless of stage or comorbid factors, while others use a more selective approach offering VLNT only in patients with early-stage disease after optimization with CDT and weight loss. Relatively few studies have reported outcomes using adjunctive quantitative or qualitative outcomes such as lymphoscintigraphy, ICG lymphography, and validated patient-reported outcomes measures. These differences in surgical techniques, patient selection, use of compression garments following surgery, and analysis of outcomes makes it challenging to compare studies critically. Nevertheless, a recent systematic review of 18 studies reporting on outcomes in 305 patients treated with VLNT for upper or lower extremity lymphedema

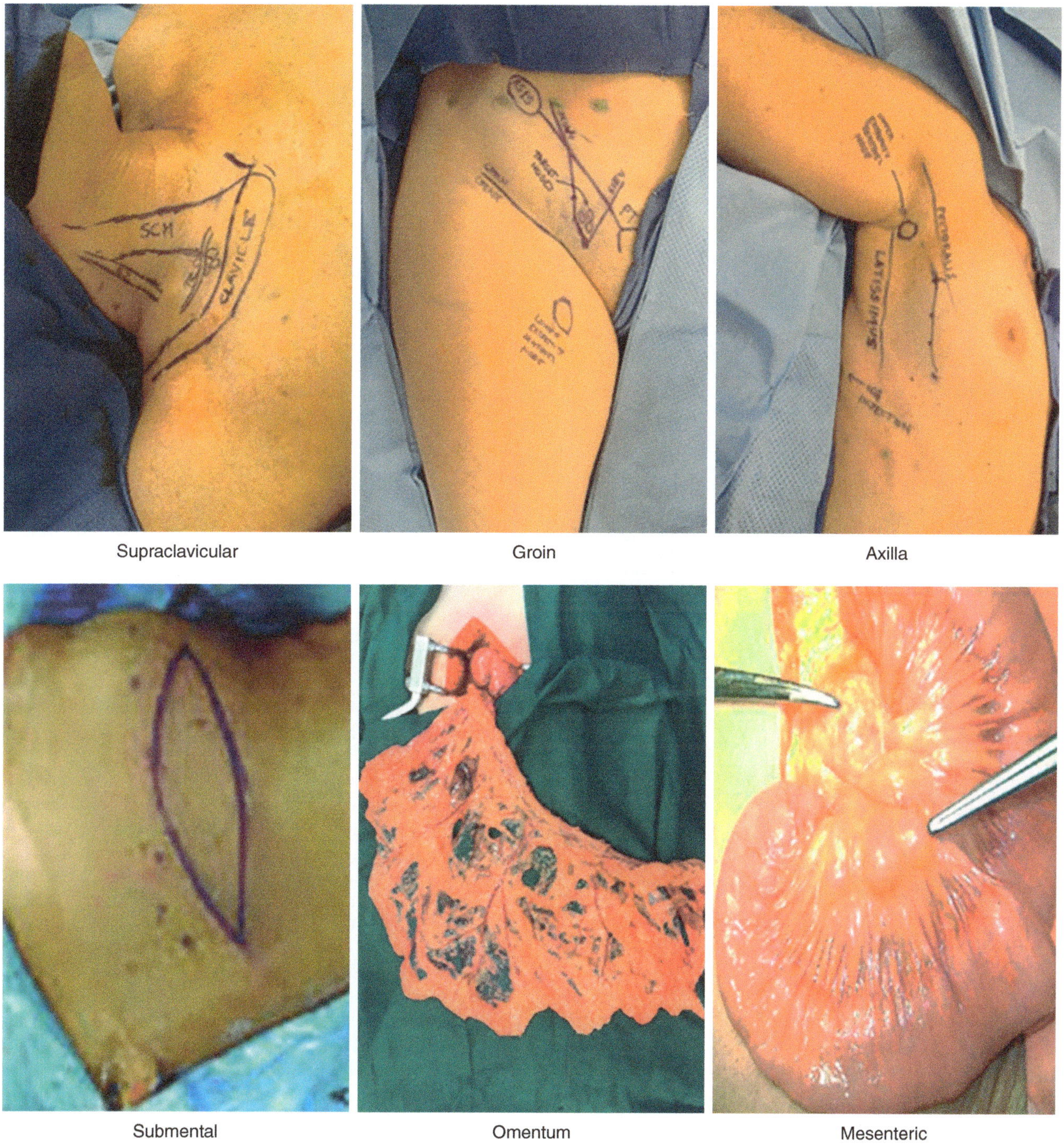

• **Fig. 44.8** Donor site options for vascularized lymph node transfer including supraclavicular, groin, axilla, submental, omentum, and mesenteric.

reported encouraging results.[40] For example, in studies that used circumference measurements (n = 182 patients), >90% of patients had improvements after surgery. Similarly, in studies that used volumetric analysis as the outcome measure, >86% of patients improved following surgery. Mean limb reduction was assessed using both circumferential change and volumetric change. The weighted average for limb reduction was 39.5% for excess circumference and 26.4% for excess volume reduction. These findings are supported by a study on vascularized omental transplants in 42 patients that were not included in the systematic review.[41] In this study, 83% of patients had a subjective improvement in upper extremity lymphedema symptoms and the authors noted a 22% reduction in mean volume. VLNT is also effective in reducing the symptoms of lymphedema. In seven studies with patient-reported outcomes (n = 105 patients), 93% of respondents were satisfied or highly satisfied with the surgery, and the remainder of patients were no better or worse following surgery.[40] More than 50% of patients were able to discontinue the use of compression

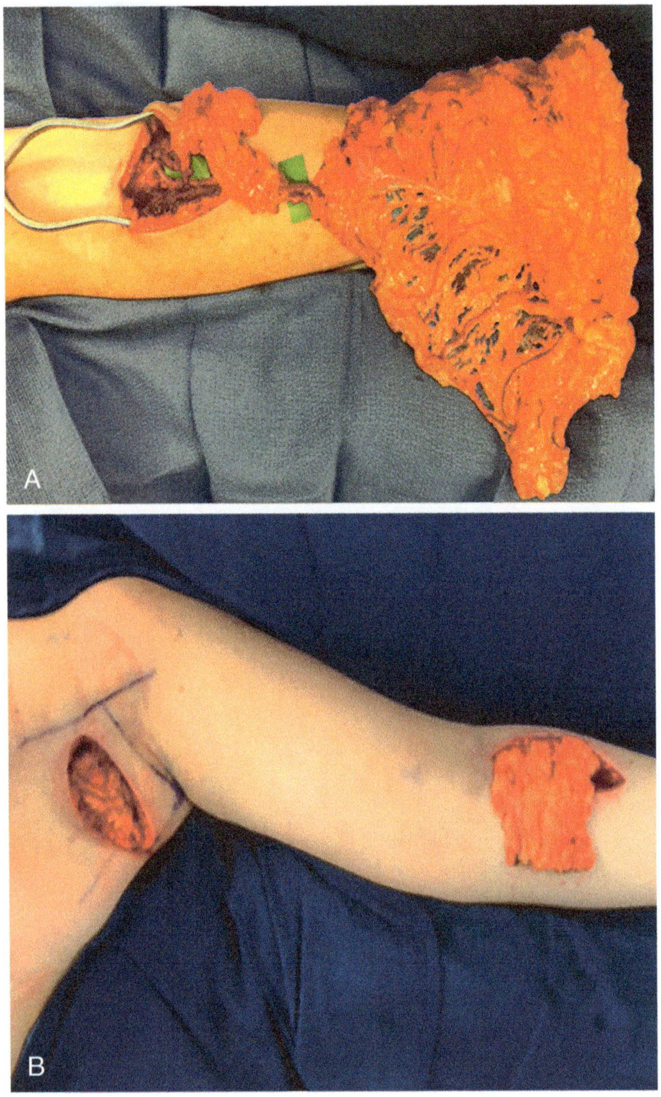

• **Fig. 44.9** (A) Omentum flap anastomosed at proximal forearm. (B) Omentum split, with anastomosis and inset at both proximal forearm and axilla.

garments and there was a 90% decrease in the incidence of cellulitis (n = 106 in six studies).[40] Taken together, these studies suggest that VLNT is a promising technique that can be used to restore lymphatic circulation in patients with lymphedema. This technique, like other physiological procedures, is most effective in patients with early-stage disease. Combination of VLNT with other procedures such as lymphovenous bypass or liposuction may be more effective depending on the patient's anatomy and degree of adipose deposition.

Conclusions

Lymphedema is a common problem and a significant source of morbidity. Recent studies have advanced our understanding of the pathophysiology of the disease and have, as a result, led to novel therapies. Medical and surgical treatments for lymphedema have provided hope for patients who previously were offered only palliative therapies. This is an exciting area of research and improvements in surgical techniques, imaging, and pharmacological interventions promise improved outcomes and additional options.

References

1. McLaughlin SA, Wright MJ, Morris KT, et al. Prevalence of lymphedema in women with breast cancer 5 years after sentinel lymph node biopsy or axillary dissection: patient perceptions and precautionary behaviors. *J Clin Oncol*. 2008;26:5220–5226.
2. Helyer LK, Varnic M, Le LW, et al. Obesity is a risk factor for developing postoperative lymphedema in breast cancer patients. *Breast J*. 2010;16:48–54.
3. Shaw C, Mortimer P, Judd PA. A randomized controlled trial of weight reduction as a treatment for breast cancer-related lymphedema. *Cancer*. 2007;110:1868–1874.
4. Arngrim N, Simonsen L, Holst JJ, et al. Reduced adipose tissue lymphatic drainage of macromolecules in obese subjects: a possible link between obesity and local tissue inflammation? *Int J Obes*. 2013;37:748–750.
5. Greene AK, Grant FD, Slavin SA. Lower-extremity lymphedema and elevated body-mass index. *N Engl J Med*. 2012;366:2136–2137.
6. Garcia Nores GD, Cuzzone DA, Albano NJ, et al. Obesity but not high-fat diet impairs lymphatic function. *Int J Obes*. 2016;40:1582–1590.
7. Kissin MW, Querci della Rovere G, Easton D, et al. Risk of lymphoedema following the treatment of breast cancer. *Br J Surg*. 1986;73:580–584.
8. Kataru RP, Baik JE, Park HJ, et al. Regulation of immune function by the lymphatic system in lymphedema. *Front Immunol*. 2019;10:470.
9. Hayes SC, Janda M, Cornish B, et al. Lymphedema after breast cancer: incidence, risk factors, and effect on upper body function. *J Clin Oncol*. 2008;26:3536–3542.
10. Finegold DN, Baty CJ, Knickelbein KZ, et al. Connexin 47 mutations increase risk for secondary lymphedema following breast cancer treatment. *Clin Cancer Res*. 2012;18:2382–2390.
11. Visser J, van Geel M, Cornelissen AJM, et al. Breast cancer-related lymphedema and genetic predisposition: a systematic review of the literature. *Lymphat Res Biol*. 2019;17(3):288–293.
12. Jensen MR, Simonsen L, Karlsmark T, et al. Higher vascular endothelial growth factor-C concentration in plasma is associated with increased forearm capillary filtration capacity in breast cancer-related lymphedema. *Physiol Rep*. 2015;3(6):e12403.
13. Nakamura K, Radhakrishnan K, Wong YM, et al. Anti-inflammatory pharmacotherapy with ketoprofen ameliorates experimental lymphatic vascular insufficiency in mice. *PloS One*. 2009;4:e8380.
14. Rockson SG, Tian W, Jiang X, et al. Pilot studies demonstrate the potential benefits of antiinflammatory therapy in human lymphedema. *JCI Insight*. 2018;3:e123775. https://doi.org/10.1172/jci.insight.123775.
15. Gardenier JC, Kataru RP, Hespe GE, et al. Topical tacrolimus for the treatment of secondary lymphedema. *Nat Commun*. 2017;8:14345.
16. Brorson H, Hoijer P. Standardised measurements used to order compression garments can be used to calculate arm volumes to evaluate lymphoedema treatment. *J Plast Surg Hand Surg*. 2012;46:410–415.
17. Fu MR, Cleland CM, Guth AA, et al. L-dex ratio in detecting breast cancer-related lymphedema: reliability, sensitivity, and specificity. *Lymphology*. 2013;46:85–96.

18. Mihara M, Hara H, Araki J, et al. Indocyanine green (ICG) lymphography is superior to lymphoscintigraphy for diagnostic imaging of early lymphedema of the upper limbs. *PloS One*. 2012;7:e38182.
19. Hassanein AH, Maclellan RA, Grant FD, et al. Diagnostic accuracy of lymphoscintigraphy for lymphedema and analysis of false-negative tests. *Plast Reconstr Surg Glob Open*. 2017;5:e1396.
20. Mihara M, Hara H, Narushima M, et al. Indocyanine green lymphography is superior to lymphoscintigraphy in imaging diagnosis of secondary lymphedema of the lower limbs. *J Vasc Surg Venous Lymphat Disord*. 2013;1:194–201.
21. Mihara M, Hara H, Hayashi Y, et al. Pathological steps of cancer-related lymphedema: histological changes in the collecting lymphatic vessels after lymphadenectomy. *PloS One*. 2012;7:e41126.
22. Chang DW, Suami H, Skoracki R. A prospective analysis of 100 consecutive lymphovenous bypass cases for treatment of extremity lymphedema. *Plast Reconstr Surg*. 2013;132:1305–1314.
23. Feldman JL, Stout NL, Wanchai A, et al. Intermittent pneumatic compression therapy: a systematic review. *Lymphology*. 2012;45:13–25.
24. Smoot B, Chiavola-Larson L, Lee J, et al. Effect of low-level laser therapy on pain and swelling in women with breast cancer-related lymphedema: a systematic review and meta-analysis. *J Cancer Survivorship: Res Pract*. 2015;9:287–304.
25. Hou C, Wu X, Jin X. Autologous bone marrow stromal cells transplantation for the treatment of secondary arm lymphedema: a prospective controlled study in patients with breast cancer related lymphedema. *Japn J Clin Oncol*. 2008;38:670–674.
26. Maldonado GE, Perez CA, Covarrubias EE, et al. Autologous stem cells for the treatment of post-mastectomy lymphedema: a pilot study. *Cytotherapy*. 2011;13:1249–1255.
27. Toyserkani NM, Jensen CH, Sheikh SP, et al. Cell-assisted lipotransfer using autologous adipose-derived stromal cells for alleviation of breast cancer-related lymphedema. *Stem Cells Translat Med*. 2016;5:857–859.
28. Baker A, Kim H, Semple JL, et al. Experimental assessment of pro-lymphangiogenic growth factors in the treatment of post-surgical lymphedema following lymphadenectomy. *Breast Cancer Res*. 2010;12:R70.
29. Brorson H, Svensson H. Liposuction combined with controlled compression therapy reduces arm lymphedema more effectively than controlled compression therapy alone. discussion 68 *Plast Reconstr Surg*. 1998;102:1058–1067.
30. Hoffner M, Ohlin K, Svensson B, et al. Liposuction gives complete reduction of arm lymphedema following breast cancer treatment-a 5-year prospective study in 105 patients without recurrence. *Plast Reconstr Surg Glob Open*. 2018;6:e1912.
31. Carl HM, Walia G, Bello R, et al. Systematic review of the surgical treatment of extremity lymphedema. *J Reconstr Microsurg*. 2017;33(6):412–425.
32. Stewart CJ, Munnoch DA. Liposuction as an effective treatment for lower extremity lymphoedema: a single surgeon's experience over nine years. *J Plast Reconstr Aesthet Surg*. 2018;71:239–245.
33. Scaglioni MF, Fontein DBY, Arvanitakis M, et al. Systematic review of lymphovenous anastomosis (LVA) for the treatment of lymphedema. *Microsurgery*. 2017;37:947–953.
34. Campisi C, Davini D, Bellini C, et al. Lymphatic microsurgery for the treatment of lymphedema. *Microsurgery*. 2006;26:65–69.
35. Boccardo F, Casabona F, De Cian F, et al. Lymphatic microsurgical preventing healing approach (LYMPHA) for primary surgical prevention of breast cancer-related lymphedema: over 4 years follow-up. *Microsurgery*. 2014;34:421–424.
36. Feldman S, Bansil H, Ascherman J, et al. Single institution experience with lymphatic microsurgical preventive healing approach (LYMPHA) for the primary prevention of lymphedema. *Ann Surg Oncol*. 2015;22:3296–3301.
37. Boccardo F, Valenzano M, Costantini S, et al. LYMPHA technique to prevent secondary lower limb lymphedema. *Ann Surg Oncol*. 2016;23:3558–3563.
38. Scaglioni MF, Arvanitakis M, Chen YC, et al. Comprehensive review of vascularized lymph node transfers for lymphedema: outcomes and complications. *Microsurgery*. 2018;38(2):222–229.
39. Dayan JH, Dayan E, Smith ML. Reverse lymphatic mapping: a new technique for maximizing safety in vascularized lymph node transfer. *Plast Reconstr Surg*. 2015;135:277–285.
40. Ozturk CN, Ozturk C, Glasgow M, et al. Free vascularized lymph node transfer for treatment of lymphedema: a systematic evidence based review. *J Plast Reconstr Aesthet Surg: JPRAS*. 2016;69:1234–1247.
41. Nguyen AT, Suami H, Hanasono MM, et al. Long-term outcomes of the minimally invasive free vascularized omental lymphatic flap for the treatment of lymphedema. *J Surg Oncol*. 2017;115:84–89.

45 Congenital Hand Differences

BRAN SIVAKUMAR, JONATHAN ADAMTHWAITE, AND PAUL SMITH

For videos accompanying this chapter see ExpertConsult.com. See inside cover for access details.

Embryology

The upper limb bud develops from the flank of the developing embryo from day 26.[1] Somatic lateral plate mesoderm forms the skeleton and mesoderm from somites migrates in to form the musculature and contributes to the vascular system. Fibroblast growth factors initiate development along three axes with the interaction of signaling centers: proximodistal axis controlled by the apical ectodermal ridge; anteroposterior (radioulnar) controlled by the zone of polarizing activity (ZPA); and the dorsoventral (or dorsovolar) controlled by the wingless gene encoded protein (Fig. 45.1). Genes and their encoded proteins control growth and differentiation and act as messengers between signaling centres and developing cells. Mutations, whether inherited or spontaneous, disrupt secreted proteins, ligand factors, and transcription factors. Environmental factors including drugs (e.g., thalidomide), radiation, nutrition, and infection can also disrupt molecular pathways.[1]

Timeline

The limb bud contains a core of proliferating mesenchymal cells covered by ectoderm which thickens at the tip to form the apical ectodermal ridge (AER). The spinal nerves grow into this and an initial capillary network coalesces into a main stem artery, which drains into a marginal vein. The mesoderm organizes into the ZPA and a progress zone (PZ). By day 33, there is a paddle-shape limb with prechondrogenic condensations at sites where cartilaginous skeletal elements will form. Chondrogenesis takes place and myoblasts migrate into the limb and aggregate into ventral and dorsal muscle masses by day 36. At 6 weeks, digital rays form giving the hand a webbed appearance, and at 7 weeks the upper limb rotates by 90 degrees and the elbow flexes bringing the palm anteriorly. Ossification occurs in parallel and apoptosis between rays leads to tissue involution and digital separation. Thus by week 8 a miniature adult upper limb is formed[1] (Table 45.1).

Limb Patterning

Research into the developing chick embryo has provided a great deal of information on the process of limb patterning. In the proximodistal axis, the AER is formed by the *Wnt7a* gene and secretes FGF 2, 4, and 8 stimulating proliferation and bud outgrowth.[2] AER resection leads to a truncated limb, whilst AER grafting extends the limb. In the anteroposterior (radioulnar) axis, the ZPA is on the ulnar side between the polarizing region (posterior limb bud mesenchyme) and limb bud tip mesenchyme. This secretes Shh, which is the product of the sonic hedgehog gene.[3] If the polarizing region is grafted anteriorly, a mirror set of digits results. In the dorsoventral axis, the somite provides a dorsal signal to the mesenchyme, which dorsalizes ectoderm. *Wnt7a* from the dorsal ectoderm and *Lmx1b* from the mesoderm coordinate tendon and ligament formation.[4] Other important genes in limb patterning include *HoxD* (*HoxD13* mutations are associated with central polydactyly) and *Gli3* (mutations lead to polydactylies).[5]

Classification

There have been multiple attempts to classify congenital hand differences, however an entirely inclusive system remains elusive. A largely morphological system, first proposed in 1968 then refined in 1976 and 1983[6] by Swanson et al, was adopted as the standard by the International Federation of Societies for Surgery of the Hand in 1976 and remains the most widely used (Table 45.2). However, approximately 10% of congenital hand differences do not fit into this classification, and some anomalies fit into more than one category. Extensions to this classification include those by Knight and Kay in 2000[7] and Upton in 2006.[8] More recently, Tonkin in 2013[9] presented a classification system based on causation taking into account the growing body of knowledge from molecular biology. He categorizes anomalies into malformations (an abnormal formation of tissue resulting from abnormal cell function), deformations (an insult to cells that have already formed normally), and dysplasias (a lack of normal organization of cells into tissue).

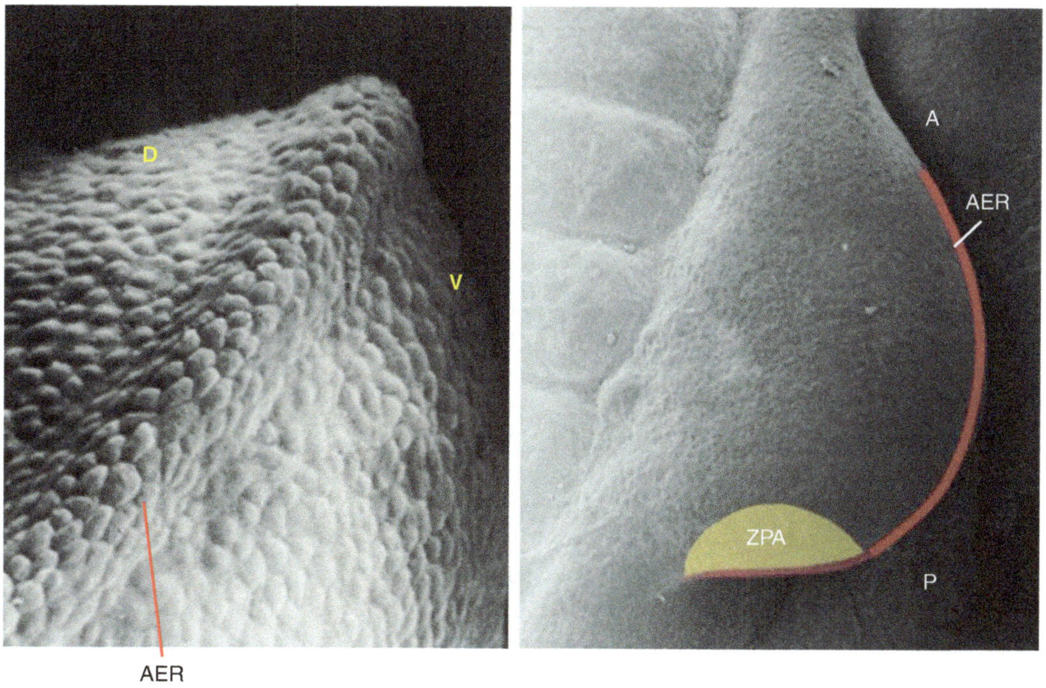

• **Fig. 45.1** Development and patterning centers of the upper limb. Limb patterning is coordinated along three axes that are intimately linked through feedback loops. Outgrowth of the limb from proximal to distal is driven by the apical ectodermal ridge (*AER*). The anteroposterior axis is controlled by the zone of polarizing activity (*ZPA*) through the morphogen sonic hedgehog (SHH). Dorsal (*D*) and ventral (*V*) patterning is controlled via engrailed–1 (EN1), which is expressed in the ventral ectoderm and WNT7A, whose expression is limited to the dorsal ectoderm.

TABLE 45.1 Timetable of Upper Limb Development

Time Point	Upper Limb Development
Day 26	Limb bud first appears
Day 33	Paddle-shaped hand present
Day 42	Digital ray present Hand assumes a webbed appearance
7th week	Upper limb rotates 90 degrees laterally to bring the palm anteriorly Elbow begins to flex Ossification begins Involution of tissue between fingers occurs by apoptosis
8th week	Upper extremity resembles miniature adult upper limb

Disruptions, alteration of tissue that is already formed, are considered alongside deformations. This system is growing in its popularity and application.

Syndactyly

A normal web ends at the midproximal phalanx on the volar side and an abnormal continuation beyond this level is termed syndactyly (Greek *syn* = together, *dactylos* = digit/finger). Syndactyly is the commonest congenital hand abnormality, with an incidence of 1 in 1000 live births. It is more common in Caucasians than Africans and affects males more than females (46%–84%). It is familial in 15%–40% and can be unilateral or bilateral (25%–50%).[10] Syndactyly may affect the fingers and/or toes and most commonly presents as an incomplete second web syndactyly in the foot. In the hand, the third web is most frequently involved (50%) (see Fig. 45.2A, B), followed by the fourth (30%), second (15%), and first (5%) %).[10] A failure of apoptosis or programmed cell death, a process mediated by BMP-4 (bone morphogenic protein), is thought responsible during digit separation from day 41–53.[11]

Syndactyly may occur in isolation. However, it also associated with a number of syndromes including Poland, Apert, and Greig syndromes. It can also occur in conjunction with other limb deformities, such as polydactyly and constriction rings.

Classification

Syndactyly is classified as follows[10] (Fig. 45.2):

- Incomplete or complete (extending to the distal phalanx)
- Simple (soft tissue only) or complex (with bony synostosis)
- Complicated (a haphazard arrangement of bones with loss of normal ray patterning)
- Acrosyndactyly (fusion of digits distally, from the Greek *acro* meaning “tip,” with proximal fenestrations commonly associated with constriction ring syndrome).

TABLE 45.2 Swanson Classification of Congenital Hand Differences

Failure of formation	Transverse arrest	Complete deficiencies
		Intercalated deficiencies
	Longitudinal arrest	Radial (preaxial)
		Central longitudinal deficiency
		Ulnar (postaxial) longitudinal deficiency
Failure of differentiation	Soft tissue	Syndactyly
		Camptodactyly
		Trigger thumb
		Clasped thumb
	Skeletal	Clinodactyly
		Symphalangism
		Synostosis
		Arthrogryposis
		Windblown hand
Duplication	Ulnar polydactyly	
	Central polydactyly	
	Ulnar dimelia	
Overgrowth	Macrodactyly	
Undergrowth	Brachydactyly	
	Thumb hypoplasia	
Constriction ring syndromes	Groups 1–4	
Generalized skeletal abnormalities	Achondroplasia	

First proposed in 1968 and adopted as the standard by the International Federation of Societies for Surgery of the Hand in 1976.

Clinical Examination

Inspect the syndactylized digits. With complete syndactyly, the nails can be fused with an inward rotation of the digits, which eludes to the presence of a complex distal bony union (Fig. 45.2C). The degree of skeletal disruption within a syndactyly tends to parallel the degree of soft tissue abnormality, including that of tendons and digital neurovasculature structures. It is important to examine for the presence of digital creases, which provides valuable information about the passive and active joint range of motions, which may also be abnormal. The status of the joints pre-separation must be established to ensure adequate counseling of patients and their families with regard to the postoperative motion and function. Often a child and family will opt for the correct complement of digital number over function in equivocal cases.

In complicated syndactyly there is more than just a bony synostosis. Often there is a haphazard arrangement including extra skeletal elements concealed within a digit with associated fusions, rudimentary bones, missing bones, abnormal joints, and sometimes cross bones, which can span several rays[12] (Fig. 45.2D). It can be uncertain which bones best match with which digits. In acrosyndactyly, there is a complex syndactyly characterized by fusion of the bone distally but not proximally with often fenestrations or sinuses proximally (Fig. 45.2E). This is discussed later under Constriction Ring Syndrome (CRS).

Surgical Principles and Management

Timing of Surgery

Timing is controversial. To reduce anesthetic risk, most surgeons operate when patients are over the age of 1. Delaying separation in this way has the added advantage of larger anatomy, including that of the vasculature. Indications for earlier surgery include syndactyly involving the border digits, i.e., between the thumb and index and the little and ring fingers where tethering of growth can occur due to marked discrepancy in digital length. This can result in compromised function, and in neglected cases flexion contractures. Early release is also advised in cases of complex and acrosyndactly, where bony fusions can also affect growth. The aim is for all possible separations to be complete by school age or around 5 years.

Technique

The aim is to achieve both optimal function and cosmesis. Release involves separation of conjoined skin and subcutaneous tissue, ligaments, and bony synostosis whilst preserving the integrity of the neurovascular bundles. Subcutaneous fat may be removed in an effort to facilitate closure and contouring.

Separation can be divided into reconstruction of the web, sides of the digits, and tips including the paronychial folds.

Web Reconstruction

Multiple techniques have been described using volar, dorsal, or a combination of flaps of varying sizes and designs. The web is generally reconstructed with a proximally-based dorsal flap. Grafts are best avoided in the webspaces as they can lead to problems of poor pliability and delayed healing with associated web creep. Large triangular flaps are practical and versatile (Fig. 45.3). They allow for adjustments to be made around abnormal distal branching of digital vessels and avoid transverse scars that can recontract in the future. They must be designed in such a way as to create a gentle slope from dorsoproximal to volar-distal.

Release of the first web involves the use of Z-plasties (four-flap, Fig. 45.4), double, double-opposing, five-flap), transposition flaps (from the dorsum of the hand and index or thumb), pedicled and free flaps depending on the defect size following thumb and index separation.[13] It is important to release the fascia on the first dorsal interosseous and the adductor muscles. Sometimes it is necessary to reinsert the adductor muscle more proximally.

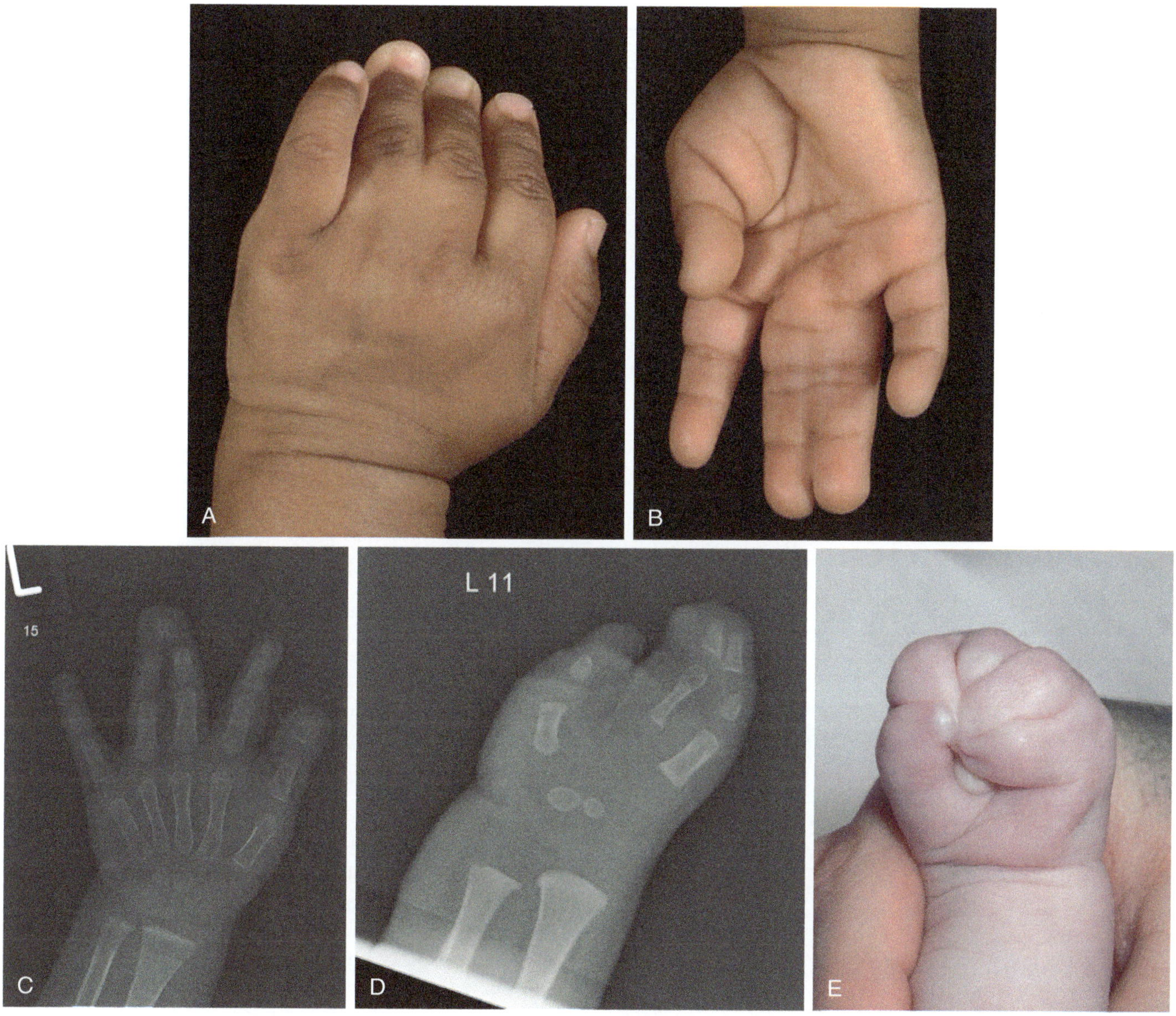

• **Fig. 45.2** Images of different types of syndactyly. (A) Complete syndactyly. (B) Incomplete syndactyly. (C) Complex syndactyly. (D) Complicated syndactyly. (E) Acrosyndactyly.

Reconstruction of the Sides of Digits

Most commonly interdigitating flaps from the volar and dorsal aspects are used to close the defects along the borders of the digits (see Fig. 45.3). Straight-line incisions along the borders should be avoided as they have a high incidence of scar contracture and subsequent digital deformity. A skin graft is usually needed in all but the most minor cases as even in a simple syndactyly skin shortage is at least 36% of the circumference.[14] The graft should be full thickness from the groin, inner arm, or antecubital fossa. Thick split-thickness grafts from the instep can be used in some cases of toe separation. Graft take may be improved with quilting onto the underlying soft tissues, and in the case of complex, directly onto bone. Graftless techniques have been advocated by some as a way of improving skin match and reducing operative time. This approach relies on thinning and undermining interdigitating flaps to permit direct closure. Care must be taken with this method to avoid excessive tension and resultant vascular compromise.[15]

Single-stage releases of both sides of a digit should be avoided as this may jeopardize digital vascularity in cases of anomalous vascular anatomy. For example, in short multiple syndactylous fingers, dominant digital vessels can only exist on the lateral sides of the conjoined fingers. Sometimes it is necessary to sacrifice one of the vessels in a distal bifurcation. The digital nerves can usually be gently separated more proximally.

Tips

In a complete syndactyly with separate nails or partly fused nails, on separation of the pulps the skin can generally be advanced to close the resultant defects. In conjoined nails without a ridge, the lateral nail fold requires reconstruction,

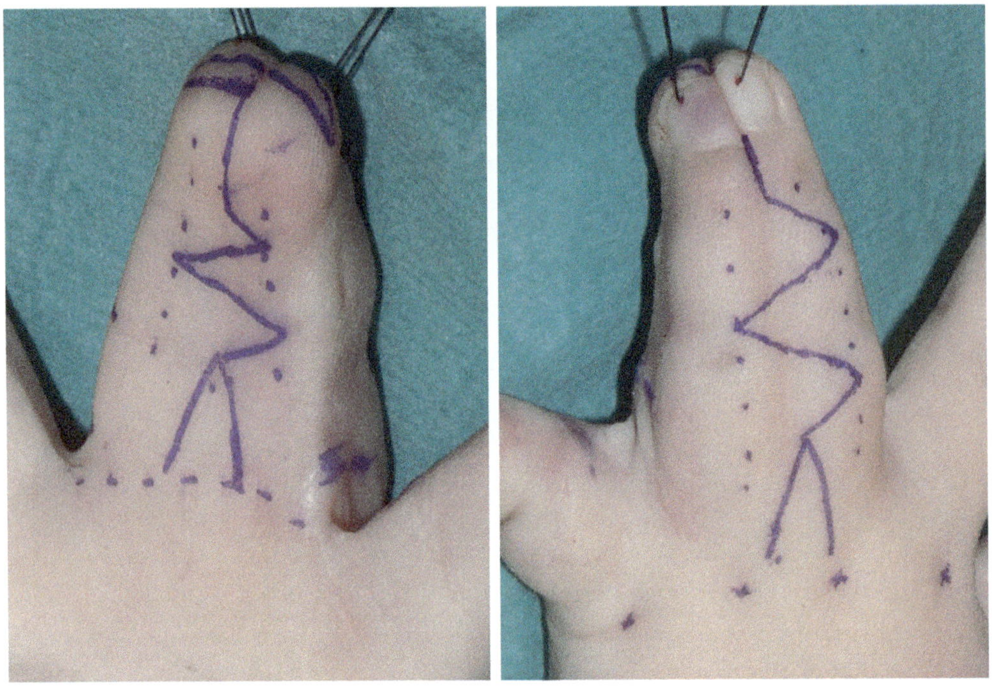

• **Fig. 45.3** Author's preferred technique for syndactyly release using interdigitating triangular flaps. Design of interdigitating flaps marked on volar and dorsal sides of simple complete syndactyly.

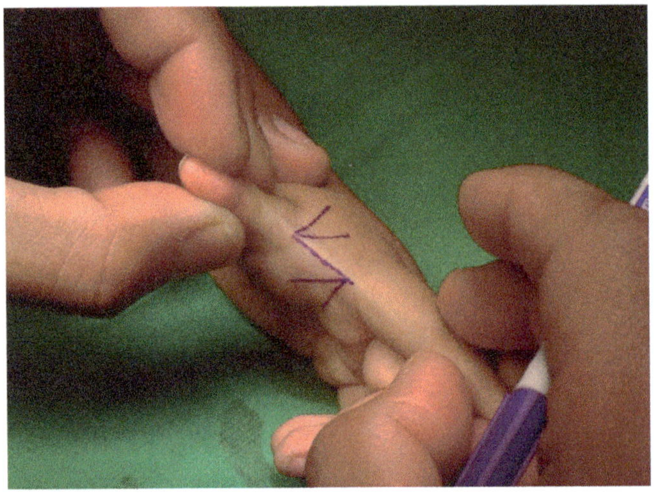

• **Fig. 45.4** Preferred method of first web release using a four-flap Z-plasty.

most commonly with interdigitating flaps from the hyponychium, e.g., Buck–Gramcko "stiletto" flaps[16] (Fig. 45.5). Care must be taken to ensure these paronychial reconstructions are not too bulky and do not leave an excessively narrow tip.

Clinodactyly

Clinodactyly (Greek *clino* = deviated, *dactylos* = digit/finger) is a congenital deformity in the radioulnar plane at the phalangeal level. Incidence is reported as 1%–19.5% depending on the degree of angulation used to define it.[17] It is inherited as an autosomal dominant trait with incomplete penetrance though the exact etiology is unknown. The angulation commonly occurs as a result of a triangular-shaped, "delta" or trapezoidal, middle phalanx (Fig. 45.6), though more rarely the proximal phalanx can be involved. This is formed by an abnormal C-shaped epiphysis (longitudinal bracketed or comma-shaped), the arm of which extends onto the ulnar side of the middle phalanx (Fig. 45.6A). The articular surface of the phalanx does not lie perpendicular to the longitudinal axis of the finger. The middle phalanx ossifies later than the other phalanges and latest in the little finger, hence clinodactyly occurs most commonly in the little finger. The thumb is the second most common. Clinodactyly most frequently occurs as an isolated familial abnormality. However, it may also be linked to syndromes including the Apert (thumb), Trisomy 21, Poland, Treacher Collins and Klinefelter syndromes.[18]

Clinical Assessment

The most common presentation congenitally is in the little finger, with radial deviation of more than 10 degrees, seen at the proximal interphalangeal (PIP) and distal interphalangeal (DIP) joints, and a positive family history.[19] An acquired deformity may occur due to growth plate injury or deviation following syndactyly release. Kirner's deformity may be mistaken for clinodactyly. However, Kirner's deformity represents a volar and radial curvature at the DIP joint. It most commonly affects females and appears between the ages of 7 and 14 years, often presenting as a painless swelling at the base of the nail.[20]

A common presenting complaint with clinodactyly is cosmesis as milder forms are not associated with any functional

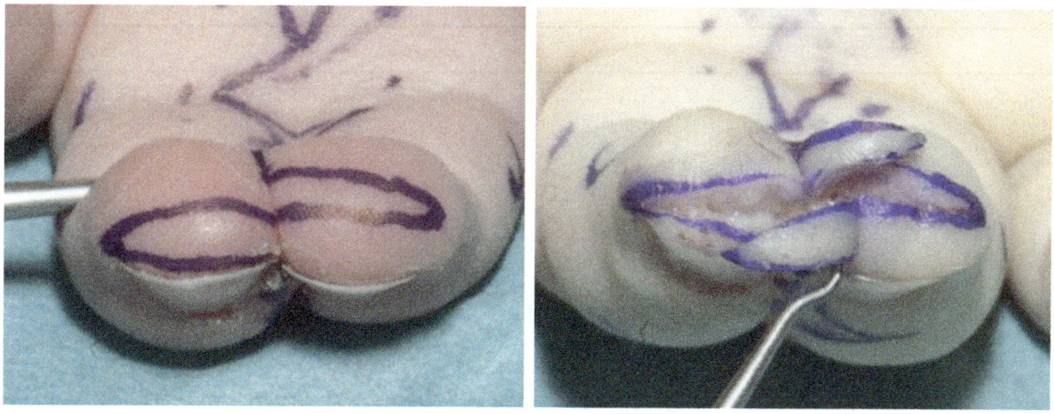

• **Fig. 45.5** Buck-Gramcko stiletto flaps used for reconstruction of paronychial folds.

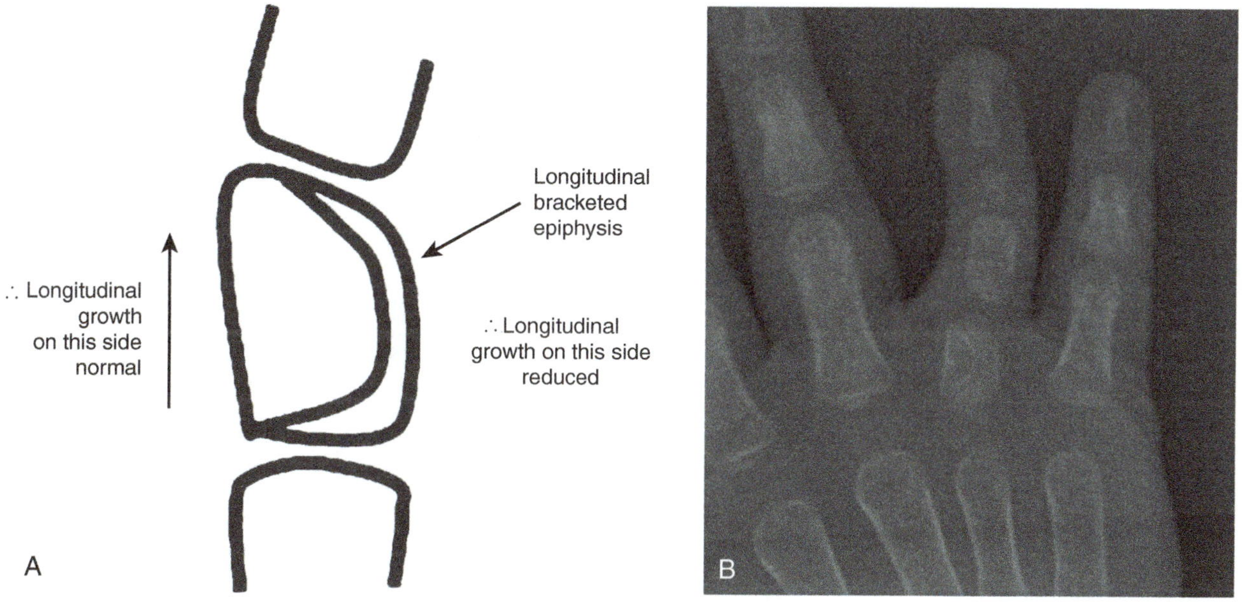

• **Fig. 45.6** Formation of a trapezoidal phalanx as the result of a longitudinal bracketed epiphysis. (A) Growth on the side of the bracketed epiphysis is compromised. (B) Radiograph of a clinodactylous digit with a trapezoidal proximal phalanx.

impairment. However, with worsening angulation, function can become impaired. Radiographic assessment allows identification of an abnormal or bracketed epiphysis. The status of the growth plate is an important factor in deciding treatment.

Surgical Principles and Management

As the abnormality is primarily skeletal and not corrected with growth, there is little role for splintage or stretches. The main indication for surgery is worsening deviation with associated functional impairment. This commonly occurs with deviations of more than 20–30 degrees. Age and the status of the epiphysis are critical factors. If growing, physiolysis with resection of the lateral physis and interposition of a fat graft can achieve good results with reliance then on the finger growing straight and correcting itself.[21] This is best done before the age of 6 years. Durability of this procedure is influenced by the extent of soft tissue release at the time of surgery.[21] Epiphyseal bar resection with fat grafting is best avoided in small triangular-shaped bones with minimal growth potential and best not repeated to avoid premature epiphyseal closure. With persistent deformity or after completion of growth, correction is best achieved via osteotomy procedures. These include a closing wedge osteotomy, where bony wegde is removed from the longer side in order to correct angulation. If length preservation is more critical an opening wedge, reverse wedge or dome osteotomy (Fig. 45.7) may be more appropriate. However, in this form of correction the soft tissue deficit on the shorter side must be addressed in order to facilitate correction and prevent recurrence in the long term. This can be achieved through techniques such as Z-plasties or local transposition flaps. Our preference whenever possible is for an opening wedge or dome osteotomy (see Fig. 45.7) with longitudinal K-wire fixation.

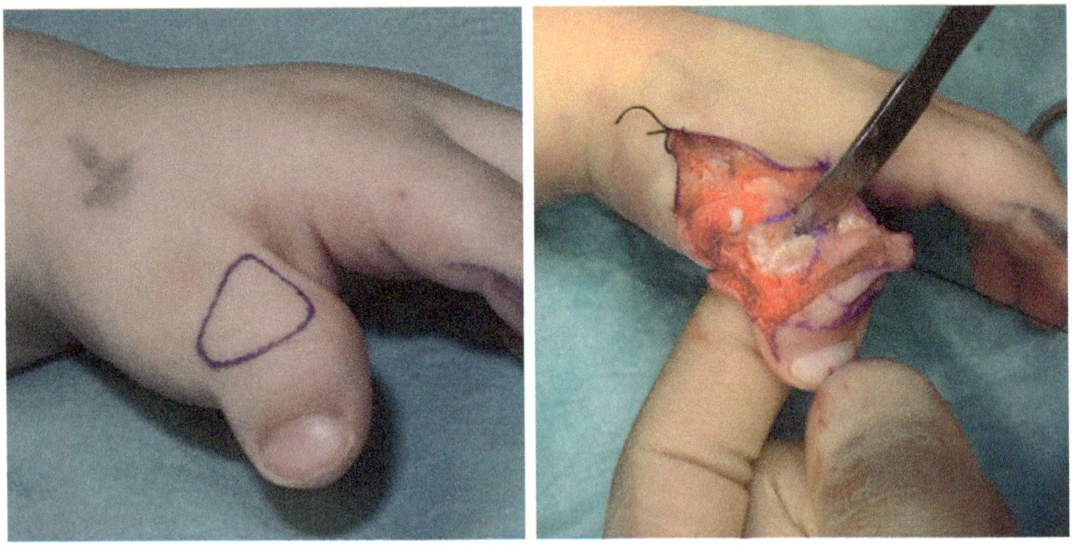

• **Fig. 45.7** A dome osteotomy for correction of clinodactyly. The dome is created via multiple K-wire holes in an arch configuration linked through the use of an osteotome or fine side-cutting burr.

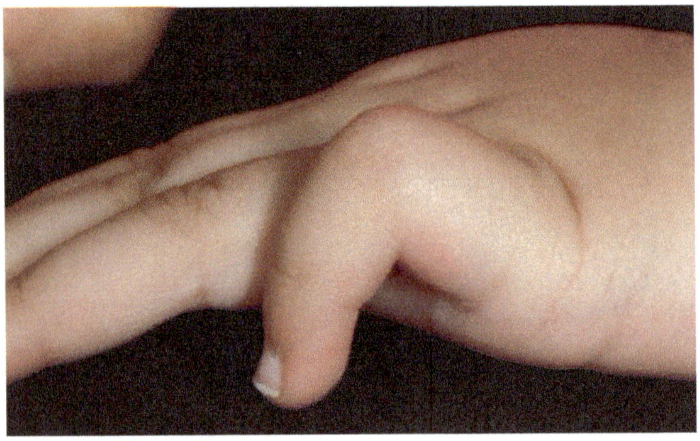

• **Fig. 45.8** Image of a camptodactylous little finger. A web can be seen across the proximal interphalangeal joint.

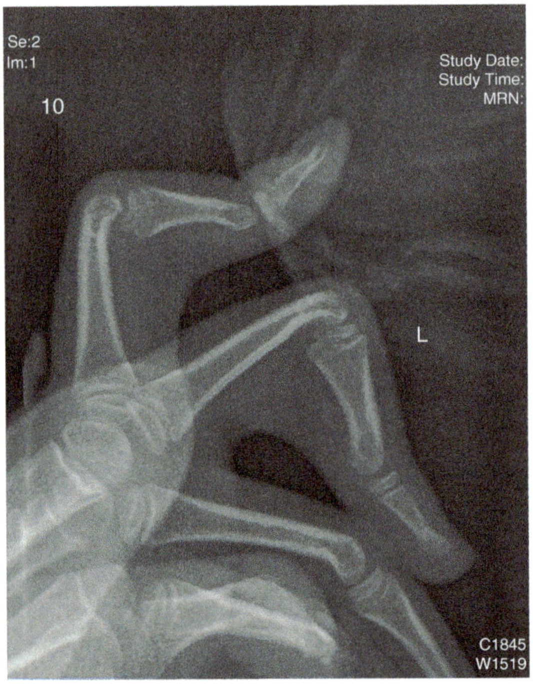

• **Fig. 45.9** Radiographic image of camptodactylous digits, demonstrating narrowing of the joint space in the proximal interphalangeal joint, flattening with volar curvature of the head of the proximal phalanx, and flattening of the base of the middle phalanx.

Camptodactyly

Camptodactyly (Greek *kampylos* = arched, *dactylos* = digit/finger) is a congenital flexion deformity of the PIP joint (Fig. 45.8). There are approximately 1 million cases in the UK per year. The little finger is affected most commonly (70%), then the ring (20%), and then the other digits (10%). Bilateral involvement is common and multiple digits can be affected. Two common patterns of presentation exist. Firstly, in the newborn age group worsening during the 1–4-year growth spurt. In this group males and females tend to be equally affected. Secondly, in the adolescent growth spurt between 10 and 14 years of age, in which there is a female preponderance. The condition tends to not progress beyond skeletal maturity. Most cases are sporadic. However in 30% of cases it is inherited as an autosomal dominant trait.[22]

Pathology

Virtually every structure crossing volar to the PIP joint has been implicated in the condition. However, abnormalities can be divided into primary causal anomalies and those that are secondary effects. The primary causes are abnormal lumbrical and flexor digitorum superficialis anatomy. Tightness and aberrant distal insertions lead to a flexor–extensor imbalance. Secondary effects include abnormalities of the retinaculum cutis, volar plate, collateral ligaments lateral bands, central slip, and skeletal changes.[22] Skeletal changes such as joint space narrowing, flexion of the proximal phalangeal head, and flattening of the base of the middle phalanx auger a poorer response to treatment and prognosis (Fig. 45.9).

TABLE 45.3 Foucher Classification of Camptodactyly

Grade	Description
Ia	Early and stiff
Ib	Early and correctable
IIa	Late and stiff
IIb	Late and correctable

Data from: Foucher G, Lorea P, Khouri RK, et al. Camptodactyly as a spectrum of congenital deficiencies: a treatment algorithm based on clinical examination. *Plast Reconstr Surg*. 2006;117(6):1897–1905.

Clinical Assessment

Functional impairment can occur when the flexion contracture exceeds 60 degrees and multiple digits are involved. Otherwise issues tend to be more cosmetic. Foucher described four types[23] (Table 45.3).

Factors associated with a poor response to treatment include skeletal changes, older patients (teenagers), with stiff joints and those who demonstrate poor compliance with hand therapy.[23]

Surgical Principles and Management

The mainstay of initial management is stretching and splintage. We reserve surgical intervention for patients with a progressive condition despite compliance to hand therapy and flexion contractures of more than 60 degrees. Outcomes from surgery range from 14% to 35% improvement.[22] Outcomes from hand therapy in young children in the Japanese population have been excellent, with an 80%–92% improvement reported[24] though poorer in Caucasian series (mean improvement of 40°).[23]

Preferred Method of Surgical Correction

All abnormal structures both primary and secondary, must be addressed. We use a volar longitudinal approach with Z-plasty lengthening as required. Steps include:

1. Release of the retinaculum cutis, lateral digital sheets, and Grayson's ligaments.
2. Release of any abnormal insertions of the lateral bands and interossei.
3. The lumbricals are inspected and abnormal insertions are released.
4. If the flexor digitorum superficialis (FDS) is functional and traction on the lateral bands produces PIP joint extension an FDS transfer to the extensor mechanism via the lumbrical canal can be performed.
5. If the FDS is deficient proximally and not useable it is released.
6. If the flexor digitorum profundus (FDP) or FDS musculotendinous units are short but functional they can be fractionally or step-lengthened in the forearm.
7. Joint release may be necessary, including release of the check rein ligaments, accessory collaterals, and volar plate in turn as required.
8. Our preference is to avoid skeletal correction as this leads to further stiffness of the PIP joint and a poorer outcome.

However, no single procedure has proved to be universally successful. Other techniques described include Glicenstein's subperiosteal release,[25] angulation osteotomy and arthrodesis.

TABLE 45.4 The Expanded Wassel Classification System of Thumb Duplication Based upon Radiographic Appearance

Grade	Description
Type I	Bifid distal phalanx
Type II	Duplicated distal phalanx (approximately 20%)
Type III	Bifid proximal phalanx
Type IV	Duplicated proximal phalanx (commonest, approximately 50%)
Type V	Bifid metacarpal
Type VI	Duplicated metacarpal
Type VII	Triphalangeal, in either or both thumbs (approximately 12%)

Data from: Wassel HD. The results of surgery for polydactyly of the thumb. *Clin Orthop Rel Res*. 1969;64:175–193; Wood VE. Polydactyly and the triphalangeal thumb. *J Hand Surg*. 1978;3(5):436–444; Hung L, Cheng JC, Bundoc R, et al. Thumb duplication at the metacarpophalangeal joint. Management and a new classification. *Clin Orthop Rel Res*. 1996;(323):31–41.

Duplication

Duplication may involve the whole limb or part of a limb. Polydactyly occurs when greater than five digits or toes are present. It may occur as an isolated anomaly, either sporadic or inherited, or syndromal with a multitude of associated syndromes described. Syndromic polydactyly may occur in combinations such as radial with ulnar and may coexist with other hand and foot anomalies. The aims of surgical intervention are to improve function, especially in terms of glove and shoe fitting, and cosmesis. Upper limb polydactyly is the focus of this section.

Radial Polydactyly

Radial, or preaxial, polydactyly occurs in 1 in 3000 live births.[17] It is usually unilateral and sporadic, with no associations. The expanded Wassel classification with contributions from Wood in 1978 and Hung in 1996 is generally the most widely used system[26–28] (Table 45.4). A significant proportion of cases may not fit completely into this classification and so additional terms such as deviation or triphalangism can be used. Chromosome 7q36, harbouring the regulatory element of the SHH protein, is implicated in the rarer dominantly inherited radial polydactyly.[29] Typically there is some degree of hypoplasia of both duplicates with the radial usually the smaller of the two (see Fig. 45.11A). The ulnar-innervated intrinsics to the thumb typically insert onto the ulnar-most duplicate and the median-innervated onto the radial duplicate.

Clinical Examination

Other anomalies may be present and so it is always important to examine all four limbs. More specifically, in radial polydactyly the thenar musculature may be hypoplastic, especially with increasing Wassel grade.[19] The extrinsics are usually Y-shaped and asymmetrical with hypoplasia or absence involving the smallest digit. Simultaneous flexion or extension may occur with or without deviation. The joints may be stiff, hypermobile or hypoplastic. Note the presence of creases and hence the chance of active movement following surgery. There may be asymmetry of the pulps and nail beds. The first web may be tight, especially with more proximal duplications.

Surgical Principles and Management

Our preference for timing of surgical correction is between 12 and 18 months of age as long as other more pressing comordities have been addressed. In an unbalanced duplication the thumb to be retained and reconstructed should be first determined. Different parts from each thumb may need to be used in order to provide the best complement of structures for stability and function.[19] Careful dissection of the intrinsic and extrinsic muscles, and tendons and ligamentous structures must be carried out. Pollex abductus – an abnormal deviating radial connection between the flexor and extensor apparatus – must be looked for and divided if present to allow for unrestricted motion and growth.[30] Preservation of an optimal neurovascular supply is important for thumb viability and the preservation of sensibility. One-stage reconstruction, including osteotomies, to ensure correct skeletal alignment is recommended.

Correction of Distal Duplications (Wassel Types I to III)

Unbalanced Distal Duplications

In unbalanced distal duplications where one side is larger with a well-formed nail, excision of the deficient partner, most commonly the radial, is best. The preserved duplicate – usually the ulnar is augmented with tissue salvaged from its radial partner. Incisions are planned high in the axial line dorsal to the junction of glabrous and non-glabrous skin. The radial border of the ulnar thumb is excised to allow insetting of the flap. During the dissection, the radial nail and bone are excised, and the tendons are sectioned at the level of their division. Only one nail is preserved. A broad proximal phalangeal head can be trimmed. Residual deviation of the thumb can be corrected via a closing wedge osteotomy of the distal phalanx in type II duplications or proximal phalanx in type III. Reconstruction of a radial collateral ligament using local tissue is important in this technique.

Balanced Distal Duplications

Decision-making becomes more complex when the duplications are hypoplastic but of equivalent size (balanced type). One approach in this situation is a modified Bilhaut–Cloquet procedure using asymmetric skeletal elements from each phalanx in an effort to preserve joint surface integrity and an entire nail bed from one duplicate to avoid a nail ridge.[31] However, this approach can still result in a broad and esthetically suboptimal thumb so the aforementioned method of retaining one duplicate and augmenting it with tissue salvaged from the other is preferred whenever possible.

Correction of Type IV Duplications

Generally, the best approach for these the most common of pre-axial duplications, is the preservation of the ulnar more developed thumb and reconstruction of motion and stability using elements from its radial partner. The principles and steps are similar to those in type II reconstruction with also initial detachment and subsequent reattachment of the intrinsic muscles. Incisions are planned around the radial duplicate to be excised, preserving skin to allow for soft tissue recontouring of the retained thumb. Decisions around which duplicate to retain becomes more complex in a balanced duplication (Fig. 45.10). Skeletal work is often necessary to achieve long-term correction of alignment. The bifid head of the metacarpal must be trimmed to prevent residual exostosis distorting the radial contour of the reconstructed thumb. An additional osteotomy of the metacarpal may be necessary to correct any residual clinodactyly. This involves the removal of a triangular wedge of metacarpal neck to create a perpendicular articular surface. The osteotomy is fixed with a longitudinal K-wire and the radial collateral ligament should be reconstructed if possible. The latter may not be possible due to the extensive dissection required for skeletal realignment, and stability relies upon correct reinsertion of intrinsic musculature in particular the abductor digiti minimi.

Correction of Proximal Duplications (Wassel Types V, VI, and VII)

The basic principles outlined above apply to those of type V, VI, and VII duplications. The ulnar more developed thumb is usually retained and reconstructed (Fig. 45.11). The intrinsic muscles must be repositioned, the lax radial collateral ligament must be tightened and the extrinsic tendons centralized if necessary. Adduction contractures in the first web must also be released to improve function. In type VI duplications where both the metacarpophalangeal (MCP)

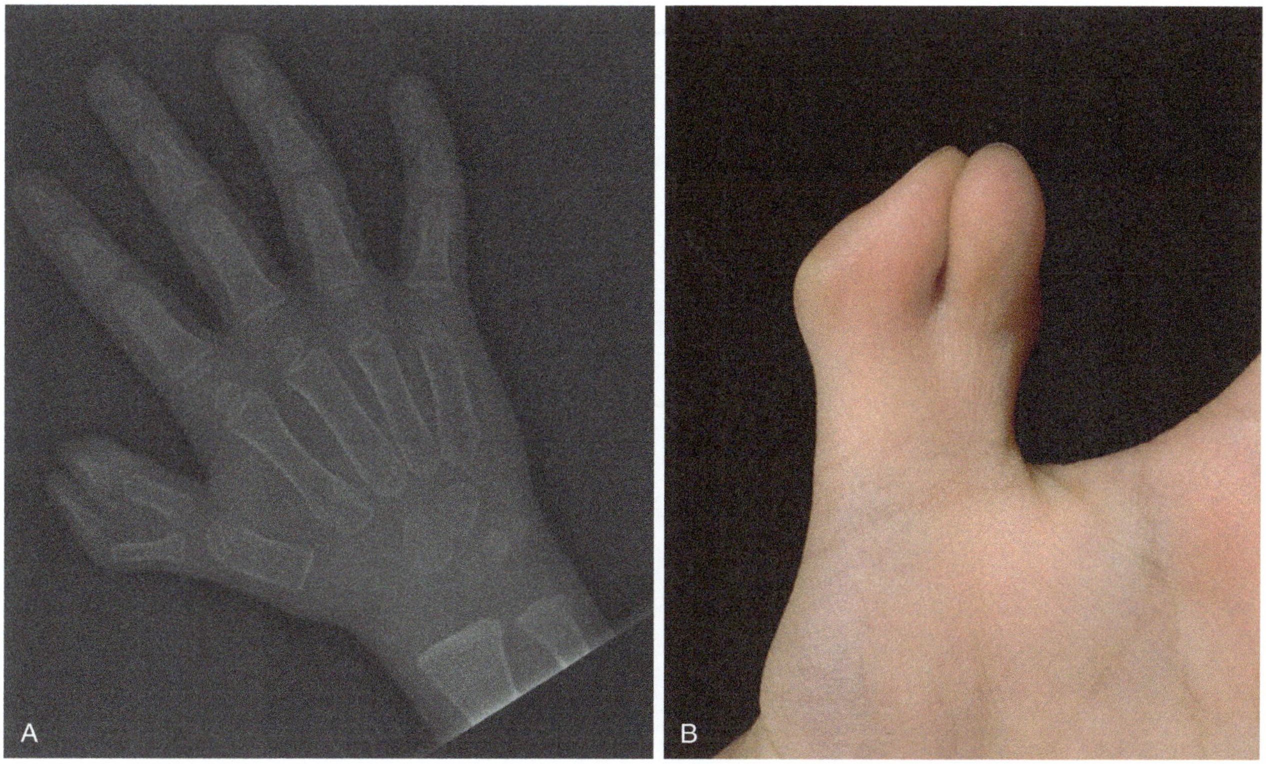

• **Fig. 45.10** Wassel IV thumb duplication. (A) Radiographic image of a balanced Wassel type IV duplication demonstrating duplication from the proximal phalangeal distally. (B) Image of a patient with a Wassel type IV thumb duplication.

and carpometacarpal (CPC) joints are abnormal an epiphyseal-sparing chondrodesis at the MCP joint will provide the necessary stability for a functional thumb. In type VII duplications the thumb with the two phalanges is retained if it is the more stable and components of the triphalangeal duplicate used for reconstruction. If the thumbs are comparable in size and functionality then preference should be given to that with the more stable ulnar collateral ligament at the MCP joint.[17] In some instances triphalangeal thumb reconstruction may require an on-top-plasty whereby the distal portion of one thumb is transferred to the proximal part of the other with the better basal joint.

Ulnar Polydactyly

Ulnar, or postaxial, polydactyly occurs in 1 in 500 live births.[17] It is the most common congenital hand anomaly. It is often bilateral and usually of autosomal dominant inheritance. Temtamy and McKusick in 1969 divided ulnar polydactyly into type A duplications, which were more developed and substantial, and type B, which were rudimentary and pedunculated.[32] Type B are ten times more common in the African population. Whereas type A is rarer and its incidence is more common across races.[33] Ulnar polydactyly, in particular the more substantial type A, is associated with a number of different syndromes, especially in Caucasian and Asian populations. These include chromosomal abnormalities such as Trisomy 13 and 18 and bone dysplasias such as Ellis–Van Creveld.

Classification

Stelling and Turek in 1963 classified ulnar polydactyly into three types based on the degree of duplication,[34] as shown in Table 45.5 and Fig. 45.12. Type I within this classification is the most common (see Fig. 45.12A). However, clinically there is a spectrum of complexity and the common small pedunculated digit usually has at least a nail and distal phalanx. A neurovascular bundle is always present, however rudimentary the appendage. The digit may autoinfarct and autoamputate prior to presentation.

Clinical Examination

Clinical assessment follows the principles of radial polydactyly. The most common site of attachment when a more developed digit is present is at the MCP joint level. It is often abducted at the MCP joint and radially deviated at the PIP joint. The extrinsics tendons are usually Y-shaped and asymmetrical, as in radial polydactyly.[19]

Surgical Principles and Management

Type I (Fig. 45.12A)

We find ligaclip ligation or crushing with diathermy to the neurovascular bundle at the base in an outpatient setting effective, being less likely to leave a residual nubbin than the more traditional tying off. Alternatively, formal excision under local anesthetic can be performed within the first 3 months of age.

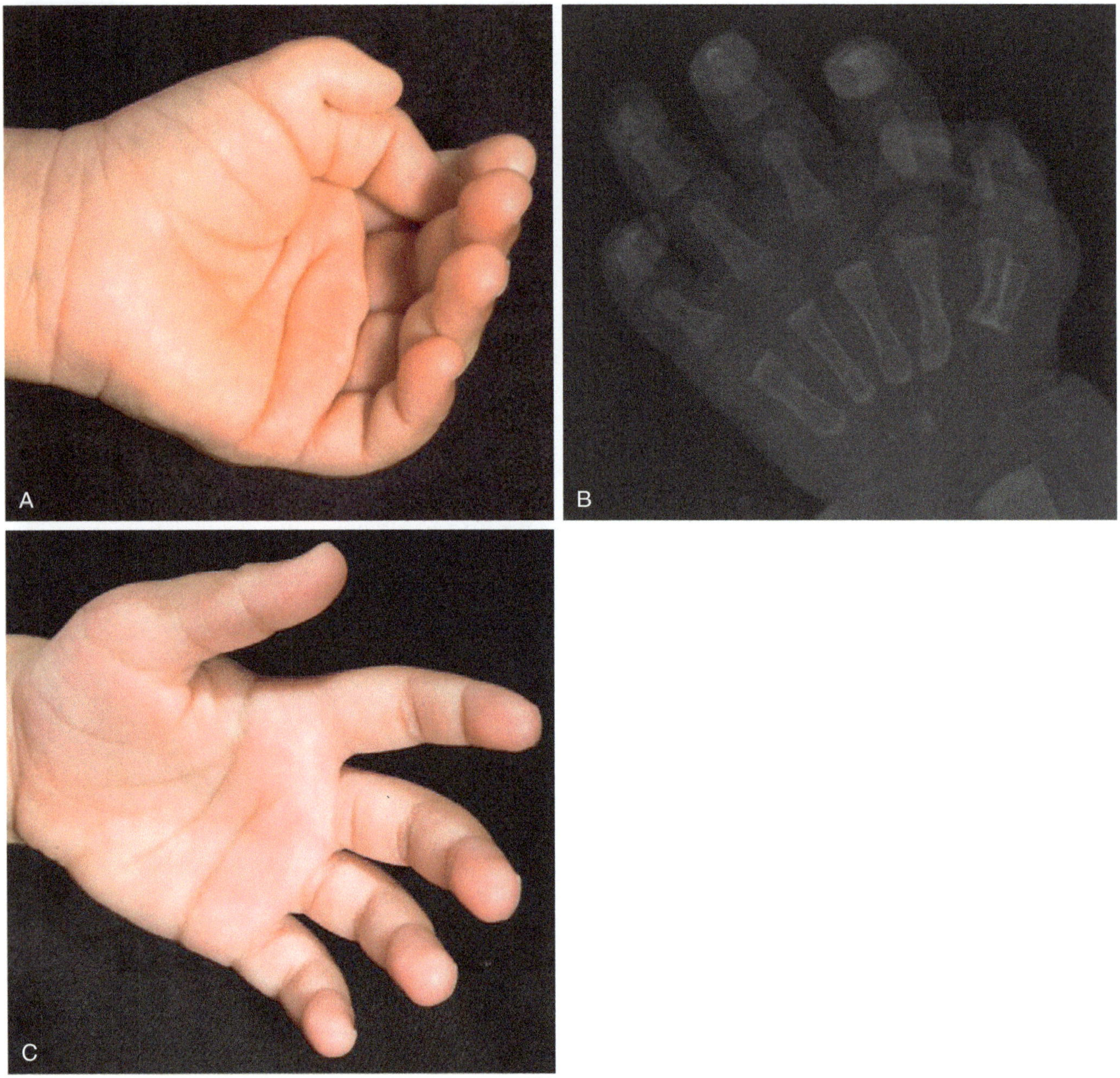

• **Fig. 45.11** Reconstruction of a Wassel type VII duplication. (A) Preoperative image of an unbalanced type VII duplication. (B) Preoperative radiograph demonstrating smaller triphalangeal radial duplicate. (C) Postoperative image of corrected type VII duplication after removal of radial duplicate.

TABLE 45.5 Stelling and Turek Classification of Ulnar Polydactyly

Grade	Description
Type I	Soft tissue mass without skeletal structure and skin bridge only (pedunculated)
Type II	Digit with all normal components and articulating with a normal or bifid metacarpal or phalanx
Type III	Complete digit articulating with an extra metacarpal

Data from: Stelling F. The upper extremity. In: Ferguson AB, ed. *Orthopedic Surgery in Infancy and Childhood*. Baltimore: Williams & Wilkins; 1963:282–402.

Type II (Fig. 45.12C)

The ulnar duplicate is usually the most hypoplstic and is therefore removed with preservation of the ulnar collateral ligament at the MCP joint if required and reinsertion of any aberrantly positioned hypothenar musculature. Trimming of a broad metacarpal head may be required to create the optimal ulnar contour. Resection of the metacarpal head and MCP joint reconstruction may be necessary.

Type III (Fig. 45.12D, E)

Principles detailed above with reference to type II corrections apply in particular with unbalanced type III polydactyly. In balanced type III situations it is preferable to retain the ulnar ray with its intact complement of hypothenar muscles.

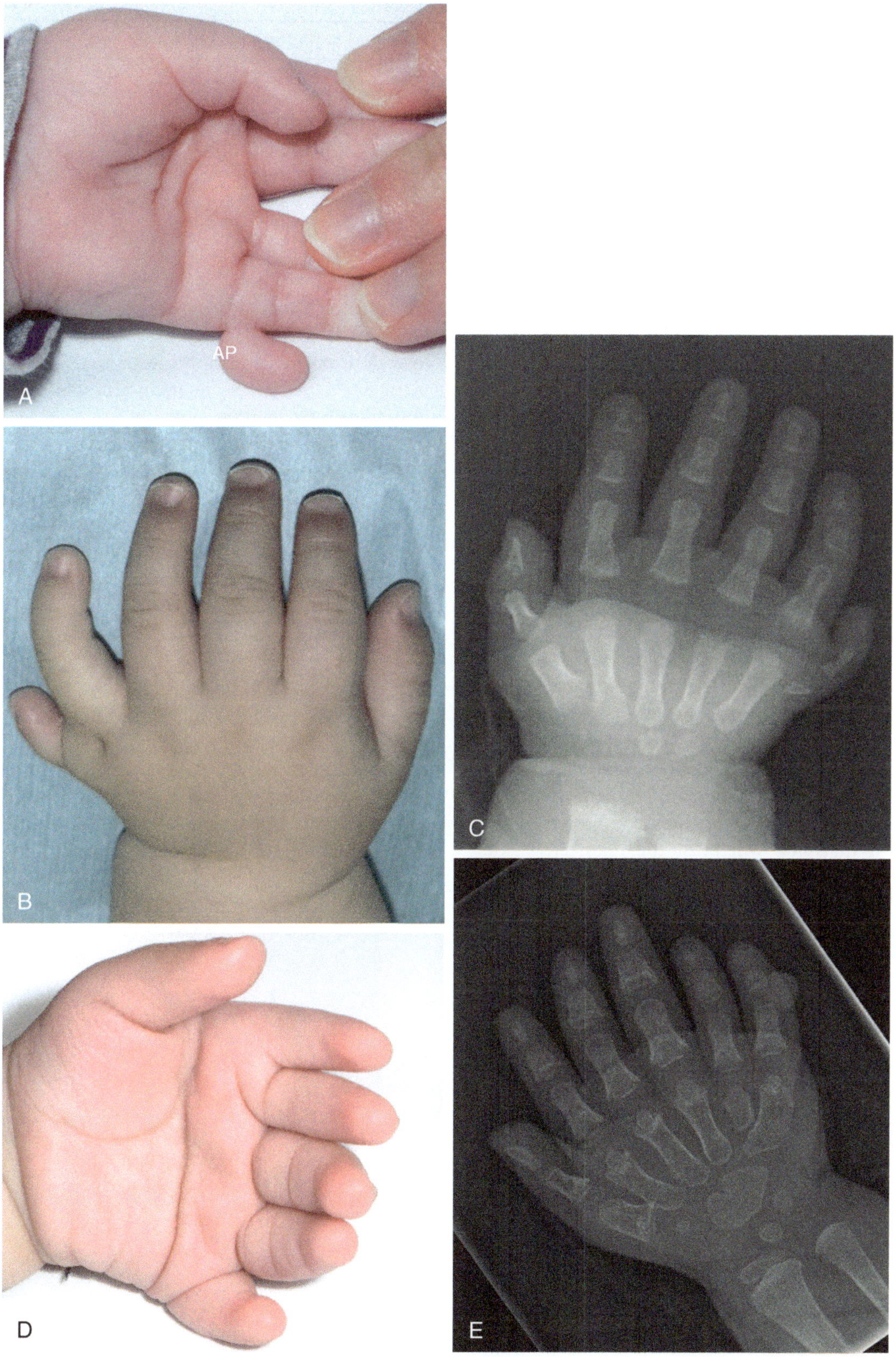

• **Fig. 45.12** Images of three Stelling grades of ulnar polydactyly.[70] (A) Type I – pedunculated soft tissue digital mass. (B,C) Type II – complete digit articulating with bifid phalanx or metacarpal. (D,E) Type III – complete digit along with extra metacarpal.

Central Polydactyly

Central polydactyly is a rare condition. The ring finger is most often involved followed by the middle, then the index. A complete extra independent digit is rare. Often the situation is more complex, involving more than one digit with aberrant bones and abnormalities of the extrinsics, intrinsics, and neurovascular supply[12] Examples include duplication of the middle finger proximally at the metacarpal level, which shifts to an apparent duplication of the ring finger within the digit. Duplication of the ring finger is often partial and hidden by a syndactyly with the middle digit. Polysyndactyly can be associated with *HOXD19* gene mutations with involvement of the little toe of the foot together with a suppressed polysyndactyly of the ring finger.[35] Surgical management should be considered carefully in central polydactyly as involved digits are often deficient, with significant soft tissue anomalies with poor function upon release.

Macrodactyly

Macrodactyly involves the localized enlargement of all structures of an affected digit (see Figs. 45.13 and 45.14). This distinguishes it from conditions where only part of the digit is involved, e.g., hemangiomas, and vascular malformations. It is rare, with an estimated incidence of 0.2 per 10,000 births. It affects the index most commonly and is usually unilateral.

The enlarged area often corresponds to the cutaneous distribution of specific nerves, i.e., nerve territory-orientated macrodactyly.[36] If one digital nerve is affected, the macrodactyly on that side will push the unaffected side away from the midline causing a clinodactyly. If the common digital nerve is affected, both sides of adjacent fingers will be involved, leading to divergent clinodactyly . Macrodactyly tends to follow two patterns of progression – a static form where growth is commensurate with the child's limb and a progressive form in which the growth is out of proportion (Fig. 45.13).[37] It can also be classified into five types according to specific disease entities as described by Flatt and expanded by Upton.[17,38] Type I is associated with lipofibromatosis (Fig. 45.14), II with neurofibromatosis, III with hyperostosis, IV with hemihypertrophy, and V with additional conditions linked to overgrowth.[38] Conditions associated with overgrowth include Proteus and Beckwith–Wiedemann syndromes.[39]

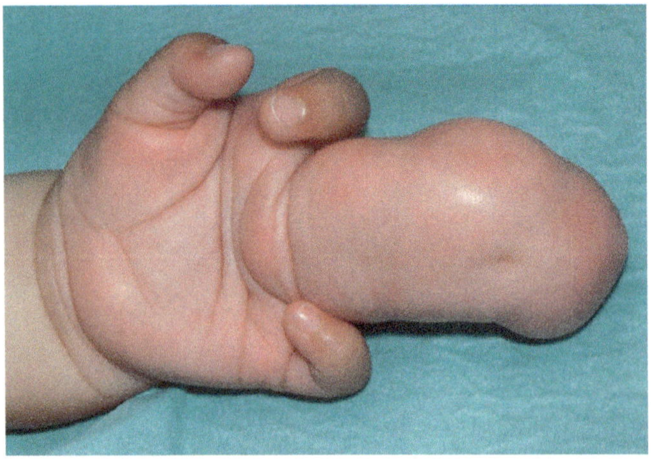

• **Fig. 45.13** Image of a patient with macrodactyly affecting predominantly the central two rays with an associated syndactyly.

Surgical Principles and Management

Management of these cases is challenging due to the extensive nature and relentless progression of the condition. Surgery can be complicated by problems of delayed healing, infection, and hypertrophic scarring.[39] The aims of treatment are to reduce bulk, maintain sensation and preserve joint motion whenever possible.[40] Careful counseling and the individualization of treatment is crucial. Psychological support is important as the psychosocial distress macrodactyly causes to patients and their families should not be underestimated. The main surgical options are epiphyseal ablation (epiphysiodesis), soft tissue debulking with or without skeletal reduction (see Fig. 45.14), and finally, amputation. Nerve stripping or resection has also been recommended by some authors in an effort to suppress the neurotrophic drive seen in cases of nerve-orientated or neurofibromatosis-type overgrowth.[41] However, the long-term results of nerve excision/neurolysis are unpredictable and do not reliably prevent overgrowth. Epiphysiodesis is carried out to control longitudinal growth. It is best carried out when the size of the affected digit reaches that of the parents. Destruction of the growth bar can be achieved with a needle, burr or osteotome under radiographic guidance. This often requires

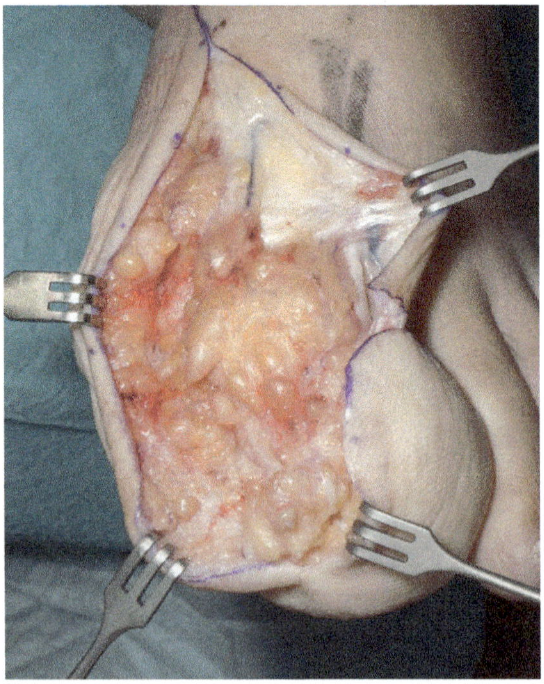

• **Fig. 45.14** Intraoperative image of a case of macrodactyly demonstrating hamartomatous overgrowth of all tissues.

repetition and can be combined with debulking procedures to control circumferental girth. However, results from serial debulking surgery can be frustrating and the endpoint, despite early and repeated intervention, is often amputation, particularly in cases with a progressive growth pattern. Amputation should not be considered a treatment failure as it can significantly unencumber the hand thereby improving overall function and cosmesis. Careful joint decision-making with the patient and family must be carried out to avoid a protracted course with repeated hospital admissions and surgical procedures.[39,40]

Thumb Hypoplasia

Thumb hypoplasia can significantly impact on hand use as the thumb contributes to at least 50% of overall hand function. Thumb hypoplasia represents a spectrum of abnormalities that range from structurally normal but small thumbs, through varying degrees of skeletal and soft tissue deficiency to complete thumb aplasia. It can exist as an isolated entity but is commonly seen as a component feature of radial ray deficiency. Its true incidence is hard to ascertain as thumb hypoplasia is present in a multitude of congenital malformations, in particular central and transverse deficiencies. Incidences of up to 37% of all congenital hand anomalies have been reported. The etiology is complex, encompassing multiple genetic and environmental factors. This is confirmed through links to many different conditions, each with distinct etiologies, including Fanconi's anemia, thrombocytopenia with absence of radius (TAR) syndome, Holt–Oram syndrome, and the vertebral, anal, cardiac, tracheal, esophageal, renal and limb association (VACTERL).[42] Therefore involvement of a geneticist is advised.

Classification

The classification of thumb hypoplasia has evolved since that first proposed by Muller in 1937.[43] Currently the most widely accepted is the Blauth classification,[44] which has been refined through contributions from Buck-Gramcko in 1981,[45] Manske et al in 1995[46] and Smith in 2002[47] (Table 45.6). Complete assessment of thumb hypoplasia must incorporate detailed analysis of its size and position in relation to the other digits, the first web space, intrinsic musculature, extrinsic tendons, and quality and stability of the thumb osseoarticular column to ensure optimal management. Accurate classification of anatomical and functional deficiency allows planning of surgical treatment.

Grade 1

There may be hypoplasia of the phalanges and metacarpal with weak intrinsics. The first web may be marginally tight. Joints are all present and stable. There is excellent function and parents may be unaware of any hypoplasia. This form is common in those with a contralateral more severe radial dysplasia.

TABLE 45.6 The Modified Blauth Classification of Thumb Hypoplasia

Grade	Features
1	Mild hypoplasia with all structures present
2	Moderate hypoplasia Thenar muscle hypoplasia MCP joint laxity Modified by Smith: 2A = ulnar collateral ligament laxity only 2B = global instability of MCP joint
3	Severe hypoplasia Metacarpal hypoplasia Thenar muscle hypoplasia Extrinsic hypoplasia Modified by Manske et al: 3A = relatively stable CMC joint present 3B = unstable CMC joint
4	No metacarpal present Floating thumb (French *pouce flottant*; German *Pendeldaumen*) Complete absence

Data from: Blauth W. [The hypoplastic thumb]. *Arch Orthop Unfallchir*. 1967;62(3):225–246; Buck-Gramcko D. Hypoplasia and aplasia of the thumb. In: Buck-Gramcko D, Nigst H, Millesi H, eds. *Hand Surgery*. Stuttgart: Thième; 1981; Manske PR, McCarroll HR Jr., James M. Type III–A hypoplastic thumb. *J Hand Surg*. 1995;20(2):246–253; Smith P. Congenital. In: Lister G, ed. *The Hand: Diagnosis and Indications*, 4th edn. Edinburgh: Churchill Livingstone; 2002:457–522.

Grade 2

The metacarpal and phalanges are present but may be narrower and smaller than usual. In addition, the radial carpus, particularly the trapezium, trapezoid, and scaphoid, may be hypoplastic. A large spectrum of soft tissue abnormalities can occur affecting both the extrinsic and intrinsic radial musculature. The median innervated thenar muscles, in particular the opponens pollicis and abductor pollicis brevis, are underdeveloped and weak. In contrast, the ulnar innervated intrinsics, particularly the adductor pollicis, are strong, which results in an abnormal adduction of the thumb and resultant narrowing of the first web space. Hypoplasia of the thenar intrinsics leads to a weakness of thumb opposition, another defining feature of type 2 hypoplasia. This in combination with instability of the MCP joint further compounds thumb dysfunction. In particular, laxity of the ulnar collateral ligament leads to radial collapse of the thumb during pinch. Grade 2A thumbs are defined by uniaxial (ulnar) instability and 2B by multiaxial instability of the MCP joint.[47] Pollex abductus may also be present, causing radial deviation distal to the MCP joint through abnormal connections between the flexors and the extensor mechanism.[30]

Grade 3

Features of grade 2 thumbs are present but with more pronounced osseoarticular and extrinsic musculature deficiency. The osseous deficiency is most significant at the proximal metacarpal level rendering the thumb even more unstable.[48] There is in addition a degree of hypoplasia of the radial carpus, in particular the scaphoid, which is often absent. The distal radius is smaller and there is hypoplasia or total absence of the radial styloid. The thumb MCP joint is unstable in all directions with severe underdevelopment of the collateral ligaments and volar plate. Intrinsic and extrinsic muscle abnormalities are pronounced. Flexors and extensors are usually present but are markedly weak. Abnormal tendinous interconnections can be present producing a pollex abductus deformity[30] Intrinsic muscles are similarly underdeveloped, particularly those innervated by the median nerve, whereas ulnar-innervated adductor is relatively spared, compounding the first web adduction contracture.[49] Manske et al subdivided this category into types 3A and B.[46] In 3A thumbs, the metacarpal, although hypoplastic, is present, forming a relatively stable articulation at the CMC joint, whereas in the 3B thumb the proximal end of the first metacarpal is absent, which leads to instability of the CMC joint. As with the subclassification of the grade 2 group, qualification of grade 3 hypoplasia in this way helps guide surgical management.

Grade 4

These "floating" thumbs (pouce flottant) arise most commonly distally along the radial midaxial line of the hand. They usually comprise two hypoplastic phalanges within a pedunculated soft tissue envelope that is connected to the hand by a narrow skin bridge containing a neurovascular pedicle. There are no metacarpal or intrinsic muscle insertions into the phalanges. A first dorsal interosseous may, however, be present.[49]

Grade 5

This is defined by complete absence of the thumb and in 50% of cases there is a degree of radial deficiency.[17] The degree of radial hypoplasia correlates with deficiency within the index finger.[49] Hence those with a normal radius may try to "autopollicize" their index finger by pronating and abducting it and widening their second intermetacarpal space.[17,49]

Surgical Principles and Management

Grade 1 function well and no intervention is required. The aims of reconstruction in grade 2 thumbs is widening of the first web space, stabilization of the MCP joint and the provision of oppostion. All three aims can be achieved through one surgery. Release of the adduction contracture allows the thumb to passively abduct and oppose, utilizing the shape of the CMC joint. Simultaneous opponensplasty adds the active ability to do so.

Addressing the first web contracture must ensure adequate release of all structures, limiting thumb abduction, including the tight investing fascia over the adductor and first dorsal interosseous musculature. In addition, in severe cases release of the musculature itself from its origin or insertion may be required. Resurfacing the new opened web can be achieved in a number of ways, depending on the degree of skin deficit. Mild to moderate contractures can be dealt with adequately using a single or four flap Z-plasty technique. These also allow access to the MCP joint to facilitate joint stabilization and opposition transfers. More severe contractures may necessitate a large dorsal rotation/advancement flap to resurface the first web.[50] More complex options include regional pedicled flaps such as the radial forearm or posterior interosseous flap or free tissue transfer with thin pliable flaps, such as the groin flap.[51,52]

Management of the lax MCP joint and the provision of opposition should be guided by the type of joint instability seen.[53] Uniaxial (usually ulnar) instability of the MCP joint (grade 2A) can be corrected in the majority of cases as part of a FDS opposition transfer[54] (Fig. 45.15A). The two slips of the FDS usually from the ring finger can be split and passed through drill holes in the base of the proximal phalanx and the head of the metacarpal, in a square configuration, as originally described by Lister.[54] Our preference, however, is to place the tendon repair on the radial side of the MCP joint so that in pinch, tension is taken off it[53] (Fig. 45.15B). The use of the superficialis transfer in this way enables both MCP joint stabilization and thumb opposition using the distal border of the carpal tunnel as a pulley. In contrast, those with poor bone stock and instability in all planes (2B) require an epiphyseal plate-sparing fusion of the MCP joint – a chondrodesis, in combination with an abductor digit minimi opponensplasty[55] (Fig. 45.16) in order to produce equivalent functional results.[53]

Grade 3A thumbs are generally reconstructable following the aforementioned principles outlined for grade 2 thumbs. But beware that even though the CMC joint may be present it may be unstable or may appear stable at rest but may not be so in pinch. This is further exacerbated by MCP joint stabilization with increased force through the joint.

Grade 3B thumbs and onwards are best treated by ablation and substitution through pollicization of the index finger.[49] Despite the advantages of a pollicization in grade 3B, some cultural and parental beliefs may preclude the use of the index finger and demand alternative forms of reconstruction to preserve total digit number. These alternatives include staged reconstruction with both vascularized and non-vascularized tissue transfers. These approaches, despite yielding some good results, are more unpredictable and generally suboptimal when compared to index finger pollicization.[56]

Pollicization

Pollicization is the transposition of the index as a vascular island into a functional thumb position. Excellent functional and esthetic results can be achieved through careful planning and surgical execution but there will be compromises due to lack of a true CMC joint, weaker intrinsic muscles, and differences in phalangeal lengths.[57] Power is diminished to approximately 30%–50% of the normal thumb. The key determinant of outcome is the quality of

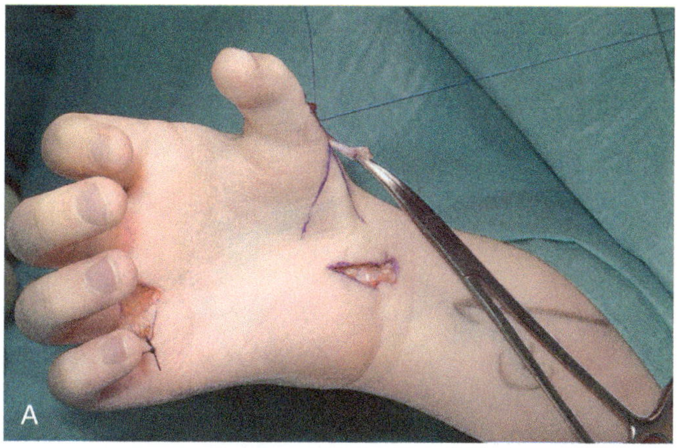

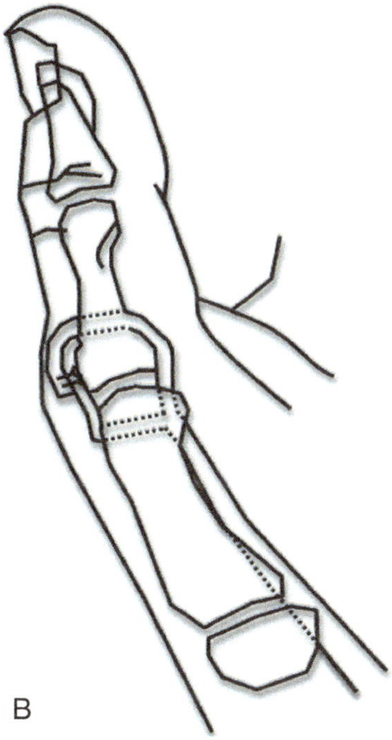

• **Fig. 45.15** Flexor digitorum superficialis tendon combined collateral ligament reconstruction and opposition transfer. The two slips of the flexor digitorum superficialis are split and passed through drill holes in the base of the proximal phalanx and the head of the metacarpal in a "box-like fashion" The tendon repair is placed on the radial side of the MCP joint so that in pinch, tension is taken off the repair site. (A) Two slips of the flexor digitorum superficialis used to stabilize the MCP joint. (B) A schematic of the "box-like" arrangement of the superficialis tendon around the MCP joint.

the index finger to be transferred. The principal stages are as follows:

1. Incisions – we prefer those described by Buck-Gramcko.[58]
2. Neurovascular dissection – commonly requires freeing of a neural ring, splitting the common digital nerve, and division of the radial digital artery to the middle finger.
3. First dorsal and first palmar interossei detachment from their insertions.
4. Second metacarpal resection from the distal physis to the CMC joint. The physis is ablated to prevent future growth of the neotrapzeium. Metaphyseal periosteum is removed to avoid new bone formation and painful bony spicules.

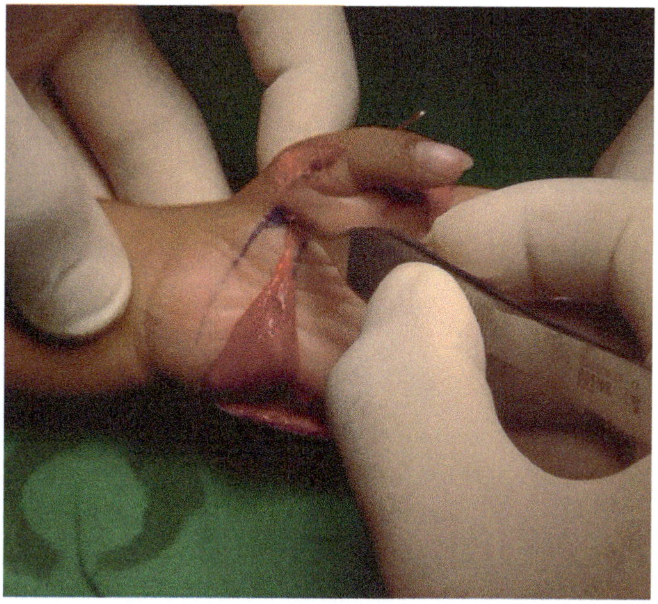

• **Fig. 45.16** Abductor digiti minimi opposition transfer. Insertions of the abductor digiti minimi muscle into the base of the little finger are released. The muscle is then transferred, maintaining its origin on the pisiform and proximally-based blood supply, to the thumb to provide opposition.

5. Fixation of the index MCP joint in maximal hyperextension to compensate for loss of the volar plate and provide stability in pinch.
6. Correct fixation of the neothumb into 100 degrees pronation and 30 degrees of abduction to allow for a degree of derotation during healing and rehabilitation.
7. Musculotendinous unit reattachment and balancing as follows:
   - Extensor digitorum communis becomes the new extensor pollicis brevis as it is the more radial
   - Extensor indicis proprius becomes the new extensor pollicis longus
     - The extensors are routinely, both shortened, advanced and sutured at the level of the thumb MCP joint. The degree of shortening is proportional to that of the index metacarpal.
   - After adjustment of the extrinsic tendons the intrinsics are inserted and tensioned appropriately
     - The first dorsal interosseous becomes the new abductor
     - The first palmar interosseous becomes the adductor
     - Balancing of the intrinsics is critical to correct posturing of the neothumb. The thumb is placed into maximal flexion at the IP joint and the intrinsics inserted on each side at maximal tension
     - Long flexor shortening is only required over 7 years of age; otherwise it tightens with growth and use.
8. Decompression of the tourniquet to allow for hemostasis and to check viability of the transfer.
9. Skin redraping and closure to contour the new thumb and first web space.

Revisional procedures are necessary in a significant proportion of patients and usually involve first web releases, extensor tenolyses, and transfers to supplement opposition.

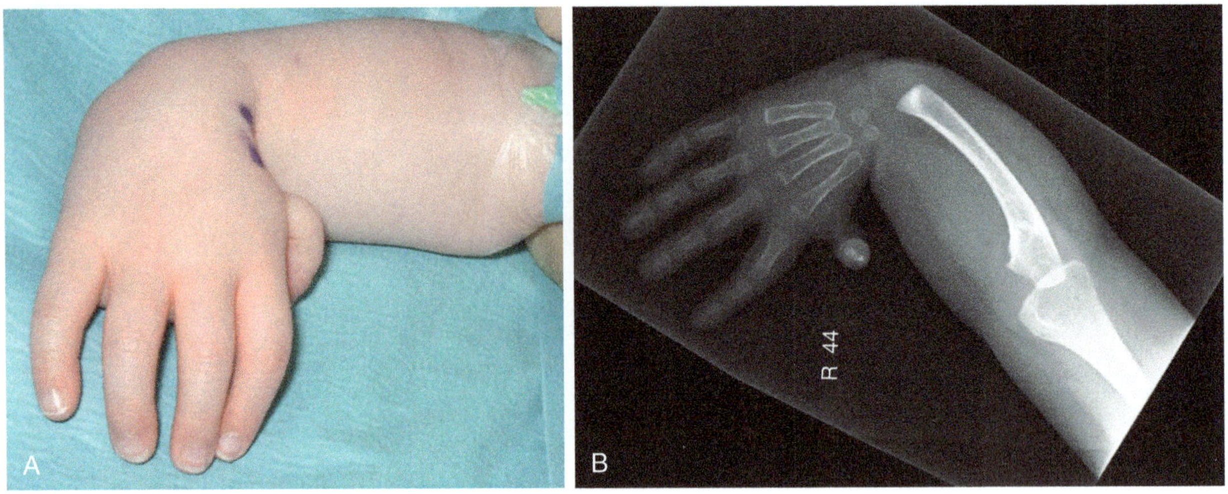

• **Fig. 45.17** (A) Image of a patient with type IV radial dysplasia showing radial deviation at the wrist and shortening of the forearm. A Blauth grade 4 pouce flottant (floating thumb) hypoplasia is also present. (B) Radiograph of the same patient demonstrating complete absence of the radius with absence of a wrist joint and bowing of the ulna.

Radial Longitudinal Deficiency

Radial longitudinal deficiency (RLD), previously referred to as radial club hand, represents a spectrum of abnormalities along the preaxial side of the upper limb. As a result of both skeletal deficiency and soft tissue abnormalities the hand adopts a radially deviated, flexed, and pronated position at the distal end of a shortened forearm[17] (Fig. 45.17A). This may be associated with abnormalities along the whole length of the upper limb, including the shoulder, elbow down to the thumb, and radial digits. There may only be a mild thumb hypoplasia or, in its severest form, complete absence of the thumb and radius. The condition may be unilateral or bilateral but is rarely symmetrical. The right side is affected twice as often as the left. RLD also occurs slightly more frequently in males. The incidence is reported at 1:30,000–1:100,000 live births.[17]

Etiology

Environmental and genetic factors play a role, though the exact etiology is unknown. Environmental causative factors include thalidomide, valproic acid, phenobarbital, and ethanol.[59] Bilateral cases are more likely to be linked to a syndrome. Most are due to sporadic mutations but some have a genetic basis and can be transmitted as either autosomal dominant or recessive disorders. Experimentally, radial dysplasia can be created in chick wings and the zone of polarizing activity (ZPA) identified as responsible for anteroposterior limb patterning. Expression of the sonic hedgehog gene and retinoic acid[60] have been shown to be critical in regulating the function of the ZPA. This is influenced by several factors, including the homeobox genes and is only induced due to signalling from the apical ectodermal ridge,[5] probably through fibroblast growth factor.[61] Abnormal limb development may be related to several different interruptions within this pathway.

Associated Syndromes

There are multiple associated syndromes, which confer a poorer prognosis. Syndromes that require early exclusion include those with hematological conditions, cardiac abnormalities, and renal defects. It is therefore important to seek early input from a clinical geneticist.

Hematological

Fanconi's anemia is an autosomal recessive pancytopenia, which is fatal without bone marrow transplantation. It is indentified through a chromosomal breakage study which is recommended for all children with radial dysplasia. Thrombocytopenia–absent radius (TAR) syndrome is a rare autosomal recessive disorder characterized by bilateral absence of the radii in the presence of both thumbs and hypomegakaryocytic thrombocytopenia.[62] The presence of functional thumbs distinguishes TAR syndrome from other conditions with radial aplasia which are usually associated with severe thumb hypoplasia or aplasia.[62] In TAR syndrome the platelet count usually improves with age so intervention is best delayed until levels normalize.

Cardiac

Holt–Oram syndrome is an autosomal dominant condition, which commonly exhibits atrial and ventricular septal defects.[63]

VACTERL Association

This is the largest individual syndromic group with associated radial dyplasia. Patients within this group vary in the severity of their presentation, demonstrating a wide spectrum of associated anomalies. The diagnosis is made on the basis of a minimum of three of the following abnormalities – vertebral, anorectal, cardiac, tracheoesophageal, renal, limb, and a single umbilical artery. Limb malformations are reported in 40%–50% of cases and mostly represent radial deficiency.[64]

Classification

Bayne and Klug classified RLD based on the degree of radial hypoplasia on radiographic assessment[65] (Table 45.7). This classification system does not encompass the degree of carpal or hand involvement.

Clinical Findings

RLD is usually identified on a routine neonatal check. Investigations should then be instigated to exclude associated anomalies. The most profound changes in radial dyplasia are seen in the hand and wrist but it is important to examine the entire upper limb. Type 1 cases can be easily missed but are often heralded by the presence of associated thumb hypoplasia. Bilateral involvement is often asymmetrical in terms of severity so careful examination of both upper limbs is important.

Upper Arm

The upper arm may be shorter than the opposite side, with distal humeral epiphysis involvement. The humeral involvement parallels the degree of radial hypoplasia.

Elbow

The elbow may demonstrate bony abnormalities. There is usually full extension but flexion is sometimes limited initially. However, this has been observed to improve over time if the wrist deformity is controlled with splintage.[66] In addition, active pronation and supination are compromised. Patients tend to compensate for this by using shoulder rotation to turn their hands.

Forearm

The forearm is short, with varying degrees of radial deficiency. The ulna is also hypoplastic and often bowed – growing to a maximum of two-thirds the length of the contralateral side (see Fig. 45.17B). Without treatment, ulna bowing can worsen. If some form of proximal radius is present its distal portion is replaced by a fibrous condensation or anlage. An additional deforming force is the presence of an abnormal combined radial muscle mass of flexor carpi radialis, extensor carpi radialis longus and brevis, and brachioradialis, which inserts into the anlage and on occasion the carpus (see Fig. 45.20). Soft tissue abnormalities, including those of musculotendinous units and neurovascular structures, tend to parallel the degree of skeletal deficiency. Affected structures such as the median nerve tend to favor an aberrant radial course towards the distal forearm, hence complicating treatment and surgical correction.[67]

TABLE 45.7 Bayne and Klug Classification of Radial Longitudinal Deficiency

Grade	Description
Type I	*Short distal radius*
Type II	*Hypoplastic radius* with distal and proximal epiphyses present but defective
Type III	*Partial absence of the radius* – most commonly of the distal one or two thirds
Type IV	*Complete absence* of the radius

Data from: Bayne LG, Klug MS. Long-term review of the surgical treatment of radial deficiencies. *J Hand Surg*. 1987;12(2):169–179.

Carpus

The radiocarpal articulation is often non-functional and may not even be present, with a hypoplastic or absent trapezium and scaphoid (see Fig. 45.17B). With ossification increasing carpal coalitions are seen.

Hand

The thumb is often either hypoplastic or absent (see Fig. 45.17A). The ulnar side of the hand is the least affected, with worsening hypoplasia and stiffness in the radial digits. Motion at the MCP joints is restricted although a degree of hyperextension is present. There are often flexion deformities of the PIP joints, particularly affecting central digits and in syndromic cases.

Surgical Principles and Management

The aims of treatment in radial club hand are to provide stable realignment of the carpus and hand on the distal ulna, improve function of the limb as a whole and maximize growth potential.[16,65,66] The soft tissue structures on the radial side of the wrist are short, therefore treatment begins with stretching and splintage carried out by the parents with the guidance of a hand therapist. Physiotherapy aims to correct wrist deviation and to improve and maintain range of motion of the digits. For type I cases, where the wrist is stable and easily corrected to neutral, no intervention is required. But if a tendancy for radial deviation remains, a tendon transfer of the tight combined dorsoradial muscle mass to the ulnar side of the carpus may be required. Type II cases are some of the most challenging to treat. Attempts have been made to distract and lengthen the radius with or without a bone graft.[68] This, however, often needs to be repeated as a child grows and results are unpredictable. In type III cases we advocate removal of the radial anlage and treatment as for type IV cases as detailed below.

Soft Tissue Distraction

The benefits of stretching and splinting on addressing radial deforming forces should not be underestimated. However, these maneuvers alone have proven insufficient in completely addressing radial tension prior to wrist correction, particularly in severe type III and IV cases. As a result, Kessler proposed the idea of soft tissue distraction.[69] Since its conception, soft tissue distraction has revolutionized the treatment of radial dysplasia and has evolved through the use of a variety of different uniplanar and multiplanar devices. Our preference is a uniplanar device with a central coaxial hinge, which is placed on the radial side of the limb and secured by pin fixation into the ulnar proximally and into the index metacarpal through to third metacarpal distally (Fig. 45.18). On-table distraction yields a significant amount after which incremental distraction is taught to parents to perform at a rate of approximately 1 mm per day. Maximizing this latter slower distraction is crucial in minimizing long-term radial tension and pressure on the ulnar physis. Distraction is stopped once the third metacarpal base is aligned with the distal ulna, at which point the soft tissue are allowed to adapt to their new position prior to a wrist corrective procedure. We have noted that this "consolidation" period of stress relaxation facilitates wrist stabilization and can produce some remodeling and straightening of the ulna.

Wrist Correction

This can be achieved through a centralization with a proximal row carpal notch or a (non-notched) stabilization procedure. Centralization involves alignment of the third metacarpal with the ulna through the creation of a notch in the carpus producing a fusion or fibrous union to the proximal carpal row (Fig. 45.19). This is more stable than a stabilization but inherently immobile. A stabilization procedure, also known as a radialization, involves rebalancing the carpus on the end of the ulna in line with second metacarpal without a carpal slot. Both procedures are combined with a tendon transfer of the dorsoradial muscles mass into the base of the fifth metacarpal or extensor carpis ulnaris tendon to rebalance forces at the wrist and prevent recurrence into radial deviation (Fig. 45.20). A dorsal approach via a longitudinal incision is all that is required, rendering complex incision patterns or flaps to address skin shortages obsolete. Repositioning through a radialization, although it preserves motion, is inherently more unstable than a centralization. Review of our series shows there is a tendency for more long-term recurrence in radialization cases. As a result we would favor a stable centralization in cases where the quality of the dorsoradial muscle mass or ulna joint congruity does not lend itself to the balance that is required for a radialization. Both types of correction are supported with longitudinal K-wire fixation for a period of 6 months to a year.

Alternative Procedures in Radial Dysplasia

We consider the outcomes from soft tissue distraction followed by centralization or radialization with a tendon transfer satisfactory and have not pursued other methods. Vascularized and nonvascularized fibular head transfers have been used to replace the radius as well as vascularized metatarsophalangeal joint transfer.[70] The cohorts in these series have been smaller and their take-up so far limited worldwide.

Following wrist correction, thumb hypoplasia can be addressed and, later, forearm lengthening. Forearm lengthening requires stability at the wrist and is fraught with

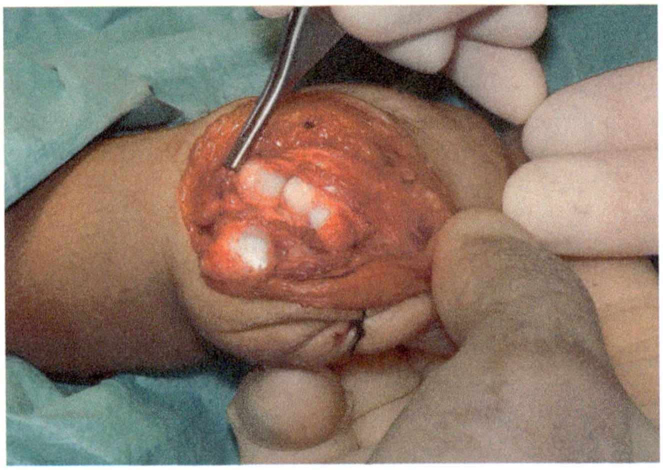

• **Fig. 45.19** Intraoperative image of a centralization procedure demonstrating creation of a carpal slot. The ulna is placed into the carpal notch and a tendon transfer is carried out of the dysplastic combined dorsoradial muscle mass.

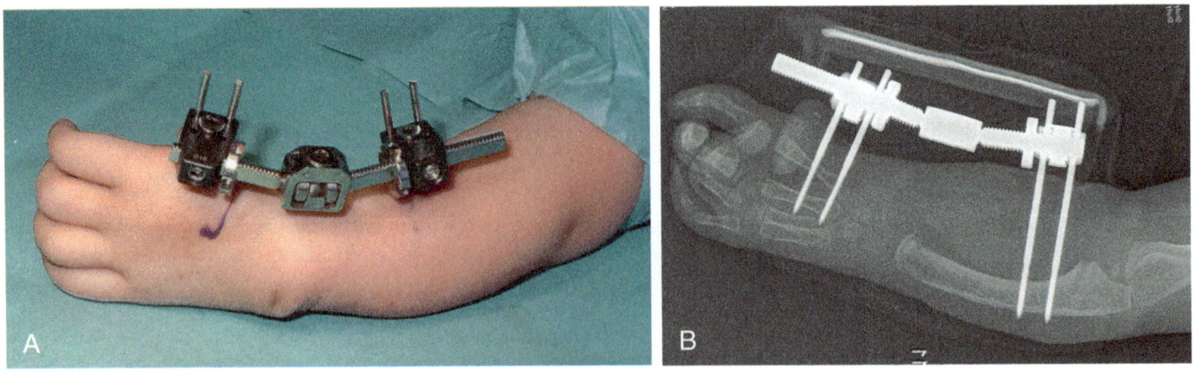

• **Fig. 45.18** Soft tissue distraction with a uniplanar minifixator device. (A) Image of a patient with type IV radial dysplasia with a Pennig Minifixator device with a central coaxial hinge in situ on the radial aspect of the limb. (B) Radiograph of the same patient demonstrating two-pin fixation across the second and third metacarpals distally and into the ulna proximally.

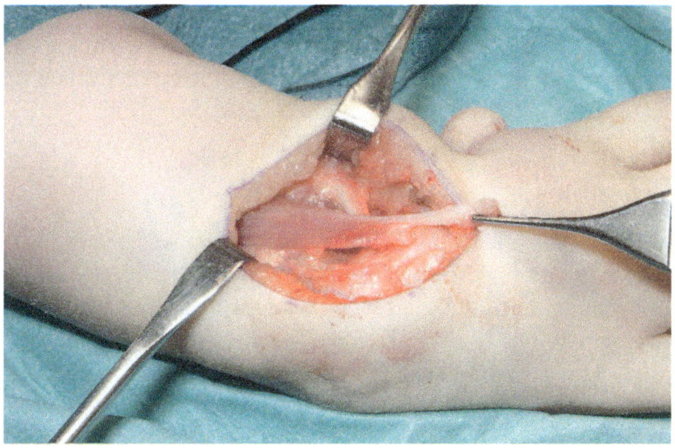

• **Fig. 45.20** Intraoperative image of a radialization procedure showing transfer of the combined dorsoradial muscle mass. No carpal slot is made in a radialization (stabilization). Stability relies upon transfer of the combined dorsoradial muscle and congruency of the ulna and carpal joint surfaces.

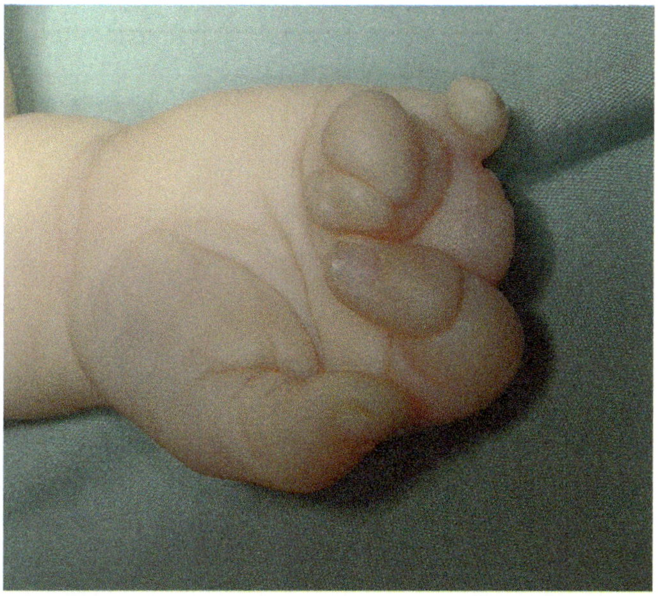

• **Fig. 45.21** Right hand showing constriction rings affecting the index, middle, and ring fingers. Circumferential ring affecting the distal index finger and further constrictions producing acrosyndactyly of the middle and ring fingers.

potential complications. In highly selected patients it may bring functional and cosmetic gains, which they consider worthwhile.[71]

Constriction Ring Syndrome

Constriction ring syndrome is a rare condition of unknown etiology. Numerous names have been used to describe this entity in the past, including annular band syndrome, constriction band syndrome, Streeter dysplasia, Torpin dysplasia, amniotic band disruption sequence, acrosyndactyly, fenestrated syndactyly, and congenital amputation syndrome.[72] The syndrome is characterized by bands of ranging severity, always present at birth, that can affect any part of the body with a particular predilection for the upper or lower extremities[73] (Fig. 45.21). The reported incidence in the literature varies from 1 in 1200 to 1 in 15,000 live births depending on the population sampled and the diagnostic criteria used.[73] When found in conjunction with significant limb involvement its incidence has been recorded as low as 0.19 per 10,000. No genetic inheritance pattern has been identified but some environmental associations have been postulated. These have included possible links with abnormal gestational histories and oligohydramnios.[59]

Etiology

Several theories have been postulated, which include an intrinsic theory of localized areas of imperfectly formed tissue due to "defective areas of germ plasm"[73] and an extrinsic theory due to the formation of mesodermic strands due to rupture of or damage to the amnion during the first or early second trimester.[74] These amniotic strands become entangled with the fetus and in particular the extremities within the sac. In addition, resultant transient oligohydramnios caused by a loss of amniotic fluid can lead to abnormal pressure on developing limb buds resulting in associated deformities such as talipes equinovarus – club foot.[75] Anomalies such as cleft palate as part of Pierre Robin sequence also appear closely linked to the effects of oligohydramnios.[76] Similarly, there is a strong association between limb ring constrictions and rare craniofacial clefts, again supporting the idea of a common causality.[77]

Clinical Presentation

No two cases of congenital ring syndrome are identical. The deformities are always present at the time of birth and prenatal ultrasonographic techniques enable early diagnosis. More than one limb is usually affected and associated musculoskeletal anomalies are commonly present[78] (Table 45.8). There is a predilection for the more distal extremities – in particular the longer central three digits and longer great toe (see Fig. 45.21). In line with an extrinsic etiology, involvement of the thumb is rare due to its flexed adducted posture during intrauterine development making entrapment more difficult. More proximal rings do occur but with much less frequency. However, it is rare for only one ring to be present as an isolated abnormality.[17] The severity of the deformity can vary dramatically even between affected limbs of the same individual. The depth of the groove can range from mild indentations with minimal involvement of subcutaneous tissue to deep deficiency with associated disruption of lymphatic channels, nerves, and blood vessels. Generally, the rings tend to be deeper on the dorsal surface of affected extremities. Deep volar involvement can be associated with tendon involvement and joint contractures. Skeletal involvement is rare because in these cases autoamputation tends to have already occurred.[72] Amputations can occur at any level and stumps tend to be tapered. Sensation tends to be normal and despite the presence of rings and

TABLE 45.8 Classification of Constriction Ring Syndrome

Grade	Description
Type 1	Simple ring constrictions
Type 2	Ring constrictions accompanied by deformity of the distal part with or without lymphedema
Type 3	Ring constrictions accompanied by fusions of distal parts ranging from mild to severe acrosyndactyly
Type 4	Intrauterine amputations

Data from: Patterson TJ. Congenital ring-constrictions. *Br J Plast Surg* 1961;14:1–31.

amputations function is generally good as proximally all soft tissue and skeletal anatomy remains unaffected.[79] Fusion of distal parts is also common in cases of constriction ring syndrome in the form of acrosyndactyly[73] (Fig. 45.2E). Distal fusions can be either simple or complex with bony fusions present between adjacent digits. Proximal fenestrations tend to lie characteristically distal to the level of the commissure.

Classification

A number of classification systems have been proposed for constriction ring syndrome. The most widely used of these is that described by Patterson,[73] a clinically useful system of four different groups which reflect a range of severity (see Table 45.8).

Surgical Principles and Management

The timing of surgery is dependent of the type and severity of presentation. In the neonatal period the main treatment that may be required is the division of small soft tissue bridges between digits and the thumb to ensure unrestricted growth.[72] In some instances it may be possible to see fibrous bands encircling the fingers and toes of newborns. These can be simply removed or unwound to release the tethered digits. Occasionally, ring constrictions can produce severe distal edema and vascular compromise, particularly in cases of delayed healing in the postnatal period. These cases represent an emergency situation which requires expeditious decompression in the early neonatal period in order to prevent impending tissue ischemia. Hemicircumferential decompression can yield a dramatic improvement in the status of the distal extremity. Once the decompression has had time to take effect resultant redundant skin and the remaining half of the ring can be dealt with as a delayed second stage.

Simple constriction rings can be dealt with non-urgently prior to school age using principles described below. Syndactyly separation is best carried out early if it involves the border digits and is tethering growth. Otherwise, it can be dealt with after 1 year of age. Bilateral procedures and those treating upper and lower limbs simultaneously are possible but best performed before the child is ambulatory. More complex procedures such as toe-to-hand transfers, skeletal lengthening, and digital transpositions can be delayed to optimize patient and family compliance and the size of surgical anatomy.[72]

Method of Constriction Ring Correction

Traditional methods of correction involved excision of grooves, mobilization of adipose tissue, and reapproximation of skin using Z-plasty- or W-plasty-based techniques.[17] However, resultant scars have a tendency to indent with time and occasional partial loss of flaps and resultant delayed healing can result in a conspicuous depressed saw-tooth appearance.[79] The ideal correction of a deep constriction ring should address the tight scar at the base of the indentation, atrophic tissue along the side walls, and indurated fatty tissue within the distal swollen segment.[72] Transverse incisions are first marked on either side of the depressed area on the limb or digit. These are marked on the shoulders flanking the constriction to ensure complete removal of all scarred tissue from within the ring (Fig. 45.22). Gentle compression of one marked side against its opposing unmarked partner guides correct incision placement. All scarred tissue is then excised from within the depth of the ring preserving large dorsal veins, volar neurovascular structures, and flexor tendons. Excess fatty tissue, usually most apparent distally, can then be excised and the remaining deeper tissue can be redraped to fill the annular contour defect. In this way final closure of the layers can be staggered to minimize the effects of vertical scar contracture. If the ring is circumferential one or two Z-plasties can be incorporated to break up the scar and are best placed in the midlateral axes to avoid the most socially visible areas of the limb or digit.[79]

Toe-to-Hand Transfers

Constriction ring amputations of the thumb and digits are ideal candidates for vascularized toe-to-hand transfers as proximal anatomy, including the neurovasculature, is normal. These techniques can dramatically improve hand function through the reconstruction of a sensate mobile thumb or digits which will show a degree of commensurate growth with the child[80] (Fig. 45.23). However, this approach can occasionally be limited by a lack of useable toes in the context of constriction ring syndrome.

Distraction Lengthening

An alternative approach is the use of distraction lengthening.[81] This method is very effective at restoring a functional prehensile unit but can be a very involved process that requires a great deal of patient and family commitment. Indications for surgery must be carefully considered. This method appears to be more effective when used at the metacarpal and forearm levels as the distracted tissue is surrounded by more soft tissue with greater vascularity.[72] Distraction at the phalangeal level is possible but is extremely challenging due to problems of poor skeletal stock and soft tissue coverage.

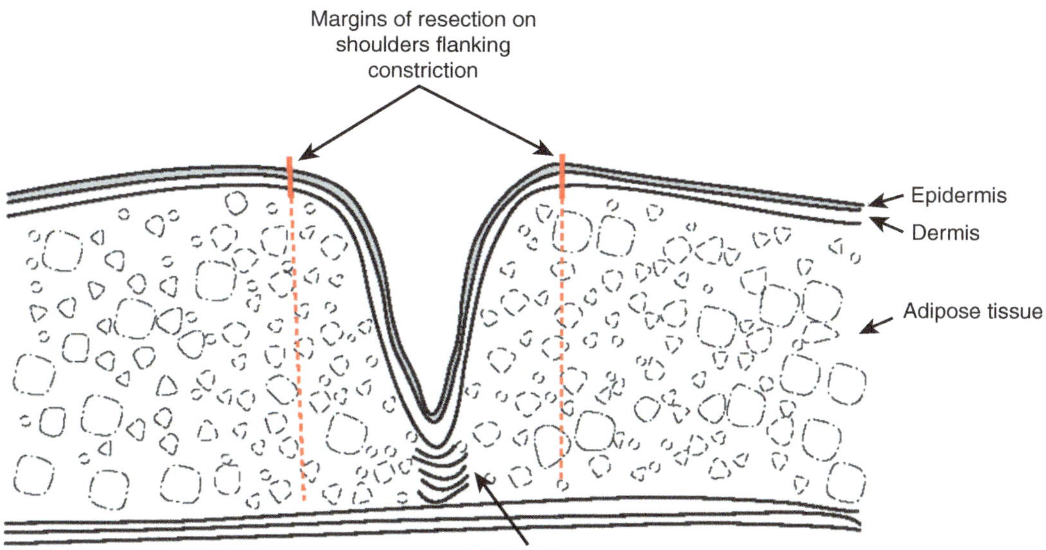

• **Fig. 45.22** Schematic demonstrating excision margins for correction of ring constriction. Transverse incisions are made on the shoulders flanking the constriction to ensure complete removal of all scarred tissue from within the ring.

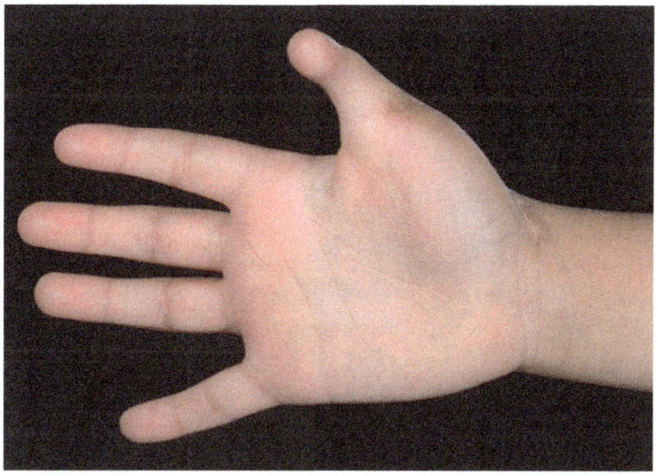

• **Fig. 45.23** Image of a free vascularized toe-to-hand transfer to reconstruct a thumb intrauterine auto-amputation secondary to constriction ring syndrome.

Digital Transposition

Transposition of a redundant digital tip based on its neurovascular pedicle as an "on-top"-plasty including its proximal phalanx can lengthen digits improving length for prehension. Transposition of a short nonfunctioning index finger in this way can also broaden a first web space.

Arthrogryposis

Arthrogryposis (Greek *arthron* = joint, *grūpōsis* = hooking) is an umbrella term encompassing more than 300 disorders in which there are congenital contractures affecting at least two different areas of the body.[82] The overall prevalence of arthrogryposis is around one in 3000 live births. The inheritance, natural history, optimum management, and prognosis varies across the disorders. Therefore ensuring a specific diagnosis and individualized treatment plan is key.[83] When the results of neurological examination are normal the most common causes are amyoplasia, one of the distal arthrogrypotic syndromes, a generalized connective tissue disorder or fetal crowding.[83] An abnormal neurological examination points towards a central nervous system disorder or a neuromuscular disease (peripheral nervous system, motor end plate or muscle).[83] Amyoplasia, also known as classic arthrogryposis or arthrogryposis multiplex congenita (AMC), is a specific disease entity characterized by congenital joint contractures and muscle wasting without evidence of any progressive neuromuscular disease. Distal arthrogryposis exhibits primarily hand and foot involvement but is a heterogeneous subset of autosomal dominant disorders.[84] For the purposes of this chapter, we will focus on amyoplasia.

Etiology

Amyoplasia is sporadic, occurring in 1 in 10,000 live births. Its exact etiology remains unclear but evidence points towards a likely cause being patchy damage of the anterior horn cells of the spinal cord in the developing fetus. Genetic factors are not significant as twin cohort studies have demonstrated discordance and no clear environmental factors have been identified.[85]

Clinical Findings

The vast majority have both upper limbs and both lower limbs affected (84%). They appear fusiform, wasted, and without flexion creases (Fig. 45.24). Lower limb involvement alone occurs in 11% and upper limb involvement alone in 5%. The joint contractures tend to be symmetrical. Characteristic features of amyoplasia include the following:[86]

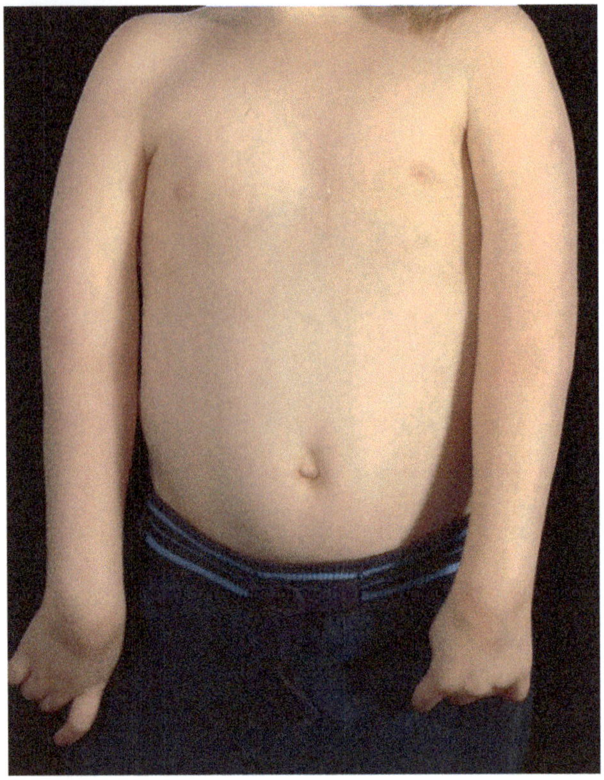

• **Fig. 45.24** Image of patient demonstrating the common features of amyoplasia. The upper limb is internally rotated at the shoulder with the elbows extended, forearms pronated, and the wrists flexed and ulnar-deviated.

Upper Limbs (Fig. 45.24)

- Shoulders adducted and internally rotated
- Elbows extended
- Forearms pronated
- Wrists flexed and ulnarly deviated
- Thumbs adducted, laxity of ulnar collateral ligament, absence of abductor pollicis brevis
- Fingers partially flexed.

Lower Limbs

- Hips flexed and abducted with dislocation of one or both sides in 30%
- Knee usually fixed in extension
- Feet held in rigid equinovarus contractures in the majority.

Other Common Features

- Deformities of face and jaw – asymmetry, flat nasal bridge, hemangiomas (frontal midline capillary hemangioma in 90% of those with all limbs involved), micrognathia and trismus
- Genital deformities, umbilical or inguinal hernias are common.

Surgical Principles and Management

Most often affected children are of above-average intelligence with the potential for independence.[86,87] The priorities are communication, activities of daily living, and mobilization.

Timing of Surgery

We advocate a coordinated multidisciplinary approach, with parallel upper and lower limb surgery where possible to reduce the number of operations the child has to endure and ensuring greatest benefit, especially as in both early surgery confers a better outcome. A protracted course of lower limb surgery focused on ambulation alone, which may involve addressing club feet, knee contractions and hip dislocations, for example, may result in significant delays to upper limb treatment.[88]

Aims of Treatment of the Upper Limb

1. Maintain and improve joint range of motion – focus on passive as this may improve function with passive assistance maneuvers.
2. Maintain and improve muscle strength.
3. Preserve bimanual function.
4. Optimize upper limb positioning to reach table tops.

These can be achieved initially with gentle manipulation and splintage with the help of occupational and physical therapy. Occupational therapy also teaches adaptive skills, trains caregivers to provide home therapy, and tailors assistive equipment to meet individual patient needs. Therapy is an ongoing process which, in the majority of patients, extends at least into their teenage years. Surgical intervention in the upper limb is recommended for fixed joint contractures that interfere with upper-limb function.

Surgical Options by Region

Shoulder

This is rarely indicated unless there is significant shoulder internal rotation to preclude functional positioning of the limb in space. In these cases a humeral rotational osteotomy to around 45 degrees will facilitate midline functioning of the hand.[87]

Elbow

The main goal is to enable elbow flexion to allow hand to mouth reach. Improvement of passive range allows assistance techniques such as trunk swaying and table top propping. A posterior elbow joint release with a Z- or W-plasty to regain 90 degrees of passive flexion with a tricepsplasty works well.[82] If active flexion is poor an elbow flexor-plasty transfer can be carried out at the same time. A variety of different options have been described for this purpose, including the use of pectoralis major, latissimus dorsi,[82] and triceps.[89] However, care must be taken to avoid development of a unwanted flexion contracture that can impair preexisting function. In this regard, transfer of the long head of triceps alone as a functional unit has been shown to produce reliable antigravity flexion whilst preserving active extension with minimal donor site morbidity.[90]

Wrist

Early carpectomy prior to ossification of the carpal bones facilitates removal of a trapezoidal wedge from the mid carpus without damage to the radius or ulnar articular surfaces.

This resection allows for correction of the wrist flexion contracture to around 40 degrees of hyperextension and relaxes volar soft tissues, including the neurovascular structures and flexor tendons. This permits the fingers to adopt a more functional empowered posture.[91] The wrist position is initially maintained with K-wire fixation and recurrence is prevented through the transfer of the flexor carpi ulnaris and radialis tendons to augment the dorsal pull on the metacarpals. Early surgery achieves more active flexion and allows greater bone remodeling.[82,91]

Thumb

Patients with tight adduction contractures who do not respond to stretching and splintage may benefit from a first web space release and either an extensor indicis transfer to improve extension or an epiphyseal-sparing chondrodesis of the MCP joint. In some cases an opposition transfer is required at the same time.[87]

Fingers

Finger position can be significantly improved with early stretching and splintage. Further improvement can be achieved through functional repositioning of the wrist contracture through wedge carpectomy, as mentioned above. In rare instances digital flexion contractures require surgical release with full-thickness skin graft reconstruction.[82]

Trigger Thumb

Trigger thumb occurs due to obstruction of the flexor pollicis longus tendon at the A1 pulley as a result of stenosing tenovaginitis.[92] Unlike the intermittent triggering seen in adult cases, children most commonly present with their thumbs locked in flexion at the IP joint. A small minority present locked in extension.

Notta's node is palpable proximal to the A1 pulley in a fixed flexion deformity. Most authors view this as secondary to bunching up of the tendon, as it appears to resolve following A1 release, rather than as a primary lesion. When the thumb is locked in extension, the failure to glide through the A1 pulley occurs distal to proximal with Notta's node abutting the distal end.

Etiology and Presentation

Trigger thumb usually presents between 6 months to 2 years. There is debate as to whether this is in fact an acquired rather than congenital condition. Most studies reporting presence at birth depend upon a retrospective history from the parents. Prospective studies with early postnatal assessment report very few cases. However, diagnosis in the newborn is unreliable as they tend to clasp their thumb and clicking or triggering is more difficult to elicit in a child than in an adult. A congenital basis is supported by the presence of trigger thumb in twins, the frequency of bilateral trigger thumb (25%) and the association with Trisomy 13.[93] Trigger thumbs occur 14 times more frequently than trigger fingers. It is usually pain-free unless attempts are made to straighten the digit. A missed diagnosis of dislocation may be made with rapid recurrence following attempted reduction.

Surgical Principles and Management

Trigger thumbs tend not to resolve spontaneously in most cases. However, there is some evidence that suggests resolution is higher in those diagnosed prior to the age of 6 months.[93] Trigger fingers have yet higher rates of spontaneous resolution. This recovery may be assisted by splinting and passive stretching programs. However, we have found compliance difficult in this age group. Furthermore, we do not advocate treatment with steroid injections in pediatric cases.

Surgical release of the A1 pulley of the thumb is very successful. We advise release prior to the age of 3 years[93] due to a risk of permanent joint deformity. Access is via a transverse incision at the base of the thumb within a skin crease. Care must be taken to avoid damage to neurovascular bundles, which tend to sit more anteriorly when compared to the digits. However, direct visualization of the bundles is not required, only care in their protection. The radial part of the A1 pulley is divided under direct vision to allow unobstructed tendon gliding and to prevent damage to the oblique pulley. Trigger fingers, however, usually do not respond to A1 division alone, requiring sacrifice of one slip of FDS also.

References

1. Tickle C. Limb development: an international model for vertebrate pattern formation. *Int J Dev Biol.* 2000;44(1):101–108.
2. Martin GR. The roles of FGFs in the early development of vertebrate limbs. *Gene Develop.* 1998;12(11):1571–1586.
3. Riddle RD, Johnson RL, Laufer E, et al. Sonic hedgehog mediates the polarizing activity of the ZPA. *Cell.* 1993;75(7):1401–1416.
4. Riddle RD, Ensini M, Nelson C, et al. Induction of the LIM homeobox gene Lmx1 by WNT7a establishes dorsoventral pattern in the vertebrate limb. *Cell.* 1995;83(4):631–640.
5. Dlugaszewska B, Silahtaroglu A, Menzel C, et al. Breakpoints around the HOXD cluster result in various limb malformations. *J Med Gene.* 2006;43(2):111–118.
6. Swanson AB, Swanson GD, Tada K. A classification for congenital limb malformation. *J Hand Surg.* 1983;8(5 Pt 2):693–702.
7. Knight SL, Kay S. Classification of congenital anomalies. In: Gupta AKS, Scheker LR, eds. *The Growing Hand: Diagnosis and Management of the Upper Extremity in Children.* London: Mosby; 2000:125–135.
8. Upton J. Classification of upper limb congenital differences and general principles management. In: Mathes SJ, ed. *Plastic Surgery. The Hand and Upper Limb.* 2nd edn. Vol 8. Philadelphia: Elsevier; 2006:25–50.
9. Tonkin MA, Tolerton SK, Quick TJ, et al. Classification of congenital anomalies of the hand and upper limb: development and assessment of a new system. *J Hand Surg.* 2013;38(9):1845–1853.

10. Flatt AE. *The Care of Congenital Hand Anomalies.* St. Louis: Mosby; 1977.
11. Bakrania P, Ugur Iseri SA, Wyatt AW, et al. Sonic hedgehog mutations are an uncommon cause of developmental eye anomalies. *Am J Med Gene Part A.* 2010;152A(5):1310–1313.
12. Upton J. Central polydactyly. In: Mathes SJ, ed. *Plastic Surgery. The Hand and Upper Limb.* 2nd edn. Vol 8. Philadelphia: Saunders Elsevier; 2006:234–244.
13. Upton J. Failure of differentiation and overgrowth. In: Mathes SJ, ed. *Plastic Surgery. The Hand and Upper Limb.* 2nd edn. Vol 8. Philadelphia: Saunders Elsevier; 2006:265–322.
14. Cronin TD. Syndactylism: results of zig-zag incision to prevent postoperative contracture. *Plast Reconstr Surg.* 1956;18(6):460–468.
15. Sharma RK, Tuli P, Makkar SS, et al. End-of-skin grafts in syndactyly release: description of a new flap for web space resurfacing and primary closure of finger defects. *Hand (NY).* 2009;4(1):29–34.
16. Buck-Gramcko D. Congenital malformations. In: Lister G, ed. *Hand Surgery.* Stuttgart: Thième; 1988.
17. Flatt AE. *The Care of Congenital Hand Anomalies.* 2nd edn. St. Louis: Mosby, Quality Medical; 1994.
18. Burke F, Flatt A. Clinodactyly: a review of a series of cases. *Hand.* 1979;11(3):269–280.
19. Hovius SER. Hand and upper extremity. In: Neligan PC, ed. *Plastic Surgery. Hand and Upper Extremity.* 3rd edn. Vol 6. Philadelphia: Elsevier Saunders; 2013.
20. Scott CE, Engber W. Kirner's deformity: a case report and review. *Iowa Orthop J.* 1996;16:167–169.
21. Vickers D. Clinodactyly of the little finger: a simple operative technique for reversal of the growth abnormality. *J Hand Surg Br.* 1987;12(3):335–342.
22. Smith PJ, Grobbelaar AO. Camptodactyly: a unifying theory and approach to surgical treatment. *J Hand Surg.* 1998;23(1):14–19.
23. Foucher G, Lorea P, Khouri RK, et al. Camptodactyly as a spectrum of congenital deficiencies: a treatment algorithm based on clinical examination. *Plast Reconstr Surg.* 2006;117(6):1897–1905.
24. Hori M, Nakamura R, Inoue G, et al. Nonoperative treatment of camptodactyly. *J Hand Surg.* 1987;12(6):1061–1065.
25. Glicenstein J, Haddad R, Guero S. [Surgical treatment of camptodactyly]. *Ann Hand Upper Limb Surg.* 1995;14:264–271.
26. Wassel HD. The results of surgery for polydactyly of the thumb. *Clin Orthop Relat Res.* 1969;64:175–193.
27. Wood VE. Polydactyly and the triphalangeal thumb. *J Hand Surg.* 1978;3(5):436–444.
28. Hung L, Cheng JC, Bundoc R, et al. Thumb duplication at the metacarpophalangeal joint: management and a new classification. *Clin Orthop Relat Res.* 1996;(323):31–41.
29. Smith PJ, Smith G. Congenital deformities and reconstruction. In: Siemionow MZ, Eisenmann-Klein M, eds. *Plastic and Reconstructive Surgery.* London: Springer-Verlag; 2010:497–502.
30. Tupper JW. Pollex abductus due to congenital malposition of the flexor pollicis longus. *J Bone Joint Surg Am.* 1969;51(7):1285–1290.
31. Bilhaut M. Guerison d'une pouce bifide par un nouveau procède operatoire. *Congrès Français de Chirurgie.* 1889;4:576–580.
32. Temtamy SA, McKusick VA. Synopsis of hand malformations with particular emphasis on genetic factors. *Birth Defects Orig Artic Ser.* 1969;3:125–184.
33. Woolf CM, Myrianthopoulos NC. Polydactyly in American negroes and whites. *Am J Hum Genet.* 1973;25(4):397–404.
34. Stelling F. The upper extremity. In: Ferguson AB, ed. *Orthopedic Surgery in Infancy and Childhood.* Baltimore: Williams & Wilkins; 1963:282–402.
35. Goodman FR, Mundlos S, Muragaki Y, et al. Synpolydactyly phenotypes correlate with size of expansions in HOXD13 polyalanine tract. *Proc Natl Acad Sci U S A.* 1997;94(14):7458–7463.
36. Kelikian H. *Congenital Deformities of the Hand and Forearm.* Philadelphia: Saunders; 1974.
37. Barsky AJ. Macrodactyly. *J Bone Joint Surg Am.* 1967;49(7):1255–1266.
38. Upton J. Treatment of congenital forearm and hand anomalies. In: May JW, Littler JW, eds. *The Hand. Plastic Surgery.* Vol 8. Philadelphia: WB Saunders; 1990:5352–5356.
39. Hardwicke J, Khan MA, Richards H, et al. Macrodactyly – options and outcomes. *J Hand Surg Eur Vol.* 2013;38(3):297–303.
40. Upton J. Overgrowth. In: Mathes SJ, ed. *Plastic Surgery. The Hand and Upper Limb.* 2nd edn. Vol 8. Philadelphia: Saunders; 2006:298–317.
41. Tsuge K, Ikuta Y. Macrodactyly and fibro-fatty proliferation of the median nerve. *Hiroshima J Med Sci.* 1973;22(1):83–101.
42. Abdel-Ghani H, Amro S. Characteristics of patients with hypoplastic thumb: a prospective study of 51 patients with the results of surgical treatment. *J Pediatr Orthop B.* 2004;13(2):127–138.
43. Muller W. Die angieboren Fehlbildungen der menschlichen Hand. *The Hand.* Thième: Leipzig; 1937.
44. Blauth W. [The hypoplastic thumb]. *Arch Orthop Unfall-Chir.* 1967;62(3):225–246.
45. Buck-Gramcko D. Hypoplasia and aplasia of the thumb. In: Buck-Gramcko D, Nigst H, Millesi H, eds. *Hand Surgery.* Stuttgart: Thième; 1981.
46. Manske PR, McCarroll HR Jr, James M. Type III-A hypoplastic thumb. *J Hand Surg.* 1995;20(2):246–253.
47. Smith P. Congenital. In: Lister G, ed. *The Hand: Diagnosis and Indications.* 4th edn. London: Churchill Livingstone; 2002:457–522.
48. Manske PR, McCarroll Jr HR. Reconstruction of the congenitally deficient thumb. *Hand Clin.* 1992;8(1):177–196.
49. Upton J. Hypoplastic or absent thumb. In: Mathes SJ, ed. *Plastic Surgery. The Hand and Upper Limb.* 2nd edn. Vol 8. Philadelphia: Saunders; 2006:323–367.
50. Woolf RM, Broadbent TR. The four-flap Z-plasty. *Plast Reconstr Surg.* 1972;49(1):48–51.
51. Upton J, Havlik RJ, Coombs CJ. Use of forearm flaps for the severely contracted first web space in children with congenital malformations. *J Hand Surg.* 1996;21(3):470–477.
52. Kay S, Coady M. The role of microsurgery and free tissue transfer in the reconstruction of the paediatric upper extremity. *Ann Acad Med Singapore.* 1995;24(4 suppl):113–123.
53. Smith P, Sivakumar B, Hall R, et al. Blauth II thumb hypoplasia: a management algorithm for the unstable metacarpophalangeal joint. *J Hand Surg Eur Vol.* 2012;37(8):745–750.
54. Lister G. Reconstruction of the hypoplastic thumb. *Clin Orthop Relat Res.* 1985;195:52–65.
55. Huber E. Relief operation in the case of paralysis of the median nerve. 1921. *J Hand Surg Br.* 2004;29(1):35–37.
56. Nishijima N, Matsumoto T, Yamamuro T. Two-stage reconstruction for the hypoplastic thumb. *J Hand Surg.* 1995;20(3):415–419.
57. Taghinia AH, Upton J. Index finger pollicization. *J Hand Surg.* 2011;36(2):333–339.
58. Buck-Gramcko D. Pollicization of the index finger. Method and results in aplasia and hypoplasia of the thumb. *J Bone Joint Surg Am.* 1971;53(8):1605–1617.

59. Sivakumar B, Adamthwaite J, Smith P. Congenital hand dfferences. In: Farhardieh R, Bulstrode N, Cugno S, eds. *Plastic and Reconstructive Surgery: Approaches and Techniques*. Oxford: Wiley–Blackwell; 2015:660–687.
60. Tickle C, Lee J, Eichele G. A quantitative analysis of the effect of all-trans-retinoic acid on the pattern of chick wing development. *Dev Biol.* 1985;109(1):82–95.
61. Niswander L, Jeffrey S, Martin GR, et al. A positive feedback loop coordinates growth and patterning in the vertebrate limb. *Nature.* 1994;371(6498):609–612.
62. Hall JG, Levin J, Kuhn JP, et al. Thrombocytopenia with absent radius (TAR). *Medicine (Baltim).* 1969;48(6):411–439.
63. Goldfarb CA, Wall L, Manske PR. Radial longitudinal deficiency: the incidence of associated medical and musculoskeletal conditions. *J Hand Surg.* 2006;31(7):1176–1182.
64. Solomon BD. VACTERL/VATER association. *Orphanet J Rare Dis.* 2011;6:56.
65. Bayne LG, Klug MS. Long-term review of the surgical treatment of radial deficiencies. *J Hand Surg.* 1987;12(2):169–179.
66. Lamb DW. Radial club hand. A continuing study of sixty-eight patients with one hundred and seventeen club hands. *J Bone Joint Surg Am.* 1977;59(1):1–13.
67. Heikel HV. Aplasia and hypoplasa of the radius: studies on 64 cases and on epiphyseal transplantation in rabbits with the imitated defect. *Acta Orthop Scand Suppl.* 1959;39:1–155.
68. Upton J. Management of transverse and longitudinal deficiencies (failure of formation). In: Mathes SJ, ed. *Plastic Surgery. The Hand and Upper Limb.* Vol 8. Philadelphia: Elsevier; 2006:51–137.
69. Kessler I. Centralisation of the radial club hand by gradual distraction. *J Hand Surg Br.* 1989;14(1):37–42.
70. Vilkki SK. Vascularized metatarsophalangeal joint transfer for radial hypoplasia. *Semin Plast Surg.* 2008;22(3):195–212.
71. Peterson BM, McCarroll Jr HR, James MA. Distraction lengthening of the ulna in children with radial longitudinal deficiency. *J Hand Surg.* 2007;32(9):1402–1407.
72. Upton J. Constriction ring syndrome. In: Mathes SJ, ed. *Plastic Surgery. The Hand and Upper Limb.* 2nd edn. Vol 8. Philadelphia: Elsevier; 2006:185–213.
73. Patterson TJ. Congenital ring-constrictions. *Br J Plast Surg.* 1961;14:1–31.
74. Torpin R. Amniochorionic mesoblastic fibrous strings and amnionic bands: associated constricting fetal malformations or fetal death. *Am J Obstet Gynecol.* 1965;91:65–75.
75. Jones MC. The spectrum of structural defects produced as a result of amnion rupture. *Semin Perinatol.* 1983;7(4):281–284.
76. DeMyer W, Baird I. Mortality and skeletal malformations from amniocentesis and oligohydramnios in rats: cleft palate, clubfoot, microstomia, and adactyly. *Teratology.* 1969;2(1):33–37.
77. Coady MS, Moore MH, Wallis K. Amniotic band syndrome: the association between rare facial clefts and limb ring constrictions. *Plast Reconstr Surg.* 1998;101(3):640–649.
78. Wiedrich TA. Congenital constriction band syndrome. *Hand Clin.* 1998;14(1):29–38.
79. Upton J, Tan C. Correction of constriction rings. *J Hand Surg.* 1991;16(5):947–953.
80. Bellew M, Haworth J, Kay SP. Toe to hand transfer in children: ten year follow up of psychological aspects. *J Plast Reconstr Aesthet Surg.* 2011;64(6):766–775.
81. Kessler I, Baruch A, Hecht O. Experience with distraction lengthening of digital rays in congenital anomalies. *J Hand Surg.* 1977;2(5):394–401.
82. Mennen U, van Heest A, Ezaki MB, et al. Arthrogryposis multiplex congenita. *J Hand Surg Br.* 2005;30(5):468–474.
83. Bamshad M, Van Heest AE, Pleasure D. Arthrogryposis: a review and update. *J Bone Joint Surg Am.* 2009;91(suppl 4):40–46.
84. Beals RK. The distal arthrogryposes: a new classification of peripheral contractures. *Clin Orthopaed Relat Res.* 2005;(435):203–210.
85. Fahy MJ, Hall JG. A retrospective study of pregnancy complications among 828 cases of arthrogryposis. *Genet Couns.* 1990;1(1):3–11.
86. Bernstein RM. Arthrogryposis and amyoplasia. *J Am Acad Orthop Surg.* 2002;10(6):417–424.
87. Ezaki M. Treatment of the upper limb in the child with arthrogryposis. *Hand Clin.* 2000;16(4):703–711.
88. Ty JM, James MA. Failure of differentiation: part II (arthrogryposis, camptodactyly, clinodactyly, madelung deformity, trigger finger, and trigger thumb). *Hand Clin.* 2009;25(2):195–213.
89. Van Heest A, Waters PM, Simmons BP. Surgical treatment of arthrogryposis of the elbow. *J Hand Surg.* 1998;23(6):1063–1070.
90. Gogola GR, Ezaki M, Oishi SN, et al. Long head of the triceps muscle transfer for active elbow flexion in arthrogryposis. *Tech Hand Up Extrem Surg.* 2010;14(2):121–124.
91. Ezaki M, Carter PR. Carpal wedge osteotomy for the arthrogrypotic wrist. *Tech Hand Up Extrem Surg.* 2004;8(4):224–228.
92. Tonkin M. Hand and upper extremity. In: Neligan PC, ed. *Plastic Surgery. Hand and Upper Extremity.* Vol 6. Philadelphia: Elsevier Saunders; 2013:647.
93. Dinham JM, Meggitt BF. Trigger thumbs in children. A review of the natural history and indications for treatment in 105 patients. *J Bone Joint Surg Br.* 1974;56(1):153–155.

46

Fingertip Injuries

DONALD SAMMUT AND ROBERT PEARL

Introduction

The hand is in harm's way. It is at the frontier of all work and contact with the environment. The fingertips, as a collective functional unit, bear the statistical brunt of such injuries. Hand injuries constitute the single most frequent surgical presentation in an average Emergency Department.[1]

The hand is unique in its dual role as a considerable gatherer of information about the environment and also as an executor. Unlike the other major sensory organ, the eye, the hand is also able to act on the information gathered, constantly modifying action by feedback of sensation and proprioception. The gathering of information about the environment is especially developed in pulp and palmar digital skin, which is not to be regarded merely as skin covering, but as a specialized organ in its own right. The dense population of sensory end organs is housed in skin with specialized, mechanical properties. The skin is robust and yet deformable – the nail complex and the skeleton provide a fixed stop, against which the pulp and palmar skin complex are deformed – without such a rigid stop, one would obtain less meaningful information about the contour and texture of a held object or touched surface.

The esthetic importance of the hand is not to be underestimated and is an important consideration in all reconstruction. Irrespective of custom and attire, in virtually all societies, the hand is always on display (the hand is exposed even in societies where the face is concealed). The back of the hand, in particular, is a significant esthetic unit. In this regard, function and appearance are closely interlinked. The hand which behaves fluently and efficiently attracts little attention, even if it carries significant scar, or is missing anatomical parts. Smooth, healthy-looking skin cover, as well as fluid, natural behavior, form important aspects of social acceptability. Hand gestures reinforce facial expression and in some spheres, hand movement and posture constitute a very specific vocabulary, interpretable by those who converse in that language. Aside from the obvious example of signing for the deaf, the orchestra conductor's hand gestures speak a clear language to musicians and culture-specific hand gestures convey meaning over distance beyond that possible through sound. Convention and social context convey specific messages with hand gestures – the extended index finger held vertically over the lips is universally interpreted as a request for quiet, for silence. It is also relevant that the hand is the most frequent acceptable point of contact; in most societies, the handshake is considered a permissible intrusion into personal space, and a permitted form of contact, irrespective of the difference in social standing of those shaking hands.

The hand is an integral part of one's identity for any individual but specific professions imbue the hand with an additional importance. The musician, for instance, has a special relationship with the hand since this forms an integral part of his/her identity and "voice." The same can be said of the craftsman or in sports that use the hand. Although these aspects form an important element of management, one must not overrate the contribution of profession to the decision-making process. While some methods of reconstruction may entail an unacceptable period off work for, say, the manual worker, whose main concern may be for strength and durability, all will require a large measure of pain-free, sensate dexterity. Irrespective of work or leisure pursuits, all will still need to perform delicate, precise tasks, such as writing and doing up fastenings and buttons, touching spouse and offspring. Most will be disturbed by an unattractive extremity on display.

Since the hand is the part most frequently involved in work-related injuries,[2] the issue of personal injury claims and the cloud of possible compensation frequently hangs over the outcome of repair and reconstruction.

The growing hand presents special challenges on a number of fronts. Any repair must take into account the facilitation of growth of soft tissues and skeletal elements. Scarring and contracture, a perennial problem in the hand, assume an added importance. To these factors must be added the factor of parental anxiety and elements of guilt and regret centered on the occurrence of the injury in the first place. In general, the management of the child's hand involves the management of the family.

These various factors should all figure in the assessment of injury, the "feel" of patient compliance and cooperation, the choice and planning of repair and reconstruction, and the required aftercare. All too often these injuries are downgraded in the queue of surgical priorities – many still consider that "all soft tissue injuries of the pulp heal" without regard to the quality of function of such healing. Injuries that can lead directly to significant loss of function, persistent pain,

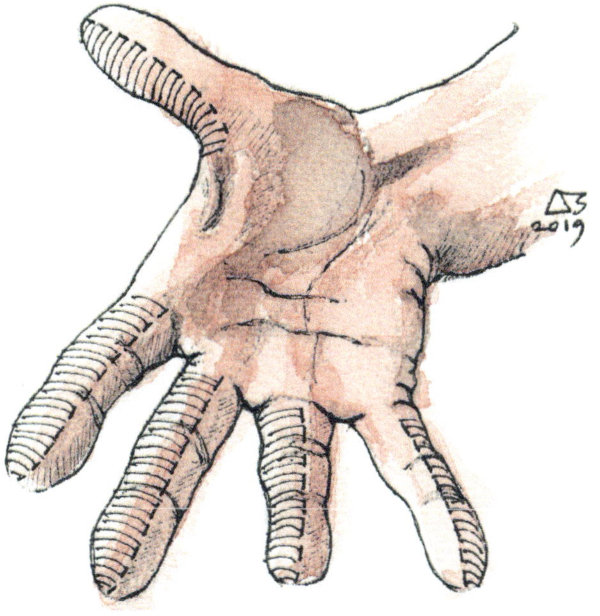

• **Fig. 46.1** The leading aspects of the digits.

and compromised appearance are still, regrettably, considered trivial and meriting little surgical input. They are often misguidedly delegated to inexperienced members of the surgical team with little appreciation of their complexity and functional significance.

Assessment

The challenge of reconstruction in the hand lies in the assessment and decision-making, not in the technique, however immaculately executed is the latter. In assessing any injury (and the patient) one brings to bear experience and a big repertoire so that, as far as possible, questions are answered before the start of surgery. This is not to say that plans may not change when the examination reveals more detail, but it is the planning and selection of technique that is the focus and the essential to a good outcome.

In the field of reconstruction, there are no recipes, only principles. In the management of reconstruction challenges of the digits, one vital principle is the appreciation that not all areas of the hand are of equal functional value.

Observation of the hand in action soon reveals that all digits have leading and trailing aspects. While one would not suggest that any part of the hand is of lesser importance, in reconstructive terms these could also be considered "high premium" and "low premium" territories (Fig. 46.1).

The leading edge is the more commonly used in contact with a held object or contact with a surface. The trailing edge is less often in contact, and tends to have less developed discriminatory abilities or needs. This principle is most true of the thumb: the ulnar pulp "leads" and is involved in virtually all dexterous activity and certainly all precision actions, since it is this area which faces the long digits most effectively. By contrast, the radial pulp "trails" during most tasks coming into play with relatively unspecialized tasks such as tapping on a horizontal surface or keyboard. The principle is least true of the index, both of whose aspects are frequently involved in common activity.

Once this principle is accepted, one can start to assess the functional significance of a specific defect and the availability of suitable methods of reconstruction:

1. High premium areas require the best possible reconstruction, preferably sensate, glabrous pulp skin taken if possible from the same digit.
2. Injury to a low premium area may be reconstructed acceptably and reliably with relatively nonspecialized cover, such as a skin graft or an insensate skin flap.
3. Low premium areas can be considered for transfer to high premium areas, preferably on the same digit, as for instance the reconstruction of ulnar pulp in the thumb using radial pulp (Fig. 46.2).

These observations are proposed as factors to be taken into account, and are certainly not absolute. They are amongst many that should be considered, including the requirements of the patient overall, likelihood of compliance, as well as special requirements for a particular patient, such as the playing of musical instruments or professional sport.

In few other areas of reconstruction is collaboration with the patient as essential. This element needs careful assessment if one is to obtain a good outcome – in this situation a good outcome is the maximum restoration of function (and hence appearance) and an acceptance by the patient of any limitations consequent on the injury.

Detailed informed consent also needs to take into account the time and effort investment required of the patient, particularly in the more complex reconstructions. The extension of the site of injury and/or the involvement of distant donor sites are all factors to be included in the detail of the process of informed consent.

Finally, in the process of assessment, the surgeon must also have a realistic and honest assessment of his/her capabilities. Many methods of reconstruction are attractive to the surgeon since they fulfill a natural mechanical neatness and challenge of construct. The seduction of such methods must be resisted in the absence of expertise or adequate guidance (and, preferably, also assistance) by those more experienced.

It cannot be overemphasized that the method selected must suit the defect and the level of expertise of the surgeon. In this regard one must mention that it may be entirely appropriate to select a temporary method known to be insufficient for long-term wear and restoration of function (such as a dressing or a split-skin graft on pulp), leaving all options open for reconstruction with the availability of appropriate expertise. If this approach is selected, it is wise to present this to the patient as a two-stage procedure so that he/she is prepared for the second surgery and it does not come as a "salvage," or adjustment, of the first.

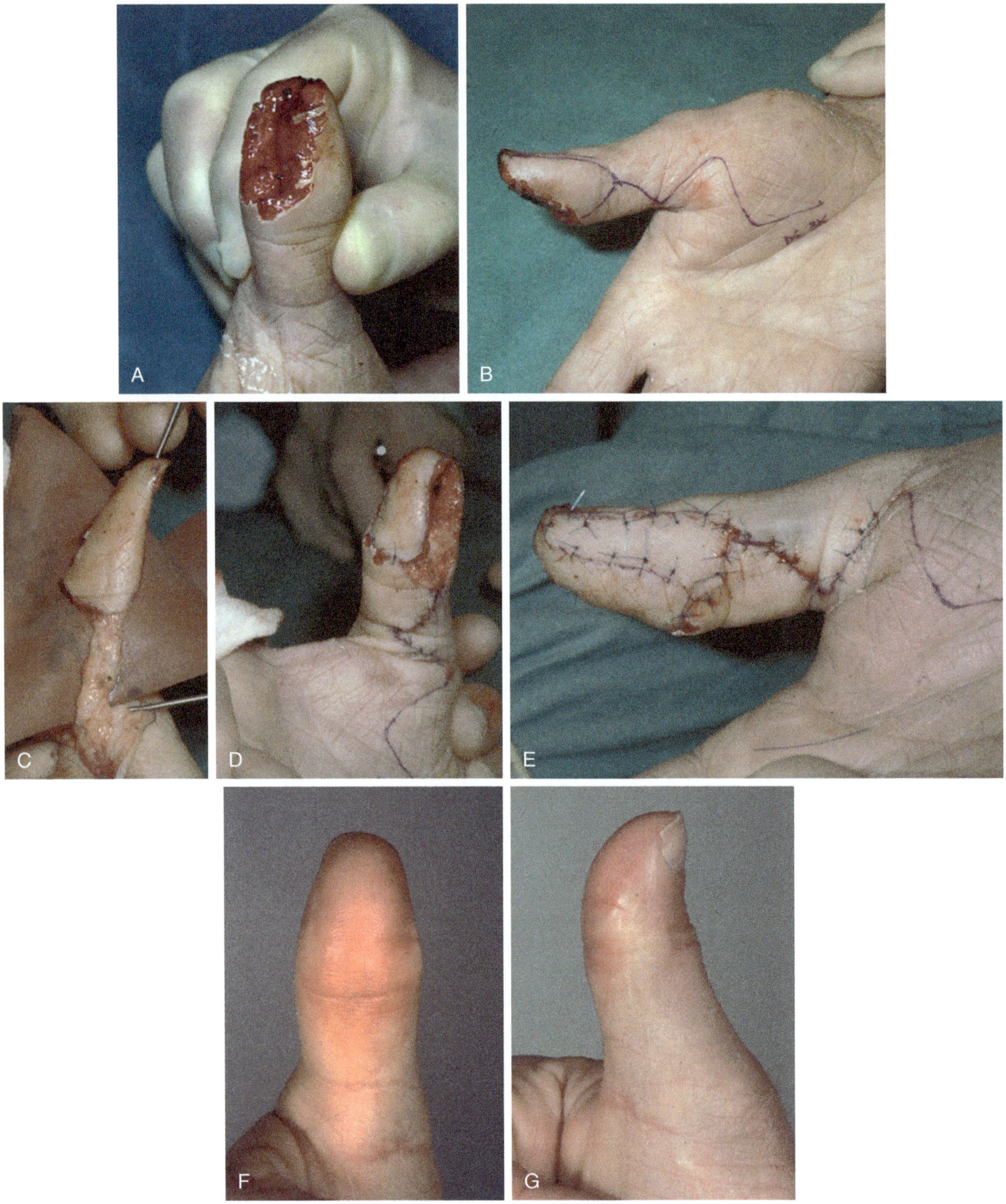

• **Fig. 46.2** Pulp exchange flap. (A) The defect involves the entire leading (ulnar)surface of the thumb pulp. (B) The trailing (radial) aspect of pulp is intact and an island flap is deigned on this pulp. (C) The flap is entirely islanded, leaving ample fat around the nerve and artery. (D) The island is transposed to reconstruct the ulnar pulp. (E) The secondary defect is resurfaced with a skin graft, in this case a full-thickness graft taken from the amputated part, which was de-fatted. (F,G) Final result at 3 months.

Healing by Secondary Intention

Both pulp and palmar skin have remarkable powers of regeneration, as evidenced by the reliable healing of the open palm technique advocated by McCash.[3]

Large defects of pulp will heal reliably provided a number of important criteria are observed:

1. The defect must be suited to this method. No vital structure, such as tendon, bone, or joint, must be exposed. Severely contaminated or crush defects must be thoroughly debrided of all contamination or necrosis.
2. The hand must be elevated.
3. The patient must understand that the method requires careful adherence to instruction and compliance with treatment. (Many patients will only remember that "It needs no surgery" and this is rapidly translated into "It needs no care").
4. Nonadherent dressings require regular change, preferably on alternate days. Exception is made for children, where it is routine to leave a dressing undisturbed for a week, after which the wound can be left exposed, in order to avoid the trauma of painful dressings.

The dressing in direct contact with the wound is a matter of personal preference. Tulle gras (paraffin impregnated gauze) is traditional. It is cheap and easily available or can be improvised, but dries rapidly and tends to adhere more than one might expect. Many, superior, alternatives are available, such as thin, perforated silicone sheeting (e.g., Mepitel, Mölnlycke Healthcare, Gothenburg, Sweden), which is resistant to all adherence. Chitin (Beschitin, Unitika, Osaka, Japan), and other natural substances, have their advocates. The important aspects are: nonadherence, a barrier to contamination, and assiduous care and compliance.

Surgical Options for Cover

Amputation

In cases where a significant part of the digit is crushed with accompanying disruption of the nail complex and/or the distal interphalangeal joint, amputation with closure of locally available skin may be the indicated option. In this situation, it may be appropriate to elect to ablate any nail elements which, regenerating, will be unsupported, nonadherent, unattractive or likely to lead to functional problems such as snagging on clothing.

Much morbidity results from amputation performed without proper regard to indications and points of technique. There is a natural tendency to preserve length at all costs. The aim should be to achieve a nontender digit covered by good-quality skin, irrespective of length. It is better to elect for a slightly shorter length, with good quality, mobile skin cover, than to preserve length at all costs but with a tight and painful digit end. A digit with tense, painful, skin cover may well be excluded from function, resulting in an effective loss of all useful length. This is particularly true of the index, which is readily substituted by the middle finger and regularly requires subsequent revision. It is a wise surgeon who seeks to prevent the cycle of pain, tenderness, and exclusion.

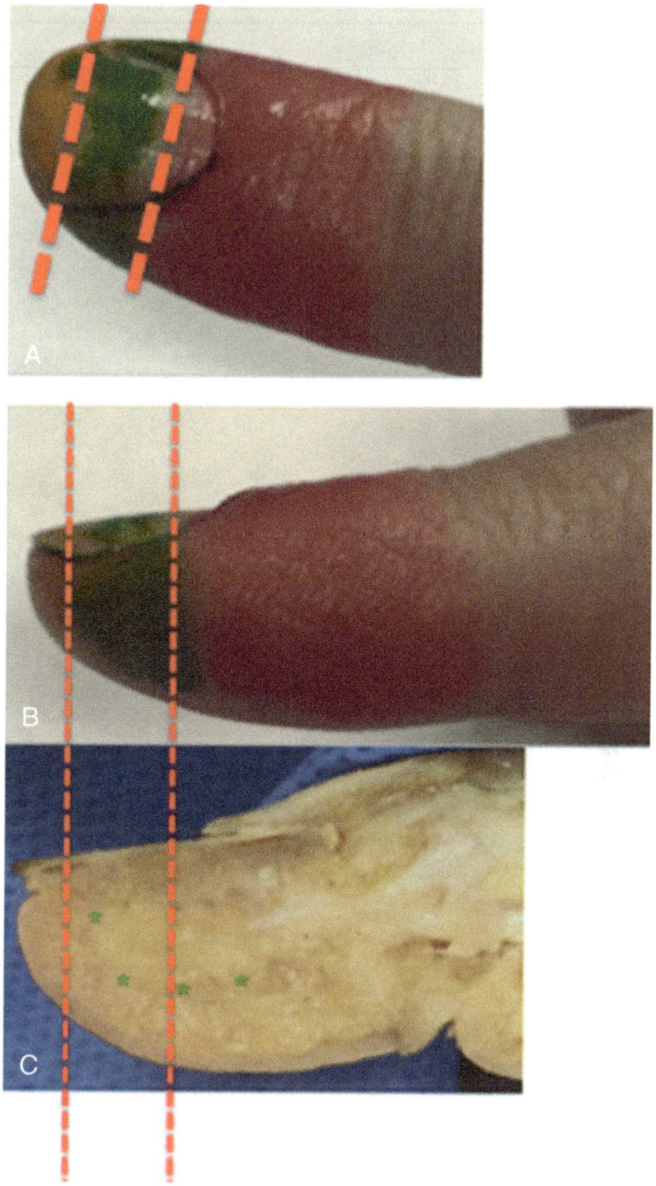

• **Fig. 46.3** The levels of amputation. *Level 1*: There is a skin defect with minimal loss of nail and no significant loss of supporting distal phalanx. Indication: Dressing or, if bone exposed, advancement of skin flap. *Level 2*: A significant portion of nail and supporting bone is lost. Indication: Ablation of nail remnant and trimming of bone so as to preserve the next vital structures, the insertion of extensor and flexor, while achieving tension free cover (direct closure or flap). *Level 3*: The tendon insertions are disrupted. Indication: Trimming of bone and removal of articular cartilage to achieve skin cover with appropriate cover (direct closure or flap). (A,B Courtesy Dr. DA Stearns, Department of Emergency Medicine, Massachusetts General Hospital, Harvard Medical School, Boston.)

There are three generally indicative levels of amputation of the fingertip (Fig. 46.3):

Level 1: involves loss of skin and only a minimal loss of nail and distal phalanx. In this case all of the tip vital structures are preserved and skin cover is indicated.

Level 2: involves loss of skin and most of the distal phalanx/nail complex. In this case the nail should be ablated and the next proximal structures to preserve are the tendon insertions. Just enough bone should be left, to preserve these insertions which will preserve power and elements of proprioception.

Level 3: has lost all nail elements and the tendon insertions. The condyles of the middle phalanx can be removed to prevent an unattractive, spatulate stump shape. The phalanx is shortened to a level where tension-free, good skin cover can be achieved. One should not be tempted to anchor the tendons, or to suture them to each other. This invariably leads to an imbalance and most frequently to a flexion contracture.

All amputations require attention to the nerve ends. One should take the opportunity of any skeletal shortening to keep the nerve ends long and to transpose them dorsally, away from contact areas.

Options for Skin Cover

If skin cover is required the options are:

1. Skin graft, or
2. Flap cover.

Reconstruction most often involves moving tissue around from one site to another, with the added, vital, phrase "and keeping it alive." Blood supply is paramount. A skin graft requires a bed capable of angiogensis, the essential process of "take." "Take" is the establishment of a blood supply to support a graft. A flap requires no such bed – it brings its own blood supply and can be placed over any surface, including metalwork. Provided this principle is observed, the decision can then be taken on what form of cover will best restore function and structure. The concept of the "reconstructive ladder" with its implications that one chooses the simplest reconstruction available, is outdated – one chooses what is appropriate and best restores form and function.

It follows that the surgeon must have in his/her repertoire as large a variety of reconstruction as possible, in order to match the reconstruction to the defect, and patient, and not the other way around. This, incidentally, is another strong reason for involvement of experienced, senior surgeons. All too often this process is left to those with one or two methods at their disposal; this invariably results in the dispensation of a method which the surgeon knows, rather than that which is appropriate.

Skin Grafts

Provided the bed will ensure take, a split-thickness skin graft (STSG) provides excellent temporary cover or permanent cover of a "low priority" area, including a secondary defect, from flap harvest. Many wounds involve crushing or bursting mechanisms and it is difficult, at first view, to be sure of viability unless one is wastefully radical with excision. In such situations, a flap may be the appropriate skin cover but its territory may itself lie in the area of trauma. Proceeding with immediate flap cover may lead to flap loss and failure with waste of a reconstructive option. A skin graft may provide comfort, initiate healing, resolve inflammation, and will keep all other options open.

In some situations, skin graft provides good definitive cover. These include the trailing aspects of digits and the secondary defects from the raising of a flap. It need hardly be added that a flap donor source is chosen from an area that can be closed directly, can take a skin graft, or can be left to heal by secondary intention.

Skin grafts do not provide good definitive cover in the pulp, where accurate, pain-free sensibility and good mechanical properties are required. In such a situation, the skin graft will lead to unacceptable hyperesthesia, poor cosmesis, and troublesome long-term fissuring.

The choice between split- and full-thickness skin graft (FTSG) is a matter of balance of various factors. A full-thickness graft requires a better quality bed, since there is a larger cell population to nourish. Take of a split-skin graft is more reliable on a poorer bed. Conversely, split-skin grafts contract more significantly than full-thickness grafts – an important factor in cover of mobile areas crossing joint creases and anywhere in the growing hand.

Points of Technique

Split-Thickness Skin Graft

1. Donor site: Small grafts can be taken from the hypothenar mound. The skin here is thick enough to permit harvest of the dermis while replacing the epidermis.[4] Larger grafts can be taken from the proximal inner aspect of the forearm, where it can be unattractive and/or tender or from the thigh. With both STSG and FTSG, the opportunity to harvest skin, or indeed any other element, from a finger that is to be discarded should not be lost (the concept of "the bank digit", see below).[5]
2. A guarded skin graft knife is used, such as the Watson, Humby, Silvers knife or, for larger areas, the electric dermatome.

Full-Thickness Skin Graft

1. Donor site: Avoid harvest from the wrist skin crease – scars here can be misinterpreted as the outcome of self-inflicted wounds and can prove tender and troublesome with the wearing of watches or bracelets. The cubital fossa provides ample skin for most needs in the hand and digits. It is usually hairless, and is in the same bloodless field, which speeds up proceedings and makes harvest more accurate. Hairy donor sites should be avoided – harvest from the groin crease in children before the distribution of pubic hair is evident provides a common pitfall.
2. The graft should be taken thin, without subcutaneous fat, or thinned just before final detachment.
3. The graft should be sutured tense over the recipient site (suture of a graft provides the only instance when suture under tension is permissible) and larger areas require a tie over dressing.

Finally, one may mention the composite graft as a form of skin grafting. This is particularly applicable in the child's hand, when the section is clean and the segment uncrushed. It is more successful the fresher the injury and the younger the child. The amputated part should be applied rapidly, with minimal dissection of either surface and with accurate alignment of landmarks, such as nail fold and even print ridges. Parents are warned that the method is not guaranteed and that reconstruction may be required if it fails. The part often appears to necrose and perish, only to reveal accurate resurfacing some 3 weeks later when the carapace falls off or is peeled off.

Flap Cover

The indications for flap cover may be summarized:

1. When bone, joint, and tendon are exposed, or when metalwork needs cover. In some situations one has no choice but to apply a skin graft to intact tendon sheath or paratenon, or even direct to cancellous bone where somewhat surprisingly, it frequently takes. These are relative indications – by and large, exposure of such structures requires flap cover.
2. When deeper structures are not exposed and the defect is capable of nourishing a graft, but sensibility, mechanical quality or cosmesis are relevant requirements.

Flaps have been classified in all manner of ways. In the hand, the most relevant classifications are two:

1. The basis of the *blood supply* – preservation of continuity of blood supply is paramount. This may be either left unidentified in the flap base (e.g., the Hueston flap[6] or the cross finger flap[7]) or formally dissected free, as in the islanded flaps. In general, the latter type of designs are the more mobile and versatile, but demand a higher level of technical expertise.
2. The presence of *sensibility* – for classification purposes, one may consider "sensate" flaps those which maintain pulp quality and replace lost pulp with sensate pulp. One should not consider adequately "sensate" the cross finger flap, which regains some sensibility despite the numerous reports of recovery of "excellent" two-point discrimination.[8,9] Nor should one consider that the transfer of an island of dorsal skin (e.g., the kite flap) to replace adequate pulp quality sensibility.

On this basis, one may classify the commonly available flaps thus:

- *Relatively insensate flaps*
  - Kite flap
  - Delayed flaps: cross finger, thenar, distant flaps, e.g., groin flaps, random flaps
  - Free venous flaps
- *Relatively sensate flaps*
  - V–Y advancements
  - Thenar advancement
  - Bipedicle homodigital
  - Homodigital islands (Segmuller,[10] Venkataswami,[11] Joshi[12])
  - Heterodigital (Littler[13])
  - Free flaps, e.g., hemipulp transfer from toe or from a bank digit. The recovery of sensation is inversely proportional to age in these examples.

This definition of sensate/insensate is a working classification serving to underline the importance of replacing like with like. It sorts out flaps rather too harshly on the basis of restoration of pulp quality sensation. Many studies report recovery of 2-point discrimination approaching normal in flaps that cannot transfer nerve continuity, such as the cross finger flap.[9,14] In this context, one should note that our methods of assessment of sensory discrimination remain relatively crude and subject to significant operator variability and subjectivity.

The description of flap qualities is not intended to label any flap superior or inferior to others. All are useful in context and the wise reconstructive surgeon will master all, and will amass a large repertoire on which to draw when analyzing each individual defect. It cannot be repeated too often that each defect will have qualities that will be met by this or that flap, and one should have all at one's disposal, so as to be able to produce a flap that matches the defect, not the other way around. In this regard, one should resist the tendency to refer to this or that flap as a "workhorse" or to apply the same, favorite, flap to a wide variety of defects. Conversely, it is also ill advised for the inexperienced to be captivated by a clever flap and to resolve to "try" it.

The account below cannot be exhaustive. Representative flaps in each category have been selected which illustrate the principles of selection, technique, flap attributes that form part of the analysis, planning, and execution of skin cover of the digit.

Flaps with Less than Pulp-Quality Sensation

The Kite Flap

This flap was originally designed, with a wide base pedicle, by Holevitch.[15] Vilain and Michon developed this design, narrowing the pedicle to about 1 cm, including the vascular axis, and this design was named the "flag flap." It was Foucher who islanded the skin flap, denuding the pedicle of skin and conferring a greater degree of mobility as well as the potential for tunneling of the pedicle.[16] The island of skin is raised in a plane just superficial to the extensor tendon parateneon (which must be left intact so as to receive a graft). The pedicle includes the first dorsal metacarpal artery, local veins, as may be found (usually plentiful), and any superficial branches of the radial nerve that are identifiable (Fig. 46.4).

The radial nerve branches provide sensation but the density of end organs in the dorsal skin never matches the density required to provide pulp-quality sensation and it is for this reason that this flap is included in the "insensate" category.

Although it is tempting to use it for resurfacing of the leading edge of thumb pulp, its use should be reserved to

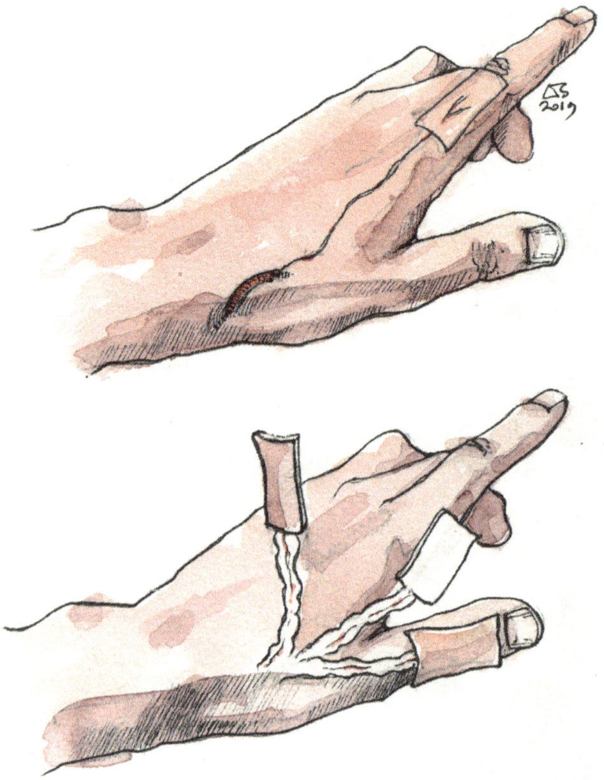

• **Fig. 46.4** The Kite flap raised on the dorsum of the index.

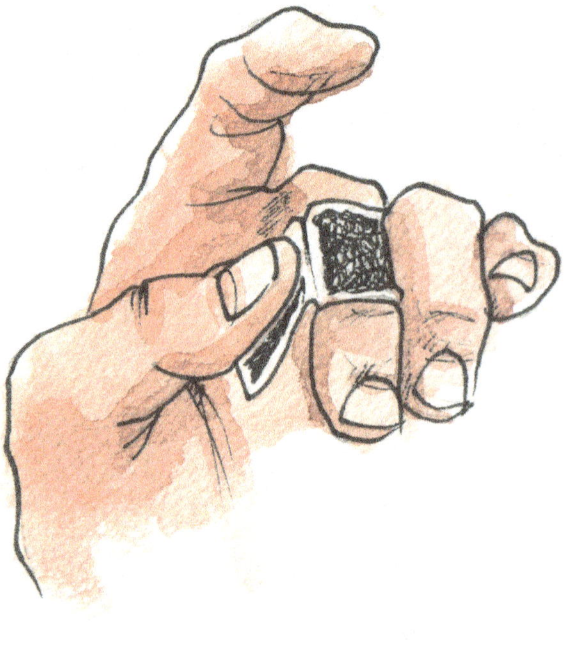

• **Fig. 46.5** Cross finger flap raised on the dorsum of the middle finger to resurface distal palmar index. The secondary defect receives a skin graft.

areas with less demanding sensory qualities, such as the dorsum of the thumb and the radial aspect.

Important Points of Technique

1. The first dorsal metacarpal artery should be identified early since it may follow a course part way through the substance or fascia of the first dorsal interosseous muscle.
2. It is prudent to include any veins that can be gathered into the pedicle – a surfeit of veins makes for a healthier flap.
3. Terminal branches of the radial cutaneous nerve are fine and must be sought and preserved.
4. If the flap is tunneled, the tunnel must be generous and without sharp kinks in its course.
5. The donor area must be carefully protected, the paratenon left intact so as to receive a graft.

Advantages

The technique is relatively unchallenging and the flap is robust provided important points of technique are observed. The loss of skin from the dorsum of the index produces no functional impairment. Care with the dissection should ensure full and immediate take, so that the cosmetic defect is minimized. The pedicle is mobile and long and permits placement of the flap in a wide radius of reach.

Disadvantages

The quality of the thin, poorly sensate, transferred skin cannot replace glabrous skin with its myriad of end organs and special mechanical qualities. This limits its application. The transferred skin may be hairy, particularly in males and, in black skin, will be darker than palmar skin. The skin graft applied to the donor site may pigment.

Delayed, Staged, Flaps

The Principle of Delay

Delayed flaps have a random design, i.e., they are not planned over a known vascular pedicle. They are inset into a recipient defect and their relative ischemia (which can be encouraged by judicious clamping) encourages ingrowth of vessels from the recipient site. The flap can then be detached from the donor site. The period required before the flap can be safely detached from its original vascular supply varies, but generally depends on the quality of blood supply in the recipient bed and the volume of flap that must be nourished. The principle of delay is discussed in more detail in Chapter 1.

The Cross Finger Flap

Gurdin and Pangman are credited with the first description of this flap, which uses a well-established principle. It is still one of the most commonly used (and abused) flaps employed for skin cover in the digits.[7] In principle, dorsal skin from a digit is raised and turned over like the page of a book. A palmar defect in an adjacent digit can be inset and receive cover. The secondary defect receives a graft. There are a number of variations, including the innervated neurovascular cross finger flap and the reverse dermis cross finger flap (Figs. 46.5 and 46.6).

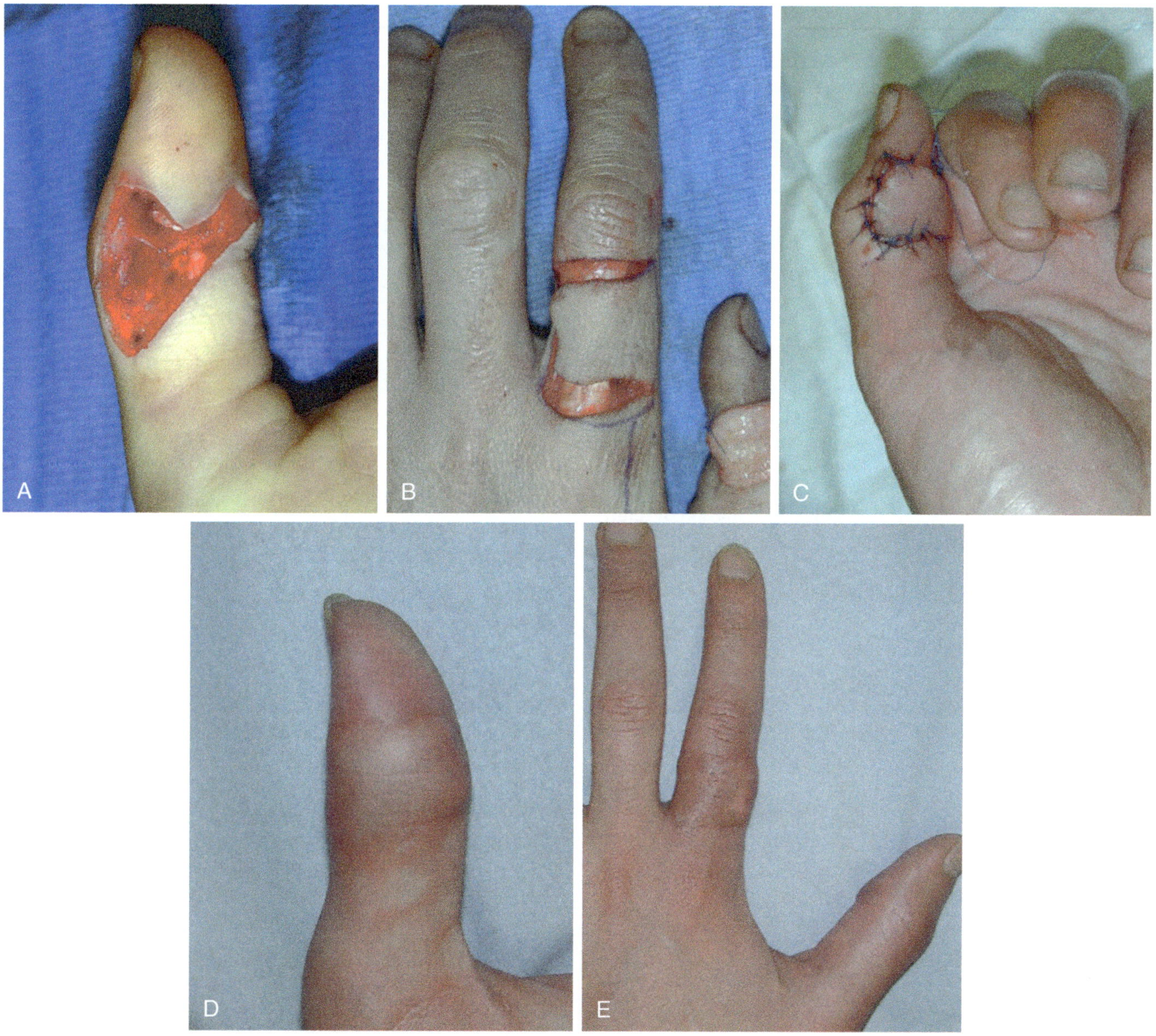

• **Fig. 46.6** Cross finger flap. (A) The defect on the anterolateral part of the thumb. (B) The cross finger flap raised from the dorsum on the index finger, leaving behind the paratenon of the extensor tendon for skin grafting. (C) The flap is inset without tension, and the pedicle left attached for 3 weeks before division. (D,E) The healed flap on the thumb and the grafted donor site on the index finger. (Courtesy Peter Burge.)

Important Points of Technique

1. The recipient defect should be thoroughly debrided before planning of the flap.
2. It is best, if possible, to design the flap over the dorsum of the finger between the interphalangeal joints.
3. The flap must be raised carefully so as to preserve its dermal plexus but also to leave behind a graftable defect.
4. The skin graft (usually full-thickness) is best secured and inset into the donor defect before the flap is sutured to the recipient. It is easier to gain access to all the borders of the graft while the fingers are still unattached.

Advantages

The flap is reliable, simple to perform, and versatile – the same digit can act as donor, giving a flap to a neighbor and as recipient, receiving a second flap from another neighbor, e.g., dorsum of middle finger to palmar index combined with dorsum index to palmar thumb.

Disadvantages

The enforced delay produces stiffness, particularly in the PIP joint of the recipient finger, which is kept flexed for some 2–3 weeks. Pigmented, or hairy, dorsal skin may be unsightly on the palmar surface (Fig. 46.7). A skin graft is required and may pigment. The flap is totally insensate

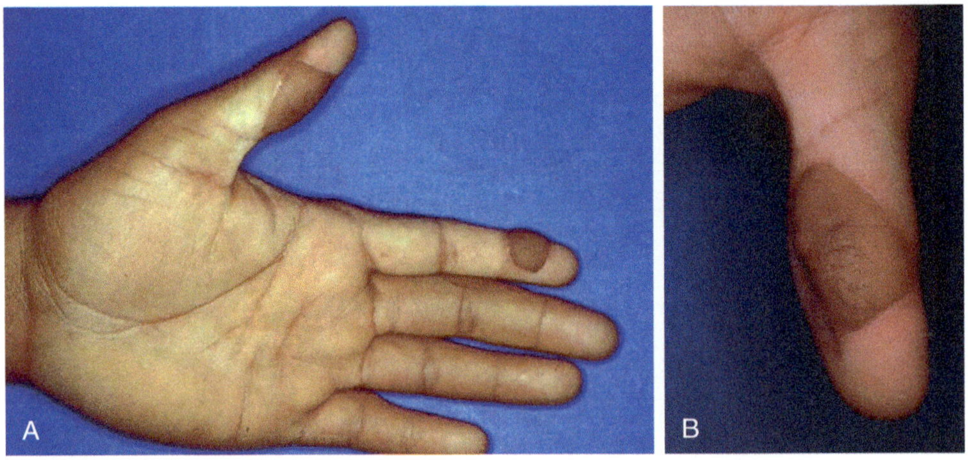

• **Fig. 46.7** Pigmented cross finger flap. (A,B) Dorsal, hairy, pigmented skin transposed to pale palmar skin. (Courtesy Peter Burge.)

unless modified in one of the described methods (e.g., Venkataswami), which are technically more demanding. Its lack of sensation should restrict its use to more proximal defects where the pulp has been preserved.

Distant, Delayed Flaps

The limited indications and disadvantages of locally sourced delayed flaps hold true for distant flaps with the added problems of immobilization and difficulties with elevation of the hand. Nevertheless, it is occasionally necessary to raise and use a random flap from abdomen or arm or an axial pattern, delayed flap from the groin. The groin flap has its application, delayed or by immediate free transfer, in larger defects, especially in staged reconstructions such as multidigit loss which may later receive free toe transfers, at which time it is a bonus to be able to transplant into good-quality trophic skin rather than dense scar.

Flaps with Pulp-Quality Sensation

The Atasoy Flap[17]

Some elements of the literature have likened this V–Y advancement of pulp flap described by Atasoy in 1970 to the Tranquili-Leali flap[18] described in 1935, to which some even attribute precedence. There is no connection between the two other than the original triangular shape of the flap (Fig. 46.8).

The Tranquili-Leali flap involved division of both vascular pedicles and flap survival depended on direct supply from the vertical connections between skin and deeper surfaces. This was sheared forward rather like a jelly and its advancement was very limited. In fact the Atasoy flap is a bipedicle island flap, raised on both, intact, vascular pedicles and nerves.

Important Points of Technique

1. Selection is crucial. Only transverse or dorsally inclined defects should be considered. At least half of the distal phalanx should be preserved to provide adequate nail support.
2. The width of the advancing edge must correspond precisely to the width of the nail plate. Too narrow a flap produces unattractive "shoulder pads" either side. Too wide a flap produces an unattractive spatulate result.
3. The flap must be completely islanded, i.e., it must remain attached only by the neurovascular pedicle.
4. The proximal V apex need not be limited to the DIP joint crease. The flap should be designed of the dimensions required and the crease line is an irrelevant landmark.
5. If, postoperatively, there seems to be tension, or congestion, only the side sutures should be considered for release. The leading edge sutures must be left intact; their division will result in retraction of the flap proximally, exposure of bone and healing with a tender, dimpled scar.

The Kutler flaps,[19] double V–Y advancements, each flap on either side of the digit tip, are mentioned because they bear a superficial resemblance to the Atasoy V–Y but, once again, the main point in common is the shape. They are technically challenging and generally unreliable, not least because the anatomy of the vasculature on this area is variable. The vascular arcade in the pulp may be U-shaped, Y-shaped or H-shaped[20] and one cannot rely on an axial vessel on either side, in the flap triangle. In practice, Kutler flaps are raised without islanding, left attached to their bed, and teased forward to obtain modest advancement, a process made more difficult by the presence, in the flap, of Cleland's ligament, which must be teased apart or divided.

The Thenar Advancement Flap

This flap consists of the entire palmar surface of the thumb, raised off the flexor sheath and skeleton, and stretched distally to cover a distal transverse defect. It enjoys the advantage of perfectly sensate, homodigital cover, which requires no re-education (Fig. 46.9).

In essence, this flap "creeps" distally, the division of septa and tethering fibers enabling the skin to cover a larger area by stretching. In practice, there is also an element of flexion

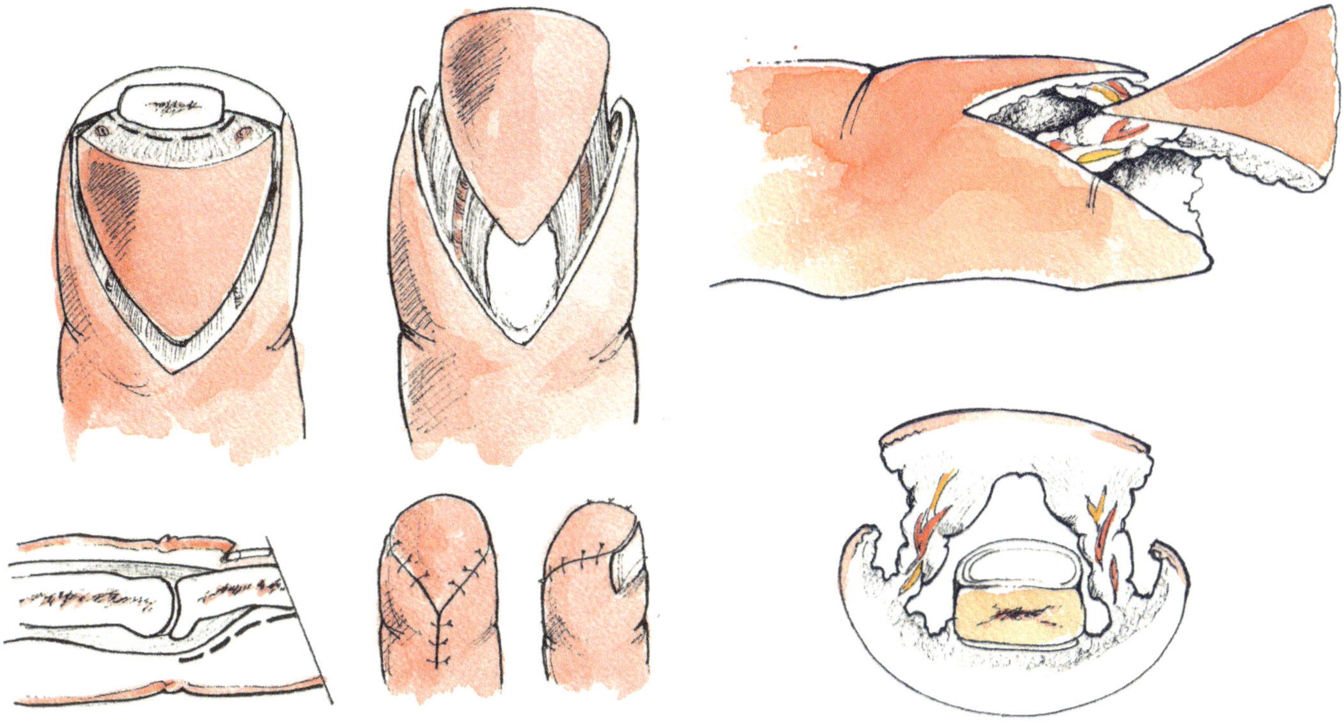

A B

• **Fig. 46.8** Atasoy flap. (A,B) The flap is raised as a V on palmar skin. The distal width of the flap must equal the width of the nail plate. The digital bundles on either side are mobilized. It is important that the flap be entirely islanded free from its bed and attached only by the pedicles with a generous sheath of fat. The flap is advanced and inset. The secondary defect can be closed as a V–Y or left to heal. In selecting an appropriate defect, it is important that the amputation be angled transversely or, preferably, with a dorsal angulation.

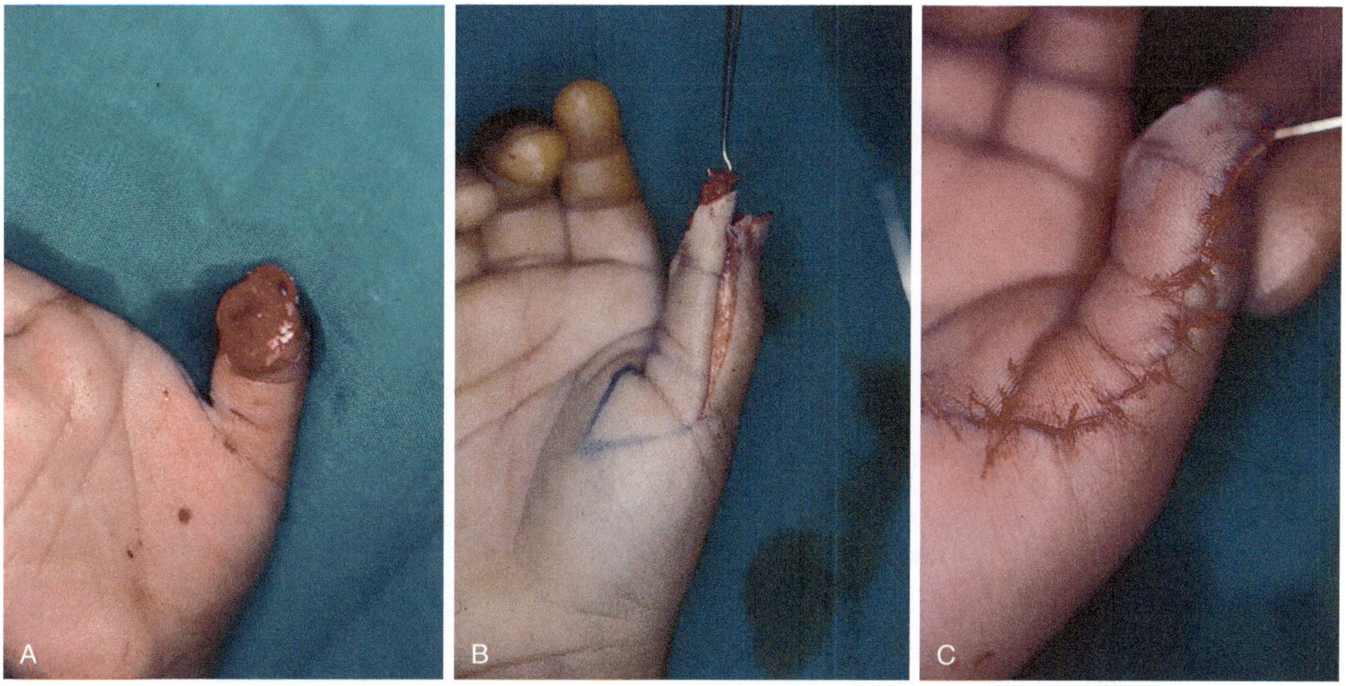

• **Fig. 46.9** The Moberg flap. The flap is raised in the plane of the flexor pollicis longus sheath and includes both digital bundles. The original flap simply advanced by "creep;" aided by some flexion of the thumb, and with no secondary defect. Further advancement can be obtained by transecting (and islanding) the base (O'Brien), and grafting or closing as a V–Y (Carroll). Clinical case: (A) The defect. (B) The flap raised in classical design. (C) The Carroll V–Y modification to close.

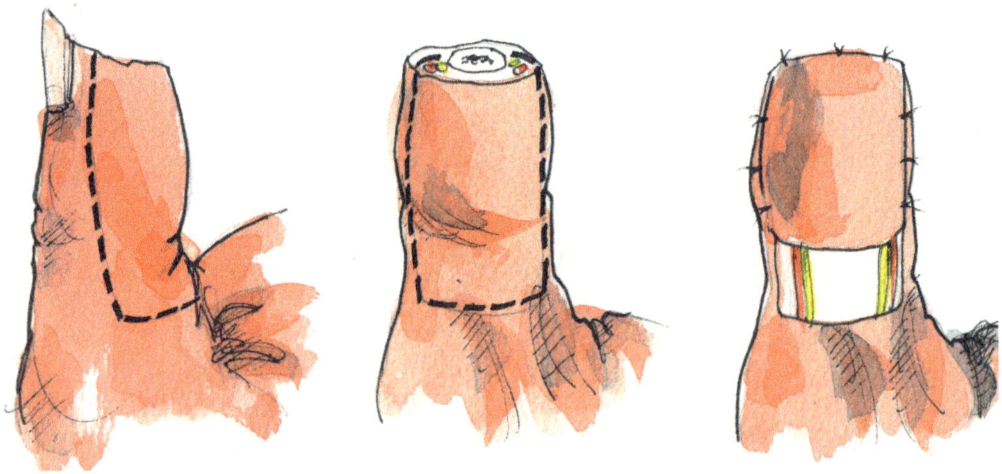

• **Fig. 46.10** The O'Brien islanded flap. O'Brien modified the Moberg flap by transection of the base and islanding.

of the IP joint in most instances, so that the defect comes to meet the flap as much as the flap advances to cover the defect. Flexion contracture of the IP joint is a common sequel to this flap and is, fortunately, not a significant functional impairment.

The flap, originally described by Moberg,[21] is applicable only to the thumb, which enjoys a dual vasculature, dorsal and palmar, so that the two can be separated. Application in other, long, digits, as advocated by Snow, runs a significant risk of necrosis of the dorsal skin.

Important Points of Technique

1. The neurovascular bundles in the thumb lie apposed to the FPL tendon sheath either side and not down the midlateral lines.
2. The parallel incisions must be strictly in the midlateral axis if one is to avoid subsequent flexion contracture.
3. If the flap does not advance enough and/or is too tense, one can join the two parallel incisions on the palmar aspect, effectively islanding the flap on its bundles as advocated by O'Brien[22] (Fig. 46.10) or close the base as a V–Y (Carroll) (see Fig. 46.9).

The Advancement Rotation Flap

This flap is based on one digital bundle, without islanding, rotating to cover a terminal defect. It was described by Hueston[6] (Fig. 46.11) as a square, or rectangular flap, raised by an L-shaped incision. It excludes the neurovascular (NV) bundle from the leading edge and is nourished by the NV bundle in the base. This means that the leading half of the flap is insensate.

Important Points of Technique

1. Selection is best reserved for transverse amputations or for oblique loss slanted towards the base. This minimizes the required arc of travel.
2. One should divide Cleland's ligament in the static base of the flap, since this base too is involved in the stretch and rotation required.

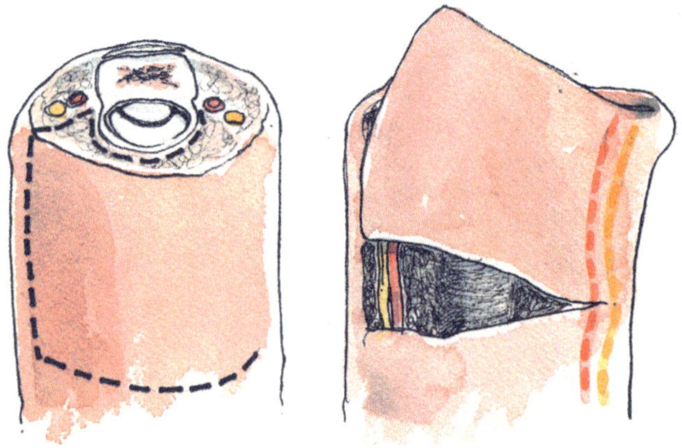

• **Fig. 46.11** The Hueston flap. The flap is square, raised palmar to the leading edge NV bundle, in the plane of the flexor sheath and nourished by the NV bundle in its base. The leading half of the flap is insensate since the leading edge bundle is not included.

3. The distal end of the base will produce a dog-ear and this should be dealt with in the manner described by Foucher, by excision of a square of skin on the dorsum (Fig. 46.12) without reducing the width of the base pedicle.
4. The secondary defect, a raw triangle at the proximal border, can be left to heal by secondary intention or may accept a STSG.
5. Provided the underlying bone is not wide (for instance including phalangeal condyles), one should not trim the skin to coat the skeleton too closely. A looser skin pocket will contract to conform to the skeleton without tension.

The issue of loss of sensation of the leading half has been addressed in various ways:

- Souquet described a modification which included the leading NV bundle in the flap and teasing it so as to permit some stretch. This maintains sensation but greatly limits the ease of rotation and movement (Fig. 46.13).

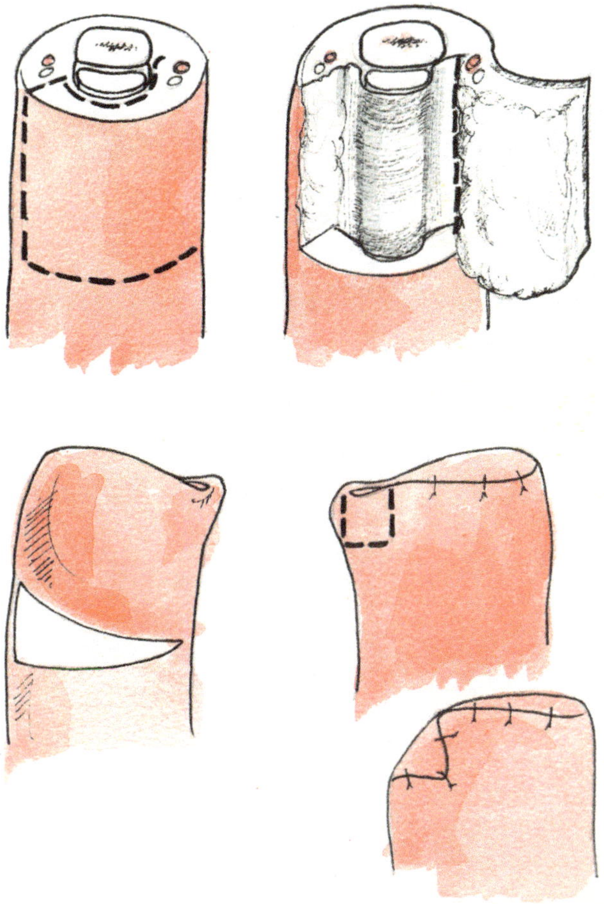

• **Fig. 46.12** Foucher elimination of the Hueston dog-ear.

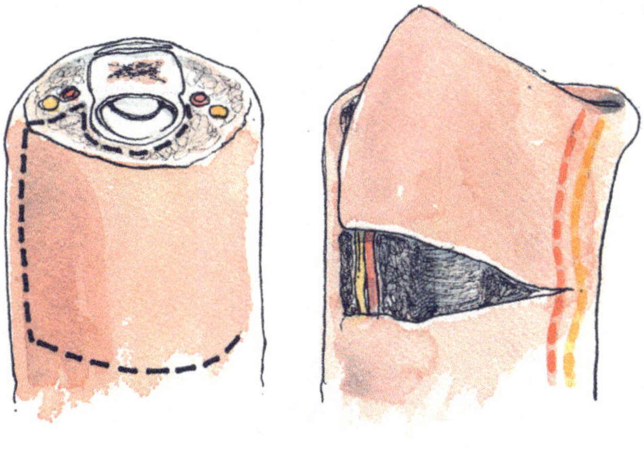

• **Fig. 46.13** The Souquet flap. Like the Hueston flap, the design is square but includes the NV bundle in the leading edge. The flap will rotate less but remains sensate in all areas.

- The flap can be based on the leading edge of a digit, so that the insensate half comes to be placed on the trailing edge and is of lesser functional consequence.
- The two techniques, Hueston and Souquet, can be combined in the manner described by Lloyd and Sammut (Fig. 46.14),[23] which includes both bundles in the flap, but mobilizes the leading NV bundle to obtain better movement.

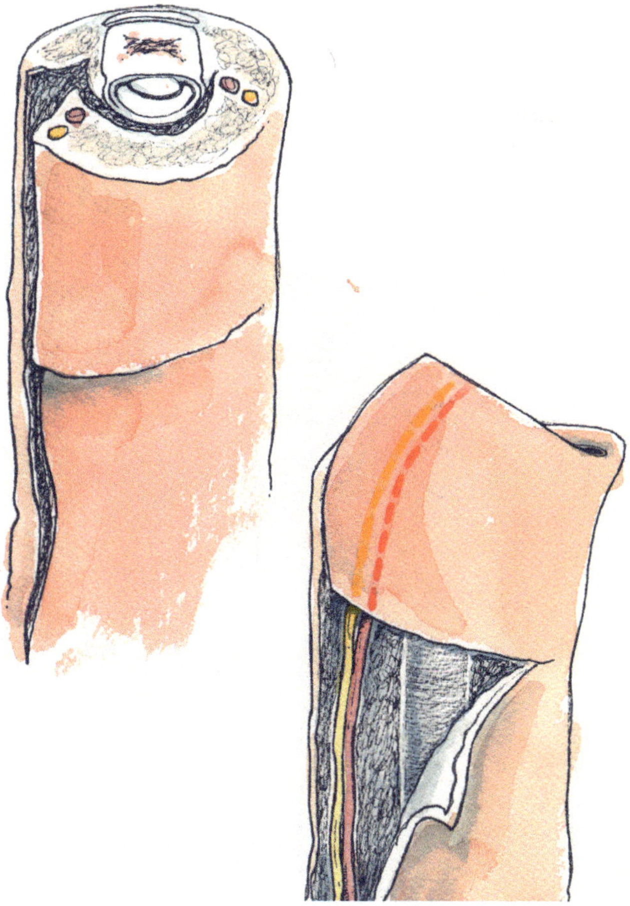

• **Fig. 46.14** Sammut modification of Souquet flap. The Hueston flap has a wide arc of rotation, but the leading edge is insensate. The Souquet flap moves far less but is entirely sensate. The Sammut achieves the best qualities of both flaps by including the leading pedicle (retaining sensibility) and mobilizing it so that it permits flap advancement.

The Island Flaps, Homodigital and Heterodigital

Numerous variations of islanded flaps have been described[10–12] but the principle is the same as that originally designed by Littler, who, in 1953, raised an island of skin from the ring finger, on its NV bundle, and transferred this to the ulnar aspect of a reconstructed thumb to confer sensation.[13]

These are amongst the most versatile flaps for reconstruction since the pedicle permits so much movement. They are technically challenging but provided important points of technique are observed, they have a safe ratio of blood supply to volume of flap. In most cases they are raised on a digital artery which could have supplied the entire digit and, in supplying an island, is now providing generous vascular input.

The homodigital flaps (Segmuller,[10] Venkataswami,[11] Joshi,[12] Evans[24]) vary in their design and orientation – the Segmuller flap is lateral, the Joshi design is predominantly dorsolateral, and the Venkataswami modification was

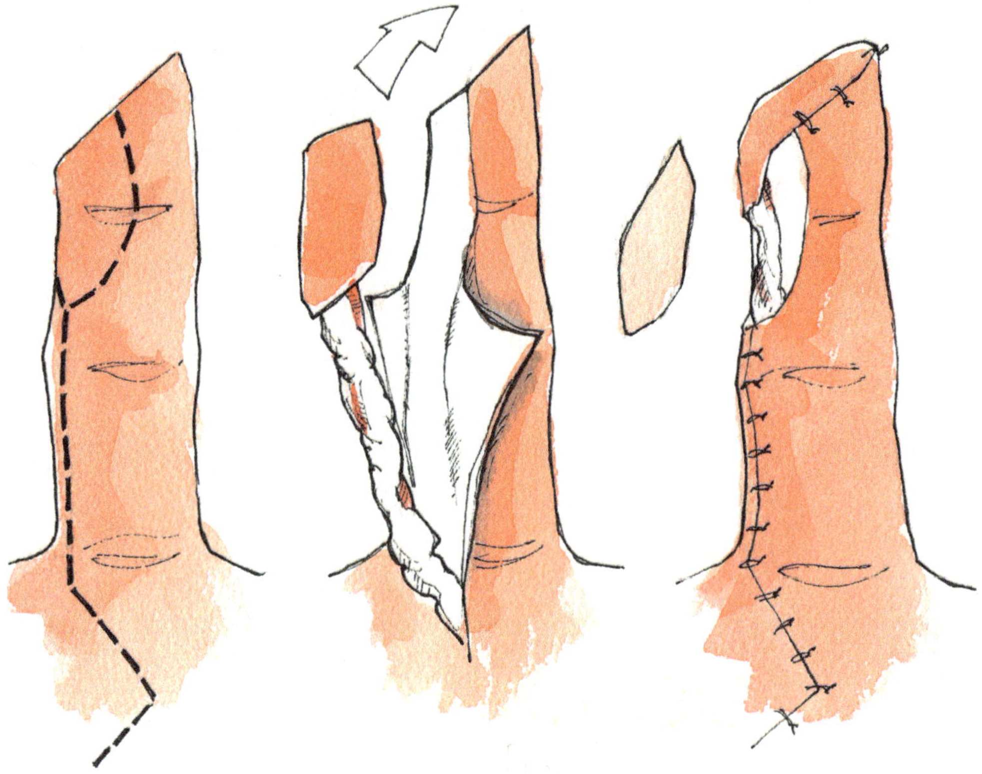

• **Fig. 46.15** Design of the homodigital island flap.

designed obliquely lateral (Figs. 46.15 and 46.16). Evans designed an ingenious version, the step advancement island flap which utilizes a series of triangular flaps each of which advances distally into the next defect, such that the most proximal secondary defect is closed directly (Fig. 46.17). Many modifications of the island flap have been described, including the exchange island flap (Foucher) (see Fig. 46.2); the technique of dividing the flap nerve and anastomosing it to the nerve in the defect in order to minimize reorientation.[25] Glicenstein proposed a retrograde perfusion flap similar in principle to the Chinese radial forearm flap, but based in the digit and rotating on the transverse arcades at the level of the joints.[26]

The vessel and nerve, with accompanying fat which contains essential venous drainage, are dissected free, as far proximally as is required. Additional advancement can be obtained by supplementary techniques such as ligation and section of the vessel to the adjacent digit at the Y bifurcation and by careful longitudinal separation of the relevant elements of the digital nerve from the common digital nerve. On the radial side of the index the digital bundle is tethered at the base – additional advancement can be obtained by releasing the bundle from this tethering (Fig. 46.18)

Important Points of Technique

1. The digital artery is not accompanied by an identifiable digital vein, since most venous drainage in the digit travels via the dorsum. It is important to include the fatty investiture of the NV pedicle since this contains important venules that later dilate and drain the flap (Fig. 46.19).
2. One must produce adequate advancement and not be tempted to flex the finger to accommodate the flap. Flexion contracture inevitably follows. The finger must leave the operating room with the flap inset and without resort to flexing splintage.
3. Any tunneling must be relaxed, ample, and there should be no points of kinking. The process of tunneling must also ensure that no twisting movement of the pedicle occurs.

Free Pulp Transfer

First described by Buncke and Rose in 1979,[27] free pulp transfer gives arguably the most "like for like" reconstruction, the subcutaneous fat, fibrous septa, and glabrous skin of the toe pulp providing an excellent pad for the fingertip. In the young, where a useful return of sensation can be expected from nerve anastomosis, free transfer provides the opportunity to customize the transferred tissue for reconstruction. Options include the contiguous hemipulps of first and second toes, toenails including germinal matrix, wrap-around flaps from first or second toes, and partial lesser toes.[28]

Pulp flaps can consist of simple skin islands or may extend to inclusion of the nail as a wrap-around flap. In this case, it is useful to include the distal phalanx of the toe to which the nail matrix adheres, to provide stability and to prevent resorption of the otherwise "open" end of the recipient skeleton.

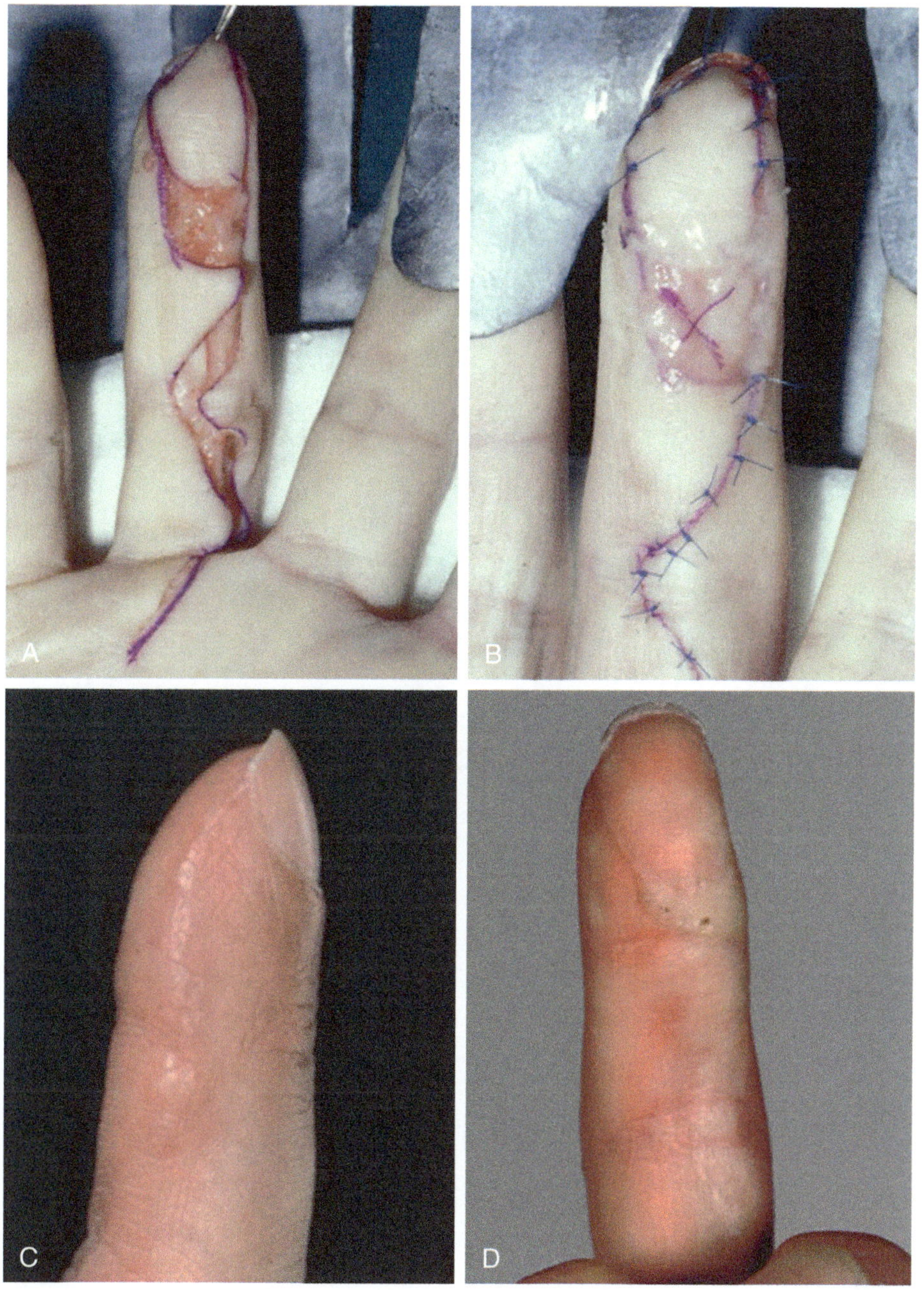

• **Fig. 46.16** The homodigital island flap. (A–D) The island is designed over the neurovascular bundle which is dissected to the base and advanced. The secondary defect receives a split-thickness skin graft.

Important Points of Technique

1. Most microsurgeons will favor distal to proximal dissection in this situation. This ensures that the island of tissue is in continuity with the vessel to be harvested and also minimizes the incursion into the donor toe.
2. The design and harvest of the flap and the preparation of the recipient should ensure that the transferred tissue is not excessively bulky to avoid the well-recognized "cobra" appearance of the recipient digit

The Bank Digit

The concept of the "bank digit" was introduced by Foucher.[5] In multidigit trauma a damaged finger might be beyond salvage but may still be capable of providing elements useful in the repair or reconstruction of other digits. These include any element ranging from split-thickness skin graft, and nail plate, to arterial grafts or a complete island (or free) flap. One should not miss the opportunity to utilize such elements.

Venous Flaps

The concept of establishing an arterial inflow to a venous flap ("arterialized" venous flap) was introduced in an experimental model by Nakayama et al in 1981,[29] and then used clinically both by Mimoun et al[30] and Yoshimura et al,[31] the latter to reconstruct a traumatic finger defect.

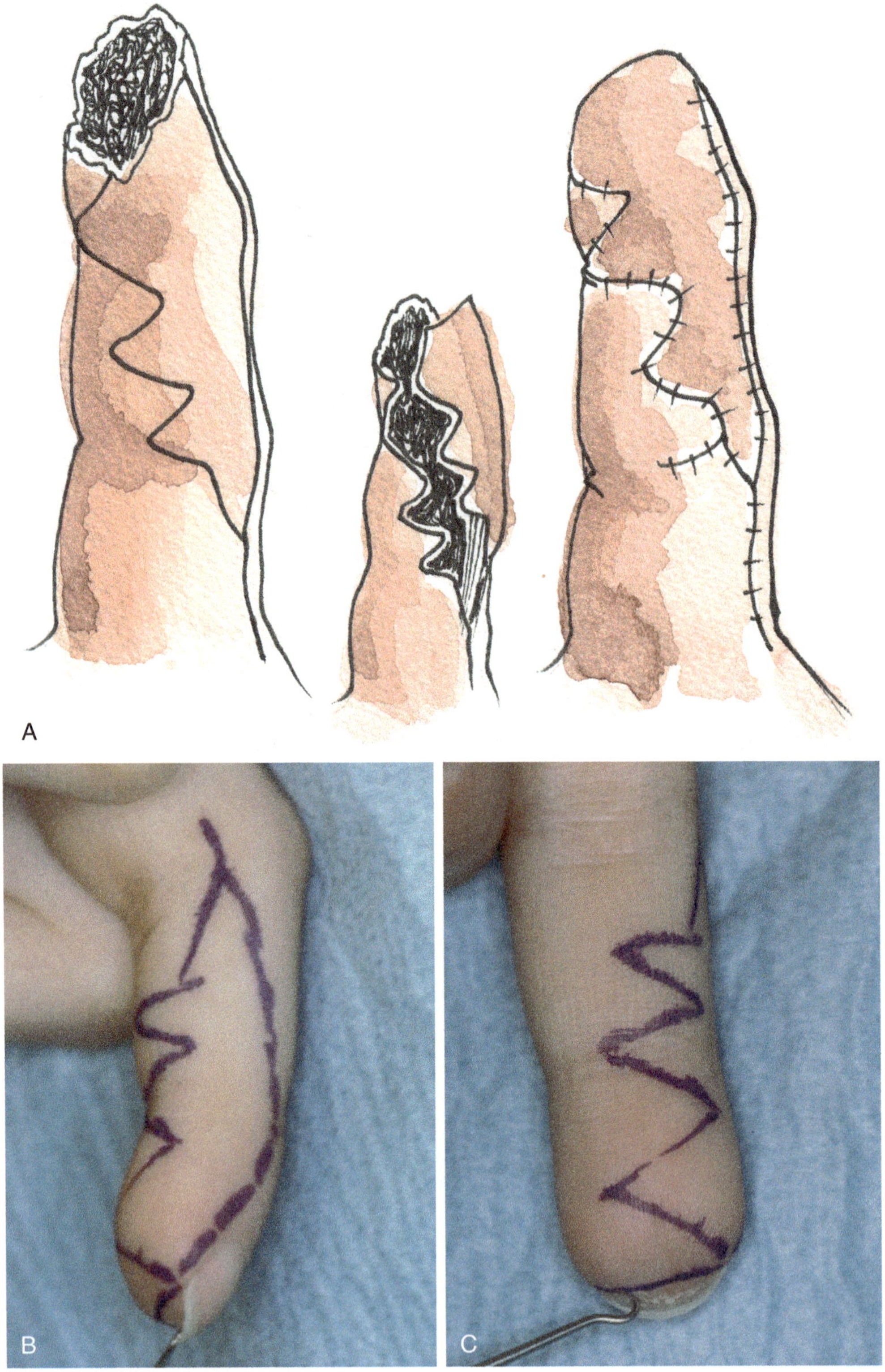

A B C

• **Fig. 46.17** The Evans step advancement island flap. (A) An island is designed with triangulated edges and the flap is advanced such that the leading portion surfaces the defect and successive triangles advance by one place. (B,C) Design of the flap. Note that the dorsal border is a straight midlateral line and that the triangles diminish in size from distal to proximal.

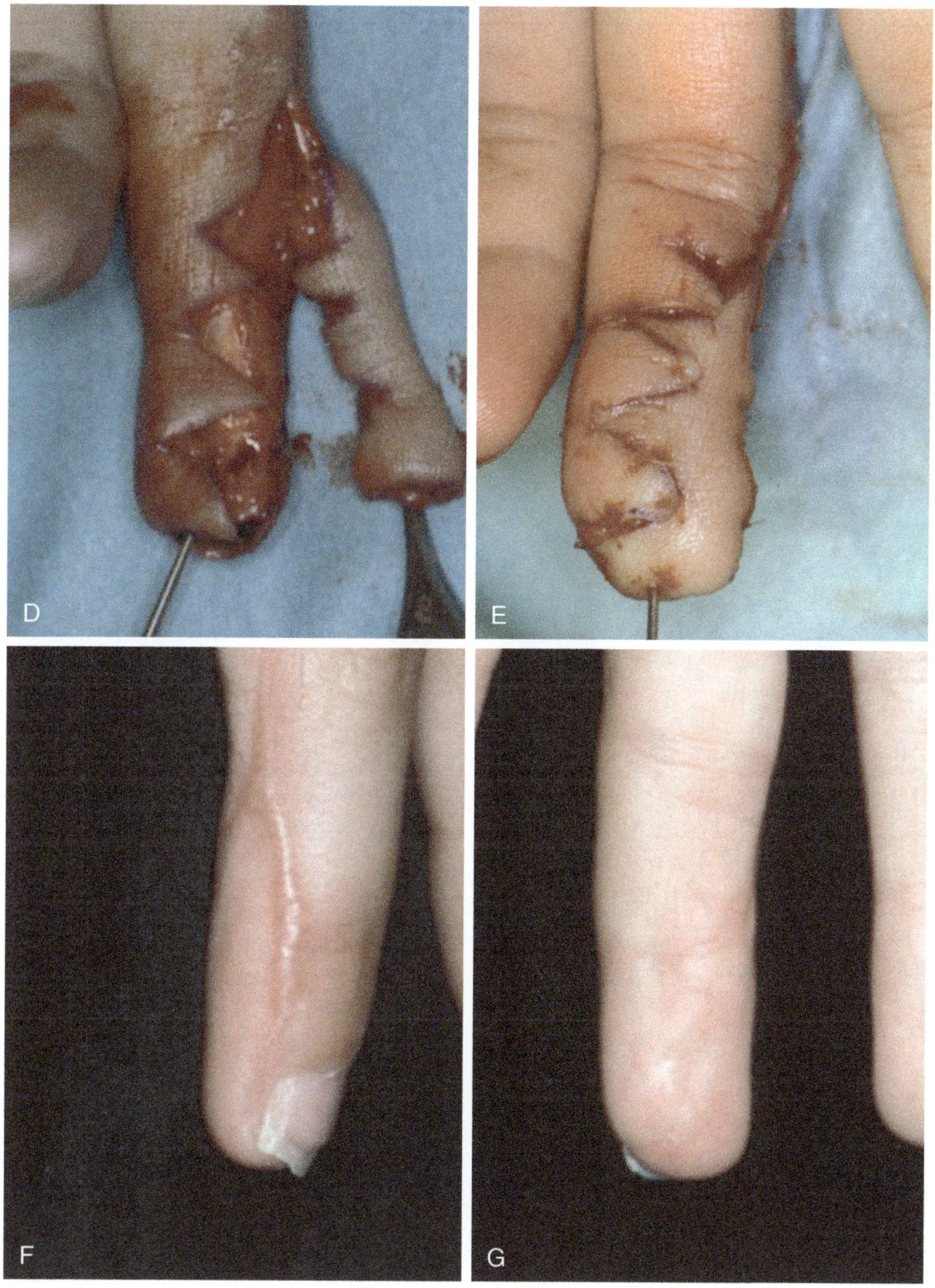

Fig. 46.17 cont'd (D) The flap is completely islanded. (E) The flap is advanced so that each triangle takes the place of the defect immediately distal. The final, proximal, defect is closed. (F,G) Result.

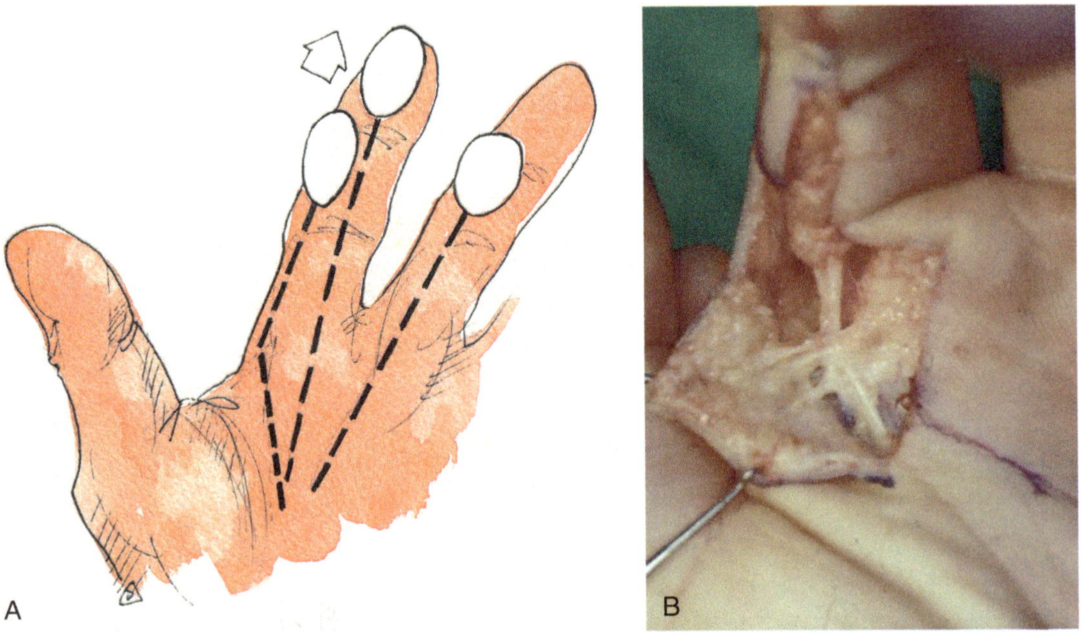

• **Fig. 46.18** Release of base of radial pedicle in the index. (A,B) The radial NV bundle in the index executes a sharp angle at the base. Useful extra advancement can be gained if these tethering bands are released, and the NV bundle straightens out.

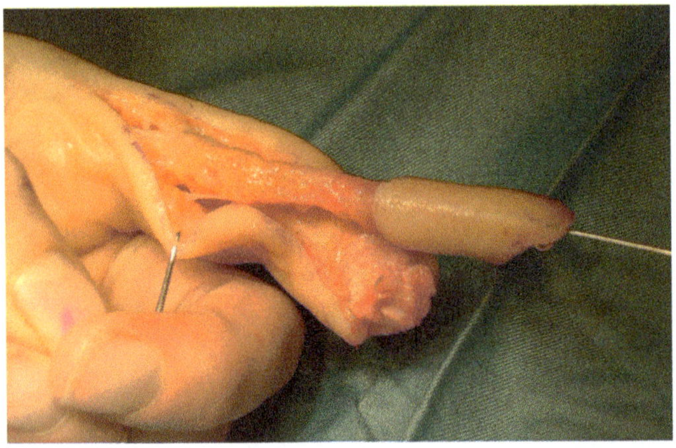

• **Fig. 46.19** Fatty pedicle. The neurovascular bundle contains no formal vein since venous drainage is mainly on the dorsum of the digit. It is important to include generous fat with the pedicle since it contains important venules and drainage.

Thatte and Thatte[32] subsequently classified venous flaps into three types:

a. venous flow-through (venous inflow, venous outflow),
b. single venous pedicle, and
c. arterialized (arterial inflow, venous outflow).

This classification is generally accepted, although it is only the arterialized venous flap which has a role in fingertip reconstruction.

Advantages

Advantages include ease of harvest and a thin versatile flap with minimal donor site morbidity are the chief advantages of the free venous flap. Several veins are usually visible through the thin skin of the volar wrist/forearm which allows a choice of pedicle whose length can be tailored and the flap orientated to suit the fingertip defect. Small cutaneous nerves invariably run with the veins and these can be anastomosed to terminal branches of the digital nerves.

Disadvantages

The veins supplying these flaps are <1 mm diameter and the anastomoses are technically challenging. Venous flaps are inevitably difficult to monitor, as their initial blueish/purple hue and gradual darkening is easily mistaken for vascular congestion. Capillary refill is always more brisk than the norm for flaps but is a reliable indicator.

Points of Technique

The afferent and efferent veins of the flap should not be in direct continuity, since blood flow may choose this low resistance route and shunt from one to the other without perfusing the capillary bed. Longer pedicle length will aid the microsurgery Some operators prefer shorter pedicles to try to limit the number of valves within the afferent veins.[33] Either way, the venous flaps should be reversed so any valves will not impede blood flow.

The Nail

The nail deserves special mention since it is often neglected in crush and amputation injuries. Deformities of nail shape or growth can compromise otherwise very successful and ingenious soft tissue reconstruction.

Many such unfavorable outcomes can be avoided if basic features of nail support and growth are borne in mind (Fig. 46.20).

1. The germinal matrix must be unscarred. If it is involved in laceration, it should be repaired as accurately as possible, preferably with microscope assistance.
2. The nail fold must be kept open – the nail plate is only plate-shaped because the nail fold permits it out of the germinal matrix in this shape, much as the outlet of a toothpaste tube dictates the round shape of the extrusion. If the nail plate is removed, detached or lost, it should be replaced and kept in the fold while a new nail plate is advancing.
3. The sterile matrix has special qualities – it allows the nail to adhere, while permitting slow progression of the plate as it grows. It is also smooth and flat, as is the plate. Any laceration of the sterile matrix must be repaired as accurately as possible, preferably with microscope assistance, in order to reduce scarring and preserve these qualities.
4. The distal phalanx is essential for support, while the pulp provides no structural support. A digit without pulp will support the nail (Fig. 46.21) while one with soft tissue but no bony support will allow the nail to curve over the end (Fig. 46.22). Even crushed elements of distal phalanx should be preserved if possible and be allowed to unite – it is often surprising how well these will remold or require minor secondary surgery while the support is maintained.
5. All surgery to an injured nail structure is best performed in the acute situation while these structures are relatively supple and, indeed, have some distinctive features that

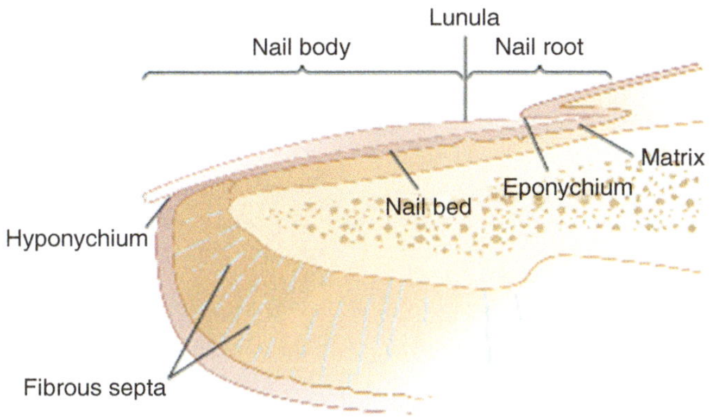

• **Fig. 46.20** Cross-section of nail complex. The germinal matrix, the nail fold, the sterile matrix, and the support provided by the phalanx are all essential elements in producing the nail complex shape and structure. (From Siegel DB, Gelberman RH. Infections of the hand. *Orthop Clin North Am.* 1988;19:779–789.)

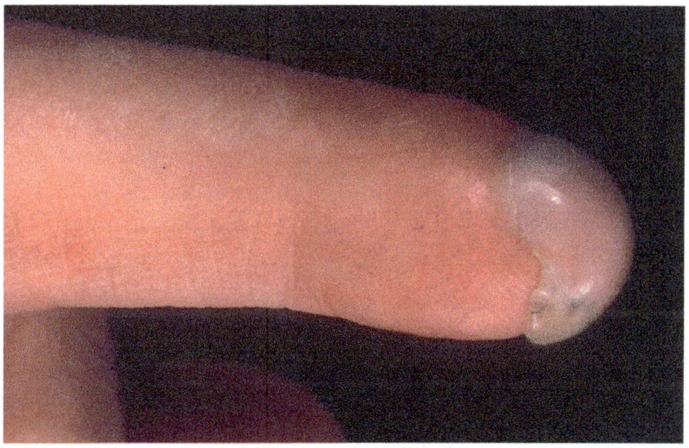

• **Fig. 46.22** Hang nail. The loss of distal phalanx length removes support for the nail.

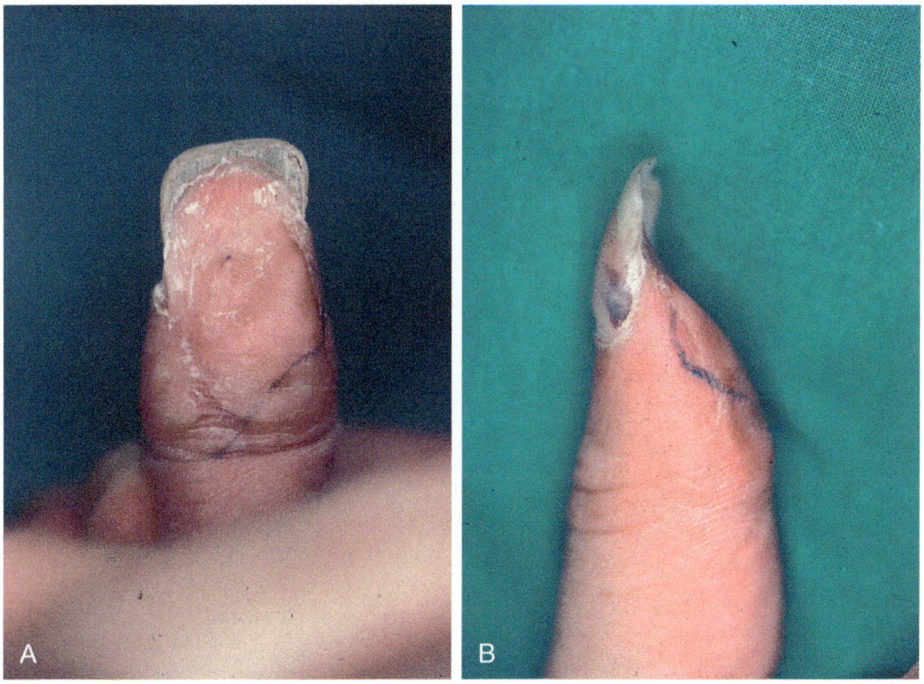

• **Fig. 46.21** Nail support. (A,B) The presence of the phalanx provides full support for the nail despite loss of all soft tissue.

aid identification. Elective secondary surgery on germinal matrix or sterile matrix is especially difficult if it has been allowed to scar.

Psychological Aspects of Hand Injuries

All injuries and surgery to the hand carry a psychological dimension. Leaving aside the special situation of the professional sportsman, the musician, the creative artist, the child, most will require their hands to earn their living and for the performance of the most elemental functions. It is part of the initial assessment of any hand injury, quickly to sense these dimensions and to incorporate them in one's analysis and plans. The manual worker who suffers a major hand injury in a repetitive, uninspiring and low-paid job also merits particular attention to this aspect. The initial attention by many professionals, and the sudden thrust into the center of attention, is unfamiliar and curiously welcome. Surgery and assiduous care follow, then discharge and increasingly spaced visits, until this person comes out at the other end of the process, back in a humdrum, low-paid job (or unemployed), now with even worse employment prospects and skills. The attention disappears and the specialized team moves on, while life is now even less inspiring and lower-earning.

Conclusions

1. Assessment of the defect, overall injury, and psychological aspects is crucial, as is the formulation of a plan based on restoration of function, not mere anatomy.
2. The managing surgeon should master as many techniques as possible, even those that seem unspecialized or unappealing. The larger the toolbox available the more likely is there to be found just the right tool for the task.
3. The patient must be as informed as possible of the issues at stake, the plan of action, the realistic outcome, and the possible complications. The need for secondary procedures should be set at the outset so that it becomes part of an anticipated plan not a remedy for initial failure.
4. If tissue is to be discarded, one should always be aware of the possibility of harvest of skin, nail, bone, etc. for use in reconstruction in other digits.
5. Points of technique for the various methods must be respected since there is usually little room for error or revision. It need hardly be added that a method should be used only if technical competence has been achieved and not merely because it is an enticing and attractive technique.

In the field of skin cover of the fingertips, restoration of function is the goal. Despite ingenious and constantly evolving methods of tissue movement and reconstruction, this field is dogged by perennial limitations, including: the relatively limited outcome of nerve repair; the incidence of neuroma and cold intolerance; the problem of scar contracture. Advances in the understanding of nerve regeneration and methods of influencing nerve recovery may one day transform our approach to these common and debilitating injuries.

References

1. British Society for Surgery of the Hand (BSSH) Hand Surgery in the UK. *Manpower, Resources, Standards and Training*. London: BSSH; 2007.
2. European Commission. *Causes and Circumstances of Accidents at Work in the EU*. Luxembourg: Office for Official Publications of the European Communities; 2009.
3. McCash CR. The open palm technique in Dupuytren's contracture. *Br J Plast Surg*. 1964;17:271–280.
4. Venkataswami R, Gnanasekaran TC. The staged island flap: a new method of repair for thumb injuries. *J Hand Surg*. 1990;15(4):425–428.
5. Foucher G, Marin-Braun F, Merle M, et al. Le doigt "banque" en traumatique de la main. *Ann Chir*. 1980;35:301–303.
6. Hueston JT. Local flap repair in fingertip injuries. *Plast Reconstr Surg*. 1966:349–350.
7. Cronin TD. The cross finger flap: a new method of repair. *Am Surg*. 1951;17:419–425.
8. Woon CY, Lee JY, Teoh LC. Resurfacing hemipulp losses of the thumb: the cross finger flap revisited: indications, technical refinements, outcomes, and long-term neurosensory recovery. *Ann Plast Surg*. 2008;61(4):385–391.
9. Lee NH, Pae WS, Roh SI, et al. Innervated cross finger pulp flap for reconstruction of the fingertip. *Arch Plast Surg*. 2012;39(6):637–642.
10. Segmuller G. Modifikation des Kutler-Lappens neuro-vaskulare Steilung. *Handchir*. 1976;8:75–76.
11. Venkataswami R, Subramanian N. Oblique triangular flap: a new method of repair for oblique amputations of the fingertip and thumb. *Plast Reconstr Surg*. 1980;66(2):296–300.
12. Joshi BB. A local dorsolateral island flap for restoration of sensation after avulsion injury of fingertip pulp. *Plast Reconstr Surg*. 1974;54(2):175–182.
13. Littler JW. Neurovascular pedicle transfer of tissue in reconstructive surgery of the hand. *J Bone Joint Surg*. 1956;38A:917.
14. Cohen BE, Cronin ED. An innervated cross-finger flap for fingertip reconstruction. *Plast Reconstr Surg*. 1983;72:688–697.
15. Holevitch Y. Use of the skin islet flap from the dorsal aspect of the index finger for restoration of the sensitivity of the thumb. *Acta Chir Plast*. 1964;6:1–8.
16. Foucher GD, Braun J-B. A new island flap transfer from the dorsum of the index to the thumb. *Plast Reconstr Surg*. 1979;63(3):344–349.
17. Atasoy E, Ioakimidis E, Kasden ML, et al. Reconstruction of the amputated finger tip with a triangular volar flap. A new surgical procedure. *J Bone Joint Surg Am*. 1970;52A:921–926.
18. Tranquili-Leali E. Ricostruzione dell'apice delle falangi ungueali mediante autoplastica volare peduncolata per scorrimento. *Inf Traum Lavoro*. 1935;1:186–193.
19. Kutler WA. A new method for finger tip amputation. *J Am Med Soc*. 1947;133:129.
20. Voche P, Merle M. Vascular supply of the palmar subcutaneous tissue of fingers. *Br J Plast Surg*. 1996;45(5):315–318.
21. Moberg E. Aspects of sensation in reconstructive surgery of the upper extremity. *J Bone Joint Surg Am*. 1964;46:817–825.
22. O'Brien B. Neurovascular island pedicle flaps for terminal amputations and digital scars. *Br J Plast Surg*. 1968;21:258–261.

23. Lloyd N, Sammut D. A modification of the Souquet advancement flap in fingertip reconstruction. *J Hand Surg*. 2013;38(4):395–398.
24. Evans DM, Martin DL. Step advancement island flap for fingertip reconstruction. *Br J Plast Surg*. 1988;41:105–111.
25. Foucher G, Braun FM, Merle M, et al. La technique de "debranchement–rebranchement" du lambeau en ilôt pedicule. *Ann Chir*. 1981;35(4):303.
26. Glicenstein J. Island flaps in hand surgery. Introduction. *Ann Chir Main*. 1988;7(2):120–121.
27. Buncke HJ, Rose EH. Free toe-to-fingertip neurovascular flaps. *Plast Reconstr Surg*. 1979;63:607.
28. Morrison WA. Thumb and fingertip reconstruction by composite microvascular tissue from the toes. *Microsurg*. 1992;8(3):537–550.
29. Nakayama Y, Soeda S, Kasai Y. Flaps nourished by arterial inflow through the venous system: an experimental investigation. *Plast Reconstr Surg*. 1981;67:328.
30. Mimoun M, Baux S, Kirsch JM, et al. Un lambeau de conception originale: le lambeau veineux arterialize. *Ann Chir Plast Esthet*. 1986;31(3):219–224.
31. Yoshimura M, Shimada T, Imura S, et al. The venous skin graft method for repairing skin defects of the fingers. *Plast Reconstr Surg*. 1987;79(2):243–250.
32. Thatte MR, Thatte RL. Venous flaps. *Plast Reconstr Surg*. 1993;91(4):747–751.
33. Wu SH, Kim KC, Lee GJ, et al. A retrospective analysis of 154 arterialized venous flaps for hand reconstruction: an 11 year experience. *Plast Reconstr Surg*. 2007;119(6):1823–1838.

47

Flexor Tendon Injuries

JIN BO TANG

Introduction

Flexor tendon injuries are among commonly seen hand trauma, and outcomes of the treatment in the fingers and thumbs are traditionally unsatisfactory. In the hand and the forearm, flexor tendons are divided into five anatomical zones. Zone 2 is the most complex area, which has attracted most attention from surgeons and investigators alike. Over the past decades, zone 2 flexor tendon repairs have evolved greatly, and outcomes have changed dramatically.[1–5] Several conceptual changes, as well as key surgical methods and postoperative hand therapy protocols, have led to the changes.[6–16] The new principles and clinical practices include: (1) using strong core sutures, typically 4- or 6-strand repairs; (2) judicious venting of the critical annular pulley; (3) ensuring that a slight tension is created by the repair to prevent gapping at the repair site; (4) performing on-table digital extension–flexion tests to confirm the quality of the surgical repair; and (5) early partial-range active motion to ensure tendon gliding, without overloading the repair.

In addition, having the patient wide awake under local anesthesia with epinephrine without use of a tourniquet during surgery is an important advance. In such settings, the patient can actively move the tendon to ascertain that after end-to-end repair the repair site has no gapping or does not impinge against the pulleys.[9,10] Wide-awake surgery also enables better intraoperative judgment of tenolysis or proper tensioning of the tendon graft during secondary surgery.

Anatomical Features

There are 12 flexor tendons in the hand and forearm regions. These tendons include finger and thumb flexors and wrist flexors. Finger flexor tendons are the flexor digitorum superficialis (FDS) and the flexor digitorum profundus (FDP). In the thumb there is only one flexor tendon, i.e., the flexor pollicis longus (FPL). The tendons of the FDP come from a common muscle belly in the mid forearm. The tendons of the FDS originate from the separate muscle bellies, which allow more independent finger flexion. Within the carpal tunnel, nine tendons (four FDS, four FDP, and one FPL) exist.

In the fingers and thumb, the digital flexor tendons glide within a closed fibro-osseous sheath with segmental, semi-rigid, constrictive bands present. Proximally, the synovial sheath ends proximal to the neck of the metacarpals, forming the proximal reflection of the digital flexor sheath. The FDS tendons lie superficial to the FDP tendons proximal to the bifurcation of the FDS tendon at the level of the metacarpophalangeal joint. Distal to the bifurcation, the FDS tendon becomes two slips coursing laterally and then deeper to the FDP tendons. This FDS bifurcation is in the middle part of the A2 pulley area. In this area, the FDS tendon also serves to constrain the FDP tendon, acting as the second sheath constricting the FDP tendon. Deep to the FDP tendon, the FDS slips rejoin to form Camper's chiasm, and insert on the middle phalanx as two separate slips. The FDP tendon inserts into the distal phalanx. Inside the flexor sheath of the thumb, the FPL tendon is the only tendon and inserts at the distal phalanx.

The digital flexor sheath consists of *synovial sheath* and segmental, condensed fibrous bands called *pulleys*. Synovial sheath, a thin layer of continuous paratenon covering the inner surface of the fibrous sheath, provides a smooth surface for tendon gliding and nutrition to the tendons. The pulley system of the fingers consists of *annular pulleys* (condensed, rigid, and heavier annular bands) and *cruciate pulleys* (filmy cruciform bands) (Fig. 47.1). In the thumb, there are two annular pulleys (A1 and A2) palmar to the two thumb joints and one oblique pulley; there are no cruciate pulleys. In the fingers, there are five annular pulleys (A1, A2, A3, A4, and A5), three cruciate pulleys (C1, C2, and C3), and one palmar aponeurosis (PA) pulley (see Fig. 47.3A). The A1, A3, and A5 pulleys attach to the palmar plates of the metacarpophalangeal (MCP), proximal interphalangeal (PIP), and distal interphalangeal (DIP) joints, and the A2 pulley attaches to the proximal two-thirds of the proximal phalange and A4 pulleys attach to the middle portion of the middle phalange.

The presence of annular pulleys is a unique anatomical feature. The A2 pulley is the largest and strongest, and the A4 pulley the second largest. The annular pulleys serve to prevent tendon bowstringing during digital flexion. The A3 and A1 pulleys also perform this function, but their role is less critical than the A2 and A4. Loss of integrity of any one

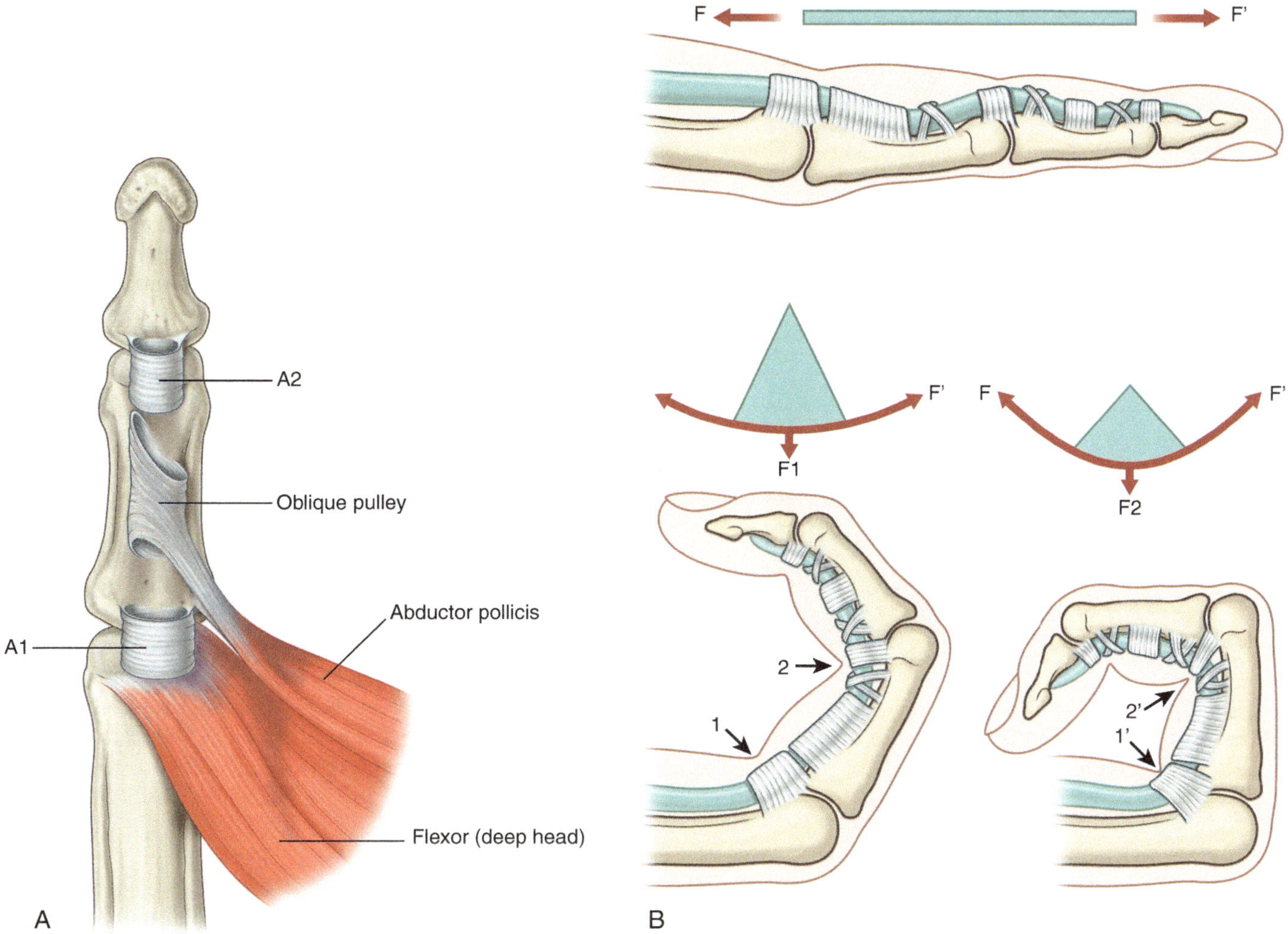

• **Fig. 47.1** The location of pulleys in the (A) thumb and (B) fingers. (A) In the thumb, there are only three pulleys: A1, oblique, and A2. (B) The cruciate and annular pulleys. When the finger flexes, the cruciate pulleys shorten ("concertina effect") but annular pulleys are more rigid and do not change their shapes. (From Tang JB. Flexor tendon injuries and reconstruction. In: Chang J, Neligan P, eds. *Plastic Surgery*: Vol 6: *Hand and Upper Extremity.* 4th edn. Elsevier; 2018: (A) Fig. 9.2; (B) Fig. 9.8C.)

of the pulleys alone has no marked functional consequence, though anatomically, minor tendon bowstringing occurs at the site of the loss.

The middle and distal part of the A2 pulley (1.5–1.7 cm long in adult middle finger) and the A4 pulley (about 0.5 cm long) are the narrowest and constricting. These sites become very compressive to the repaired tendons because of postoperative tendon swelling. These narrow pulley sites can be incised to allow the repaired tendons to glide more freely.

Zones and Subzones of Flexor Tendons

In the 1960s, the flexor tendons were divided into five zones by Verdan. In the 1990s, subdivisions of zone 1 by Moiemen and Elliot[17] and zone 2 by Tang[18] were added into the zoning system, in order to describe the location of injuries and repairs more specifically. These zoning and subzoning systems provide surgeons with the nomenclature to document the injuries and outcomes, and describe treatment methods.

The zoning of flexor tendons is described below and seen in Figs. 47.2 and 47.3:

Zone 1: From the insertion of the FDS tendon to the terminal insertion of the FDP tendon
Zone 2: From the proximal reflection of the digital synovial sheath to the FDS insertion
Zone 3: From the distal margin of the transverse carpal ligament to the digital synovial sheath
Zone 4: Area covered by the transverse carpal ligament
Zone 5: Proximal to the transverse carpal ligament.

In the thumb, zone 1 is distal to the interphalangeal joint, zone 2 is from the interphalangeal joint to the A1 pulley, and zone 3 is the area of the thenar eminence.

The subdivisions of zone 1 by Moiemen and Elliot are:

1A: The very distal FDP tendon (usually <1 cm), not possible to insert a core suture

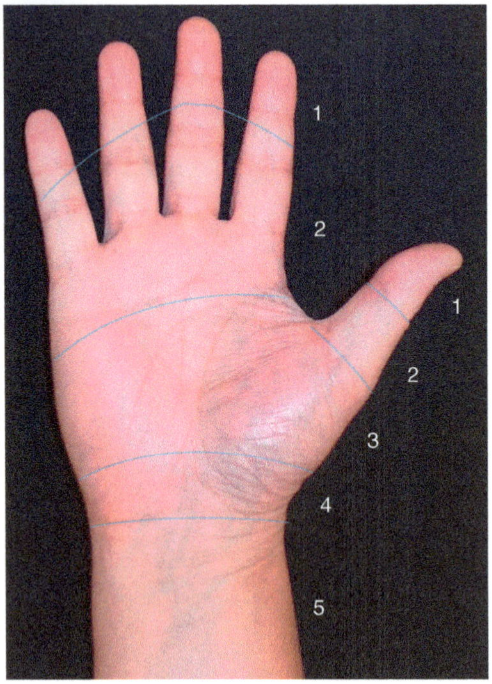

• **Fig. 47.2** Location of the five zones of the flexor tendons in the hand and forearm.

1B: From zone 1A to the distal margin of the A4 pulley
1C: The FDP tendon within the A4 pulley

The subdivisions of zone 2 by Tang are:

2A: The area of the FDS tendon insertion
2B: From the proximal margin of the FDS insertion to the distal margin of the A2 pulley
2C: The area covered by the A2 pulley
2D: From the proximal margin of the A2 pulley to the proximal reflection of the digital sheath.

Biomechanical Considerations

Two major considerations are factors affecting the strength of repaired tendons as well as contributing to the resistance to active digital flexion.

Factors Affecting the Strength of Repaired Tendons

The following factors affect the strength of repaired tendons: (1) the number of core suture strands across the repair sites – strength is roughly proportional to the number of core sutures; (2) the tension of repairs – most relevant to gap formation and stiffness of repairs; (3) the core suture purchase; (4) the types of tendon–suture junction – locking or grasping; (5) the diameter of suture locks in the tendons – a small diameter of locks diminishes anchor power; (6) the suture calibers (diameter); (7) the material properties of suture materials; (8) the curvature of tendon gliding paths – the repair strength decreases as tendon curvature increases; and (9) above all, the holding capacity of a tendon, affected by varying degrees of trauma and posttraumatic tissue softening, plays a vital role in repair strength.

It must be realized that tendon curvature during finger flexion greatly effects the repair strength. A tendon under curvilinear tension is subjected to both linear pulling and bending forces. Therefore, a repair in a tendon under a curvilinear load is weaker than that under a linear load. The repair strength decreases progressively as the curvature increases.[19,20] Therefore, the repair fails more easily in the flexed finger and when the finger moves to approach full flexion, a bent tendon is particularly prone to fail. This is the mechanical basis of current partial active finger flexion protocols and one reason why a full fist should be avoided in the initial few weeks post surgery (Table 47.1).

Factors Affecting the Resistance to Tendon Gliding after Surgery

Fig. 47.4 summarizes the breakdown of contributors to postoperative resistance to tendon gliding,[21] which should be considered in planning and adjusting the active motion protocols. The safety margin of early active digital flexion can be enhanced by a strong surgical tendon repair or appropriately decompressing the tendon during surgery through releasing restricting pulleys, limiting the lengths of skin incisions, and minimizing the trauma to the tendon and sheath. After surgery, delicate adjustments in early active flexion to fit individual patients by therapist or surgeon is also important.

Clinical Diagnosis

Open injuries are the most common cause of flexor tendon injuries in the hand and upper extremity. Less commonly the rupture of the tendons is found with a closed injury, such as forceful finger flexion. After injury, the natural resting posture of the wounded digits are usually changed, with the affected fingers seen in a relatively extended position and loss of active finger flexion at PIP and DIP joints. During clinical examination, if the patient can actively flex the DIP joint while the motion of the PIP joint is blocked, the FDP tendon has no injuries or has only a partial disruption (Fig. 47.5). To assess the continuity of the FDS tendon, the adjacent fingers must be held in full extension by the examiner. The FDS tendon is severed completely if the patient cannot actively flex the PIP joint (Fig. 47.6).

The FDS in 30%–35% of little fingers has connection with the FDS in the ring or middle fingers, and the FDS tendon is missing in 10%–20% of the little fingers. These patients have limited or no PIP flexion of the little finger during testing.

Weakness and pain during resisted finger flexion indicates a possible partial tendon cut. Loss of active flexion at the interphalangeal (IP) joint indicates complete severance of the FPL tendon.

Primary and Delayed Primary Repair

Nowadays the majority of lacerated flexor tendons in the hand and forearm are repaired at the same day of injury or

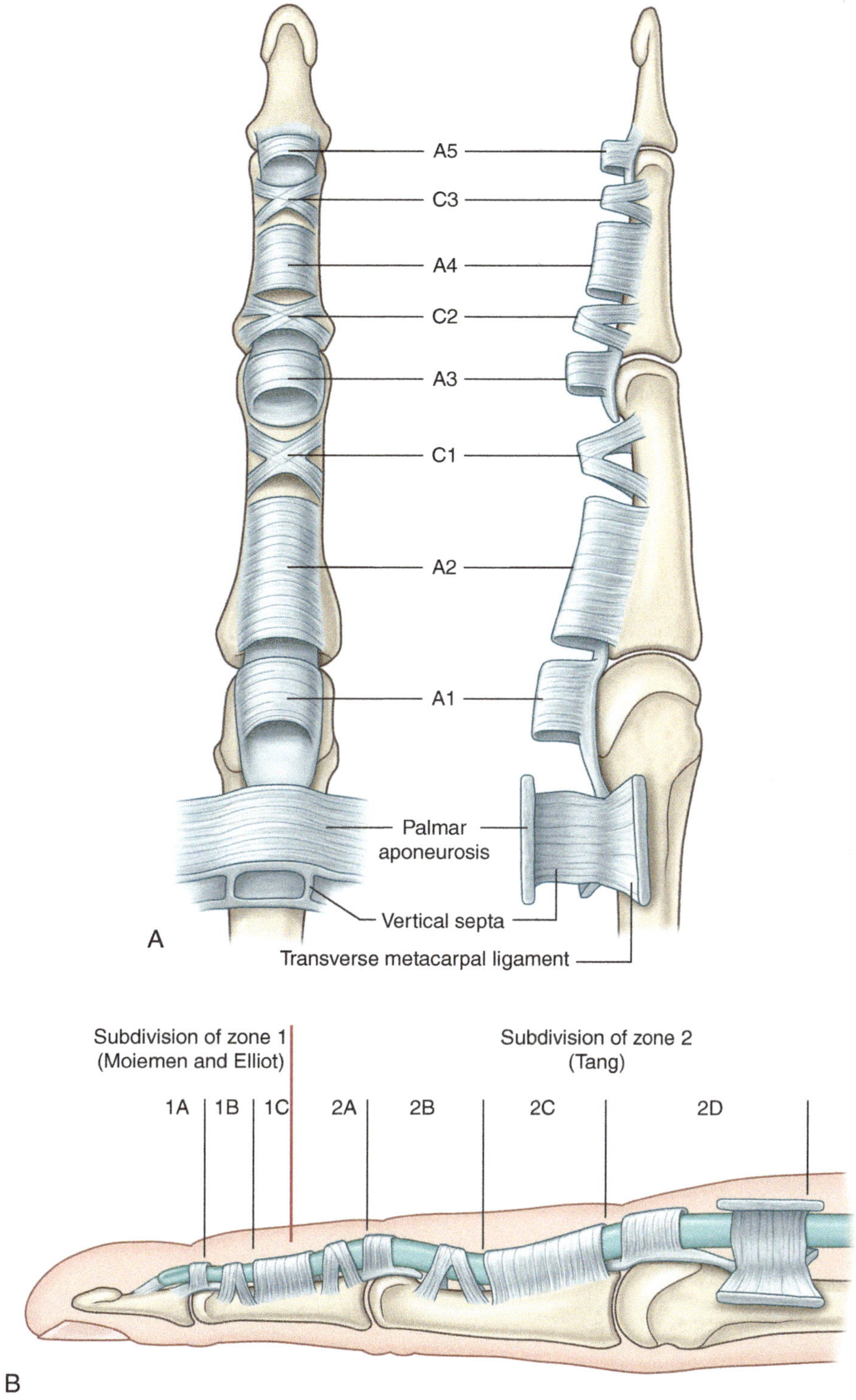

• **Fig. 47.3** (A) Locations of the annular and cruciate pulleys of the fingers. (B) The subdivisions of zone 1 and 2. (From Tang JB: Flexor tendon injuries and reconstruction. In: Chang J, Neligan P, eds. *Plastic Surgery*. Vol 6: *Hand and Upper Extremity*. 4th edn. Elsevier; 2018: (A) Fig. 9.1; (B) Fig. 9.5.)

a few days later. Primary repair indicates end-to-end repair performed within 24 hours after tendon injury. When an experienced surgeon is not available at the day of injury, the repair can be deliberately delayed and delayed primary repair is performed in a selective surgical setting. The delay usually has no adverse effects on outcomes, but in this period of delay antibiotic use reduces the risk of infection of the wound. Delayed primary repair is a repair performed within 3 or even 4 weeks after injury. The end-to-end repair is often still possible 5 weeks after injury. Because zone 2 is the most complex and demanding, the repair methods for zone 2 injuries are given in detail below.

Repair in Zone 2

Exposure and Finding Tendon Ends in Zone 2

The surgical incision to access the tendons is usually a Bruner's skin incision of 1.5–2 cm (Fig. 47.7). We keep the skin incision as limited as possible to decrease edema of the digit and resistance to tendon gliding after surgery. Retraction of the proximal tendon stump is very common, especially in delayed primary repair. If the FDP tendon end has not retracted far proximally, flexion of the MCP or PIP joints can deliver the proximal end into the incision site.

If the proximal FDP tendon end retracts into the palm, it is preferable not to extend the incision to the palm, but instead to make an additional incision in the distal palm. In the author's experience, the retracted tendon end can always be found in the distal palm. From this small incision, the proximal tendon end is pushed distally within the synovial sheath bit by bit using two forceps, like pushing a rope until the distal end is seen out of the distal opening in the sheath.

TABLE 47.1 Resistance to Tendon Gliding during Active Finger Flexion in Initial Weeks of Tendon Healing

Active Flexion	Resistance to Tendon Gliding	Healing Tendons during Active Motion
None to mild	Low	Not easily disrupted
Mild to moderate	Low or moderately high	Not easily disrupted
Moderate to full	Very high	Easy to disrupt. Should avoid such motion

The forceps instrument is used to pull the exposed proximal stump distally out of the preserved sheath for about 1 cm. Then the finger is held in slight flexion, a 25G needle is inserted at the base of the finger through the proximal tendon stump to hold it during repair (Fig. 47.8).

Surgical Repair Techniques

At the cut ends the tendon tissue is often ragged, which should be conservatively shaved with a scalpel or sharp scissors. Basic requirements of direct end-to-end repair are: (1) sufficient strength of the repair methods; (2) smooth tendon gliding surface, with fewer suture exposures; (3) prevent gapping of the repair site under tension; and (4) easy to perform. Different configurations of the suture strands in the tendon may produce good outcomes given all the requirements are met. Surgeons in different centers use different multistrand repairs (Fig. 47.9).[22] In the author's patients, a 6-strand M-Tang method is used as the core suture (Figs. 47.10 and 47.11).[12] Then a simple running epitendon suture or 3 or 4 stitches of separated peripheral stitches are added sparsely over the palmar repair site with 6-0 nylon, to smoothen the junction of the two tendon ends (Fig. 47.12).

Surgical essentials for making a strong tendon repair are, firstly, we must ensure core suture purchase of at least 0.7–1.0 cm to generate maximal holding power and a sufficiently large size (2 mm in diameter) of locks if a locking suture is used. Surgical repair strength decreases as the length of the purchase decreases. Tendon cut surfaces tend to soften after trauma. The repair is at great risk of rupture if the suture purchase is short. The second key to successful repair is that a certain amount of tension across the repair site should be maintained. To prevent gapping, it is very important to ensure the repair has tension or bulkiness that results in 10%–20% shortening of the tendon parts

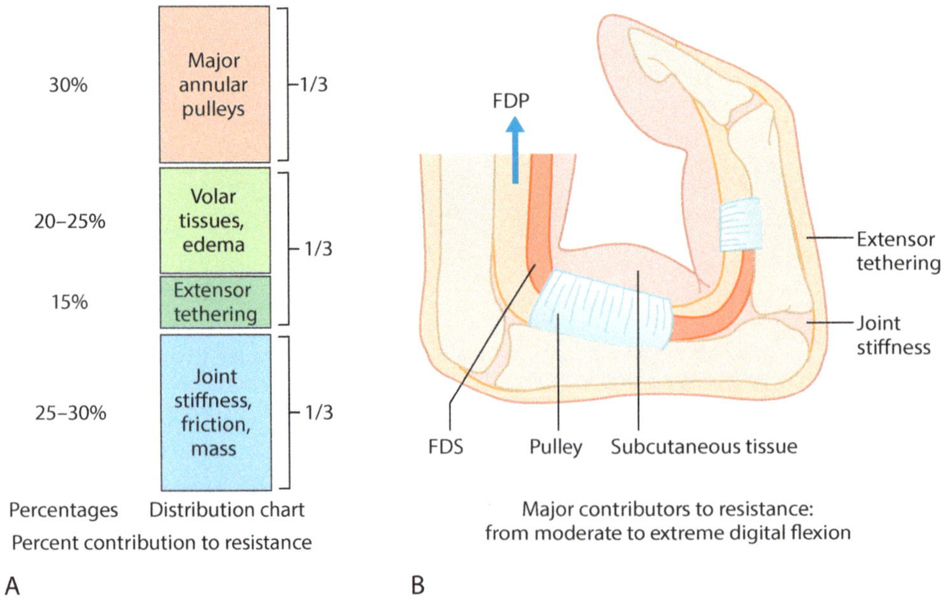

• **Fig. 47.4** The breakdown of contributors to postoperative resistance to active gliding of the flexor tendons.

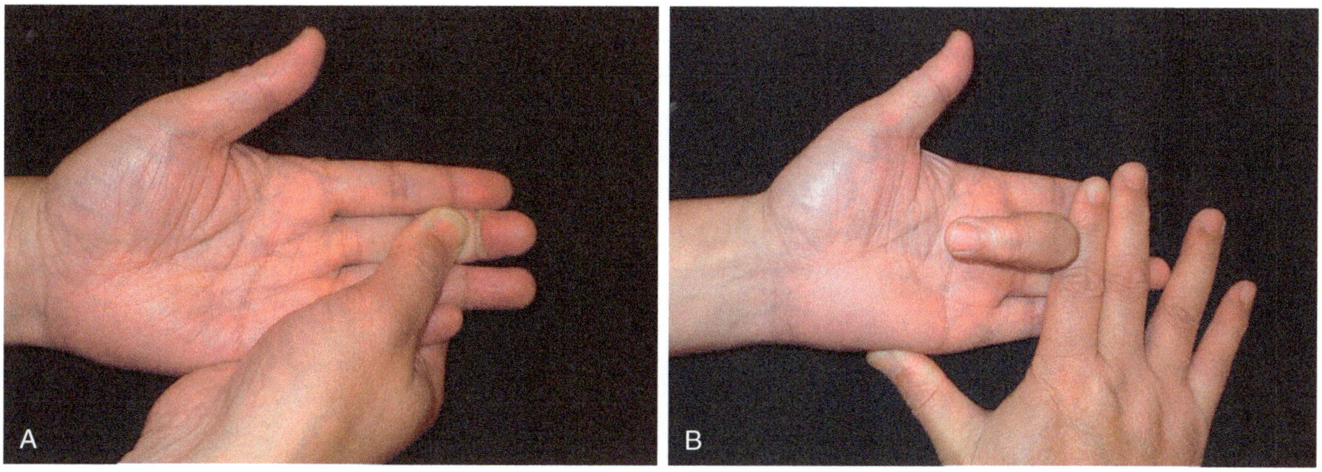

• **Fig. 47.5** Examination of function of the flexor tendons in fingers. (A) No injuries or only partial injuries to the FDP tendon can be diagnosed if the patient can actively flex the DIP joint while the motion of the PIP joint is blocked. (B) To assess the continuity of the FDS tendon, the adjacent fingers are held in full extension. The FDS tendon is severed completely if the patient cannot actively flex the PIP joint.

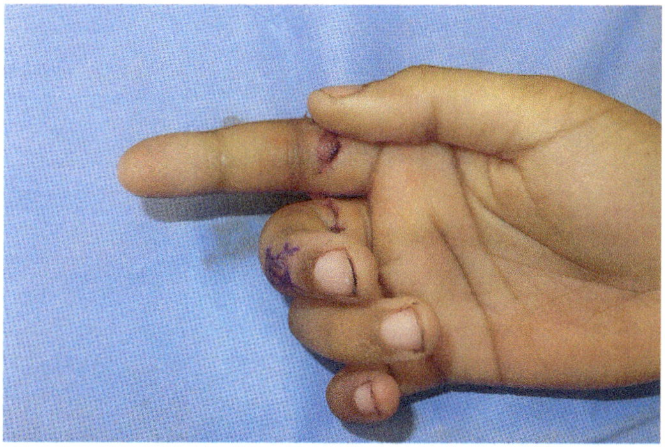

• **Fig. 47.6** The index finger has complete laceration of both flexor tendons, and resting position of the finger is different from that of the other fingers.

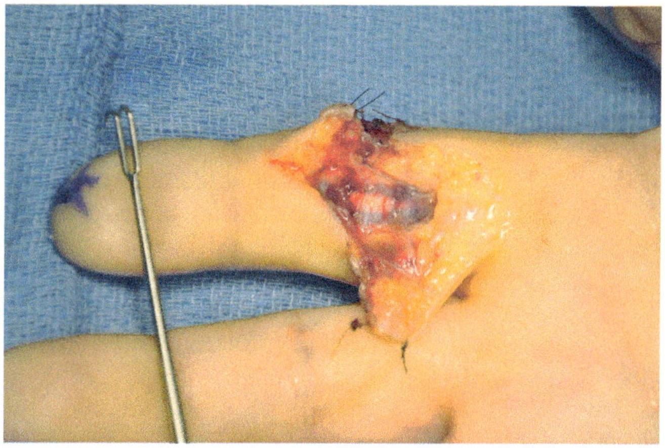

• **Fig. 47.7** A Bruner skin incision of 1.5–2 cm for exposure of the laceration site. A limited skin incision is preferred to decrease postoperative swelling of the finger.

encompassed by core sutures, or a 20%–30% increase in the diameter of the junction site of the two tendon ends (Fig. 47.13).[23] A small amount of baseline tension would counteract the tension of the flexor muscles during resting or active motion. The repair site becomes more flattened once it is under the load of active digital flexion. Such degrees of bulkiness do not hamper tendon gliding with proper pulley venting. Thirdly, at least a 4-strand core suture is required; a 6-strand core suture is ideal. The caliber of suture used in adults is either 4-0 or 3-0. Key clinical technical points for achieving repair are summarized in Box 47.1.

Locking suture-junction in the tendon is not a must, though locking anchors are slightly more secure. If the locks are incorporated, the locking circles of the suture in the tendon should be of a sufficient size (approximately 2 mm in diameter).

Epitendon sutures mainly serve to tidy up the repaired tendon stumps. Most surgeons now choose to insert only simple or sparse peripheral stitches. Some surgeons even do not supplement epitendinous sutures when multistrand core sutures have been used.[24,25] In the presence of a strong core repair that has been tensioned over the repair sites, peripheral sutures are less important (Box 47.2).

The author does not usually repair the FDS tendon unless the FDS injury is partial or the wound is very clean. The author's practice is not to repair the FDS tendon during delayed primary repair or if the injury is in the area of the A2 pulley (zone 2C).

Venting of the Critical Pulleys

It was previously believed that the A2 and A4 pulleys should not be divided. One of the important improvements in tendon repair in recent decades is the understanding that clinically significant bowstringing does not occur when the A2 pulley is released up to two-thirds of its length and that the A4 pulley can be entirely released, given the integrity of the other critical pulleys.[12] A part of the synovial sheath including cruciate pulleys is often released together with the annular pulleys (Fig. 47.14). The release is a longitudinal cut

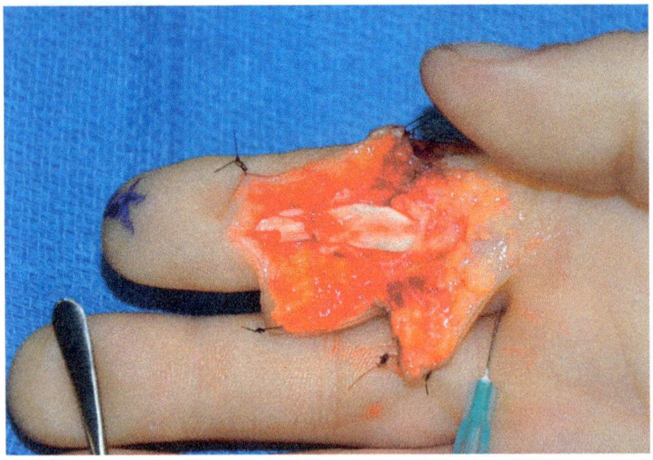

• **Fig. 47.8** After pulling the retracted FDP tendon to approximate the distal tendon stump, a needle is inserted at the base of the finger to transfix the FDP tendon to reduce tension during repair.

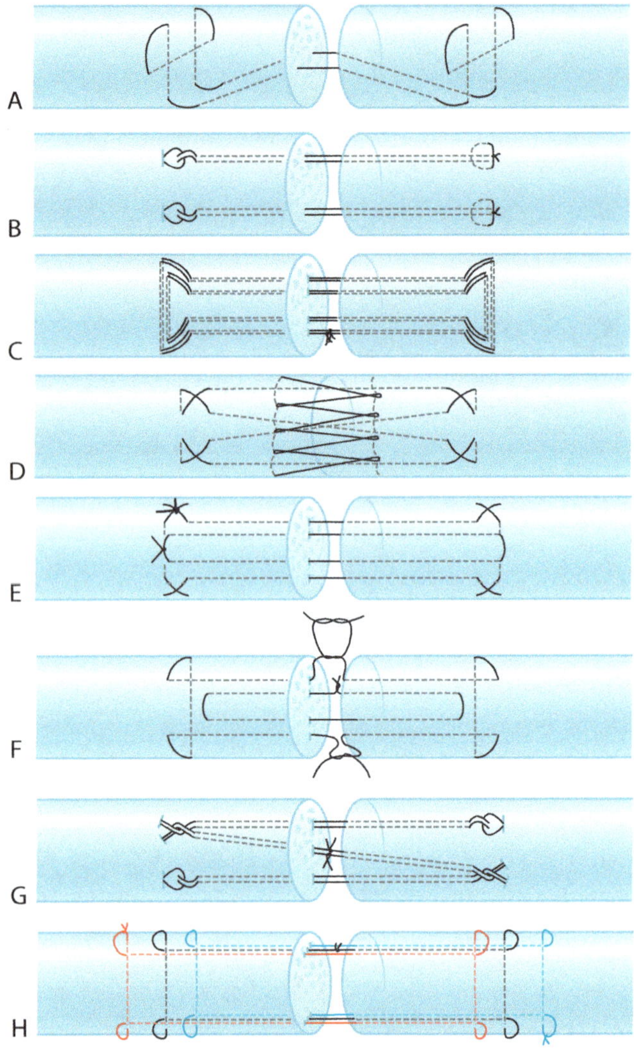

• **Fig. 47.9** Different multistrand repairs used in different centers. (A,B) Mayo Clinic. (C) 8-strand repair used in Washington University in St. Louis. (D) Cruciate repair plus cross-stitch repair used in The Hospital for Special Surgery in New York. (E) 4-strand repair used in Stanford University, USA. (F) 4-strand repair used in Indiana Hand Center. (G) 4-strand repair used in Bern University, Switzerland. Looped sutures (one needle carrying two suture strands) are used for repair methods shown in (B), (C), and (G). (H) A 6-strand repair made from three groups (each in a different color) of the Kessler repair in asymmetric placement in two tendon stumps, which is sometimes used by the author.

through the midline with scissors. Clinically, the A4 pulley needs complete venting, but the A2 pulley should be vented partially only (Fig. 47.15).

Usually no more than 1.5–2 cm length of the pulleys with the synovial sheath should be released.[12] In fact, such a release does not need to be over 2 cm, because in the proximal part of a finger of an average adult, the flexor tendons glide only 1.5–2 cm. This judicious pulley venting permits unimpeded gliding of a strong, yet slightly bunched or edematous tendon repair site during active tendon motion postoperatively.

Venting the A4 pulley entirely does not lead to clinically significant bowstringing, though anatomically there is minor tendon bowstringing, this is of no clinical consequence. In some patients, where the tendons are cut just distal to the A3 pulley, the A3 pulley has to be vented together with the A4 to allow surgical repair or gliding of the tendon.[23,24] Venting of the two pulleys has been found to have minor tendon bowstringing at the PIP joint, but it did not impair finger function.[24]

Performing Digital Extension–Flexion Test

After repairing the tendon and venting of pulleys, it is always necessary to verify the quality of the repair and adequate venting through an on-table *digital extension–flexion test.*[1,13,23] The test has three steps: (1) The repaired finger is held at full extension to confirm that no gaps are seen between the two cut ends. (2) The finger is moderately flexed to make sure the repaired tendon moves smoothly. (3) Finally, the finger is further pushed to marked flexion to confirm that the repair site does not bunch against the pulleys and that venting of the pulley is adequate (Fig. 47.16).

With sedation, brachial plexus blocks, or general anesthesia, the above test is performed with the surgeon's hand holding the repaired finger to obtain passive finger motion. Under local anesthesia without a tourniquet and no sedation, the patient can actively move the tendon to ascertain repair quality,[26] which is an even more powerful way to validate quality of the repair (Box 47.2).

During the testing, if gapping is found between tendon ends, the repair is too loose and should be revised with additional core or peripheral sutures. If the pulley is found to block smooth tendon gliding, it should be further released. However, such additional release should be progressive, 1–2 mm at a time, with repeated digital extension–flexion tests, to ensure the release is just enough to let the repair site glide smoothly, rather than making one unnecessary lengthy cut.

Postoperative Active Motion Protocols

A short dorsal splint is usually sufficient for postoperative protection. The splint extends from the distal forearm to the fingertips. Some other surgeons use an even shorter splint, which ends at the wrist proximally.[27] The exact wrist

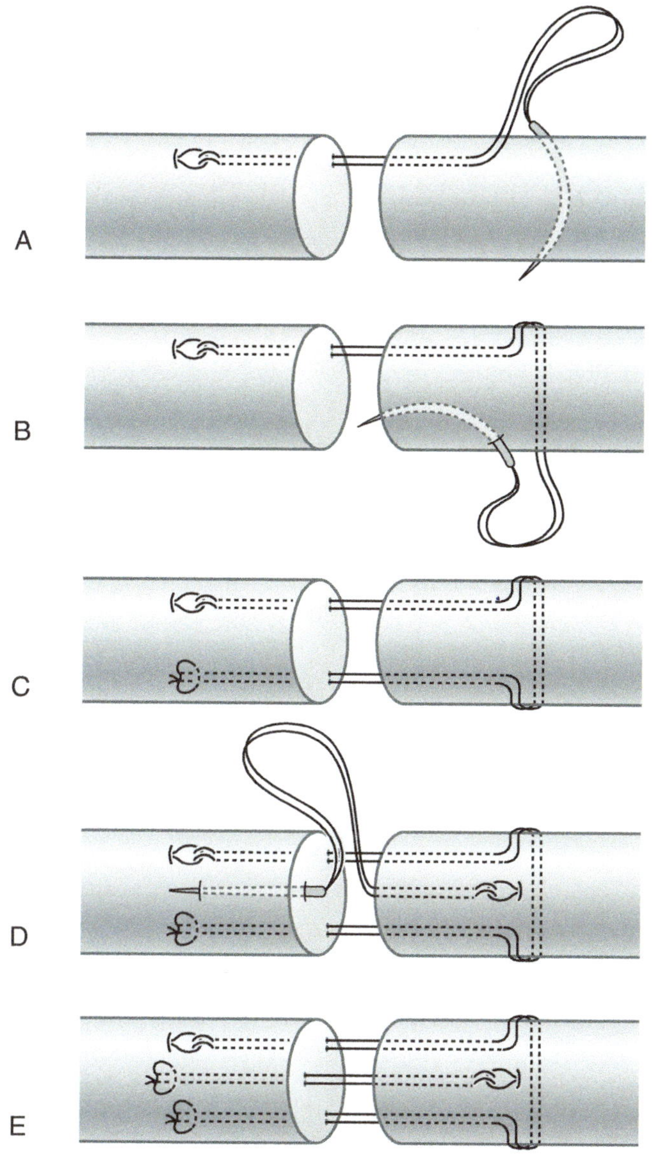

• **Fig. 47.10** (A–E) The method of making a 6-strand M-Tang repair, which the author uses for the FDP and PFL repair in almost all zone 2 and proximal zone 1 repairs. (From Tang JB. Flexor tendon injuries and reconstruction. In: Chang J, Neligan P, eds. *Plastic Surgery*. Vol 6: *Hand and Upper Extremity*. 4th edn. Elsevier; 2018: Fig. 9.19.)

position is unimportant. The wrist can be in neutral, mild flexion, or mild extension as long as the patient is comfortable. The splint should be slightly flexed at the MCP joint, usually for 30–40 degrees, and be straight beyond this joint. The wrist position for splinting should avoid marked flexion (which is uncomfortable) or marked extension (which adds a lot of tension to the repaired tendon).

There is no need to start motion or therapy in the first 3 or 4 days after surgery, which also avoids pain and discomfort.[1,12] From day 4 or 5, the patient performs at least a few sessions of digital motion exercises. In each session, to lessen resistance of joint stiffness, full passive finger motion – usually 20 to 40 repetitions – should be performed before active digital flexion (Fig. 47.17). Then active digital flexion should proceed gradually[1,12]. In the first 3–4 weeks, only one-third to two-thirds active motion range should be the goal. Extreme digital flexion should be avoided, because marked finger flexion would overload the repaired tendons, risking repair disruption (Fig. 47.18). Most patients have marked swelling at this time; a full range of active motion of the operated finger is difficult to achieve. Aiming at full active flexion of the finger is both unnecessary and unrealistic. However, full passive finger flexion and extension should always be performed to make the hand and finger as supple as possible.

From the end of week 3 or 4, a full range of active flexion is the goal. Some patients who have difficulty with full active flexion at week 4 or 5 may gradually achieve full flexion in later weeks. However, exercise to reduce joint stiffness and prevent extension lag should always be performed for eventual recovery of active finger flexion. The splint protection can be removed at the end of week 5 or 6, but therapy usually should persist for a few weeks to get rid of often-seen remaining stiffness of the DIP joint, with or with nighttime splint protection. After week 6, the author sometimes urges patients to wear a splint only when they go outside, which prevents unintentional use or injury.

More Recent Evolution of Methods

The major conceptual changes in the past three decades in repairing flexor tendons are summarized in Table 47.2. Some of the recent trends and evolution are further highlighted here.

1. *Placing the knots between the two tendon ends may not favor the repair.* Most current multistrand repairs have knots over the tendon surface, and no adverse clinical consequences have been noted. It is now believed that placement of the knots between tendon ends is not important.[28]
2. *Asymmetric suture configurations may be preferable to symmetric designs.* Recent investigations have revealed that asymmetry in the configuration of sutures attaching two tendon stumps are better than symmetric suture placement.[29,30] Asymmetric placement likely favors gap resistance, and this design can be found in some popular suture methods.
3. *A tensioned slightly bunched repair is better than a flat tension-free repair.* A flat, tension-free repair should be avoided. A tensioned slightly bunched repair favors gap resistance and does not hamper tendon gliding as the narrow pulleys are released.[28]
4. *Slightly extended pulley venting to benefit finger flexion outweighs the drawbacks of minor tendon bowstringing.* In case of need to allow gliding of the repaired tendons, slightly extended release favors gliding of the repaired tendon, and the bowstringing caused by slightly extended release is noticeable but still mild. This practice appears especially beneficial at the PIP joint area, where we may extend the venting of the sheath and pulleys from the A4 to A3.[24]
5. *Epitendinous suture is unnecessary when a strong core suture (a 6-strand repair) is used.* This is a recent observation.

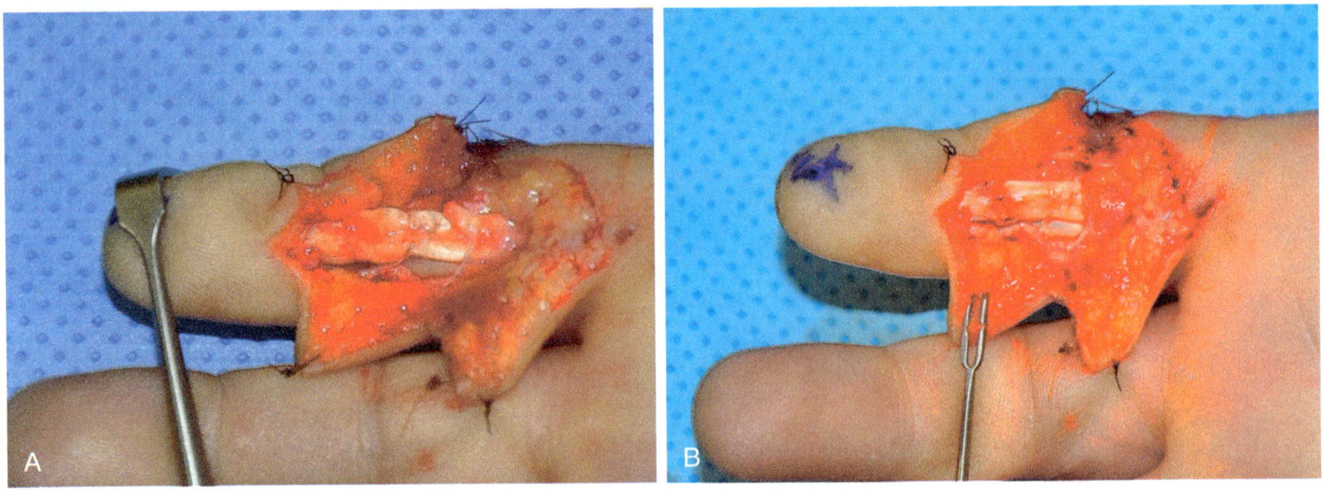

• **Fig. 47.11** (A) The tendon of the patient shown in Fig. 47.8 was repaired with a 6-strand M-Tang repair. Note the core suture was made with some tension to resist tendon gapping, but the tendon should not be too bulky after core suture. The allowed bulkiness at the repair site is a 20%–30% increase in tendon diameter at the repair site. (B) Separate peripheral stitches were sparsely added at three sites – two at the lateral aspect, one at the volar center – where the approximation of tendon ends may be further smoothened by these sparse stitches.

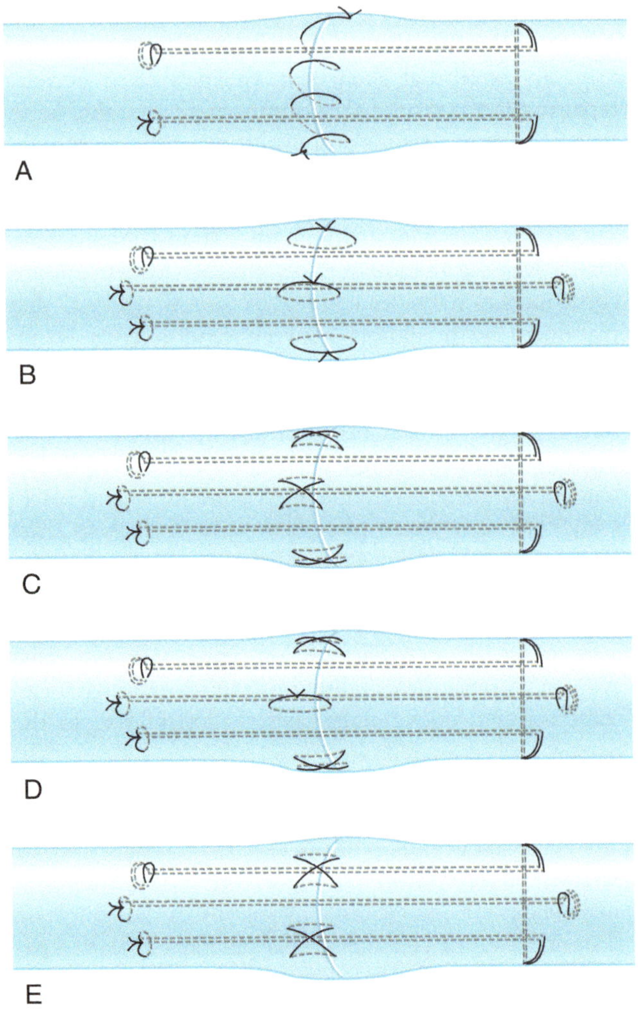

• **Fig. 47.12** (A–E) The simpler, sparse peripheral stitches that can be used after completion of a strong and tensioned core suture that has already approximated the tendon ends closely and tightly.

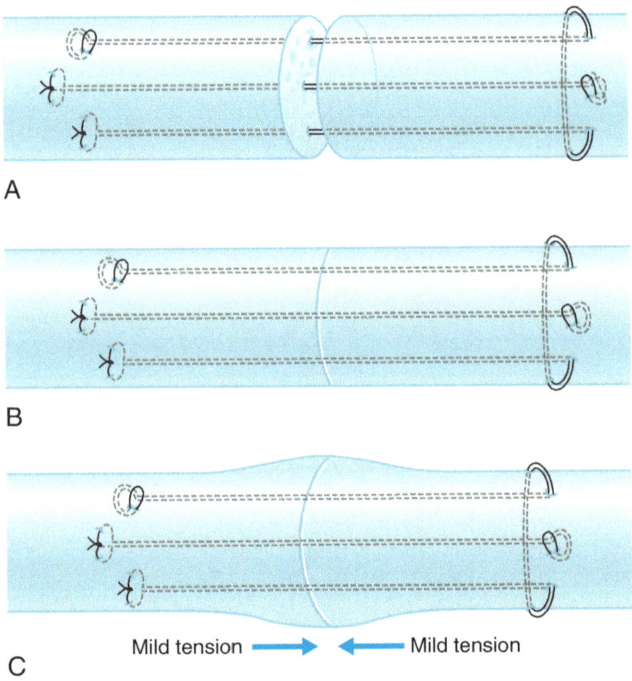

• **Fig. 47.13** (A–C) Appropriately tensioning the repair site is key to preventing gap formation during active finger flexion. The recommended degree of bunching up is 20%–30% increases in diameter of the tendons at the junction of the two tendon ends.

A few surgeons have reported not adding epitendinous sutures when a strong 6-strand repair is made with tension; no repair ruptures were reported.[25,26,31]

6. *Wrist positioning is unimportant and a short splint is safe.* It is now understood that if the tendon repair is strong, the wrist does not have to be placed in a specific position; this allows considerable freedom in wrist positioning.
7. *Out-of-splint exercise is safe.* In the author's practice, out-of-splint motion has been safe for compliant patients; it

• BOX 47.1 Clinical Technical Keys for Achieving Ideal Repair Outcomes

Zone 2 flexor tendon repair has evolved greatly over the past three decades. Some key clinical techniques for ideal outcomes are:

1. Using strong core sutures, typically 4- or 6-strand repairs
2. Judicious venting of the critical annular pulley
3. Ensuring that a slight tension is created by the repair to prevent gapping
4. Performing digital extension–flexion tests to confirm the quality of the surgical repair
5. Early partial-range active motion to ensure tendon gliding without overloading the repair

• BOX 47.2 Repair Techniques that Have Become Popular

1. Direct strong repair of the terminal FDP tendon to any tissues available distally to repair tendon cut close to the distal insertion. Similar methods can be used in making the distal junction of the grafted tendon.
2. Using strong core-suture-only repair or a strong core suture plus separate simple peripheral stitches.
3. Venting the A3 together with A4 pulleys if greater range of motion of the finger is needed.
4. Using a wide-awake setting for tendon repair, including grafting.

is actually more efficient. Splinting compliant patients mainly serves to protect them from getting hurt or unintentional hand use. For this reason, the splint should be worn only between exercise sessions and at night.

Repair in Other Zones and the Thumb

Zone 1

The methods of proximal zone 1 (zone 1B and 1C) repairs are similar to those of zone 2. The postoperative therapy methods are the same as those of zone 2 as well. When the FDP tendon is cut in distal zone 1 (zone 1A), pull-out sutures through the finger nail have been a common treatment (Fig. 47.19). The pull-out suture is reliable, but it passes through the nail. More recently, the author's preference is a direct repair using several strong core suture, i.e., up to 10- or 12-strand core suture repair, which connects the proximal stump to the remnant of the distal stump and tissues such as periosteum adjacent to the tendon insertion on the distal phalanx (Fig. 47.20). This direct repair from proximal tendon stump to any distal tendon tissue and those around it can be applied to the cut close to tendon insertion (zone 1A). There are a variety of bone anchors, including small-sized anchors, which some surgeons use for tendon–bone junction. Large anchors may not fit the fingertip area. The author has no experience with them.

A strong tendon-to-bone junction can be achieved without conventional pull-out suture. The fact is that the terminal tendon just proximal to its insertion to the distal phalanx is distal to the DIP joint, which does not require motion. Adhesions are allowed to develop to help strengthen the repair. Therefore, as much as possible, suture strands can be used to achieve a strong and somewhat bulky repair, which favors both healing and strength. After such a repair, the finger is protected with a dorsal splint for 2 weeks without early mobilization. From week 3, passive finger motion is started. From week 5, active motion of the finger is started and the splint can be discarded at the end of week 6.

Zone 3, 4, and 5

The FDP tendons in zone 3 are repaired using the same technique as in zone 2. The repairs are easier because of lack of sheath covering the tendon. The injuries in the carpal tunnel area (zone 4) are rare and are accompanied by lacerations in the median nerve and arteries. The transverse carpal ligament has to be opened to facilitate repairs. Zone 5 injuries often involve multiple tendons with neurovascular injury. Repair of the FDS and FDP tendons is preferred, and early postoperative motion is advised.

Thumb Flexor Tendon

The FPL tendon repairs follow the same methods of repair as the FDP tendon in fingers. The surgical incision should usually be less than 2 cm. The oblique pulley has to be vented to allow performing the repair. The author uses the 6-strand M-Tang repair for all FPL tendons (Fig. 47.21). The proximal tendon frequently retracts into the thenar muscles, which can be retrieved through an incision in the thenar muscles or the carpal tunnel.

Repair of Partial Tendon Laceration

Treatment of the partially-lacerated tendon depends on the extent of the injury. Any laceration through less than 60% of the diameter of the tendon does not necessitate a repair by core sutures. The lacerated ends can be trimmed to reduce the chance of entrapment by pulley edges and friction against the sheath. Alternatively, the cut portion of the tendon may be repaired with epitendinous stitches to smooth the tendon surface and to strengthen the tendon. If the laceration is over 60% of the tendon diameter, risk of triggering, entrapment, or ruptures is increased. A core suture is necessary to prevent tendon entrapment and disruption. Lacerations of 60%–80% require an epitendinous repair and are better repaired using a 2-strand core suture through the cut portion. Lacerations of 80%–90% are treated as complete lacerations with strong core suture supplemented with a epitendinous sutures as described earlier.

Flexor Tendon Repairs in Children

The repair techniques of flexor tendons used for children are the same as in adults. In children, it is more difficult to recognize the pulleys. Therefore, care must be taken not to vent the pulleys unnecessarily or incorrectly. Tendon healing

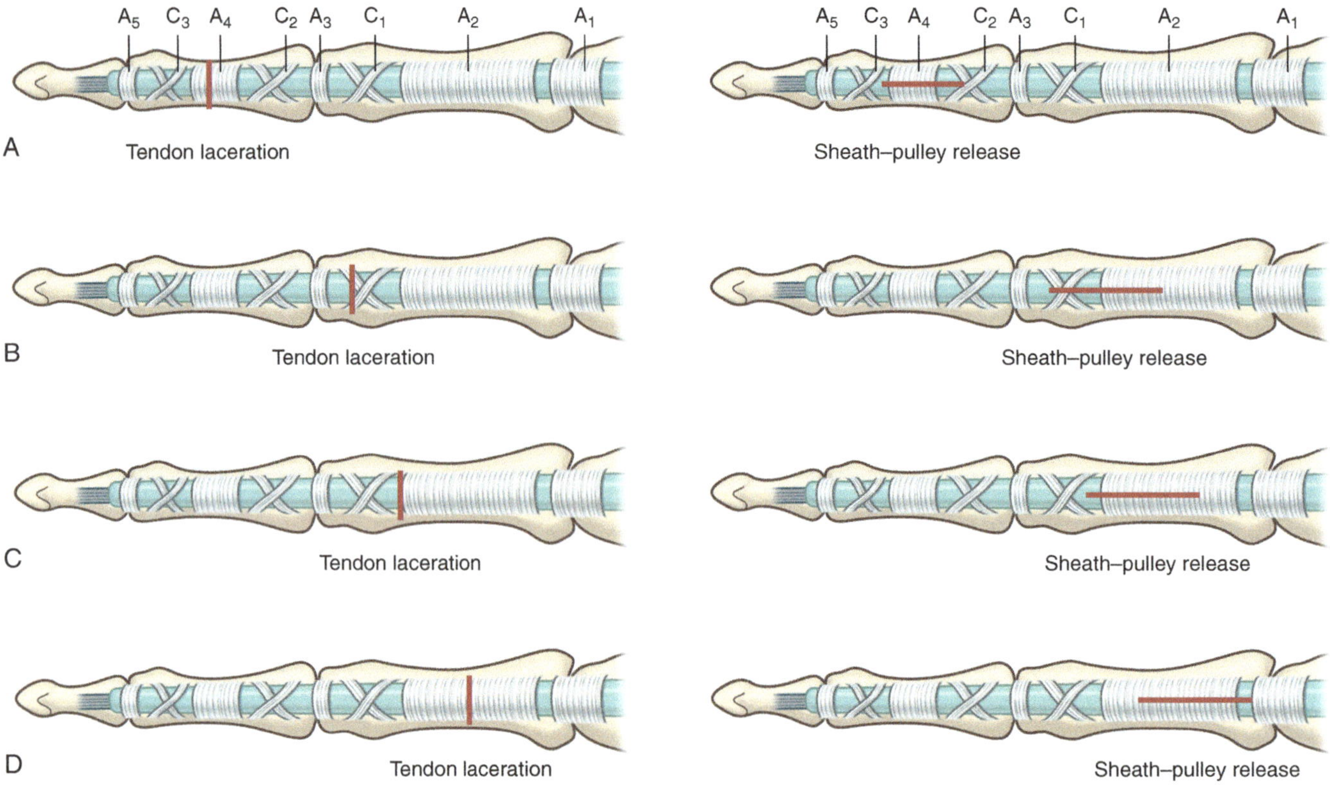

• **Fig. 47.14** Drawings depicting the length and areas of release of the sheath–pulley complex to decompress the repaired tendons, without bowstringing and loss of tendon function. (A) Release of the entire A4 pulley when the FDP tendon has been cut around the A4 pulley and the tendon cannot pass easily beneath this pulley. (B) Release of a part of the sheath distal to the A2 pulley and the distal half of the A2 pulley, when the tendons are cut a little distal to the A2 pulley. (C) Release of a short part of sheath distal to the A2 pulley and the distal two-thirds of the A2 pulley when repairing tendons cut at the edge of, or in the distal part, of the A2 pulley. (D) Release of the proximal two-thirds of the A2 pulley when repairing a cut in the middle, or proximal part of, the A2 pulley. The allowed length of venting is indicated with red lines. (From Tang JB. Flexor tendon injuries and reconstruction. In: Chang J, Neligan P, eds. *Plastic Surgery*. Volume 6: *Hand and Upper Extremity*. 4th edn. Elsevier; 2018: Fig. 9.38.)

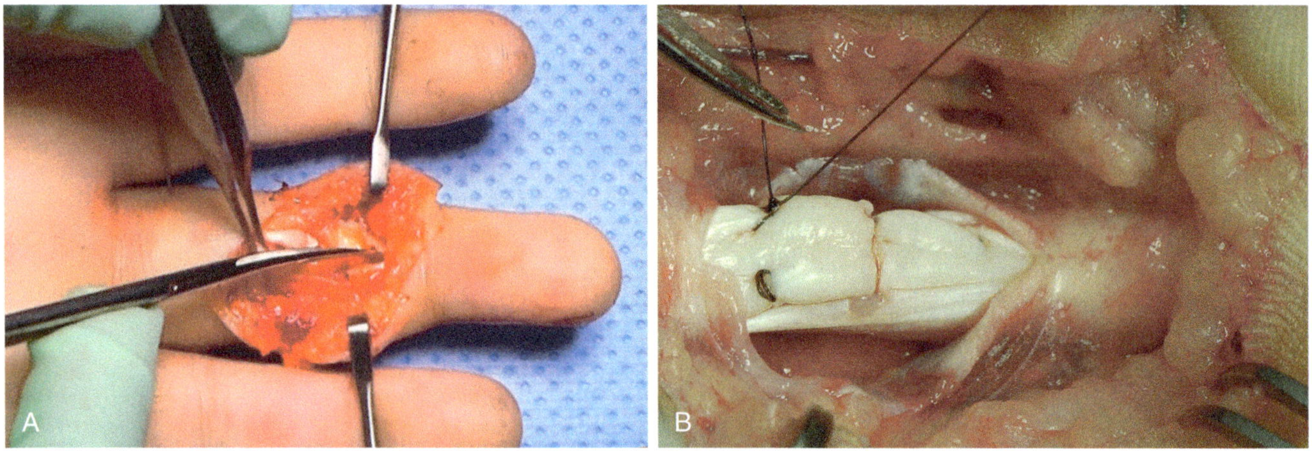

• **Fig. 47.15** Operative pictures showing the complete venting of the A4 pulley and partial venting of the A2 pulley. (A) The entire A4 pulley is vented through a midline cut with scissors to facilitate surgical repair. (B) The distal 60% of the A2 pulley is vented through a midline cut. The tendon is repaired with a 6-strand M-Tang repair.

in children is quicker with less adhesions. It is important to avoid lengthy pulley venting. In children younger than 10 years old, the tendons can be repaired with a 2-strand or, at most, a 4-strand core suture, plus some epitendinous sutures. The fingers or the thumb are protected with a dorsal short-arm splint with the wrist in moderate flexion for 5–6 weeks. Early mobilization of the tendons is not necessary in children.

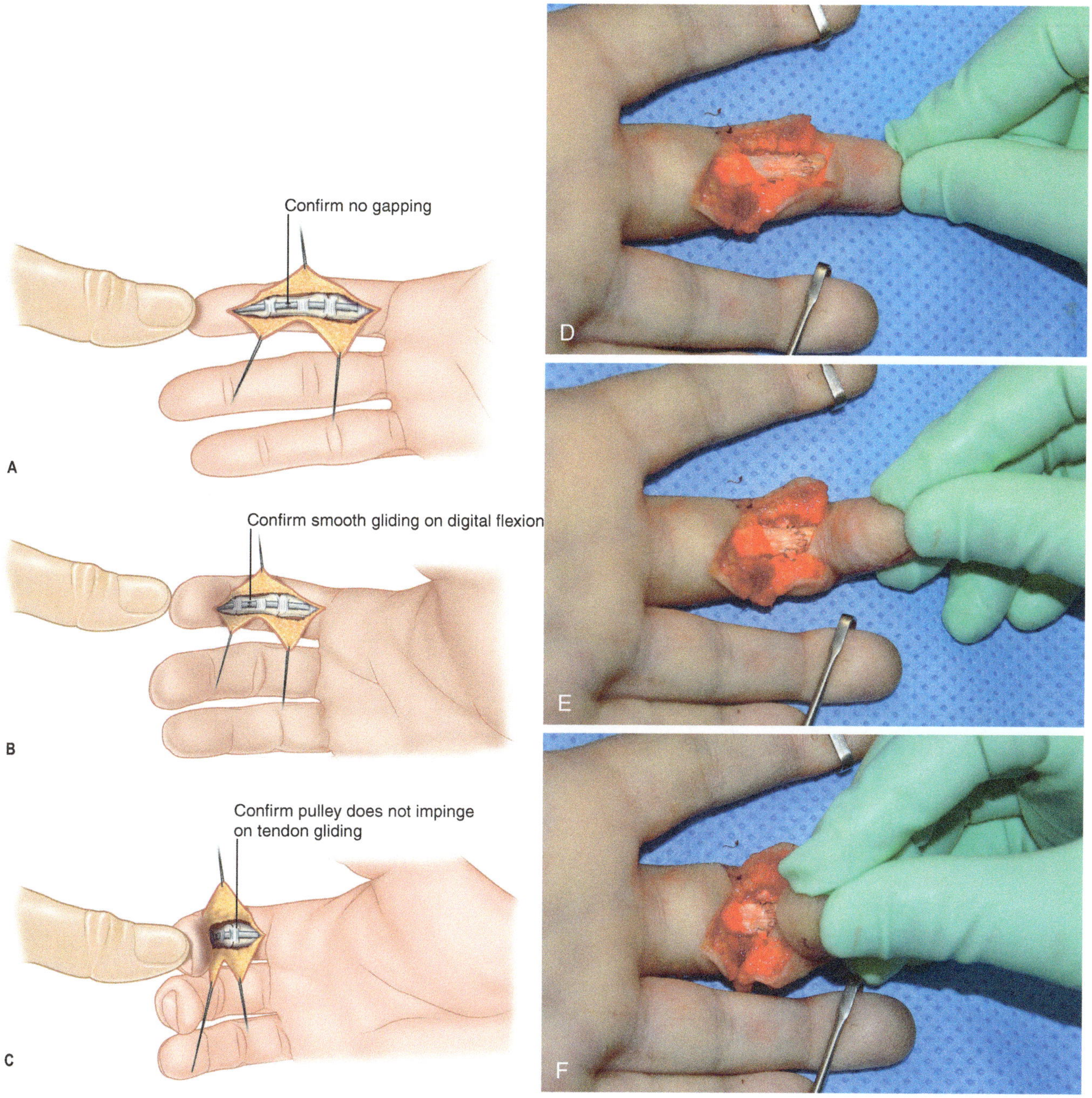

• **Fig. 47.16** (A–C) The extension–flexion test has three steps, performed immediately after completion of the tendon repair to check quality of the repair. (A) *Part I*: passive full extension of the digit to ensure the tendon repair site shows no gapping (above). (B) *Part II*: passive flexion of the digit to confirm that gliding is smooth (middle). (C) *Part III*: pushing the digit to almost full flexion to check whether the tendon repair site impinges against the edge of the sheath or a pulley. (D–F) Operative photos showing the three steps of the test after a repair in the border area of zone 1 and 2. (A–C, From Tang JB. Flexor tendon injuries and reconstruction. In: Chang J, Neligan P, eds. *Plastic Surgery*. Vol 6: *Hand and Upper Extremity*. 4th edn. Philadelphia: Elsevier; 2018: Fig. 9.39; D–F, courtesy Celeste Ryfa.)

Closed Rupture of the Flexor Tendons

The FDP tendon can be avulsed from the insertion to the distal phalanx during forceful extension of the DIP joint, which is called *jersey finger*. During examination, the patient has pain and tenderness over the volar distal finger. The finger lies in slight extension relative to other fingers in resting position, with no active flexion of DIP joint. It may be possible to palpate the flexor tendon retracted proximally along flexor sheath. Radiographs may reveal avulsion fracture in the distal phalanx in the patient with bony avulsion. Three types of closed avulsion are seen:

I. *Tendon avulsion only*: the tendon is avulsed from its insertion site and retracts to the palm or within the finger.
II. *Bony avulsion only*: the tendon insertion site is intact, but the bone attaching to the FDP tendon end is avulsed with limited retraction.
III. *Double avulsion*: both the FDP tendon and the bone attaching to it are avulsed.

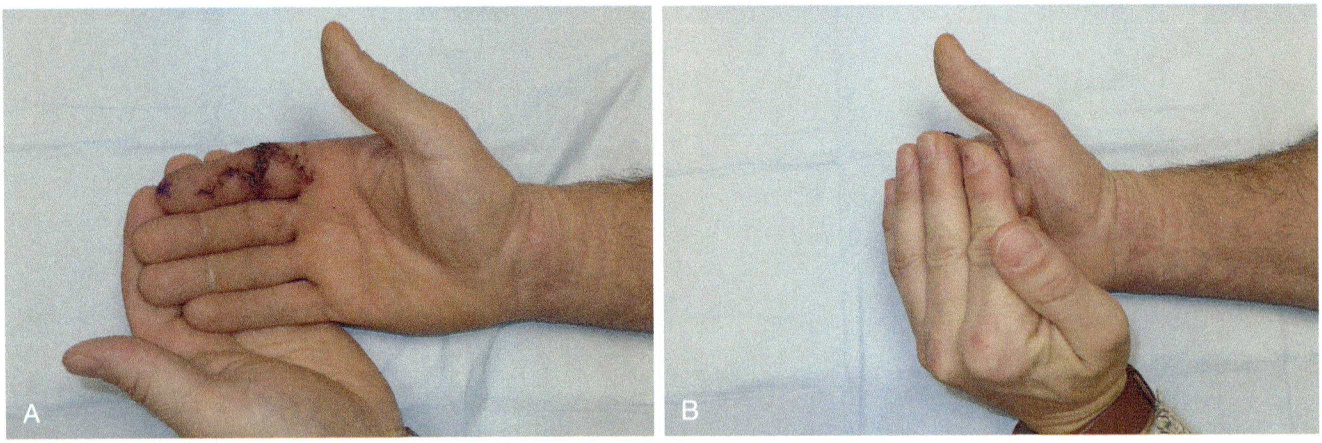

• **Fig. 47.17** (A,B) Full passive motion of the repaired finger should be performed to lessen the stiffness of the joint before active flexion exercise. Patient is shown at postoperative day 7.

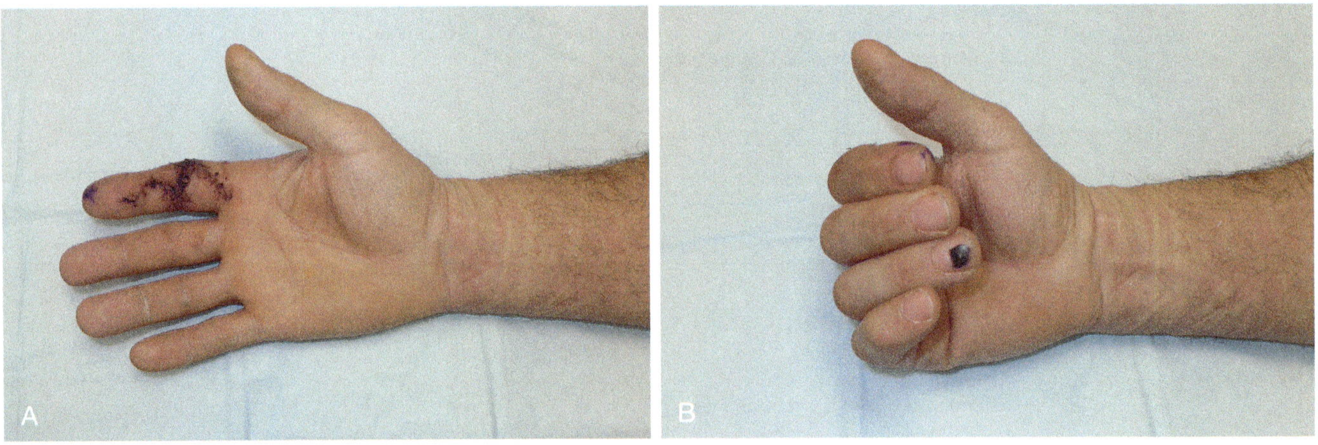

• **Fig. 47.18** (A,B) Partial-range active motion in the initial 2–3 weeks after surgery. Only partial active finger flexion is allowed. Full fist or marked active finger flexion should be avoided to prevent repair rupture.

The three types are easier to use than the Leddy and Packer classification, without loss of detail. Once diagnosed, the tendon needs to be repaired through the volar approach and the avulsed tendon is repaired with sutures, or a pullout suture, or a bone anchor followed by protected finger joint motion after surgery.

The FDP or FDS tendons can be disrupted by a fractured hamate. The closed rupture can be associated with other fractures or surgical plating. The disrupted tendon should be repaired directly or with a graft once surgical exploration has confirmed the diagnosis.

Outcomes

When they followed an updated protocol, young or junior hand surgeons were able to obtain good outcomes in the majority of patients with very few or no repair ruptures.[23] Surgeons have also reported zero ruptures in a case series of more than 50 tendons.[25,26] Repair rupture appears to no longer be a major concern if all modern guidelines are carefully followed. Rupture occurs only in patients who actively use the fingers in the first few weeks after surgery and there are rare instances (estimated to be less than 1%) of unexplained ruptures of ordinarily reliable repairs.[23] With early active motion after surgery, cases of tenolysis have dropped. However, severe tissue damage always poses the risk of developing dense adhesions, which remain a concern.

Strickland criteria have been popular in evaluation of outcomes. In recent years, the criteria have been modified to include stringent criteria for "excellent" and a category of "failure" (Table 47.3).[13,32]

Tenolysis

Tenolysis is indicated when the passive range of digital motion greatly exceeds that of active flexion, several months after direct end-to-end tendon repair or tendon grafting. Tendon trauma with severe damage to peritendinous tissues or compound injuries (such as digital or palm replantation) have greater chances of adhesion formation, thus are more likely to require tenolysis as a later surgery. Children may also be candidates for this surgery.

The prerequisites for this operation are: (1) all fractures are healed; (2) wounds have reached equilibrium

TABLE 47.2 The Major Conceptual Changes in Repairing Flexor Tendons over the Past Three Decades

	1980s and 1990s	2010s
Surgical Techniques		
Tendon repair	Zone 2 2-strand suture	Multistrand suture (4 or 6 strands)
A2 pulley	Should not be violated	Can be partially vented if needed
A4 pulley	Should not be violated	Can be entirely vented if needed
Synovial sheath	Closure recommended	Do not need to repair the sheath
Suture purchase of repair	Not been stressed	Should be more than 0.7–1 cm
Tension across repair site	Not been discussed	An essential key of surgical repair
Extension–flexor test	None	A common quality check point
Wide-awake surgery	Not incorporated	A better approach for tendon repair
After Surgery		
Wrist position in protection	Wrist flexion stressed	Flexible, from mild flexion to extension
Starting motion within 4 days	Common	Unnecessary; no motion is better
Active flexion: first 2–3 weeks	Not popular	Popular
Avoid extreme flexion	None	A key to ensure safety of active flexion
Place-and-hold motion	Popular	Not a useful or efficient exercise
Out-of-splint motion	None	Advocated for reliable patients

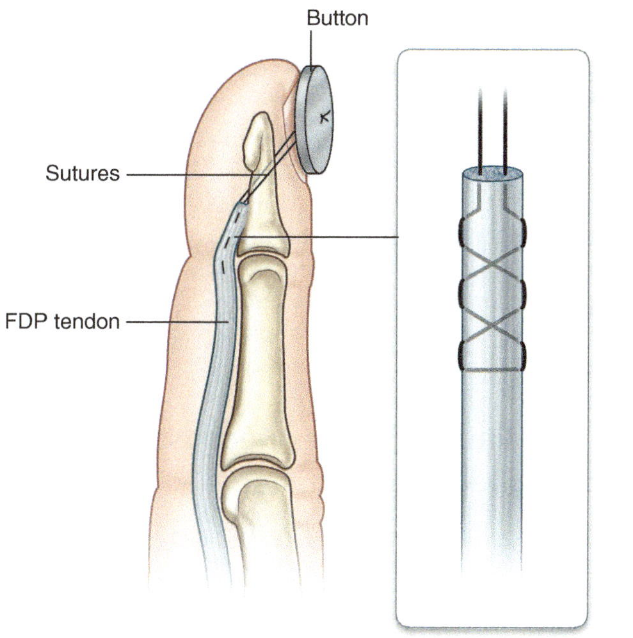

• **Fig. 47.19** A conventional method to anchor the FDP tendon to the bone by pull-out sutures through the nail and tied over a button. (From Tang JB. Flexor tendon injuries and reconstruction. In: Chang J, Neligan P, eds. *Plastic Surgery.* Vol 6: *Hand and Upper Extremity.* 4th edn. Elsevier; 2018: Fig. 9.14A.)

with soft, pliable skin and subcutaneous tissues, and minimal reactions around the incision scars; and (3) joint contractures must have been corrected and a normal or near-normal passive range of digital motion achieved. The exact optimal timing of tenolysis remains controversial. It is reasonable to consider tenolysis if the desired range of motion is not achieved after 3 months of therapy or if there is no improvement of active range of motion for 3 months of therapy. However, surgery should only be considered at the very least 3–6 months following primary repair or graft, to allow necessary healing and revascularization of tendons; this helps to avoid endangering tendon strength.

There is no absolute criterion for how poor the range of motion ranges must be to indicate tenolysis. Surgeons should consider the patient's age, occupational requirements, and functionality of the hand in decision of the operation. Preoperatively, the patients should be informed that intraoperative findings may be incompatible with intended tenolysis; thus the surgeon may need to proceed to the first step of staged reconstruction on finding serious destruction of pulleys or a lengthy lysed tendon segment. It is estimated that about 10%–20% of patients need tenolysis after primary or delayed primary repair.

Anesthesia

Tenolysis is best performed in the wide-awake setting without tourniquet. The patient should move actively during the procedure to demonstrate ample active tendon motion. In addition, the patient is asked to forcefully flex the finger and wrist to break any remaining adhesions after surgical release of adhesions. Axillary block, sedation, or general anesthesia

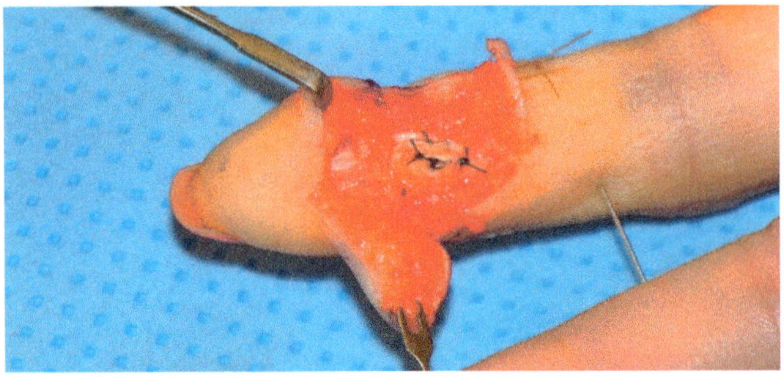

• **Fig. 47.20** An operative picture showing the robust direct repair of the lacerated FDP tendon at the insertion site, with 12 core strands across the cut sites to connect the proximal stump with the very short distal stump, periosteum, and other soft tissue which could be found adjacent to the insertion site. (Courtesy Celeste Ryfa.)

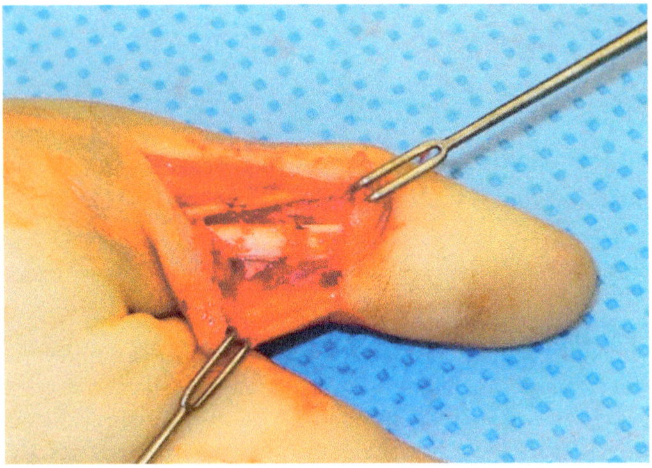

• **Fig. 47.21** Harvesting a tendon graft through a small skin incision and using a tendon tripper.

are used if the surgeon expects an extensive operation, such as tenolysis in multiple digits, a staged reconstruction procedure, or if the patient is unlikely to tolerate surgery with local anesthesia.

Operative Techniques

Through either a Bruner's or midlateral incision, dissection proceeds from the unaffected area to the affected area. Tenolysis requires wider surgical exposure. All limiting adhesions are meticulously divided. Care is taken to define the borders of the flexor tendons. During dissection, the major pulleys should be maintained, and the synovial sheath embedded within the scar is removed. However, if other sheath and major pulleys are intact, it is acceptable to excise a part of the A2 pulley or the A4 pulley. It is vital to avoid any sheath defect over 2 cm. If possible, the A3 pulley and its adjacent sheath are also preserved. Whenever possible, the FDS and FDP tendons are separated from one another. Dissection is continued until normal tissues are revealed and no scar around the tendon is visible. Adequacy of the release is then checked by active digital flexion of the patient or by a gentle proximal traction in the palm through a separate proximal incision.

After surgery, the patient is protected with a dorsal splint and should proceed to early active tendon motion starting from day 3 or 4 after tenolysis.

TABLE 47.3 The Strickland Criteria and Tang Criteria Based on Active Range of Motion (ROM) of the Repaired Finger

Grade	Strickland (1980)[a]	Tang (2013)[b]
Excellent	85–100%	90–100%
Good	70–84%	70–89%
Fair	50–69%	50–69%
Poor	0–49%	30–49%
Failure[c]	–	0–30 %

[a]This criterion is mostly used in zone 2 repair. The normal active ROM of the PIP and DIP joints is considered 175 degrees. The ROM of the repaired finger is divided by 175 degrees to compute percentage return of ROM.
[b]Percentage total active motion of the contralateral side is used in this criterion after repair in any zone. For zone 2 injury, only the PIP and DIP joints are measured; 175 degrees is the sum of the motion of the normal PIP and DIP joints. For zone 2 injury, either 175 degrees or measured actual ROM of the contralateral hand is used to compute percentage return of ROM.
[c]No failure grade in Strickland criteria.

Intraoperative Judgment of Tendon and Pulley Quality

During the surgery, it is important to check the quality of the tendon and integrity of the pulleys. If direct evaluation shows that tendon continuity is maintained only by scar, or greater than one-third of the tendon width is lost, the tendon is unlikely to function properly. Silicone tendon rod is inserted, as the first stage operation of staged reconstruction. Similarly, if the critical pulleys are destroyed, it is appropriate to proceed to pulley reconstruction.

Tendon Grafting, Pulley Reconstruction, and Staged Reconstruction

One-Stage Tendon Grafting

Traumatic lacerations of the digital flexor tendons are usually treated with end-to-end repair. Only those patients who are not treated primarily or have tendon defects that prevent direct end-to-end repair require secondary repairs. In the presence of severe contamination, infection, lengthy loss of tendon substance, extensive destruction of the pulleys, or accompanying injuries, primary tendon repairs are not indicated.[33,34] These patients should be treated secondarily with a tendon graft.

Secondary tendon repairs are achieved mainly by one-stage free tendon grafting, or in some instances by staged tendon reconstruction. Patients who have failed primary surgery or previous efforts at one-stage tendon grafting, or serious scarring are appropriate for a staged tendon reconstruction, rather than one-stage tendon grafting. The surgeon may make this decision intraoperatively based on findings, such as severity of scarring and pulley loss, as described earlier.

Before one-stage tendon grafting or staged tendon reconstruction is attempted, the soft tissue wound should be well healed, with supple passive motion of the hand. Physical therapy is prescribed to improve the range of motion of the digits if passive joint motion is limited substantially. Lack of passive range of joint motion is a contraindication for one-stage tendon grafting, but may be suitable for staged tendon reconstruction. The timing of tendon grafting is usually at least 3 months after injury.

The donors are palmaris longus, plantaris, long toe extensors, or in rare instances the FDS tendon from a normal finger. The palmaris longus tendon (about 15 cm) from the ipsilateral limb is frequently used as donor and is appropriate for a palm-to-fingertip graft. It can be easily harvested through a short transverse incision over the tendon just proximal to the flexion crease of the wrist. The tendon is divided and grasped with a hemostat, while a tendon stripper is advanced slowly into the proximal forearm. Care must be taken to protect the median nerve trunk and its cutaneous lying beneath the tendon. This tendon is absent in about 15% of all hands, examination to confirm its presence is essential prior to surgery. The plantaris tendon is another option for a graft; it is obtained by an incision medial to the Achilles tendon and with a tendon stripper (Fig. 47.22). The length of this tendon (25 cm) is well suited for a long distal forearm–fingertip graft. However, this tendon is absent in 7%–20% of limbs, and its presence cannot be predicted preoperatively except with imaging. Extensor digitorum longus tendons to the second, third, and fourth toes, the extensor indicis proprius, the extensor digit quinto proprius, and the FDS tendon to the fifth finger can be used as well. The author uses the palmaris longus tendon most frequently.

The flexor tendon is exposed through a palmar Bruner's incision or the midlateral approach. Integrity of the major annular pulleys is important to the function of the tendon graft. At least the A2 and A4 pulleys should be preserved. If possible, other annular pulleys such as A1 or A3 and a part of the synovial sheath are preserved to foster better gliding of the grafted tendon.

The distal junction of the graft is placed at the fingertip. The most common method is to suture the graft directly to the residual FDP stump or bury it under an osteoperiosteal flap in the volar phalanx. In the latter case, the straight needles are passed through the distal phalangeal drill hole and exit over the proximal portion of the nail. After emerging from the nail surface, the needles are passed through a gauze pad or a sponge, and

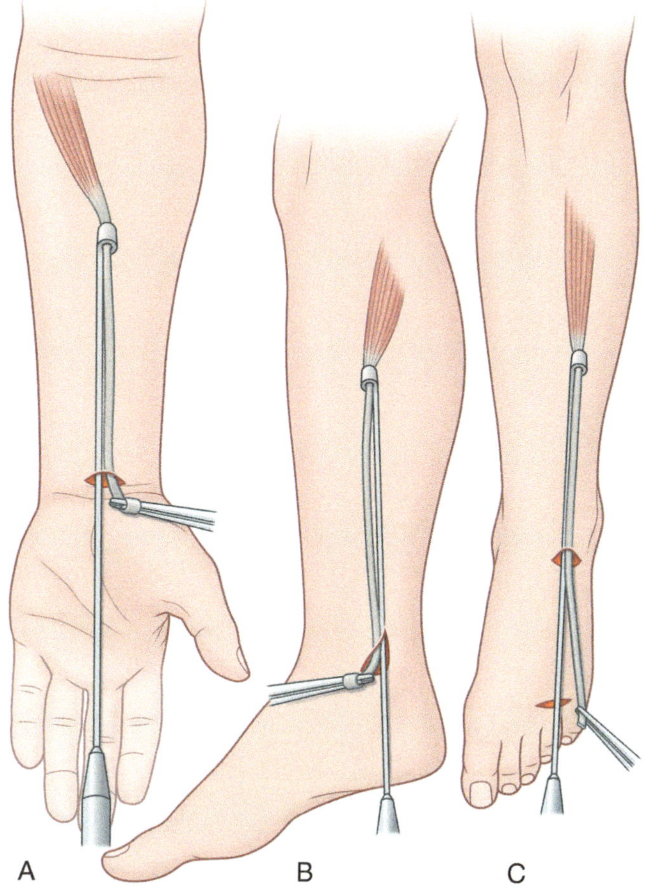

• **Fig. 47.22** Three common donors of tendon grafts. (A) Palmaris longus tendon. (B) Plantaris. (C) Toe extensors. (From Tang JB. Flexor tendon injuries and reconstruction. In: Chang J, Neligan P, eds. *Plastic Surgery*. Vol 6: *Hand and Upper Extremity*. 4th edn. Elsevier; 2018: Fig. 9.47A–C.)

through the holes of an overlaying button. The sutures are tied over the button to anchor the graft. Additional sutures are used to secure the FDP tendon stump to the graft. In children, drill-holes at the distal phalanx may damage the open epiphyses; the graft is sutured directly to the stump of the profundus instead. The author now uses direct suture of the graft to the remnants of the FDP tendon repair using strong repair methods as described earlier for zone 1 tendon repair. The author no longer uses a pull-out suture and has not used bone anchors.

The proximal junction of the graft can be made either at the palm or in the forearm. Placement of the junction at the palm requires only a shorter graft and preserves the function of lumbrical muscles. Care is taken to avoid suturing the tendon to the lumbrical muscle, because this tends to increase the tension in the muscle. Placement of the junction proximal to the wrist allows easy adjustment of the tension of the graft, and scar may be less severe. In the author's experience, a Pulvertaft weave suture is

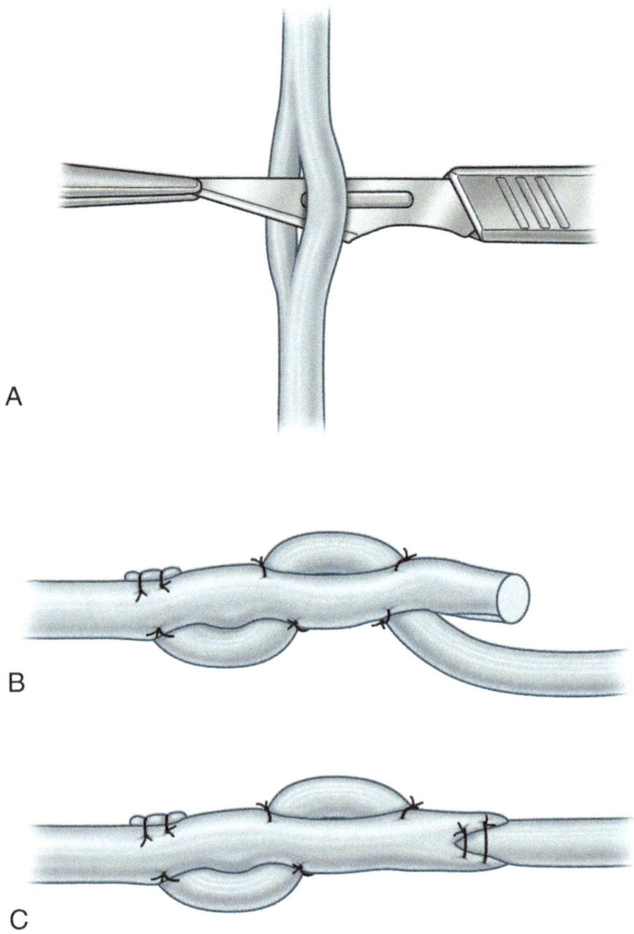

• **Fig. 47.23** A Pulvertaft weave junction of the grafted tendon. (A) A blade is used to split the tendon through the midline. (B) The graft is passed through the opening in the middle of the recipient tendon and sutured together. (C) The graft and the recipient tendon are weaved together through 2–3 weaves. The sutures are added to secure the connection of two tendons as shown in the drawings. (From Tang JB. Flexor tendon injuries and reconstruction. In: Chang J, Neligan P, eds. *Plastic Surgery*. Vol 6: *Hand and Upper Extremity.* 4th edn. Elsevier; 2018: Fig. 9.48B.)

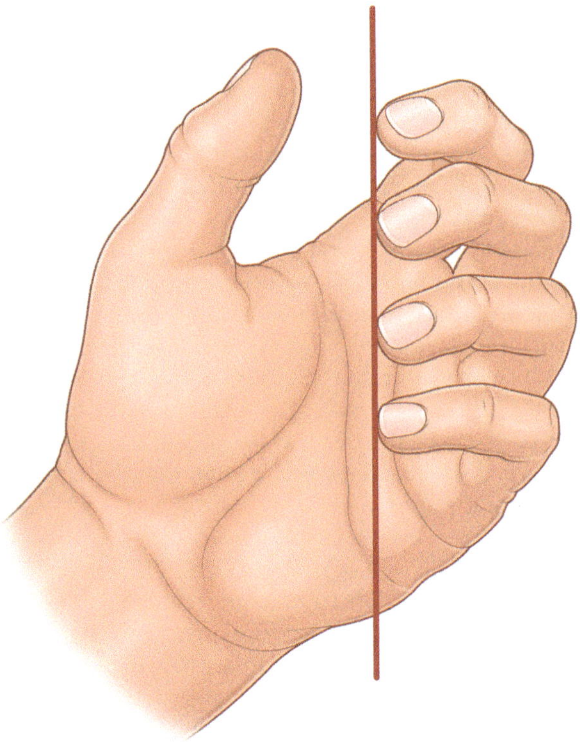

• **Fig. 47.24** Tension status of the fingers at the time of suturing the proximal tendon junction of a graft. With the wrist in neutral position, the fingers are slightly more flexed than at the resting position, with each finger falling into slightly more flexion than its radial neighboring fingers. (From Tang JB. Flexor tendon injuries and reconstruction. In: Chang J, Neligan P, eds. *Plastic Surgery*: Vol 6: *Hand and Upper Extremity*. 4th edn. Elsevier; 2018: Fig. 9.50.)

appropriate for the proximal junction in both areas (Fig. 47.23), and the finger is held in slightly greater flexion than in the resting position when the proximal stump is sutured (Fig. 47.24).

Pulley Reconstructions

If a series of annular pulleys are found to be destroyed, reconstruction of the A2 and A4 pulleys is required. Some surgeons do not think that the A4 pulley should be reconstructed; they feel the A2 needs reconstruction, but the A4 does not. Various materials can be used. A portion of an excised flexor tendon or the palmaris longus tendon may be used. This is wrapped around the phalanx twice to obtain sufficient width, and has to be placed deep to the extensor mechanism. Another method is to make use of one rim of a residual pulley, and a tendon graft, a portion of an excised flexor tendon, or a part of the extensor retinaculum is woven back and forth to form a volar part of the residual pulley, or the grafted tendon is sutured to the rim of residual pulleys without weaving (Fig. 47.25). Most cases requiring pulley reconstruction need to be preceded by staged tendon reconstruction.

When the FDS tendon is fully functional, but the FDP tendon is cut and has not been repaired directly within 3–4 weeks after trauma, the need of tendon graft or reconstruction is controversial. There is a risk of losing function if a profundus graft fails. However, such operations are worth the risk in selected cases, such as in young people with a reasonable need for active DIP joint flexion. The procedures are similar to those described above. A thinner donor tendon is preferable. Alternatively, one slip of the FDS tendon can be removed to favor passage of the graft. Overall, caution must be exercised with patient selection. Patients with intact superficialis tendon may adapt nicely and require no treatment. The surgeon should fully inform patients about the expected gain of function as well as the risks of this operation.

Staged Tendon Reconstruction

The staged reconstruction is indicated in cases with severely scarred digits, because of injury or multiple failed attempts

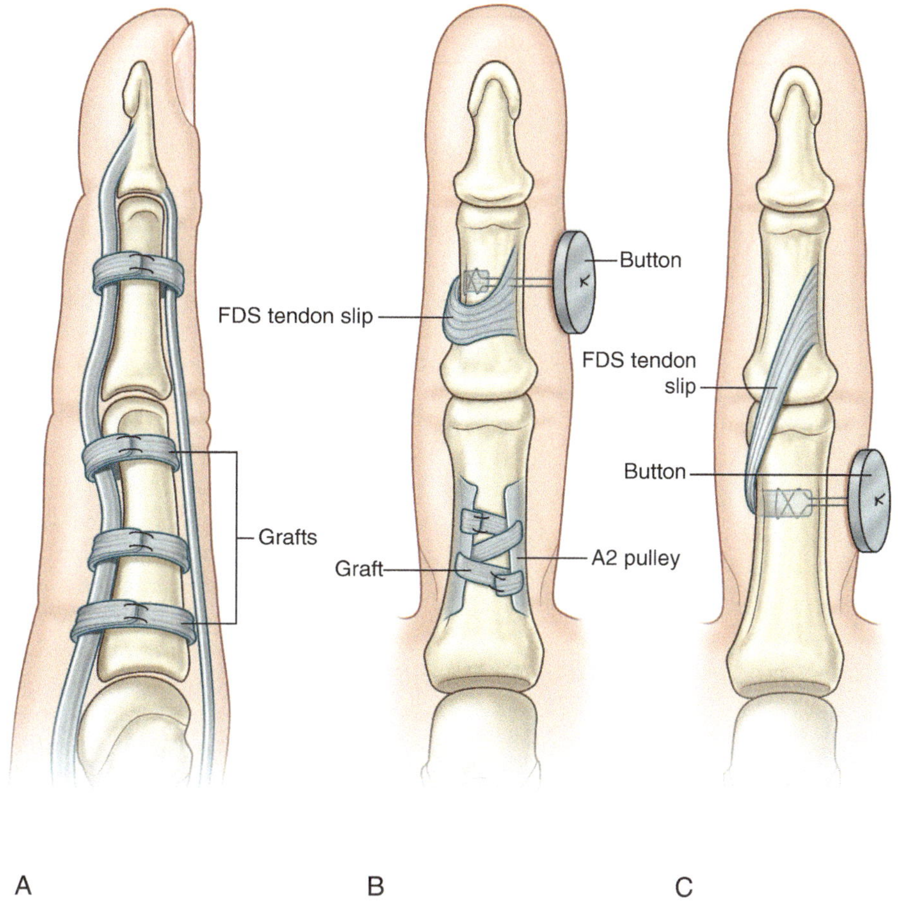

• **Fig. 47.25** Several methods of flexor pulley reconstruction. (A) Reconstruction of the A4 and A2 pulleys using flexor tendon grafts passed circumferentially around proximal and middle phalanges. The tendon graft passes deeper to the extensor apparatus at the proximal phalangeal level and superficial to the extensors at the middle phalangeal level. (B) A tendon graft is weaved through remnant of the A2 pulley to reconstruct the A2 pulley. (C) Use of a slip of FDS tendon for middle digital pulley reconstruction. (From Tang JB. Flexor tendon injuries and reconstruction. In: Chang J, Neligan P, eds. *Plastic Surgery*: Vol 6: *Hand and Upper Extremity*. 4th edn. Elsevier; 2018: Fig. 9.52AB.)

to restore tendon continuity and tendon gliding. This operation is divided into two stages. The first stage consists of excising the tendon and scar from the tendon bed, preserving or reconstructing pulleys. A silicone gliding implant (Hunter rod) is inserted into the scarred tendon bed to maintain the tunnel and to stimulate the formation of a pseudosheath. Following maturation of the pseudosheath a tendon is grafted to replace the implant in the second stage.[35]

The Surgery at the First Stage

The approach to the tendons is similar to that for tendon grafting. The tendons are excised with a 1-cm stump of the profundus tendon retained at its distal insertion. Unscarred portions of the flexor pulleys are carefully preserved. In the presence of flexion contracture of the finger joint, check-rein extensions of the palmar plate and the accessory collateral ligaments are divided to release the contracture. The profundus tendon is transected at the midpalm. The size of the Hunter rod is determined by the tightness of the digital pulleys. In adults, smaller (4 mm) Hunter rods are often preferable, which are closer in size to the tendon graft. After insertion of the implant underneath the pulleys, the implant should be able to glide freely. The distal end of the Hunter rod is sutured to the FDP tendon stump using 2–3 stitches of nonabsorbable sutures. The author places the proximal end of the rod to the palm, not extending it to the distal forearm. However, the rod can be passed from the proximal palm into the distal forearm using a tendon passer. After the Hunter rod is seated, traction is placed on the proximal end of the Hunter rod to make sure that it glides smoothly beneath the pulleys (Fig. 47.26).

The Surgery at the Second Stage

The second stage surgery should follow in 3 months. A small incision is made adjacent to the DIP joint, exposing the implant–tendon junction. After disconnecting the implant from the tendon, the implant is tagged. Proximal incision of about 2 cm is made in the palm to find the proximal end of the implant. A free tendon graft is harvested and inserted

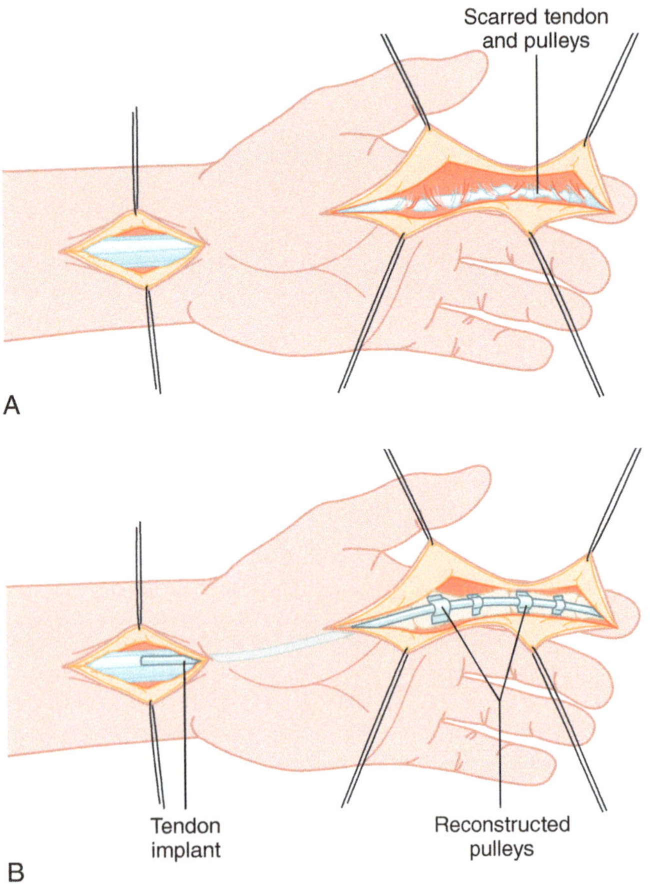

• **Fig. 47.26** (A) In stage 1 of the staged reconstruction, the Hunter rod is placed into the scarred tendon bed. The annular pulleys are preserved. (B) Proximal end of the tendon implant is left free without suturing to any tendons. (From Tang JB. Flexor tendon injuries and reconstruction. In: Chang J, Neligan P, eds. *Plastic Surgery*. Vol 6: *Hand and Upper Extremity*. 4th edn. Elsevier; 2018: Fig. 9.53A–C.)

into the pseudosheath tunnel from the incision in the palm (Fig. 47.27A). The Hunter rod is then pulled from the distal incision until the entire grafted tendon sits inside the digit. The distal tendon junction is made as previously described for free tendon grafting (Fig. 47.27B).

Care is taken not to open the pseudosheath proximal to the DIP joint. In the palm a suitable profundus tendon stump is chosen for a Pulvertaft suture with the finger held in moderate flexion. The author prefers to put the proximal repair in the palm. It can be placed in the distal forearm, however the tendon graft is usually not long enough. Correct tension on the graft is essential for good function.

Postoperative Care

After one-stage tendon grafting or after stage 2 of the staged reconstruction, the wrist is held in slight flexion (30 degrees) and the MCP joint in marked flexion with a short arm splint. Some surgeons immobilize the hand for 3–4 weeks; others favor an early protected motion program initiated days after surgery. The author prefers a less aggressive early active finger flexion program with passive finger motion. Therapy proceeds carefully through passive and light active motion until at least 6 weeks, when the tensile strength of the tendon and its junctures are sufficiently strong to tolerate more vigorous motion. By 8 weeks, full activity is permitted, except powerful grip until 12 weeks.

After stage 1 of the staged reconstruction, passive finger motion should start a few days postoperatively. The hand should not be immobilized for a period of weeks. In cases with pulley reconstruction over the Hunter rod, the fingers must be protected by circumferential taping or Orthoplast rings and passive finger motion should be instructed. In cases with pulley reconstruction over an intact tendon, only very gentle active flexion of the digit is allowed in the first few weeks.

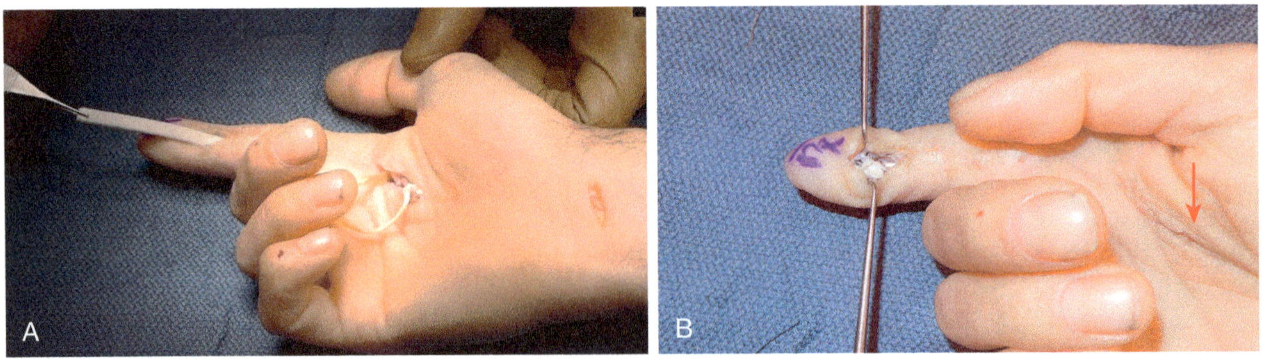

• **Fig. 47.27** In stage 2, the Hunter rod is replaced by a tendon graft. (A) The Hunter rod is exposed through a small incision at the distal part of the finger. After the rod is disconnected from the FDP tendon stump, it is sutured to the tendon graft. The distal end of the Hunter rod is pulled from the distal incision to lead the grafted tendon into the newly formed sheath. The incision in the distal forearm is for harvesting a palmaris longus tendon. (B) The graft has been tunneled in the finger, with the proximal junction site indicated with a red arrow. The proximal tendon junction is completed with a Pulvertaft weave suture. Distally, the graft is repaired to the residual FDP tendon stump through a robust direct repair as used for repair of the terminal zone 1 FDP tendon.

References

1. Tang JB. New developments are improving flexor tendon repair. *Plast Reconstr Surg*. 2018;141:1427–1437.
2. Giesen T, Calcagni M, Elliot D. Primary flexor tendon repair with early active motion: experience in Europe. *Hand Clin*. 2017;33:465–472.
3. Wong JK, Peck F. Improving results of flexor tendon repair and rehabilitation. *Plast Reconstr Surg*. 2014;134:913e–925e.
4. Elliot D, Giesen T. Primary flexor tendon surgery: the search for a perfect result. *Hand Clin*. 2013;29:191–206.
5. Tang JB. Recent evolutions in flexor tendon repairs and rehabilitation. *J Hand Surg Eur*. 2018;43:469–473.
6. Wu YF, Tang JB. Recent developments in flexor tendon repair techniques and factors influencing strength of the tendon repair. *J Hand Surg Eur*. 2014;39:6–19.
7. Savage R. In vitro studies of a new method of flexor tendon repair. *J Hand Surg Br*. 1985;10:135–141.
8. Tang JB. The double sheath system and tendon gliding in zone 2C. *J Hand Surg Br*. 1995;20:281–285.
9. Lalonde DH. Conceptual origins, current practice, and views of wide awake hand surgery. *J Hand Surg Eur*. 2017;42:886–895.
10. Lalonde DH, Martin AL. Wide-awake flexor tendon repair and early tendon mobilization in zones 1 and 2. *Hand Clin*. 2013;29:207–213.
11. Tang JB. Clinical outcomes associated with flexor tendon repair. *Hand Clin*. 2005;21:199–210.
12. Tang JB. Indications, methods, postoperative motion and outcome evaluation of primary flexor tendon repairs in zone 2. *J Hand Surg Eur*. 2007;32:118–129.
13. Tang JB. Outcomes and evaluation of flexor tendon repair. *Hand Clin*. 2013;29:251–259.
14. Kwai Ben I, Elliot D. "Venting" or partial lateral release of the A2 and A4 pulleys after repair of zone 2 flexor tendon injuries. *J Hand Surg Br*. 1998;23:649–654.
15. Tang JB. Release of the A4 pulley to facilitate zone II flexor tendon repair. *J Hand Surg Am*. 2014;39:2300–2307.
16. Wu YF, Tang JB. Effects of tension across the tendon repair site on tendon gap and ultimate strength. *J Hand Surg Am*. 2012;37:906–912.
17. Moiemen NS, Elliot D. Primary flexor tendon repair in zone 1. *J Hand Surg Br*. 2000;25:78–84.
18. Tang JB. Flexor tendon repair in zone 2C. *J Hand Surg Br*. 1994;19:72–75.
19. Tang JB, Xu Y, Wang B. Repair strength of tendons of varying gliding curvature: a study in a curvilinear model. *J Hand Surg Am*. 2003;28:243–249.
20. Tang JB, Cao Y, Xie RG. Effects of tension direction on strength of tendon repair. *J Hand Surg Am*. 2001;26:1105–1110.
21. Wu YF, Tang JB. Tendon healing, edema, and resistance to flexor tendon gliding: clinical implications. *Hand Clin*. 2013;29:167–178.
22. Tang JB, Amadio PC, Boyer MI, et al. Current practice of primary flexor tendon repair: a global view. *Hand Clin*. 2013;29:179–189.
23. Tang JB, Zhou X, Pan ZJ, et al. Strong digital flexor tendon repair, extension-flexion test, and early active flexion: experience in 300 tendons. *Hand Clin*. 2017;33:455–463.
24. Giesen T, Reissner L, Besmens I, et al. Flexor tendon repair in the hand with the M-Tang technique (without peripheral sutures), pulley division, and early active motion. *J Hand Surg Eur Vol*. 2018;43:474–479.
25. Pan ZJ, Chen J. Zone 2 flexor tendon repairs using a tensioned strong core suture, sparse peripheral stitches, and early active motion: results in 60 fingers. *J Hand Surg Eur*. 2019;44:361–366.
26. Tang JB. Wide-awake primary flexor tendon repair, tenolysis and tendon transfer. *Clin Orthop Surg*. 2015;7:275–281.
27. Howell JW, Peck F. Rehabilitation of flexor and extensor tendon injuries in the hand: current updates. *Injury*. 2013;44:397–402.
28. Tang JB. Flexor tendon injuries. *Clin Plast Surg*. 2019;46(3):295–306.
29. Wu YF, Tang JB. The effect of asymmetric core suture purchase on gap resistance of tendon repair in linear cyclic loading. *J Hand Surg Am*. 2014;39:910–918.
30. Kozono N, Okada T, Takeuchi N, et al. A biomechanical comparison between asymmetric Pennington technique and conventional core suture techniques: 6-strand flexor tendon repair. *J Hand Surg Am*. 2018;43:79. e1–79.e8.
31. Giesen T, Sirotakova M, Copsey AJ, et al. Flexor pollicis longus primary repair: further experience with the Tang technique and controlled active mobilization. *J Hand Surg Eur Vol*. 2009;34:758–761.
32. Tang JB. Outcomes of flexor tendon repairs and methods of evaluation. In: Tang JB, Amadio PC, Guimberteau JC, et al., eds. *Tendon Surgery of the Hand*. Philadelphia: Elsevier; 2012: 246–258.
33. Tang JB. Flexor tendon injury and reconstruction. In: Chang J, Neligan PC, eds. *Plastic Surgery*. Vol. 6: *Hand and Upper Extremity*. 3rd edn. Philadelphia: Elsevier Saunders; 2013:178–209.
34. Boyes JH, Stark HH. Flexor tendon grafts in the fingers and thumb. A study of factors influencing results in 1000 cases. *J Bone Joint Surg Am*. 1971;53:1332–1342.
35. Hunter JM, Salisbury RE. Flexor-tendon reconstruction in severely damaged hand. A two-stage procedure using a silicone-Dacron reinforced gliding prosthesis prior to tendon grafting. *J Bone Joint Surg Am*. 1971;53:829–852.

48

Extensor Tendon Injuries

KRISHNA RAO AND GREGORY McCARTEN

Extensor Tendon Injuries

Unlike flexor tendons, the extensor tendons are not constrained in a sheath, but nevertheless have a complex and intricate anatomy. The dorsal skin being thinner and pliable is more susceptible to trauma. As extensor tendon repairs are perceived to be a lot easier, they end up being delegated to junior surgical trainees.

Although the surgical repair itself may be simple, thorough understanding of extensor tendon dynamics is necessary to optimize hand function after repair. In contrast to flexor tendon injuries some extensor injuries like closed mallet and closed boutonnière-type injuries are best treated conservatively. Some of the extensor tendon injuries have associated joint injuries and require careful debridement and lavage to prevent joint infections. Associated nerve injuries may be present, usually the sensory branches of the radial nerve and occasionally the posterior interosseous nerve, requiring microsurgical repair.

The cross-sectional morphology of extensor tendons varies significantly according to the site of the injury. Thin flat tendons encountered over the dorsum of the fingers require a different suture technique in comparison to the more rounded thicker counterparts encountered over the dorsal wrist joint. Appropriate and postoperative splinting, mobilization, and hand therapy are essential to avoid early tendon ruptures and joint contractures and to minimize adhesions to overlying skin.

Anatomy

Long extensors arise from the lateral epicondyle of the humerus and the dorsal surface of the forearm (radius, ulna, and interosseous membrane). Wrist extensors, which include extensor carpi radialis longus (ECRL), extensor carpi radialis brevis (ECRB), and extensor carpi ulnaris (ECU) originate from the lateral epicondyle, as do the extensor digitorum communis (EDC) and extensor digiti minimi (EDM).

The dorsal surface of the radius, ulna, and the interosseous membrane give origin to extensor indicis (EI), abductor pollicis longus (APL), extensor pollicis brevis (EPB), extensor pollicis longus (EPL), and extensor indicis proprius (EIP).

Brachioradialis (elbow flexor, forearm mid-pronator with no action on the wrist) and ECRL are innervated by the radial nerve while the remaining extensors are supplied by the posterior interosseous nerve (in addition to the supinator).

Wrist and Hand

At the level of the wrist the extensor tendons pass under a synovial-lined condensation of the deep fascia called the extensor retinaculum (Fig. 48.1). The extensor retinaculum has transverse and vertical fibers which form septae separating six compartments. From radial to ulnar the first dorsal compartment contains the APL and EPB while the second contains ECRL and ECRB. The third compartment contains EPL while the fourth contains EDC and EIP. The fifth compartment contains EDM and the sixth, ECU.

Over the dorsum of the hand, the EDC tendons contain several short oblique interconnecting tendinous slips called juncturae tendinum.[1] These intricate interconnections prevent significant tendon retraction following complete division of a single EDC tendon in zone V/VI (see below). The EIP tendon has no attached juncturae and this can help distinguish it from EDC to index.[1]

At the level of the metacarpal heads the EDC tendons are stabilized by sagittal bands which keep them in close relation to the metacarpophalangeal (MCP) joint while preventing ulnar or radial subluxation.[2] At this level the extensor tendons tend to sublux ulnarly and this renders the radial sagittal band extremely important in preventing such subluxation.[3] The EDC (and EIP) are the primary extensors of MCP joints.

Fingers

Distal to the MCP joints the EDC divides into a central slip and paired lateral slips which are joined by tendons of intrinsic muscles (interossei and lumbricals) to form the lateral band.[4] The central slip inserts into the dorsal aspect of the base of the middle phalanx and is joined by medial slips from the lateral bands (Figs. 48.2 and 48.3). The lateral bands continue and insert into the dorsal aspect of the base of the distal phalanx as the conjoint lateral bands before which they are joined by the oblique retinacular ligament of Landsmeer.[5]

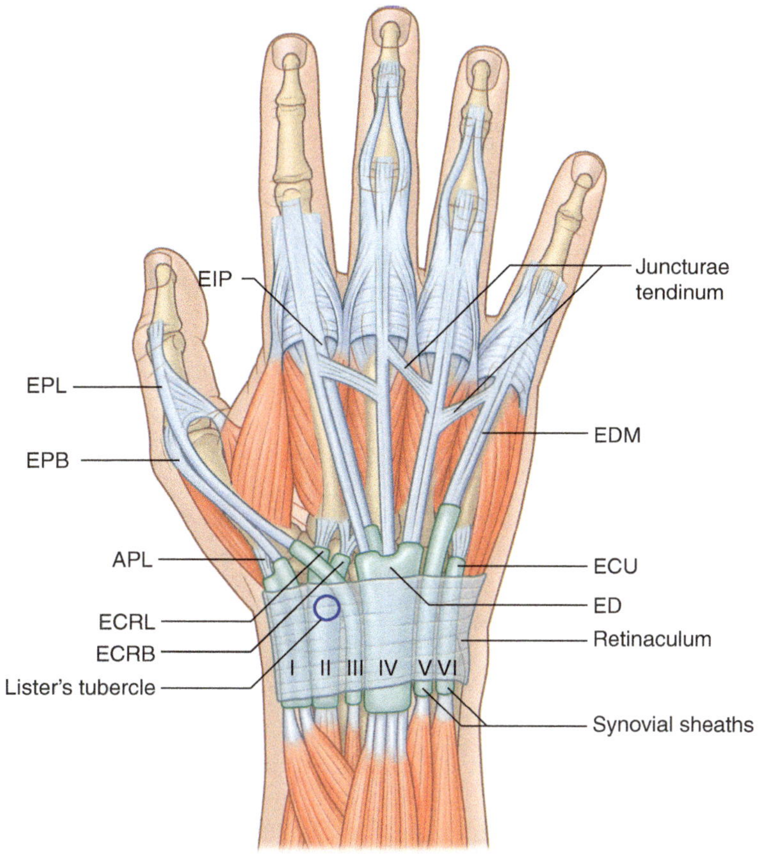

• **Fig. 48.1** Extensor tendons over dorsum of hand and wrist. For abbreviations see text. (From Megerle K, Prommersberger KJ. Extensor tendon injuries. In: Chang J, Neligan PC, eds. *Plastic Surgery*. Vol 6: *Hand and Upper Extremity*. 4th edn. Philadelphia: Elsevier Saunders; 2018.)

Extension at the proximal interphalangeal (PIP) and distal interphalangeal (DIP) joints is primarily a function of intrinsic muscles (4 lumbricals, 3 palmar, and 4 dorsal interossei).[6] The intrinsic muscles arise in the hand and course distally dorsal to the deep transverse metacarpal ligaments at which point they are volar to the joint axis. Hence these intrinsic muscles act as the primary flexors of the MCP joints. Once the intrinsic tendons join the lateral slip of the EDC, they are dorsal to the axis of PIP and DIP joints, thus becoming the extensors of PIP and DIP joints.[7] Although the dorsal aspect of the base of the middle phalanx is the primary bony insertion of the EDC, the intrinsic muscles extend the PIP joint through medial slips which join the central slip. EDC can act on the PIP joint only while the MCP joint is flexed.

The transverse retinacular ligament extends from the conjoint lateral bands to the flexor sheath at PIP joint level, and acts to prevent dorsal dislocation of the lateral bands.[8] The oblique retinacular ligament (ORL) connects the conjoint lateral band from the dorsum of the distal phalanx to the volar check rein ligaments at the PIP joint. The ORL thus lies volar to the PIP joint and sits dorsal to the axis of the DIP joint, allowing coordination of flexion and extension within those joints.[5] The triangular ligament a fascial band connecting the conjoint lateral bands and the terminal tendon. It prevents volar subluxation of the conjoint lateral bands during PIP joint flexion.[9]

Thumb

APL, EPB, and EPL all play separate roles in thumb extension. APL inserts into the base of the first metacarpal, EPB attaches to the base of the proximal phalanx, while EPL maintains a broad area of contact with the base of the distal phalanx. As it traverses the dorsum of the MCP joint, EPL is anchored on the ulnar side by the aponeurosis of adductor pollicis, whereas radially, abductor pollicis brevis (APB) performs a similar role. Consequently, EPL is held securely in a centralized position as it courses over the metacarpal head. Consequently, proximal stump retraction is found only when EPL division occurs proximal to the MCP joint.

Presentation and Management by Zone

Kleinert and Verdan proposed a division of extensor tendon injuries into eight zones with an additional more proximal ninth zone proposed later by Doyle.[10] The management of extensor tendon injuries is dependent on the zone of the

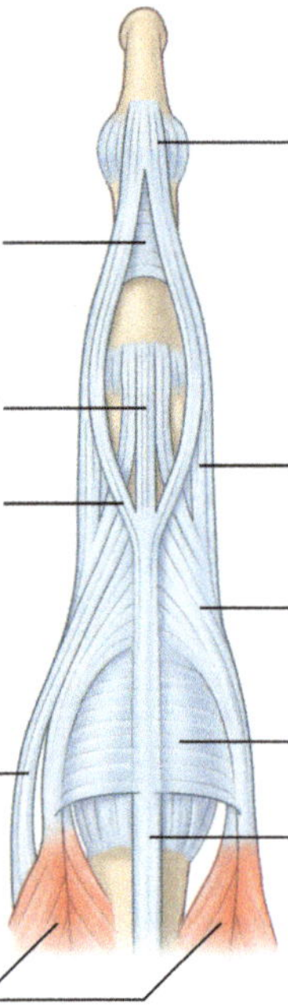

• **Fig. 48.2** Extensor apparatus over fingers showing the contribution of intrinsic musculature. (From Megerle K, Prommersberger KJ: Extensor tendon injuries. In: Chang J, Neligan PC, eds. *Plastic Surgery*. Vol 6: *Hand and Upper Extremity*. 4th edn. Philadelphia: Elsevier Saunders; 2018.)

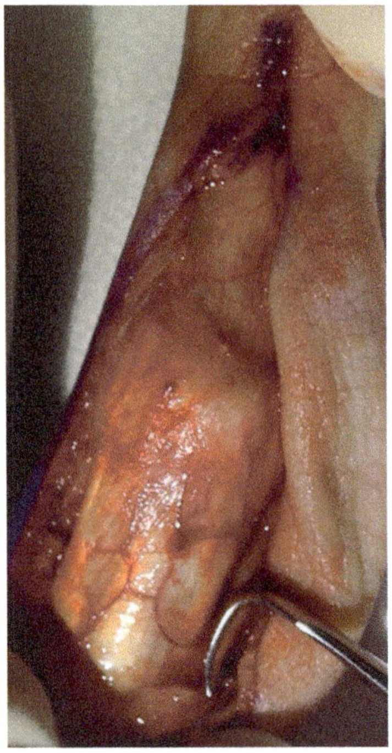

• **Fig. 48.3** Intraoperative view showing normal extensor tendon over zones III and IV. The medial slips from lateral bands can be seen.

injury. As an aide-memoire, excepting zone IX, odd-numbered zones are located over joints (Fig. 48.4).

- Zone I – DIP joint
- Zone II – middle phalanx
- Zone III – PIP joint
- Zone IV – proximal phalanx
- Zone V – MCP joint
- Zone VI – dorsum of hand
- Zone VII – extensor retinaculum
- Zone VIII – distal forearm
- Zone IX – muscular area, middle and proximal forearm

The anatomical zone of extensor injury in the thumb are as follows:

- Zone TI – IP joint
- Zone TII – proximal phalanx
- Zone TIII – MCP joint
- Zone TIV – metacarpal
- Zone TV – carpometacarpal joint

Zone I: Dorsal Interphalangeal Joint

Zone I extensor tendon injuries result in a mallet finger, a deformity characterized by persistent flexion at the DIP joint.

Open injuries require a repair of zone I and as the tendon itself lacks substance, a variety of methods have been described. The tendon repair can be made more robust by inclusion of dermis. This procedure, called dermotenodesis or tenodermodesis, can be done using interrupted external polypropylene sutures or buried sutures using PDS (polydioxanone dermal suture). The authors prefer to protect open tendon repairs using a transarticular Kirchner wire (K-wire) (1.25 mm). The wire may be removed once the healed wound is robust enough to withstand pressure from splinting.

Closed injuries involving extensor tendon (soft tissue mallet) are best treated nonoperatively in a well-fitting splint which holds the DIP joint in neutral to full hyperextension.[11] The splinting needs to be continuous for approximately 8 weeks and continued for a further 2–4 weeks at night or during strenuous use. Up to 10 degrees lag post treatment may be

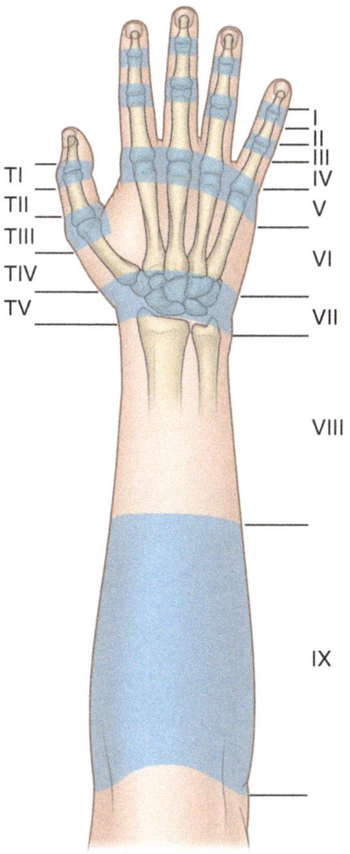

• **Fig. 48.4** Extensor tendon zones of hand. (From Megerle K, Prommersberger KJ. Extensor tendon injuries. In: Chang J, Neligan PC, eds. *Plastic Surgery*. Vol 6: *Hand and Upper Extremity*. 4th edn. Philadelphia: Elsevier Saunders; 2018.)

accepted and usually causes little functional problem.[12] Persistent lag may cause a secondary swan-neck deformity due to a proximal shift in the extensor mechanism. If noted early this can be prevented and treated using an oval-8-type splint which allows full PIP joint flexion but prevents hyperextension. Extensor lag unresponsive to splinting may be improved by central slip Fowler tenotomy, which allows the entire extensor mechanism to shift proximally. This proximal shift of the extensor mechanism corrects the lag caused by the lax terminal extensor tendon. This is best done at least 6 months after injury in order to allow the scar tissue to mature.

Closed extensor tendon avulsion fractures (mallet fractures) can be associated with volar subluxation of the distal interphalangeal joint. Subluxation is frequent in mallet fractures involving more than 50% of the articular surface of the base of the distal phalanx. Mallet fractures with no subluxation can be suitably treated nonoperatively by continuous splinting in full extension or slight hyperextension for 6 weeks followed by mobilization and night splinting for 2–4 weeks. Mallet fractures with subluxation are best treated surgically using a transarticular K-wire[13] alone or in combination with a dorsal blocking wire[14] (Fig. 48.5). Rarely, if the fragment is substantial, other methods like interfragmentary screw, hook plate fixation or interosseous wire fixation can be used.

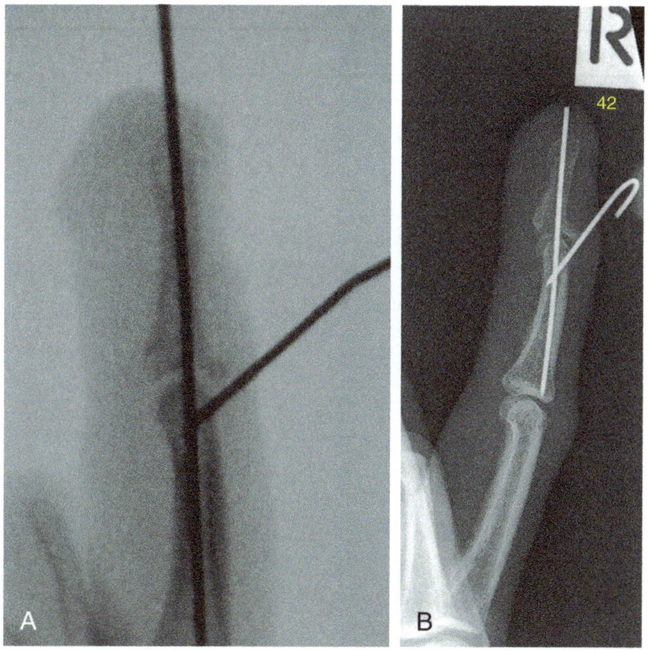

• **Fig. 48.5** (A,B) Extension block wiring for mallet fracture. The oblique dorsal wire blocks the mallet fragment in place.

Recurrent chronic mallet finger with secondary swan-neck deformities are difficult to treat and often DIP joint fusion may be necessary with postoperative splinting for correction of swan-neck deformity. Especially in the radial digits DIP joint fusion is well tolerated and causes little functional impairment. Alternatively, a spiral oblique retinacular ligament reconstruction using tendon graft may be considered. Thompson described this in 1978[15] and this involves an oblique tendon graft from EDC insertion to the volar plate/flexor sheath complex, mimicking the ORL.

Zone II Injuries: Middle Phalanx

Injuries in Zone II, i.e., between the DIP and PIP joint, cause a mallet-type deformity if both lateral bands and the ORLs (oblique retinacular ligament) are divided. The tendon can be repaired with either simple continuous or a figure-of-8-type suture using delayed or nonabsorbable suture. Splinting protocol is similar to that for Zone I injuries.

Extensor tendon excursion in Zone I and II is only 1–2 mm. Hence static splinting is sufficient at these levels.[16]

Zone III Injuries: Proximal Interphalangeal Joint

These injuries cause a boutonnière-type deformity, which initially starts as a passively correctable flexion deformity that progresses to a fixed flexion deformity of the PIP joint with an extension deformity of the DIP joint (Fig. 48.6). The genesis of this deformity is a buttonhole-type displacement of the PIP joint between the two lateral bands with a volarward displacement of the lateral bands.[17]

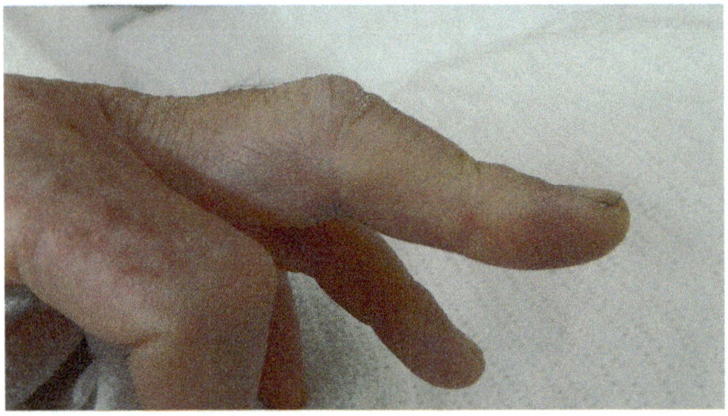

• **Fig. 48.6** Boutonniere deformity with flexion at the PIP and hyperextension at the DIP joint.

Acute Closed Injuries

These are best treated by continuous splinting of the PIP joint in full extension.[18] The DIP joint should be left free for regular active and passive flexion exercises. At approximately 6 weeks the splinting strategy should be changed to static night splinting in extension and a short arc motion splint for limited PIP flexion exercises during the day. Alternatively, a dynamic PIP extension splint can be used. These injuries frequently result in residual stiffness and flexion deformity of the PIP joint.

Acute Open Injuries

The central slip should be repaired using a continuous or a figure-of-8 delayed or nonabsorbable suture. An initial period of K-wire stabilization of the PIP joint should be considered to allow skin healing robust enough for splinting. Segmental defects of the central slip may be reconstructed using a distally-based turnover flap of the central slip.[19,20] If the lateral bands are intact, they may be sutured in the dorsal midline to mimic the central slip.[21] At 3–4 weeks short arc motion should be started aiming for full flexion exercises after 8 weeks post injury.

Chronic Closed Injuries

An established boutonnière deformity can be a frustrating problem if managed surgically. Secondary anatomical abnormalities include volar migration of lateral bands with contraction of transverse retinacular ligament and attenuation of triangular lamina. Many surgeons prefer to treat them nonoperatively with serial splinting to correct the PIP joint and passive DIP flexion exercises to correct the lateral band position.

Surgical correction of established boutonnière deformity may be done by tenotomy of lateral bands just distal to the PIP joint (proximal zone II) to reconstruct the central slip.[22] The division of lateral bands allows the hyperextended DIP joint to flex while the intact ORL preserves active extension. In chronic deformity it may be better to prioritize DIP flexion over PIP extension and accept an extension lag.

Zone IV Injuries: Proximal Phalanx

The extensor tendon at this level is characterized by a broad flat tendon expansion. Injuries at this level are best repaired by continuous or figure-of-8 sutures using delayed or nonabsorbable sutures. Nonabsorbable sutures can sometimes need late removal for suture knot irritation or recurrent infection. Splinting in the POSI (position of safe immobilization) position in the immediate postoperative period should be followed by early active motion (EAM). This can be done using a relative motion splint that holds the affected finger in 30 degrees relative extension compared to other fingers. No studies have shown substantial long-term differences in outcomes between immobilization and early mobilization protocols,[23] but early mobilization results in a faster return of function in the form of total active motion (TAM).[24]

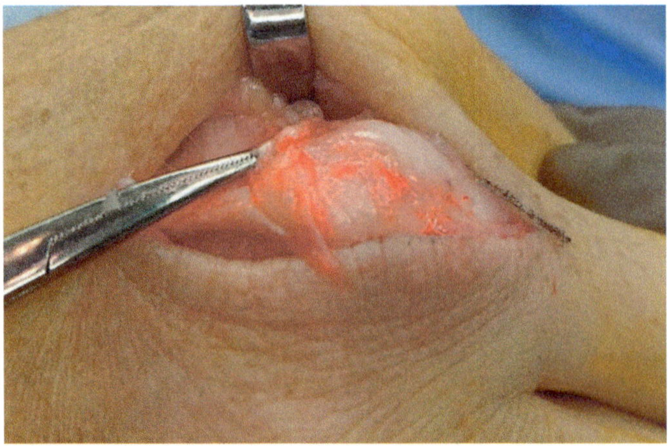

• **Fig. 48.7** Extensor tendon centralization for chronic sagittal band rupture. A distally based slip of extensor tendon/junctura has been passed around the transverse metacarpal ligament.

Zone V Injuries: MCP Joint

Closed Injuries

Closed injuries in zone V usually take the form of sagittal band rupture. The patient is able to maintain MCP joints in extension once passively extended. On flexion, the extensor tendon subluxes (usually ulnarly) and active MCP extension is not possible. Acute sagittal band rupture can be treated conservatively using a relative motion splint for approximately 6 weeks.[25] Non-acute injuries and those that fail conservative treatment need surgical centralization of the extensor tendon. This can be done using a slip of junctura or part of the extensor tendon that can then be lassoed around the transverse metacarpal ligament or neighboring EDC or repaired to the remnant of the sagittal band (Fig. 48.7). Repair of the sagittal band may be possible in rare cases.

Open Injuries

At this level the extensor tendon usually has sufficient substance for preferably a 4-strand core suture using nonabsorbable or delayed absorbable sutures and epitenon sutures (Fig. 48.8). Care should be taken to avoid a tight repair or excessive shortening. Acute open injuries involving the radial sagittal bands should always be repaired to prevent subluxation, and in the event of excessive tension, the ulnar

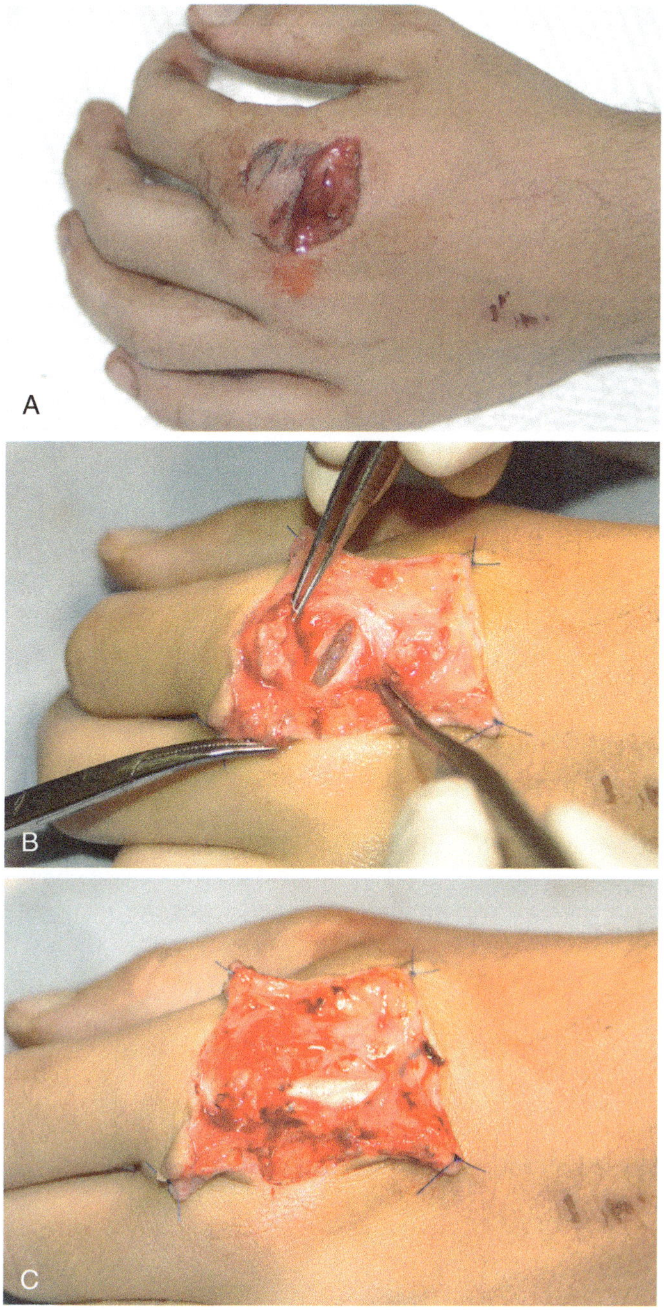

• **Fig. 48.8** (A–C) Chainsaw injury to proximal zone V of the index finger with a breach of the dorsal cortex of the second metacarpal. The EIP and EDC have been repaired using cruciate core sutures (4-strand) and running epitenon sutures. An accessory EIP was present at the radial aspect of the EDC and has been repaired.

sagittal band may be divided. Of special significance are fight bite injuries caused by impact of a flexed MCP joint in a clenched fist against a tooth. As soon as the MCP joint extends, the inoculum (frequently intraarticular) gets contained and significant suppurative infection then follows from streptococci and staphylococci.[26] When seen early, the wound may appear insignificant but needs careful exploration and meticulous lavage. In established infection or septic arthritis, it may be necessary to delay the repair to address infection.

Postoperative therapy can be done using a relative motion splint[27] (Fig. 48.9). In multiple injuries, the hand and wrist should be splinted in a POSI (Fig. 48.10) and early passive and assisted active extension exercises can be started.

Zone VI: Dorsum of Hand

In comparison to more distal zones, zone VI injuries undergo little retraction as the proximal cut end is held in place by juncturae. The tendon can usually be repaired with a core and epitenon suture using nonabsorbable or delayed absorbable suture. In a static splint the wrist is placed in 30° of extension, with the MCP joints in 20°–30° of flexion with IP joints in full extension. Dynamic mobilization is appropriate in compliant patients. In late presentations, direct repair may not be possible, in which case end-to-end or end-to-side transfer to an adjacent tendon (EDC or EIP) is appropriate.

Zone VII: Wrist

Acute Injuries

Penetrating trauma at this level usually injures both the extensor retinaculum and the underlying extensor tendons. When the cross-sectional diameter of the tendon permits, a core suture repair using a 3-0 or 4-0 nonabsorbable suture is performed. Frequently, the proximal tendon ends are markedly retracted, requiring extensive exposure. Severe wounds, such as those from a chain saw, cause problems not only with tendon identification, but also with ragged tendon ends and significant segmental loss of tendon. Tendon grafting or tendon transfer may be necessary under these circumstances. Where possible, the extensor retinaculum should be repaired to prevent subluxation or bowstringing of the tendons, except for EPL which can be completely exteriorized. The surgeon should be aware of anatomical variations within APL, frequently in one, two or four slips, creating the potential for confusion when attempting to repair proximal and distal stumps. Repairs of APL and EPB are commonly associated with repair of sensory branches of the radial nerve. Of the wrist extensors, ECRB is the most important as it acts as a central wrist stabilizer.

Chronic/Attrition Injuries

Extensor synovitis, wrist fractures, and chronic wrist arthritis all predispose EDC and EPL to attrition ruptures. EPL rupture is best managed with an EIP tendon transfer. This is necessary because the EPL being a single muscle–tendon unit is prone to myostatic contracture and a tendon graft does not restore function. Ruptures of EDC are treated with suture of the distal stump to adjacent extensor tendons. If all EDCs are divided it is still possible to use a tendon graft from toe extensor or strips of fascia lata as tenodesis effect (passive extension of MCP joints on wrist flexion) alone provides useful function.

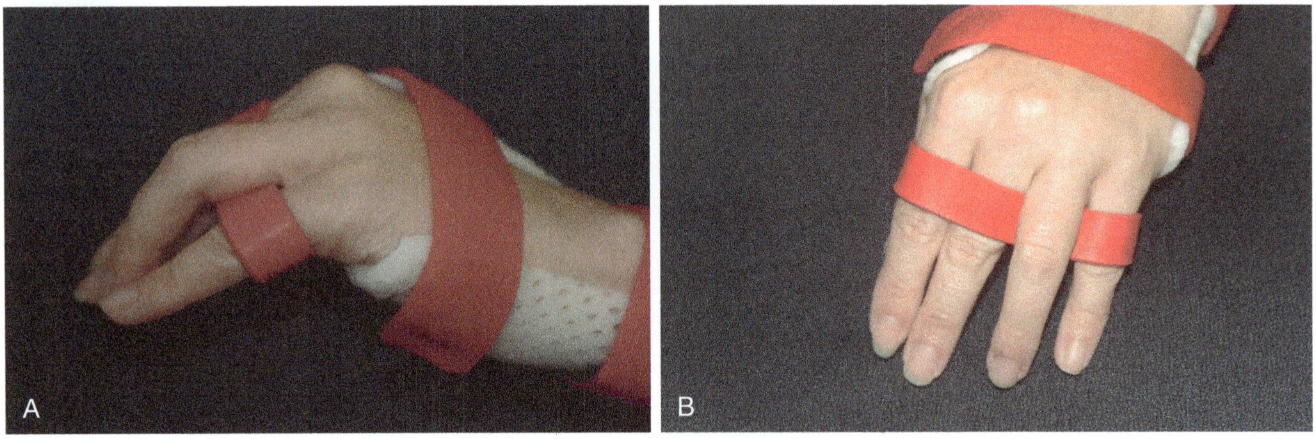

• **Fig. 48.9** (A,B) Relative motion splint, useful for zone IV–VI injuries involving a single tendon. This splint permits active mobilization and should be supplemented with a volar splint keeping the wrist in dorsiflexion.

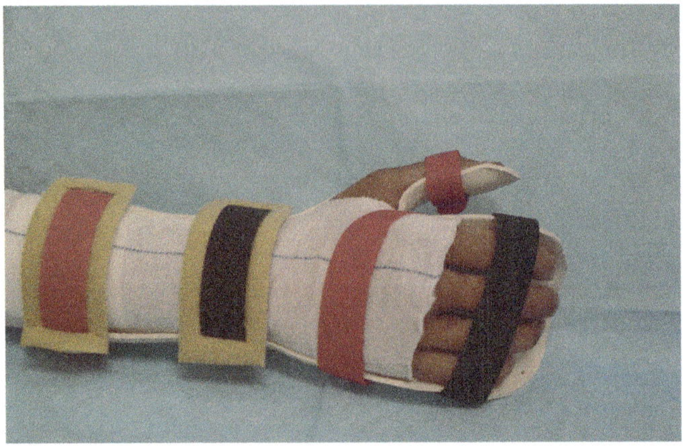

• **Fig. 48.10** POSI (position of safe immobilization) splint for injuries involving multiple tendons or for more proximal injuries (zones VII–IX).

Zone VIII: Proximal and Distal Forearm

Open distal forearm injuries produce disruption around the musculotendinous junction. Achieving adequate strength of repair using conventional tendon repairs is difficult. Frequently the best repair possible is a figure-of-8 or a Bunnell-type repair using monofilament sutures. Postoperative splinting is necessary to ensure adequate wrist dorsiflexion to protect the repair. Penetrating injuries to the proximal half of the forearm, usually the result of glass, chain saws or knives, result in partial or total muscle belly divisions. Intramuscular fibrous septa may help with orientation of muscle bellies, and also provide the most robust structures for suture placement. Concomitant injury to the posterior interosseous nerve at this level is frequent and should be meticulously repaired.

Injuries to Extensor Tendons of the Thumb

Zone TI: Interphalangeal (IP) Joint

Open Injuries

Direct repair of tendon ends is usually possible as proximal retraction is minimal. Of greater concern is damage to the underlying capsule with exposure of the DIP joint. Vigorous lavage of the joint is required prior to capsular and tendon repair, and a single K-wire is used to hold the joint in extension. Bone-anchoring devices are appropriate for reattaching EPL when division has occurred at its insertion.

Closed Injuries

In the absence of a significant fracture or subluxation, acute closed injuries resulting in EPL disruption, "mallet thumb," are treated with 8 weeks of splinting.[28] Indications for operative intervention extend to those cases with a large bone fragment or volar subluxation. These cases are managed using the dorsal blocking wire technique. Treatment is generally similar to a mallet finger.

Zone TII: Proximal Phalanx of the Thumb

The EPL tendon runs over the dorsoulnar aspect of the proximal phalanx of the thumb. The tendon is usually amenable to repair using a figure-of-8 or continuous suture.

Zone TIII: Metacarpophalangeal (MCP) Joint of the Thumb

MP joint lacerations in the dorsum of the thumb can result in division in any or all of EPL, EPB, and the joint capsule. The tendon, in this zone, is usually flat and may not be suitable for a core and epitendinous-type repair.

For Zone II and Zone III injuries the repair can be treated with static splinting for 4 weeks followed by intermittent gradual mobilization. EPL repairs have a higher risk of dehiscence than EDC.

Zones TIV and TV: First Metacarpal and Carpometacarpal Joint

Injuries sustained over the first metacarpal may incur injury to EPL, APL (zone V only) and EPB. The cross-sectional morphology of APL and EPL allows for a core suture in a modified Kessler configuration. EPB tendon is much smaller and may only accommodate a 2-strand repair or a simple continuous or figure-of-8 suture. Sensory branches of the radial nerve are numerous and require preservation or repair as appropriate.

Open Injuries

Retraction of the proximal stump of EPL in these zones is likely. The repair is usually tight and the third compartment of the extensor retinaculum should be released (the entire EPL tendon can be exteriorized). If found to be excessively damaged or delayed presentation does not allow it be pulled out to length, an extensor indicis (EIP) transfer produces better results than a tendon graft.

Closed Injuries

Ruptures of EPL are well described in patients with rheumatoid arthritis or previous plating of distal radius fractures. The etiology of the rupture is usually due to ischemic necrosis of the EPL tendon.[29] Inability to retropulse the thumb while held in abduction is the diagnostic sign of EPL rupture. Minimal IP joint extension may still be present, despite EPL rupture. EIP to EPL tendon transfer is the preferred method of choice for EPL attrition ruptures.[29,30] This procedure requires harvest of the EIP tendon at the level of the second MCP joint (EIP is the more ulnar tendon) and a Pulvertaft-type weave into the EPL tendon. This technique is usually well tolerated and produces predictable results.

Summary

Extensor tendon injuries are common and unless treated promptly can result in a significant loss of function with secondary deformities that can be difficult to treat. These injuries do not have a one-size-fits-all approach and some of the injuries, in contrast to flexors, are better treated nonoperatively. Although the surgical repair is an important part of treatment, postoperative hand therapy is essential for optimal result and preservation of hand function.

References

1. Wehbe MA. Junctura anatomy. *J Hand Surg*. 1992;17:1124–1129.
2. Kettelkamp DB, Flatt AE, Moulds R. Traumatic dislocation of the long finger extension tendon. A clinical, anatomical and biomechanical study. *J Bone Joint Surg Am*. 1971;53A:229–240.
3. Young CM, Rayan GM. The sagittal band: anatomic and biomechanical study. *J Hand Surg*. 2000;25:1107–1113.
4. Kaplan EB. Anatomy, injuries and treatment of the extensor apparatus of the hand and fingers. *Clin Orthop Relat Res*. 1959;13:24–41.
5. Landsmeer JM. The coordination of finger–joint motions. *J Bone Joint Surg Am*. 1963;45:1654–1662.
6. Backhouse KM, Catton WT. An experimental study of the functions of the lumbrical muscles in the human hand. *J Anat*. 1954;88:133–141.
7. Harris C, Rutledge GL. The functional anatomy of the extensor mechanism of the finger. *J Bone Joint Surg Am*. 1972;54A:713–726.
8. Kleinman WB, Petersen DP. Oblique retinacular ligament reconstruction for chronic mallet finger deformity. *J Hand Surg*. 1984;9:399–404.
9. Landsmeer JM. The anatomy of the dorsal aponeurosis of the human finger and its functional significance. *Anatom Rec*. 1949;104:31–36.
10. Kleinert HE, Verdan C. Report of the committee on tendon injuries. *J Hand Surg*. 1983;8:794–798.
11. Lin JD, Strauch RJ. Closed soft tissue extensor mechanism injuries (mallet, boutonniere, and sagittal band). *J Hand Surg*. 2014;39(5):1005–1011.
12. Abouna JM, Brown H. The treatment of mallet finger: the results in a series of 148 consecutive cases and a review of the literature. *Br J Surg*. 1968;55:653–667.
13. Posner MA, Green SM. Diagnosis and treatment of finger deformities following injuries to the extensor tendon mechanism. *Hand Clin*. 2013;29(2):269–281.
14. Pegoli L, Toh S, Arai K, et al. The Ishiguro extension block technique for the treatment of mallet finger fracture: indications and clinical results. *J Hand Surg*. 2003;28:15–17.
15. Thompson JS, Littler JW, Upton J. The spiral oblique retinacular ligament, SORL. *J Hand Surg (Am)*. 1978;3:482–487.
16. Howell JW, Peck F. Rehabilitation of flexor and extensor tendon injuries in the hand: current updates. *Injury*. 2013;44(3):397–402.
17. Mason ML. Rupture of tendons of the hand. *Surg Gynecol Obstetr*. 1930;50:611.
18. Lutz K, Pipicelli J, Grewal R. Management of complications of extensor tendon injuries. *Hand Clin*. 2015;31(2):301–310.
19. Snow JW. Use of a retrograde tendon flap in repairing a severed extensor tendon in the PIP joint area. *Plast Reconstr Surg*. 1973;51:555–558.
20. Türker T, Hassan K, Capdarest-Arest N. Extensor tendon gap reconstruction: a review. *J Plast Surg Hand Surg*. 2016;50(1):1–6.
21. Amirtharajah M, Lattanza L. Open extensor tendon injuries. *J Hand Surg*. 2015;40(2):391–397.
22. Fowler SB. The management of tendon injuries. *J Bone Joint Surg Am*. 1959;41:579–580.
23. Khandwala AR, Webb J, Harris SB, et al. A comparison of dynamic extension splinting and controlled active mobilisation of complete division of extensor tendons in zones 5 and 6. *J Hand Surg*. 2000;25:140–146.
24. Wong AL, Wilson M, Girnary S, et al. The optimal orthosis and motion protocol for extensor tendon injury in zones IV–VIII: a systematic review. *J Hand Ther*. 2017;30(4):447–456.
25. Kleinhenz BP, Adams BD. Closed sagittal band injury of the metacarpophalangeal joint. *J Am Acad Orthop Surg*. 2015;23(7):415–423.
26. Mann RJ, Hoffeld TA, Farmer CB. Human bites of the hand: twenty years experience. *J Hand Surg*. 1977;2:97–104.
27. Hirth MJ, Howell JW, O'Brien L. Relative motion orthoses in the management of various hand conditions: a scoping review. *J Hand Ther*. 2016;29(4):546–557.
28. McCarten GM, Bennett CS, Marshall DR. Treatment of mallet thumb. *Aust N Z J Surg*. 1986;56(3):285–286.
29. Gelb RI. Tendon transfer for rupture of the extensor pollicis longus. *Hand Clin*. 1995;11(3):411–422.
30. Magnussen PA, Harvey FJ, Tonkin MA. Extensor indicis proprius transfer for rupture of the extensor pollicis longus tendon. *J Bone Joint Surg*. 1990;72(5):881–883.

49 Tendon Transfers

ADAM C. GASCOIGNE AND STEPHEN FLOOD

For video accompanying this chapter see ExpertConsult.com. See inside cover for access details.

Introduction

Tendon transfer is the surgical transplantation of a normal muscle–tendon unit (MTU) into a new location to restore function of a nonfunctioning MTU. This may be distinguished from a tendon graft, as in tendon transfer the donor tendon remains connected to its native muscle.

In 1770 Missa, a French surgeon, repaired a middle finger extensor tendon injury by grafting the index and ring finger extensor tendons to the middle finger extensor tendon, thus performing the first recorded tendon transfer. However, the modern technique of tendon transfer as defined above was pioneered by Carl Nicoladoni in 1881, and further developed by Tomasz Drobnik with particular reference to radial nerve palsy in 1894.

There was subsequently a dramatic expansion in the number and use of tendon transfer techniques by surgeons such as Bunnell, Brand, and Boyes (Fig. 49.1), faced with the polio epidemics and war injuries of the early 20th century. In this chapter we present the approach of the senior author (S.F.) to tendon transfers in the upper limb for peripheral nerve injury and tetraplegia. See Table 49.1 for definitions of terms used in this chapter.

Indications

The essential indication for tendon transfer is the functional impairment of an MTU, either through direct injury, denervation, or developmental abnormality of muscle (Table 49.2). Specific indications for tendon transfer are delayed presentation or direct injury resulting in loss of tendon length rendering primary repair impossible, direct nerve injuries not amenable to repair, late presentation of nerve injury with motor endplate fibrosis, failed nerve transfers, plexus injuries, nerve root avulsions, spinal cord injuries, central neurological insults, and certain congenital or developmental disorders.

Burkhalter has also advocated the use of early tendon transfer as an adjunct to nerve repair to retain function and reduce development of contractures during nerve recovery.[1] Such a transfer serves to improve function during nerve regeneration, reducing the need for external splinting, supplements the power of the muscles being reinnervated, and may serve as a definitive procedure where nerve regeneration is limited. However, such transfers should not themselves cause significant loss of function, or result in deformity following recovery of function in the affected nerve.

Biomechanics

The majority of tendon transfers performed routinely are known to be based on sound biomechanical principles. However, an understanding of basic biomechanics is helpful for the surgeon, particularly when faced with a difficult case where the standard approach may not be feasible. The ultimate aim of a tendon transfer is the creation of a new MTU capable of generating torque sufficient to move a target joint through a useful range of motion. Torque is determined by the power, or force-generating ability, of the muscle, and its mechanical advantage, or leverage. Other relevant biomechanical characteristics are the degree of tendon excursion, and tensioning of the muscle during transfer.

Power and Leverage

The power, or force-generating ability, of a muscle is proportional to its physiological cross-sectional area (PCSA).[2] Leverage is a measure of the mechanical advantage of a muscle. It is determined by the moment arm, which is the perpendicular distance from the target joint's axis of rotation to the line of pull of the muscle (Fig. 49.2). It should be noted that the moment arm may vary depending on joint position, and any measurements should be taken with the joint in a useful position. Muscles with a larger moment arm have relatively more leverage, and hence exert greater torque.[3] For an MTU to be useful for a transfer, it must have adequate power and leverage to move the target joint.

Tendon Excursion

Excursion is the distance a tendon can move from when it is relaxed to its fully contracted position. Tendon excursion and contraction velocity are proportional to muscle fiber length.[2] An appropriate donor MTU must have adequate excursion to move the target joint through a useful range of motion. The moment arm is again relevant here (see above). As the moment arm increases, the amount of joint movement produced by a given amount of tendon

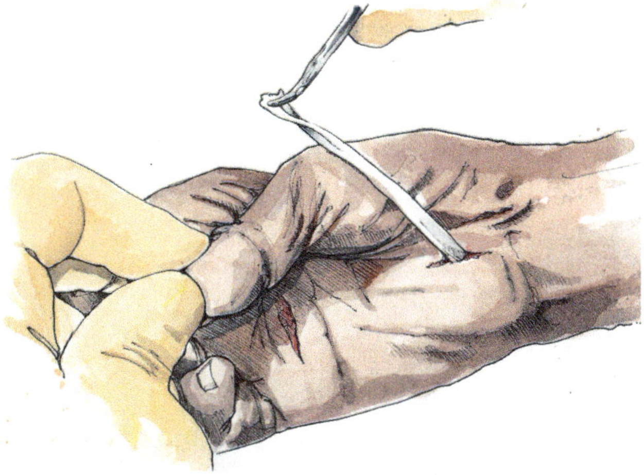

• **Fig. 49.1** Flexor digitorum superficialis (FDS; Royle, Thompson, Bunnell) opponensplasty. (© Mr Donald Sammut.)

excursion decreases. Hence, adjusting the moment arm of a transferred MTU is a tradeoff between range of motion and leverage.

Tensioning

Normal contraction of an MTU requires overlap of actin and myosin filaments in the sarcomeres of the muscle fibers. An excessively tight or loose muscle will not contract effectively, as is expressed by the Blix curve.[4] Hence, it is critical for the surgeon to put the transferred MTU under appropriate tension. It has been suggested that it may be preferable to place the transferred MTU under excess tension, relying on postoperative relaxation and lengthening to correct any errors.[5] However, studies have demonstrated that this may overestimate the degree to which the muscle may remodel to accommodate its new length and result in a significant loss of muscle power.[6] Ultimately, the surgeon should aim to neither over- nor undertension the transferred MTU by setting it as close to its optimal length as possible. However, this is not easy to establish intraoperatively, as the muscle's slack length once it has been released from its insertion is not reliably related to its optimal length. Nevertheless, an on-table estimate of the tension on a transferred tendon remains the usual method of determining the amount of tension to put on the transferred MTU. The senior author uses a comparison of distance from MTU origin to previous and new insertion as a guide.

Principles

General principles guiding tendon transfer have been developed and refined since the early 20th century.[7] It should be borne in mind that these are not strict rules that need to be followed in all cases (Table 49.3). For example, though Steindler proposed that the "gliding apparatus" of the tendon should be preserved or reconstructed as much as possible, to minimize the risk of adhesions developing,[8] this is not possible for every patient. However, if the transferred tendon's course passes through scarred, inflamed, or edematous tissues, then it may be desirable to revise the soft tissue bed using flaps or grafts prior to transfer. Nevertheless, these principles are useful guidelines for both assessing patients' suitability for tendon transfers, and also in selecting the best procedure for an individual patient.

TABLE 49.1 Definitions

Tendon transfer: surgical transplantation of normal muscle–tendon unit (MTU) into a new location to restore function of a non-functioning MTU (only at one end)
Arthrodesis: surgical immobilization of a joint by fusion of adjacent bones
Tenodesis: surgical anchoring of a tendon to bone
Tenodesis grip: passive grip due to finger flexor shortening with wrist extension

TABLE 49.2 Indications for Tendon Transfer

Primary
Traumatic loss of muscle or tendon
Irreparable peripheral nerve injury
Brachial plexus injury
Secondary
Motor endplate fibrosis
Failed nerve transfer
Adjunct to nerve transfer
Central
Spinal cord injury including root avulsion
Central neurological injury including stroke
Congenital or developmental disorders

General Approach

Patients presenting with peripheral nerve palsies should have a comprehensive history taken, recording the symptoms, etiology, time course, and any investigations or procedures performed. A complete neurological examination is required to document the motor and sensory deficit. The limb should be further assessed for soft tissue injuries, especially for any areas of scarring, edema, or inflammation along the path of any tendon transfers.

Measurements of the passive and active range of motion of all affected joints should be taken. Further imaging and investigation by means of nerve conduction studies and electromyography may be performed where the diagnosis of the original injury is not clear, or to identify potential confounding anatomical variants such as Martin–Gruber, Marinacci, Riche–Cannieu, and Berretini anastomoses.[9] Once the problem has been clearly defined, reconstruction may be planned.

It is the senior author's preference to wait for neurological recovery to plateau prior to considering tendon transfers. Based on the works of Sunderland and Seddon, nerve

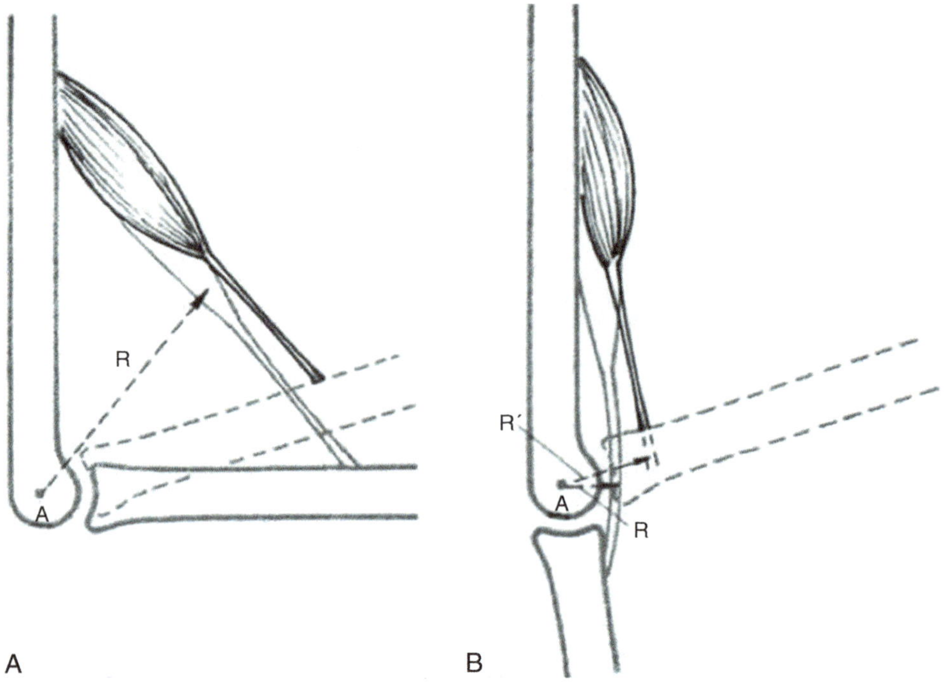

• **Fig. 49.2** Moment arm. (A) The moment arm of a muscle whose line of pull passes distant from the axis of the joint has great mechanical advantage but acts through a relatively small range of motion. (B) By comparison, a muscle with a line of pull that passes close to the axis of the joint acts through a large range of motion but has little leverage. (From Brand PW. Biomechanics of tendon transfer. *Orthop Clin North Am*. 1974;5(2):205–230.)

regeneration progresses at approximately 1 mm a day.[10] Depending on the location of the injury, this may mean delaying surgery for 12–18 months.

Surgical Technique

A number of different techniques have been developed for the coaptation of tendons. The Pulvertaft weave, Kessler grasping suture, and Mason/Nicoladoni side-to-side repair have all been used historically. Recently, newer alternatives have been developed, such as the lasso and spiral linking repairs, which demonstrate comparable strength and may be easier and quicker to perform.[11] The senior author's preference is to use the Pulvertaft weave (Fig. 49.3).

Radial Nerve Palsy

Anatomy[5,10,12]

The posterior cord of the brachial plexus continues as the radial nerve after having given off its terminal branches in the axilla. It comprises motor and sensory fibers from the ventral rami of C5 to T1. While in the axilla it gives off its first two branches to triceps, to the long and medial heads. It crosses the lower border of teres major to enter the anterior compartment of the arm and immediately dives into the posterior compartment via the triangular interval. It then runs in the spiral groove (aka radial groove) of the humerus. While in the posterior compartment it gives its last two branches to triceps, one to the lateral head, and a second to the medial head, as well as two sensory branches: the lower lateral and posterior cutaneous nerves of arm. Approximately halfway down the arm the radial nerve pierces the lateral intermuscular septum to re-enter the anterior compartment of the arm. Here it gives off a medial branch to brachialis and lateral branches to brachioradialis and extensor carpi radialis longus (ECRL). It then enters the cubital fossa under cover of brachioradialis, before dividing into deep and superficial branches. The deep branch passes between the two heads of supinator to become the posterior interosseous nerve, while the superficial branch continues down the anterior compartment of the forearm under cover of brachioradialis. The posterior interosseous nerve immediately divides into branches to the extensor musculature of the forearm. The superficial branch of the radial nerve emerges on the radial side of brachioradialis at the wrist to cross the anatomical snuffbox and provide the sensory supply to the dorsum of the hand and the radial three and a half digits.

Clinical Findings[12]

The characteristic sign of radial nerve palsy is wrist drop. Due to the loss of the extensor musculature of the forearm, the patient is unable to extend the wrist or digits. In addition, grip strength is lost due to the weakness of finger flexion with the wrist in a flexed position. Low radial nerve lesions are defined as those below the elbow, thus sparing supply to brachioradialis and ECRL. In these cases, wrist extension is relatively preserved, though with radial deviation. Due to

TABLE 49.3 General Principles of Tendon Transfer

Appropriate strength	The donor MTU should be of comparable strength to the recipient, in order to provide useful movement at the target joint
Adequate power	The donor MTU should be capable of contraction against resistance, which corresponds to a grading of 4 or greater on the Medical Research Council (MRC) scale
Amplitude of excursion	The donor MTU must have adequate amplitude of excursion to be effective at moving the target joint
Anatomical location	The donor MTU should contract in parallel with the recipient, and be located such that its transfer results in a functionally useful line of pull. This may be optimized during the procedure by redirecting the tendon using anatomical pulleys
Control	The donor MTU must be under voluntary control. Transferring a spastic muscle will result in a negative outcome
Supple joints	Preoperatively, maximum range of motion must be achieved for the joints to be moved by the transferred MTU. Ideally soft tissue contracture should be prevented from developing, otherwise they must be dealt with during or prior to any tendon transfer
Expendability	The functional benefit gained from the tendon transfer must be greater than the impairment caused by losing the donor MTU's original action. Muscles with redundant functions are hence ideal, e.g., ECRL/ECRB or FCR/FCU
Single function per transfer	Each tendon transfer should be used to restore a single function to avoid compromising on strength and movement
Tissue equilibrium	The transferred MTU should not pass through scarred, inflamed, or edematous tissues in which development of adhesions is likely
Synergism	The patient will find it easier to learn to use an MTU whose original function is synergistic with the function it is replacing. If this is not practical, muscles that are usually activated together are also suitable for transfer, for example wrist flexors and finger extensors

the proximal origin of the majority of the branches of the radial nerve, triceps function is only affected in very proximal lesions. The sensory deficit of radial nerve injury is less significant, only affecting the less sensitive dorsum of the hand and radial three and a half fingers.

Approach[5,12,13]

The key reconstructive aims are: wrist extension, metacarpophalangeal (MCP) joint extension, and thumb extension and abduction (Table 49.4). These are generally performed

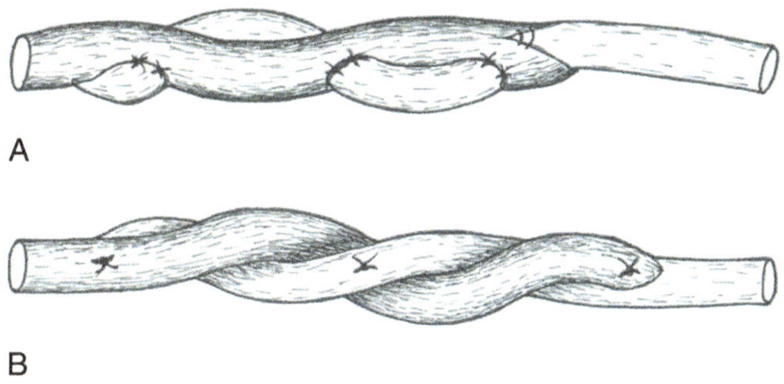

• **Fig. 49.3** Tenorrhaphy technique. (A) Pulvertaft weave. The donor tendon is interlaced with the recipient tendon, and sutured in place. Usually three or four weaves are performed. (B) Spiral linking. The donor tendon is wound around the recipient tendon, with mattress sutures in each spiral. Again, a variable number of spirals may be performed. (From Kulikov YI, Dodd S, Gheduzzi S, et al. An in vitro biomechanical study comparing the spiral linking technique against the Pulvertaft weave for tendon repair. *J Hand Surg Eur.* 2007;32(4):377–381.)

TABLE 49.4 Approach to Radial Nerve Palsy

Reconstructive Aim	Preferred Options	Alternatives
Wrist extension	PT → ECRB	Rarely consider BR (if function preserved) or FCR → ECRB
Metacarpophalangeal joint extension	FCR → EDC (Starr, Brand, Tsuge)	FDS → EDC (Boyes, Chuinard) FCU → EDC (Jones)
Thumb extension and abduction	PL → EPL	Ring finger FDS → EPL (Boyes)

in set combinations for ease of access and operative technique, with the main difference being the choice of MTU to be used for restoration of MCP joint extension.[12] As discussed above (see Indications), some authors advocate using an early tendon transfer procedure to preserve function and prevent contractures in cases of radial nerve injury. Where this is not done, the use of a dynamic outrigger splint (Fig. 49.4) results in greatly improved grip strength by fixing the wrist in extension.[14]

Wrist Extension

For reconstruction of wrist extension, the pronator teres (PT) to extensor carpi radialis brevis (ECRB) transfer is ideal (Fig. 49.5), and other options are rarely considered. If radial nerve recovery is not anticipated, this should be performed end-to-end to achieve a more direct line of pull. If radial nerve recovery is anticipated, the transfer should be performed by an end-to-side technique, to allow ECRB to resume wrist extension once it regains function.[5] PT should be released from its insertion with a strip of periosteum to provide a robust attachment. It is tunneled subcutaneously superficial

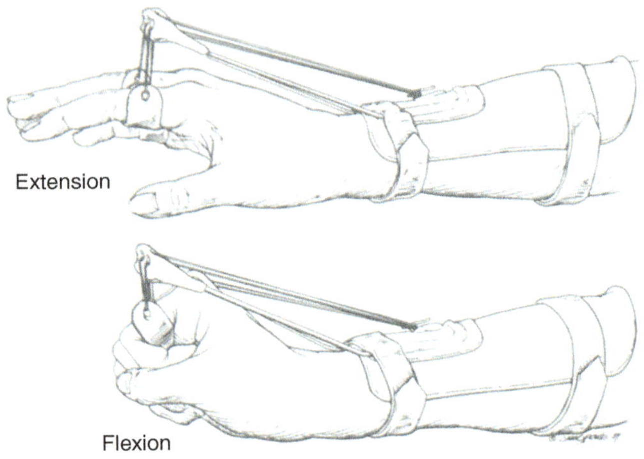

• **Fig. 49.4** Splinting for radial nerve palsy. Use of a dynamic outrigger splint to enable finger grip by fixing the wrist in extension. This is an application of the tenodesis effect: the synergistic action of wrist extension with finger flexion. (From Colditz JC. Splinting for radial nerve palsy. *J Hand Ther*. 1987;1(1):18–23.)

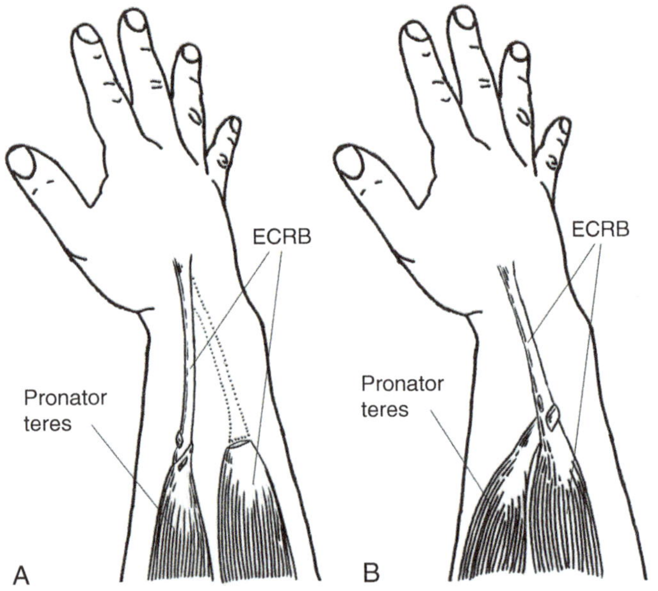

• **Fig. 49.5** Pronator teres to ECRB transfer. (A) End-to-end transfer. (B) End-to-side transfer. (From Sammer DM, Chung KC. Tendon transfers: Part I. Principles of transfer and transfers for radial nerve palsy. *Plast Reconstr Surg*. 2009;123(5):169e–177e.)

to brachioradialis and ECRL, and inserted into the tendon of ECRB.[12] If desired, ECRL may be synchronized to ECRB, with PT redirected to the new extensor complex.

Metacarpophalangeal Joint Extension

To restore MCP joint extension, a tendon transfer to extensor digitorum communis (EDC) is required. The surgeon is presented with a number of alternatives for this purpose (see Table 49.4). Of these, the flexor carpi radialis (FCR) transfer is generally preferred in low radial nerve palsy (Fig. 49.6), as its loss is balanced on the radial side of the wrist by the preserved function of ECRL.[5] By comparison, use of the flexor carpi ulnaris (FCU) transfer necessitates sacrifice of the only

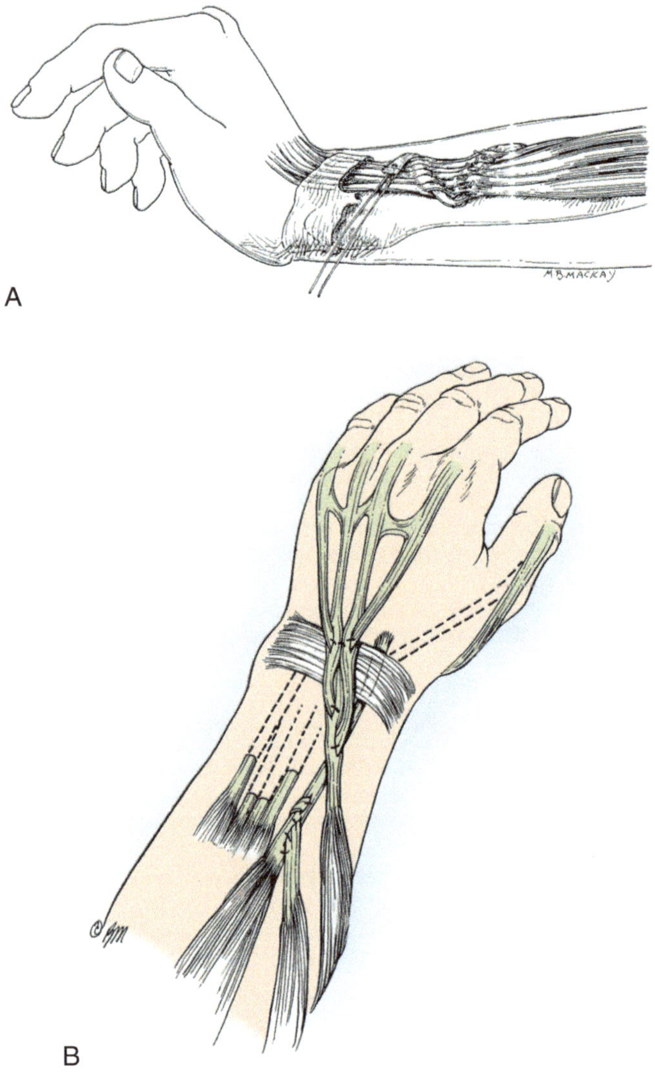

• **Fig. 49.6** FCR to EDC transfer. (A) EDC left in continuity. (B) EDC divided. (A, From Richards RR. Tendon transfers for failed nerve reconstruction. *Clin Plast Surg*. 2003;30(2):223–45. B, From Ingari JV, Green DP. Radial nerve palsy. In: *Green's Operative Hand Surgery E-Book*. Elsevier Health Sciences; 2010:1075–1092.)

remaining muscle acting on the ulnar side of the wrist, resulting in radial deviation. However, both of these transfers suffer from the major drawback of having relatively low excursion for their intended function. For this reason, flexor digitorum superficialis (FDS) transfer as described by Boyes is sometimes preferred, as it has significantly greater excursion, allowing full extension of the digits without requiring wrist flexion. Whichever donor is used, it may be attached to EDC either by leaving it in continuity, or by dividing the tendons of EDC to allow end-to-end attachment of the transferred tendon. If the tendons are divided, they may be passed superficial to the extensor retinaculum to optimize the line of pull.

Thumb Extension

Extensor pollicis longus (EPL) is the common target for tendon transfers to restore thumb extension. It is divided at its musculotendinous junction and transposed to the radial aspect of Lister's tubercle. PL is divided at the wrist and freed up proximally, passed over the radial side of the wrist, then inserted into the distal stump of EPL (Fig. 49.7). The line of pull of the transferred tendon should cross the anatomical snuffbox, resulting in combined extension and abduction with muscle contraction. An alternative is to use the ring finger FDS tendon to power EPL. This is usually done during a Boyes transfer, when other parts of FDS are also being transferred to extensor indicis (EI).

Median Nerve Palsy

Anatomy[5,10,15]

The median nerve is formed by a root from each of the medial and lateral cords of the brachial plexus. The larger lateral root carries the contribution from C5, C6, and C7, and the smaller medial root carries the contribution from the C8 and T1. It thus receives motor and sensory fibers from the ventral rami of all the segments contributing to the brachial plexus. It initially lies anterolateral to the third part of the axillary artery, but after crossing the lower border of teres major to enter the anterior compartment of the arm it crosses in front of the artery to lie on its medial side. The median nerve lies medially in the cubital fossa, entering the forearm by passing between the two heads of pronator teres. The nerve then runs under the fibrous arch of the origin of FDS, continuing down the forearm bound to the deep surface of FDS by areolar tissue. It is accompanied in its course by the median branch of the anterior interosseous artery. Within the forearm it gives off the anterior interosseous nerve, which supplies the deep layer of forearm flexors. Injuries above where the anterior interosseous nerve is given off are usually defined as high median nerve lesions. Proximal to the wrist the median nerve gives off its palmar cutaneous branch, and then enters the carpal tunnel on the radial side of the tendons of FDS. The recurrent motor branch supplies the thenar muscles, and the remainder of the nerve provides the palmar digital nerves for the radial three and a half digits, and also supplying the radial two lumbricals. Note that there is some variation in the supply of the thenar muscles (see below, under Ulnar nerve palsy). There is also frequently variation in the pattern of innervation due to median to ulnar connections in the forearm, such as the Martin–Gruber anastomosis. An ulnar to median connection, or Marinacci anastomosis, is less common. It is important for the surgeon to recognise the presence of these connections as they may result in of unusual presentations of peripheral nerve injury.

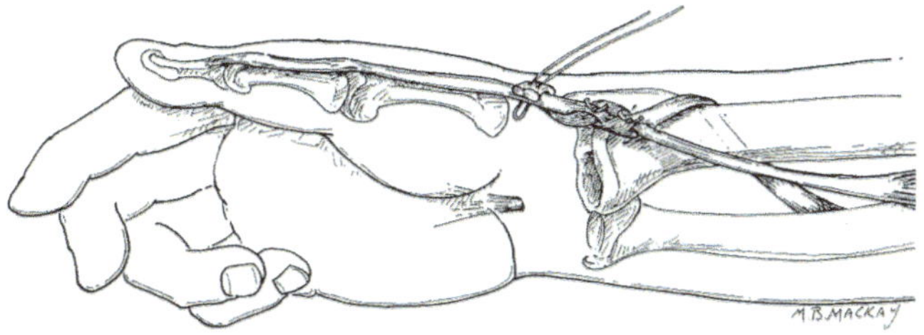

• **Fig. 49.7** Palmaris longus to EPL transfer. (From Richards RR. Tendon transfers for failed nerve reconstruction. *Clin Plast Surg*. 2003;30(2):223–245.)

Clinical Findings[15–17]

"Low" injury to the median nerve occurs distal to the origin of the anterior interosseous nerve and results in loss of thumb abduction and opposition, with preservation of interphalangeal joint flexion and forearm flexor function. In proximal "high" injuries these are also lost, with the exception of wrist and finger flexion provided by FCU and the part of flexor digitorum profundus (FDP) supplied by the ulnar nerve, usually to the ring and little fingers. Sensation is lost over the volar surface of the palm and radial three and a half digits. This has great functional significance, as sensation in this distribution is essential for precision movement. Palmar sensation is preserved in compression of the median nerve in the carpal tunnel due to sparing of the palmar cutaneous branch.

Approach[13,15–17]

The key reconstructive aims are: thumb opposition, thumb interphalangeal (IP) joint flexion, and index distal interphalangeal (DIP) joint flexion (Table 49.5). However, it should be noted that even with restoration of thumb opposition, many patients' hand function remains poor due to the debilitating sensory deficit.[15] For this reason, opponensplasty may not be appropriate for every patient.

TABLE 49.5 Approach to Median Nerve Palsy

Reconstructive Aim	Preferred Options	Alternatives
Thumb opposition	EIP opponensplasty (Burkhalter) ADM opponensplasty (Huber)	FDS opponensplasty (Royle, Thompson, Bunnell) Palmaris longus opponensplasty (Camitz)
Thumb IP joint flexion	BR to FPL	ECRL to FPL ECU to FPL
Index DIP joint flexion	FDP side-to-side (lose independent flexion of fingers)	ECRL to FDP

Thumb Opposition (Opponensplasty)

The usual target of opponensplasty procedures is the tendinous insertion of abductor pollicis brevis (APB) at the proximal phalanx of the thumb. Bunnell stated that any tendon transfer intended to restore thumb opposition should be passed "through a tendon pulley constructed at the pisiform bone or by passing it around the tendon of the flexor carpi ulnaris," and be "inserted into the dorso-ulnar aspect of the base of the proximal phalanx of the thumb to give pronation."[18] Any donor MTU that satisfies these requirements may be used for opponensplasty. The extensor indicis proprius (EIP) opponensplasty provides effective thumb opposition with the least sacrifice of function for the loss of the donors original function. It is also effective even in high median nerve lesions where other candidates for transfer are paralysed. The EIP tendon is identified on the ulnar aspect of the index finger EDC tendon and is divided immediately proximal to the extensor expansion (Fig. 49.8). Alternatively, if further length is desired it may be harvested with a length of extensor expansion, though this is usually unnecessary for opponensplasty. The tendon should be freed from its attachments in the distal forearm and passed around the ulnar aspect of the forearm to the tendinous insertion of APB at the proximal phalanx of the thumb.

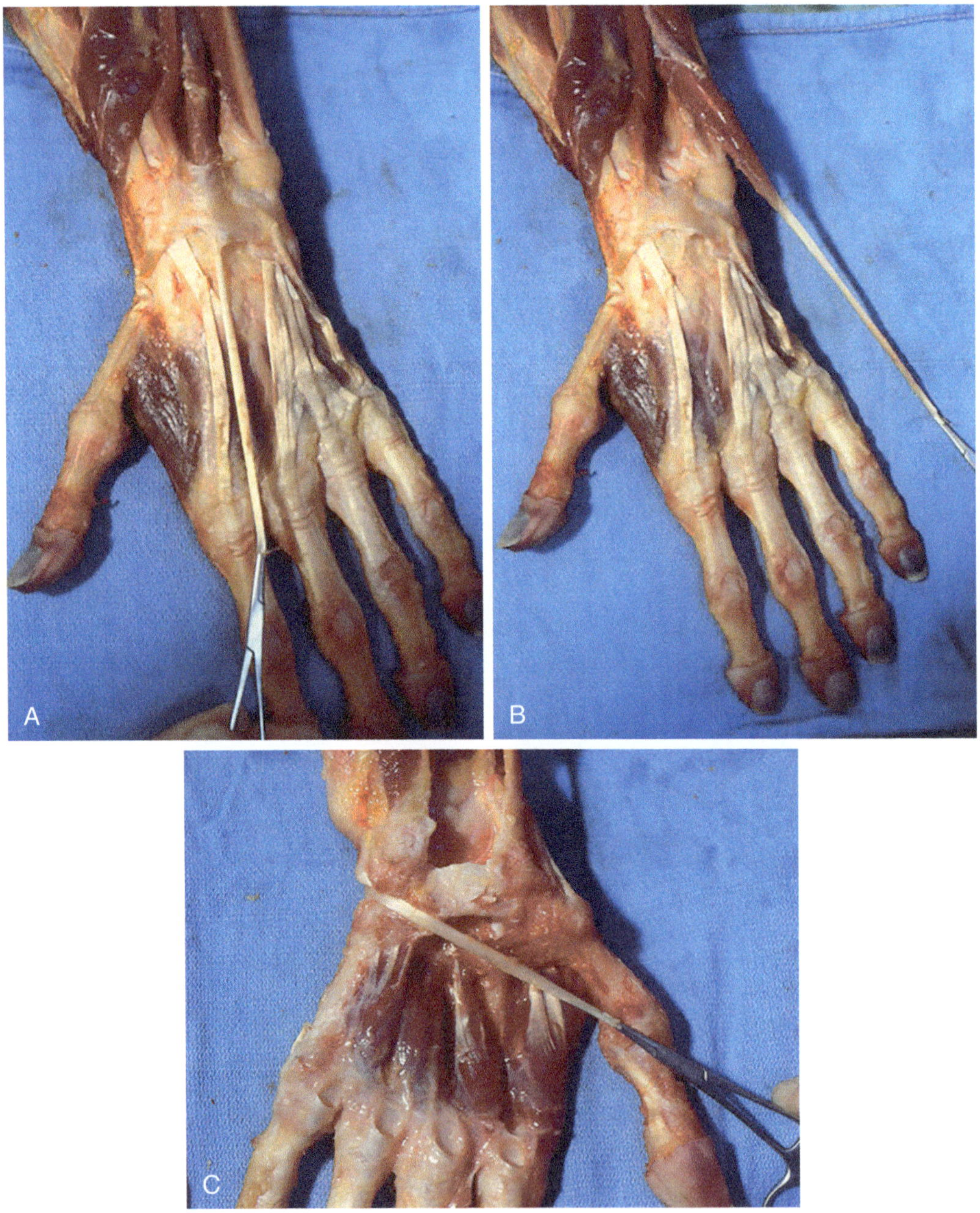

• **Fig. 49.8** EIP (Burkhalter) opponensplasty. (A) EIP identified immediately ulnar to the index finger EDC tendon. (B) EIP divided immediately proximal to the extensor expansion and freed from attachments in distal forearm. (C) EIP passed around ulnar aspect of wrist to the tendinous insertion of APB at the proximal phalanx of the thumb. (All images © Mr Donald Sammut.)

Alternatives to the EIP opponensplasty include the palmaris longus, superficialis, and abductor digiti minimi (ADM) opponensplasties. The palmaris longus opponensplasty may incorporate palmar fascia in continuity with the tendon or the contralateral palmaris longus as a free tendon graft in order to gain sufficient length to reach the APB insertion. It is tunneled subcutaneously from distal forearm to the thumb. This method is best for a low median nerve lesion with an intact palmaris longus. One drawback is its line of pull, which results in less effective opposition than that offered by other options.[15] This may be partially overcome by passing the tendon via a pulley created at the pisiform.

The FDS opponensplasty utilizes the tendon to the ring finger. The line of pull may be optimized by bringing the tendon through a window in the flexor retinaculum. This is also more secure than simply diverting the tendon at the distal end of the carpal tunnel. The tendon is divided via a distal incision in the finger or palm, and transferred across the palm to the tendinous insertion of APB (Fig. 49.9). One shortcoming of this method is a significant rate of complications, including deformity and extensor lag of the donor digit.[15] Harvesting the FDS via a palmar rather than digital incision may reduce this risk.

The ADM opponensplasty offers the further benefit of restoring the appearance of bulk to the thenar eminence. It is released from its insertion and transferred across the palm to APB (Fig. 49.10). This may be complicated by compression of the ulnar nerve by edema or scar where it is crossed by the transferred tendon. To overcome this, ADM may be partially or completely detached from its proximal origin.

Thumb IP and Index DIP Joint Flexion

In high median nerve injury, thumb IP and index DIP joint flexion may require restoration. For thumb IP joint flexion, ECRL or extensor carpi ulnaris (ECU) may be transferred to flexor pollicis longus (FPL). For index finger DIP joint flexion, ECRL may be transferred to FDP, or a side-to-side synchronization of FDP may be performed, relying on the ulnar-innervated component of the muscle.

Ulnar Nerve Palsy

Anatomy[5,10,15]

The ulnar nerve commences as the continuation of the medial cord of the brachial plexus in the axilla, comprising fibers from the ventral rami of spinal segments C8 and T1. It also usually receives a contribution composed of C7 fibers from either the lateral cord of the brachial plexus or the median nerve in the axilla, these are destined for FCU in the forearm. The nerve lies on the medial side of the axillary artery, and enters the posterior compartment of the arm by piercing the medial intermuscular septum. It then passes

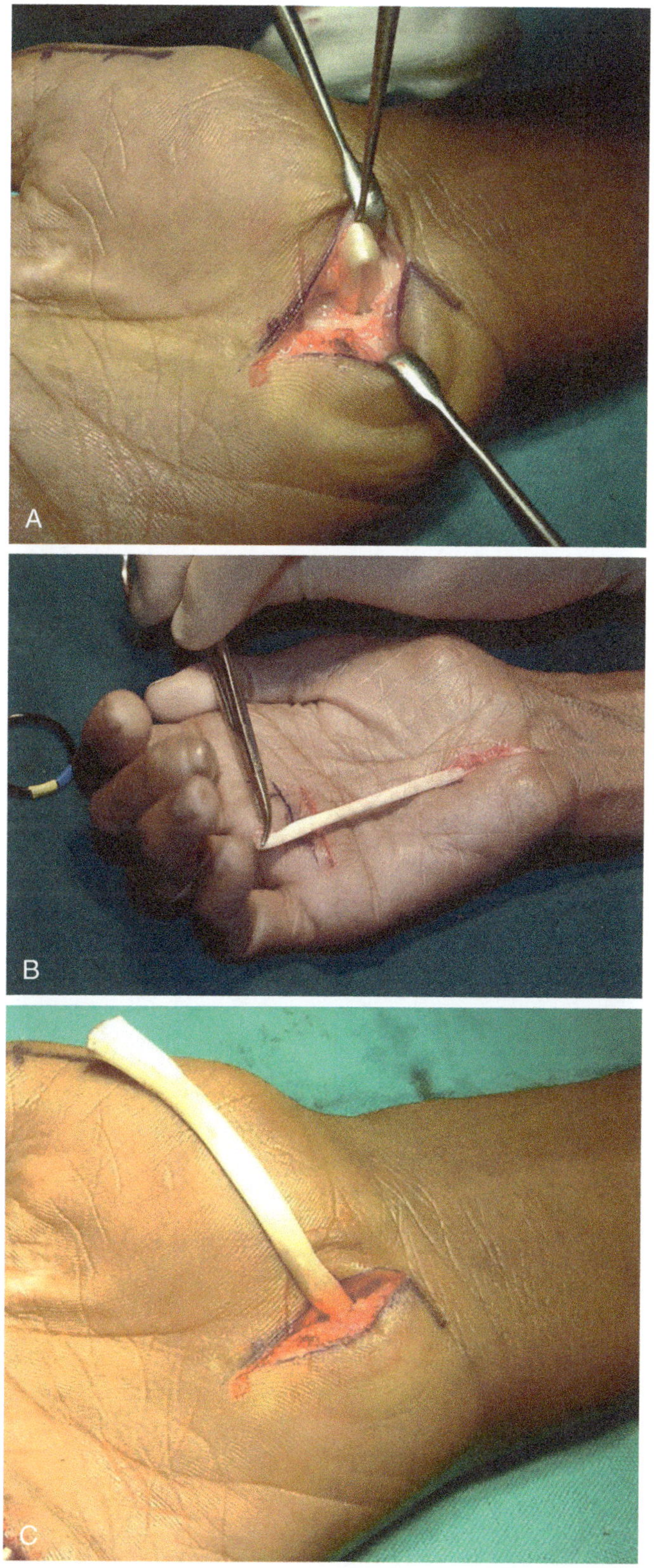

• **Fig. 49.9** FDS (Royle, Thompson, Bunnell) opponensplasty. (A) The FDS tendon to the ring finger being brought out through a window in the flexor retinaculum. (B) The tendon is divided through a distal incision in either the finger or palm. (C) The tendon is tunneled subcutaneously and attached to the tendinous insertion of APB via an incision on the radial aspect of the thumb. (All images © Mr Donald Sammut.)

between the medial epicondyle and the olecranon, through the cubital tunnel, and enters the anterior compartment of the forearm by passing between the two heads of FCU. It passes down the forearm beneath FCU and superficial to FDP, giving branches to those muscles, and accompanied by the ulnar artery. High ulnar nerve injuries are those that occur above where these branches originate. Just proximal to the wrist, the nerve emerges from beneath FCU and gives off volar and dorsal sensory branches. At the wrist, it passes through the ulnar (Guyon's) canal, superficial to the transverse carpal ligament, to enter the hand. It then divides into superficial and deep branches. The superficial branch provides the palmar digital nerves for the little finger and the ulnar aspect of the ring finger, and supplies the palmaris brevis muscle when present. The deep branch innervates the intrinsic muscles of the hand with the exception of the thenar muscles and two of the lumbricals. This pattern is variable, however, with the supply to the lumbricals shared unevenly between median and ulnar nerves in some cases. Frequently opponens pollicis and FPB may also receive a branch, receiving either a sole supply from the ulnar or dual innervation from both ulnar and median nerves.

Clinical Findings[15–17]

The claw or intrinsic minus hand is virtually pathognomonic of ulnar nerve injury. The loss of the intrinsic muscles of the hand and unopposed pull of the long extrinsic tendons result in hyperextension of the MCP joints and flexion at PIP and DIP joints. Specific testing may elicit Froment's sign: flexion of the thumb IP joint when holding a piece of paper between thumb and index finger, indicating weakness of adductor pollicis and the first dorsal interosseous. High ulnar nerve lesions are proximal to the origin of the branches to FCU and FDP, resulting in reduced grip strength and radial deviation of the hand. An ulnar nerve palsy also results in loss of sensation over the ulnar one and a half digits.

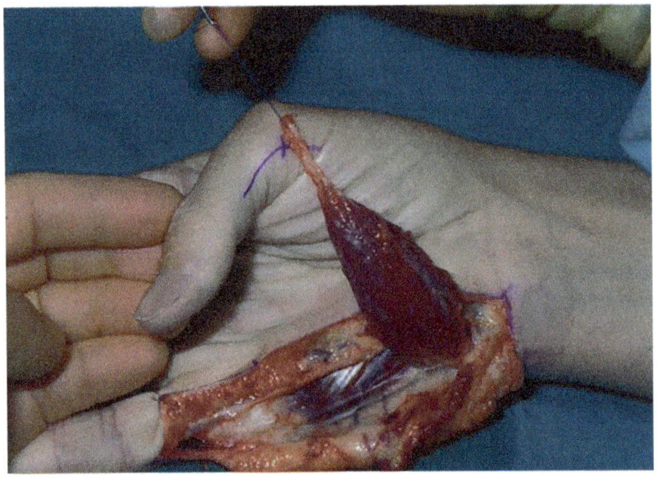

• **Fig. 49.10** ADM (Huber) opponensplasty. If desired, FDM may be transferred together with ADM for greater strength, as shown. (© Mr Donald Sammut.)

Approach[13,15–17]

The key reconstructive aims are: restoration of key grip by thumb adduction, and correction of clawing (Table 49.6). It is usually not necessary to reconstruct index finger abduction to achieve a useful key grip, as the patient is able to stabilize the index finger against adjacent digits. Where fixed contractures have developed, joint fusion may be employed to fix the affected digit in a more functional position.

Thumb Adduction (Adductorplasty)

The common target for restoration of thumb adduction is, unsurprisingly, adductor pollicis. Again, a variety of donor MTUs may be used. Common choices include the ring or middle finger FDS, the ECRB, or EIP (Fig. 49.11). In the case of ECRB and EIP, additional length may be required in order to reach adductor pollicis (Fig. 49.12). For EIP this may be achieved by harvesting a length of the central tendon of the extensor expansion in continuity with the tendon, but ECRB requires a free tendon graft. Whichever donor is used, in order to recreate the line of pull of adductor pollicis, a pulley is required. This may most easily be achieved by passing the tendon around the second or third metacarpal.

Correction of Clawing

The essential problem in the intrinsic minus digit is the hyperextension instability of the MCP joint, with flexion of the PIP and DIP joints (Fig. 49.13). Procedures for correction of clawing thus focus on correction of this deformity.

Stiles and Forrester-Brown first described transferring a single slip of each FDS tendon to EDC to correct clawing. Their technique was modified by Bunnell, who transferred

TABLE 49.6 Approach to Ulnar Nerve Palsy

Reconstructive Aim	Preferred Options	Alternatives
Thumb adduction	EIP adductorplasty (Brown) FDS adductorplasty (Edgerton and Brand)	ECRB adductorplasty (Smith, Omer)
Correction of clawing	FDS of middle or ring finger to A1 pulley of affected digit (modified Stiles–Bunnell)	FCR or ECRB to radial lateral bands of ring and little fingers (Brand)

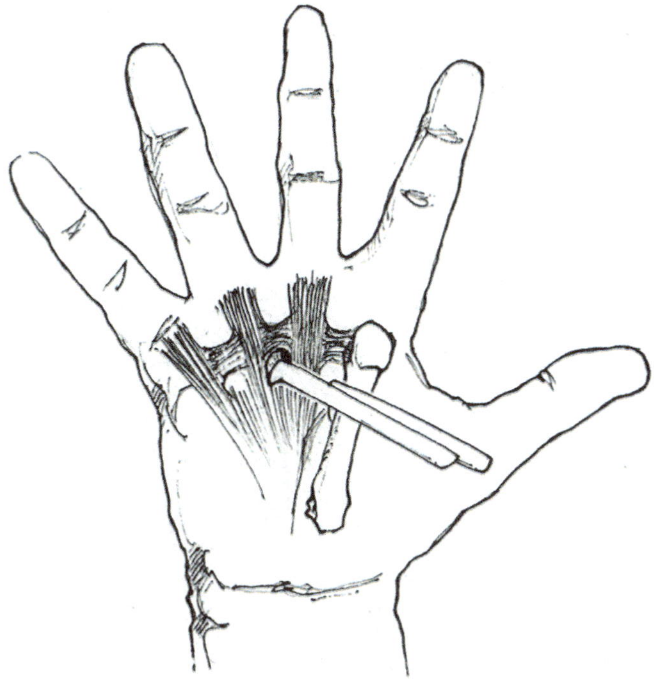

• **Fig. 49.11** Adductorplasty. Both FDS and EIP tendons are shown. It should be noted that when using EIP it is desirable to hook the tendon around the second metacarpal, as shown. (© Mr Donald Sammut.)

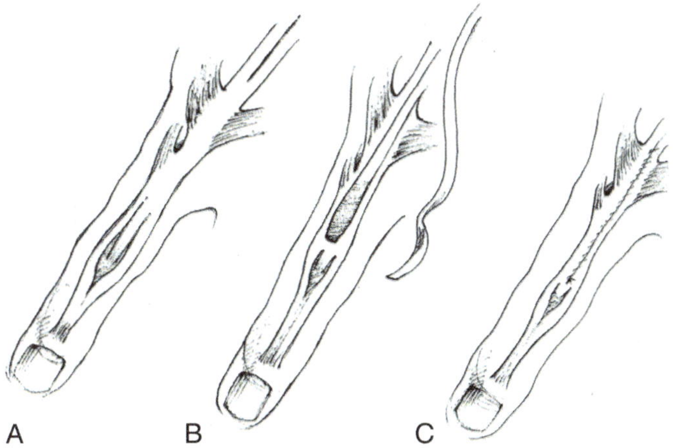

• **Fig. 49.12** Extension of EIP length for adductorplasty. (A) Appearance of extensor tendon insertions into dorsum of left index finger, note the EIP tendon on the ulnar aspect of the EDC tendon to the index finger. (B) EIP tendon released from insertion, including part of central tendon of extensor expansion, redirected to target adductor pollicis. (C) Lateral slips sutured to central tendon of extensor expansion. (© Mr Donald Sammut.)

each slip onto each of the lateral bands of the extensor expansion. However, this frequently resulted in complications due to adhesion formation and overcorrection.[15] Bunnell's procedure was further modified by Littler, whose technique is now widely known as the modified Stiles–Bunnell procedure. The FDS tendon of the middle or ring finger is divided over the PIP joint and split into four slips. Each slip is then passed through the lumbrical canals and inserted into the radial lateral band only. There have subsequently been many further modifications to the technique, though

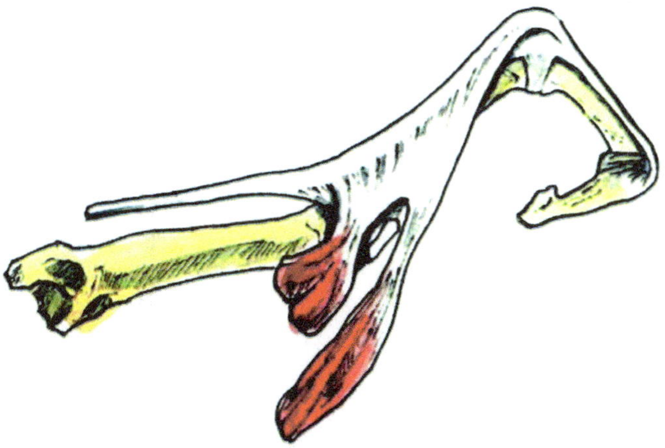

• **Fig. 49.13** The intrinsic minus digit. Unopposed action of the long extrinsic tendons and weakness of the intrinsic muscles results in instability and hyperextension of the MCP joint, with flexion of PIP and DIP joints. (© Mr Donald Sammut.)

the essential elements – the division of a single FDS tendon into four and the attachment of the resulting slips into the individual digits – remain the same. The senior author's preferred method is that described by Riordan[19] and Zancolli,[20] in which the A1 pulley is used as the insertion of the slips of FDS (Fig. 49.14). Alternative donors include wrist flexors and extensors, though these require free tendon grafts to provide adequate length to reach their targets.

Combined Palsy

Patients presenting with combined peripheral nerve palsies should have their individual problems and severity carefully characterized. This requires a detailed examination and further investigation with electromyography and nerve conduction studies with an aim to establishing both remaining function as well as deficiencies. Once this is done, a tailored approach to the individual patient may be planned. Innervated free muscle transfer may be considered for difficult situations where there are no suitable donor tendons, or where a standard transfer would result in unacceptable loss of function.

Tetraplegia

Restoration of upper limb function is a priority for tetraplegic patients, comparable to or of higher significance than bladder, bowel, sexual, and lower extremity function.[21] It allows the tetraplegic patient some autonomy, permitting completion of some personal activities of daily living (ADLs) independently or with the aid of appliances. Surgical restoration of upper limb function by means of tendon transfers originated with the work of Bunnell in the mid-20th century. Significant advances in the approach were made by Moberg, who abandoned the prior focus on providing the patient with a tip-to-tip tripod pinch grip in favor of a lateral pinch or key grip between the thumb and index finger.[22] This gave the patient a functional grip without the stiff hand resulting from the multiple tenodeses required to achieve a thumb fixed in opposition.[23] Even more recently, single-stage reconstructions aimed at reducing hospital stay and improving patient outcomes have been described. The approach to the surgical reconstruction of upper limb function in tetraplegia used at a major spinal unit in Australia is described in this section.

Classification

The commonest levels of cervical spinal cord injury are between the C4 and C7 vertebral levels. Generally speaking, injuries above the fifth cervical cord segment are not amenable to surgical restoration of upper limb function by means of tendon transfers due to lack of transferable muscles with useful function. However, Moberg recognized that spinal level of injury may not accurately reflect the degree of motor impairment and residual function. He devised a classification system for use in planning surgical restoration of upper limb function based on which muscles remained with strength of grade 4 or greater according to the familiar Medical Research Council scale, that is a muscle of either full strength or whose strength is reduced but may still move the joint against resistance.[22]

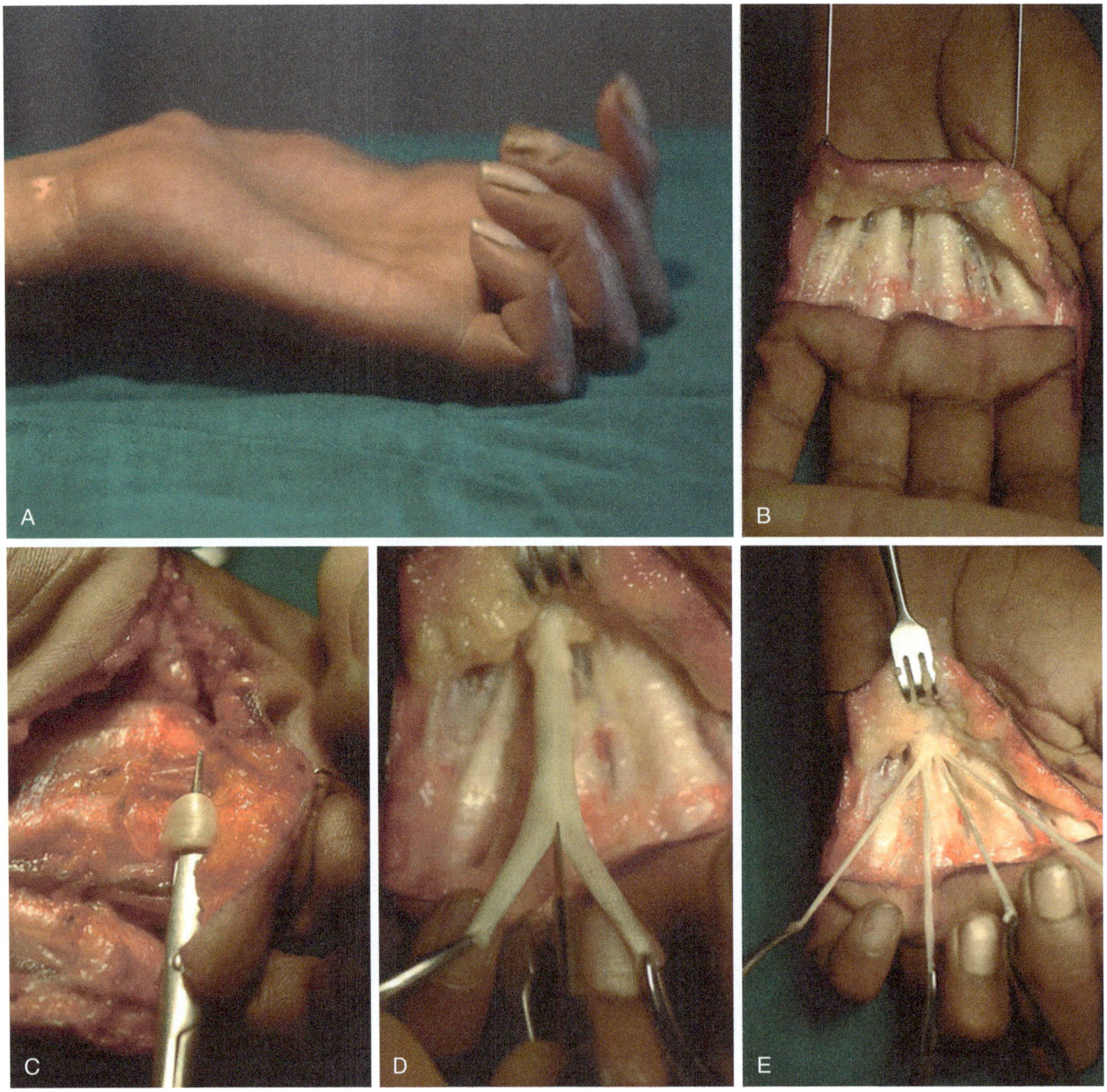

• **Fig. 49.14** Correction of clawing using four tail division of FDS transferred into A1 pulleys. (A) Preoperative deformity. (B) Skin incised at the distal palmar crease and reflected proximally. (C) Exposure of FDS tendon to ring finger. (D) The tendon is divided over the MCP joint, and incised longitudinally. (E) Division of the tendon into four slips, one for each finger.

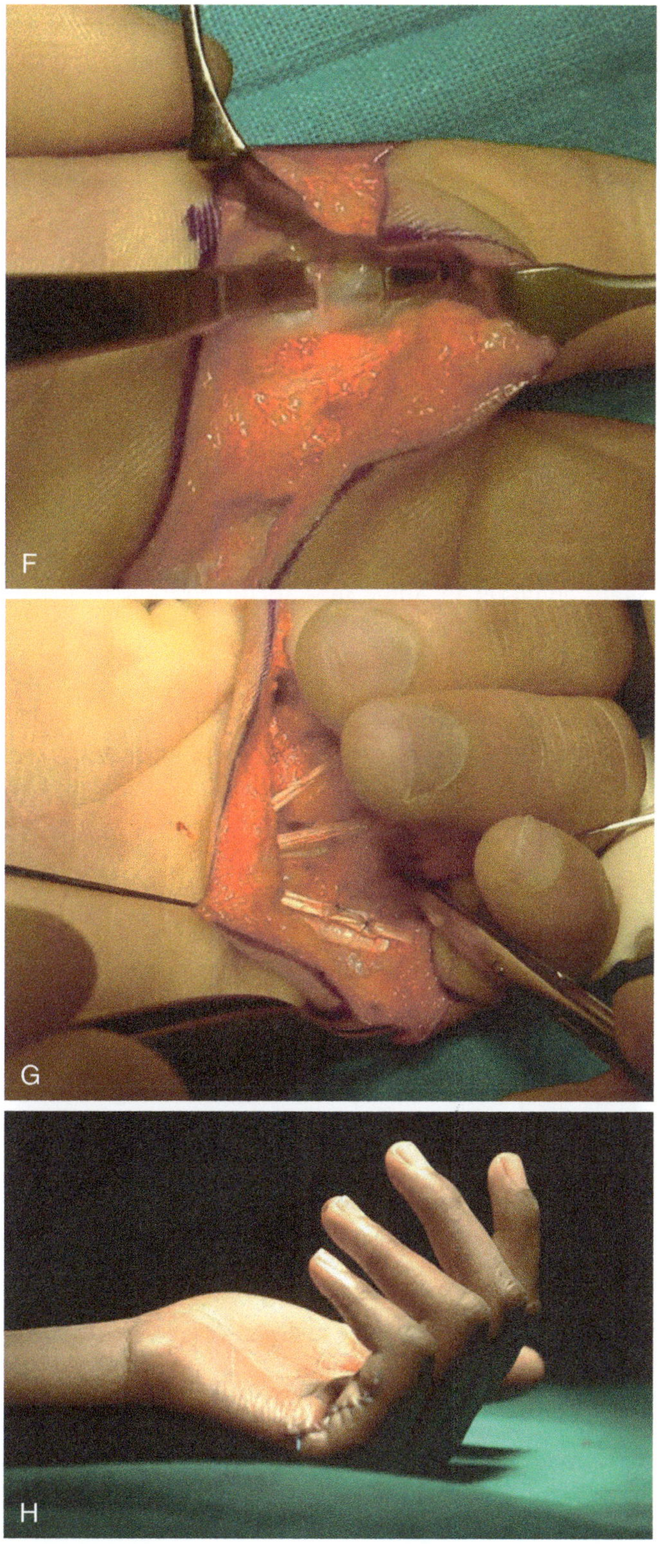

Fig. 49.14 cont'd (F) The A1 pulley is identified over the flexor aspect of the PIP joint. (G) The individual slips are transferred into the A1 pulleys. (H) Postoperative appearance. (All images © Mr Donald Sammut.)

This classification system was adopted and improved at the first International Conference on Tetraplegia in Edinburgh in 1978, the result of which is international classification for surgery of the hand in tetraplegia, the Giens

TABLE 49.7 International Classification for Surgery of the Hand in Tetraplegia (Giens Classification 1984, adapted from Edinburgh Classification 1978)

Sensitivity Group	Motor Characteristics	Description of Function
0	No muscle below elbow suitable for transfer	Flexion and supination of elbow
1	Brachioradialis	
2	Extensor carpi radialis longus	Extension of wrist (weak or strong)
3	Extensor carpi radialis brevis	Extension of wrist
4	Pronator teres	Extension of wrist and pronation of forearm
5	Flexor carpi radialis	Flexion of wrist
6	Finger extensors	Extrinsic extension of fingers (partial or complete)
7	Thumb extensors	Extrinsic extension of thumb
8	Partial digital flexors	Extrinsic flexion of fingers (weak)
9	Lacks only intrinsics	Extrinsic flexion of fingers

Source: Zancolli EA. History of surgery in the rehabilitation of the tetraplegic upper limb. *Hand Clin*. 2002;18(3):369–376.

revision of which is still in widespread use (Table 49.7). The patient receives a separate classification for each arm, and sensory function is recorded, together with the sensitivity group as either O (ocular input only), or Cu (intact tactile function, defined as 10 mm or better two-point discrimination at the thumb). This system is useful to provide a quick summary of a patient's residual function in order to help plan surgery. In general, relatively high lesions that result in absent triceps and intact biceps and brachioradialis with one or both of ECRL and ECRB fit into groups 1 to 3. These patients will require reconstruction of elbow extension in addition to forearm reconstruction. Mid-level lesions with intact triceps function with or without PT and FCR occupy groups 3 to 5, and these groups generally have a good outcome from tendon transfers. Elbow extension is preserved, and the surgeon may proceed directly to forearm reconstruction. PT function also allows supination/pronation, which is otherwise difficult to restore. The remaining groups (6 to 9) are only lacking function in the intrinsic muscles of the hand, with or without the long extensors of the fingers and thumb. There are many surgical options for these patients, who may even be treated as for an ulnar nerve palsy.

TABLE 49.8 Contraindications to Surgical Reconstruction of Upper Limb Function in Tetraplegia

Unavailability of suitable muscles for transfer
Severe pressure sores/generally unwell
Severe muscle spasticity or joint contractures
Inadequate patient preparation or motivation

Multidisciplinary Team

Input from surgeons, physicians, nursing and allied health staff during planning and postoperatively is crucial for the care of these complex patients. This reduces postoperative complications and streamlines rehabilitation and retraining of muscle groups in their new function. As such, the ideal environment for tetraplegic patients undergoing tendon transfers is within a established program with a multidisciplinary team, comprising reconstructive surgeons experienced in tendon transfers, rehabilitation medicine physicians, hand therapists, physiotherapists, and on a ward staffed by specially trained nurses.

Timing of Surgery

Patients must be neurologically stable in order to determine what their level of impairment is. Furthermore, the post-injury period is fraught for patients managing difficult psychological and social changes, and significant motivation required to achieve a good outcome from tendon transfers. However, the appropriate amount of time to wait post-injury before embarking on surgical restoration of upper limb function will differ considerably between patients. As such, firm cutoffs are misleading, and may under- or overestimate the amount of time required for an individual. Generally, a minimum of 6 to 12 months is required for the patient to reach neurological stability following injury, as prior to this significant gains may still be made with rehabilitation alone.

Assessment

Careful assessment is of key importance, in particular for any contraindications to surgery (Table 49.8). Neurological stability should be ascertained, and the functional level clearly established. Current functional capabilities should also be reviewed, including bed mobility and transfers, and use of occupational aids or appliances, including wheelchairs. Any psychological issues should be addressed, and the patient's motivation and expectations assessed. Patient must be highly motivated and involved in their treatment and postoperative rehabilitation to allow recruitment of transferred muscles and any previous issues with compliance should be examined in detail. Unrealistically high expectations regarding the level of function attainable post procedure should be gently corrected. A general medical history should be taken, as significant current medical problems are a relative contraindication.

Examination

Careful examination and recording of upper limb function is important in the preoperative period, both for patient selection purposes and to compare pre- and postoperative function. Residual muscle function is assessed and the patient given a categorization for each upper limb according to the international classification (see Classification, below). Potential donor muscle groups should be assessed for spasticity and range of motion of elbow, wrist, and hand joints measured. Standard preoperative examination should be undertaken to screen for any medical issues that may be problematic in the perioperative period.

Preparation

Preparing the tetraplegic patient for tendon transfers to restore upper limb function should begin as early as possible. Splinting of joints in a useful position to prevent problematic contractures should commence at an early stage. The patient and members of their social support network, including spouse, family, and carers, should be educated regarding the operation and rehabilitation. Allied health reviews regarding these topics should be performed, and any appliances required for the postoperative period ordered, including electric wheelchairs. If there are any outstanding medical issues these should be addressed and optimized in the preoperative period. The procedures for a given patient should be individualized according to their residual function and goals. Use of a "one-size-fits-all" approach to tendon transfers in tetraplegics is a recipe for disaster. As a general rule, the less functional upper limb is operated on first.

Approach

The goal of surgical restoration of upper limb function in tetraplegia is the improvement in quality of life and enabling independent completion of ADLs. The means by which this is achieved is by restoration of elbow and wrist extension by means of tendon transfers and augmentation of the passive tenodesis effect to enable hand grip.[22]

Elbow Extension

Restoration of triceps function allows improvements in bed mobility, transfers and stability, wheelchair skills, operating reach, ability to push off bedclothes, social contact, and enables further tendon transfers for reconstruction of forearm function. There are two established options for donor muscles: posterior deltoid and biceps.[24]

The posterior deltoid to triceps transfer for restoration of elbow extension in the tetraplegic patient is a procedure pioneered by Moberg in the 1970s.[22] This takes advantage of the mechanically advantageous position of the deltoid muscle and its proximal innervation by the axillary nerve. However, there is a significance distance that must be bridged between the deltoid insertion and triceps tendon, necessitating the use of a graft. Various donors have been used historically, including extensor digitorum longus, tibialis anterior, fascia lata, and synthetic polyethylene terephthalate (Dacron). The senior author's current preference is the use of hamstring tendon (gracilis and semitendinosis) with a slip of tibial periosteum, given its low morbidity and proven effectiveness.[25] The donor tendons are harvested with the patient positioned prone, via a longitudinal incision over their insertion into the tibia. A curvilinear incision is then made over the posterior border of deltoid (Fig. 49.15). The deep fascia is incised, the muscle is dissected out and the posterior third mobilized, with care taken to protect the axillary nerve and its branches. The slip of tibial periosteum is then sutured to the posterior deltoid and the donor tendons are secured to the triceps insertion by a weave technique.

Biceps brachii to triceps transfer has been used to restore elbow extension in tetraplegia since the 1950s.[26] It is generally less preferred than posterior deltoid transfer due to the loss of elbow flexion power, increased difficulty in rehabilitation and retraining, and the risk of radial nerve injury during biceps transfer.[24] However, some research has suggested that biceps transfer provides stronger elbow extension, resulting in antigravity movement in a greater proportion than in posterior deltoid transfers.[27] It should be noted that an intact and functional brachialis is required for a biceps transfer to be considered as an option. The approach is made through a transverse incision in the cubital fossa. The biceps tendon is released from its insertion into the radial tuberosity, with care taken not to injure the lateral or medial cutaneous nerves of forearm. A second incision is made on the medial side of the arm and the medial intermuscular septum divided to allow the biceps tendon to be passed posteriorly. A further incision is made over the olecranon, through which the biceps tendon is fixed to the tendinous insertion of triceps and the olecranon using sutures with or without a tenodesis screw.

Forearm Reconstruction

With intact elbow extension, forearm function may be reconstructed. Through a combination of tendon transfers and tenodeses it is possible to achieve wrist extension, finger grasp, and lateral key pinch between thumb and index finger. Finger grasp is achieved by augmenting the tenodesis grip associated with wrist extension. The Alphabet procedure was devised by Fridén et al as a combination of procedures consisting of seven individual operations done as a single-stage reconstruction for hand function tetraplegics (Table 49.9). It has been shown to be effective in providing hand function in patients with C6 tetraplegia.[28] It comprises a number of procedures that may be performed together or separately. The split FPL to EPL tenodesis (aka New Zealand tenodesis) is designed to stabilize the interphalangeal joint of the thumb. Free grafting of the ring finger FDS tendon to the extensor hood by looping it under the EDC tendons results in the fingers assuming an intrinsic plus

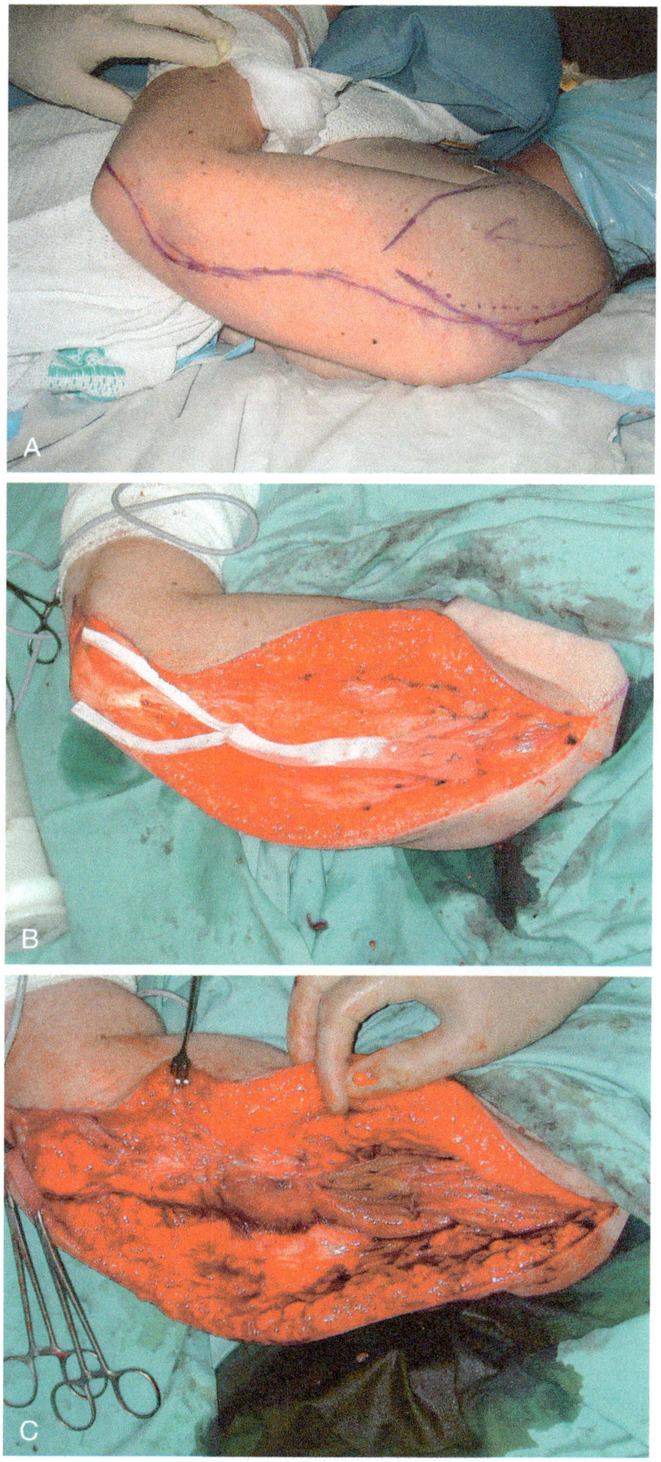

• **Fig. 49.15** Posterior deltoid to triceps transfer. (A) Preoperative markings. (B) Synthetic graft secured to posterior deltoid proximally (note that autologous tissue such as hamstring tendon is now more commonly used). (C) Graft secured to triceps insertion distally.

position. Thumb CMC joint arthrodesis fixes the thumb in a position useful for a lateral key grip. An alternative to this favored by the senior author is a silicon interpositional spacer (Swanson implant) in the first webspace between the first and second metacarpals (Fig. 49.16). Brachioradialis to FPL and ECRL to FDP tendon transfers are to restore thumb and finger flexion respectively. EPL is rerouted to

TABLE 49.9 Alphabet Procedure (Advanced Balanced Combined Digital Extensor Flexor Grip Reconstruction)

Split FPL to EPL tenodesis
Free tendon graft (FDS4) to extensor hood digits 2–3 and 4–5
Thumb CMC joint arthrodesis*
BR to FPL tendon transfer
ECRL to FDP tendon transfer
EPL to dorsal forearm fascia tenodesis
ECU to ulnar head tenodesis

*Alternatively, a synthetic spacer in the first webspace may be used (see Fig. 49.16).
Source: Fridén J, Reinholdt C, Turcsányii I, et al. A single-stage operation for reconstruction of hand flexion, extension, and intrinsic function in tetraplegia: the Alphabet procedure. *Tech Hand Up Extrem Surg*. 2011;15(4):230–235.

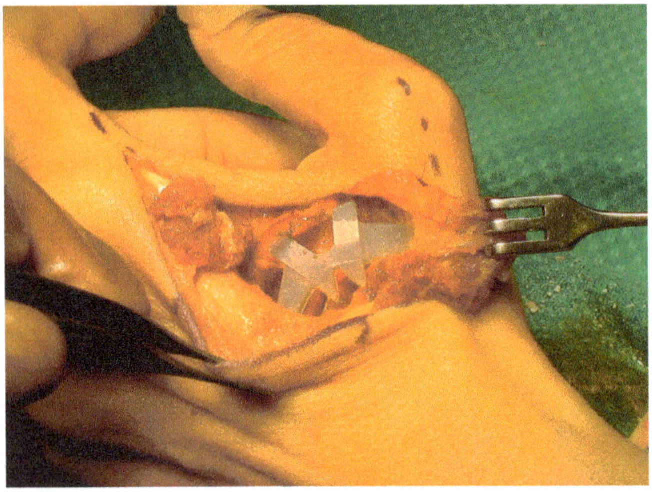

• **Fig. 49.16** Swanson spacer interposed between first and second metacarpals.

the dorsal forearm fascia to passively extend the thumb during wrist flexion, and finally ECU is shortened and attached to the ulnar head to stabilize the wrist. The senior authors preference is to substitute free grafting of FDS with instead using it to enable passive tenodesis of the metacarpophalangeal joints by releasing it from its insertion, delivering it from the flexor sheath proximally superficial to the A1 pulley, and suturing it to itself.

Recent Advances

Nerve transfer surgery established in the treatment of brachial plexus injuries has been trialed in the treatment of tetraplegia. Early results have shown transfer of the branch to supinator into the posterior interosseous nerve result in excellent finger and thumb extension,[29] and combined transfer of multiple nerves has been demonstrated to be effective for restoring overall upper limb function.[30] Other nerve transfers that show promise in case series include transfer of the motor nerve to ECRB to the anterior interosseous nerve, and the motor branch to teres minor or posterior division of the axillary nerve to the triceps motor nerve.[31] It is likely that a combined approach utilizing nerve and tendon transfers in concert will be most effective.

Postoperative Care

Patients who have undergone tendon transfer procedures, particularly those who are tetraplegic or immobilized, require high-quality postoperative care to prevent complications, and allow rehabilitation and retraining to commence when able. It is important for all these patients to be on prophylactic anticoagulation due to the high risk of venous thromboembolism in the postoperative period. Traditional teaching dictates that a 3–4 week period of static immobilization must follow any tendon transfer procedure, to allow tendon healing and reduce risk of early rupture.[5,16] However, early active mobilization has become widespread practice following tendon repair procedures,[32,33] and there is mounting evidence that such rehabilitation protocols may improve outcomes following tendon transfers.[34] Such protocols may reduce edema and development of adhesions, and allow earlier commencement of rehabilitation and retraining.[28]

Benefits of such protocols include reduced cost of rehabilitation, improved function in the short term, similar long-term outcomes, and no increase in risk of complications such as tendon pull-out.[34] It is important to emphasize that careful patient selection is essential when deciding on a rehabilitation program. For success with early active mobilization patients must be particularly motivated, compliant, and able to follow complex instructions from hand therapists. In both early or delayed mobilization protocols, mobilization should be introduced in a gradual fashion by hand therapists experienced in managing patients following tendon transfer or repair procedures, followed by progressive strengthening exercises and finally, full activity.

Devices such as electrical stimulators and biofeedback may be used for muscle re-education, though studies of their effectiveness have been disappointing.[35] The senior author's preference is to reserve early active mobilization for selected patients. Otherwise, the protocol requires immobilization for 2 weeks followed by passive ROM exercises, and then a gradual return to normal activity after 6–8 weeks. Following restoration of elbow extension with either deltoid to triceps or biceps to triceps transfer it is our routine to immobilize the elbow in a Bedsloe caliper splint for 12 weeks. Initially the caliper should be set to allow a range of motion of 0–15 degrees, to be gradually increased each fortnight if the previous increase is tolerated.

Conclusion

Tendon transfers have been used since the late 19th century to restore function for patients suffering irreversible neurological or musculoskeletal injury. Recently, with the development of microsurgical techniques and improvement in our understanding of neuroanatomy, nerve repair and transfer, and innervated free muscle transfer have become the usual treatment of choice for many of these problems. However, there remains a role for tendon transfer, either for early function during nerve recovery, or for those whose pathology is no amenable to nerve repair or transfer. This chapter should equip the surgeon with the essential knowledge of tendon transfer: the principles, approach, and techniques required to perform these procedures.

Acknowledgments

The authors would like to acknowledge the generous assistance of Mr Donald Sammut in the preparation of this chapter.

References

1. Burkhalter WE. Early tendon transfer in upper extremity peripheral nerve injury. *Clin Orthopaed Relat Res.* 1974;104:68–79.
2. Lieber RL, Fridén J. Functional and clinical significance of skeletal muscle architecture. *Muscle Nerve.* 2000;23(11):1647–1666.
3. Brand PW. Biomechanics of tendon transfer. *Orthop Clin North Am.* 1974;5(2):205–230.
4. Blix M. Die Länge und die Spannung des Muskels1. *Scand Archiv Physiol.* Wiley Online Library. 1894;5(1):173–206.
5. Sammer DM, Chung KC. Tendon transfers. Part I: principles of transfer and transfers for radial nerve palsy. *Plast Reconstr Surg.* 2009;123(5):169e–177e.
6. Fridén J, Lieber RL. Evidence for muscle attachment at relatively long lengths in tendon transfer surgery. *J Hand Surg.* 1998;23(1):105–110.
7. Wilbur D, Hammert WC. Principles of tendon transfer. *Hand Clin.* 2016;32(3):283–289.
8. Steindler A. Tendon transplantation in the upper extremity. *Am J Surg.* 1939;44(1):260–271.
9. Dogan NU, Uysal II , Seker M. The communications between the ulnar and median nerves in upper limb. *Neuroanatomy.* 2009;8:15–19.
10. Sunderland SS, Walshe F. *Nerves and Nerve Injuries.* Edinburgh: E. & S. Livingstone; 1968.
11. Kulikov YI, Dodd S, Gheduzzi S, et al. An in vitro biomechanical study comparing the spiral linking technique against the Pulvertaft weave for tendon repair. *J Hand Surg Eur.* 2007;32(4):377–381.
12. Ingari JV, Green DP. *Radial nerve palsy. Green's Operative Hand Surgery E-Book.* Elsevier Health Sciences; 2010:1075–1092.
13. Richards RR. Tendon transfers for failed nerve reconstruction. *Clin Plast Surg.* 2003;30(2):223–245.
14. Colditz JC. Splinting for radial nerve palsy. *J Hand Ther.* 1987;1(1):18–23.
15. Davis TRC. *Median and ulnar nerve palsy. Green's Operative Hand Surgery E-Book.* Elsevier Health Sciences; 2010:1093–1137.
16. Sammer DM, Chung KC. Tendon transfers. Part II: transfers for ulnar nerve palsy and median nerve palsy. *Plast Reconstr Surg.* 2009;124(3):212e–221e.
17. Seiler JG, Desai MJ, Payne SH. Tendon transfers for radial, median, and ulnar nerve palsy. *J Am Acad Orthop Surg.* 2013;21(11):675–684.
18. Bunnell S. Opposition of the thumb. *J Bone Joint Surg Am.* 1938;20(2):269–284.
19. Riordan DC. Tendon transfers for median, ulnar or radial nerve palsy. *Hand.* 1969;1(1):42–46.
20. Zancolli EA. Claw-hand caused by paralysis of the intrinsic muscles a simple surgical procedure for its correction. *J Bone Joint Surg Am.* 1957;39(5):1076–1080.
21. Wagner JP, Curtin CM, Gater DR, et al. Perceptions of people with tetraplegia regarding surgery to improve upper-extremity function. *J Hand Surg.* 2007;32(4):483–490.
22. Moberg E. Surgical treatment for absent single-hand grip and elbow extension in quadriplegia. Principles and preliminary experience. *J Bone Joint Surg Am.* 1975;57(2):196–206.
23. Hentz VR, Curtin CM, Leclercq C. Functional restoration of the upper extremity in tetraplegia. In: Lin VW, Bono CM, eds. *Spinal Cord Medicine.* 2nd edn. Demos Medical Publishing; 2010.
24. Leclercq C, Hentz VR, Kozin SH, et al. Reconstruction of elbow extension. *Hand Clin.* 2008;24(2):185–201.
25. Dunn JA, Mohammed KD, Beadel GP, et al. A comparative outcome study of hamstring versus tibialis anterior and synthetic grafts for deltoid to triceps transfers. *J Hand Surg.* 2017;42(10):833.
26. Friedenberg ZB. Transposition of the biceps brachii for triceps weakness. *J Bone Joint Surg Am.* 1954;36(3):656–658.
27. Mulcahey MJ, Lutz C, Kozin SH, et al. Prospective evaluation of biceps to triceps and deltoid to triceps for elbow extension in tetraplegia. *J Hand Surg.* 2003;28(6):964–971.
28. Fridén J, Reinholdt C, Turcsányii I, et al. A single-stage operation for reconstruction of hand flexion, extension, and intrinsic function in tetraplegia: the Alphabet procedure. *Tech Hand Up Extrem Surg.* 2011;15(4):230–235.
29. Bertelli JA, Ghizoni MF. Transfer of supinator motor branches to the posterior interosseous nerve in C7–T1 brachial plexus palsy. *J Neurosurg Am Assoc Neurol Surg.* 2010;113(1):129–132.
30. van Zyl N, Hahn JB, Cooper CA, et al. Upper limb reinnervation in C6 tetraplegia using a triple nerve transfer: case report. *J Hand Surg.* 2014;39(9):1779–1783.
31. Cain S, Gohritz A, Fridén J, van Zyl N. Review of upper extremity nerve transfer in cervical spinal cord injury. *J Brachial Plex Peripher Nerve Inj.* 2015;10(01):e34–e42.
32. Starr HM, Snoddy M, Hammond KE, et al. Flexor tendon repair rehabilitation protocols: a systematic review. *J Hand Surg.* 2013;38(9):1712–1714.
33. Ng CY, Chalmer J, Macdonald DJM, et al. Rehabilitation regimens following surgical repair of extensor tendon injuries of the hand – a systematic review of controlled trials. *J Hand Microsurg.* 2012;4(2):65–73.
34. Sultana SS, MacDermid JC, Grewal R, et al. The effectiveness of early mobilization after tendon transfers in the hand: a systematic review. *J Hand Ther.* 2013;26(1):1–21.
35. Glinsky J, Harvey L, van Es P, et al. The addition of electrical stimulation to progressive resistance training does not enhance the wrist strength of people with tetraplegia: a randomized controlled trial. *Clin Rehabil.* 2009;23(8):696–704.

50

Digital Replantation and Thumb Reconstruction

WAYNE A.J. MORRISON, ROSTAM D. FARHADIEH, AND OLIVIA M. PEROTTI

For videos accompanying this chapter see ExpertConsult.com. See inside cover for access details.

Introduction

Vascular surgeons Jacobson and Suarez introduced the microscope to perfect microvascular small vessel anastomosis in 1960,[1] which rapidly led to its application in revascularizing digits and replantation.[2,3] It was promptly adopted in Taiwan, the USA, Australia and, later, Europe. China independently and unbeknown to the West had been achieving remarkable successes despite primitive instrumentation and facilities. The need for small animal models for transplantation research led to laboratories being equipped for microvascular surgery and they doubled as training centers for skilling budding young surgeons enthused by the potential of this new technique. Establishing "replant services" became an achievable and desirable goal worldwide. Unsurprisingly, the enthusiasm of reconstructive teams was not met with equal passion from anesthetists, hospital administrators, and other surgical disciplines whose routine was often disturbed by seemingly unending theater occupation and repeat operations for what many saw in the overall scheme of things as a trivial pursuit. Microvascular surgery was here to stay, and there quickly evolved a divide between the older generation of surgeons who were skeptical or intimidated by the technical expertise demanded and those of a younger set who relished the challenge, the new anatomy, and the vistas that were on offer.

Indications for Replantation

Like all surgical procedures, the indication for replantation is when the estimated benefit outweighs the possible risks. The more extensive the injury, the greater the likely benefits of replantation, because in the severely damaged hand a little is a lot.

Intuitively, replanting everything seems the best solution to restoring lost function and this will be the desire of most patients, but it presupposes that the results from replantation will be close to the original. Sadly, experience shows that this is often not the case. The experienced surgeon needs to estimate the outcome taking into account the general fitness of the patient, the extent of injury of the parts, their capacity for repair and functional potential, and the suitability of the patient to commit to the arduous postoperative therapy required to maximize this potential. Having balanced these expectations and limitations, the surgeon must present the patient with an honest as well as a compassionate opinion regarding the wisdom of replantation including the potential need for multiple procedures, flap coverage, ultimate poor result, and later amputation. Mostly the patient in a state of shock will plead that the parts are reattached, and mostly this will be the correct decision. With major limb or multiple digit amputations, rational decisions cannot be made until a thorough assessment in theater is performed. What initially looks to be hopeless can sometimes prove quite feasible; alternatively, the opportunity to prioritize salvageable digits to essential sites, use segments of nonreplantable digits for spare parts, and even banking in ectopic sites, presents itself only at the time of initial surgery. Resuscitation and management of concurrent life-threatening injuries take priority and guide decision-making regarding amputation or replantation and its timing. More severe crush and avulsion mechanisms have less likelihood of overall success compared to guillotine-type injuries. Age, general medical health, occupation, handedness, and expectations are also essential considerations guiding decision-making.

Proper handling of the amputated part is imperative to a successful outcome. The severed part is stored in moist saline gauze inside a watertight bag, placed in a container of ice. Care must be taken to avoid direct contact with ice, which can irreversibly damage the microvascular anatomy. Although the expedient transfer to a microsurgical center is critical, multiple reports have shown successful replantation after more than 24 hours of cold ischemia.[4]

Functional Loss Assessment

If the guiding principle of replantation is to restore lost function then a well-grounded understanding of the basic functions of the hand and the expected outcomes of hand surgery

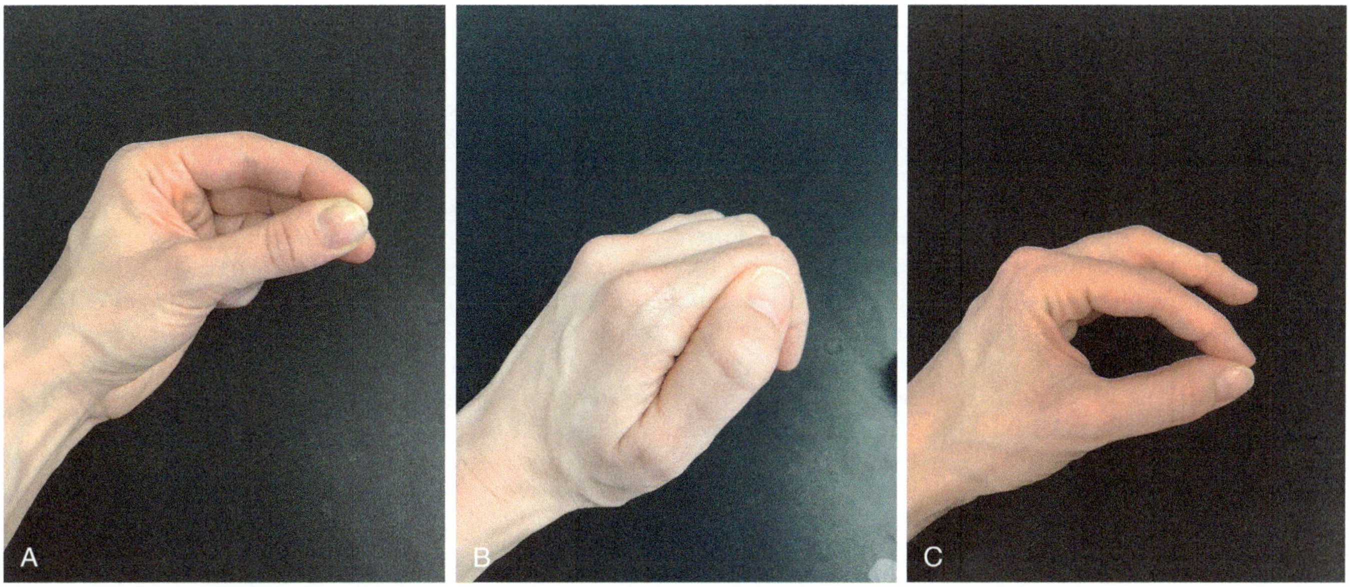

• **Fig. 50.1** Basic hand function. (A) Pollico-digital pinch grip and palmar digital grip. (B) Lateral key pinch, requires thumb adduction, mobile basal joint, and stable opposition post. (C) Pulp pinch, requires intrinsics for joint stabilization. (Courtesy Professor Wayne AJ Morrison.)

are essential. It follows that a hand surgeon with microvascular expertise should be the director of the expedition and not an enthusiastic microsurgeon whose pinpoint focus may be technical vascular gymnastics in the face of big picture stupidity. Because of the daytime injury leading often to nighttime surgery queues, too often the task of replantation is given to junior trainees who have to reinvent the wheel in the trenches at night without supervision. Anesthetists and nursing staff have to suffer interminable time wasting as the resident's indecision lapses into mesmerizing Brownian movement. It should be remembered that secondary surgery on replanted digits is the most challenging of all hand surgery so that meticulous primary repair of all structures is the goal.

Normal Hand Function

The functional role of the digits can be looked at from the individual finger point of view and from their role as a partner in group hand functions, pinch grip, palmar grip, global pinch etc. Rarely do they function in isolation except perhaps in keyboard practice (Fig. 50.1).

The radial three digits function as a unit to achieve the manipulative, dextrous function of pulp pinch or radial tripod or chuck grip, typically a dominant hand function. Sensation is preeminent. The pulps convey multiple sensory modalities that in concert allow the brain to interpret what the fingers are feeling, they are the eyes of the hand. This is tactile gnosis and is considerably more sophisticated than what is assessed by simple sensory two-point discrimination. Pinch between index and thumb uses a dominant radial side of the index whereas holding a pen or using fine instruments in the tripod fashion demands sensory acuity of the ulnar side of the index pulp and radial side of the middle. The basal joint is the key to allowing the mobile thumb ray to range variably across the digits to perform the range of pinch grip options from lateral (key) pinch against the stable proximal side of the index where the thumb is in full adduction and retropulsion, to pulp pinch and tripod pinch with index and long finger pulps where the thumb moves into maximum abduction and opposition. The pill rolling motion of the thumb pulp against the finger members is performed by circumduction (abduction, adduction, flexion, and extension) of the metacarpophalangeal joint. At the moment of final application of forced tripod pinch the proximal joints of the three rays must be stabilized by their intrinsic muscles to allow transmission of the flexor tendon force to flex the distal joints. Fortunately, intrinsics are protected in most digital amputations. By understanding the essential elements of this radial pinch grip according to each digit's contribution we can better make decisions about the residual potential of the amputated part and the value or otherwise of replanting it.

It is estimated that the thumb, which has no substitute, contributes 40% of hand function and it should take priority for replantation. Provided the amputation does not involve the basal joint, and this is very rare, then even a relatively badly damaged thumb that is shortened and stiff can still perform most functions provided adequate sensation returns. In contrast, the index finger is readily substituted for by the middle if it has inferior function, especially sensory, and replantation can hinder residual hand function. Most of the unique function of the index resides beyond the distal joint (glabrous skin with finger printed sweat traction grip, padded stable pulp, multiple modality sensory nerve endings, and a finger nail acting as an exoskeleton to stabilize the pulp against its bony platform and to magnify sensation) so that with the exception of guillotine injuries proximal amputations of the index are likely to be numb and stiff because of tendon adhesions and joint damage and are arguably contraindicated for replantation.

The middle finger functions as a partner in the tripod pinch team but is also the most powerful palmar flexor because of its central position and the size of its tendons. Thus in combination with the ring and little fingers it also participates in the ulnar-sided palmar grip function. Here movement and length of digit rather than sensation are critical to function. All the joints must fold into full flexion for power grip and to prevent objects falling out of the open palm. The little finger is more valuable than the ring in this regard because it exploits full width of the palm and facilitates the stable and secure gripping of long-handled brooms, axes, etc. The torque power is augmented by the hypothenar muscles and the mobile carpometacarpal joints of these two digits.

Replantation of the middle finger proximal to the proximal interphalangeal (PIP) joint in isolation has considerable merit because its sensory need is relative, and even with limited mobility it will contribute to tripod pinch while its mere presence prevents small objects, coins, etc. falling through the cupped hand. A truly successful replant will serve both functions. The isolated ring finger replantation can also contribute usefully for the same reasons even if the result is mediocre although it is possible that flexor tendon adhesions may also limit adjacent finger tendon gliding and produce the quadriga effect. Little finger replants have theoretical logic and limits for the reasons mentioned but for some reason regain less function.

Single digit replantations distal to superficialis insertion were previously thought to be too difficult and not cost-efficient, but with greater experience they have been shown to be technically straightforward, and if nerves are repairable, afford a good outcome even if the distal joint is stiff. Likewise, fingertip amputations through the distal phalanx, although technically more challenging, can often be replanted by joining an artery and vein if possible and give a meaningful sensory return. They are the ultimate local flap, unlike some local flap options which add insult to injury.[1] Terminalization often necessitates further bone shortening which may convert a usable into a nonusable digit. Here replantation may be the better option.

Where multiple digits are injured and/or amputated then the disruption to both radial and ulnar hand functions can be dire and every attempt to replant as many digits as is feasible is called for on the basis that something, even if compromised, is better than nothing. The best replantable digits should be strategically targeted to the most important sites so that elements of both radial pinch and ulnar grip can be restored. In severe mutilations, digits may be transposed for maximal function but when the index or little fingers are not replanted their metacarpal head stumps should not be resected for cosmetic reasons because torque (rotational) grip is reduced by more than 50%. Spare parts from nonreplantable digits can be used to salvage other damaged digits and in extreme cases parts can be banked in anticipation of later use, for example large pieces of innervated glabrous volar digit or palmar flap skin. An isolated index amputation in association with a middle finger pulp loss or divided radial digital nerve now becomes a strong indication for replantation. A compound PIP joint injury to a viable ring finger that will result in stiffness strengthens the indication for replanting the otherwise debatable adjacent little finger. The ulnar digits institute the power grip by fully flexing their terminal phalanges into the palm. Whereas a single proximal ulnar digit replantation risks restricting movement of the other, distal ulnar digit, replantation, which will not interfere with proximal tendon gliding, would restore full length of the digit to accomplish palmar closure even if the distal interphalangeal joint is stiff. Similarly, replantation of a single distal ring or little finger may be thought to be a trivial indication but if both are amputated then the critical locking of objects into the palm is lost and replantation of at least one becomes strongly indicated.

A rudimentary listing of indications to justify the resources to patient, surgeon, and health system would look something like: the thumb, single digits distal to superficialis insertion, multiple digits, and any pediatric digit. With the only reservations being single digits proximal to the PIP joint, which because of the circumferential injury to extensor and flexor tendon systems inevitably risk unyielding stiffness and reduced sensitivity requiring prolonged costly therapy, secondary surgery, and extended time from work. In reality, when confronted with a patient bringing with them their amputated part and immense hope, an honest conversation regarding the realistic likelihood of a functioning, noninterfering digit is paramount but not likely heard.

Assessment of the Functional Capacity of the Amputated Part

Successful proximal digit replantation demands that all repaired structures at the level of injury must function. The bone fixation should be rigid to allow early mobilization; the periosteum should be repaired to facilitate extensor and flexor tendon gliding; The extensor mechanism over the proximal phalanx is complex, being a confluence of intrinsic and extrinsic tendons that lasso the phalanx and must glide as a sleeve over the site of the osteosynthesis. Both flexor tendons must glide independently within the tight fibrous flexor sheath and nerves must generate over a significant distance. Arterial and venous repairs must be from "normal" vessels, and finally, the skin must be closed without tension over the repairs to prevent vascular compression and tendon exposure. The experienced hand surgeon will be able to estimate the likely function after evaluation of the nature of the injury to the various structures. Shattered missing bone and periosteal loss impede fixation and tendon gliding, prolong immobilization, imbalance the tendon units and carry the risk of nonunion. Extensor tendon adherence at the proximal phalanx prevents passive flexion and active extension of both distal joints. Joint obliteration in the ulnar digits compromises their vital purpose of palmar grip. Metacarpophalangeal joint destruction impacts on adjacent fingers if replanted. Avulsed digital nerves have little hope of critical sensory recovery. Segmental injury, although sometimes technically feasible, will rarely allow useful function.

Contraindications

Contraindications apply to the digit and the patient.

Patient Factors

Age exclusion for replantation is not automatic. Preoperative stiffness may mean that a minimally functional outcome may replicate their pre-injury state well. Terminalization, especially for single digits, is more likely appropriate as functional and cosmetic requirements are often less, sensory recovery reduced, and thrombosis risk higher. For these reasons, many elderly patients avoid a prolonged operation, hospital stay, and rehabilitation in preference for a quick solution.

Significant associated injuries and premorbid status will impact on anesthesia and the required lengthy rehabilitation before embarking on replantation. Life- and limb-threatening injuries take precedence over digit replantation. Cold storage is a feasible option for 24 hours and buys time for reassessment. Temporizing soft tissue coverage may be more suitable acutely, with reconstruction offered once patients recover from other injuries. Poorly controlled diabetes, small vessel disease, thromboembolic disease, and smoking all adversely affect microvascular patency.

In a series of 4483 replantations, failure as high as 53.3% was reported when the platelet count exceeded 300×10^9 cells/liter. Another series of 211 demonstrated a 42.8% failure rate, compared with 14% in patients with normal platelet counts ($81–299 \times 10^9$ cells/liter).[5] This evidence suggests that augmenting anticoagulation in patients with high platelet counts should be adopted to improve survival, and those suffering from thrombocytosis.[5]

Patients with severe psychological problems who are unable to cooperate with the required postoperative monitoring and rehabilitation may be contraindicated.

Digit Factors

Fortunately, there is no muscle tissue in fingers and ischemia time is less critical than with major limbs. There is no significant survival benefit in amputated digits replanted within the first 12 hours compared to first 24 hours. While there are documented cases of successful replantation up to 33 hours of warm ischemia and 94 hours of cold ischemia, after 24 hours survival rates drop to 66.7%, far below accepted success rates of greater than 90%.[6] Muscle starts to undergo irreversible ischemia after 6 hours at room temperature. For this reason, proximal limb amputations require rapid cooling. Initial arterial perfusion through an arterial shunt before venous connection allows for a reduction of possible toxic myoglobin breakdown products entering the circulation.

Significant deep infection is rare in replanted digits despite the sometimes unsavoury nature of their amputation. It is more relevant for high energy injuries and massive contamination in industrial or agricultural settings. Meticulous debridement and appropriate Gram-negative antibiotic coverage, as well as consideration of terminalization in patients with systemic immunosuppression or diabetes mellitus, is necessary.

Multiple level, segmentally injured digits, and severe avulsions may be impossible to replant, or if they survive will inevitably lead to a poor outcome. When multiple digits are amputated, spare parts surgery is possible where the best proximal stump is matched with the least damaged amputated part. It is better to have fewer well-functioning digits than multiple stiff, unusable digits. In addition to digit transposition, digits unsuitable for replantation can offer vascularized small joints, nerve grafts, and innervated or venous free flaps.

Technique and Principles

Replantation requires disciplined leadership and continued momentum, which quickly wanes in the early hours of the morning. There needs to be communication with anesthetics regarding thromboembolism prophylaxis, a warmed theatre to prevent vasospasm, adequate warming and hydration to maximize peripheral vasodilatation, appropriate antibiotics (usually cephazolin with the occasional addition of Gram-negative and aerobic cover for agricultural mechanisms), pressure area prevention, and an indwelling catheter.

The techniques of digital replantation have been described in innumerable texts, and personal preferences determine the surgeon's specific routine. Several principles, however, should guide the procedure involving identification and meticulous primary repair of each component of the severed digit.

1. **Supervision by a person with hand experience.** Upper limb replantation is hand surgery, not microsurgery. The indication for surgery should not just be technical feasibility but the estimated functional potential, which requires experienced intraoperative assessment.
2. **Primary repair of every structure.** Revisional surgery in replants is exceptionally difficult, hazardous, and often unrewarding. Take time and care to perfect each step. Early postoperative mobilization is the key to achieving maximum functional recovery, and this demands skeletal stability and primary wound healing. Where tendon damage demands a staged reconstruction, it is probably wiser despite infection risk to insert a silicone rod at the primary operation to avoid secondary reopening of the digit at the replantation level.
3. **Predetermined routine.** Random repair of one structure and then another and back to the first wastes time and confuses assistants. Two teams are ideal, especially if multiple digits are being repaired. Replantation is a time and motion study.
4. **Debridement rarely needs to be radical, especially of the skin.** Infection is rare and primary skin closure is the ideal without grafts or flaps.
5. **Skin access incisions should ideally be Bruner type.** Avoid midlateral, so that if the wound is too tight to

close the neurovascular repairs will be flap covered. Bruner incisions can be extended safely, as is often required for avulsion injuries where vascular resection may be extensive. Precious time is wasted because of inadequate exposure to the proximal vascular bundle, so avoid hesitation in gaining greater access proximally.

6. **Tag vessels, nerves, and tendons in the amputated segment and at the proximal stump.** The proximal exploration is best under tourniquet control until arterial assessment, when it should be released to assess for pulsatile flow.
7. **Bone shortening facilitates primary skin closure.** It also allows judicious debridement of damaged nerve to enable tension-free end-to-end coaptation. Bone shortening is not to avoid vein grafting the artery. The arterial debridement should not be compromised by concerns with end-to-end repair but determined by pulsatile forward flow from the proximal vessel, and this may require aggressive resection proximal to the next branch point. Aim to shorten bone from the amputated end because if the replant fails, at least the stump length is preserved.
8. **Rigid bone fixation is key to early active movement of the replant.** Care should be taken to perfect this step as it lays the foundation both intraoperatively and postoperatively.[7,8] A dorsal meshed plate is ideal where possible, leaving the adjacent joints free. Unfortunately, abandoning these ideals for the ease and speed of Kirschner wire (K-wire) fixation is standard; K-wire fixation also requires minimal periosteal dissection and allows flexibility in rotational correction. K-wire can risk infection, tethers joints and tendons, and creates movement at the fracture site. In a Korean study of 1247 successful replantations, single axial K-wire was not associated with poorer outcomes compared to rigid fixation.
9. **Periosteal repair** where possible facilitates tendon gliding, especially dorsally beneath the broad expanse of the extensor tendon complex at middle and proximal phalangeal levels. Bone shortening often enables periosteal repair.
10. **Dorsal structures repaired first** – periosteum, extensor tendon including the intrinsics, veins, and skin. Venous repair before arterial avoids unnecessary blood loss from open veins or the need to clamp the artery post repair or maintain tourniquet. Veins tend to rupture rather than avulse, and for that reason rarely require vein grafts. If bony fixation is correctly aligned, dorsal veins should line up directly. K-wire fixation allows slight rotational correction if required. Subcutaneous bruises and blood clot provide clues to their location, also applying circumferential pressure to the cut edge should encourage them into vision. Lastly, if these methods fail, an arterial repair can be performed first to force them open. At least two veins must be repaired. With very distal replants the veins will be necessarily volar, most likely in the 4 and 8 o'clock regions, but anastomosable vessels may be absent.[9] When no suitable veins exist, temporary venous outflow by leech therapy, subcutaneous heparin, topical heparin to the sterile matrix or subdermal pocketing of the de-epithelialized pulp into palm or chest will help. Venous anastomosis improves the overall success rate in distal replantation by 15%. However, substantial evidence suggests it carries no survival benefit distal to the lunula. Even when venous anastomosis proves impossible, published success rates over 75% justify attempts at replantation in distal amputation.[5] Following venous repair, the skin is loosely approximated avoiding kinking of the veins. Epithelial only sutures will avoid distortion of the tissues.
11. **Volar repair begins at the periosteum, flexor tendons, arteries, nerves and skin.** The periosteum is again repaired where possible to reduce adhesions. The tendons should be repaired before the vessels and nerves to restore the preinjury elastic tension-length of the volar digit. This then determines the tension-length of the vessel repair and is especially important in assessing the length of interpositional vein grafts, which will elongate once flow is restored in the artery. Judgment will guide whether one or both flexors are repaired.
    a. *Arterial repair under tourniquet control allows the vessels to be identified in their anatomical sites.* The ulnar artery of the thumb is dominant and must be selected. Access to its proximal reaches is difficult and requires appropriate assistance and positioning. The radial vessels of the index and little fingers are usually dominant. Relevant to distal amputations, just distal to the level of the DIP joint the digital arteries merge from their lateral location into one central vessel which passes deep along the periosteal surface of the distal phalanx. Once located the vessel ends are inspected for signs of intimal tears and medial splits, bruising or delamination of the wall or intraluminal thrombus. Distal damage is challenging to judge beyond gross retraction, coiling or delamination. Once debridement is done the tourniquet is released to evaluate pulsatile flow from the proximal artery. If reperfusion fails, start investigating proximally for the underlying cause. If the patency test demonstrates no flow up to the anastomosis, then the explanation is spasm, proximal vessel damage or central causes. Aggressive resection of the proximal vessel and grafting may be required. If the flow goes up to but not across the anastomosis, then the diagnosis is thrombus and requires reanastomosis or grafting. In both of these situations, a stat dose of IV heparin is helpful before application of the vessel clamps. If the flow passes across the anastomosis, but the finger does not perfuse then the explanation is distal or intrinsic microvascular damage due to crush, spasm, or prolonged ischemia causing reperfusion injury. This problem may respond to Trinitrin patches, intravenous heparin, dependent positioning of the hand to increase arterial inflow pressure or thrombolytics such as urokinase.[8] Beyond these, fate will determine the outcome.
    b. *Nerve repair; if a nerve graft is required it should be done at the primary operation.* Use the posterior interosseous

or medial antebrachial cutaneous nerve of the forearm or, if another digit is to be discarded, then nerve from this digit is ideal. However, where possible trade skeletal shortening for direct nerve coaptation. The neural recovery is vital for meaningful function of radial-sided digits.

c. *Skin closure is the key to early healing and pos-operative mobilization.* It should be as loose as possible with the minimum number of stitches in the knowledge that the tissues will swell in the initial postoperative period. Where the skin cannot be closed thin fenestrated grafts for small defects will take, even over vascular repairs, but this compromises the use of heparin. More substantial defects require flap coverage, especially if tendon or bone is exposed. Thumb or mutilating hand injuries may require regional flaps or distant free flaps including venous flow-through flaps.[10]

Multiple Digital Replantation

Multiple digit loss is an absolute indication for replantation, despite sometimes limited expectations and increased surgical time and resources. In the mutilated hand a little can mean a lot and be the critical difference between employability or functional independence.

Replanting all digits in their intended positions is not always possible or desirable, and decision-making depends on the quality of amputated parts and stumps. When amputated parts are not all replantable, the guiding principle is thumb replantation is prized above all; the dominant hand should take priority and strive to restore primary hand function; either radial pinch or ulnar power grip. Theoretically, the dominant hand should favor radial pinch grip for dextrous work and the nondominant hand ulnar grip for power to stabilize objects while being manipulated by the dominant hand. Transposing ulnar digits to a radial position may mean the dominant digital arteries are reversed so that anastomosis may require vein grafting across the flexor sheath[11] (Table 50.1).

The operative sequence should be cognizant of time and motion. Addressing one component of all the digits, i.e., all bone fixation, then all dorsal repairs and finally volar structures, is time-efficient rather than doing one complete finger at a time. It means the bones and tendons are stabilized before microsurgical repair and has the advantage of reduced risk of accidental injury to delicate adjacent microsurgical repair and multiple applications of the tourniquet. This method is likely to lead to higher survival rates. The distinct disadvantage is prolonged warm ischemia, alleviated by keeping the amputated parts in cold storage until required.[11]

TABLE 50.1 Considerations for Prioritized and Transpositional Replantation[12]

Multiple digit amputations: With or without thumb amputation	Where the thumb is not replantable, replant the best-preserved digit in place of thumb Following this, target the next available digit to the middle finger site if required, as this is central and strongest and can perform both radial and ulnar functions Next to replant is ulnar side to preserve hand span and power grip If one more digit is salvageable, position it on the index stump for stable three-point tripod grip
Bilateral thumb amputations	Where the thumb of the dominant hand is irreversibly damaged, transfer the less injured thumb of the nondominant to dominant thumb
Symmetric digital amputations	Transpose digits from nondominant hand to the dominant hand

Ring Avulsion Injury

Ring avulsions can be the most challenging injuries for hand surgeons to treat, and the decision to attempt salvage for high-grade injuries remains difficult.

Kay[13] and Adani[14] have expanded Urbaniak's original classification,[15] shown in Table 50.2. Although classifications do not seem to add anything to what is obvious, assess avulsions according to the layer(s) involved from superficial to deep.

Skin breach alone with dorsal vein disruption needs venous repair only and has an excellent prognosis.[16]

Deeper more severe degloving without amputation will involve vascular bundle damage, frequently with extensive proximal arterial and nerve injury. The skin is sleeved distally to a variable degree in which case the veins are also divided but not always depending on the angle of incidence of the ring injury; these require arterial vein grafting but have a good prognosis.

TABLE 50.2 Ring Avulsion Injury Classification

I	Circulation adequate	
II	Circulation inadequate, no skeletal injury	
	a	Arterial circulation inadequate
	v	Venous circulation inadequate
	av	Arterial and venous circulation inadequate
III	Circulation inadequate, skeletal injury	
	a	Arterial circulation inadequate
	v	Venous circulation inadequate
	av	Arterial and venous circulation inadequate
IV	Complete amputation	
	i	Complete degloving with intact tendons
	d	Amputation distal to FDS insertion
	p	Amputation proximal to FDS insertion

Sources: Urbaniak JR, Evans JP, Bright DS. Microvascular management of ring avulsion injuries. *J Hand Surg Am*. 1981;6:25–30; Kay S, Werntz J, Wolff TW. Ring avulsion injuries: classification and prognosis. *J Hand Surg Am*. 1989;14:204–213; Adani R, Castagnetti C, Busa R, et al. Ring avulsion injuries: microsurgical management. *J Reconstr Microsurg*. 1996;12:189–194.

The next stage involves skeletal fracture/dislocation at the DIP joint or neck of the middle phalanx distal to the superficialis tendon insertion leaving the digit attached by the intact flexor profundus. Here the extensor tendon is destroyed, the joint damaged, nerves variably avulsed, and the skin sleeve on the degloved segment devascularized over a considerable distance and relies on retrograde fill following arterial reconstitution. Venous flaps may provide a vascularized paddle of skin as well as a segment of a vein to bridge arterial or venous defects.[16] It is evident that the functional potential of these injuries is restricted even if they can be revascularized.

The final stage is complete avulsion/amputation with proximal disruption of the flexor profundus tendon. In the process of disruption, the muscle belly with the tendon is destroyed as it is drawn through the carpal tunnel and presents as a delayed carpal tunnel syndrome. Attempted salvage of these injuries is mainly for cosmetic reasons.

Postoperative Care

Keep the patient warm, hydrated, and pain-free with the limb elevated to avoid vasospasm. Antibiotics are given intravenously for a surgeon-specified period.

Monitoring and Reexploration

In most units still, circulatory monitoring is most reliably done using clinical observation by the experienced nursing staff looking for a change in vascular status. Strict processes for swift escalation of concerns should be in place at a departmental level, to allow for early reexploration. Approximately 10% of cases require take-back. The operated part should be protected by bulky dressing or splint, with great care to avoid constricting on the operated part itself. It must be loose enough to allow for the inevitable swelling but supportive for delicate anastomoses and bony fixation.[17]

Smoking

Every attempt should be made to counsel patients against smoking in the immediate postoperative period. An extensive series of digital replantations demonstrated smoking was associated with a lower success rate (92% vs. 61%), although free flap research has failed to show such equivocal results relating to microvascular complications despite increased wound-healing complications.[18]

Anticoagulation

No consensus exists on the ideal anticoagulation protocol for microsurgery; however, most microsurgeons use prophylactic anticoagulants following replantation, and almost all use direct heparin irrigation at the time of vessel anastomosis. Thrombosis risk is highest within the first 48 hours and decreases to 10% after 72 hours. Ninety percent of arterial thrombi occur within the first 24 hours and usually result from platelet aggregation at the anastomoses. Forty-two percent of venous thrombi occur after 24 hours and usually result from fibrin clotting. Therefore, inhibiting platelet aggregation and thrombin effects as well as decreasing blood viscosity are goals of anticoagulation, and strengthen the argument for heparin and aspirin. In the few prospective studies comparing anticoagulation versus no anticoagulation or aspirin versus heparin, no statistical significance has been shown in microvascular thrombosis or hematoma, and given the risks of troublesome bleeding, many centers do not give heparin.[19] Proton pump inhibitors should be added to postoperative drug regimens including antiplatelet medication to avoid iatrogenic gastric complications. A Cochrane review comparing low molecular weight heparin (LMWH) such as enoxaparin to unfractionated heparin (UFH) showed no differences in success rates of replantation, but a lower risk of postoperative bleeding and hypocoagulability after the use of LMWH.[20]

Rehabilitation

The rehabilitation post replantation is in equal parts unsexy and essential. Indeed, one could argue that without a suitable hand therapy department, transfer of such microsurgical endeavors to appropriate centers is advisable. Therapy should commence as early as possible, once the replanted or transferred digit is viable and the operating team comfortable. Goals of rehabilitation are to increase the range of motion, encourage sensory restoration, and facilitate coordination of the reconstructed hand. Appropriately aggressive rehabilitation decreases secondary procedures for adhesions and stiffness. Digits and thumbs should be splined in slight flexion to favor the flexor repair. A protected gentle active motion should be commenced 4–7 days postoperatively, assuming stable bone fixation — a gradual increase in active and gentle passive exercises over 4–6 weeks to avoid excessive tension. The gentle compression from 3 weeks to control edema is necessary. Introduce sensory reintegration early to maximize sensory return and optimize pain management.

Psychosocial Aspects of Replantation

Early identification and appropriate referral of psychosocial aspects are imperative to the rehabilitation period, most notably for significant amputations of the upper limb where 80% of patients suffer posttraumatic stress disorder and require treatment 6 months after the injury.[21] Also, many patients are of working age and require social work involvement for loss of income and return to work assistance.

Complications

Early

Prolonged ischemia and the "no-reflow" phenomenon: The "no-reflow" phenomenon, first described in association with post cardiac intervention, refers to the clinical observation during replantation that there is no venous outflow despite a patent arterial anastomosis and is a sign of irreversible injury and microcirculatory collapse within the amputated part. Following prolonged ischemia, endothelial cell injury reaches a critical point whereby reperfusion brings activators of prothrombotic cascades which further constrict circulation within the part, eventually obstructing microcirculation and inflow.[18]

Microvascular complications: Recognition of vascular compromise is a learned art and requires instinct and courage to make the demoralizing call to return to theater. While troubleshooting is imperative, not only to avoid unnecessary return but also to understand the underlying cause, it must not delay the expedient return. Salvage rates are directly related to how soon the compromised replant is recognized. Address extrinsic reasons by releasing dressings and sutures. Exclude intrinsic factors with blood pressure optimization, position changes or giving a bolus of heparin.[18]

Late

Infection rates are low and rarely severe. They may be related to leech use (2.4%–20% reported *Aeromonas hydrophilia* infection) and can present with abscess or cellulitis to sepsis. Antibiotic coverage is obligatory. Pin site infection is common, but usually presents later and requires removal of wire.[22] Nonunion is also unusual and along with rotational or angular deformity are attributable to deficient bone stock, poorly vascularized bone and inadequate or poor choice of fixation. Limited range of movement and tendon adhesions are not unsurprising considering the nature of the injury and the total severance of all structures. Early active movement may prove unrealistic but must always be the goal. It depends on the robust repair of structures and primary healing and patient motivation. Internal rigid fixation where possible avoids the risk of K-wires limiting early mobilization because of pain and joint or tendon tethering and infective complications.

Sensory recovery is critical to the overall hand function and is dependent on the nature of injury and age of the patient. In a series of 367 fingers and 87 thumbs, where mean follow-up was 33.5 months only 61% of thumbs and 54% of fingers achieved a useful sensory return. Intermittent cold intolerance is a complaint of the majority of replanted patients.[23]

Thumb Reconstruction

The thumb accounts for approximately 40% of hand function and its loss is devastating. The most basic and valuable form of pollico-digital grip is lateral or key pinch against the radial side of the index. It is secure but relatively imprecise compared to the increasingly sophisticated more distal pulp-to-pulp pinch against the index or both index and middle (tripod or chuck). Finally, nail pinch is the most distal precision pinch and requires flexion of the distal thumb

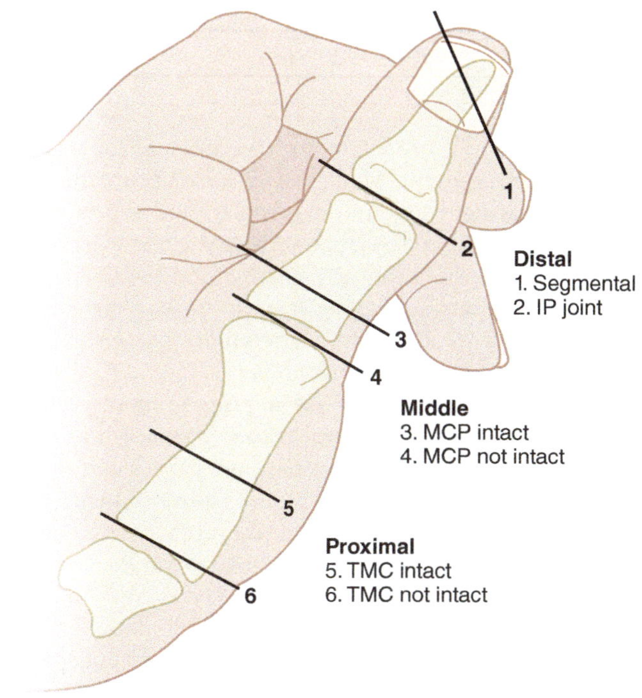

• **Fig. 50.2** Levels of amputation determining reconstructive options.

joint. The anatomical requirements to achieve these radial-sided hand functions have been discussed earlier in this chapter. The principles that guide thumb reconstruction are considerations of length, padded nonshear pulp, sensibility, mobility, stability, and cosmetic issues. Thumb defects are classified according to soft tissue loss or amputations.

- Soft tissue loss
  - Dorsal surface
  - Volar surface
  - Both (degloving)
- Amputation levels (Fig. 50.2)
  - Distal
    - 1. Segmental
    - 2. At the IP joint
  - Middle
    - 3. Distal to MCP
    - 4. MCP joint not intact
  - Proximal
    - 5. Distal to TMC
    - 6. TMC joint not intact

Soft Tissue Loss

Dorsal

Most dorsal injuries can be at least in part grafted with good esthetic and functional results, but exposed bone and joint need flap cover. Options include transposition of proximal phalangeal or distally-based first web skin, de-epithelialized cross-finger flaps and proximally- or retrograde-based first dorsal metacarpal artery flaps (FDMA). However, flaps from the radial side of the index, especially those inclusive of nerve, are unwise as they add insult to injury by denervating and scarring the opposition post for thumb pinch. More substantial defects extending over the first web region may require reverse perforator or free radial artery flaps or posterior interosseous artery flaps.

Volar

The thumb pad is unique for its large area and sophisticated structure and content. Manage small areas of superficial skin loss by allowing the wound to granulate and contract in the hope that it will epithelialize with specialized neighboring glaborous skin. Grafting prevents wound contracture and replaces unique skin leaving it prone to chronic keratosis and fissuring. When grafts are required, harvest from the medial plantar or hypothenar areas.

Full-thickness loss and de-pulping injuries need flap replacement. For small distal defects, because the thumb is broader than fingers, transposition flaps based laterally have a greater arc of rotation for distal advancement.[24] They require grafting to the proximal secondary defect. Alternatively, and for defects 1–1.5 cm, island advancements on single[25] or double neurovascular pedicles with proximal grafting[26] are appropriate, or cross-finger flaps for larger areas still. Where the whole of the distal thumb is depulped, the only satisfactory method of reconstruction is by hemipulp toe transfer because of its large area and uniquely similar sophisticated properties. The only remaining sensory feedback for the damaged thumb is the radial side of the index finger, and so sacrificing radial index finger with kite flaps or equivalent is contraindicated, and in any event, these flaps will not reach the distal thumb.

Neurovascular island flaps[27] from the ring or middle fingers are too small in area and lead to a confusing interpretation of pinch unless the nerve is transferred to the proximal thumb nerve.

Total Degloving

This is the indication par excellence for the wrap-around toe flap method of reconstruction, discussed below.[28]

Amputation Level

Replantation yields the best functional outcome even in the face of extensive damage, but when this is not achievable, reconstruction with like tissue is the aim. The level of amputation dictates the reconstructive options (Table 50.3).

Principles of Reconstruction

Length: The principle that most thumb functions are still possible after the loss of the distal phalanx and that lengthening is not an essential part of the repair is generally accepted. Further bone shortening to achieve stump closure will critically exacerbate the defect so that appropriately chosen flaps must be advanced to preserve length.

The innervated, non-shear, padded pulp: Despite acceptance that length can be compensated for, the soft tissue of the distal thumb is the essence of its function. It is not the length per se that affects function but the loss of this unique tissue. Here lives the thick fingerprinted glabrous skin which traps the sweat for traction grip, and the non-shear, padded fibrofatty pulp, dense with sensory receptors which are stabilized by septa anchoring it to the spatulated distal phalanx tuft. The dorsal nail is an exoskeleton to prevent pulp swivel and a platform which amplifies sensation during pinch via dense sensory receptors in the nail bed. There is no automatic transfer of these pivotal functions to the soft tissue of the proximal phalanx when an amputation occurs. They are lost forever; hand span is shortened, pulp and nail pinch lost, fine sensation dulled and opposition between index finger and thumb contorted for a pinch grip. An absent nail means diminished two-point discrimination, loss of nail pinch, and a cosmetic deformity. It is for these reasons that distal thumb reconstruction using toe replicates, by some measures a luxury, warrants discussion with many patients.

Mobility: The basal joint is essential to positioning the thumb for distal function. One other joint is also necessary, either MCP or IP, for the thumb to passively reach the opposition posts. Otherwise, the thumb is awkward, with undue rigidity of the skeletal column, and it is easily injured. Amputations at or distal to the IP joint are generally considered adequate for most functions and do not need lengthening as discussed. Fortunately, thumb amputations rarely involve the basal joint so that the assessment of what type of reconstructions are suitable to depend on the integrity of the metacarpophalangeal joint. If this is intact, then a joint is not essential to the reconstruction plan. Here bone lengthening by distraction or osteoplastic graft are feasible considerations. If the amputation is at or proximal to the MCP joint, then a joint should be ideally included with the reconstruction. This limits options to pollicization or toe transfer. It goes without saying that if the base of the proximal phalanx is present, it is sacrosanct and must not be removed at primary surgery to facilitate direct stump closure. For the rare proximal and basal joint level injuries pollicization and second toe transfers are the only techniques likely to restore function significantly.

Stability: A short stable thumb is preferable to a long unstable one. The fusion of either the MCP or IP joint is acceptable but ideally not both. Reconstructions usually suffer from stiffness rather than instability but multijointed second toes or pollicizations may need intrinsic tendon reconstitution to prevent collapse deformities.

Cosmesis: The thumb is a significant cosmetic aspect of the hand, visible in the natural midprone habitat and conspicuous during all fine manipulative actions. To some, the deformity is as much an issue as the loss of function. Toe tissue has unparalleled functional and esthetic similarities with the thumb. Despite this, performing a technically challenging, lengthy, and risky operation with potential donor morbidity for a perceived small injury leads to a justifiable hesitance in surgeons and patients. Patients with strong esthetic concerns, demanding

TABLE 50.3 **Amputation Levels and Suggested Hierarchy of Reconstructive Procedures**

	Level	Objective	Options in Order of Senior Author's Preference
Distal	Segmental	Predominantly cosmetic	Local homodigital flaps Cross-finger flaps If substantial, is also ideal for segmental matching pulp or pulp/nail/bone composite toe flap
	IP joint	Predominantly cosmetic	Local flaps to preserve residual length with good function. Can consider wrap-around flap for lengthening and nail reconstruction. No bone graft required
Middle	MCP intact Amputation through the proximal phalanx	No joint required	Wrap-around flap with short iliac bone graft (functional and cosmetic) Trimmed toe, distraction lengthening of metacarpal, or other osteoplastic methods (tubed skin around bone graft with neurovascular island flap from ring – poor functional results) Hemipulp free neurovascular flap from the big toe for larger pad and greater stability
	MCP not intact At or proximal to the MCP joint	Requires a joint. May require skin flap	Pollicization (especially if index finger damaged) Whole toe transfer (hallux) Trimmed toe if through the joint or distal metacarpal Pollicization or second toe with metatarsal bone for more proximal amputations; patient preference
Proximal	TMC intact	Needs preliminary or simultaneous skin flap cover, metatarsal lengthening ± tendon transfers	Pollicization or second toe transfer
	TMC not intact		Fuse the basal joint or reconstitute it with the MCP joint of the index (pollicization) or a stemmed silicone joint prosthesis (Swanson type) stemmed into the scaphoid proximally and metatarsal shaft distally if second toe is chosen. Finger or toe long and short tendons are brought for stabilization and functional transfers

functional requirements, and who have the discipline required for postoperative rehabilitation are suitable candidates for toe transfer.

Distal Thumb Reconstruction

(1) *Distal to the IP joint/segmental*: Retain length by soft tissue flap closure of the stump with flaps as suggested above for soft tissue only injuries.

(2) *At the IP joint*: As discussed above, extra length per se is not required, and local flap closure is acceptable provided there is no further bone shortening. Whole phalangeal and segmental distal phalangeal loss including a portion of the nail are well suited to reconstruction with toe replicates for the reasons mentioned above and with minimal donor site morbidity but for these distal defects most patients will reasonably shirk from such suggestions and accept more conservative closures.

Mid-thumb Reconstruction

(3) *MCP joint intact (distal to the base of the proximal phalanx)*: This is the most commonly encountered thumb amputation requiring reconstruction. If the MCP joint is intact, then the reconstruction does not require an added joint so that simple bone graft skeleton and soft tissue cover (osteoplastic) are theoretically appropriate. Here the key to satisfactory reconstruction is a well-padded, stable, and innervated pulp. Without an IP joint, the skeleton should be designed shorter than the original, but bone grafts will be prone to resorption because of poor vascularity. The soft tissue sleeve cover must be non-swivel and pedicled forearm, or free flaps cannot achieve this aim. Furthermore, the volar surface must be innervated, and neurovascular island pulp flaps from the fingers[27] are small in size and difficult to cortically reorientate. The only satisfactory way to stabilize and innervate this soft tissue sleeve is with a toe hemi-pulp which will anchor to the bone graft and reinnervate appropriately following nerve repair. If it is accepted that this is the minimum that is required to restore function, then it is not a great leap to convert this pulp transfer to the "wrap-around" flap procedure which brings with it the nail and a portion of toe nail–distal phalanx complex. This vascularized bone from the toe reduces the length of required interposition iliac crest bone graft (maximum 2 cm), prevents bone graft resorption and stabilizes the pulp. The soft tissue sleeve from the toe replicates the missing thumb cosmetically and functionally, and the skeleton is shaped to ensure size match with the

opposite thumb. The toe defect is closed by folding the remaining medial skin flap around the tip and a cross-toe flap from the dorsum of the second toe. The dorsal defect is skin grafted. Some advocate trimmed toe transfer[29] as an alternative procedure for this level injury, but it is essentially a whole toe transfer with a primary cosmetic reduction; it sacrifices the whole toe, the avoidance of which being the primary rationale for the wrap-around flap.

(4) *MCP joint not intact (at or proximal to the MCP joint)*: This level amputation ideally needs a new joint so that osteoplastic procedures including the wrap-around are no longer options. Whole toes, including the Trimmed toe technique which retains a joint, or pollicization are appropriate.

Proximal Thumb Reconstruction

(5,6) *Trapezio-metacarpal (TMC) joint intact AND (6) TMC joint not intact*: Such injuries are often associated with major damage to the web region, including thenar and interosseous intrinsic muscles and adjacent digits. Salvage will likely require initial generous flap cover anticipating pollicization or toe and metatarsal inset and first web reconstruction. Again, it is critical to retain any potentially mobile basal joint remnants at primary surgery. Depending on the retained length of the metacarpal, distal reconstructions may be managed in the same way as in (4) above, but may need bone grafts for lengthening. The hallux transfer can include a sliver of the dorsal aspect of the metatarsophalangeal (MTP) joint, including the collateral ligaments, but the plantar bony platform is sacrosanct. This adds length to the transfer usually sufficient to avoid an extra bone graft, otherwise select the second toe with its metatarsophalangeal joint and shaft or index pollicization, which has ample bone length. For the most proximal levels, which include the basal joint and thenar muscles, index pollicization is attractive because of the potential for its MTP joint to become the basal thumb joint. Unlike in the congenital 4-finger hand, however, where the first dorsal interosseous muscle becomes the new abductor, these motors are unlikely to be functional in this proximal injury so that the second toe with its metatarsal and multiple tendons for stabilization is probably a less morbid solution. As stated above, frequently proximal and/or first web skin cover will be needed in association with the digital transfer and it is essential that with toes no skin is taken from the foot proximal to the level of the first web to avoid morbid skin grafting over the working parts of the foot, especially the MTP joint region. A separate islanded dorsal foot flap more proximal on the same vascular pedicle leaving the distal foot skin intact is acceptable. Otherwise, the hand skin deficiency should be addressed by other means. Whether the hallux or a second toe is chosen is the patient's and surgeon's choice. The second toe is less morbid to the foot but has a more inferior function and distinctly poorer cosmesis.

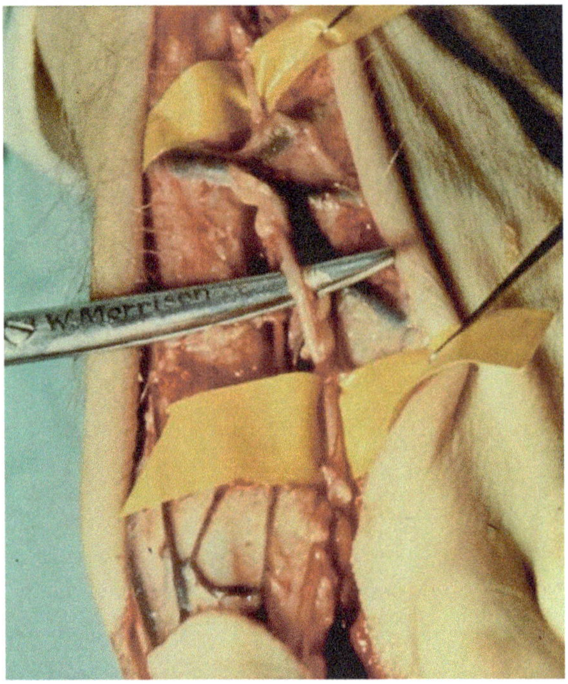

• **Fig. 50.3** Dorsal dissection showing dorsalis pedis/dorsal metatarsal artery and dorsal venous system. (Courtesy Professor Wayne AJ Morrison.)

Toe Transfer Technique

Whole Toes

The ipsilateral hallux and contralateral second toe are chosen so that the first dorsal metatarsal vascular pedicle neatly courses through the first web region of the hand towards the dominant ulnar artery of the thumb or more proximally to the snuff-box region. All toes and toe segments are ideally transferred on their dorsal arterial and venous system (Fig. 50.3).

The dorsal metatarsal artery extending from the dorsalis pedis may be superficial, within the interosseous muscle or occasionally absent in which case the plantar arterial system is dominant and must be used. Access to this vessel is then limited so that it is generally shorter and will need vein grafting to reach the snuff-box, the preferred site for anastomosis.

Incisions for whole toes are racket-shape design at the level of the web, the handle extending proximally in a straight line over the first intermetatarsal space to assess the dorsal arterial and venous systems. No skin should be included with the toe proximal to the level of the web to avoid long-term morbidity from skin grafts (Fig. 50.4). The metatarsal artery is best identified initially at the first web space level to confirm its presence and the site of bifurcation to each toe. Clip the digital branch to the second toe for hallux transfer and the vice versa for the second toe as is the plantar

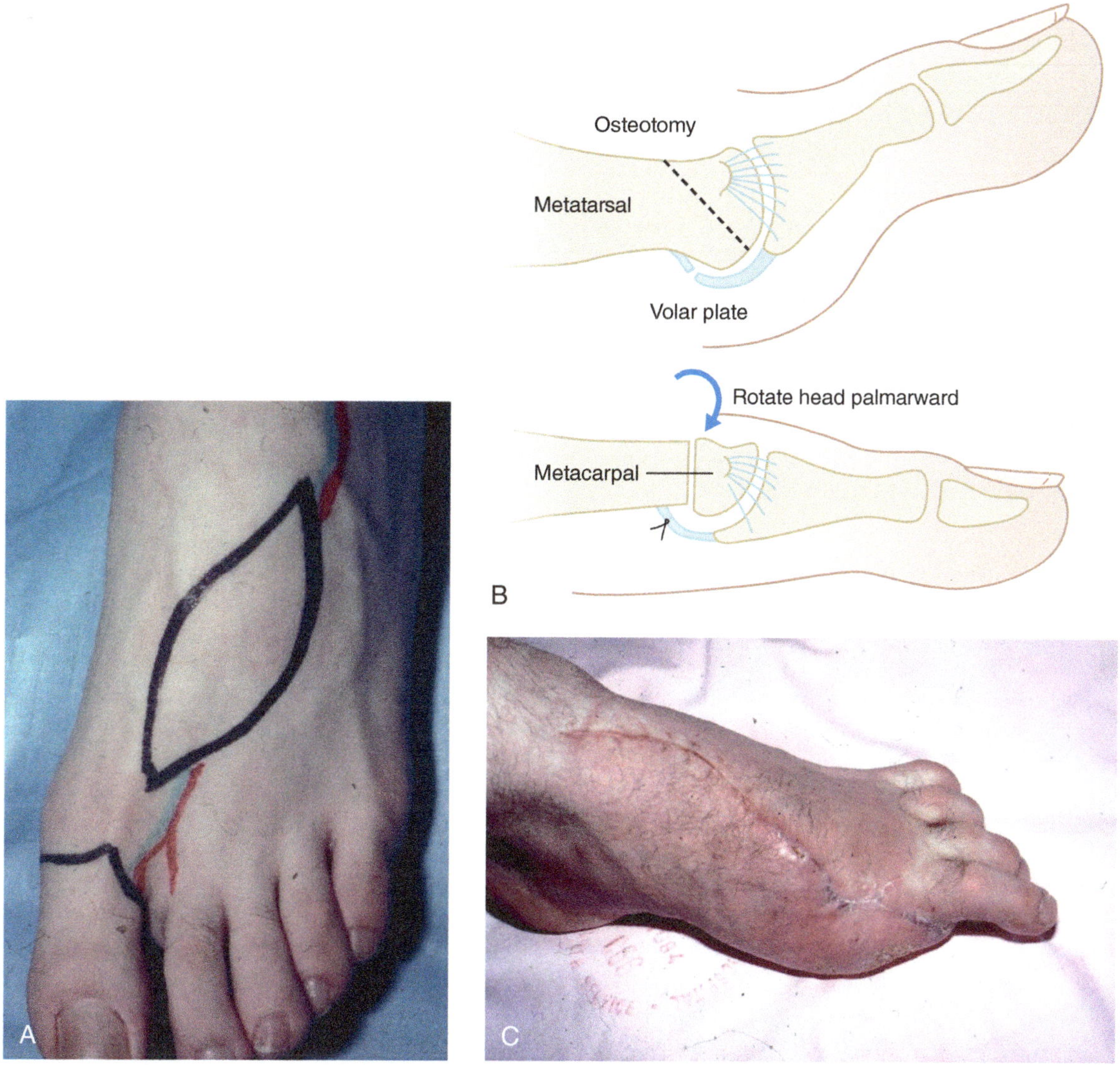

• **Fig. 50.4** (A) Incisions for whole toe preserving the skin over the metatarsophalangeal joint. If extra skin is required a separate conservative island of skin overlying the same dorsalis pedis vascular pedicle can be safely taken and the defect grafted. (B) Oblique osteotomy to include a functional component of the MTP joint and facilitate skin closure. (C) Standard skin closure with good flap cover over MTP joint. (A and C, Courtesy Professor Wayne AJ Morrison.)

extension into the sole. With the hallux an oblique osteotomy of the metatarsal head preserving the plantar platform but including the collateral ligaments allows a functioning MTP joint to be included with the transfer although its range of movement is small. It also extends the length of the skeleton and facilitates foot skin closure. When the second toe is taken it usually includes the MTP joint, so the distal metatarsal is resected to narrow the foot gap. An osteotomy of the metatarsal head angled volarly and the shortening the plantar plate will convert the mainly extended second MTP joint into a useful flexed position. Take both digital nerves as proximally as possible and tendons chosen according to need. Close the skin directly.

Hemi-pulps

The lateral half of the hallux from the web space proximally to the tip can be harvested simply without significant morbidity. The distal limit of the flap should not extend to the very tip to preserve protective padded pulp at this site. The key to the dissection is to be sure to include veins in the flap. The flap design should be moved more proximally into the web if need be to maximize the capture of veins. The same arterial and venous anatomy applies as for whole toes, but the same pedicle length may not be needed. Raise the flap as for neurovascular island flaps in the hand, but care must be taken to avoid damage to the artery at the point where a large and constant branch arising just proximal to the IP joint passes under the volar plate supplying joint and the vincular system. The defect is closed partially by direct suture and the remainder with a split-thickness skin graft.

Wrap-around Flap

The flap is designed to deglove the whole of the big toe except for a medial skin bridge which extends along the

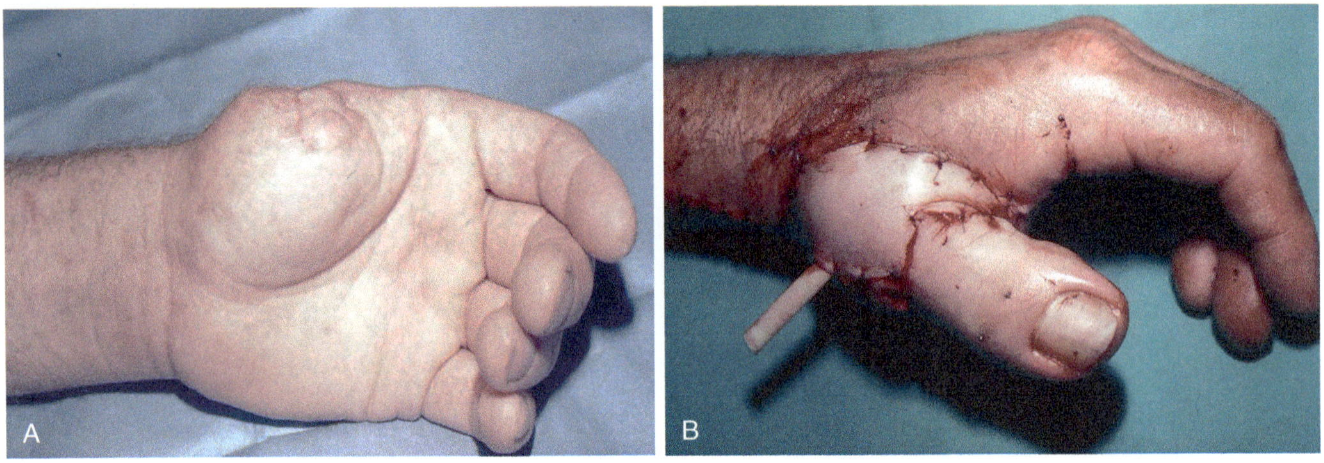

• **Fig. 50.5** (A) Pre and (B) post great toe transfer with islanded dorsal foot flap for proximal skin cover. (Courtesy Professor Wayne AJ Morrison.)

medial border of the toe and around the toe tip (Fig. 50.5). The width of this medial flap is the difference between the circumference of the opposite thumb and that of the toe. The ipsilateral toe is chosen so that the dominant ulnar neurovascular pedicle of the thumb will align with the dominant lateral vessels of the toe and the seam closure of the flap around the bone graft will be on the nonworking radial side of the new thumb. The proximal limit of the flap design in the foot is to the level of the web and plantar crease and no more.

The dorsal arterial and venous systems are defined, and the dorsal skin then elevated taking care to include its venous system but preserving the underlying extensor tendon paratenon. At the point of termination of the extensor the proximal limit of the germinal matrix is identified and carefully elevated subperiosteally with the dorsal skin flap to the level of the eponychial fold (sterile matrix level). Elevate the plantar pulp flap from the flexor sheath, and distal phalanx as opening a book, and the exposed phalanx is osteotomized at the level of the eponychial fold (approximately mid phalanx). The toe flap with its composite nail and distal half of the distal phalanx remains attached by its vessels and nerves (Fig. 50.6). Do not include tendon or joint. Divide the nerves as proximally as needed and the tourniquet is released to ensure that the flap vascularizes before it is removed for transfer. Spasm is common, and vascularization can be delayed. An iliac bone graft is harvested, which is tricortical. The maximum length required should be no more than 2.5–3 cm if the procedure is limited to amputations distal to an intact MCP joint as it is interposed between the proximal phalanx base and the toe distal phalanx. The design length should be deliberately shorter than the original because no joint is included. The volume of the bone graft must fill the cavity of the flap sleeve to achieve the best esthetic appearance. It must be considerably larger in diameter than the natural phalanges (unlike in the original description) to compensate for the absence of flexor and extensor tendon bulk. The bones are fixed with axial and crossed K-wires and the skin flap wrapped around the skeleton and loosely sutured. The vessels are anastomosed and nerves repaired. The toe defect is closed by folding the medial tip flap around the shortened phalanx, the plantar surface closed with a cross-toe flap from the dorsum of the second toe, and the remaining exposed big and second toes grafted (Figs. 50.7 and 50.8).

There is inherent discrepancy between normal great toe two-point discrimination (2PD) and thumb (12 mm vs. 3 mm), however sensory re-education is possible with some patients reportedly achieving up to 4 mm 2PD (average of 10 mm) upon toe transfer.[30] There has been no discernible difference in 2PD between methods of toe transfer. However, replanted thumb 2PD is statistically better than toe transfer (mean 8.8 mm vs. 10 mm).[30] The same review records toe transfers achieving 75% pinch strength and 70% grip strength compared to the contralateral hand, although this will depend almost entirely on the residual basal joint function rather than the method of reconstruction which simply lengthens the thumb ray to enable it to engage with an opposition post. When compared with other forms of thumb reconstruction via M2-DASH scores, second toe transfer performed best at 8.32 when compared to free lateral arm osteocutaneous flap (19.44), pollicization (31.01), and no reconstruction (32.77). A systematic review comparing outcomes between four methods of toe transfer (second, great, wraparound, trimmed) no statistical difference in survival, motion, grip, pinch or 2PD were noted.[30]

Ultimately the decision whether to reconstruct a thumb and the type of reconstruction is based on the patient's perception of disability and willingness to commit to further surgery, especially the risks of further morbidity with toe tissue transfers. In children, growth requirements preclude bone graft techniques so that toe or pollicizations are needed. The ability for nerve regeneration underpins microvascular reconstruction and precludes the elderly from a complete functional recovery. Compensating for loss of length by web space deepening is sometimes an appropriate reconstruction in the elderly.[31]

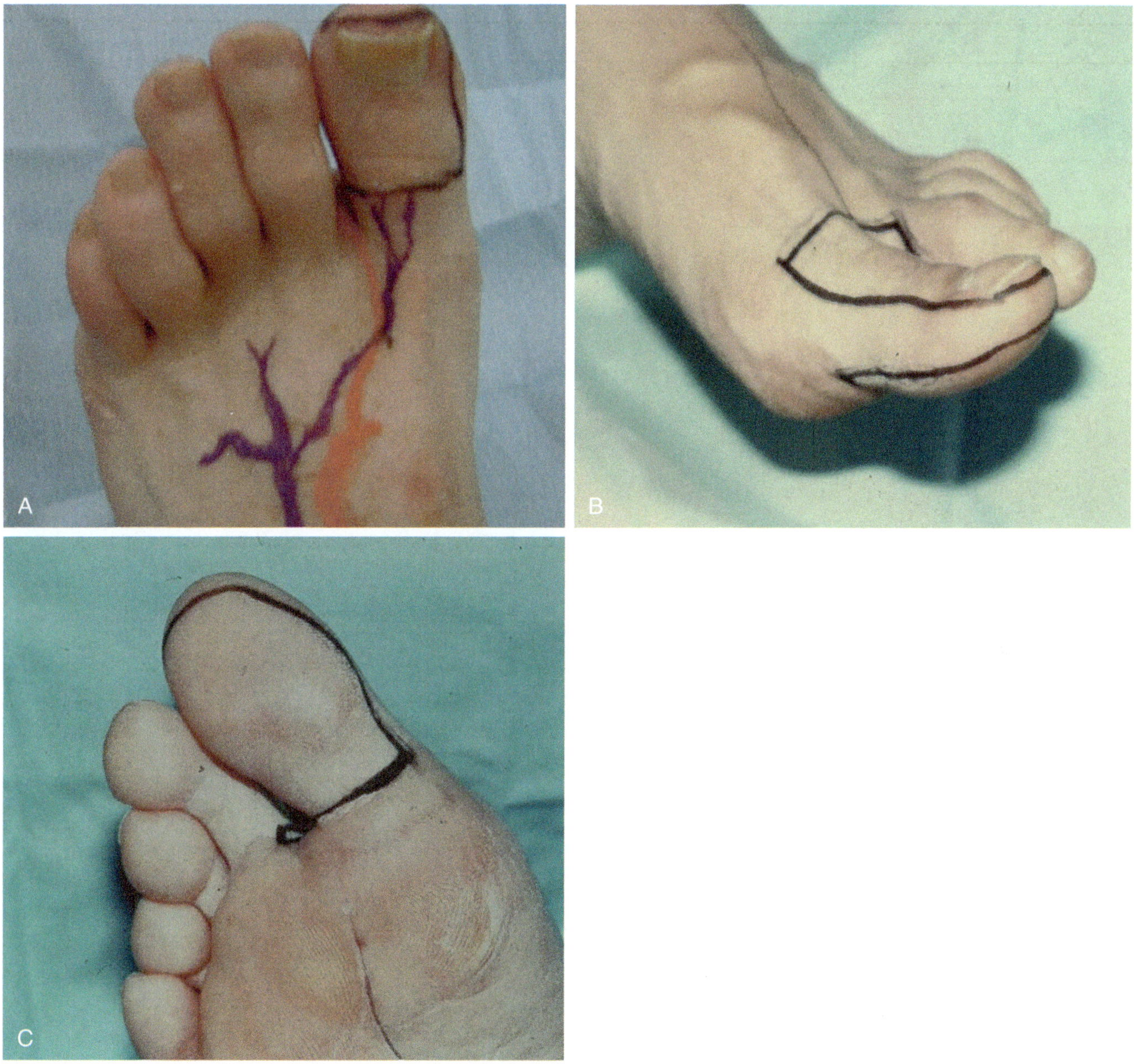

• **Fig. 50.6** (A) Dorsal, (B) medial, and (C) plantar skin markings of wrap-around flap. (Courtesy Professor Wayne AJ Morrison.)

Distraction Lengthening

Distraction osteogenesis is a method of increasing the first metacarpal length by up to 3 cm. Matev[32] independently and unaware of the Ilizarov technique devised a lengthening device held in place by transfixion wires proximal and distal to a subperiosteal metacarpal osteotomy. By rotating a bridging screw, the patient self-distracts the osteotomy up to 1 mm per day until the desired length is obtained. The fixator remains for a further 4 months or until visualization of trabeculae signifying radiological union appears. Bone grafting may still be required in older patients or if the gap is more substantial than 3 cm. Potential complications include pin-track infection, loosening, nonunion, and flexion deformity at the expense of lengthening due to tethering of the volar soft tissue and ligamentous restraints, especially if a remnant of the MCP joint remains. A standard limitation is the thinning of the distal thumb stump skin and soft tissue with increasing tension which may require a more complex padded flap cover. No joint is created so that it is rigid and clumsy, but unlike osteoplastic lengthening, the sensation is retained.

Pollicization

Pollicization, the movement of a finger, usually the index, into the position of the thumb, is classically indicated when the index itself has been partially injured. It involves isolating the digit on its neurovascular pedicle and transposing it onto the thumb stump. Even more so than toes, it is uniquely appropriate for digital reconstruction. Depending on the level of amputation the index is osteotomized to match the missing thumb length. The proximal phalanx becomes the metacarpal, and the middle and distal phalanges become

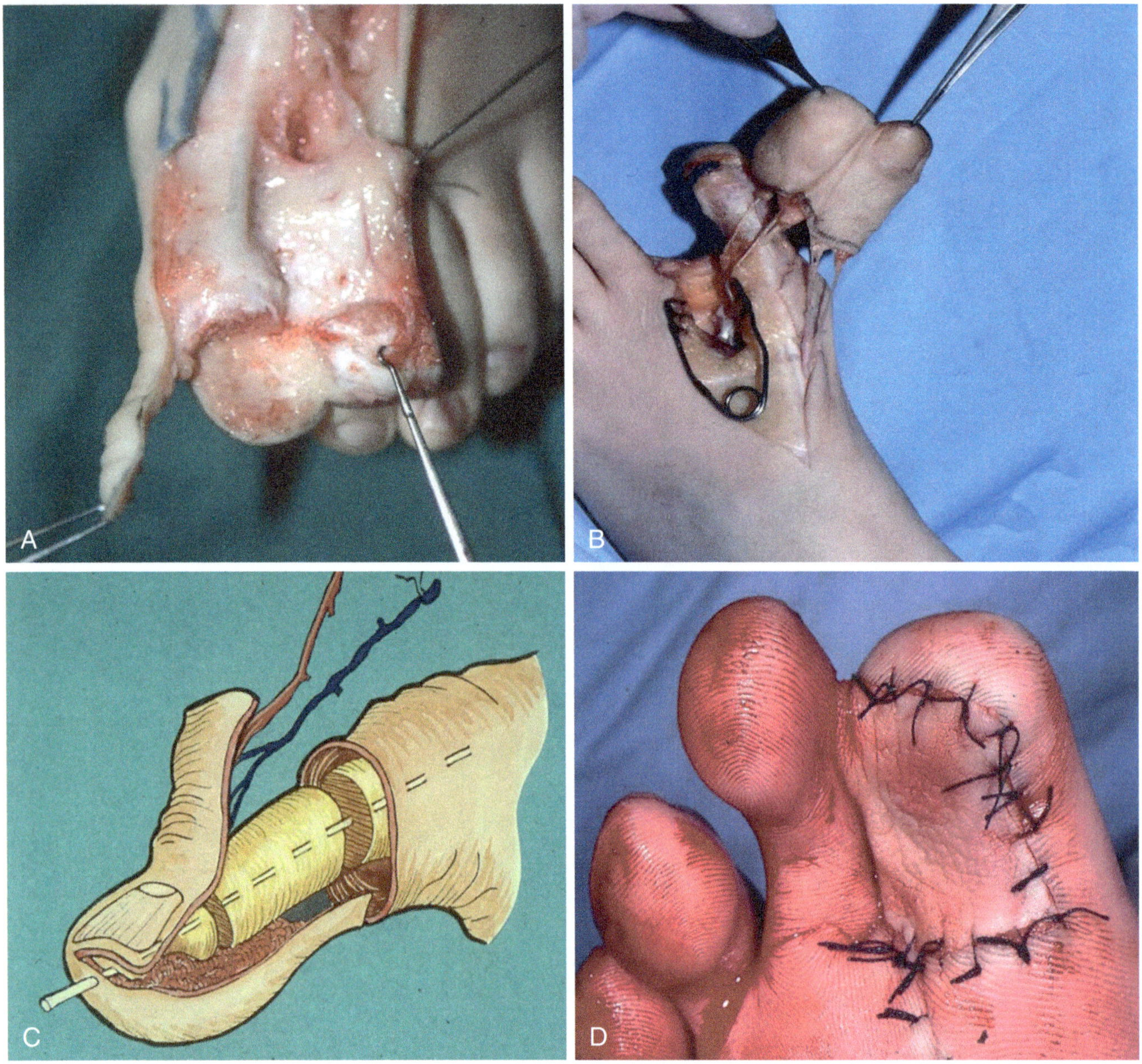

• **Fig. 50.7** Wrap-around toe technique. (A,B) Distal half of the distal phalanx remains attached with nerve and vessels. (C) Schematic of composite flap. (D) Plantar donor surface closed with a cross-toe flap from the second toe. (Courtesy Professor Wayne AJ Morrison.)

the proximal and distal thumb phalanges. For basal joint injuries, the MCP joint of the finger becomes the new trapeziometacarpal joint. If the distal phalanx has been amputated on the index, the remaining phalanges transpose to become the thumb counterparts. If the thumb amputation is proximal to the MCP joint then the index MCP will be included with the transfer; if the MCP of the thumb is intact, then the index is osteotomized through the proximal part of the proximal phalanx. The index metacarpal head is an integral part of pronation grip strength and when not used in the thumb reconstruction should be left intact rather than shaving it down for merely cosmetic reasons. Reconstructing a thumb by sacrificing another digit is often anathema to the patient, and transfer of the ring finger can be more palatable, less functionally debilitating and is more convincing cosmetically as a thumb. Its venous drainage may not reach the thumb without division and reanastomosis. Tendons lengths are adjusted or transferred to their thumb counterparts while the nerves are traditionally left intact. This will lead to confusion and particularly if the ring is chosen it is preferable to transfer its nerves to those of the proximal thumb. Depending on levels often a large skin flap is needed to facilitate inset of the finger.

Pollicization is functionally useful with high patient satisfaction, return to work, 75% average grip strength compared to contralateral hand, and 2PD from 4–6 mm.[30]

Phalangization

Phalangization is the deepening of the first web space, often in association with removal of remnant second metacarpal bone to accommodate objects in an adductor type grasp. It is indicated for amputations through the distal half of the

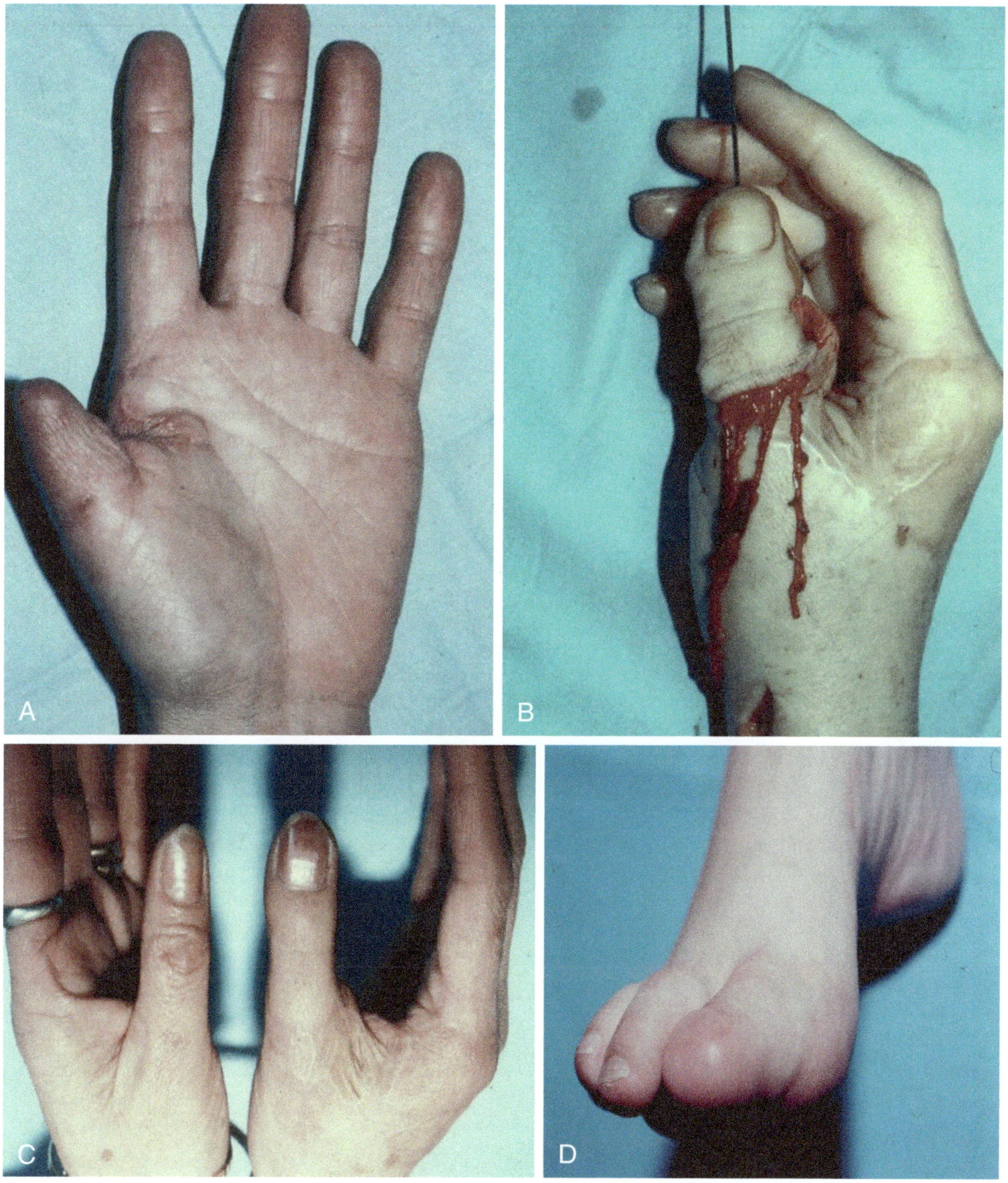

• **Fig. 50.8** Wrap-around flap to reconstruct thumb defect. (A) Preoperative. (B) Intraoperative. (C) Postoperative. (D) Toe defect. (Courtesy Professor Wayne AJ Morrison.)

middle third of the thumb in selected patients unable or unwilling to undergo a more major reconstruction. Requirements include a mobile first metacarpal base and some functioning thenar muscle/adductor function. Although no bone length is gained a functional space is created in the first web with minimal morbidity via simple two-flap, four-flap or jumping-man type Z-plasty technique. When extensive scarring is present, locoregional flaps can be used such as the dorsal hand or reverse radial forearm flap. The first dorsal interosseous muscle can be released, as well as the proximal transfer of the insertion of the adductor pollicis for additional deepening, but this will weaken the potential adductor power. Phalangization may be combined with distraction lengthening to gain absolute length to the thumb.[30]

Web Space Reconstruction

The first web space is vital for full thumb function and is often involved in proximal thumb injuries resulting in debilitating contracture. Classically presenting as an adducted, supinated thumb metacarpal with metacarpophalangeal joint flexion, Sandzen's classification[33] described mild, moderate, and severe contracture. Mild contractures involve skin only, moderate involve the skin and partial damage to underlying structures, and severe contractures involve the skin, muscle, and joint capsule. Correction potentially involves serial release of all layers of the web from skin, dorsal, and palmar fascia, muscles and or joint capsule. Remember all these layers when undertaking formal release. Contracture of adductor pollicis, flexor pollicis brevis or first dorsal

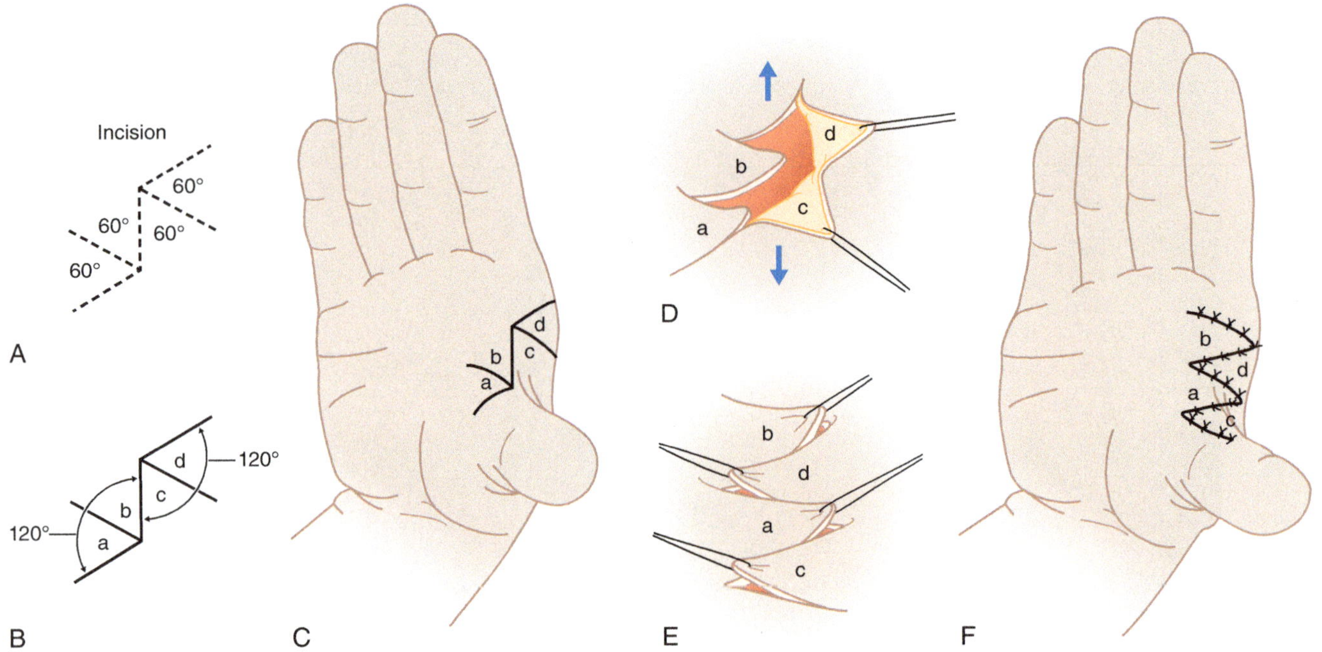

• **Fig. 50.9** Different Z-plasty technique to improve web space contracture. (Modified from Woolf RM, Broadbent TR. The four-flap Z-plasty. *Plast Reconstr Surg.* 1972;49:48–51.)

interosseous muscles requires a release from their origin or insertion and tendon lengthening techniques. Once the complete release is achieved, the often underestimated soft tissue defect requires resurfacing. Skin grafts are inappropriate due to their eagerness to contract. Mild contractures can be managed with Z-plasty variants (Fig. 50.9). Moderate contractures necessitate local flap options including dorsal hand rotation flaps with or without secondary grafting; severe contractures require pedicled radial or posterior interosseous perforator flaps or thin free flaps such as a radial artery or lateral arm. Foot first web space flaps should never be taken in conjunction with a toe transfer for reasons previously discussed. Groin flaps are advocated but are usually too bulky except in children and continually adapt to the patient's dietary habits.[34]

Metacarpal Hand

Metacarpal hand is the term used where both thumb and all digits are lost and only metacarpal stumps remain. Less destructive injuries may spare whole or partial digits and the deformity is then referred to as the mutilated hand. The principles of reconstruction of both are essentially the same as those discussed above for assessing multiple digit amputations for replantation. The core elements of essential hand function are three digits, the most important of which is the thumb, whose basal joint should be intact.[35] A spared thumb basal joint and some thenar motor remnants are the key to potentially useful reconstructive possibilities and must be protected at primary surgery with conservative debridement and generous flap cover. The priority aim is to restore radial (pollico-digital) pinch and if possible the ulnar-sided functions of palmar (pollico-digital) grip and breadth of palm. Reconstructions require length, mobility, sensation, and stability. These can only be realistically furnished from digital transfer from the foot and/or the opposite hand. The radial thumb needs basal joint mobility, length sufficient to engage with an opposition post, and innervation for sensory feedback. Stability is also vital for surety of pinch. The new thumb should, therefore, be shorter than the original and provided there is some remnant metacarpal, the big toe is the ideal to meet these needs; it is innervated and short, broad, and relatively stiff for stability. Its long tendons are sutured to flexor and extensor pollicis longus respectively and extensor hallucis brevis to abductor pollicis longus. An opponensplasty may be required if the basal joint is mobile, but no active motors remain. If the basal joint is absent or stiff, then the toe base should be fused, usually via a lengthening bone graft, in the fully abducted and opposed position and movement will then rely purely on flexion and extension of its two distal joints. The toe may be powered by as many synergistic tendons as are available rather than the original single flexor and extensor recipient tendons to maximize the range of movement and power of the thumb. In the case of very proximal bone loss with trapezium, it is preferable to use a second toe with its metacarpal to achieve the desired thumb length rather than the more challenging bone graft and hallux, but this limits donor options for finger reconstruction.

The opposition post/s for radial pinch should also be innervated, short, and stable, and the second toe fits these requirements unlike those of the ulnar side where length and mobility are key to full flexion into the palm. The toe will come with its MTP joint and metacarpal shaft and is oriented so that the central/radial aspect of the pulp will oppose the flexed thumb. Its equivalent long tendons motorize it. Ideally, if the thumb can retropose (extensor pollicis longus function) and abduct, then it will also be able to reproduce a degree of lateral pinch against the side of the second toe as well as an end-to-end pinch. "Radial tripod" pinch involves three digits coming together as the chuck in a drill, which greatly increases the stability of grip by reducing swivel as is prone to occur when only two digits oppose, especially end on. It is challenging to convince patients to sacrifice one toe let alone potentially three, but three-point pinch is the ideal. If two second toes are an option, then they are best taken from opposite feet as the toes require metatarsal extensions and taking two adjacent metatarsals from the same foot causes significant deformity and risks long-term morbidity. The question then arises where should these toes be sited in the hand. If two second toes are available, they are best sited as a pair on the original index and middle metacarpals, but a similar argument can be made for their positioning on the middle and ring rays in an attempt to gain both radial pinch and a component of ulnar grip. If only one, then it should be more central in the hand on the middle ray.

The ulnar palmar–digital grip cannot be achieved from second toes because of their inadequate flexion range and consequent open palm, but they do present a broader platform to hold and balance objects in the supinated hand. The ring finger from the opposite hand leaves relatively little disability and sited on the middle ray is the only realistic way of restoring true palmar grip to the metacarpal hand. It can equally function as a radial opposition post for a pinch (Fig. 50.10).[36]

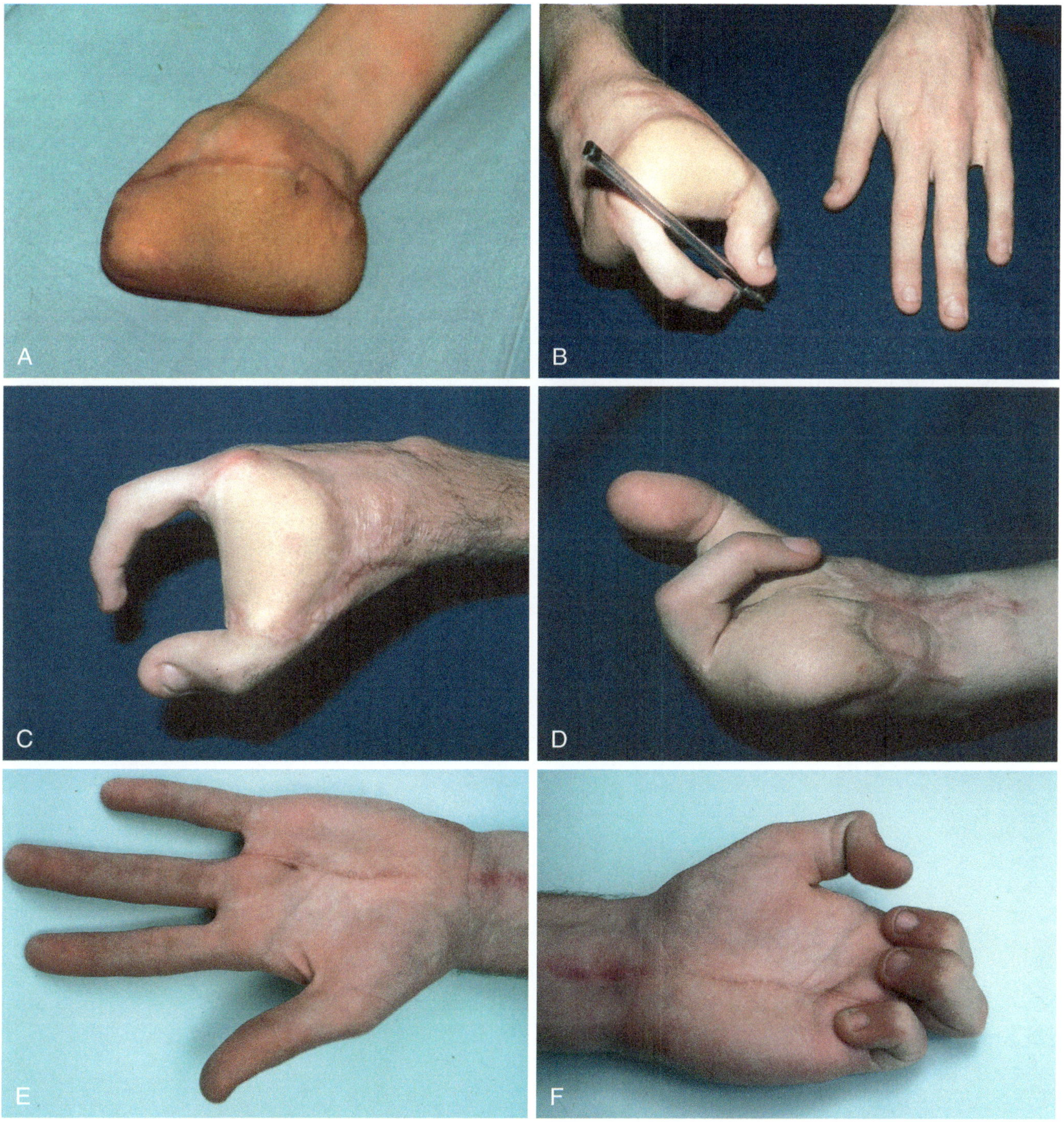

• **Fig. 50.10** (A–D) Cross-hand ring finger transfer combined with hallux for reconstruction of radial and ulnar sided functions. (E,F) Secondary defect in the opposite hand. (Courtesy Professor Wayne AJ Morrison.)

References

1. Jacobson JH, Suarez EL. Microsurgery in anastomosis of small vessels. *Surg Forum*. 1960;11:243.
2. Kleinert HE, Kasdan ML. Anastamosis of digital vessels. *J Ky Med Assoc*. 1965;63:106–108.
3. Komatsu S, Tamai S. Successful replantation of a completely cut-off thumb: case report. *Plast Reconstr Surg*. 1968;142:374–377.
4. Lin CH, Aydyn N, Lin YT, et al. Hand and finger replantation after protracted ischemia (more than 24 hours). *Ann Plast Surg*. 2010;64:286–290.
5. Li J, Guo Z, Zhu Q, et al. Fingertip replantation: determinants of survival. *Plast Reconstr Surg*. 2008;122:833–839.
6. Yu H, Wei L, Liang B, et al. Nonsurgical factors of digital replantation and survival rate: a metaanalysis. *Indian J Orthop*. 2015;49:265–271.
7. Lee SW, Lee DC, Kim JS, et al. Analysis of bone fixation methods in digital replantation. *Arch Plast Surg*. 2017;44(1):53–58.
8. Morrison WA, McCombe D. Digital replantation. *Hand Clin*. 2007;23:1–12.
9. Aksoy A, Gungor M, Sir E. Fingertip replantation without and with palmar venous anastomosis: analysis of the survival rates and vein distribution. *Ann Plast Surg*. 2017;78(10):62–66.
10. Tang JB, Wang ZT, Chen J, et al. A global view of digital replantation and revascularization. *Clin Plast Surg*. 2017;44:189–209.
11. Chim H, Maricevich MA, Carlsen BT, et al. Challenges in replantation of complex amputations. *Semin Plast Surg*. 2013;27:182–189.
12. Soucacos PN, Beris AE, Malizos KN, et al. Transpositional microsurgery in multiple digital amputations. *Microsurgery*. 1994;15:469–473.
13. Kay S, Werntz J, Wolff TW. Ring avulsion injuries: classification and prognosis. *J Hand Surg Am*. 1989;14:204–213.
14. Adani R, Castagnetti C, Busa R, et al. Ring avulsion injuries: microsurgical management. *J Reconstr Microsurg*. 1996;12:189–194.
15. Urbaniak JR, Evans JP, Bright DS. Microvascular management of ring avulsion injuries. *J Hand Surg Am*. 1981;6:25–30.
16. Bamba R, Malhotra G, Bueno RA, et al. Ring avulsion injuries: a systematic review. *Hand*. 2018;13:15–22.
17. Buncke Jr HJ. Microvascular hand surgery – transplants and replants – over the past 25 years. *J Hand Surg*. 2000;45:415–428.
18. Shores JT, Andrew Lee WP. Microsurgical complications in the upper extremity. *Hand Clini*. 2010;26:291–301.
19. Levin LS, Cooper EO. Clinical use of anticoagulants following replantation surgery. *J Hand Surg Am*. 2008;33:1437–1439.
20. Chen YC, Chi CC, Chan FC, et al. Low molecular weight heparin for prevention of microvascular occlusion in digital replantation. *Cochrane Database Syst Rev*. 2013;7:CD009894.
21. Solarz MK, Thoder JJ, Rehman S. Management of major traumatic upper extremity amputations. *Orthoped Clin North Am*. 2016;47:127–136.
22. Woo SH, Kim YW, Cheon HJ, et al. Management of complications relating to finger amputation and replantation. *Hand Clin*. 2015;31:319–338.
23. Glickman LT, Mackinnon SE. Sensory recovery following digital replantation. *Microsurgery*. 1990;11:236–242.
24. Hueston J. Local flap repair in finger tip injuries. *Plast Reconstr Surg*. 1966;2:261–277.
25. Venkataswami R, Subramanian N. Oblique triangular flap: a new method of repair for oblique amputations of the fingertip and thumb. *Plast Reconstr Surg*. 1980;66:296–300.
26. O'Brien B. Neurovascular island pedicled flaps for terminal amputation and digital scars. *Br J Plast Surg*. 1968;21:258–261.
27. Littler J. Neurovascular pedicle method of digital transposition for reconstruction of the thumb. *Plast Reconstr Surg*. 1953;12:303–319.
28. Morrison WA, O'Brien BM, MacLeod AM. Thumb reconstruction with a free neurovascular wrap-around flap from the big toe. *J Hand Surg Am*. 1980;5:575–583.
29. Wei FC, el-Gammal TA, Lin CH, et al. Metacarpal hand: classification and guidelines for microsurgical reconstruction with toe transfers. *Plast Reconstr Surg*. 1997;99(1):122–128.
30. Graham DJ, Venkatramani H, Sabapathy SR. Current reconstruction options for traumatic thumb loss. *J Hand Surg*. 2016;41:1159–1169.
31. Morrison WA. Thumb reconstruction: a review and philosophy of management. *J Hand Surg (Br Eur. Vol)*. 1992:383–390.
32. Matev IB. Thumb reconstruction through metacarpal bone lengthening. *J Hand Surg Am*. 1980;5:482–487.
33. Sandzén Jr SC. Thumb web reconstruction. *Clin Orthop Relat Res*. 1985;195:66–82.
34. Moody L, Galvez MG, Chang J. Reconstruction of first web space contractures. *J Hand Surg*. 2015;40:1892–1895.
35. del Piñal F. Severe mutilating injuries to the hand: guidelines for organizing the chaos. *J Plast Reconstr Aesthet Surg*. 2007;60:816–827.
36. Morrison WA, O'Brien BM, MacLeod AM. Ring finger transfer in reconstruction of transmetacarpal amputations. *J Hand Surg Am*. 1984;9:4–11.

51 Compartment Syndrome in the Extremities

STEVEN E.R. HOVIUS AND TIM H.J. NIJHUIS

Introduction

Compartment syndrome in either upper or lower extremity is often underestimated and may have detrimental consequences for functioning of the involved extremity. Muscle groups in the extremities are separated by fascial sheaths to ensure that muscles move in the right vector and achieve maximal efficiency during contraction. Fascial sheaths also provide additional surface area for muscle origins because bone alone does not offer enough surface area. Fascial sheaths protect neurovascular bundles.

Groups of muscles in the arms and legs, together with blood vessels and nerves, are contained in compartments surrounded by non-elastic fascia and/or bone; therefore, whenever bleeding and/or edema occur, increased pressure is inevitable. This increased pressure can harm the intracompartmental soft tissues, leading to detrimental consequences. Focusing on the different compartments in both the upper and lower extremities a distinct architecture can be recognized.

In this chapter we address the anatomy of both upper and lower extremities to illustrate the rationale for the occurrence of compartment syndrome, its consequences, and management strategies.

Anatomy

Fascia

The thickness of the fascia is determined by the amount and direction of the applied force. Comparing the fascia of the lower leg (i.e., fascia cruris) to the fascia of the forearm (i.e., fascia anti-brachii), not only can a significant difference in thickness be noted, favoring the fascia cruris, but also a difference in the direction of the fascia fibers. The fascia cruris fibers run in a circular direction, whereas the fibers of the fascia antibrachii do not have a uniform shape or direction. This difference can be explained by the constant contraction and relaxation of the calf muscles, which is of much higher amplitude than that of their forearm counterparts.

Upper Extremity

Forearm

The forearm contains three compartments: dorsal, volar, and mobile wad compartments. The *dorsal compartment* contains the abductor pollicis, extensor pollicis longus, extensor carpi ulnaris, extensor digiti minimi, and extensor digiti communis muscles. Inferior to the muscles, the radius and ulna can be found, separated by the interosseous membrane. The *volar compartment* is separated into superficial and deep muscles. The deep muscles include the flexor pollicis longus, flexor digitorum profundus, and pronator quadratus. The superficial muscles are the palmaris longus, pronator teres, flexor digitorum superficialis, flexor carpi ulnaris and radialis. The ulnar and radial bone and the interosseous membrane border the compartment dorsally. Volar borders are the subcutaneous antebrachial fascia. This fascia also separates the volar compartment from the *lateral compartment* (i.e., the *mobile wad*), which holds the brachioradialis, extensor carpi radialis brevis and longus muscles (Fig. 51.1A–C).

Hand

Looking at the different osteofascial compartments of the hand, 10 separate compartments can be distinguished: four dorsal interossei compartments, three palmar interossei compartments, the adductor pollicis compartment, and the thenar as well as hypothenar compartments (Fig. 51.1D, E).

Lower Extremity

Lower Leg

Anatomically, the lower leg can be divided in four compartments: the deep and superficial posterior compartments and the lateral and anterior compartments.

The fascia cruris, tibia, fibula, and interosseus membrane surround the *anterior compartment*. The anterior tibial muscle, extensor hallucis longus, and extensor digitorum longus are the muscles in this compartment. The anterior tibial artery and veins run along these muscles distally and the deep peroneal nerve innervates them. The *lateral compartment*

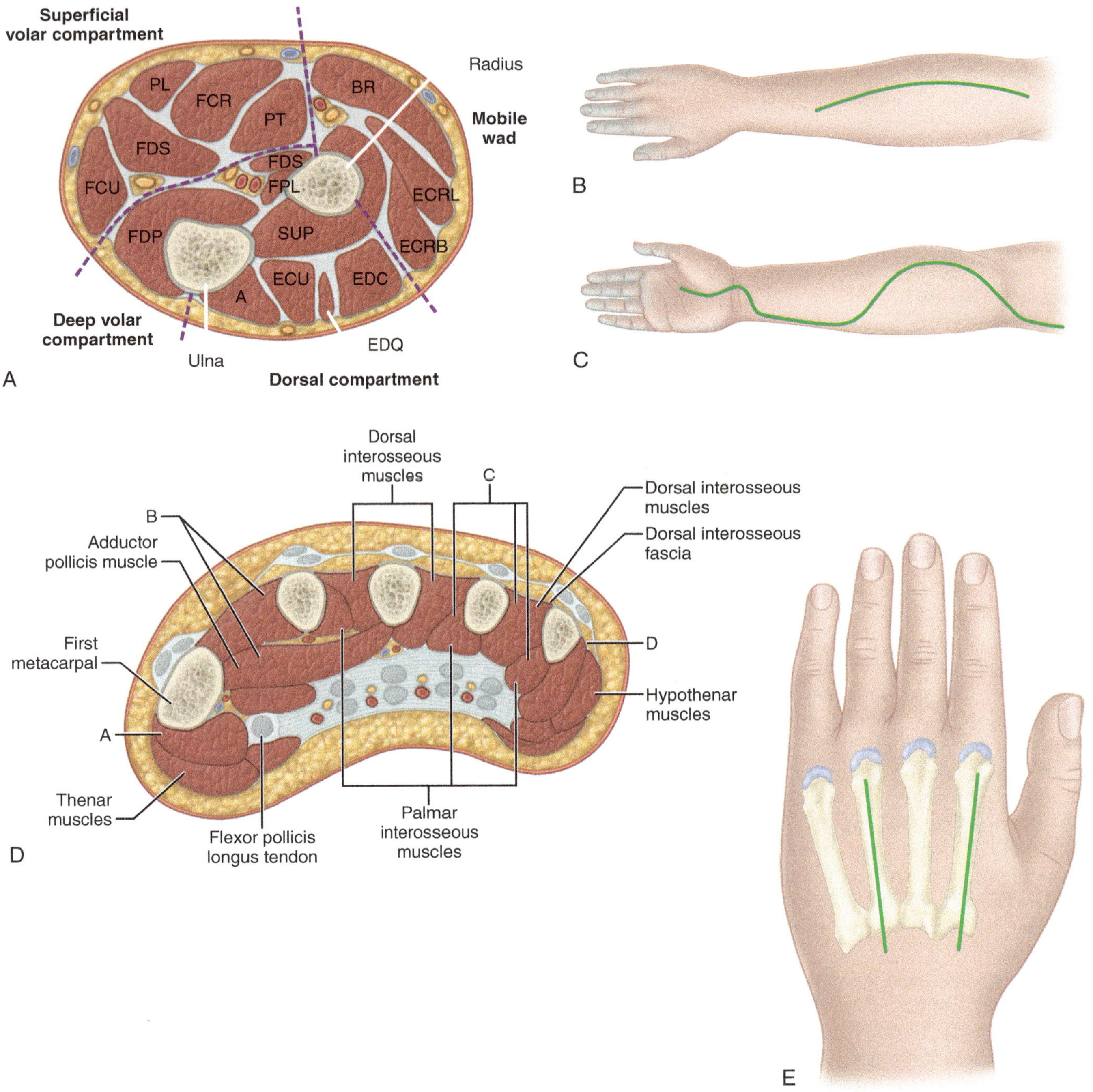

• **Fig. 51.1** (A) Cross-section through upper third of forearm. *A*, anconeus muscle; *BR*, brachioradialis; *ECRB*, extensor carpi radialis brevis; *ECRL*, extensor carpi radialis longus; *ECU*, extensor carpi ulnaris; *EDC*, extensor digitorum communis; *EDQ*, extensor digiti quinti; *FCR*, flexor carpi radialis; *FCU*, flexor carpi ulnaris; *FDP*, flexor digitorum profundus; *FDS*, flexor digitorum sublimis; *FPL*, flexor pollicis longus; *PL*, palmaris longus; *PT*, pronator teres; *SUP*, supinator. (B) Extensive opening of fascia of the forearm dorsum in dorsal compartment syndromes. (C) Incision used for anterior forearm compartment syndromes in which skin and underlying fascia are released completely throughout. (D) Cross-section through hand. Dorsal and volar interosseous compartments and adductor compartment to thumb (B and C in illustration); thenar and hypothenar compartments (A and D in illustration). (E) Longitudinal incisions over second and third metacarpals. (From Jobe MT. Compartment syndromes and Volkmann contracture. In: Azar FM, Beaty JH, Canale ST, eds. *Campbell's Operative Orthopaedics.* 13th edn. Philadelphia: Elsevier; 2017.)

comprises the long peroneal and brevis muscles and the common peroneal nerve proximally. The crural fascia, intermuscular septum fascia, and fibula compartmentalize these structures. The *superficial posterior compartment* is separated from the deep compartment by the transverse intermuscular septum and is ensheathed by the fascia cruris. This compartment holds space for the plantar, soleus, and gastrocnemius muscles. The *deep posterior compartment* is encircled by the already mentioned transverse septum, the tibial and fibular bones, and the interosseus membrane; it also contains the tibial nerve and posterior tibial and peroneal arteries and veins. Muscles that are located in this compartment are the posterior tibial, flexor hallucis longus, and flexor digitorum longus muscles.

Foot

Three compartments cover the full length of the foot: medial, lateral, and superficial compartments. In addition, six intrinsic compartments are described (i.e., four interossei compartments and an adductor compartment) and a calcaneal compartment.

The *medial compartment* holds the flexor hallucis brevis and the abductor hallucis muscle. The *lateral compartment* contains the abductor digiti quinti and the flexor digiti minimi muscles. In the *superficial compartment* the flexor digitorum brevis, the flexor digitorum longus tendons, and the lumbrical muscles are located. Also, the medial plantar nerve is running through this compartment. The interossei and adductor compartments hold the interossei muscles and the adductor muscle, respectively. The calcaneal compartment not only comprises the quadratus plantae muscle, but also the posterior tibial, medial, and lateral plantar nerves. All vessels of the foot run through this compartment: the posterior tibial, medial, and lateral plantar arteries and veins.

Pathophysiology

Each compartment has an ideal pressure for optimal tissue perfusion, based on the balance between the hydrostatic and osmotic pressure. The intracapillary hydrostatic pressure normally varies between 20 mmHg and 30 mmHg and relates to the difference between venous and arterial pressures.[1] The osmotic pressure or interstitial fluid pressure ensures prevention of outflow and ranges between –5 and +5 mmHg.[2]

Disturbance of this pressure balance can occur as a result of an increase of intracompartmental pressure (ICP) or a decrease of compartmental volume caused by bleeding or swelling of the tissue or a reduction of external volume due to high-pressure compression or casting. It is generally accepted that an increase of the interstitial fluid pressure above the intraluminal pressure of the capillary will prohibit adequate perfusion of the intracompartmental structures.[3]

Translated to a clinical decision tool, different authors choose to have a threshold within 10–30 mmHg of the diastolic blood pressure for surgical fasciotomy in adults.[4–6] Others state that a fasciotomy is indicated with absolute compartment pressures of >30–45 mm Hg.[7,8]

These threshold values may help decide the necessity for a decompression of a compartment in children. Tharakan et al published their work on compartment pressures in children with normal and fractured forearms. They describe a mean compartmental pressure of 10.22 mmHg (range 3–33 mmHg), which is similar to those reported in adults.[9]

As soon as the perfusion is jeopardized, hypoxia will lead to edema and the initiation of anaerobic metabolism. This cascade leads to a further increase of ICP and thus an even greater decrease of capillary flow. Subsequently, only an intervention can halt this process. If intervention is not performed within 3 hours after the onset of ischemia, an impaired muscle response will occur. Six to eight hours after ischemia the muscle and soft tissue will have suffered irreversible damage.

Subjective

Compartment syndrome is a clinical challenge where the clinical history foretells the physician the problem. Classically, pain, pallor, pulselessness, paresthesia, and paralysis (also called "the five Ps") are described as the clinical symptoms related to compartment syndrome. Although pain and loss of sensibility are not universal findings, in our survey only one of our patients was asymptomatic (see the section discussing ischemic contracture, below). In all other patients symptoms were present but unfortunately not adequately recognized or treated.

The review by Wall et al confirmed "the five Ps," except their observation that pulses may be present. Moreover, the pain may be out of proportion to the injury and there is a palpable painful tenseness or swelling of the compartment.[10] Also important is pain on passive stretch of wrist and fingers in the developing compartment syndrome of the upper extremity. Progressively, the increased pressure will lead to ischemia of the nerves, resulting in late-onset clinical signs as sensory and motor deficits.

In the upper extremity a supracondylar fracture of the humerus is the most frequent cause for the development of an ischemic contracture, followed by a fracture of the forearm. These fractures should be monitored carefully with regard to compartment syndrome, especially in children.

It is important to note that compartment syndrome is often missed or discovered later because of modern early treatment with drugs to diminish pain. In most modern hospitals it is supposed to be a medical mistake if patients have pain. At our unit and in our hospital compartment syndromes have been missed for this reason. To prevent this misdiagnosis Schmidt et al have initiated a multicenter prospective study to develop a prediction model for the likelihood of acute compartment syndrome. They have completed their inclusion and published their collected data and are currently developing their prediction model.[11]

Objective

Intracompartmental Pressure

An objective measurement for the diagnosis of compartment syndrome is evaluation of ICP. Aside from the decision of evaluating pressure, one should perform a fasciotomy immediately if there is any doubt about compartment syndrome. In our medical practice, working in a trauma referral center dealing with substantial injuries to the extremities, it is common practice to perform preventive open fasciotomies, especially if vascularization is compromised more proximally.

All techniques described for the assessment of pressure monitoring are based on the same concept, which is, in fact, an intracompartmental placement of a specific measuring device (i.e., the subtle difference between the different techniques), a fluid column, and a transducer for measurement of ICP. As such, either a continuous or a repeated ICP measurement can be established. Ideally, the same clinician monitors the ICP with an interval range between every 30 minutes to 12 times a day.[12]

A recent experimental study by Hammerberg et al compared the reliability of different devices, both digital and analog, using three different terminal devices.[13] The devices investigated were the 18-gauge bevel-tipped needles, the side-ported bevel-tipped needles, and the slit catheters. They concluded that the differences between these three terminal devices are small and unlikely to have an impact on clinical decision-making for fasciotomy. However, when the electronic measurement approach is compared with the analog Whitesides' technique, the electronic technique is favored because it does not require prior preparation. Nevertheless, Hammerberg et al recommended using the slit catheter for continuous monitoring of one compartment. In the event multiple compartments are at risk or multiple measurements in the same compartment are required, the clinician is advised to use either a standard 18G or side-port bevel-tipped 18G needle.[13]

Near-Infrared Spectroscopy

Near-infrared spectroscopy uses a differential light absorption to measure the level of hemoglobin, thus providing a measure of oxygenation. Recognizing decreased muscle oxygenation is correlated to the intracompartmental tissue perfusion gradient and thus could be helpful in the diagnosis of acute compartment syndrome.[14] Furthermore, Reisman et al showed an inverse correlation between tissue perfusion and ICP. They noticed an 8% difference, with the perfusion dropping below 10 mmHg.[15] As near-infrared spectroscopy can scan at different depths intracompartmentally, it seems to be useful for monitoring patients at risk of compartment syndrome. However, Shuler et al have recently published their innovative work on continual near-infrared spectroscopy and could not find a strong correlation between presence of compartment syndrome and deviated values. They advised additional interventional studies.[16]

Treatment

If a compartment syndrome is not adequately released, necrosis with all its consequences will be unavoidable. In the presence of the aforementioned symptoms our advice is to act with aggressive decompression of compartments without delay. Surgery is the only treatment that can prevent the disastrous consequences of compartment syndrome by restoring the microcirculation and preventing further damage to the muscles and nerves. Measures such as opening of the plaster cast and elevation of the extremity are not sufficient in these cases. Sheridan and Matsen found that the frequency and severity of complications of decompression were directly related to the promptness with which it was performed.[17] In cases of a suspected vascular injury, decompression has to be combined with vascular exploration and restoration of blood flow. At our unit most decompressions are performed preventively. This is especially the case in crush injuries of the extremities, and particularly if vascularization of the involved extremity is at risk. We do not have a wait-and-see policy and thus do not use this objective evaluation on a regular basis. Table 51.1 provides an overview of fasciotomies carried out in our unit between 2002 and 2012 in order to prevent compartment syndrome or further damage due to ischemia in cases of compartment syndrome. This table well illustrates our policy not to wait and see.

Upper Extremity

Forearm

When addressing compartment syndrome, the superficial and deep flexor compartments, the dorsal compartment and mobile wad in the forearm, the carpal tunnel and the intrinsic compartments should be released (Fig. 51.1A). The most affected muscles in compartment syndrome of the forearm are the deep muscles in the volar compartment. Different approaches have been reported to release the compartments. They all share, however, the same principle of placing a long longitudinal incision over the forearm (Fig. 51.1B, C). Ronel et al investigated the best approach for releasing the compartments of the forearm.[18]

To open the volar compartment, a radial approach was described. An incision is made radial to the volar midline, starting at the proximal wrist crease and extended to the antecubital fossa. In this way the superficial fascia can be seen and opened to enter the deep muscles radial to the flexor carpi radialis.

Central and ulnar approaches were also investigated. For the central approach the volar incision is planned in the midline, the fascia is opened and, approaching either ulnar or radial to the palmaris longus, the deep muscles can be inspected. The ulnar approach requires an incision radial to the flexor carpi ulnaris. The dorsal compartment is opened through a midline incision in the dorsum of the arm. After opening the superficial fascia the compartment should be adequately decompressed.

Gelberman et al described incisions that were prolonged over the carpal tunnel and introduced a curved incision for easy access to the muscles without harming the brachial artery or major nerves.[19] The authors use a similar approach as described by Gelberman.

Hand and Wrist

A well-executed study by DiFelice et al illustrated the compartments of the hand and proposed a protocol for releasing them[20] – placing two incisions on the dorsum of the hand, one in the thenar region and one in the hypothenar region allowing access to all compartments (Fig. 51.1D).

TABLE 51.1 Overview of Fasciotomies Executed in the Preventive (i.e., Primary) Trauma Setting and Fasciotomies Performed with Evident Symptoms of Compartment Syndrome to Prevent Permanent Damage due to Ischemia (Secondary)[a]

Upper Extremity (*n* = 231)	CTR	GR	IR	HHT	DF	VF
Primary (*n* = 186)						
Crush (76)	76	57	54	33	40	41
Multitrauma (44)	41	24	26	17	16	17
Deglovement injury (24)	21	10	13	8	6	5
Glass/stab injury (31)	31	11	2	1	5	7
Burn injury (6)	6	5	6	5	4	4
Circular saw injury (5)	5	2	0	0	0	0
Secondary (*n* = 45)						
Extravasation (12)	12	9	6	5	8	10
Postoperative bleeding (20)	18	9	6	1	6	7
Infection (13)	11	6	6	6	6	6

Lower Extremity (*n* = 48)	Anterior Compartment	Superficial Posterior Compartment	Deep Posterior Compartment	Lateral Compartment	Foot	Upper Leg
Primary (*n* = 33)						
Crush (15)	9	8	8	9	9	
Deglovement injury (13)	5	5	5	5	8	
Fracture (5)	3	3	3	3	3	1
Secondary (*n* = 15)						
Extravasation (4)	1	1	2	2	4	
Postoperative bleeding (5)	1	1	1	1	3	1
(Postoperative) swelling (5)	5	1	1	1	3	1
Infection (1)	1	1	1	1	1	

[a]Fasciotomies in upper and lower extremity, October 2002 to October 2012.

CTR, carpal tunnel release; DF, dorsal forearm release; GR, Guyon release; HHT, hypo- and hyperthenar release; IR, intrinsic release; VF, ventral forearm release.

Another incision over the carpal tunnel allows release of the carpal tunnel as well as Guyon's canal. Regarding the dorsal incisions, the incisions should be made over the second and fourth metacarpals. The incision over the second metacarpal creates access to the first dorsal interosseous muscle, the adductor pollicis, the second dorsal interosseous, and the second palmar interosseous. In contrast to our experience, DiFelice advises release of interossei from their origin (i.e., the connection to the second metacarpal bone) as well. The adductor pollicis fascia can be found radial and inferior to the first dorsal interosseous. The incision over the fourth metacarpal logically gives access to the fourth and third interosseous compartments using a similar approach to that described over the second metacarpal.

To release the hypothenar fascia a longitudinal incision should be placed just ulnar to the fifth finger. This will prevent harming the motor nerve bundles. The thenar incision should be parallel to the first metacarpal bone. Be careful not to lacerate the motor bundles innervating the thenar muscle. To open the carpal tunnel, the well-accepted longitudinal incision is placed at the centre of the tip of the fourth metacarpal in full flexion, running distal towards the flexing point of the wrist. The flexor retinaculum is the roof of the carpal tunnel and the floor of Guyon's channel. After opening the skin, the retinaculum is followed ulnar to the point where the ulnar nerve is visualized. Subsequently, the tendon sheath between the os pisiforme and os hamatum can be opened to release Guyon's channel. To release the carpal tunnel the flexor retinaculum can be opened.

The senior author opens the thenar and hypothenar sheaths via the carpal tunnel incision and not via separate incisions, therefore using only three incisions – two dorsal for the interosseous muscles and one volar in the hand – to adequately release the compartments.

Lower Extremity

Lower Leg

Exposure of all four compartments is required to prevent (further) necrosis in the acute compartment syndrome, including the tarsal tunnel and compartments in the foot.

Either a single lateral incision can be made or a two-step anterolateral and posteromedial approach can be used. Both authors favor the two-step approach and therefore we choose to discuss this technique in detail.

Two-Step Anterolateral and Posteromedial Approach

The first incision is anterolateral, which allows exposure of the anterior and lateral compartments. The incision should be placed over the anterior intermuscular septum. The fascia is then opened and, moving laterally, the lateral compartment can be decompressed. Be aware of the superficial peroneal nerve, which exits the lateral compartment 10 cm cephalad from the lateral malleolus. The anterior compartment can be decompressed by opening the fascia medial from the intermuscular septum. The anterior tibial and extensor hallucis longus muscles protect the deep peroneal nerve and peroneal artery. This paradigm, as described by Kashuk et al, allows an easy and safe dissection.[21] The posteromedial incision is placed medial from the tibia, and over a length of 15 cm sufficient exposure is created for a safe decompression. Some promote extending the incision with a medial retromalleolar incision, which evidently will release the tarsal tunnel.[22] After placement of the first incision, the fascia can be opened and anterior retraction will prevent laceration of the saphenous vein and both the saphenous nerve and vein. After the superficial compartment is decompressed, approaching the insertion of the soleus muscle can expose the deep compartment. Retraction of this muscle exposes the fascia of the long flexor digitorum, which can then be opened. It is important to identify the neurovascular bundle (i.e., posterior tibial nerve and artery), which is located between the soleus, flexor hallucis longus, and posterior tibial muscle.

Recommendation

The posteromedial incision is designed to create a safer decompression of the deep and superficial posterior compartments. In our practice, the two-step incision technique is mostly used to prevent inadequate deep flexor compartment release and unnecessary damage, as this technique opens the compartments under direct vision. This is especially important in a training institution.

Foot

For the foot, various techniques have been described and a nice overview is given by Frink et al in which the dorsal fasciotomy is promoted.[23] This approach uses two incisions medial to the second metatarsal bone and lateral to the fourth metatarsal bone. Taking care of the superficial veins and nerves, the fascia can be located and should be opened longitudinally over each interosseous compartment. Subsequently, the medial compartment is decompressed with an incision parallel to the plantar surface, starting just caudal to the insertion of the Achilles tendon (i.e., tarsal tunnel). The incision exposes the medial and abductor compartment. Lifting the abductor compartment opens the calcaneal compartment. The superficial and lateral compartments can be opened, consequently, through the calcaneal compartment. The superficial compartment is found just lateral to the medial compartment and after opening the medial fascia longitudinally, the flexor digitorum brevis can be retracted inferior and the medial fascia of the lateral compartment exposed.

Our approach to foot compartmental release is to use two dorsal incisions for the dorsal compartments. The incision over the tarsal tunnel is further lengthened distally on the medial side parallel to the plantar fascia to open the abductor, calcaneal, superficial, and lateral compartments of the foot.

Late Sequelae

Volkmann's Contracture of the Upper Extremity

The classic case of a patient with an ischemic Volkmann's contracture is a child sustaining a supracondylar humeral fracture treated with a cast. The following days the child is in considerable pain and although the cast is changed the pain is not relieved. Subsequently the fingers start clawing gradually and the wrist is no longer able to extend. Passively the fingers can only be stretched when the wrist is flexed completely. Furthermore, the sensibility of the hand is severely impaired.

In 1881, Richard von Volkmann described a condition of muscle ischemia, necrosis, and subsequent contracture of the forearm. This condition was the result of diminished arterial blood supply due to the application of tight, constricting bandages to the injured arm. In 1908, J.J. Thomas collected 107 cases with ischemic contracture from the literature. He reported that contractures were also possible in patients without treatment with splints or bandages; extrinsic pressure could therefore not be the only cause of Volkmann's contracture. The deep flexor compartment of the forearm is the first to be damaged as it is closest to the bone, with a tight surrounding fascia.[24] Also the flexor digitorum profundus is most distant from the arterial anastomotic pathways available to re-establish circulation. The centre of the muscle of the deep flexor tendons to the middle and ring finger is particularly vulnerable.[25]

In more severe cases or when the trauma is more in the vicinity of other compartments, the infarction can also encompass the superficial flexor muscles, the extensor muscles, and the intrinsic hand musculature. When ischemia is prolonged, the muscles become necrotic and are eventually replaced by fibrous tissue and fat. In addition, the initial ischemia can cause nerve damage, which becomes worse when the surrounding muscle becomes fibrotic.

If compartment syndrome is not treated adequately, Volkmann's ischemic contracture will occur (Fig. 51.2).

Unfortunately ischemic contracture still occurs as a result of an underestimation of the symptoms, with serious consequences for the function of the involved extremity. Not only is a fully developed contracture of the flexor muscles with impaired sensibility in the forearm extremely incapacitating, it can also cause psychological trauma. In the USA, failure to diagnose an acute compartment syndrome is a well-known cause of litigation against the medical profession.[26]

In regard to classification, Seddon introduced a classification in 1964, later modified by Tsuge in 1975.[27] The contractures are divided into three types: mild, moderate, and severe.

In the *mild* type the deep flexor muscles are partially affected. Mostly the ring and the long fingers are involved and, when more extensive, the index and little finger are also involved. The muscle of the pollicis longus is less affected. None to slight sensory disturbances can be present. Flexion of the fingers at the IP joints can be pronounced with extension of the wrist (tenodesis effect).

In the *moderate* type the deep flexors are involved as well as the flexor pollicis muscle and partially also the more superficial flexor muscles of fingers and wrist can be affected leading to contracture. Sensory deficits are always detectable.

In the *severe* type all the flexor muscles are involved with partially affected extensor muscles leading to severe contractures with severe sensory disturbances.

Other classifications are also designed, such as by Zancolli in 1965 or later by Holden.[28,29]

The first author has treated contractures with a great variety in the manifestation of the contractures and was more inclined to describe the contractures and sensory deficits.

An established contracture varies from a few affected deep flexor muscles with no nerve damage to a complete infarction of one or more muscle compartments with extensive nerve damage. Treatment should therefore be custom-made and directed to improve overall function. Although several methods of treatment have been reported, long-term results in different treatment regimens are rarely described.[27,30]

In our study we analyzed our cases (25 patients) and reported on the long-term results of the different treatment methods for Volkmann's contractures.[31] Patients filled in questionnaires concerning their disability, together with their satisfaction with the treatment. They were examined physically, including arm length, and tests were performed to measure strength and sensibility. In addition, motor function was classified based on Buck Gramcko's classification. Most patients sustained supracondylar fractures and the mean age was 13 (range 2–60) years. Follow-up had a mean of 7 (range 3–29) years. Posttrauma severe pain was encountered in 88%, loss of sensation 80%, blue fingers 60%, and skin necrosis in 28%. In the majority, sensibility, motion, and strength improved in the first months. In five patients sensibility did not improve.

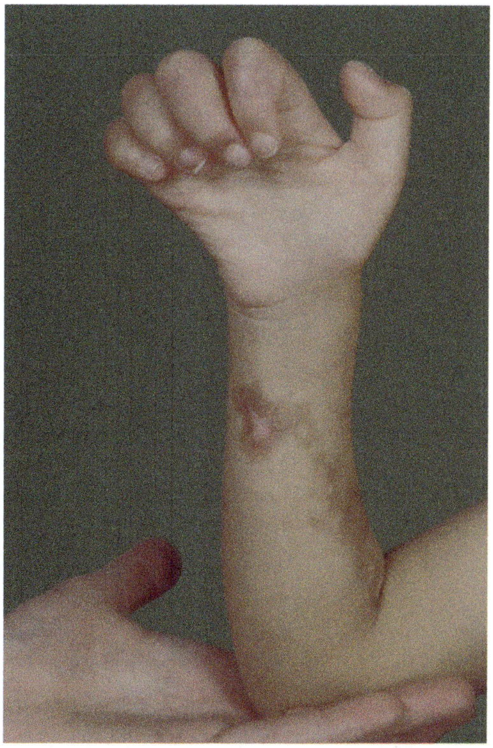

• **Fig. 51.2** This 4-year-old girl sustained a supracondylar fracture (6 months earlier) resulting in a severe Volkmann's ischemic contracture with PIP contractures and loss of motion in fingers and wrist as well as sensibility loss in both ulnar and median nerve distribution. (From Hovius SE, Ultee J. Volkmann's ischemic contracture. Prevention and treatment. *Hand Clin.* 2000;16(4):647–657. Reproduced with permission of Elsevier.)

Treatment varied, ranging from conservative splinting through excision of fibrous tissue, neurolysis, tenolysis, proximal "muscle slide," tendon lengthening, tendon transfers, and nerve grafting to free vascularized, innervated musculocutaneous flaps.

The treatment of an established contracture depends strongly on the severity of the infarction and the affected muscle and nerve tissue. Decisions about when and how to operate are not easy and are often discussed in literature.

Based on our study, we operate on patients with poor or insufficient hand function, with severe muscle necrosis diagnosed by MRI and with neurological signs in an earlier stage to prevent further joint stiffness and nerve damage by fibrosis.[31] Severe muscle necrosis is easily differentiated from viable muscle tissue at an early stage, and can subsequently be removed. In patients with a so-called "prolonged pain syndrome" we strongly advise early neurolysis and excision of fibrotic tissue, as in our experience it will immediately resolve the pain.

In patients with good to reasonable hand function we suggest initial conservative treatment with hand therapy and splinting and then waiting for spontaneous improvement of sensibility and motor function. If after 3 months hand function does not improve or diminishes, surgical intervention has to be considered.

In patients with insufficient hand function with infarction of a considerable part of the deep and superficial flexors and neurological signs, excision of fibrotic muscle tissue, neurolysis, and tenolysis is advised.[31] Good results can be obtained if excision and neurolysis are combined with tendon transfer, specifically in the early cases. We do not recommend tendon lengthening only, due to the high recurrence rate of the contractures and possible loss of power grip strength.

In patients with poor hand function with extensive infarction diagnosed by MRI, we advise a free vascularized innervated muscle transfer. We prefer a two-stage procedure with early excision in the first stage followed by the flap and if necessary a nerve graft in the second stage a few months later. If in the first stage the nerve is in continuity without deformity, a neurolysis is performed. In our experience, quite often a substantial recovery of sensory function will occur in these cases. If in the first stage the nerve is deformed, a nerve graft is planned in the second stage, combined with the free muscle transfer (Fig. 51.3). The nerve is mostly deformed when a substantial number of the forearm flexor muscles are fibrotic. In the majority of our patients both hand mobility and sensory function improved tremendously after free muscle transfer (Fig. 51.4). Although the contractile force of the gracilis muscle will stay limited for grip strength, a considerable increase of power grip strength was noticed in our cases.

We have described the difference in length of the forearm and hand on the affected side in relation to the healthy side in our patients who still had open growth plates.[31] Reasons for this length difference might be impaired oxygenation of growth plates, impaired muscle function, and damaged nerve tissue. We therefore recommend informing children and/or parents or caregivers about the possibility of a length

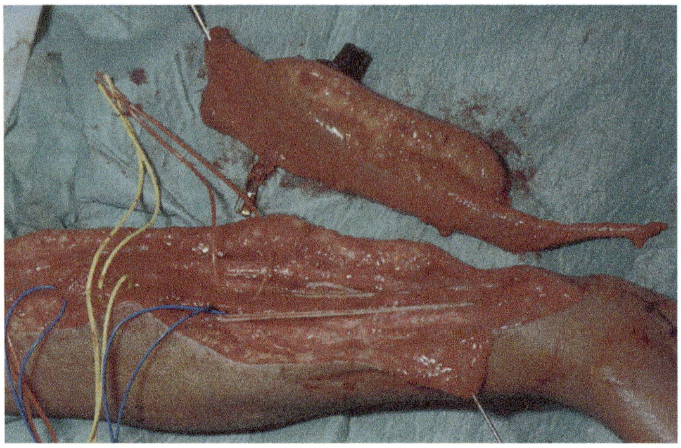

• **Fig. 51.3** Second phase: median and ulnar nerve reconstruction with sural cable grafts and a free vascularized innervated gracilis flap for flexor function (same patient as Fig. 51.2). In the first phase, scar tissue excision, neurolysis, and flexor tenotomy was performed. (From Hovius SE, Ultee J. Volkmann's ischemic contracture. Prevention and treatment. *Hand Clin*. 2000;16(4):647–657. Reproduced with permission of Elsevier.)

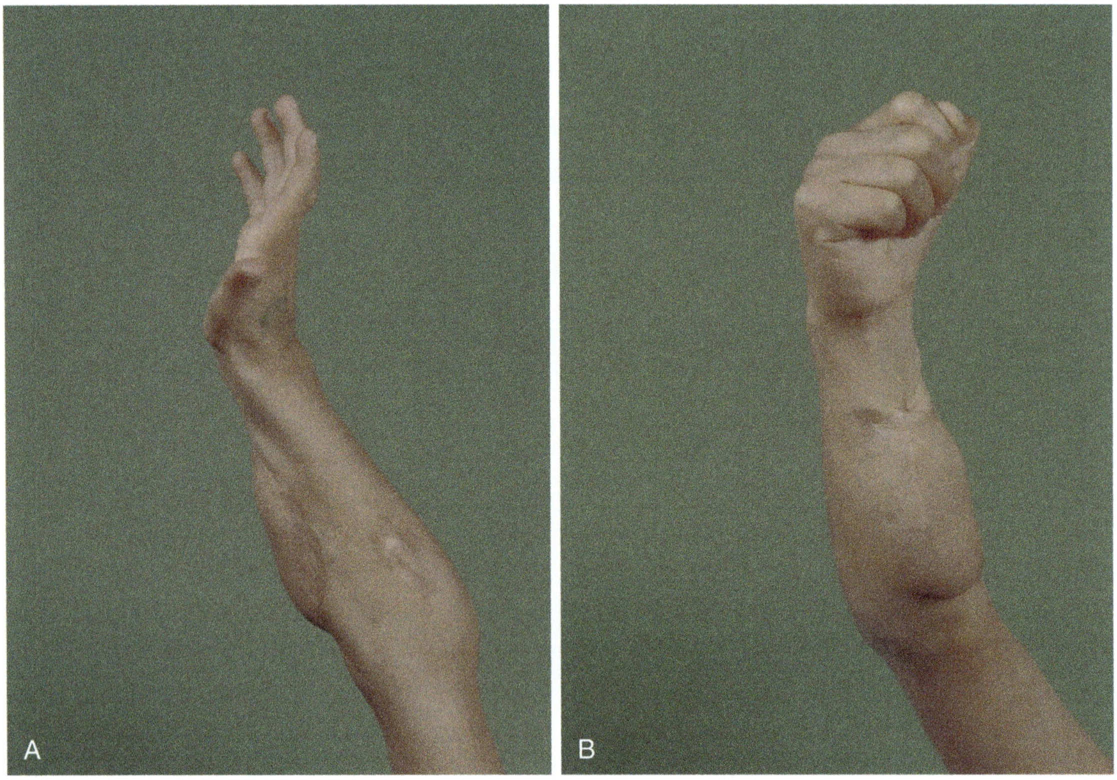

• **Fig. 51.4** Extension (A) and flexion (B) of fingers following free vascularized innervated flap 2 years postoperative (same patient as Fig. 51.2). (From Hovius SE, Ultee J. Volkmann's ischemic contracture. Prevention and treatment. *Hand Clin*. 2000;16(4):647–657. Reproduced with permission of Elsevier.)

difference of the forearm developing when they have sustained an ischemic contracture of the forearm.

A recent anatomical study by Taylor et al illustrated the potential advantage of treating Volkmann's ischemia using angiosome-based allografts. They state that current approaches are unable to fully address the structural and functional demands of Volkmann's ischemia. A tailored vascularized composite allotransplantation could provide a solution to replace the missing or destructed anatomical elements.[32] Although this study enlightens the potential gain in reconstructive surgery, one should not underestimate the major downside, especially in young children, which is the lifelong requirement of immunosuppressive drug therapy.

Volkmann's Contracture of the Lower Leg

Zwipp discussed the late sequelae after compartment syndrome in the lower leg and foot.[33] The contractures can be subdivided into five groups. Group I consists of small toe contractures, including hammertoes (i.e., intrinsic muscle necrosis and contractures of the m. flexor brevis) and claw toes (ischemic damage of the m. flexor brevis and flexor digitorum longus). Group II comprises the pathology of the hallux, which can be either isolated muscle necrosis of the flexor hallucis longus (resulting in a claw deformity during knee bending) or a contracture of the flexor hallucis longus. Group III is the combination deformity of groups I and II. Group IV is the pes equinus deformity based on the contractures of the superficial dorsal compartment (without nerve dysfunction) or based on dysfunction of the anterior compartment (either muscle necrosis or nerve paralysis). Group V is the pes equinovarus deformity, which is caused by the tibial, peroneal or combined ischemic nerve injury.

There is little information about the surgical options in the literature. The group of Hansen proposed scarred muscle excision (including the respective tendon),[34] but the recent work of Zwipp et al promotes a percutaneous release of tendons by Z-plasties, which can adequately correct the contracted toes and/or foot. In the experience of the first author most cases have sustained an ischemic event of the anterior compartment with or without the lateral compartment. The lack of extension of the forefoot and toes is corrected by tendon transfers if possible, such as the transfer of the viable posterior tibial tendon to create either extension of the forefoot or extension of the toes. Other examples we have encountered include contracture of the toes following extension at the ankle joint. Release of fibrosis and tendon transfers is mostly performed in these cases.

References

1. Levick JR, Michel CC. The effects of position and skin temperature on the capillary pressures in the fingers and toes. *J Physiol.* 1978;274:97–109.
2. Guyton AC, Granger HJ, Taylor AE. Interstitial fluid pressure. *Physiol Rev.* 1971;51(3):527–563.
3. Balogh ZJ, Butcher NE. Compartment syndromes from head to toe. *Crit Care Med.* 2010;38(9 suppl):S445–S451.
4. Matava MJ, Whitesides Jr TE, Seiler 3rd JG, et al. Determination of the compartment pressure threshold of muscle ischemia in a canine model. *J Trauma.* 1994;37(1):50–58.
5. Whitesides TE, Haney TC, Morimoto K, et al. Tissue pressure measurements as a determinant for the need of fasciotomy. *Clin Orthop Relat Res.* 1975;(113):43–51.
6. Whitesides TE, Heckman MM. Acute compartment syndrome: update on diagnosis and treatment. *J Am Acad Orthop Surg.* 1996;4(4):209–218.
7. Cohen MS, Garfin SR, Hargens AR, et al. Acute compartment syndrome. Effect of dermotomy on fascial decompression in the leg. *J Bone Joint Surg Br.* 1991;73(2):287–290.
8. Matsen FA 3rd, Winquist RA, Krugmire Jr RB. Diagnosis and management of compartmental syndromes. *J Bone Joint Surg Am.* 1980;62(2):286–291.
9. Tharakan SJ, Subotic U, Kalisch M, et al. Compartment pressures in children with normal and fractured forearms: a preliminary report. *J Pediatr Orthop.* 2016;36(4):410–415.
10. Wall CJ, Lynch J, Harris IA, et al. Clinical practice guidelines for the management of acute limb compartment syndrome following trauma. *Aust N Z J Surg.* 2010;80(3):151–156.
11. Schmidt AH, Bosse MJ, Frey KP, et al. Predicting Acute Compartment Syndrome (PACS): the role of continuous monitoring. *J Orthop Trauma.* 2017;31(suppl 1):S40–S47.
12. Tiwari A, Haq AI, Myint F, et al. Acute compartment syndromes. *Br J Surg.* 2002;89(4):397–412.
13. Hammerberg EM, Whitesides Jr TE, Seiler JG 3rd. The reliability of measurement of tissue pressure in compartment syndrome. *J Orthop Trauma.* 2012;26(9):e166; author reply.
14. Shuler MS, Reisman WM, Kinsey TL, et al. Correlation between muscle oxygenation and compartment pressures in acute compartment syndrome of the leg. *J Bone Joint Surg Ser A.* 2010;92(4):863–870.
15. Reisman WM, Shuler MS, Kinsey TL, et al. Relationship between near infrared spectroscopy and intra-compartmental pressures. *J Emerg Med.* 2013;44(2):292–298.
16. Shuler MS, Roskosky M, Kinsey T, et al. Continual near-infrared spectroscopy monitoring in the injured lower limb and acute compartment syndrome. *Bone Joint Lett J.* 2018;100-B(6):787–797.
17. Sheridan GW, Matsen FA 3rd. Fasciotomy in the treatment of the acute compartment syndrome. *J Bone Joint Surg Am.* 1976;58(1):112–115.
18. Ronel DN, Mtui E, Nolan WB 3rd. Forearm compartment syndrome: anatomical analysis of surgical approaches to the deep space. *Plast Reconstr Surg.* 2004;114(3):697–705.
19. Gelberman RH, Zakaib GS, Mubarak SJ. Decompression of forearm compartment syndromes. *Clin Orthop Relat Res.* 1978;134:225–229.
20. DiFelice Jr A, Seiler JG 3rd, Whitesides Jr TE. The compartments of the hand: an anatomic study. *J Hand Surg Am.* 1998;23(4):682–686.
21. Kashuk JL, Moore EE, Pinski S, et al. Lower extremity compartment syndrome in the acute care surgery paradigm: safety lessons learned. *Patient Saf Surg.* 2009;3(1):11.
22. Masquelet AC. Acute compartment syndrome of the leg: pressure measurement and fasciotomy. *Orthop Traumatol Surg Res.* 2010;96(8):913–917.
23. Frink M, Hildebrand F, Krettek C, et al. Compartment syndrome of the lower leg and foot. *Clin Orthop Relat Res.* 2010;468(4):940–950.
24. Seddon HJ. Volkmann's contracture: treatment by excision of the infarct. *J Bone Joint Surg Br.* 1956;38-B(1):152–174.

25. Inoue Y, Taylor GI. The angiosomes of the forearm: anatomic study and clinical implications. *Plast Reconstr Surg.* 1996;98(2):195–210.
26. Mabee JR. Compartment syndrome: a complication of acute extremity trauma. *J Emerg Med.* 1994;12(5):651–656.
27. Tsuge K. Treatment of established Volkmann's contracture. *J Bone Joint Surg Am.* 1975;57(7):925–929.
28. Zancolli E. Tendon transfers after ischemic contracture of the forearm. Classification in relation to intrinsic muscle disorders. *Am J Surg.* 1965;109:356–360.
29. Holden CE. The pathology and prevention of Volkmann's ischaemic contracture. *J Bone Joint Surg Br.* 1979;61-B(3):296–300.
30. Matsen 3rd FA. Compartmental syndrome. An unified concept. *Clin Orthop Relat Res.* 1975;(113):8–14.
31. Ultee J, Hovius SE. Functional results after treatment of Volkmann's ischemic contracture: a long-term followup study. *Clin Orthop Relat Res.* 2005;(431):42–49.
32. Taylor GI, Sparks DS, Gascoigne AC, et al. Angiosome-based allografts: vascularized composite allotransplantation for tailored subunit reconstruction with Volkmann ischemic contracture as a case in point. *Plast Reconstr Surg.* 2017;139(6):1291e–1304e.
33. Zwipp H. Reconstructive surgery of sequelae of compartment syndrome of the lower leg and/or foot. Presentation of a new classification. *Unfallchirurg.* 2008;111(10):776–784.
34. Manoli 2nd A, Smith DG, Hansen Jr ST. Scarred muscle excision for the treatment of established ischemic contracture of the lower extremity. *Clin Orthop Relat Res.* 1993;(292):309–314.
35. Hovius SE, Ultee J. Volkmann's ischemic contracture. Prevention and treatment. *Hand Clin.* 2000;16(4):647–657.

52

Nerve Injury, Repair, and Reconstruction

EMILY M. KRAUSS, RENATA V. WEBER, AND SUSAN E. MACKINNON

For videos accompanying this chapter see ExpertConsult.com. See inside cover for access details.

Nerve injury, repair, and reconstruction describes the traditional classification of nerve injuries as well as a clinical grouping of nerve injuries according to the mechanism of injury. A clinical grouping of open versus closed and crush versus traction/avulsion or penetrating injuries has implications on the severity of associated soft tissue and bony injury, and impacts diagnosis and the timing of surgical treatment. Preoperative adjunct studies are reviewed and their usefulness in surgical decision-making for different injury patterns is discussed. The clinical classifications also provide guidance to the peripheral nerve surgeon about realistic expectations for recovery.

Specifics on nerve repair techniques, usefulness of pre- and postoperative imaging and electrical studies and their role in the assessment of the nerve injury and recovery, and therapy modalities to assist in the clinical recovery are discussed.

New additions to the chapter include the appropriate use of newer technology such as acellular human nerve allografts and biodegradable conduits, a discussion of the treatment of neuromas, and an updated guideline for treatment of complex regional pain syndrome.

Introduction

Nerve injury and its sequelae have posed countless challenges to surgeons and patients over the past centuries. Since the development of microsurgical techniques in the 1960s, a relative explosion of innovation and knowledge has occurred to provide surgeons with greater tools to treat nerve injury.

Nerve injury classification remains the same, and the original principles of repair (early repair of complete injury, anatomical and tension-free coaptation, use of autologous nerve grafts), are still considered the gold standard. Improved understanding of microfascicular anatomy and the internal neural topography now enables surgeons to not only perform a microfascicular repair, but has led the way to the development of nerve transfers in nerve reconstruction. Nerve transfers can restore distal function and critical sensation in difficult nerve injuries, including proximal injury or those with large nerve gaps.

Despite these innovations, the major limitation to peripheral nerve recovery is still the time it takes for the nerve to regenerate. This remains true regardless of the technique used for the repair. Without prompt motor nerve input, denervated muscle after a prolonged period of time becomes resistant to nerve regeneration. Although avoidance of tension at the neurorrhaphy site and improvements in suturing techniques have improved the process to some extent, the ultimate success is dependent on innervation time, number of neurorrhaphy sites, supply and type of donor nerves, and the condition of the surrounding tissue. At every coaptation site, a percentage of nerve fibers are lost.[1]

New technology is being developed to assist in evaluating the nerve injury and providing alternative solutions for nerve repair. This technology includes improved nerve stimulators, nerve conduits, and acellular nerve allografts. Alternatives to standard treatment for short, small-diameter nerve gaps include commercially available nerve conduits and acellular human-processed nerve allografts. Schwann cell-lined nerve conduits and tissue-engineered substitutions are still experimental, but may offer the solution for enhanced nerve regeneration in the future. It is important, however, to remember that even the "gold standard" nerve autograft gives functional results typically deserving of a "bronze" award, and no nerve substitute to date equals the results of an autograft. Nerve transfer techniques have largely replaced nerve grafts for many proximal-level nerve injuries in our practice. A careful evaluation of the patient, nerve injury, and available options, including their limitations, is important in enabling the modern surgeon to restore function and reduce post-injury complications.

Even with new advances, post-injury neuroma and complex regional pain syndrome continue to affect patients. Ongoing research into successful management strategies can offer these patients new possibilities for improved pain control and quality of life.

TABLE 52.1 **Classification of Nerve Injury**

Mackinnon	Sunderland	Seddon	Injury	Recovery	
Degree I	Degree I	Neurapraxia	Conduction block resolves spontaneously	Favorable	Fast/excellent
Degree II	Degree II	Axonotmesis	Axonal rupture without interruption of the basal lamina tubes	Favorable	Slow/excellent
Degree III	Degree III		Rupture of both axons and basal lamina tubes, some scar	Favorable	Slow/incomplete
Degree IV	Degree IV		Complete scar block	Unfavorable	None
Degree V	Degree V	Neurotmesis	Complete transection	Unfavorable	None
Degree VI			Combination of I–V ± normal fascicles	Mixed	Mixed

Source: Weber R, Boyd K, Mackinnon S. Repair and grafting of peripheral nerve. In: Gurtner G, Neligan P, eds. *Plastic Surgery*. Volume 1: *Principles*. Elsevier; 2013. Reproduced with permission of Elsevier.

Nerve Injury Classification

Sir Herbert Seddon's classification system was the first to classify peripheral nerve injuries and is based on gross and histological anatomical changes rather than the mechanism of injury.[2] He described three types of nerve injuries. (a) *Neurapraxia* involves a local conduction block at a discrete area along the course of the nerve. Wallerian degeneration does not occur and the recovery is excellent within a "short" time period. (b) *Axonotmesis* implies axonal damage, while (c) *neurotmesis* is the equivalent of a peripheral nerve transection. In both axonotmesis and neurotmesis, Wallerian degeneration occurs distal to the site of injury. Although an axonotmetic injury will recover, a neurotmetic injury cannot. Within axonotmesis, Seddon described a degree of injury associated with scarring and less complete recovery. Within neurotmesis, he described injury of "in continuity" scar and an inability to recover.

Sunderland emphasized Seddon's expanded description of axonotmesis and neurotmesis with a classification that emphasized five degrees of nerve injury.[3] Sunderland's classification system is widely used today due to the improved clarity in describing partial injuries and its ability to communicate the probability of recovery. (Table 52.1 and Fig. 52.1). First-degree (neurapraxia) and second-degree (axonotmesis) injuries recover spontaneously, the latter at a rate of 1–1.5 mm/day or 1 inch/month (2.5 cm/month).[4] Third-degree injuries have partial recovery through the fascicles that are not affected by scar. Surgical correction of third-degree injuries is challenging, as identifying scarred fibers while preserving undamaged fascicles with the potential for spontaneous recovery is technically challenging. Fourth- and fifth-degree injuries do not recover spontaneously and require surgical reconstruction. Mackinnon later described a sixth-degree injury that could include normal fascicles with various degrees of injury to other fascicles.[5] The sixth-degree injury is the surgeon's most technically challenging injury.

It is clinically helpful, and simpler, to classify peripheral nerve injuries into "favorable" and "unfavorable." Favorable injuries recover fully and quickly (neurapraxia, first degree) or slowly (axonotmesis, second degree), or only partially and slowly (axonotmesis, third degree). "Unfavorable" injuries will not recover (neurotmesis, fourth and fifth degrees).

Clinical Classification of Nerve Injuries by Mechanism

Nerve injuries may alternatively be classified by mechanism of injury or by open versus closed injury. This clinical classification is useful in determining the likelihood for spontaneous recovery, and provides an algorithm for managing these injuries. Table 52.2 lists the typical nerve injury patterns and their significance with respect to assessment and treatment. For simplicity, nerve injuries can be grouped as: (a) crush and compression injuries; (b) stretch and avulsion injuries; and (c) penetrating injuries. Although avulsion and crush injuries tend to be closed injuries, they may be open. When the skin is violated, a significant force was exerted to the body and thus it is not unusual to have associated soft tissue, vascular, and orthopedic injuries. The extent of soft tissue loss, especially muscle and skin, will ultimately influence the outcome of the nerve repair. More extensive soft tissue damage, with or without concomitant bony injuries, raises the complexity and the likelihood for a staged reconstruction. Often, the nerve reconstruction is appropriately delayed in light of more acute vascular and orthopedic injuries.

Crush Injuries

The most common peripheral nerve injury in the extremities is from external forces crushing the tissue. In the case of light compressive forces, a self-limiting neurapraxia occurs,

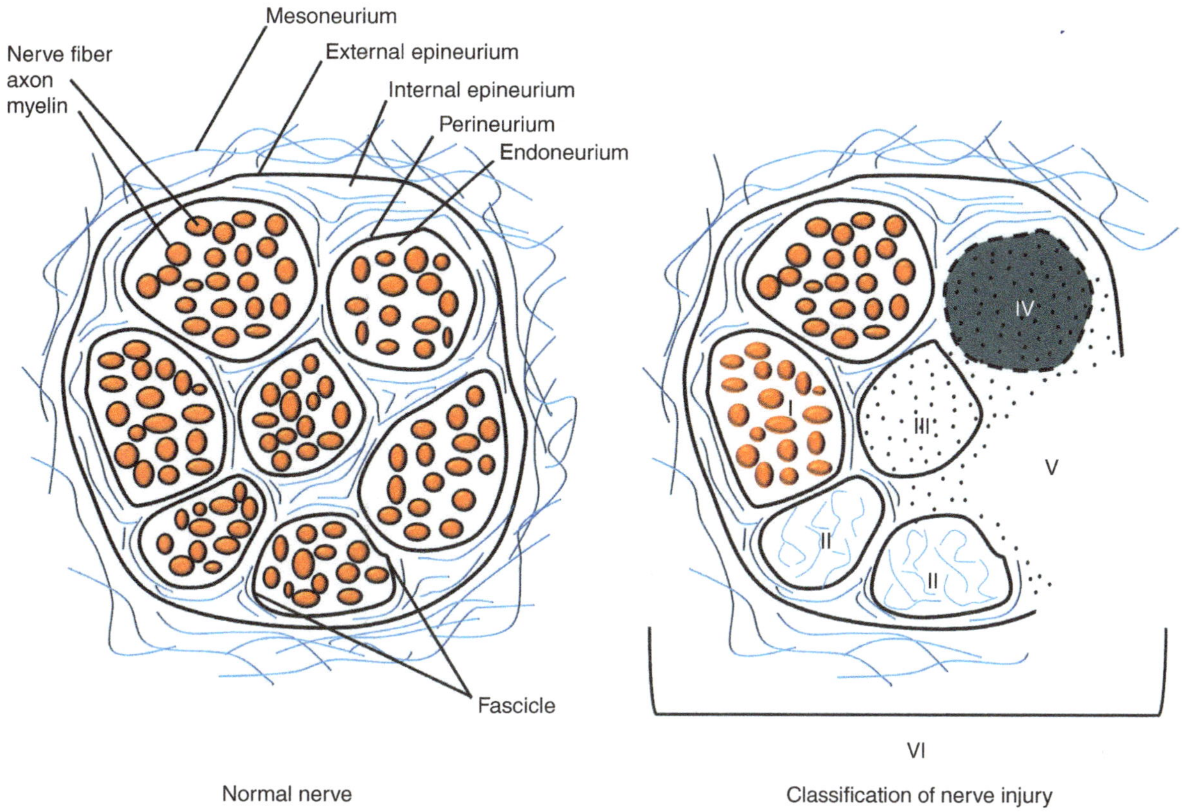

• **Fig. 52.1** Schematic representation of the cross-section of a normal peripheral nerve showing the connective tissue and nerve tissue components. The cross-section of the peripheral nerve on the right demonstrates a mixed, or sixth-degree, injury pattern. The fascicle at the top left is normal. Moving in a counterclockwise direction, fascicle I is a first-degree injury (neuropraxia) with segmental demyelination. Fascicle II is a second-degree injury (axonotmesis). The second degree involves both the axon and the myelin. The endoneurial tissue is not damaged. Fascicle III demonstrates a third-degree injury, with injury to the axon, myelin, and endoneurium. The perineurium is intact and normal. Fascicle IV demonstrates a fourth-degree injury, with injury to the axon, myelin, endoneurium, and perineurium. The fascicle is marked by scarring across the nerve, with only the epineurium being intact. Fascicle V is a fifth-degree injury in which the nerve is not in continuity and is transected. The surgeon will separate the fourth- and fifth-degree injury patterns, which will require reconstruction from the normal fascicles and the fascicles demonstrating first-, second-, and third-degree injury patterns. These latter patterns of injury require, at most, neurolysis. (From Mackinnon S. *Nerve Surgery*. New York: Thieme. 2015.)

but with increased force, the higher the probability of irreparable damage. In addition to external force, increased internal pressure from a hematoma, fracture, and local tissue edema may increase the compressive injury to the nerve. Compartment syndrome is the extreme of the spectrum and constitutes a surgical emergency. An early sign of impending compartment syndrome is a decrease in vibration sensibility. The complications of a missed compartment syndrome are so devastating that the standard of care is to err on the side of caution and release the muscle compartment if clinical suspicion is high.

Although nerves are fairly resistant to injury, especially when the surrounding tissue is not significantly damaged, a mixed nerve injury can occur. The connective tissue surrounding larger nerves can contract as it heals, causing an additional compression of the nerve as well as a tethering effect to the surrounding tissue. In addition, local soft tissue damage, especially to muscle, which is much less resilient to pressure than skin, nerve, and tendon, can lead to fibrosis. Thus a relatively minor nerve injury may produce enough muscle swelling to cause irreparable damage without clinical evidence of a compartment syndrome, leading to more extensive permanent damage than one would anticipate.

This mechanism of nerve injury is usually treated conservatively and exploration is warranted if the nerve recovery does not follow an expected pattern. Along with traction injuries, crush injuries are followed with serial exams prior to 3 months post injury, and electromyograms (EMGs) at 3 months if no clinical evidence of neurological recovery is noted.

Traction and Avulsion Injuries

Stretch or traction injuries to a nerve occur when the strain exerted on a particular nerve exceeds the maximum limit that nerve diameter can accept. The internal structure of the nerve becomes injured, usually without any appreciable external evidence of injury. High-velocity or high-impact injury can often lead to a proximal avulsion of the nerve

TABLE 52.2 Classification of Nerve Injury by Mechanism

Type	May Be Injured	Significance
Stretch/Avulsion Injury		
Avulsion	Nerve roots	Unable to be repaired primarily
	Nerves exiting	Indication for nerve transfer
	Foramen, bony fracture	
Stretch	Any nerve	Mixed nerve injury (degree VI)
Crush and Compression Injury		
Complex crush	Skin, subcutaneous tissue, muscle, nerve ± bone	Varying degree of depth, loss of function is related to amount of tissue destruction
Chronic compression	Nerve	Slow onset, reversible
Acute compression	Nerve ± muscle	Quick onset, reversible muscle ischemia, variable recovery of both muscle and nerve
Compartment syndrome	Nerve + muscle	Quick onset, reversible muscle ischemia if ischemia less than 6 h; no or variable recovery of muscle if released after 6 h
Penetrating Injury		
Sharp	Skin, subcutaneous tissue, muscle, nerve ± bone. All levels	Needs surgical exploration because of high probability for nerve disruption
Blunt	Variable	Injury may extend further then expected
Blast	Variable	Injury pattern depends on ballistic makeup and velocity
Electrical	Variable	Neuropathy is from damage to myelin sheath and ranges from neuropathy to causalgia

Source: Weber R, Boyd K, Mackinnon S. Repair and grafting of peripheral nerve. In: Gurtner G, Neligan P, eds. *Plastic Surgery*. Volume 1: *Principles*. Elsevier; 2013. Reproduced with permission of Elsevier.

or nerve root. Soft tissue attachments around joint or bony foramina act as tethering points along the nerve's path. If arteries and veins run in parallel to the nerves, which is often the case, a severe injury can compromise the circulation.

Even at major medical centers with ample resources and personnel it is rare to see a multispecialty surgery occur in the emergency setting at the time the limb-threatening injury is addressed. The nerve injury is usually addressed at a later date.

Nerve injuries in which the proximal nerve is accessible are repaired directly or with a graft. Nerve transfer and possible tendon transfers can be performed to complement and augment the nerve reconstruction. Nerves avulsed distally at the neuromuscular junction present a different problem, as there is no distal end available for repair. For motor nerves, the proximal nerve can be directly implanted into the muscle belly. Some clinical studies show as good as Medical Research Council (MRC) grade 4 motor recovery 1–2 years after direct nerve-to-muscle neurotization; however, experimental studies do not support these findings; rather, recovery is much less than a nerve coaptation would produce and we rarely use this technique in preference to tendons or muscle transfers.

Penetrating Injuries

Penetrating trauma can be a result of sharp or blunt penetration, and will often have concomitant vascular and tendons injury in addition to the nerve injury. A sharp laceration, such as a hand laceration from a knife or piece of glass, necessitates exploration if a nerve deficit is present. The likelihood that the nerve is partially or completely transected is high. It is recommended to explore these injuries semi-electively within the first week. The more time that passes from the injury date, the less likely the two ends of the nerve can be mobilized to perform a primary repair. More than likely a gap will result after the traumatized nerve is trimmed to healthy nerve and a graft will be needed. In our practice, acute nerve grafting is performed if there is concern about a degree of injury that would make it difficult to reoperate in the future.

In the event of a penetrating trauma with an associated vascular injury, immediate exploration is warranted. Occasionally in proximal injuries with large arterial injuries with or without underlying fractures, the nerve injury is overlooked in the face of more urgent vascular and orthopedic injuries. Rather, the deficit is noticed postoperatively, when it is unclear if the nerve injury is from the inciting event, iatrogenic during the repair of the vascular injury, or secondary to edema or hematoma. Although a CT scan or MRI may be helpful to evaluate for the latter, internal scarring of the nerve may not always be clearly determined. As with traction injuries, a very proximal penetrating nerve injury may benefit from distal nerve transfers to augment recovery in addition to the acute repair or grafting.

Blunt penetrating and blast injuries are usually treated conservatively, similar to closed crush and stretch injuries, because they may recover spontaneously. The local tissue trauma often causes a neurapraxia that resolves; however, following the same algorithm for traction or crush injury, those injuries that do not recover clinically after 3 months should be evaluated by electrodiagnostic studies.

Evaluation of Nerve Injuries

A thorough history and clinical examination with an understanding of anatomy is the cornerstone of evaluating nerve injuries. Mechanism of injury can raise or lower the clinical suspicion of irreversible nerve injury requiring reconstruction, as described above for crush, traction, avulsion, and sharp and blunt penetrating injuries. An open injury is easier to assess, as surgical exploration is most often justified except in the case of a blast injury. Typically, we recommend that a sharp injury with associated motor or sensory deficits be explored within 7 days if possible. Conventionally, it is accepted that primary neurorrhaphy should be possible up to 2 weeks after an injury. With injuries that present later than 3 weeks, the surgeon should be prepared to do a nerve graft repair.

Determining spontaneous sensory or motor nerve recovery in closed injuries may be difficult and intervention is guided by serial physical examination. For sensory nerve injuries, an advancing Tinel's sign signals sensory recovery. Sensation may be tested using two-point static and moving discrimination, the Semmes–Weinstein filament test, or the "10 test." This quick and easy screening test uses the patient's own subjective perception to moving light touch to elicit differences in sensation between the right and left sides of the mirror digit.[6] For example, both index fingers are stroked at the same time and patients are asked if the sensation is the same or different between the two digits. This technique is particularly useful in young children and in patients who have some underlying neuropathy. If in doubt that the patient has a nerve injury after the "10 test," two-point discrimination is a more sensitive test to determine severity of injury.

In motor nerve injuries, serial physical examination of affected muscle groups is performed and graded using the Medical Research Council (MRC) scale.[7] Muscle groups are tested against gravity and against resistance. Other muscle groups unaffected in the extremity by the nerve injury can also be assessed for strength and may provide options for future nerve transfer donor fascicles.

In addition to serial physical examination, electrodiagnostic studies are performed generally at 3 months post injury to evaluate for recovery as EMG changes indicating recovery precede clinical recovery.

Signs of ongoing acute denervation include positive sharp waves, fibrillations, and fasciculations on EMG. Motor unit potentials (MUPs) are the EMG equivalent of active muscle activation. There are three commonly encountered scenarios in electrodiagnostic testing at 3 months post injury:

1. No acute denervation, normal MUPS – This electrodiagnostic pattern corresponds to a neuropraxic injury, or Sunderland I, and will recover fully
2. No acute denervation, abnormal MUPS – This pattern represents a slightly higher level of injury, Sunderland II, which has begun to heal and will recover fully
3. Acute dennervation, some abnormal MUPS – There is ongoing denervation of the muscle but there are some recovering MUPs. These patients may benefit from distal decompression to enhance recovery (preventing the "double crush phenomenon"). Clinical recovery will be partial
4. Acute dennervation, no MUPS – This electrodiagnostic pattern represents a severe injury. The prognosis for recovery is guarded and surgical intervention and reconstruction is recommended.

We recommend early evaluation of nerve injury and close follow-up. This strategy enables clinical identification of those patients whose mechanism of injury warrants early exploration, and avoids delay in recognizing a nerve deficit that will not resolve spontaneously. It also enables us to order the electrodiagnostic testing to evaluate both injured nerves and potential donors if we are considering nerve or tendon transfers in the reconstruction. There are clinical investigations using newer ultrasound machines that can detect nerve pathology; however, these studies are still investigational and are highly operator-dependent.

Factors Affecting Nerve Recovery in Nerve Repair

Many factors besides technique affect nerve repair and age of the patient seems to be the most important factor. From historical data, we know that nerve repair in children and young adults yields better results than in adults. One reason is that the nerve has a shorter distance to travel. Nerves regenerate at 1–1.5 mm/day, and in a child the nerve recovery would be expected to reach the intended target organ earlier than in an adult and thus have a quicker recovery. Secondly, a child's brain has greater plasticity and more neural activity than an adult, thus the child has an enhanced ability to process the reinnervated motor and sensory input within the brain cortex.

Type of Injury

The type of injury, the location, and the degree or depth of the injury affect the outcome. A sharp laceration will have less associated soft-tissue trauma as a crush or avulsion injury at the same level. Proximal injuries may affect larger muscle or sensory domains. The reconstruction can be more challenging and a minor misalignment of fascicles has greater consequences than a more distal injury. Sensory nerve lacerations in the finger repaired a few days after the injury usually have excellent outcomes while sensory nerve neuromas from an original crush injury may require reconstruction with grafts months after the injury and do not recover as well. Often the internal damage is underestimated and if care is not taken to be outside the zone of injury, the repair may be suboptimal.

When considering the surgical intervention, timing, type of repair, tension and alignment of fascicles have an equally important role in the outcome of nerve recovery. Earlier repair usually results in better outcomes and the best results occur if the repair can be performed within 3 weeks. A good result can still be expected if the repair occurs before 6 months, although a nerve graft will most likely be needed. Functional recovery is directly proportional to the number of motor axons reaching the target endplate and inversely proportional to the time of denervation: "Time = muscle."

$$\text{FR} \propto \frac{\text{Number of motor axons reaching target endplate}}{\text{Time of denervation}}$$

Timing of Repair

In the case of a nerve transection, patients who are clinically stable should be taken to the operating room for exploration and repair of the nerve within the first 7–10 days. Repair within the first 72 hours is preferable in large motor and mixed nerves, as a nerve stimulator can be used to map motor fascicles in the distal segment. Nerves repaired acutely within the first 2 days are considered repaired primarily. A delayed primary repair occurs between 2 and 7 days. In either case, the proximal and distal ends of the nerve are freshened and an end-to-end coaptation performed. Nerves repaired after the first week are considered repaired secondarily. The cut-off days of 2 and 7 are arbitrary because even at 2–3 weeks from injury, the nerve can occasionally be coapted without need for a graft; however, the longer the time from injury, the less likely it is that a primary neurorrhaphy can be achieved, even with significant mobilization of the proximal and distal nerve ends.

Tension and Nerve Repair

Excessive tension can result in impaired regeneration from scarring at the neurrorhaphy site. Studies on an uninjured nerve show that a 15% stretch of the nerve causes a reduction in microvascular flow. For the hour after relaxation the peak conduction velocity is decreased to 66% of its normal velocity.[8] Any repair that withstands gentle range of motion is considered a "tension-free" repair. In a cadaveric study comparing suture size to the strength of an acute repair of the median nerve, 9-0 nylon withstood the greatest distractive forces.[9] At a lower tension 10-0 snapped, and 8-0 sutures pulled out of the nerve tissue. However, in clinical practice, 10-0 and 8-0 sutures are often used based on the size of the nerve, the thickness of the epineurium, and the amount of inflammation. Fibrin glue may be used in place of suture repair when there is no tension. Experimentally, lasers have been used to coapt the epineurium; however, the heat produced causes tissue damage and a suboptimal tensile strength at the repair site.

In clinical practice we do not formally measure the tension across a neurorrhaphy; however, we prefer to have a completely tension-free repair (Fig. 52.2). Each nerve end is mobilized in order to reapproximate the two ends in a reasonable manner. A single 8-0 or 9-0 nylon suture is used to bring the newly fresh nerve ends together. If the nerve remains together after the limb is manipulated in its normal range of motion, the tension is deemed to be appropriate and the remainder of the repair completed with 9-0 nylon.

When primary neurorrhaphy is not possible, decompression, mobilization, and elongation of both nerve ends can bridge small gaps usually less then 5 mm in size because of the inherent elasticity of a nerve.[10] We do not recommend using postural manipulation, such as positioning the arm in abduction or the wrist and fingers in flexion, in order to force primary repair. Not only can dehiscence occur when the joint near the repair is moved too early, but it may create significant stiffness from prolonged immobilization. An immobilized nerve also results in scarring at the repair site. If the nerve ends cannot be brought into reasonable proximity, reconstruction with a nerve graft is recommended.

Techniques: Epineural versus Fascicular Repair

Microsuture of 8-0, 9-0 or 10-0 nylon placed with the use of loupe or microscopic magnification remains the gold standard in nerve repair. Approximately two-thirds of surgeons use a combination of microsutures and glue, whereas one-third use one or the other. A personal preference of the senior author is not to use a nerve wrap.

External markers, such as a vessel on the surface and matching the fascicular patterns, assist in aligning the two nerve ends (Fig. 52.3). Overlap should be avoided. By placing the sutures in the epineurium after the fascicles have been trimmed back behind the level of the epineurium, a sleeve is created with the external connective tissue. For larger nerves, a fascicular repair is possible, where the perineurium acts as the epineurium. As long as the fascicles do not overlap, both techniques give similar results.[11] Neither repair technique seems to be superior to the other. The more critical issues are tension and alignment to avoid fibrosis.

Our preferred method for repair is a grouped fascicular repair with the aim of aligning the sensory and motor groups appropriately. The least number of epineural sutures, using 9-0 nylon to approximate the ends and keep the repair intact through a full range of motion, is used. If there is a slight mismatch in size, as in the setting of a nerve transfer, we can improve that size mismatch by going more proximally on the recipient nerve to make the diameter smaller and more distally on the donor nerve to make a cross–sectional area greater. We will occasionally also use fibrin glue, but do not use nerve wraps as we have seen these remain present years after placement in some patients presenting with neural ischemia and pain.

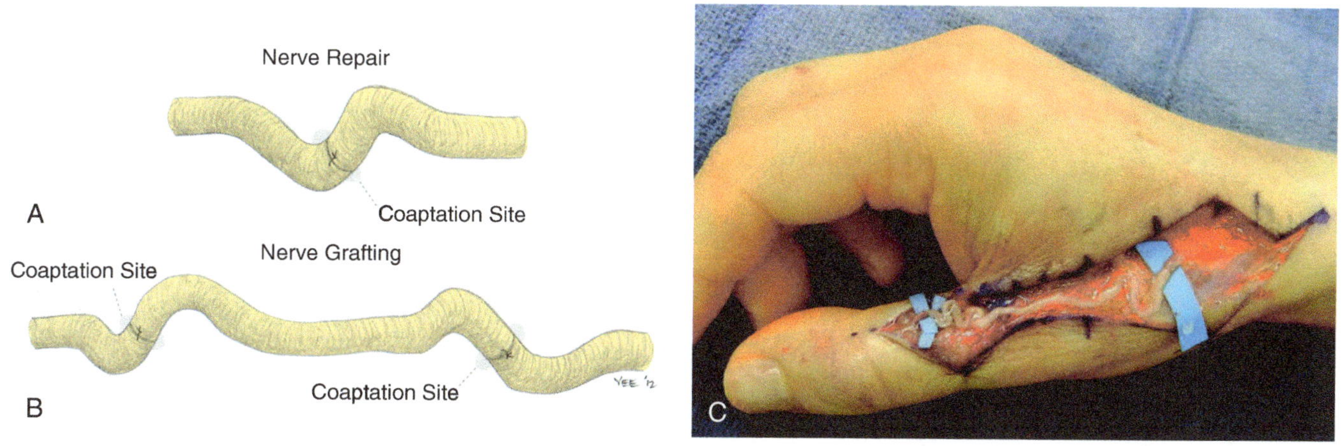

• **Fig. 52.2** Tension-free nerve repair. A nerve repair without tension is important for optimal recovery, as tension on the nerve repair will significantly downgrade the functional results. In addition, it is important to have redundancy at the coaptation sites. Tension is checked by performing range-of-movement on the extremity. (A) Nerve repair without tension at single coaptation site. (B) Nerve grafting without tension at two coaptation sites. (C) This patient had a radial sensory neuroma that was grafted with a lateral antebrachial cutaneous nerve graft in the hand. The tension-free repair sites with redundancy occurred at both ends of the nerve graft. (From Mackinnon S. *Nerve Surgery*. New York: Thieme. 2015.)

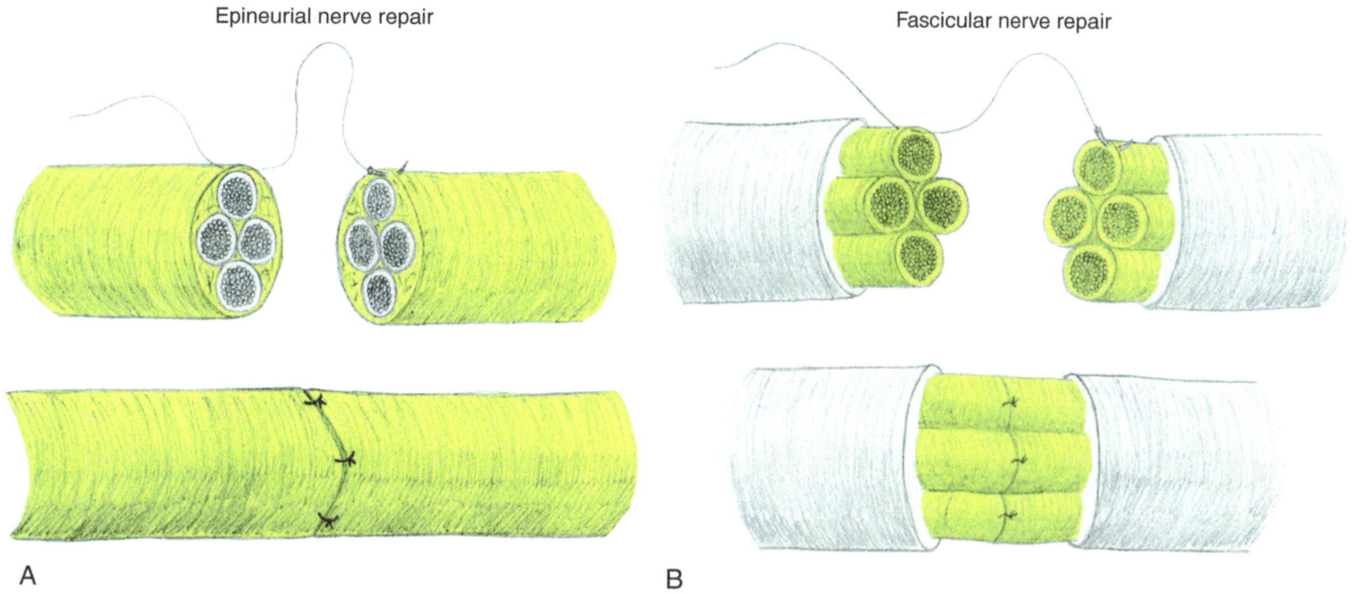

• **Fig. 52.3** Epineurial and fascicular nerve repair. (A) Epineurial nerve repair. (B) Fascicular nerve repair. (From Mackinnon S. *Nerve Surgery*. New York: Thieme. 2015.)

Technology: Intraoperative Nerve Stimulation

In our practice, a detailed clinical examination, combined with preoperative electromyogram/nerve conduction studies (EMG/NCS) completed by our skilled and experienced neurologists have made intraoperative nerve monitoring unnecessary. We do routinely, however, use a handheld nerve stimulator in the operating room. It provides muscle contraction, but no information about sensory recovery and is used when motor nerve transfers are performed. Intraoperative nerve stimulation allows us to identify redundant motor nerve fascicles, which will be transferred into nonfunctioning motor nerves to restore function (Fig. 52.4). For routine acute lacerations that require grafting or primary repair, there is no additional benefit to the use of nerve stimulation, unless it is performed in motor and mixed motor nerves transected and repaired within 72 hours. For a partial nerve injury with neuroma involving only a portion of the nerve's cross–sectional area, a nerve stimulator can help determine which motor nerve fascicles to preserve, while resecting the damaged tissue. In nerves that are purely or mostly sensory fibers, a handheld nerve stimulator is not useful.

Nerve Reconstruction

Nerve Grafting

The gold standard for a nerve injury repair is a primary neurorrhaphy within the first few days. The belief that a primary nerve repair with a single coaptation site is superior

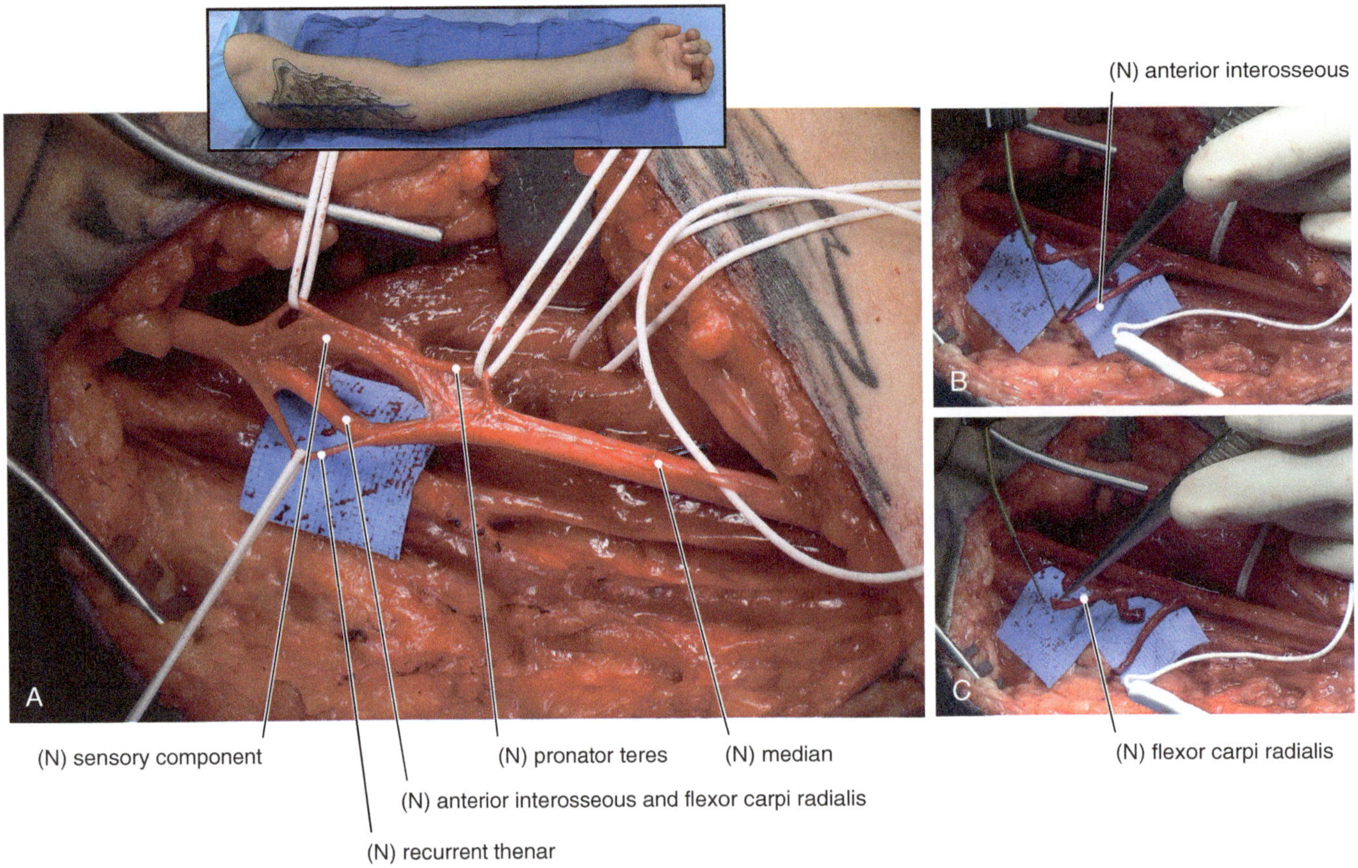

• **Fig. 52.4** Intraoperative electrical stimulation of nerve for identification. Intraoperative electrical stimulation allows for identifying motor and sensory components of a normal nerve, in addition to determining whether a motor nerve has innervated a muscle following an injury. Evaluation within 72 hours post injury will allow electrical stimulation of the distal injured nerve for identification. After 72 hours, the distal injured nerve will not respond to electrical stimulation due to the degeneration process. (A) This patient had a C7 spinal cord injury, where the peripheral neurons were intact and the central neurons were compromised, and underwent a nerve transfer. Interfascicular neurolysis of the median nerve revealed its fascicular component that were identified through electrical stimulation. (B,C) After proximal transection of the flexor carpi radialis and anterior interosseous nerve fascicles, the nerve fascicles continued to respond to electrical stimulation and are expected to respond for another 72 hours post transection. (From Mackinnon S. *Nerve Surgery*. New York: Thieme. 2015.)

to a nerve reconstruction with a graft involving two neurorrhaphy sites is supported by multiple animal studies (Fig. 52.5).[12] A percentage of fibers may be lost at each neurorrhaphy site; some studies suggest that as much as 50% of regenerating sensory or motor axons may never reach the correct end organ.[1] Tension at the repair should be avoided and a primary repair should never be forced together. When there is extreme tension and contamination, scarring of the repair site will invariably occur, and a proximal neuroma will develop.

Where tension is unavoidable despite proximal and distal mobilization of a nerve, a graft repair should be performed. We recommend reconstructing the nerve with a graft and rather accept two neurorrhaphy sites than perform a single neurorrhaphy under unfavorable conditions. Making sure to be outside the zone of injury is essential (Fig. 52.6) as well as using meticulous microneurosurgical technique, accurately matching the sensory and motor nerve fascicles, and early postoperative protected motion to allow neural gliding.

Several options for gap reconstruction are listed below with the pros and cons for each option (Table 52.3).[13]

Short Nerve Gaps (≤6 cm)

An autologous nerve graft remains the most common technique for repairing defects in peripheral nerves. The purpose of the nerve graft is to guide the regenerating axons to target. Choice of donor autologous nerve graft is a balance between donor site morbidity and quality of regeneration. Experimental studies indicate that motor or mixed donor nerve grafts yield superior clinical results when repairing a motor nerve defect.[14,15] That being said, expendable motor nerves are limited in clinical practice. Two possible motor nerve grafts with limited morbidity include the obturator nerve branch to the gracilis muscles and the anterior interosseous nerve branch to pronator quadratus.

The most common harvested nerve graft is the sural nerve; however, when working in the upper limb we prefer to use an expendable sensory nerve in the field such as the

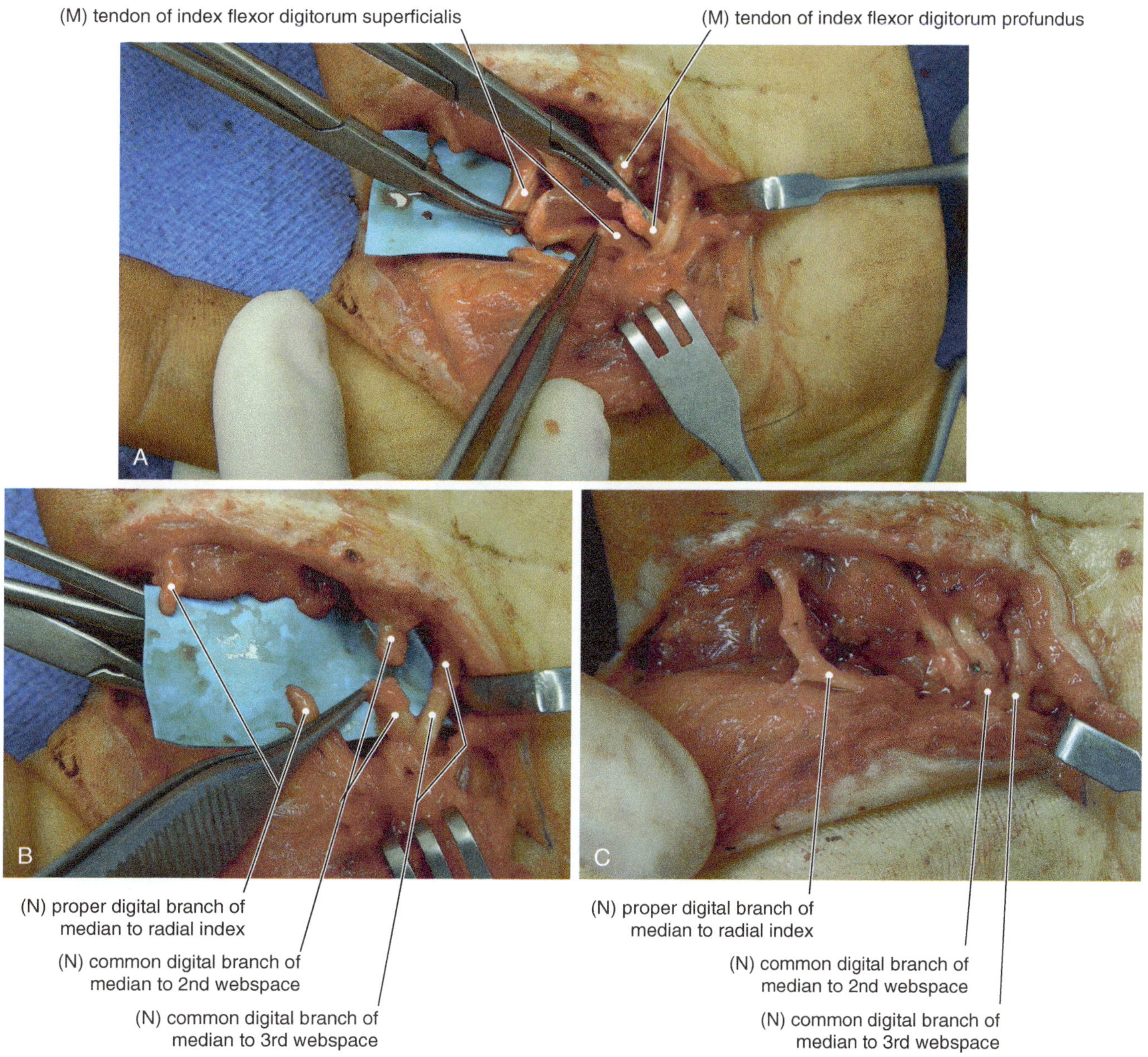

• **Fig. 52.5** Primary nerve repair of a sharp lacerating nerve injury. Nerve injuries that are sharp and lacerating induce a small zone of injury, which can allow for a tension-free primary repair. (A) This patient had a sharp lacerating injury to the right palm, which involved the digital nerves and tendons of the flexor digitorum superficialis and profundus. These tendons were repaired in zone 3. (B) Digital nerves of the median nerve were identified transected. (C) The proximal and distal ends of the digital nerves were trimmed by evenly transecting the ends for healthy nerve fibers. Primary repairs were performed without tension in all range of motion of the fingers, wrist, and hand. (From Mackinnon S. *Nerve Surgery*. New York: Thieme. 2015.)

lateral or medial antebrachial cutaneous nerve or the distal anterior or posterior interosseous nerve.[16] Sural nerve is still our graft of choice if performing cable grafts to a critical nerve, such as the median nerve, due to the length of available donor in a sural nerve.

Nerve grafts typically are less than 3 mm in diameter, which is a consequence of the historically poor results achieved when full-thickness nerve trunks were used as grafts. When necessary, the grafts may be cabled together. It is believed that smaller grafts will revascularize more easily, ultimately contributing to the success of the graft.

The gold standard for repairing a nerve gap injury is with an autologous nerve graft (Figs. 52.7 and 52.8). Because the major disadvantage of autografts is the donor site morbidity and the limited number of donor nerves available, new approaches to repairing the gap defect have been created. This has led to the use of vein grafts, biological and synthetic conduits, and nerve allograft as substitutes for short gap injuries. The current consensus is that for a sensory deficit in a non-critical, small-diameter nerve less than 3 cm, any of these options is equally reliable, although more recent literature supports the fact that while nerve allografts offer

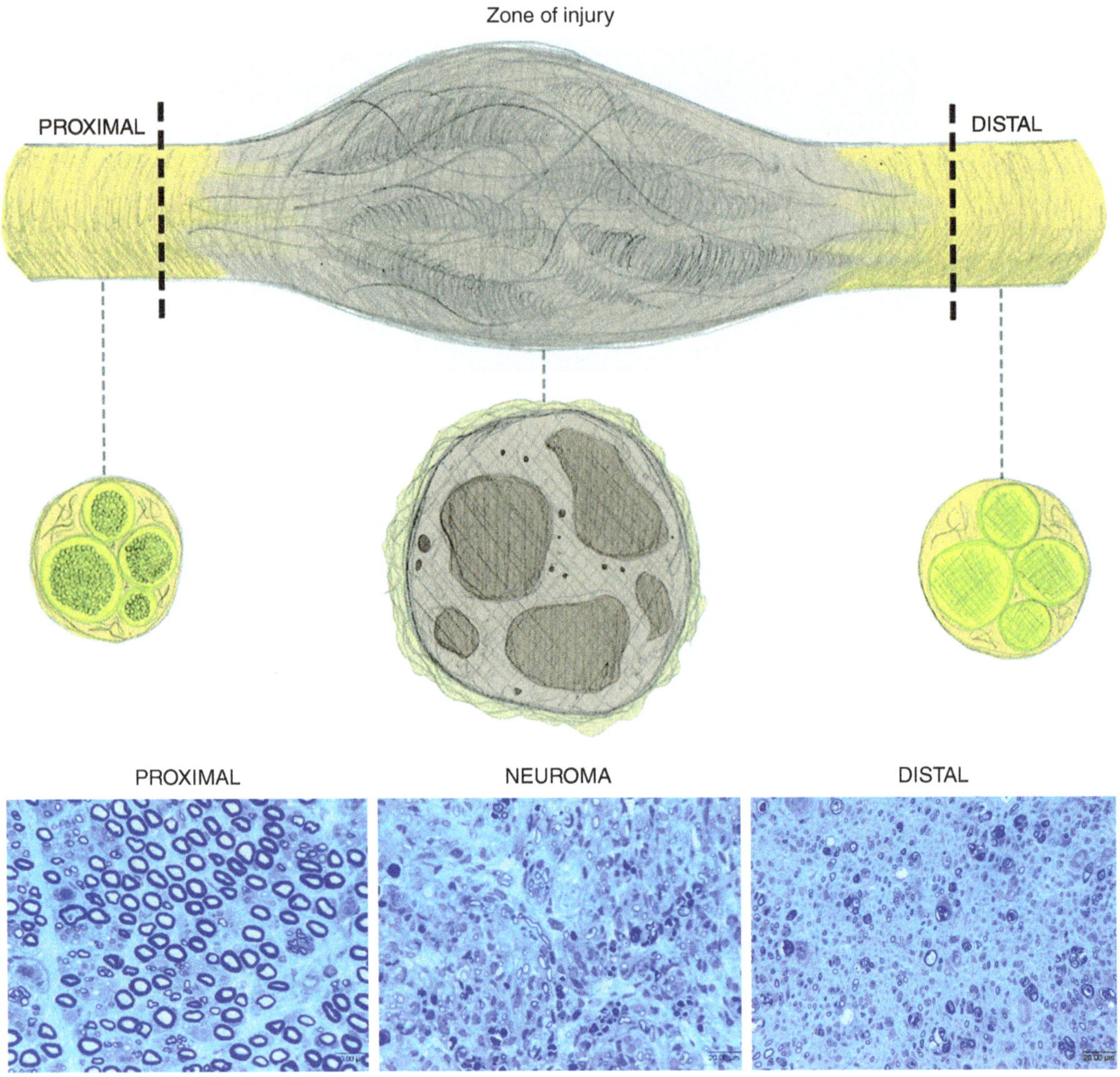

• **Fig. 52.6** Zone of injury within a nerve. The zone of injury is dependent on the mechanism of injury. A sharp lacerating injury will have a small zone of injury, while blunt, stretch, gunshot and traumatic injuries will have large zones of injury. It is important to excise the injured nerve outside the zone of injury (*dotted lines*) to allow proximal nerve fibers to regenerate distal without inhibitory factors from the injury. Histological section of proximal nerve exhibits normal nerve fibers. Histological section of neuroma exhibits disorganized patterns of fibers in a dense stroma of connective tissue. Histological section of distal nerve, distal to the injury, exhibits degenerating nerve fibers. Magnification × 400, toluidine blue. (From Mackinnon S. *Nerve Surgery*. New York: Thieme. 2015.)

excellent results in this gap range, the conduit results can vary greatly depending on type of material when the gap is greater than 15 mm.[17] Neither conduits nor allografts are currently recommended for gaps longer than 3 cm or for gaps in motor and mixed motor defects, although clinical trials are in progress assessing the role of allografts in some of these situations.

Acellular human processed nerve allografts have been available for clinical use since 2008 as an alternative to conduits (Fig. 52.9). In an animal study, Whitlock showed that the acellular allograft was superior to an empty conduit because of its extracellular matrix, but inferior to an autograft, which provides Schwann cells in addition to the extracellular matrix.[18] Initial clinical trials using allografts for short sensory gaps show recovery comparable to autografts and better than a conduit.[19] Because this is human tissue, it retains its three-dimensional structure, including epineurium, fascicles, endoneural tubes, and laminin, and it is believed that the scaffold allows for repopulation of the host cells, as in autologous nerve tissue. The product is expensive; however, since it shortens operative time, it allows the surgeon to be more efficient if working without assistance and may save overall operating room costs. The patient benefit is no morbidity of an additional scar and associated sensory loss. It handles similarly to autologous nerve and comes in various widths ranging from 1 to 5 mm in diameter and up to 70 mm in length. Interestingly, research studies have not shown successful regeneration at a distance of 40 mm or 60 mm (Fig. 52.10).[20,21]

TABLE 52.3 Options for Management of a Nerve Gap

Type	Advantage	Disadvantage
Autograft	Gold standard for reconstruction Schwann cells in extracellular matrix	Second operative site Results in donor sensory loss Potential for neuroma formation/pain Sensory nerve autograft do not support motor regeneration as well as motor or mixed sensory nerves Limited available length
Acellularized allograft	Functional recovery is almost equivalent to autograft No donor site morbidity Nonimmunogenic	Length limitation (<7 cm) No Schwann cells
Allograft	Functional recovery is almost equivalent to autograft No donor site morbidity	Requires patient systemic immunosuppression (about 18 months) Patient vulnerable to opportunistic infections
Conduit	Guides regenerating nerve to intended target No donor site morbidity	Length limitation (<5 cm) Only for small-diameter sensory nerves
End-to-side	No length limitation	Poor sensory results Motor requires donor neurectomy
Reverse end-to-side	Augment partial motor/sensory nerve injury	Requires knowledge of topography Requires knowledge of expendable donors May need nerve autograft or acellular graft
Nerve transfer	Earlier motor/sensory target recovery	Requires expendable donor Requires motor (sensory) re-education Requires knowledge of topography

Source: Weber R, Boyd K, Mackinnon S. Repair and grafting of peripheral nerve. In: Gurtner G, Neligan P, eds. *Plastic Surgery*. Volume 1: *Principles*. Elsevier; 2013. Reproduced with permission of Elsevier.

An acellular nerve allograft can be used for short nerve gaps ≤3 cm for small diameter/noncritical nerves.[18,20,21] In the senior author's opinion, based on laboratory findings, if an acellularized allograft ≥4 cm is used, it will not consistently drive axons across the allograft. In a noncritical digital nerve this would be an acceptable result, as collateral sprouting of an adjacent sensory nerve will occur to provide some sensation.

Autologous vein grafts are the oldest conduit and are still used both as a primary conduit and as a wrap. Biological conduits, including bone, artery, and muscle, have been used, but not as conventionally as vein, collagen or small intestine submucosa (SIS). Biodegradable synthetic conduits such as polyglycolic acid are currently used, while nondegradable nerve guides made from silicone have fallen out of favor. Their major disadvantage is leaving foreign material that potentially causes a chronic reaction with excessive scarring (Fig. 52.11).

Of the commercial conduits in use today, collagen and polyglycolic acid are biodegradable, while the SIS conduits are resorbed and replaced by the body's natural tissue. Like the original vein graft, they are used as primary conduits or as nerve wraps. They provide at least protective sensation and, in some cases, good sensory recovery.[22] Since the conduit is essentially a hollow tube with no structure, experimental studies have shown that placing morselized nerve into the tube can help to augment nerve growth.[23] When using a conduit, we recommend placing a small portion of the proximal nerve into the conduit to provide a source of Schwann cells.

Long Nerve Gaps (>6 cm)

There is no consensus on what is the maximum length an autologous nerve graft may be and still achieve regeneration of the nerve, although there are a few studies that have shown success with grafts as long as 20 cm. In general, nerve autografts ≤6 cm seem to be more reliably successful if close to the target, compared with longer nerve autografts. Failure of the long nerve autografts was the stimulus to move towards nerve transfer techniques in the 1990s, just as failure with nerve repair done under tension to overcome longer gaps was the stimulus to the shift towards the nerve grafts by Millesi in the 1970s.

Free vascularized nerve grafts were introduced in 1976 by Taylor and Ham in order to treat these longer gaps.[24] For smaller defects, a vascularized graft and conventional graft do not appear to differ in clinical outcome; however, Doi et al recommend using free vascularized nerve grafts when the gap distance is greater than 6 cm with associated soft tissue loss over the repaired area.[25] Currently the indication for a free vascularized nerve graft is for reconstruction of large-diameter nerve grafts, such as the ulnar nerve in brachial plexus avulsion surgery.

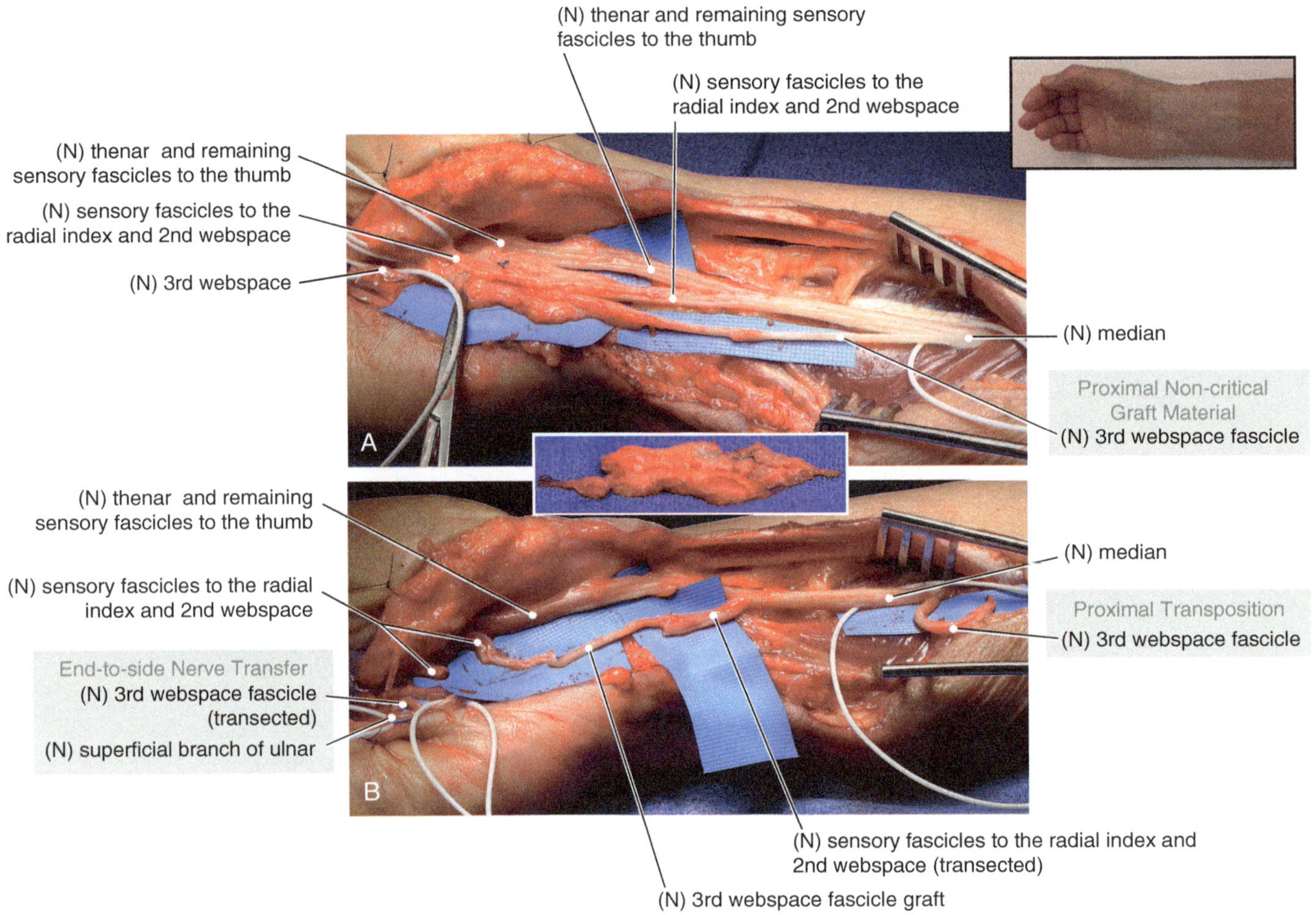

• **Fig. 52.7** Case of median nerve reconstruction at the wrist with third webspace graft. This patient had a significant injury to the median nerve at the wrist that involved the sensory components. (A) The zone of injury was identified and the neuroma was resected with proximal and distal median nerve components identified. The third webspace was further neurolysed proximally to mobilize graft material. (B) The proximal end of the third webspace fascicle was transected and used as a nerve graft to repair a portion of the median nerve. The proximal remainder of the third webspace was transposed proximally to prevent a painful neuroma. The distal third webspace was end-to-side transferred to the sensory component of the ulnar nerve to provide rudimentary sensation for donor deficit. (From Mackinnon S. *Nerve Surgery*. New York: Thieme. 2015.)

Nerve Transfers

The introduction of nerve transfers in the early 1990s has resulted in a paradigm shift in how nerve injuries are managed. In severe proximal injuries, nerve transfers have resulted in marked improved functional results. Nerve transfers offer the advantage of converting a proximal high-level nerve injury to a low-level nerve injury by moving the reconstruction closer to the target muscle or sensory territory of the affected nerve. In high ulnar and high median nerve injuries this is critical. A donor nerve close to the injured nerve is used in nerve transfers and usually nerve grafts are not needed. The donor and recipient nerves are neurolysed from the main nerve so that an end-to-end repair between donor and recipient fascicles can be done. Nerve transfers are also well suited to injuries with a large nerve gap, by providing distal reconstruction outside of the zone of injury where a long nerve graft is unlikely to have successful results (Table 52.4).

Tendon transfers set the stage for the development of motor nerve transfers. The principles are similar except that a single nerve transfer can innervate more than one muscle, unlike a tendon transfer. Unlike tendon transfers, muscle excursion and vectors of pull do not need to be considered in nerve transfers, although the number of axons in the donor nerve will affect the overall strength of the recovery. The ideal donor nerve has a similar number of motor axons as the recipient nerve. Expendable nerves and redundant fascicles or branches are used, avoiding nerves that innervate critical functions. Nerve transfers have evolved because of our understanding of the internal topography and the redundancy built into the human nerve. Intraoperative electrical stimulation with a handheld nerve stimulator identifies the motor

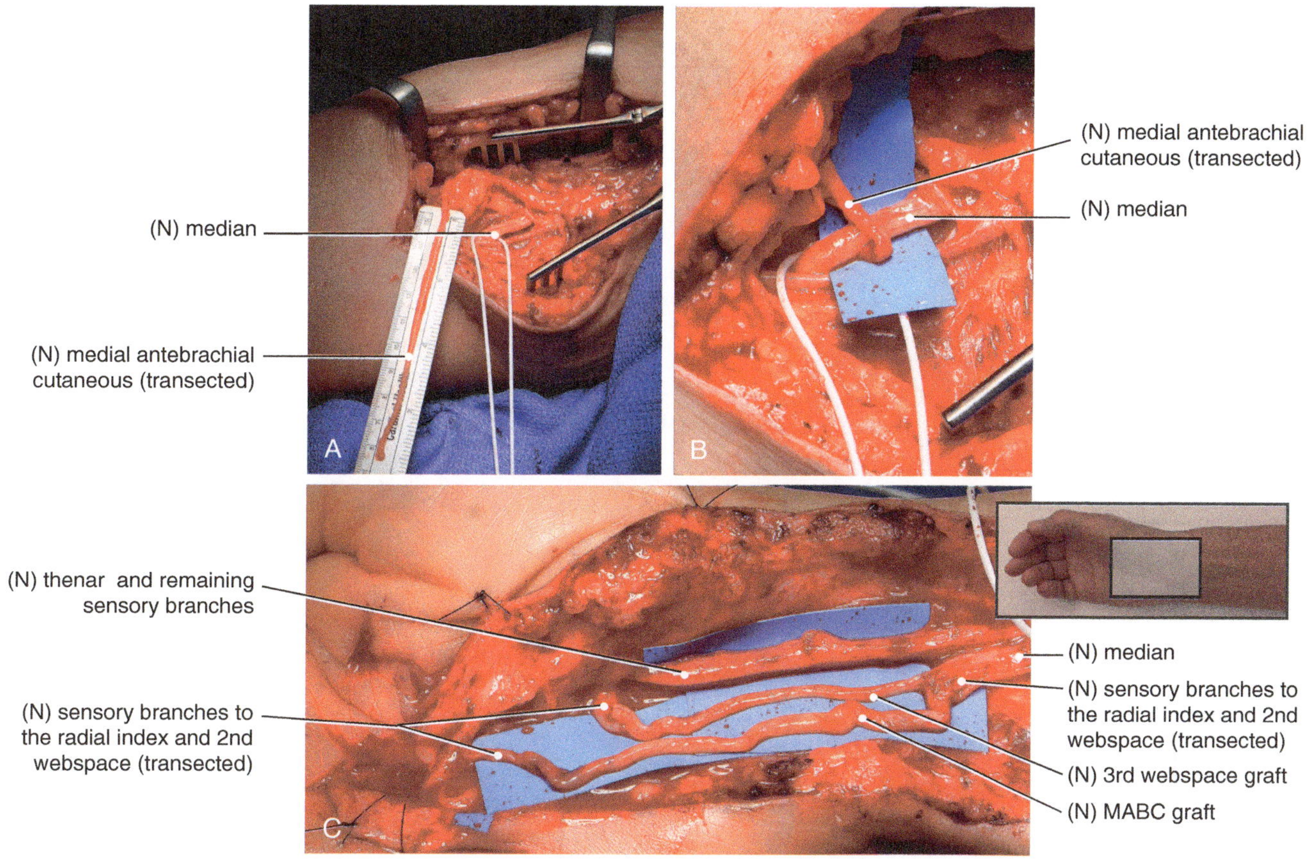

• **Fig. 52.8** Second webspace grafted with a medial antebrachial cutaneous nerve graft. (A) The medial antebrachial cutaneous nerve (MABC) was isolated within the arm for donor material. (B) The MABC was then transected with the distal end transferred to the sensory component of the median nerve through an end-to-side epineural window fashion. The sensory component of the median nerve is located on the superior aspect of the median nerve. Note that in this image, the median nerve has been rotated so that it appears to be on the inferior portion. (C) The MABC graft was used to repair the remaining portion of the median nerve. The thenar branch and remaining sensory branches to the thumb were protected and were found to be not injured. (From Mackinnon S. *Nerve Surgery*. New York: Thieme. 2015.)

TABLE 52.4 Indications for Nerve Transfer

1. Brachial plexus injury with only very proximal or no nerve available for grafting
2. High proximal injury that requires a long distance for regeneration
3. Scarred areas in critical locations with potential for injury to critical structures
4. Major limb trauma with segmental loss of nerve tissue requiring several grafts
5. Prolonged time from injury to reconstruction as an alternative to nerve grafting
6. Partial nerve injury with a defined functional loss
7. Spinal cord root avulsion injury
8. Idiopathic neuritides, radiation trauma, and nerve injuries where the level of injury is uncertain

donor fascicles, allowing for selection of the donor nerve without extensive neurolysis. Fascicle groups can easily be cleaved from the main nerve even in the proximal extremity without injuring unintended fascicle groups because the nerves do not merge distally as once thought. Instead, the fibers course parallel to each other via an extensive plexus pathway. This enables the surgeon to use "redundant" donor nerve fascicles for nerve transfer while maintaining enough fascicles to prevent loss of function in the donor muscle.

The major advantages of a nerve transfer over a tendon transfer are that: (a) sensory nerve transfers can restore sensibility; (b) a nerve that innervates multiple muscle groups can be restored with a single nerve transfer; and (c) the insertion and attachments of the muscle(s) in question are not disrupted, thus the original muscle function and tension are maintained. When choosing donor nerves for transfer, a nerve that innervates a synergistic muscle group is preferable, as it facilitates postoperative re-education. Although a nerve supplying a nonsynergistic, or even antagonistic, muscle group may be used, more motor retraining may be necessary to learn to contract the newly reinnervated muscle. Although a synergistic nerve transfer is ideal, antagonistic nerve transfers can be successfully utilized in some cases, such as branches of radial nerve used to restore median nerve function. In median to radial nerve transfers we are careful to transfer flexor carpi radialis to the posterior

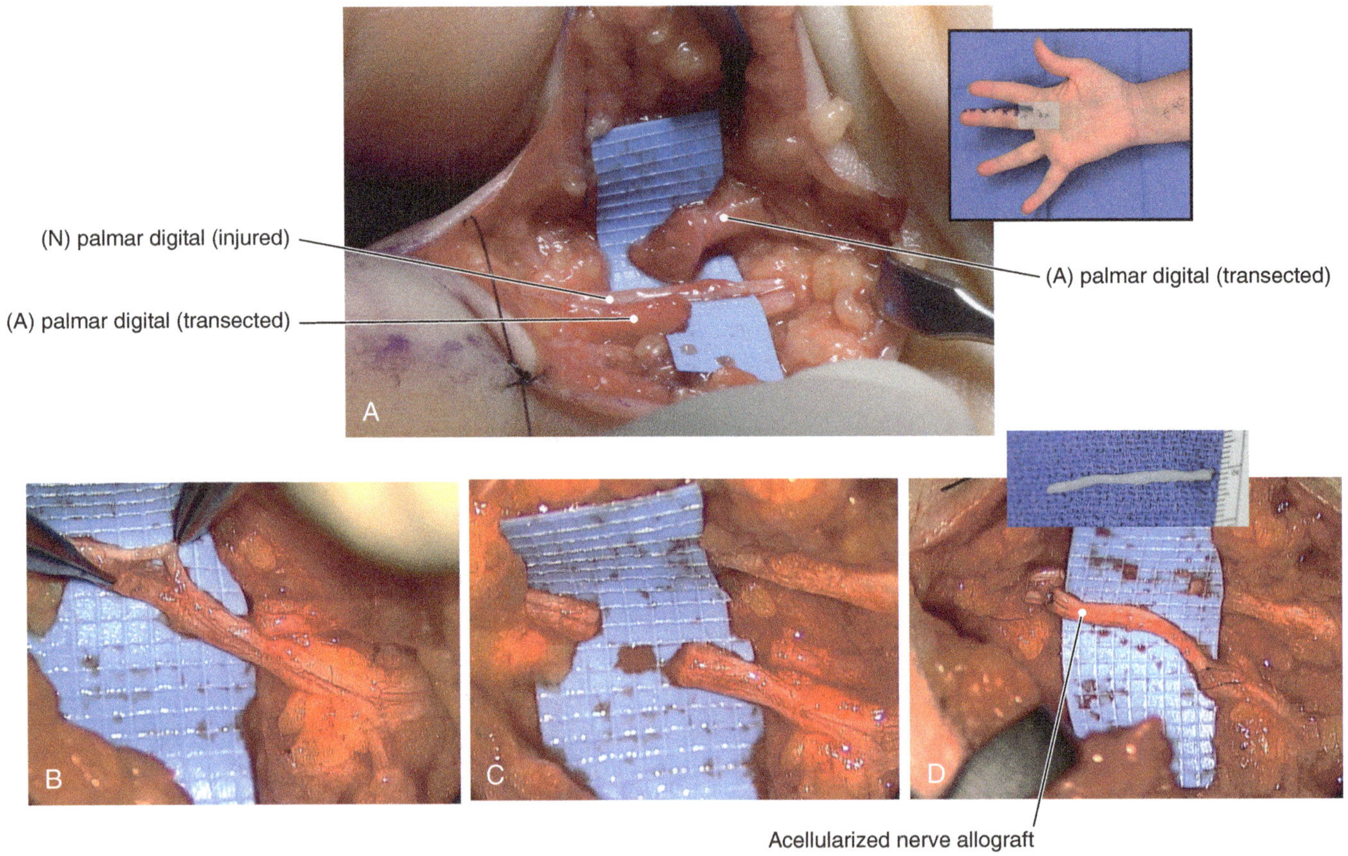

• **Fig. 52.9** Reconstruction of a noncritical sensory nerve with acellularized nerve allograft. This patient had a lacerating injury at the base of the long finger. (A) Upon exploration, the palmar digital artery was found to be transected. The palmar digital nerve to the radial aspect of the long finger was found to be intact but injured. (B) The digital nerve had been longitudinally injured by the sharp object. (C) The zone of injury was identified and resected until healthy nerve was seen at both proximal and distal ends. (D) A 2 cm acellularized allograft was used to bridge the nerve gap for a tension-free repair. The nerve repair was tested for tension by putting the long finger through full flexion and extension. (From Mackinnon S. *Nerve Surgery*. New York: Thieme. 2015.)

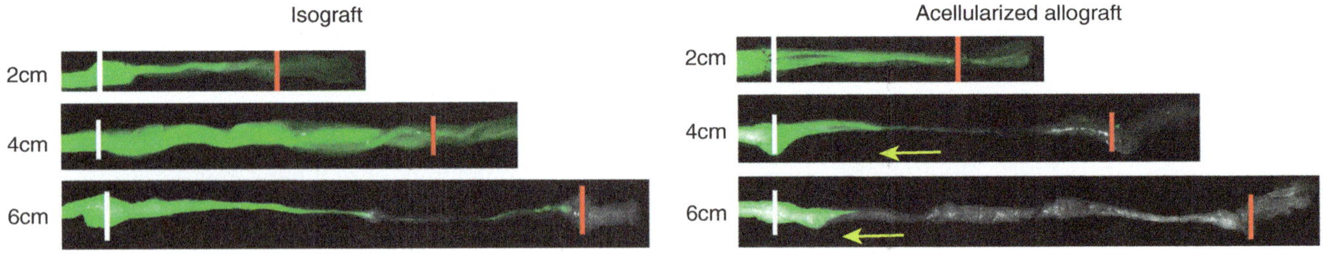

• **Fig. 52.10** Nerve regeneration through various lengths of isografts and acellularized nerve allografts (ANA) in a fluorescent GFP rat model. Regeneration through a short 2 cm graft was similar between an isograft and ANA, however as the graft length increased, the regeneration distance of the ANA decreased in comparison to an isograft. (From Mackinnon S. *Nerve Surgery*. New York: Thieme. 2015.)

interosseous nerve and flexor digitorum sublimus nerve to the extensor carpi radials brevis nerve (Fig. 52.12). Similarly, when we do a double fascicular transfer (DFT) for elbow flexion we will try to always use the median fascicle to transfer to the brachialis nerve and the ulnar fascicle to transfer to the biceps nerve for faster motor reeducation (biceps supinates and median nerve pronates, so it is a bit harder to re-educate if done the opposite way). Nerve transfers for specific nerve reconstructions are discussed in greater detail in Chapter 53.

End-to-Side and Reverse End-to-Side Nerve Transfers

Most nerve transfers are done with an end-to-end repair. The circumstances in which an end-to-side neurorrhaphy is utilized continues to evolve.

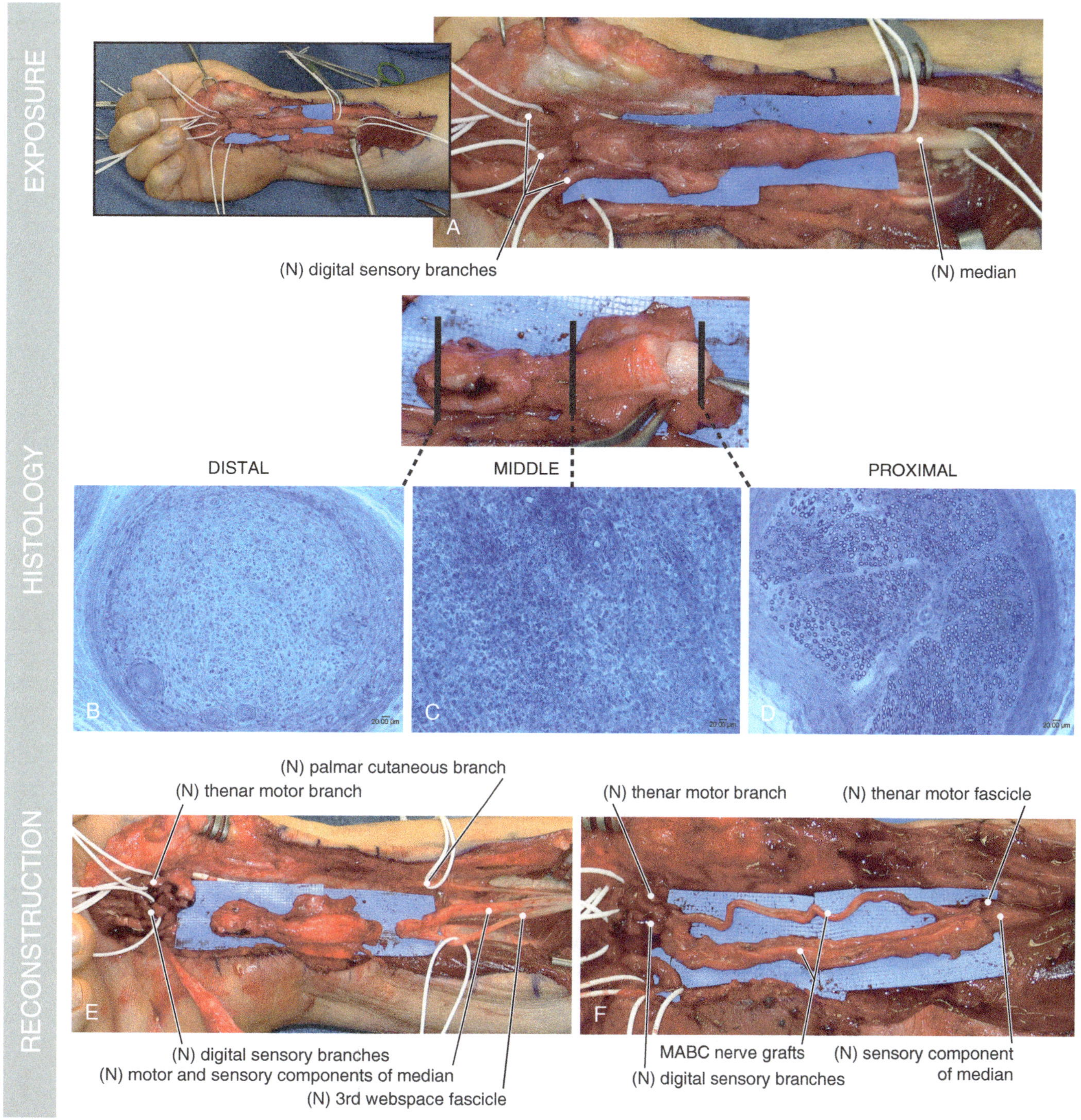

• **Fig. 52.11** Failed nerve wrap case. Patient presented with a right median nerve injury following a carpal tunnel release that was repaired with a nerve wrap 2 years postoperatively. The sensory component of the median nerve was injured and repaired with a nerve wrap. (A) Upon exposure, the median nerve was identified with a large neuroma. (B) Histological evaluation revealed scarce nerve fibers in the distal segment. (C) The middle segment displayed significant disorganized architecture with no axonal organization, consistent with neuroma. (D) The proximal segment revealed healthy nerve fibers. (E) The neuroma was resected and the motor and sensory components of the median nerve identified. (F) The gap was reconstructed with several medial antebrachial cutaneous nerve cable grafts with an individual graft for repair of the motor component. (From Mackinnon S. *Nerve Surgery*. New York: Thieme. 2015.)

End-to-side nerve repairs involve coapting the distal end of the injured nerve into the side of a healthy donor nerve without disrupting the donor nerve target. In our practice we reserve an end-to-side nerve repair technique for nerve transfers for non-critical sensory nerves (Fig. 52.13). Noncritical sensory nerves include the dorsal cutaneous branch of the ulnar nerve, or a donor sensory nerve graft territory after that graft has been taken for reconstruction. For example, when restoring critical distal ulnar nerve sensation, we use fascicles from the median nerve innervating

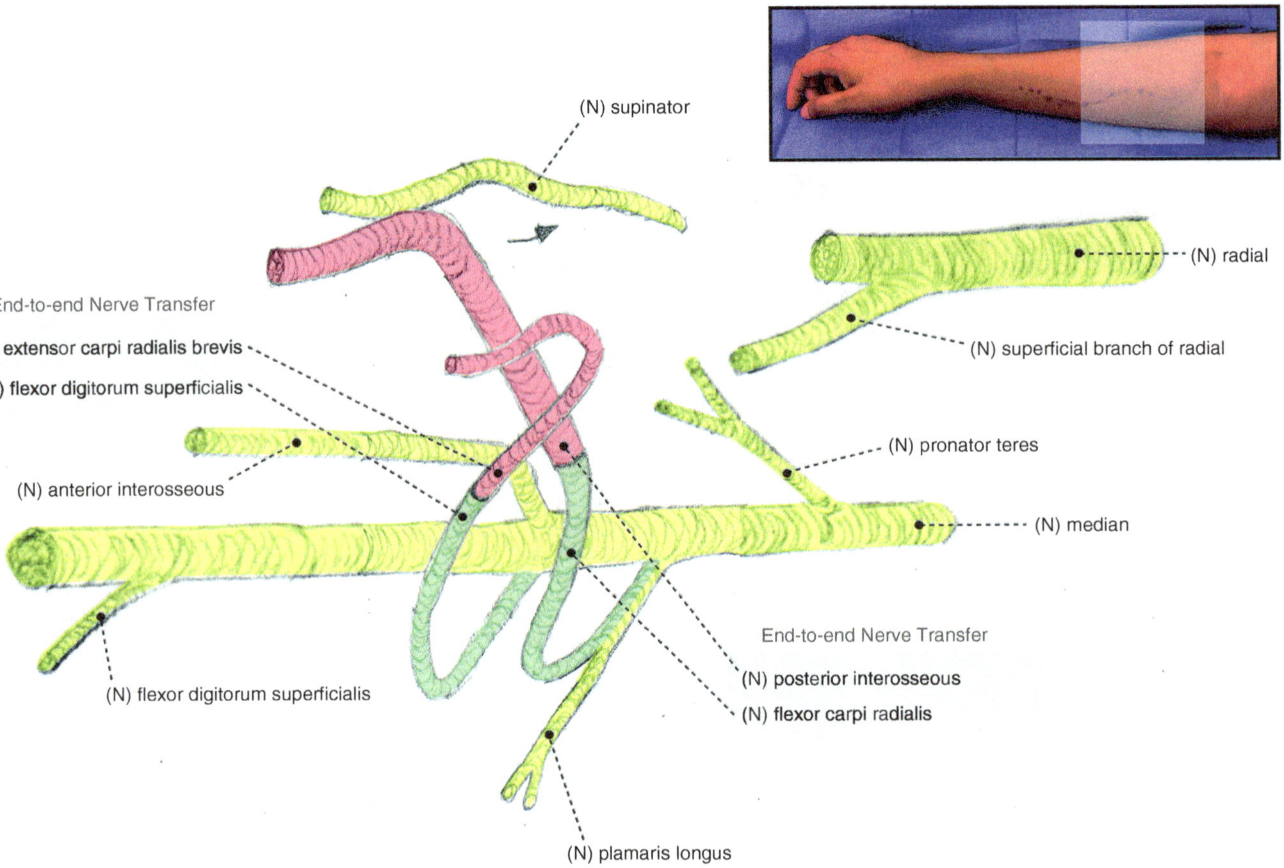

• **Fig. 52.12** Illustrative median to radial nerve transfer. Two nerve transfers occur in the median to radial nerve transfer for restoration of wrist/finger extension. The donors (green) and recipients (pink) occur in the following specific sets for optimal results with postoperative rehabilitation: (1) flexor carpi radialis to posterior interosseous (PIN) and (2) flexor digitorum superficialis (FDS) to extensor carpi radialis brevis. PIN and FDS are antagonistic. (From Mackinnon S. *Nerve Surgery*. New York: Thieme. 2015.)

the third webspace and perform an end-to-end nerve transfer into the distal ulnar nerve. We then commonly use an end-to-side transfer of the distal third webspace nerve into the side of the recovering ulnar nerve to restore some sensation in the donor nerve distribution (third webspace median).

Reverse end-to-side nerve transfers involve coapting the distal end of a donor nerve into the side of a recipient nerve to augment or support recovery. The primary example of a reverse end-to-side nerve transfer is the distal anterior interosseous motor nerve branch to the pronator quadratus into the side of the ulnar nerve. We use this nerve transfer in severe ulnar compression neuropathy which has created a second- or third-degree injury in the ulnar nerve. Based on our experimental studies, the normal anterior interosseous motor nerve branch to the prontator quadratus is transferred to the side of the motor component of the ulnar nerve, about 8–9 cm proximal to the wrist crease. Each of the 2–3 distal anterior interosseous nerve branches is sewn to the side of the ulnar motor fascicular group, which in general includes 2–3 fascicles. We believe these anterior interosseous nerve axons both innervate and "babysit" the ulnar intrinsic muscles, in essence creating a Martin–Gruber anastomosis while the nerve recovers from its proximal injury. Results have been very encouraging.[26]

While sensory axons can spontaneously sprout collateral axons in an end-to-side repair, motor axons need to have a proximal injury in order for "traumatic" sprouting to occur (Fig. 52.14). One setting where we employ this technique is for the spinal accessory to suprascapular nerve transfer. The suprascapular recipient nerve is transferred end-to-side to the spinal accessory donor nerve via a partial neurectomy in the donor nerve. An area of the spinal accessory nerve proximal to the repair is crushed with micro forceps to initiate sprouting into both the suprascapular recipient nerve and the spinal accessory donor nerve to minimize deficit of the donor nerve.

Postoperative Management and Long-Term Sequelae

Postoperative Mobilization

We recommend immobilizing for 1–2 weeks after a simple nerve repair; however, gentle protected range of motion can be started as early as 2–3 days. No consensus exists on what

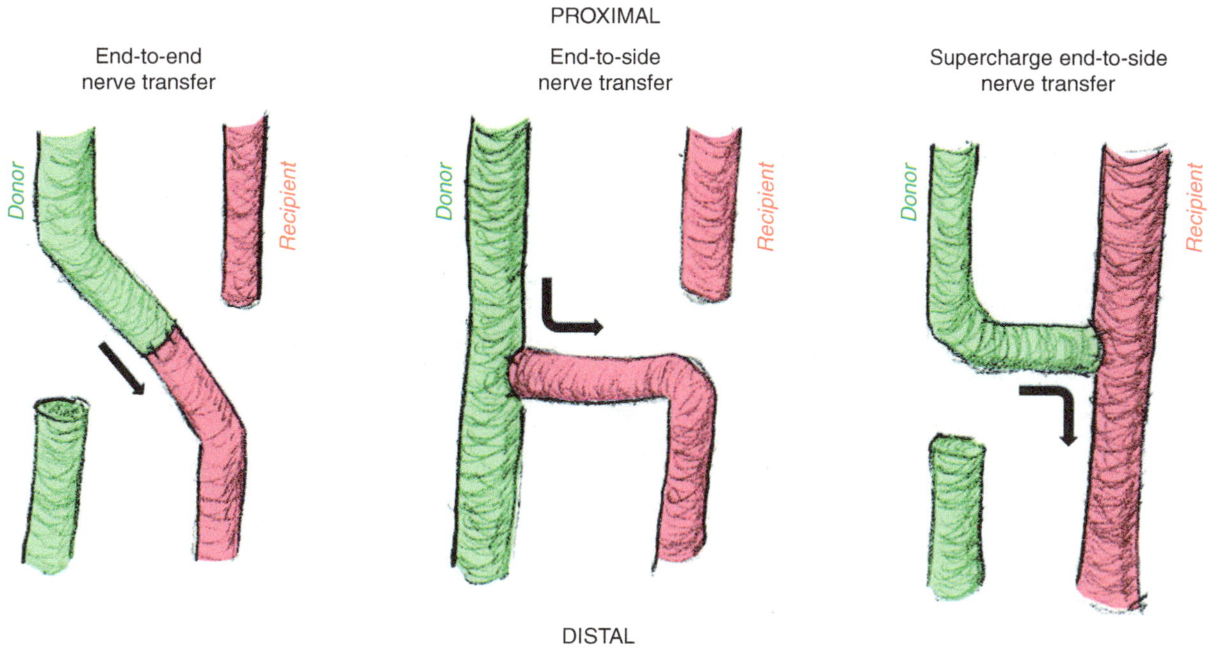

• **Fig. 52.13** Types of nerve repairs. Primary nerve repairs and nerve grafting occur in a traditional end-to-end fashion with its native nerve. When a nerve is transposed to another nerve, it is described as a nerve transfer. Nerve transfers can have a coaptation of an end-to-end, end-to-side or supercharge end-to-side fashion. Traditional nerve transfers occur from donor to recipient in an end-to-end fashion. End-to-side nerve transfer is described as the recipient nerve end being transferred to the side of the donor nerve. Opposite of an end-to-side, supercharge end-to-side nerve transfers is described as the donor nerve end being transferred to the side of a recipient nerve. (From Mackinnon S. *Nerve Surgery*. New York: Thieme. 2015.)

length of time for immobilization is necessary. However, we believe that early, protected range of motion is critical for neural gliding and an excellent result. In patients with concomitant tendon or bony injuries, the postoperative protocol is guided by the injury most difficult to rehabilitate. For example, in finger lacerations in which both tendon and nerves are transected, a flexor tendon protocol is followed postoperatively in order to maximize tendon gliding. The nerve repair, while important, is easier to reconstruct if necessary later. In the case of fractures, in addition to nerve and soft tissue injures, the bony fixation takes precedence.

Postoperative Neuropathic Pain

Most patients complain in the postoperative period of paresthesia and electric shocks, which extend beyond the area of the injury. Most of these can be controlled with neurotropic medications such as nortriptyline or pregabalin. In patients with neuropathic pain, prompt involvement of a pain specialist is critical. Physical therapy and occupational therapy continue for an extended rehabilitative period to prevent joint contractures while the nerve recovery is in progress, to fabricate and adjust protective splints, and to assist in motor and sensory re-education as the recovery process is underway. Whenever possible, our hand therapists evaluate and advise patients preoperatively and re-education begins within the first month of surgery, long before results of regeneration are anticipated. Similarly, mirror training is used to keep the "brain open" and receptive for eventual sensory recovery and has helped patients cope with their neuropathic pain. Mirror therapy and graded motor imagery, a pain program directed primarily by a hand therapist, has been successfully used at our institution in the treatment of neuropathic pain.[27,28]

Neuroma

Early primary repair or reconstruction of nerve injuries serves the main purposes of: (1) restoring distal function or sensibility and (2) preventing neuroma formation. Unfortunately, in every nerve surgeon's practice there are patients who are either a delayed presentation from injury or have developed postreconstruction neuroma. Neuroma can be a difficult problem to treat. Recent technology and laboratory studies have provided new surgical interventions for the treatment of neuroma with improved success in reducing pain symptoms.[29]

In neuroma resulting from a nerve injury where both the proximal and distal cut nerve ends are available, consensus is to excise the neuroma to healthy fascicles and reconstruct across the defect to provide a target for regenerating nerve fibers, thus reducing pain, recurrence of neuroma, and potentially restoring distal function or sensation. Due to scarring and loss of elasticity in the cut nerve, neuroma excision almost always requires a strategy to bridge a nerve gap.

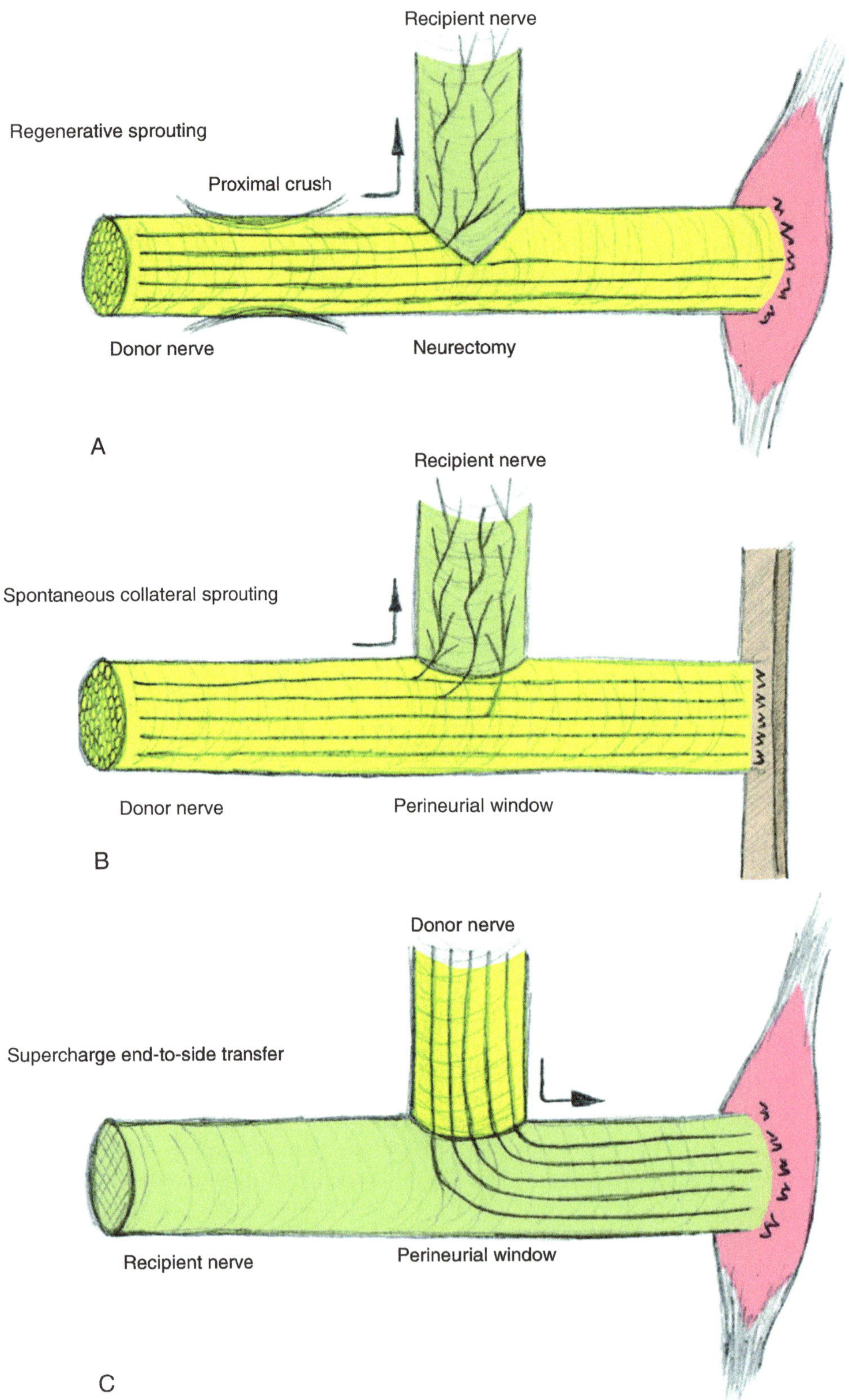

• **Fig. 52.14** Nerve regeneration in end-to-side nerve repairs. The two types of end-to-side nerve repairs or transfers are the traditional end-to-side and supercharge end-to-side. End-to-side nerve transfers have two sprouting mechanisms that are characteristic of either motor or sensory nerves. (A) Regenerative sprouting occurs in motor nerves in response to an injury. In order to elicit regenerative sprouting for a nerve transfer, a partial neurectomy and a proximal crush is required. The proximal crush causes an axonometric injury and creates a proximal regenerative front that regenerates into the recipient nerve and backfills the donor nerve. (B) Spontaneous collateral sprouting occurs in sensory nerves. Due to the spontaneous sprouting, no injury is required except for a perineurial window for the nerve fibers to regenerate through. (C) Supercharge end-to-side nerve transfer is where the donor nerve end is transferred into the side of a recipient nerve. This allows nerve fibers to regenerate into the recipient nerve through a perineurial window without sacrificing the integrity of the donor nerve. (From Mackinnon S. *Nerve Surgery*. New York: Thieme. 2015.)

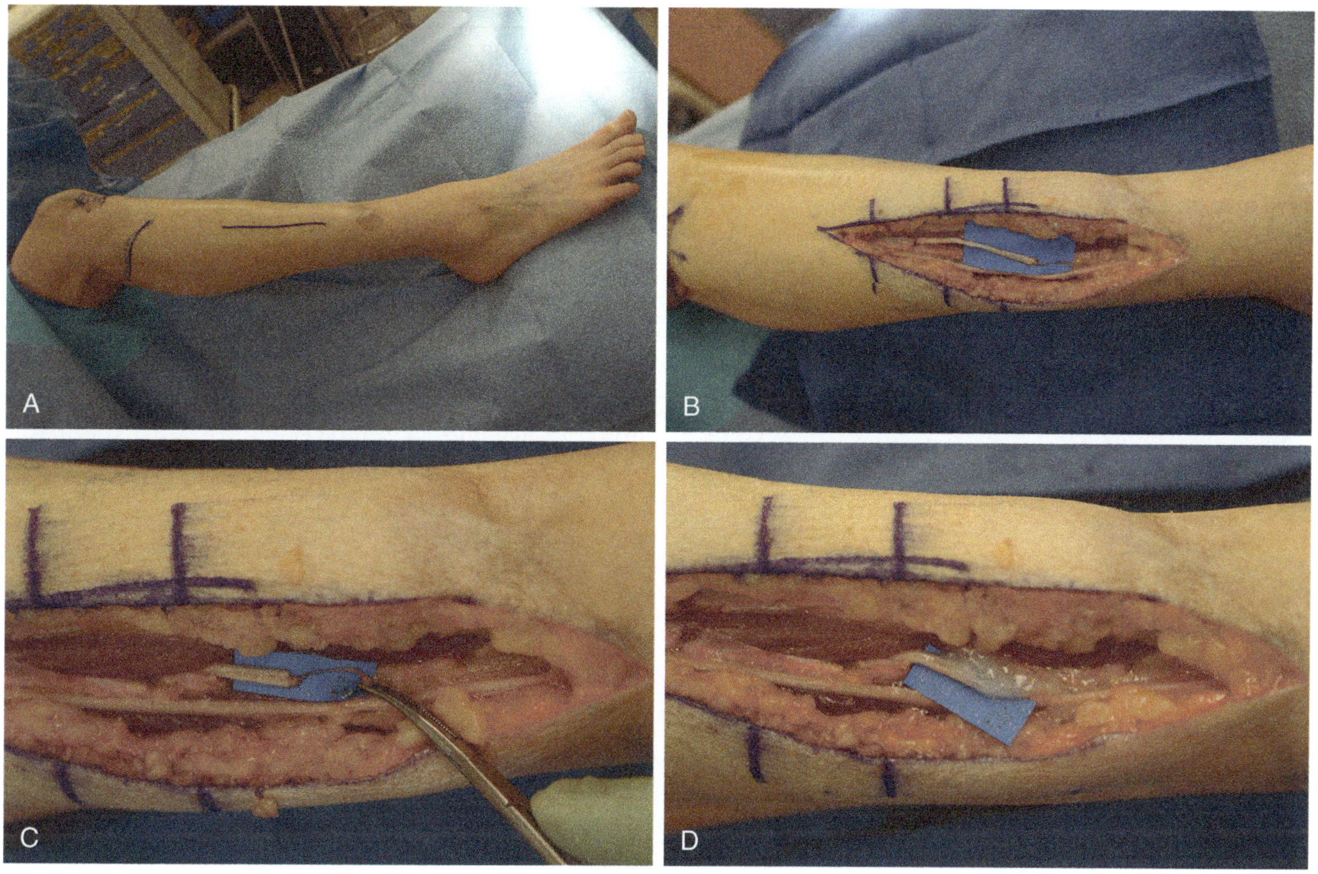

• **Fig. 52.15** Acellular nerve allograft in the treatment of neuroma. (A–D) After excision of the proximal neuroma, a 5-cm acellular nerve allograft is coapted to the free end of the nerve. The nerve is then transposed under no tension proximally. Use of the acellular nerve allograft provides a scaffold for regenerating nerve fibers which will grow and eventually "dwindle" with no distal target.

We have not had great success in using conduits, and suggest either autograft or acellular nerve allograft for appropriate short nerve gaps, or autograft from longer nerve gaps as outlined in the section on nerve grafting.

In patients with a neuroma-in-continuity, scarring occurs around the injured or repaired segment producing pain, but the nerve fibers are in continuity to the target. Variable function can be preserved distal to the neuroma, creating a treatment dilemma. Surgical treatment of a neuroma in continuity is reserved for clinical situations where the potential improvement of pain symptoms in the patient outweighs the risk for possible loss of distal function. To surgically remove a neuroma in continuity when some distal function is intact, we suggest using a handheld nerve stimulator to avoid injury to transmitting motor fascicles while performing a microneural dissection. Once the neuroma is trimmed to healthy-appearing fascicles, cable grafting across the defect is one surgical option. In patients with sensory or motor neuroma-in-continuity of a critical nerve (e.g., median nerve), distal end-to-side nerve transfers can be performed to restore or augment return of function or sensation, while grafting across the neuroma defect can provide a target for regenerating axons from the nerve stump.

Neuroma involving the proximal stump of a nerve without anatomic continuity to target can be treated with either ablative surgical strategies or with reconstructive strategies.[30] Traditionally, ablative treatments of neuroma involve neuroma excision and implantation in a variety of tissues, including muscle, bone, and vein, with variable results. The principle behind these treatments is to move the regenerating neuroma away from the subcutaneous tissue. The cut nerve end itself continues to have the potential to form another neuroma, as the regenerating axons still have no target. The centro-central neurorrhaphy technique was developed to redirect fascicular growth along intraneural fascicular coaptations by creating a looped coaptation within a large nerve or between small adjacent nerve branches.[31] This technique is not commonly used. Nerve caps, including the use of synthetic resin, vein, and silicone, have also been used to reduce axonal sprouting and recurrence of neuroma.

Findings in the laboratory of disappointing axonal growth across an acellular nerve graft longer than 4 cm encouraged us to use acellular nerve grafts to treat the proximal neuroma stump. After excising the neuroma from the proximal nerve stump, a 5 cm acellular nerve graft is coapted to the free nerve end and the nerve is transposed proximally, tension free, in a new plane away from the subcutaneous tissue (Fig. 52.15). This technique provides a target tissue for regenerating nerve fibers to grow; however, the lack of distal neurotrophic factors causes the axonal growth to "dwindle" within the acellular nerve allograft. Preliminary results in lower extremity neuroma have shown improved pain symptoms using this technique. This technique has also been called "relocation nerve grafting" in a recent review.[30]

Reconstructive treatments of neuroma provide distal living tissue to act as a target for regenerating axons in the prevention of neuroma recurrence. Reconstructive techniques include end-to-side neurorrhaphy, regenerative peripheral nerve interface (RPNI), and targeted muscle reinnervation (TMR).

In our practice, an end-to-side neurorrhaphy is a useful and commonly employed technique to treat the proximal or distal end of a less critical sensory nerve after neuroma excision or after harvesting a donor nerve graft. We most commonly use this technique to treat the "free" end of the donor nerve after it is used for a reconstruction (e.g., the distal or proximal end of a lateral antebrachial cutaneous (LABC) nerve after a segment has been taken as nerve graft). In this technique, an epineural window is created on the side of an adjacent nerve or nerve branch, and the available end of the injured nerve is microsurgically coapted into the window. This technique directs regenerating nerve fibers down the nerve allowing for more organized axonal growth.

Regenerative peripheral nerve interface (RPNI) wraps a small free muscle graft around the terminal nerve stump after neuroma excision.[32] The free muscle graft becomes reinnervated by the regenerating nerve fibers. This technique has the opportunity for functional interface in a myoelectric prosthesis, and pilot studies in amputees have reported significantly improved pain scores.[32]

Targeted muscle reinnervation (TMR) was developed to improve function in myoelectric prostheses and has been found incidentally to improve pain in amputees. After excision of the distal neuroma to healthy fascicles, adjacent muscles that have been rendered functionless by the amputation are identified, and their nerve branches are used as distal targets for coaptation with the neuroma stump. A recent randomized clinical trial in 28 major limb amputees found a clinical significant reduction in phantom limb pain, and a trend toward improved pain scores in the residual limb.[33]

Complex Regional Pain Syndrome

Complex regional pain syndrome (CRPS) was documented as early as 1864 during the American Civil War by Silas Weir Mitchell in his book titled *Gunshot Wounds and Other Injuries of Nerves*, where he describes "long after the trace of the effects of a wound has gone … neuralgic symptoms are apt to linger, and too many carry with them throughout long years this final reminder of the battlefield." In 1900, Sudeck noted muscle atrophy and demineralization of bone described as "patchy osteoporosis of the small bones of the hands or feet and the distal metaphysis of the forearm or tibial bones." This gave rise to the term *Sudeck's dystrophy*. Almost 50 years later, the term *reflex sympathetic dystrophy* was used to describe what Evans assumed to be sympathetic nervous system involvement with the abnormal activity observed in the affected extremities. However, the signs and symptoms of this disease did not consistently show sympathetic involvement, a reflex mechanism or the presence of dystrophy. For this reason, the Special Consensus Group of the International Association for the Study of Pain (IASP) created the term *complex regional pain syndrome* in 1994 to allow for a more broad inclusion of patients that showed varying levels of the disease process.

CRPS is a rare disease, with a prevalence of less than 2%. It is more common in younger adults, with a mean age of 41.8 years and with greater frequency in females than males (2.3–3:1). CRPS more commonly occurs as a result from work–related injuries or surgery and is associated with functional impairment, sleep disturbance, and suicidal ideation.

Clinical Features and Diagnosis

Although there is currently no gold standard to test the diagnosis of CRPS, it is imperative to perform a thorough history and physical examination. In 2007, the Budapest Criteria were developed to refine and create strict guidelines for research studies and clinical diagnosis of CRPS (sensitivity 0.99, specificity 0.68).[34]

1. Presence of continued disproportional pain from the known inciting event.
2. Must report at least one symptom in three of the following four categories:
   - Sensory: hyperesthesia, allodynia
   - Vasomotor: temperature asymmetry, changes in skin color
   - Sudomotor/edema: edema, changes in sweating, sweating asymmetry
   - Motor/trophic: decreased range of motion, motor dysfunction (tremor, weakness, dystonia), trophic changes (hair, nail, skin).
3. Must report at least one sign in two or more of the following categories at the time of evaluation:
   - Sensory: hyperalgesia to pinprick, allodynia to touch or joint movement
   - Vasomotor: temperature asymmetry, colour asymmetry
   - Sudomotor/edema: edema, asymmetrical sweating, sweating changes
   - Motor/trophic: decreased range of motion, motor dysfunction, trophic changes
4. No other condition that would otherwise explain the degree of pain or dysfunction.

CRPS is further divided into two groups (CRPS 1 and CRPS 2), with the distinction being that CRPS 2 has the presence of a definable nerve lesion nerve injury.

Other common diagnostic tests to aid in the diagnosis of CRPS include three-phase bone scintigraphy, which can detect alterations in bone metabolism, quantitative sensory testing, which can show impaired mechanical pain thresholds, and infrared thermography, which can show differences in temperature in the affected region.

Pathophysiology

Although the majority of patients who develop this syndrome have an initiating inciting event such as trauma, surgery, ischemia or nerve compression, it is unclear why only some patients develop CRPS. It is becoming increasingly apparent that multiple mechanisms may be involved in the development of this disease. Some of these mechanisms include an alteration to cutaneous sensory innervation with a reduction in C and A-delta fiber density, central and peripheral sensitization, an increase in the release of proinflammatory cytokines and neuropeptides, alterations in sympathetic nervous system function, and altered processing of nociceptive stimuli from cortical reorganization.

Treatment

Unfortunately, there is limited evidence as to the most effective treatment regimens for CRPS, with very few randomized controlled trails. Current recommendations are based on treatment modalities for other neuropathic pain conditions, favoring a multimodal, multidisciplinary approach. Of utmost importance is that earlier recognition and diagnosis with earlier initiation of targeted therapy typically achieves greater results. A recent review has provided a helpful treatment algorithm in CRPS for both acute CRPS, CRPS that persists greater than 6 months, and chronic CRPS.[35]

All patients with CRPS benefit from a thorough discussion of the pathophysiology of CRPS, as well as physical and occupational therapy including mirror therapy or graded motor imagery. Physical and occupational therapy targeting functional restoration continues to be the benchmark for successful CRPS treatment. Exercises that target myofascial release, isometric strengthening, and increased range of motion as well as desensitization techniques should be instituted as soon as possible for the best results. As an increasing amount of evidence supports cortical reorganization as a component of CRPS, there is also an increasing amount of evidence that supports the beneficial effects of graded motor imagery (GMI). Graded motor imagery is a three-stage program consisting of implicit motor imagery (left/right handedness), explicit motor imagery (imagined movements), and mirror therapy.[58] A randomized controlled study showed that at 6 and 12 weeks those patients who underwent GMI had significantly less pain and swelling.

Treatment of the neuropathic pain accompanying CRPS includes the use of antidepressants such as tricyclic antidepressants (TCAs) and serotonin noradrenaline reuptake inhibitors (SNRIs). Anticonvulsants and membrane stabilizers such as gabapentin and pregabalin have been shown to be effective in diabetic neuropathy and postherpetic neuralgia.

Acute Treatments

New evidence suggests that corticosteroids may decrease the acute inflammatory process that occurs during CRPS, and have shown clinical success when started early and given at high doses for 4 weeks. Bisphosphonates have been advocated for use in patients with CRPS to counteract the features of bone demineralization. Several studies using either intravenous or oral bisphosphonates have shown improvement in both reported pain scores as well as functional assessment in both short-term as well as medium-term outcomes. More novel pharmacological approaches include the use of free radical scavengers such as dimethyl sulfoxide (DMSO) 50% applied in a topical cream and *N*-acetylcysteine, which have shown medium-term benefit.

There is a role for nerve surgery in the management of CRPS, particularly in patients with a superimposed compression neuropathy, or whose CRPS is the result of a nerve injury (causalgia). We have had success in improving pain relief in patients with CRPS 1 when a nerve injury is the inciting factor (e.g., carpal tunnel syndrome following wrist fracture) and of course in CRPS 2 when pain is localized to a specific nerve injury.

CRPS Persisting Greater than 6 Months

Interventional strategies include sympathetic nerve blocks, stellate ganglion or lumbar sympathetic, for both diagnostic and treatment purposes. As a diagnostic tool, these blocks help differentiate sympathetically maintained pain from sympathetically independent pain. Should these blocks provide relief, they typically do not last greater than 7 days. These injections should not be performed as the sole form of treatment, but as part of a multidisciplinary regimen that includes physical therapy and desensitization.

CRPS-associated dystonia can be treated with botulinum toxin to reduce posturing. Dosing of botulinum toxin to reduce pain associated with dystonia requires doses large enough to reduce muscle strength in multiple affected muscles. For this reason, botulinum toxin to treat CRPS dystonia tends to be used at specialized centers only.

In this group of patients antiinflammatories, including corticosteroids, are currently not indicated and limiting pharmacological therapies with side-effects is suggested.

Treatment of Chronic Persistent CRPS

There is some evidence that intrathecal baclofen can be useful for otherwise treatment-resistant dystonia that may develop as a result of CRPS. Spinal cord stimulation (SCS) has been shown to be beneficial in patients with CRPS who have failed conventional therapy. In a 5-year follow-up study, SCS plus physical therapy showed a greater reduction in pain than physical therapy alone at 2 years, though at 5-years both groups had similar results. In the lower extremity, dorsal root ganglion stimulators are indicated instead of SCS.

Summary

Primary neurorrhaphy remains the gold standard for all nerve repair techniques, whereas an autologous nerve autograft is the gold standard for bridging a nerve defect. Since the first implementation of a nerve allograft in 1870 by Philipeaux and Vulpian, significant contributions regarding suturing technique, neural topography, and the biology of nerve regeneration have transformed the way we approach nerve reconstruction. Although primary neurorrhaphy and autografts are the most common methods for repair, several newer options are at our disposal. Nerve transfers have revolutionized the approach for treating devastating brachial plexus injuries, converting them to highly-selected upper and lower motor and sensory nerve injuries.

Nerve allografts and conduits offer alternatives to autologous nerve grafting when needed. However, after decades of research towards defining the best nerve substitutes, we still struggle to find an alternative as good as a nerve autograft even for small diameter/short gap injuries. For these short injuries, autograft material is readily available. Intuitively, culturing recipient Schwann cells to repopulate a conduit or acellularized nerve allograft is appealing. This concept has, however, been explored for decades in the laboratory without clinical translation. It is unlikely that modifications of nerve conduits or acellularized allografts are going to provide a nerve graft alternative in the near future for injuries where the need is greatest (long-gap/large-diameter nerve injury). It is likely that other avenues of basic research will lead to the "next" meaningful advance in this field.

References

1. Trumble TE, Archibald S, Allan CH. Bioengineering for nerve repair in the future. *J Am Soc Surg Hand.* 2004;4:134–142.
2. Seddon HJ. Three types of nerve injury. *Brain.* 1943;66:237–288.
3. Sunderland S. *Nerves and Nerve Injuries.* 2nd edn. Edinburgh: Churchill Livingstone; 1978.
4. Seddon HJ, Medawar PB, Smith H. Rate of regeneration of peripheral nerves in man. *J Physiol.* 1943;102:191–215.
5. Mackinnon SE. New directions in peripheral nerve surgery. *Ann Plast Surg.* 1989;22:257–273.
6. Strauch B, Lang A, Ferder M, et al. The ten test. *Plast Reconstr Surg.* 1997;99:1074–1078.
7. *Aids to the Examination of the Peripheral Nervous System – MRC Memorandum No. 45 Superseding War Memorandum No. 7.* Medical Research Council; 1976.
8. Driscoll PJ, Glasby MA, Lawson GM. An in vivo study of peripheral nerves in continuity: biomechanical and physiological responses to elongation. *J Orthop Res.* 2002;20:370–375.
9. Giddins GE, Wade PJ, Amis AA. Primary nerve repair: strength of repair with different gauges of nylon suture material. *J Hand Surg.* 1989;14:301–302.
10. Millesi H. The nerve gap. Theory and clinical practice. *Hand Clin.* 1986;2:651–663.
11. Cabaud HE, Rodkey WG, McCarroll Jr HR, et al. Epineurial and perineurial fascicular nerve repairs: a critical comparison. *J Hand Surg.* 1976;1:131–137.
12. Myckatyn TM, Mackinnon SE. A review of research endeavors to optimize peripheral nerve reconstruction. *Neurol Res.* 2004;26:124–138.
13. Ray WZ, Mackinnon SE. Management of nerve gaps: autografts, allografts, nerve transfers, and end-to-side neurorrhaphy. *Exp Neurol.* 2010;223:77–85.
14. Brushart TM. Preferential reinnervation of motor nerves by regenerating motor axons. *J Neurosci.* 1988;8:1026–1031.
15. Moradzadeh A, Borschel GH, Luciano JP, et al. The impact of motor and sensory nerve architecture on nerve regeneration. *Exp Neurol.* 2008;212:370–376.
16. Novak CB, Mackinnon SE. Distal anterior interosseous nerve transfer to the deep motor branch of the ulnar nerve for reconstruction of high ulnar nerve injuries. *J Reconstr Microsurg.* 2002;18:459–464.
17. Wangensteen KJ, Kalliainen LK. Collagen tube conduits in peripheral nerve repair: a retrospective analysis. *Hand (NY).* 2009;5:273–277.
18. Whitlock EL. Processed allografts and type I collagen conduits for repair of peripheral nerve gaps. *Muscle Nerve.* 2009;39(6):787–799.
19. Karabekmez FE, Duymaz A, Moran SL. Early clinical outcomes with the use of decellularized nerve allograft for repair of sensory defects within the hand. *Hand (NY).* 2009;4:245–249.
20. Saheb–Al–Zamani M, Yan Y, Farber SJ, et al. Limited regeneration in long acellular nerve allografts is associated with increased Schwann cell senescence. *Exp Neurol.* 2013;247:165–177.
21. Moore AM, MacEwan M, Santosa K, et al. Acellular nerve allografts in peripheral nerve regeneration: a comparative study. *Muscle Nerve.* 2011;44:221–234.
22. Weber RA, Breidenbach WC, Brown RE, et al. A randomized prospective study of polyglycolic acid conduits for digital nerve reconstruction in humans. *Plast Reconstr Surg.* 2000;106:1036–1045. discussion 1046–1048.
23. Lloyd BM, Luginbuhl RD, Brenner MJ, et al. Use of motor nerve material in peripheral nerve repair with conduits. *Microsurg.* 2007;27(2):138–145.
24. Taylor GI, Ham FJ. The free vascularized nerve graft. A further experimental and clinical application of microvascular techniques. *Plast Reconstr Surg.* 1976;57:413–426.
25. Doi K, Tamaru K, Sakai K, et al. A comparison of vascularized and conventional sural nerve grafts. *J Hand Surg.* 1992;17:670–676.
26. Davidge KM, Yee A, Moore AM, et al. The supercharge end-to-side anterior interosseous-to-ulnar motor nerve transfer for restoring intrinsic function: clinical experience. *Plast Reconstr Surg.* 2015;136:344e–352e.
27. Cacchio A, De Blasis E, Necozione S, et al. Mirror therapy for chronic complex regional pain syndrome type 1 and stroke. *N Engl J Med.* 2009;361:634–636.
28. Moseley GL. Graded motor imagery is effective for long-standing complex regional pain syndrome: a randomised controlled trial. *Pain.* 2004;108:192–198.
29. Poppler LH, Parikh RP, Bichanich MJ, et al. Surgical interventions for the treatment of painful neuroma: a comparative meta-analysis. *Pain.* 2018;159:214–223.
30. Eberlin KR, Ducic I. Surgical algorithm for neuroma management: a changing treatment paradigm. *Plast Reconstr Surg Glob Open.* 2018;6:e1952.
31. González-Darder J, Barberá J, Abellán MJ, et al. Centrocentral anastomosis in the prevention and treatment of painful terminal neuroma. An experimental study in the rat. *J Neurosurg.* 1985;63:754–758.

32. Woo SL, Kung TA, Brown DL, et al. Regenerative peripheral nerve interfaces for the treatment of postamputation neuroma pain: a pilot study. *Plast Reconstr Surg Glob Open*. 2016;4:e1038.
33. Dumanian GA, Potter BK, Mioton LM, et al. Targeted muscle reinnervation treats neuroma and phantom pain in major limb amputees. *Ann Surg*. 2019;270(2):238–256.
34. Harden RN, Bruehl S, Perez RS, et al. Validation of proposed diagnostic criteria (the "Budapest Criteria") for complex regional pain syndrome. *Pain*. 2010;150(2):268–274.
35. Birklein F, Dimova V. Complex regional pain syndrome-up-to-date. *Pain Rep*. 2017;2:e624.

53

Brachial Plexus Injuries and Reanimation

SHELLEY S. NOLAND, KIRSTY BOYD, AND
SUSAN E. MACKINNON

For videos accompanying this chapter see ExpertConsult.com. See inside cover for access details.

The brachial plexus comprises a complex grouping of nerve fascicles, giving function and sensation to the upper extremity. Progressing from proximally to distally, the plexus is divided into regions termed roots, trunks, divisions, cords, and branches. Within these nerves, there is a clearly defined internal topography that will guide future reconstructive efforts (Fig. 53.1).

Roots

The traditional brachial plexus has contributions from cervical roots C5–C8 and thoracic root T1. Anatomical variations of this included a prefixed plexus (additional contribution from C4) and a postfixed plexus (additional contribution from T2). The spinal roots pass between the anterior and middle scalene muscles. There are three nerve branches exiting from the root level. The dorsal scapular nerve arises from the C5 nerve root and supplies the rhomboid muscles and the levator scapulae muscle. The long thoracic nerve arises from roots C5, C6, and C7 and supplies the serratus anterior muscle, which stabilizes the scapula. The nerve to subclavius arises from the distal C5 and C6 nerve roots. This nerve supplies the subclavius muscle, which is unable to be tested on clinical examination.

Trunks

In the inferior portion of the posterior cervical triangle, the roots combine to form trunks. The upper trunk is formed from C5 and C6. The middle trunk is a continuation of the C7 root. The lower trunk is formed from C8 and T1. There is a single branch off the upper trunk, the suprascapular nerve, that is critical for shoulder function. It departs from the upper trunk, travels deep to the trapezius muscle and runs through the suprascapular notch of the scapula to supply the supraspinatus and infraspinatus muscles.

Divisions

Passing deep to the clavicle, each trunk divides into an anterior and posterior division. There are no extraneous branches at the level of the divisions.

Cords

The divisions pass deep to the pectoralis minor muscle and combine in a predictable fashion to form the cords. The cords are named in relation to their anatomical location around the axillary artery. The anterior divisions of the upper and middle trunks combine to form the lateral cord. The medial cord is the continuation of the anterior division of the lower trunk. All of the posterior divisions combine to form the posterior cord.

Branches

There are several branches that arise from the cords. The lateral cord gives off the lateral pectoral nerve, which innervates the clavicular head of the pectoralis major. The medial cord gives off the medial pectoral nerve, which innervates the sternocostal head of the pectoralis major muscle. The medial brachial cutaneous and medial antebrachial cutaneous nerves also branch from the medial cord supplying sensation to the medial aspect of the upper arm and forearm. More distally, the lateral and medial cords each contribute to the median nerve, supplying the sensory and motor functions of the nerve respectively. This relationship continues distally and is useful for understanding the internal topography of the median nerve, where motor fascicles are located on the medial side of the nerve and sensory fascicles remain more lateral. Following its contribution to the median nerve, the lateral cord becomes the musculocutaneus nerve. This nerve innervates the coracobrachialis, biceps brachii, and brachialis. The terminal portion of this nerve is the lateral cutaneous nerve of the forearm. After contributing to

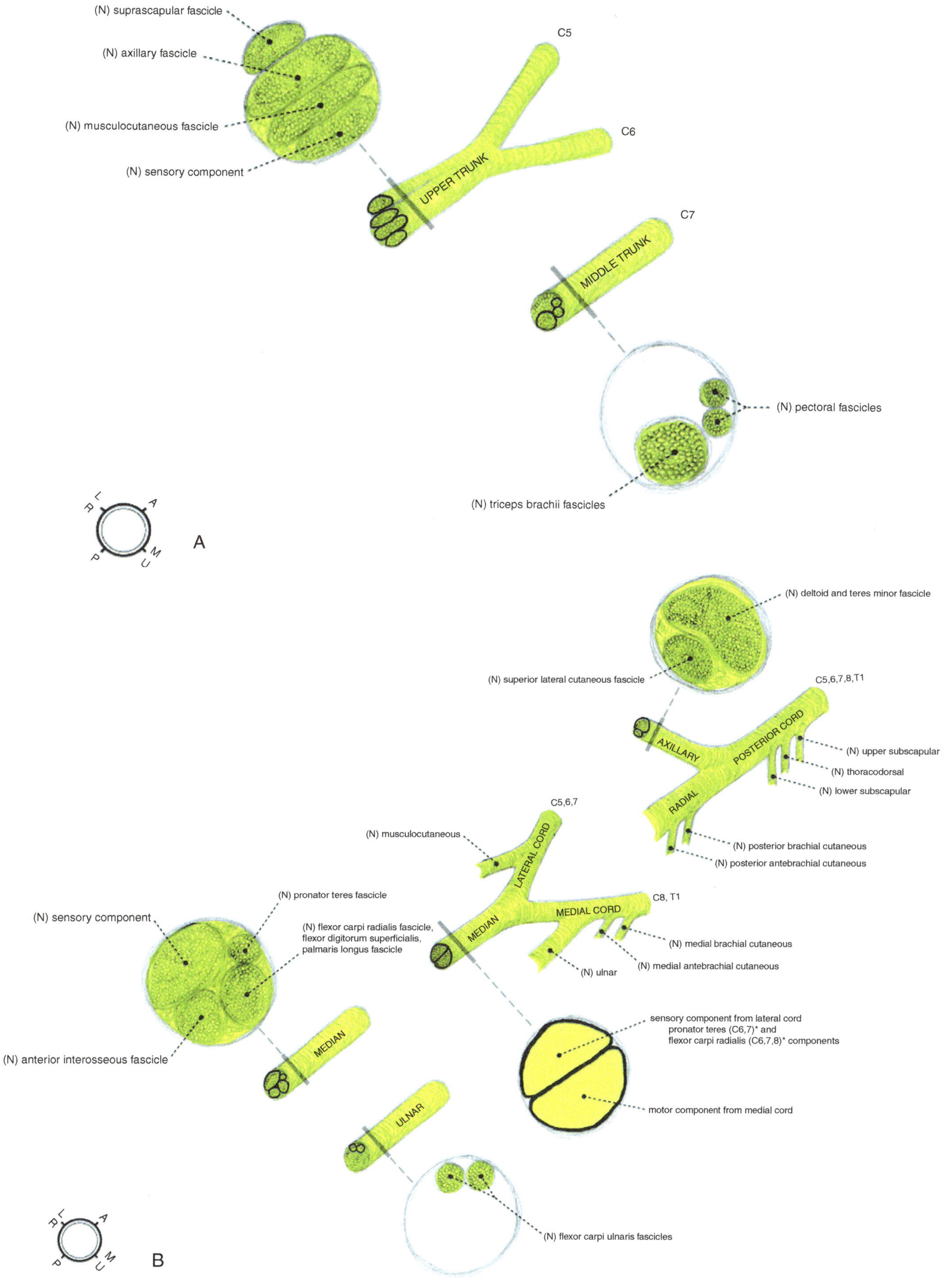

• **Fig. 53.1** Internal topography of the brachial plexus. (A) Cross-sections of the upper and middle trunks delineating fascicular grouping. (B) Internal topography at the level of the cords and branches. (From Mackinnon SE. *Nerve Surgery*. New York: Thieme; 2015. Reproduced with permission.)

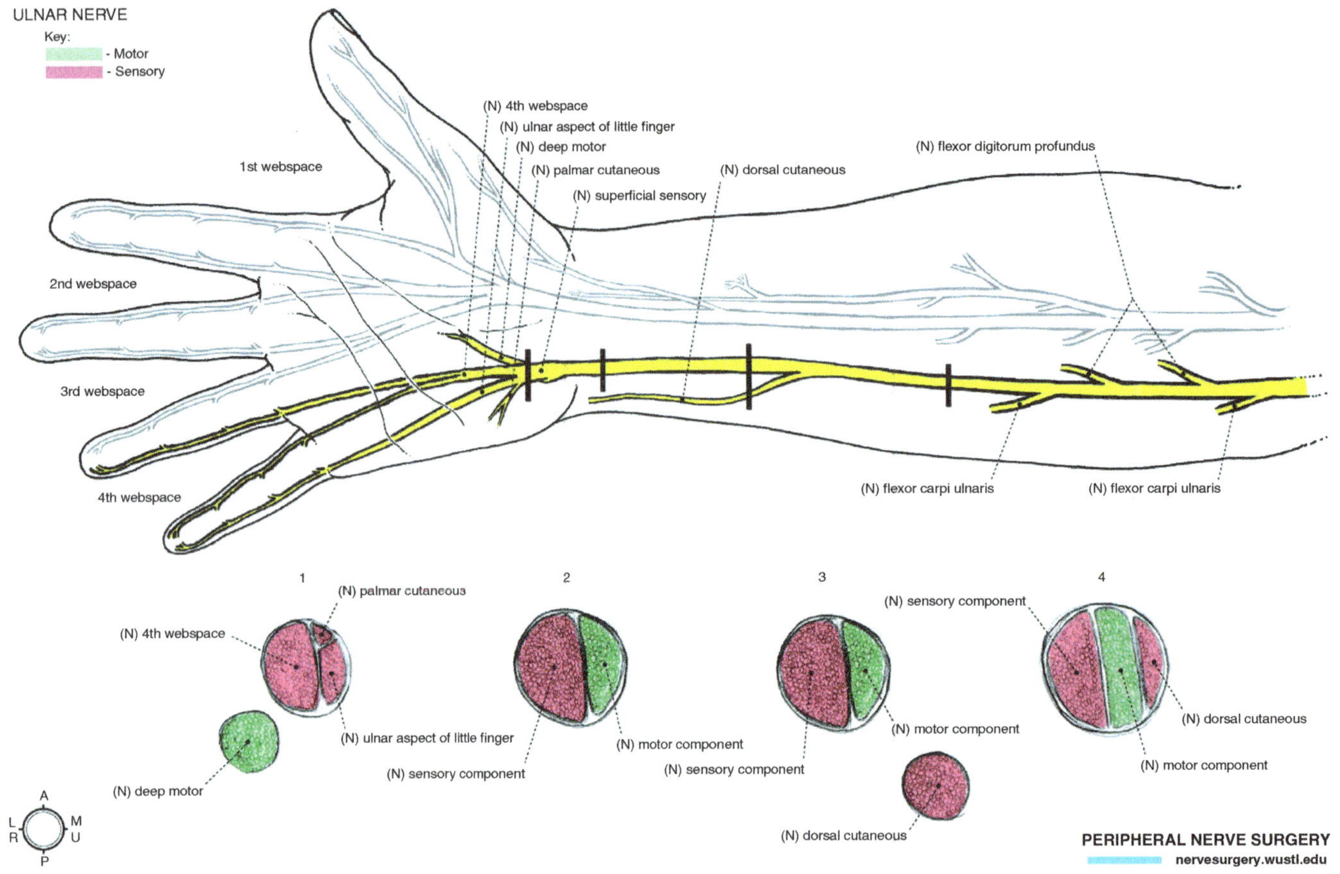

• **Fig. 53.2** The internal topography of the ulnar nerve. (From Mackinnon SE. *Nerve Surgery*. New York: Thieme; 2015. Reproduced with permission.)

the median nerve, the medial cord becomes the ulnar nerve, which, after innervating the flexor carpi ulnaris and the small and ring flexor digitorum profundus muscles, is primarily responsible for the intrinsic musculature of the hand.

The internal topography of the ulnar nerve can best be remembered as sensory–motor–sensory, where the most medial portion of the nerve will eventually contribute to the dorsal cutaneous ulnar branch, exiting the main portion of the ulnar nerve approximately 9 cm proximal to the wrist crease and providing sensation to the dorsal ulnar aspect of the hand. After this division, the more medial 40% of the ulnar nerve will pass through Guyon's canal to become the deep motor branch and the more radial 60% will contribute to the superficial sensory branch (Fig. 53.2).

The posterior cord gives off the upper subscapular nerve, the thoracodorsal nerve, and the lower subscapular nerve. These branches innervate the superior portion of the subscapularis muscle, the latissimus dorsi muscle, and the lower subscapularis/teres major muscles, respectively. The two most terminal branches of the posterior cord are the axillary nerve and the radial nerve. The axillary nerve travels through the quadrangular space (bounded by the humerus, the long head of triceps brachii, teres minor, and teres major) with the posterior circumflex humeral artery. It innervates the deltoid and the teres minor, but also provides sensation to a patch of skin overlying the deltoid, sometimes known as the "soldier's patch." This sensory component is located at the most inferior portion of the axillary nerve. The radial nerve travels through the triangular interval (bounded by the teres major and the lateral and long heads of triceps brachii) with the profunda brachii artery. Wrapping around the spiral groove, the radial nerve goes on to supply the elbow, wrist, finger, and thumb extensors.

Clinical History and Assessment

Brachial plexus injuries occur in approximately 1% of polytrauma victims, most frequently in young males. The vast majority are due to motor vehicle collisions and of these, up to 84% may involve motorcycles. Due to these circumstances, many patients present with multisystem trauma requiring resuscitative procedures. Associated closed head injuries including loss of consciousness can occur in almost three-quarters of patients, which can often result in a delay of recognition of a brachial plexus injury. It is not uncommon for the patient to be the first to identify the injury. In the obstetrical population, approximately 1.6% of deliveries have a shoulder dystocia and of these, almost 20% experience a brachial plexus palsy.

Acquiring a thorough history is critical in the investigation of a patient with a brachial plexus injury. The mechanism of injury may provide information to recognize a pattern of injury or to estimate the degree of injury. For a trauma, details about a motor vehicle collision, including the speed, direction of impact, use of safety equipment such as seatbelts or helmets, and concomitant injury may be useful in ascertaining risk to certain structures. In the event of a blow or a fall, knowing the direction and weight of impact, location of impact, and arm position can contribute valuable information. Knowledge of preexisting upper extremity injuries and medical comorbidities is also useful. The patient's general medical status may contribute to candidacy for surgical intervention. In an obstetrical brachial plexus injury, information about birth weight, gestational age, shoulder dystocia, delivery aides such as forceps, and duration of labor are useful.

An important component of the history is evaluation of pain. Patients should be questioned regarding the severity, location, and nature of their pain to assist in determining musculoskeletal versus neuropathic components. Severe pain can be suggestive of root avulsions. Inclusion of a pain questionnaire at the initial assessment and then at subsequent visits can provide both quantitative and qualitative assessment of pain. Having a low threshold for starting neuropathic pain medications or involving a pain specialist is crucial for these patients, as pain management can be a significant problem. In addition, patients should be screened for depression and mood disorders, as the incidence in this patient population can be as high as 40%.

In this patient population, serial clinical examination is crucial to determine spontaneous recovery. At the initial physical examination, a complete upper extremity sensory and motor examination should be performed with care to document both peripheral and central nervous system examination. Atrophy may not initially be present but will later mark denervated muscle groups. Having a systematic approach to the brachial plexus examination will allow for determination of patterns of injury and more specifically about level of injury. A thorough knowledge of the anatomy of the plexus can help to localize lesions simply by physical examination.

The location of scars on the upper extremity, shoulder, and neck should be noted, from either trauma or surgical intervention. Joint mobility should be assessed for the entire extremity, and, in the setting of any decreased passive range of motion or stiffness, early intervention with an occupational or physiotherapist should be arranged to optimize overall outcome. Assessment should be carried out for concomitant findings such as a Horner's sign (ptosis, miosis, and anhydrosis), which occurs due to injury to the cervical sympathetic fibers during avulsion of the C8 and T1 roots.

Perhaps the most critical part of the physical examination is accurate documentation. Careful recording of the Medical Research Council (MRC) scale for muscle strength for each muscle group in an organized fashion will allow comparison over time. Given the known rate of recovery following nerve injury of 1 mm/day, this allows for assessment of whether spontaneous recovery is progressing at the expected rate, or whether surgical intervention may be appropriate. It should be remembered that examination for potential donors is as important as identifying nonfunctioning muscle groups. The preparation for surgical reconstruction of brachial plexus injuries is the biggest determinant of success.

Etiology

The etiology of brachial plexopathy can be traumatic, iatrogenic, compressive, neuralgic amyotrophy or radiation.

Traumatic

The majority of brachial plexopathies secondary to trauma occur in young males, with up to 90% of cases comprising this patient population. Traumatic injuries to the brachial plexus can be divided into open and closed injuries. Open injuries are those secondary to penetrating injury, such as knives or other sharp objects. These necessitate immediate surgical exploration. The majority of traumatic brachial plexus injuries are closed, and these can be composed of crush injuries or traction injuries. Crush injuries tend to occur after motor vehicle accidents, whereas traction injuries are more likely to be related to motorcycle accidents, skiing, falls, and sports injuries. In traction injuries, displacement of the upper extremity inferiorly combined with neck flexion contralaterally causes an increase in the neck–shoulder angle, which results in injury to the upper roots and trunks. This commonly occurs in both high-velocity injuries such as motorcycle collisions and also in lower-velocity accidents such as sports injuries. The opposite can occur with strong upward force or traction on the upper extremity increasing the scapula–humoral angle and causing injury to the lower plexus. The brachial plexus is susceptible to these injuries due to limited mobility secondary to prevertebral fascia and attachment of the cervical roots to the vertebrae. Traction injuries are also responsible for obstetrical brachial plexopathies, most commonly following shoulder dystocia. Risk factors for obstetrical plexus injury include high birth weight, fetal acidosis, posterior arm involvement, and narrow pelvis.

Iatrogenic

During long operations, positioning of the upper extremity can contribute to a traction palsy. Most commonly these injuries are neuropraxic in nature and will recover spontaneously; occasionally, however, a more severe injury will occur. There are patient factors that contribute to the propensity for developing these injuries, including diabetes, hypothyroidism, prior injury, hereditary neuropathy with liability to pressure palsy (HNPP), and obesity.

Compression

Compression can be secondary to structures adjacent to the plexus in an enclosed space such as malignancy, callous formation, hematoma or pseudoaneurysm. Anatomical variants may be responsible for compression primarily or may increase the propensity for trauma to the brachial plexus. These variants include cervical ribs, prominent transverse processes, and congenital fibrous bands.[1] Compression often occurs in the costoclavicular space as the brachial plexus travels between the clavicle and the first rib. Traumatic injuries can result in swelling or hematoma that cause compression of the brachial plexus. Occupational injuries where a heavy object lands on the shoulder or neck are an example.

Neuralgic Amyotrophy

Brachial neuritis, or Parsonage–Turner syndrome, is a brachial plexopathy of unclear etiology that most commonly involves the lower brachial plexus; the axillary nerve is implicated in up to 70% of patients. Most commonly, these nontraumatic plexopathies present with a history of severe neuropathic pain that resolves and then is followed by patchy weakness. Possible contributory factors are viral disease, infection, immunization, trauma, surgery, and autoimmune mechanisms. The majority of these plexopathies will have a full spontaneous recovery within approximately 3 years, however the prognosis is more guarded in the setting of other medical comorbidities such as diabetes.

Radiation

Transient or permanent brachial plexopathy can occur as a result of radiation therapy. Approximately 1.2% of women receiving radiation as adjuvant therapy for breast cancer will present with clinical manifestations anywhere from 6 months to 20 years following treatment (median 1.5 years).

Investigations

Imaging

Brachial plexopathy and level of injury are primarily a clinical diagnosis supported by electrodiagnostic studies, however there are several circumstances where imaging contributes valuable information.

Plain films are useful for identifying fractures that might be associated with certain patterns of brachial plexopathy. For example, a transverse process fracture is more likely associated with a root avulsion injury because of the deep cervical fascia that tethers cervical root to transverse process. Clavicular fractures can cause sharp injuries to the plexus on bony fragments, or can contribute to compression injuries related to either hematoma acutely, or callus formation in a more delayed fashion.

CT myelography is a useful investigation for assessing for root avulsion. The use of contrast material allows for visualization of the dural sheath around the nerve root, which is not pathognomonic for a root avulsion, but can be suggestive. The absence of a root at a particular level is diagnostic. When obtained at least 1 month post injury, which allows time for the dural sheath to heal improving distribution of the dye, CT myelography is associated with a sensitivity of 95% and a specificity of 98% for root avulsion injuries.

MRI is becoming a more valuable tool for the imaging of the brachial plexus due to newer techniques and protocols. The advantage of MRI is that it can directly visualize the entire brachial plexus and is noninvasive. Soft tissue injury is more easily assessed and three-dimensional imaging is possible.

Electrodiagnostic Studies

It is crucial that all patients presenting with brachial plexopathies receive electrodiagnostic studies, and in many cases serial studies will confer helpful information in the decision to proceed with surgery. Electrodiagnostic studies are not useful before Wallerian degeneration has occurred and fibrillation potentials have appeared, therefore delaying investigation for approximately 6 weeks is beneficial. There are two components to the electrodiagnostic study: nerve conduction and electromyography. Nerve conduction studies are traditionally more useful for compression neuropathies, although they can portray valuable information in the setting of a preganglionic lesion to the brachial plexus. In these injuries, the dorsal root ganglion remains intact and the peripheral sensory nerve does not undergo Wallerian degeneration. The motor nerve, however, arising more proximally in the spinal cord, will still be affected. The resultant nerve conduction studies will demonstrate intact sensory nerve action potentials (SNAPs) but no volitional activity.

The electromyography portion of the study also has several components. On insertion of the needle, a denervated muscle will exhibit spontaneous discharges or fibrillations and positive sharp waves. In contrast, a normal muscle will not have any waveform on insertion alone. When the patient is asked to voluntarily contract the designated muscle, the presence of motor unit potentials (MUPs) signifies that the action potential is reaching the desired motor endplate. Nascent units are representative of connections to the motor endplates from regenerating injured axons, while MUPs signify distal motor sprouting from uninjured axons. Both are good prognosticators of a spontaneous recovery without surgical intervention. Electromyography often precedes clinical signs of recovery by 1–2 months, and the presence of new MUPs and nascent units can be a promising prognostic sign before the patient notices any changes. In addition, electrodiagnostic studies can be valuable in preoperative planning, especially where nerve or tendon transfers are being contemplated.

Patterns of Injury

Brachial plexus injuries can occur in any potential combination, however there are several common patterns of injury that warrant mention, as the approach to treatment can be dictated by the predictable deficits.

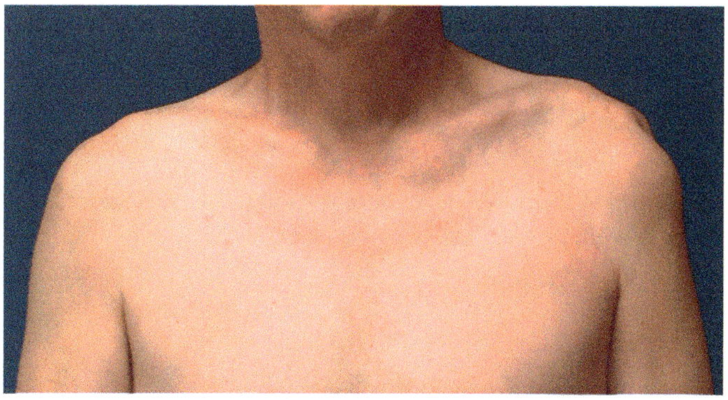

• **Fig. 53.3** A sulcus sign secondary to denervation of the left axillary and suprascapular nerves. (From Mackinnon SE. *Nerve Surgery*. New York: Thieme; 2015. Reproduced with permission.)

Upper Plexus Injuries

These injuries comprise injuries to the C5 and C6 roots or to the upper trunk. This occurs when the shoulder is wrenched away from the head and neck. Classically these patients will present with deficits of shoulder abduction, external rotation, and loss of elbow flexion. There will be a concomitant loss of sensation over the deltoid muscle. A sulcus sign may be present, identifying the inability of the shoulder girdle to support the weight of the arm (Fig. 53.3). Priorities are to reestablish elbow flexion and then to restore shoulder stability and function.

Lower Plexus Injuries

Injuries to the lower plexus typically involve C8 and T1 roots or the lower trunk. This occurs when the arm is forcefully abducted above the head. In this pattern of injury, wrist and hand flexion will be the most greatly affected, with intrinsic muscle paralysis and potential clawing. Loss of sensation in the ulnar nerve distribution accompanies the lower plexus injury. Priorities include restoration of hand function.

Posterior Cord Injury

Injury to the posterior cord involves contributions from C5–T1. When injured, extension of the elbow, wrist, thumb, and fingers are affected, as is shoulder abduction from the axillary nerve, which is a terminal branch of the posterior cord. Priorities are to restore shoulder abduction and wrist, finger, and thumb extension. Restoration of elbow extension is more controversial.

Pan-Plexus Injuries

This injury involves the entire plexus (C5–T1) and presents with a flail, insensate upper extremity. Associated with a poor prognosis, this extremity will likely be a 'helper extremity' at best. Priorities to restore function include elbow flexion, shoulder stability and abduction/external rotation, and hand function. Often associated procedures such as wrist arthrodesis will be considered given the lack of potential donor nerves or tendons for surgical intervention.

Obstetrical Brachial Plexus Injuries

Classically, these patients present with an Erb's palsy, which is injury to the upper plexus. This leads to loss of shoulder abduction, external rotation, and loss of elbow flexion. These patients are often described as presenting in the "waiter's tip" position, where the arm hangs by the child's side with the shoulder internally rotated, the elbow extended, and the forearm pronated. Alternatively, these children can present with a Klumpke's palsy, which is a lower plexus lesion. These children present with paralysis of multiple muscle groups, including the hand and wrist flexors and the intrinsic muscles of the hand. They will often have an associated claw deformity and potentially an associated Horner's syndrome (triad of ptosis, miosis, and anhydrosis). They will have a sensory deficit in the ulnar nerve distribution.

Management Principles and Operative Approach

Timing

The management of brachial plexus injuries is determined by the mechanism, level, and degree of injury. Open injuries of the brachial plexus should be explored within 72 hours to allow for intraoperative stimulation of the distal nerve segment. Depending on the mechanism, acute nerve repair may be warranted. If, however, the mechanism is not a sharp, transecting injury, it is important to consider the zone of injury. In the event of a crush or avulsion, identification and intraoperative tagging of the nerve may be prudent, followed by reexploration approximately 3 weeks after the injury (when the zone of injury is well demarcated). If acute repair is desired, both the distal and proximal nerve ends should be resected to ensure healthy fascicular nerve ends. The authors advocate the use of a bread-loafing technique to ensure that adequate scar is resected while preserving optimum nerve length, by sequentially cutting the nerve in thin slices until clearly past the zone of injury and able to visualize healthy cut fascicular ends.

In the event of resection of the damaged nerve, a nerve gap will be present. Addressing the nerve gap is critical to avoid tension on the nerve repair. The nerve gap can be addressed with nerve grafting. Potential donors include the medial antebrachial cutaneous nerve (MABC) or the sural nerve. Our preference is to use the MABC given that it is located within the injured extremity, is expendable, has a larger caliber than the sural nerve, and sensation can potentially be restored into the donor deficit by transferring the distal end to an intact sensory donor in the upper arm. Although nerve grafts can be used to span the distance of a nerve gap, such as following neuroma resection, debridement of nerve ends, or for nerve transfers where the donor and recipient are not in close enough proximity, they involve two coaptations, which reduces the number of successfully traversing axons.

Another potential option for addressing the nerve gap is to use distal nerve transfers. There are several advantages conferred by this technique, including avoiding operating within the zone of injury, conversion of a proximal injury to a more distal one with axon regeneration closer to the motor endplates, and a single coaptation.[2–5] Tendon transfers and functional muscle transfers are options for dealing with injuries that present in a delayed fashion or that have minimal donor options.[6,7]

Closed injuries, such as traction or crush injuries, are significantly more common than open injuries to the brachial plexus. These injuries are not immediately explored, but are instead followed with serial clinical examination and electrodiagnostic studies to evaluate for any spontaneous functional recovery.[8] With these injuries, it is imperative to be cognizant of timing. Peripheral nerve regeneration occurs at a rate of approximately 1 mm/day. The distance from injury to the first expected nerve branches to show recovery in an injured nerve should be documented and serially examined for signs of recovery within the anticipated time period. Permanent atrophy and fibrosis of denervated muscle occurs between 12 and 18 months following nerve injury and therefore it is necessary to intervene surgically in a timely manner to achieve reinnervation to the motor endplates prior to this occurring.[2,3,9]

Priorities to Establishing Function

The first priority in a complete brachial plexus injury is to restore elbow flexion. This is followed by shoulder stability/range of motion and subsequently restoration of hand and wrist function.

Exploration of the Brachial Plexus

Exploration of the proximal brachial plexus takes place through a hockeystick-shaped incision along the posterior border of the lower sternocleidomastoid muscle and extending transversely above the clavicle. This allows access to the roots with careful dissection and mobilization of the supraclavicular fat pad. The roots travel between the anterior and middle scalene muscles. Caution to avoid the phrenic nerve, which runs longitudinally along the anterior surface of the anterior scalene muscle, is imperative. To explore the more distal plexus, an infraclavicular exposure is performed, with an incision extending from the clavicle to the anterior axillary fold in the deltopectoral groove. We perform this incision in a zig-zag fashion to allow for improved exposure to prevent scar contracture. The pectoralis major muscle is temporarily divided and reflected medially, as is the pectoralis minor. The patient should be positioned supine with the chest and ipsilateral upper extremity prepped and the arm abducted to 90° and the head turned gently to the contralateral side. Paralytic agents are avoided on induction to allow for intraoperative nerve stimulation. Traditionally, exploration and grafting at the level of the plexus was the gold standard for these injuries, but more recently, there has been a momentum to more distal nerve transfers.[10] The authors' preference is for distal nerve transfer.

Restoring Elbow Flexion

There are a number of different potential donors to re-establish elbow flexion.[5,11] This necessitates exposing the musculocutaneous nerve in the upper arm. A longitudinal incision is made along the brachial sulcus on the medial upper arm. The musculocutaneous nerve travels deep to this sulcus in between the biceps brachii and brachialis muscles and can often be palpated against the humerus in the proximal incision. Once this nerve is identified, the branch to the biceps brachii, which branches laterally into the muscle at approximately the upper third/lower two-thirds junction of the upper arm, and the brachialis branch, which branches medially closer to the mid-upper arm, can be localized and stimulated. The continuation of the musculocutaneous nerve becomes the lateral antebrachial cutaneous nerve, which can be confirmed by the "tug test," which will put traction on the skin of the proximal forearm when the nerve is gently tugged.

When it has been confirmed that the musculocutaneous nerve does not stimulate, appropriate donors can be selected for nerve transfer. Our preference would be to perform the double fascicular nerve transfer (DFT), which restores function to both the brachialis and biceps brachii branches of the musculocutaneous nerve (Fig. 53.4).[5] This procedure involves borrowing redundant fascicles from the flexor carpi radialis or palmaris longus from the median nerve and the flexor carpi ulnaris from the ulnar nerve as donors.[5] If the median and ulnar nerves are involved distally, other potential donors include the medial pectoral nerve or the thoracodorsal nerve. In patients presenting with a pan–plexus injury, extraplexal donors are required. The most commonly used extraplexal donor to restore elbow flexion is the intercostals, which can be harvested through a curvilinear incision in the inframammary fold. Approximately three levels are selected as donors and often the nerve to the rectus abdominis is taken as an additional source of motor fascicles. With meticulous dissection distally, the use of a nerve graft can be prevented as the donor nerves are passed through a subcutaneous tunnel in the axilla to the recipient musculocutaneus nerve in the upper arm. Remembering the mantra "donor distal, recipient proximal" to maximize length and avoid tension on the transfer is essential.[9]

The use of other extraplexal donors has been described, including the phrenic nerve and the contralateral C7, however these are less favorable options due to distance from the recipient nerve and donor deficit.

Restoring Shoulder Function

Restoration of shoulder function is the next priority and involves regaining shoulder stability, abduction, and external rotation. In order to accomplish this, reinnervation of the axillary nerve distribution (deltoid, teres minor) and suprascapular nerve (supraspinatus, infraspinatus) are required.[4,12] Our preference for addressing the suprascapular nerve is the spinal accessory to suprascapular nerve transfer (Fig. 53.5). This transfer is possible from either an anterior or posterior approach. The anterior approach has the advantages of supine patient positioning and the ability to perform the transfer in an end-to-side manner, which preserves spinal accessory nerve function.[13] With the posterior approach, release at the suprascapular notch, preserving more innervation to the trapezius, and a wider exposure are advantages.[14,15]

The spinal accessory nerve is located on the deep surface of the trapezius muscle approximately 44% of the way along a line drawn from the spine to the acromion at the level of the superior scapular border.[2] The suprascapular nerve travels through the suprascapular notch at the midway point along the superior scapular border and is most

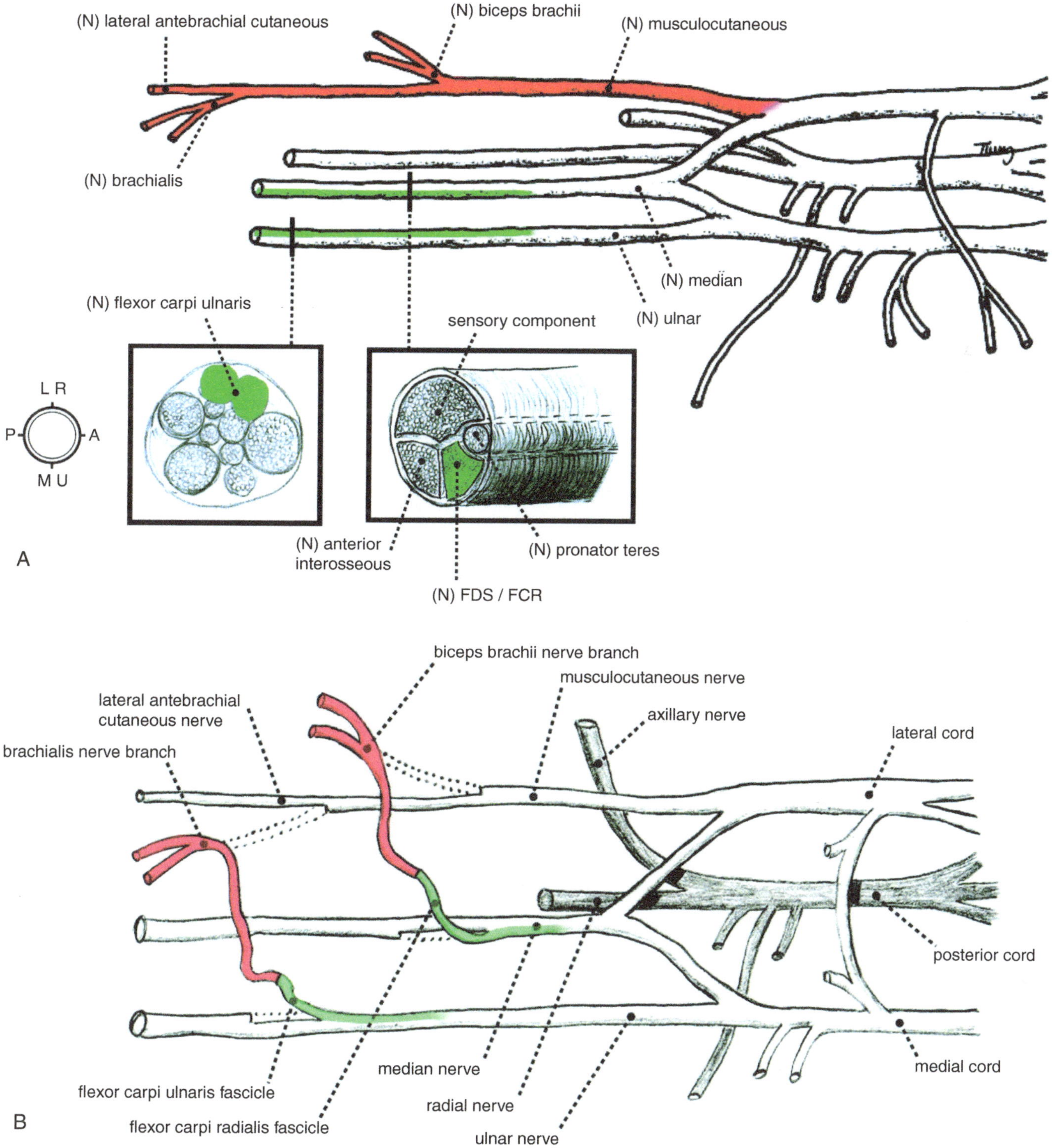

• **Fig. 53.4** The double fascicular nerve transfer (DFT). (A) The internal topography of the median and ulnar nerves delineating the desired motor donors (green) and the injured musculocutaneous nerve recipients (red). (B) A schematic illustrating the donor and recipient pairings of the DFT.

(Continued)

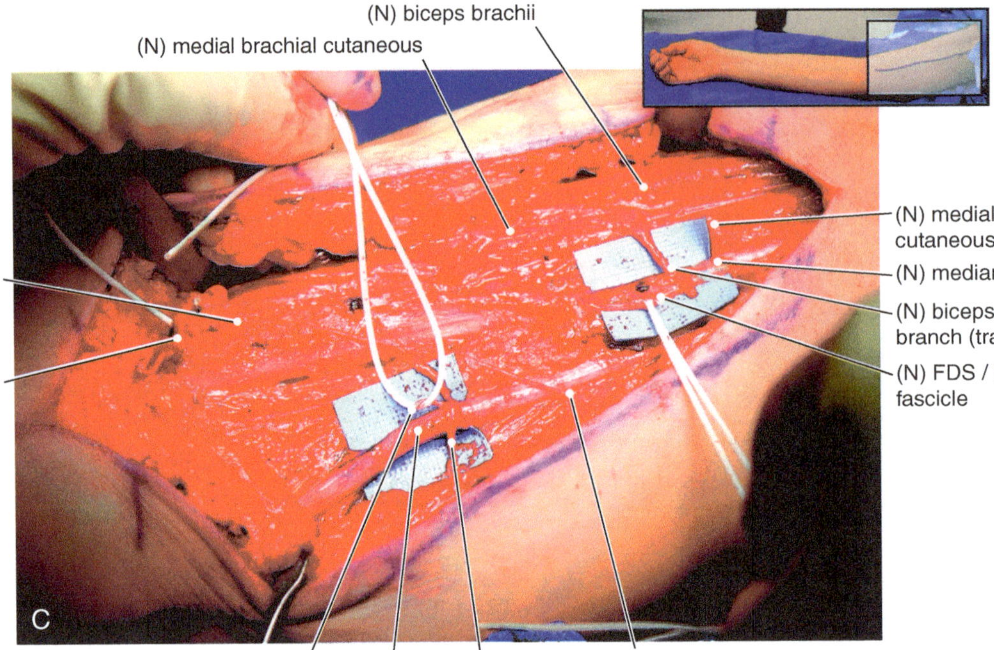

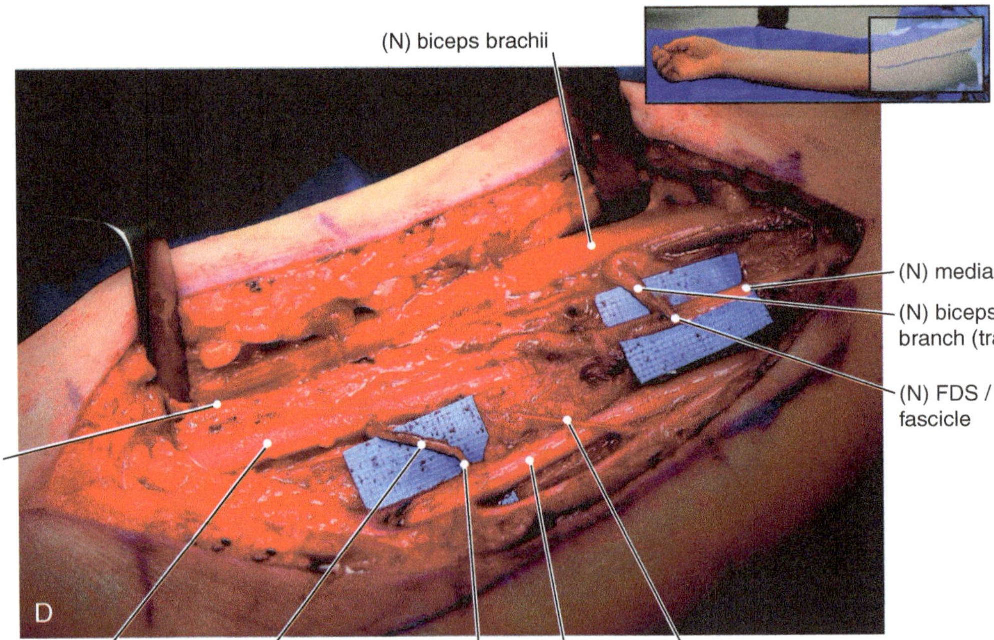

• **Fig. 53.4 cont'd** (C) Intraoperative photo illustrating the isolated motor donor fascicles from the median and ulnar nerve and the divided musculocutaneous recipients draped over to facilitate deciding on location of coaptation. (D) Intraoperative photo illustrating the two transfers coapted with no tension. (From Mackinnon SE. *Nerve Surgery*. New York: Thieme; 2015. Reproduced with permission.)

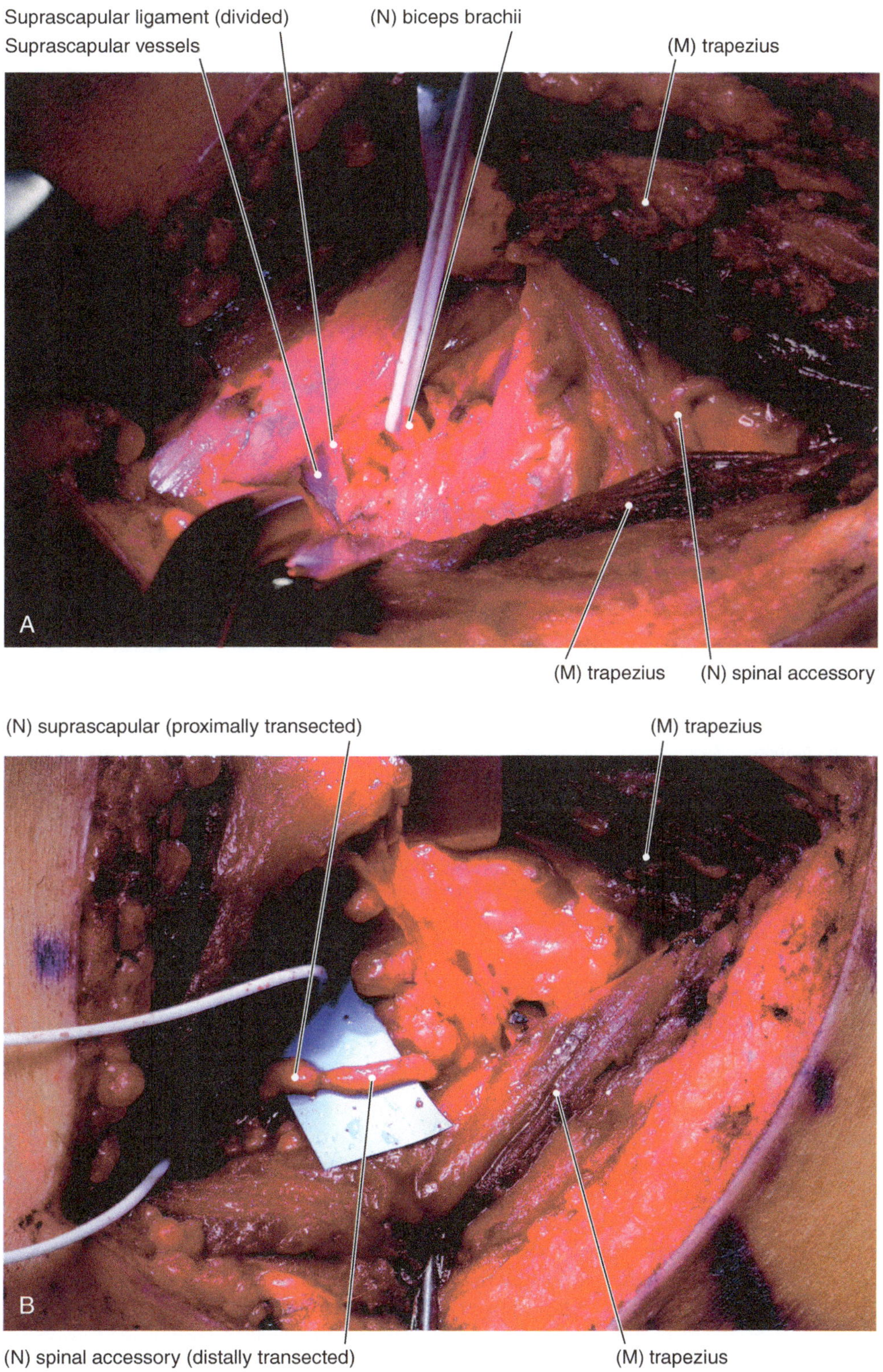

• **Fig. 53.5** Spinal accessory to suprascapular nerve transfer from posterior approach. (A) Intraoperative photo documenting the location of both donor spinal accessory and recipient suprascapular nerves. (B) Coaptation under no tension. (From Mackinnon SE. *Nerve Surgery*. New York: Thieme; 2015. Reproduced with permission.)

easily accessed by release of the ligament that travels over the notch.

Shoulder abduction is addressed by reinnervation of the deltoid and teres minor. Our preference is to transfer the medial branch of triceps, which travels along the superficial surface of the radial nerve as its own fascicular group, to the axillary nerve (Fig. 53.6).[15,16] This can be performed by an incision on the posterior arm that extends from the quadrangular space, where the axillary nerve can be located, to the distal upper arm. It is easily performed in conjunction with a spinal accessory to suprascapular nerve transfer as a double nerve transfer.[15] Other potential donors include the

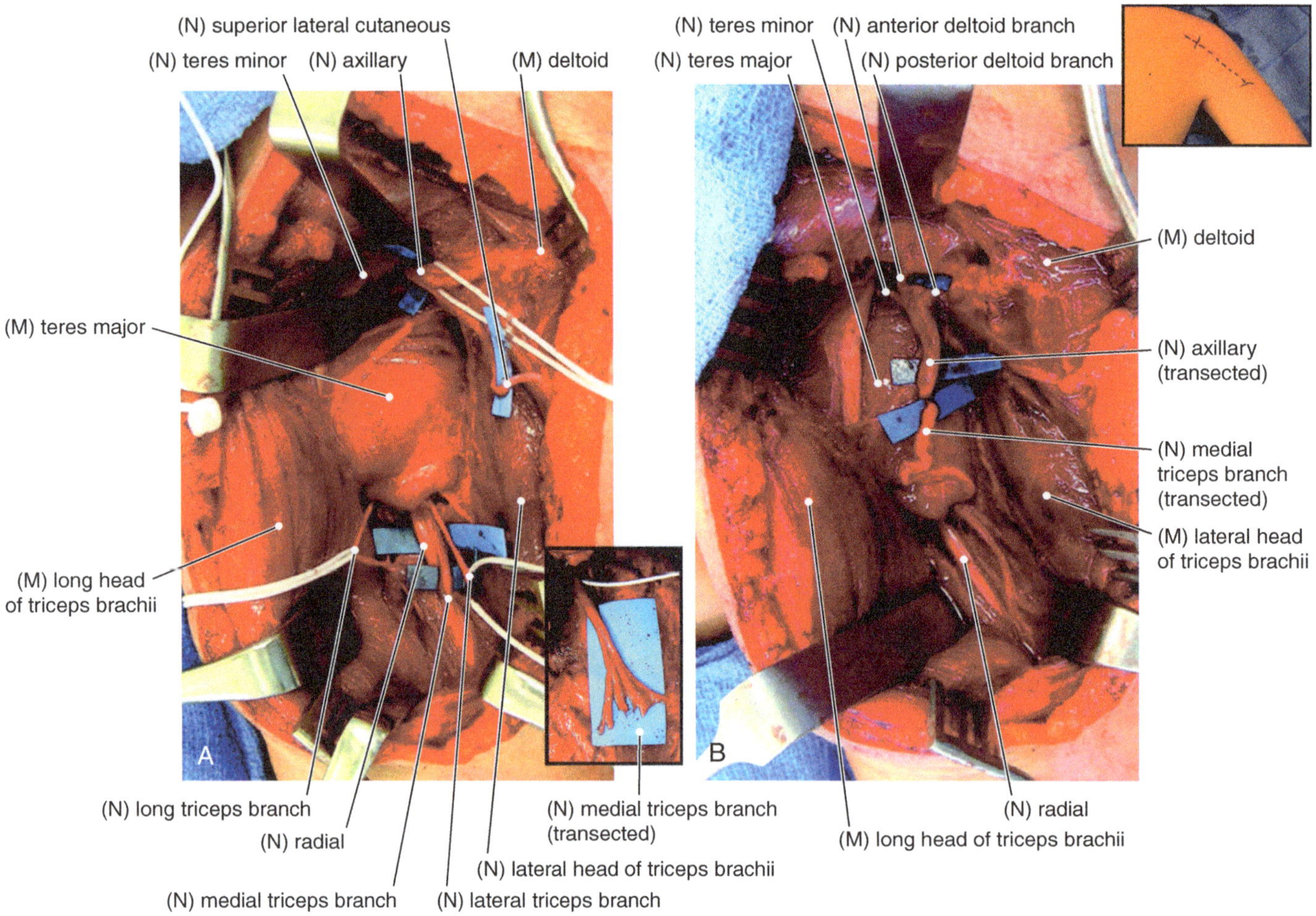

• **Fig. 53.6** Medial triceps to axillary nerve transfer. (A) Intraoperative photo documenting the location of both the donor medial triceps branch and the recipient axillary nerve. (B) Nerves prepared for coaptation under no tension. (From Mackinnon SE. *Nerve Surgery*. New York: Thieme; 2015. Reproduced with permission.)

contralateral C7, the medial pectoral nerve, and the thoracodorsal nerve, although the thoracodorsal nerve is harder to rehabilitate.

Restoring Hand Function

In a pan–plexus injury, restoring hand function is a challenging problem. With limited donors and with priority going to restoring elbow and shoulder function, there are few options for donors to the hand. Although use of the contralateral C7 with a long nerve graft to median nerve transfer has been described, the long distance from the motor endplates and the multiple coaptations results in suboptimal restoration of function.[17–19] The authors' preference in that setting is to use a free functioning muscle transfer, most commonly gracilis, to restore extrinsic hand function.[20–22] The first stage of this transfer can be performed at the time of the original plexus reconstruction with inset of a long graft from the intercostal donors. Once enough time has passed to allow sufficient regeneration, the second stage transfer of the muscle to restore finger flexion can be performed.

In lower plexus injuries, where patients present with isolated nerve palsies, more distal nerve transfer is accomplished using synergistic donors. For recovery of a median nerve palsy, establishing anterior interosseous nerve function is a priority and can be performed with a number of potential donors. Options include the brachialis branch,[23] and expendable branches of the radial nerve.[24] The internal topography of the median nerve is now well understood. In the proximal arm, the anterior interosseous nerve fascicles can be found located on the posterior medial aspect of the nerve. More distally, the fascicles wrap under the nerve and become the only branch to exit from the radial side of the median nerve, distal to the branches to flexor carpi radialis, palmaris longus, and flexor digitorum superficialis. For exposure, the nerve can be isolated in the upper arm through the same brachial sulcus incision. More distally, the anterior interosseous nerve can be exposed through a curvilinear incision on the volar forearm.

Following ulnar nerve paralysis, recovery of intrinsic muscle function is a priority and is often accomplished by making use of the terminal branch of the anterior interosseous nerve as a donor to the deep motor branch of the ulnar nerve (Fig. 53.7).[25] This terminal branch can be located on the anterior surface of the interosseous membrane as it penetrates into the pronator quadratus muscle. Harvesting it at its most terminal branching point will allow for enough length to transfer it to the side of the ulnar nerve, allowing this procedure to be used as a supercharging or babysitting option.[25] The internal topography of the ulnar nerve at the level of the distal forearm is such that after the dorsal cutaneous ulnar branch exits the ulnar aspect approximately 9 cm proximal to the wrist crease, the more ulnar 40% of the nerve is motor and the more radial 60% is sensory. It is important to make the epineurotomy window at the motor aspect of the nerve to allow the anterior interosseous fascicles to reach the intrinsic muscles of the hand. If the anterior interosseous nerve is not available, other options include the extensor digiti quinti or extensor carpi ulnaris, both of which will require a nerve graft.

Radial nerve deficits can be addressed by borrowing redundant fascicles from the median nerve as donors. Priorities are to re-establish posterior interosseous and extensor carpi radialis brevis functions.[26]

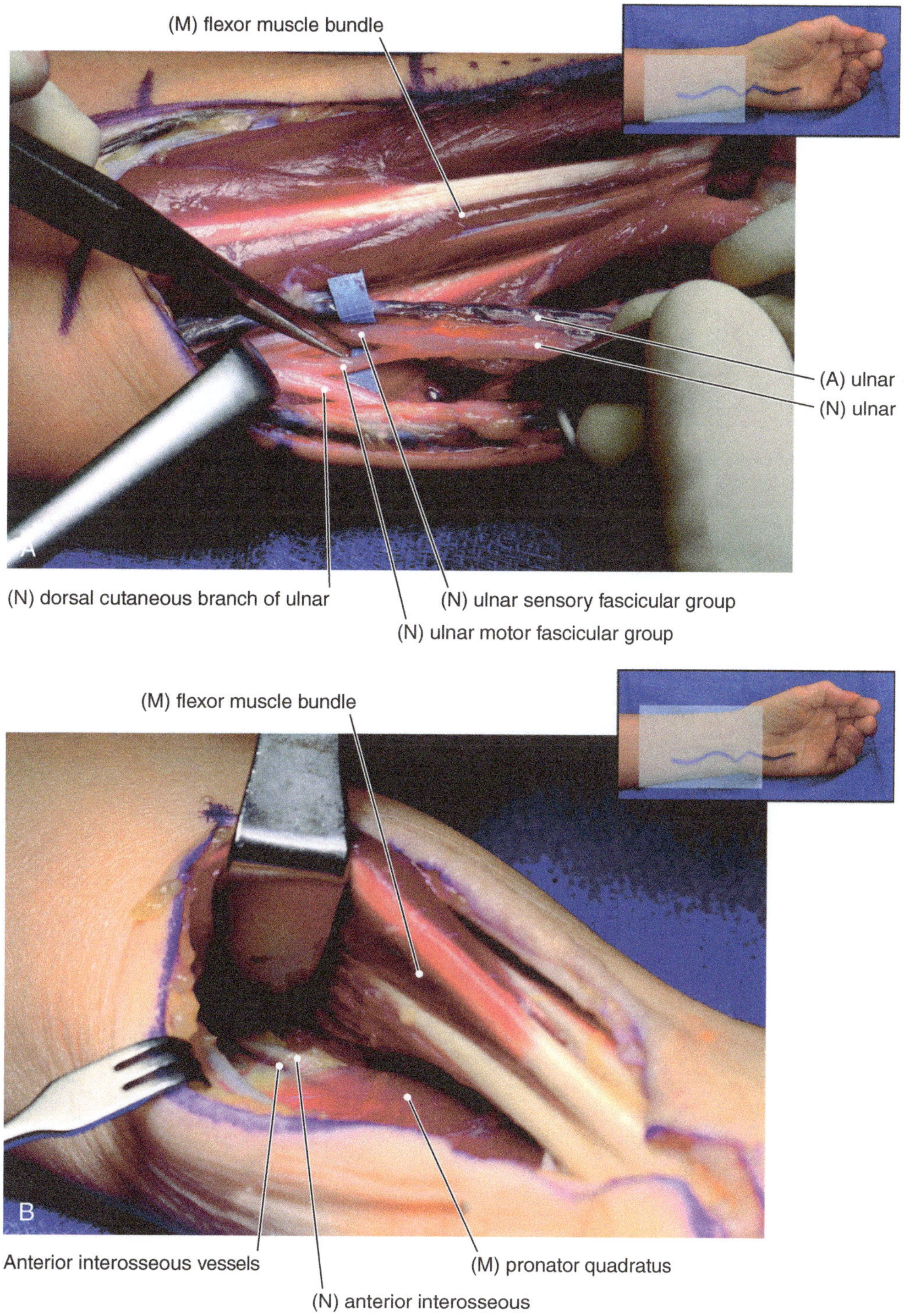

• **Fig. 53.7** Anterior interosseous to deep motor branch ulnar nerve transfer. (A) Intraoperative photo illustrating the topography of the ulnar nerve at the level of the distal forearm and wrist with isolation of the motor fascicles. (B) Intraoperative photo of the anterior interosseous nerve lying on the interosseous membrane just deep to pronator quadratus.

(Continued)

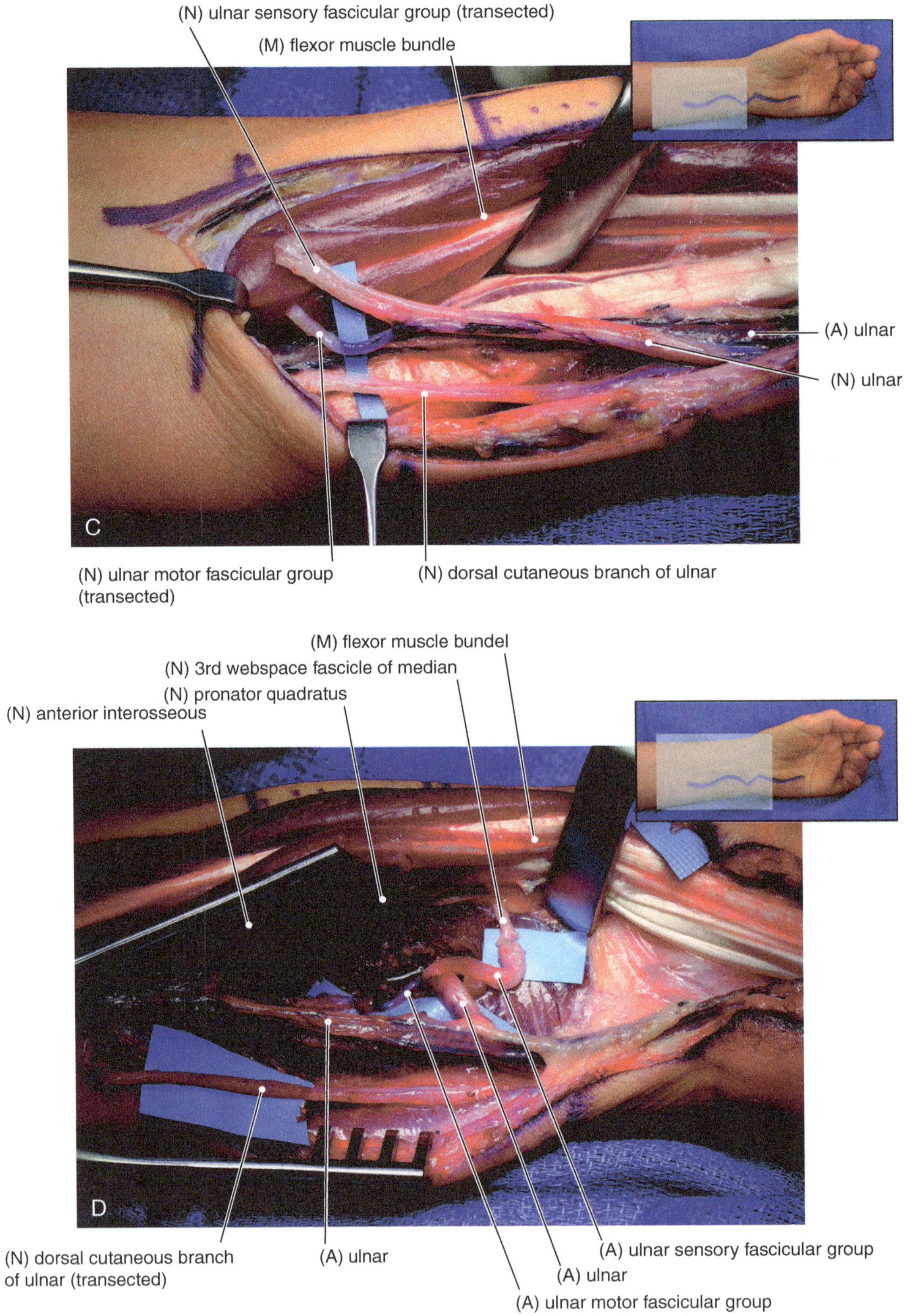

• **Fig. 53.7 cont'd** (C) Recipient ulnar nerve divided proximally (donor distal, recipient proximal). (D) Donor and recipient nerves prepared for coaptation under no tension. (From Mackinnon SE. *Nerve Surgery*. New York: Thieme; 2015. Reproduced with permission.)

Restoring Function after Obstetrical Brachial Plexus Palsy

The approach to the brachial plexus in the obstetrical population is slightly different than in adults. Here there remains a significant role for exploration of the plexus and nerve grafting.[27] Neuroma excision and sural nerve grafting to obtain sufficient graft length are standard of care. The recent addition of motor nerve transfers, either in combination with nerve grafting or independently, has potentially augmented clinical recovery by providing a source of motor axons closer to the neuromuscular junction.[27]

Restoring Sensation

Significantly improved clinical recovery is achieved in the sensate hand. Similar to options for motor nerve transfers, the authors advocate for the use of sensory nerve transfers to restore sensation to critical areas such as the first web space for improving pinch. Unlike the motor nerve transfers, these sensory transfers can be performed independent of time.[9]

Postoperative Care

The majority of brachial plexus reconstructions can be performed on an outpatient or brief hospital stay basis. Postoperative pain control is critical and surgeons should have a low threshold for starting patients on an aggressive postoperative pain regimen, including targeting neuropathic pain.

The period of immobilization following surgery is largely dependent on operative procedure, but also factors in patient compliance and age. Given that primary repair or nerve grafting should only be performed in the setting of no tension, a brief period of immobilization less than one week is all that is required postoperatively. Similarly, nerve transfers require minimal immobilization so long as they are taken through a full range of motion for the joint above and below at the time of coaptation and there is no evidence of tension. Tendon transfers require a more prolonged period of immobilization, ranging from 3 to 6 weeks depending on the transfer. Early gentle passive range of motion is encouraged to prevent adhesion formation and joint stiffness. Where the plexus has been fully exposed by dividing the pectoralis major tendinous insertion, the patient should be kept in a sling for 4 weeks to avoid tension on the repair. Elbow, wrist, and hand range of motion within the sling are encouraged. Hand therapy and physical therapy are critical for optimizing recovery and the role of the therapist cannot be overstated. In addition, cortical retraining, motor re-education, and strengthening will be part of the longer term rehabilitation.

Complications

As with any surgery, the complications associated with brachial plexus surgery can be divided into acute, short term, and long term. The majority of these patients are young and otherwise healthy, making their anesthetic risks significantly less; however, given that they often require multiple surgical procedures, the risk cannot be completely discounted. Other acute complications include injury to adjacent structures, bleeding, and inability to complete the procedure. Locating a paralysed nerve can be humbling, given that the nerve does not function, cannot be stimulated, and often the surrounding musculature is denervated and abnormal in appearance. Having an excellent knowledge of nerve anatomy is critical to these transfers and it is not unusual for the authors to bring an anatomy atlas into the operating theatre.

Short-term complications include infection, wound healing problems or dehiscence, seroma, and hematoma. Long-term complications include scarring, joint stiffness, pain, and ineffective or unsuccessful results from the surgery. For tendon transfers, additional complications would include tendon rupture or adhesion, although using a Pulvertaft weave should make rupture less probable.

Donor deficit, for either nerve or tendon transfer, is a consideration. For the majority of nerve transfers, a transient donor deficit is a possibility, but almost no long-term deficits are reported.[9] Similarly, for tendon transfers, the selection of an expendable donor means that overall function should not be significantly affected.

Outcomes

Outcomes for brachial plexus injuries are related to the level and severity of the injury, the method and timing of reconstruction, and the patient's degree of compliance with postoperative rehabilitation. Due to the proximal level of these injuries, outcomes have been notoriously poor and prior to the advent of nerve transfers, when results were dependent on plexus exploration and grafting, "good" outcomes were achieved in only 20%–33% of patients.[10] Many of these earlier studies, however, lack an objective outcome measure, and thus it is difficult to compare degree of recovery. A recent publication comparing almost 300 patients with upper trunk lesions found significantly better outcomes following dual nerve transfers than traditional nerve grafting in establishing shoulder function.[10]

The Medical Research Council (MRC) grading system for strength, along with other objective measures such as grip strength, pinch strength, and potentially maximum weight lifted, provides a more acceptable way to compare outcomes.

For recovery of elbow flexion, the results following single or double nerve transfer are generally quite good.[5,11,28–31] Using a double fascicular nerve transfer, 28 of 29 patients regained elbow flexion and, of these, 23 regained MRC 4/5 strength or greater.[28] Liverneaux et al reported MRC 4/5 recovery of elbow flexion in all patients using the same procedure.[32] There was no permanent donor deficit in either of these studies. In the obstetrical brachial plexus population, 67% of patients showed good or excellent recovery following nerve reconstruction for the elbow and the results were significantly better for those patients with a C5 to C7 palsy than those with a pan–plexus palsy.[33]

When comparing extraplexal donors, one study found better success when three or more intercostal nerves were harvested as compared to two.[34] In addition, results were better when the lower intercostal nerves T7–T10 were used compared to the upper intercostals of T3–T6. They report good to excellent results in almost three-quarters of patients undergoing intercostal to musculocutaneous nerve transfer.[34] However another more recent study found that the number of intercostal nerves transferred did not change the ultimate outcome.[21]

Recovery of shoulder function is not as successful as elbow flexion, however it is significantly better than results achieved with shoulder arthrodesis. Reports of the outcomes of the spinal accessory to suprascapular nerve transfer are mixed. Songcharoen reported on 577 patients undergoing spinal accessory to suprascapular and/or axillary nerve transfer and reported that 80% of patients regained at least MRC 3/5 motor recovery. Reinnervation of both the suprascapular and axillary nerves results in improved results compared to transfer to a single nerve. Leechavengvongs described seven cases where a triceps branch was transferred to the axillary nerve and all patients regained MRC 4/5 deltoid function and 5 of 7 had an excellent result.

Recovery of hand function has been less successful. Gu reported on 32 patients undergoing contralateral C7 root transfer.[35] Fourteen of the patients had median nerve recipients and half regained MRC 3/5 motor function and 12 regained MRC 3/5 sensory function. Ray and Mackinnon report on 12 of 19 patients with good to excellent (MRC 4/5 or greater) recovery of finger and thumb extension following median to radial nerve transfers. In the same population 18/19 had meaningful recovery of wrist extension.[26]

Regardless of the clinical recovery, patient satisfaction and return to work are important determinants of the success of brachial plexus reconstruction. Of 32 patients with brachial plexus injuries, over three-quarters reported at least moderate overall life satisfaction and no patients reported extreme dissatisfaction.[36] Ten of the 32 patients reported that the injury greatly affected their overall quality of life. Approximately half returned to work following their injury and of these, 70% reported moderate to high satisfaction with their job. This compares to 85% of the general population.

In a later study, Kretschmer et al[37] revealed that 87% of patients undergoing brachial plexus reconstruction were satisfied with their results and 83% would undergo surgery again. This was interesting in light of the fact that 52% of patients who had been gainfully employed prior to injury returned to their former occupation, pain since the injury was expressed in 86% of patients, and 21% suffered from depression and anxiety. The group did find that occupational retraining was successful for 70% of patients, suggesting that this is an effective option in the patient with a brachial plexus injury.

Summary

Brachial plexus injuries are devastating and have a significant impact on quality of life and upper extremity function. Although traditionally surgical intervention has resulted in relatively poor recovery of function, the implementation of new surgical techniques such as nerve transfers, combined with significantly improved knowledge of internal nerve topography, has dramatically improved outcomes. Although there remains a role for surgical interventions such as nerve grafting and tendon transfer, especially in the obstetrical brachial plexus palsy population, nerve transfers are rapidly emerging as the standard of care for the treatment of these difficult patients.

References

1. Mackinnon SE, Novak CB. Evaluation of the patient with thoracic outlet syndrome. *Semin Thorac Cardiovasc Surg.* 1996;8(2):190–200.
2. Boyd KU, Nimigan AS, Mackinnon SE. Nerve reconstruction in the hand and upper extremity. *Clin Plast Surg.* 2011;38(4):643–660.
3. Fox IK, Mackinnon SE. Adult peripheral nerve disorders: nerve entrapment, repair, transfer, and brachial plexus disorders. *Plast Reconstr Surg.* 2011;127(5):105e–118e.
4. Leechavengvongs S, Malungpaishorpe K, Uerpairojkit C, et al. Nerve transfers to restore shoulder function. *Hand Clin.* 2016;32(2):153–164.
5. Mackinnon SE, Novak CB, Myckatyn TM, et al. Results of reinnervation of the biceps and brachialis muscles with a double fascicular transfer for elbow flexion. *J Hand Surg Am.* 2005;30(5):978–985.
6. Doi K. Management of total paralysis of the brachial plexus by the double free-muscle transfer technique. *J Hand Surg Eur.* 2008;33(3):240–251.
7. Zuker RM, Manktelow RT. Functioning free muscle transfers. *Hand Clin.* 2007;23(1):57–72.
8. O'Shea K, Feinberg JH, Wolfe SW. Imaging and electrodiagnostic work-up of acute adult brachial plexus injuries. *J Hand Surg Eur Vol.* 2011;36(9):747–759.
9. Tung TH, Mackinnon SE. Nerve transfers: indications, techniques, and outcomes. *J Hand Surg Am.* 2010;35(2):332–341.
10. Garg R, Merrell GA, Hillstrom HJ, et al. Comparison of nerve transfers and nerve grafting for traumatic upper plexus palsy: a systematic review and analysis. *J Bone Joint Surg Am.* 2011;93(9):819–829.
11. Oberlin C, Ameur NE, Teboul F, et al. Restoration of elbow flexion in brachial plexus injury by transfer of ulnar nerve fascicles to the nerve to the biceps muscle. *Tech Hand Up Extrem Surg.* 2002;6(2):86–90.
12. Merrell GA, Barrie KA, Katz DL, et al. Results of nerve transfer techniques for restoration of shoulder and elbow function in the context of a meta-analysis of the English literature. *J Hand Surg Am.* 2001;26(2):303–314.
13. Baltzer HL, Wagner ER, Kircher MF, et al. Evaluation of infraspinatus reinnervation and function following spinal accessory nerve to suprascapular nerve transfer in adult traumatic brachial plexus injuries. *Microsurgery.* 2017;37(5):365–370.

14. Bhandari PS, Deb P. Dorsal approach in transfer of the distal spinal accessory nerve into the suprascapular nerve: histomorphometric analysis and clinical results in 14 cases of upper brachial plexus injuries. *J Hand Surg Am.* 2011;36(7):1182–1190.
15. Bhandari PS, Deb P. Posterior approach for both spinal accessory nerve to suprascapular nerve and triceps branch to axillary nerve for upper plexus injuries. *J Hand Surg Am.* 2013;38(1):168–172.
16. Desai MJ, Daly CA, Seiler JG 3rd, et al. Radial to axillary nerve transfers: a combined case series. *J Hand Surg Am.* 2016;41(12):1128–1134.
17. Songcharoen P, Wongtrakul S, Mahaisavariya B, et al. Hemi-contralateral C7 transfer to median nerve in the treatment of root avulsion brachial plexus injury. *J Hand Surg Am.* 2001;26(6):1058–1064.
18. Sammer DM, Kircher MF, Bishop AT, et al. Hemi-contralateral C7 transfer in traumatic brachial plexus injuries: outcomes and complications. *J Bone Joint Surg Am.* 2012;94(2):131–137.
19. Yang G, Chang KW, Chung KC. A systematic review of outcomes of contralateral C7 transfer for the treatment of traumatic brachial plexus injury: part 2. Donor-site morbidity. *Plast Reconstr Surg.* 2015;136(4):480e–489e.
20. Barrie KA, Steinmann SP, Shin AY, et al. Gracilis free muscle transfer for restoration of function after complete brachial plexus avulsion. *Neurosurg Focus.* 2004;16(5):E8.
21. Maldonado AA, Kircher MF, Spinner RJ, et al. Free functioning gracilis muscle transfer versus intercostal nerve transfer to musculocutaneous nerve for restoration of elbow flexion after traumatic adult brachial pan-plexus injury. *Plast Reconstr Surg.* 2016;138(3):483e–488e.
22. Maldonado AA, Kircher MF, Spinner RJ, et al. Free functioning gracilis muscle transfer with and without simultaneous intercostal nerve transfer to musculocutaneous nerve for restoration of elbow flexion after traumatic adult brachial pan-plexus injury. *J Hand Surg Am.* 2017;42(4):293.e291–293.e297.
23. Mackinnon SE, Yee A, Ray WZ. Nerve transfers for the restoration of hand function after spinal cord injury. *J Neurosurg.* 2012;117(1):176–185.
24. Hsiao EC, Fox IK, Tung TH, et al. Motor nerve transfers to restore extrinsic median nerve function: case report. *Hand (NY).* 2009;4(1):92–97.
25. Barbour J, Yee A, Kahn LC, et al. Supercharged end-to-side anterior interosseous to ulnar motor nerve transfer for intrinsic musculature reinnervation. *J Hand Surg Am.* 2012;37(10):2150–2159.
26. Ray WZ, Mackinnon SE. Clinical outcomes following median to radial nerve transfers. *J Hand Surg Am.* 2011;36(2):201–208.
27. Borschel GH, Clarke HM. Obstetrical brachial plexus palsy. *Plast Reconstr Surg.* 2009;124(1 suppl):144e–155e.
28. Ray WZ, Pet MA, Yee A, et al. Double fascicular nerve transfer to the biceps and brachialis muscles after brachial plexus injury: clinical outcomes in a series of 29 cases. *J Neurosurg.* 2011;114(6):1520–1528.
29. Martins RS, Siqueira MG, Heise CO, et al. A prospective study comparing single and double fascicular transfer to restore elbow flexion after brachial plexus injury. *Neurosurgery.* 2013;72(5):709–714; discussion 714–715; quiz 715.
30. Ladak A, Spinner RJ. Double fascicular nerve transfer for elbow flexion: is 2 better than 1? *Neurosurgery.* 2013;72(6):1055–1056.
31. Carlsen BT, Kircher MF, Spinner RJ, et al. Comparison of single versus double nerve transfers for elbow flexion after brachial plexus injury. *Plast Reconstr Surg.* 2011;127(1):269–276.
32. Liverneaux PA, Diaz LC, Beaulieu JY, et al. Preliminary results of double nerve transfer to restore elbow flexion in upper type brachial plexus palsies. *Plast Reconstr Surg.* 2006;117(3):915–919.
33. Terzis JK, Kokkalis ZT. Restoration of elbow extension after primary reconstruction in obstetric brachial plexus palsy. *J Pediatr Orthop.* 2010;30(2):161–168.
34. Terzis JK, Kostopoulos VK. The surgical treatment of brachial plexus injuries in adults. *Plast Reconstr Surg.* 2007;119(4):73e–92e.
35. Gu YD, Wu MM, Zhen YL, et al. Phrenic nerve transfer for brachial plexus motor neurotization. *Microsurgery.* 1989;10:287–289.
36. Choi PD, Novak CB, Mackinnon SE, et al. Quality of life and functional outcome following brachial plexus injury. *J Hand Surg Am.* 1997;22:605–612.
37. Kretschmer T, Ihle S, Antoniadis G. Patient satisfaction and disability after brachial plexus surgery. *Neurosurgery.* 2009;65:A189–A196.

54 Nerve Compression

HOLLIE A. POWER, KRISTEN M. DAVIDGE, AND SUSAN E. MACKINNON

For videos accompanying this chapter see ExpertConsult.com. See inside cover for access details.

Nerve compression syndromes are a common clinical presentation in plastic surgery practice. The upper extremity is most commonly affected, with carpal tunnel syndrome being most frequent followed by cubital tunnel syndrome. The etiology of these disorders is usually multifactorial, with systemic disorders, prolonged postural changes, and repetitive activities contributing to their development. The increasing prevalence of obesity, metabolic disorders, and an aging population has resulted in increased numbers of patients seeking care for compression neuropathies. Surgeons treating these conditions must rule out neurological disorders that can mimic nerve compression, such as brachial neuritis, mononeuritis, and polyneuropathy. A subset of patients may have a genetic predisposition to multiple nerve compressions. Effective diagnosis and management require a detailed understanding of the anatomy and pathophysiology of nerve compression. A multidisciplinary approach to clinical evaluation, diagnosis, and management are key in attaining favorable outcomes.

Pathophysiology

Response to Chronic Compression

The clinical presentation of patients with nerve compression is variable and dependent upon a spectrum of changes that occur within the nerve in response to a complex interplay of mechanical and ischemic forces applied over a period of time. This results in a classic constellation of symptoms, including pain, paresthesiae, and weakness (Fig. 54.1). The histopathological response to chronic compression has been difficult to study in human patients for ethical reasons, and thus much of what we know originates from animal studies.[1] As the nerve travels through a given compartment, the available volume is finite. Any reduction in compartment volume or increase in nerve size may result in compression of the nerve. External compression may occur from structures such as the transverse carpal ligament, bony prominences or the tendinous leading edge of muscles. Prolonged changes in limb position may reduce the overall size of the compartment and increase pressure on the nerve (e.g., prolonged wrist or elbow flexion).[2,3]

Chronic compression leads to breakdown of the blood–nerve barrier, followed by endoneurial edema and perineurial thickening and fibrosis.[1] Increased endoneurial pressure may restrict blood flow to the nerve, making it susceptible to dynamic ischemia.[4] If not corrected, areas of focal demyelination develop, followed by diffuse demyelination. This progresses to axonal injury and Wallerian degeneration in the absence of intervention.[1] These changes may not be uniform across the nerve, and are related to the compressive forces applied to different areas of the nerve. For example, patients with early carpal tunnel syndrome often present with paresthesiae to the long and ring finger, owing to the superficial location of these fascicles relative to those of the thumb and index finger.[5]

Classification of Nerve Injury

Accurate determination of the type of nerve injury is critical when approaching a patient with compression neuropathy as it guides management and helps to determine their prognosis. The Sunderland and Seddon classifications of nerve injury were originally described for acute nerve injuries,[6] but can also be applied to compression neuropathy (Table 54.1). A first-degree injury (neurapraxia) has areas of focal demyelination, with no axonal loss. Recovery is expected to be complete once the compressive insult is corrected. A second-degree injury (axonotmesis) has mild axonal loss and complete recovery is anticipated, whereas a third-degree injury (axonotmesis) has significant axonal loss with recovery that is variable and incomplete. Fourth- and fifth-degree injuries (neurotmesis) have no functional recovery because the axonal loss is complete. Fourth-degree injuries are uncommon in compression neuropathy but may occur with severe compression or iatrogenic injury. Fifth-degree injuries occur following traumatic or iatrogenic injury. When axonal injury occurs, any surrounding healthy axons collaterally sprout to innervate territories up to five times their original size.[7] Therefore, weakness detected on clinical examination may not directly correspond with the degree of axonal loss. When linked to the classification of nerve injury, this concept can be used to better relate electrodiagnostic findings with the clinical examination (Fig. 54.2).

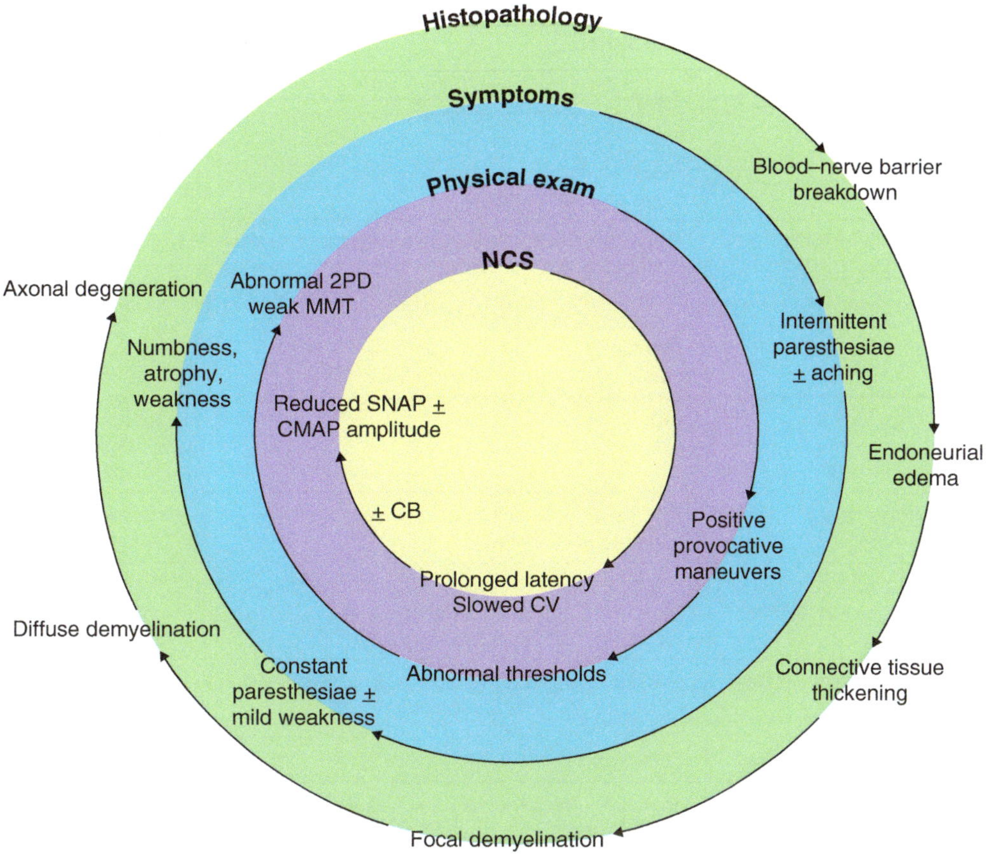

• **Fig. 54.1** The histopathology of chronic nerve compression and its correlation with symptoms, physical exam and electrodiagnostic findings. 2PD, two-point discrimination; CB, conduction block; CV, conduction velocity; CMAP, compound muscle action potential; MMT, manual muscle testing; NCS, nerve conduction study; SNAP, sensory nerve action potential. (Modified with permission from Mackinnon SE, Novak CB. Compression neuropathies. In: Wolfe SW et al, eds. *Green's Operative Hand Surgery*. 7th edn. Philadelphia: Elsevier Inc; 2017.)

Clinical Evaluation

A thorough history and physical examination is essential to identify all potential points of compression and musculoskeletal disorders contributing to patient symptomatology. The history should explore the nature and time course of symptoms, and address all relevant comorbidities, medications, and risk factors for nerve compression. Typical symptoms of compression neuropathy include numbness, paresthesiae, pain, and/or weakness in the distribution of the affected nerve(s). A pain questionnaire is a useful adjunct, especially in patients with diffuse symptomatology.

The physical examination should consist of a complete sensory and motor evaluation of both upper extremities, to localize the site of compression and determine the severity of neuropathy. All potential entrapment sites should be evaluated, owing to the double crush mechanism, wherein compression of a nerve at one site renders it more susceptible to compression at a second site.[8] Failure to identify and address all involved compression points can lead to ongoing or residual symptoms following treatment.

Numerous methods are available to evaluate sensation and there is no accepted gold standard. These include assessment of light touch (e.g., the Ten Test[9]), vibration, pressure detection thresholds (e.g., Semmes–Weinstein monofilament testing), and two-point discrimination (static and dynamic). Abnormal sensory thresholds are an early finding in compression neuropathy, whereas abnormal two-point discrimination is typically found later.

Provocative tests using percussion (i.e., Tinel's test), direct pressure, or joint movement can elicit patient symptoms by increasing compression at known nerve entrapment sites (see Table 54.1). The scratch collapse test (SCT) is a useful tool to identify areas of compression, and can be performed in hierarchical fashion to identify multilevel nerve compression.[10]

Motor testing should include inspection of both upper extremities for atrophy and abnormal posture, as well as quantification of muscle strength using the Medical Research Council grading system, dynanometers (e.g., key pinch and grip strength), and special tests specific to each nerve. Weakness is usually a late finding in compression neuropathy.

Further details regarding symptomatology and exam findings unique to each compression neuropathy can be found in their respective sections.

TABLE 54.1 **Provocative Tests for Nerve Compression**

Nerve	Site of Compression	Test	Conservative Therapy
Median	Carpal tunnel	Carpal compression test Phalen test Reverse Phalen test	Splint wrist in neutral at night
	Proximal forearm	Pressure over pronator teres with the forearm supinated Resisted elbow flexion with the forearm supinated (lacertus fibrosus) Resisted forearm pronation (PT) Resisted long finger flexion (FDS)	Stretching of pronator teres
Ulnar	Cubital tunnel	Elbow flexion Pressure proximal to cubital tunnel	Splint elbow in extension at night Elbow pad use
	Guyon's canal	Pressure proximal to Guyon's canal Reverse Phalen test	Splint wrist in neutral at night
Radial	Proximal forearm (Radial tunnel/PIN)	Pressure over supinator (arcade of Fröhse) Resisted forearm supination Resisted long finger and wrist extension	Favor positioning in supination Avoid repetitive forearm rotation
	Distal forearm (Radial sensory)	Pressure over brachioradialis and extensor carpi radialis longus tendinous junction Forearm pronation with wrist flexion and ulnar deviation	
Brachial plexus	Supraclavicular	Pressure over brachial plexus at the level of the scalenes Elevated arm stress test	Stretching of shortened muscles Strengthening of weak scapula stabilizing muscles
	Infraclavicular	Pressure over pectoralis minor	

Modified from Mackinnon SE, Novak CB. Compression neuropathies. In: Wolfe SW, Hotchkiss RN, Pederson, WC et al, eds. *Green's Operative Hand Surgery*, 7th edn. Philadelphia: Elsevier; 2017: Table 28.1.

Investigations

Electrodiagnostic Studies

Electrodiagnostic studies help to accurately localize the site of compression, assess the severity and progression of neuropathy, and exclude alternate diagnoses (e.g., cervical radiculopathy, systemic polyneuropathy, or disuse atrophy). However, they should be interpreted with an awareness of their limitations. Nerve conduction studies (NCS) evaluate the large, myelinated fibres and not smaller unmyelinated pain fibres. Since the latter are affected first in compression neuropathy, NCS may be normal early in the disease process.[1] Similarly, dynamic ischemia resulting from compression cannot be detected on electrophysiological studies. History and physical examination therefore remain a critical component in the diagnosis of compression neuropathy.

Initial changes seen on NCS relate to focal demyelination and/or conduction block and include prolonged latency and slowing of conduction velocity. Axonal loss occurs in later stages of compression and results in decreased compound muscle action potential (CMAP) and sensory nerve action potential (SNAP) amplitudes (see Fig. 54.1).[11] Electromyography (EMG) provides a qualitative assessment of muscle function and is a sensitive indicator of axonal injury. Increased insertional activity, the presence of spontaneous activity (e.g., fibrillation potentials, positive sharp waves), and changes in the morphology and recruitment of motor unit potentials (MUPs) signify axonal injury. In the setting of compression neuropathy, the presence of spontaneous activity provides evidence that denervated muscle is capable of receiving reinnervation. In very late stages of compression neuropathy, the sensory and motor NCS may have absent responses and EMG may demonstrate no MUPs.[5]

Imaging

Imaging is used as an adjunct to clinical examination and electrodiagnostic testing and generally does not establish the diagnosis of compression neuropathy on its own. It is most useful for identifying pathology contributing to the development of nerve compression at a specific location. Plain radiographs and/or computed tomography are useful for any compression neuropathy where trauma or bony abnormalities (i.e., a supracondylar process in pronator syndrome) are suspected. Ultrasonography and magnetic resonance imaging (MRI) can determine if cysts or other space-occupying lesions (e.g., ganglion or peripheral nerve sheath tumor) are present. Both ultrasound and MRI

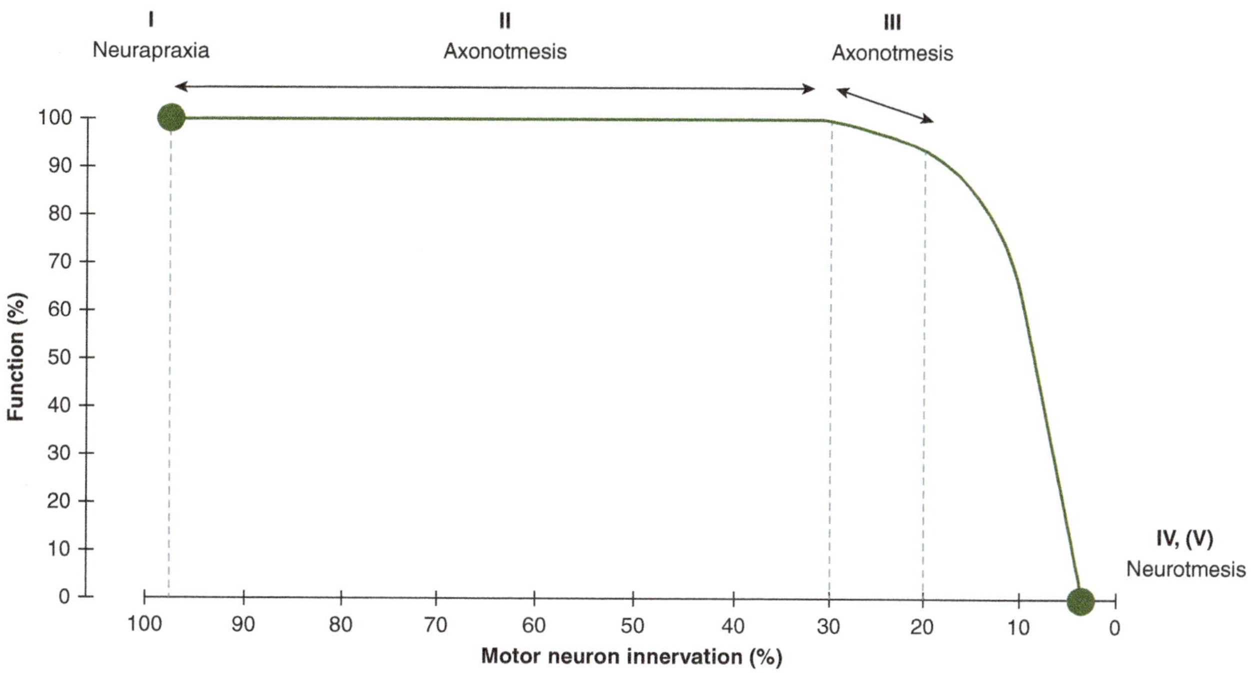

• **Fig. 54.2** Relationship between muscle function, percentage of intact motor neurons and the classification of nerve injury. While the relationship between function and motor neuron connection has been recognized by researchers for some time,[7] its correspondence to the Sunderland and Seddon classifications of nerve injury[6] has not been linked to this physiological relationship. For example, a Sunderland first-degree injury (I) (Seddon neurapraxia) has no axonal loss and therefore should recover full function. A second-degree injury (II) (axonotmesis) has variable axonal loss and complete recovery is anticipated, whereas a third-degree injury (III) has significant axonal loss with functional recovery that is variable and incomplete. Fourth (IV) and fifth-degree (V) injuries (neurotmesis) usually have no functional recovery as the axonal loss is complete. Fourth-degree injuries can occur with severe compression neuropathy or as a complication of surgery, and fifth-degree injuries occur with traumatic peripheral nerve injuries. Note: This figure depicts the anticipated functional recovery with appropriate correction of compression. (Reproduced with permission from Power HA, Sharma K, Haj El M, Moore AM, Patterson MM, Mackinnon SE. Compound muscle action potential (CMAP) amplitude predicts the severity of cubital tunnel syndrome. *J Bone Joint Surg*. 2019;101(8):730–738.)

have also been used for the diagnosis of cubital tunnel syndrome with reasonable sensitivity and specificity: ultrasound evaluates the cross-sectional area of the ulnar nerve at the elbow, whereas MRI also looks at ulnar nerve hyperintensity.[12]

Median Nerve Compression

Anatomy

The median nerve is formed by the medial (motor) and lateral (sensory) cords of the brachial plexus, then crosses superficial to the brachial artery and courses distally along its medial aspect. In the upper arm, the median nerve lies between the medial intermuscular septum and brachialis and then runs distally through the antecubital fossa deep to the lacertus fibrosis. It then passes between the superficial and deep heads of the pronator teres (PT). Less commonly, the median nerve will pass deep to both heads of the PT or through the substance of the superficial head.[13]

The median nerve passes under the fibrous edge of the flexor digitorum superficialis (FDS), traveling in the forearm between the FDS and flexor digitorum profundus (FDP). It gives off four groups of branches in the proximal forearm: branches to PT (proximal, superficial); branches to flexor carpi radialis (FCR) and palmaris longus (PL) (deep, ulnar); branches to FDS (deep, ulnar, more distal); and, the anterior interosseous nerve (AIN), which arises from the radial aspect of the median nerve, approximately 3 cm distal to the intercondylar line, and innervates the FDP to the index and long fingers, the flexor pollicis longus (FPL), and the pronator quadratus.

In the distal forearm, the median nerve becomes more superficial and courses just deep to the FCR and PL tendons. The palmar cutaneous branch (PCM) arises from the volar–radial aspect of the median nerve 5 cm proximal to the wrist flexion crease and may course distally up to 6 mm ulnar to the thenar crease. The PCM usually crosses the wrist as a single branch and then arborizes in the palm superficial to the palmar fascia.[13]

At the wrist the median nerve enters the carpal tunnel along with nine tendons (FDS ×4, FDP ×4, FPL). The carpal tunnel is bordered dorsally by the carpal bones, ulnarly by the hamate and triquetrum, and radially by the scaphoid, trapezium, and FCR sheath. The volar roof of the carpal tunnel is formed by the transverse carpal ligament (TCL), with contributions from the antebrachial fascia proximally and the thenar/hypothenar aponeuroses distally.

At the distal aspect of the carpal tunnel, the median nerve divides into the common digital nerves to the thumb and radial border of the index finger, and the common digital nerves to the second and third webspaces. The recurrent motor branch typically arises from the radial border of the median nerve just distal to the flexor retinaculum (extraligamentous course), turning back to innervate the abductor pollicis brevis (APB), opponens pollicis, and superficial head of the flexor pollicis brevis. The recurrent branch may also take a subligamentous (31%) or transligamentous course (23%).[14] Other anatomic variations include an accessory median nerve branch that can arise distal or proximal to the carpal tunnel, and a bifid or duplicated median nerve.[14]

The Riche–Cannieu anastomosis is an anomalous motor connection from the ulnar to median nerve in the palm that contributes an average 28% of the innervation to APB.[13] When present, thenar function may be preserved in the setting of severe carpal tunnel syndrome.

There are four main compression syndromes associated with the median nerve: carpal tunnel syndrome (CTS), pronator syndrome, AIN syndrome, and PCM compression.

Carpal Tunnel Syndrome

CTS is the most common compression neuropathy in the upper extremity, with an annual incidence of 0.5–5.1 per 1000 people.[13] The etiology of CTS is thought to relate to compression of the median nerve within the carpal tunnel resulting in impaired microcirculation, subperineurial edema, and eventually fibrosis. Any condition that reduces the volume of the carpal canal or increases the volume of its contents can initiate this process. Several risk factors for the development of CTS have been proposed including: female gender, advanced age, diabetes, thyroid disease, pregnancy, rheumatoid arthritis, obesity, and smoking.[15] Positioning the wrist in flexion or extension during sleep may exacerbate many of these risk factors.[3] Occupational factors such as repetitive hand use and prolonged vibration exposure have also been associated with CTS.[16] Anatomical causes are identified in a minority of cases. Most commonly, this involves a space occupying lesion within the carpal tunnel, but lumbrical incursion into the carpal tunnel can also occur.[13]

Clinical Presentation

CTS classically presents with pain and paresthesiae in the volar aspect of the thumb, index, long, and radial border of the ring fingers. This may progress to constant numbness over time. Thenar sensation is generally preserved since the PCM courses outside the carpal tunnel. Symptoms are often exacerbated by gripping and wrist flexion and are usually worse at night. With severe or long-standing compression, weakness and atrophy of the thenar muscles may occur.

Provocative tests for CTS include the SCT, Tinel's test, Phalen test (wrist flexion to 90 degrees for up to 60 seconds), the carpal compression test, and the fist test for lumbrical incursion (gentle flexion of the fingers into the palm) (see Table 54.1). Clinical tests for CTS tend to have high specificity and moderate sensitivity.[13,17]

Patients often have normal electrodiagnostic studies early in the disease, with symptoms attributed to dynamic ischemia of the median nerve. As the disease progresses, demyelination occurs first in a focal pattern, followed by diffuse demyelination. The majority of patients with carpal tunnel syndrome present with demyelinating disease and respond well to surgical treatment.[18] However, axonal loss may be seen in longstanding disease.

Management

Initial management of mild-to-moderate CTS should be nonoperative and include activity modification, wrist-neutral splints, oral antiinflammatory agents, and/or corticosteroid injection. Wrist-neutral nighttime splinting can significantly improve symptoms, and there is no advantage to wearing splints full time.[19] Corticosteroid injection into the carpal tunnel is effective at relieving CTS symptoms and may also be used for diagnosis and prognosis. The results tend to be short-lived and injection is most useful for patients requiring temporary relief (e.g., pregnancy-related CTS).[20] A Cochrane review of other nonoperative modalities in CTS showed no benefit.[21]

Surgery is indicated when conservative measures fail, and in severe CTS with thenar involvement. Patients with significant weakness and/or dense numbness should be advised that surgical intervention will prevent progression but is unlikely to yield complete recovery. An opponensplasty may be needed to restore thumb opposition in severe cases.

Carpal tunnel release (CTR) can be performed via endoscopic or open techniques. Multiple randomized controlled trials have been performed comparing open versus endoscopic CTR, none of which has demonstrated significant differences in outcomes or complications.[22] The potential advantages of endoscopic CTR include less postoperative pain, which may allow earlier return to work. However, there is a learning curve to the endoscopic approach during which time there is increased risk of injury to the median nerve and a longer operative time. Limited-incision open techniques also carry an increased risk of nerve injury owing to the reduced visualization afforded by the small incision, and have no proven advantage over full-length open CTR.[22] Since even a small injury to the median nerve can be life-altering for the patient, the senior author's preferred approach remains open CTR with a full-length incision.

Open Carpal Tunnel Release (Fig. 54.3)

The procedure is performed under tourniquet control, with a Bier block or local anesthesia plus sedation. A 3-cm incision is made in the palm, with the proximal extent abutting the wrist crease. In obese patients, the incision is extended proximal to the wrist crease in a zig-zag fashion to allow complete visualization. The incision is placed 5 mm ulnar to the interthenar depression to avoid injury to the PCM

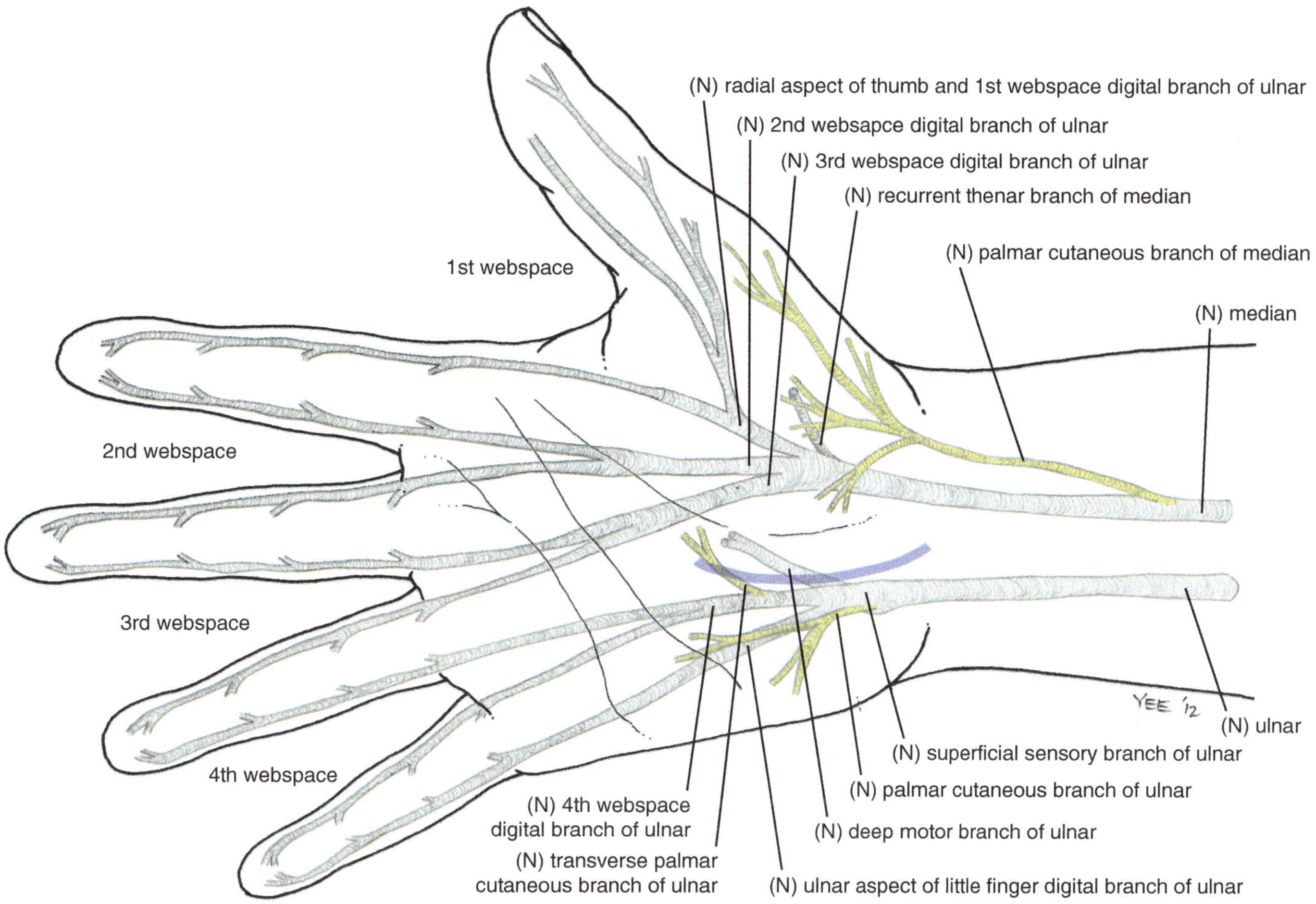

A

• **Fig. 54.3 (A–F)** Author's preferred technique for open carpal tunnel release. (A) Relationship of the skin incision to the underlying median and ulnar nerve anatomy.

Continued

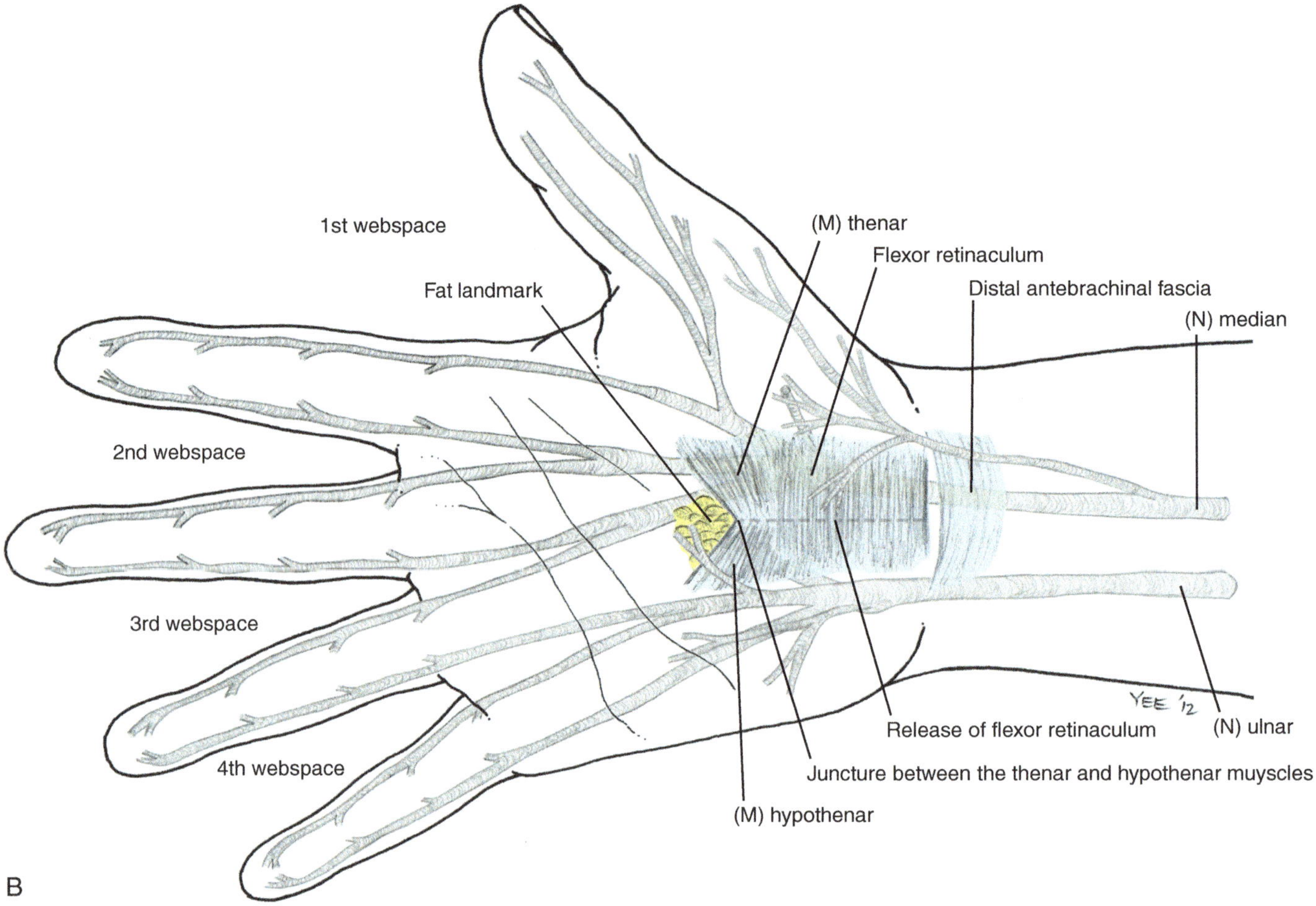

B

• **Fig. 54.3, cont'd.** (B) Landmarks for complete release of the transverse carpal ligament (TCL) (flexor retinaculum). The distal extent of the TCL is the "V" intersection of the hypothenar and thenar musculature, distal to which is the mid-palmar fat pad. The proximal extent of the TCL is the antebrachial fascia.

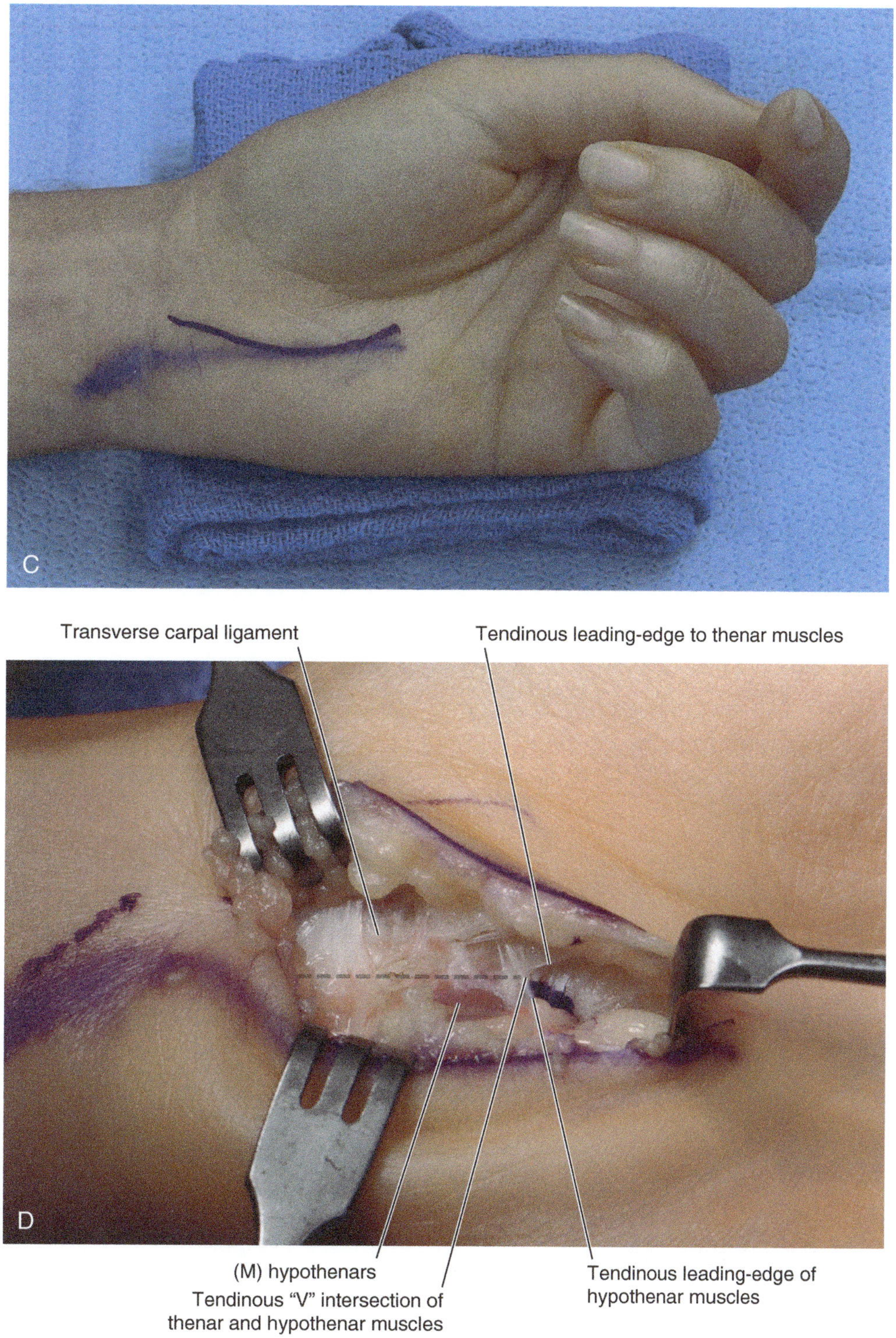

• **Fig. 54.3, cont'd.** (C) Design of the skin incision approximately 5 mm ulnar to the interthenar depression on the left hand. (D) Longitudinal division of the palmar aponeurosis. The TCL lies immediately dorsal (posterior) to this aponeurosis.

Continued

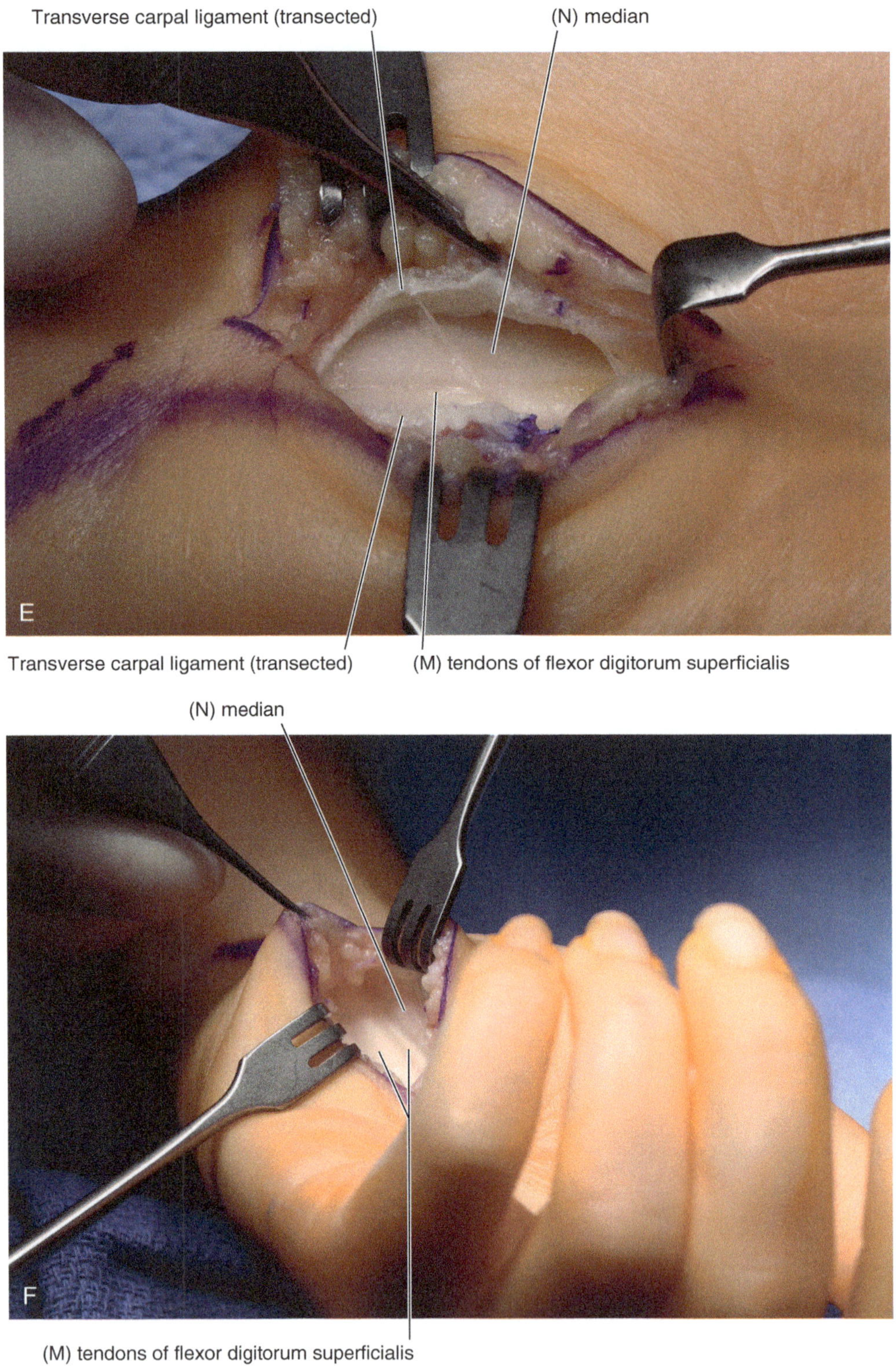

• **Fig. 54.3, cont'd.** (E) Following transection of the TCL, the median nerve and tendons within the carpal canal are visualized. (F) With good retraction, the proximal extent of the TCL should be clearly visualized to ensure an adequate, complete release. The surgeon should be positioned at the end of the hand table for the most ideal view. (Reproduced with permission from Susan E. Mackinnon, ed. *Nerve Surgery.* New York: Thieme; 2015.)

and to avoid dividing the TCL directly over the median nerve. The skin is incised, and dissection is carried through the subcutaneous tissue to the palmar aponeurosis, which is divided longitudinally. Care is taken to identify and protect any crossing cutaneous nerve branches, as these may be a source of prolonged "pillar" pain postoperatively. The TCL is identified and sharply divided along its ulnar border. The distal extent of the release is the "V" junction between the hypothenar and thenar muscles. The proximal aspect of the palmar fat pad is also visible at this level. Proximally, the antebrachial fascia is divided under direct vision. Neurolysis of the median nerve, epineurotomy, and tenolysis is not routinely performed.[13] Hemostasis is achieved with bipolar cautery, and the skin closed with nonabsorbable interrupted sutures. A well-padded wrist splint is applied for comfort and removed after 2–3 days. Immediate range of motion (ROM) of the digits and light hand use are encouraged. The wrist is splinted at night for 2–3 weeks postoperatively to prevent bowstringing of the flexor tendons. Sutures are removed at 14 days and a gradual return to full activity is permitted after 5–6 weeks.

Pronator Syndrome

Pronator syndrome is a sensory neuropathy resulting from compression of the median nerve in the proximal forearm and is much less common than CTS. Risk factors include female gender, advanced age, and repetitive pronation activities (which can result in a short, tight PT).[23]

There are several potential compression points along the median nerve that can contribute to pronator syndrome. Proximally, there may be a supracondylar process (present in <5%, located 3–6 cm above the medial epicondyle) and ligament of Struthers, a fibrous band between the medial epicondyle and the supracondylar process.[13] When present, the median nerve separates from the brachial vessels and passes posterior to these structures, where it can be compressed. Distally, the lacertus fibrosis, fibrous bands between the superficial and deep heads of the PT, a tendinous deep head of the PT, and the fibrous leading edge of the FDS can also compress the median nerve.[24] Less common causes of compression include an anomalous PT, snapping brachialis, accessory FPL (Gantzer's muscle), palmaris profundus, and FCR brevis.[24]

Clinical Presentation

Unlike CTS, sensory abnormalities in pronator syndrome include the PCM distribution and the radial three and a half digits. Patients frequently describe pain in the volar forearm, exacerbated by direct pressure and resisted pronation. Less commonly, patients report weakness or difficulty with small object manipulation.

On examination, pain is reproduced by passive supination with direct pressure over the median nerve at the leading edge of PT. The PT may be tender and occasionally a ligament of Struthers may be palpated.[5] A positive Tinel's sign and SCT may be present. Success in eliciting a positive SCT at this site requires firm pressure over the median nerve, owing to its deep location. Additional provocative maneuvers for pronator syndrome include resisted forearm pronation (PT), resisted elbow flexion with the forearm supinated (lacertus fibrosis), and resisted long finger PIP flexion (FDS).

Management

Nonoperative management consists of stretching exercises for PT, activity modification, splinting, and antiinflammatory medications. Surgery is indicated when conservative measures fail. The senior author's preferred technique is as follows.

Median Nerve Decompression in the Forearm (Fig. 54.4)

A longitudinal S-shaped incision is made in the proximal third of the volar forearm, extending to the antecubital fossa proximally. Dissection is carried down to the lacertus fibrosis, which is sharply divided. The radial artery and superficial radial sensory nerve (SRN) are identified under the brachioradialis and the tendon of the superficial head of PT is identified by dissecting between these structures. The PT is step-lengthened to decompress the median nerve and also to allow ease of access. The superficial head of PT is then retracted ulnarly and the median nerve is identified proximally, medial to the brachial vessels. The deep head of PT is identified, and its tendinous portion resected. Care is taken to preserve median nerve branches to the PT. The tendinous leading edge of FDS is divided. Any crossing vessels compressing the median nerve are ligated and divided. Proximally, the surgeon should be able to easily run a finger along the median nerve. If any compression is felt or if a ligament of Struthers or supracondylar process is identified preoperatively, the incision should be extended above the antecubital fossa to allow resection of these structures. Following hemostasis and a layered closure, a sterile dressing and well-padded splint keeping the elbow in slight flexion are applied. The splint is removed in 2–3 days, and the patient is instructed to perform full ROM exercises as tolerated.

Anterior Interosseous Nerve Syndrome

The AIN can be selectively compressed by the same anatomic structures described for pronator syndrome. However, unlike pronator syndrome, AIN syndrome is a motor neuropathy with no loss of sensory function. The hallmark feature is atrophy and weakness of the FPL, FDP of the index and long fingers, and pronator quadratus. The syndrome usually occurs spontaneously, but in some cases can result from trauma or a tumour. A history of severe pain for several weeks followed by weakness in the AIN distribution suggests neuritis (i.e., Parsonage–Turner syndrome) rather than mechanical compression.[5] The majority of these cases recover spontaneously without operative intervention.

Palmar Cutaneous Nerve Compression

The PCM pierces the antebrachial fascia 2 cm proximal to the wrist flexion crease and travels through a tunnel 3 mm to 2 cm in length. The tunnel may pass through the thickened antebrachial fascia or TCL. PCM compression results in altered sensation over the thenar eminence and radial aspect of the palm. Rarely, these symptoms occur from distal compression, but are more commonly secondary to proximal compression (i.e., pronator syndrome) or iatrogenic injury to the PCM (e.g., after volar distal radius fracture fixation).

Ulnar Nerve Compression

Anatomy

The ulnar nerve is formed from the medial cord (C8–T1), lying medial to the axillary artery at its origin. In the middle third of the arm, the ulnar nerve pierces the medial intermuscular septum and travels distally between this septum and the medial head of the triceps. At the elbow, the ulnar nerve enters the cubital tunnel. This fibro-osseous tunnel is bordered superficially by Osborne's band (a fascial band spanning the olecranon and medial epicondyle), on its deep surface by the ulnar groove of the medial epicondyle proximally, and the ulnohumeral joint capsule and medial collateral ligament distally.

The ulnar nerve enters the forearm between the two heads of the flexor carpi ulnaris (FCU), coursing distally between FCU and FDP on the medial aspect of the ulnar artery. The most proximal motor branch innervates the FCU approximately 1.6 cm distal to the medial epicondyle.[13] Subsequent branches to the FCU and ulnar two FDPs originate from both the medial and lateral sides of the ulnar nerve. The dorsal cutaneous branch (DCU) of the ulnar nerve, which gives sensation to the dorsal aspect of the ring and small fingers, originates 10 cm proximal to the wrist crease.

At the wrist, the ulnar nerve enters Guyon's canal along with the ulnar vessels. Gross and Gelberman divided this area into three zones according to the internal topography of the ulnar nerve.[25] In Zone 1 (proximal), the ulnar nerve lies superficial to the TCL, deep

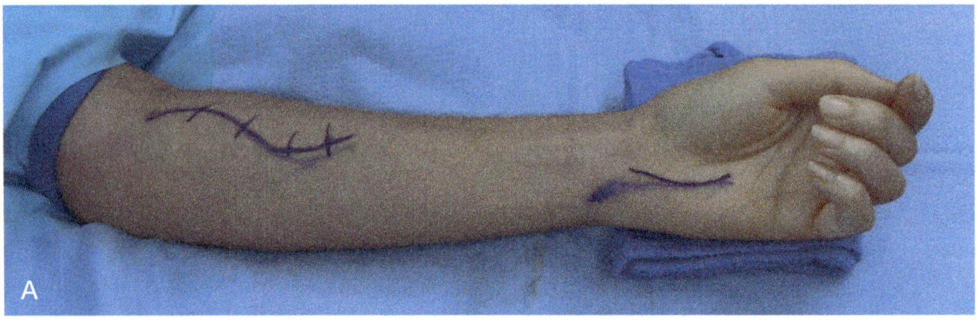

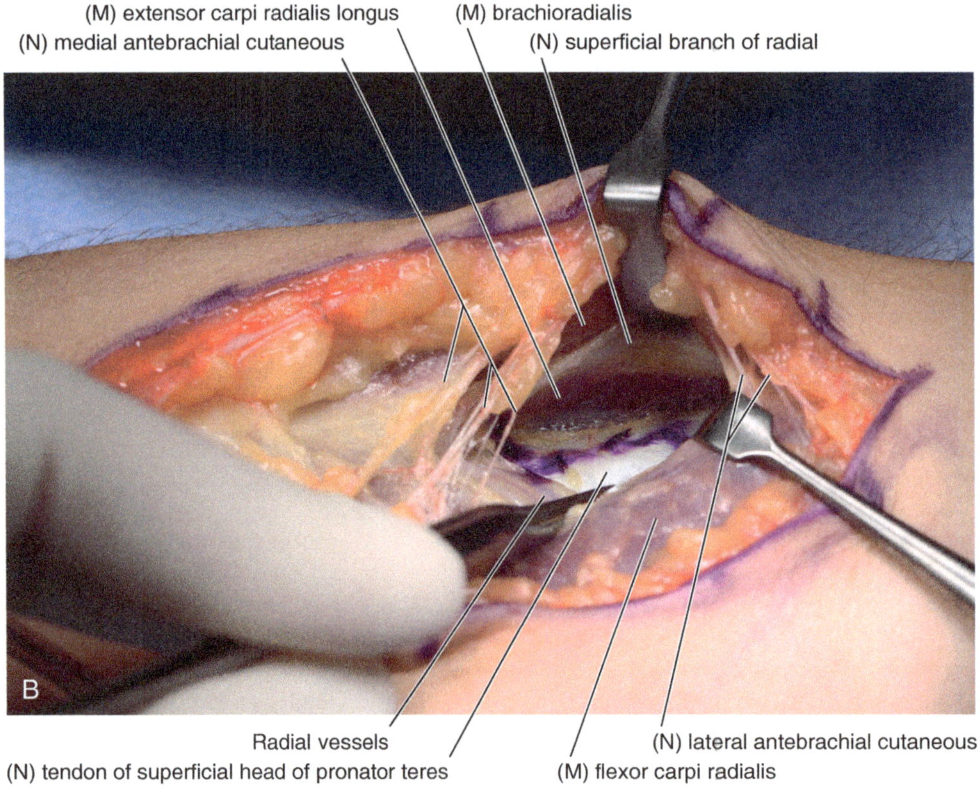

• **Fig. 54.4 (A–F)** Author's preferred technique for decompression of the median nerve in the forearm. (A) Design of the skin incision in the proximal volar left forearm. A carpal tunnel release is simultaneously performed if there is evidence of distal median nerve compression on clinical evaluation. (B) The pronator teres (PT) tendon is identified between the radial vessels and SRN in the mid-forearm.

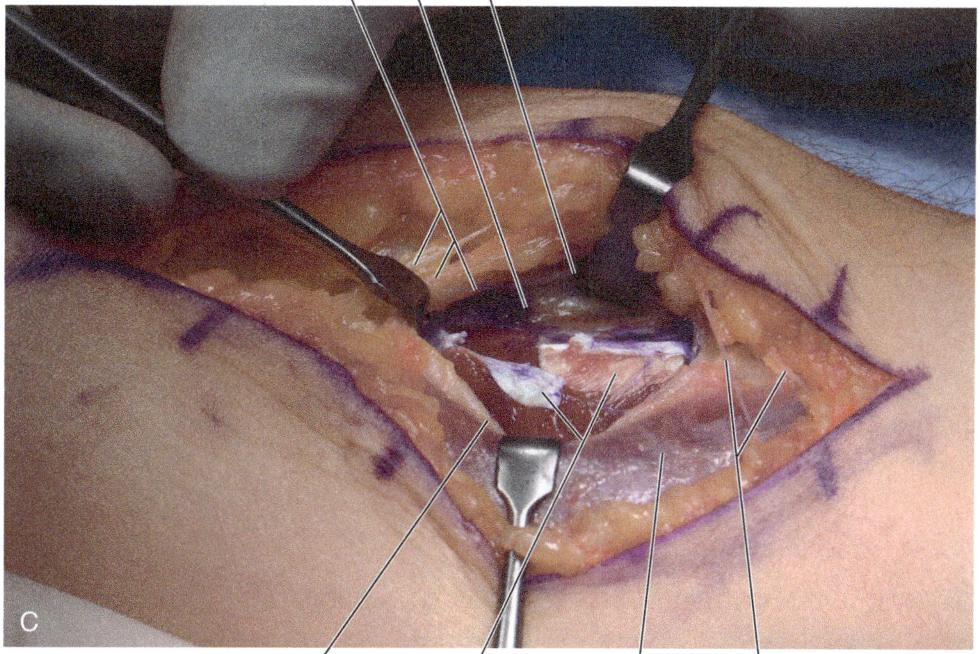

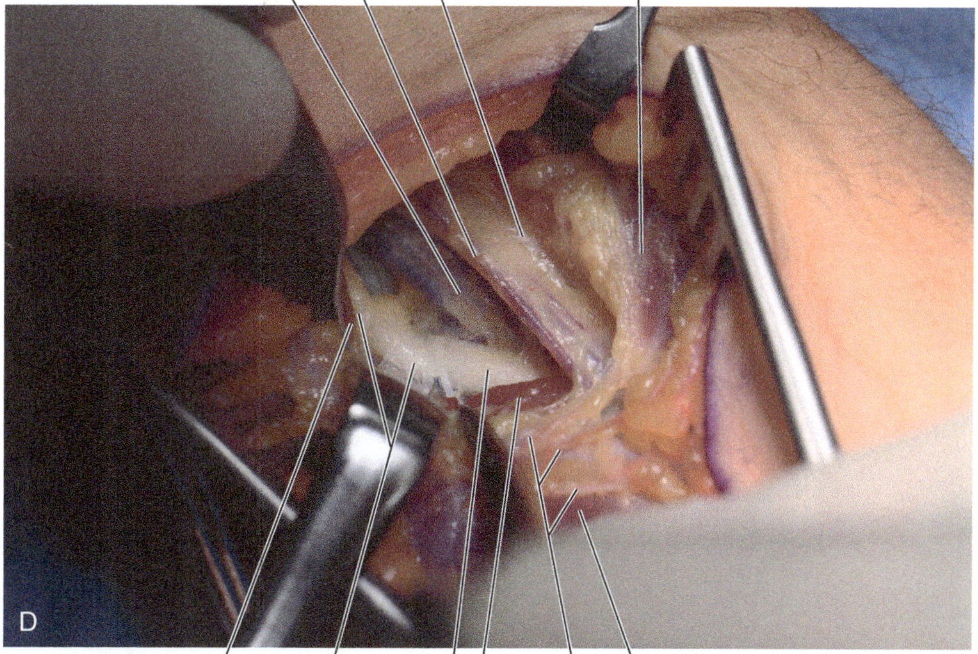

• **Fig. 54.4, cont'd.** (C) Step-lengthening of the PT tendon. (D) With retraction of the superficial head of PT, the median nerve can be identified on the ulnar side of the radial vessels. The tendinous portion of the deep head of PT can be seen compressing the median nerve.

Continued

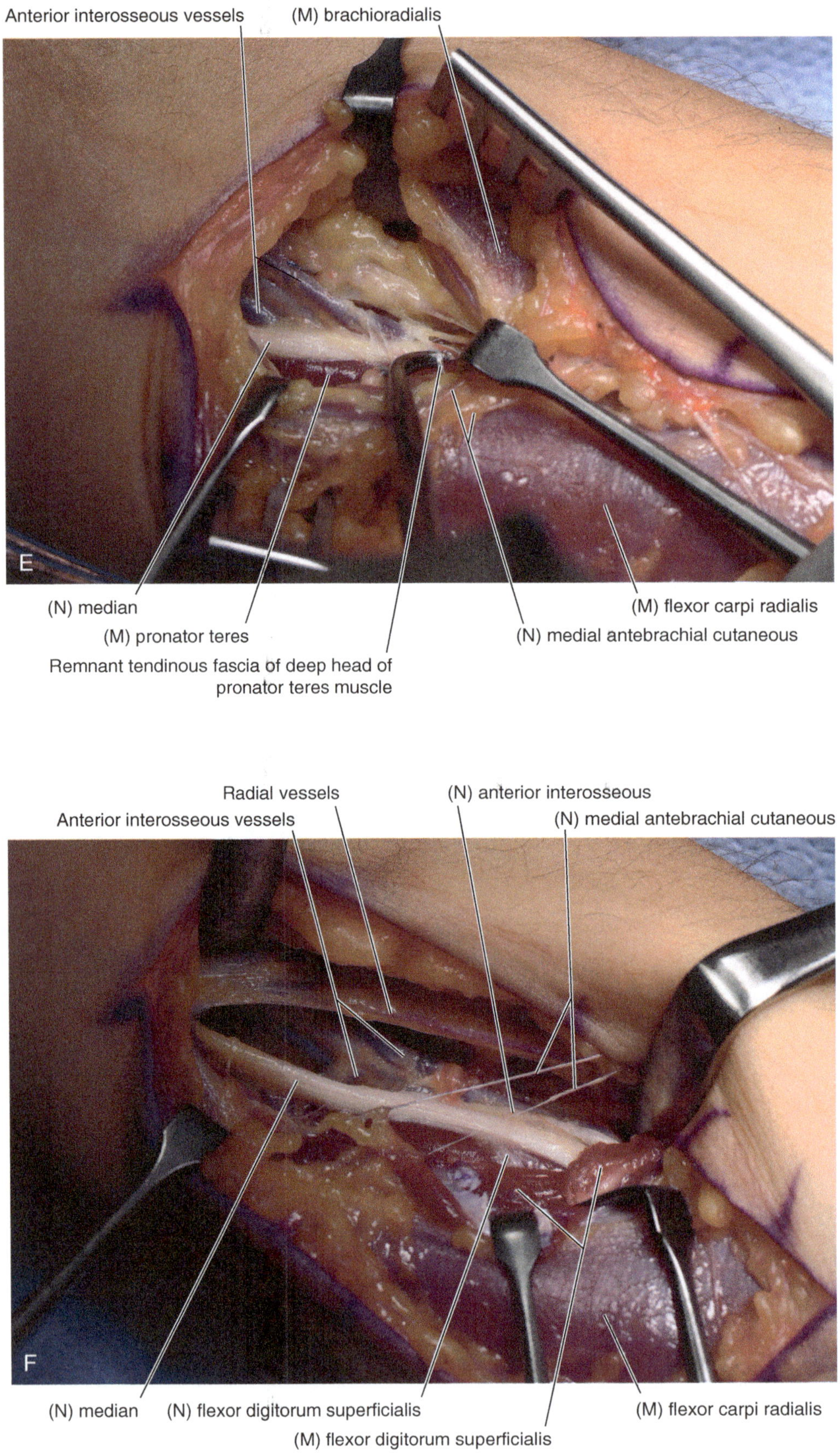

• **Fig. 54.4, cont'd.** (E) Resection of the tendinous portion of the deep head of PT. (F) Division of the tendinous leading edge of flexor digitorum superficialis and any crossing vessels completes the decompression of the proximal median nerve. (Reproduced with permission from Susan E. Mackinnon, ed. *Nerve Surgery.* New York: Thieme; 2015.)

to the antebrachial fascia, and radial to the FCU tendon. Just distal to the pisiform, the motor and sensory fascicles of the ulnar nerve separate. In Zone 2 (distal motor), the motor component courses radially around the hook of the hamate and deep to the leading edge of the flexor digiti minimi to innervate the intrinsic muscles of the hand. At this level, the floor of Guyon's canal is formed by the opponens digiti minimi, the ulnar border by the abductor digiti minimi, and the roof by the volar carpal ligament and palmaris brevis. In Zone 3 (distal-sensory), the sensory component of the ulnar nerve travels superficial to the hypothenars to innervate the volar aspect of the small finger and ulnar half of the ring finger. The ulnar artery and its tributaries remain radial and superficial to the ulnar nerve as it travels distally into the wrist and palm.

The Martin–Gruber anastomosis is an anomalous median to ulnar connection in the proximal forearm, present in 10%–25% of cases.[13] The "anastomotic" nerve branch may arise from the median nerve proper or the AIN and when present, can result in preserved ulnar intrinsic function despite severe proximal ulnar neuropathy.

Cubital Tunnel Syndrome

Cubital tunnel syndrome is the second most common compression neuropathy. Potential sites of entrapment include: the arcade of Struthers (a thick fascial connection between the medial head of the triceps and the medial intermuscular septum located approximately 8 cm proximal to the medial epicondyle), the medial intermuscular septum, the bony retrocondylar groove (which may be altered by trauma, arthritis, and heterotopic ossification), and the arcuate ligament of Osborne (a thickened confluence of fascia between the two heads of FCU) (Fig. 54.5). The ulnar nerve may also be compressed where it exits the FCU, by fibrovascular bands coursing over the nerve from the ulnar artery to the distal FCU, and by a fascial aponeurosis between the FCU and FDS to the ring finger (ligament of Spinner).

Congenital anatomical variations, such as cubitus valgus, the presence of an anconeus epitrochlearis, a prominent medial triceps, and a hypoplastic roof of the cubital tunnel (allowing subluxation of the ulnar nerve) may also contribute to ulnar compression. Other associated risk factors include female gender, advanced age, systemic neuropathy (e.g., diabetic), external compression (e.g., above-elbow cast), occupations involving repetitive or persistent elbow flexion, and sleeping with the elbows flexed.[13] Several mechanisms have been proposed to explain why elbow flexion contributes to ulnar neuropathy, including dynamic compression, traction, ischemia, extraneural scar, and recurrent nerve subluxation.[26]

Clinical Presentation

Cubital tunnel syndrome presents with sensory changes in the ulnar nerve distribution, and hand weakness that often manifests as clumsiness, cramping, difficulty opening jars, and difficulty manipulating small objects. These changes are initially intermittent and may become continuous if not addressed. Symptoms tend to be worse at night and with activities requiring prolonged elbow flexion.

Sensory testing will reveal diminished sensation in both the volar and dorsal aspects of the ring and small fingers. Provocative tests include Tinel's sign in the retrocondylar groove, the SCT, and the elbow flexion test with or without simultaneous digital pressure over the ulnar nerve (see Table 54.1). Provocative maneuvers should also evaluate for compression proximal and distal to the cubital tunnel.

Motor examination may demonstrate atrophy and weakness of the interossei, ulnar-innervated lumbricals, hypothenars, FDP to the ring and small fingers, and FCU. Specific findings related to ulnar intrinsic weakness include clawing of the ring and small fingers (Duchenne's sign), abducted posture of the small finger (Wartenburg's sign), compensatory FPL flexion when attempting key pinch (Froment's sign), inability to cross the long and index fingers, reduced key pinch strength, and weakness of index and small finger abduction against resistance.

When evaluating a patient with cubital tunnel syndrome, a systemic sensory neuropathy should be considered if sensory loss is much worse than motor loss. If motor deficits predominate, a C8–T1 cervical radiculopathy or systemic motor neuropathy should be excluded. Combined thenar and ulnar intrinsic wasting is also indicative of cervical radiculopathy.

Management

A 2–4-month trial of nonoperative management is recommended for patients with mild symptoms. Patient education, consistent nocturnal splinting using an elbow pad or rolled towel to maintain the elbow in extension, and modifications to reduce elbow flexion during daytime activities can effectively reduce symptomology. Corticosteroid injections are not recommended due to risk of intraneural injection or subcutaneous placement.

Operative management is indicated when nonoperative measures fail and when symptoms are moderate to severe. These patients should have electrodiagnostic testing to determine the urgency of surgical intervention and to allow the surgeon to predict the time course and potential for recovery. Patients with atrophy, significant weakness, and where NCS demonstrates reduced CMAP amplitude(s), significant conduction block and/or abnormal MUPs may warrant expedited operative intervention to preserve the remaining healthy motor units and optimize functional outcomes.[27]

Multiple surgical techniques have been described for the treatment of cubital tunnel syndrome and no single technique has proven superior.[28] Surgical options include in situ decompression, medial epicondylectomy, and anterior transposition in a subcutaneous, transmuscular, intramuscular or submuscular position. In the case of severe weakness and/or sensory neuropathy, the senior author often performs adjunctive procedures in addition

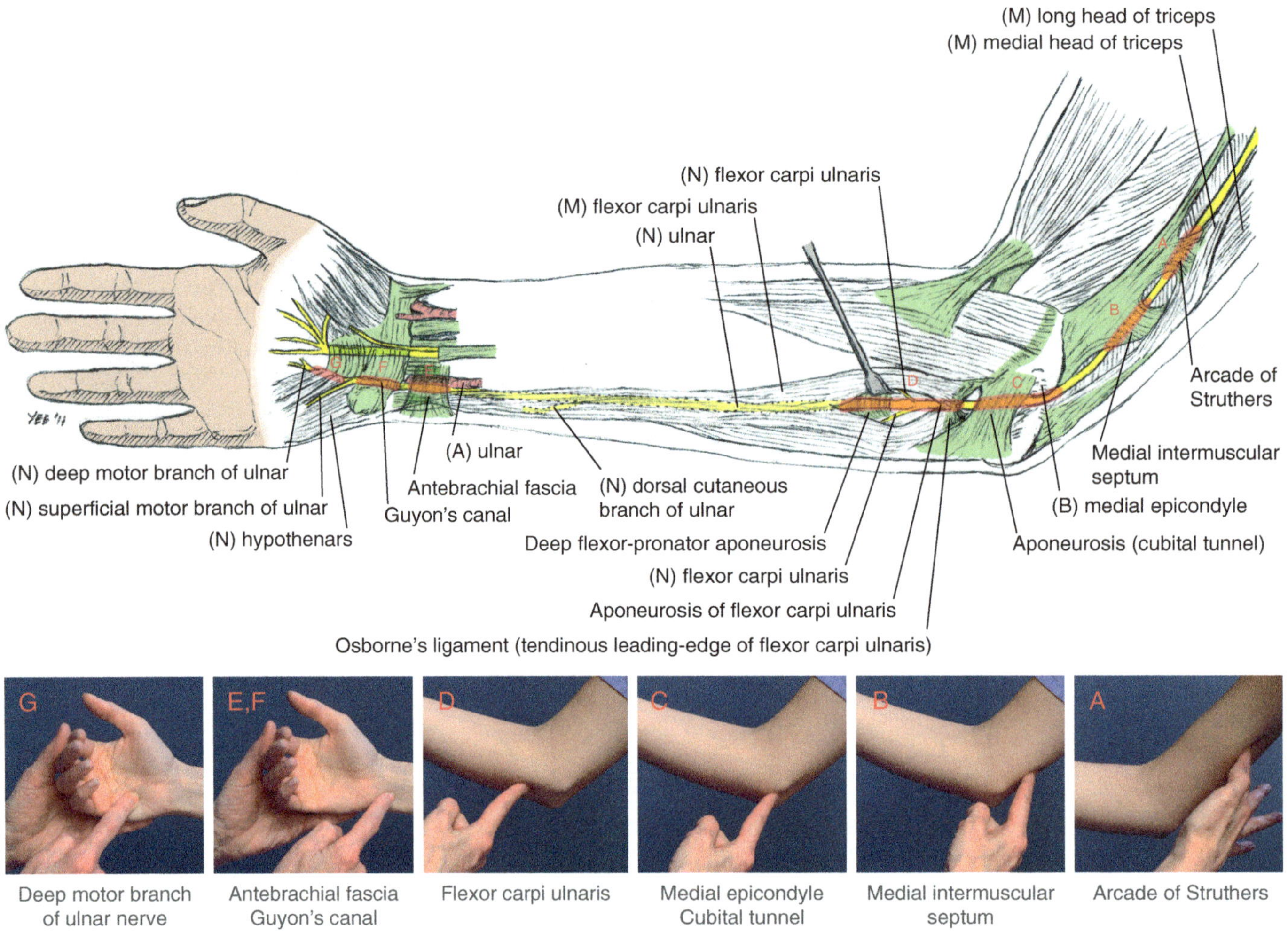

• **Fig. 54.5** Potential sites of compression along the course of the ulnar nerve. The lower photos illustrate the potential entrapment points along the course of the ulnar nerve at the (A) arcade of Struthers, (B) medial intermuscular septum, (C) medial epicondyle and cubital tunnel, (D) flexor carpi ulnaris, (E) antebrachial fascia, (F) Guyon's canal, and (G) the leading edge of the hypothenar muscles for the deep motor branch of the ulnar nerve. (Reproduced with permission from Susan E. Mackinnon, ed. *Nerve Surgery*. New York: Thieme; 2015.)

to primary surgery at the elbow. Procedures to consider include decompression of Guyon's canal with specific release of the deep motor branch, supercharge end-to-side AIN to ulnar motor nerve transfer, side-to-side profundus tenodesis and/or cross-palm nerve grafts from the median to ulnar sensory nerve.[26,29,30]

In situ decompression of the ulnar nerve entails releasing all relevant entrapment sites through a 6–10 cm incision posterior to the medial epicondyle, without disturbing the ulnar nerve from its bed and without performing neurolysis. Endoscopic and limited incision techniques have been described, although the risk of hematoma, nerve injury, and inadequate release are increased.[5] Potential advantages of in situ decompression over transposition include reduced technical complexity, lower complication rates, and lower risk of nerve devascularization, yet it does not address instability or tension on the nerve during elbow flexion. A revision surgery rate of up to 19% has been reported.[31]

Medial epicondylectomy or ulnar nerve transposition should be considered if intraoperative subluxation of the ulnar nerve is seen following decompression. Complications of medial epicondylectomy include pain, weakness, and instability of the elbow joint,[5] and this technique is not commonly used. Alternatively, some authors advocate the use of a stabilizing flap when ulnar nerve instability is encountered following in situ decompression.[32]

Proponents of transposing the ulnar nerve anterior to the medial epicondyle cite several benefits, including reduced tension and compression forces on the ulnar nerve during elbow flexion, definitive treatment of nerve instability, and provision of a well-vascularized bed for the nerve.[26] In a subcutaneous transposition, the anterior position of the ulnar nerve can be maintained by suturing the dermis to a fascial flap elevated off the flexor–pronator mass.[13] The subcutaneous technique involves less muscle dissection, but extensive mobilization of the ulnar nerve is required to avoid proximal or distal kinking.

An intramuscular transposition requires creation of a groove in the flexor–pronator mass in line with the transposed position of the ulnar nerve, and a soft tissue or fascial sling is then created to maintain the nerve position.[13] Relative to subcutaneous transposition, the intramuscular technique offers greater protection and places the ulnar nerve in a straighter axis. It also necessitates less dissection than submuscular transposition but carries a risk of iatrogenic nerve compression.

Submuscular transposition of the ulnar nerve under the flexor–pronator mass is advocated as the definitive procedure for cubital tunnel syndrome, especially in revision cases.[33] The flexor/pronator mass is directly reattached to the medial epicondyle, with or without step-lengthening to minimize compression on the transposed nerve. Disadvantages of the submuscular technique include a longer incision, more extensive muscle dissection, new symptoms from heterotopic bone formation, and the potential for iatrogenic nerve compression.[5]

Ulnar Nerve Transposition (Fig. 54.6)

The senior author's preferred technique is transposition of the ulnar nerve in a transmuscular plane, which minimizes nerve tension during elbow motion and requires less muscle dissection than submuscular techniques. The procedure is performed under regional or general anesthesia using a sterile tourniquet. A 6–10-cm incision is made overlying the ulnar nerve centered at the medial epicondyle. During subcutaneous dissection, care is taken to protect the medial antebrachial cutaneous (MABC) nerve branches. The ulnar nerve is identified proximally posterior to the medial intermuscular septum, which is then excised over a 1–2-cm segment. The nerve is followed distally as it enters the retrocondylar groove, where the roof of the cubital tunnel and Osborne's band are released. Distal to the elbow, there is a distal medial intermuscular septum between the ulnar-innervated FCU and the median-innervated flexor/pronators; this is removed to avoid kinking of the nerve after transposition.[34] Motor branches to the FCU and FDP are identified and preserved.

A step-cut incision in the flexor/pronator origin is made. The proximally-based flap elevates easily with some muscle attached, whereas the distally-based flap must be elevated with sharp dissection and close to the medial epicondyle to preserve innervation. Enough muscle should be released distally so that it does not kink the ulnar nerve when the nerve is transposed anteriorly. Intermuscular fascia must also be excised to avoid compression.[34]

The ulnar nerve is then transposed anterior the medial epicondyle. Motor branches to the FCU or FDP that inhibit tension-free transposition should be neurolysed proximally. The entire course of the nerve is re-evaluated to ensure it lies in a straight line with no proximal or distal sites of compression. The fascial flaps are then secured loosely over the nerve with nonabsorbable sutures.

The tourniquet is then removed, and meticulous hemostasis achieved. The ulnar nerve is palpated proximally to assess for an arcade of Struthers, which is released if present. The MABC branches are inspected and if inadvertent injury has occurred, the injured branch should be crushed proximally, the end cauterized and then transposed proximally to a protected location away from the incision. A layered closure is performed over a Jackson–Pratt drain. The arm is immobilized for 2–3 days with a well-padded splint to maintain the wrist in neutral, forearm pronated, and elbow flexed at 45–60 degrees. ROM exercises are then initiated. Progressive strengthening starts at 1 month postoperatively, with return to full activities at 2 months.

Guyon's Canal Syndrome

Compression of the ulnar nerve at the wrist is the second most common site of ulnar nerve impingement but is substantially less common than cubital tunnel syndrome. A thickened antebrachial fascia can compress the ulnar nerve at the wrist (Zone 1), whereas the tendinous leading edge of the hypothenar musculature can cause isolated compression of the deep motor branch (Zone 2). Additional etiologies include compression by extra-anatomical structures (e.g., ganglion cysts, tumors, vascular malformations, anomalous musculature) and trauma (e.g., hypothenar hammer syndrome, hook of hamate fractures, distal radius fractures, carpal dislocations).[5]

Clinical Presentation

Patients may give a history of hand trauma or fullness in the hypothenar region, and often report worse hand function than patients with cubital tunnel syndrome. Sensory testing will demonstrate loss of sensation on the volar aspect of the ring and small fingers, but sensation on the dorsal–ulnar hand (DCU distribution) is spared. Signs and symptoms of ulnar-innervated intrinsic weakness may be present, but FCU and ring/small finger FDP function are preserved. The examiner may also elicit a positive Tinel's sign, SCT, and pressure provocation test at the wrist (see Table 54.1). Holding the wrist in extension may aggravate patient symptoms. In patients presenting with cubital tunnel syndrome, it is important to assess for secondary compression at Guyon's canal related to the double-crush phenomenon.[8] With the exception of compression by extra-anatomical structures (where imaging is needed), the diagnosis of Guyon's canal compression is mainly clinical as electrodiagnostic confirmation requires specialized testing not performed on routine NCS.[11]

Management

Management of ulnar nerve compression at the wrist is primarily surgical, as wrist-neutral splinting has no proven benefit. Compression of the ulnar nerve by extraanatomic structures requires surgical management of the offending structure, in addition to decompression of the ulnar nerve through Guyon's canal.

Guyon's Canal Release (Fig. 54.7)

In the senior author's preferred technique for Guyon's canal release, a Taleisnik incision is made approximately

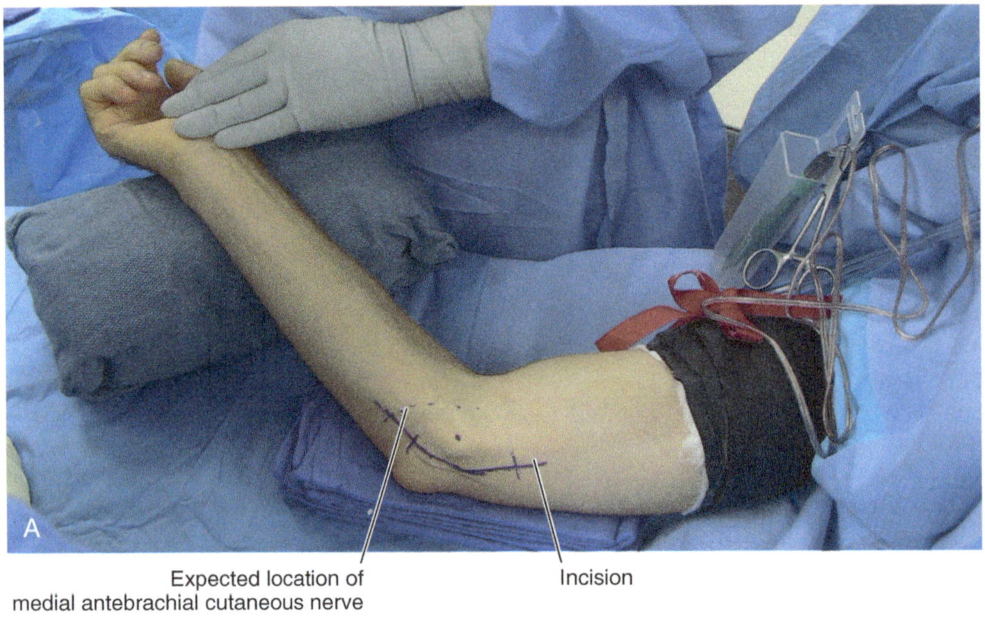

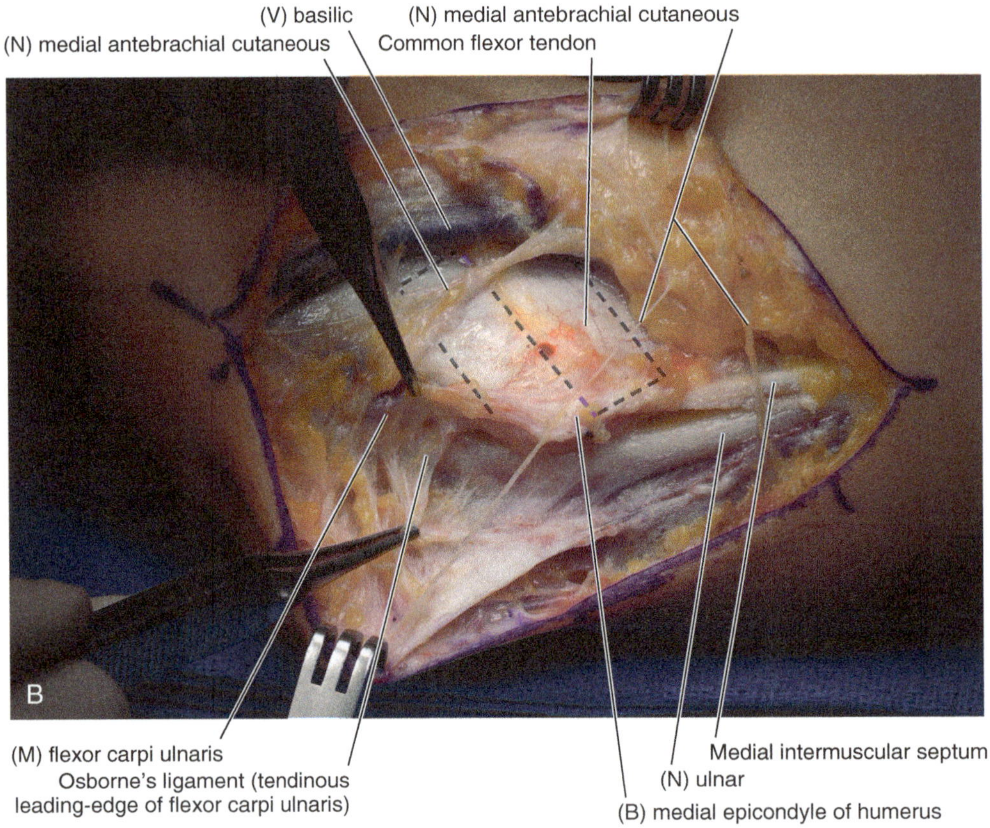

• **Fig. 54.6 (A–F)** Author's preferred technique for ulnar nerve transposition. (A) Design of the skin incision just posterior to, and centered over, the medial epicondyle on the right upper extremity. (B) The medial antebrachial cutaneous nerve should be preserved during subcutaneous dissection. The ulnar nerve is identified posterior to medial intermuscular septum above the elbow and is decompressed through the cubital tunnel. Design of the step-cut incision in the fascia of flexor/pronator mass.

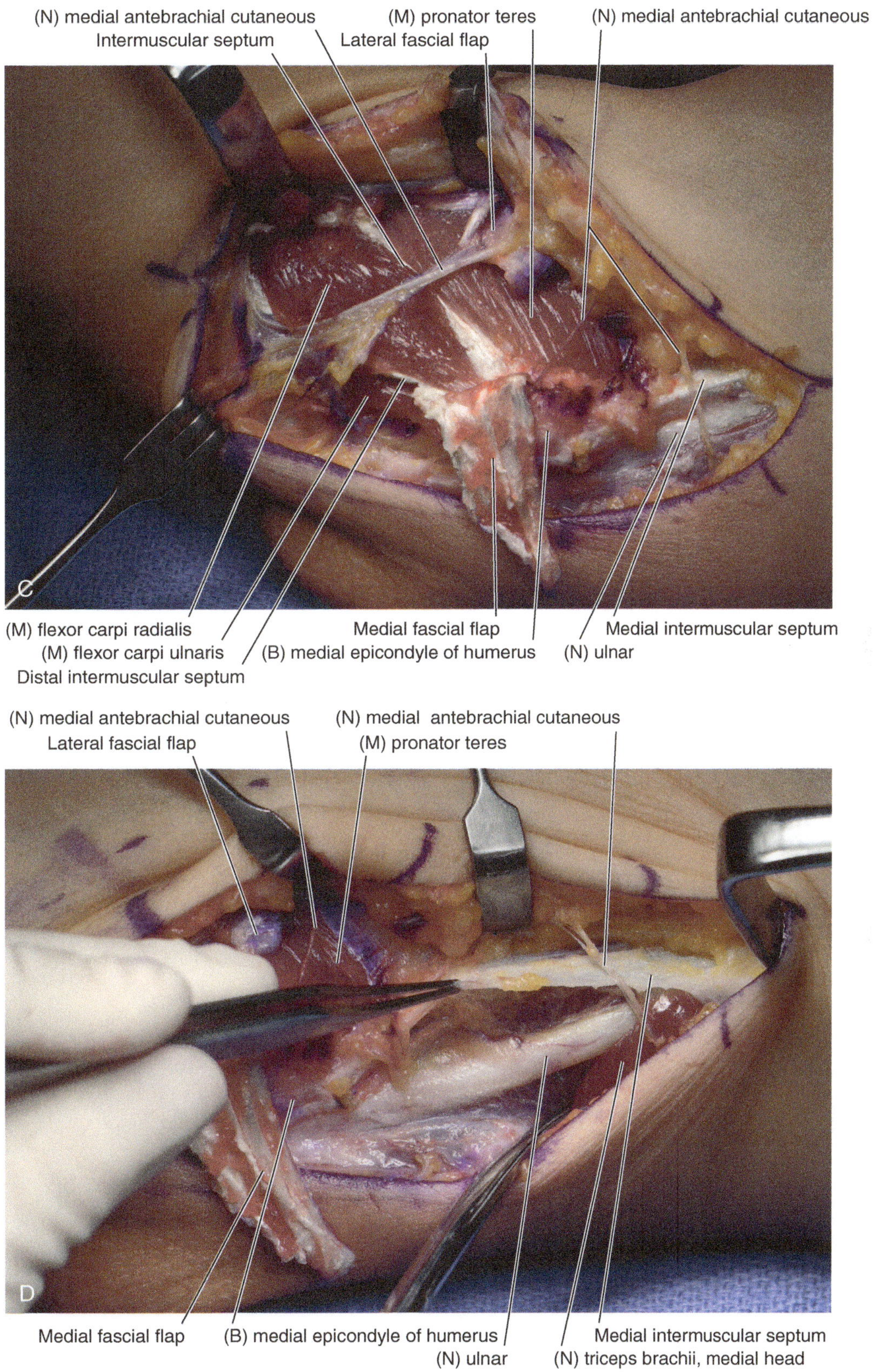

• **Fig. 54.6, cont'd.** (C) Elevation of the fascial flaps at the flexor/pronator origin allows visualization of the intermuscular fascia that should be excised prior to transposition of the ulnar nerve. (D) Proximally, the medial intermuscular septum is exposed and resected prior to nerve transposition.

Continued

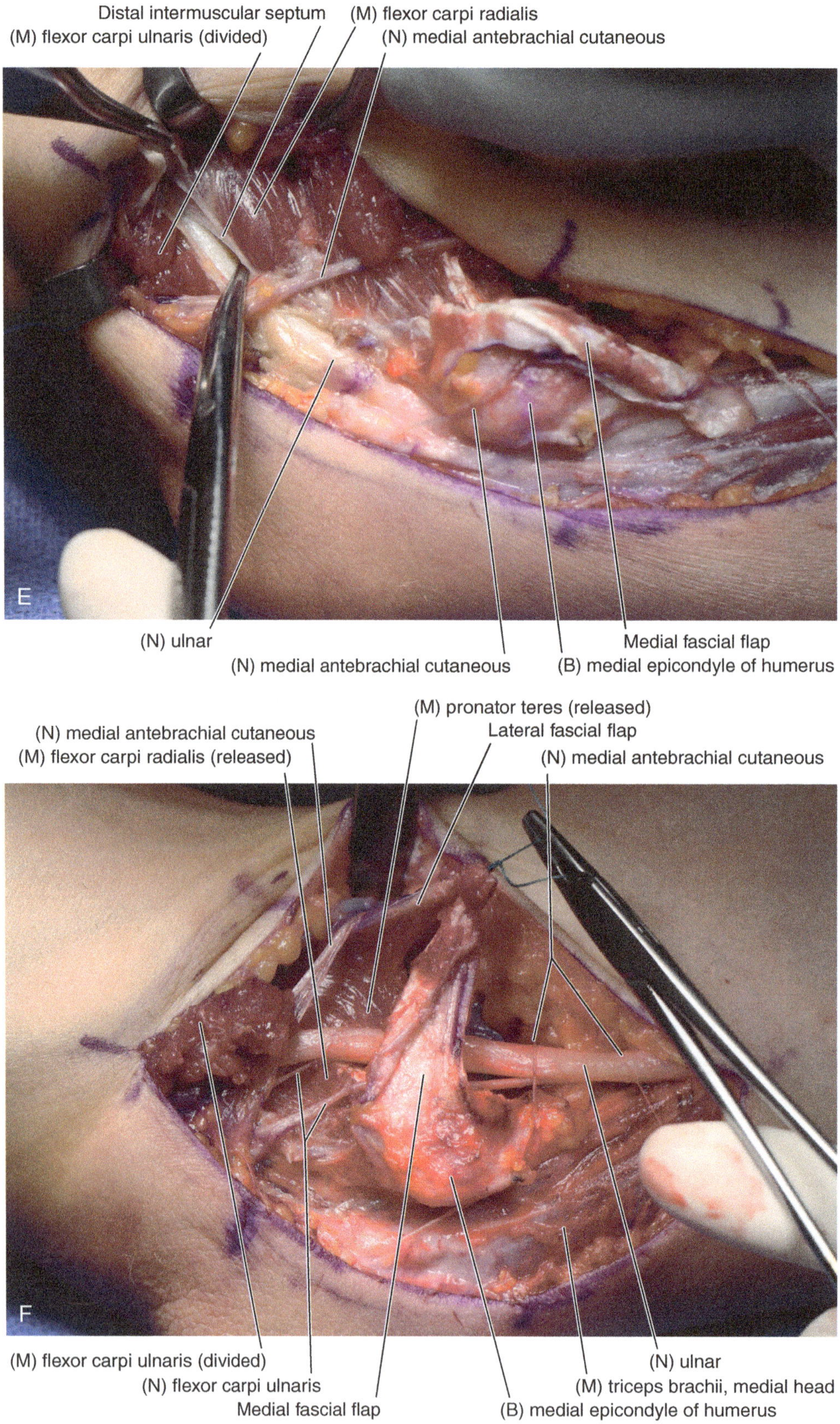

• **Fig. 54.6, cont'd.** (E) The ulnar nerve is followed as distally as possible to ensure it is completely decompressed, so that it will not be kinked when it is transposed anteriorly. (F) Anterior transposition of the ulnar nerve. The fascial flaps are very loosely closed over the ulnar nerve to maintain its new position. (Reproduced with permission from Susan E. Mackinnon, ed. *Nerve Surgery.* New York: Thieme; 2015.)

1 cm ulnar to the thenar crease, crossing the wrist in a zigzag fashion; dissection is carried through the subcutaneous tissue and palmaris brevis, while preserving the cutaneous branch that is often present in the distal third of the palmar incision. The ulnar neurovascular bundle is identified and retracted ulnarly. The tendinous leading edge of the hypothenar musculature is identified just ulnar to the hook of hamate, with the deep motor branch travelling deep to it. The tendinous leading edge is carefully released under direct vision. Often the deep motor branch is not visible until the initial 2–3 mm of the leading edge is divided. Division of the hypothenar fascia proceeds until the deep motor branch is completely decompressed. In order to adequately visualize and release the antebrachial fascia, the surgeon must incise

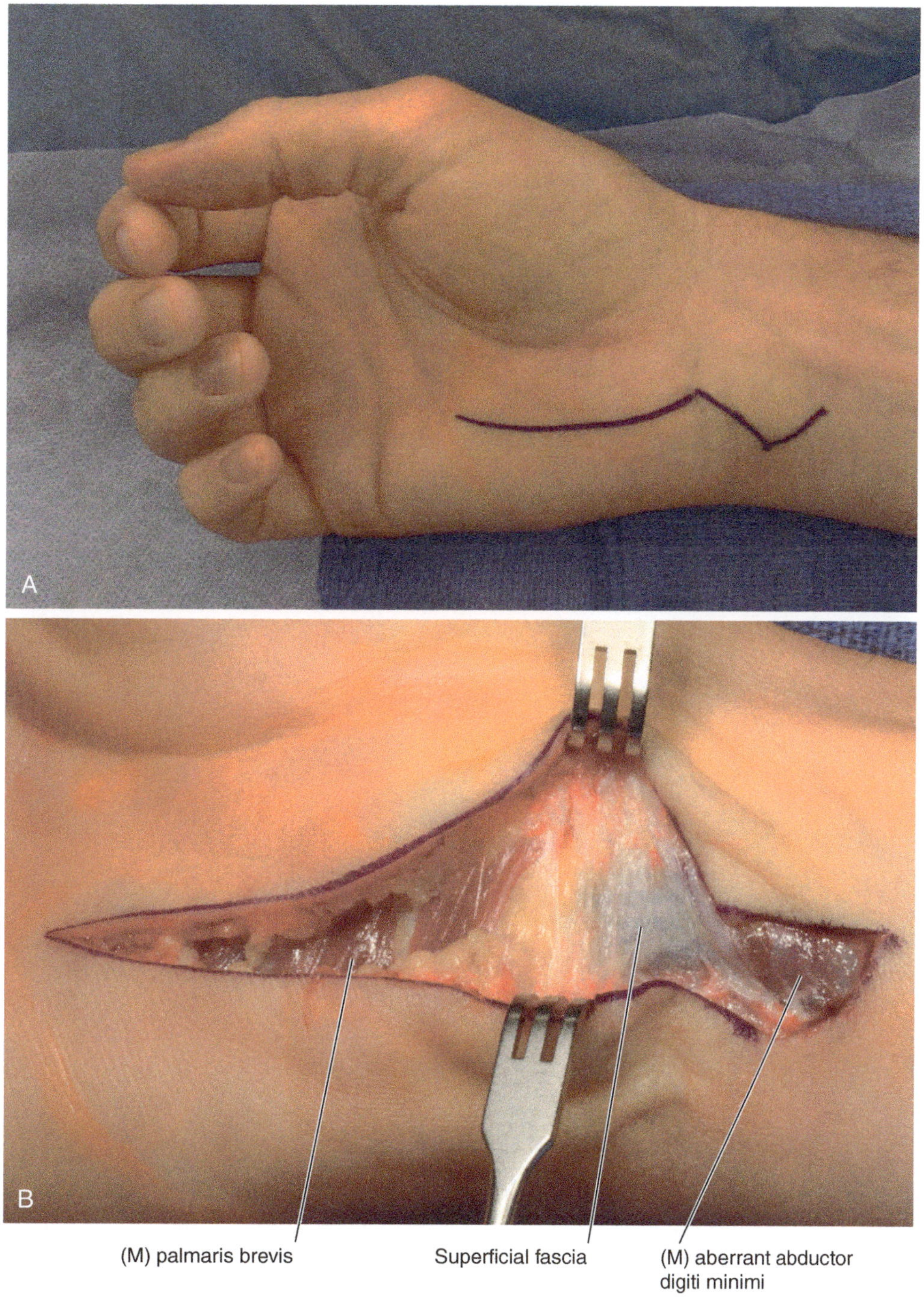

• **Fig. 54.7 (A–D)** Author's preferred technique for Guyon's canal release. (A) Design of the skin incision on the right hand. (B) Deep to the subcutaneous tissue, the palmaris brevis and fascia overlying the ulnar neurovascular bundle are identified and subsequently divided.

Continued

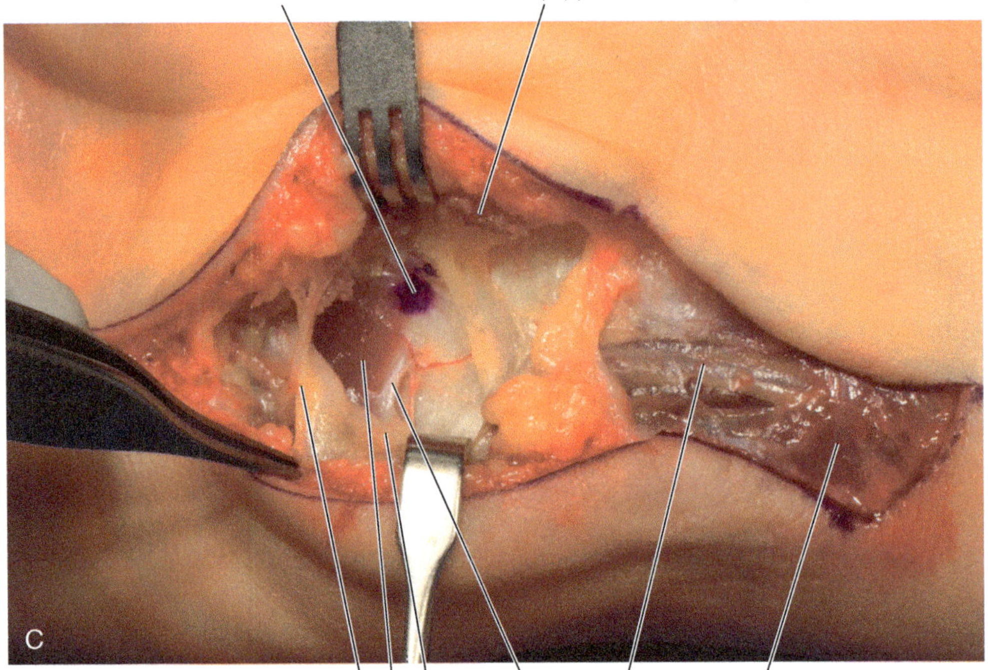

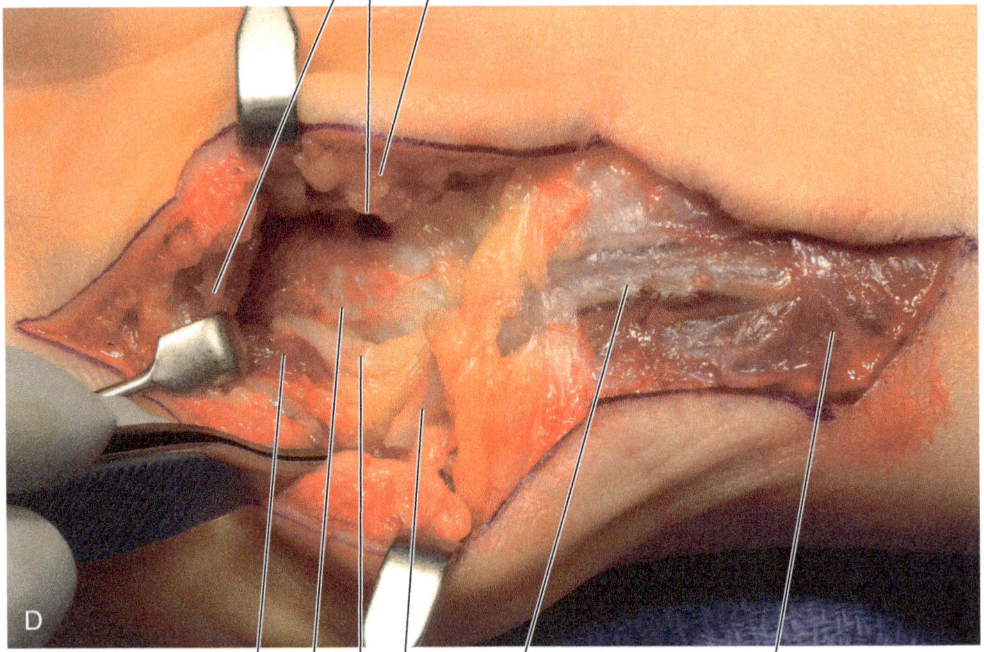

• **Fig. 54.7, cont'd.** (C) The ulnar nerve is retracted ulnarly, and the tendinous leading edge of the hypothenar musculature is identified just radial to the hook of the hamate. (D) The deep motor branch of the ulnar nerve is decompressed by carefully dividing the tendinous leading edge of the hypothenar muscles. The motor branch is often not visualized until the initial 2–3 mm of this leading edge is divided. Proximally, the antebrachial fascia overlying the ulnar nerve is divided to complete the decompression. (Reproduced with permission from Susan E. Mackinnon, ed. *Nerve Surgery.* New York: Thieme; 2015.)

and dissect proximal to the wrist crease. The ulnar nerve is then inspected proximally and distally to ensure there are no further sites of compression. The incision is closed with interrupted sutures, and a well-padded wrist-neutral splint is applied. Immediate ROM exercises of the fingers are encouraged. The splint is removed in 2–3 days, and a gradual return to full activity is permitted over 6–8 weeks.

Radial Nerve Compression

Anatomy

The radial nerve is a terminal branch of the posterior cord (C5–T1). It lies dorsal to the axillary vessels at its origin, then courses beneath the lateral head of the triceps, where it gives off the motor branches to the triceps, the posterior cutaneous nerve of the arm, and posterior cutaneous nerve of the forearm. At the mid-humeral level, the radial nerve travels within the spiral groove of the humerus, crossing from the posteromedial to posterolateral aspect of the upper arm. It pierces the lateral intermuscular septum approximately 10 cm proximal to the lateral humeral epicondyle and can be found between the brachialis and the origin of the brachioradialis just above the antecubital fossa.[35] Here, motor branches to the brachioradialis and extensor carpi radialis longus (ECRL) arise. The radial nerve then bifurcates into the posterior interosseous nerve (PIN; motor component) and the superficial radial nerve (SRN; sensory component).

The radial tunnel is a region of the proximal forearm and elbow approximately 5 cm in length, starting distal to the motor branches to the brachioradialis and ECRL and ending distal to the supinator.[5] Here, the radial nerve is bordered medially by the brachialis and biceps tendon, laterally by the brachioradialis, and posteriorly by the lateral epicondyle.

The PIN courses dorsolaterally over the radiohumeral joint, around the radial head through the substance of the supinator, and distally along the dorsal surface of the interosseous membrane. The PIN supplies the extensor carpi radialis brevis (ECRB), supinator, extensor digitorum communis (EDC), extensor digiti minimi, (EDM), extensor carpi ulnaris (ECU), abductor pollicis longus (APL), extensor pollicis longus (EPL) and brevis (EPB), and extensor indicis proprius (EIP). The nerve branch to ECRB arises as a separate branch proximal to where the PIN enters the supinator. The terminal branch of the PIN travels at the base of the fourth extensor compartment to provide sensation to the dorsal wrist capsule and intercarpal ligaments.

The SRN travels distally on the undersurface of the brachioradialis in the radial aspect of the forearm. About 10 cm proximal the radial styloid, the SRN exits dorsally between the brachioradialis and ECRL tendons and travels subcutaneously to provide sensory innervation to the dorsal-radial aspect of the hand.

Radial Tunnel/Posterior Interosseous Nerve Syndrome

Compression of the radial nerve and its branches in the proximal forearm is usually anatomical in nature, although other etiologies such as fractures of the radial head have been reported. The anatomical structures responsible for radial tunnel syndrome and PIN syndrome are similar, but symptomatology differs: radial tunnel syndrome is predominately sensory in nature whereas PIN syndrome causes motor deficits.

Structures that may compress the radial nerve or PIN include fibrous adhesions at the radiocapitellar joint (i.e., from lateral epicondylitis), the tendinous leading edge of the ECRB, the tendinous superficial head of the supinator (arcade of Fröhse), the distal fascial edge of the supinator, and the vascular leash of Henry. Rare anatomical variations, such as fusion of the brachioradialis and brachialis, may also predispose the radial nerve and PIN to compression.[13]

Clinical Presentation

Radial Tunnel Syndrome

Patients with radial tunnel syndrome typically describe aching pain in the proximal forearm that is worse with activity, and tenderness over the radial tunnel. Distal sensation is normal and weakness of the extensors is uncommon. The main differential diagnosis of radial tunnel syndrome is lateral epicondylitis. In lateral epicondylitis, pain is maximal at the bony lateral epicondyle and is aggravated by resisted wrist extension. In radial tunnel syndrome, tenderness is present over the mobile wad and is worsened by resisted long finger extension.[5] The SCT is also routinely positive in radial tunnel syndrome.

Provocative tests may help localize the site of radial nerve compression: compression due to fibrous bands at the radial neck will be aggravated by elbow flexion plus forearm supination with the wrist in neutral; compression by the ECRB will be aggravated by forearm pronation, elbow flexion to 45–90 degrees with the wrist in full flexion; and compression at the arcade of Fröhse will be aggravated by isometric active supination from a fully pronated position (see Table 54.1).[5]

PIN Syndrome

PIN syndrome presents as weakness of finger metacarpophalangeal joint (MCPJ) extension (EDC function), and inability to extend the thumb when resting flat on a table (EPL function). Finger interphalangeal joint (IPJ) extension is preserved owing to the intact intrinsics, and weak thumb IPJ extension may be present due to preserved function of the thumb intrinsic muscles. Wrist extension is present but may be radially deviated due to preserved ECRL function with weakness of the PIN-innervated ECU and ECRB. No sensory deficits are present, and the same provocative maneuvers used for radial tunnel syndrome can help to localize the site of compression.

Management

Conservative measures should always be attempted first, especially in radial tunnel syndrome, and include splinting and activity modification to help limit elbow extension, forearm pronation, and wrist flexion. Antiinflammatories and corticosteroid injections have also been utilized, especially if concomitant lateral epicondylitis is thought to be contributing to patient symptoms.[5] A wrist cock-up splint and ROM exercises are also useful in PIN syndrome.

Radial Tunnel Decompression (Fig. 54.8)

Preoperatively, the patient is asked to flex the elbow against resistance with the forearm in neutral to identify the borders of the brachioradialis. In the senior author's preferred technique, a 7-m incision is marked on the posterior border of the brachioradialis in the proximal forearm. Dissection is carried through the subcutaneous tissues to fascia, where the interval between the brachioradialis and ECRL is identified. Two landmarks are used: (1) the posterior cutaneous nerve of the forearm runs longitudinally along this interval, superficial to the fascia; and (2) the brachio*R*adialis fascia appears more *R*ed (thinner fascia) and the ECR*L* fascia appears *L*ighter (thicker fascia). The posterior cutaneous nerve of the forearm is protected, and the avascular plane between the two muscles is finger dissected down to the radial nerve.

The branches of the radial nerve are found in consistent orientation: the SRN is volar/radial and large, the ECRB branch is thinner and lies between the SRN and PIN, and the PIN is large and most dorsal/ulnar. The PIN is also obliquely oriented as it courses under the superficial head of the supinator. The fascial edge of the ECRB is divided first, which allows visualization of the supinator. The fascia of the superficial head of the supinator (arcade of Fröhse) is completely released, which decompresses the underlying PIN. Any crossing vessels (vascular leash of Henry) compressing the PIN are ligated and divided.

If the preoperative history and physical examination suggest radial nerve compression in the proximal radial tunnel (as indicated by aching pain over the radial nerve above the elbow), more proximal dissection and release may be required to release conjoined fibres of the brachioradialis and brachialis. Occasionally, a second incision is required to achieve adequate visualization and release. If there is associated lateral epicondylitis, then a proximal tenotomy of the ECRB tendon is also performed.

The radial nerve and its three branches should then be inspected to ensure no residual points of compression are present. Neurolysis should be considered in patients with significant weakness, especially if scarring of the nerve is identified intraoperatively. Neurolysis should proceed until a normal fascicular pattern and bands of Fontana are seen.

Postoperatively, the patient is placed in a well-padded dressing. This is removed in 2–3 days and gentle ROM exercises are encouraged. Strengthening begins at 1 month and return to full activities with no restrictions at 2 months postoperatively.

Superficial Radial Nerve Compression

Compression of the SRN is known as Wartenberg syndrome or *cheiralgia paresthetica*.[13] This can occur by the brachioradialis tendon and may be aggravated by activities requiring hyperpronation. However, the superficial location of the SRN distally and its numerous branches render it highly susceptible to traumatic and iatrogenic injury (e.g., DeQuervain's tenosynovitis release, thumb carpometacarpal joint arthroplasty). Other, less common etiologies include compression by space occupying lesions, hematomas, thrombosis of radial recurrent vessels, muscle anomalies, and external compression from a watchband or bracelet.[13]

Clinical Presentation

SRN compression presents as isolated sensory complaints in the dorsal–radial hand and wrist. A Tinel's sign, SCT, and digital pressure test may be positive where the SRN exits between the brachioradialis and ECRL tendons. Motor examination is normal. Use of local anesthesia can help differentiate symptoms related to the lateral antebrachial cutaneous (LABC) nerve.

Management

Conservative management is often effective, and surgery is rarely necessary. This includes avoidance of repetitive pronation activities and constriction of the forearm (e.g., with a watch). Corticosteroid injection at the entrapment site can be effective. Splinting is generally not used, owing to the difficulty of splinting the forearm in supination.

Superficial Radial Nerve Decompression (Fig. 54.9)

Decompression of the SRN is generally performed in conjunction with tenotomy of the brachioradialis tendon. In the senior author's preferred technique, the most prominent site of the Tinel's sign is marked preoperatively. A 3–4-cm longitudinal incision is made just volar to the musculotendinous junction of the brachioradialis, approximately 10 cm proximal to the radial styloid. The branches of the LABC nerve are identified and protected. The fascia between the ECRL and brachioradialis tendons is opened and the SRN is identified and decompressed along its length. A portion of the brachioradialis tendon is divided to completely decompress the SRN. After hemostasis is obtained, the incision is closed in layers. A well-padded soft dressing is applied. The dressing is removed 3 days following surgery and gentle ROM exercises are encouraged. Desensitization therapy is initiated as needed.

Proximal Radial Nerve Compression

Proximal compression of the radial nerve in the arm is uncommon. It may be compressed by the lateral intermuscular septum or a fibrous arch formed by the lateral head of triceps.[5] More commonly, the proximal radial nerve is compressed by external forces, such as prolonged pressure over the radial nerve in the spiral groove, resulting in a "Saturday night palsy" or a pneumatic tourniquet.

Clinical Presentation

Radial nerve compression in the arm results in loss of sensation in the SRN distribution as well as weakness of the

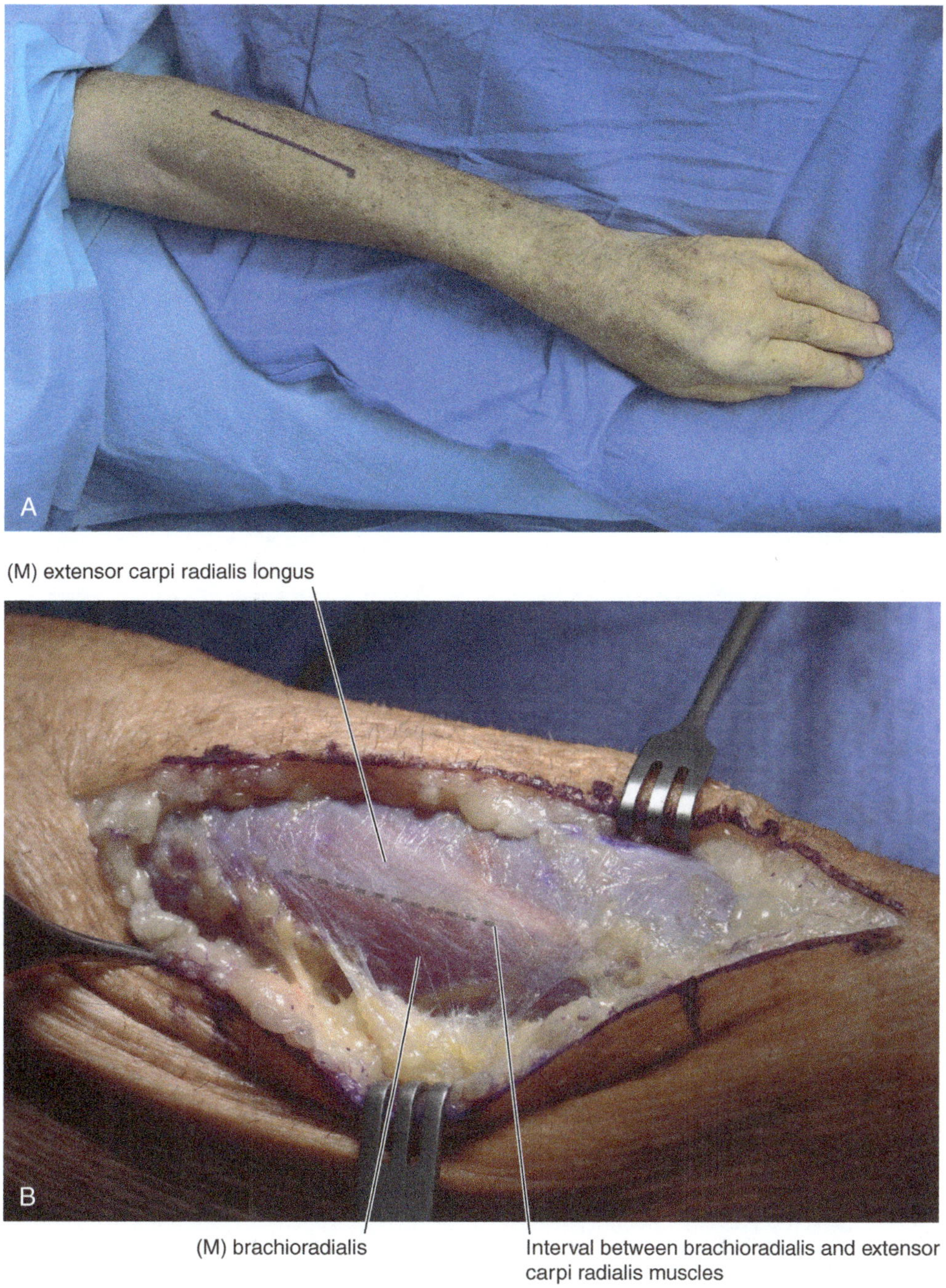

• **Fig. 54.8 (A–G)** Author's preferred technique for decompression of the radial tunnel and posterior interosseous nerve (PIN). (A) A straight incision is designed along the posterior margin of the brachioradialis in the left proximal forearm. (B) The interval between the brachioradialis and extensor carpi radialis longus (ECRL) is identified, and the fascia is divided longitudinally at this location.

Continued

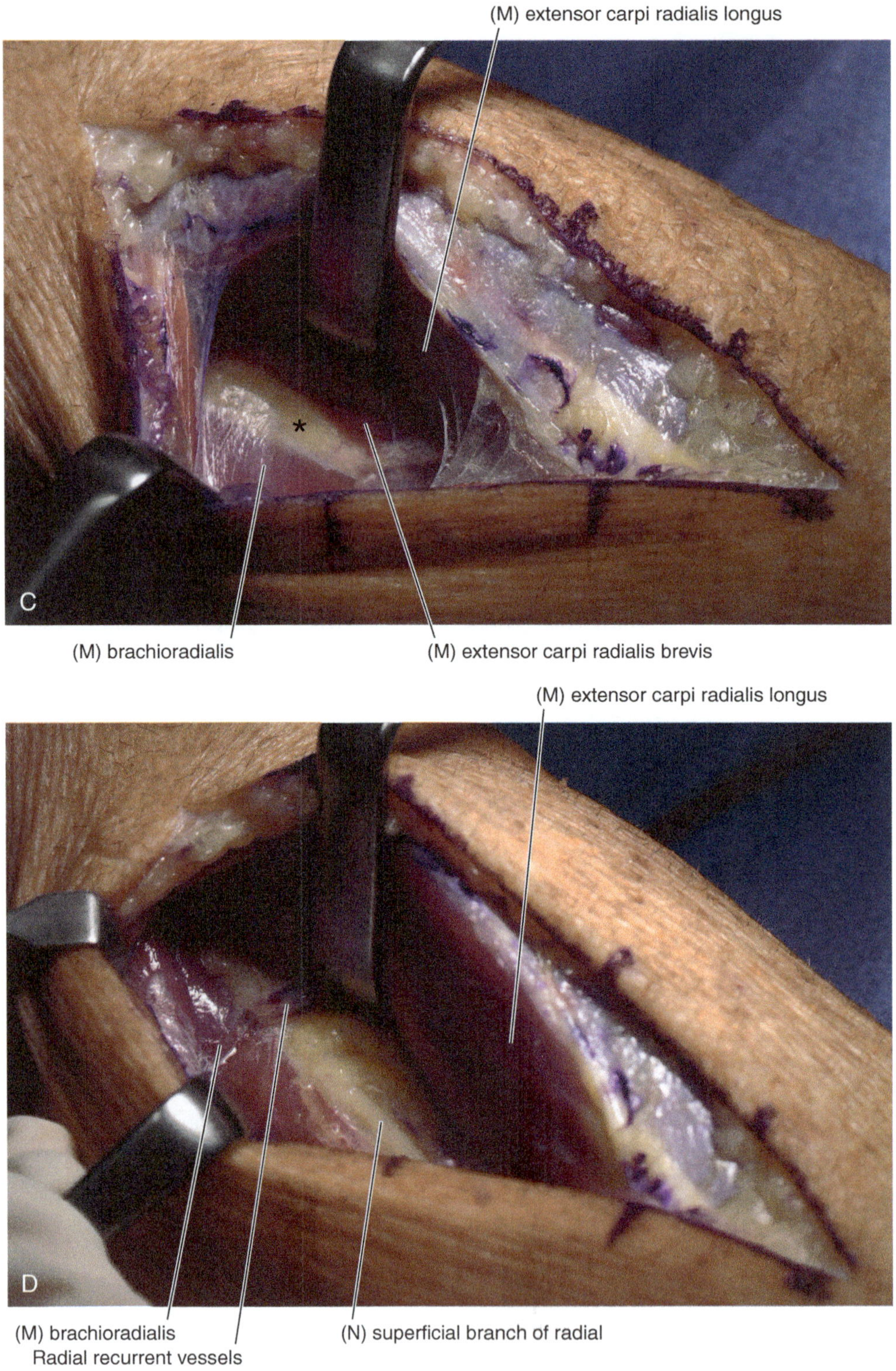

• **Fig. 54.8, cont'd.** (C) Finger dissection is performed in the interval between brachioradialis and ECRL down to the radial nerve (*). (D) The radial recurrent vessels (vascular leash of Henry) may be seen compressing the radial nerve proximally. These are ligated and divided.

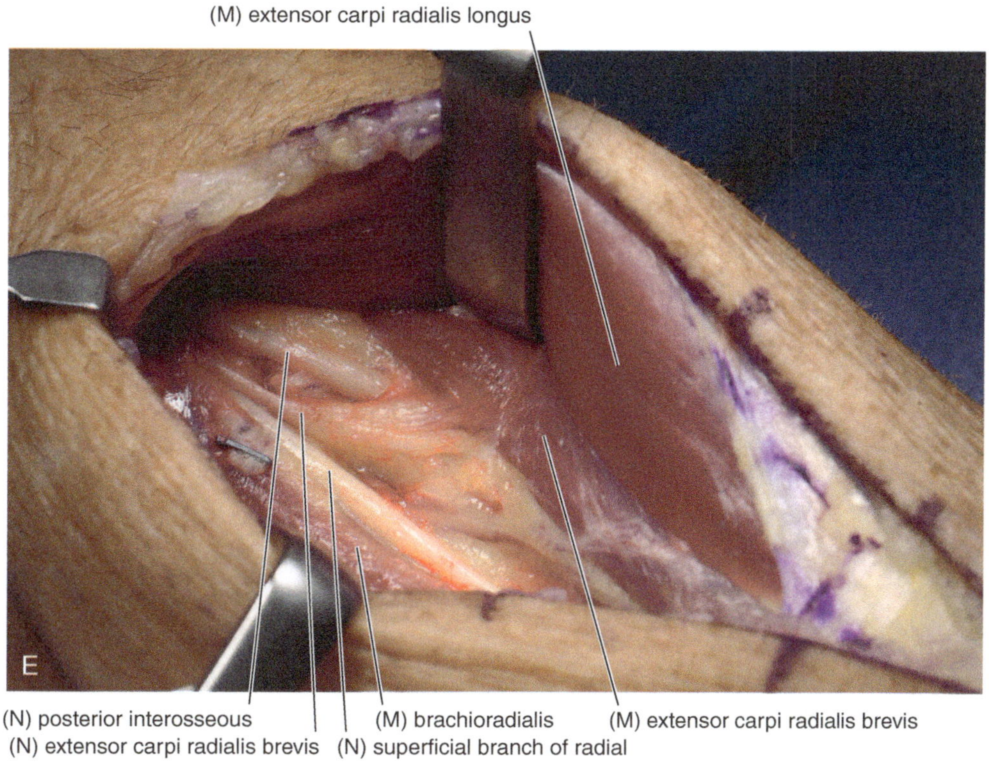

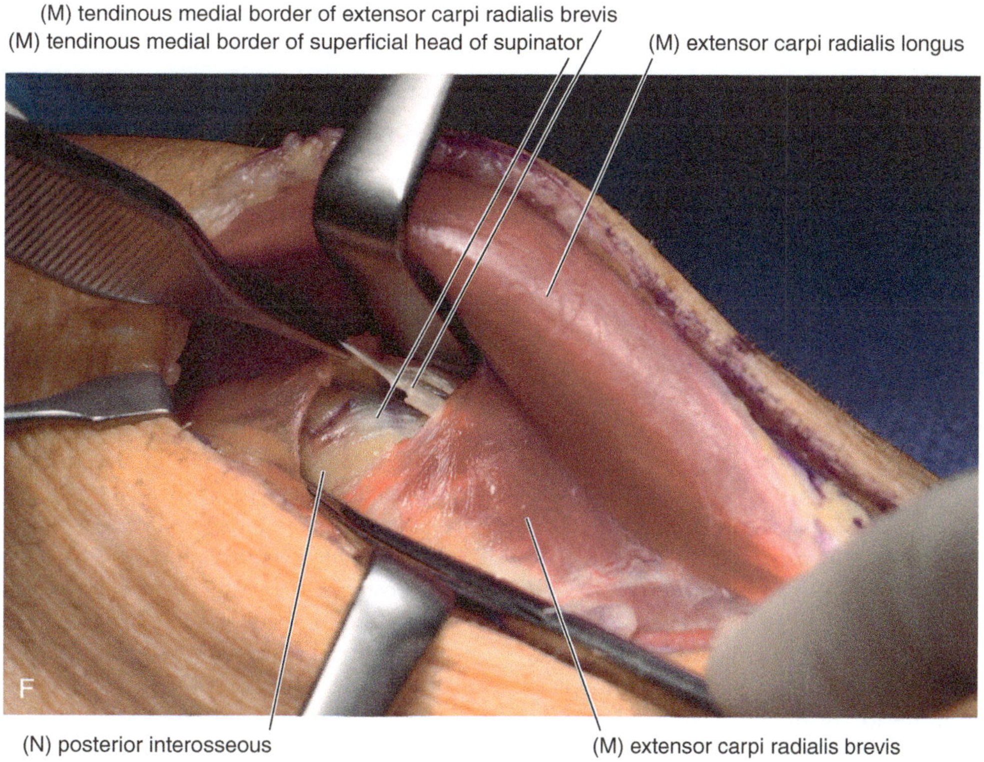

• **Fig. 54.8, cont'd.** (E) The orientation of the branches of the radial nerve at this level: the superficial radial sensory nerve (large) is most radial, the PIN (large) is most ulnar, and the extensor carpi radialis brevis (ECRB) nerve (small) lies between these. (F) Division of the tendinous edge of the ECRB allows visualization of the arcade of Fröhse (tendinous leading edge of the supinator).

Continued

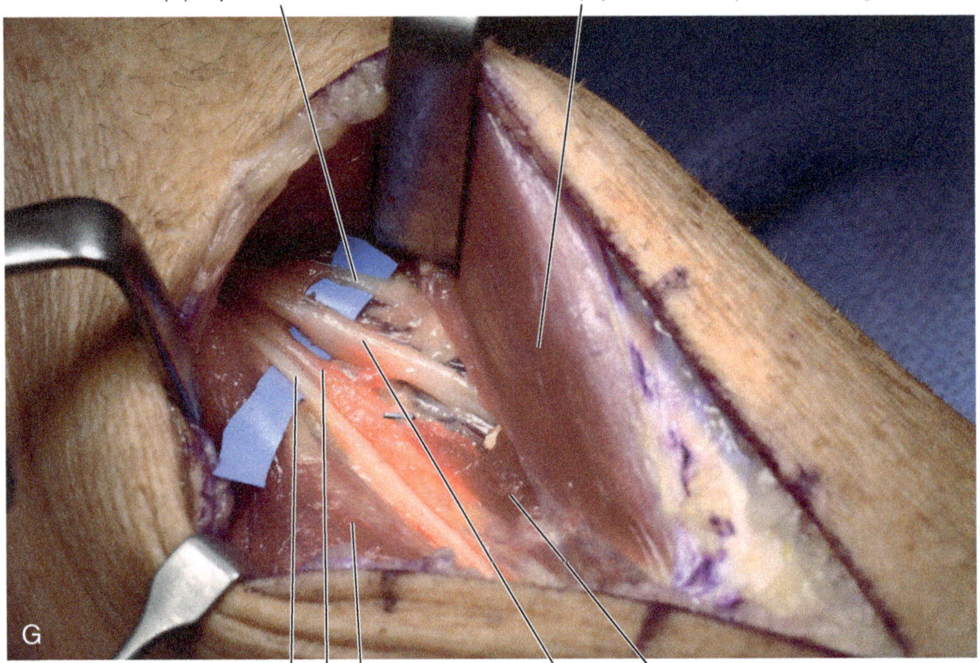

• **Fig. 54.8, cont'd.** (G) Complete transection of the arcade of Fröhse decompresses the underlying PIN. The nerve branch to the supinator can be seen exiting from the PIN on its posterior aspect. (Reproduced with permission from Susan E. Mackinnon, ed. *Nerve Surgery*. New York: Thieme; 2015.)

brachioradialis, ECRL, and PIN-innervated muscles. If there is sensory loss in the distribution of the posterior cutaneous nerves of the arm and forearm, and/or weakness in the triceps, the site of compression is even more proximal. A posterior cord lesion should be considered if there is axillary or thoracodorsal nerve involvement, and a C7 radiculopathy should be suspected if altered sensation is present in both the palmar and dorsal aspects of the middle finger and if there is concomitant weakness in muscles innervated by the median nerve (i.e., PT, FCR, FDS, FPL).

Management

Compression neuropathies caused by transient forces tend to resolve spontaneously without surgical intervention.[13] If no recovery occurs within 3 months, electrodiagnostic testing should be performed. If there is no evidence of reinnervation, and provocative testing indicates entrapment in the arm, then decompression of the radial nerve should be considered.[5] The senior author's preferred technique is as follows.

Radial Nerve Decompression at the Spiral Groove

This procedure is an uncommon decompression. It is often performed in conjunction with radial tunnel decompression and/or SRN decompression, in which case we suggest performing these procedures first to allow use of a tourniquet and to orient the surgeon to the radial nerve's proximal location. The tourniquet should then be removed to allow proximal dissection. A 7–8-cm incision is marked in the interval between the brachioradialis and brachialis just above the elbow. The skin is incised, and care is taken to protect the crossing cutaneous branches. Blunt dissection in the interval between brachioradialis and brachialis leads to the radial nerve. The nerve is followed proximally to the lateral intermuscular septum and this entrapment point is divided. The radial collateral vessels and posterior cutaneous nerves are identified and protected. The incision is extended and the radial nerve is followed further proximally, deep to the lateral head of the triceps to ensure complete decompression of the nerve at the spiral groove. The incision is closed in layers over a drain and a soft bulky dressing is applied. Gentle ROM exercises are initiated after 3 days with full return to activity anticipated within 4–6 weeks.

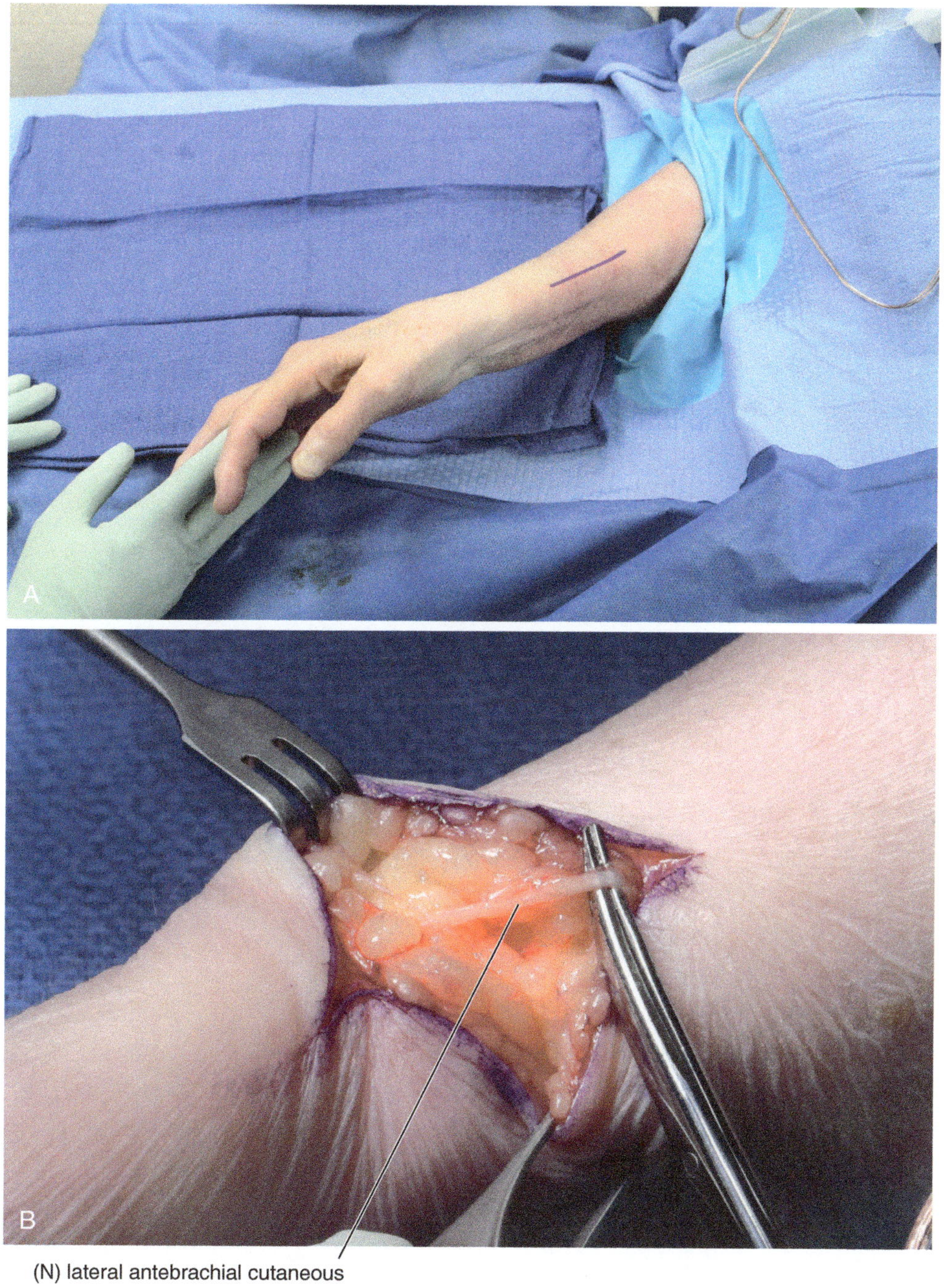

• **Fig. 54.9 (A–D)** Author's preferred technique for decompression of the superficial radial nerve (SRN). (A) A longitudinal incision is made 10 cm proximal to the radial styloid over the radial border of the distal forearm. (B) Branches of the lateral antebrachial cutaneous nerve are identified and protected.

Continued

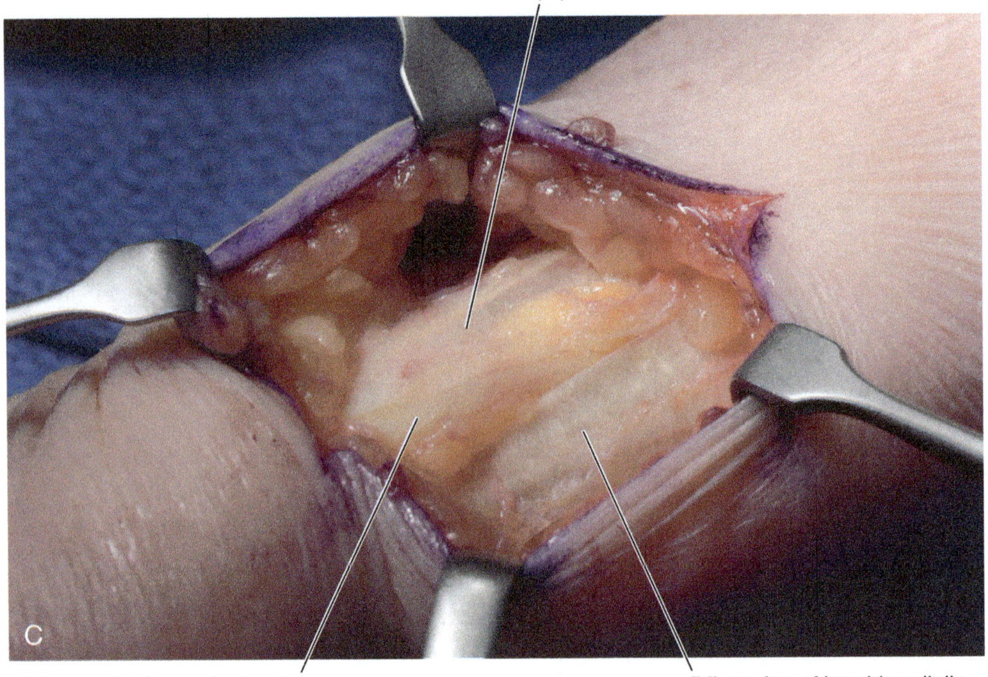

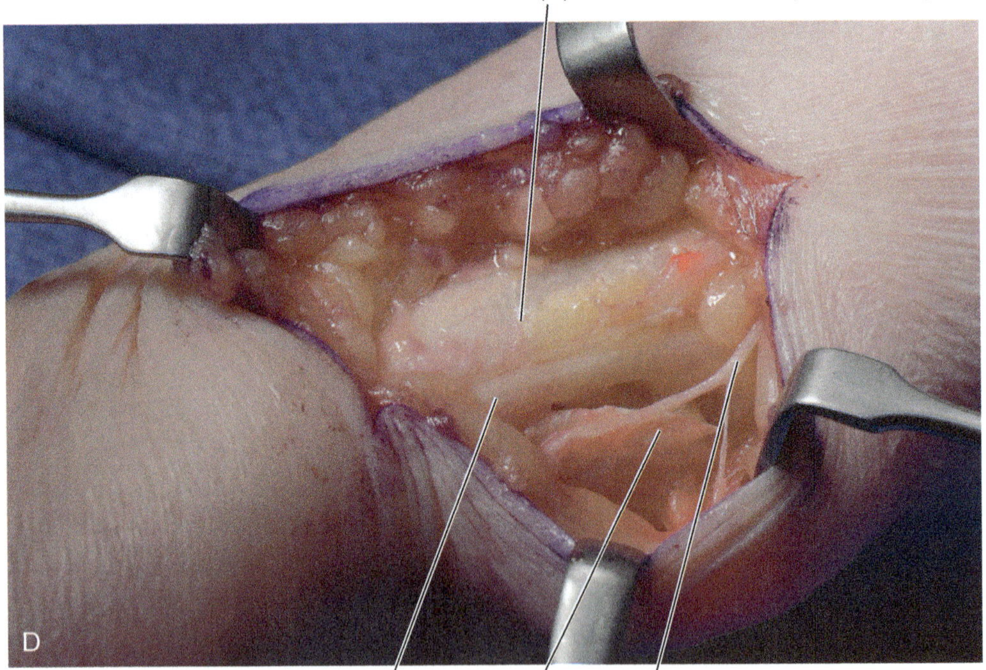

• **Fig. 54.9, cont'd.** (C) The fascia between the extensor carpi radialis longus and brachioradialis tendons is divided. The SRN is identified as it emerges between the two tendons and is decompressed along its length. (D) Tenotomy of a portion of the brachioradialis tendon is performed to completely decompress the SRN.

References

1. Mackinnon SE. Pathophysiology of nerve compression. *Hand Clin*. 2002;18(2):231–241.
2. Gelberman RH, Yamaguchi K, Hollstien SB, et al. Changes in interstitial pressure and cross-sectional area of the cubital tunnel and of the ulnar nerve with flexion of the elbow. An experimental study in human cadavera. *J Bone Joint Surg Am*. 1998;80(4):492–501.
3. McCabe SJ, Uebele AL, Pihur V, Rosales RS, Atroshi I. Epidemiologic associations of carpal tunnel syndrome and sleep position: is there a case for causation? *Hand (NY)*. 2007;2(3):127–134.
4. Jung J, Hahn P, Choi B, Mozaffar T, Gupta R. Early surgical decompression restores neurovascular blood flow and ischemic parameters in an in vivo animal model of nerve compression injury. *J Bone Joint Surg*. 2014;96(11):897–906.
5. Mackinnon SE, Novak CB. Compression neuropathies. In: Wolfe SW, Hotchkiss RN, Pederson WC, Kozin SH, Cohen MS, eds. *Green's Operative Hand Surgery*. 7th edn. Philadelphia: Elsevier Inc.; 2017:921–958.
6. Sunderland S. A classification of peripheral nerve injuries producing loss of function. *Brain*. 1951;74(4):491–516.
7. Gordon T, Yang JF, Ayer K, Stein RB, Tyreman N. Recovery potential of muscle after partial denervation: a comparison between rats and humans. *Brain Res Bull*. 1993;30(3–4):477–482.
8. Upton AR, McComas AJ. The double crush in nerve entrapment syndromes. *Lancet*. 1973;2(7825):359–362.
9. Strauch B, Lang A, Ferder M, et al. The ten test. *Plast Reconstr Surg*. 1997;99(4):1074–1078.
10. Davidge KM, Gontre G, Tang D, et al. The "hierarchical" Scratch Collapse Test for identifying multilevel ulnar nerve compression. *Hand (NY)*. 2015;10(3):388–395. https://doi.org/10.1007/s11552-014-9721-z.
11. Landau ME, Campbell WW. Clinical features and electrodiagnosis of ulnar neuropathies. *Phys Med Rehabil Clin North Am*. 2013;24(1):49–66.
12. Terayama Y, Uchiyama S, Ueda K, et al. Optimal measurement level and ulnar nerve cross-sectional area cutoff threshold for identifying ulnar neuropathy at the elbow by MRI and ultrasonography. *J Hand Surg Am*. 2018;43(6):529–536.
13. Davidge KM, Mackinnon SE. Nerve compressions. In: Farhadieh R, Bulstrode N, Cugno S, eds. *Plastic and Reconstructive Surgery: Approaches and Techniques*. Chichester: Wiley; 2015:813–837.
14. Lanz U. Anatomical variations of the median nerve in the carpal tunnel. *J Hand Surg Am*. 1977;2(1):44–53.
15. Nathan PA, Istvan JA, Meadows KD. A longitudinal study of predictors of research-defined carpal tunnel syndrome in industrial workers: findings at 17 years. *J Hand Surg Br*. 2005;30(6):593–598.
16. Wieslander G, Norbäck D, Göthe CJ, Juhlin L. Carpal tunnel syndrome (CTS) and exposure to vibration, repetitive wrist movements, and heavy manual work: a case-referent study. *Br J Ind Med*. 1989;46(1):43–47.
17. Ghavanini MR, Haghighat M. Carpal tunnel syndrome: reappraisal of five clinical tests. *Electromyogr Clin Neurophysiol*. 1998;38(7):437–441.
18. Kronlage SC, Menendez ME. The benefit of carpal tunnel release in patients with electrophysiologically moderate and severe disease. *J Hand Surg Am*. 2015;40(3):438–444.
19. Walker WC, Metzler M, Cifu DX, Swartz Z. Neutral wrist splinting in carpal tunnel syndrome: a comparison of night-only versus full-time wear instructions. *Muscle Nerve*. 2000;81(4):424–429.
20. Marshall S, Tardif G, Ashworth N. Local corticosteroid injection for carpal tunnel syndrome. *Cochrane Database Syst Rev*. 2007;2:CD001554.
21. O'Connor D, Marshall S, Massy-Westropp N. Non-surgical treatment (other than steroid injection) for carpal tunnel syndrome. *Cochrane Database Syst Rev*. 2003;1:CD003219.
22. Scholten RJPM, Mink van der Molen A, Uitdehaag BMJ, Bouter LM, de Vet HCW. Surgical treatment options for carpal tunnel syndrome. *Cochrane Database Syst Rev*. 2007;4:CD003905.
23. Hartz CR, Linscheid RL, Gramse RR, Daube JR. The pronator teres syndrome: compressive neuropathy of the median nerve. *J Bone Joint Surg Am*. 1981;63(6):885–890.
24. Fuss FK, Wurzl GH. Median nerve entrapment. Pronator teres syndrome. Surgical anatomy and correlation with symptom patterns. *Surg Radiol Anat*. 1990;12(4):267–271.
25. Gross MS, Gelberman RH. The anatomy of the distal ulnar tunnel. *Clin Orthop Relat Res*. 1985;196:238–247.
26. Davidge KM, Boyd KU. Ulnar nerve entrapment and neuropathy. In: Mackinnon SE, ed. *Nerve Surgery*. New York: Thieme; 2015:262–271.
27. Power HA, Sharma K, Haj El M, et al. Compound muscle action potential (CMAP) amplitude predicts the severity of cubital tunnel syndrome. *J Bone Joint Surg*. 2019;101(8):730–738.
28. Caliandro P, La Torre G, Padua R, Giannini F, Padua L. Treatment for ulnar neuropathy at the elbow. Padua L, ed. *Cochrane Database Syst Rev*. 2012;7:CD006839.
29. Davidge KM, Yee A, Moore AM, Mackinnon SE. The supercharge end-to-side anterior interosseous-to-ulnar motor nerve transfer for restoring intrinsic function: clinical experience. *Plast Reconstr Surg*. 2015;136(3):344e–352e.
30. Felder JM, Hill E, Power HA, Hasak JM, Mackinnon SE. Cross-palm nerve grafts to enhance sensory recovery in severe ulnar neuropathy. *Hand (NY)*. *2020*;15:526–533. https://doi.org/10.1177/1558944718822851.
31. Krogue JD, Aleem AW, Osei DA, Goldfarb CA, Calfee RP. Predictors of surgical revision after in situ decompression of the ulnar nerve. *J Shoulder Elbow Surg*. 2015;24(4):634–639.
32. Tang P. The blocking flap for ulnar nerve instability after in situ release: technique and a grading system of ulnar nerve instability to guide treatment. *Tech Hand Up Extrem Surg*. 2017;21(4):137–142.
33. Ehsan A, Hanel DP. Recurrent or persistent cubital tunnel syndrome. *J Hand Surg Am*. 2012;37(9):1910–1912.
34. Felder JM, Mackinnon SE, Patterson MM. The 7 structures distal to the elbow that are critical to successful anterior transposition of the ulnar nerve. *Hand (N Y)*. 2019;14(6):776–781.
35. Carlan D, Pratt J, Patterson JMM, et al. The radial nerve in the brachium: an anatomic study in human cadavers. *J Hand Surg Am*. 2007;32(8):1177–1182.

55

Dupuytren Disease

PAUL M.N. WERKER AND ILSE DEGREEF

Introduction

Definition

Dupuytren disease (DD) is a benign fibromatosis of the palmar fascias in which nodules and skin pits in the distal palm are usually the first signs. As it progresses, cords are formed which in time may contract limiting extension of the fingers and causing webspace contractures. The disease usually starts in the ring finger and little finger ray, but may affect any ray in a variable pattern. The same is true for the age at which the first symptoms occur. In the majority of cases the disease emerges in people of over 50 years of age. In the younger age groups, males are more affected than females. Systematic meta-analysis of the published work on prevalence has revealed it to range from 0.6 to 31.6%.[1] The disease may affect all races, although prevalence of DD has not been studied extensively in other than Caucasian races (only incidence reports).

Similar fibromatoses may affect the fascias in the instep area of the foot (Ledderhose disease (LD)), the penis (Peyronie disease (PD)), and the knuckles of the finger joints (Garrod pads). LD can cause pain during walking. Toe contractures are only sporadically seen. In PD contraction of plaques formed within the tunica albuginea may cause penile curvature during erection, sometimes hampering sexual intercourse.

Impact of DD and its Reflection in Patient-Rated Outcome Measures

The impact of DD on the patient varies with the demands the patient has. Awkwardness and functional incapacity are usually direct consequences of increasing contracture, especially when the total extension deficit of a finger exceeds 90 degrees, turning the finger into a hook that inadvertently catches objects, that cannot be easily released. Specific common complaints may be difficulty to put on gloves or getting one's hand into a pocket, eye poking with the bent fingers during facial wash and embarrassment in social hand shaking. Dupuytren contractures may interfere with various job-specific tasks and functionally impair in numerous ways.[2] Primary DD in general does not limit finger flexion.

It is not easy to quantify the disabilities, since most general upper limb impairment scores do not reflect the specific impairment of the contractures, nor their effect on performance of activities or quality of life. There are a few disease-specific questionnaires, but they have been found to have their limitations in use too.[3]

Variable Disease Course of DD

In the majority of DD cases contractures do not develop and it is good to realize that in clinics a subset of the affected population is seen; those who become patients do so mostly because they have developed contractures. Within this group, a further subset of patients can be distinguished that challenges surgeons the most, due to an aggressive disease course (Dupuytren diathesis): in these patients, whose family members often also are affected, the disease typically starts at a young age, affects both hands, also involves the radial side of the hand and is commonly associated with fibromatoses such as knuckle pads, PD and LD.[4] Since these patients develop contractures earlier in life, treatment is often needed at a younger age. Because the disease activity is higher, they often develop (early) recurrences – especially of the little finger – which may demand additional and repeated surgery, which ultimately may inflict damage to neurovascular (NV) bundles and even gangrene.

In the symptomatic population in general, DD is often found to recur or progress and should therefore be regarded as a chronic disease that at present cannot be cured. Therefore, a thoughtful individually tailored treatment strategy is indispensable. On one hand, the aim is to correct the disabling contractures with as minimally invasive treatment options as possible. On the other hand, more aggressive measures sometimes need to be considered in those cases, where recurrence is almost inevitable. This chapter aims to summarize the current knowledge of the various aspects of this disease and give some guidelines for treatment.

Surgical Anatomy of the Palmar Fascia and Changes Found in DD

McFarlane and McGrouther have to be credited for pointing out the anatomical basis of most of the fascial structures relevant for DD and for relating them to what may be expected at surgery.[5,6]

Palmar and Digital Fascias

In the palm the normal fascial structures form a three-dimensional network consisting of longitudinally, transversely, and sagittally running fibers. The longitudinal fibers are organized in a triangle and form the palmar aponeurosis. In this triangle, pretendinous and prelumbrical bands can be distinguished, the former being more condensed than the latter. They all pass superficial to the transverse ligament of the palmar aponeurosis (TLPA), which is situated at a line joining the proximal and distal palmar crease. The ulnar border of the TLPA forms a crossroad with fibers of the hypothenar fascia and the radial border is continuous with the proximal commissural band, which runs through the first webspace and ends in the thenar fascia at the level of the first metacarpophalangeal joint. Just beyond TLPA, the pretendinous bands divide into three layers (Fig. 55.1). Layer 1 is the most superficial layer, which has its insertion in either the skin of the distal palm or the proximal phalanx. Layer 2 fibers form the so-called "spiral band," since it spirals around the NV bundle on its course towards the finger. This band is present on both sides in all long fingers, except for the ulnar side of the little finger. Layer 3 is the deepest layer of fibers, which takes a sagittal course into the hand on both sides of the flexor tendon sheath to insert on either side of the corresponding metacarpophalangeal (MCP) joint.

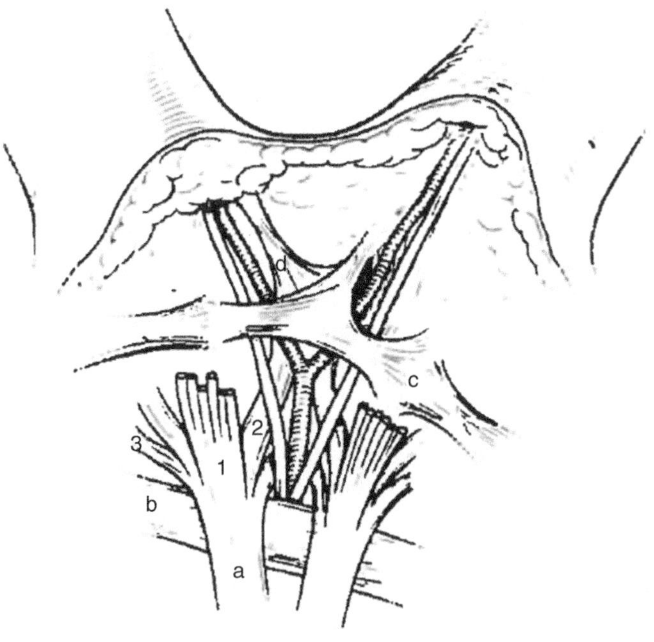

• **Fig. 55.1** Schematic drawing of the relevant palmar fascial structures at the palmo-digital junction. The pretendinous fibers can be seen to divide in three layers. Layer 2, the spiral band, courses around the neurovascular bundle. *a*, pretendinous band (PT); *b*, Transverse ligament of the palmar aponeurosis (TLPA); *c*, natatory ligament (NL); *d*, continuation of the spiral band as it extends into the digit. *1*, layer 1; *2*, layer 2 or spiral band; *3*, layer 3. (From McGrouther DA. The palm. In: Flint MH, McGrouther DA, McFarlane DA. *Dupuytren Disease: Biology and Treatment*. Edinburgh: Churchill Livingstone; 1990: Fig. 12.3.)

Another important transverse fascial structure is the natatory ligament (NL). This ligament lies just underneath the skin in the distal palm and is situated superficial to the NV bundles (see Fig. 55.1). On its ulnar end it is continuous with the hypothenar fascia, and on the radial side with the distal commissural band. NL has attachments to the flexor tendon sheet, lines the webs, and has extensions along the lateral sides of the digits. It also blends with fibers from the spiral band and is continuous with the lateral digital sheet. It is important not only because it may be affected, but also because its proximal border defines the place where a spiral nerve superficially crosses a spiral cord, making it vulnerable during surgery.

The vertical or sagittal ligaments in the palm worth mentioning are the septa of Legueu and Juvara that are usually just as wide as TLPA and, except in the thumb, connect the longitudinal fibers at the level of the TLPA, and TLPA itself with the deep transverse palmar ligament that runs between the volar plates of all MCP joints. On cross-section, the TLPA and the deep transverse ligament, together with the ligaments of Legueu and Juvara, form nine boxes, which on an alternating basis hold either the lumbrical muscle and NV bundles, or the flexor tendons of each ray. Much smaller vertical fibers are dispersed throughout the palmar aponeurosis and anchor it to the overlying skin.

The digital fascial structures relevant to Dupuytren disease bear the names of Cleland and Grayson. Their detailed anatomical description has undergone significant changes over time and drawings depicting the exact course of their fibers have been conflicting. Recently their microanatomy has been redefined (Fig. 55.2).[7,8] Grayson ligament as it was described in 1941 appears to be the most condensed part of a trabecular network of fibers that is located volar to the NV bundle and consists of fibers that originate from the outside of the flexor tendon sheet and end in the deep dermis on the contralateral side of the finger. The fibers have an inverted V-shaped orientation, which becomes less pointed during flexion. Since the trabecular network encompasses

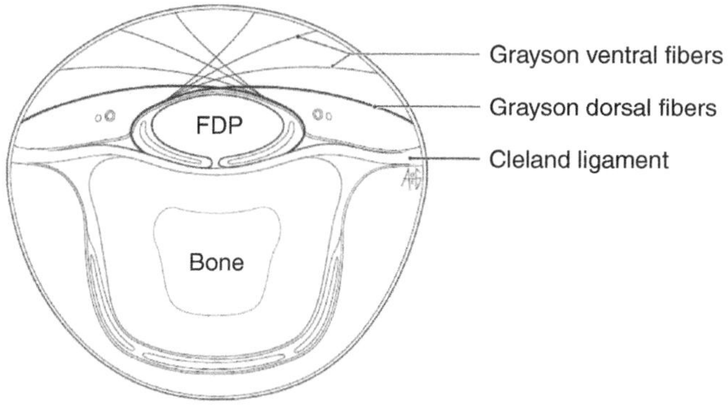

• **Fig. 55.2** Schematic cross-section through the distal proximal phalanx, showing Cleland ligament and Grayson trabecular network. (From Zwanenburg RL, McGrouther DA, Werker PMN. Grayson ligament: a revised description of its anatomy and function. *J Hand Surg Am*. 2019:44(4):341e1–341e6:Fig. 4.)

fat lobules, it seems to accommodate the adaptation of the skin to objects held in the flexed finger hands.

Regarding Cleland ligaments, they have been found to be oriented in pairs located on each side and originating at the level of the proximal interphalangeal (PIP) and distal interphalangeal (DIP) joints, and from there they course proximally and distally. Three layers have been distinguished: the most volar layer emerges from the fibers of the C1 and C3 pulleys of the flexor tendon sheet, the middle layer from the volar plate, and the most dorsal layer, which actually is a double layer, circumvents the extensor apparatus. After joining just lateral from the volar plate, they fan out proximally and distally, and run dorsal to the NV bundles.

At the place where the hypothenar muscles pass into the little finger there is a blending of fibers that run in all three directions, and they all seem to play a role in Dupuytren disease. At the thenar and in the first webspace there is also a complex three-dimensional network of bands, which may also play a part in the disease.

Band and Cords

There is consensus about the role of most of these fascial structures in the disease (Table 55.1). If a well-defined band becomes affected by disease, it is no longer called "band" but becomes "cord."

At present it is believed that the transverse ligament of the palmar aponeurosis (TLPA) is not affected by DD. Because of this, and since this structure lies palmar to the NV bundles but dorsal to the pretendinous and prelumbrical cords, most surgeons agree that it can be left in situ, and as such serves as a reference point during secondary surgery. Distal to TLPA, however, the dissection always needs to be performed with great care as the NV bundle may be displaced by a spiral cord medially and volarly and may become so intimately related to it that only the experienced eye can discern it. Fat present between a cord and the skin in between TLPA and NT, should raise a high suspicion of a spiral cord.[9] In 2010, Hettiaratchy et al described a number of cases in which a *double* spiral around the digital nerve was encountered, and in these cases, at least one of the spirals was found in the finger.[4] McFarlane tried to simplify the often complex phenotype of the disease in the finger by defining three anatomical patterns of disease: the central cord, the lateral cord, and the spiral cord.[6] Further work is required to be able to explain all these findings, including those of Hettiaratchy et al, during surgery.

Etiology

The etiology of DD has still not been fully clarified, but it is clear that an interplay of genetic and environmental factors sets the stage for the emergence of the disease. Additionally, the disease occurs more frequently when other diseases such as diabetes mellitus, liver disease or epilepsy needing long-term barbiturate use are present.[10] In addition, there is an association between high levels of exposure to manual labor and vibration (metanalysis odds ratio (OR) for manual work: 2.0 [1.6;2.6] and for vibration exposure: 2.9 [1.4;6.1]) and the development of Dupuytren disease in certain cases.[4] Vibration exposure may also be the reason that DD was found more often in field hockey players.[11]

As for the genetic basis for the disease, a number of older population studies suggesting an autosomal dominant trait with variable penetrance have been set aside by recent Genome Wide Association Studies (GWAS). Using this technology first Dolmans et al and later Ng et al have shown that DD is a polygenetic disease.[12,13] It has been calculated that the sibling recurrence risk for DD is 4.5. From a recent Danish study in twins it was concluded that the heritability of Dupuytren's disease was approximately 80%, showing that genetic factors play a major role in the development of DD.[14]

Pathophysiology and Histology

The cells that have a key role in DD and deposit the superfluous extracellular matrix proteins are called myofibroblasts. They have contractile properties and express α-smooth muscle actin that is known from smooth muscles cells of vascular origin.[15] Much basic research is being devoted to this cell type in DD and it is clear now that myofibroblasts derived from DD nodules exhibit an abnormal response to mechanical tension[4]: they pull back harder than control fibroblast when lattices in which they have been seeded are put under tension. Contracture formation in DD seems to start with fixation of extended myofibroblasts to their extracellular matrix (ECM) followed by their active contraction. The shortened situation is thereafter fixated by the secretion of collagen type I and III and other ECM molecules. The collagen acts to stabilize the contracture, allowing the myofibroblast to relax again and repeat the cycle.[4] Recently, researchers also revealed an influence of adipocytes and macrophages on myofibroblast behavior in laboratory settings.[4,16]

In this respect the classic work of Luck in 1959 and the newer work of Lam et al in 2010 still has some relevance.[4] Luck analyzed the histopathology of Dupuytren disease and proposed a quite artificial subdivision in three phases and Lam analyzed the changes in collagen content over time:

1. During the proliferating phase an abundance of disorganized cells are found in nodules. In this phase Lam et al found that over 35% of the collagen that is deposited is of type III.
2. During the involutional phase the number of cells declines but alignment along lines of stress becomes obvious. The amount of collagen type III diminishes (20%–35%), whereas the amount of type I collagen increases.
3. In the residual phase the pathology resembles a scar and is hypocellular and consists of less than 20% of collagen type III.

The relevance of the presence of nodules with an abundance of proliferating cells is that it has been found to be a predictor for early recurrence.[4] It is, however, good to realize

TABLE 55.1 **Various Fascial Structures in Palm and in Fingers of Interest in Dupuytren Disease**

Anatomical Structure	Name if Affected by DD	Clinical Relevance
Fascial Structures in the Palm		
Pretendinous band (PTB), prelumbrical band (PLB)	Pretendinous cord (PTC), prelumbrical cord (PLC)	Situated immediately beneath the skin in the palm. Responsible for earliest signs of disease in most patients. Divides in three layers distal to transverse ligament of palmar aponeurosis
Layer 1 of PTB	PTC in palm, central cord in finger	Situated immediately beneath the skin, distal to line joining proximal and distal palm crease. May cause MCP joint and PIP joint contracture. Does not displace NV bundle
Layer 2 of PTB (spiral band)	Spiral cord	Contracture causes displacement of NB bundle medially and palmarly. May cause MCP joint contracture. Warning sign: Short–Watson sign[9]
Layer 3 of PTB	Vertical cord	Dives deep into the hand on both sides of MCP joint. May cause painful triggering
Transverse ligament of palmar aponeurosis (TLPA)	–	Runs along line joining proximal and distal palmar crease, deep to PTB/PLB. Not affected by DD. Can be left behind during fasciectomy. Will facilitate subsequent surgery when left intact
Ligaments of Legueu and Juvara	–	Connect TLPA to deep transverse ligament
Natatory ligament (NTL)	Natatory cord	Situated immediately beneath the skin and superficial to NB bundle. May cause web contracture
Proximal/distal commissural band	Proximal/distal commissural cord	Proximal band is extension of TLPA; distal band is extension of NTL. Situated immediately beneath the skin in the first web; may cause first web contracture
Abductor digiti minimi fascia	Abductor digiti minimi cord (ADMC)	Forms Y-shape together with PTB and ulnar NV bundle can always be found proximal to junction. ADMC may have multiple levels
Deep transverse ligament (DTL)	–	Connects volar plates of MCP joint. Together with ligaments of Legueu and Juvara and TLPA forms nine boxes through which flexor tendons and lumbrical muscles and NV bundles pass
Fibers of Gosset	– / nodules in palm?	Dispersed over palmar aponeurosis. Anchor palmar skin to TLPA
Fascial Structures in the Digits		
Lateral digital sheet	Lateral digital cord	Situated immediately under the skin on each side of each finger; may displace NV bundle towards midline. May cause MCP joint and PIP joint contracture when involved together with spiral cord and Grayson's ligament inserting to A4 pulley. May also cause DIP joint contracture as lateral cord
Grayson's ligament	Central cord (CC)	Harbors nodules and cords at proximal phalanx. May cause PIP contracture
Cleland's ligament	Cleland cord	Not easily visualized, since situated behind NV bundle. May cause PIP and DIP joint contracture
Transverse retinacular ligament	–	Connects mid slip of the extensor apparatus at PIP joint to the lateral bands and the volar plate. Palmar portion may shorten in severe PIP joint contractures, preventing the lateral bands to slide back after contracture release
Oblique retinacular ligament (Landsmeer)	–	Connects volar plate of PIP joint to dorsal capsule of DIP joint. May shorten and cause boutonnière deformity

Abbreviations: see text.

that nodules and cords may occur simultaneously and that nodules may even be found within cords, and that therefore the prognostic value of histological analysis of Dupuytren tissue remains controversial today, as compared to clinical parameters for fibrosis diathesis.[17]

Clinical Assessment and Differential Diagnosis

The early signs of DD are subtle irregularities in the palm under the skin, which may be difficult to discern, even for specialists. Such nodules and skin pits suggest the diagnosis, but the differential diagnosis in that stage should include ganglia and inclusion cysts, occupational hyperkeratosis, callous formation, tenosynovitis, giant cell tumors, and epitheloid sarcoma or even metastatic disease.[4] Once contractures emerge, the diagnosis is usually clear, although one may confuse DD with burn scars, congenital conditions (such as camptodactyly), stuck trigger finger, tendon bowstringing after pulley rupture as in rock climbers, tendon adhesions following infection or repair, tendon imbalance (as in sagittal band rupture), intrinsic joint contractures, CRPS 1 and cerebral or psychogenic spasticity.

The speed at which the disease progresses from nodules to cords to contractures has been subject of research by Lanting and Broekstra, who followed more than 250 people with early DD for 20 months and found that 75% of the participants had either stable disease or showed regression. Regression was correlated with a smaller surface area of pathology as projected on the skin.[18]

Notwithstanding this, once cords have formed, contracture formation is more likely to follow an exponential course than a linear one. Cords in the fingers can be central, and/or on either side and may be short, or extend from the palm to beyond the DIP joint. They can cause extension deficits of any finger joint, although DIP joint contracture is rare. More often, a longstanding PIP joint flexion position leads to an attenuation of the central slip, resulting in a proximal migration of the extensor apparatus, forcing the DIP joint into hyperextension and thereby causing a boutonnière deformity of the affected finger. DD often affects both hands, but often in dissimilar phases.

Grading Systems

The most practical grading systems for research purposes are those of Iselin, and Tubiana and Michon (Table 55.2).[4] Iselin's staging system is very practical for quick scoring such as during prevalence studies. Tubiana's system is more sophisticated and the modification suggested by Tubiana in 1986 makes the system relatively complex, hampering its widespread application. The downside of this system is that progression into a higher stage may take 5–40 degrees and is therefore not linear, but stepped. Therefore, for follow-up studies it is better to register and report the active or passive extension deficit (AED or PED) by joint and its sum by ray (TAED/TPED).

Management Principles, Operative and Nonoperative Options, and their Outcome

At present, both surgical and nonsurgical treatment options are available for the management of DD. Since the first reported fasciotomy in 1821 by Cooper, the pendulum of surgical treatment has swung from open fasciotomy (the demonstration of which made Baron Dupuytren famous),

TABLE 55.2 Grading Systems for Dupuytren Disease: Every Ray is Given a Stage Number

Described by	Stage	Meaning
Iselin	1	DD nodules and cords without contracture
	2	MCP joint contractures
	3	MCP joint and PIP joint contracture
	4	Boutonnière deformity with MCP and PIP joint contracture and DIP joint hyperextension
Tubiana	0	No signs of Dupuytren disease
	N	Nodules only. No contracture
	I	Total passive extension deficit (TPED) smaller than 45 degrees
	II	TPED between 46 and 90 degrees
	III	TPED between 91and 35 degrees
	IV	TPED between 136 and 180 degrees

Abbreviations: see text.

to radical surgery in an – unsuccessful – attempt to prevent extension and recurrence, and then back to minimally invasive percutaneous needle fasciotomy. In between the extremes of the pendulum's swing, treatments of intermediate aggressiveness such as selective or limited fasciectomy of pathology only, segmental fasciectomy, a procedure in which only small segments of cords are removed, and dermofasciectomy, the excision of both diseased fascia and skin and replacement of skin by skin grafting, have been promoted. In addition to all this, and still ongoing, there is research into the optimization of fasciectomy with interposition materials and a potential role of disease control with adjuvant peri-interventional pharmacotherapy with substances such as fluorouracil or tamoxifen to improve surgical outcome and reduce recurrence risk. The nonoperative treatments include injection therapy of nodules with steroids, or cords with collagenase and radiotherapy.

In the comparison of these treatment strategies, a number of aspects need to be addressed. These include: how the method manages (if at all) affected and adjacent skin, fascia, and the joints; the indication for and best timing of the treatment; specific treatment risks and complications; aftercare; immediate outcome (efficacy) and time of reconvalescence; late outcome (including its definition), also named durability, rate of recurrence, and treatment options for recurrences. The discussion will start with the description of each treatment, its short-term outcome and complications.

Operative Treatments

If surgery is considered, the skin, the fascia, and the affected joints should each be addressed.

Skin Management

When there is no or only limited shortage of skin, and the skin needs to be opened, a longitudinal incision from the distal palm into finger, a Bruner type incision, or a transverse incision at the level of TLPA and at all affected joint creases or a combination of these can be used. For segmental fasciectomy (SF), small C-shaped incisions are used.

Transverse incisions, especially in the palm, can be left open to heal secondarily, as long as not too big areas of bare tendon are exposed. To gain extra length for closure in the fingers, Z-plasties can be used to lengthen longitudinal incisions, and YV-plasties to lengthen zig-zg insicions. Z-plasties are best planned between the proximal finger crease and the PIP joint crease, since at that level there is usually the greatest abundance of skin. Attention should be paid not to transpose the flaps too far and stitch the flaps so tight that they hamper flexion.

If skin transposition is not sufficient to close a defect, or if the skin has been removed, it can be augmented or replaced using skin grafts. Skin grafts have also been advocated as firebreaks and in some hands proved very successful in the prevention of recurrence.[19] Full-thickness skin grafts (FTSGs) are usually recommended because they are more durable and undergo less secondary contracture than split-thickness skin grafts (STSGs). FTSGs are usually taken from the ipsilateral extremity, or the groin. Donor sites are closed primarily but leave scars, one of the downsides of this treatment. Others are: increased duration of the procedure, prolonged rehabilitation period, and increased risk for complications: a graft may not take, extending the reconvalescence period.

Apart from grafts, a great variety of local (homo- or heterodigital), regional flaps have been reported to manage skin shortage and even free flaps were used in severe diathesis cases to prevent recurrence with very good long-term results in one case report.[4]

Fascia Management: Transsection, Partial Excision, Total Excision

Of the surgical treatment modalities, radical fasciectomy (RF) is only listed here for completeness. It involved the attempt at complete removal of all palmar fascia of the hand and fingers with the intention to cure the patient. It was abandoned because this latter goal was usually not achieved and because of a high complication rate, particularly hematoma formation, pain, stiffness, cold intolerance, and skin slough.

Due to the association of these complications with extensive surgery, selective or limited fasciectomy (LF) still is the most commonly performed surgical procedure for DD. Only the diseased fascia is removed, usually with a small margin of normal fascia. The generally accepted indication for treatment is a painful nodule that does not respond to conservative measures or a progressive flexion contracture of MCP joint of 20–30 degrees or any PIP joint contracture. A PIP joint contracture of more than 60 degrees is at higher risk for both incomplete correction and early recurrence. It should therefore be addressed without delay.

SF is a less invasive variant of LF in which only 1-cm pieces of diseased tissue at strategic places are removed.[4] Open fasciotomy, the method employed by Dupuytren himself, is also still employed by some: through transverse incisions, cords responsible for contractures are identified, isolated from the NV bundles and divided.

All above-mentioned procedures for the management of the fascia are usually employed under wide-awake-local-anesthesia-no-tourniquet (WLANT), regional or general anesthesia. This is one of the major differences with needle aponeurotomy (NA), also named percutaneous needle fasciotomy (PNF), which is one of the least invasive surgical procedures for DD treatment. During PNF, cords are *percutaneously* divided with a fine (27–28G) needle under local anesthesia. PNF may be performed at multiple levels along the cords during the same session.[20] Since cords are insensate, only very small aliquots of intradermal local anesthesia are needed at the site of skin puncture to allow the procedure. By doing this, nerve conduction is maintained, enabling the patient to warn the surgeon if the needle touches a nerve.

Combined Removal of Skin and Fascia

Dermofasciectomy (DF) is the removal of both skin and underlying pathology. Most authors apply it in cases with aggressive disease with clearly affected skin and (early) recurrence, especially in young patients. Logan advocates the removal of all palmar skin and pathology from the distal palm all the way to the DIP joint crease, leaving the flexor tendon sheet and NV bundles behind. The wound is subsequently covered using a full-thickness skin graft and the hand is immobilized using a cast for a week to allow the graft to take.[19] The skin graft in general adapts well, becomes sturdy, and regains sensibility, which is similar to that of thinly elevated skin flaps in LF.

PIP Joint Management

Removal of the DD cords can virtually always correct MCP joint contractures. Using PNF some contractures may persist, since they are caused by cords that run behind the NV bundles and cannot easily be reached without damaging the NV bundles. PIP joint contractures on the other hand can be more difficult to redress by removal of cords only, since in contrast to the MCP joint the PIP joint capsule itself may be affected by DD. One approach for persistent PIP joint contractures at the end of cord removal is sequential transverse division of the flexor tendon sheath, the check rein ligaments of the palmar plate, and the release of the accessory collateral ligaments, until full release of the contracture is accomplished.[4] Alternatively, and with similar results, intraoperative gentle manipulation can be applied. In fact, this is what probably takes place during continuous traction via an external fixator.

Attenuation of the central slip of the extensor apparatus may also be a significant factor in the inability to preserve correction of PIP joint contractures greater than 60 degrees.

Postoperative Management

After PNF, a very small dressing for just one day suffices. Following LF and SF, the treated hand is usually put in a soft bulky dressing for a few days to a week, sometimes reinforced by a splint, which is standard after DF and skin grafting. Following graft take and suture removal, patients begin flexion and extension exercises and this process is often supervised by hand therapists.

Early Outcome, Complications, and Reconvalescence Time After Surgery

With LF an average reduction of total passive extension deficit (TPED) of 79% at 6 weeks postoperatively has been reported. Results were best at the MCP joint (87% reduction of PED) and less good at the PIP joint (49% reduction of PED), which is a common finding with any surgical technique applied.

Treatment-specific complications of surgery are common.[4] The cumulative complication rate for LF has been found to be 19% and even higher in DF and RF. Skin slough can usually be treated conservatively. Hematomas should be evacuated before settling and causing fibrosis and early recurrence. Joint stiffness is most difficult to treat and functionally sometimes worse than the original flexion deformity. Nerve injury occurs in approximately 1% of primary cases and should be handled by direct repair, if feasible. Surgery may also cause injury to the digital arteries, the incidence of which is most likely underreported. In a worst-case scenario, especially after repeated surgery, vascular injury may result in gangrene of the operated finger, necessitating partial or complete amputation of a finger. The mean recovery period to normal hand use after surgery is for LF on average 6–12 weeks and for DF 2 weeks longer. During this period, the achieved functional result measured at 1 week will gradually improve.[21]

Overall, PNF is similarly effective than the more invasive surgical procedures for MCP joint, but less so for PIP joint contractures. Early outcome of PNF is therefore similar as for LF when the initial TPED is less than 90 degrees.[4] Complications are limited to skin tears and the risk of damaging nerves or tendons is far less than 1%. Skin fissures are more likely to occur with adherent skin, although one can try to prevent this by releasing the skin from the cord. Since they heal without leaving a trace, they usually do not bother the patient. The cumulative risk of serious complication of PNF is much less than that of the more invasive treatments and this is one of the reasons for its popularity.

Medicinal Treatment as Adjunct to Surgery: Interposition Materials after SF

Since DD is a disease wherein myofibroblast activation plays a key role, any pharmaceutical influence of this process may alter or even control disease progression. Several studies have assessed possible future options of disease control in association with surgery. 5-Fluorouracil in vitro was able to delay fibroblast proliferation. Unfortunately, systemic treatment with 5-fluorouracil in a randomized controlled trial (RCT) proved ineffective.[4]

Short-term surgical outcome improvement was achieved with neoadjuvant highly dosed tamoxifen, but long-term effects were lost after cessation of the drug.[19]

Nonoperative Treatments: Steroid and Collagenase Injections, Radiotherapy, Splinting

Treatment in early DD (Tuniana stage N) is rarely indicated. DD nodules may be painful but no unequivocal effective treatment for this is available. Patients may be advised to wear padded (biking) gloves to disperse pressure and limit pain during power grip. Steroid injection is also advocated by some to relieve pain and discomfort, and was found to reduce the size of 40% of the treated nodules after 6 months and in 56% of cases after 5 years.[22]

Collagenase injection is a popular nonoperative treatment modality for contractures, although not available in all countries. The technique was developed by Hurst and Badalamente and is a classic example of a "bench-to-bed" development of a new therapy.[23] It degrades the collagen in cords to obtain an enzymatically induced fasciotomy effect. Two types of collagenase derived from the microorganism *Clostridium histolyticum* are injected. The action of these enzymes is limited to types I and III collagen, present in cords but also in pulleys and tendons, so injection with care is needed. Since digital nerves and arteries primarily contain type II and IV collagen, they are not at risk for enzymatic damage. The collagenase is strategically injected into a cord causing a minimum of 20 degrees contracture, to weaken and rupture it by manipulation afterwards. This manipulation can be painful and is most often performed under local anesthesia. If the obtained result is not satisfactory, the treatment may be repeated after 30 days. Recently, successful results of simultaneous multiple injections in multiple cords using a double enzyme dose have been reported.[24] In 77% of the MCP joints and in 40% of the PIP joints, collagenase injection[4] released the contracture to 0–5 degrees. Serious adverse events (SAEs) such as tendon ruptures and complex regional pain syndrome are rare complications, but adverse events (AEs) such as swelling, hematoma, and pain occur almost always (97% of cases) but resolve spontaneously.

Halfway through the 20th century, the first report on radiotherapy (RTX) emerged as a possible treatment modality for early DD. It is based on the idea of possible ionizing radiation-induced DNA damage and consequent apoptosis of rapidly growing cells.[19] Early reports were ambiguous. This changed in subsequent series, but available evidence on the efficacy of radiotherapy in DD remains weak since all studies were performed in early and mild DD and only retrospective cohort analysis is reported to emphasize a possible reduction in disease progression.[19] High-quality RCTs are missing to substantiate the benefit of RTX and the risks in DD are unclear. Next to its mild local toxicity, an absolute 0.02% risk increase for malignancies is estimated.[25] Lastly, late radiation fibrosis, a known side-effect of radiotherapy, remains an uncertain long-term risk whereof the patient also needs to be informed before considering this option.

Therapeutic splinting in DD is controversial.[26] With intensive splinting (traction or compression orthotic devices are available), correction of contractures can be achieved without surgery. Nevertheless, the splinting is intense and not always tolerated by the patient. Moreover, after successful corrective splinting, recurrence of contractures is expected, unless long-term (night-)splinting is continued.

Long-Term Outcome

Definition of Recurrence

When fasciectomy was the predominant treatment option, recurrence was defined as the occurrence of new fibromatosis in previously cleared areas and extension as the occurrence of fibromatosis in new areas. Gradually and powered by other treatment regimens, a wide disparity in definitions came into use, hampering the comparison of case studies.[27]

Durability of Operative Treatments

An RCT comparing LF and PNF with a follow-up duration of 5 years showed a recurrence rate following LF of 21% using a definition of any increase of TPED of over 30 degrees relative to the result at 6 weeks postop.[21] Others, using the LeClercq definition, have published recurrence figures of up to 73%, 7 years after LF.[4]

For the long-term outcome of skin grafting in DD, the work of Ketchum is instructive.[19] He found no recurrent disease under the skin grafts in 36 hands of 24 patients an average of 4 years after fasciectomy and "firebreak" skin grafting. The incidence of extension of disease outside the grafts was 8%. It is, however, critical to distinguish the above technique of simple intercalated "firebreak" skin grafting and dermofasciectomy and skin grafting. Armstrong et al reported a recurrence rate under the grafts with the latter technique of 8.4% of 143 treated rays at 6 years.[4] The recurrence rates of SF appear similar to those of LF.[4]

PNF recurrence rates are relatively high compared to more aggressive treatment modalities. The 5- year recurrence rates of PNF in the earlier-mentioned RCT of LF versus PNF were 85%.[21] Selles et al have failed to reduce this high recurrence rate by adding autografted fat by means of lipofilling to cords that had been extensively divided.[28]

Degreef et al have demonstrated a delay in recurrence following SF by placing cellulose implants in the gap created by segmental fasciectomy.[19] Long-term results of OF are scarce, but recurrence rates of 41% after an average of 5.6 years' follow-up seem to match outcome reports of LF.[4]

Long-Term Outcome of Nonoperative Treatments

Ketchum also investigated the durability of triamcinolone injections. Fifty percent of his patients did experience reactivation of disease in the nodules 1–3 years after the last injection, necessitating one or more injections.[4]

The recurrence rate in collagenase studies is defined as loss of more than 20 degrees of PED in joints that had initially complete correction. Because this definition excludes recurrence in joints that were not initially fully corrected (and have higher recurrence rates[4]), it skews results favorably and makes comparison to studies in which other definitions of recurrence are used difficult. Using this definition of recurrence, recurrence following collagenase was 47% after 5 years.[29]

The reported progression rates of radiotherapy are as follows: After a mean of 10 years, 87% of the patients that had been treated with Tubiana Stage N and 70% of the patients treated while in Tubiana Stage N/I remained stable or regressed. In more advanced stages, the rate of disease progression increased to 62% (Stage I) or 86% (Stage II). Sixty-six percent of the patients showed a long-term relief of initially reported side effects (i.e., burning sensations, itching and scratching, pressure and tension).[4] The basic issue that needs further study, however, is the time versus progression relation in Dupuytren disease. This relation seems more likely exponential than linear and since radiotherapy has only been found to be effective in early stages of the disease, it is unclear what actually is being accomplished.

Efficacy and Durability of Surgical Methods in Comparative Studies

Recently, a number of comparative studies have appeared that shed more light on the efficacy and durability of the various surgical treatments. Two approaches can be distinguished: one in which an RCT design was chosen in which consecutive participants were randomly assigned to a treatment, and one in which surgeons together with their patients chose what they thought was the best treatment at that moment, while what later statistical methods called "propensity score matching" was applied to create groups with comparable age, sex, diathesis, and other characteristics. Both designs have their specific advantages and disadvantages: RCTs usually have difficulties recruiting participants and therefore take relatively long to execute; propensity score matching removes all participants that do not match on the previously decided items and may inadvertently filter out cases that would have influenced ultimate comparison.

Representatives of the RCT design are the Scandinavian studies from Strömberg, Skov et al and Scherman et al, in which the efficacy and durability of PNF was compared to that of collagenase.[30–32] Statistical analyses of their data revealed that the short-term as well as the long-term results of both treatments are not significantly different. Another example is the earlier cited RCT of the Rotterdam group, in which they compared LF with extensive percutaneous needle fasciotomy in combination with lipofilling (PALF). Although the one-year results were promising, since PALF results were still not statistically significantly different from LF, the durability of PALF was clearly less good than that of LF and in our view very similar to those of PNF studies that did not use lipofilling as an adjunctive (although not statistically analyzed).[28]

Using the propensity matching approach, the Rotterdam group has found no differences in efficacy between PNF and collagenase *Clostridium histolyticum* (CCH), and PNF and LF.[33]

Treatment of Recurrence

Evidence for the best treatment for recurrence is scarce. What is known is that PNF can also be used safely for the treatment of recurrences and is just as effective as during primary PNF, which makes it an even more interesting treatment modality: at least it postpones more aggressive treatment to a higher age, where recurrence may occur after a longer time frame.[21] Collagenase can also be used safely in recurrences.[4]

Surgery following PNF is not more difficult than virgin surgery. No unequivocal opinion exists as to surgery after treatment with collagenase.[4]

The role of radiotherapy for recurrent disease is yet unclear.

In repeated limited fasciectomy there is a greater risk of complications,[4] most likely because the anatomy is severely altered following the first LF and it is much more difficult to identify and preserve the NV bundles. For this reason, the number of LF procedures should be limited to the minimum, and for the treatment of early recurrence DF and skin grafting has our preference.

Rehabilitation

Splinting and hand therapy are commonly advised after surgery for DD and a great variety of protocols is being employed.[4] Evidence for the use of either of them is lacking, however.[4] Compression therapy does seem to be beneficial to reduce edema and enhance functional recovery. Some are of the opinion that only patients with rapidly reoccurring extension deficits may benefit from night splints, but research is missing that can substantiate this.

Conclusions/Personal View

Dupuytren disease is a chronic disease with variable penetrance, phenotype, and disease course for which at present a cure is lacking. Since the turn of the century the body of knowledge on the basics of the disease, especially on genetic and molecular level, has increased substantially. Additionally, new treatment modalities have emerged and gradually high-quality trials are emerging in the literature that compare treatment regimens. Gradually, an evidence-based treatment algorithm can be drawn. Nonetheless, no treatment at present is universally the best for every patient with DD.

Following counselling the patient about all surgical and nonsurgical treatment modalities, we advise him or her primarily based on: (1) age, (2) progressiveness, (3) extent of disease, and (4) diathesis characteristics. In the most extreme forms, a young (<40 years) patient with aggressive disease with PIP contractures will be warned for early recurrence with minimally invasive (PNF of collagenase) and standard technique (LF) and is offered DF and skin grafting. In patients of over 75 years of age with contracture and mild progression, PNF or collagenase will be advised, based on the work of van Rijssen et al and Peimer et al.[21,29]

All others are offered either PNF of limited fasciectomy, stating that PNF is less invasive and thus gives less trouble after treatment on the short run, but is hampered by earlier recurrence, that can be treated again with PNF, while LF may have a more cumbersome reconvalescence but has better durability.[21,34] Although PNF can often be repeated,[34] at some point it is not effective any more and maybe there is a role for CCH there.

For recurrence in general, the choice for the best treatment is even more difficult. As said before, PNF can be effectively applied again for recurrences.[34] Only if the fibromatosis is very adherent to the skin, it may become difficult to achieve an acceptable result without skin rupture. If the patients accept skin rupture and a small flap or graft to close the defect, it can be offered. When PNF is no longer possible or desired, LF is the next step and DF for very early recurrences. Collagenase also has a role in the treatment of recurrence, maybe especially in those cases where PNF is no longer an option, because of diffuse disease and maybe even in recurrences following LF, but that is yet to be proven.

Given the increasing body of evidence that splinting does not improve the result of surgery, we advise splints only for all those with extensive disease, and primarily aim to help regain flexion as soon as possible, but do continue to send patients to hand therapists for compression therapy and early active mobilization.

References

1. Lanting R, Broekstra DC, Werker PM, et al. A systematic review and meta-analysis on the prevalence of Dupuytren disease in the general population of Western countries. *Plast Reconstr Surg.* 2014;133(3):593–603.
2. Wilburn J, McKenna SP, Perry-Hinsley D, et al. The impact of Dupuytren disease on patient activity and quality of life. *J Hand Surg Am.* 2013;38(6):1209–1214.
3. Rodrigues JN, Zhang W, Scammell BE, et al. Recovery, responsiveness and interpretability of patient-reported outcome measures after surgery for Dupuytren's disease. *J Hand Surg Eur.* 2017;42(3):301–309.
4. Werker PMN. Dupuytren disease. In: Farhadieh RD, Bulstrode NW, Cugno S, eds. *Plastic and Reconstructive Surgery: Approaches and Techniques.* Oxford: Wiley; 2015:838–849.
5. McGrouther DA. The microanatomy of Dupuytren's contracture. *Hand.* 1982;14(3):215–236.
6. McFarlane RM. Patterns of the diseased fascia in the fingers in Dupuytren's contracture: displacement of the neurovascular bundle. *Plast Reconstr Surg.* 1974;54(1):31–44.
7. Zwanenburg RL, Werker PM, McGrouther DA. The anatomy and function of Cleland's ligaments. *J Hand Surg Eur.* 2014;39(5):482–490.
8. Zwanenburg RL, McGrouther DA, Werker PMN. Grayson ligament: a revised description of its anatomy and function. *J Hand Surg Am.* 2019;44(4):341.
9. Short WH, Watson HK. Prediction of the spiral nerve in Dupuytren's contracture. *J Hand Surg Am.* 1982;7(1):84–86.
10. Broekstra DC, Molenkamp S, Groen H, et al. A systematic review and meta-analysis on the strength and consistency of the associations between Dupuytren disease and diabetes mellitus, liver disease and epilepsy. *Plast Reconstr Surg.* 2018;141(3):367e–379e.
11. Broekstra DC, van den Heuvel ER, Lanting R, et al. Dupuytren disease is highly prevalent in male field hockey players aged over 60 years. *Br J Sports Med.* 2018;52(20):1327–1331.
12. Dolmans GH, Werker PM, Hennies HC, et al. Wnt signaling and Dupuytren's disease. *N Engl J Med.* 2011;365(4):307–317.
13. Ng M, Thakkar D, Southam L, et al. A genome-wide association study of Dupuytren disease reveals 17 additional variants implicated in fibrosis. *Am J Hum Genet.* 2017;101(3):417–427.
14. Larsen S, Krogsgaard DG, Aagaard Larsen L, et al. Genetic and environmental influences in Dupuytren's disease: a study of 30,330 Danish twin pairs. *J Hand Surg Eur.* 2015;40(2):171–176.
15. Tomasek JJ, Gabbiani G, Hinz B, et al. Myofibroblasts and mechano-regulation of connective tissue remodelling. *Nat Rev Mol Cell Biol.* 2002;3(5):349–363.
16. Verjee LS, Verhoekx JS, Chan JK, et al. Unraveling the signaling pathways promoting fibrosis in Dupuytren's disease reveals TNF as a therapeutic target. *Proc Natl Acad Sci U S A.* 2013;110(10):E928–E937.
17. Degreef I, De Smet L, Sciot R, et al. Beta-catenin overexpression in Dupuytren's disease is unrelated to disease recurrence. *Clin Orthop Relat Res.* 2009;467(3):838–845.
18. Lanting R, van den Heuvel ER, Werker PM. Clusters in short-term disease course in participants with primary Dupuytren disease. *J Hand Surg Am.* 2016;41(3):354–361; quiz 361.
19. Werker PMN, Degreef I. Alternative and adjunctive treatments for Dupuytren disease. *Hand Clin.* 2018;34(3):367–375.
20. Eaton C. Percutaneous fasciotomy for Dupuytren's contracture. *J Hand Surg Am.* 2011;36(5):910–915.
21. van Rijssen AL, ter Linden H, Werker PM. Five-year results of a randomized clinical trial on treatment in Dupuytren's disease: percutaneous needle fasciotomy versus limited fasciectomy. *Plast Reconstr Surg.* 2012;129(2):469–477.
22. Yin CY, Yu HM, Wang JP, et al. Long-term follow-up of Dupuytren disease after injection of triamcinolone acetonide in Chinese patients in Taiwan. *J Hand Surg Eur.* 2017;42(7):678–682.
23. Hurst LC, Badalamente MA, Hentz VR, et al. Injectable collagenase *Clostridium histolyticum* for Dupuytren's contracture. *N Engl J Med.* 2009;361(10):968–979.
24. Gaston RG, Larsen SE, Pess GM, et al. The efficacy and safety of concurrent collagenase *Clostridium histolyticum* injections for 2 Dupuytren contractures in the same hand: a prospective, multicenter study. *J Hand Surg Am.* 2015;40(10):1963–1971.
25. Kadhum M, Smock E, Khan A, et al. Radiotherapy in Dupuytren's disease: a systematic review of the evidence. *J Hand Surg Eur.* 2017;42(7):689–692.
26. Brauns A, Van Nuffel M, De Smet L, et al. A clinical trial of tension and compression orthoses for Dupuytren contractures. *J Hand Ther.* 2017;30(3):253–261.
27. Werker PM, Pess GM, van Rijssen AL, et al. Correction of contracture and recurrence rates of Dupuytren contracture following invasive treatment: the importance of clear definitions. *J Hand Surg Am.* 2012;37(10):2095–2105. e7.
28. Selles RW, Zhou C, Kan HJ, et al. Percutaneous aponeurotomy and lipofilling versus limited fasciectomy for Dupuytren's contracture: 5-year results from a randomized clinical trial. *Plast Reconstr Surg.* 2018;142(6):1523–1531.
29. Peimer CA, Blazar P, Coleman S, et al. Dupuytren contracture recurrence following treatment with collagenase *Clostridium histolyticum* (CORDLESS [collagenase option for reduction of Dupuytren long-term Evaluation of safety study]): 5-year data. *J Hand Surg Am.* 2015;40(8):1597–1605.
30. Scherman P, Jenmalm P, Dahlin LB. One-year results of needle fasciotomy and collagenase injection in treatment of Dupuytren's contracture: a two-centre prospective randomized clinical trial. *J Hand Surg Eur.* 2016;41(6):577–582.

31. Skov ST, Bisgaard T, Sondergaard P, et al. Injectable collagenase versus percutaneous needle fasciotomy for Dupuytren contracture in proximal interphalangeal joints: a randomized controlled trial. *J Hand Surg Am.* 2017;42(5):321–328. e3.
32. Strömberg Joakim J. Percutaneous needle fasciotomy versus collagenase treatment for Dupuytren contracture: a randomized controlled trial with a two-year follow-up. *J Bone Joint Surg Am.* 2018;100(13):1079–1086.
33. Zhou C, Hovius SE, Slijper HP, et al. Collagenase *Clostridium histolyticum* versus limited fasciectomy for Dupuytren's contracture: outcomes from a multicenter propensity score matched study. *Plast Reconstr Surg.* 2015;136(1):87–97.
34. van Rijssen AL, Werker PM. Percutaneous needle fasciotomy for recurrent Dupuytren disease. *J Hand Surg Am.* 2012;37(9):1820–1823.

56

Fractures and Dislocations in the Hand

BARBARA JEMEC AND NICOLA BURR

Introduction

"Many handis make light warke"

John Heywood (1497–1580)

Hand surgery is always teamwork between the surgeon, the patient, and the therapist. One cannot get a successful outcome without the cooperation of the other two.

Interestingly there are exceedingly few randomized controlled trials in the management of hand fractures despite this being a common injury. Hand fractures are often considered to be a soft tissue injury with an underlying bone injury.[1]

This chapter deals with the diagnosis and management of fractures of the phalanges and metacarpal bones in adults and children. The majority of these digit injuries can be treated effectively with conservative management and early therapy intervention. This chapter identifies the injuries that may need surgical intervention and the options available.

Pediatric Fractures of the Digits

Assessment, Classification, Management, and Complications

The differences between pediatric and adult hand fractures lie in the elasticity of children's bones and the potential disruption of their growth.

Children's bones have increased water content and plasticity, and tend to fracture incompletely with trauma. Incomplete fractures are seen as bows (bending forces), buckle fractures (one cortex buckles with compression), or green-stick fractures (one cortex ruptures under tension, the other is intact or buckles). The plastic deformation may prevent complete reduction of the fracture when manipulated, but most fractures still do not require open operations, but can be managed with closed or percutaneous techniques, due to the remodeling potential.

The assessment of the fracture is clinical and radiological. The child will have point tenderness in the nondisplaced fracture over the physis, which should increase suspicion of a fracture. If plain X-rays in two, if not three planes, cannot explain pain or deformation, MRI or CT will. The tenodesis test adequately demonstrates any rotational deformity, as the fingers should all be pointing towards the scaphoid tubercle. If in doubt, compare with the other hand. Angular deformities in children may remodel, rotational will not and needs to be corrected.

Any fracture interfering with the growth-plate has a potential for disrupting normal growth. Pediatric fractures involving growth plates are classified according to Salter and Harris. Ogden expanded the classification in 1984 (Table 56.1).[2,3]

The most common fracture pattern encountered in the fingers is a Salter–Harris II, which is satisfyingly corrected with a simple maneuver with a pen, over which the finger is manipulated (Fig. 56.1).

Crush distal phalanx fractures and nailbed injuries are the most common pediatric fracture. These occasionally need a Kirschner-wire (K-wire) or an orange needle to pin a larger distal fragment in place, but often the fragment is too small. A special type of nailbed injury is the Seymour fractures, which are displaced distal phalanx Salter I or II fractures, with avulsion of the proximal edge of the nail from the eponychial fold and the germinal matrix often interposed in the fracture itself (Fig. 56.2). Accurate and timely debridement and repositioning of all tissues is therefore paramount to allow adequate growth of both digit and nail. The clinical presentation can be confused with a mallet finger (because the extensor tendon inserts itself in the epiphysis whilst the flexor tendon inserts itself in the metaphysis), but a true lateral X-ray and a thorough examination under anesthetic should reveal the injury.

Fractures through the neck of the phalanges are usually only found in children and mostly involve some unfortunate interface between fingers and doors. Al-Qattan[4]

TABLE 56.1 The Pediatric Fracture: Management and Potential Complications According to the Salter–Harris Classification, Including Later Additions

Classification	Clinical	Configuration	Management	Complication
I: through physis, showing increased width of physis	Point tenderness only	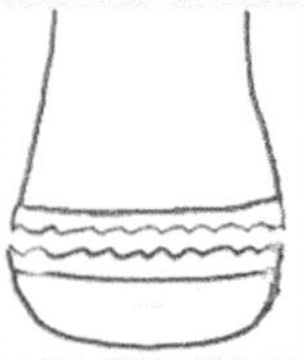	Conservative	Possible shortening
II: through physis and metaphysis	Occurs >10 years old	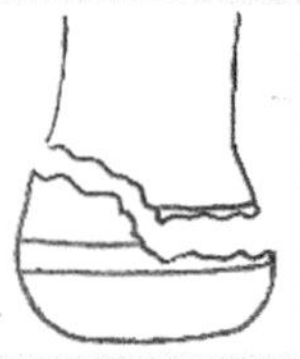	Manipulation under anesthetic if displaced	Minimal shortening
III: through physis and epiphysis	>10 years old	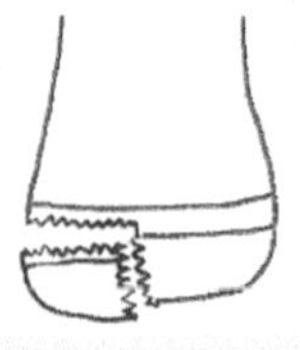	Accurate surgical reposition	Can result in chronic disability as extending into joint
IV: metaphysis, physis and epiphysis	Any age, rare in hand	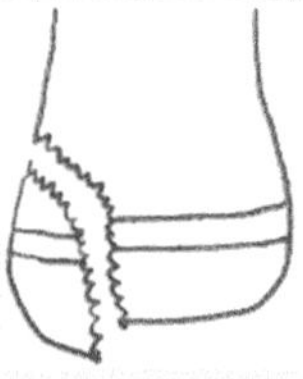	If displaced consider ORIF	Intraarticular so can result in chronic disability and can cause premature focal fusion of the joint
V: compression of the epiphyseal plate	Usually from axial loading	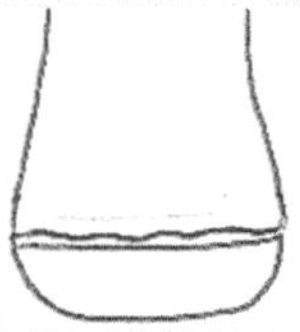	Conservative	Growth disturbances
VI: open fracture in which part of the physis is missing	Open fracture	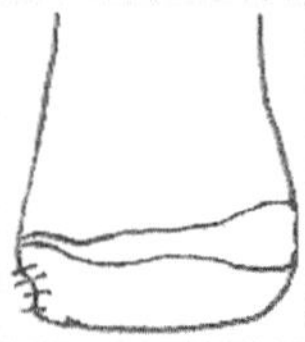	Initial fat grafting to prevent physeal bar, later reconstruction with bone graft	Growth disturbances
VII: epiphyseal plate only		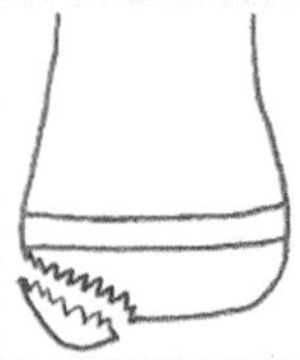	Requires accurate re-positioning as intraarticular fracture	No impact on growth
VIII: Isolated injury to the metaphysis		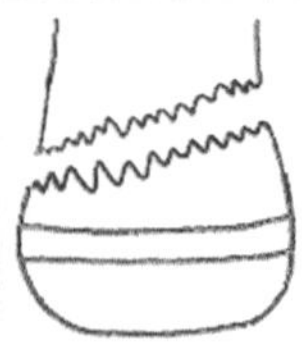	Usually can be manipulated under anesthetic or if necessary fixed with K-wire	Potential injury related to endochondral ossification
IX: Injury to the periosteum		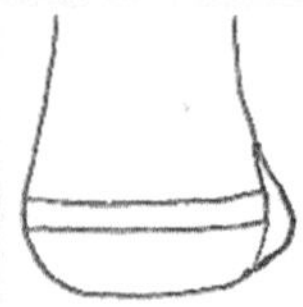		May interfere with membranous growth

K-wire, Kirschner wire; ORIF, open reduction internal fixation.
Figures redrawn after Salter RB, Harris R. Injuries involving the epiphyseal plate. *J Bone Joint Surg Am*. 1963;45:587–621.

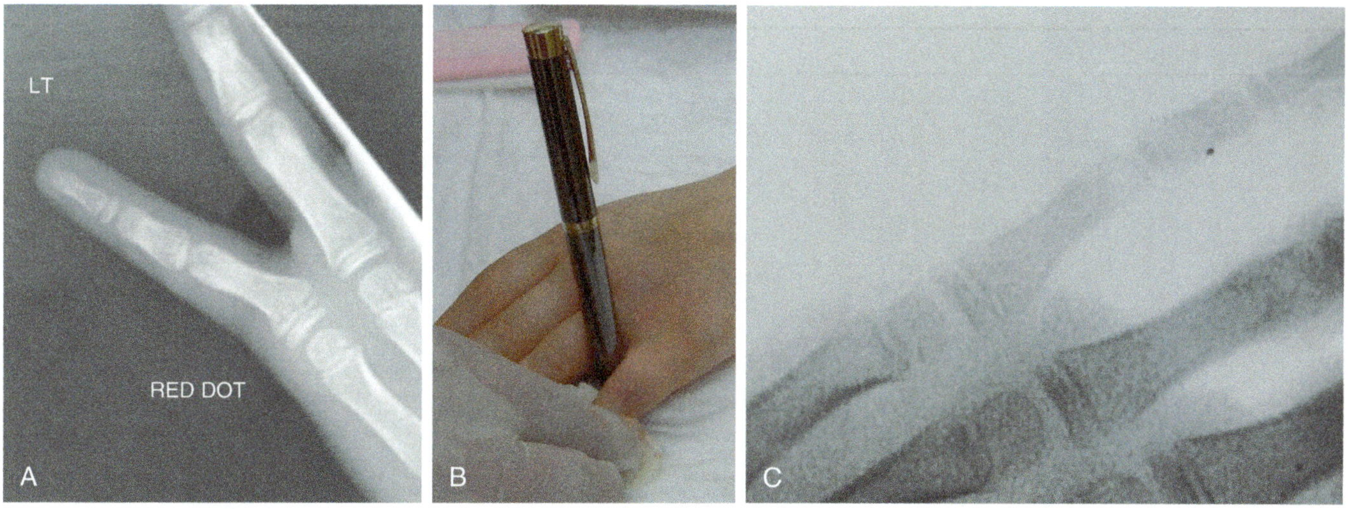

• **Fig. 56.1** Example of Salter–Harris II. (A) Pre-reduction radiograph; (B) mode of reduction; (C) post-reduction radiograph.

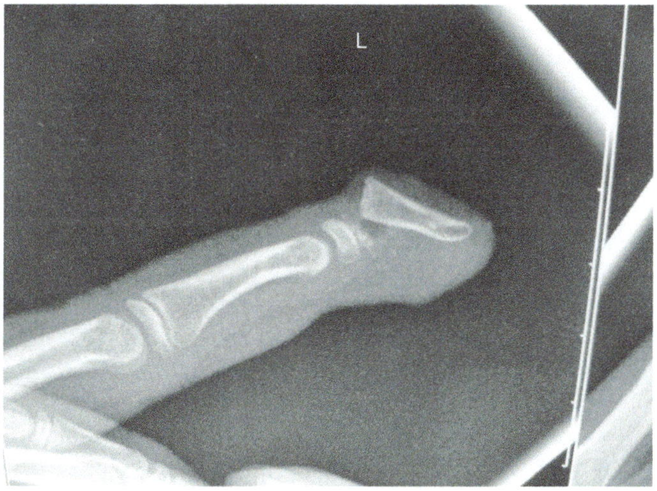

• **Fig. 56.2** Seymour fracture.

divided them into three categories, which determined prognosis and treatment: type I fractures are undisplaced, type II fractures are displaced, but maintain some bone-to-bone contact, whilst type III fractures have no bone-to-bone contact. Type III is furthermore subdivided according to the location of the distal fragment, type IIID especially being associated with an avascular fingertip (Fig. 56.3). Since the smallest displacement is poorly tolerated, all types apart from type I require open reduction and K-wiring, but have progressively worse prognoses.

Hand therapy intervention for these patients is minimum as younger children rarely become stiff at the DIP joint and instinctively start functional use once the bulky bandage or splint has been removed. Older children may require a volar splint of the affected digit until pain has settled alongside edema control work.

It is worth remembering that there is no gain in changing the dressings in nailbed injuries before 10 days, unless you are worried about infections, which of course is a different matter.

Adult Fractures

Hand fractures account for ~17% of all fractures in adults, with 59% of hand fractures occurring in the phalanges, 33% in the metacarpals, and 8% in the carpal bones.[5]

It is the authors' practice always to speak to patients about bone grafts and obtain consent for this option before the operation, even though it is rarely needed.

Metacarpal Fractures

Metacarpal fractures can be divided into their anatomical location or configuration, but most commonly occur in the little or ring fingers and the thumb.

Neck

Neck fractures of the fourth and fifth metacarpal are usually treated conservatively and many surgeons now state they will never treat these surgically, whatever the angulation of the fracture is. They can be manipulated and the digit neighbor-strapped, accepting that the patient will lose the knuckle and may have some extensor lag. If there is rotation of the digit this should be corrected surgically.

Neck fractures where the head is completely off the metacarpal and involves the index or little fingers may be fixed with minicondylar plates. In other fingers, H-plates or T-plates (the two-hole fixation on each side of the fracture can be transverse remember) can be used or perhaps even better, intramedullary K-wiring.

Intraarticular

Intraarticular metacarpal head fractures are best seen on Brewerton's views and can be fixed with countersunk screws, if the fragments are large enough. The fragment must be three times the size of the screw head to hold it. If this is not possible a primary joint replacement or a free joint from the second toe may be considered at a later date if function is

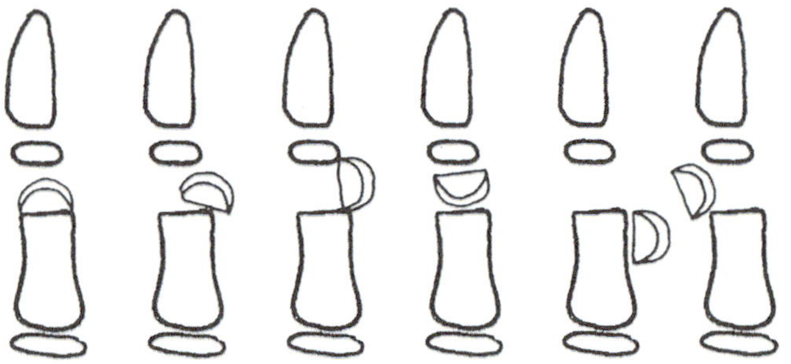

• **Fig. 56.3** Classification of fractures of neck of proximal phalanx in children. (Modified from Al-Qattan MM. Phalangeal neck fractures in children: classification and outcome in 66 cases. *J Hand Surg Br.* 2001;26:112–121.)

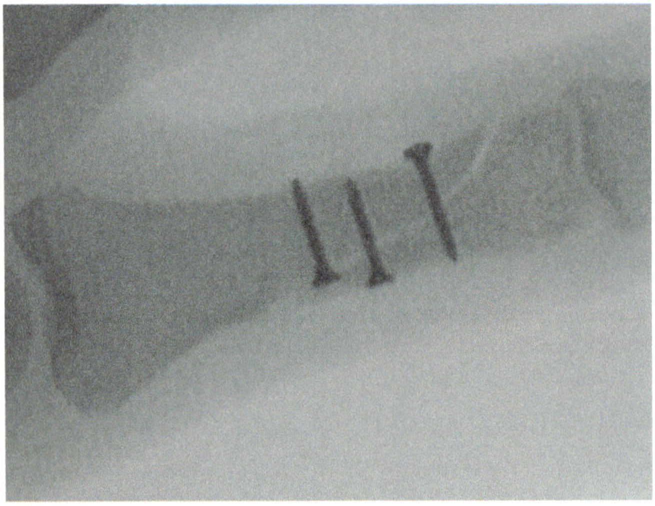

• **Fig. 56.4** Screw fixation of spiral fracture, note the spiral placement of screws.

compromised. Very rarely does this joint get considered for fusion in the fingers.

Shaft

Metacarpal shaft fractures can be divided according to their configuration into transverse, spiral, short and long oblique, butterfly fragments, and comminuted.

If the fracture can be held in position with one, or two bone-holding forceps, you can fix it with screws (which must be placed perpendicular to the fracture, not perpendicular to the bone) (Fig. 56.4).

If you cannot maintain position with a bone-holding forceps, you must consider a fracture fixation which involves a plate (or even an external fixator for the first or fifth metacarpal). For a simple transverse fracture intramedullary K-wiring or an intramedullary screw is also a possibility. Be aware that crossed K-wires can distract the fragments rather than compressing the fracture. Moon et al[6] compared intramedullary versus percutaneous K-wiring of distal third metacarpal fractures and found that the intramedullary group of patients returned to work 2 weeks earlier than the K-wire group, which was the only group to suffer any complications.

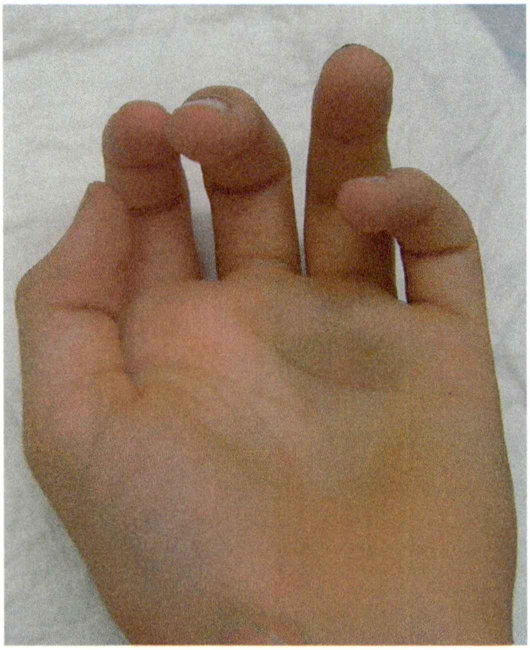

• **Fig. 56.5** Rotation: spot the odd one out.

It is important to keep checking the position of the fingers, even when the fracture looks to be perfectly aligned when using plates, before drilling and inserting screws, to avoid rotation (Fig. 56.5).

When applying plates to fractures it is important to understand the difference between locking and nonlocking plates. Conventional plates require precise adaptation of the plate to the aligned bone. The bone is pulled towards the plate when the screws are tightened and screw insertion can therefore alter the fracture position if everything is not precisely positioned. In locking plates the threaded screw head fits into the threaded plate hole and locks when tightened, thus providing a stable constellation of plate and screws. The bone is therefore not pulled towards the plate when the screws are tightened: the underlying cortical bone perfusion is not disrupted and the screws are unlikely to loosen from the plate, even if they have been inserted into a bone graft or fracture gap.

There are three plates to consider in metacarpal shaft fractures: a normal plate, a compression plate, and a bridging plate (= a locking plate). If the fracture is a simple short or long oblique, a normal plate can be used with or without a lag-screw, but must be bent appropriately to contour the bone. A compression plate is used for transverse fractures and must be slightly overbent to produce the compression of the fracture at the far cortex. A bridging plate is best viewed as an extramedullary splint, which "bridges" the part of the bone which is unsuitable for direct fixation, as in very comminuted or bone grafted fractures. With a dorsally placed locking plate, it is not necessary for the screws to reach the far cortex, so the fixation becomes unicortical and therefore quite quick as you do not have to measure the screw length.

Plates may be placed on the lateral cortex of the metacarpals, to avoid the adherence of the extensor

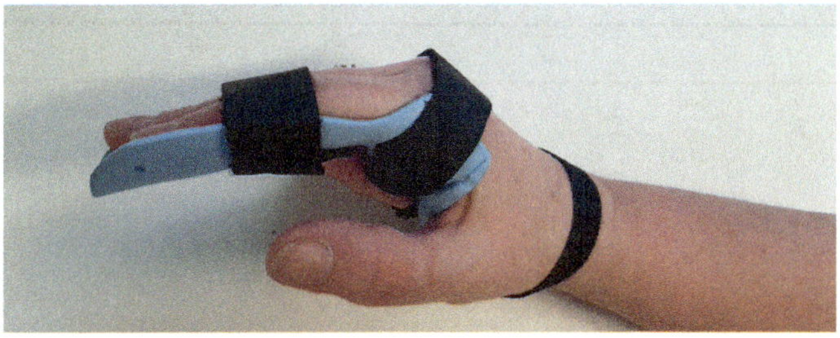

• **Fig. 56.6** Volar hand splint

mechanism, though this flies in the face of fracture fixation principles which are based on counteracting the forces exerted on the dorsal aspect of the fracture when the fist is clenched.

Intramedullary headless screw fixation of metacarpal fractures (and phalangeal fractures) is also possible and this method allows for very early mobilization, no periosteal stripping with dissection (and hence no potential subsequent tendon adhesion) or sticky-out metal work (K-wires), though it does violate the articular cartilage.[7]

If unsure whether a fracture needs operative intervention, splint the fracture and re-X-ray after one week. If the position is not maintained, it needs to be surgically corrected, but remember to act on the X-ray no later than a week to 10 days post fracture.

Base

A reversed oblique view is a useful additional view to a true lateral and three-quarter radiograph in demonstrating injury at the base of the fourth and fifth metacarpals (in addition to the adjacent carpal bones and CMC joints). Have a low threshold for requesting a CT scan of these fracture, especially the fifth metacarpal base fractures. It is often difficulty to see whether there also is an associated impacted hamate fracture with this injury. It must be disimpacted by pulling the metacarpal out to length (ligaments will ensure that the hamate follows suit so to speak) and this reduction held in place, easiest with K-wires.

Metacarpal base fractures, which cannot maintain position, are almost always fixed with percutaneous K-wires, rarely plates, as there is not enough proximal bone for a plate.

In general, stable simple metacarpal fractures can be treated with buddy strapping, compression bandage and reduced function for 3–4 weeks until the fracture is pain-free and stable. Patients must limit their function otherwise they will develop large amounts of callus as the fracture heals.

Many patients experience swelling and pain. Resting in a custom-made Thermoplastic volar or dorsal splint in the position of safe immobilization if possible (Fig. 56.6) can help ease this and allow the patient some light hand-function using the unaffected digits whilst fracture healing occurs.

Feehan and Bassett[8] discuss how custom-made splints reduce complications compared with off-the-shelf splints or plaster of Paris. Hand-based splints are made for head and neck metacarpal fractures and longer splints for shaft and base fractures. Unfortunately, despite the high incidence of these fractures the research on rehabilitation is still limited.[9] Most therapists would recommend early motion (3–5 days post operation) of the hand, especially if open surgical intervention has occurred. A Cochrane review by Poolman et al[10] showed there was no research consensus of which splint was most effective to protect a fifth metacarpal neck fracture.

Feehan[11] discusses how experienced hand therapists can mobilize the adjacent joints around a potentially unstable fracture, as an alternative to immobilization, in the first 3 weeks post fracture to achieve good long-term function. Early referral is essential.

Midgely and Toeman[12] illustrated an example of an evidence-based patient pathway which is often used within trauma centers. For example, hand therapists use tendon gliding exercises within a splint that stabilizes the fracture. These techniques prevent stiffness and allow good tendon glide. Passive exercises will be introduced once healing has occurred normally, around 6 weeks, and patients will have movement controlled until this time.

After surgical repair scar management is essential, to avoid adhesions of the extensor mechanism. Depending on the nature of the fracture, an extensor lag at the MCP joint may be evident and the therapist can work with the patient to resolve this.

After basal fractures of the little and ring finger metacarpal bones some patients complain of discomfort when shaking hands. This is due to intermetacarpal stiffness and the inability to arch the hand and oppose the little finger to the thumb utilizing the hypothenar muscles. This motion must always be restored with targeted exercises.

Thumb Metacarpal Fractures

Two base-of-thumb fracture patterns must be mentioned separately: Bennett's and Rolando's.

A Bennett's fracture is an intraarticular fracture dislocation of the thumb metacarpal base, which has a fragment, attached to the palmar beak ligament, and is usually fixed with K-wires (remember no need to spear the actual bony fragment!). Do remember that Bennet's fractures can also be treated in a plaster or scotch cast, though long-term studies suggest the rate of pain seems higher in conservatively treated Bennet's, but obviously complications only occur in the surgically treated group.

A Rolando's fracture is also an intraarticular fracture of the base of the thumb metacarpal, but consists of three fragments, with a T or Y, configuration and is usually fixed with a T or Y plate, but can be K-wired.

Thumb metacarpal fractures, which are treated conservatively, are usually put in a forearm-based thumb splint/cast immobilizing the fracture for 3–4 weeks and protecting the thumb for 6 weeks. This splint must maintain the first web space so patients do not develop adduction contracture. All finger joints are mobilized fully.

Phalanges

Distal Phalanx

Distal phalanx fractures are classified into tuft, shaft or intraarticular fractures. They account for about half of all digital fractures seen.

Tuft fractures rarely need treatment themselves, but are often associated with nail-bed injuries, which must be treated as open fractures and the nail-bed matrix meticulously apposed.

Shaft fractures can usually be treated conservatively, but a longitudinal K-wire for a transverse fracture or the occasional cerclage wire or even screw may be necessary for the longitudinal fracture.

The treatment of intraarticular fractures depends on the size of the fragment and therefore the potential degree of subluxation. Small fragments must be treated conservatively in a mallet splint immobilizing the joint for at least 6 weeks. The concern has always been that larger dorsal fragments will become unstable due to the pull of the attached collateral ligaments. The decisive size of the fragment used to be quoted as one-third of the distal phalanx joint surface, but more recently studies have established that even fragments up to 50% of the articular surface did not necessarily subluxate.[13,14] Effective splintage is required for a good prognosis. The degree of subluxation can be assessed by lateral extension radiograph, though it remains unclear what level of subluxation requires treatment.

In volar fractures the flexor digitorum profundus (FDP) pulls the attached fragment away from the distal phalanx and will need surgical reattachment and a flexor tendon rehabilitation regimen. In dorsal fractures the fragment is held in place by the extensor tendon, whilst the FDP pulls the distal phalanx volarly, the latter resulting in a bony mallet or a mallet fracture. If surgery is required and the fragment is dorsal, Ishiguro's method of fixation is a good solution.[15] The dorsal wire supports the dorsal fragment and is placed first with the DIP joint in flexion; the fracture dislocation is then reduced and the longitudinal wire is placed under image-intensifier (II) guidance (Fig. 56.7). In volar fractures the fragment, if large enough, can be secured with a screw. If, however it is too small to withstand instrumentation, then the FDP can be fixed to the distal phalanx by bony anchors, pull-out sutures, or by sutures passed through the distal phalanx transversely, using a white needle drilled through the bone. The DIPJ will become somewhat stiff whatever you do.

If the joint is unsalvageable, a primary fusion is best. There are numerous options for fusion of this joint. Solutions that include internal metal work or memory staples seem to produce quicker stability and obviously obliviate the necessity for removal of any metal work or the chance of protrusion of same.

Therapy for tuft fractures often includes a small volar splint if this helps settle the pain and rest the DIP joint (Fig. 56.8).

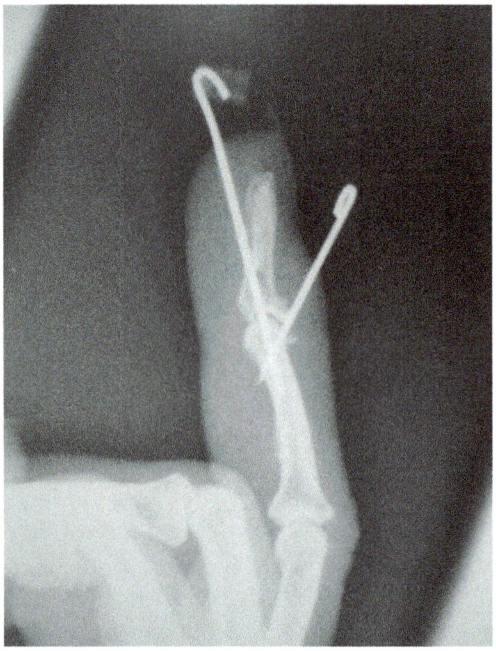

• **Fig. 56.7** Ishiguro frame.

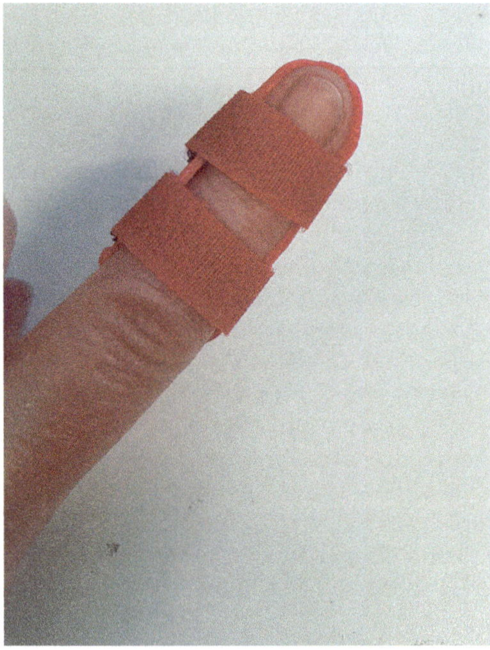

• **Fig. 56.8** Volar gutter DIP joint splint.

Patients should not perform strong gripping with this digit until the fracture has healed. Active motion at the DIP/PIP joints and edema control is commenced as soon as possible. Desensitization techniques and scar management are also often needed before the patient feels comfortable enough to use the digit normally.[16]

Mallet fractures must be treated with DIP joint immobilization for 6 weeks, followed by a weaning period of 2 weeks. The splint used varies from center to center but a small dorsal splint seems to be the most affective at holding

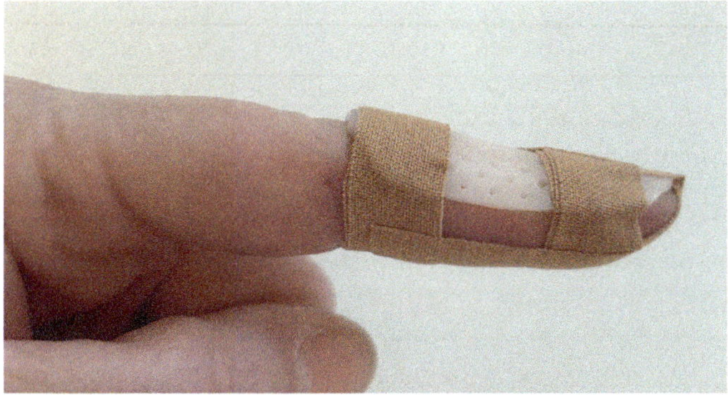

• **Fig. 56.9** Dorsal mallet splint.

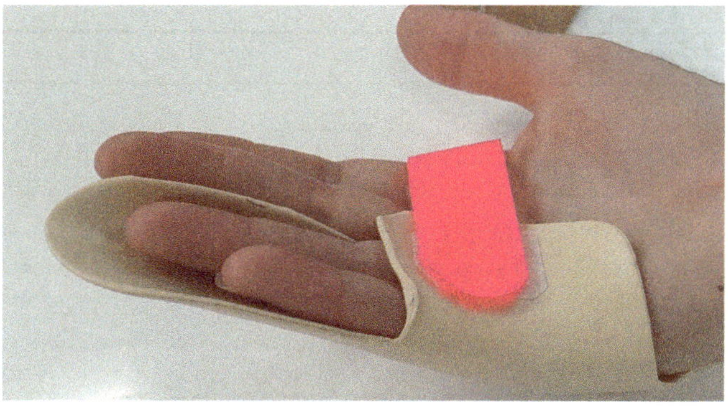

• **Fig. 56.10** Example of a dorsal splint for proximal phalanx fractures.

full DIP joint extension and preventing complications like skin maceration (Fig. 56.9). Off-the-shelf stack splints often provide suboptimal correction of DIP joint extension and are often so long that they limit PIP joint flexion. This can lead to unnecessary stiffness of this joint.

Proximal and Middle Phalanx

Proximal phalanx fractures are more common than middle phalanx fractures and can be the most challenging to treat. They can lead to deformities due to soft tissue imbalance from alteration of bone length. Shaft fractures of the proximal and middle phalanges are managed according to their configuration, though splinting and percutaneous screw fixation (dissect as little as possible) or K-wiring is preferred (try not to pin the extensor apparatus in the process, so that the joints can be mobilized early). Plates can be used, but complication rates are high, probably due the extensor mechanism getting irretrievably stuck to the scar tissue.[17]

Stable proximal and middle phalanx fractures are often placed in a custom-made hand splint for protection, pain relief, and to ensure that the IP joints do not contract whilst edema resolves. The splint keeps the IP joints in neutral and cohesive bandage wrap is often used as the first line of intervention for edema control and prevention of joint contractures. Early motion and tendon glide of both the flexor and extensor mechanism is essential. Protection splints are worn until fracture union occurs clinically. Dorsal blocking splints are very useful if there is also soft tissue damage or instability at the PIP joint as the patient can easily mobilize the joint within this splint.

It makes no sense in fixing these fractures and then keeping them immobile, as tendon adherence occurs quickly.[18] Patients must be referred to therapy early to prevent known complications occurring.

The most common complications found are PIP joint extensor lag leading to fixed flexion deformity and once these occur it is very difficult, if not impossible, to correct fully with therapy, especially if over 30 degrees. This most commonly occurs after little and ring finger proximal phalanx fractures especially when the patient can easily hyperextend their MCP joint and after surgical repair when the tendons become adhered. MCP joint hyperextension must be controlled by a dorsal blocking splint (Fig. 56.10) or strapping to allow the extensor mechanism to improve the lag. Longer-term night splintage may be required for PIP joint fixed flexion deformities.

If the PIP joint has a very tight end-feel many therapists use serial casting to improve passive range of motion. These fractures take at least 6 weeks to heal so protection is required for longer than most metacarpal fractures. Many patients experience intrinsic tightness and will require flexion strapping to improve flexibility of the digit into a fist once healing has occurred.

Intraarticular Proximal Interphalangeal (PIP) Joint Fractures

PIP joint fractures are difficult, can potentially lead to severe disability, multiple operations and therefore have many surgical options and potential interventions. Many patients with these injuries will not restore normal motion of this joint despite the therapist's/surgeon's and patient's best efforts.

Some patients with a severely comminuted fracture may be best provided with a dorsal blocking splint to prevent subluxation and given early motion in an attempt to regain any PIP joint flexibility.

External frames rely on the principle that the periosteal sleeve of the fractured bone, when pulled, will push the bony fragments together rather like a Chinese finger-trap and are classically used for pilon fractures, which are comminuted, centrally depressed, and splayed (both sagittally and coronally) fractures of the articular surface of the base of the middle phalanx. (*Pilon* is French for a pestle, as in pestle and mortar.)

There are many methods. Some rely on elastic band pulling on the frame (Suzuki frame[19]) and the Banjo frame,[20] some rely on the bend in the K-wires to put the periosteum under tension,[21] and yet again others rely on springs or hinges to achieve the same effect (S-Quattro)[22] (Fig. 56.11).

The success of these frames relies on the joints involved being mobilized early and effectively, whilst maintaining the fracture in a stable position. However, for the majority of these fixators the degree of traction exerted depends on how much the finger is flexed (the head of the proximal phalanx is not round) which is, to some degree, compensated for by the elastic element of the frame. The Banjo addresses this point as the wire frame is made so that the forces pulling on the digit are constant through the whole range of motion.

If the fracture-dislocation of the PIP joint still tends to dislocate after the two main K-wires have been inserted in a rubber band or spring system, a third transverse wire (reduction wire) can be placed through the base of the middle phalanx. When the finger is bent, the long proximal wire of the frame pushes against the reduction pin and the dislocation is reduced.

Unicondylar fractures have been classified according to their radiological appearance and on the four different types of forces exerted hypothesized to produce the fractures by Weiss and Hastings[23] (Fig. 56.12). All fractures were treated with screws, single or multiple-wires: the statistical analysis revealed no difference in outcome between the fracture types or how long after the operation they were mobilized, though screw fixation seemed to give better results.

For unstable dorsal fracture-dislocations of the PIP joint (dorsal coronal, Class III, Weiss Hastings), a method similar to the Ishigura method described for the DIP joint has been described by Vitale et al.[24] The primary K-wire is passed through the fragment from the volar surface of the middle phalanx after the fracture has been reduced percutaneously with a bone-holding forceps; the K-wire is then retracted dorsally until it is flush with the volar cortex, and then finally a dorsal blocking wire is inserted through the head of the proximal phalanx.

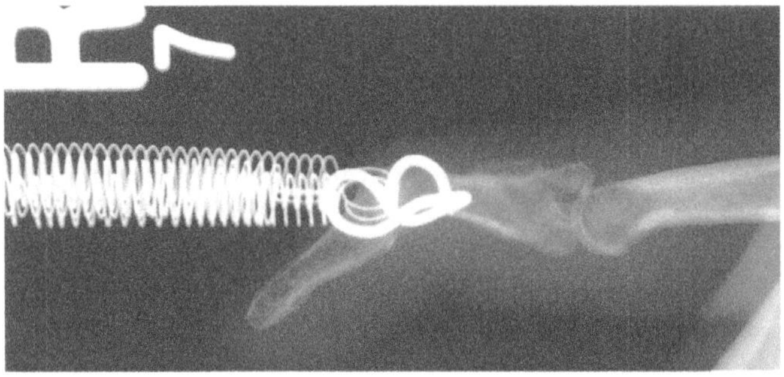

• **Fig. 56.11** Spring-based traction frame for intraarticular fracture.

For middle phalangeal fractures with large fragments, especially where the bone has been split in the coronal plane, single screw fixation can convert an unstable fracture to an injury that can be mobilized. A volar approach is easier than it intuitively might appear.

For the PIP joint which has an unsalvageable fracture, there are a few other options: fusion, volar arthroplasty, hemi-hamate, a joint replacement or a free joint transfer.

A volar arthroplasty[25] is used when the volar lip is beyond salvage: through a volar incision all (but the most volar collateral ligaments), are excised, the joint hyperextended, an incision between the volar plate and collaterals is made and the volar plate is advanced into the joint to cover the defect (usually up to 5 mm). The volar plate is secured through pull-out sutures, taking care to avoid pinning down the lateral bands.

A hemihamate graft[26] is employed because the dorsal portion of the hamate looks like the volar lip of the PIP joint: the joint is approached from the volar side, the volar plate is detached distally, and the ruined volar lip is excised (with a saw) to make room for the dorsal portion of the hamate (taken with an osteotome). The graft is secured with a couple of screws and the position checked with a lateral X-ray (the hamate graft must provide adequate volar support (lip)). The volar plate is then reattached.

The choices for PIP joint replacements are many: proximal interphalangeal replacement (PIPRTM),[27] total metacarpophalangeal replacement (TMPRTM), the Saffar, the

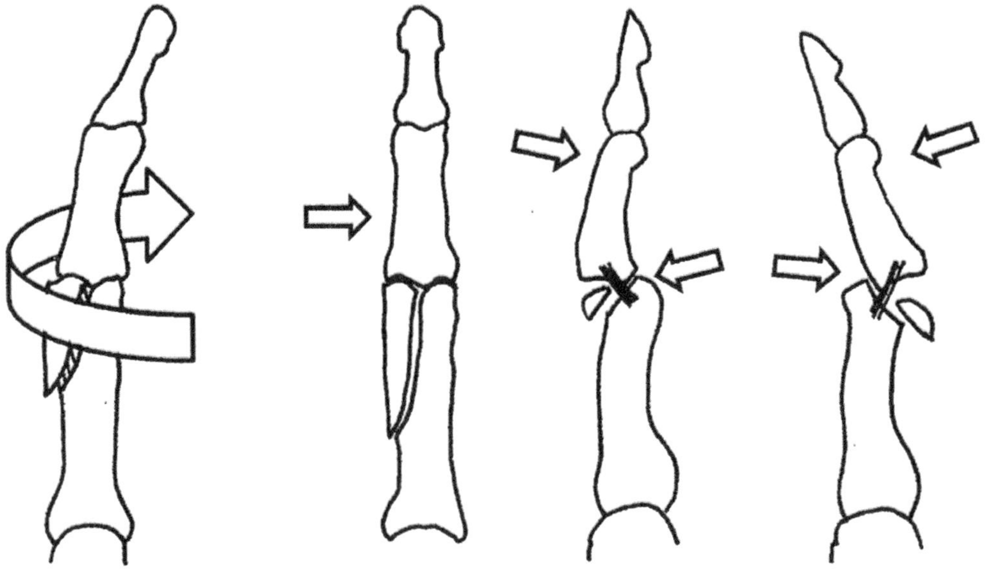

• **Fig. 56.12** Weiss–Hastings classification of unicondylar fractures of the proximal phalanx. Arrows indicate direction of force. (Modified from Weiss APC, Hastings HH. Distal unicondylar fractures of the proximal phalanx. *J Hand Surg Am.* 1993;18:594–599.)

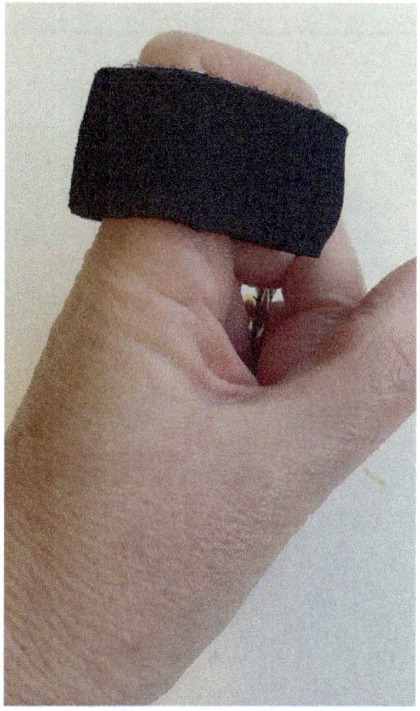

• **Fig. 56.13** Example of a flexion strap to increase IP joint flexion.

Digitos,[28] DJO3A, the Mathy, Avanta PIP SRA, RM finger joint replacement system,[29] and Swanson's.[30] Some joint replacements do well; some have failed repeatedly and been taken off the market, confirming the PIP joint as one of the hardest joints to replace well. Even with extensive rehabilitation most patients only achieve their preoperative range of motion after 6 months, but hopefully it will be pain free, making the digit more functional. Free joints, taken from the second toe, are a life-long solution and give useful movement, though not a full range.[31]

Early hand therapy after any PIP joint injury is essential for a good outcome. Small fractures within the PIP joint can be treated with a dorsal blocking splint that prevents hyperextension, cohesive bandage wrap for early edema control, and early mobilization. Controlling edema is important as if it persists in this joint it can limit joint motion for many months. As well as PIP joint motion it is essential for the patient to perform good DIP joint motion as often intrinsic tightness occurs and remains a concern for months. Flexion straps are often utilized to try to resolve this tightness once the fracture has healed (Fig. 56.13).

If external fixation has been utilized to stabilize the fracture, again edema control around the fixation is important and cohesive bandage works well for this. Early motion and tendon gliding of both the PIP joint and DIP joint is important. Patients are generally supplied with a custom-made splint to protect the fracture, fixation, and prevent flexion deformities.

Management of Other Soft Tissue Injuries

Volar Plate Injuries

Volar plate injuries can occur at any of the digit joints but are most commonly diagnosed at the PIP joint with pinpoint tenderness, if not a dorsally unstable joint. Ninety percent of these injuries occur dorsally and are common in ball sports. Severe volar plate avulsion can occur after dislocation of the PIP joint and may require surgical repair to restore stability of the joint. This type of injury commonly occurs together with other PIP joint soft tissue structure injury, like the collateral ligaments. If untreated these can lead to flexion contractures of the affected joint.

Most injuries are treated conservatively and the healing time is usually 4–6 weeks.

In adults with stable PIP joints buddy strapping may be enough to protect the volar plate and collateral ligaments whilst healing. Edema control around the affected joint is essential as is early motion of all the digit joints.

In children and hyperextending adults a dorsal blocking splint prevents hyperextension and tension on the volar plate whilst it heals. This blocking splint may start in slight flexion at the injured joint but should be straightened as pain eases so the patient does not develop a flexion deformity. Early active motion of the digit is essential to prevent adherence of the flexor tendons, especially in more severe injuries (Fig. 56.14).

A volar PIP joint injury will need treating in an extension splint if the central slip attachment has been damaged.

Ulnar and Radial Collateral Ligament Injuries to the MCP Joint

All ligamentous injuries can be classified into three grades:

I: Pain, but no laxity
II: Laxity, but a firm endpoint, stable arc of motion
III: Grossly unstable, no firm endpoint.[32]

The most common ligament to be injured in the hand is the thumb ulnar collateral ligament (UCL). Thumb radial collateral ligament (RCL) damage can occur, but it is uncommon; however, RCL tears of the finger MCP joints can occur if lateral force is applied to the digits when in MCP joint flexion.

When the thumb UCL is injured, X-rays and high resolution ultrasound will show whether there is an associated fracture and Stener lesion, indicating a complete tear of the ligament. The clinical diagnosis is made by stressing the ligament with the thumb MCP joint in flexion and comparing with the other side. Incomplete injuries are treated by 4–6 weeks of splinting, complete injuries by bony anchor fixation of the ruptured ligament, and screw fixation of the bone if the fragment is large enough. It is important to fix the concomitant tear in the capsule as well to obtain stability. Complete tears will never heal by splinting alone as interposition of the adductor aponeurosis prevents apposition of the torn ends (Stener lesion).

Protection of the thumb MCP joint UCL is essential irrespective of conservative or surgical intervention, as stability is required at this joint. A custom-made thumb spica splint which immobilizes only the MCP joint is the splint of choice for most hand therapists. This is worn full time

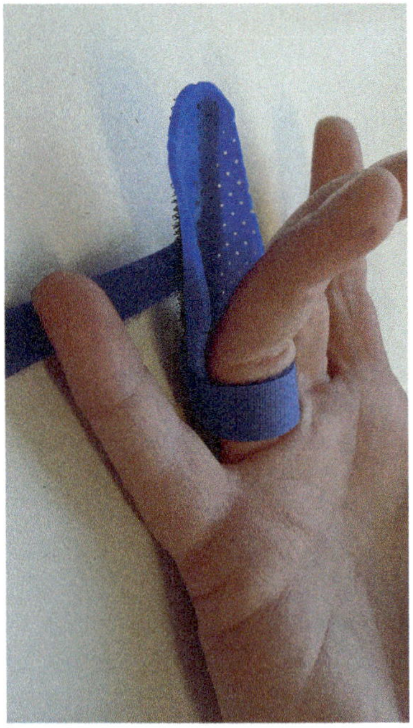

• **Fig. 56.14** Dorsal blocking splint and exercises.

for 4–6 weeks. Commonly after surgical repair the splint is removed after 2 weeks for scar massage as this area often becomes sensitive. Gentle MCP joint exercises may commence after 4 weeks depending on pain. The same regimen is also used if a RCL injury is diagnosed.

In chronic UCL tears the thumb acquires a Z-deformity, which may be repaired surgically using a bony anchor, free tendon graft or adductor advancement (adductor pollicis in detached and reattached to the ulnar side of the proximal phalanx at the MCP joint). Many patients will achieve good function if an unstable/painful MCP joint is fused.

RCL digit injury is diagnosed by passive flexion of the MCP joint and ulnar pressure causing pain. An X-ray (Brewerton's views) may show a small avulsed bone fragment. Grade I and II can usually be treated conservatively with buddy-strapping and splinting, whilst the ligament with grade III damage is fixed with a bone anchor with the MCP joint at 45 degrees when tensioning the repair or splinted in radial deviation.

Chronic injuries can be repaired with tendon grafts or the joint fused, but this is uncommon.

Collateral injuries of the digits are effectively managed by buddy strapping of the affected digit with its neighbor until stability and pain improves, usually 4–6 weeks at least.

Sometimes a small thermoplastic splint is made to support the affected joint if extra protection is required, especially at work. Good tendon glide at all joints is essential.

Ulnar and Radial Collateral Ligament Injuries to the PIP and DIP Joints

PIP joint collateral ligament injuries are usually treated conservatively, may lead to stiff joints, but rarely unstable joints. If the resulting joint becomes unstable, however, several reconstructive options exist utilizing palmaris longus or a slip of the FDS tendon.[33]

Collateral injuries of the digits are effectively managed by buddy strapping of the affected digit with its neighbor until stability and pain improves, usually 4–6 weeks at least.

Sometimes a small thermoplastic splint is made to support the affected joint if extra protection is required, especially at work. Good tendon glide at all joints is essential.

Old unstable DIP joint ligamentous injuries are best treated with fusion.

Conservative management involves buddy strapping, good range of motion and avoiding twisting of the digit until stability achieved. Early edema control is also essential to prevent fixed flexion deformities and reduced flexion.

Management Principles and Operative Options and Tips

As a rule any major injury starts with the bony fixation to provide stability for the finer neurovascular repairs and for the forces exerted by the repaired tendons. This stabilization is ideally so stable that it allows immediate active mobilization. Therapy aims must include early controlled motion, pain management, and edema control to prevent joint stiffness, digit tightness, joint contracture, and tendon adherence. The therapy program/intervention must be tailored to the individual needs of the patient and their injury. Patients with hand injuries wish to return to work as soon as possible, even when the injury is still healing, so they need protection which allows this if possible without compromising their prognosis. If surgical intervention occurs the surgeon must be confident that they can stabilize a fracture well enough to allow early motion before intervening otherwise a longer period of immobilization can lead to a poor result. Immobilization of the hand/digit after soft tissue injuries or digital fractures can lead to very poor functional outcomes for the patient. Although the literature on early mobilization of fractures is limited and not always robust,[8,9] hand therapists would agree that early referral and early controlled mobilization has a direct positive effect on final outcome after these injuries.

If immobilization of a hand fracture is requested by the hand surgeon for a high-risk unstable fracture it should be limited to a period of less than 4 weeks and preferably 3 weeks.[9,34]

All fractures that can be stabilized with a bone-holding forceps can be stabilized by screws, but the bony fragment must be three times the size of the screw-head to hold it. Otherwise it will shatter when the screw is inserted and tightened.

Periosteal stripping must always be held at a minimum, and always interpose soft tissue (periosteum) between metal and tendons in an attempt to avoid adhesions.

Do not make the patients' outcome worse by damaging the soft tissues more.

Positioning of the reduced fracture must be checked on I-I and rotation must be checked before the first screw hole is drilled. Always try to get the "worst" view on the I-I, to make sure your fracture is optimally reduced; if necessary, use the continuous mode and scan the fracture from all angles.

It is possible to have an excellent X-ray, but a bad fixation.

It is possible to have an unfavorable X-ray and a great range of motion so do not rely on X-rays for decision making.

Deviation usually remodels in children, but not rotation, which must be corrected.

Closed vs. Open

All open fractures should be washed out immediately and given antibiotics. They should, of course, be fixed on the next list.

The most important open fracture involving the metacarpal bone *not* to misdiagnose is a "fight bite." This is when the tooth of the person your patient punched, breeches the cartilage of your patient's metacarpal head. If this is not recognized and appropriately washed out and treated with antibiotics it will result in septic arthritis and possibly osteomyelitis.

Complications

Complications from fractures can be in the bones itself, such as osteomyelitis, in the fracture itself, such as nonunion and malunion, including rotation, and more generalized problems, such as cold intolerance, complex regional pain syndrome (CRPS), and overall persistent swelling and pain which results in a reduced range of movement and ultimately functional use. Thankfully, with a good patient pathway, adequate diagnosis and early intervention these are all rare with hand fractures.

Importantly, a badly managed hand fracture can mean the end of an occupation and the beginning of chronic disability. Luckily, however, most fractures heal well and the majority of patients return to near preinjury functional levels.

Osteomyelitis most commonly involves the distal phalanx, and is often the result of an open fracture, septic arthritis or severe soft tissue infection. When foreign material is present organisms form a surface biofilm, which antibiotics cannot penetrate, making the infection very difficult to eradicate while the foreign body remains in-situ. If a fracture has been internally fixed it is necessary to remove metalwork to facilitate successful treatment. Debridement of infected and/or necrotic bone is also a key part of the management. A positive bone biopsy confirms the diagnosis, which is usually due to beta-hemolytic streptococci or *Staphylococcus aureus*. If metal fixation is present, *Staphylococcus epidermidis* is common. Acute osteomyelitis should be treated with a minimum of 6 weeks of antibiotics. As for septic arthritis, there is no defined length for intravenous treatment and clinicians may choose to switch to oral antibiotics if there are suitable options as guided by the culture. The antibiotics must be well absorbed by the enteric route and penetrate well into bone, as exemplified by ciprofloxacin and clindamycin. Rifampicin is often added to treat ongoing biofilm infection as it has excellent penetration, but it cannot be used on its own as bacteria develop resistance very quickly. Other specialists prefer to treat for the full 6 weeks using intravenous therapy and referral to an outpatient antibiotic team who can administer the antibiotics via a peripherally inserted central or midline catheter may be appropriate.

The imaging of choice is X-rays and MRI, which show osteolysis and soft tissue swelling, with sequestra and involucra less common in the hand.

Nonunions of digit fractures are rare but need to be opened again and bone grafted, to bring growth factors and scaffolding material to the site. Malunions may not cause any functional issue but can be corrected at the fracture site itself, but more often, if there is a rotational element at the level of the digits, this is corrected with a derotational osteotomy of the metacarpal.

The overall chance of getting CRPS after hand trauma is unknown, and the only known factor to reduce the likelihood of getting CRPS postoperatively, is to ingest large doses of vitamin C a minimum of 6 weeks preoperatively. It is of course rare that one can predict injury with this accuracy, but it is a useful tool in elective surgery. The earlier CRPS is diagnosed and treated the better the outcome. When suspecting the diagnosis, the patient is issued with an increasing dose of gabapentin or pregabalin, possibly amitriptyline for nighttime and enough simple analgesia to tidy them over, before they are seen by the expert pain consultant, who can design an individualized treatment plan. Adequate primary postoperative analgesia and early therapy intervention are key.

Cold intolerance affects up to 38%[35] of digital fractures and can be worse if metal work is left in. This usually improves after a couple of winters, but can be permanent and is best treated by local heat and warm gloves in winter.

Therapy complications as indicated in each section range from:

- Persistent edema, which influences joint deformities and reduces range of motion of these small joints
- Joint stiffness, which can mostly be prevented by early motion but may occur in some intraarticular fractures despite extensive therapy
- Intrinsic muscle tightness, which often occurs in digit injuries and may take many months to be completely resolved helped by normal function and intrinsic stretch exercises
- Weakness of grip, which needs to be assessed and treated with strengthening work once the fracture or soft tissue injury has healed
- Reduced function and delayed return to work, which can be improved with early rehabilitation for most patients

- Scarring and tendon adhesion, which can often be alleviated by early scar management and tendon gliding exercises but sometimes requires tenolysis or removal of any internal fixation
- Complex regional pain syndrome is generally prevented by early referral to hand therapy, good early pain relief, and extensive patient advice and education.

Outcomes

Outcomes can be objectively measured using goniometry and assessing total range of motion or using DASH scores, or subjective, such as pain analog score and discussion about functional ability and return to work.

The aim for therapy is to prevent chronic edema, restore normal range of motion by the time the fracture has healed, allowing early return to function and work following these injuries. The patient can then concentrate on increasing strength with the aim of returning to work/function in full capacity as their job or lifestyle requires. Many patients will have been able to return to work in some reduced capacity much earlier due to the fact that the therapists can make much smaller bespoke splints for them and they do not need plaster of Paris casts for their whole hand.

Final Comments

As you will have gathered, close liaison with the hand therapy team is essential as early therapy intervention is crucial to ensure the best outcomes and prevent stiffness. The therapists are extremely good at assessing the injuries and the functional requirements of the patients whilst they recover from their injuries. Patient education and understanding is essential for compliance and good prognosis and the hand therapist will spend a large amount of their therapy time educating and assessing the patient and their needs.

Surgeons should only intervene surgically if they are certain they can improve digit stability, fracture configuration or if the injury is open. Immobilizing hand fractures post surgery because the surgeon is anxious about stability will lead to poorer outcomes, more stiffness, and potential tendon tethering. Gentle early controlled motion 36 hours post injury/surgery is ideal for the best functional outcomes.

Although hand fractures may be forgiving, soft tissue injuries are not.[35] Providing hand splints that rest and protect only the affected digits/joints, instead of full plaster casts, should always limit complications and improve outcomes.

Hand surgeons should always be in constant communication with their therapy team to ensure the patients have the potential of the best outcomes.

References

1. Haughton D, Jordan D, Malahias M, et al. Principles of hand fracture management. *Open Orthop J*. 2012;6:43–53.
2. Salter RB, Harris WR. Injuries involving the epiphyseal plate. *J Bone Joint Surg Am*. 1963;45:587–622.
3. Ogden JA. Skeletal growth mechanism injury patterns. *J Pediatr Orthop*. 1984;2(4):371–377.
4. Al-Qattan MM. Phalangeal neck fractures in children: classification and outcome in 66 cases. *J Hand Surg Br*. 2001;26:112–121.
5. Houwelingen AV, McKee MD. Management and complications of humeral shaft fractures. *Univ Toronto Med J*. 2004;81:96–102.
6. Moon SJ, Yang J-W, Roh SY, et al. Comparison between intramedullary nailing and percutaneous K-wire fixation for fractures in the distal third of the metacarpal bone. *Arch Plast Surg*. 2014;41(6):768–772.
7. Tobert DG, Klausmeyer M, Mudgal CS. Intramedullary fixation of metacarpal fractures using headless compression screws. *J Hand Microsurg*. 2016;8(3):134–139.
8. Feehan L, Bassett M. Is there any evidence for early mobilization following an extra articular hand fracture. *J Hand Ther*. 2004;17:300–308.
9. Giddins G. Nonoperative management of hand fractures. In: Boeckstyns MEH, Richter M, eds. *Fractures of the Hand and Carpus. FESSH 2018 Instructional Course Book*. Stuttgart: Thieme; 2018:15–28.
10. Poolman RW, Gosling JC, Lee J, et al. Conservative management for closed 5th metacarpal fractures. *Cochrane Database Syst Rev*. 2005;(3):CD003210.
11. Feehan L. Early controlled mobilisation of potentially unstable extra articular hand fractures. *J Hand Ther*. 2003;116:61–170.
12. Midgely R, Toeman A. Evaluation of an evidence-based patient pathway for non-surgical and surgically managed metacarpal fractures. *Hand Ther*. 2011;16(1):19–25.
13. Kim JK, Kim DJ. The risk factors associated with subluxation of the distal interphalangeal joint in mallet fracture. *J Hand Surg*. 2015;40(1):63–67.
14. Giddins GE. Bony mallet finger injuries: assessment of stability with extension stress testing. *J Hand Surg*. 2016;41(7):696–700.
15. Ishiguro T, Itoh Y, Yabe Y, et al. Extension block with Kirschner wire for fracture dislocation of the distal interphalangeal joint. *Techn Hand Upper Extrem Surg*. 1997;1(2):95–102.
16. Cannon N. Rehabilitation approaches for distal and middle phalanx fractures of the hand. *J Hand Ther*. 2003:105–116.
17. Kurzen P, Fusetti C, Bonaccio M, et al. Complications after plate fixation of phalangeal fracture. *J Trauma*. 2006;60(4):841–843.
18. Freeland A, Hardy M, Singletary S. Rehabilitation for proximal phalanx fractures. *J Hand Ther*. 2003;16:129–142.
19. Suzuki Y, Matsunaga T, Sato S, et al. The pins and rubbers traction system for treatment of comminuted intraarticular fractures and fracture-dislocations in the hand. *J Hand Surg Br*. 1994;19(1):98–107. Erratum in. *J Hand Surgery Br*. 1994;19(3):408.
20. Schenck RR. The dynamic traction method. Combining movement and traction for intra-articular fractures of the phalanges. *Hand Clin*. 1994;10:187–198.
21. Hynes MC, Giddins GE. Dynamic external fixation for pilon fractures of the interphalangeal joints. *J Hand Surg Br*. 2001;26B(2):122–124.
22. Fahmy NR. The Stockport Serpentine Spring System for the treatment of displaced comminuted intra-articular phalangeal fractures. *J Hand Surg Br*. 1990;15:303–311.
23. Weiss APC, Hastings HH. Distal unicondylar fractures of the proximal phalanx. *J Hand Surg Am*. 1993;18:594–599.
24. Vitale MA, White NJ, Strauch RJ. A percutaneous technique to treat unstable dorsal fracture-dislocations of the proximal interphalangeal joint. *J Hand Surg Am*. 2011;36A(9):1453–1460.

25. Eaton RG, Malerich MM. Volar plate arthroplasty of the proximal interphalangeal joint: a review of ten years' experience. *J Hand Surg Am*. 1980;5:260–268.
26. Williams RMM, Thomas KR, Sommerkamp TG, et al. Treatment of unstable dorsal proximal interphalangeal fracture/dislocations using a hemi-hamate autograft. *J Hand Surg Am*. 2003;28(5):856–865.
27. Watts AC, Trail IA. Anatomical small joint replacement in the hand. *J Bone Joint Surg Br*. 2011:1–6.
28. Gülke J, Wachter NJ, Hoss H, et al. DIGITOS-fingermittelgelenkprothese – Langzeitergebnisse. *Handchir Mikrochir Plast Chir*. 2007;39(4):257–262.
29. Middleton A, Lakshmipathy R, Irwin LR. Failures of the RM finger prosthesis joint replacement system. *J Hand Surg*. 2011;36E(7):599–604.
30. Swanson AB. Flexible implant for replacement of arthritic or destroyed joints in the hand. *Inter-Clinic Information Bulletin*. 1966:16–19.
31. Hjerner R, Berger AK. Long-term results after vascularised joint transfer for finger joint reconstruction. *J Plast Reconstr Surg*. 2008;61(11):1338–1346.
32. Merrel G, Slade JF. Dislocations and ligament injuries in the digits. In: Wolfe SW, Hotchkiss RN, Pederson WC, et al., eds. *Green's Operative Hand Surgery*. 6th edn. Philadelphia: Saunders; 2011:292.
33. Carlo J, Dell PC, Matthias R, et al. Collateral ligament reconstruction of the proximal interphalangeal joint. *J Hand Surg Am*. 2016;41(1):129e–132.
34. Stickland JW, Steichen JB, Kieinman WB. Phalangeal fractures, factors influencing digital performance. *Orthop Rev*. 1982;11:39–50.
35. Meals C, Meals R. Hand fractures: a review of current treatment strategies. *J Hand Surg Am*. 2013;38:1021–1031.

57

Osteoarthritis and Prosthetic Joints in the Hand

ANTONIO J. FORTE AND PETER M. MURRAY

Introduction

Osteoarthritis (OA) is the most common debilitating joint disorder worldwide, and its prevalence is likely to increase as life expectancy increases, creating a substantial economic burden.[1] Risk factors such as sex, radiographic features, and scintigraphy have not been specifically associated with the condition.[2] Commonly, patients will report pain, decreased function, deformity, and challenges undertaking simple tasks such as activities of daily living as well as essential occupational tasks.[3]

As patients age, the progressive wear and tear of the cartilage and bone compromise the overall joint integrity. As osteoarthritis develops and progresses, joint reconstruction may become a reasonable option. In this patient population, thumb carpometacarpal (CMC) reconstruction is among the most commonly performed surgeries, and while arthrodesis of the small joints of the hand remains a predictable and durable approach, arthroplasty procedures have become more popular in recent decades.

Osteoarthritis of the Small Joints of the Hand

Preoperative Evaluation

Physical examination starts with careful inspection and palpation of the involved digits. Joint swelling, pain, and instability can be found at the metacarpophalangeal (MCP) joint, the proximal interphalangeal (PIP) joint and the distal interphalangeal (DIP) joint. Inflammation associated with osteoarthritis can produce erythema, warmth, effusion, and soft tissue swelling.[3] A more distinguishing feature is the presence of Bouchard and Heberden nodes at the PIP and DIP, respectively. The range of motion may also be restricted due to concomitant MCP or PIP flexion contracture. Furthermore, the tendon integrity may be compromised, especially of the extensor tendons, with ulnar subluxation at the MCP secondary to failure of the sagittal bands. However, this is more commonly recognized in inflammatory disorders such as rheumatoid arthritis of the hand.

Multiple modalities of imaging can be used to assess osteoarthritis of the small joints of the hand. A 3-view radiograph, including PA, lateral, and oblique angles, are the views preferred for imaging patients suspected of having osteoarthritis of the hand.[4] Computed tomography (CT) and magnetic resonance imaging (MRI) are rarely used for assessment of MCP, PIP, and DIP OA with the possible exception of the CT evaluation of intraarticular fracture malunion or the MRI assessment of articular cartilage. Additionally, radiographic scores do not precisely correlate with clinical evaluation.[5]

Due to the diverse presentation, OA treatment is tailored to specific individual needs. Nonoperative treatment options include education about hand therapy techniques to protect hand joints during activities of daily living.[6] Heat modalities, orthoses, gloves, as well as pharmacological agents such as paracetamol/acetaminophen, nonsteroidal antiinflammatory agents (NSAIDs) and intraarticular corticoid injections[5,7] may also be of therapeutic benefit. Kroon et al performed a systematic review and meta-analysis on the topic and found that the data indicated that intraarticular steroid injection might be effective in interphalangeal joint OA, but no compelling evidence has been presented.[8] Similarly, strengthening exercises under the supervision of a hand therapist are commonly prescribed. However, as indicated by Magni et al in a meta-analysis published in 2017, despite low-level evidence that exercise may reduce joint stiffness and pain,[9] there is no definite evidence showing that resistance training carries any substantial benefit on hand OA pain and overall hand joint function.[10]

Distal Interphalangeal Joint Arthrodesis

Indications for DIP joint arthrodesis include pain related to either primary degenerative arthritis or posttraumatic arthritis. Contraindications include active infection or an open wound over the joint, atrophic skin, and digital ischemia. Dickson et al[11] highlight three essential considerations that will help with surgical planning:

1. The angle of arthrodesis – typically no or slight flexion and fixation with a variable pitch compression screw
2. Adequate bone stock
3. Size of the distal phalanx – important when considering compression screw fixation as threads of the variable pitch compression screw are at risk to cut out dorsally, potentially damaging the nail bed and ultimately producing an unsightly nail plate

Fowler et al recommend using Kirschner wires (K-wires) and a single loop of surgical steel wire if the distal phalanx diameter is less than 2 mm larger than the width of the variable pitch compression screw to be used.[12]

Surgical Technique

The procedure can be performed under regional or general anesthesia. Through a skin H incision, the terminal tendon is transversely incised, and the joint is exposed. Using a rongeur or a 2-mm high-speed bur, the articular cartilage is denuded, and a flush contact surface is created. Either K-wires, K-wires with a surgical steel wire loop or a headless variable pitch compression screw (Fig. 57.1) can be used to achieve appropriate fixation. Care is taken to avoid inside-out injury of the nail bed which may lead to nail plate deformity. Complications include infected and aseptic nonunions, nail deformity, and prominent hardware distally at the tip of the finger.[13]

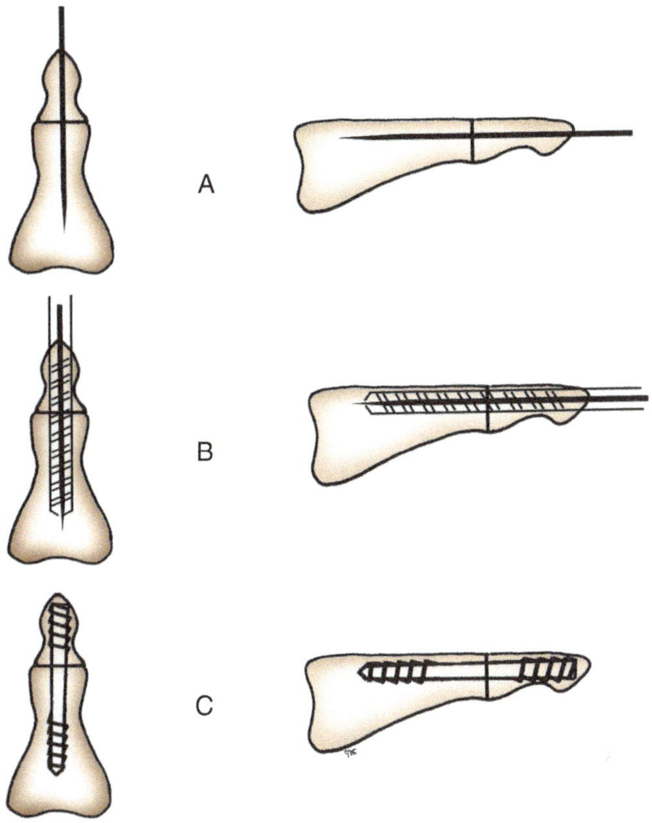

• **Fig. 57.1** (A–C) Distal interphalangeal joint arthrodesis (Used with permission of Mayo Foundation for Medical Education and Research. All rights reserved.)

Proximal Interphalangeal Joint Arthrodesis

Indications for PIP arthrodesis include symptomatic idiopathic or posttraumatic osteoarthritis.[14] Contraindications include infection, inadequate bone stock, and poor skin envelope.[15]

Surgical Technique

The procedure can be performed under regional or general anesthesia. A longitudinal skin incision is made on skin and extensor mechanism.[16] The articular surface is visualized and the collateral ligaments released. An oscillating saw is then used to cut the bone just proximal to the condylar flares of the proximal phalanx and just distal to the articular surface of the middle phalanx. Only a very small wafer of bone should be removed from the proximal aspect of the middle phalanx. It is essential to make these cuts perpendicular to the longitudinal axis of the digit to prevent digit angulation.

K-wire figure-of-8 tension band wire technique is generally preferred. The degenerative articular surfaces of the PIP joint are osteotomized. The osteotomy of the middle phalanx articular base is performed perpendicular to the long axis of the bone while the osteotomy of the head of the proximal phalanx is done at a progressive angle (30, 40, 50 or 60 degrees) for the index, long, ring or small fingers, respectively. Two parallel 0.035-inch K-wires are drilled first in a retrograde fashion perpendicular to the osteotomy cut of the proximal phalanx then in an antegrade direction across the osteotomized surface of the middle phalanx. The tips of the K-wires should stop about 5 mm shy of the distal articular aspect of the middle phalanx for later advancement. Once the articular surfaces are stabilized, another 0.035-inch K-wire is drilled transversely to the axis of the middle phalanx through the dorsal cortex at the junction of the proximal and middle thirds of the shaft. A figure-of-8 loop using a 20G surgical steel wire is passed through the drill hole in the middle phalanx shaft then just proximal to the K-wires exiting the proximal phalanx. Next, the exposed K-wires are cut approximately 1 cm superficial to the dorsal cortex of the proximal phalanx and are bent 90 degrees to capture and secure the figure-of-8 wire loop after the wire loop has been tightened down by twisting with a needle driver or needle nose pliers. The twist of the figure-of-8 wire is then cut and gently driven down over the middle phalanx with a small bone tamp and mallet[17] (Fig. 57.2). Complications of the figure-of-8 tension band arthrodesis technique for the PIP joint include nonunion (3%), malunion (1%), hardware prominence (9%), phalangeal fracture, hardware failure, and skin necrosis (3.5%).[13,15]

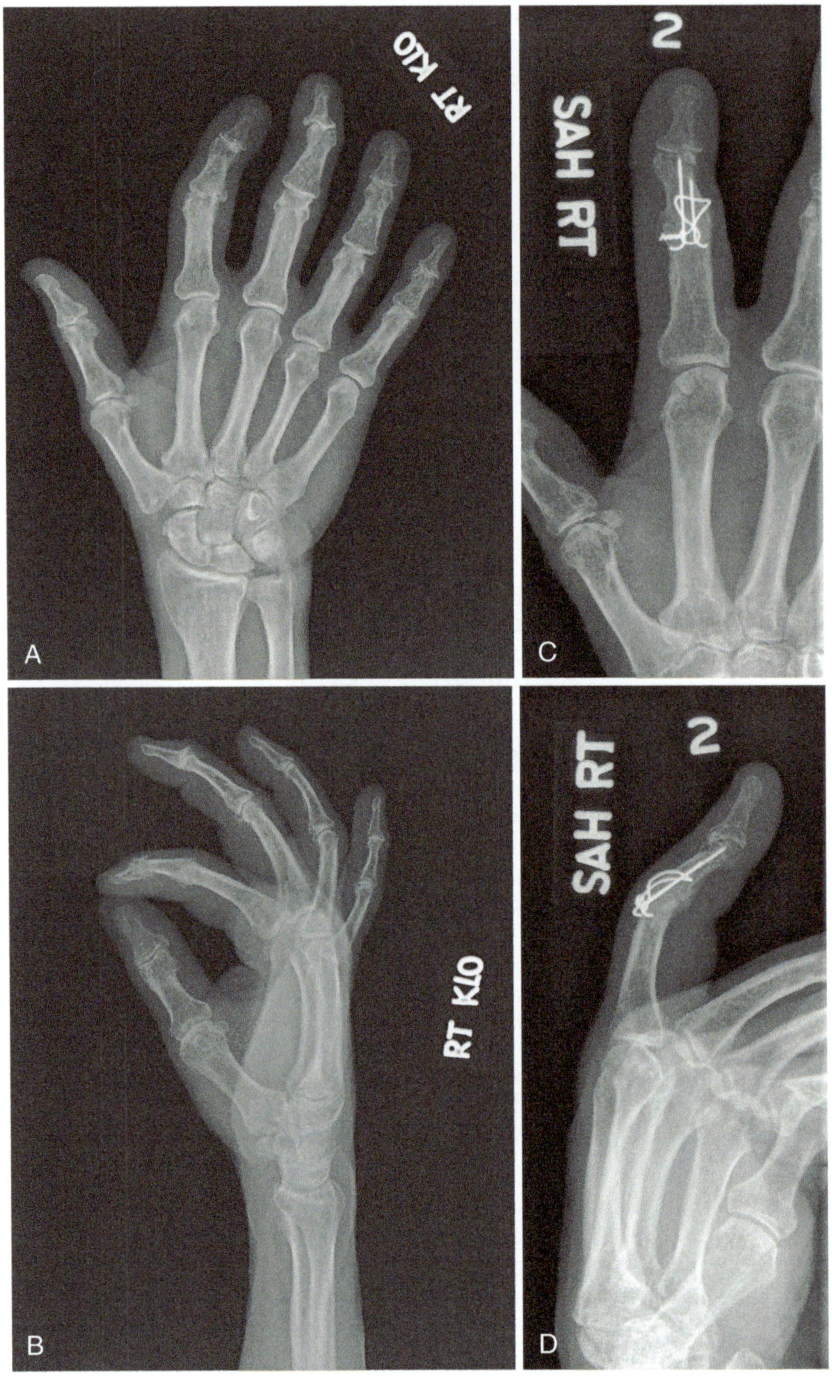

• **Fig. 57.2** (A–D) Proximal interphalangeal joint arthrodesis. (From Murray PM. Treatment of the osteoarthritic hand and thumb. In: Wolfe SW, Hotchkiss RN, Pederson WC, eds. *Green's Operative Hand Surgery*. 7th edn. Elsevier; 2018:Fig. 11-7.)

Proximal Interphalangeal Joint Arthroplasty

According to Zhu et al,[18] replacement arthroplasty aims to eliminate pain, restore motion, and maintain joint stability. If an implant does not recreate normal joint kinematics, it provides no benefit, no matter how anatomically accurate. Implant stability is achieved through appropriate implant design and bone interface, as well as the presence of intact soft tissue structures.[18] PIP joint implant arthroplasty includes silicone spacers and semiconstrained devices such as pyrocarbon implant arthroplasty and metal–plastic surface replacement arthroplasty (SRA).[19]

Silicone PIP joint implant arthroplasty was first introduced by Dr. Albert Swanson in the 1970s.[20] This hinged Silastic implant is designed to act as a spacer, and generally provides excellent pain relief.[19] Yamamoto et al report that in this modality of arthroplasty, using a volar approach, better restoration of motion, less extension lag, and fewer complications were gained when compared to other types of implants or surgical implantation methods.[21] Similar results with Silastic implant arthroplasty have also been shown using either the dorsal or the lateral approaches.

Pyrocarbon implants are nonconstrained and do not allow bony ingrowth. Even though pyrocarbon does not undergo degradation due to cyclic loading and presents high breaking strength,[18] its use remains controversial and overall high complication rates have been observed with its use in the PIP joints with more favorable results from pyrocarbon implants realized in the MCP joints of the hand.[19]

SRA implant arthroplasty (Fig. 57.3) is also a nonconstrained device that was designed by Ronald Linscheid based on his analysis of anthropomorphic data determined from cadaveric specimens.[19] Murray et al followed 47 patients that had 67 prostheses, with a mean follow-up of 8.8 years finding 59/67 joints still in service at follow-up with a cumulative failure rate of 16% at 15–25 years. The authors found no association of failure, radiolucency surrounding the implant or subsidence of the implant whether cement was or was not used. There was also no association of implant failure based on the diagnosis of OA or RA. There were 22 complications among 14 patients. There were no infections. The authors concluded that this modality of

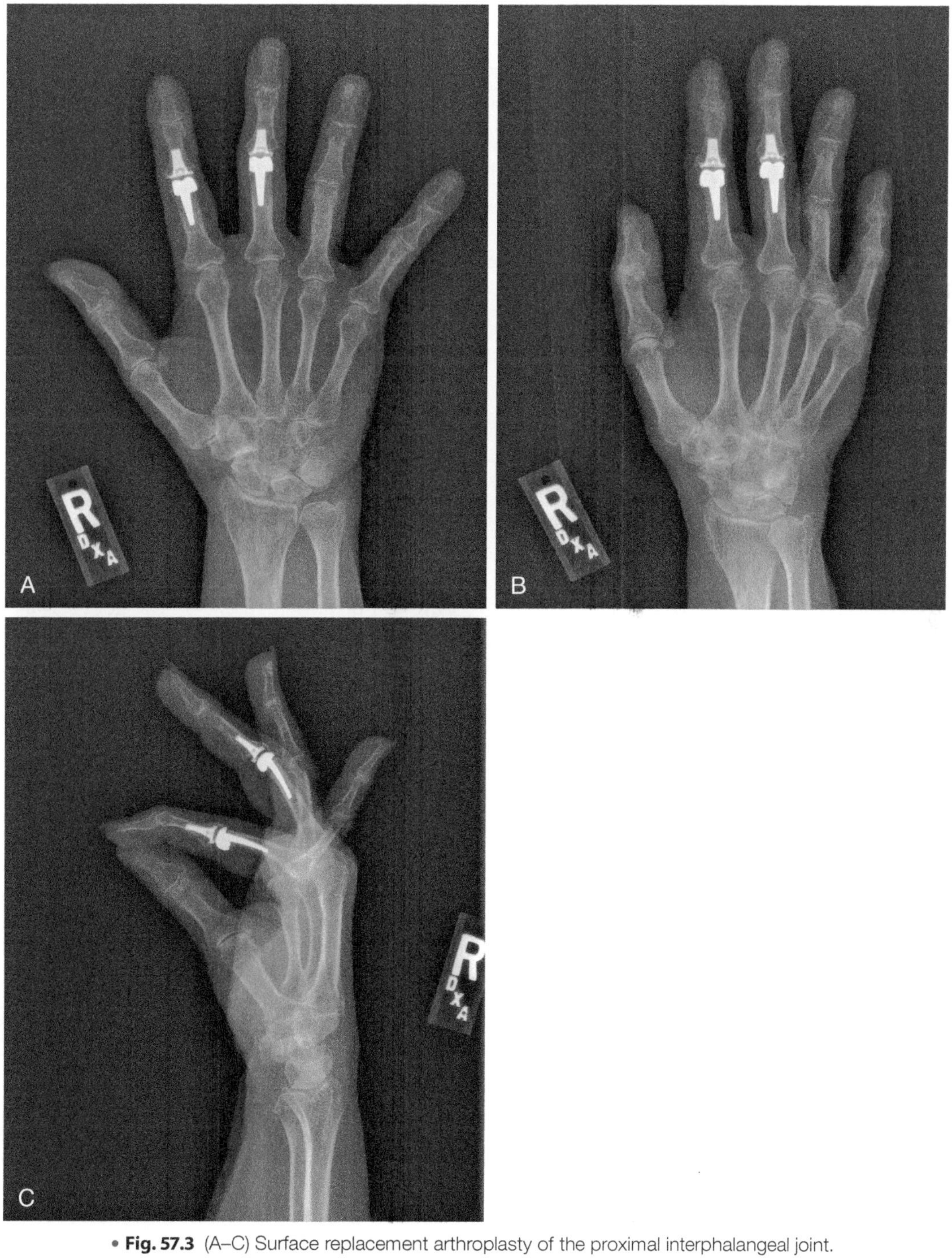

• **Fig. 57.3** (A–C) Surface replacement arthroplasty of the proximal interphalangeal joint.

arthroplasty is a reliable option to address pain and deformity, both in osteoarthritis and in rheumatoid arthritis.[22]

Indications for PIP joint implant arthroplasty include degenerative or posttraumatic arthritis of the PIP in an elderly, low demand patient who desires to maintain joint motion and reduce pain. Contraindications include poor soft tissue envelope, swan neck or boutonnière deformity, infection, and absence of extensor tendon or collateral ligament integrity.

Surgical Technique

The procedure can be conducted under regional or general anesthesia. A dorsal midline approach allows the extensor mechanism to be incised and retracted according to the technique of Chamay whereby a distally based flap of the extensor mechanism is created at the central slip insertion on the base of the middle phalanx (Fig. 57.4).[16] Alternative approaches favored by some are the volar approach and the lateral approach. Once the joint is exposed, the collateral ligaments are protected, and perpendicular osteotomies are placed just proximal to the proximal phalangeal head articular surface and just distal to the origin of radial and collateral ligaments from the head of the proximal phalanx. A back, camphor cut is also performed on the posterior aspect of the head of the osteotomized proximal phalanx to better accommodate the phalangeal component An osteotomy is performed at the base of the middle phalanx, and it should be no more than 2 mm thick, depending on the preexisting subsidence of the proximal articular surface of the middle phalanx. The most important factor is removal of the proximal and middle phalanx articular surfaces in their entirety, as this can be a source of continued pain. Then, both proximal and middle phalanges are broached to the largest best fit with care taken to prevent implantation of undersized components (Fig. 57.5). Once the joint motion is satisfactory after placement of trial components, the permanent components are chosen. Press fitting of the components is preferred, however cement is considered in overly capacious canals or when a "snug" press fit cannot be achieved.

Complications include instability, implant subsidence or loosening, dislocation, extensor mechanism failure resulting in boutonnière deformity, extensor tenodesis, collateral ligament failure or incompetence resulting in instability, joint contracture, and phalangeal fracture.[18,19] Salvage procedures including implant revision or arthrodesis have been described for both silicone and SRA implants.[23]

Rehabilitation

Multiple protocols are available, but the authors recommend removal of the initial dressing at 1 week postoperative, and placement of a dynamic extension outrigger splint. This allows graduated increasing active flexion every 2 weeks until the sixth postoperative week. At that point, full extension and flexion is expected without the splint but the splint is maintained at bedtime for an additional 6 weeks. Heavy lifting or gripping is discouraged long term for concerns over implant loosening.

Metacarpophalangeal Joint Arthroplasty

Indications for this procedure include painful osteoarthritis of the MCP joints of the hand, refractory to nonoperative management. The most commonly affected joints are the index and middle fingers. Osteoarthritis of the MCP joints of the hand is unusual, being more common in patients with inflammatory arthritis. The procedure should only be considered in the less active individual following the sixth decade of life. Contraindications include poor bone stock, poor skin envelope, and infection. Improvement in pain, arc of motion as well as pinch and grip strength after this procedure can be anticipated.[19,24] The gold standard for implant arthroplasty of the MCP joints of the hand remains the Silastic implant although pyrocarbon and surface replacement implants are available.[17]

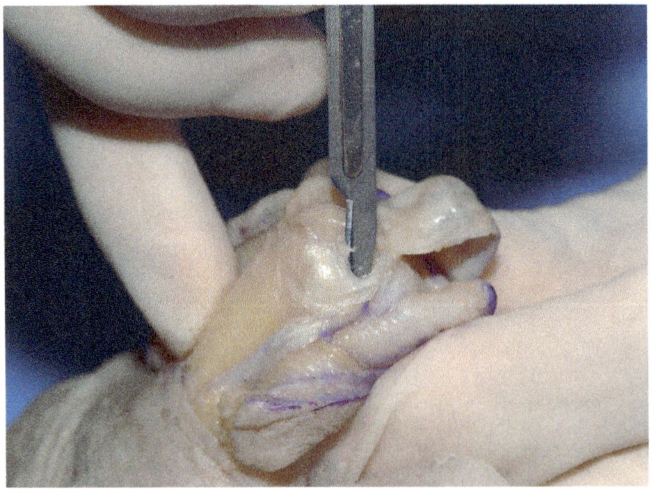

• **Fig. 57.4** Dorsal Chamay approach to the proximal interphalangeal joint of the finger with the creation of a distally based flap of the extensor mechanism.

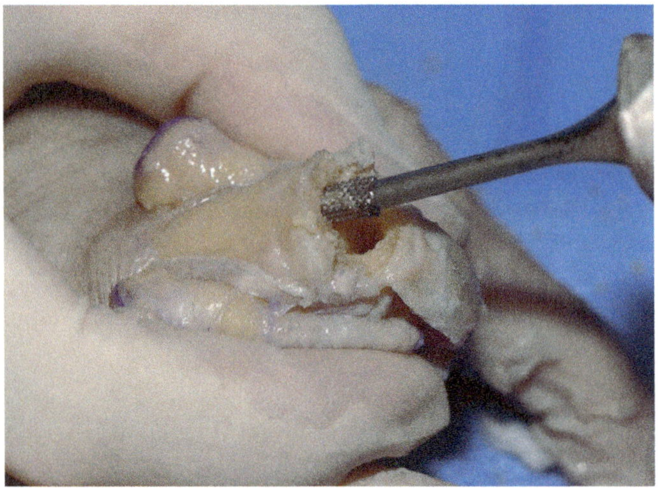

• **Fig. 57.5** Broaching of the proximal phalanx during preparation for implant arthroplasty with the surface replacement components.

Surgical Technique

A transverse incision is preferred for multiple metacarpal arthroplasties while a longitudinal skin incision is used for single joint replacements. Typically, the sagittal band is incised along the ulnar aspect of the extensor tendon and the extensor tendon is then separated from the underlying capsule. The capsule is then incised longitudinally and the joint exposed. Articular wear is commonly seen on the dorsal aspect of the articular base of the proximal phalanx (Fig. 57.6) and the articular surface of the metacarpal head (Fig. 57.7) given that there is frequent volar and ulnar subluxation of the middle phalanx relative to the metacarpal head. The base of the proximal phalanx is prepared first. A thin wafer of bone is removed containing the remains of the proximal articular surface.

The collateral ligaments are identified and released with a small blade at their origin from the sulcus of the metacarpal head (when performing MCP surface replacement arthroplasty, it is imperative to preserve the origins of the collateral ligaments). The radial collateral ligament is released from metacarpal head and tagged with a 2-0 absorbable suture.

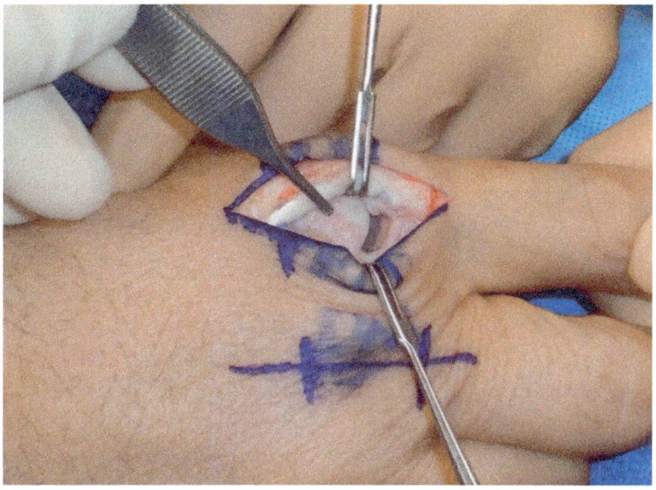

• **Fig. 57.6** Articular wear on the base of the proximal phalanx, typically seen in advanced osteoarthritis of the metacarpal phalangeal joint.

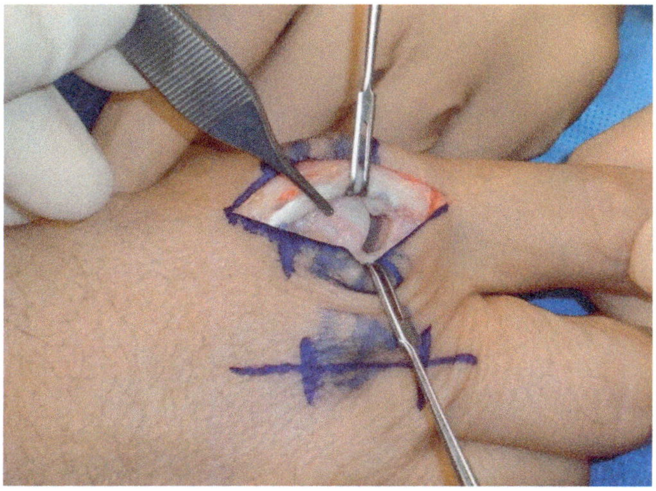

• **Fig. 57.7** Articular wear on the metacarpal head, typically seen in advanced osteoarthritis of the metacarpal phalangeal joint.

Using an oscillating saw, the metacarpal head is resected at the proximal extent of the articular surface. Next, a small wafer of bone is removed from the base of the proximal phalanx, such that a 1-cm gap is created for the implant (Fig. 57.8). The proximal phalanx and then the metacarpal are progressively broached to accept the largest trial Silastic implant. The trial is inserted and intraoperative radiographs obtained to assess the restoration of digital length and coverage of the metacarpal and proximal phalanx bone ends. Range of motion of the digit and stability of the digit are also assessed. The radial collateral ligament is repaired to bone and the permanent implants implanted with a "no touch" technique.

Rehabilitation

Our preferred rehabilitation protocol includes a low-profile extensor outrigger splint, allowing both MCP graduated flexion as well as unrestricted PIP flexion. The outrigger splint is maintained during the day for approximately 6 weeks and a night time extension splint is maintained for a total of 12 weeks. Heavy lifting and gripping with the hand is discouraged long term.

Osteoarthritis of the Thumb

Preoperative Evaluation

At least 50% of overall hand function depends on proper thumb function. Thumb CMC OA radiographic prevalence is approximately 7% in men and 15% in women.[25] Despite the lack of distinction between thumb and interphalangeal OA in the proposed criteria of the American College of Rheumatology (ACR), thumb CMC OA is defined as a separate subset in the European League Against Rheumatism (EULAR) criteria.[26–28]

Notable symptoms include pain at the thumb base, decreased range of motion in thumb abduction and reduced strength, including key pinch and cylindrical grasp. Interestingly, pinching maneuvers may increase forces that are

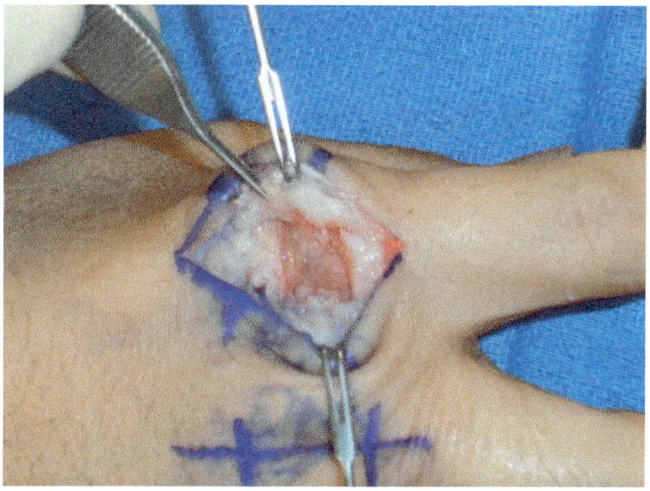

• **Fig. 57.8** Following resection of the metacarpal head and proximal phalanx, a 1-cm gap for the implant arthroplasty is created.

translated to the CMC joint by a factor of 12. Traditional stress tests during a physical examination include the grind test (pressure application while joint rotation is performed to detect pain or crepitus) and traction-shift or "lever test" (examiner provokes CMC joint subluxation and passive relocation to test for pain).[3] Additionally, on inspection, thumb adduction contracture coupled with compensatory thumb MCP joint hyperextension can be observed. In addition to the imaging modalities described previously in this chapter, a Robert view of the thumb CMC allows a better posteroanterior view of this joint. The Bett's view (true lateral) can be obtained with a neutral forearm position, ulnar wrist deviation, and thumb abduction.[29]

The most adopted radiographic staging system for CMC arthritis is the Eaton–Glickel classification[30,31]:

Stage 1. Minimal joint widening
Stage 2. Minimal joint narrowing, minimal subchondral sclerosis, and joint debris (osteophytes or loose bodies) less than 2 mm
Stage 3. Noticeable narrowing or obliteration of joint space, cystic changes, sclerotic bone, varying degrees of dorsal subluxation, and joint debris greater than 2 mm
Stage 4. Stage 3 deterioration plus scaphotrapezial joint narrowing with sclerosis and cystic changes

Nonoperative treatment relies on activity modification, analgesics, NSAIDs, neoprene orthoses (thumb stabilizers), and steroid injections.[32] High-quality evidence-based studies show that hand therapy treatments may lead to less pain and functional improvement in patients with basilar thumb OA.[33] Orthoses may also provide some pain reduction up to 1 year without a clear benefit to overall hand function or strength.[34]

A variety of surgical reconstructive procedures have been described for thumb CMC joint osteoarthritis. They include trapeziectomy with or without ligament reconstruction/tendon interposition, CMC joint arthrodesis and implant arthroplasty. In general, similar results can be expected with trapeziectomy alone or in combination with ligament reconstruction. Arthrodesis of the thumb CMC joint is favored for young, active individuals who have sustained posttraumatic osteoarthritis or in those individuals engaged in heavy labor. Nonunion of the arthrodesis is unusual as is arthrodesis malpositioning.

The results of implant arthroplasty for the thumb CMC joint have been largely disappointing. Complications ranging from implant failure to implant dislocation have been seen. Complications of the trapeziectomy procedure, with or without ligament reconstruction, include carpal instability, tendon rupture/irritation, superficial radial nerve neuritis, first metacarpal proximal migration resulting in scaphometacarpal impingement and tendon interposition herniation.[35]

Resection Arthroplasty

Trapeziectomy is one of the most common surgical procedures of the upper limb.[32] It can be performed in combination with ligament reconstruction, which we will describe below, or it can be performed in isolation with good results and is also termed the hematomaplasty by some authors. Despite the multiple available techniques, loss of trapezial space height does not seem to correlate with loss of pinch or grip strength directly, and no additional advantage was reported in prospective studies comparing simple trapeziectomy and trapeziectomy with combined soft tissue reconstruction.[25,36,37]

Surgical Technique

The procedure can be performed through either a dorsal or volar-radial/anterior approach (Wagner approach) to the thumb CMC joint. The dorsal approach consists of a straight dorsal incision over the joint, between the abductor pollicis longus and extensor pollicis brevis. The deep branch of the radial artery is isolated and protected as it courses between the base of the first and second metacarpals. The CMC joint capsule is incised and preserved when possible, and the trapezium is resected in a piecemeal fashion using a ¼-inch osteotome and a small ronguer. The anterior approach is an L-shaped incision at the junction between volar and dorsal skin and provides better exposure of the thumb metacarpal base.[38,39]

Trapeziectomy with Ligament Reconstruction and Tendon Interposition

Popularized by Burton and Pelligrini, this procedure seeks to provide additional stability to the CMC joint arthroplasty by reconstructing the intermetacarpal ligament. Other tendon reconstruction techniques include the Weilby procedure, whereby the FCR tendon (either whole or one-half) is woven around the APL tendon to create a lattice support for the thumb axis post trapeziectomy. Both procedures as well as simple trapeziectomy alone have enjoyed good mid-term results in terms of pain relief and overall patient satisfaction.

Surgical Technique

The procedure can be performed under regional or general anesthesia. A volar radial, also known as Wagner, incision is used. The branches of the radial sensory nerve are identified and protected. The trapezium is exposed and resected using either rongeur or osteotome. Advanced degenerative changes are typically seen on the volar aspect of the base of the first metacarpal as well as the distal articular surface of the trapezium (Fig. 57.9). Care must be taken to prevent flexor carpi radialis (FCR) injury. With a 2-mm bur, an oval window is made over the proximal dorsoradial aspect of the base of the first metacarpal through the metacarpal shaft to the base of the first metacarpal, and exits into the space previously occupied by the trapezium (Fig. 57.10). A 1-cm transverse incision is placed on the forearm approximately 10 cm proximal to the wrist flexion crease, at the level of the myotendinous junction of the flexor carpi radialis tendon (FCR). The FCR tendon is transected proximally then delivered into the

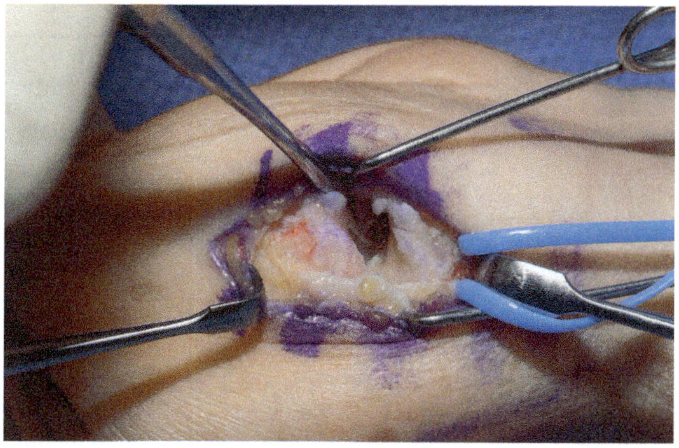

• **Fig. 57.9** Advanced articular changes are typically on the volar aspect of the base of the first metacarpal as well as the distal articular surface of the trapezium.

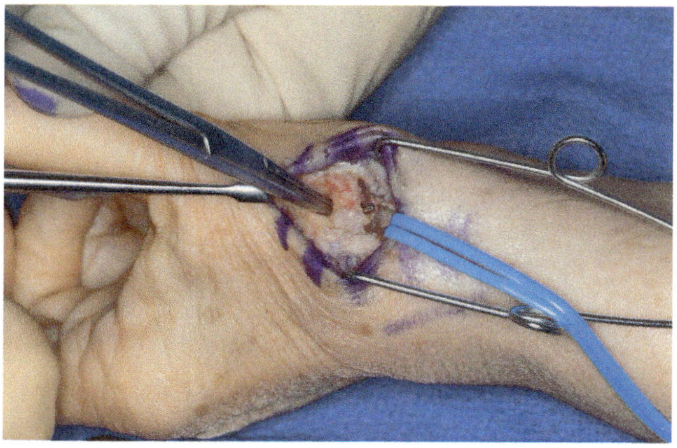

• **Fig. 57.10** Oval window made on the dorsal radial aspect of the base of the metacarpal communicating with the shaft of the first metacarpal and the void created by trapeziectomy (demonstrated with an angled forceps).

distal wound overlying the thumb metacarpal base (Fig. 57.11). Either the complete FCR or the radial one-half of the FCR tendon may be harvested. The FCR is delivered through the base of the first metacarpal and through the oval window with the aid of a small right-angle forceps. The FCR tendon is then sutured back to itself using 2-0 nonabsorbable sutures (Fig. 57.12). A second 2-0 nonabsorbable suture is placed deep into the anterior CMC joint capsule. The suture attached in the joint capsule is then woven through the remaining FCR tendon to create an anchovy by collapsing the FCR tendon down (Fig. 57.13) and then delivering the tendon mass into the trapezium space (Fig. 57.14). This filler FCR tendon or anchovy can be further supplemented with the use of heparin-soaked Gelfoam which can be packed around the tendon mass. The capsule of the thumb CMC joint is closed using a 4-0 absorbable suture. This is critical to prevent herniation of the tendon mass and Gelfoam, if used.

At this point an examination under anesthesia of the thumb MCP joint is performed. If hyperextension of the thumb MCP joint beyond 30 degrees exists (Fig. 57.15),

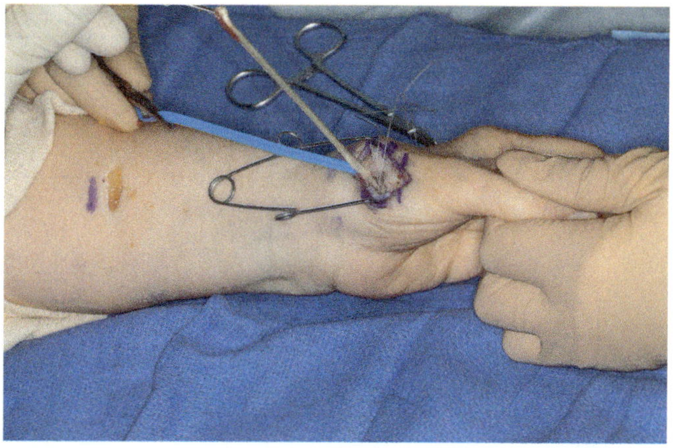

• **Fig. 57.11** Flexor carpi radialis tendon delivered into the distal void created by the resection of the trapezium.

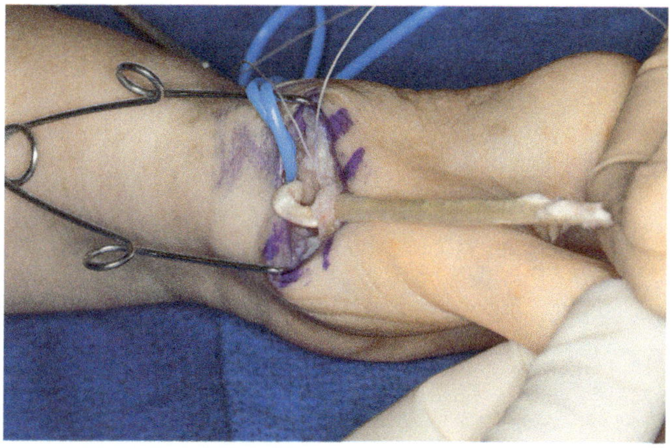

• **Fig. 57.12** Flexor carpi radialis tendon is passed through the metacarpal base then out the oval hole on the dorsal aspect of the base of the first metacarpal, stabilized on itself using a 2-0 absorbable suture.

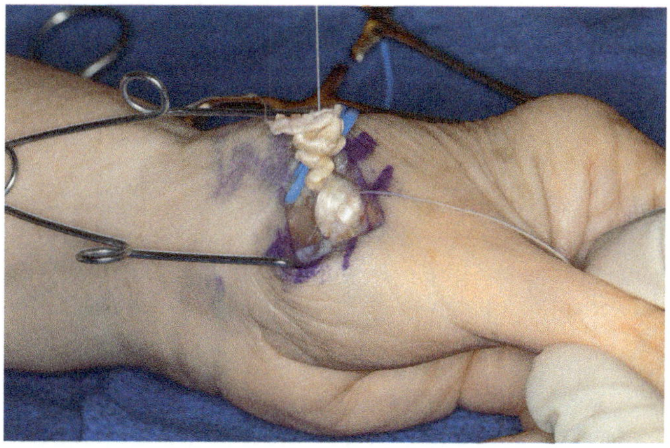

• **Fig. 57.13** Using a 2-0 nonabsorbable suture placed in the base of the void, the flexor carpi radialis tendon is then collapsed on itself, thereby creating an anchovy for the void created by the trapeziectomy.

then some form of stabilization of the thumb MCP joint is performed due to concerns over the metacarpal phalangeal joint instability ultimately leading to failure of the CMC joint reconstruction. The authors prefer stabilization of the thumb MCP joint with a single 0.045-inch K-wire

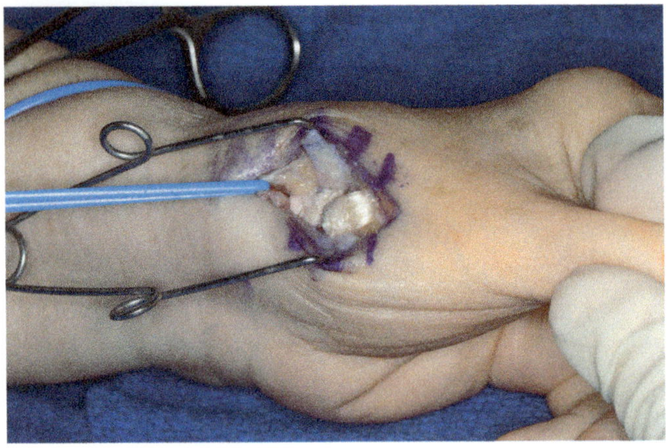

• **Fig. 57.14** Flexor carpi radialis anchovy in place.

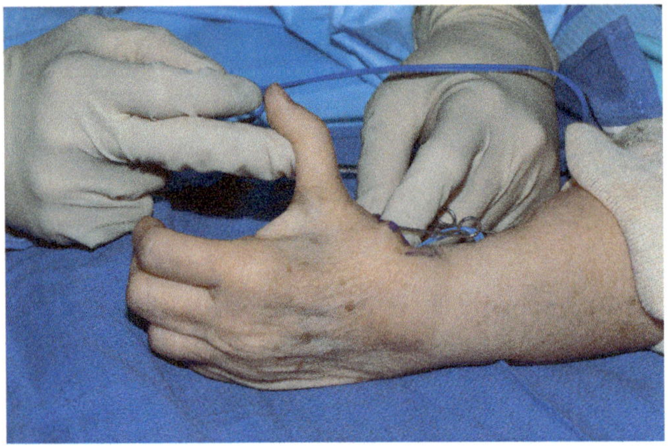

• **Fig. 57.15** Hyperextension instability of the thumb metacarpal phalangeal joint.

with the joint in the 45-degree flexed position for 6 weeks. Alternatives include advancement of the thumb MCP joint volar plate or, under some circumstances, thumb MCP joint arthrodesis.

Thumb CMC Arthrodesis

Indications for thumb CMC joint arthrodesis include idiopathic or posttraumatic arthritis in young, active patients or manual laborers. The procedure has a reported satisfaction rate of approximately 90%.[25]

Surgical Technique

We prefer a dorsal longitudinal incision centered on the projection of the CMC joint on the skin. The articular base of the first metacarpal and the distal articular surface of trapezium are denuded of cartilage using a rongeur. Ideally, two matching opposing surfaces are created. If this is not possible, consider autologous bone grafting. Osteosynthesis is then conducted with either crossing 0.045-inch K-wires, screws or 2.4-mm low-profile T-plate.[17] Optimal position for the carpometacarpal fusion is 35 degrees of palmar abduction, 10 degrees of radial abduction, and 15 degrees of pronation.

Rehabilitation

A thumb spica cast is applied for a total of 6 weeks. If K-wires are used, they are removed at the sixth postoperative week. A removable splint is then used until radiographic arthrodesis is achieved. Once the arthrodesis is deemed radiographically solid, graduated strengthening and return to activities is permitted.

References

1. Leung GJ, Rainsford KD, Kean WF. Osteoarthritis of the hand I: aetiology and pathogenesis, risk factors, investigation and diagnosis. *J Pharm Pharmacol.* 2014;66(3):339–346.
2. Kwok WY, Plevier JW, Rosendaal FR, et al. Risk factors for progression in hand osteoarthritis: a systematic review. *Arthr Care Res.* 2013;65(4):552–562.
3. Marshall M, Watt FE, Vincent TL, et al. Hand osteoarthritis: clinical phenotypes, molecular mechanisms and disease management. *Nat Rev Rheumatol.* 2018;14(11):641–656.
4. Hayashi D, Roemer FW, Guermazi A. Recent advances in research imaging of osteoarthritis with focus on MRI, ultrasound and hybrid imaging. *Clin Exp Rheumatol.* 2018;36(suppl)114(5):43–52.
5. Gabay O, Gabay C. Hand osteoarthritis: new insights. *Joint Bone Spine Rev Rhum.* 2013;80(2):130–134.
6. Bennell KL, Hall M, Hinman RS. Osteoarthritis year in review 2015: rehabilitation and outcomes. *Osteoarthritis Cartilage.* 2016;24(1):58–70.
7. Lue S, Koppikar S, Shaikh K, et al. Systematic review of non-surgical therapies for osteoarthritis of the hand: an update. *Osteoarthritis Cartilage.* 2017;25(9):1379–1389.
8. Kroon FP, Rubio R, Schoones JW, et al. Intra-articular therapies in the treatment of hand osteoarthritis: a systematic literature review. *Drugs Aging.* 2016;33(2):119–133.
9. Osteras N, Kjeken I, Smedslund G, et al. Exercise for hand osteoarthritis: a Cochrane systematic review. *J Rheumatol.* 2017;44(12):1850–1858.
10. Magni NE, McNair PJ, Rice DA. The effects of resistance training on muscle strength, joint pain, and hand function in individuals with hand osteoarthritis: a systematic review and meta-analysis. *Arthr Res Ther.* 2017;19(1):131.
11. Dickson DR, Mehta SS, Nuttall D, et al. A systematic review of distal interphalangeal joint arthrodesis. *J Hand Microsurg.* 2014;6(2):74–84.
12. Fowler JR, Baratz ME. Distal interphalangeal joint arthrodesis. *J Hand Surg.* 2014;39(1):126–128.
13. Satteson ES, Langford MA, Li Z. The management of complications of small joint arthrodesis and arthroplasty. *Hand Clin.* 2015;31(2):243–266.
14. Herren DB. Current European practice in the treatment of proximal interphalangeal joint arthritis. *Hand Clin.* 2017;33(3):489–500.
15. Jung J, Haghverdian B, Gupta R. Proximal interphalangeal joint fusion: indications and techniques. *Hand Clin.* 2018;34(2):177–184.
16. Cheah AE, Yao J. Surgical approaches to the proximal interphalangeal joint. *J Hand Surg.* 2016;41(2):294–305.
17. Murray PM. Treatment of the osteoarthritic hand and thumb. In: 7th edn. *Green's Operative Hand Surgery.* Vol. 1. Elsevier; 2017.
18. Zhu AF, Rahgozar P, Chung KC. Advances in proximal interphalangeal joint arthroplasty: biomechanics and biomaterials. *Hand Clin.* 2018;34(2):185–194.

19. Srnec JJ, Wagner ER, Rizzo M. Implant arthroplasty for proximal interphalangeal, metacarpophalangeal, and trapeziometacarpal joint degeneration. *J Hand Surg*. 2017;42(10):817–825.
20. Adkinson JM, Chung KC. Advances in small joint arthroplasty of the hand. *Plast Reconstr Surg*. 2014;134(6):1260–1268.
21. Yamamoto M, Malay S, Fujihara Y, et al. A systematic review of different implants and approaches for proximal interphalangeal joint arthroplasty. *Plast Reconstr Surg*. 2017;139(5):1139e–1151e.
22. Murray PM, Linscheid RL, Cooney 3rd WP, et al. Long-term outcomes of proximal interphalangeal joint surface replacement arthroplasty. *J Bone Joint Surg Am*. 2012;94(12):1120–1128.
23. Aversano FJ, Calfee RP. Salvaging a failed proximal interphalangeal joint implant. *Hand Clin*. 2018;34(2):217–227.
24. Martin AS, Awan HM. Metacarpophalangeal arthroplasty for osteoarthritis. *J Hand Surg*. 2015;40(9):1871–1872.
25. Bakri K, Moran SL. Thumb carpometacarpal arthritis. *Plast Reconstr Surg*. 2015;135(2):508–520.
26. Altman R, Alarcon G, Appelrouth D, et al. The American College of Rheumatology criteria for the classification and reporting of osteoarthritis of the hand. *Arthritis Rheum*. 1990;33(11):1601–1610.
27. Zhang W, Doherty M, Leeb BF, et al. EULAR evidence-based recommendations for the diagnosis of hand osteoarthritis: report of a task force of ESCISIT. *Ann Rheum Dis*. 2009;68(1):8–17.
28. Kloppenburg M, van Beest S, Kroon FPB. Thumb base osteoarthritis: a hand osteoarthritis subset requiring a distinct approach. *Best Pract Res Clin Rheumatol*. 2017;31(5):649–660.
29. Melville DM, Taljanovic MS, Scalcione LR, et al. Imaging and management of thumb carpometacarpal joint osteoarthritis. *Skeletal Radiol*. 2015;44(2):165–177.
30. Berger AJ, Meals RA. Management of osteoarthrosis of the thumb joints. *J Hand Surg*. 2015;40(4):843–850.
31. Eaton RG, Glickel SZ. Trapeziometacarpal osteoarthritis: staging as a rationale for treatment. *Hand Clin*. 1987;3(4):455–471.
32. Baker RH, Al-Shukri J, Davis TR. Evidence-based medicine: thumb basal joint arthritis. *Plast Reconstr Surg*. 2017;139(1):256e–266e.
33. Ahern M, Skyllas J, Wajon A, et al. The effectiveness of physical therapies for patients with base of thumb osteoarthritis: systematic review and meta-analysis. *Musculoskeletal Sci Pract*. 2018;35:46–54.
34. Spaans AJ, van Minnen LP, Kon M, et al. Conservative treatment of thumb base osteoarthritis: a systematic review. *J Hand Surg*. 2015;40(1):16–21. e11–16.
35. Rhee PC, Shin AY. Complications of trapeziectomy with or without suspension arthroplasty. *J Hand Surg*. 2014;39(4):781–783; quiz 784.
36. Wajon A, Vinycomb T, Carr E, Edmunds I, Ada L. Surgery for thumb (trapeziometacarpal joint) osteoarthritis. *Cochrane Database Syst Rev*. 2015;(2):CD004631.
37. Li YK, White C, Ignacy TA, et al. Comparison of trapeziectomy and trapeziectomy with ligament reconstruction and tendon interposition: a systematic literature review. *Plast Reconstr Surg*. 2011;128(1):199–207.
38. Gay AM, Cerlier A, Iniesta A, et al. Surgery for trapeziometacarpal osteoarthritis. *Hand Surg Rehabil*. 2016;35(4):238–249.
39. Mahoney JD, Meals RA. Trapeziectomy. *Hand Clin*. 2006;22(2):165–169.

58
Wrist Pathology

ODED BEN-AMOTZ, SHAUN D. MENDENHALL,
JASON WINK, AND L. SCOTT LEVIN

Physical Examination of the Wrist

When performing a physical examination of the wrist, it is helpful to approach the wrist in a systematic fashion based on anatomical regions. Knowledge of anatomical landmarks will help the practitioner develop a differential diagnosis, while several exam maneuvers can help in making the correct diagnosis. The importance of wrist palpation based on anatomical region cannot be understated. Imaging can then be used to aid in the diagnostic process. In this chapter, we will use an anatomical approach to the wrist to identify and better understand commonly seen wrist pathologies and their treatments.

Radial-Sided Wrist Pain

The bones, tendons, and ligaments that lie on the radial side of the wrist can all be sources of pain for the patient. The first extensor compartment contains the extensor pollicis brevis (EPB) and abductor pollicis longus (APL) tendons and can be a source of significant pain, known as De Quervain's tenosynovitis. These tendons can be identified making up the lateral/radial border of the anatomical snuffbox at the level of the radial styloid. Pain with palpation over this compartment or a Finkelstein's test – clasping the thumb in the palm with ulnar deviation of the wrist – will confirm the diagnosis. Pain elicited with this maneuver more proximal in the forearm can be the result of intersection syndrome. Palpating just distal to the radial styloid in the anatomical snuffbox can indicate scaphoid pathology. The distal pole of the scaphoid can be palpated at the base of the thenar eminence. This can be confirmed by ranging the wrist from radial to ulnar deviation and feeling the scaphoid flex and extend. Palpating just distal to the anatomical snuffbox can elicit tenderness in the scaphoid–trapezium–trapezoid (STT) or trapezium–metacarpal (carpometacarpal, CMC) joint of the thumb. Pain in this region is commonly seen in CMC arthritis.

Central Wrist Pain

Just ulnar to the anatomical snuffbox on the dorsal side of the wrist is the "soft spot," which is the region of the scapholunate (SL) ligament. The Watson shift test can be performed to assess the integrity of the SL ligament; this is performed by moving the wrist from ulnar hyperextension to radial flexion while pressing on the scaphoid tubercle volarly and assessing for a "clunk." The contralateral wrist should always be assessed for comparison. Pain in the dorsal midline of the wrist can also be the result of Kienböck's disease. The distal radioulnar joint (DRUJ) is assessed more proximally. A radioulnar ballottement test can be used to test for congruency of the DRUJ.

Ulnar-Sided Wrist Pain

The ulnar-sided wrist exam should start by palpating the ulnar head and ulnar styloid. Pain with palpation of the ulnar soft spot or fovea can be an indication of triangular fibrocartilage complex (TFCC) pathology. Injury to the TFCC can be confirmed with magnetic resonance imaging (MRI) or arthroscopy. Pain elicited by pushing the distal ulna in a radial direction like a "piano key" is a sign of DRUJ instability or injury. Immediately dorsal to the ulnar soft spot lies the extensor carpi ulnaris (ECU) tendon. Pain and snapping while performing ulnar flexion and supination of the wrist indicates ECU tendinitis and subluxation respectively. Pain on the volar side of the ulnar wrist is likely due to injury to the pisiform or hook of the hamate. This can be seen from both arthritic and traumatic pathologies.

Kienböck's Disease

Pest first described avascular necrosis of the lunate based on cadaveric dissections although the disease gets its name from radiologist Robert Kienböck. Despite Kienböck's disease being described over 100 years ago, the etiology and natural history are not clearly understood and it is thought to result from a vascular etiology.[1] Kienböck's disease presents in patients as wrist pain, usually located centrally over the dorsum of the wrist, and is rarely bilateral. Pain is usually present with wrist motion, but as the disease progresses, pain at rest is frequent. This diagnosis is commonly seen in men 20–40 years of age. It was originally thought that trauma to the lunate likely results in Kienböck's disease, although long-term follow-up studies have shown that lunate fractures do not reliably develop avascular necrosis, even with an ulnar negative variance.[2] Ulnar negative variance has been associated with Kienböck's disease, prompting many to point to this anatomical feature as a possible etiology. Hulten's classic study in 1928 showed an association between ulnar negative variance and Kienböck's disease but more recent studies do not demonstrate a clear correlation.[3]

Clinical Evaluation

The clinical evaluation of the patient with Kienböck's disease starts with a thorough physical exam of the wrist. However, the exam findings for Kienböck's disease are usually nonspecific. Dorsal wrist pain, often with motion or activity, is the main physical exam finding. Radiographic evaluation is followed by the physical exam. Kienböck's disease can be diagnosed by correlating the physical exam with radiographs, however imaging using MRI is often necessary for definitive diagnosis. Radiographs are evaluated for sclerosis of the lunate and negative ulnar variance.

Staging and Treatment

Radiographs and MRI are used to stage Kienböck's disease. The staging system as presented by Lichtman and associates is the most popular and helps guide treatment and determine prognosis.[4] The treatment of Kienböck's disease is based on the staging and will be discussed together. Treatments of Kienböck's disease are evolving with advances in microsurgery and 3D printing technology.

Stage I

Symptoms of stage I Kienböck's disease are usually nonspecific and mimic wrist sprains or synovitis. Radiographs are usually normal in stage I Kienböck's and represent precollapse and early appearance of the disease. MRI will demonstrate low signal on T1- and T2-weighted images in the entirety of the lunate. If the low signal is localized to a specific area of the lunate on T1-weighted images then other more focal diagnoses are more likely. If T2-weighted images show increased signal, this can be a sign of revascularization and MRI can be used to monitor resolution of disease. Stage I disease is best treated nonoperatively with a splint. Most people advocate for at least 3 months of splint use. If symptoms do not improve a radial shortening osteotomy in the setting of negative ulnar variance would then be considered.

Stage II

Radiographs become diagnostic or at least suggestive of Kienböck's disease during stage II. One typically finds increased sclerosis of the lunate with possible fracture lines or early collapse. MRI continues to be diagnostic with the entire lunate showing low T1 and T2 signal intensity. Lunate height is maintained and symptoms usually mimic chronic wrist synovitis. Treatment usually involves a trial of splinting, although at this stage a radial shortening osteotomy is more aggressively pursued to prevent advancement of the disease and collapse of the lunate.

Stage IIIA

Stages II and IIIA are usually discussed together because the treatment options are the same. Stage IIIA Kienböck's disease demonstrates collapse of the lunate; however, there is maintenance of carpal height and no signs of arthritis. The anterior–posterior distance of the lunate is usually increased on the lateral radiograph. Sclerosis is present and MRI findings of low signal intensity on T1- and T2-weighted images remain consistent. The treatment of stage II and stage IIIA disease should start with initiating supportive care and immobilization. A surgeon should not rush to surgery during this stage of treatment and a course of nonoperative treatment should be initiated. The severity of the patient's symptoms should dictate whether to proceed with surgical treatment or continue with nonoperative management. The surgical treatment options differ based on ulnar variance.

Stage II and IIIA with Ulnar Negative Variance

When ulnar variance is negative, it is thought that increased pressure from the lunate fossa of the distal radius is the cause of the symptoms. Unloading and decreasing the pressure on the lunate through a radial shortening osteotomy is usually the treatment of choice. One study demonstrated 93% of patients had diminished pain after a radial shortening osteotomy.[5] Ulnar lengthening osteotomy has been described for stage II and IIIA disease with ulnar negative variance but this is generally considered a more difficult procedure with higher complications. Ulnar lengthening requires bone grafting and healing at two osteotomy sites, both the proximal and distal ends.

Stage II and IIIA with Ulnar Positive or Neutral Variance

Revascularization procedures are most appropriate in stage II and IIIA with ulnar positive or neutral variance. A number of revascularization procedures have been described, including vascularized pedicle transfer from the distal radius, vascularized pisiform transfer, vascularized bone graft from the metacarpal, and free vascularized grafts from the iliac crest, medial femoral condyle or medial femoral trochlea. The most popular vascularized pedicle transfer is from the distal radius and is the 4,5 extensor compartment artery (ECA)[6] (Fig. 58.1). In more advanced disease, coronal fractures of the lunate can be fixated in preparation for a vascularized osteochondral graft.[7] These procedures may be accompanied by joint leveling procedures such as capitate shortening, radius osteotomy or external fixation.

Stage IIIB

Stage IIIB is characterized by lunate collapse, rotation of the scaphoid, and loss of carpal height. Revascularization procedures are usually not considered after lunate collapse and

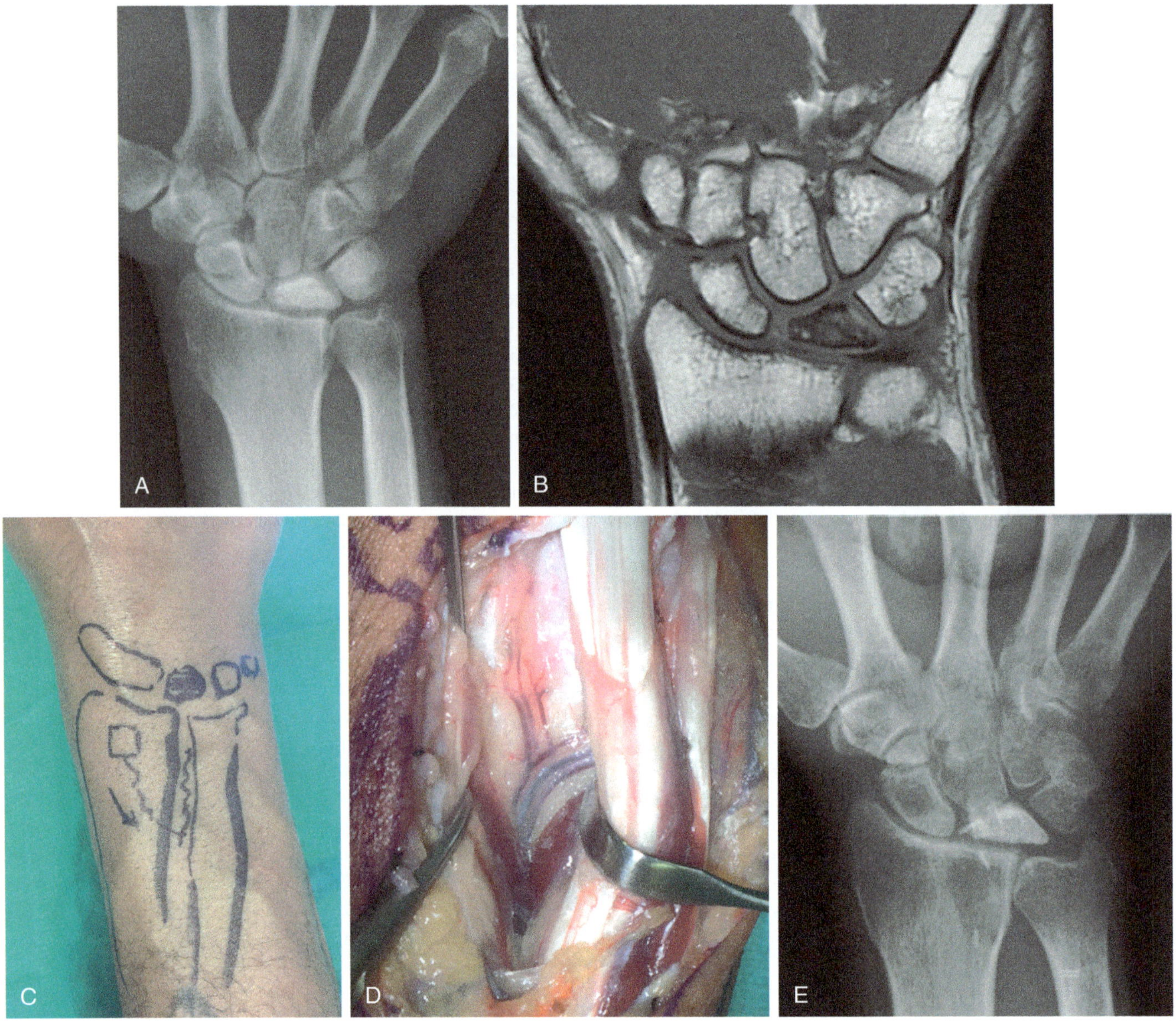

• **Fig. 58.1** This is a case of a 38-year-old laborer with stage IIIA Kienböck's disease in his dominant hand which was treated with a 4,5 ECA pedicled bone graft. (A) Plain radiograph shows increased opacity of the lunate with an ulnar neutral wrist and (B) MRI reveals presence of avascular necrosis. (C) Preoperative markings. (D) The flap was dissected and the vascular arcade perfusing the distal radius where the graft was taken is clearly visualized. (E) Postoperative radiographs after K-wire fixation was removed. (Case courtesy L. Scott Levin, MD.)

loss of carpal height because of the destruction of normal anatomical architecture. There is some controversy about the best way to treat stage IIIB disease and some authors have had good results with limited wrist arthrodesis, including scaphocapitate arthrodesis and scaphotrapezium–trapezoid arthrodesis. Although controversial, other authors have had good results with radial shortening osteotomies.[8] Lunate excision with interposition arthroplasty or proximal row carpectomy are additional salvage procedures that have been described. A recent case report has been published describing the implantation of a 3D-printed lunate prosthesis with near normal recovery of wrist motion at 12 months postoperatively.[9] Another very promising new treatment for stage II and III Kienböck's is the free medial femoral trochlea flap. In a report by Bürger et al, 13 of 16 patients went on to have complete pain relief with similar range of motion as before surgery. Grip strength was 85% of the contralateral hand.[10,11]

Stage IV

Stage IV is characterized by collapse of the lunate and degenerative changes in the radiocarpal and midcarpal joints. Joint leveling or revascularization procedures are not performed once degenerative changes appear. Many patients can be managed nonoperatively with supportive care such as splints, antiinflammatory medications, and activity modification. In patients who have failed nonoperative management, salvage procedures can be considered such as limited or total wrist arthrodesis or proximal row carpectomy. For a proximal row carpectomy to reliably provide pain relief, the proximal capitate and lunate fossa must be free from degenerative changes since they will make up the new radiocarpal articulation.

De Quervain's Tenosynovitis

De Quervain's tenosynovitis causes pain on the radial side of the wrist, centered over the first extensor compartment. Active radial deviation of the wrist or passive ulnar deviation causes severe pain over the tendons of the first dorsal compartment. This presentation is commonly seen with new mothers or more recently with frequent cell phone texting users.[12] The first dorsal compartment tendon sheath can be up to five times its normal size due to fibrous tissue deposition and may feel like a mass over the radial styloid. De Quervain's tenosynovitis is a myxoid degeneration of the first dorsal compartment. Although nonsteroidal antiinflammatory medications are a first-line treatment, it is not an acute inflammatory process. Often the tendon sheath can be easily palpated due to its enlarged size. There is known to be significant anatomical variation of the first extensor compartment that is associated with increased risk for developing tenosynovitis, including multiple slips of APL. A septum within the first compartment has also been found in 50% of individuals in cadaver studies.[13]

Intersection syndrome should be ruled out during the diagnosis of De Quervain's tenosynovitis. Intersection syndrome causes pain in an area about 4 cm proximal to the radial styloid and there are subtle differences. It is caused when pain, swelling, and sometimes crepitus occurs because the outcropping muscle bellies of the APL and EPB intersect with the long wrist extensors on the dorsum of the forearm. This should also not be confused with a neuropathy of the radial sensory nerve as it exits the deeper tissues between brachioradialis and extensor carpi radialis longus. This is known as Wartenberg's syndrome.

Diagnosis of de Quervain's tenosynovitis is usually done with a patient history and physical exam. Imaging studies are usually not required. Pain over the first dorsal compartment on the radial aspect of the wrist, which is made worse with palpation, is the first physical exam finding. A thickened tendon sheath and pain with active radial deviation are also common symptoms. Finkelstein's maneuver is the classic physical exam maneuver used to aid in the diagnosis, although this can also be positive in intersection syndrome. Ultrasound can also be used to visualize the tendons and inflammation present within the tendon sheath, and can aid in steroid injection directly into the sheath, but is rarely used.

Initiation of nonsurgical treatments such as watchful waiting, splinting, nonsteroidal antiinflammatory medication, and steroid injections into the first extensor compartment should be considered. Multiple studies have shown successful treatment with each of these nonsurgical techniques. The authors recommend nonsurgical treatment be initiated upon diagnosis. We recommend a removable thumb spica splint, nonsteroidal antiinflammatory medications, and steroid injection into the compartment. Cases that are refractory to nonsurgical management should be considered for surgical release.

Surgical release of the first extensor compartment is very successful and produces reliable, long-term pain relief. Open surgery through a small horizontal incision is the authors' preferred method of treatment. Care is taken to make incision through the sheath as dorsal as possible to decrease the risk of volar tendon subluxation postoperatively. Branches of the radial sensory nerve are in or near the operative site and should be carefully identified and/or avoided. These branches lie deep to the venous structures of the forearm. If a branch of the radial sensory nerve is cut during surgery, a painful neuroma can result. When performing the surgery, it is necessary to thoroughly explore the first extensor compartment due to significant anatomical variation, including presence of a septum and multiple slips of APL.

Scaphoid Fractures

The scaphoid is most commonly injured by a fall on an outstretched hand, resulting in radial-sided wrist pain and, classically, snuffbox tenderness. Scaphoid fractures represent 60% of all carpal bone fractures. They can occur as isolated trauma or in association with other bony or ligamentous injuries of the distal radius and carpal bones. The triquetrum is the second most commonly fractured carpal bone.

The distally based blood supply of the scaphoid makes fractures notoriously difficult to heal. The result is a high incidence of delayed union, nonunion, and avascular necrosis. Eighty percent of the scaphoid is covered in articular cartilage, which limits its blood supply entry points. The majority of the blood supply to the scaphoid comes from the dorsal scaphoid branches of the radial artery, with a minority of the blood supply from the volar scaphoid branches. These vessels enter the scaphoid relatively distally, resulting in purely intraosseous perfusion of the proximal pole. The tenuous blood supply of the proximal pole explains the reported avascular necrosis that occurs in 13%–50% of scaphoid fractures.

Early diagnosis and treatment are important since scaphoid fractures that are left untreated have a higher incidence of nonunion, malunion, and avascular necrosis. Scaphoid nonunion is difficult to treat and if left untreated will progress to carpal collapse and degenerative arthritis, specifically, scaphoid nonunion advanced collapse (SNAC wrist).

Diagnosis begins with a good history and physical exam as most patients report a recent history of trauma to the hand and wrist. Patients typically have pain on the radial side of the wrist, specifically in the anatomical snuffbox, decreased range of wrist motion, decreased grip strength, and pain with thumb motion. Adequate radiographs, including posteroanterior (PA), lateral, pronated oblique, supinated oblique, and a PA with ulnar deviation (scaphoid view), are essential. However, X-rays often show no evidence of fracture. It is thought that initial radiography misses 15%–20% of scaphoid fractures.[14] When there are signs of scaphoid fracture on history and physical exam but no radiographic evidence, the traditional algorithm would be to cast the patient in a short arm thumb spica cast and repeat the X-rays in 2 weeks. After 2 weeks, there is usually sufficient resorption at the fracture site to visualize a scaphoid fracture on radiographs. Advanced imaging studies, such as MRI and computed tomography (CT) scans, can help in the diagnosis and in surgical planning. MRI is the preferred test if the diagnosis of a scaphoid fracture is in question. The sensitivity and specificity of diagnosing a fracture is 90%–100% with MRI. CT scans show bone structure better than MRI and are therefore better in determining displacement of a fracture or in visualizing bony healing. However, a CT scan should be used with caution in diagnosing an occult scaphoid fracture because there is a high rate of overdiagnosis with CT (false-positives), most likely due to normal vascular foramina appearing as a fracture. Therefore, a CT scan is better used in surgical decision-making to determine if a fracture seen on radiographs is displaced or not and for operative planning.

Cast immobilization for 8–12 weeks can successfully treat most nondisplaced or minimally displaced scaphoid fractures. There is no consensus on whether to use a short arm or long arm cast, although data from a small randomized trial suggests an initial period of long arm casting can decrease time to union and decrease the nonunion rate.[15] A long arm cast theoretically prohibits wrist rotation and shear stresses on the scaphoid. If treating a scaphoid fracture nonoperatively, the authors recommend using a long arm cast for the first 4–6 weeks and then changing to a short arm cast for the duration of the treatment. The disadvantages to cast treatment are increased time to healing, frequent office visits, increased need for radiographs, potential for skin breakdown, and stiffness. There is high-level data that suggests immobilization of the thumb is not necessary and may in fact be detrimental to healing.[16]

Some authors have advocated immediate percutaneous internal fixation of minimally displaced and nondisplaced scaphoid fractures. The reasons behind the trend to immediate percutaneous fixation of these fractures are a decreased time to healing, faster return to sports or work, and a favorable economic analysis in terms of social life and return to work.[17,18] There appear to be similar functional outcomes at 2 years of cast versus percutaneous treatment of nondisplaced or minimally displaced scaphoid fractures.

Internal fixation is indicated in scaphoid fractures with displacement of more than 1 mm on any radiographic view. Scaphoid fractures with displacement have a much higher probability of progressing to a nonunion with cast immobilization compared with internal fixation. The headless compression screw is the most accepted technique for fixation of scaphoid fractures. It has the advantage of being recessed below the articular surface of the scaphoid. The scaphoid is a curved bone, shaped much like a cashew, although there can be significant variability. The shape of the scaphoid makes screw fixation challenging; for the best results, the screw should be placed down the central axis of the scaphoid in all dimensions. Breaching of the scaphoid with the screw during fixation should be avoided since it will lead to early degenerative arthritis. Healing rates of 95% have been reported with adequate screw fixation.

Scaphoid Nonunions

Scaphoid nonunions develop in about 5% of scaphoid fractures and are usually the result of inadequate immobilization, displacement, or delayed diagnosis. Scaphoid nonunions are difficult because of the tenuous blood supply of the proximal pole and resultant avascular necrosis, the tendency for the scaphoid to collapse into a "humpback deformity," and the systematic progression to a SNAC wrist.

Successful treatment of scaphoid nonunions without collapse, using open and percutaneous techniques, has been described. Percutaneous fixation of scaphoid nonunions without collapse or displacement has been described with a cannulated compression screw.[19] Even with resorption of bone at the fracture site, the union rates of percutaneous screw fixation is high. The Matti–Russe technique has traditionally been the treatment of choice for scaphoid nonunions without collapse.[20] This technique uses corticocancellous pieces of bone taken from the iliac crest and placed into the scaphoid after the fibrous tissue from the nonunion has been removed. Modifications of the Matti–Russe technique have taken the graft from the distal radius instead of the iliac crest[21] or placed a corticocancellous graft with either screw or Kirschner wire (K–wire) fixation. The Matti–Russe technique has been reported to provide union in up to 90% of patients. The majority of patients who did not achieve union were reported to have avascular necrosis of the proximal pole, and this technique is not generally recommended for patients with avascular necrosis.

Treatment of scaphoid nonunions with collapse ("humpback deformity") is more difficult since this requires a need for reduction of the deformity, replacement of the lost bone, and stable fixation. Volar wedge fixation with a tricorticocancellous bone graft taken from the iliac crest has been a successful way to correct a humpback deformity and replace lost bone. This technique is usually augmented with screw fixation down the central axis of the scaphoid. Recently, there have been published reports of treating scaphoid nonunions with humpback deformity without structural bone graft and only placing cancellous bone graft. The reduction is performed open through a volar approach and assisted with K-wires, while a screw fixation provides a stable construct for healing. Bone graft is then harvested from the distal radius or iliac crest and packed around the screw to replace the bone lost from the collapse.[22] The good results reported with these techniques have not been duplicated when the proximal pole has gone onto avascular necrosis.

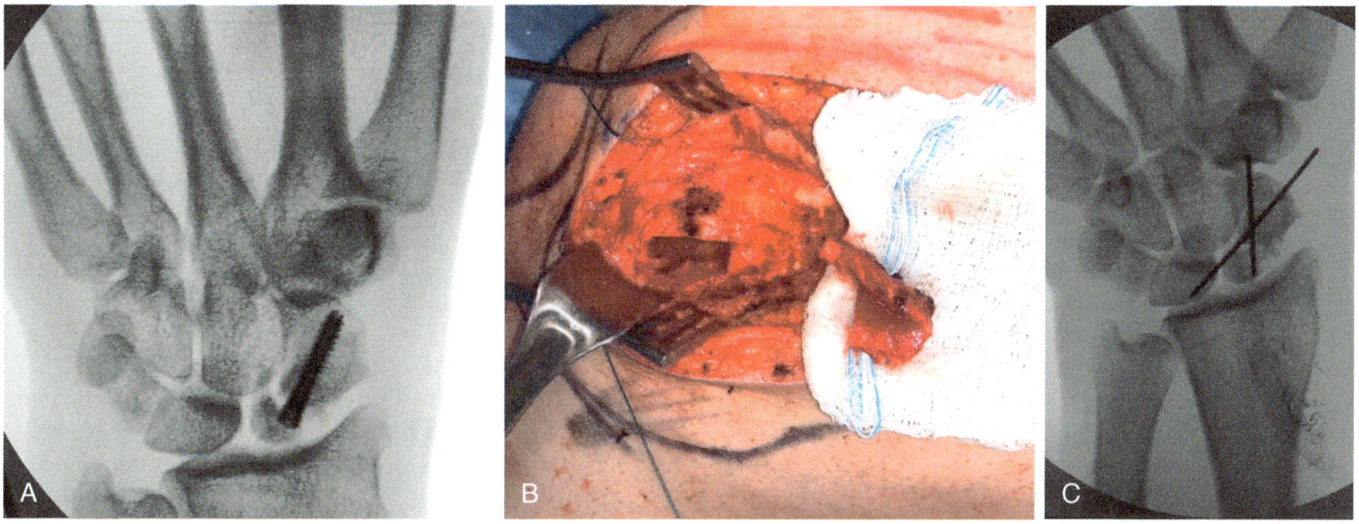

• **Fig. 58.2** Representative case of a patient presenting with scaphoid nonunion after a proximal pole scaphoid fracture originally treated with cannulated screw fixation. (A) PA X-ray view of the wrist clearly displays the nonunited fracture. (B) A free medial femoral condyle vascularized bone flap was performed. Note the corticocancellous bone flap dissected on the descending geniculate vessels prior to final ligation and the resulting defect in the medial femoral condyle. (C) The flap was then fixated within the bony defect with two K-wires and anastomosis was performed to the radial artery and venae comitantes. (Case courtesy Shaun Mendenhall, MD.)

Treatment of scaphoid nonunions with avascular necrosis of the proximal pole have been most successfully treated with vascularized bone grafts. The most popular vascularized bone graft is the 1,2 intercompartmental supraretinacular artery (1,2 ICSRA) bone graft taken from the dorsal aspect of the distal radius.[23] The vascular anatomy of the 1,2 ICSRA is consistent, but very small. Recent reports have shown about a 75% union rate with use of the 1,2 ICSRA vascularized graft. A capsular-based vascularized bone graft has been described by Sotereanos et al and based off the artery of the base of the fourth dorsal compartment.[24] This technique has been praised for its simplicity. However, both these techniques provide only a small amount of bone for reconstructing a humpback deformity and the vascular pedicles are tenuous. Recently, free vascularized bone grafts taken from the medial femoral condyle (MFC) or trochlea (MFT) and based off either the longitudinal (MFC) or transverse (MFT) branches of the descending geniculate artery has been described.[25] The free vascularized medial femoral condyle flap can be taken without articular cartilage or with articular cartilage as a medial femoral trochlea flap utilizing the transverse branch of the descending geniculate artery, with or without a chimeric skin paddle.[26] The vascular pedicle of these flaps is sufficiently robust and is usually anastomosed end-to-side into the radial artery in the anatomical snuffbox or volar wrist. The donor sites of each of these flaps appear to be well tolerated, with patients returning to normal lower extremity function[27] (Fig. 58.2). In the setting of proximal pole avascular necrosis, we prefer to core out the proximal pole bone, preserving the cartilaginous cap and the scapholunate ligament, and place the bone graft as a dowel into the scaphoid.[28]

Scapholunate Dissociation

Injuries to the scapholunate (SL) joint are part of a broader category of pathology termed carpal instability dissociative (CID). CID is a dissociation between two bones of the same carpal row. Common injuries such as SL dissociation (SLD), lunotriquetral (LT) dissociation (discussed later), unstable scaphoid fractures, inflammatory arthritis, or advanced Kienböck's disease can cause CID. Carpal instability nondissociative (CIND) describes pathology between the bones of two separate carpal rows.

SLD is caused by an injury to the SL ligament. It represents a wide spectrum of pathology, ranging from minor sprain of the scapholunate ligament to total acute perilunate dislocation. The severity of the perilunate injury is described using the Mayfield classification. Complete SLD results in the lunate-triquetrum rotating into an extended position while the scaphoid assumes a flexed position as it rotates around the radioscaphocapitate ligament without the constraint of the SL ligament. These classic pathological positions of the scaphoid and the lunate–triquetrum are termed dorsal intercalated segmental instability (DISI) and is best identified on a lateral radiograph with an increased SL angle (normal SL angle = 30–60 degrees). The DISI deformity caused by SLD is in contrast to the resultant volar intercalated segmental instability (VISI) caused by LT dissociation (see later). This results in the scaphoid and lunate taking a flexed position and the triquetrum in an extended position without the constraint of the LT ligament. SLD is part of a process of carpal destabilization that can lead to scapholunate advanced collapse (SLAC) and severe degenerative arthritis. The SL ligament is thought to be stronger on the dorsal side, while the LT ligament is thought to be stronger on the volar side of the hand.

SLD is usually caused by a fall on a hyperextended and ulnar deviated hand. A low index of suspicion is needed for diagnosis since many of these injuries go undiagnosed because of the subtle physical exam and radiographic findings. Low-grade (predynamic) sprains to the SL ligament may have no discrete physical exam or radiographic finding and are usually diagnosed on arthroscopy. Patients with acute or chronic SLD usually have pain localized at the scapholunate ligament when palpated over the dorsal wrist soft spot just distal to Lister's tubercle. Some patients will also have pain in the anatomical snuff box and over the scaphoid tubercle.

The scaphoid shift test is a dynamic test that aids in the diagnosis of complete SL ligament tears. The scaphoid shift test, or Watson test, produces abnormal scapholunate motion and pain when positive. The examiner places the thumb over the scaphoid tubercle (volar) and the other four fingers on the distal radius (dorsal) and pushes the scaphoid in a dorsal direction with the thumb. The examiner then moves the patient's wrist from ulnar deviation (scaphoid extended) to radial deviation (scaphoid flexed). If there is a tear in the scapholunate ligament with instability, the scaphoid will be unable to be flexed and will instead be subluxated from the dorsal aspect of the distal radius. When the pressure is released from the scaphoid, the scaphoid will reduce back into anatomical position with a classic "clunking" sound. This test is helpful in diagnosis but one should be aware of the low specificity of the maneuver. The contralateral side should also always be tested for comparison.

The scapholunate ballottement test is performed by holding the lunate firmly with thumb and index finger of one hand and the scaphoid with the thumb and index of the other hand. The scaphoid and lunate are then shifted volar and palmar opposite to each other. An excessive amount of motion, pain, and crepitus are signs of a positive result.

The classic radiographic sign of SLD is an increased distance between the scaphoid and the lunate. An increased scapholunate distance on radiographs has been called the "Terry Thomas" sign (in reference to the English film comedian's space between his two front teeth). This often can only be seen in the more chronic setting as the other stabilizing ligaments of the carpal bones have become attenuated. However, the normal three views of the wrist (posteroanterior (PA), oblique, lateral) may not show an increased distance and as a result there is a high false-negative incidence. Special radiographic views have been described that center the X-ray beam tangentially to the SL joint and therefore show the true extent of the SL distance. The clenched fist view and the Moneim view (PA with 20 degrees of hyperpronation) are both helpful in better visualizing the scapholunate distance. A distance of 5 mm or more is diagnostic of SLD. The clenched fist view forces the capitate to press down on the SL interval and can cause widening if an injury is present.

The lateral radiograph should be examined carefully for DISI. An increase in the SL angle compared to the contralateral side or a unilateral SL angle of 70 degrees (normal range is 30–60 degrees) usually indicates increased flexion or rotatory subluxation of the scaphoid. A DISI deformity is seen in advanced stages of SLD and may not be present in occult or predynamic SLD.

Often, advanced imaging is needed to confirm a suspected SLD. MRI is the advanced imaging of choice used by the authors. The gold standard of SL injury diagnosis would be direct visualization during arthroscopy.

Treatment

The treatment of SLD is based on the stage of the injury at the time of treatment. SLD is separated into six different stages which progress from occult SL injury to SLAC wrist. When determining the severity of the injury and subsequent treatment, there are five questions proposed by Garcia-Elias et al[29] that help the surgeon understand the pathology and provide a framework for treatment.

1. Is the dorsal SL ligament intact?
2. Does the dorsal SL ligament have enough tissue to repair?
3. Is the scaphoid posture normal?
4. Is any carpal malalignment reducible?
5. Is the cartilage on the radiocarpal and midcarpal surfaces normal?

Stage I SLD presents as an occult SL injury with only a partial tear of the SL ligament. The dorsal SL ligament is usually intact. Many stage I SLD injuries are diagnosed late, but if they are diagnosed early they may benefit from temporary pinning or nonoperative treatment, including casting, splinting, nonsteroidal antiinflammatory medications, and therapy.

Stage II SLD is characterized by dynamic instability, a complete tear of the SL ligament, and enough SL ligament tissue remaining to repair. Patients typically have pain and instability under loading conditions. By definition, there is no fixed deformity. Patients are treated with open repair of the SL ligament, which can be accomplished by a number of methods. Commonly, the SL ligament tears off of the scaphoid and remains attached to the lunate. Direct repair can be done with suture using transosseous suture holes, bone tunnels or suture anchors. K-wires are helpful in reducing the scaphoid and lunate, and providing temporary fixation or headless screw fixation of the scapholunate joint is often helpful. It is important to note the three-dimensional nature of the SL ligament, and that the strongest fibers lie on the dorsal side of the wrist.

Stage III SLD is characterized by a dynamic instability, complete tear and an irreparable SL ligament without DISI deformity. For a patient to be a candidate for the reconstructive surgeries required to address this problem, there must not be collapse of the carpal bones or degenerative changes. The modified Brunelli procedure has become a popular ligament reconstruction that has had some success,[30] but the preservation of motion and the maintenance of alignment continue to be a problem, likely due to the attenuation of the ligament reconstruction over time. A technique called the reduction and association of the scaphoid and lunate

(RASL) attempts to make a pseudarthrosis between the scaphoid and lunate.[31] There have been some positive short-term results, but no long-term results are available. Loosening of the screw and symptomatic hardware have been a problem with this technique.

The scaphoid will naturally fall into a flexed position, or a DISI deformity, when it is dissociated from the lunate. To counteract this flexion deformity of the scaphoid, a dorsal capsulodesis is performed. The traditional capsulodesis was performed by Nathan and Blatt[32] and is proximally based. There have been a number of modifications to the original Blatt technique,[33] which theoretically will allow for more motion. A drawback of the Blatt dorsal capsulodesis is the common 20 degree loss of flexion.

Stage IV SLD is characterized by a complete tear of the SL ligament, an irreparable ligament, and a DISI deformity that is reducible. Rotatory subluxation with the scaphoid in flexion and the lunate in extension is the hallmark of stage IV. SLD with associated DISI deformity represents a severe acute injury, as seen in perilunate dislocation, or a chronic attritional process that has destroyed the secondary stabilizers of the scaphoid. If left untreated, these injuries will predictably progress to degenerative arthritis and SLAC. The progression to SLAC is predictable and starts with degeneration of the radial styloid, progresses to the entire scaphoid fossa, and then begins to affect the midcarpal joint. However, the time course to SLAC is unpredictable and in many patients is very slow. Some patients will choose to be treated with splinting and activity modification instead of a ligament reconstruction which limits motion. Treatment of stage IV SLD is similar to stage III with the use of a modified Brunelli ligament reconstruction, RASL and/or dorsal capsulodesis. New techniques are being developed using augmented tendon grafts anchored directly into bone tunnels placed into the carpal bones. Reduction of the SL joint is performed with the aid of K-wires and the ligament reconstruction is completed. Temporary K-wires between the scaphoid and capitate are used to reinforce the repair during the healing process (Fig. 58.3).

Stage V SLD is characterized by a complete tear of the scapholunate ligament, an irreparable ligament, and a fixed DISI deformity. There have been a number of limited intercarpal fusions recommended for a symptomatic SLD with DISI deformity. However, few patients fall into this category since degenerative changes usually accompany symptomatic, fixed DISI deformities. There are limited trials or results that support the use of scaphoid–sparing intercarpal arthrodesis. SL arthrodesis has largely been abandoned because of the low fusion rate.

Stage VI SLD is represented by carpal collapse and degenerative arthritis. SLAC wrist is the term used to describe this deformity. Patients should first be given a trial of nonoperative treatment consisting of activity modification, splinting, steroid injections, and nonsteroidal antiinflammatory medications. If nonoperative intervention fails, then surgery may be indicated. Radial styloidectomy, radioscaphoid arthrodesis, scaphoid excision four-corner fusion, and proximal row carpectomy have all been described for SLAC. If the midcarpal joint is involved in the arthritic process, then a proximal row carpectomy usually has poor results, due to the inability to articulate on the proximal lunate. If the lunate facet and midcarpal joint show degenerative changes, then a total wrist arthrodesis may be the best option for the patient.

Perilunate and Lunate Dislocations and Fracture Dislocations

Perilunate dislocations (PLDs) are a spectrum of injuries represented by the carpal bones dislocating around the lunate. These injuries start on the radial aspect of the wrist with a SL ligament tear, then progress to the articulation between the lunate and the capitate. The spectrum of injury severity progresses with tearing of the lunotriquetral ligament, dislocation of the capitate from the lunate (usually the capitate migrates dorsally), then finally the lunate dislocates into the carpal canal and possibly rotates on its own axis. These injuries are often missed because they are rare and the X-ray findings are not often seen by general medical providers, although these injuries usually occur due to high-energy trauma (Fig. 58.4). PLD can be purely ligamentous as noted above, or can have associated fractures (usually the scaphoid). Lesser and greater arc injuries refer to PLDs that are purely ligamentous (lesser arc) or associated with a scaphoid fracture (greater arc), respectively.

Radiographic evaluation of a PLD starts with standard, high-quality images. A decrease in carpal height, disruption of Gilula's lines, increased distance between carpal bones, and fractures of the carpal bones or distal radius may be seen on the PA radiograph. Ulnar migration of the carpus can also present with PLD since these injuries are such high energy and contain both intercarpal (intrinsic) ligament and intracarpal (extrinsic) ligament disruption (carpal instability complex). The lateral may show the capitate dislocated from the lunate or possibly the lunate dislocated volarly into the carpal tunnel (termed a lunate dislocation, in contrast to a perilunate dislocation where the lunate stays in the lunate fossa). MRI and CT scans are often helpful in diagnosing ligamentous injuries and the extent of carpal fractures, respectively.

Nonoperative treatment of PLDs or fracture dislocations has been shown to have poor results and is not recommended. Urgent closed reduction to relieve pressure on the median nerve is the first line of treatment, with open repair of ligament injury and pinning to follow. Dorsal spanning plates can be used to offload the carpus during the healing period and can be removed 3–4 months after repair. Closed reduction of a perilunate dislocation can be performed by doing a wrist block with local anesthetic, placing the wrist in traction with finger traps and weights for 15 minutes, and then pulling traction on the wrist, extending the wrist, and then pulling the hand up and over into flexion while placing dorsal pressure on the capitate to reduce it back

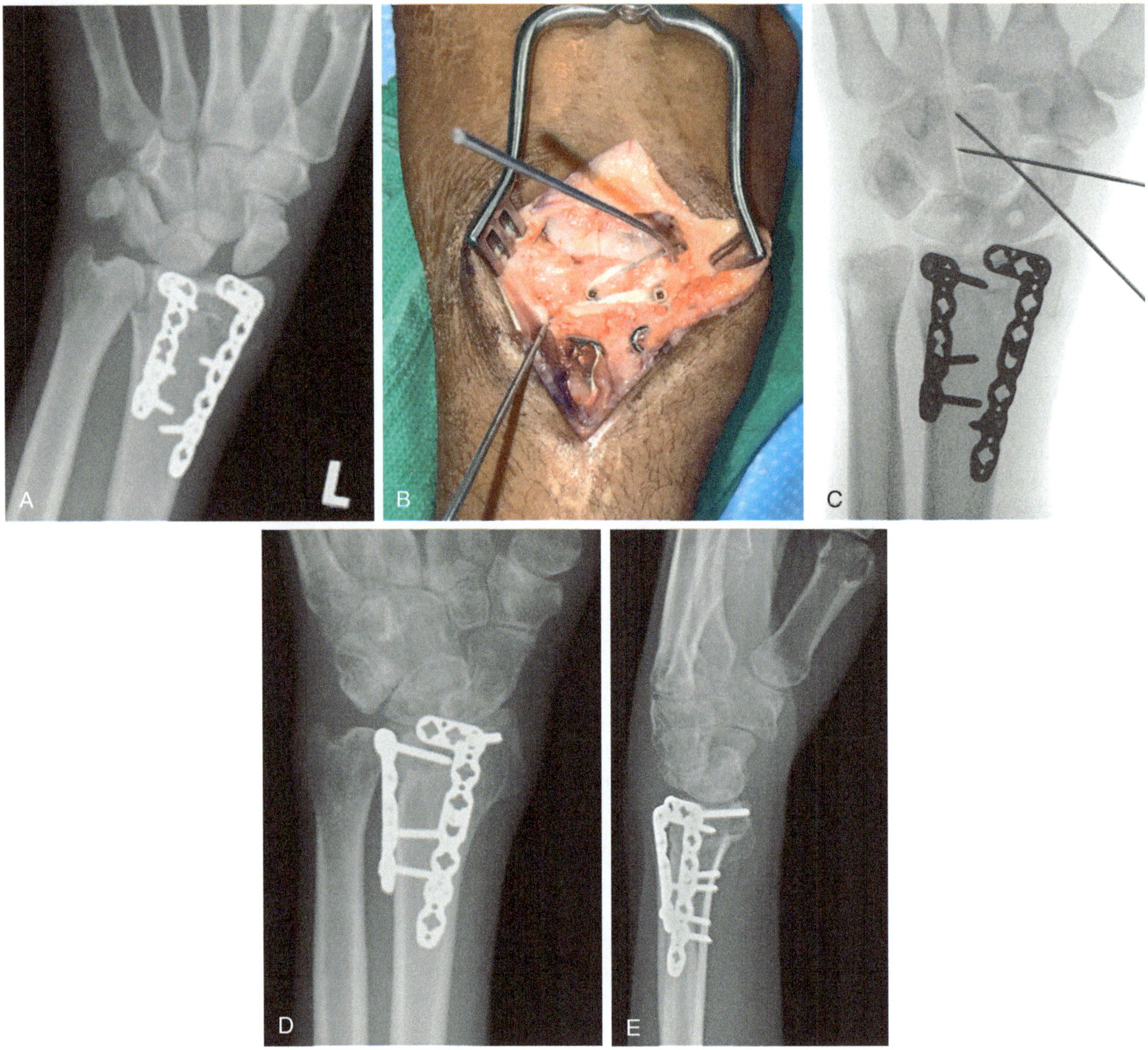

• **Fig. 58.3** Representative case of a patient with chronic SL dissociation after distal radius fracture. (A) A widened SL gap can clearly be visualized on the PA view of the X-ray. (B) The dorsal wrist is exposed and ligament reconstruction was performed utilizing the Arthrex dorsal SL reconstruction technique with suture tape augmented tendon graft placed using 3.5-mm swivel locks. K-wires were used as joysticks to aid in the SL reduction. Postoperative imaging confirms reduction of the SL joint. (C) Temporary K-wires are in place between the scaphoid and capitate and are left for 8 weeks. (D,E) Radiographs taken 7 months postoperatively confirming the stability of the SL ligament repair. (Case courtesy David Steinberg, MD.)

into position on the lunate. Fluoroscopy should be used if available to confirm the reduction. The median nerve must be monitored for progressive symptoms of dysfunction. If closed reduction cannot be obtained, then open reduction in the operating room should be performed. Regardless of the success of reduction the patient should be brought to the operating room on an urgent basis to fix associated bony and ligamentous injuries.

Both dorsal and volar approaches have been described for treatment. The dorsal approach gives good access to the proximal carpal row, midcarpal joint, and for repair of the SL ligament. The volar approach has the advantage of being able to decompress the carpal tunnel (especially important in lunate dislocations) and assist in reduction of the lunate if needed, and allows visualization with possible repair of the volar ligaments and capsule. Greater arc injuries with fractures of the scaphoid usually have an intact SL ligament and a disruption of the LT ligament. Whenever PLD are associated with fractures, most authors recommend fixation with

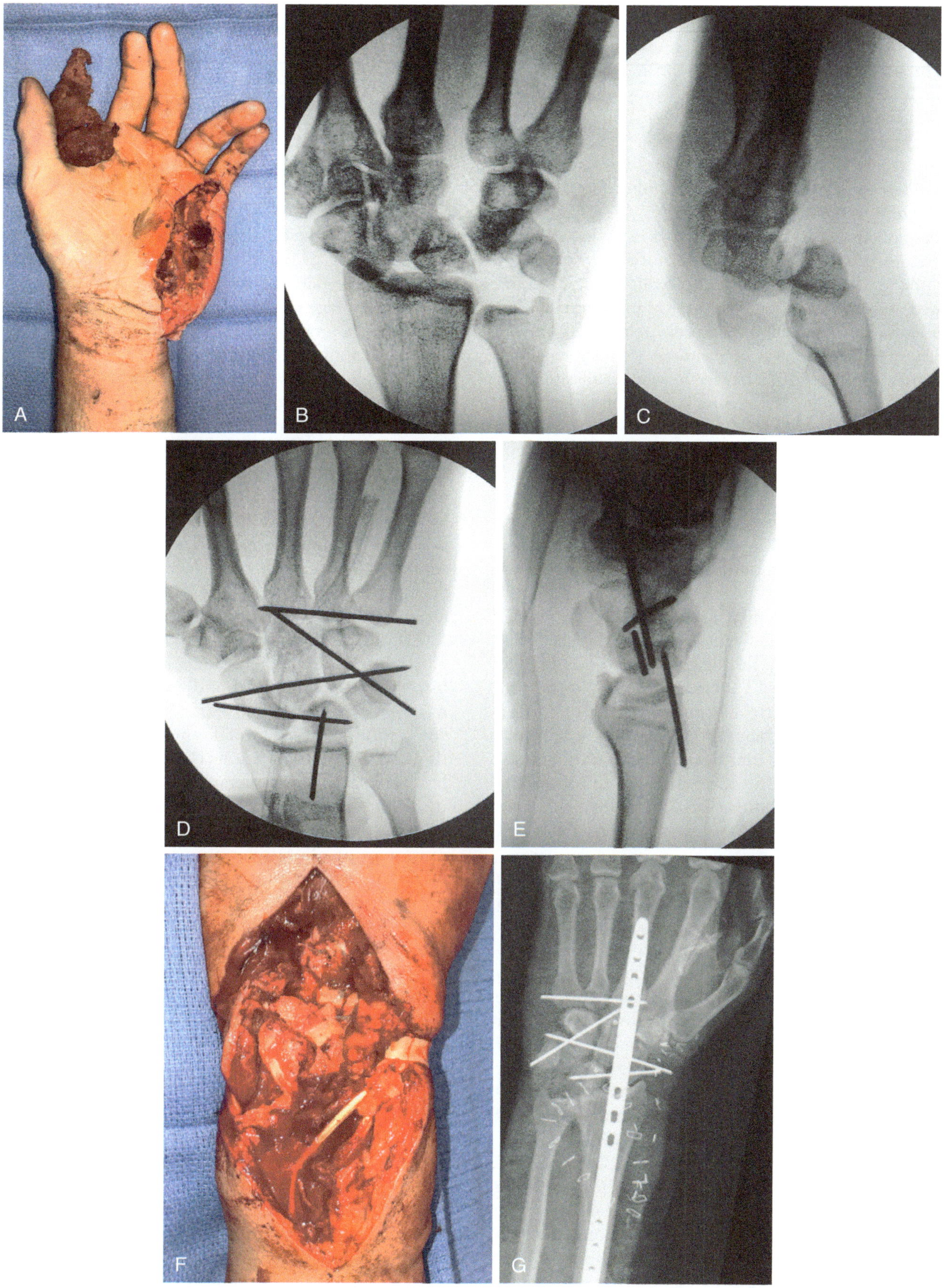

• **Fig. 58.4** A 37-year-old male who suffered a traumatic injury to his right hand at a log mill. (A) He presented with significant soft tissue injury, including exposure of the ulnar neurovascular bundle and extrusion of the thenar musculature through a wound in the first webspace. (B,C) Bony injury included a perilunate dislocation with the lunate remaining in the lunate fossa and a perihamate dislocation as seen on intraoperative fluoroscopy. (D,E) Open reduction was performed with a dorsal approach and K-wires were used to hold the carpus in proper alignment. (F) Ligamentous repair was attempted with a bone anchor and the remaining soft tissue that was present. (G) A dorsal bridging plate was also used to offload the carpal bones due to the severity of the injury. (Case courtesy of Shaun Mendenhall, MD.)

headless compression or cannulated screws. K-wire stabilization of ligamentous injuries is advocated by some, with or without augmentation by primary ligamentous repair. Intercarpal screws have been compared to K-wire stabilization of ligamentous injuries without significant difference in outcome, except for fewer pin site-related complications with intercarpal screws. This can usually be avoided by burying the pins and removing them at least 8 weeks later.

The outcome of PLD treated after a delay in diagnosis (around 4 weeks or more) is worse than those treated soon after injury. There is no surgical procedure that is recommended above another, but the surgical procedure chosen should provide adequate visualization, repair of ligamentous injuries, and fixation of fractures. Primary repair of ligaments, suture anchor repair, K-wire stabilization or intercarpal screws are all accepted treatments of unstable ligamentous injuries.

Lunotriquetral (LT) Dissociation

LT dissociation is an often-missed tear of the ligament connecting the lunate and triquetrum. This is usually caused by a fall backwards on an outstretched hand in supination and radial deviation. This position concentrates the force on the pisiform, which acts as a punch against the triquetrum. The resulting ulnar-sided wrist pain is often misdiagnosed as a TFCC tear. This diagnosis can be confirmed on MRI or arthroscopy. LT dissociation can also be part of a more severe perilunate dislocation injury. It follows a familiar pattern of wrist deformity, with the scaphoid and attached lunate rotating into flexion and the triquetrum rotating into extension. The deformity is called volar intercalated segmental instability (VISI). The lunate follows the scaphoid and rotates into flexion (opposite to DISI deformity).

Physical exam findings of lunotriquetral dissociation are often sensitive but not very specific. Lunotriquetral ballottement and a triquetral shear test are often positive. Radiographic evaluation will often show a subtle disruption of Gilula's lines and a possible increased lunotriquetral distance if secondary stabilizers have become attenuated. Dynamic radiographs with the wrist in ulnar and radial deviation can be helpful in showing the disruption between the lunate and triquetrum. At times the radiographs will be normal and MRI or arthroscopic evaluation of the ligamentous structures will show evidence of LT ligament injury.

If nonoperative treatment of an acute LT dissociation is initiated, a long arm cast should be applied to inhibit wrist supination and pronation. Failure of nonoperative management is not uncommon. The indications for surgical treatment of LT dissociation are varied and not very clear. There are many ways to address LT dissociation surgically, including arthroscopic debridement, ligament repair or reconstruction, capsulodesis, K-wire stabilization, and arthrodesis. LT ligament injuries are often associated with other injuries that may need addressing at the time of surgery.

Scapholunate Advanced Collapse (SLAC) and Scaphoid Nonunion Advanced Collapse (SNAC)

SLAC and SNAC are arthritic changes that take place in the wrist with typical progression. They are both caused by trauma, but SLAC can also be caused by nontraumatic chronic degenerative changes of the wrist such as gout. SLAC wrist stage I arthritic changes begin at the radial styloid and then progress to (stage II) the proximal radioscaphoid articulation. Arthritic changes next advance to the midcarpal joint between the capitate and the lunate (stage III). The lunate fossa rarely shows arthritic changes. SNAC wrist arthritis begins at the radioscaphoid articulation and follows a similar predictable pattern.

The diagnosis of SLAC and SNAC is made through history, physical exam, and radiographs. The patient usually has a painful wrist with decreased range of motion. Radial-sided wrist pain predominates and dorsal wrist swelling is common. Bilateral radiographs are helpful for comparison. Staging the arthritic changes will help in determining treatment options.

Nonoperative treatment will be beneficial for many patients. There are no studies delineating the natural history of the diagnosis and many patients will have minimal symptoms for years. Symptomatic treatment with splints, nonsteroidal antiinflammatory medications, and steroid injections is the first line of treatment. If a patient fails nonoperative treatment and continues to have a painful, arthritic wrist, salvage surgical procedures are an option to reduce pain at the expense of wrist motion. Surgical options for SLAC and SNAC include partial wrist arthrodesis (scaphoid excision and four-corner fusion (Fig. 58.5), complete wrist arthrodesis, proximal row carpectomy, posterior/anterior interosseus nerve denervation, and radiostyloidectomy. SNAC can also be treated with excision of the distal scaphoid fragment. Traditional teaching states that a proximal row carpectomy should not be performed in patients with capitate arthritis, due to the inability to articulate on the proximal capitate. However, outcomes comparing scaphoid excision four-corner fusion with proximal row carpectomy show similar results.[34] Proximal row carpectomy has the added benefit of lower cost, no need for hardware, no need to wait for fusion, and no extended postoperative immobilization. There has been some question about the lasting durability of proximal row carpectomy with younger patients (<35 years) and patients who are very active or manual laborers.[35] Total wrist arthrodesis reliably relieves pain in the arthritic wrist but sacrifices wrist motion. Total wrist arthrodesis can be performed after a failed proximal row carpectomy or partial wrist fusion.

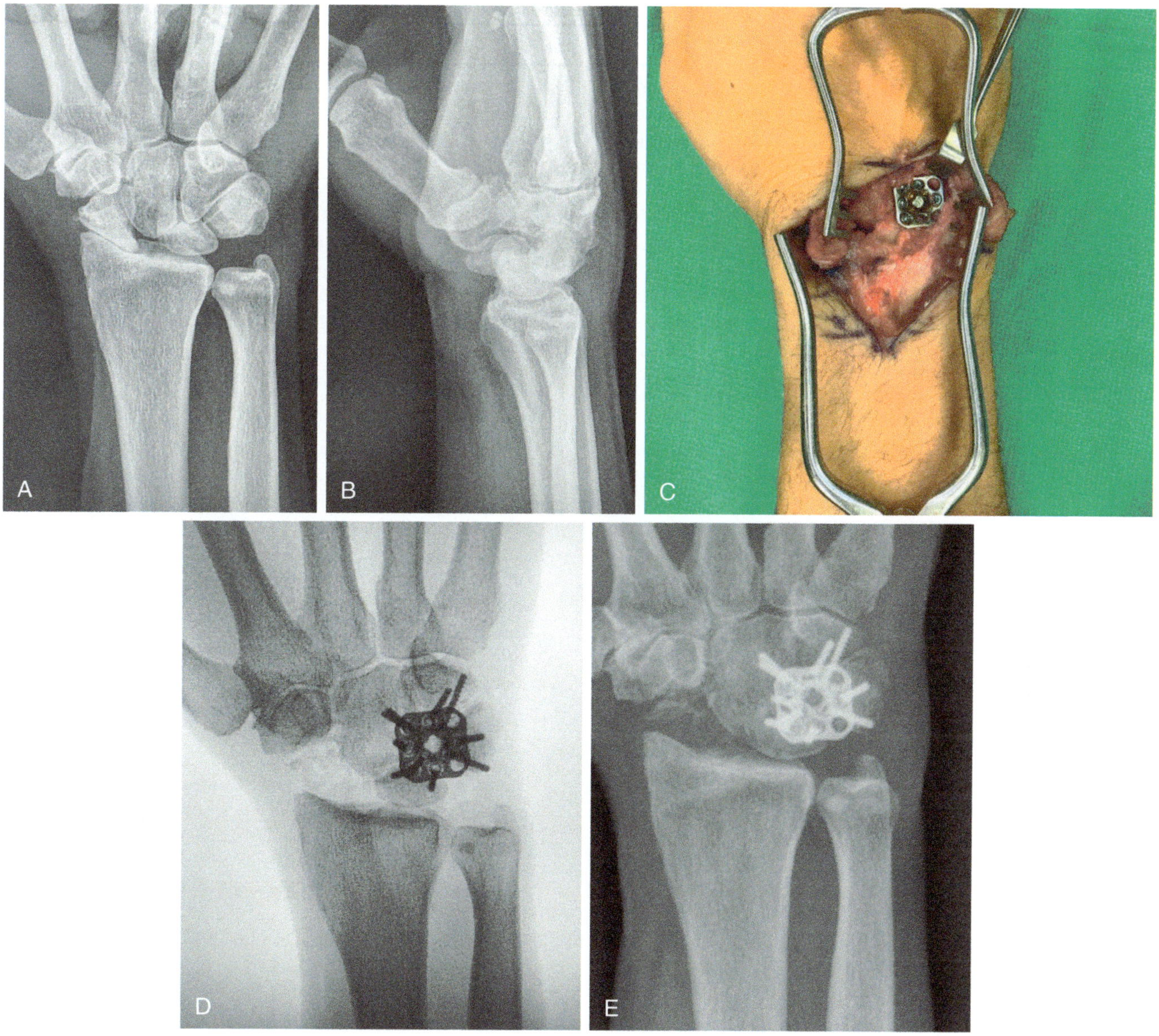

• **Fig. 58.5** Representative case of a SLAC wrist managed with scaphoid excision and four-corner fusion. (A) PA X-ray view of the wrist reveals a widened SL gap with significant arthritic change at the radioscaphoid joint. (B) Lateral view of the wrist is significant for a DISI deformity. (C) A dorsal approach to the wrist was performed. The scaphoid was removed and a four-corner fusion plate was placed. (D) Postoperative PA X-ray confirms complete excision of the diseased scaphoid bone and four-corner fusion. (E) Follow-up radiograph 2 months postoperatively, confirming stable bony fusion. (Case courtesy David Steinberg, MD.)

Acknowledgments

The authors would like to thank the previous authors of this chapter, Owen L. Ala, MD and T. Shane Johnson, MD, for their contributions.

References

1. Williams CS, Gelberman RH. Vascularity of the lunate. Anatomic studies and implications for the development of osteonecrosis. *Hand Clin*. 1993;9(3):391–398.
2. Teisen H, Hjarbaek J. Classification of fresh fractures of the lunate. *J Hand Surg Br*. 1988;13(4):458–462.
3. Chung KC, Spilson MS, Kim MH. Is negative ulnar variance a risk factor for Kienbock's disease? A meta-analysis. *Ann Plast Surg*. 2001;47(5):494–499.
4. Lichtman DM, Mack GR, MacDonald RI, et al. Kienbock's disease: the role of silicone replacement arthroplasty. *J Bone Joint Surg Am*. 1977;59(7):899–908.
5. Quenzer DE, Dobyns JH, Linscheid RL, et al. Radial recession osteotomy for Kienböck's disease. *J Hand Surg Am*. 1997;22(3):386–395.
6. Kakar S, Shin AY. Vascularized bone grafting from the dorsal distal radius for Kienböck's disease: technique, indications and review of the literature. *Chir Main*. 2010;29(suppl 1):S104–S111.
7. Gillis JA, Higgins JP. Coronal fracture of the lunate in advanced Kienböck disease: reestablishing midcarpal congruency to enable

osteochondral reconstruction: a case report. *JBJS Case Connect.* 2018;8(2):e37.

8. Calfee RP, Van Steyn MO, Gyuricza C, et al. Joint leveling for advanced Kienböck's disease. *J Hand Surg Am.* 2010;35(12):1947–1954.
9. Xie MM, Tang KL, Yuan CS. 3D printing lunate prosthesis for stage IIIc Kienböck's disease: a case report. *Arch Orthop Trauma Surg.* 2018;138(4):447–451.
10. Burger HK, Windhofer C, Gaggl AJ, et al. Vascularized medial femoral trochlea osteochondral flap reconstruction of advanced Kienböck disease. *J Hand Surg Am.* 2014;39(7):1313–1322.
11. Higgins JP, Burger HK. Medial femoral trochlea osteochondral flap: applications for scaphoid and lunate reconstruction. *Clin Plast Surg.* 2017;44(2):257–265.
12. Ashurst JV, Turco DA, Lieb BE. Tenosynovitis caused by texting: an emerging disease. *J Am Osteopath Assoc.* 2010;110(5):294–296.
13. Gao Z-Y, Tao H, Xu H, et al. A novel classification of the anatomical variations of the first extensor compartment. *Medicine.* 2017;96(35):e7875–e7875.
14. Baldassarre RL, Hughes TH. Investigating suspected scaphoid fracture. *Br Med J.* 2013;346:f1370.
15. Gellman H, Caputo RJ, Carter V, et al. Comparison of short and long thumb-spica casts for non-displaced fractures of the carpal scaphoid. *J Bone Joint Surg Am.* 1989;71(3):354–357.
16. Buijze GA, Goslings JC, Rhemrev SJ, et al. Cast immobilization with and without immobilization of the thumb for nondisplaced and minimally displaced scaphoid waist fractures: a multicenter, randomized, controlled trial. *J Hand Surg Am.* 2014;39(4):621–627.
17. Papaloizos MY, Fusetti C, Christen T, et al. Minimally invasive fixation versus conservative treatment of undisplaced scaphoid fractures: a cost-effectiveness study. *J Hand Surg Br.* 2004;29(2):116–119.
18. Alnaeem H, Aldekhayel S, Kanevsky J, et al. A systematic review and meta-analysis examining the differences between nonsurgical management and percutaneous fixation of minimally and nondisplaced scaphoid fractures. *J Hand Surg Am.* 2016;41(12):1135–1144. e1131.
19. Saint-Cyr M, Oni G, Wong C, et al. Dorsal percutaneous cannulated screw fixation for delayed union and nonunion of the scaphoid. *Plast Reconstr Surg.* 2011;128(2):467–473.
20. Russe O. Fracture of the carpal navicular. Diagnosis, non-operative treatment, and operative treatment. *J Bone Joint Surg Am.* 1960;42:759–768.
21. Zoubos AB, Triantafyllopoulos IK, Babis GC, et al. A modified Matti–Russe technique for the treatment of scaphoid waist nonunion and pseudarthrosis. *Med Sci Monit.* 2011;17(2):MT7–M12.
22. Cohen MS, Jupiter JB, Fallahi K, et al. Scaphoid waist nonunion with humpback deformity treated without structural bone graft. *J Hand Surg Am.* 2013;38(4):701–705.
23. Steinmann SP, Bishop AT, Berger RA. Use of the 1,2 intercompartmental supraretinacular artery as a vascularized pedicle bone graft for difficult scaphoid nonunion. *J Hand Surg Am.* 2002;27(3):391–401.
24. Sotereanos DG, Darlis NA, Dailiana ZH, et al. A capsular-based vascularized distal radius graft for proximal pole scaphoid pseudarthrosis. *J Hand Surg Am.* 2006;31(4):580–587.
25. Jones Jr DB, Burger H, Bishop AT, et al. Treatment of scaphoid waist nonunions with an avascular proximal pole and carpal collapse. Surgical technique. *J Bone Joint Surg Am.* 2009;91(suppl 2):169–183.
26. Burger HK, Windhofer C, Gaggl AJ, et al. Vascularized medial femoral trochlea osteocartilaginous flap reconstruction of proximal pole scaphoid nonunions. *J Hand Surg Am.* 2013;38(4):690–700.
27. Mehio G, Morsy M, Cayci C, et al. Donor-site morbidity and functional status following medial femoral condyle flap harvest. *Plast Reconstr Surg.* 2018;142(5):734e–741e.
28. Kazmers NH, Thibaudeau S, Levin LS. A scapholunate ligament-sparing technique utilizing the medial femoral condyle corticocancellous free flap to reconstruct scaphoid nonunions with proximal pole avascular necrosis. *J Hand Surg Am.* 2016;41(9):e309–315.
29. Garcia-Elias M, Lluch AL, Stanley JK. Three-ligament tenodesis for the treatment of scapholunate dissociation: indications and surgical technique. *J Hand Surg Am.* 2006;31(1):125–134.
30. Talwalkar SC, Edwards AT, Hayton MJ, et al. Results of tri-ligament tenodesis: a modified Brunelli procedure in the management of scapholunate instability. *J Hand Surg Br.* 2006;31(1):110–117.
31. Rosenwasser MP, Miyasajsa KC, Strauch RJ. The RASL procedure: reduction and association of the scaphoid and lunate using the Herbert screw. *Tech Hand Up Extrem Surg.* 1997;1(4):263–272.
32. Nathan R, Blatt G. Rotary subluxation of the scaphoid. Revisited. *Hand Clin.* 2000;16(3):417–431.
33. Linscheid RL, Dobyns JH. Treatment of scapholunate dissociation. Rotatory subluxation of the scaphoid. *Hand Clin.* 1992;8(4):645–652.
34. Vanhove W, De Vil J, Van Seymortier P, et al. Proximal row carpectomy versus four-corner arthrodesis as a treatment for SLAC (scapholunate advanced collapse) wrist. *J Hand Surg Eur.* 2008;33(2):118–125.
35. Wall LB, Didonna ML, Kiefhaber TR, et al. Proximal row carpectomy: minimum 20-year follow-up. *J Hand Surg Am.* 2013;38(8):1498–1504.

59

Rheumatoid Arthritis of the Hand and Wrist

REBECCA AYERS AND MARK PICKFORD

Definition

Rheumatoid arthritis (RA) is a chronic inflammatory disease characterized by symmetrical polyarticular arthritis, typically affecting the wrist and small joints of the hands and feet. Inflammation progresses to joint destruction with pain, deformity, and disability.

Nonarticular manifestations include rheumatoid nodules, pulmonary fibrosis, renal amyloidosis, pericarditis, endocarditis, atherosclerosis, Felty's syndrome, keratoconjunctivis sicca, hemolytic anemia and generalized systemic symptoms such as malaise, anorexia, anemia, and weight loss. The course of RA is variable and unpredictable; premature mortality is well recognized.

The incidence of RA is generally quoted across European and North American literature as affecting 1% of the population. RA is two to four times more common in females than males, with a peak age of incidence in the seventh decade. RA may have a significant social and economic impact on the people afflicted with this disease. The UK National Institute for Health and Care Excellence (NICE) has estimated that approximately one-third of people stop work within 2 years of diagnosis and the total cost to the UK economy is £3.8 billion to £4.75 billion per year.[1]

Diagnostic Criteria

In 2010 the American College of Rheumatology (ACR) and the European League Against Rheumatism (EULAR)[2] revised the classification schema for RA (Table 59.1). Diagnosis is confirmed by affecting one or more joints, not explained by another cause and a total score of 6 or greater (out of 10) in four domains: joint involvement, serology, acute phase reactants, and duration of symptoms. A key aim was to identify patients with RA early, especially those with persistent or erosive disease, in order to allow early medication.[3]

Pathophysiology

The cause of RA is unknown and tremendously complex. Antigen presenting cells (APCs) bind and present an as yet unknown arthritogenic antigen to T-cells. The binding of co-stimulatory ligands, also on the APCs, such as CD80 and CD86, assists in activation of T-cells. T-cells, fibroblasts, and macrophages secrete numerous proinflammatory cytokines, such as IL-1, IL-6, and TNF-α. These recruit and activate neutrophils, lymphocytes, macrophages, synovial cells, fibroblasts, and B-cells. Inheritance of certain HLA-II loci may mediate antigen presentation, T-cell reactivity and other immune relationships.

B-cells differentiate into plasma cells that secrete antibodies and autoantibodies. This process is abetted by IL-6. Autoantibodies include those to IgG (rheumatoid factor, RF) and citrullinated peptides (anticitrullinated protein antibody, ACPA), amongst others. The autoantibodies form immune complexes that drive the secretion of proinflammatory cytokines, augmenting the inflammatory process. Activated B-cells also act as APCs. In conjunction with cells of the innate and acquired immune system there are numerous other chemokines that guide and control this intricate process.

The final stage in the pathogenesis is swollen synovium full of macrophages, T-cells, B-cells, plasma cells, and synovial fibroblasts. This synovial pannus then erodes cartilage, bone, and supporting soft tissues leading to joint destruction, deformity, and pain. Synovial proliferation around tendons (tenosynovitis) may cause tendon attrition and rupture. Joint destruction begins early and erosive changes may occur within months.

Rheumatoid nodules are typically cutaneous, demonstrating central fibrinoid necrosis surrounded by macrophages and fibroblasts and a cuff of connective tissue containing lymphocytes and plasma cells. Rheumatoid nodules typically occur at sites of repeated mechanical stress or over bony prominences such as the olecranon, the calcaneum, and the metacarpophalangeal joints; they are associated

TABLE 59.1 The 2010 American College of Rheumatology/European League Against Rheumatism Classification Criteria for RA

Patients with at Least One Joint with Clinical Synovitis, not Explained by Another Disease	Score (out of 10)
A. Joint Involvement	
1 large joint	0
2–10 large joints	1
1–3 small joints	2
4–10 small joints	3
>10 joints (at least one small joint)	5
B. Serology	
Negative RF and negative ACPA	0
Low positive RF or low positive ACPA	2
High positive RF or high positive ACPA	3
C. Acute-Phase Reactants	
Normal CRP and normal ESR	0
Abnormal CRP or abnormal ESR	1
D. Duration of Symptoms	
<6 weeks	0
≥6 weeks	1

ACPA, anti-citrullinated protein antibody; CRP, C-reactive protein; ESR, erythrocyte sedimentation rate; RF, rheumatoid factor.

with more aggressive disease. Due to generalized dysfunction of the immune system RA patients have an increased susceptibility to infection.

Management Principles and Operative Options

Assessment and Evaluation

Referral to a rheumatologist should be made for any patient with persistent and unexplained synovitis. This includes patients with normal inflammatory markers and those who are RF-negative. Referral should be expedited if the synovitis affects multiple joints, or if the duration of symptoms has been longer than 3 months. There is an urgency to diagnose RA since prompt treatment has been shown to reduce permanent joint damage.

RA should be managed by a multidisciplinary team (MDT), which may include a rheumatologist, occupational therapist, hand surgeon, besides other allied health professionals.

General Assessment

Assessment includes examination for joint synovitis and extraarticular manifestations (Box 59.1). Blood tests should include inflammatory markers such as erythrocyte sedimentation rate (ESR) and C-reactive protein (CRP). Serology should include RF and ACPA, the latter being more specific for RA. Baseline full blood count (FBC), liver, and renal biochemistry are useful for planning treatment.

• BOX 59.1 Initial Assessment of Rheumatoid Arthritis

Clinical evaluation
  Joint synovitis and extraarticular manifestations
Blood work
  ESR, CRP, RF, ACPA, complete blood count, liver and renal biochemistry
X-rays of hands and feet

Abbreviations as Table 59.1.

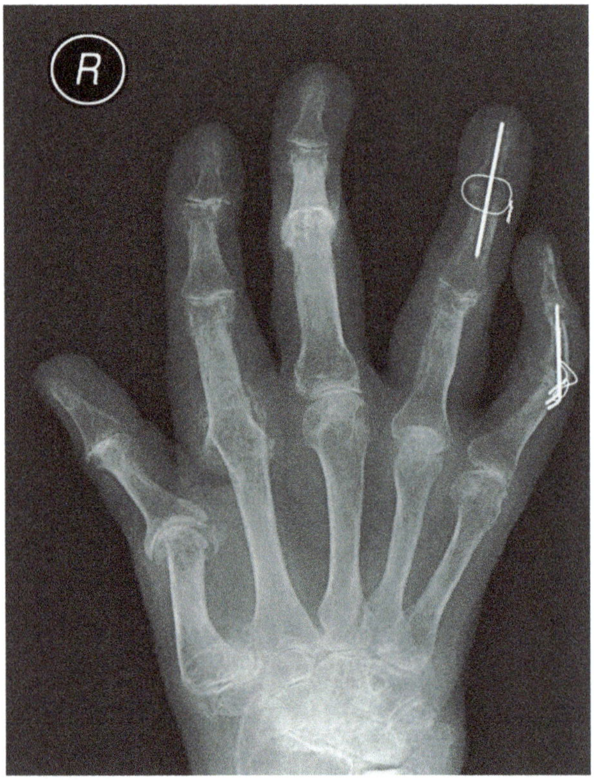

• **Fig. 59.1** Various rheumatoid deformities of the hand including a swan neck deformity of thumb, subluxation of the index metacarpophalangeal joint (MCPJ), and generalized arthritic change throughout the hand and wrist. Note fusion of distal interphalangeal joint (DIPJ) of the ring and proximal interphalangeal joint (PIPJ) of the little fingers.

Radiological Features

X-rays provide a record of the permanent damage of RA (Fig. 59.1 and Box 59.2). Changes include: surface erosions, cystic changes, cortical thinning, osteoporosis, and progressive joint narrowing through to frank ankylosis, subluxation, and dislocation. In mutilans arthropathy there is bony destruction, which may progress rapidly.

• BOX 59.2 Radiological Features of Rheumatoid Arthritis

Joint narrowing and destruction progressing to ankylosis
Erosions
Cortical thinning
Osteoporosis
Subluxation/dislocation
Bony destruction (mutilans)

• BOX 59.3 Poor Prognostic Features on Diagnosis of Rheumatoid Arthritis

Positive RF or ACPA
Early functional limitations
Multiple swollen or tender joints
Early bony erosions on X-ray
Extra-articular manifestations
High ESR or CRP

Abbreviations as Table 59.1.

The Sharp and Larsen scores are the most widely used radiological assessments for RA. Each scores X-rays of the hands, wrists, and feet; higher scores indicate greater bony destruction. The Sharp method scores bony erosions and joint space narrowing separately over 31 areas to give a score from 0 to 448. The Larsen score assesses 20 joints to give a score out of 100. Although the Larsen score is more widely used, the Sharp assessment is more sensitive for detecting changes over time. The Sharp and Larsen assessments have significant correlation with each other[4] and with the extent of joint and cartilage destruction.[5]

Magnetic resonance imaging (MRI) is increasingly used to detect pre-erosive synovitis, and early bone damage not seen on standard radiography. Fat-suppressed gadolinium-enhanced T1-weighted images will demonstrate pre-erosive synovitis, tenosynovitis, and bony erosions. The presence of bone marrow edema, seen on T2-weighted images, is also predictive of the development of bony erosions.[6] Identification and treatment of subclinical synovitis and prevention of bony erosions are the aims of more aggressive medical management regimes.[7]

Identifying Patients with Aggressive Disease

One of the key goals of initial assessment is to identify those patients with signs that suggest an aggressive disease process (Box 59.3). Such patients are monitored closely; a poor response to first-line medical treatment may warrant early use of biologic therapies to gain early control of the disease.

Assessment of Disease Activity

People with newly-diagnosed RA require regular assessment of disease activity until the disease is stable. Usually this consists of monthly to trimonthly review, including CRP and a Disease Activity Score (DAS28). The DAS28 is a measure of disease activity in RA; an online tool collates a clinical assessment of 28 specified joints, serum inflammatory markers, and a visual analog scale (0–10) of the patient's global function. A score greater than 5.1 indicates active disease and less than 3.2 indicates well-controlled disease. A score of less of than 2.6 indicates remission. Alteration in the DAS28 can be used to assess response to treatment. Until the disease is well controlled repeat radiography of the extremities is recommended every 6–12 months. Persistent erosive disease despite good symptom control may warrant a change in medication regime. Stable disease only requires annual review.

Assessment of Disability Status and Health Status

RA is a chronic illness and it is crucial to document both the disability and health status of each patient.

The most common measure of disability status is the Stanford Health Assessment Questionnaire Disability Index (HAQ – DI), which has eight categories covering dressing, arising, eating, walking, hygiene, reach, grip, and activities. For each domain, a score of 0–1 represents mild to moderate disability, 1–2 moderate to severe disability, and 2–3 severe to very severe disability.

Health status is frequently assessed via the Short Form 36 (SF-36). The SF-36 has eight domains covering vitality, physical functioning, bodily pain, general health, ability to perform social roles, ability to perform physical roles, ability to perform emotional roles, and mental health. Each of the eight sections are scored from 0 to 100, with 100 being normal health status.

Surgical Options

The benefits of surgery include relief of pain, recovery of function, and cosmetic improvement. Rheumatoid deformities are frequently multifactorial and they must be assessed within the context of the patient's rheumatoid pathology and global function. The decision to offer surgery requires evaluation of the surgical problem and functional limitations. There are general principles when creating a rheumatoid management plan: operate on the lower limb before the upper limb, operate proximally then distally, offer reliable procedures with the highest chance of success first. Souter presented his personal reflections on the relative merits of different rheumatoid hand procedures and felt that the three most efficacious procedures were extensor synovectomy combined with excision of the ulna head, wrist stabilization, and thumb metacarpophalangeal joint fusion.[8] Critical analysis of different surgical procedures is, however, not evidenced in the literature and randomized controlled trials comparing different surgical treatments are rare. There is also considerable discrepancy between the views of surgeons and rheumatologists, hence the benefits of managing rheumatoid patients within the confines of a MDT.[9]

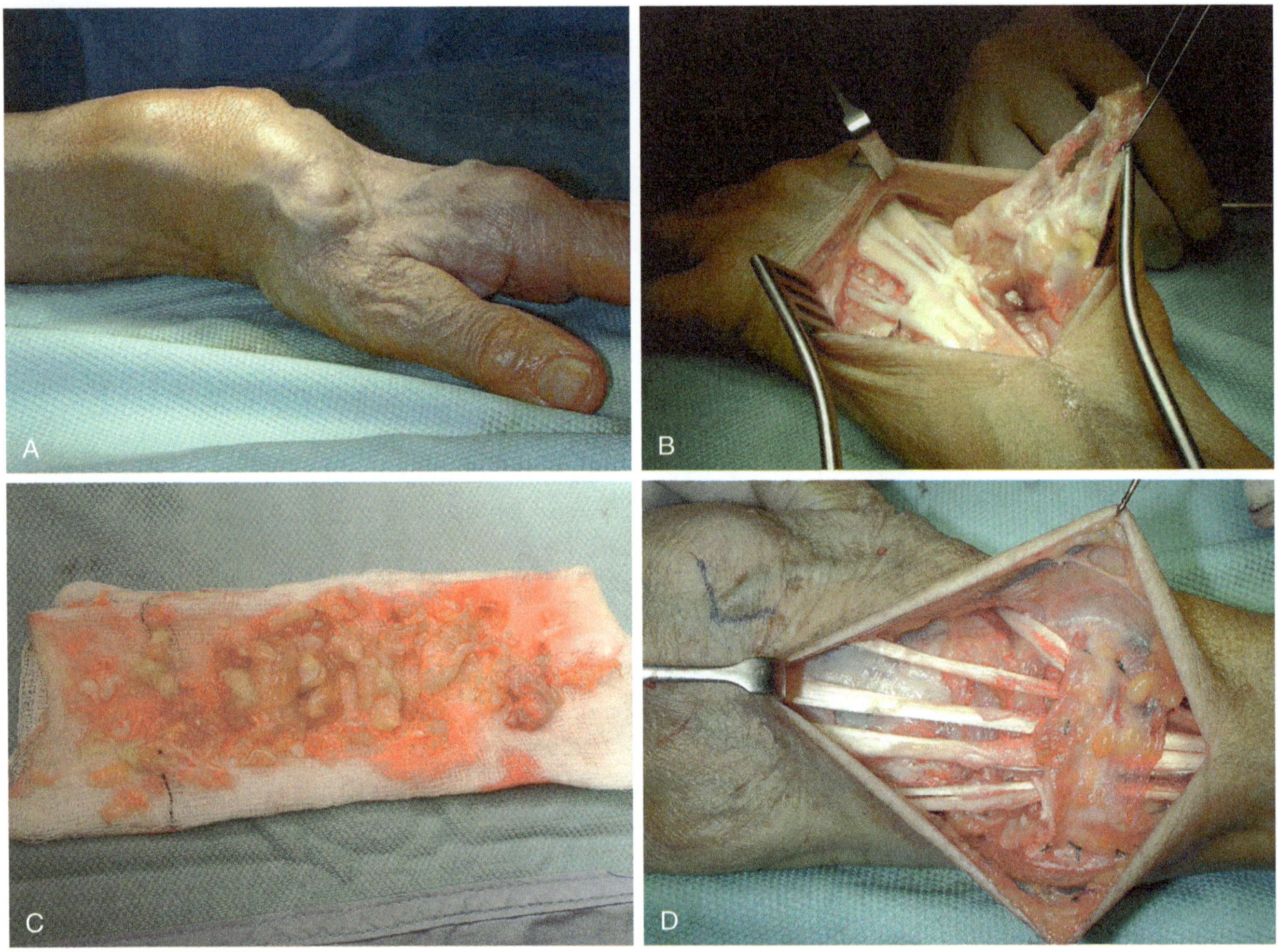

• **Fig. 59.2** (A) Bulging synovitis is seen extending from proximal to distal under the extensor retinaculum. (B) The latter is elevated from the sixth compartment as far as the first compartment if needed; synovitis and rheumatoid nodules can be seen attached to the retinaculum. (C) Synovectomy tissue is seen on the swab. (D) The retinaculum has been split, with half lying across the radiocarpal and distal radioulnar joints and half lying across the tendons to prevent bow stringing.

Synovectomy and Tenosynovectomy

Synovectomy is the excision of inflamed synovial tissue within a joint and tenosynovectomy implies excision of inflamed synovial tissue affecting tendons. The benefits and roles of synovectomy and tenosynovectomy are quite different; refractory tenosynovitis benefits more clearly from surgical treatment.

Synovitis is typically managed with systemic medications, although isolated persistent synovitis may benefit from intraarticular steroid injection. Recalcitrant synovitis or incidental synovitis, discovered during the course of a surgical procedure may be excised but there is no evidence that synovectomy alters disease course or reduces intraarticular cartilage destruction. Synovectomy may relieve pain[10] and may be complicated by stiffness.

Tenosynovitis may affect any tendon surrounded by synovium. Extensor tenosynovitis typically causes dorsal wrist swelling, extending beneath and restrained by the extensor retinaculum. The synovial pannus may cause tendon attrition and rupture. Extensor tenosynovectomy is recommended to prevent tendon rupture when synovitis persists for more than 3–6 months despite aggressive medical management. A dorsal longitudinal incision allows exposure of all extensor compartments (Fig. 59.2). The extensor retinaculum is elevated from the sixth to second compartments; the tendons are examined for rupture and tenosynovectomy performed. The distal radioulnar joint (DRUJ) should be examined and treated (synovectomy/capsular repair/Darrach procedure) if required. The retinaculum may then be split in half transversely, with one half being placed beneath the tendons to provide protection from the DRUJ and the other used to reconstitute the extensor retinaculum and prevent bowstringing. Brumfield et al[1] reviewed 78 rheumatoid patients, with 102 dorsal wrist tenosynovectomies, intraarticular synovectomies, and a Darrach (ulnar head) resection. With an average follow-up of 11 years, pain was improved in 83% of wrists, with a 13-degree loss in wrist movement. Synovitis recurred in 16% of patients, subsequent tendon ruptures occurred in 5% of patients but radiologically the disease progressed unchecked. Twenty-seven wrists required revision surgery, including tendon transfers, partial and total wrist fusion, and wrist arthroplasty.

There are three principal types of flexor tenosynovitis: isolated carpal tenosynovitis, palmodigital tenosynovitis, and diffuse tenosynovitis. Synovial proliferation within the carpal tunnel may cause carpal tunnel syndrome. Wrist tenosynovectomy is performed through an extended carpal tunnel incision preserving the palmar cutaneous branch of the median nerve. Bony protrusions on the floor of the carpal tunnel should be smoothed. Palmodigital tenosynovitis typically causes diffuse swelling, triggering, and restriction of flexion, and may progress to rupture of flexor tendons. Again, if there is no improvement after 3 months of intensive medical treatment then tenosynovectomy is indicated. Palmar synovectomy requires broad exposure and may necessitate extension into the digits. Digital triggering may be improved by synovectomy, nodule excision, and A1 pulley release. Adrian Flatt[1] recommended release of the radial side of the A1 pulleys and cautioned against the release of multiple A1 pulleys, which may potentiate ulnar drift. In this situation resection of the one slip of flexor digitorum superficialis (FDS) is a reasonable alternative.

Wrist

The wrist is the major load-bearing joint of the hand, therefore pain or instability may significantly impair function. Wrist involvement affects up to 50% of patients within 2 years of disease onset, increasing to 90% after 10 years[11]; wrist surgery is both common and beneficial to rheumatoid patients.

Pathogenesis of Rheumatoid Wrist Disease

The wrist is inherently unstable and relies on an extensive collection of extrinsic and intrinsic ligaments to preserve stability between the forearm bones and carpus. Extrinsic ligaments extend from the radius and ulna to the carpus; palmar ligaments are stronger than dorsal ligaments. Intrinsic ligaments link the carpal bones only. The scapholunate and lunotriquetral ligaments secure the proximal carpal row and are key in maintaining the mechanics of force transmission through the wrist. Further stability is provided by the flexor and extensor retinaculi, and the 23 extrinsic extensor and flexor tendons that surround the wrist. The triangular fibrocartilage complex provides stability to the DRUJ. Normally, 80% of load is transmitted through the capitate, scaphoid, and lunate to the radius. Pathological weakening of ligaments distorts the biomechanics of the wrist, initially during loading and later at rest. Weakening of the important volar radiocarpal ligaments (radioscaphocapitate and radiolunotriquetral) contributes to ulnar translation and volar subluxation of the carpus. The ulna remains in its original position and becomes relatively prominent as the carpus subluxes. This collection of signs is termed a caput ulnae deformity (Box 59.4). Bony destruction and intrinsic ligament failure, especially scapholunate ligament disintegration, leads to carpal dissociation and loss of carpal height. With ulnar translation of the carpus the metacarpals fall into radial deviation.

• BOX 59.4 Classic Patterns of Rheumatoid Wrist Deformity – Caput Ulnae Deformity

Ulnar translation and radial deviation of the carpus
Palmar subluxation of carpus
Supination of carpus
Prominent ulnar head

• BOX 59.5 Key Features to Document on Radiographs of a Rheumatoid Wrist

General features of rheumatoid arthritis: osteoporosis, erosion, diminished joint space
Focal area of arthritis: radiocarpal joint, midcarpal joint
Features of caput ulnae deformity
Carpal height
Ulnar translation
Status of the DRUJ/ulnar head

X-ray Assessment of the Rheumatoid Wrist

Standard posteroanterior (PA) and lateral wrist X-rays should be assessed for features of RA and caput ulnae deformity. Two further aspects should be assessed: carpal height ratio and ulnar translation. The key features to document are listed in Box 59.5.

The carpal height ratio as described by McMurtry et al in 1978 is the distance from the third carpometacarpal joint (CMCJ) to the lunate fossa divided by the length of the third metacarpal. The average carpal height ratio is 0.53 (range 0.45–0.60). Other methods of calculation are also available.

A rapid semiquantitative measure of ulnar carpal translation can be made by assessing the position of the lunate relative to the radius; approximately 50% of the lunate should reside over the radius. A formal measure, described by Chamay and Della Santa,[1] can be made by calculating the distance from the center of the capitate head to the long axis of the ulna, divided by the length of the third metacarpal; the average is 0.3 (range 0.27–0.33).

Classifications of Rheumatoid Wrist Disease

There have been several classification systems for RA of the wrist. The Larsen classification is a radiographic descriptive classification (Table 59.2).[12]

The Wrightington classification is another radiographic classification system, designed to codify wrist pathology and guide treatment (Table 59.3). This scheme lacks the ability to anticipate the progression of wrist disease.[13]

Simmen and Huber[1] proposed an alternative classification system to try to predict the pattern of disease development (Table 59.4). Identifying the broad progression of RA can be of assistance in planning surgical procedures,

TABLE 59.2 The Larsen Classification for Rheumatoid Arthritis of the Wrist

0	No changes
1	Soft tissue swelling, demineralization
2	Marginal erosions, radial deviation
3	Articular erosions, joint space narrowing, mild radiocarpal instability
4a	Midcarpal ankylosis, major radiocarpal instability
4b	Radiocarpal ankylosis, stable
5a	Destruction of carpus, radiocarpal dislocation
5b	Destruction of carpus, complete ankylosis

TABLE 59.3 The Wrightington Classification of Rheumatoid Wrist X-rays

Grade 1	Wrist architecture is preserved Periarticular osteoporosis Early cyst formation Mild rotatory instability of scaphoid
Grade 2	Ulnar carpal translation Marked scaphoid flexion Radiolunate arthritis
Grade 3	Midcarpal arthritis Radioscaphoid arthritis Volar subluxation of the carpus on the radius
Grade 4	Significant loss of bone stock from distal radius

TABLE 59.4 Simmen's Classification for Rheumatoid Arthritis of the Wrist

Type I – Ankylosis	Spontaneous tendency to fuse Stable
Type II – Arthrosis	Articular loss and arthrosis (similar to osteoarthritis) Stable
Type III – Disintegration	Progressive destruction Loss of alignment Unstable

especially for type III patients, whom the authors felt should be followed closely and offered reliable stabilization of the wrist with the onset of ulnar translation or loss of carpal height.

Partial Wrist Arthrodesis

Partial wrist arthrodesis in RA may be performed for two reasons: isolated radiocarpal arthritis and ulnar translation. Options include radiolunate fusion and radioscapholunate (RSL) fusion. The benefit of partial arthrodesis is to preserve movement at the midcarpal joint; most activities of daily living can be accomplished with satisfactorily using a relatively limited range of wrist movement. Should it be necessary, subsequent conversion of partial arthrodesis to total arthrodesis is not technically difficult.[14]

Chamay introduced radiolunate (RL) fusion in 1983 after it was observed that spontaneous ankylosis of the radiolunate joint prevented continued distortion of the wrist and preserved a reasonable range of movement.[15] Partial fusion may be combined with synovectomy and ulna head resection. The radiolunate joint is debrided, then the lunate is positioned in a neutral position of 10–15 degrees flexion and secured with K-wires, screws, or staples. It is important to place the lunate in a neutral position to allow maximal extension of the wrist. Bone graft may or may not be used. RL fusion is one of the classic and reliable operations for rheumatoid wrist pathology; it provides pain relief and maintains wrist motion. Linscheid et al[16] reviewed 19 wrists, an average of 28 months post RL fusion; the average wrist extension and flexion were 25 degrees and 30 degrees respectively, pain and grip strength were generally improved. Progression of arthritis at the midcarpal joint may still occur due to alteration of carpal kinetics or disease progression. Borisch and Haussmann retrospectively reviewed 91 wrists post RL fusion with a mean follow-up of 60 months. RL fusion was often accompanied by synovectomy, ulna head resection, and division of the posterior interosseous nerve. Radiologically ulnar translation was effectively reduced. Most patients were pain free and content with the overall result, despite disease progression in 37% of midcarpal joints. There was an 8% complication rate, comparable with other studies; this consisted mainly of problems with osteosynthesis, either displacement or malplacement of metal ware or subsequent fractures. Of note, the authors recommend that in wrists with a fixed carpal collapse, repositioning of the lunate and restoration of carpal height should not be attempted as this seemed to precipitate secondary arthrosis and cause midcarpal dislocation.[17]

RSL arthrodesis is a less commonly performed operation, but may be appropriate for patients with extensive involvement of the radioscaphoid joint. Gordon and King reported the first RSL arthrodesis in 1961. Via a dorsal midline incision and through the fourth extensor compartment, the wrist joint is exposed, preserving the dorsal wrist ligaments; the articular surfaces of the radius, scaphoid, and lunate are debrided and osteosynthesis performed with or without bone graft. RSL arthrodesis reduces pain and preserves some motion, however the incidence of serious complications is significant, including nonunions, subsequent scaphoid fractures, and midcarpal arthritis, probably a consequence of altered carpal kinematics. Distal scaphoid resection may improve postoperative wrist flexion-extension; McCombe et al demonstrated an 86% increase in passive midcarpal motion in a cadaver model following distal scaphoid excision with RSL fusion.[1]

Total Wrist Arthrodesis

Total wrist arthrodesis is a reliable option for patients with severe painful rheumatoid wrist destruction, flexion deformity secondary to extensor tendon rupture, and as a salvage procedure following failed arthroplasty or partial wrist fusion. The radius, scaphoid, lunate, capitate, and third CMCJ should be fused. The suggested position of arthrodesis is 0–30 degrees extension, with or without a small amount of ulnar deviation. Reliable arthrodesis was established in the 1960s; Hazewinkel et al (1962) introduced wrist fusion with a Rush pin and bone graft, Clayton et al (1965) used a Steinmann pin, Mannerfelt et al (1971) modified this with the addition of staples, and Benkeddache et al (1984) used staples in isolation. Internal fixation with an intramedullary nail through the third metacarpal is well known for being a fast and reliable method of fixation, especially in the presence of osteopenic bone; bone grafting is not essential. Wrist fusion using plates and screws absolutely relies on decent bone stock; it is suitable for osteoarthritic wrists and seldom used in RA.

Solem et al reviewed 42 wrist fusions, 34 for rheumatoid wrist disease, over a mean 10.5-year period.[1] There were 21 Mannerfelt fusions (Rush pin and staples) and 21 plate fusions. There were two nonunions in the Mannerfelt group. The mean position of the wrist following Mannerfelt and plate fusions was 0 degrees and 8 degrees of extension respectively ($P<0.02$). There was no significant difference in key pinch, grip strength, pain in the wrist, and patient satisfaction between the two methods of fusion, although scores in the plate fixation group were slightly better.

There is no clear consensus on the position of fusion in bilateral arthrodesis. Suggestions within the literature range from 10 degrees extension of both wrists, neutral position both wrists or 5–10 degrees flexion of the nondominant wrist and a neutral position of the dominant wrist. Slight flexion does assist with some activities of daily living, e.g., perineal hygiene.

Total Wrist Arthroplasty

Total wrist arthroplasty (TWA) is an attractive option for rheumatoid patients with painful wrists, reasonable range of movement, and well-preserved hand function. It is especially appealing in patients requiring surgery for bilateral wrist disease. Contraindications include an active RA flare, infections, high demand patients, patients requiring the use of walking aids, poor hand function, poor bone stock or previous carpal resections and inadequate wrist control, especially poor wrist extension. The surgeon should document the current disease activity, status of the skin and extensor tendons (especially extensor carpi radialis brevis, ECRB), presence or absence of carpal tunnel syndrome, and range of movement.

The first wrist replacement implant was designed by Swanson and consisted of a simple silicone spacer.[18] Despite similar implants being successful within the small joints of the hand, Swanson wrist replacements are no longer used due to a high rate of complications. Jolly et al reviewed 23 Swanson wrist implants, an average of 72 months following surgery.[1] Complications included implant fracture (58%), revision surgery (30%), radiographic changes consistent with particulate synovitis (30%), and prosthetic settling and bone resorption (75%).

A number of surface replacement arthroplasties for the wrist have been introduced since Swanson's silicone spacer. The Menon prosthesis/Universal Wrist Implant, was developed by Jay Menon in the 1980s. Titanium stemmed protheses are inserted into the radius and carpus, with a broad ellipsoid articulation between a contoured cobalt chrome surface on the radial component and a polyethylene carpal component. Limited resection of the carpus and intercarpal fusion aids in prosthetic stability. Radial inclination and volar offset improve joint stability and wrist extension. The ulna head may be retained or a Darrach procedure performed. The Universal-2 Total Wrist Implant System is a later modification with reduced radial inclination and a porous coating to encourage osseous integration.

Kailash et al reviewed 92 Universal-2 wrist replacements, 83 for rheumatoid wrist disease. With a mean follow-up of 51 months, 91% of patients had satisfactory pain relief with 23 degrees extension and 21 degrees of flexion. Complications included joint stiffness (10%), wrist pain (9%), and superficial infection (2%). Almost 5% of patients required revision surgery and 3.5% needed salvage arthrodesis.[19] Salvage options for failed total wrist joint replacement include revision surgery or arthrodesis. Beer and Turner followed 12 patients who underwent salvage arthrodesis after TWA using tricortical bone graft and an intramedullary Steinmann pin. Seven patients united and five had a painless pseudoarthrosis, with 17 complications in nine patients.[1]

For patients with severe bilateral wrist involvement, wrist arthroplasty of the nondominant wrist and fusion of the dominant wrist may confer a functional advantage. Vicar and Burton noted that patients who had a wrist fusion on one side and a wrist arthroplasty on the other prefer the arthroplasty.[1]

Distal Radioulnar Joint

The DRUJ is often affected early in RA. Caput ulnae syndrome is present in 25% of patients, whereby the head of the ulna appears prominent due to carpal subluxation and supination plus DRUJ subluxation. Clinically this generates the piano key sign on examination: downward pressure on the head of the ulna temporarily relocates the ulna head. DRUJ arthritis occurs in 31%–75% of patients and causes pain during forearm rotation (especially with compression of the distal forearm).

Ulna head prominence and associated tenosynovitis can cause tendon attrition and rupture (typically extensor digiti minimi (EDM) is affected first). Surgical treatment requires synovectomy and either stabilization or excision of the ulna head.

Ulna head resection, as described by Darrach in 1912, gives good results in the majority of low demand rheumatoid

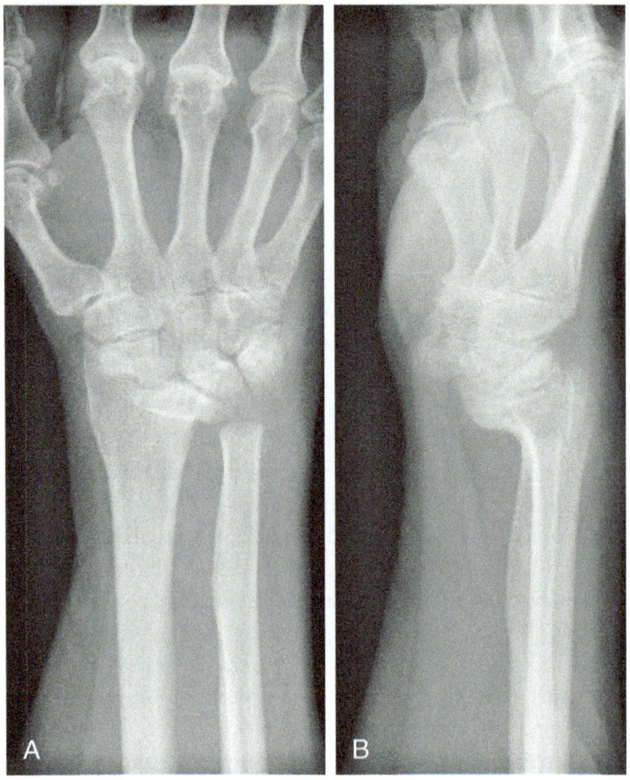

• **Fig. 59.3** (A) AP view of wrist post Darrach procedure with marked degenerative change within carpus. (B) Lateral view of wrist demonstrating palmar subluxation of the carpus.

patients (Fig. 59.3). It is easily combined with other procedures on the dorsum of the wrist, such as synovectomy, partial or total wrist arthrodesis, and TWA. The surgical approach is dorsal via the fifth compartment, preserving the extensor carpi ulnaris (ECU) subsheath of the sixth compartment. An osteotomy of the ulna is performed just proximal to the sigmoid notch, thus preserving the attachments of the pronator quadratus, which acts as a dynamic stabilizer. There is no evidence that surgical stabilization of the stump with part of pronator quadratus muscle or flexor carpi ulnaris or extensor carpi ulnaris tendons improves results. Ulnar carpal translation is not a complication of ulna head resection; most patients achieve excellent pain relief.

Rasker et al followed 40 RA patients following Darrach procedures. After 35 months, 38 patients had complete or almost complete resolution of pain. Functional use, supination, pronation, and strength all improved.[20] It is clear this symptomatic benefit applies to rheumatoid patients rather than patients with posttraumatic DRUJ pathology. Fraser et al reviewed patients following resection of the distal ulna for rheumatoid and posttraumatic conditions. While 83% of rheumatoid patients were pain free, only 36% of patients with post-traumatic DRUJ problems had similar benefit.[1]

The Sauve–Kapandji procedure involves DRUJ arthrodesis and segmental resection of the ulna; it is seldom indicated in RA. Via a dorsal incision, the DRUJ is exposed and debrided and arthrodesis is performed with compression screws or K-wires. The ulna head is placed in a position of neutral or slight negative variance. A narrow wafer of ulna shaft is resected just proximal to the arthrodesis site to create a pseudoarthrosis. Complications include painful radioulnar impingement, nonunion, tendon rupture, and union of the ulna.

Ulna head arthroplasty is a relatively recent option for rheumatoid DRUJ pathology although it is mainly used in osteoarthritis; there are hemi or total ulnar head implants available. Currently it is mainly used as a salvage option for failed Darrachs or Sauve–Kapandji procedures. The benefits of arthroplasty include improved stability of the forearm axis and prevention of impingement. The contraindications to ulna head arthroplasty include poor bone stock, infection, advanced joint destruction, and significant instability of the DRUJ. The surgical approach is similar to that for a Darrach or Sauve–Kapandji; soft-tissue stabilizers such as the dorsal radioulnar ligaments, ECU and dorsal capsule are carefully preserved. A cutting guide marks the amount of ulna resection and after broaching the canal the implant is inserted. The sigmoid notch may be deepened to facilitate stability of the DRUJ; soft tissues are carefully repaired to provide support. Berger and Cooney used the Avanta U-Head prosthesis in 22 patients, including some with RA, and followed them for 2 years. Clinical results were good to excellent in 18 of 22 patients; two patients were successfully revised after prosthetic loosening.[21]

• **BOX 59.6 Possible Causes of Loss of Digital Extension**

Extensor tendon rupture
Posterior interosseous nerve (PIN) palsy
Subluxation of extensor tendons
Volar subluxation of metacarpal heads

Digital Extensor Deficiency

Loss of digit extension is a common problem in RA and has a number of possible causes: extensor tendon rupture, posterior interosseous nerve (PIN) palsy, extensor tendon subluxation, and volar subluxation of metacarpal heads (Box 59.6).

Extensor tendon rupture always occurs at the wrist and is due to tendon attrition by proliferative synovium. Vaughan-Jackson first described sequential rupture of digital extensor tendons at the level of the DRUJ. Usually the EDM tendon ruptures first followed by other digital and wrist extensors. Surgery has a reparative and prophylactic role and involves tenosynovectomy and surgical treatment of the ulnar head/DRUJ plus tendon repair or transfer as required.

Due to gradual attrition and retraction of tendon ends, direct repair is usually not feasible. For isolated ruptures an end-to-side transfer or intercalated grafting are options. Multiple ruptures require intercalated grafts or tendon transfers of extensor indicis proprius (EIP) or adjacent extensor digitorum communis (EDC) tendons (Table 59.5). If all the digital extensors are ruptured then an FDS transfer (middle

TABLE 59.5 Suggested Extensor Tendon Transfers

Ruptured Tendon	Transfer
EPL	EIP to EPL
EDM	Tenosynovectomy and treatment of the DRUJ
EDM and EDC 5	EIP to EDC 5 or EDC 5 to EDC 4
EDM and EDC 4 and 5	EIP to EDM, EDC 4 to EDC 3
EDM and EDC 3–5	EIP to EDM and EDC 4, EDC3 to EDC 2
Multiple EDC, EDM and EIP	FDS 4 to EDM and EDC 4, FDS 3 to EDC 2 and 3 and EIP
Thumb and all fingers	FDS 4 to EDC 3–5, FDS 3 to EPL and EIP

For abbreviations see text.

and ring) is required[22]; the latter are transferred through the interosseous membrane or around the radius to the digital extensors. Intercalated tendon grafts can be used with reasonable results in recent ruptures; excursion of greater than 2 cm of the proximal muscle–tendon unit is required for this to work. Results are always best in those who maintain good wrist mobility (because of the beneficial tenodesis).

Rupture of the extensor pollicis longus (EPL) tendon on Lister's tubercle is common, but the functional deficit depends on the function of the extensor pollicis brevis (EPB) and the condition of the interphalangeal joint (IPJ). Often EPB and the intrinsic thumb muscles are too weak to fully extend the metacarpophalangeal joint (MCPJ), which causes difficulties with opening the hand for grasp. The treatment of choice is extensor indicis proprius (EIP) transfer, however with multiple extensor ruptures the EIP may be needed to reconstruct digital extension and so other options need to be considered. An interposition tendon graft may be used for fresh ruptures with sufficient excursion of the proximal muscle–tendon unit. EPL to EPB transfer provides simultaneous extension of the IPJ and MCPJ and the functional limitations are minimal.

Extension of digits is achieved by combined action of the EDC tendons and sagittal bands; sagittal bands are crucial for maintaining the position of the extensor tendons over the MC heads. Radial sagittal band attenuation or rupture causes rheumatoid digits to move into a position of ulnar drift. A zig-zag deformity of the wrist and digits is common as RA progresses; the metacarpals fall into radial deviation and the digits into ulnar deviation. Subluxation of extensor tendons between the heads of the metacarpals ultimately causes them to behave as MCPJ flexors.

Extensor tendon subluxation requires rebalancing of the extensor tendons. The extensor hood is opened to allow access to the joint for synovectomy, the radial sagittal band is then imbricated to centralize the extensor tendon over the head of the metacarpal. A crossed intrinsic transfer may be performed; the tight ulnar lateral band is transferred to the adjacent radial lateral band or MCPJ collateral ligament.[23]

Flexor Tendon Rupture

Flexor tendon rupture is also due to synovial infiltration and attrition and may occur within the wrist, palm or digits. The Mannerfelt lesion is a rupture of the flexor pollicis longus (FPL) tendon at the wrist and is frequently followed by ruptures of other long digital flexors.[24] Surgical treatment incorporates an extended carpal tunnel exposure, synovectomy, and debridement of bony prominences. Tendon ruptures are reconstructed on an individual basis and after consultation with the patient. Isolated FPL rupture may be treated by IPJ fusion, tendon graft or FDS transfer. Flexor digitorum profundus (FDP) ruptures may be treated with distal interphalangeal joint (DIPJ) fusion, tendon grafting or side-to-side transfer. Ruptured FDS tendons are typically ignored.

Ertel at al reviewed 115 flexor tendon ruptures in 36 rheumatoid patients; 80% of ruptures occurred at the wrist, 17% within the digits, and 3% within the palm. At the wrist level most FPL ruptures are due to bony prominences causing infiltrative tenosynovitis. While active motion was achieved in 88% of tendon reconstructions, the range of motion was poor; average movement was just 23 degrees at the thumb IPJ and 55 degrees at the digital PIPJs. Isolated ruptures within the palm or wrist had the best results. The authors highlighted the importance of early surgery, if only to debride tenosynovium and bony spurs that may cause further ruptures.[1]

Rheumatoid Digital Joint Replacements

The classic end-stage MCPJ deformity is one of flexion, ulnar deviation, and subluxation or dislocation. Proliferative synovitis attenuates or destroys supporting capsuloligamentous structures around the joint. Proximal deformities, such as carpal translation and radial deviation of the metacarpals plus the relatively ulnar pull of long flexor and extensor tendons and the intrinsic musculature all contribute to the ulnar drift. The established surgical practice has been to offer MCPJ arthroplasty only when function is severely limited. Recently the benefits of pain relief and cosmetic improvement, as well as range of movement have altered the indications for MCPJ arthroplasty.[25] Indications include pain, a significant extensor lag, ulnar deviation, and functional impairment, although some patients with advanced changes may remain pain free and function well. These patients may still consider surgery for cosmesis but should be warned that function may not be improved and grip strength may be weakened.[26] Correction of proximal wrist deformities and extensor tendon ruptures should ideally be performed prior to arthroplasty.

Silicone interposition implants are still the preferred choice due to their intrinsic stability and durability.

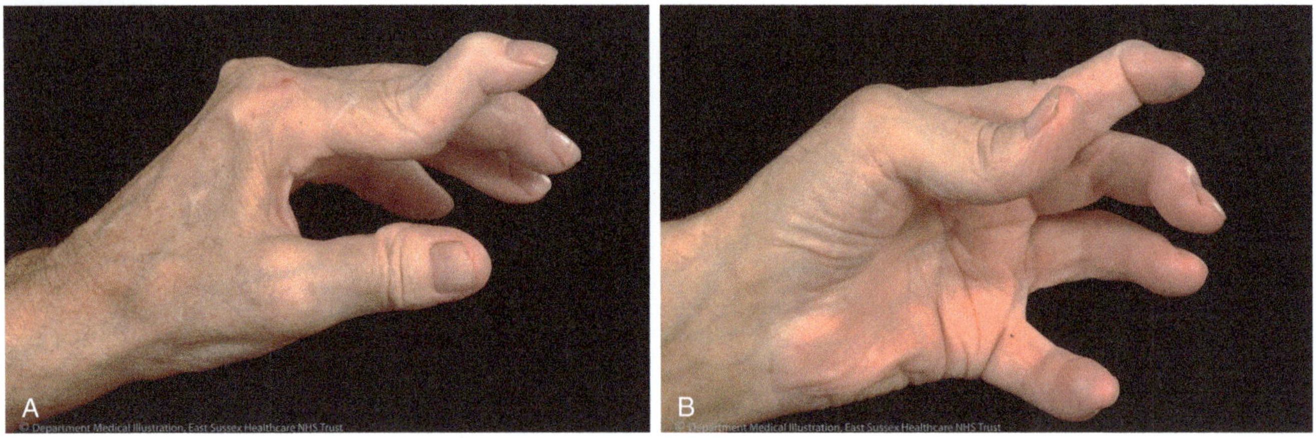

• **Fig. 59.4** (A) Swan neck deformity of index finger. (B) Boutonnière deformity of thumb.

Swanson's implants encapsulate in scar like all implants; they are not fixed to bone, a fact that almost certainly contributes to their long-term survival.[27] Encapsulation may mean that implant failure does not necessitate revision of the arthroplasty but implant failure may be associated with increased ulnar drift and poorer outcome. Pain relief is good but the subsequent range of motion, of about 40 degrees, is not significantly changed. Improved extension allows the MCPJ to function in a more useful arc and facilitates opening of the hand for grasp. Complications include recurrence of deformity, implant failure, implant dislocation, osteolysis, instability, stiffness, and silicone synovitis.[28]

Rothwell et al confirmed significant improvement in hand function following silicone arthroplasty; benefits were maintained for at least 3–4 years following surgery.[29] Chung et al prospectively followed 16 patients following Swanson MCPJ arthroplasty. At 6 and 12 months functional measures such as grip- and pinch-strength were unchanged but significant improvements in subjective hand function, activities of daily living, pain, esthetics, and patient satisfaction were reported. Ulnar drift significantly improved too (mean 24 degrees). The arc of motion (mean 46 degrees) was unchanged.[1] The initial benefits of arthroplasty appear to diminish with time. Goldfarb and Dovan[26] assessed long-term follow-up of 208 silicone MCPJ arthroplasties over a mean of 14 years. The mean arc of movement improved from 30 degrees preoperatively to 46 degrees postoperatively but this decreased to 36 degrees at final follow-up. The MCPJs were placed in a better position for grip with improved extension lag; preoperative extension lag was 57 degrees, postoperative extension lag was 11 degrees but this decreased to 23 degrees at final follow-up. Initial improvement in ulnar drift was not maintained. Implant fractures were reported in 63% of arthroplasties and were associated with increased ulnar drift. Only 27% of patients were pain free at the time of final follow-up. Different silicone implants may have different longevity and outcome measures. Sutter implants used a modified design and had a 45% failure rate by 3 years.[30] Analysis demonstrated that the stress of flexion was concentrated, rather than distributed diffusely as with a Swanson implant, resulting in a high rate of implant failure at the central portion of the hinge.

A newer option is surface replacement arthroplasty (SRA). The indications for these implants are as above but their use is typically contraindicated by inadequate soft tissue stabilizers and poor bone stock. Cook et al followed 71 pyrolytic carbon unrestrained MCPJ arthroplasties, for a mean of 11 years in 26 patients, 19 with RA. The replacements were all used in patients with minimal deformity of the MCPJ. At follow-up, 94% of implants were in a reduced position, with an improved range of motion and 13–16 degrees reduction in extensor lag. There was no change in ulnar deviation. The 10-year implant survival rate was 81%.[1] Pyrocarbon arthroplasty is a suitable and wear-resistant implant for mild MCPJ deformity in patients complaining of pain.

Flexible silicone implant arthroplasty can also be performed at the PIPJ. Ashworth et al[1] followed 99 Swanson PIPJ replacements after an average 5.8-year follow-up. Sixty-seven percent of patients were pain free. The average postoperative arc of motion was 29 degrees, which was less than the preoperative arc of motion of 38 degrees. Nineteen percent of the implants required revision at 9 years. Surface replacement arthroplasty for the PIPJ of rheumatoid patients is rare and typically contraindicated due to instability. Murray et al reviewed 67 protheses in 47 patients with a mean follow-up of 8.8 years: 75% of patients had osteoarthritis and 25% rheumatoid arthritis. The average range of movement was 40 degrees. There was a 15% failure rate by 15 years, and there were 22 complications requiring four PIPJ fusions and two amputations. The failure rate was not different in osteoarthritis and rheumatoid patients.[31] The alternative and reliable option is fusion of the PIPJ.

Rheumatoid Digital Deformities

The two classic digital deformities are a boutonnière deformity (BND) and swan neck deformity (SND; Fig. 59.4). In established RA the approximate incidence of BND is 36% and SND 14%. Both conditions have PIPJ deformity due

TABLE 59.6 Summary Treatment Guide for Swan Neck Deformity

	Fully Correctable	Partially Correctable	Fixed
MCPJ	Correction ulnar deviation Arthroplasty and/or Soft tissue correction	Soft tissue release and Arthroplasty and/or Intrinsic release	As for partially correctable
PIPJ	FDS tenodesis or Lateral band transfer	Soft tissue release and FDS tenodesis or Lateral band transfer	Arthrodesis or Arthroplasty
DIPJ	Arthrodesis	Arthrodesis	Arthodesis

to rheumatoid synovitis but the mechanical etiology is quite different. Deformities may be classified as fully correctable, partially correctable or fixed. Surgery for rheumatoid digital deformities usually occurs towards the end of the rheumatoid treatment sequence.

BND is characterized by flexion of the PIPJ and hyperextension of the DIPJ. The primary pathology is synovitis of the PIPJ leading to attenuation or rupture of the central slip insertion, and with time, volar subluxation of the lateral bands; the latter then act to flex the PIPJ and hyperextend the DIPJ. Secondary contracture of the accessory collateral ligaments, transverse retinacular ligaments, oblique retinacular ligament, and volar plate creates a fixed deformity. While patients often dislike the appearance of BNC, function remains relatively well preserved.

Results of BND surgery are often disappointing; treatment should avoid converting a bent digit into a stiff extended one. A fully correctable BND usually has an extensor lag of less than 15 degrees and is best treated with splintage. The PIPJ is held straight in the splint and flexion of the DIPJ is encouraged to allow lateral band glide. If the DIPJ cannot be flexed with the PIPJ in neutral then a "Dolphin" extensor tenotomy may be used, in which the extensor tendon is divided at the mid portion of the middle phalanx, while preserving the oblique retinacular ligament (ORL). A partly correctable BND usually has an extensor deficit of 30–40 degrees. Splintage is used initially to convert the partly correctable deformity back to a flexible deformity; extensor tendon reconstruction may then be attempted.

The central slip can be reconstructed using various techniques, including transfer of a distally-based FDS slip through the middle phalanx base, which can then be woven through the extensor in zone 4.[32] A fixed BND may require fusion in an improved position, especially if X-rays show PIPJ destruction. Kiefhaber et al performed 21 reconstructions for rheumatoid BNDs. Tendon reconstructions included either reefing of the central slip, coaptation of the lateral bands, use of a free tendon graft, a Matev procedure or flexor digitorum sublimis transfer.[33] At a mean follow-up of 2 years the results of were variable and unpredictable; the mean final extensor deficit was 39 degrees and the average loss of flexion was 12 degrees.

SND is characterized by hyperextension of the PIPJ and flexion of the DIPJ. While the hyperextension of the PIPJ is the most obvious clinical finding, the primary pathology may occur at the MCPJ, PIPJ or DIPJ. Determining which joint is responsible for the SND guides treatment. Secondary contracture of intrinsic muscles may also contribute to the deformity. SND causes difficulty in initiating grasp and can prove a functional problem for patients.

Treatment of SND depends on the joint pathology that initiates the disease (Table 59.6). As with other rheumatoid conditions it is important to treat proximal deformities first. Correctable SND requires treatment of the abnormal anatomy. Thus MCPJ dislocation or ulnar subluxation of tendons should be corrected and tight intrinsic muscles should be released. At the PIPJ a palmar restraint to prevent hyperextension may be achieved by FDS tenodesis. The latter involves division of one slip of FDS proximal to the A1 pulley, which is then secured to the proximal phalanx or to the A1 or A2 pulley, keeping the PIPJ in 20 degrees of flexion and preventing hyperextension. Another option is lateral band transfer (Zancolli) in which both lateral bands are mobilized from the midpoint of the proximal phalanx to the midpoint of the middle phalanx; the flexor sheath is opened between the A2 and A4 pulleys and the radial lateral band is routed palmarward under a pulley created between the FDS tendon slip and palmar plate. Lateral band transfer has the added benefit of improving DIP flexion. Tonkin et al performed lateral band transfer in 30 digits with SND, the majority with RA. Mean preoperative hyperextension of 16 degrees was corrected to a mean flexion contracture of 11 degrees; all deformities were corrected with no recurrences or complications.[34] Deformities that are not passively correctable may imply contracture of soft tissues around the joint, which require release before surgical correction of the primary deformity may be performed. This typically involves mobilization of the dorsally subluxed lateral bands off the central slip and dorsal capsulectomy or capsulotomy. Absence of movement may indicate articular damage, which requires either arthrodesis or arthroplasty.

Rheumatoid Thumb Deformities

The thumb is commonly involved in RA; 60%–80% of patients are affected. Nalebuff developed a classification system for the rheumatoid thumb by identifying the joint primarily responsible for deformity (Table 59.7).[35] In type I

TABLE 59.7 Nalebuff Classification of Rheumatoid Thumb Deformity

I	Boutonnière deformity
II	Boutonnière deformity with CMCJ involvement
III	Swan deformity
IV	Gamekeeper's thumb
V	Swan neck deformity due to MCPJ involvement
VI	Arthritis mutilans

For abbreviations see text.

(BND) the primary pathology is synovitis at the MCPJ with attenuation of the EPB insertion and subluxation of the EPL ulnarly. Extensor force concentrates on the IPJ, causing hyperextension. It is the most common thumb deformity.

In type II thumbs, a BND is also present but originates due to pathology at the CMCJ. In a type III thumb (SND) the problem originates with synovitis at the CMCJ causing dorsal and radial subluxation of the MC base, adduction of the first MC, narrowing of the first web, and reciprocal MCPJ hyperextension and IPJ flexion.

In a type IV thumb (gamekeeper deformity) attenuation of the ulnar collateral ligament creates lateral instability of the MCPJ. Type V deformity is a SND due to volar plate laxity at the MCPJ with a normal CMCJ. Type VI deformity is arthritis mutilans with extensive bony resorption.

While the Nalebuff classification provides a mechanical explanation for the zig-zag deformities found in rheumatoid thumbs, it is the two concepts of BND and SND that are of value to surgeons.

A BND classically requires treatment at the MCPJ and occasionally at the IPJ. Terrono et al followed 53 rheumatoid patients with BNDs of the thumb over 7 years.[36] The authors classified type I deformities into early, moderate, and advanced to aid assessment and treatment. Early deformities had fully correctable MCPJ and IPJs; treatment was MCPJ synovectomy and EPL–EPB rerouting as described by Nalebuff.[35] In moderate deformities the MCPJ was destroyed and fixed but the IPJ was correctable; surgical options were MCPJ arthroplasty or arthrodesis. Advanced deformities were fixed at both joints, which were radiologically destroyed and both joints required treatment; options included MCPJ arthroplasty or fusion and IPJ release or fusion. For moderate deformities MCPJ arthrodesis provided a high degree of satisfaction (4.7/5), and a pinch-strength of 6 pounds; 13% had subsequent IPJ collapse. MCPJ arthroplasty patients experienced a lower satisfaction rate (4.1/5), and a 3.5 pound pinch-strength; 23% subsequently had IPJ collapse. In advanced cases 85% of IPJ releases failed. Combined MCPJ and IPJ fusion were recommended for high demand patients and MCPJ arthroplasty and IPJ fusion for low demand patients.

EPL re-routing can be performed with numerous variations. Nalebuff's original description divides the EPL just distal to the MCPJ and attaches it either into the dorsal capsule of the MP joint or to the proximal phalanx, EPL then extends the MCPJ. The EPB is reattached to the EPL and extension of the IPJ is performed by the intrinsic muscles via the lateral bands. Another option is the EPB-plasty; the thinned or ruptured EBP is dissected free from the extensor hood and reattached to the proximal phalanx. The extensor hood is plicated over the tendon repair. Both procedures required immobilization of the MCPJ for 4–6 weeks postoperatively.

MCPJ arthroplasty is performed through a curved dorsal incision with arthrotomy between EPB and EPL. A minimal amount of bone is resected, preserving the collateral ligaments The largest silicone implant that fits is inserted, capsular structures are repaired, and the attenuated EPB and EPL are restored to their anatomical position. Average range of movement is about 25 degrees, with an improved flexion arc of 15–40 degrees.[37] Complications include implant failure and instability. Arthroplasty is not suitable for high demand patients or patients with gross instability around the MCPJ. Conversion to arthrodesis may require bone graft.

Arthrodesis of the MCPJ is a reliable procedure for disorders of the rheumatoid thumb, especially if CMCJ or IPJs are intact. The position of fusion is usually 15 degrees flexion, 5 degrees abduction, and 20 degrees pronation.[35] Fusion rates range from 80% to 100%. Bone grafting may be required, particularly for arthritis mutilans.

Surgical treatment of SND usually involves trapeziectomy, in order to improve the metacarpal base position; ligament reconstruction and tendon interposition, as described by Burton and Pellegrini,[1] is optional. Persistent hyperextension of the MCPJ may warrant sesamoid arthrodesis, or even formal fusion, depending on X-ray appearances. Very occasionally, restriction of the first web may require deepening or release. Arthrodesis of the CMCJ is rarely indicated.

Fortunately RA does not usually affect all three thumb joints to the same degree. Soft tissue procedures often do not provide long-term correction but may be performed, cognizant that further surgery may be required. When more than one joint is affected it is best to preserve mobility in as many joints as possible; arthroplasty is preferable at the CMCJ, the MCPJ may have either arthroplasty or arthrodesis depending on patient demand and the IPJ is usually fused.

References

1. Ayers R, Pickford M. Rheumatoid arthritis of the hand and wrist. In: Farhadieh RD, Bulstrode NW, Cugno S, eds. *Plastic and Reconstructive Surgery: Approaches and Techniques.* Oxford: Wiley–Blackwell; 2015:890–903.
2. Kay J, Upchurch K. ACR/EULAR 2010 rheumatoid arthritis classification criteria. *Rheumatology*. 2012;51:15–19.

3. Aletaha D, Neogi T, Silman AJ, et al. Rheumatoid arthritis classification criteria: an American College of Rheumatology/European League against rheumatism collaborative initiative. *Ann Rheum Dis.* 2010;69:1580–1588.
4. Sokka T. Radiographic scoring in rheumatoid arthritis. *Bull NYU Hosp Joint Diseases.* 2008;66:166–168.
5. Van der Heijde DM. Plain X-rays in rheumatoid arthritis: overview of scoring methods, their reliability and applicability. *Ballieres Clin Rheumatol.* 1996;10:435–453.
6. Boutry N, Morel M, Flipo R-M, et al. Early rheumatoid arthritis: a review of MRI and sonographic findings. *AJR Am J Roentgenol.* 2007;189:1502–1509.
7. Peterfy C. MRI of wrist in early rheumatoid arthritis. *Ann Rheum Dis.* 2004;63:473–477.
8. Souter WA. Planning treatment of the rheumatoid hand. *Hand.* 1979;11:3–16.
9. Burke FD, Miranda SM, Owen VM, et al. Rheumatoid hand surgery: differing perceptions amongst surgeons, rheumatologists and therapists in the UK. *J Hand Surg.* 2011;36E:632–641.
10. Arthritis Foundation Committee on evaluation of synovectomy. Multicenter evaluation of synovectomy in treatment of rheumatoid arthritis. *Arthr Rheum.* 1977;20:765–771.
11. Klemens T. Treatment of the wrist in rheumatoid arthritis. *J Hand Surg.* 2008;33A:113–123.
12. Larsen A. Radiological grading of rheumatoid arthritis: an interobserver study. *Scand J Rheumatol.* 1973;2:136–138.
13. Hodgson SP, Stanley JK, Muirhead A. The Wrightington classification of rheumatoid wrist Xrays: a guide to surgical management. *J Hand Surg.* 1989;14B:451–455.
14. Herren DB, Ishikawa H. Partial arthrodesis for the rheumatoid wrist. *Hand Clin.* 2005;21:545–552.
15. Chamay A, Della Santa D, Vilaseca A. Radiolunate arthrodesis. Factor of stability for the rheumatoid wrist. *Ann Chir Main.* 1983;2:5–17.
16. Linscheid RL, Dobyns JH, Yourn Y, et al. Radiolunate arthrodesis. *J Hand Surg.* 1985;10A:821–829.
17. Borisch N, Haussmann P. Radiolunate arthrodesis in the rheumatoid wrist: a retrospective clinical and radiological follow-up. *J Hand Surg.* 2002;27B:61–72.
18. Swanson AB. Flexible implant arthroplasty for arthritic disabilities of the radiocarpal joint. *Orthop Clin North Am.* 1973;4:383–394.
19. Kailash K, Raza A, Mahalingham S, et al. Outcome of universal-2 total wrist arthroplasty for rheumatoid arthritis: our experience at Wrightington. *J Bone Joint Surg.* 2012;94B(suppl XXXIX):143.
20. Rasker JJ, Veldhuis EF, Huffstadt AJ, et al. Excision of the ulna head in patients with rheumatoid arthritis. *Ann Rheum Dis.* 1980;39:270–274.
21. Berger RA, Cooney WP. Use of an ulnar head endoprosthesis for treatment of an unstable distal ulnar resection: review of mechanics, indications and surgical technique. *Hand Clin.* 2005:603–620.
22. Nalebuff EA. Surgical treatment of tendon rupture in the rheumatoid hand. *Surg Clin North Am.* 1969;49:811–823.
23. Schindele SF, Herren DB, Simmen BR. Tendon reconstruction for the rheumatoid hand. *Hand Clin.* 2011:105–113.
24. Mannerfelt L, Norman O. Attrition rupture of flexor tendons in rheumatoid arthritis caused by bony spurs in the carpal tunnel. *J Bone Joint Surg Br.* 1969;51:270–277.
25. Chung KC, Kotsis SV, Kim HM. A prospective outcome study of Swanson metacarpophalangeal joint arthroplasty for the rheumatoid hand. *J Hand Surg Am.* 2004;29:646–653.
26. Goldfarb CA, Dovan TT. Rheumatoid arthritis: silicone MCPJ arthroplasty indications, techniques, and outcomes. *Hand Clin.* 2006;22:177–182.
27. Swanson AB. Flexible implant arthroplasty for arthritic finger joints: rationale, technique, and results of treatment. *J Bone Joint Surg.* 1972;1972:435–455.
28. Trail IA. Metacarpophalangeal joint silicone implant arthroplasty. *J Hand Surg Am.* 2005;5:201–208.
29. Rothwell AG, Cragg KJ, O'Neill LB. Hand function following Silastic arthroplasty of the metacarpal joint in the rheumatoid hand. *J Hand Surg Br.* 1997;22:90–93.
30. Bass RL, Stern PJ, Nairus JG. High implant fracture incidence with Sutter silicone metacarpophalangeal joint arthroplasty. *J Hand Surg Am.* 1996;21:813–818.
31. Murray PM, Linscheid RL, Cooney WP, et al. Long-term outcomes of PIPJ surface replacement arthroplasty. *J Bone Joint Surg Am.* 2012;94:1120–1128.
32. Ahmad F, Pickford M. Reconstruction of the extensor central slip using a distally based flexor digitorum superficialis slip. *J Hand Surg Am.* 2009;34:930–932.
33. Kiefhaber TR, Strickland JW. Soft tissue reconstruction for rheumatoid swan-neck and boutonnière deformities: long term results. *J Hand Surg Am.* 1993;18:984–989.
34. Tonkin MA, Hughes J, Smith KA. Lateral band translocation for swan neck deformity. *J Hand Surg Am.* 1992;17:260–267.
35. Nalebuff EA. The rheumatoid thumb. *Clin Rheum Dis.* 1984;10:589–607.
36. Terrono A, Millender L, Nalebuff EA. Boutonnière rheumatoid thumb deformity. *J Hand Surg Am.* 1990;15:999–1003.
37. Figgie MP, Inglis AE, Sobel M, et al. Metacarpal-phalangeal joint arthroplasty of the rheumatoid thumb. *J Hand Surg Am.* 1990;15:210–216.

60

Lesions of the Hand

KAREEM HASSAN AND PATRICK L. REAVEY

Introduction

Masses of the upper extremity are among the most common reasons for referral to a hand surgeon, with ganglions alone representing the second most frequent cause of referral. The vast majority of these lesions are benign, however the average hand surgeon will encounter a few malignant sarcomas during their career. For this reason, when evaluating any mass of the upper extremity it is imperative that the surgeon maintains a high level of suspicion and performs a thorough history and examination. With a systematic approach and strict adherence to standard principles of management, surgeons can provide optimal care to patients.

History, Examination, and Diagnosis

A thorough history and physical examination can provide a careful clinician with an accurate diagnosis in many cases. Targeted questions regarding an upper extremity mass should include: the length of time the mass has been present, the presence and quality of pain, any change in size/symptoms, a history of trauma in the area, and any systemic symptoms. The patient's age, history of weight loss, personal/family history of malignancy, tobacco use, exposure to radiation/other carcinogens, and medications should all be elicited.

A thorough standard hand examination should be performed and documented in order to uncover any potential functional deficits due to mass involvement. This is especially important for medical-legal reasons prior to surgical intervention. When focusing on the lesion, the size, shape, color, consistency, and mobility of the lesion should be noted. Transillumination can be helpful in determining if a mass is cystic (Fig. 60.1). The approximate depth of the mass relative to other tissues in the area can also frequently be assessed through palpation. Additionally, manipulating the mass in both transverse and proximal to distal directions can elucidate any adherence to the overlying skin or deeper structures (tendon, bone). Lastly, the function of adjacent structures should be carefully assessed; a Tinel's sign in nearby nerves should be noted if present, and nearby joints should be a assessed for their range of motion. Any patient with a lesion determined to be high risk for malignancy requires a thorough pulmonary and lymphatic examination.

Imaging

Plain radiographs are the mainstay of work-up for hand masses. The majority of soft tissue lesions will not be directly visualized, however radiographs can help diagnose underlying pathology causing soft tissue manifestations or demonstrate soft tissue calcification as well as distortion or erosion into the bone (Fig. 60.2). Plain radiographs will demonstrate any primary osseous tumor. Well-circumscribed lesions are generally benign and slow-growing, while those that demonstrate periosteal reaction without signs of infection or trauma are worrisome for malignancy.

Magnetic resonance imaging (MRI) provides the highest definition of soft tissue lesions and provides the best information regarding soft tissue planes. MRI's utility is greatest prior to biopsy, as surgical changes will distort borders of the structures. Generally, intravenous contrast is required in order to truly characterize masses; this is especially true in vascular malformations.

Computerized tomography (CT) is helpful in assessing extent of involvement of masses as well as providing multiplane information for assessment of smaller lesions. This is especially true for lesions that involve the carpal bones, as their relatively small size requires the higher resolution provided by CT. Additional CT scans of distant areas (e.g., chest CT) may also be required to determine the presence of metastatic disease in cases of malignancy.

Ultrasound, while incredibly helpful in imaging soft tissue, is limited by the availability of a skilled technologist and radiologist. Newer ultrasonography machines can provide high-resolution images when available.

Principles of Biopsy

Once a lesion has been thoroughly evaluated, the majority of lesions of the hand are definitively managed with excisional biopsy. In the case of suspected malignancy, the preferred method of tissue diagnosis is incisional biopsy. The possibility of malignancy should be considered whenever performing a

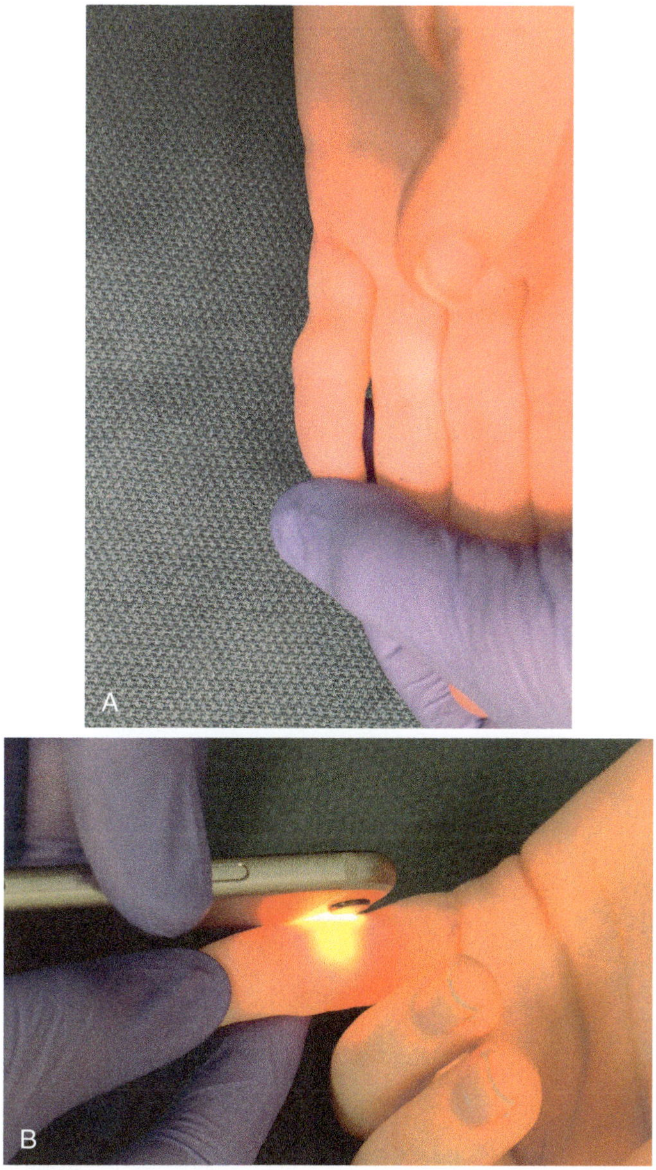

• **Fig. 60.1** (A) Volar mass of a small finger. (B) Diffuse glow of mass during transillumination with "flashlight" of a smart phone indicates cystic lesion, consistent with retinacular cyst.

biopsy, and planning should be done so that any biopsy performed does not hinder the definitive surgery. The incision should be placed longitudinally in a way that it can be excised in the definitive surgery and should be directly over the lesion to prevent creation of a contaminated tunnel. Exsanguination should be through elevation not with the use of an Esmarch bandage. Spreading should be avoided to avoid nearby contamination; infection and gouty tophi (Fig. 60.3) should always be considered as part of the differential, and cultures and cell count should be collected when indicated.

Narrowing the Differential

When considering any hand lesion there are a multitude of ways to formulate a differential diagnosis. It is frequently helpful to think of the most common lesions by the location on the hand and the depth of tissue. For instance, a painful lesion under the nail bed with some erosion into the distal phalanx on X-ray is likely to be a glomus tumor. Similarly, the dorsal hand has a high exposure to the sun, consequently skin lesions such as squamous cell carcinoma or basal cell carcinoma are frequently found there. A summary of frequently encountered masses organized by their location on the hand and depth within tissue is found in Table 60.1.

This chapter aims to discuss the most common masses of the upper extremity. For simplicity, masses are categorized by tissue type and by histologic cell of origin. It is important to note that this organization is primarily pathologic. Clinically, masses of different tissue types are found at varying depths and within other tissue types. For instance, epidermal inclusions cysts, while a mass of skin origin, are most commonly found subcutaneously.

Soft Tissue

Skin

Epidermal Inclusion Cysts

Epidermal inclusion cysts (EIC) are extremely common throughout the body, representing one of the most common lesions of the skin. EICs are also known as inclusion cysts, sebaceous cysts, epithelial cysts, or keratin cysts. However, the name sebaceous cyst implies it is from sebaceous etiology; that is a misnomer and can generate some confusion. The accepted theory of pathogenesis of EICs is the traumatic or embryologic burying of epithelial cells leading to a walled off shedding of keratin with in the affected tissue. Although human papillomavirus (HPV) and exposure to ultraviolet light have also been recently implicated.[1] EICs represent approximately 1%–16% of masses of the hand, with the vast majority – approximately over 70% – presenting on the glabrous skin of the palm and fingers.[2–4]

EICs generally present as small firm, slowly growing subcutaneous masses that do not transilluminate. The masses may be bothersome but are not generally tender, unless infected. Asymptomatic lesions require no treatment. The preferred treatment of symptomatic EICs is excision of the whole cyst including its capsule without perforating the mass. Complete excision is imperative, as cells that are left behind may continue to shed keratin and lead to recurrence. Excision of the cysts is not recommended when they are acutely infected. In this scenario, open drainage of the cyst followed by a short course of antibiotics is the recommended treatment. Once the acute inflammation has subsided (at least 4 weeks), a smaller excision can be performed with less chance of postoperative infection.

Warts

Warts represent one of the most common lesions of the hand in children and young adults. Warts represent infection of human papilloma virus (HPV), which occurs through direct inoculation of the infection from an infected individual or through self-infection. Approximately 70% of warts resolve

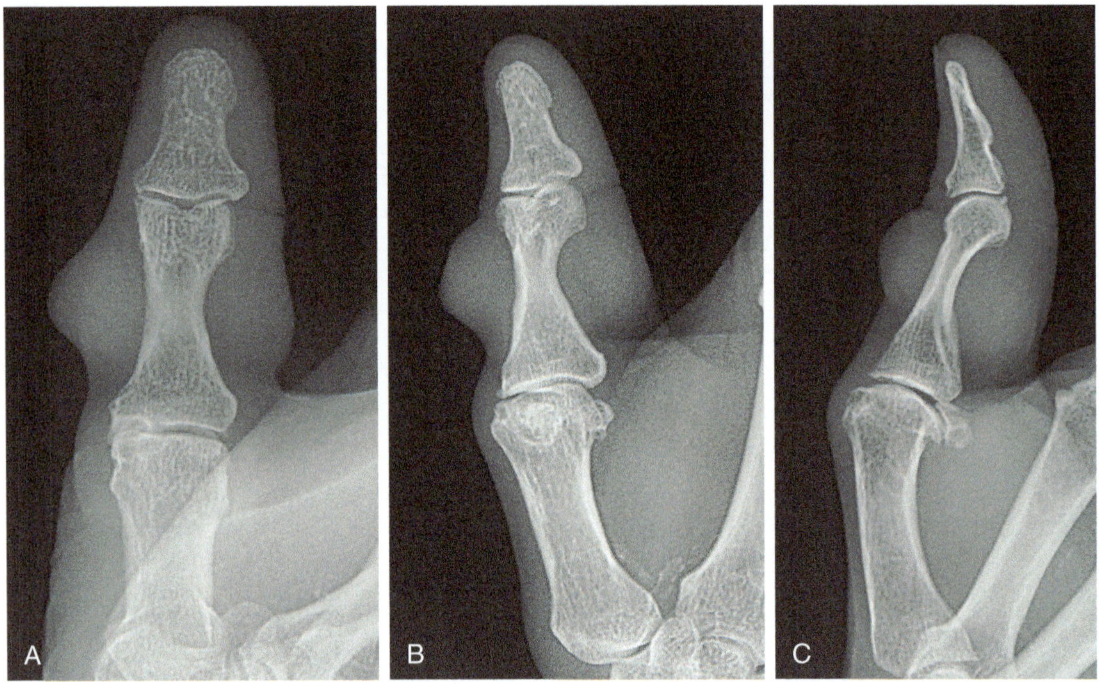

• **Fig. 60.2** (A–C) Plain X-rays of thumb soft tissue mass demonstrating distortion of proximal phalanx from slow growth, but no bony erosion.

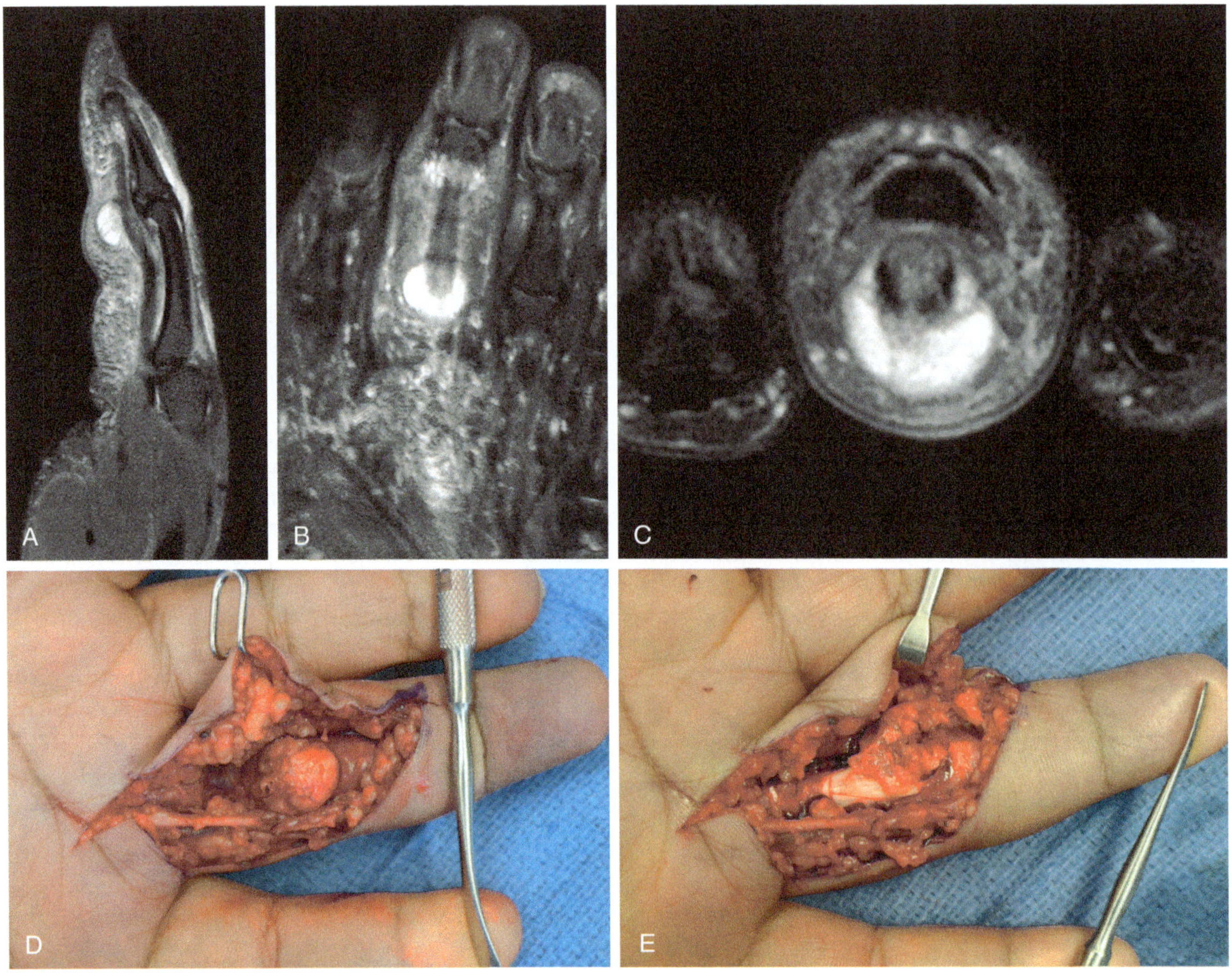

• **Fig. 60.3** (A–C) MRI of a patient presenting with a painful volar finger mass, demonstrating a fluid-filled lesion of the tendon sheath. On exploration, the lesion was found to be (D) a gouty tophus, with (E) direct invasion into the flexor tendons.

TABLE 60.1 Common Lesions by Location and Depth

	Skin	Key Findings	Subcutaneous	Key Findings	Bone	Key Findings	Other
Distal finger	Warts	Rough irregular papules	Mucous cyst	Nail deformity, arthritis of DIP	Glomus tumor	Pain, cold intolerance	Most common site of metastatic disease
Finger	Epidermal inclusion cyst	Chronic, occasional inflammation, "cheeselike" discharge	**Volar:** Giant cell tumor Fibroma	Firm fixed nodule along tendon course	Enchondroma	Pathologic fracture, lytic bone lesion on radiograph	Nerve sheath tumors along course of Neurovascular bundle
	Pyogenic granuloma	Bleeding, pedunculated lesion					
Hand	**Dorsal:** Actinic keratosis	Scaly, crusting lesions	Lipoma	Soft, compressible, freely mobile, no transillumination	Enchondroma	Pathologic fracture, lytic bone lesion on radiograph	
	Squamous cell carcinoma	Scaly, crusting, bleeding	**Volar:** Giant cell tumor Fibroma	Firm fixed nodule along tendon course			
	Basal cell carcinoma	Waxy, pearly papules, Telangiectases					
Wrist			Ganglion cyst	Transillumination	Giant cell tumor	Swelling and pain of wrist, large lytic lesion of distal radius	

spontaneously within 2 years, however rarely they can degenerate into a low-grade squamous cell carcinoma known as verrucous carcinoma.[5,6] Treatment options shown to decrease time to resolution include topical salicylic acid, topical dinitrochlorobenzene and intralesional immunotherapy.[7] No strong evidence exists for use of cryotherapy despite its widespread use.[7] Recurrent or long-lasting lesions which have been biopsy proven to not represent malignancy may be treated with excision with closure with grafts or secondary intention.

Primary Malignancies of the Skin

Several primary malignancies of the skin may present as masses in the upper extremity. The most common of these include actinic keratosis, squamous cell carcinoma, basal cell carcinoma, and melanoma. These are discussed in more detail separately in this text, however it is important when evaluating any hand mass that these diagnoses remain within the surgeon's differential.

Fat

Lipoma

Lipomas represent the most common soft tissue tumor of fat origin, representing approximately 3%–5% of all hand tumors.[8,9] While they are most commonly found in other more fatty parts of the body, lipomas can occur anywhere in the hand, including within muscle, nerve, bone or within the deep spaces (Fig. 60.4). Clinically, lipomas present as a slow-growing painless mass that is homogenous, freely mobile, and soft. It does not transilluminate. Generally, they are asymptomatic unless their size causes irritation, or if their location causes compression/irritation of nerves or tendons in the area. Radiographically, lipomas represent a homogenous radiolucent area on plain radiographs. MRI is the preferred imaging modality in order to determine extent of involvement and to rule out malignancy. Heterogeneity or ill-defined borders on MRI suggests possible presence of malignancy. If symptomatic, surgical excision of the lipoma is the preferred treatment method. Generally, lipomas are well encapsulated and surrounded by a layer of loose areolar tissue, allowing them to be easily bluntly excised. Sarcomatous degeneration of lipomas is extremely rare.

Lipoblastoma

Lipoblastomas are rare benign lipomatous tumors found in children less than 7 years of age.[10] They are generally found in the extremities and present similarly to lipomas; however, they are frequently lobulated and histologically are characterized by the presence of a varying range of immature adipose

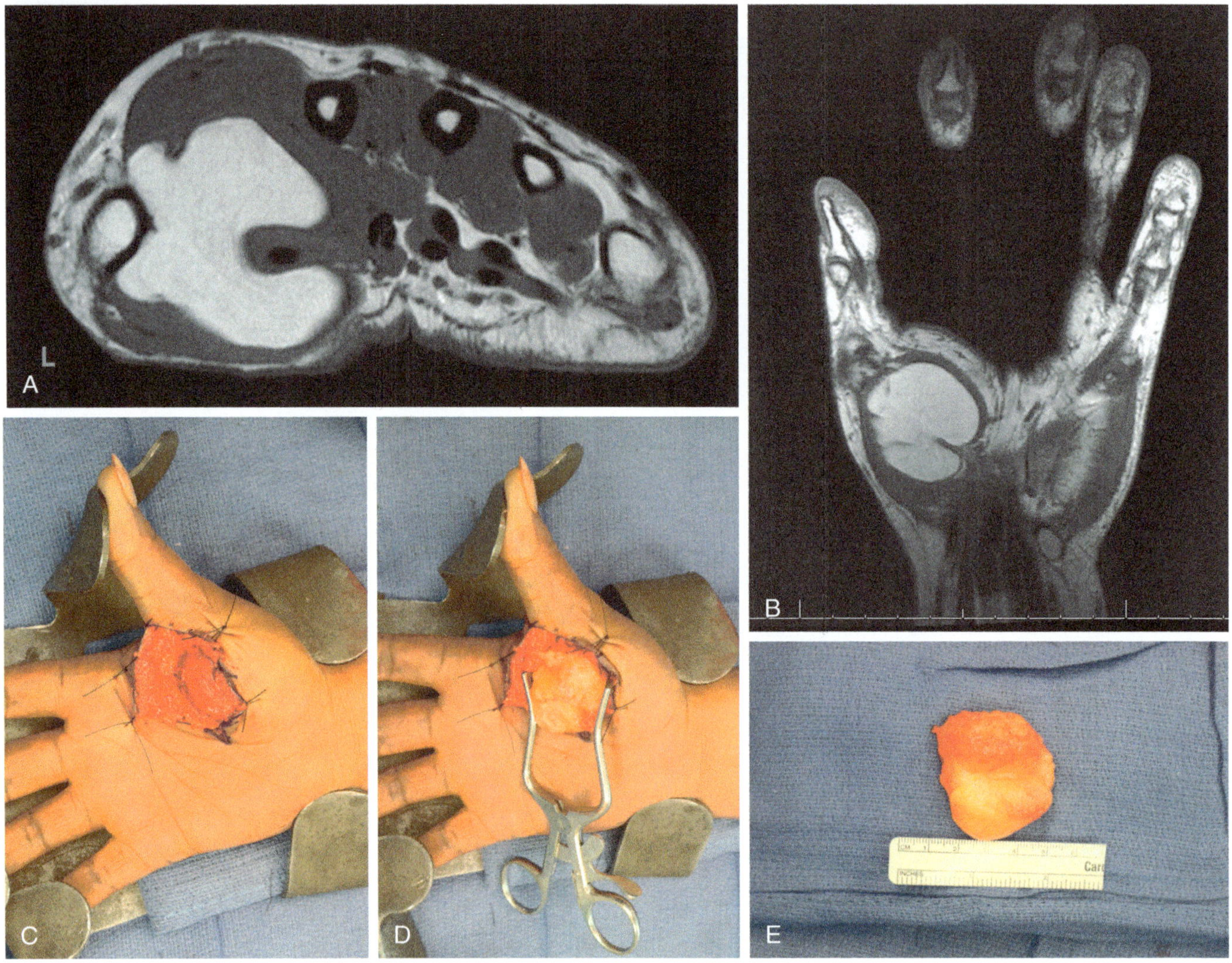

• **Fig. 60.4** (A,B) MRI of a patient with a significant thenar mass demonstrating a lipoma within the thenar compartment. (C–E) A well-encapsulated lipoma was removed by direct excision.

tissue. Excision is generally curative and is recommended in order to definitively rule out the presence of a liposarcoma. Another variant of this condition, known as lipoblastomatosis, is characterized by lack of encapsulation and local infiltration; recurrence is more common in this variant.[10]

Other

Angiolipomas are another tumor of adipose origin, however as the name implies they also contain vascular sinuses. Angiolipomas are benign masses, however they may be locally infiltrative and generally are painful.[11] Lipofibromatous hamartomas or fibrolipomas are rare benign fatty tumors closely associated with a nerve. They have been reported in close association with the radial, ulnar, and median nerves. Given their close association and infiltration of nerves, they frequently cause symptoms of nerve compression. Treatment involves decompression of the nerve without resection, as resection is frequently impossible without sacrifice of the nerve itself. If the diagnosis is not clear, biopsy should performed to confirm the etiology before the tumor is left in situ.

Connective Tissue

Ganglion Cyst

Ganglion cysts represent the most common mass of the hand and wrist.[12] Ganglion is both a general term and the name of a cyst occurring on the dorsum of the wrist. However, ganglion cysts may also be known as mucous cyst when found near the distal interphalangeal (DIP) joint or retinacular cyst when found along the flexor tendon sheath. Despite their high incidence, the pathogenesis of ganglions remains unconfirmed. The name ganglion cyst itself is a misnomer as ganglions lack an epithelial lining and therefore are not true cysts.[13] Ganglions are collagen-lined sacks filled with mucinous material. In the past it was thought ganglion cysts represented synovial herniation from the associated joint, however the lack of synovial lining weakens this theory.[13] Currently, the most accepted theory is that repetitive damage and stretching to the joint capsule creates a one-way valve, which allows synovial fluid to leak. As this leak becomes sealed off, the water component of the fluid is reabsorbed leaving the gelatinous substance that fills the cysts.[13] The fact that ganglions frequently appear at sites of microtrauma such as the scapholunate ligament, the ability to treat ganglions arthroscopically and the need to excise the stalk to prevent recurrence all give credence to this theory.

The vast majority of wrist ganglions present as atraumatic, slow-growing, painless masses, with over 70% located on the dorsal wrist (Fig. 60.5) and approximately 20% located on the volar wrist. Typically, ganglions are asymptomatic, although dorsal ganglions may cause discomfort when extending the wrist. Patients frequently describe the mass swelling with activity and decreasing in size with rest. On examination ganglion cysts typically are firm, round lesions that transilluminate. Dorsally, ganglion cysts most frequently arise from the scapholunate ligament; volarly they commonly originate from the scaphotrapezium–trapezoid joint. Asymptomatic ganglion cysts require no treatment, however when treatment is indicated, management is through direct surgical excision. Aspiration of the cyst has a high recurrence rate. During surgical excision, it is essential to locate and remove the stalk of the lesion to prevent recurrence; cauterizing the base of the lesion is also recommended to devitalize any microscopic remnants left behind. When treating volar ganglions, care must be taken to avoid the radial artery, as the lesions are frequently intimately associated with the artery (Fig. 60.6). For this reason, we routinely obtain MRI on volar ganglions to assist with surgical planning.

Mucous cysts typically present as a lesion on the dorsal distal phalanx proximal to the nail fold. Patients may complain of pain in the DIP joint as mucous cysts are associated with DIP joint arthritis. X-rays of the finger will often demonstrate dorsal osteophytes of the joint. Occasionally the only presenting symptom may be an abnormal nail plate when the cyst is located over the germinal matrix (Fig. 60.7). When removing mucous cysts, excision of any associated osteophytes should be performed to prevent recurrence.

Retinacular cysts occur volarly along the flexor tendon sheath (see Fig. 60.1). Diagnosis can often be made by transillumination. Repeated aspiration of retinacular cysts has an approximately 80% cure rate. Surgical excision is reserved for cases of recurrence.

Giant Cell Tumor

Giant cell tumors of the tendon sheath are relatively uncommon lesions, which present as firm painless masses

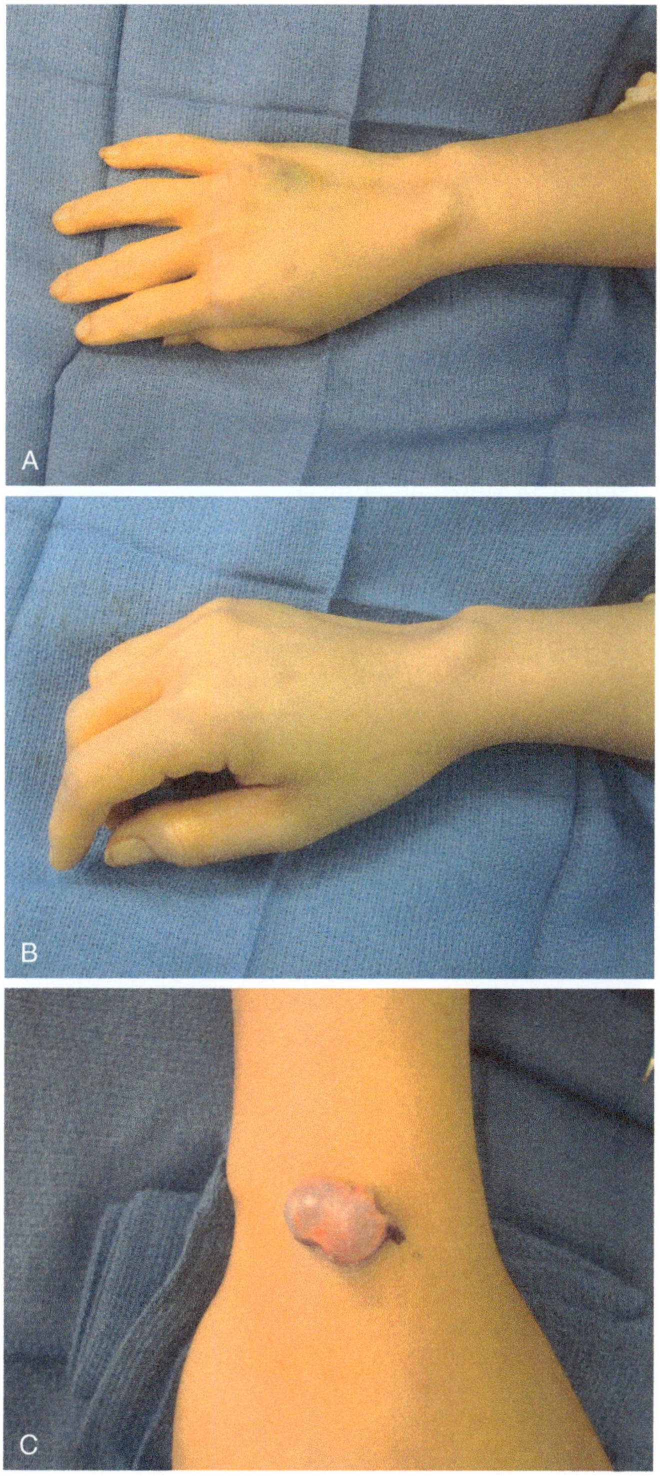

• **Fig. 60.5** (A,B) Dorsal wrist mass over the scapholunate interval consistent with a ganglion cyst. (C) Intraoperative photo during excision.

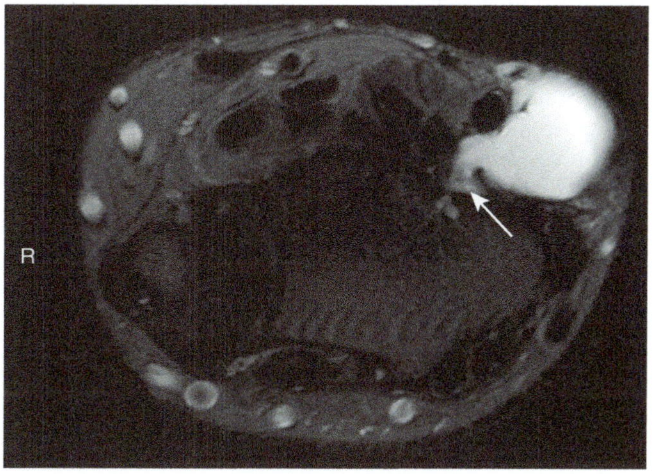

• **Fig. 60.6** MRI of volar wrist ganglion in close proximity to radial artery and stalk extending to radial carpal joint (*arrow*).

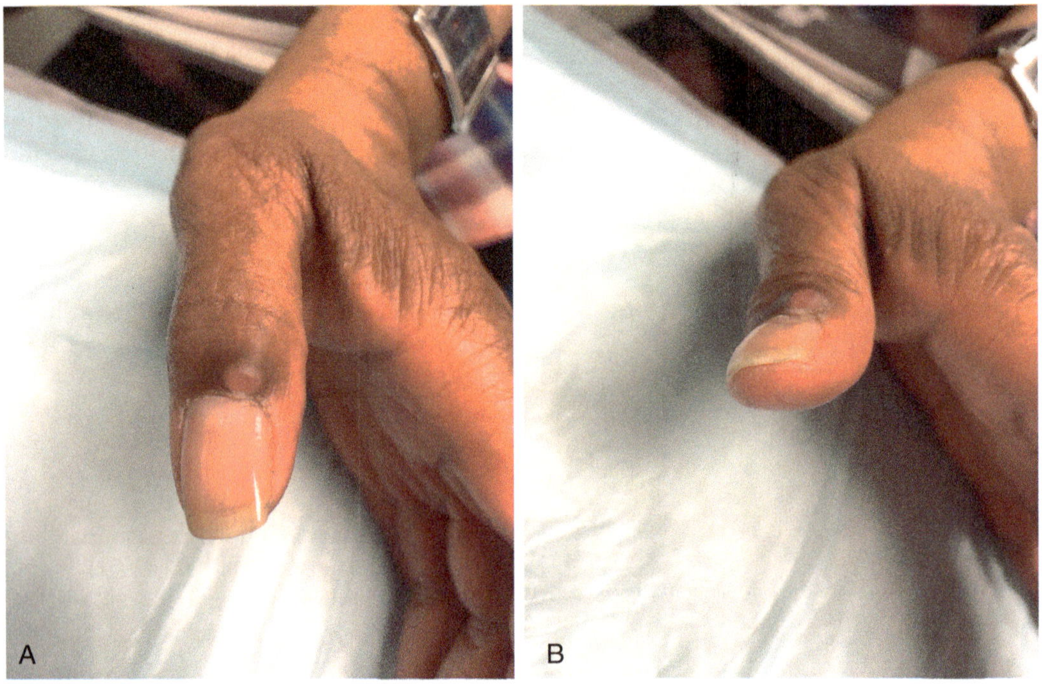

• **Fig. 60.7** (A) Mucous cyst of thumb proximal to nail fold. Note thinning of skin overlying the cyst. (B) Pressure on the germinal matrix resulted in flattening of the nail distal to the cyst.

most commonly on the volar surface of the digits (Fig. 60.8) or palm. They have a slightly higher incidence in women when compared to men.[13] The etiology of giant cell tumors remains largely unknown, they comprised largely of multinucleated giant cells, foam cells, and hemosiderin deposits (which are responsible for their characteristic brown color). The most common origin is the flexor tendon sheath, and while cortical invasion is rare it has been described. Malignant transformation has also never been reported in the literature. Management of these lesions is by direct complete excision. Complete excision can be facilitated by identifying the brown color of the mass and ensuring that no brown tissue is left behind. This is especially important as recurrence is reportedly between 4% and 44%, with higher incidence with incomplete resection. While the marginal excision is essential, it is also important to explore joints, which may be involved, and care must be taken to preserve the neurovascular bundles to the digits, which are frequently intimately related to the mass.

Fibroma

Fibromas of the tendon sheath are clinically nearly indistinguishable from giant cell tumors of the tendon sheath. They generally present as firm, painless masses of the volar finger arising from the flexor tendon sheath, however unlike giant cell tumors, they are slightly more common in men.[14] Treatment of fibromas is identical to giant cell tumors; however, grossly they appear more white and microscopically lack the hemosiderin deposits.[14] Likewise, fibromas have a high recurrence rate, with the largest series reporting a recurrence rate of approximately 24%.[14]

Vascular

Pyogenic Granuloma

Pyogenic granulomas – also known as lobular capillary hemangiomas – are common benign vascular lesions of the skin. Their name is a misnomer as the lesions are not infectious in origin or granulomatous in nature. The exact cause of these lesions remains unknown, however trauma, *BRAF* mutations, and probably herpes virus type 1, Orf virus, and/or HPV type 2, as well as numerous medications, have all been implicated.[15] Pyogenic granulomas present as rapidly growing pedunculated lesions with a friable red–purple apex which often easily bleeds (Fig. 60.9). The development can be classified into: (i) cellular phase, (ii) capillary phase or vascular phase, and (iii) involutionary phase. Treatment ranges from symptomatic relief of bleeding by cautery or silver nitrate application to surgical excision, which provides resolution in the vast majority of cases; medical treatment with beta-blockers and selected *BRAF* inhibitors have shown success recently.[15]

Glomus Tumor

The glomus body is a specialized arteriovenous shunt that functions to aid in thermoregulation by responding to temperature changes. The highest density of these structures is found in the fingertips and nailbeds in the body. Glomus tumors are characterized by pain, cold intolerance, and exquisite point tenderness over the mass.[15] Pain that resolves after application of a tourniquet, known as Hildreth's test, is very characteristic of the lesion. The mass may also appear as a blue discoloration to the skin or nailbed. Plain radiographs may reveal a lytic bone lesion of the distal

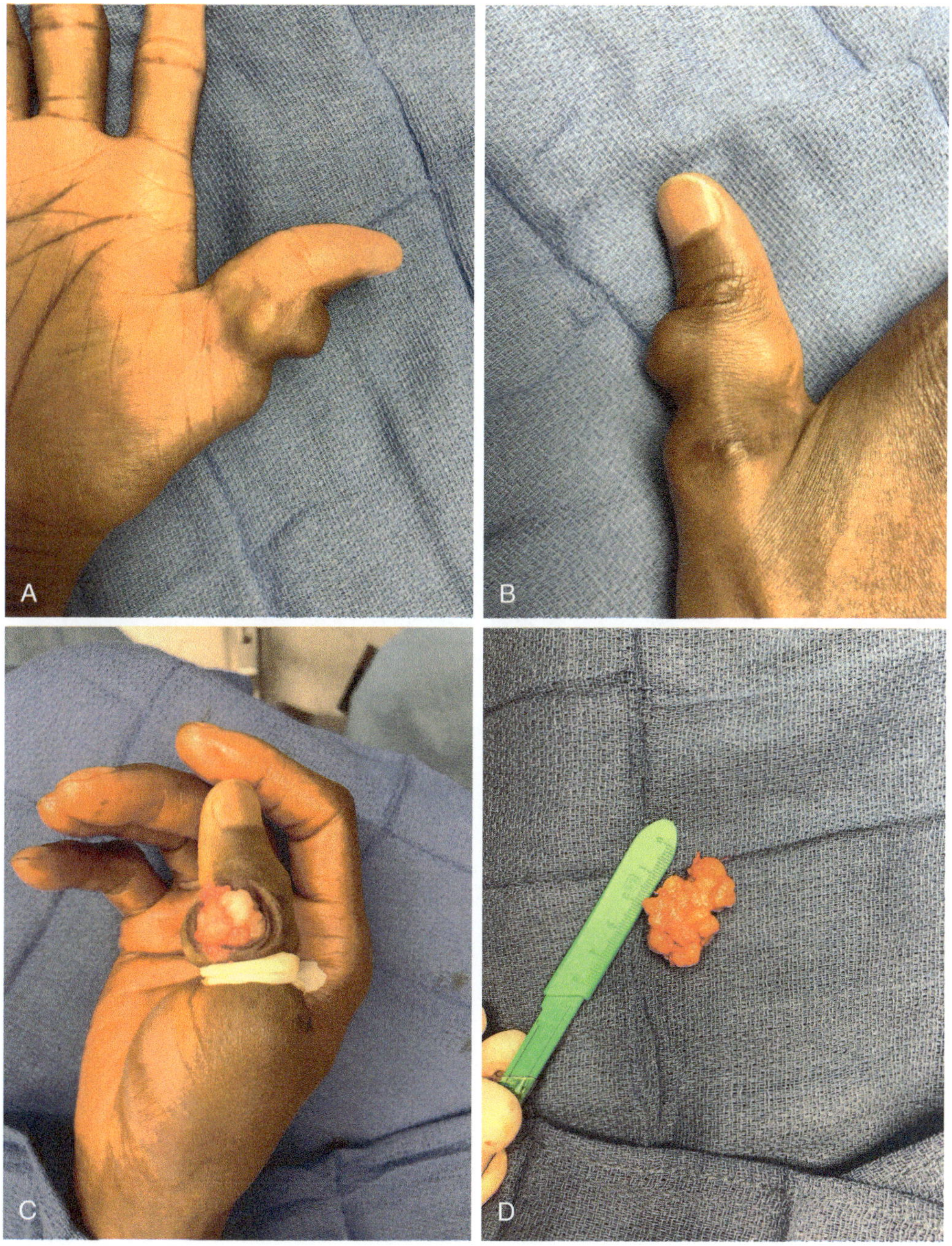

• **Fig. 60.8** (A,B) Large soft tissue mass of thumb. X-rays of mass seen in Fig. 60.2 demonstrate distortion of the proximal phalanx from slow growth of the tumor. (C,D) Brown, lobulated appearance of the lesion during excision typical of giant cell tumor of the tendon sheath.

phalanx; MRI can also be useful in confirming the diagnosis or identifying multicentric disease. Direct surgical excision is curative in nearly all cases.[16] Malignant glomus tumors are rare, and require wide excision to prevent recurrence.[17]

Hemangioma

Hemangiomas are idiopathic tumors generally found in infants around 4–6 weeks of age. The appearance of these lesions varies depending on their depth, ranging from a superficial red plaque-like lesion to deeper lesions appearing as a blue discoloration. This is covered in detail in Chapter 15, Vascular Anomalies. Classically there is no sign of these lesions at birth, and they then undergo their proliferative phase, which is marked by rapid growth. Following this there is a phase of slow involution in which the hemangioma slowly is replaced by fibrofatty tissue, and finally the resolution phase which is marked by a 10% reduction in size per year.[18] Generally 50% of the tumors have regressed by age of 5 and 90% by 9 years of age.[15] Given their self-limited nature, treatment is largely through observation. Resolution of large lesions that are cosmetically bothersome may be hastened with oral or topical beta-blockers, or intralesional steroids.[19] Systemic steroids and more recently beta-blockers form the basis of medical therapies. Surgery is also an option for small lesions which would allow for primary closure, or if ulceration and bleeding is causing recurrent issues.

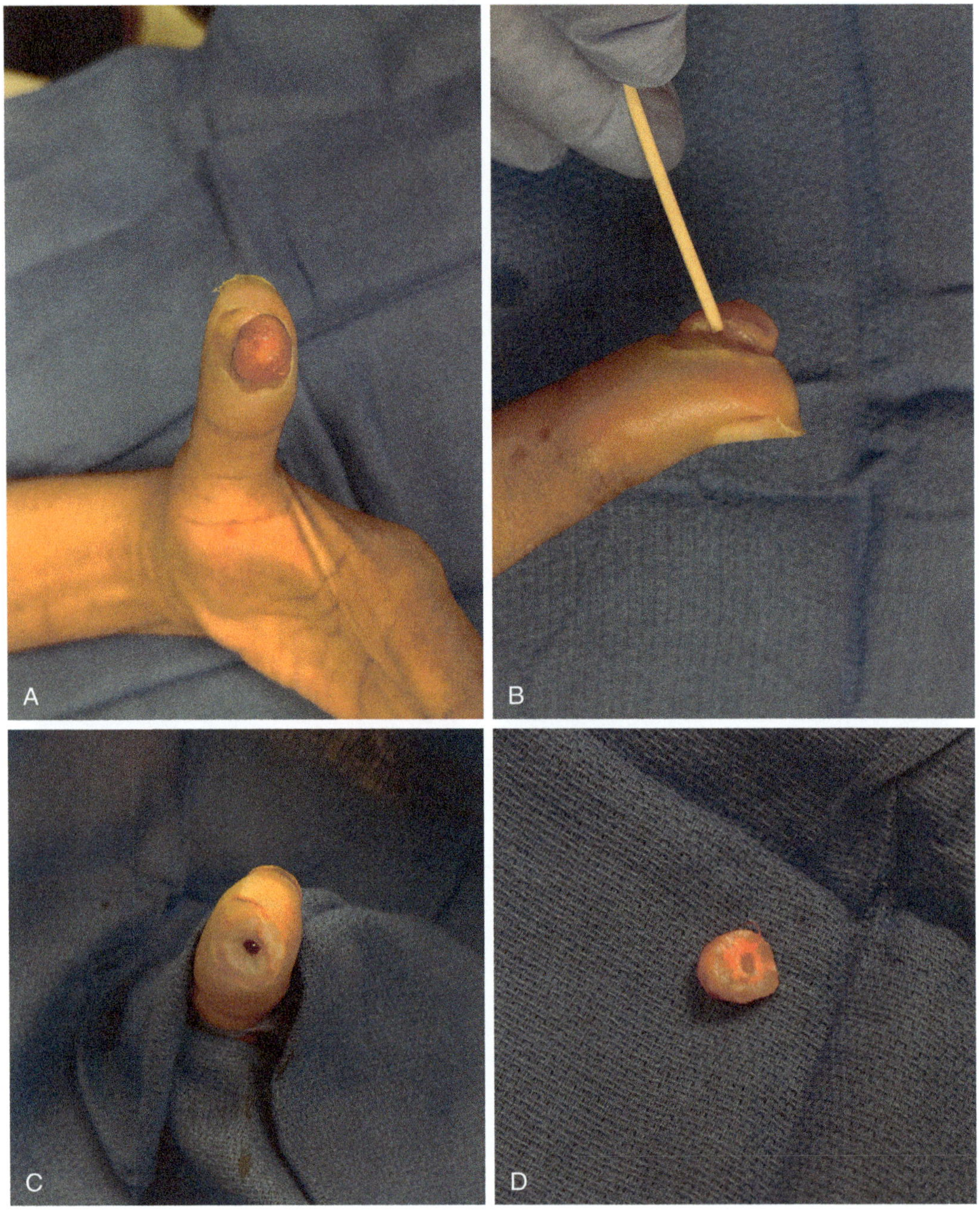

• **Fig. 60.9** (A) Pyogenic granuloma of the thumb with (B–D) characteristic hypervascular appearance and small stalk. The granuloma was removed and the small wound in the thumb cauterized to prevent recurrence.

Vascular Malformations

Vascular malformations are commonly seen in the extremities. Unlike hemangiomas, they are generally apparent at birth and their growth rate is proportional to the child's growth rate.[20] Mulliken and Glowacki, and Upton et al developed a widely accepted system to classify these lesions based on a combination of their flow state and histological origins respectively; these principles are covered in detail in Chapter 15.[20,21]

Low-Flow Lesions

Venous, capillary, and lymphatic malformations are all categorized as low-flow lesions.[21] Combined malformations also exist, such as lymphatic venous malformations. The vast majority of the low-flow lesions are diagnosed at birth, with the remaining usually diagnosed early in childhood.

Venous malformations can vary widely in size, with variation in size with dependency as well as compression. Generally, they present as soft blue pulseless lesions. They may be accompanied with pain when they are associated with thrombosis. Plain radiographs may demonstrate calcified densities representing thrombosed veins; ultrasounds may be helpful in larger masses to identify flow within the lesions; and MRI is useful to analyze the extent of the lesions (Fig. 60.10). Aspirin can be used to avoid painful thrombosis. Compression garments and symptomatic control are the

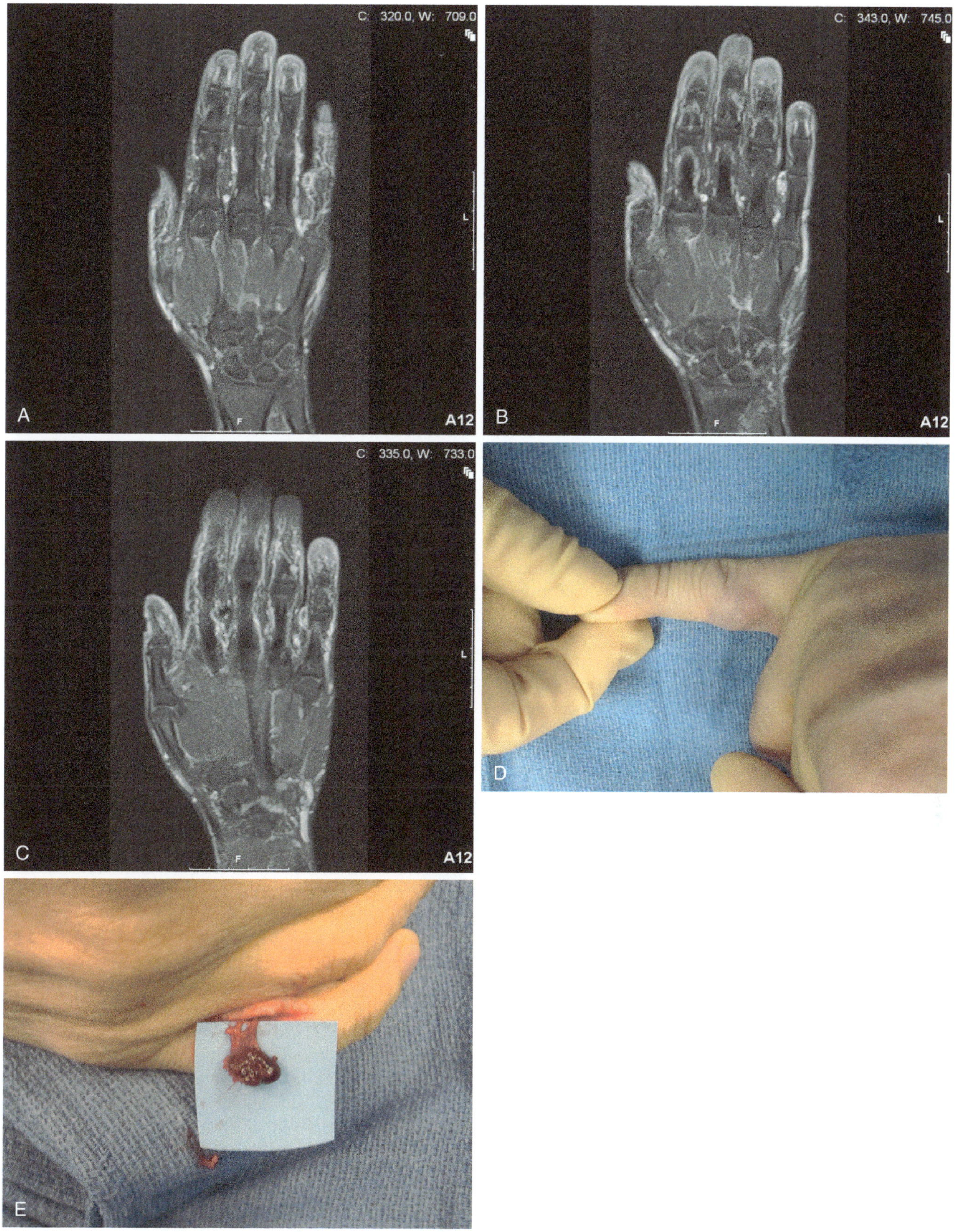

• **Fig. 60.10** (A–C) Venous malformation of the small finger demonstrated on MRI. (D) Note the blue coloration of the lesion on clinical exam and (E) communication with normal-appearing veins during excision.

mainstay of treatment. Sclerotherapy can also be useful in reducing the size of the lesion.

Lymphatic malformations, like venous malformations, are nonpulsatile lesions of variable size. However, unlike venous malformations, they feel rubbery and do not acutely decrease in size with elevation of the limb. Lymphatic malformations frequently can become infected with bacteria, likely due to impaired immune activity within the lesion. MRI is the mainstay for imaging. Compression and sclerotherapy are also effective in lymphatic malformations.

Capillary malformations present as small areas of erythematous discoloration and are frequently confused as bruises from trauma. They are also known as port wine stains. Typically, these lesions are superficial within the dermis, however deeper involvement is also possible. Unlike venous and lymphatic malformations, imaging and compression are of little utility in capillary malformations. The mainstay of treatment is pulse-dye laser, which targets oxyhemoglobin through control of wavelength.

Surgical management of the low-flow lesions is limited to lesions refractory to conservative measures.

High-Flow Lesions

High-flow lesions are arterial or arteriovenous malformations (AVM). Unlike low-flow lesions, only 40% of these lesions are diagnosed at birth.[21] AVMs are two times more common in females than males, and are most frequently found in the right arm and hand.[21] These lesions appear to respond to hormones, as a majority of patients report increasing size and pain during pregnancy and puberty.[21] These lesions have a palpable thrill or pulse and may present with distal symptoms of ischemia.

High-flow lesions can be further divided into type A lesions which are arteriovenous fistulas, type B which are arteriovenous anomalies in addition to the fistulas in a single artery, and type C lesions which is defined by diffuse AV anomalies and fistulas of the entire limb. Imaging is needed to confirm the diagnosis of these lesions. Doppler ultrasound is useful to determine the flow characteristics as well as number of vessels involved, MRI is also extremely helpful. Formal angiography can be used diagnostically as well as therapeutically through embolization.

When all conservative measures have failed, resection of these lesions can be performed; however, doing so has significant risks. Perioperative bleeding is a large risk in these cases; preoperative embolization is a useful adjunct for resection. In type B and C lesions, excision has significant risk of causing distal ischemia and possible embolic events. In the case of type C lesions amputation may be needed.

Nerve

Schwannoma

Schwannomas, or neurilemomas, are benign overgrowths of Schwann cells and represent the most common solid nerve tumor. They most commonly affect middle-aged adults.[22] Schwannomas are associated with neurofibromatosis types 1 and 2, however type 1 is more associated with schwannomas of the extremity and trunk. Occasional schwannomatosis has been reported where multiple schwannomas have been found without a diagnosis of neurofibromatosis.[22]

Schwannomas present as slow-growing, painless masses found alongside the course of a nerve. While neurological deficits and pain are possible, they are not the typical presentation. Tinel's sign can be found, however it is not consistent, with reports in the literature ranging from 4% to 79% of schwannomas having a positive Tinel's sign.[22]

Grossly, schwannomas appear firm with whirls of yellow-gray tissue.[23] Schwannomas are usually well encapsulated and distinct from the nerve fascicles. Excision can usually be performed by bluntly shelling the schwannoma away from the nerve fascicles. Operative microscopy should be utilized to identify and protect the source nerve. If concern exists due to inconsistent appearance of the mass, frozen section or incisional biopsy should be performed prior to formal excision. While it is possible to maintain function of the origin nerve, recent reports have suggested that deficits may exist in up to half of patients following excision.[23] Malignant degeneration of schwannomas is extremely rare.

Neurofibroma

Neurofibromas are another benign tumor of Schwann cell origin, however they are distinguished from schwannomas by the presence of fibroblasts and in that they are frequently intertwined within nerve fascicles. Three types of neurofibromas exist: localized, diffuse, and plexiform. Localized neurofibromas occur sporadically in individuals without neurofibromatosis and usually present as a solitary cutaneous lesion. When diffuse neurofibromas are encountered, with or without the presence of café-au-lait spots, neurofibromatosis should be considered (Fig. 60.11). Neurofibromatosis is divided into type 1 (NF1) and type 2 (NF2). Both types are caused by an autosomal dominant mutation,:type 1 is caused by alterations in the *NF1* gene while type 2 is caused by the *NF2* gene. Boxes 60.1 and 60.2 summarize diagnostic criteria for NF1 and NF2. Localized lesions generally arise from the terminal branches of sensory nerves; excision of these lesions generally is straight forward. Plexiform lesions occur in continuity with main nerve branches; excision of these lesions while maintaining nerve function is extremely difficult or impossible[24] (Fig. 60.12). Malignant degeneration of plexiform neurofibromas ranges from 2% to 13% in patients with neurofibromatosis.[23] It is therefore important to monitor for acute increases in growth rate of lesions, increased pain, or development of new neurological deficits as this may indicate malignant degeneration (see Malignant peripheral nerve sheath tumors, below). As such, patients with neurofibromatosis are best referred to and monitored in the setting of a multidisciplinary care team.

Granular Cell Tumor

Granular cell tumors are relatively rare soft tissue tumors, with early descriptions and case reports focused primarily on their occurrence in the head and neck, particularly the

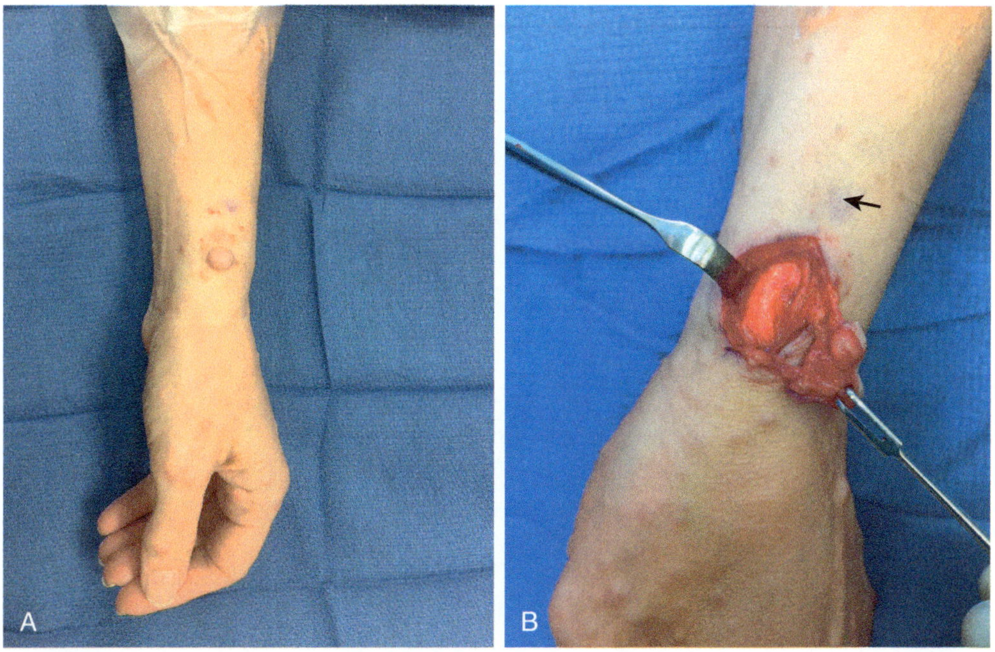

• **Fig. 60.11** (A) Typical appearance of a diffuse cutaneous neurofibromas in a patient with neurofibromatosis type 2. (B) The cutaneous lesion is intimately involved with the overlying skin and well encapsulated within the subcutaneous tissues. *Arrow* demonstrates a small plexiform neurofibroma involving a branch of the superficial radial nerve, which was left in place.

• BOX 60.1 Diagnostic Criteria for NF1

Presence of two or more of the following features:

- One plexiform neurofibroma *or*
- Two or more neurofibromas
- First-degree relative with NF1
- Optic glioma
- Freckling of the axilla or groin
- Six or more café-au-lait macules

• BOX 60.2 Criteria to Evaluate for NF2

Presence of one or more of the following features:

- Multiple spinal tumors
- Solitary meningioma in childhood
- A schwannoma in childhood
- First-degree relative with NF2
- Bilateral vestibular schwannomas
- Multiple meningiomas combined with neurofibromas

tongue. However, approximately 10%–20% of granular cell tumors are found in the upper extremity.[23] While their exact etiology is not precisely known, their tendency to be located near or within nerves (Fig. 60.13), as well as their histological staining, suggest that they originate from Schwann cells.[23] The vast majority present as superficial nodules, with up to 25% being multifocal.[25] Diagnosis requires excision or biopsy, which can be performed similar to schwannomas, preserving the surrounding nerve. Granular cell tumors can be observed once the diagnosis is confirmed, given that over 97% are benign. However, malignancy has been described in the upper extremity.[23]

Perineurioma

The name perineurioma may refer to either the soft tissue perineurioma or the intraneural perineurioma, which are clinically distinct from one another. Both types of perineuriomas occur primarily in children and young adults.[26] Soft tissue perineurioma are rare, and can occur anywhere in the body.[26] They present as painless, asymptomatic nodules and are not found in association with nerves.[26] Excision of soft tissue perineuriomas carries little risk as they are not associated with a source nerve, rarely recur, and malignant transformation has not been reported.

As their name suggests, intraneural perineuriomas arise within peripheral nerves, frequently with associated loss of function of the nerve.[26] The etiology of these tumors is not understood, however recent research has linked their underlying pathology with meningiomas.[26] While most commonly found in the sciatic nerve, intraneural perineuriomas may be found in the brachial plexus or any of the nerves of the upper extremity.[26] While perineuriomas do not undergo malignant degeneration, resection and reconstruction of the nerve may be indicated to restore function.[26]

Other Benign Nerve Tumors

Several other benign peripheral nerve tumors exist, however they are all rare. Neurothekeoma, originally described as a nerve sheath myxoma, are dermal tumors with three pathological variants – cellular, myxoid, and mixed.[23] Neurothekeomas are small, benign cutaneous lesions that occur mostly on the face or upper extremities of young adults with

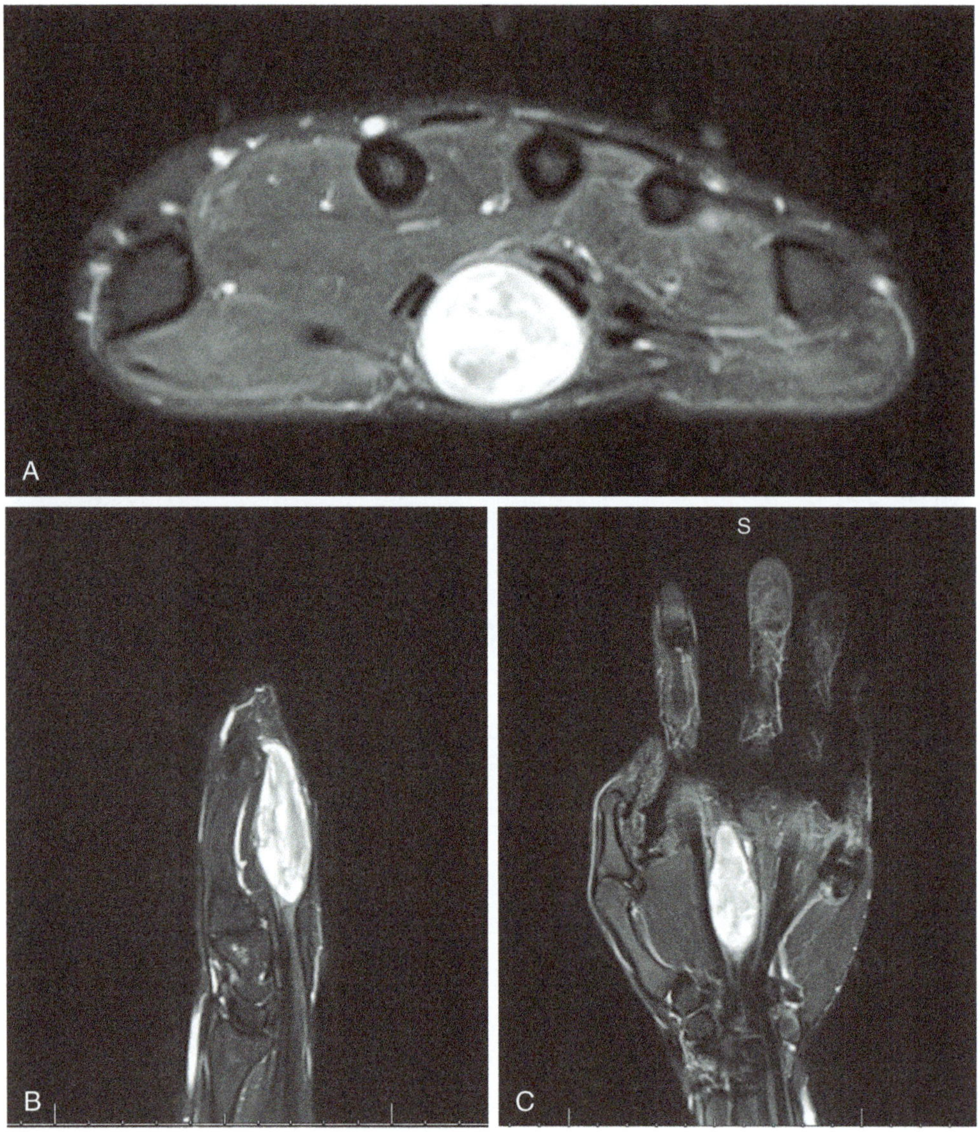

• **Fig. 60.12** (A–C) MRI of a large plexiform neurofibroma involving the median nerve.

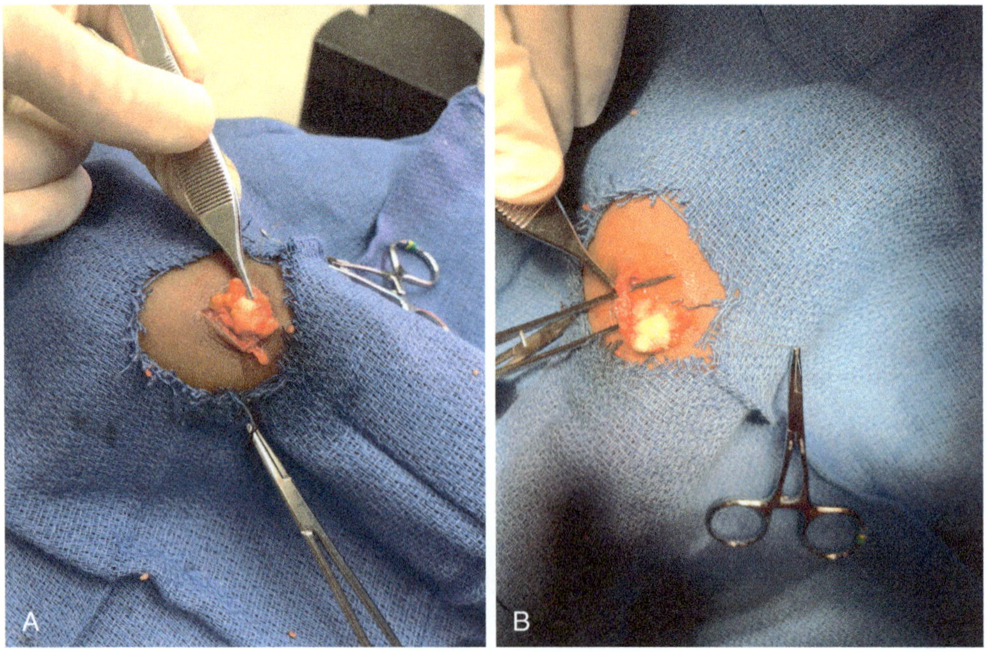

• **Fig. 60.13** (A) Granular cell tumor on the dorsum of the hand. The tumor was originating from a branch of the dorsal cutaneous ulnar nerve. (B) The tumor was dissected off the nerve, leaving the fascicles intact.

slight predominance in females; their appearance is similar to neurofibromas.[23] Excision of these lesions is curative.

Neuromuscular hamartomas, or benign triton tumors, are extremely rare tumors of mixed skeletal muscle and nerve.[23] These tumors most frequently are found in the large nerves of young children, such as the brachial plexus and trunk. Excision may cause disability and spontaneous regression has been reported, therefore excision is not recommended.[23]

Pacinian neuromas are benign overgrowths of Pacinian corpuscles, typically presented as painful masses on the digit of an adult.[23] These growths are also extremely rare. They may be found adhered to a digital nerve, however, excision and nerve preservation is possible and curative.

Malignant Peripheral Nerve Sheath Tumors

Malignant peripheral nerve sheath tumors (MPNST) are rare, aggressive soft tissue sarcomas of Schwann cell origin. Over 50% of these lesions arise from patients with NF1, with the rest occurring de novo or rarely from malignant degeneration of schwannomas or solitary neurofibromas.[27] Most commonly these arise from plexiform neurofibromas, and involve large deeper nerves.[23] Clinically these present as a rapidly enlarging mass, which may be accompanied by pain or neurological deficits. At time of presentation, mass is over 5 cm with metastatic disease already present in up to 50% of patients.[23] MRI is the preferred imaging modality to determine extent of tumor involvement. Diagnosis can be difficult, especially in cases where neurofibromatosis is not present, as histological characteristics are nonspecific.[23] Treatment is with en bloc radical resection or with amputation; no clear consensus exists for margins for resection, however amputation is generally reserved for cases where negative margins cannot be achieved. Radiation therapy may provide some benefit, however no chemotherapy has shown definitive benefits.[23] The 5-year survival of MPNSTs is 20%–50%.[28] The presence of neurofibromatosis has classically been considered a negative prognosticator, however the difference of survival of patients with and without neurofibromatosis has narrowed.[28]

Soft Tissue Sarcomas

Soft tissue sarcomas are rare, however due to their aggressive nature it is imperative that surgeons maintain a high level of awareness of the warning signs of a potential sarcoma. Approximately 14% of all soft tissue sarcomas arise in the upper extremity.[29] Warning signs of potential malignancy that should warrant further work-up include masses greater than 5 cm in size, rapid enlargement, and painful lesions. Patients with any of these signs should have a thorough physical examination including vascular, lymph node, and pulmonary examinations.

These lesions should be investigated adhering to the general principles mentioned earlier. MRI should be performed prior to biopsy to avoid imaging of surgical changes. Open biopsy is the preferred method of confirming diagnosis, when compared with needle biopsy.[29] The patient should be exsanguinated using elevation rather than Esmarch. The biopsy incision should be planned anticipating its inclusion in any formal resection. Biopsy should be performed at the institution that will perform the definitive surgery, as this has been linked to better outcomes.[29] It is therefore essential to consider the oncological resources available in the treating facility prior to proceeding. Once diagnosis is confirmed, basic laboratory studies should be performed, as well as chest radiography with whole body scintigraphy.[29] Early consultation with medical and radiation oncologists should be encouraged. The basic staging system for soft tissue sarcomas is summarized in Table 60.2.

In the upper extremity, the most common soft tissue sarcomas are synovial cell sarcoma, epithelioid sarcoma, and malignant fibrous histiocytoma. Synovial sarcomas are one of the most common soft tissue sarcomas of the hand and wrist.[29] Typically they present as slow-growing painless masses, and are thus commonly diagnosed late.[29] Synovial cell sarcomas are most commonly found near the

TABLE 60.2 American Joint Committee on Cancer Staging for Soft Tissue Sarcoma

TNM		Staging	
T1	Tumor <5 cm	Stage IA	T1, N0, M0, G1
T2	Tumor 5–10 cm	Stage IB	T1–4, N0, M0, G1
T3	Tumor 10–15 cm	Stage II	T1, N0, M0, G2–3
T4	Tumor >15 cm	Stage IIIA	T2, N0, M0, G2–3
N0	No nodal involvement	Stage IIIB	T3–4, N0, M0, G2–3
N1	Regional node involvement	Stage IV	Any nodal involvement or metastasis
M0	No distant metastasis		
M1	Distant metastasis		

carpal bones. Epithelioid sarcoma typically present as slow-growing firm nodules of the digits, palm or volar forearm of a young adult.[29] These tumors may be mistaken for Dupuytren's nodules, palmar fibromas, or even infection as they may become necrotic and drain. Treatment is unique in that spread to lymph node basins is common, therefore lymph node sampling is recommended.[29]

Malignant fibrous histiocytoma is the most common soft tissue sarcoma of the upper extremity in the elderly.[29] These masses initially start as painless growths, and may be first diagnosed following trauma which may be followed by rapid growth.[29] Rhabdomyosarcomas are the most common soft tissue sarcoma of children and young adults.[29] These are tumors of the deep muscles, and patients may report a history of trauma. Adjuvant chemotherapy has improved survival in these patients significantly.

Treatment of soft tissue sarcomas has moved away from amputation and towards en bloc wide local resection as outcomes have been shown to be equivalent.[29] It is imperative that functional deficits not be considered when performing the resection. Some argue for the use of a two-team approach in order to separate the resection and reconstruction. Radiation therapy may be performed preoperatively or postoperatively, with equivalent results in these patients.[29] Postoperative short interval surveillance with imaging and physical examination is an essential part of care.

Cartilage

Enchondroma

Enchondromas are the most common bone tumor in the hand, with the hand representing the majority of all diagnoses. Enchondromas are found most commonly in the proximal phalanges, metacarpals, and middle phalanges.[30] These are tumors of young adults, with presentation typically occurring in the second or third decade of life. Multiple enchondromas are characteristically found in Ollier's disease and Maffuci's syndrome, and are associated with increased risk of malignant degeneration. Generally enchondromas are asymptomatic, however pain or pathological fractures may occur. Plain radiographs are typically all that are needed to diagnose these lesions. Characteristically enchondromas present on radiographs as well-defined lucency in the central portion of the bone with possible calcifications. As the enchondroma increases in size, the surrounding cortex may thin or remodel. Signs of cortical bone destruction, demineralization, proliferation or soft tissue invasion should raise concern for potential malignant transformation.

Lesions which are minimally symptomatic may be treated with observation, with some advocating for annual radiographs to ensure stability of the lesion. Surgical management of symptomatic enchondromas is first with incisional biopsy with frozen suction to confirm diagnosis. Following confirmation, curettage of the entirety of the lesion followed by mechanical or chemical ablation of the lesion's margins is generally curative. Intraoperative fluoroscopy is helpful to ensure adequate curettage. Bone grafting of the defect may be necessary if insufficient bone stalk exists, however treatment without bone grafting has been successful.[30] Following treatment surveillance, radiographs should be obtained due to risk of recurrence, which is reported to be approximately 2%–15%.[30] Although rare, recurrence should raise suspicion for possible malignant transformation or misdiagnosis.[30]

Extraskeletal Chondroma

Extraskeletal chondroma is a rare benign lesion which is found most frequently in the hand.[30] These frequently present as slow-growing, painless masses on the volar hand. These occur entirely separately from the bone, and may arise from the tendon sheath.[30] Extraskeletal chondromas are well circumscribed and may appear as circular calcifications on radiographs. Direct excision is generally straightforward, with recurrence occurring in about 10% of cases and treated with repeat excision.[30]

Periosteal Chondromas

Periosteal chondromas are benign lesions which occur at the level of the periosteum of the phalanges or metacarpals. Presentation is classically in young to middle-aged adults with pain or swelling of the affected bone. Radiographs demonstrate eccentric scalloping of the bone from its outer margin.[31] Histologically these can be difficult to differentiate from chondrosarcoma, and therefore excision is recommended en bloc to avoid recurrence.[30]

Osteochondroma

Osteochondromas are relatively common benign overgrowths of bone covered in cartilaginous tissue, however they rarely occur in the hand.[32] As such, when an osteochondroma is diagnosed in the hand, the patient should be evaluated for multiple osteochondromatosis (multiple hereditary exostosis).[32] Osteochondromas are associated with brachydactyly of the affected digit, however are otherwise generally asymptomatic. Treatment is with observation, as malignant transformation is less than 1%. There is a slight increase risk of degeneration in the case of multiple osteochondromatosis. Growth during adulthood should warrant investigation as osteochondroma growth stops with closure of the physis.[32]

Chondrosarcoma

While the exact incidence of chondrosarcoma of the hand is unknown, it represents the most common malignant lesion of the hand and upper extremity.[30] It is believed that the majority of cases of chondrosarcoma are from malignant degeneration of other lesions, however primary or secondary chondrosarcoma remains rare.[30] Presentation of these lesions occurs later in life, and most frequently affects the proximal phalanx. Clinically, they are difficult to distinguish from benign masses, as they are generally painless and slow growing. Cortical destruction, extension beyond periosteum, and involvement of the soft tissue are all concerning signs for chondrosarcoma.[30] Standard treatment is with wide local excision. However, metastatic disease rarely occurs, therefore some have argued that treatment with curettage may be sufficient.[30]

Bone

Benign

Giant Cell Tumor

Giant cell tumors of the bone are one of the most common benign bone tumors. While they are histologically benign tumors, they do have a tendency to be locally aggressive and may even metastasize.[33] The peak incidence of giant cell tumors occurs between 20 and 45 years of age, with a slight predominance in women.[33] The third most common site overall is the wrist, with presentation in the hand itself being extremely rare.[33] Patients present with pain and swelling of the wrist, or sometimes following a pathological fracture. Radiographs demonstrate a lytic, eccentric lesion of the epiphysis of the bone.

Grading of giant cell tumors is done with the Campanacci staging system.[33] Lesions are divided into three stages: in stage I there is no distension of the cortex; in stage II there is distension of the cortex; and in stage III there is cortical perforation with extension to the soft tissue. Stage I and II lesions can be treated with wide curettage and adjuvant chemical or mechanical ablation, however local recurrence rates can be up to 25%.[33] Stage III lesions that do not involve the articular surface or extensively invade the soft tissues can be similarly treated with possible addition of bone grafting, otherwise they are treated with wide en bloc resection.[33] Local recurrence in these lesions can be as high as 50%.[33] When these lesions occur in the hand, resection of the whole bone is generally advocated.[33] Due to high recurrence rates, close surveillance following resection is necessary.

Aneurysmal Bone Cyst

While common throughout the body, aneurysmal bone cysts are rare in the hand.[33] Literature on aneurysmal bone cysts in the hand is limited to small case series, and when they do occur in the hand they are most frequently encountered in the metacarpals.[33] Similar to giant cell tumors of the bone, these are lytic lesions, however they occur mostly in children or young adults and have no metastatic potential.[33] These can be differentiated from giant cell tumors by their characteristic fluid levels found on radiographs. Treatment is very similar to giant cell tumors, with curettage and ablation when possible, and resection for larger lesions.

Osteoid Osteoma

Osteoid osteomas are small, benign osteoblastic lesions that occur mostly in the lower extremity; however they do occur in the upper extremity.[34] The most common location in the upper extremity is the humerus; within the hand, the scaphoid, capitate, and proximal phalanx are the most common sites of involvement.[34] The central core of these lesions is generally less than 1 cm in size, surrounded by reactive bone formation. They are typically found in young adult males, and characteristically present with focal nighttime pain that is frequently relieved by aspirin.

Radiographs may demonstrate cortical thickening, however generally unless deformity is present plain radiographs are not remarkable. Computerized tomography and bone scans are generally very sensitive for diagnosis of these lesions.[34] Treatment can be with observation and nonsteroidal pain relievers, as in some cases osteoid osteomas can be self-limited. However, the time for these lesions to burnout is highly variable and may take years, so many opt for surgical management. Treatment with curettage with or without bone grafting is generally very successful.[34]

Malignant

Osteosarcoma

Osteosarcomas are exceedingly rare, in the upper extremity; they most commonly occur in the humerus, compromising 10%–15% of all cases, followed by the distal radius.[34] When seen in the hand, it is generally found later in life secondary to radiation, while cases seen in the humerus and radius are more in commonly in children and adolescents.[34] Radiographically, osteosarcomas are marked by their characteristic "sun burst pattern" of radial ossification with associated periosteal elevation.[34] Treatment is with either wide local resection, when possible, or amputation. Survival between these two treatment methods are equivalent, with 5-year survival being approximately 70%.[34] Neoadjuvant and adjuvant chemotherapies have had numerous recent advances in controlling disease.[34]

Ewing's Sarcoma

While Ewing's sarcoma is the second most common malignancy of children, it is exceedingly rare in the hand.[34] Case reports suggest that the phalanges and metacarpals are the most commonly involved bones of the hand.[34] Presentation of Ewing's sarcoma is frequently sinister, with rapid onset of swelling, pain, and fever often leading to misdiagnosis of infection. Radiographically, these appear as lytic, destructive lesions with cortical violation. Following confirmation of diagnosis with incisional biopsy, current treatments focus on neoadjuvant therapy followed by wide resection.[34]

Metastatic Disease

Metastatic disease involving the hand is very rare, constituting 0.1% of all skeletal metastases.[35] Most commonly these present late in the disease process, with the patient already diagnosed with carcinoma, however hand metastates as the presenting symptom of an occult neoplasm has been reported.[35] The most common site of occurrence is the distal phalanges, with lung, renal, and breast cancers being the most common primary sites of malignancy.[35] At time of diagnosis, the patient is generally late in their course of the disease, so treatment should be tailored to reduce and palliate symptoms rather than for local disease control.

Conclusion

Lesions of the upper extremity and hand are relatively common, with the vast majority of these lesions being benign. When considering any lesion, it is essential that care be taken to systematically evaluate the patient to ensure recognition of potential malignancy. With a thoughtful approach to each lesion, it is possible to treat each patient in a way that safely maintains function of their hand.

References

1. Egawa K, Egawa N, Honda Y. Human papillomavirus-associated plantar epidermoid cyst related to epidermoid metaplasia of the eccrine duct epithelium: a combined histological, immunohistochemical, DNA-DNA in situ hybridization and three-dimensional reconstruction analysis. *Br J Dermatol.* 2005;152:961–967.
2. Lincoski CJ, Bush DC, Millon SJ. Epidermoid cysts in the hand. *J Hand Surg (Eur Vol).* 2009;34:792–796.
3. Butler ED, Hamill JP, Seipel RS, et al. Tumors of the hand. A ten-year survey and report of 437 cases. *Am J Surg.* 1960;100:293–302.
4. Carroll RE. Epidermoid (epithelial) cyst of the hand skeleton. *Am J Surg.* 1953;85:327–334.
5. McLaughlin JS, Shafritz AB. Cutaneous warts. *J Hand Surg Am.* 2011;36:343–344.
6. Miller DJ, Strauch RJ. Evidence-based medicine management of cutaneous warts of the hand. *J Hand Surg Am.* 2015;40(11):2274–2276.
7. Sterling JC, Handfield-Jones S, Hudson PM. Guidelines for the management of cutaneous warts. *Br J Dermatol.* 2001;144:4–11.
8. Marty F-L, Marteau E, Rosset P, et al. Étude rétrospective d'une série de 623 tumeurs de la main et du poignet chez l'adulte. *Chir Main.* 2010;29:183–187.
9. Cavit A, Ozcanli H, Sancmis M, et al. Tumorous conditions of the hand: a retrospective review of 402 cases. *Turkish J Pathol.* 2018;34(1):66–72.
10. Shen LY, Amin SM, Chamlin SL, et al. Varied presentations of pediatric lipoblastoma: case series and review of the literature. *Pediatr Dermatol.* 2017;34:180–186.
11. Walling AK, Companioni GR, Belsole RJ. Infiltrating angiolipoma of the hand and wrist. *J Hand Surg Am.* 1985;10:288–291.
12. Head L, Gencarelli JR, Allen M, et al. Wrist ganglion treatment: systematic review and meta-analysis. *J Hand Surg Am.* 2015;40:546–553.
13. Nahra ME, Bucchieri JS. Ganglion cysts and other tumor related conditions of the hand and wrist. *Hand Clin.* 2004;20:249–260.
14. Ingari JV, Faillace JJ. Benign tumors of fibrous tissue and adipose tissue in the hand. *Hand Clin.* 2004;20:243–248.
15. Walsh JJ, Eady JL. Vascular tumors. *Hand Clin.* 2004;20(3):261–268.
16. Chou T, Pan SC, Shieh SJ, et al. Glomus tumor. *Ann Plast Surg.* 2016;76:S35–S40.
17. Woodward JF, Jones NF. Malignant glomus tumors of the hand. *Hand.* 2016;11:287–289.
18. Willard KJ, Cappel MA, Kozin SH, et al. Congenital and infantile skin lesions affecting the hand and upper extremity. Part 1: vascular neoplasms and malformations. *J Hand Surg.* 2013;38:2271–2283.
19. Azzopardi S, Wright TC. Novel strategies for managing infantile hemangiomas. *Ann Plast Surg.* 2012;68:226–228.
20. Mulliken JB, Glowacki J. Hemangiomas and vascular malformations in infants and children: a classification based on endothelial characteristics. *Plast Reconstr Surg.* 1982;69:412–422.
21. Upton J, Coombs CJ, Mulliken JB, et al. Vascular malformations of the upper limb : a review of 270 patients. *J Hand Surg Am.* 1999;24(5):1019–1035.
22. Rockwell GM, Thoma A, Salama S. Schwannoma of the hand and wrist. *Plast Reconstr Surg.* 2003;111:1227–1232.
23. Forthman CL, Blazar PE. Nerve tumors of the hand and upper extremity. *Hand Clin.* 2004;20:233–242.
24. Rinaldi E. Neurilemomas and neurofibromas of the upper limb. *J Hand Surg Am.* 1983;8:590–593.
25. Maher DP. Granular cell tumor in the hand. *J Hand Surg Am.* 1987;12:800–803.
26. Balarezo FS, Muller RC, Weiss RG, et al. Soft tissue perineuromas in children: report of three cases and review of the literature. *Pediatr Dev Pathol.* 2003;6:137–141.
27. Ducatman BS, Scheithauer BW, Piepgras DG, et al. Malignant peripheral nerve sheath tumors. A clinicopathologic study of 120 cases. *Cancer.* 1986;57:2006–2021.
28. Kolberg M, Holand M, Agesen TH, et al. Survival meta-analyses for >1800 malignant peripheral nerve sheath tumor patients with and without neurofibromatosis type 1. *Neuro Oncol.* 2013;15:135–147.
29. Murray PM. Soft tissue sarcoma of the upper extremity. *Hand Clin.* 2004;20:325–333.
30. O'Connor MI, Bancroft LW. Benign and malignant cartilage tumors of the hand. *Hand Clin.* 2004;20:317–323.
31. Nojima T, Unni KK, McLeod RA, et al. Periosteal chondroma and periosteal chondrosarcoma. *Am J Surg Pathol.* 1985;9:666–677.
32. Ostrowski ML, Spjut HJ. Lesions of the bones of the hands and feet. *Am J Surg Pathol.* 1997;21:676–690.
33. Athanasian EA. Aneurysmal bone cyst and giant cell tumor of bone of the hand and distal radius. *Hand Clin.* 2004;20:269–281.
34. Sforzo CR, Scarborough MT, Wright TW. Bone-forming tumors of the upper extremity and Ewing's sarcoma. *Hand Clin.* 2004;20:303–315.
35. Hayden RJ, Sullivan LG, Jebson PJL. The hand in metastatic disease and acral manifestations of paraneoplastic syndromes. *Hand Clin.* 2004;20:335–343.

61 Nonoperative Facial Rejuvenation

EBBY ELAHI AND SUSAN ZOLTAN

Introduction

Over the past decades, significant advances in our understanding of the mechanisms underpinning the aging process have coincided with immense advances in the tools and technologies available to address these changes. No longer is the face seen as a monolithic entity that needs to be pulled or lifted. Changes in the bone structure, fat compartments, myofascial layers, and skin all contribute to restoring esthetic beauty and harmony. Rather than simply effacing lines, practitioners need to be attentive to the subtleties such as facial dynamic function, curvatures, transitions, and congruence. While surgery is effective in restoring many of the elements of facial aging, increasingly, patients seek interventions with less risk and downtime. It is estimated that by 2028, the US demand for minimally invasive treatment for facial rejuvenation will surpass $39 billion.

Facial rejuvenation procedures have been traditionally thought of as those that address the skin (texture, color, tone, dynamic function) and those that primarily address structure and volume. Increasingly the frontier between these approaches is effaced as the interdependence of skin appearance and volume becomes evident.

Botulinum Toxin

Initially used for the temporary treatment of strabismus, botulinum toxin (BoNT)-A has become a mainstay tool to address the aging face. BoNT is derived from *Clostridium botulinum*. Botulinum toxin blocks neuromuscular transmission by binding to presynaptic receptor sites on motor nerve terminals and inhibiting the release of acetylcholine. Initially synthetized as a single 150 kD chain, it is then cleaved into heavy and light chain molecule held by a disulfide bond. The cholinergic specificity of the heavy chain allows for binding to the presynaptic receptor while the proteolytic light chain acts as a zinc endopeptidase. When injected intramuscularly at therapeutic doses, BoNT produces temporary chemical denervation of the muscle, resulting in decrease in muscle activity. The paralytic effects of the toxin are dose- and site-related. The initial effects usually occur within 2–3 days and peak approximately 1 week after treatment. Effects generally last around 3 months, with repeated injections extending the clinical effect.

In 1992, the Carruthers and Carruthers[1]published the first report of the cosmetic use of BoNT-A for the treatment of glabellar frown lines, which was approved for cosmetic usage in the USA in 2002.

Formulations

To date, the FDA has approved three distinct formulations of BoNT-A for both therapeutic and cosmetic purposes, and one formulation of BoNT-B for therapeutic use only. The original formulation of BoNT-A, onabotulinumtoxin-A (BOTOX/BOTOX Cosmetic/Vistabel/vistabex; Allergan, CA, USA), has been joined by abobotulinumtoxin-A (Dysport or Azzalure; Galderma, TX, USA), and icobotulinumtoxin-A (Xeomin/NT-201; Merz Pharma GmBH & Co., Frankfurt, Germany). Only one formulation of BoNT-B-rimabotulinumtoxinB (Myobloc/Neurobloc; Solstice Neurosciences, CA, USA) is available in North America. All products differ in their pharmokinetics and therefore clinical doses vary and are not interchangeable.

Cosmetic Uses of BoNT-A

Initially approved only for injection into the glabellar rhytids, BoNT now is used for dozens of off-label applications on the face (Fig. 61.1). These include controlled paresis of hyperkinetic lines of the face and neck, elevation of various facial subunits by altering muscle equilibrium between depressor and elevator muscles, and reestablishing facial symmetry by selective blockade of muscles of facial

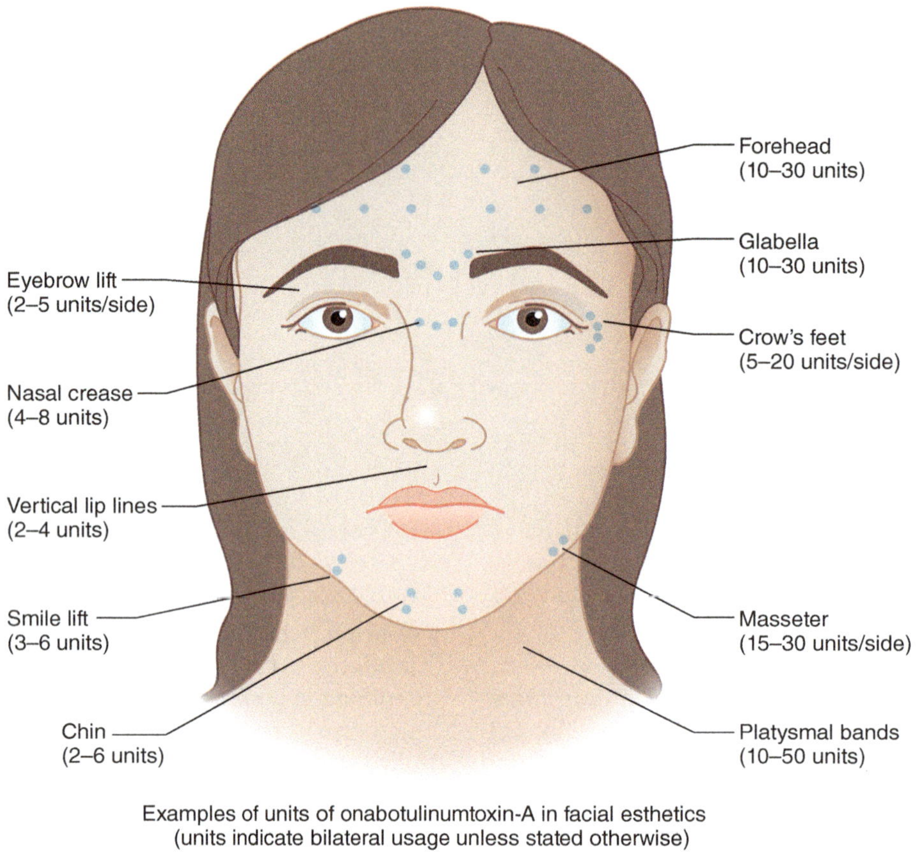

• **Fig. 61.1** Suggested map and dosage for injection of onabotulinumtoxin-A.

expression. BoNT is also increasingly used perioperatively to help with scar management or to stabilize brow position following brow elevation.

A number of technical factors can contribute to a comfortable and more predictable experience:

- Topical anesthetic is applied 30 minutes prior to the procedure (the authors prefer a triple anesthetic preparation of lidocaine, tetracaine, and benzocaine).
- Ice or cold compresses is applied immediately prior to injection.
- If a marker is used, we prefer removable white ink markers (Viscot, NJ).
- A 32G (or 33G) short needle is used on a hubless 0.5 syringe. Larger syringes provide less tactile feedback to the injector and can be more uncomfortable to patients.
- The depth of penetration of the needle follows the esthetic goals and specific muscle anatomy. When injecting the corrugators, for instance, the depth of penetration is more superficial laterally and becomes deeper medially.
- Injection is always made with low pressure and in small aliquots. It is preferable to inject multiple times than to inject a large quantity of fluid in a single push.
- It is preferable to distribute the toxin across several syringes in order to maintain tip sharpness and thus diminish patient discomfort.
- Where a large quantity of toxin is required (e.g., in men with a heavy corrugator complex), it may be preferable to increase the concentration of the toxin to diminish diffusion. In most instances with BoNT, the authors create a 2-mL solution of 5 u/0.1 mL for routine cases and 10 u/0.1 mL for cases where a higher concentration is required.
- Not all toxins have the same clinical characteristics. Abobotulinumtoxin-A for instance appears to have a wider diffusion circle. This can be advantageous in the forehead where multiple entries are often required to achieve meaningful reduction of rhytides. On the other hand, where targeting a specific muscle, highly concentrated onabotulinumtoxin-A may yield more reliable results.
- The areas injected are carefully mapped and the patient is seen between 7 and 14 days following injection for follow-up.

Adverse Effects and Complications

While adverse effects of BoNT are rare, they include watery, dry or crossed eyes. It may also include an incompetent mouth, the inability to whistle, dysphagia, and neck weakness. Most dissatisfaction from BoNT stems from unexpected changes in facial appearance or expression. Common complaints in include:

- Ptosis of the eyelid from injection into the forehead or corrugator complex.
- Ptosis of the brow from forehead injection.

- Overarching eyebrows from injection of the corrugator complex.
- Lower lid festoon formation from injection of crow's feet and secondary loss of orbicularis tone.
- Changes in phonation or smile from perioral injection.

While these adverse effects are not entirely avoidable, they could be minimized by gaining better knowledge of the underlying facial anatomy and physiology as well as paying close attention to individual anatomic variability.

Soft Tissue Fillers

The recent decades have seen substantial increase in the use of dermal fillers to address the aging face. Fillers have been used to augment the facial skeleton, soft tissue, as well as diminish fine lines and wrinkles. Increasingly fillers are used not only to address age-related changes in the face, but also as a means to enhance appearance in youth. While the injection of autologous fat continues to be a mainstay treatment of the aging face, this chapter concentrates primarily on the use of synthetic fillers, specifically fillers based on hyaluronic acid, calcium hydroxyapatite/carboxymethyl cellulose and poly-lactic acid.

Historic Context

The era of absorbable dermal fillers was ushered in in the latter part of the 20th century with the introduction of collagen fillers. Initially made of bovine collagen, fillers based on human collagen became popular in the late 1990s. Products such as Zyderm and Zyplast that were animal-derived collagen required prior skin testing, with hypersensitivity reactions observed in as much as 10% of patients.[2] In 2003 the US Food and Drug Administration approved the use of Restylane (Galderma), a hyaluronic-based product as a class III device to treat facial rhytids. Dozens of products have since been introduced to address a variety of facial volumetric needs.

Rheological Properties

Rheology refers to the physics of deformation and flow of materials, typically in a state between solid and liquid. An understanding of rheological properties of various injectable fillers is critical to the appreciation of their clinical behavior. G′ or elastic modulus refers to the resistance of the material to an applied strain and is commonly used as a measure of hardness or softness of a given material. G″, or the viscous modulus, refers to the energy dissipation due to friction. Other valuable measurements include resistance to compression and maximum water uptake. These properties, when combined with experimental data from human or animal models, provide valuable insight with regard to the actual in vivo behavior of various materials.[3] It is important to note that physical properties of the filler may not always correlate with their performance in the face over time.

Nonbiodegradable Fillers

Liquid Injectable Silicone (Purified Polydimethylsiloxane)

Primarily used in vitreoretinal surgery, liquid silicone has been used as a facial filler on an off-label basis. Silicone oil induces neocollagenesis through fibroplasia in addition to direct volume restoration. While the permanence of silicone is a highly desirable effect, the possibility of late granuloma formation and the inability to reverse the product make it a less desirable product compared to alternative options on the market. Furthermore, long-term studies are lacking on the safety and efficacy of subdermal silicone. In certain instances where the affected tissue could be excised if needed – such as a limited depressed scar – the injection of silicone may provide a valuable tool for near permanent correction of the defect without surgical intervention. However, such benefits must be weighed against significant risks of granulomas, allergic reaction, and even embolisms.[4]

Polymethylmethacrylate (PMMA)

PMMA (ArteFill; Suneva Medical Inc., CA, USA) was approved by the FDA in 2006 for the correction of nasolabial folds. It is a third-generation filler comprising 20% PMMA microspheres and 80% bovine collagen. After implantation, the carrier solution dissipates within 1–3 months, leaving behind the nonresorbable microspheres that induce fibroplasia and become encapsulated by collagen. Since it contains bovine collagen it also requires skin testing to prevent an allergic reaction. Similar to silicone, late nodule formations are observed and can be difficult to treat in highly visible areas of the face.

Biodegradable Fillers

Calcium Hydroxyapatite (CaHA) Microspheres

CaHA microspheres (RADIESSE; Merz Aesthetics, Inc., CA, USA) comprise of biocompatible smooth CaHA spherical particles that are identical in composition to bone material and suspended in an aqueous carboxymethylcellulose gel carrier. The microspheres induce a histolytic and fibroblastic response, stimulating the production of collagen around the implant while the gel carrier is absorbed. CaHA generally lasts about 15 months before the microspheres are broken down into calcium and phosphate ions and excreted. Although CaHA has a great long-term safety profile, nodules and foreign body reactions have been reported. It has both on-label uses such as the treatment of nasolabial folds and HIV-related facial lipoatrophy as well as off-label uses for cheek augmentation and contouring. One advantage of CaHA is its ability to retain its shape over time which is why it is often used for enhancement of the facial skeleton. Unlike HA fillers, however, there is no mechanism to reverse the injection of CaHA. If injected superficially, CaHA can project as a yellow discoloration under the skin. This is why its usage is not recommended in superficial zones of the eyelid and lips.

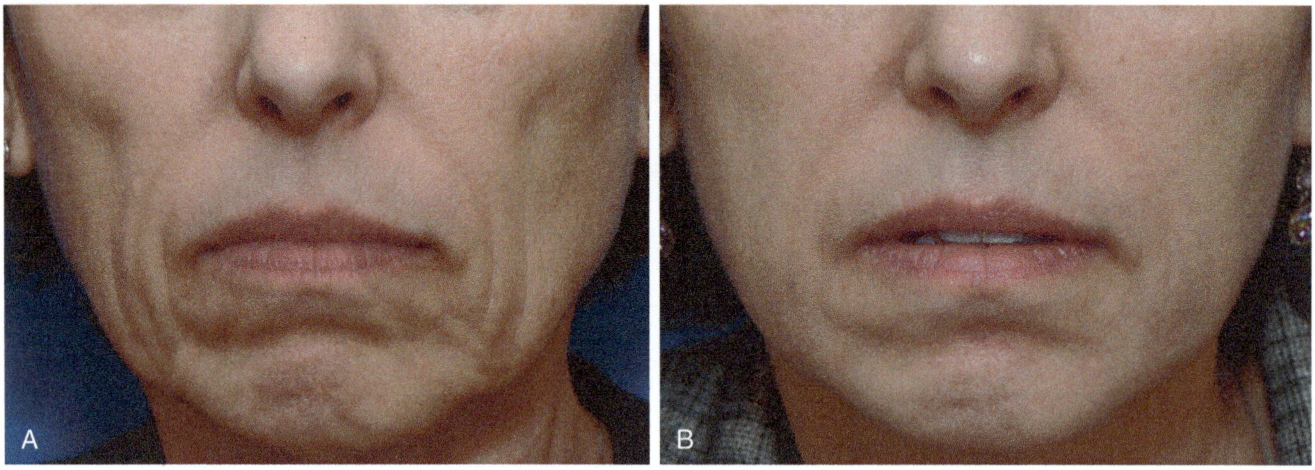

• **Fig. 61.2** Result of poly-L-lactic acid injection to the lower face, (A) before, (B) after.

Poly-L-lactic acid (PLLA)

PLLA (Sculptra; Galderma) is a biocompatible and biodegradable synthetic polymer from the alpha-hydroxy-acid (AHA) family. When injected into the skin, PLLA stimulates fibroblasts to produce collagen, resulting in an increase in volume (Fig. 61.2). The particles are eventually metabolized to lactic acid monomers that are further broken down by the body. Most side effects are due to the injection procedure, although late-onset papules and nodules have been reported. PLLA must be diluted prior to injection with sterile preserved water to allow adequate time for polymer hydration, and patients require a series of three injections over several months. Patients must be informed that volumetric change occurs with time and is often not observed with the first injection. Below are other practical considerations to take into account when injecting PLLA:

- Preparation of PLLA 5–7 days before the procedure may improve hydration and injection characteristics.
- The patient should be injected in a sitting position.
- A 25G 1–1/2-in needle is preferable as it minimizes particle blockage.
- Individual 1-mL Leuer lock syringes are preferable to larger syringes both because of flow control and precision.
- It may be valuable to slightly bend the needle with the bevel facing up for better control.
- Multiple cross-hatch passages are recommended to avoid overfilling a particular spot and to avoid granulomas.
- Small aliquots of less than 0.1 mL are placed per passage.
- PLLA is ideal for large areas of fat loss and is best avoided in areas with thin skin such as the periocular region (Fig. 61.3).
- We adhere to the "rule of 5s:" massage all the areas of injection 5 times a day for 5 minutes and for 5 days to improve even distribution and avoid granuloma formation.

Hyaluronic Acids (HA)

Currently the most common form of filler, HA devices are expected to reach a market exceeding $6 billion by 2025. HA is a naturally occurring polymer of disaccharides linked via alternating beta-glycosidic bonds and one of the chief components of the extracellular matrix in eukaryotic cells. It is thus significantly less immunogenic compared to previous human- or bovin-derived collagen preparations. A chief component of HA is a long, hydrophilic, cross-linked glycosaminoglycan that acts as a scaffold for collagen and elastin and contributes to cell proliferation and migration, as well as tissue repair. The HA molecule is stabilized through cross-linking with hydroxyl groups – allowing it to resist digestion by hyaluronidase – a characteristic that largely determines its clinical behavior and longevity in the body. All HA fillers are unique in terms of concentration of HA, cross-linking, particle size, and manufacturing processes.

When injected into the skin, HA combines with the body's own HA and binds to water, increasing skin turgor, elasticity, and volume for a period of 4–12 months, depending on the product used and the location placed. Most formulations are approved for the correction of facial rhytids and nasolabial folds but are also used off-label for volume replacement in the cheeks and midface. Side effects are generally mild and transient. More troublesome complications are rare but include granulomatous reactions and vascular ischemic complications.

Hyaluronic Acid Preparations The choice of a particular form of HA largely depends on the esthetic concern of the patient. Uses of HA include volume augmentation of the bony support of the face (e.g., malar area or mandible), replenishment of atrophic zones of the face (e.g., temple and cheek), enhancement or effacement of discreet lines of the face (nasolabial fold, vermilion line), elevation of the facial soft tissue (e.g., jowls) or filling of scars (e.g., acne). In many instances more than one goal is achieved through 3-dimensional facial contouring (e.g., tear trough area). Below are some general considerations to optimize HA injections.

- The choice of the filler must be driven by the goal at hand. As a general rule, fillers with good dispersion properties (e.g., Restylane Silk; Galderma) are best used for superficial filling while those with better structural properties (e.g., Juvéderm Voluma; Allergan) are better

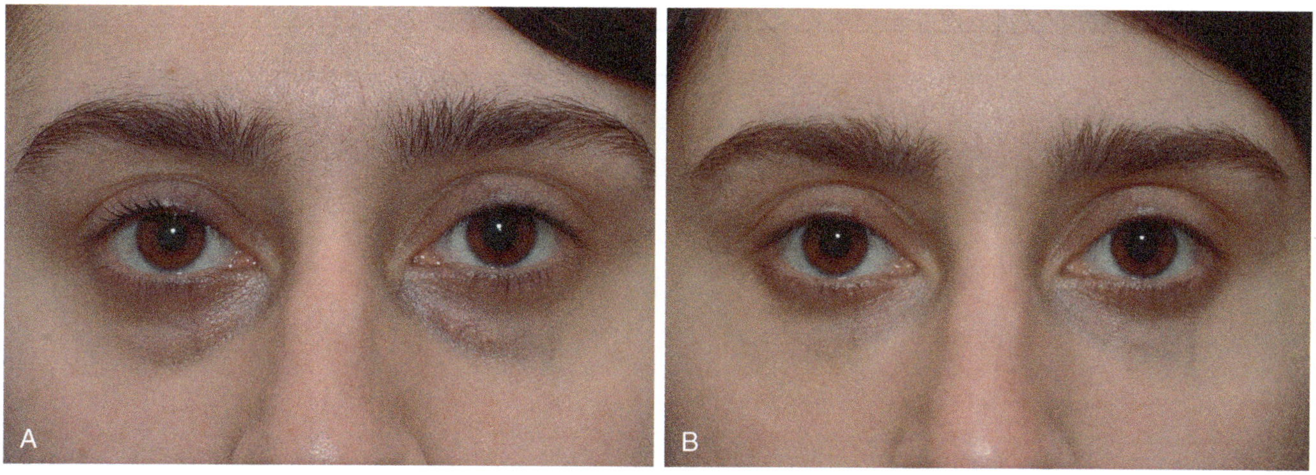

• **Fig. 61.3** Result of injection of filler to the periocular hollows, (A) before, (B) after.

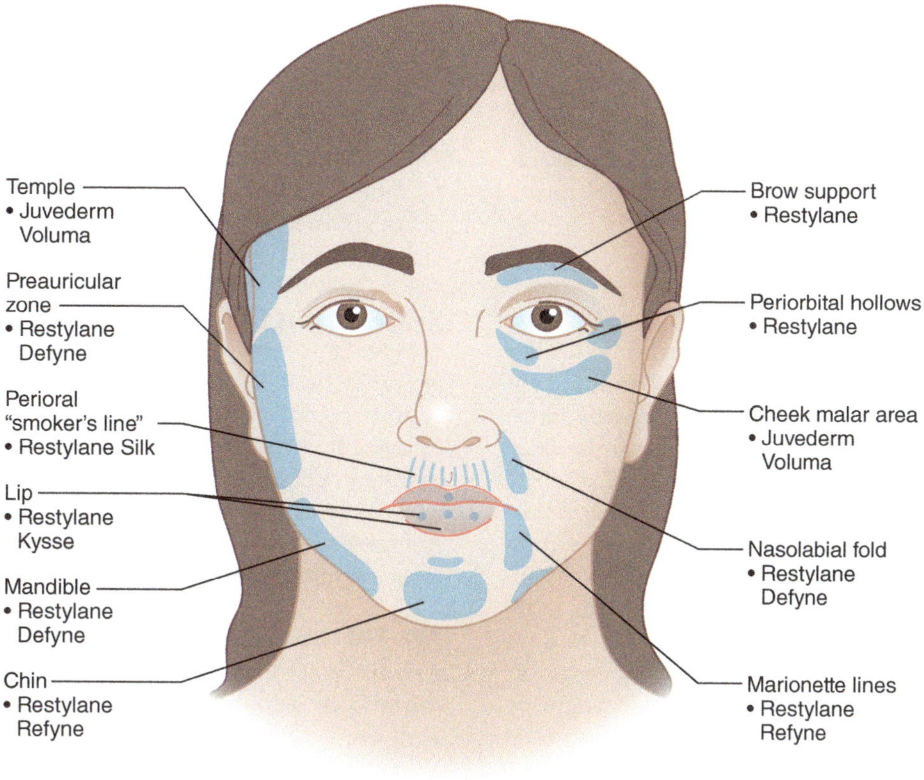

• **Fig. 61.4** Suggested map for injection of author's preferred hyaluronic acid preparations.

at addressing structural support. The author's preferences are shown in Fig. 61.4.

- "Superficial" fillers tend to have less longevity than structural fillers, which can last over 12 months.
- Fillers with intermediate rheological properties are best used for dermal filling in areas of moderate to severe wrinkles such as the nasolabial folds and the marionette lines.
- Careful cleansing and sterile technique are critical to avoid inadvertently introducing bacteria to the implant and to reduce the potential for bioactivity and biofilm formation. Recent reports suggest the use of hypochlorous as a potentially more efficient method of skin disinfection. Other options include chlorhexidine, alcohol, and povidone iodine preparations. Only disposable and sterile skin markings are used.
- In areas where the overlying tissue is thin or if filler is placed too superficially, HA may produce a bluish discoloration. Initially thought to be due to the Tyndall phenomenon, the discoloration is now postulated to be due to blue–gray dyschromia.[5] This effect is particularly

noticeable in the periocular region and may present months after treatment. The authors prefer the use of Restylane L in this region where the product is placed deep to the orbicularis muscle in small aliquots.
- Bruising and discomfort is a common complaint following facial injections. The use of cannula/s has significantly improved patient experience during the procedure. The authors prefer the use of straight 25G or 27G cannulas (TSK, Japan) depending on the material used. The cannulas also allow for multiple passages and better multiplanar distribution of the filler material.
- Injection technique should be informed by the keen understanding of facial anatomy and neurovascular structures. High-risk areas such as the interbrow region with terminal blood vessels may best be avoided. When filling lines or discreet depression, it is best to fill the area vertical or oblique to the depression with multiple passages of the canula. "Parallel" threading techniques can at times result in accentuation of the depression, particularly in the nasolabial fold.
- The use of cold compresses before and after the procedure can reduce bruising. If large volume of filler is needed, it may be preferable to spread the injections over several visits in order to minimize the edema and subsequent recovery.

Complications

Esthetic complications include overfilling, misplaced or displaced filler or dyschromia. Careful attention to the standards of facial harmony and beauty can avoid a commonly dreaded complication of "filler face" whereby facial transition zones are effaced in an attempt to elevate or erase age-related changes. Many such complications occur when fillers are inappropriately used as substitute for surgery in order to "lift" the face. Fortunately, HA can be reversed by the injection of hyaluronidase, a soluble protein enzyme that breaks down and hydrolyses HA. The effects of hyaluronidase are dose-dependent and observed hours to days following injection. Various forms of hyaluronidase exist on the market, including those of bovine or human origin. A proposed rule of thumb is to begin with 5 units of hyaluronidase for each 0.1 mL of Restylane products and 10 units for 0.1 mL of Juvéderm products.[6] Furthermore, delayed onset nodules (DON) can occur weeks or months following an injection. There is controversy as to the true nature of DONs as immunoreactivity or biofilm formation have been implicated. The responsiveness of the nodules to oral antibiotic treatments with tetracyclines or macrolides suggest bioactivity as a possible cause.

Non-esthetic complications include allergic hypersensitivity and local injection site reactions, such as bruising, edema, and pain. Vascular complications of HA injections are fortunately rare but can be devastating. To date, dozens of cases of blindness or stroke associated with dermal fillers have been reported.[7] A number of precautions and interventions have been proposed to address this complication[8]:

- Thorough knowledge of the vascular anatomy of the face. Certain zones such as the interglabellar space may best be avoided altogether.
- Injection of small amounts of filler, without pressure and in a retrograde manner can reduce the risk of vascular occlusion.
- The use of a cannula is especially recommended around areas in proximity to the facial artery.
- Digital pressure may decrease the risk of inadvertent intravascular injection.
- If blindness were to occur, it is paramount to have sufficient quantity of hyaluronidase available. Generally, 1500 units are considered a minimum dose. Thrombotic occlusions of the retina are thought to be reversible for up to 90 minutes.
- An ophthalmic examination is critical. Retrobulbar injection of hyaluronidase has been reported to aid in reversing the occlusion. Intraocular pressure reduction should be achieved, with pressure reducing drops such as timolol 0.5% and oral carbonic anhydrase inhibitors as well and digital massage. An anterior chamber paracentesis can also be performed by the ophthalmologist at the slit lamp or microscope.
- While not proven, the use of anticoagulants, intraocular pressure-lowering medication, high-flow oxygen and hyperbaric chamber have also been advocated.

Submental Fullness

Accumulation of fat in the submental and preplatysmal compartments of the neck is a common cause of undesired fullness. In a recent study, up to two-thirds of respondents reported being dissatisfied with "excess fat under the chin/neck."[9] In 2015 Kybella (Kythera Biopharmaceuticals, Allergan) was introduced in the USA as a potential alternative to surgical liposuction.

ATX-101 (Deoxycholic Acid) (Kybella)

Kybella is a nonhuman and nonanimal formulation of deoxycholic acid, a naturally-occurring molecule that aids with the body's breakdown and absorption of dietary fat. When injected into subcutaneous fat, Kybella causes the destruction of fat cells. In clinical trials, patients experienced visible results in two to four treatments, although up to six treatments may be administered. The most common adverse reactions include erythema, ecchymosis, pain, numbness, and hardness at the injection sites. Kybella has also been associated with more serious side effects including trouble swallowing and facial nerve trauma. Given the costs, potential discomfort, and the need for multiple sessions, it is important to carefully discuss with patients the value of this intervention relative to the more invasive surgical alternatives. In addition to standard techniques described above for all injectables, specific considerations include:

- Marking the skin with a grid to allow even distribution of the product.

- Using a short 30G (or smaller) needle to inject perpendicular to the fat compartments. The use of short needles is critical to avoid damage to the critical neurovascular structure of the neck.
- Avoiding injection superficially close to the skin surface as this can lead to necrosis or ulceration.
- Spacing injection sessions at least one month apart. As many as six sessions can be considered in order to obtain optimal results.

Cryolipolysis

Cryolipolysis is a noninvasive technology used to reduce adipose tissue by freezing fat cells. Commercial cryolypolysis vacuum applicators target submental fullness (CoolMini applicator, Coolsculpting System; Zeltiq Aesthetics, Allergan). Relatively high satisfaction rates are reported with the procedure although large randomized prospective controlled trials are lacking.[10] Results may not be evident for up to 1–4 months following the procedure. Most common adverse effects include local irritation at the site of treatment including erythema, firmness, edema, ecchymosis, and site tenderness.

Cutaneous Remodeling

Numerous devices continue to enter the marketplace that attempt to rejuvenate skin or erase signs of aging or sun damage. They all share in common the need to selectively target tissue while minimizing collateral damage, downtime, and adverse effects. While no single device to date has achieved all of these goal, increased understanding of the science of aging as well as advancements in engineering are transforming the landscape of device-based facial rejuvenation.

Microdermabrasion

Microdermabrasion was first introduced in 1985 by Marini and Lo Brutto as a less aggressive alternative to chemical peels. These devices propel abrasive crystals against the skin surface via a handheld vacuum device. Aluminum oxide is the most commonly used abrasive. Other crystals available include sodium chloride, sodium bicarbonate, and magnesium oxide. The crystals cause gentle mechanical abrasion to the stratum corneum layer of the epidermis and it is subsequently replaced with remodeled epidermis. Microdermabrasion is generally considered safe for all Fitzpatrick skin types although it has limited effectiveness in the long run.[11] Adverse events are unusual and include mild edema and erythema, pain, burning, and dyspigmentation. This treatment is widely used and there are various combinations of dermabrasion and chemical peels that have been published to work in concert.[12]

Chemical Peels

Chemical exfoliation involves the topical application of caustic agents to the skin with the goal of inciting a healing response and subsequent improved appearance. They have been used for a variety of applications, including pigmentary disorders (lentigines, melasma), inflammatory disorders (acnes, rosacea), scarring, precancerous lesions or aging. Peels are often categorized as superficial, medium, and deep; Superficial peels affect the upper layers of the epidermis. The most common agents for superficial peels include trichloroacetic acid (TCA, 10%–20%), glycolic acid (GA), and beta-hydroxy-acids (BHAs), such as salicylic acid (Blue Peel Radiance 20% salicylic acid; Obagi, CA, USA). Beta-lipohydroxy acid (LHA) is a derivative of salicylic acid that provides excellent exfoliation with antibacterial, antiinflammatory and antifungal properties. Results are usually seen in 3–5 days with very minimal downtime.

Medium-depth peels can contain a variety of solutions, including those described by Brody (solid carbon dioxide and TCA), Monheit (Jessner's solution and TCA), and Coleman (70% GA and TCA). The medium depth Blue Peel by Obagi contains TCA which the authors prefer to use as the blue base included in the product helps to monitor and slow the penetration of the peel. The basal cell layer of the epidermis and upper dermis are targeted. Finally, deep peels are usually performed with Baker–Gordon phenol in the surgical setting and are usually reserved for scars or lesions.

Complications of chemical peels primarily depend on the depth of peel used. Superficial peels can cause pain and burning. Prolonged sun exposure, inadequate application of sunscreen, use of topical retinoid or glycolic acid should be avoided. Erythema or hypopigmentation are more common after medium–deep peels which can lead to irregular pigmentation when healed. This is most common in individuals with type 3–4 Fitzpatrick skin types. Women on estrogen containing medications such as oral contraceptives and hormone replacement therapy are also more at risk for pigment abnormalities. The prophylactic use of antiviral medications such as valacyclovir or acyclovir is strongly advised to avoid herpetic reactivation. Broad spectrum sunscreens/bleaching agents (hydroquinone) singly or in combination can be applied following the procedure.[13]

Studies also suggest that using combination chemical peels are more effective than single treatments in mild–moderate acne vulgaris.[14] Caution should be used when applying chemical peels on Fitzpatrick skin type VI or higher as they are at a higher risk for developing post inflammatory hyperpigmentation (PIH).[15]

Platelet-Rich Plasma (PRP)

Platelet-rich plasma (PRP) is an autologous blood-derived product enriched in platelets, growth factors, and cytokines delivered in a concentrated volume of plasma. Since the 1970s, PRP has received significant attention as applied to tissue repair and regeneration. Initial studies focused predominantly on orthopedic uses for PRP; in recent years, it has been used for a range of facial rejuvenation indications including wound healing, fat grafting, scar management as well as soft-tissue volume augmentation.[16,17] PRP is prepared either manually or using automated devices. In the manual method, blood is withdrawn from the patient, an anticoagulant is added, and the mixture is centrifuged at varying speeds. Many centrifuges are available on the market today and the literature does not suggest any as a superior product. Blood is collected and centrifuged and separated into three layers: platelet-poor plasma (PPP), PRP, and red blood cells. Subsequently, the yellow plasma (the top coat containing platelets and leukocytes) is taken up using a micropipette. A second round of centrifugation is performed for 5 min at 4000 rpm. The pellet containing platelets accumulates at the bottom and the platelet-poor plasma surfaces to the top. It is best to use two spins. The first spin ("hard spin") separates the platelet-poor plasma (PPP) from the red fraction and platelet-rich plasma (PRP). The second spin ("soft spin") separates the red fraction from the PRP. The material with the highest specific gravity (PRP) will be deposited at the bottom of the tube.[18] The second centrifugation allows for better separation of the platelets.[19] PRP can be applied as an isolated modality or as an adjunct to minimally invasive and surgical interventions given its potential to improve, repair and regenerate.[20] The authors find it very safe and very easy to integrate in combination treatments such as microneedling, fillers and/or chemical peels.[21]

Plasma-rich fibrin (PRF) is a natural fibrin-based solution prepared from an anticoagulant-free blood harvest without any artificial biochemical. One study comparing the two found that PRP has significantly higher growth factors (TGF-B1) as compared to PRF.[22] Research is still needed to best determine which preparation provides better cosmetic outcomes.

Microneedling

Microneedling is a minimally invasive procedure involving superficial and controlled puncturing of the skin via miniature fine needles.[23] The concept was introduced in 1995 by Orentreich for scar treatment and then independently in 1997 for postsurgical scars.[24] Traditionally used as a collagen induction therapy for facial scars and skin rejuvenation, it has also been used as a transdermal delivery system for anesthetics during esthetic procedures as well as deepening the penetration of superficial peels without changing to more abrasive products. This procedure works by two approaches. It induces neocollagenesis as well as increases skin permeability by creating reversible microchannels in the skin. Traditional microneedling devices, such as stamps and rollers, feature needles that are arranged at fixed depths. More recently, pen-like mechanical devices that can be programmed to administer treatment to varying depths have allowed clinicians to easily customize each procedure to a patient's needs. Actual needle penetration varies from 0.5 mm to 2.0 mm with deeper penetrations reserved for dark/deep scar removal. Histological examination of the skin treated with four microneedling sessions one month apart have shown as much as 400% increase in collagen and elastin deposition at 6 months postoperatively.[25] Liebl et al have postulated that when the microneedling effect may be due to a change in cellular resting potential from -70mV to -100 mV, with a resultant release of growth factors and other proteins inducing collagen formation.[26]

The combination of microneedling with radiofrequency has further expanded the use of this technology. Insulated needles are used to penetrate the skin and release radiofrequency currents from the needle tips without damaging the overlying epidermis. Because this process does not damage the epidermis, it is safe to use on darker skin types. Studies also suggest that microneedling with PRP yields superior results than microneedling alone.[27] It has been suggested to use the platelet-poor plasma from the second spin as the buffer for rolling the microneedling device on the skin while injecting the platelet-rich plasma into wrinkles or scars.

Radiofrequency

Radiofrequency (RF) is electromagnetic radiation in the frequency range of 30–300 GHz. This technology aims to deliver uniform heat to the dermis at a controlled depth while cooling the epidermis. Because RF energy is not dependent on specific chromophore interaction, epidermal melanin is not at risk of destruction and treatment of all skin types is possible.[28] A number of manufacturers of RF devices exist including D-Finitive Evo by Beco Medical, V-form by Viora, Thermage by Solta Medical, Venus Freeze by Venus Concept, VelaShape by Syneron, Exilis by BTL, and 3DEEP by Endymed. Typically, treatment requires a series of sessions. Devices have different penetration depths depending on the number of electrodes (monopolar, bipolar, or unipolar). Some patients require sedation due to discomfort during the procedure. Cutaneous scarring and ulceration as well as loss of subdermal fat are potential adverse effects of this technology.[29]

RF has been introduced in conjunction with microneedling. In addition to the benefits seen with the microinjury provided by the microneedles, RF microneedling also delivers RF energy deep into the dermis further enhancing skin remodeling.

Microfocused Ultrasound (MFU)

MFU has been introduced into the esthetic market since 2009 to meet the public demand for achieving significant, noninvasive skin lifting and tightening. MFU can be focused on subcutaneous tissue where the temperature briefly exceeds 60°C, producing small thermal coagulation points to a depth of up to 5 mm within the mid-to-deep reticular layer of the dermis and subdermis. The intervening papillary dermal and epidermal layers of the skin remain unaffected. The application of heat at these discrete thermal coagulation points causes collagen fibers to form at different facial depths allowing for contouring of the face. Commercially available devices combine MFU with high-resolution ultrasound imaging (MFU-V), enabling visualization of tissue planes to a depth of 8 mm (Ultherapy; Ulthera Inc., AZ, USA). Using different transducers, MFU-V treatment can be customized to meet the unique needs of each patient by adjusting energy and focal depth of the emitted ultrasound. Recent studies suggest that this treatment does not alter the epidermal barrier function or physiology of skin. Brief discomfort is the most common adverse effect that can be minimized with oral nonsteroidal antiinflammatory drugs. Other adverse events include erythema, edema, and occasional ecchymosis. MFU-V is best suited for patients with mild–moderate skin and soft tissue laxity.

Lasers and Intense Pulsed Light (IPL) Technology

The role of light-based technologies in esthetics has expanded in the past few years. Lasers and IPLs have been used to treat vascular and pigmented lesions, tattoos, scars, and undesired hair as well as for cosmetic rejuvenation. These systems continue to evolve and provide enhanced therapeutic outcomes with improved safety profiles. Laser light is monochromatic and can be further classified by their mode of light emission. Continuous wave (CW) lasers produce a continuous beam of light with long exposure durations that can cause nonselective tissue damage. Pulsed laser systems emit high-energy laser light in ultrashort pulse durations with relatively long interpose time intervals.

Within laser technology there are ablative and nonablative lasers as well as fractionated and nonfractionated lasers. Fractionated lasers target an equally distributed portion of the projected area, nonfractionated lasers act on the entire projected surface area of the treated skin. Ablative lasers vaporize the epidermis and are considered more aggressive than nonablative lasers that leave the epidermis intact.

IPL is a nonlaser filtered flash lamp device. Unlike lasers, IPL devices emit polychromatic, noncoherent, and noncollimated light (420–1400 nm) with varying pulse durations. The light may be filtered to target a specific chromophore and render the device more specific.

There are few direct studies comparing IPLs and lasers. One study comparing IPL and long-pulse pulsed dye laser found that both treatments are equally effective in facial rejuvenation in Asians, but that the laser was significantly better for lentigines.[30]

Laser skin resurfacing has evolved significantly over the past two decades. It was first popularized in the mid-1990s following the introduction of the pulsed carbon dioxide (CO_2) laser system for the treatment of facial rhytids and atrophic acne scars. Subsequently erbium (Er:YAG) ablative lasers for facial rejuvenation were introduced. While extremely effective, prolonged side effects and complications associated with ablative laser resurfacing were reported. These included PIH, erythema, and edema, which could last several weeks to months. Laser application causes skin destruction at specific depths and secondary collagen formation. Erbium laser induces wound contracture while the CO_2 laser causes heat-induced collagen contraction. Although wound contraction may result in nearly the same tightening as heat-induced collagen contraction there is potentially increased cicatrization seen with erbium laser wound contracture.[31] Nonablative laser resurfacing was developed in an effort to allow for laser modalities to be utilized for facial rejuvenation without extensive downtime. These lasers were developed to primarily reduce the risk of adverse effects and the extensive postoperative recovery period associated with ablative laser resurfacing.

There are several nonablative lasers, some of which emit infrared light. They include the Nd:YAG (1064 and 1320 nm), diode (980 and 1450 nm), and erbium:glass (Er:glass, 1540 nm). Similar to ablative lasers, they primarily target dermal water, which causes collagen heating and dermal remodeling. Unlike their ablative counterparts, however, epidermal injury and tissue vaporization do not occur.

Fractional laser skin resurfacing was introduced in 2004. Fractional photothermolysis targets tissue water and produces microscopic treatment zones of controlled depth, width, and densities in the skin. These three-dimensional thermal damage zones are referred to as "microscopic thermal zones" (MTZs) and are the fundamental units of fractional photothermolysis. In contrast to full-field nonfractionated resurfacing, only a fraction of the skin is targeted. The energy in the fractionated columns (1470nm) induce thermal damage with minimal collateral damage. Adjacent unaffected tissue serves as a source for healing and rapid epidermal repair. As a result, fractionated photothermolysis minimizes the risk of complications and reduces recovery times. Another significant advantage of fractionated lasers is reduced incidence of epidermal and superficial dermal damage and reduced incidence of PIH. However, more randomized controlled studies are needed in skin types V and VI.[32] Refinement of existing devices and the development of new technologies will continue to expand the roles of lasers and IPLs.[33,34]

Conclusion

The landscape of noninvasive options for facial rejuvenation continues to rapidly expand. Increasingly patients look for ways to delay or reverse the aging process and enhance facial appearance without the downtime and potential complications associated with surgery. As such, a comprehensive understanding of noninvasive treatment options and how they can be combined with other noninvasive treatments or surgical options remains paramount to the practice of facial plastic surgery.

References

1. Carruthers JD, Carruthers JA. Treatment of glabellar frown lines with C. botulinum-A exotoxin. *J Dermatol Surg Oncol.* 1992;18(1):17–21.
2. Basta SL. Cosmetic fillers: perspectives on the industry. *Facial Plast Surg Clin North Am.* 2015;23(4):417–421.

3. Hee CK, Shumate GT, Narurkar V, et al. Rheological properties and in vivo performance characteristics of soft tissue fillers. *Dermatol Surg.* 2015;41(suppl).
4. Kontis TC, Rivkin A. The history of injectable facial fillers. *Facial Plast Surg.* 2009;25(2):67–72.
5. Rootman DB, Lin JL, Goldberg R. Does the Tyndall effect describe the blue hue periodically observed in subdermal hyaluronic acid gel placement? *Ophthalmic Plast Reconstr Surg.* 2014;30(6):524–527.
6. Jones D, Tezel A, Borrel M. In vitro resistance to degradation of hyaluronic acid dermal fillers by ovine testicular hyaluronidase. *Dermatol Surg.* 2010;36:804–809.
7. Belezenay K, Carruthers J, Humphrey S, et al. Avoiding and treating blindness from fillers: a review of the world literature. *Dermatologic Surg.* 2015;41:1097–1117.
8. de Lacerda D. Prevention and management of iatrogenic blindness associated with aesthetical filler injections. *Dermatol Ther.* 2018;31(6).
9. Shah GM, Greenberg JN, Tanzi EL, et al. Noninvasive approach to treatment of submental fullness. *Semin Cutan Med Surg.* 2017;36(4):164–169.
10. Kilmer SL, Burns AJ, Zelickson BD. Safety and efficacy of cryolipolysis for non-invasive reduction of submental fat. *Lasers Surg Med.* 2016;48(1):3–13.
11. Shah M, Crane JS. Microdermabrasion. *StatPearls.* https://www.ncbi.nlm.nih.gov/books/NBK535383/.
12. Dayal S, Sahu P, Jain VK, et al. Clinical efficacy and safety of 20% glycolic peel, 15% lactic peel, and topical 20% vitamin C in constitutional type of periorbital melanosis: a comparative study. *J Cosmet Dermatol.* 2016;15(4):367–373.
13. Nikalji N, Godse K, Sakhiya J, et al. Complications of medium depth and deep chemical peels. *J Cutan Aesthet Surg.* 2012;5(4):254–260.
14. Nofal E, Nofal A, Gharib K, et al. Combination chemical peels are more effective than single chemical peel in treatment of mild-to-moderate acne vulgaris: a split face comparative clinical trial. *J Comet Dermatol.* 2018;17(5):802–810.
15. Vermula S, Maymone MBC, Secemsky EA, et al. Assessing the safety of superficial chemical peels in darker skin: a retrospective study. *J Am Acad Dermatol.* 2018;79(3):508–513.
16. Alser O, Goutos I. The evidence behind the use of platelet-rich plasma (PRP) in scar management: a literature review. *Scars Burn Heal.* 2018;4: 2059513118808773.
17. Lynch MD, Bashir S. Applications of platelet-rich plasma in dermatology: a critical appraisal of the literature. *J Dermatolog Treat.* 2016;27(3):285–289.
18. Kim DH, Je YJ, Kim CD, et al. Can platelet-rich plasma be used for skin rejuvenation? Evaluation of effects of platelet-rich plasma on human dermal fibroblasts. *Ann Dermatol.* 2011;23(4):424–431.
19. Marx R. Platelet-rich plasma (PRP): what is PRP and what is not PRP? *Implant Dent.* 2001;10:225–228.
20. Mosca MJ, Rodeo SA. Platelet-rich plasma for muscle injuries: game over or time out? *Curr Rev Musculoskelet Med.* 2015;8:145–153.
21. Lee H, Yoon K, Lee M. Full-face augmentation using tissue fill mixed with platelet-rich plasma: "Q.O.Fill". *J Cosmet Laser Ther.* 2018;1–5.
22. Arora S, Kotwal U, Dogra M, et al. Growth factor variation in two types of autologous platelet biomaterials: PRP versus PRF. *Indian J Hematol Blood Transfus.* 2017;33(2):288–292.
23. Singh A, Yadav S. Microneedling: advances and widening horizons. *Indian Dermatol Online J.* 2016;7(4):244–254.
24. Camirand A, Doucet J. Needle dermabrasion. *Aesthetic Plast Surg.* 1997;21(1):48–51.
25. Aust MC, Fernandes D, Kolokythas P, et al. Percutaneous collagen induction therapy: an alternative treatment for scars, wrinkles, and skin laxity. *Plast Reconstr Surg.* 2008;121(4):1421–1429.
26. Liebl H, Kloth LC. Skin cell proliferation stimulated by microneedles. *J Am Coll Clin Wound Spec.* 2012;4(1):2–6.
27. Asif M, Kanodia S, Singh K. Combined autologous platelet-rich plasma with micro needling versus micro needling with distilled water in the treatment of atrophic acne scars: a concurrent split-face study. *J Cosmet Dermatol.* 2016;15(4):434–443.
28. Elsaie ML. Cutaneous remodeling and photorejuvenationusing radiofrequency devices. *Indian J Dermatol.* 2009;54(3):201–205.
29. Paasch U, Bodendorf MO, Grunewald S, et al. Skin rejuvenation by radiofrequency therapy: methods, effects and risks. *J Dtsch Dermatol Gets.* 2009;7(3):196–203.
30. Kono T, Groff WF, Sakurai H, et al. Comparison study of intense pulsed light versus a long-pulse pulsed dye laser in the treatment of facial skin rejuvenation. *Ann Plast Surg.* 2007;59(5):479–483.
31. Fitzpatrick RE, Rostan EF, Marchell N. Collagen tightening induced by carbon dioxide laser versus erbium:YAG laser. *Lasers Surg Med.* 2000;27(5):393–403.
32. Kaushik S, Alexis A. Nonablative fractional laser resurfacing in skin of color: evidence based review. *J Clin Aesthet Dermatol.* 2017;10(6):51–67.
33. Abdel Aal AM, Ibrahim IM, Sami NA, et al. Evaluation of autologous platelet-rich plasma plus ablative carbon dioxide fractional laser in the treatment of acne scars. *J Cosmet Laser Ther.* 2018;20(2):106–113.
34. Moradi A, Weinere SF. Effectiveness of combining high-intensity focused radio frequency and non-ablative fractional laser for improving the appearance of the aging face and neck. *J Drugs Dermatol.* 2019;18(1):59–64.

62 Facial Aging and Anatomy of the Facial Nerve

CHIN HO WONG AND BRYAN MENDELSON

Introduction

The pathogenesis of facial aging may be explained on an anatomical basis. An anatomical approach to surgical rejuvenation of the face provides the way to obtaining a "natural" result that is lasting and with minimal morbidity. Fundamental to safety when operating in the face is a firm grounding in the principles on which the facial soft tissue layers are constructed.[1–4] Understanding the relations of the facial nerve branches to these facial soft tissue layers, retaining ligaments, and soft tissue spaces is crucial in predicting and anticipating the location of the facial nerves. This is most important in addressing the overriding concern about the location and course of the facial nerve branches when performing surgical sub-SMAS (superficial musculoaponeurotic system) facelifts.

Five-Layered Anatomy, Facial Soft Tissue Spaces, and Retaining Ligaments of the Face

The five concentric layers of the face are: (1) skin; (2) subcutaneous tissue; (3) musculoaponeurotic layer; (4) loose areola tissue; (5) deep fascia. This five-layered arrangement is most clearly seen in the scalp and forehead (due to expansion of the soft tissues as a result of evolutionary expansion of the underlying cranial vault necessary to accommodate the highly developed frontal lobe in humans). Accordingly, the scalp is an excellent place to study the principles of the layered anatomy (Fig. 62.1). Layer 4 (the loose areolar tissue) is the layer that allows the superficial fascia (defined as the composite flap of layers 1 through 3) to glide over the deep fascia (layer 5). This arrangement enables facial expressions by the frontalis and orbicularis oculi to function independent of the deeper muscle of mastication, the temporalis located deep to the deep fascia. The simplified anatomy over the scalp gives the basic prototype of layer 4. There are not any structures crossing this plane, which is essentially an avascular gliding space. At the boundaries of the scalp along the superior temporal line and across the supraorbital rim, the scalp and the forehead are firmly anchored by retaining ligaments. Vital structures such as nerves and vessels are always located in close proximity to the retaining ligaments when transitioning from deep to superficial in their course. In other parts of the face, the principles of this construction remain the same, albeit with considerably greater complexity. This is due to the compaction resulting from the reduction of forward projection of the mid and lower face (as occurs in other species) and the predominance of the orbital and oral cavities that limit the availability of a bony platform for attachment of retaining ligaments and muscles. To secure the mobile superficial layers to the facial skeleton, an elaborate system of retaining ligaments bind the dermis to the skeleton (or deep fascia where the facial skeleton is covered by skeletal muscles for mastication); the components of this system pass through all layers (Figs. 62.2 and 62.3).[4,5]

Layer 1 – Skin

The epidermis is a cell-rich layer composed mainly of differentiating keratinocytes and a smaller number of pigment-producing melanocytes and antigen-presenting Langerhans cells. A rich vascular plexus is an important component of the dermis. The thickness of the dermis relates to its function and tends to be inversely proportionate to its mobility. The dermis is thinnest in the eyelids and thickest over the forehead and the nasal tip.

Layer 2 – Subcutaneous Tissue

The subcutaneous layer has two components: the subcutaneous fat, which provides volume, and the fibrous retinacular cutis that binds the dermis to the underlying superficial musculoaponeurotic system (SMAS) of the face. Of note, the retinacular cutis is the name given to that portion of the retaining ligament that passes through the subcutaneous tissues. The amount, proportion, and arrangement of

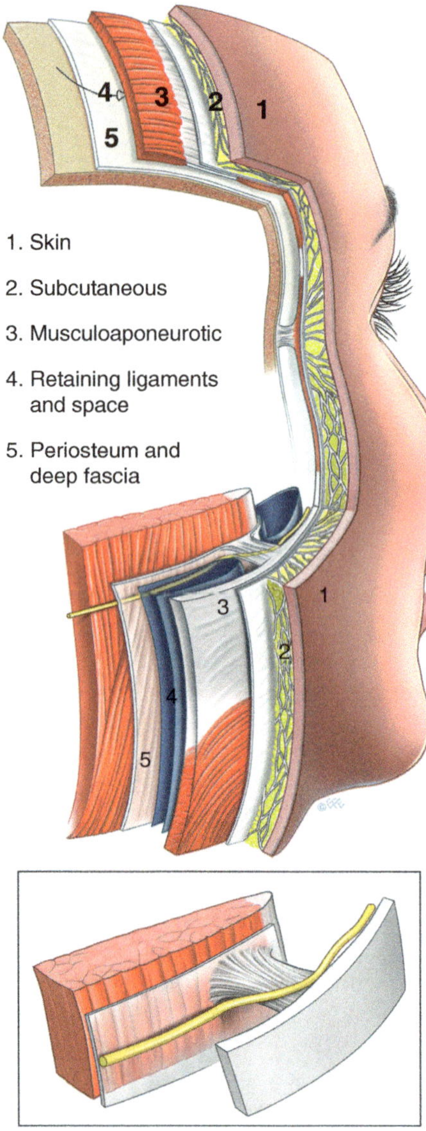

• **Fig. 62.1** The five-layered basic construct of the facial soft tissues is most readily understood in the scalp. While this same construct continues over the entire face, there are significant regional modifications for functional purposes. Layer 4, the most variable layer, contains soft tissue spaces alternating with retaining ligaments. In addition, the facial nerve branches travel through layer 4, where they remain outside the spaces and then ascend to layer 3 in close relationship with retaining ligaments. (From Mendelson B, Wong C-H. Facelift: Facial anatomy and aging. In: Rubin JP, Neligan PC, eds. *Plastic Surgery*. Volume 2: *Aesthetic Surgery*. 4th edn. Philadelphia: Elsevier; 2018: Fig. 6.1.2. © Dr. Levent Efe, CMI.)

each component varies in different regions of the face. In the scalp, the subcutaneous layer has uniform thickness and consistency of fixation to the overlying dermis. In contrast, in the face proper, the subcutaneous layer has significant variation in thickness and attachments. In specialized areas such as the eyelids and lips, this layer is significantly compacted such that fat may appear non-existent. In other areas, such as the nasolabial segment, it is very thick. In areas with thick subcutaneous tissue, the retinacular cutis lengthens significantly, predisposing its fibers to weakening and distension with aging. Within the subcutaneous tissue, the overall attachment to the overlying dermis is stronger and denser than the attachment to the underlying SMAS. This is a result of the tree-like arrangement of the retinacular cutis fibers (see Fig. 62.2), with fewer but thicker fibers deep as its rises through the SMAS that progressively divide into multiple fine microligaments as they reach the dermis. This explains why it is easier to perform subcutaneous dissection in the deeper subcutaneous level (just on the surface of the underlying SMAS) than more superficially nearer the dermis, as there are fewer retinacular cutis fibers and the subcutaneous fat here does not attach directly to the outer surface of the underlying SMAS.

Furthermore, the retinacular cutis fibers are not uniform across the face, but vary in orientation and density according to the anatomy of the underlying deeper structures. As will become apparent when the anatomy of the underlying layer 4 is described, at the location of the retaining ligaments, the vertically orientated retinacular cutis fibers are the most dense and are the most effective in supporting the overlying soft tissues. In so doing, they form the boundaries that compartmentalize the subcutaneous fat. These areas, such as the so-called McGregor's patch over the body of the zygoma, often require sharp release to mobilize. In between these retaining ligaments in layer 4 are located the soft tissue spaces of the face, that facilitate the mobility of the superficial fascia over the deep fascia. Where the subcutaneous fat overlies a layer 4 space, the retinacular fibers are less dense and orientated more horizontally, as a result of which, the tissues tend to separate with relative ease, often with just simple blunt finger dissection (Fig. 62.4). This variation in the density and orientation of the retinacular cutis fibers in the subcutaneous fat is the anatomical basis for the so-called "superficial subcutaneous fat compartments" recently described.[6] In these studies, injection of dyes into the subcutaneous fat results in staining of the fat in discrete compartments. While the relevance of superficial subcutaneous fat compartments remains debated, anatomically, they reflect the anatomy of layer 2, with diffusion of the injected dye being limited by the retaining ligaments at the boundaries of these compartments.

Layer 3 – Musculoaponeurotic Layer

The muscles of facial expression are unique and fundamentally different from skeletal muscles beneath the deep fascia because they are situated within the superficial fascia and they move the soft tissues of which they are a part. All muscles of facial expression have either all or the majority of their course within layer 3 and they are predominantly located over and around the orbital and oral cavities. In the prototype scalp, the occipital-frontalis moves the overlying soft tissue of the forehead, while its undersurface glides over the subgaleal aponeurotic space (layer 4). Layer 3 is continuous over the entire face, although for descriptive purposes, different names are given to certain parts according to the superficial muscle within. It is called the galea aponeurotica over the scalp, the temporoparietal (superficial

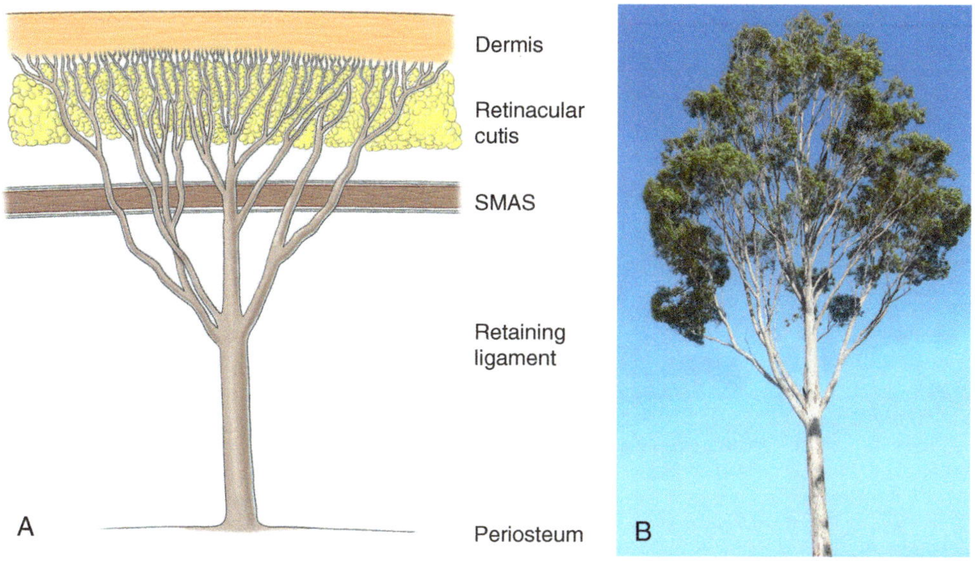

• **Fig. 62.2** The form of the retaining ligaments can be likened to a tree. The "trunk" of the ligaments attach the soft tissues to the periosteum of the facial skeleton or deep muscle fascia. The ligaments pass through all soft tissue layers, fanning out as multiple branches through the SMAS to eventually insert into the dermis. The ligamentous component in the subcutaneous layer is seen as the retinacular cutis. (From Mendelson B, Wong C-H. Facelift: Facial anatomy and aging. In: Rubin JP, Neligan PC, eds. *Plastic Surgery.* Volume 2: *Aesthetic Surgery*. 4th edn. Philadelphia: Elsevier; 2018: Fig. 6.1.3AB. © Dr. Levent Efe, CMI.)

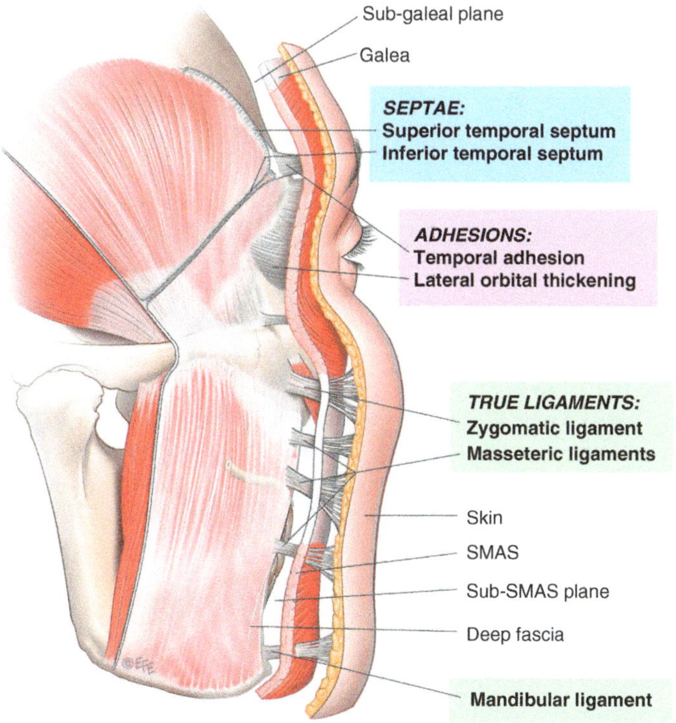

• **Fig. 62.3** The retaining ligaments of the face appear in three morphological forms, adhesions, septae, and true ligaments. (From Mendelson B, Wong C-H. Facelift: Facial anatomy and aging. In: Rubin JP, Neligan PC, eds. *Plastic Surgery.* Volume 2: *Aesthetic Surgery*. 4th edn. Philadelphia: Elsevier; 2018: Fig. 6.1.4. © Dr. Levent Efe, CMI.)

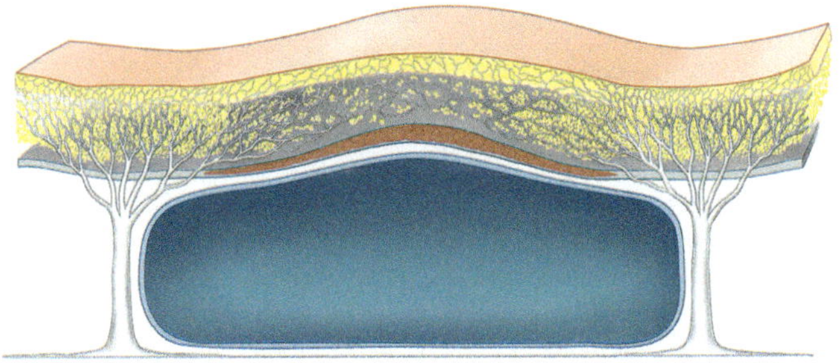

• **Fig. 62.4** The effective strength of the retinacular cutis fibers varies in different areas of the face. Overlying the retaining ligaments, the fibers are more densely arranged and vertically oriented. As a result, to surgically develop a subcutaneous flap here usually requires sharp release. In contrast, in the subcutaneous compartments overlying the sub-SMAS spaces the retinacula fibers are less dense and more horizontally oriented so that a relatively easy blunt dissection is usually sufficient to elevate the subcutaneous facelift flap here. (From Mendelson B, Wong C-H. Facelift: Facial anatomy and aging. In: Rubin JP, Neligan PC, eds. *Plastic Surgery.* Volume 2: *Aesthetic Surgery*. 4th edn. Philadelphia: Elsevier; 2018: Fig. 6.1.5. © Dr. Levent Efe, CMI.)

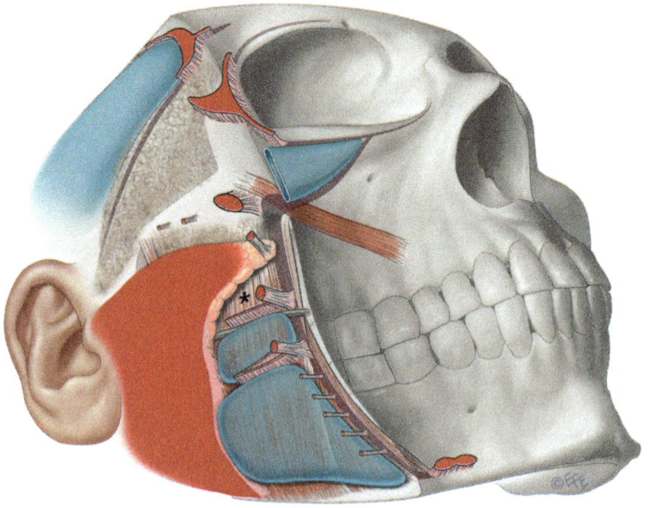

• **Fig. 62.5** Topographical anatomy of layer 4 over the lateral face: spaces (*blue*), ligaments (*red*), and the areas of important anatomy (*stippled*). The largest area of ligamentous attachment, the platysma auricular fascia, overlies the parotid, including its accessory lobe and dominates the posterior part of level 4 in the least mobile part of the face. At the vertical line of retaining ligaments the lateral face transitions into the anterior face. The spaces over the zygoma and over the lower masseter allow for intermediate mobility. The triangular-shaped areas immediately above and below the arch of the zygoma contain important anatomy, namely the temporal and zygomatic branches of the facial nerve respectively, that proceed from lateral into the anterior face. The asterisk indicates the uppermost premasseteric area. (From Mendelson B, Wong C-H. Facelift: Facial anatomy and aging. In: Rubin JP, Neligan PC, eds. *Plastic Surgery.* Volume 2: *Aesthetic Surgery*. 4th edn. Philadelphia: Elsevier; 2018: Fig. 6.1.6. © Dr. Levent Efe, CMI.)

temporal) fascia over the temple, the orbicularis fascia in the periorbital region, the superficial musculoaponeurotic system (SMAS) over the mid and lower face, and platysma in the neck.[7]

Within layer 3, the facial muscles themselves have a layered configuration, with the broad, flat muscles forming the superficial layer that covers the anterior aspect of the face. The frontalis covers the upper, obicularis oculi the middle, and the platysma the lower thirds, respectively. The muscles of this superficial layer have minimal direct attachment to the bone, stabilized to the skeleton at their periphery indirectly by the vertically orientated retaining ligaments as noted earlier. The frontalis is fixed along the superior temporal line by the superior temporal septum, the obicularis oculi laterally by the lateral orbital thickening and the main zygomatic ligament at its inferolateral border and the platysma at its upper border by the lower key masseteric ligament.[8–10] The deeper muscles in layer 3 provide greater functional control of the sphincters over the bony cavities. For the upper third, these are the corrugators and procerus and around the oral cavity, the elevators (zygomaticus major and minor, levator labii superioris, levator angulari oris) and levator labii superioris alaeque nasi, and the depressors (depressor angulari oris, depressor labii inferioris) around the oral sphincter and the mentalis.

Layer 4

Layer 4 is the plane in which dissection is performed in sub-SMAS facelifts. It is an area of significant complexity and contains the following structures: (1) soft tissue spaces, (2) retaining ligaments, (3) deep part of the intrinsic muscles where passing from their bone attachment to their more superficial soft tissue origin, and (4) facial nerve branches, transitioning from deep to superficial. Functionally, a series of soft tissue spaces exist in layer 4 to allow independent movement of the periorbital and perioral muscle of facial expressions (located in the roof of the facial soft tissue spaces) over the deep fascia on the major muscles for mastication directly beneath (located beneath the floor of the facial soft tissue spaces).[11,12] The retaining ligaments of the face are strategically placed within the boundaries between the soft tissue spaces (Fig. 62.5). In the lateral face, immediately in front of the ear, extending 25–30 mm forward of the ear cartilage to the posterior border of the platysma, is a diffuse area of ligamentous attachment, described by Furnas as the platysma auricular fascia (PAF). As no facial expression occurs here, the dermis, subcutaneous tissue, SMAS and the underlying parotid capsule (layers 1–5) are bound together as an area of diffuse retaining ligament. Layer 4 here is reduced to a fused layer, leaving it without a soft tissue space. There is no muscle in layer 3 here for mobility of this area of the superficial fascia. In contrast, in the anterior face where there is considerable movement over and around the bony cavities, the ligaments are significantly compacted and arranged around the edges of the bony cavities. These boundaries provide the last position where there is underlying deep fascia for the mobile shutters of the eyelids and lips to be supported. Importantly for the surgeon, the retaining ligaments also act as transition points for the facial nerve branches to pass from deep to superficial on their way to innervate their target muscles.

The soft tissue spaces of the face are in two forms: (1) those overlying bony cavities, such as the preseptal space of the eyelid over the orbit and the vestibule of the oral cavity under the lips and the lower nasolabial segment of the cheek and (2) those overlying bone, where the spaces allow the overlying superficial fascia to glide freely over the deeper layer 5.

Layer 5

The deep fascia, the deepest soft tissue layer of the face is formed by the periosteum where it overlies bone. Over the lateral face, where the muscles of mastication (temporalis and masseter) overlie the bone, the deep fascia is instead the fascial covering of the muscles, the deep temporal fascia and masseteric fascia, above and below the zygomatic arch respectively. The parotid fascia is also part of the deep fascia. The investing deep cervical fascia is the corresponding layer in the neck where it covers the supraomohyoid muscles and splits to form the submandibular space that contains the submandibular gland. The deep fascia, although thin, is tough and unyielding and gives attachment to the retaining ligaments of the face. In the mobile shutters over the bony cavities, the lids and lips, deep fascia is absent, being replaced by a mobile lining derived from the cavities, that of the conjunctiva or oral mucosa. The recently described "deep fat compartments" is fat located in layer 5, having more generally been called preperiosteal fat.[6]

Facial Spaces

A large part of the sub-SMAS layer 4 consists of soft tissue "spaces." These spaces have defined boundaries that are strategically reinforced by retaining ligaments. Significantly, from a surgical perspective, these areas are by definition anatomically "safe spaces" to dissect, as no structures cross within and all branches of the facial nerve are outside these spaces. As the roof of each space is the least supported part, laxity is more prone to develop here with aging, compared to their ligament-reinforced boundaries. This differential laxity accounts for much of the characteristic changes that occur with aging. Once a space has been surgically defined to its boundaries, the retaining ligaments in the boundary can then be precisely released under direct vision to achieve the desired mobilization while preserving the vital structures closely associated with the ligaments. A brief description of surgically significant facial soft tissue spaces is given below.

1. Upper Temporal Space

Overlying the temple are two compartments that are separated by the obliquely oriented inferior temporal septum (Fig. 62.6).[10] The upper compartment is a true space and the lower compartment is not a space, but an area containing important anatomy. Both compartments are interposed between the superficial temporal fascia (temporoparietal fascia) and the deep temporal fascia (temporalis muscle fascia). Anatomically, the upper compartment is an extension of the forehead anatomy down into the upper temple and the lower compartment is an upward extension of the upper cheek anatomy into the lower temple.

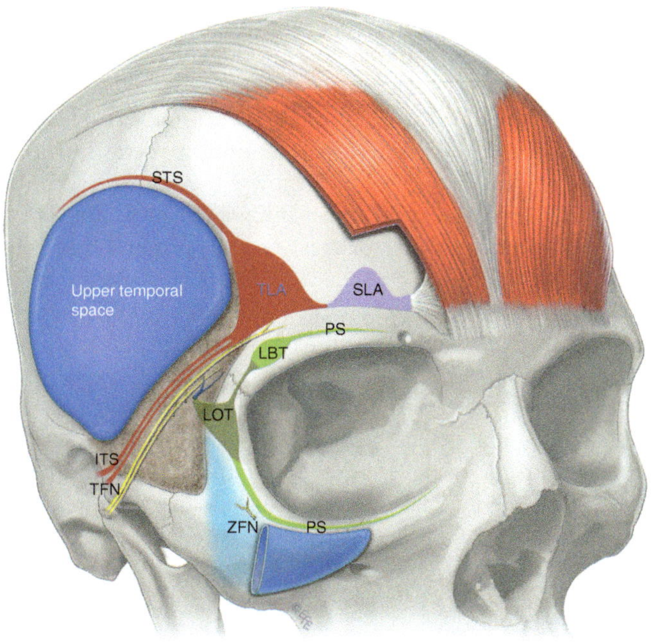

• **Fig. 62.6** Structures around the orbital cavity in layer 4. Above is the upper temporal space between the retaining ligaments of the temple; the superior temporal septum (STS) and the inferior temporal septum (ITS), both being extensions of the temporal ligamentous adhesion (TLA). There are no structures in the upper temporal space. The TLA continues medially as the supraorbital ligamentous adhesion (SLA). Below the bilaminar inferior temporal septum is the triangular-shaped lower temporal area, of important anatomy (*stippled*), where the temporal branches of the facial nerve (TFN) course immediately inferior to the septum on the underside of the temporoparietal fascia. Also crossing layer 4 in this area are the medial and lateral branches of the zygomaticfacial nerve (ZFN) and the sentinel vein. The periorbital septum (PS, *green*) just outside the orbital rim contains two areas of thickenings, the lateral orbital thickening (LOT) and the lateral brow thickening (LBT). (From Mendelson B, Wong C-H. Facelift: Facial anatomy and aging. In: Rubin JP, Neligan PC, eds. *Plastic Surgery.* Volume 2: *Aesthetic Surgery*. 4th edn. Philadelphia: Elsevier; 2018: Fig. 6.1.9. © Dr. Levent Efe, CMI.)

The upper temporal space is separated from the forehead by the superior temporal septum (STS) along the superior temporal line. Anteroinferiorly, the upper space is separated from the lower triangular temporal compartment, by the inferior temporal septum (ITS). These two septae merge at the triangular-shaped zone of adhesion called the temporal ligament. The upper temporal space provides safe surgical access to the lateral brow and upper midcheek. The space can be readily opened by blunt dissection to its boundaries. Once identified, the boundaries are then released by precise dissection. The superior temporal septum can be released sharply, taking care only to preserve the lateral (deep) branch of the supraorbital nerve, which runs parallel to the septum about 0.5 cm medial to it. The inferior temporal septum provides a marker to the important anatomy here as the temporal branches of the facial nerve are located parallel to and immediately inferior to this septum. To release the inferior temporal septum, the ceiling of the space is gently lifted off the deep temporal fascia floor, which three dimensionalises the septum in preparation for gentle release at the level of the floor, bearing in mind the frontal branches are located on the underside of the temporoparietal fascia in the ceiling, under the roof of the lower temporal area. Once released, the sentinel vein comes into view. The sentinel vein is not a good landmark for locating the temporal branches as they course cephalad to the vein, between it and the inferior temporal septum, where they travel in a layer of fat suspended on the underside of the temporoparietal fascia.

2. Prezygomatic Space

This triangular-shaped space overlies the body of the zygoma, its floor covering the origins of the zygomatic muscles.[11,12] The space allows independent movement of the obicularis oculi (pars orbitale) in its roof from the zygomatic muscles under the floor. Contraction of the overlying orbicularis elevates the prezygomatic soft tissues, which results in zygomatic smile lines (below the crow's feet) (Fig. 62.7). With aging laxity the roof of the space rests at a lower level. As a result, there is now a greater amplitude of movement on orbicularis contraction, which exaggerates the zygomatic lines with aging. This aging of the prezygomatic space, with bulging over its roof accentuated by its well-supported boundaries, is the anatomical basis for the clinical entity variously described as malar mounds, bags or malar crescent. This deformity indicates the presence of significant laxity and the treatment is directed to tightening the laxity of the roof.

3. Premaxillary Space

This quadrangular-shaped space (medial to the prezygomatic space) overlies the maxilla.[13] The space allows the independent displacement of the obicularis oculi in its roof from the lip elevators (levator labii superioris) under the floor. Fig. 62.8 details the anatomical relations of the premaxillary space. This space is clinically significant in that laxity over its roof contributes to the deepening of the nasolabial fold with aging. More importantly, it provides a safe sub-SMAS plane of dissection in the medial midcheek for surgical correction of the tear trough deformity.

4. Lower Premasseter Space

This space overlies the lower half of the masseter and is analogous to the temporal space in that it overlies the deep fascia of a muscle of mastication (Fig. 62.9).[14] This gliding soft tissue plane allows opening of the jaw without restriction and avoids excessive distortion of the overlying soft tissues. The roof of this space is formed by the platysma. The lower premasseter space has profound clinical significance as it is the anatomical basis for the development of jowls with aging. Laxity in the roof of the space, particularly where it

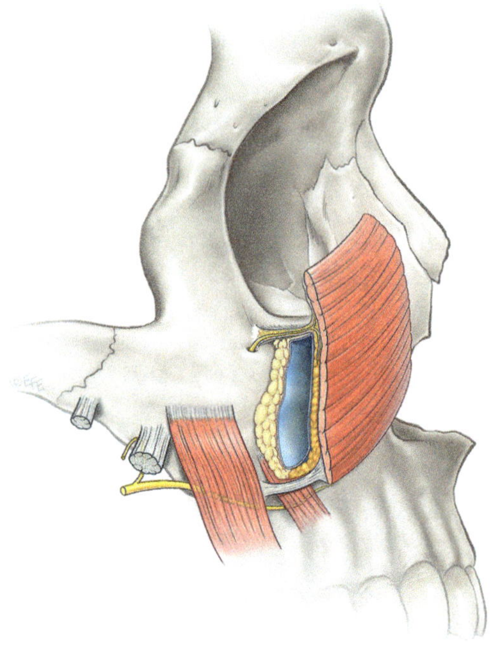

• **Fig. 62.7** The prezygomatic space overlies the body of the zygoma. The origins of the zygomatic muscles extend under the floor between preperiosteal fat. The roof is formed by the orbicularis oculi lined by the thin SOOF (suborbicularis oculi fat). The upper ligamentous border, formed by the orbicularis retaining ligament, is not as strong as the zygomatic ligament reinforced lower border. (From Mendelson B, Wong C-H. Facelift: Facial anatomy and aging. In: Rubin JP, Neligan PC, eds. *Plastic Surgery.* Volume 2: *Aesthetic Surgery*. 4th edn. Philadelphia: Elsevier; 2018: Fig. 6.1.10. © Dr. Levent Efe, CMI.)

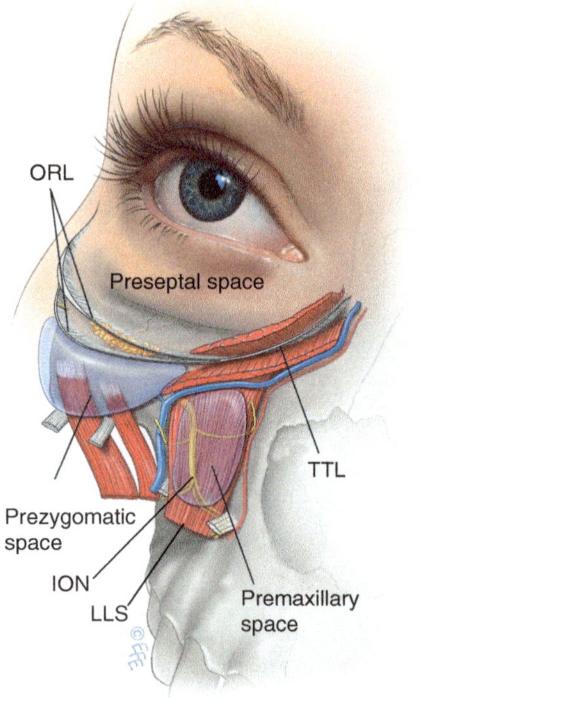

• **Fig. 62.8** The anatomy and key relations of the premaxillary space: levator labii superioris (LLS), infraorbital nerve (ION), tear trough ligament (TTL), and orbicularis retaining ligament (ORL). (From Mendelson B, Wong C-H. Facelift: Facial anatomy and aging. In: Rubin JP, Neligan PC, eds. *Plastic Surgery.* Volume 2: *Aesthetic Surgery*. 4th edn. Philadelphia: Elsevier; 2018: Fig. 6.1.11. © Dr. Levent Efe, CMI.)

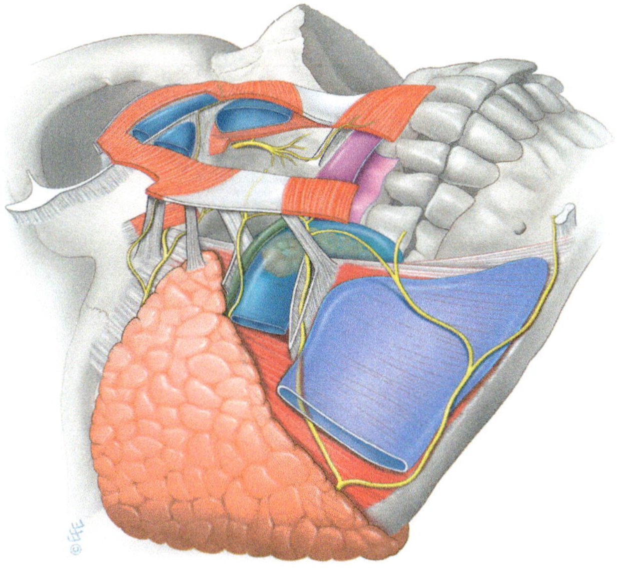

• **Fig. 62.9** The rhomboidal-shaped lower premasseter space overlies the lower half of the masseter. The platysma forms the roof of the lower space but does not extend over the middle space. The posterior border of the space is defined by the anterior edge of the parotid, while the anterior border is reinforced by the masseteric ligaments near the anterior edge of the masseter. The inferior boundary is mobile, mesentery-like, and does not contain any ligament. Weakness of attachment of the platysma roof at the lower anterior and inferior boundaries leads to the formation of the jowl, which is immediately behind the strong mandibular ligament. The buccal space containing the buccal fat is anterior to the key masseteric ligaments. All facial nerve branches course around and outside the space. The surgically important mandibular branch, after leaving the fixed platysma auricular fascia, courses under the inferior boundary of the space then rises onto the mobile outer surface of the membranous inferior border before reaching the mandibular ligament. (From Mendelson B, Wong C-H. Facelift: Facial anatomy and aging. In: Rubin JP, Neligan PC, eds. *Plastic Surgery.* Volume 2: *Aesthetic Surgery*. 4th edn. Philadelphia: Elsevier; 2018: Fig. 6.1.12. © Dr. Levent Efe, CMI.)

has a weakened attachment to the anterior masseter by the masseteric ligaments and its inferior boundary where there is no ligament, manifests as the labiomandibular fold and jowl respectively. The relatively stable fixation at the anteroinferior corner of the premasseter space provided by the mandibular ligament accounts for the dimple that is commonly seen separating the labiomandibular fold above and the jowl below.

5. *Middle Premasseter Space*

The middle premasseter space is a rectangular space cephalad to the lower premasseter space (Fig. 62.10).[15] Its floor is formed by the masseteric fascia and its roof by the SMAS, but the platysma in the roof of the lower space does not extend up to this level. It is an important facial soft tissue space in sub-SMAS facelift as it is an anatomical safe area to dissect, with the facial nerve branches located immediately outside the space within its superior and inferior boundaries. The parotid gland and the duct are closely associated with the upper boundary of the middle premasseter space.

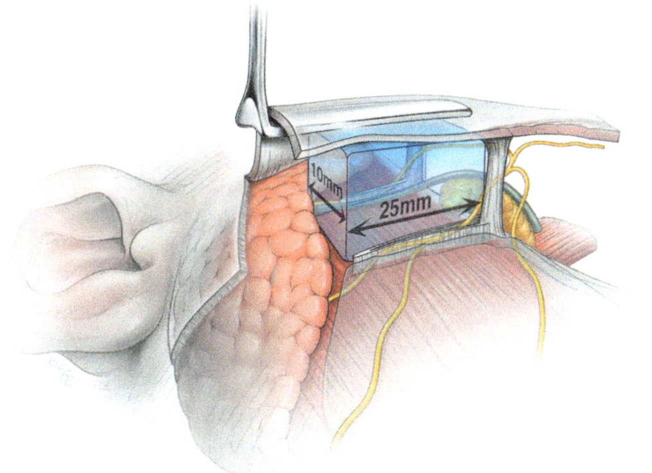

• **Fig. 62.10** The middle premasseter space is located within the concavity of the parotid overlying the anterior masseter, above the lower space. The upper and lower buccal trunks of the facial nerve course outside the space within its upper and lower boundaries. The masseteric process of the buccal fat pad is the only content and is variable. (From Mendelson B, Wong C-H. Facelift: Facial anatomy and aging. In: Rubin JP, Neligan PC, eds. *Plastic Surgery.* Volume 2: *Aesthetic Surgery*. 4th edn. Philadelphia: Elsevier; 2018: Fig. 6.1.13. © Dr. Levent Efe, CMI.)

Retaining Ligaments of the Face

To illustrate key concepts that retaining ligaments function to bind all five layers of the facial soft tissues together and that they are the anatomical basis for cutaneous grooves (seen between areas of laxity/bulges), we can examine the midcheek. The tear trough–orbicularis retaining ligament complex is the key retaining ligament of the upper midcheek. It is located just outside the orbital rim and closely follows the edges of the rim. This retaining ligament system separates the bony cavity (the orbit) from the bony platform (that of the midcheek skeleton) below, functioning to stabilize and secure the soft tissues of the lower eyelid where it transitions from the relative stability over the bone to the mobile area over the orbital cavity.

The *tear trough ligament* is a true osteocutaneous ligament originating from the maxilla and inserting into the dermis of the tear trough, passing through and binding all five soft tissue layers together.[16] As previously shown, this retaining ligament is the anatomical basis for the tear trough deformity (Fig. 62.11). Laterally, the tear trough ligament continues as the orbicularis retaining ligament (ORL). The orbicularis retaining ligament has previously been demonstrated to be the anatomical basis for the palpebromalar groove. The continuity of the tear trough ligament with the orbicularis retaining ligament then explains the observation that with more advanced aging, the tear trough becomes continuous with the palpebromalar groove, forming the prominent cutaneous groove sometimes called a prominent "lid–cheek junction." This demonstrates the key role that facial soft tissue retaining ligaments play in the cutaneous grooves seen with aging.

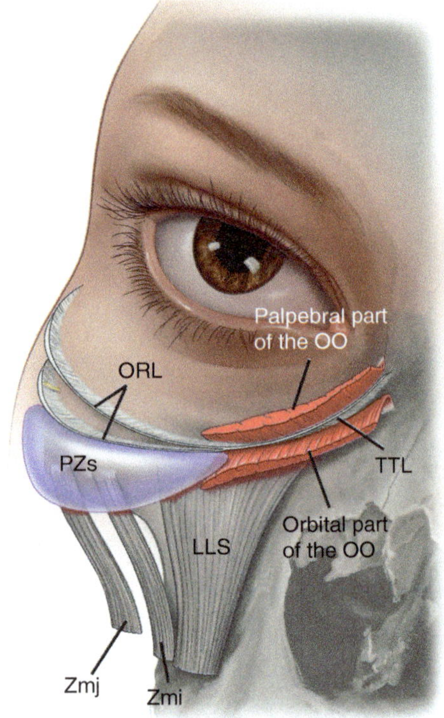

• **Fig. 62.11** The tear trough ligament, the anatomical basis for the tear trough deformity. TTL, tear trough ligament; ORL, orbicularis retaining ligament; OO, orbicularis oculi; PZs, prezygomatic space; LLS, levator labii superioris; Zmj, zygomaticus major; Zmi, zygomaticus minor. (From Mendelson B, Wong C-H. Facelift: Facial anatomy and aging. In: Rubin JP, Neligan PC, eds. *Plastic Surgery.* Volume 2: *Aesthetic Surgery*. 4th edn. Philadelphia: Elsevier; 2018: Fig. 6.1.14 © Dr. Levent Efe, CMI.)

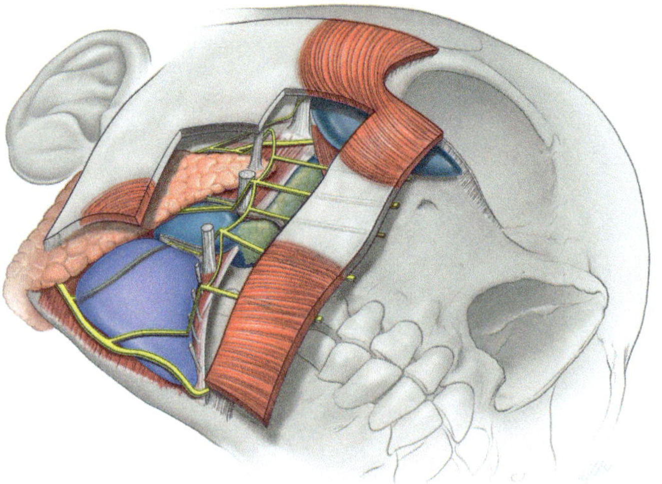

• **Fig. 62.12** Illustration to emphasize the location of the facial nerve branches and the alteration of their course relative to the spaces and ligaments. The nerves stay deep to and outside the spaces at all times in the lateral face. As they approach the ligamentous boundary into the mobile anterior face, the facial nerve branches transition from beneath layer 5 to enter layer 3, always in close relationship with the retaining ligaments forming the boundary. The interconnecting nerve branches between adjacent nerve trunks are located immediately sub-SMAS. (From Mendelson B, Wong C-H. Facelift: Facial anatomy and aging. In: Rubin JP, Neligan PC, eds. *Plastic Surgery.* Volume 2: *Aesthetic Surgery*. 4th edn. Philadelphia: Elsevier; 2018: Fig. 6.1.15. © Dr. Levent Efe, CMI.)

Facial Nerve Branches

The danger zones for facial nerve injury have been well described in the literature, but this is of limited value to the surgeon due to the topographical 2-dimensional perspective this gives of the expected course of the nerve relative to surface landmarks. Confidence when approaching the nerve surgically comes from (1) an understanding of the 3-dimensional course of the nerve relative to the layered anatomy as described above and by (2) visually identifying the nerves in relation to defined landmarks (Fig. 62.12). The facial nerve branches exit the parotid gland and remain deep to Layer 5 in the lateral face. As they approach the anterior face, the branches traverse layer 4, ascending to reach the underside of the mimetic muscles of the face. It is at these transition points across layer 4 that the nerves are at greatest risk of injury. The transitions occur at predictable locations, in close association with retaining ligaments that, being immobile, provide stability and protection for the nerves. The surgical release of these ligaments to gain the needed mobility should be performed with extreme care on account of the proximity of the nerves.

The surface marking of the temporal branch of the facial nerve is along the Pitanguy line, from a point 0.5 cm below the tragus to a point 1.5 cm lateral to the supraorbital rim. It is traditional teaching that once the temporal branch exits the parotid, it immediately runs superficially from the deep fascia and come to lie just deep to the SMAS as it crosses the arch of the zygoma. Because of its superficial location, surgical transection of the SMAS here, so-called high SMAS transection (i.e., at or above the arch) has been traditionally discouraged. It is now apparent that the nerve is deeper than was previously thought as it crosses the zygomatic arch. A histological study confirmed that the temporal branches transition from where they exit the parotid below the zygomatic arch, to where they enter the underside of the temporoparietal fascia some 2 cm above the arch.[17] The branches of the temporal branch run in a tissue layer (layer 4), just deep to the temporoparietal fascia (layer 3) and immediately superficial to the periosteum (layer 5) all along protected by a fascial layer, which is an upward prolongation of the parotid–masseteric fascia and named the parotid–temporal fascia. In another study, the temporal branch was noted to transition to under the temporoparietal fascia (layer 3) at a distance of 1.5–3 cm above the zygomatic arch. The temporal branch transitions to the underside of the temporoparietal fascia before the nerve crosses the sentinel vein more cephalically. Thus, once the sentinel vein is visualized from the temporal incision, the temporal branches would be located in the roof of the lower temporal compartment, in the wafer-like layer under the temporoparietal fascia.

The zygomatic branch exits the parotid gland deep to the deep fascia just below the zygoma and cephalad to the parotid duct. It travels horizontally on the masseter with the transverse facial artery. The strong zygomatic retaining ligament arises from the lower border of the body of the zygoma, immediately lateral to the origin of zygomaticus major, Here, the main zygomatic nerve continues beneath the muscle, and runs under zygomaticus major and minor, which it supplies from the deep aspect. At the lateral border of the zygomatic ligament, a small motor branch is usually given off to supply the orbicularis oculi, entering the muscle at its inferolateral corner. Careful dissection by vertical spreading of the scissors is crucial to avoid damaging this branch here.

The upper buccal trunk exits the parotid, about in line with, but superficial to the parotid duct, and continues deep to the investing masseter fascia, close to but outside the upper boundary of the middle premasseter space. Approaching the anterior edge of the masseter, this branch leaves the floor under the masseter fascia in close association with the upper key masseteric ligament. The lower buccal trunk leaves the parotid lower down, at about the level of the earlobe, and remains under the masseter fascia floor of the lower premasseter space and approaches the lower boundary of the middle premasseter space. Similarly, upon approaching the anterior edge of the masseter, the lower buccal trunk transitions from deep to gain the underside of the SMAS in close association with the lower key masseteric ligament. After the nerves reach level 3, the zygomatic, upper and lower buccal trunks and mandibular branch send an interconnecting branch with their neighboring trunks before continuing their course to innervate the mimetic muscles of the anterior face. This accounts for the overlap in muscles innervated by these nerves.

The temporal and mandibular branches are the most significant in terms of surgical risks because of the lack of cross-innervation of their target muscles. The marginal mandibular nerve is at risk where it is fixed by its close association with the retaining ligaments, both early in its course near the angle of the mandible, where it is within the PAF, and then well anteriorly close to the mandibular ligament. Over most of its course, the mandibular branch is mobile, being in relation to the inferior boundary of the premasseter space. It is not necessary to dissect in the vicinity of the nerve because of the inherent mobility of the platysma where it overlies the jaw and submandibular area. The mobility of the nerve as it travels within the inferior membranous boundary of the lower premasseter space accounts for the reported variability of the location of this part of its course (occasionally below the mandible).[18]

Aging Changes of the Face

Changes with aging occur at every level of the facial structure, including the facial skeleton. Changes of the skin are readily observable while changes in the skeleton effecting layer 5 can be observed radiologically. A correlation of the surface anatomy changes of aging with the anatomy of layers 2, 3, and 4 indicates that bulging occurs over the roof of soft tissue spaces, which stand out in contrast to the absence of bulging of the adjacent cutaneous grooves. The grooves reflect the restriction imposed by the dermal insertions of the retaining ligaments at the boundaries of the spaces. The extent to which the bulging reflects true elongation from primary tissue degeneration and laxity and how much it is "apparent" laxity secondary to loss of volume (skeletal and soft tissue) has yet to be defined.

Skin

Skin aging is influenced by genetics, environmental exposure, hormonal changes, and metabolic processes. With aging, the supple skin of youth becomes thinned and flattened, with loss of elasticity and architectural regularity. Atrophy of the extracellular matrix is reflected by the decreased number of fibroblasts and decreased levels of collagen (especially types I and III) and elastin in the dermis. While chronological skin aging and photoaging can be readily distinguished and considered separate entities, both share important molecular features, that of altered signal transduction that promote matrix-metalloproteinase (MMP) expression, decreased procollagen synthesis, and connective tissue damage. Oxidative stress is considered of primary importance in driving the aging process, resulting in increased hydrogen peroxide and other reactive oxygen species (ROS) and decreased antioxidant enzymes. These changes result in gene and protein structure alterations. Other environmental factors, notably smoking, accelerate skin aging, by between 10 and 20 years. Increased collagenase and decreased skin circulation have been suggested as possible mechanisms. The muscles of facial expression flex the skin in a specific pattern. As the underlying collagen weakens and the skin thins, the dermis loses its capacity to resist the constant force of the muscles and these lines becomes etched in the skin and ultimately even at rest.

Subcutaneous Tissue

The fibrous and fat components in the subcutaneous tissue are not uniform but arranged in discrete compartments. Due to the prominence of the subcutaneous fat in particular sites, they have specific names, such as the malar fat pad and nasolabial fat. The boundary of these subcutaneous compartments corresponds to the location of the retaining ligaments, which pass superficially to insert into the dermis. In youth, the transition between compartments is smooth and nondiscernible. With aging, a series of concavities and convexities develop which separates these compartments. These changes have been attributed to a number of causes, including fat descent, selective atrophy and hypertrophy, and attenuation of the retaining ligaments that causes fat compartments malpositioning. It is, however, now apparent that fat descends minimally with aging. Distinct compartmentalization by the retaining ligaments holds the fat in its relative position.

Muscle Aging

Skeletal muscles, in general, have been noted to atrophy up to 50% with age.[19] This is presumably applicable to the muscle of mastication such as the temporalis and masseter as a result of decreased demand and deterioration of the dentition with aging. As yet, no specific study on the effect of aging on these muscles has been reported. The mimetic muscle of the face, in contrast to skeletal muscles, may not undergo the same degree of degeneration with aging because of their constant use with facial expression. The orbicularis oculi has been noted to remain histologically unchanged with no loss of muscle fibers, adherence to surrounding tissues or ptosis with aging. The upper lip elevators, zygomaticus major, and levator labii superioris were also noted to remain unchanged with aging, based on magnetic resonance imaging (MRI) of their length, thickness, and volume. In contrast, the upper lip orbicularis atrophies with aging, with decreased muscle thickness, smaller muscle fascicles, and increase in surrounding epimysium.

Aging of the Facial Spaces and Retaining Ligaments

The multilinked fibrous system attenuates with aging, with decreasing strength of the ligaments and increasing laxity. In general, the spaces expand with aging in proportion to the amount of movement. This is greatest with the lower premasseter space and the related mandibular movement, and least over the zygoma. Expansion is related to the laxity that develops in the ligamentous boundaries and results in bulges between areas of relative fixation. Accordingly, the spaces dissect easily in older patients, and the boundaries widen as the ligaments weaken.[20] In young people, the spaces are more potential than real and do not open as readily with blunt dissection (Fig. 62.13).

Bone Changes

The facial skeleton changes dramatically with aging (Fig. 62.14) and this has a profound impact on the appearance of the face with aging (Fig. 62.15).[21,22] At birth, the facial skeleton is underdeveloped and rudimentary. This explains why infants and toddlers often transiently have visibly distinct midcheek segments (despite excellent tissue quality), which disappear with the expansion of the midcheek skeleton as they grow older. Peak skeletal projection is probably attained in early adulthood. Thereafter, while certain areas continue to expand, selective areas of the facial skeleton undergo significant resorption. Areas with strong predisposition to resorption include, the midface skeleton, particularly that part contributed by the anterior maxilla including the pyriform area of the nose, the superomedial and inferolateral aspects of the orbital rim,

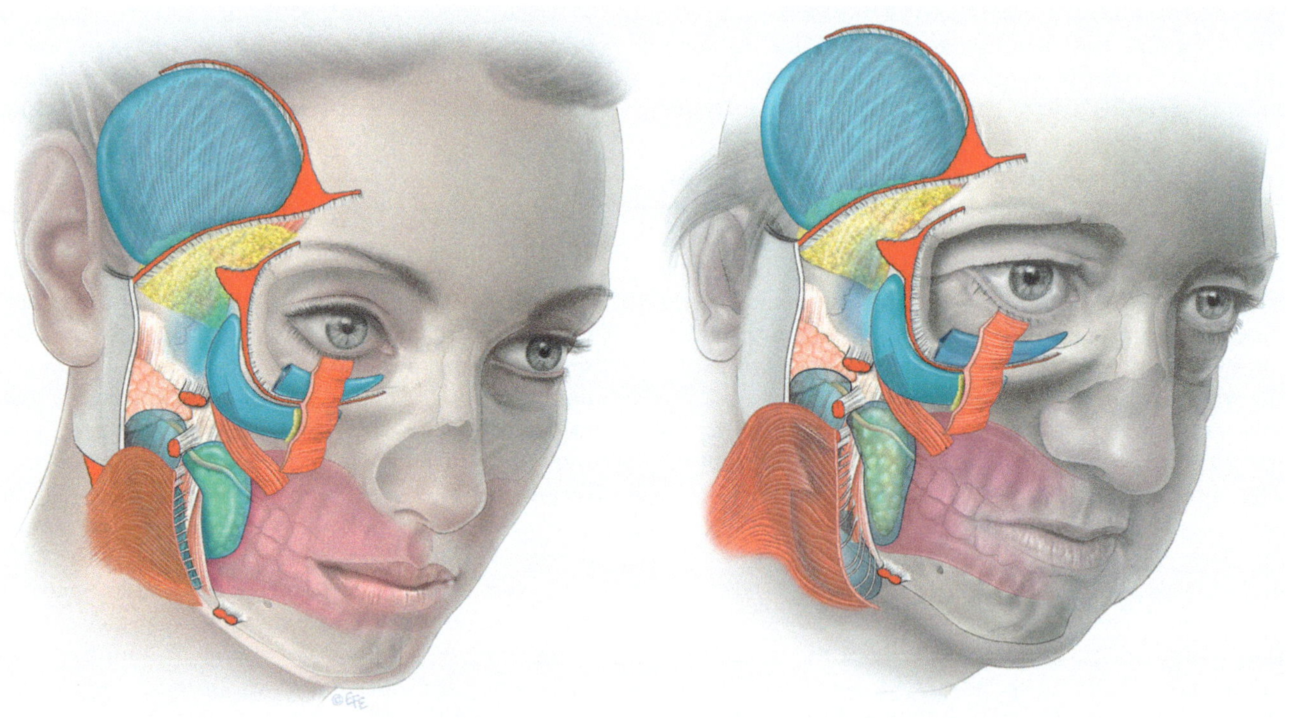

• **Fig. 62.13** In youth, the spaces are tight glide plane spaces. With aging, the spaces expand, and to a greater extent where facial movement is greater, namely in the lower face where the lower masseteric ligament fence distends the most. The weakened attachment of the platysma to the masseter here allows this corner of the lower premasseter space to expand to form the jowl. The reduction of ligament tone also allows the buccal fat to descend inferiorly into the labiomandibular fold. (From Mendelson B, Wong C-H. Facelift: Facial anatomy and aging. In: Rubin JP, Neligan PC, eds. *Plastic Surgery.* Volume 2: *Aesthetic Surgery*. 4th edn. Philadelphia: Elsevier; 2018: Fig. 6.1.16. © Dr. Levent Efe, CMI.)

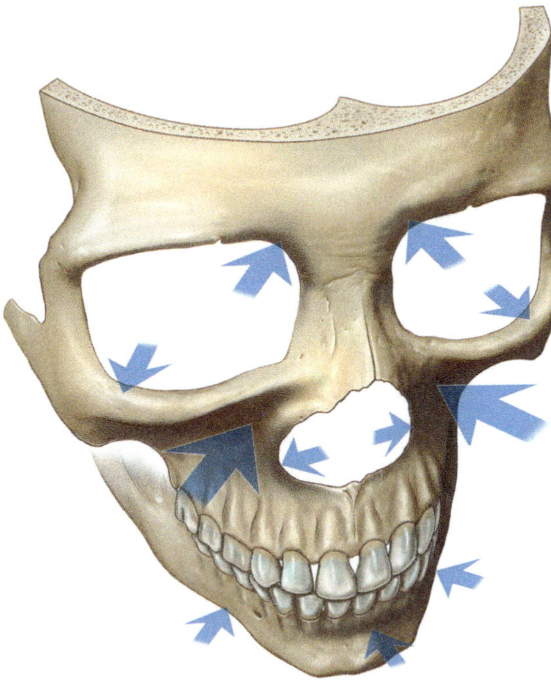

• **Fig. 62.14** The arrows indicate the areas of the craniofacial skeleton most susceptible to resorption with aging and the relative degree according to the arrow size. (From Mendelson B, Wong C-H. Facelift: Facial anatomy and aging. In: Rubin JP, Neligan PC, eds. *Plastic Surgery.* Volume 2: *Aesthetic Surgery*. 4th edn. Philadelphia: Elsevier; 2018: Fig. 6.1.17. © Dr. Levent Efe, CMI.)

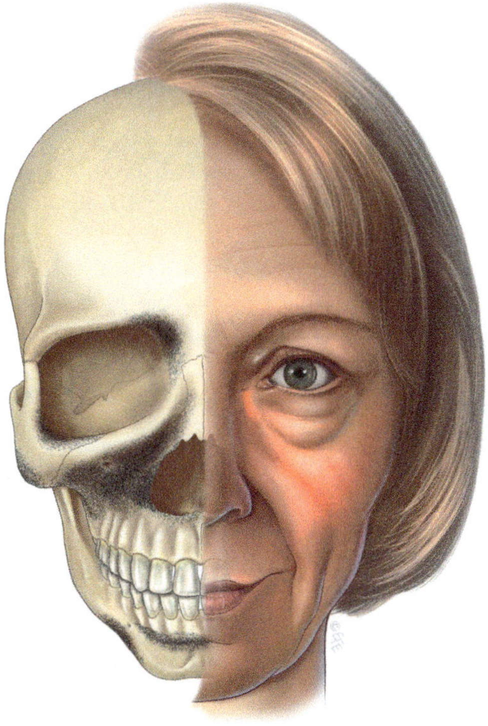

• **Fig. 62.15** Skeletal aging and its consequences. The stippled areas on the skeleton indicate where bone is resorbed and the relative amount. On the right, the stigmata of aging present in the facial soft tissues correspond to the areas of weakened skeletal support as a result of bone loss. (From Mendelson B, Wong C-H. Facelift: Facial anatomy and aging. In: Rubin JP, Neligan PC, eds. *Plastic Surgery.* Volume 2: *Aesthetic Surgery*. 4th edn. Philadelphia: Elsevier; 2018: Fig. 6.1.18. © Dr. Levent Efe, CMI.)

and the prejowl area of the mandible. The resultant deficiencies in the skeletal foundation have a significant effect on the overlying soft tissues. In the midcheek in particular, retrusion of the maxilla causes increased prominence of the tear trough and the nasolabial folds. The retrusion of the facial skeleton causes the origin of the multilinked fibrous retaining ligaments to be displaced posteriorly. This pulls the skin inwards, exaggerating the concavity between the areas of relative convexity that develop with aging. Retrusion of the midcheek with loss of projection gives the visual impression of tissue descent with aging.[23] Some patients have a congenitally weak, meaning inadequately projecting, skeletal structure. In such cases, the skeleton may be the primary cause of the manifestations of premature aging. Accordingly, in patients who suffer premature facial aging, a weakness of the relevant part of the underlying skeleton is immediately suspect and should be addressed in order to obtain better esthetic results.

Regional Changes Observed with the Aging Face

Temple and Forehead

The skin of the temple differs from that of the forehead, being thinner and less firmly supported to the underlying layers. The loose attachment reflects the underlying temporal space, which is extensive, as well as the nature of the surrounding temporal ligaments. These are unlike other facial ligaments being septal-like and do not continue through the thin, loose subcutaneous layer 2 over the temple. This explains why deep layer procedures in the temple are not as effective in toning the overlying skin as they are, for example, in the cheek.

The oblique head of the corrugator, the depressor supercilia, and the medial fibers of the obicularis oculi act in concert to depress the medial brow and produce oblique glabella frown lines. Laterally, the action of the lateral fibers of the orbicularis oculi with the transverse head of the corrugator supercilii promotes lateral brow ptosis. The ptosis of the lateral brow together and to a lesser extent the laxity of the skin with aging produces a pseudoexcess of the upper eyelid skin. Frontalis muscle hypertonicity from lateral brow skin hooding and its reaction to the action of antagonistic muscles (corrugator supercilii, obicularis oculi, and procerus) results in the development of transverse forehead skin lines. The medial brow in contrast seldom descends with aging and in fact may rise. The mechanism responsible for this includes the chronic activation of the frontalis muscle. This may either be to elevate the brow/eyelid complex associated with clinical or subclinical levator system weakness or to relieve visual field obstruction due to excess lateral upper eyelid skin. Anatomically, the frontalis muscle ends at approximately the temporal fusion line (superior temporal septum). Lateral to this, there is not an upward vector to counteract the downward pull of the medial and lateral brow depressors and gravity on the lateral brow, which may explain why more descent occurs at the lateral brow.

The Midcheek

The midcheek is the anterior part of the midface. It is triangular in shape and bounded superiorly by the pretarsal part of the lower eyelid, medially by the side of the nose and the nasolabial groove below, and laterally around the lateral cheek where the arch of the zygoma meets the body. A smooth rounded midcheek is a powerful image of youth. With aging, the three midcheek segments become clearly discernible, as they become separated by the three cutaneous grooves of the midcheek: the nasojugal, palpebromalar, and midcheek grooves. This "segmentation" of the midcheek has a profound impact on appearance that is responsible for giving the "tired" look associated with aging.

The skeletal foundation of the midcheek borders the three bony cavities of the anterior face, the orbital, nasal, and oral cavities The soft tissues of the midcheek are structurally composed of three segments or "modules," each having its own soft tissue space, and each overlying a specific part of the midcheek skeleton (Fig. 62.16). The lid–cheek segment overlies the prominence of the inferior orbital rim, from which it is partially separated by the lower part of the preseptal space of the lid. The malar segment overlies the body of the zygoma, from which it is separated by the prezygomatic space, and the nasolabial segment overlies the anterior surface of the maxilla, from which it is separated by the upper gingivobuccal recess of the vestibule of the oral cavity and the premaxillary space. Because of the many spaces and limited area of exposed bone for ligamentous support, the midcheek has some intrinsic structural weaknesses. Three factors make the midcheek susceptible to aging changes. These are (1) the wedge shape of the soft tissue of the midcheek, which are thin above and thicker below, (2) the natural posterior incline of the midcheek skeleton, from the relative prominence of the infraorbital rim, and (3) the significant retrusion that occurs with aging as a result of resorption of the maxilla. This is not uniform, as the maxilla recedes more medially and inferiorly. With early aging, the retrusion of the maxilla, along with a slight descent of the wedge-shaped cheek soft tissue results in an appreciable reduction of volume of the upper cheek. The result is that the small amount of orbital fat over the prominent edge of the infraorbital rim (originally concealed by the volume of the upper cheek), now becomes revealed, especially the underside of the lid fat bulge over the middle part. The visual impression is of a "lengthened" lower lid. At the same time, the increased thickness of the soft tissue mass over the lower cheek tends to conceal the degree of maxillary resorption and gives the profound visual impression that the soft tissue mass has descended into the lower part of the midcheek.

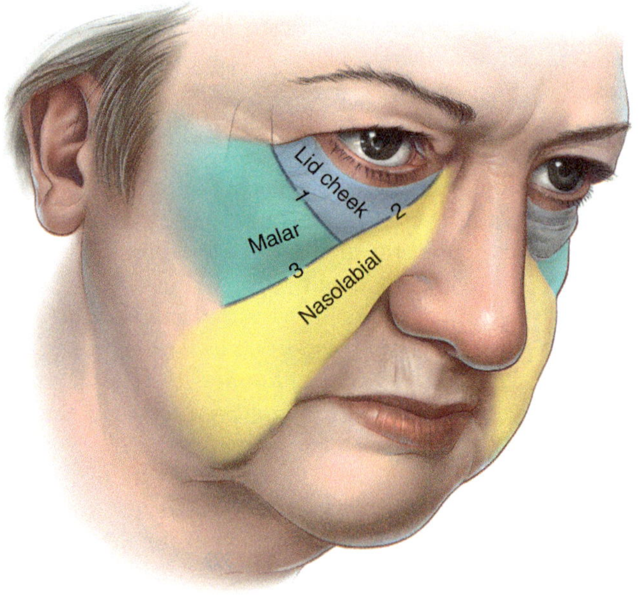

• **Fig. 62.16** The midcheek has three segments, of which the lid–cheek segment (*blue*) and the malar segment (*green*) are within the periorbital part. These are adjacent to the nasolabial segment (*yellow*), which is in the perioral part overlying the vestibule of the oral cavity. The boundaries of the three segments form three grooves, which interconnect like the italic letter *Y*. The palpebromalar groove (1) overlies the inferolateral orbital rim and the nasojugal groove (2) overlies the inferomedial orbital rim, then continues into the midcheek groove (3). (From Mendelson B, Wong C-H. Facelift: Facial anatomy and aging. In: Rubin JP, Neligan PC, eds. *Plastic Surgery.* Volume 2: *Aesthetic Surgery*. 4th edn. Philadelphia: Elsevier; 2018: Fig. 6.1.19. © Dr. Levent Efe, CMI.)

Of the three segments of the midcheek, the lower lid segment changes the most dynamically with aging. It has two distinct grooves across its surface that vary in their expression during the aging process, often coexisting. The upper is the infratarsal groove at the junction of the pretarsal and preseptal parts of the eyelid. It defines the lower boundary of the pretarsal bulge. The pretarsal bulge in youth is the visual separation of the lid above and the cheek below. This so-called "high lid–cheek junction" is located well above the infraorbital rim and is a characteristic of youth. The infratarsal groove location does not change with aging, although its contour usually fades. The lower groove is the lid–cheek junction that relates to the lower edge of the preseptal part of the lid. It is not usually present in youth and appears with aging and then progressively deepens and descends slightly over time. Its shape when it first appears is a gentle C contour but as it "descends," more so in its central portion, its shape changes to a progressively more angulated V shape with the medial side being formed by the developing nasojugal groove and the lateral side by the palpebromalar groove. The centre of the V, the lowest and deepest part, has the nasojugal groove continuing down the cheek as the midcheek groove that separates the cheek into the malar and nasolabial segments. The reason why this contour demarcation changes while the skin itself does not descend is explained by difference in the tissue layers. In level 4, the orbicularis retaining ligament is not rigid where it is over the center of the inferior orbital rim, so distension results in relative sliding between it and layer 3, the orbicularis oculi. As the lid–cheek junction becomes more prominent, it visually takes over from the infratarsal groove and becomes the new separation between the lower eyelid and the cheek. This is the basis for the commonly used but inaccurate phrase "lengthening of the lid–cheek junction with aging," which is in fact the result of a visual shift from the prominence of the infratarsal groove in youth to the lid–cheek junction with age. Correction of the aging of the lid–cheek segment of the midcheek, the visibly descended contour of the lid–cheek junction and long lower lid, has gained the colloquial name of "blending the lid–cheek junction."[24,25]

Lower Face

The jowl and the labiomandibular fold in the lower face are not present in youth and develop with aging. With the description of the concept of soft tissue spaces of the face, and specifically the premasseter space, the mechanism for the formation of the jowl can now be understood on an anatomical basis. With the onset of aging, laxity develops in the roof of the premasseter space associated with attenuation of the anterior and inferior boundaries. The major retaining ligaments (the key masseteric and mandibular) in contrast remain relatively strong and at these locations the superficial fascia remains firmly fixed to the underlying deep fascia. Distension of the weaker masseteric ligaments at the anterior border of the lower premasseter space (below the key masseteric ligament) allows inferior displacement of the buccal fat (within the buccal space), the anatomical basis for the development of the labiomandibular fold. The mandibular ligament demarcates the transition from the labiomandibular fold above and medial, and the jowl below. The jowl develops as a result of distension of the roof of the lower premasseter space with resultant descent of the tissues below the body of the mandible. The more prominent the jowl, the more apparent will be the cutaneous tethering provided by the mandibular ligament. Accordingly, the anatomical solution to correcting these aging changes is to reduce the inferiorly displaced buccal fat and to tighten the roof of the premasseter space.

Summary

This chapter has been structured to assist the reader to develop a conceptual understanding of facial anatomy and how it changes with aging. It is the framework that unifies the detailed anatomical information now available in the literature. Once understood, this knowledge will serve as the anatomical foundation for the logical and sound selection of surgical techniques for rejuvenation of the aging face.

References

1. Mendelson BC. Facelift anatomy, SMAS, retaining ligaments and facial spaces. In: Aston SJ, Steinbrech DS, Walden JL, eds. *Aesthetic Plastic Surgery*. Philadelphia: Saunders; 2009:53–72.
2. Mendelson BC. Correction of the nasolabial fold: extended SMAS dissection with periosteal fixation. *Plast Reconstr Surg.* 1992;89(5):822–833.
3. Mendelson BC, Jacobson SR. Surgical anatomy of the midcheek; facial layers, spaces, and midcheek segments. *Clin Plast Surg.* 2008;35:395–404.
4. Stuzin JM, Baker TJ, Gordon HL. The relationship of the superficial and deep facial fascias: relevance to rhytidectomy and aging. *Plast Reconstr Surg.* 1992;89(3):441–449.
5. Furnas D. The superficial musculoaponeurotic plane and the retaining ligaments of the face. In: Psillakis JM, ed. *Deep Face-Lifting Techniques*. New York: Thieme; 1994.
6. Rohrich RJ, Pessa JE. The fat compartments of the face: anatomy and clinical implications for cosmetic surgery. *Plast Reconstr Surg.* 2007;119(7):2219–2227.
7. Mitz V, Peyronie M. The superficial musculo-aponeurotic system (SMAS) in the parotid and cheek area. *Plast Reconstr Surg.* 1976;58:80.
8. Muzaffar AR, Mendelson BC, Adams Jr WP. Surgical anatomy of the ligamentous attachments of the lower lid and lateral canthus. *Plast Reconstr Surg.* 2002;110(3):873–884.
9. Furnas DW. The retaining ligaments of the cheek. *Plast Reconstr Surg.* 1989;83:11.
10. Moss CJ, Mendelson BC, Taylor GI. Surgical anatomy of the ligamentous attachments in the temple and periorbital regions. *Plast Reconstr Surg.* 2000;105(4):1475–1490.
11. Mendelson BC, Muzaffar AR, Adams Jr WP. Surgical anatomy of the midcheek and malar mounds. *Plast Reconstr Surg.* 2002;110(3):885–896; discussion 897–911.
12. Yousif NJ, Mendelson BC. Anatomy of the midface. *Clin Plast Surg.* 1995;22(2):227–240.
13. Wong CH, Mendelson B. Facial soft-tissue spaces and retaining ligaments of the midcheek: defining the premaxillary space. *Plast Reconstr Surg.* 2013;132(1):49–56.
14. Mendelson BC, Freeman ME, Wu W, et al. Surgical anatomy of the lower face: the premasseter space, the jowl, and the labiomandibular fold. *Aesthetic Plast Surg.* 2008;32(2):185–195.
15. Mendelson BC, Wong CH. Surgical anatomy of the middle premasseter space and its application in sub-SMAS face lift surgery. *Plast Reconstr Surg.* 2013;132(1):57–64.
16. Wong CH, Hsieh MK, Mendelson B. The tear trough ligament: anatomical basis for the tear trough deformity. *Plast Reconstr Surg.* 2012;129(6):1392–1402.
17. Trussler AP, Stephan P, Hatef D, et al. The frontal branch of the facial nerve across the zygomatic arch: anatomical relevance of the high-SMAS technique. *Plast Reconstr Surg.* 2010;125(4):1221–1229.
18. Nelson DW, Gingrass RP. Anatomy of the mandibular branches of the facial nerve. *Plast Reconstr Surg.* 1979;63:479.
19. Gosain AK, Klein MH, Sudhakar PV, et al. A volumetric analysis of soft-tissue changes in the aging midface using high-resolution MRI: implications for facial rejuvenation. *Plast Reconstr Surg.* 2005;115(4):1143–1152; discussion 1153–1155.
20. Mendelson BC. Surgery of the superficial musculoaponeurotic system: principles of release, vectors and fixation. *Plast Reconstr Surg.* 2001;107(6):1545–1552.
21. Mendelson BC, Hartley W, Scott M, et al. Age-related changes of the orbit and midcheek and the implications for facial rejuvenation. *Aesthetic Plast Surg.* 2007;31(5):419–423.
22. Mendelson BC, Wong CH. Changes in the facial skeleton with aging: implications and clinical applications in facial rejuvenation. *Aesthetic Plast Surg.* 2012;36(4):753–760.

23. Lambros V. Observations on periorbital and midface aging. *Plast Reconstr Surg.* 2007;120(5):1367–1376.
24. Wong CH, Mendelson BC. Mid cheek lift utilizing facial soft tissue spaces of the mid cheek. *Plast Reconstr Surg.* 2015;136(6):1155–1165.
25. Wong CH, Mendelson BC. Extended transconjunctival lower eyelid blepharoplasty with release of the tear trough ligament and fat redistribution. *Plast Reconstr Surg.* 2017;140(2):273–282.

63 Forehead Lift

TIMOTHY J. MARTEN AND DINO ELYASSNIA

Introduction

The first forehead lift procedures were performed using an "open" technique in which long incisions on the scalp or along the frontal hairline were made, a forehead flap was turned inferiorly, and modifications were made to corrugator supercilii and other muscles under direct vision. These breakthrough procedures served several generations of patients well and, while still performed by many surgeons today, they have been rejected by many patients and abandoned by some surgeons who view them as too aggressive too time-consuming to perform, and/or too difficult to market.

As endoscopic techniques made inroads into esthetic surgery, one of the first procedures they were adapted to by plastic surgeons was the forehead lift. Although a decade or more of technical refinements had to pass before the "closed" forehead lift procedure finally came of age, it has since come to be widely accepted and continues to be a viable alternative to open procedures for many patients. Experience has since shown that a "closed" technique without an endoscope can be used to mobilize and release the forehead and modify the corrugator supercilii muscles if the anatomy is understood and the operation is appropriately planned. In addition, transpalpebral corrugator myectomy, when used in conjunction with closed mobilization and resuspension of the forehead, not only provides a scheme for the performance of closed foreheadplasty without the need for an endoscope, but a method by which medial brow elevation can be minimized or avoided. Unesthetic medial brow elevation as a result of releasing the central brow to access the corrugator supercili muscles has been the "Achilles heel" of the endoscopic procedure and at least part of the reason endoscopic forehead lifts have fallen in popularity, and may, indeed, be one of the nonendoscopic short-scar procedure's most appealing and important merits.

Patient Options in Forehead Rejuvenation

Patients seeking improvement of their forehead appearance have four general categories of procedures available to them:

1. Open procedures using a bicoronal incision
2. Open "hairline-lowering" and "forehead-shortening" procedures using an incision or partial incision along the hairline
3. Closed, "limited-incision" or "short-scar" endoscopic procedures
4. Direct eyebrow lift using a supraciliary (upper edge of eyebrow) or forehead crease incision.

Selection of the "best" procedure depends on the patient's specific characteristics, including quantity of hair, hairline position, the quality of tissues, the condition of the scalp, the amount of improvement sought, and the overall degree of the aging changes that are present.

Identifying the Patient in Need of a Forehead Lift

Recognizing the changes that occur in the aging upper face is fundamental to rejuvenation of the forehead, and a requirement to communicating the need for the procedure to the patient. More detail on facial aging is available in Chapter 62. Typical changes seen in the aging forehead include eyebrow ptosis, lateral brow ptosis, pseudoblepharochalasis, glabellar "frown lines," transverse forehead creases, corrugator muscle hypertrophy, transverse upper nasal creases, and hairline recession (Fig. 63.1A). Each of these problems can potentially be improved with a foreheadplasty (Fig. 63.1B).

The forehead, eyebrow, and the upper eyelid are functionally and esthetically linked and it is *not* possible to appropriately rejuvenate the upper eyelid without performing forehead surgery in many cases. The eyebrow is the key to an attractive and appealing upper orbital appearance. The assumption that forehead ptosis is *not* present because eyebrow position appears satisfactory is the most common error in evaluating and treating the upper orbit and forehead ptosis must be suspected in any patient who appears to have *excess upper eyelid skin* – even if eyebrow position appears normal. If forehead ptosis is not recognized and appropriately treated upper blepharoplasty will result in esthetic and functional problems.

Transverse forehead creases and chronic frontalis spasm are the hallmark of forehead ptosis (Fig. 63.2). These are the result of the patient subconsciously trying to clear obstruction of their upper lateral fields of vision and to lift ptotic brow skin off their eyelids. Often these signs are not evident on initial examination, as patients learn to conceal them

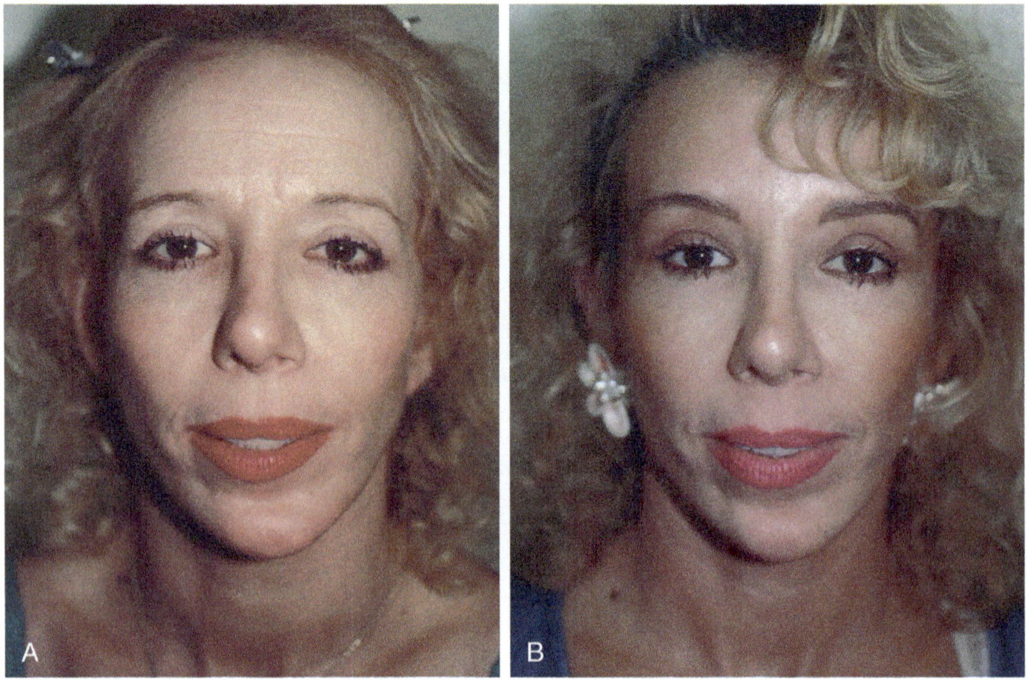

• **Fig. 63.1** Changes in the aging forehead. A patient seen before and after foreheadplasty. She has undergone previous facelift, upper and lower blepharoplasties, and chin implant placement performed by an unknown surgeon. A forehead lift was not performed. (A) Typical changes seen in the aging forehead include: eyebrow ptosis, lateral brow ptosis, pseudoblepharochalasis, glabellar "frown lines," transverse forehead creases, corrugator muscle hypertrophy, transverse upper nasal creases, and hairline recession. The patient's upper face appears older than her lower face and she has a "young face–old forehead" appearance. (B) The same patient after foreheadplasty. No eyelid or other surgery has been performed. The patient's eyebrows can be seen to have better position and configuration and the brow shape imparts a more alert, attractive, and feminine appearance. While preoperatively it might appear that excess skin is present on her upper eyelids repositioning her brows has revealed that this was pseudoblepharochalasis and that her upper lids are actually short on skin. Glabellar frown lines and transverse forehead crease have been effectively treated creating a less tense and more agreeable appearance. The frontal hairline has been lowered to a more youthful and esthetic position, creating better balance with other facial features. (Courtesy Timothy Marten, MD, FACS and the Marten Clinic of Plastic Surgery, San Francisco, CA; with permission.)

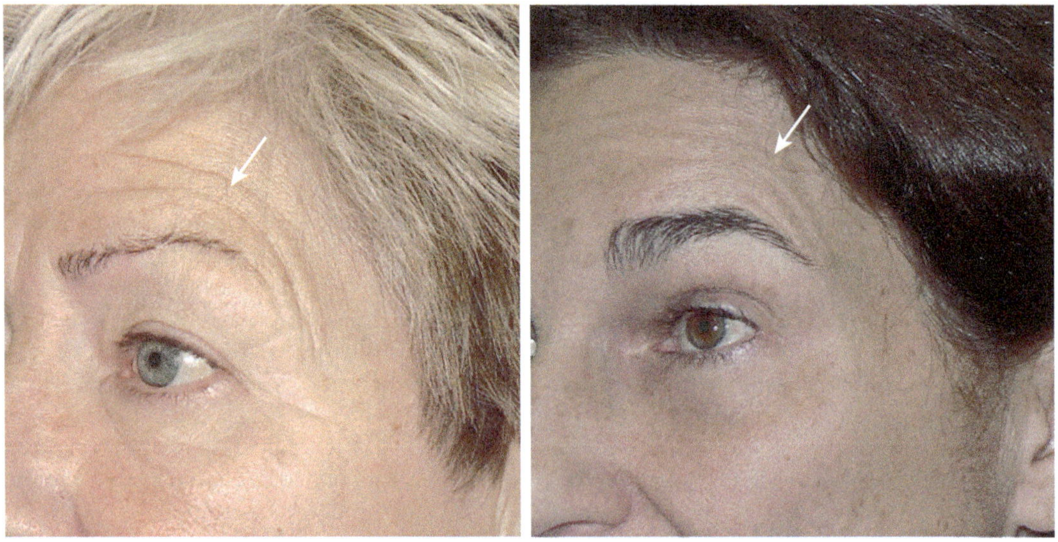

• **Fig. 63.2** Chronic frontalis spasm is a hallmark of forehead ptosis. Chronic frontalis spasm (*white arrows*) is a hallmark of forehead ptosis and is the result of the patient subconsciously trying to clear obstruction of their upper lateral fields of vision and to lift ptotic brow skin off their eyelids. It should be looked for in every patient requesting eyelid surgery. Often patients conceal its presence with their hairstyle and it is thus imperative to examine the patient with their hair off their forehead. Chronic frontalis spasm gives the false impression that the eyebrow is in an appropriate position and this further diverts suspicion that forehead ptosis is present. If eyelid skin is removed in these patients the stimulus for eyebrow raising is removed, the frontalis relaxes, and the eyebrow will drop. (Courtesy Timothy Marten, MD, FACS and the Marten Clinic of Plastic Surgery, San Francisco, CA; with permission.)

with their hairstyles. Chronic frontalis spasm gives the false impression that the eyebrow is in an appropriate position and this further diverts suspicion that forehead ptosis is present. Because the patient's hairstyle can hide important signs of forehead aging, and that compensatory frontalis spasm can give the false impression that the eyebrows are in an appropriate position, it is imperative that the patient's face be examined with their hair pushed well back off their forehead. In addition, because patients who wear forehead-concealing hairstyles often do not see the full extent of these problems, it is helpful, as it is during the rest of their evaluation, if they hold a hand mirror during this part of the examination. They can then be shown these important findings and counseled as to how they are the product of, and related to, forehead ptosis.

An upper lid skin fold that extends off the eyelid and onto the lateral periorbital area is a key sign of forehead ptosis and an important finding in differentiating forehead from eyelid problems ("Connell's sign") (Fig. 63.3). In many cases this sign will be evident only after the patient's forehead is relaxed and their brow descends to its "resting" position. For this reason it is important to examine the patient's forehead in repose with the frontalis relaxed. Often this will take some coaxing, as patients with significant forehead ptosis commonly develop compensatory chronic frontalis spasm and unconsciously hold their eyebrows up in an elevated position. Lightly stroking the forehead until the frontalis relaxes well help uncover the full extent of these patients' problems.

Frequently, patients seeking upper blepharoplasty will unknowingly signal the need for forehead surgery during their consultation by holding up their eyebrow with a fingertip while requesting eyelid surgery ("Flower's sign") (Fig. 63.4). For patients who fail to provide this sign, the surgeon should reposition the patient's brow and observe the effect produced while the patient watches holding a hand mirror. Often this simple maneuver will show that it is obvious that significant forehead ptosis is present and that little, if any, eyelid skin will need to be removed. In other cases it will be evident a combined problem is present and that both eyelid and forehead surgery is indicated. If eyebrow repositioning results in limited improvement of the upper eyelid and little improvement in the patient's overall appearance, eyelid surgery alone may be appropriate.

The erroneous assumption that forehead ptosis is not present because the eyebrow appears to be in a normal position is the most common mistake in evaluating the forehead for patients and surgeons alike. Patients are accustomed to optimizing the appearance of their face when looking at their reflection by unconsciously raising their eyebrows (Fig. 63.5). This is often further compounded by the fact that many women aggressive pluck the inferolateral portion of their eyebrow to give the illusion that it is higher and more arched. In many cases the entire outer half of the eyebrow is missing and has been drawn on in a higher position with an eyebrow pencil. The all too commonly observed circumstance is one in which the patient with marked frontalis spasm and marked transverse forehead wrinkling holds a hand mirror during their consultation and sees only that their eyebrows appear to be in a normal position. In these situations it is essential that the surgeon explain the dynamics at work (Fig. 63.6).

Many patients requesting upper blepharoplasty will have unrecognized forehead ptosis as a significant part of their "eyelid" problem, but compensatory frontalis spasm will make the eyebrow appear to be in a normal position. For these patients the goal of foreheadplasty will be to fix the eyebrow in the position the patient holds it preoperatively and to prevent the eyebrow from dropping when eyelid skin

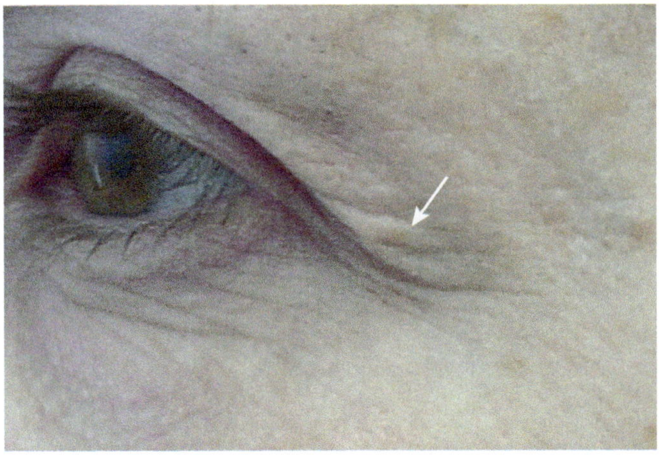

• **Fig. 63.3** "Connell's sign." An upper lid skin fold that extends off the eyelid and onto the lateral periorbital area is a key sign that forehead ptosis is present and an important finding in differentiating forehead from eyelid problems. In many cases this sign will be evident only after the patient's forehead is relaxed and their brow descends to its resting position. For this reason it is important to examine the patient's forehead in repose with the frontalis relaxed. (Courtesy Timothy Marten, MD, FACS and the Marten Clinic of Plastic Surgery, San Francisco, CA; with permission.)

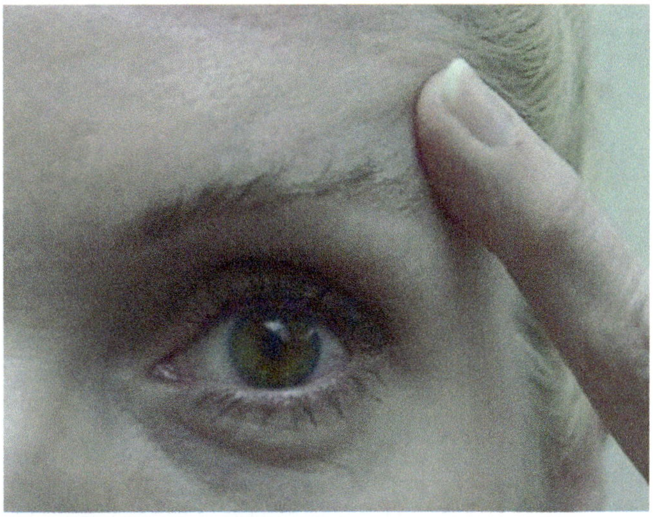

• **Fig. 63.4** "Flower's sign." Frequently, patients will unknowingly signal the need for forehead surgery during their consultation by holding up their eyebrow with a fingertip while requesting eyelid surgery. (Courtesy Timothy Marten, MD, FACS and the Marten Clinic of Plastic Surgery, San Francisco, CA; with permission.)

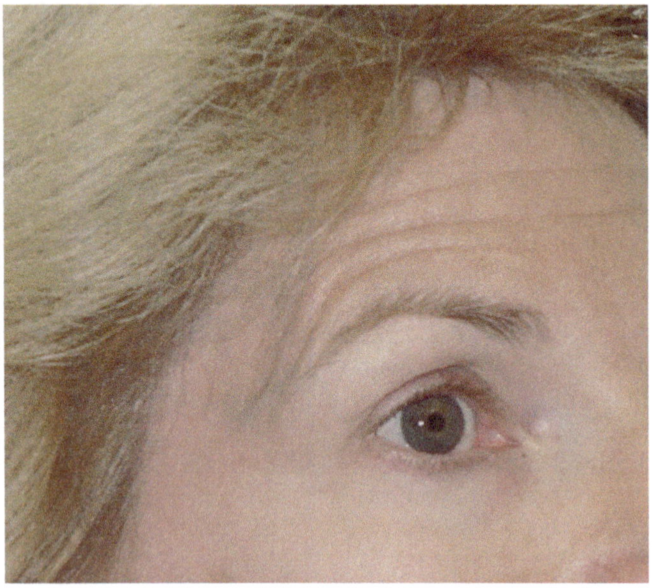

• **Fig. 63.5** Brow ptosis disguised by eyebrow raising. Patients often optimize their appearance when looking at their reflection by unconsciously raising their eyebrows. The all too commonly observed circumstance is one in which the patient with marked frontalis spasm and marked transverse forehead wrinkling holds a hand mirror during their consultation and sees only that their eyebrows appear to be in a normal position. In these situations it is essential that the surgeon explain the dynamics at work, and that forehead ptosis is present. (Courtesy Timothy Marten, MD, FACS and the Marten Clinic of Plastic Surgery, San Francisco, CA; with permission.)

is removed. In many properly performed foreheadplasties, the eyebrow will be in the *same position after surgery* as it was before, compensatory frontalis spasm, however, will be eliminated, transverse forehead wrinkles will be reduced, and the eyebrow will not drop when upper eyelid skin is removed. These facts and the need for forehead surgery must be communicated to the patient if esthetically appropriate outcomes are to be obtained.

Glabellar creases ("frown lines"), usually the result of repeated squinting to aid failing eyesight or to shield the eyes from the glare of the sun, are yet another sign of the aging upper face. These creases falsely convey expressions of pain and sadness when present in conjunction with frontalis activation (Fig. 63.7A), or anger and disapproval when present in conjunction with procerus contraction (Fig. 63.7B,C).

Upper Facial Aging and Inappropriate Expressions

In the late nineteenth century Duchenne conducted landmark electrophysiological studies of the human face and proposed that the contraction of certain muscles produced specific and characteristic facial appearances that were universally understood by others to represent the expressions of human emotion. His assertion was later embraced by Darwin and his identification of the particular muscles producing specific changes in facial appearance provided the groundwork for those who study facial behavior and perform esthetic facial surgery today. While some anthropologists reject the

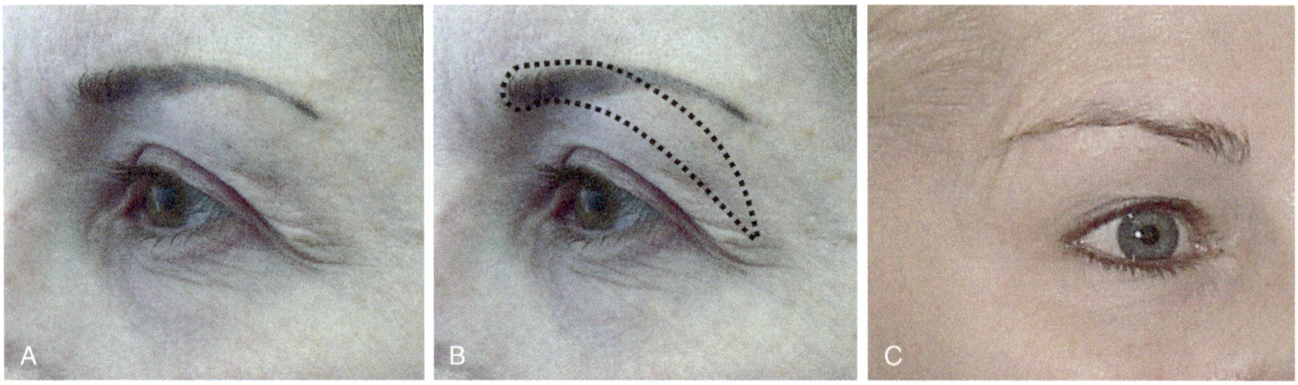

• **Fig. 63.6** (A,B) Do these patients have brow ptosis? (A) A patient whose eyebrow ostensibly appears to be in good position and configuration. A closer look shows that Connell's sign can be seen (see Fig. 63.3), indicating that brow ptosis is present. Even closer consideration shows that the patient's eyebrow is merely applied make-up and that the lateral part of her eyebrow has been plucked or shaved to hide its ptotic position (see also B). (B) In the same patient the dashed line shows the actual position of the eyebrow and the portion that has been plucked or shaved off. (C) A different patient who upon casual consideration appears to have good eyebrow position and configuration. A closer look shows she has chronic frontalis spasm and upper lateral forehead transverse wrinkles indicating that forehead ptosis is present. On yet closer examination it can be seen that the inferior portion of her lateral eyebrow has been plucked or shaved, giving the illusion that it is higher than it really is. This patient has brow ptosis and needs forehead surgery even though her eyebrow position appears to be normal. If isolated upper blepharoplasty is performed the stimulus for eyebrow raising will be removed, the frontalis will relax, and the eyebrow will drop. A well-performed foreheadplasty will fix her brow in the position she is holding it and her eyebrow may appear to be in the same position after surgery as before but the frontalis will relax and transverse forehead wrinkling will not be present. (Courtesy Timothy Marten, MD, FACS and the Marten Clinic of Plastic Surgery, San Francisco, CA; with permission.)

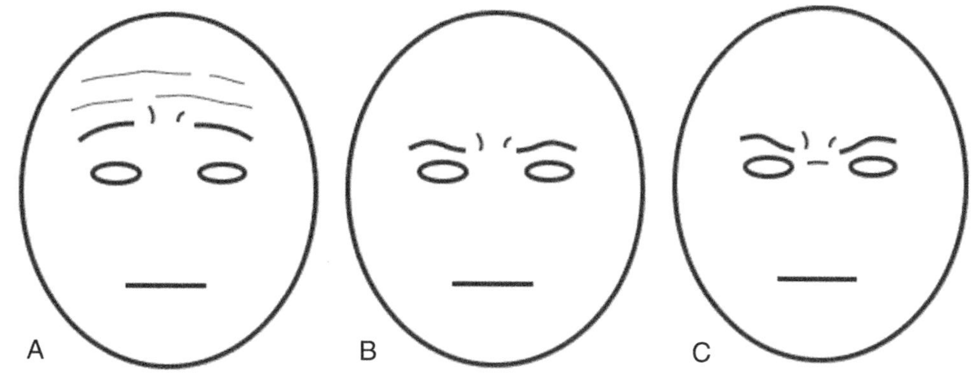

• **Fig. 63.7** Forehead aging and inappropriate expressions. (A) Typical appearance of patient with forehead aging and blepharochalasis *before* surgery. In an effort to clear upper-lateral visual field obstruction the patient uses frontalis muscles to hold up the eyebrows. Because the majority of the frontalis muscle is situated medially, this produces an exaggerated elevation of the medial eyebrow. Eyebrow elevation, in conjunction with corrugation of the forehead, results in a sad, tired, and melancholic appearance. Note that glabellar frown lines in this situation do not appear menacing and add a pained element to the melancholic appearance. (B) Typical appearance of a patient with unrecognized forehead ptosis after upper blepharoplasty alone. Upper blepharoplasty has removed the eyelid skin that provided the stimulus for frontalis muscle action, the frontalis has relaxed, and the full extent of forehead ptosis is now evident. This results in a lowering of the eyebrows. Note that the glabellar frown lines now convey a stern or angry appearance. (C) Same face and circumstances as in (B) but with the addition of a transverse upper nasal crease. Chronic procerus contraction amplifies an angry appearance and creates a look of disapproval and aggression. (Courtesy Timothy Marten, MD, FACS and the Marten Clinic of Plastic Surgery, San Francisco, CA; with permission.)

assertion that facial muscles exist solely as a dedicated system by which to communicate emotion, there appears to be a clear neurophysiological link between our emotional state, the activity of our facial muscles, and our facial expressions.

Artists, actors, illustrators, cartoonists, and others who draw or communicate with the face are all keenly aware of the key role the movements, lines, and creases produced by the muscles of facial expression on the forehead play in conveying feelings. It is also a fact that most people can instantly recognize expressions of fear, anger, sadness, disdain, surprise, and fatigue when shown only the emoting subject's upper face. Unfortunately, many of the changes that occur naturally over time in the aging forehead closely resemble features of these expressions, and these changes may thus be misinterpreted by others who instinctively, but mistakenly, assume we feel the way we look. Because of this, the aging face may appear inappropriately tired, disinterested, angry, disapproving, distressed or sad, even if its wearer is not (see Fig. 63.1 and Fig. 63.8). The *"pseudoexpressions"* that appear on our faces as we age affect how others perceive us and impacts significantly upon our interactions with them. Business people may appear angry or disinterested to associates and/or potential clients. Their appearance can provoke comments such as "You look like you're having a bad day" or "What's wrong with you?" Parents and grandparents may appear inappropriately angry or disapproving to their children and grandchildren and their appearance may compel those around them to ask "Are you mad at me?" or "Did I do something wrong?" Others may appear tired, unhealthy or lacking in vitality and their friends and family may ask or comment "You look so tired all the time," "I hope everything is OK," or "You look like you need to get some rest." It is not uncommon for patients to mention at the time of their consultation that they have heard these comments, or others like them. Although they may attribute these to be the result of changes in their eyelids, the discerning surgeon will recognize them as likely to be of forehead origin and will carefully evaluate the patient's upper face and advise her or him accordingly.

To appreciate pseudoexpressions resulting from changes in the aging forehead, the surgeon must consider the way in which the patient's appearance might make others *feel.* This is often best accomplished during the consultation by pushing one's chair back, viewing the patient's face in its entirely and, momentarily, deferring to intuition.

One of the most frequent errors made by plastic surgeons and other surgeons seeking to rejuvenate the aging upper face is performing upper blepharoplasty where a foreheadplasty is needed. This results in part from traditional emphasis on technique rather than analysis, and misconceptions as aging of the upper face ages. It is also, in part, the result of our own artistic failings when examining patients, planning procedures, and evaluating surgical outcomes.

As the forehead ages the brow descends and infra-brow skin moves into the upper orbit producing an *illusion* of upper eyelid skin redundancy. This occurrence is known as *"pseudoblepharochalasis"* and the term's etymology emphasizes the deceptive origins of eyelid skin "excess" and draws attention to the need to consider forehead surgery.

Attempts to treat pseudoblepharochalasis with an isolated upper blepharoplasty alone will at best result in a sad,

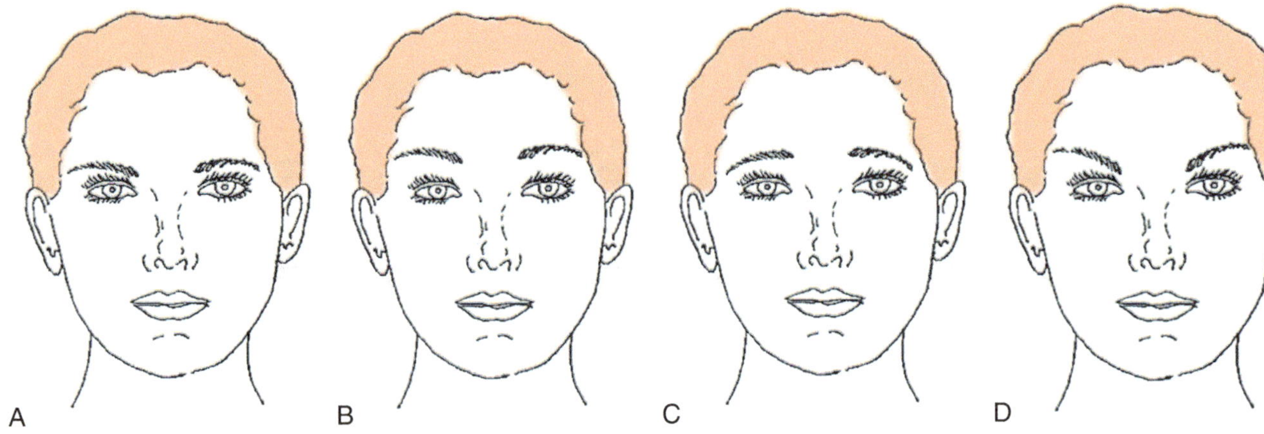

• **Fig. 63.8** Eyebrow position and configuration and its influence on expression. Many of the changes that occur naturally with age in the forehead resemble features of certain expressions, and these changes may thus be misinterpreted by others who instinctively, but mistakenly, assume we feel the way we look. Because of this, the aging face may appear inappropriately tired, disinterested, angry, disapproving, distressed, sad or conniving, even if the individual is not. (A) A prototypical face with a low, flat eyebrow. The face appears tired and disinterested. (B) A prototypical face with a high, elevated medial and lateral eyebrow. The face appears startled and surprised. (C) A prototypical face with a low, lateral and high medial eyebrow. The face appears sad and melancholic. (D) A prototypical face with a high lateral and low medial eyebrow. The face appears devilish and diabolical. (Courtesy Timothy Marten, MD, FACS and the Marten Clinic of Plastic Surgery, San Francisco, CA; with permission.)

tired-appearing patient with smoother eyelids and a long scar extending off the eyelid onto the lateral periorbital skin. More likely, however, isolated upper blepharoplasty performed where significant forehead ptosis is present usually results in a loss of the stimulus for brow elevation, further descent of the eyebrow as the frontalis muscle relaxes, and the reappearance of a pseudo skin excess in the superolateral orbit and across the upper eyelid. This, in turn, results in an exacerbation of a falsely sad, tired or disinterested appearance (Fig. 63.9).

If glabellar frown lines are also present and/or a transverse wrinkle exists over the upper nose, this "pseudo-sad"/"pseudo-tired" appearance is accentuated and will take on an angry or menacing cast. This sequence of events explains why both patients and their surgeons may be disappointed with the patient's overall appearance after upper blepharoplasty alone, despite technical proficiency in the excision of upper eyelid tissue (see Fig. 63.7).

Facial Asymmetry

Although it is true that facial beauty is correlated with symmetry of features and that most individuals regarded as attractive, fall within certain parameters in this regard, it is a fact that the attractive human face is inherently asymmetrical. Facial asymmetry should not, however, be regarded as an aberration, but as an inherent characteristic of beauty that makes the individual interesting, distinctive, and unique. In addition, it must be accepted by both patient and surgeon that precise right to left symmetry is not a realistic or desirable surgical goal and that forcing symmetry surgically on the face can result in esthetic imbalances and unusual, uninteresting, and unnatural appearances.

All patients undergoing surgery to rejuvenate their forehead will be found to have varying degrees of facial asymmetry and a careful examination will show each to have a "large" and a "small" eye, a "low" and a "high" orbit, and corresponding differences from right to left in hairline configuration, eyebrow position, pretarsal skin show, tarsal crease configuration, palpebral aperture opening, intercanthal tilt, and the like. These are the results, not only of subtle differences in the size of the ocular globe and adjacent structures, but differences in the position of the orbits and skeletal anatomy of the forehead and maxilla. Because of these differences, it will be artistically appropriate in many cases for the eyebrows to be at different heights after properly performed forehead lift surgery, if proper proportion and balance are to be maintained. Forcing the eyebrow situated over the smaller eye sitting in a lower, more deep-set orbit to the same height as the eyebrow situated over the larger eye often situated in a higher orbit, can make the smaller eye appear startled or surprised. In such cases it is arguably more appropriate to place the eyebrow over the smaller, lower eye in a lower position proportionate to it. Pointing out existing asymmetries and these facts preoperatively will prevent confusion on the part of the patient after surgery, when their face will inevitably be subject to closer scrutiny.

Eyebrow Esthetics and Planning Eyebrow Elevation

A traditional step in planning rejuvenation of the forehead is determining the desired position and configuration of the eyebrows. This decision should be made in conjunction

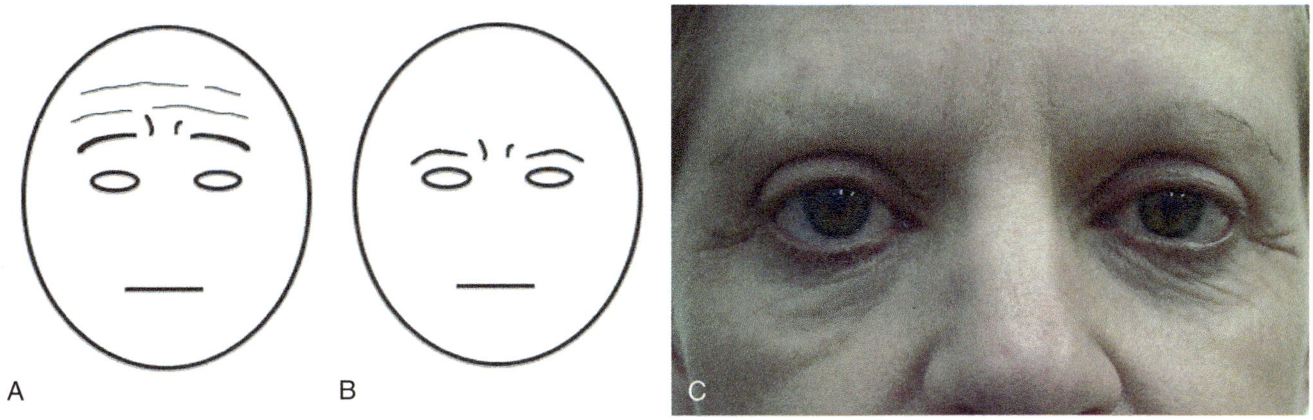

• **Fig. 63.9** Eyebrow position and configuration and their influence on expression. Mistaken attempts to treat pseudoblepharochalasis with an isolated blepharoplasty alone when significant forehead ptosis is present usually results in a loss of the stimulus for brow elevation, descent of the eyebrow as the frontalis muscle relaxes, and the reappearance of a pseudo skin excess in the lateral orbit. This, in turn, results in an exacerbation of a sad, tired or disinterested appearance. (A) Schematic of face with forehead ptosis. Brow skin resting on the eyelid triggers frontalis activation and the surgeons and patient may erroneously think that brow ptosis is not present. (B) Schematic of face of patient with unrecognized brow ptosis after isolated blepharoplasty. The stimulus for frontalis activation has been removed and the brow drops. The face takes on a tired, sad, and disinterested appearance. Often it appears as if eyelid skin had not been removed. (C) Patient example of sequence of events seen in (A) and (B). While the surgeon was technically successful at removing upper eyelid skin, the eyebrows sit in a low position and an unesthetic configuration, and the procedure is an artistic failure. (Courtesy Timothy Marten, MD, FACS and the Marten Clinic of Plastic Surgery, San Francisco, CA; with permission.)

with the patient and recorded on the preoperative record. Each patient should be informed, however, that these determinations represent a goal and a guideline, and not necessarily the outcome of their surgery.

Proper position and configuration of the eyebrow is ultimately a subjective judgment influenced by racial, cultural, and other factors that cannot be determined precisely by a fixed mathematical formula or arbitrary measurement. Marks, measurements, and published parameters should be regarded as guidelines only in planning surgery.

The amount of eyebrow elevation needed is usually neither the same at each point along the brow nor on each side of the face. In all but the unusual case, the majority of elevation will be needed laterally to restore attractive eyebrow configuration. *The artistic imperative in most patients is to tilt up the lateral eyebrow, not to lift it* and to achieve proportion and balance with other features, not precise right to left symmetry.

Accepting the fact that attractive eyebrow configuration and position are subjective and open somewhat to individual interpretation, the artist, illustrator or surgeon seeking to draw, restore or improve the appearance of the face can still benefit from guidelines as to how to proceed and a mathematical basis of beauty exists, and certain parameters can be used to assist in establishing esthetic goals.

Traditionally, most surgeons have tried to define what is attractive and beautiful in simple linear and absolute terms. Often it is said that the eyebrow should sit 25 mm over the mid-pupil in relaxed forward gaze (Fig. 63.10). While convenient, and useful to some extent, any such analysis is intrinsically flawed in that rigid linear measurements are ultimately inaccurate in that they assume each subject's head and facial features to be the same size.

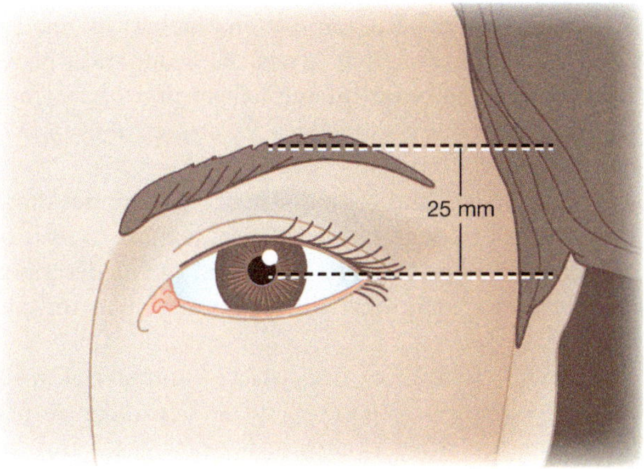

• **Fig. 63.10** Traditional guideline for attractive eyebrow position. Traditionally, surgeons have defined attractive eyebrow height in simple linear and absolute terms and often it is said that the eyebrow should sit 25 mm over the mid-pupil in relaxed forward gaze. While convenient, and useful to some extent, any such analysis is intrinsically flawed in that rigid linear measurements are ultimately inaccurate in as much as they assume each subject's head and facial features to be the same. (Courtesy Timothy Marten, MD, FACS and the Marten Clinic of Plastic Surgery, San Francisco, CA; with permission.)

A more accurate and appropriate guide to what is attractive is a model based on proportion and the interrelationships

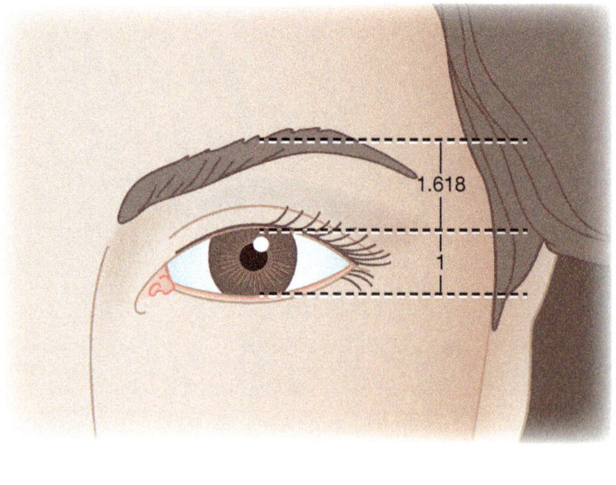

• **Fig. 63.11** The "golden eyebrow." An analysis of the attractive upper face will show that the aperture of the eye (the vertical distance between the upper and lower eyelids in forward gaze) and the distance between the margin of the upper lid and arch of the eyebrow are related to one another by the "golden proportion." Because the size of the globe and the height of the palpebral aperture will vary from patient to patient, so too must the height of the attractively positioned eyebrow. (Courtesy Timothy Marten, MD, FACS and the Marten Clinic of Plastic Surgery, San Francisco, CA; with permission.)

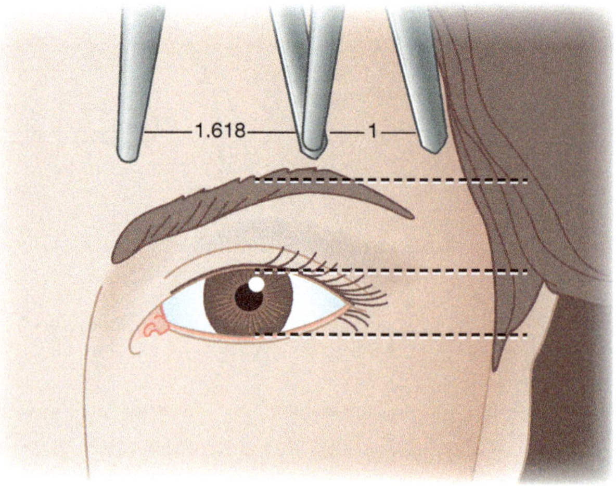

• **Fig. 63.12** The "golden eyebrow" arch. The position of the arch of the attractive eyebrow is also described by the golden ratio. (Courtesy Timothy Marten, MD, FACS and the Marten Clinic of Plastic Surgery, San Francisco, CA; with permission.)

of facial features. A useful system of analysis in this regard is the "divine proportion". Also known as the "golden proportion" and sometimes referred to as the "golden cut" or "golden ratio," this simple mathematical relationship defines a proportion that forms the foundation of what is considered to be beautiful and harmonious. As such, it can be used to establish guidelines for attractive eyebrow position and configuration.

Simply stated, the golden proportion specifies that when the proportions of an object or facial feature, or relationship between two objects or facial features, can be described by a ratio of 1 to 1.618, they will appear attractive and pleasing to the eye.

A careful analysis of the attractive upper face will show that the aperture of the eye (the vertical distance between the upper and lower eyelids in forward gaze) and the distance between the margin of the upper lid and arch of the eyebrow are related to one another by the golden proportion (Fig. 63.11). Further study will show that the position of the arch of the attractive eyebrow is well described by this ratio as well (Fig. 63.12).

Because the size of the globe and the height of the palpebral aperture will vary from patient to patient, so will the height of the attractively positioned eyebrow. As a practical matter, linear guidelines remain useful, if not entirely accurate, in that for the average face the height of the palpebral aperture will be approximately the same. And while calculating ideal eyebrow height from measurements of the patient's facial features is useful and instructive in establishing surgical goals, in time the experienced and artistic surgeon will intuitively come to recognize when features fall into the golden proportion. For these surgeons, "seeing" becomes more important than measuring.

It is a commonly observed fact that male and female eyebrow positions are not the same, and intuitively obvious that eyebrow position connotes sex differences. Interestingly, for many men, the attractive eyebrow will fall in inverse relation to that of the female but remain in golden proportion to the palpebral aperture (Fig. 63.13).

The golden proportion should be recognized as a guideline to eyebrow position and not an absolute ideal. Under certain circumstances a higher or lower position may be regarded as attractive. It should also be noted that the golden proportion defines classical standards of beauty. Models, actresses, celebrities and others in the public spotlight often seek to draw attention to themselves through exaggeration of what is traditionally thought of as attractive. While perhaps a professional imperative for them, the average plastic surgery patient is usually better served by setting goals more closely aligned with traditional definitions of beauty.

Eyebrow Position and Shape, and Influence on Expression

The position and shape of the eyebrow imparts the face with the appearance of certain emotions, even if the patient's feelings are neutral (see Fig. 63.8). If the eyebrows are lowered, the face appears tired and disinterested. Conversely, if the eyebrows are raised, the face takes on a startled or surprised look. If the lateral brow is depressed the face appears sad and melancholic. If the lateral brow is raised, the face takes on a devilish or diabolical appearance. As such, understanding the effect of eyebrow position and shape on expression is vital to performing esthetically appropriate foreheadplasty procedures and avoiding the creation of inappropriate expressions.

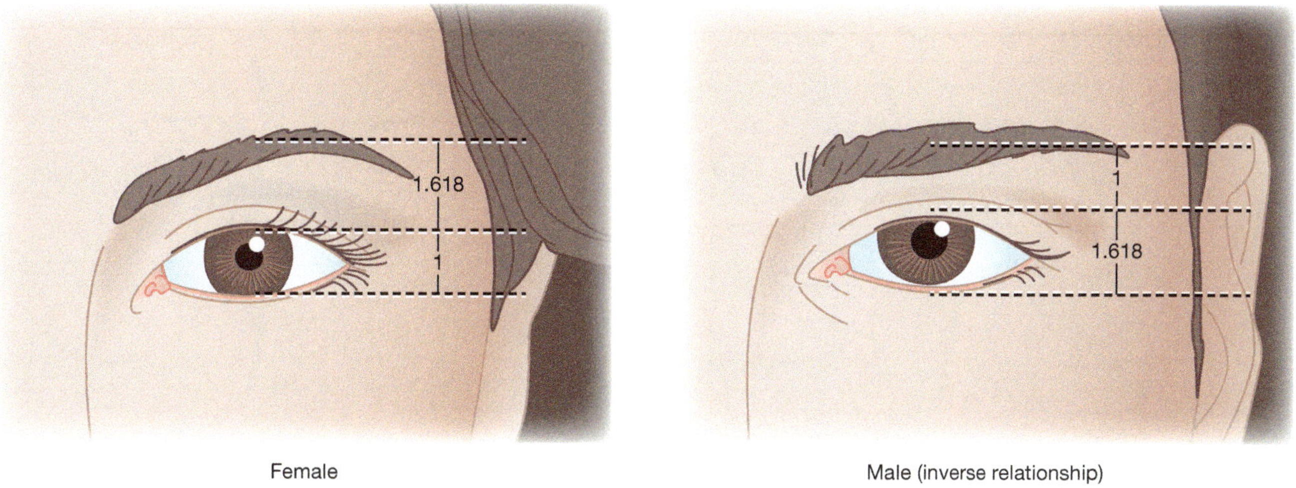

• **Fig. 63.13** The male "golden eyebrow." For many men, the attractive eyebrow will fall in inverse relation to that of the female but remain in golden proportion to the palpebral aperture. (Courtesy Timothy Marten, MD, FACS and the Marten Clinic of Plastic Surgery, San Francisco, CA; with permission.)

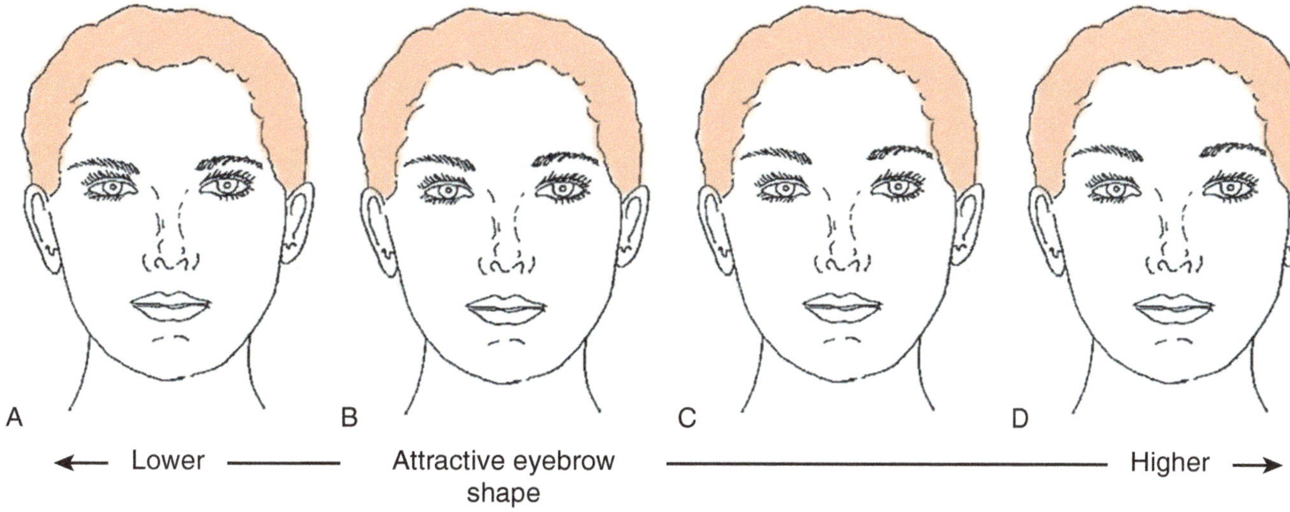

• **Fig. 63.14** The effect of brow height when eyebrow shape is *good*. Careful consideration of the attractive eyebrow will reveal that *both height and shape* are important. (B) shows a schematic of a prototypical face with attractive eyebrow shape and position. If the eyebrow is lowered (A), an attractive appearance is still present. When the eyebrow is raised (C), even when raised aggressively (D), an attractive appearance is arguably still present. All faces throughout the spectrum can be said to appear esthetic and consistent with an attractive appearance, and one can conclude that if eyebrow shape is good, the face will appear attractive at a *variety of eyebrow heights.* (Courtesy Timothy Marten, MD, FACS and the Marten Clinic of Plastic Surgery, San Francisco, CA; with permission.)

What Is More Important – Eyebrow Height or Shape?

Careful consideration of the attractive eyebrow will reveal that both height and shape are important and that it is simply short sighted to define the ideal brow strictly in terms of height only. So which is more important – height or shape? This question can be answered by exploring the effect of eyebrow height in two scenarios: one in which eyebrow shape is good, and one in which eyebrow shape is poor (Fig. 63.14). In Fig. 63.14, (B) shows a schematic of a prototypical face with attractive eyebrow shape and position (eyebrow in golden proportion to the aperture of the eye). When the eyebrow is lowered, as seen in (A), an attractive appearance is still present. When the eyebrow is raised, as shown in (C), even when raised aggressively, as shown in (D), an attractive appearance is arguably still present. In fact, all faces throughout the spectrum in Fig. 63.14 arguably appear esthetic and consistent with an attractive appearance and one can conclude that if eyebrow shape is good, the face will appear attractive at a *variety of eyebrow heights*.

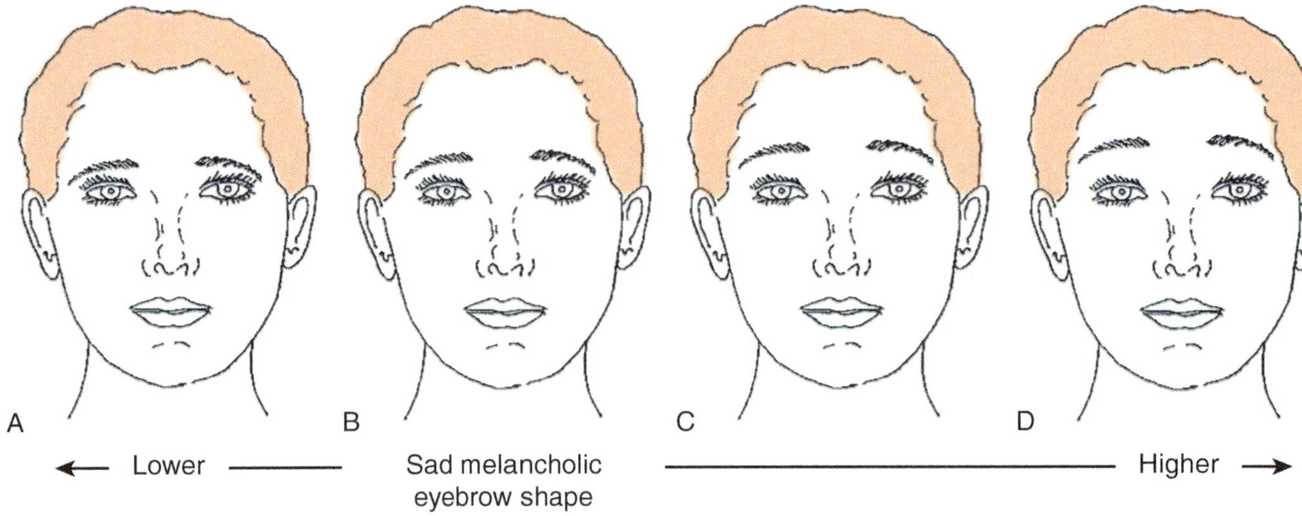

• **Fig. 63.15** The effect of brow height when eyebrow shape is *poor*. Shown in (B) a prototypical face with sad, melancholic shape and neutral position. If the eyebrow is lowered (A) a sad, melancholic appearance is still present. When the eyebrow is raised (C), even when raised aggressively (D), a sad, melancholic appearance is arguably still present. In fact, all faces throughout the spectrum shown arguably appear unesthetic and inconsistent with an attractive appearance, and one can conclude that if eyebrow shape is poor, the face will appear unattractive *regardless of eyebrow height*. (Courtesy Timothy Marten, MD, FACS and the Marten Clinic of Plastic Surgery, San Francisco, CA; with permission.)

What about the effect of eyebrow height when eyebrow shape is poor? See Fig. 63.15 for details.

In summary, if eyebrow shape is good, esthetic appearance will be present – regardless of eyebrow height– but if eyebrow shape is poor, an unesthetic appearance will be present – regardless of eyebrow height (Fig. 63.16). These observations, in turn, lead to the conclusion that eyebrow *shape* supersedes eyebrow height in importance in establishing an esthetic and attractive appearance, and that our surgical and artistic goal is to "tilt" the eyebrow – *not* "lift" it. If the foreheadplasty procedure does *not* produce good eyebrow *shape*, an attractive appearance will not be obtained.

In light of this analysis, it can be seen that the golden proportion, while a useful guideline in defining attractive eyebrow position, is not an absolute ideal. Under certain circumstances it will be seen that a higher or lower eyebrow position will be regarded as attractive. The golden proportion in particular does *not* explain the observation that a more highly placed eyebrow often appears attractive on the mature female face – or that young faces appear attractive with a more inferiorly situated eyebrow. Why does a high eyebrow appear more attractive on the older face? Why does a low eyebrow appear appropriate on the young face? Why does a low eyebrow appear less attractive on the mature face? The answer to these questions lies in the fact that the golden proportion system of analysis only positions the eyebrow in relation to the eye and it does not position it in relation to the orbit or take into account the characteristics of the adjacent midface or cheek. The characteristics of these structures contribute to a "young" or "old" appearance and thus are relevant in any method of analysis used to determine age-appropriate eyebrow position. The question can then be raised, is it possible that ideal eyebrow position is correlated with the overall appearance of the face and is influenced by orbital volume?

Is There a Relationship Between *Lower* Orbital Volume and Eyebrow Position?

To explore this assertion we can use orbital oval analysis – a method used by estheticians and makeup artists to create attractive and esthetically pleasing eyebrows. Orbital oval analysis stipulates that the eyebrow should be situated so that the eye sits in the center of an oval defined by the brow and the lid–cheek junction (Fig. 63.17).

When the lid–cheek junction is low a higher eyebrow will be necessary to maintain esthetic balance (Fig. 63.18). This may explain why a high eyebrow looks better on a mature face. The mature face typically has a low lid–cheek junction as a result of midface atrophy and descent. And why a *low* eyebrow looks better on a young face – a young face typically has a high lid–cheek junction and when the lid–cheek junction is high a *lower* eyebrow may be artistically appropriate (Fig. 63.19).

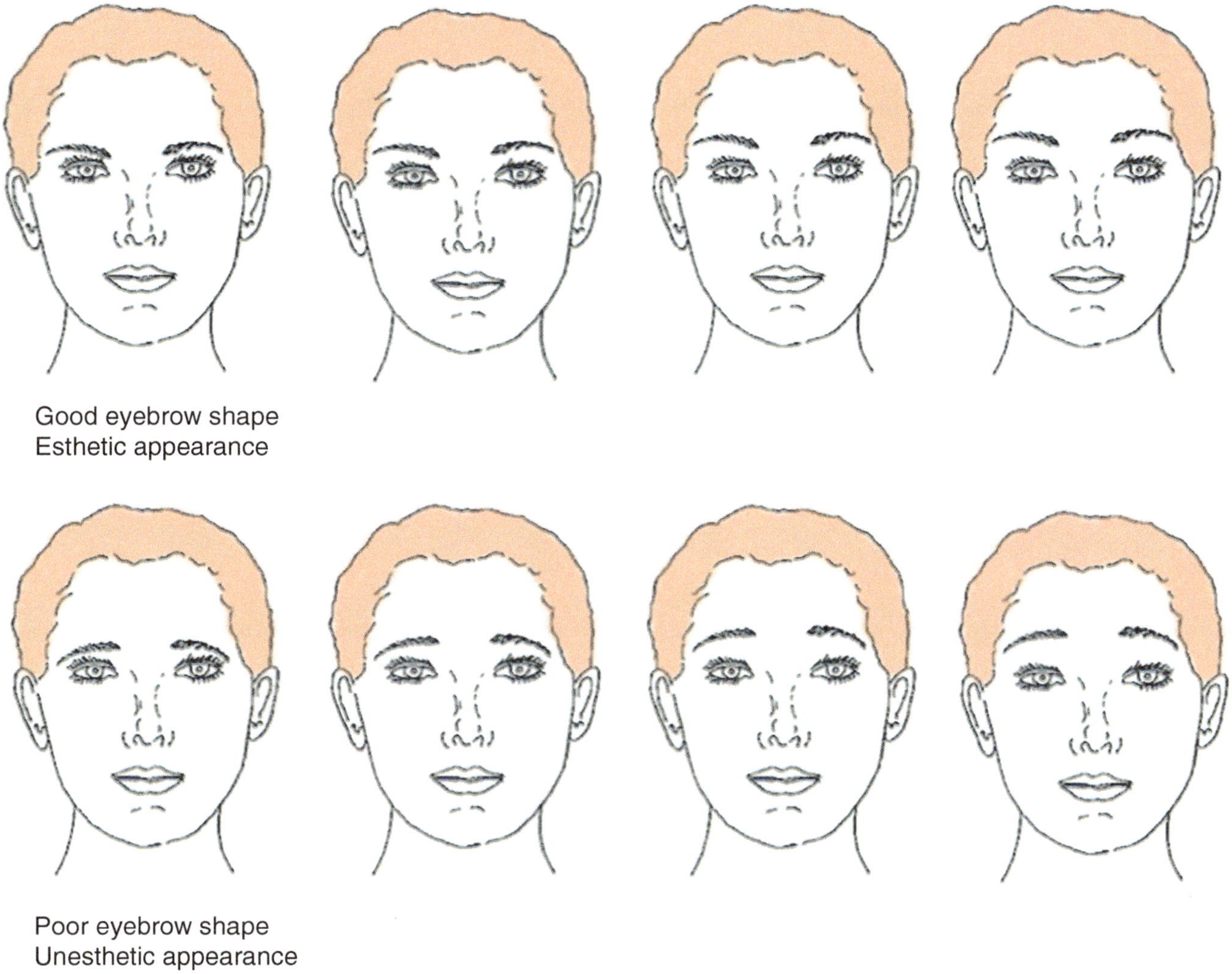

• **Fig. 63.16** Summary of eyebrow shape and appearance. If eyebrow shape is good an esthetic appearance will be present regardless of height, but if shape is poor an unesthetic appearance will be present regardless of eyebrow height. Therefore *shape* supersedes *height* in importance in establishing an esthetic appearance. The surgical and artistic goal is to "tilt" the eyebrow – *not* "lift" it. If a foreheadplasty procedure does *not* produce good eyebrow shape an attractive appearance will not be obtained. (Courtesy Timothy Marten, MD, FACS and the Marten Clinic of Plastic Surgery, San Francisco, CA; with permission.)

It can be seen that filling the lower orbit makes the eyebrow appear higher, even when its position is unchanged, and thus we must take into consideration the characteristics of the lower orbit and midface when performing esthetically nuanced foreheadplasty procedures. And once this is understood we can see that as we treat the lower eyelid more conservatively in our blepharoplasty procedures by removing less fat, and as we improve our results in the midface and as we learn to better replenish lost lower orbital volume, we may be able to treat the brow more conservatively and more closely simulate a truly youthful appearance.

Is There a Relationship Between *Upper* Orbital Volume and Eyebrow Position?

One is likely surprised to learn that there is a relationship between lower orbital volume and eyebrow position as described above, and this begs the question – is there a relationship between upper orbital volume and eyebrow position? To answer this question we can consider the effects of filling the upper orbit and the effect this has on observed eyebrow position. Fig. 63.20A (left) shows a patient after aggressive foreheadplasty and upper blepharoplasty that was performed by an unknown surgeon. The lid crease is high and the upper lid appears long – neither of which are features of a young attractive orbit. But when the lower face is masked as shown in Fig. 63.20B (left) the eyebrow appears to be in satisfactory position relative to the supraorbital rim – even though the eyebrow appears to be *too high* when considered relative to the pupil and *not* in golden proportion with the aperture of the eye. Fig. 63.20A (right) shows the same patient after periorbital fat grafting. The lid crease is now lower and the upper eyelid appears shorter (both good), but when the lower face is masked off, as shown in Fig. 63.20B (right) the eyebrow appears higher – too high – even though no foreheadplasty has been performed and

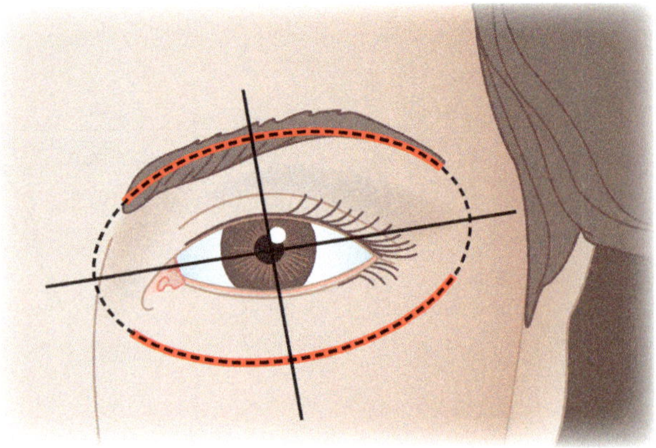

• **Fig. 63.17** Orbital oval analysis is a method used by estheticians, make-up professionals, and artists to design and draw attractive and esthetically pleasing eyebrows. Orbital oval analysis stipulates that the eyebrow should be situated so that the eye sits in the center of an oval defined by the lid–cheek junction and the eyebrow. (Courtesy Timothy Marten, MD, FACS and the Marten Clinic of Plastic Surgery, San Francisco, CA; with permission.)

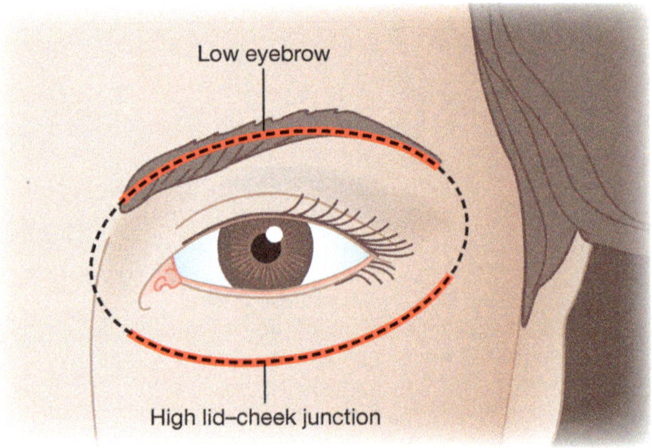

• **Fig. 63.18** Orbital oval analysis – young face. When the lid–cheek junction is high, as it is typically on the young attractive face, a lower eyebrow position will be necessary to maintain the orbital oval and esthetic balance. This may explain why a low eyebrow looks better and may be artistically appropriate on a young face, and why a higher eyebrow looks better on a mature face (see Fig. 63.19). (Courtesy Timothy Marten, MD, FACS and the Marten Clinic of Plastic Surgery, San Francisco, CA; with permission.)

the eyebrow position has not changed (white horizontal line). While the patient's upper facial appearance has been improved by filling her upper orbit she now has a somewhat startled or surprised look. It can be seen that filling the upper orbit makes the eyebrow appear higher, even when its position is unchanged, and thus we must take upper orbital volume into consideration when performing esthetically nuanced foreheadplasty procedures. And once this is understood it can be seen that as we treat the upper eyelid more conservatively in our blepharoplasty procedures by

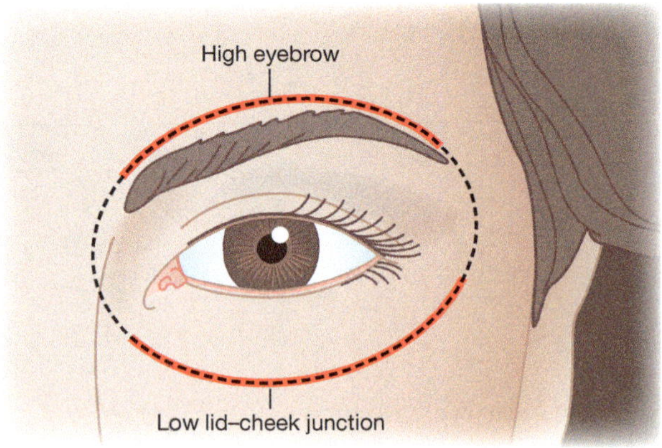

• **Fig. 63.19** Orbital oval analysis – mature face. When the lid–cheek junction is low, as it is typically on the mature attractive face, a higher eyebrow position will be necessary to maintain the orbital oval and esthetic balance. This may explain why a high eyebrow looks better and may be artistically appropriate on an older face, and why a lower eyebrow looks better on a young face (see Fig. 63.18). (Courtesy Timothy Marten, MD, FACS and the Marten Clinic of Plastic Surgery, San Francisco, CA; with permission.)

removing less skin and fat, and as we learn to better replenish lost upper orbital volume, we may be able to treat the brow more conservatively and more closely simulate a truly youthful appearance.

To summarize the relationship of eyebrow position to orbital volume:

- The volume of both the upper and lower orbit impacts the apparent height of the eyebrow
- Removing fat from the upper or lower orbit can make the eyebrow appear *lower* even if its position is not changed
- Adding fat to the upper or lower orbit can make the eyebrow appear *higher* even if its position is not changed
- An empty orbit (mature face) requires a more superiorly situated eyebrow, and thus a higher eyebrow may be more appropriate for the mature face if orbital volume is not restored
- A full upper orbit allows a lower eyebrow position, and thus a lower eyebrow may be more appropriate for the younger face
- As we treat the upper eyelid and orbit more conservatively by sacrificing less skin and fat and as we learn to replenish lost upper orbital volume using fat grafting and like techniques we may be able to place the eyebrow more inferiorly than we traditionally have and more closely simulate a truly youthful appearance.

The Attractive Eyebrow – Authors' Personal Guidelines

How does one make sense of the preceding discussion and conclusions? The following comprises the simple guidelines that we use in our practices in our own procedures.

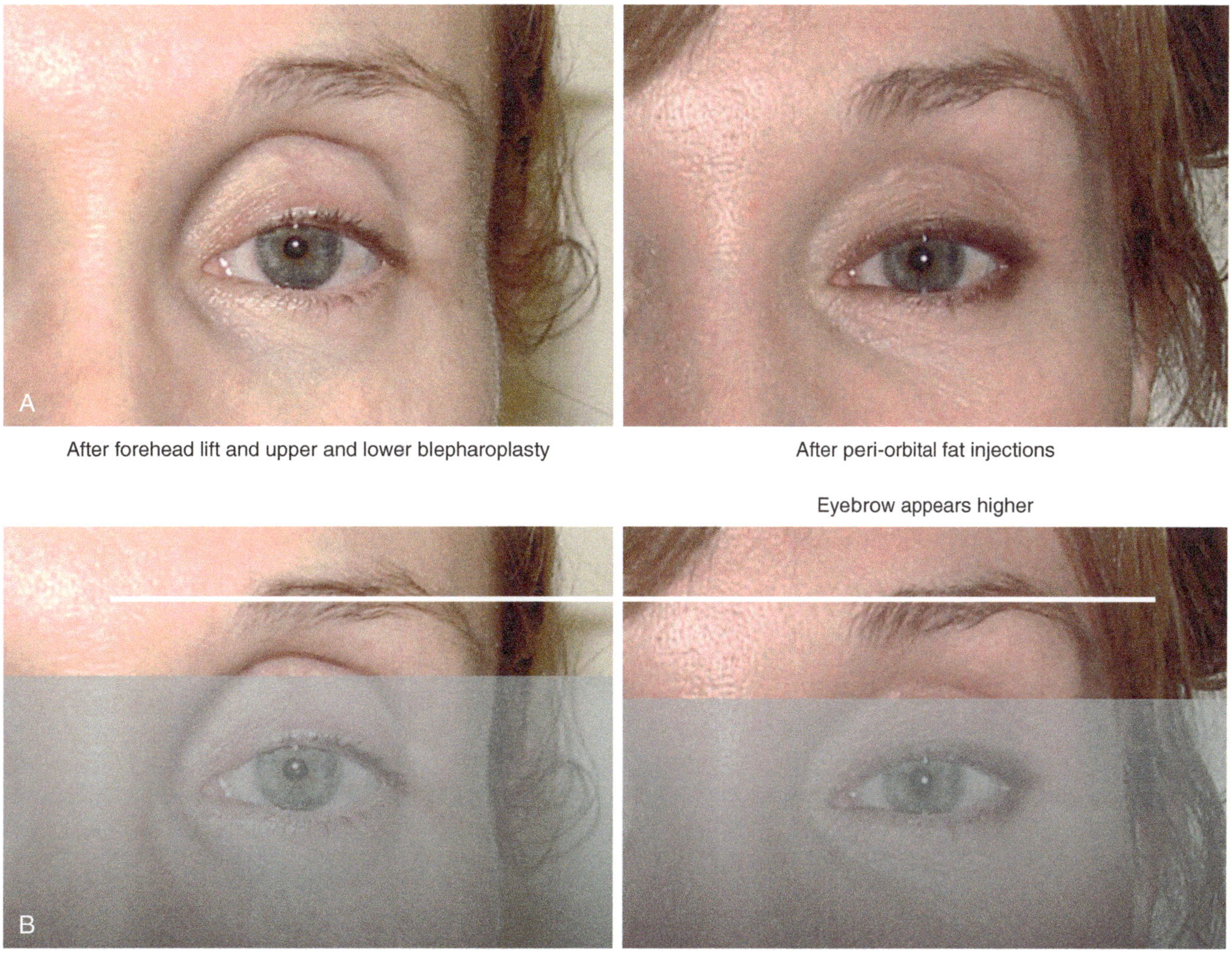

• **Fig. 63.20** Effect of increasing upper orbital volume on eyebrow position. Photographs showing a patient after foreheadplasty and upper blepharoplasty (A, left) and after periorbital fat grafting (A, right). For details, see text. It can be seen that filling the upper orbit makes the eyebrow appear higher, even when its position is unchanged (as shown by the white line, in B), and thus we must take upper orbital volume into consideration when performing esthetically nuanced foreheadplasty procedures. (Courtesy Timothy Marten, MD, FACS and the Marten Clinic of Plastic Surgery, San Francisco, CA; with permission.)

- The female eyebrow will appear attractive at a *variety of heights* if it is in an arched configuration, with its tail lying superior to its medial aspect (Fig. 63.21A). If a surgeon is able to meet this simple and straightforward objective the majority of their female patients will be happy.
- The male brow will appear attractive at a *variety of heights* if it is in a near horizontal configuration, with its tail at the same height as its medial aspect, or slightly superior to it (Fig. 63.21B). If a surgeon is able to meet this simple and straightforward objective the majority of their male patients will be happy.
- Recognize that the youthful face has a full upper and lower orbit and be conservative when excising eyelid skin and fat.
- Acknowledge that replenishing lost orbital volume has artistic merit and is often more appropriate than traditional excisional eyelid surgery.
- Removing fat from the upper or lower orbit can make the eyebrow appear *lower* even if its position is not changed, while adding fat to the upper or lower orbit can make the eyebrow appear *higher* even if its position is not changed.

Foreheadplasty Techniques

Bicoronal Incision Foreheadplasty

Foreheadplasty techniques using a bicoronal incision (Fig. 63.22) offer certain advantages over closed procedures and should result in an inconspicuous scar and few complications if skillfully performed. These advantages include that they provide an actual reduction in forehead scalp and/or skin redundancy, and as such many surgeons feel that this translates into better brow elevation and a more durable and sustained improvement. Procedures performed through

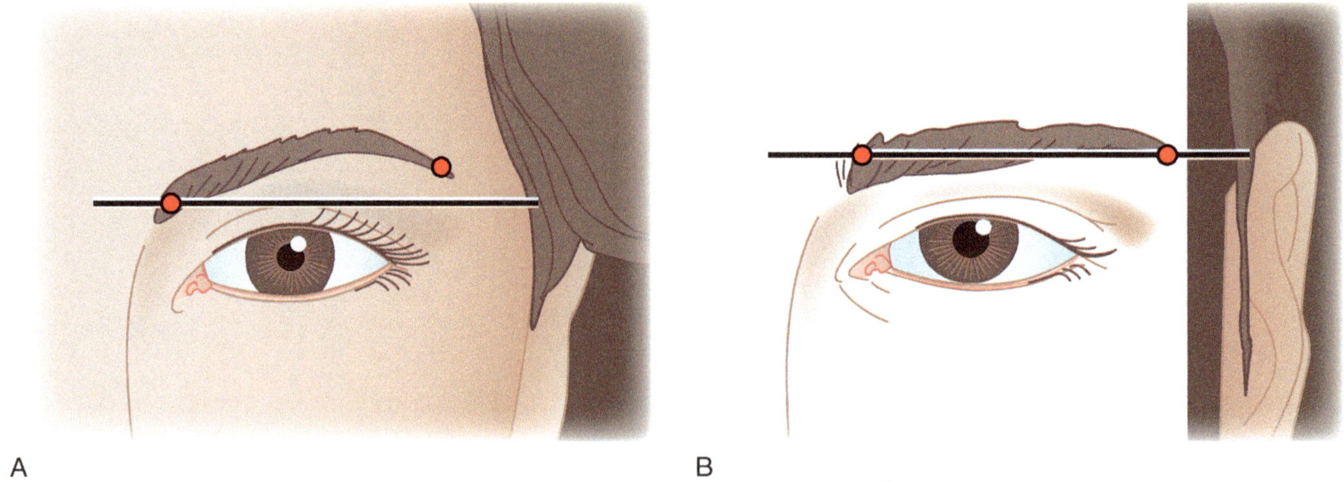

• **Fig. 63.21** Authors' personal guidelines for the attractive eyebrow. (A) The female eyebrow will appear attractive at a variety of heights if it is in an arched configuration, with its tail lying superior to its medial aspect. (B) The male brow will appear attractive at a variety of heights if it is in a near horizontal configuration with its tail at the same height as its medial aspect, or slightly superior to it. (Courtesy Timothy Marten, MD, FACS and the Marten Clinic of Plastic Surgery, San Francisco, CA; with permission.)

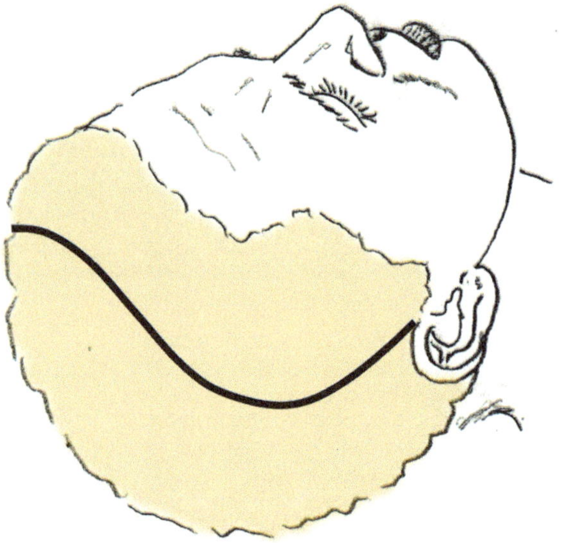

• **Fig. 63.22** Plan for coronal forehead lift. If a coronal location for the foreheadplasty incision is chosen, the incision should be planned three fingerbreadths posterior to the patient's frontal hairline in a curvilinear fashion in most cases, as opposed to the more posteriorly situated traditional straight "ear-to-ear" incision. This plan keeps the incision well within dense scalp hair but moves it closer to the brow. In addition, it provides for an easier dissection, a better mechanical effect on the brow, and it places the incision in the watershed between the deep and superficial branches of the supraorbital nerves. (Courtesy Timothy Marten, MD, FACS and the Marten Clinic of Plastic Surgery, San Francisco, CA; with permission.)

a bicoronal incision also provide optimal access for modification of the frontalis muscles, if necessary, and numbness, dysesthesias and related problems can be minimized if the anatomy of the sensory nerves is understood and appropriate nerve branches are protected during the procedure.

Practically speaking, a procedure using a bicoronal incision may be the procedure of choice for patients with abnormally low hairlines who wish their hairline to be raised and placed in better proportion with the rest of their face, and this is the most common circumstance in which the procedure is still performed in the authors' practices (Figs. 63.23–63.25).

Procedures using bicoronal incisions have certain well-known possible problems and complications, however, including hair loss, poor scars, hairline elevation, numbness, and dysesthesias, and patients generally have the notion that these procedures will result in a "surprised" or "startled" appearance. Although these problems should be uncommon if the procedures are skillfully performed by a surgeon with artistic vision, and can occur when limited-incision and endoscopic techniques are used, patients are nonetheless understandably attracted to "short-scar" techniques, and perceive them to be less likely to precipitate problems or result in unnatural appearances. In addition, because of the influence of the media, the internet, or mischaracterizations of the procedure by other physicians, many patients today arrive in the plastic surgeon's office already convinced that they only wish to undergo an "endoscopic" forehead lift, and thus, most surgeons will have to offer their patients some kind of limited-incision or endoscopic procedure as an option.

Hairline and Partial Hairline Incision Foreheadplasty

Many patients seeking rejuvenation of their foreheads are troubled by hairline recession or high hairlines and the prospect that surgery will make this problem worse. Hairline elevation occurs in both bicoronal and closed endoscopic

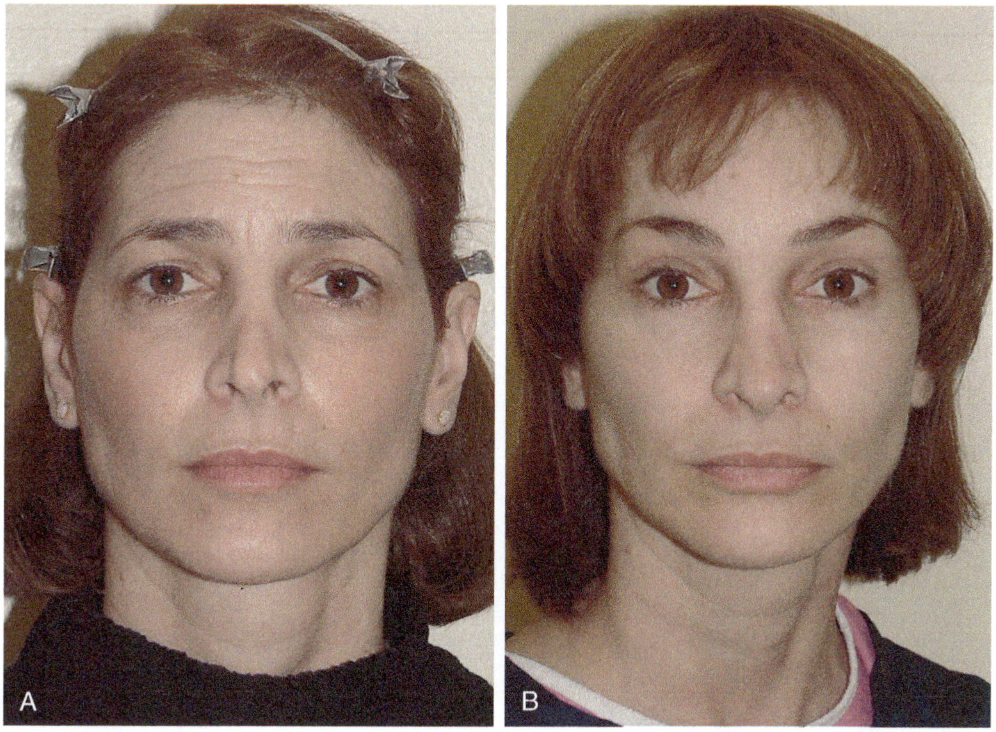

• **Fig. 63.23** Bicoronal forehead lift procedure. Patients with low hairlines and advanced forehead aging are ideal candidates for coronal incision plans because these procedures provide for maximum improvement in eyebrow position and configuration and produce the most elevation of the hairline. (A) Patient, age 49, preoperatively. Note that suboptimal eyebrow position and configuration impart a sad and melancholic appearance. Note also the low frontal hairline. (B) Same patient seen 14 months following coronal forehead lift. Note that suboptimal eyebrow position and configuration seen preoperatively have been corrected and that hairline retrodisplacement has expanded the forehead and placed it in better overall proportion with the rest of the face (see also Figs. 63.24 and 63.25). (The patient has also undergone upper and lower blepharoplasty, trichloroacetic acid peel of the lower eyelids, and secondary rhinoplasty). (Courtesy Timothy Marten, MD, FACS and the Marten Clinic of Plastic Surgery, San Francisco, CA; with permission.)

techniques, and hairstyles cannot practically conceal an overly-high forehead in all situations. A high forehead also appears aged, unnatural, and masculine, and detracts from an otherwise attractive and agreeable appearance. Hairline elevation can be particularly objectionable after surgery in the older patient with an existing receded hairline who has marked forehead and scalp redundancy.

Unlike procedures using a bicoronal or endoscopic technique, procedures using an incision or partial incisions along the hairline allow hairline position to be maintained or lowered and hairline shape to be optimized and the improvement thus gained may outweigh the drawback of the resulting scar. As such, procedures in this category will ostensibly always remain relevant and an integral part of the artistic surgeon's array of procedures used to optimize patient appearance (see Fig 63.1, and Figs. 63.26–63.28).

Patients with high hairlines generally are well aware of their own problem and are more than willing to accept the associated tradeoffs, including the scar, when informed of this option. In some such situations, hairline lowering is arguably of more overall benefit to the patient than is

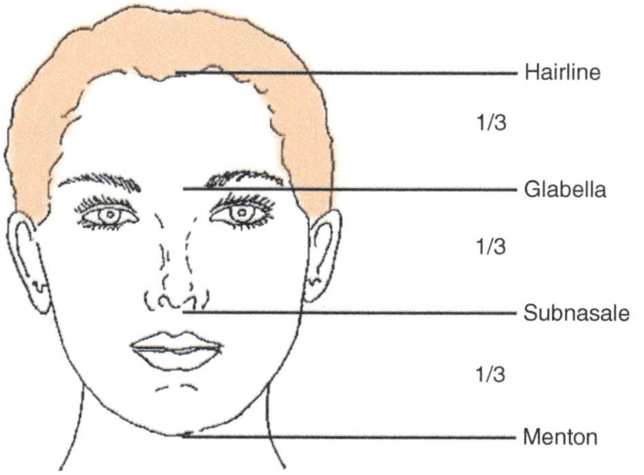

• **Fig. 63.24** The attractive and proportionate face. The artist's canon of "equal facial thirds" specifies that in the attractive and proportionate face the forehead height should be one-third the total facial height and equal, or approximate the height of, both the mid and lower face. (Courtesy Timothy Marten, MD, FACS and the Marten Clinic of Plastic Surgery, San Francisco, CA; with permission.)

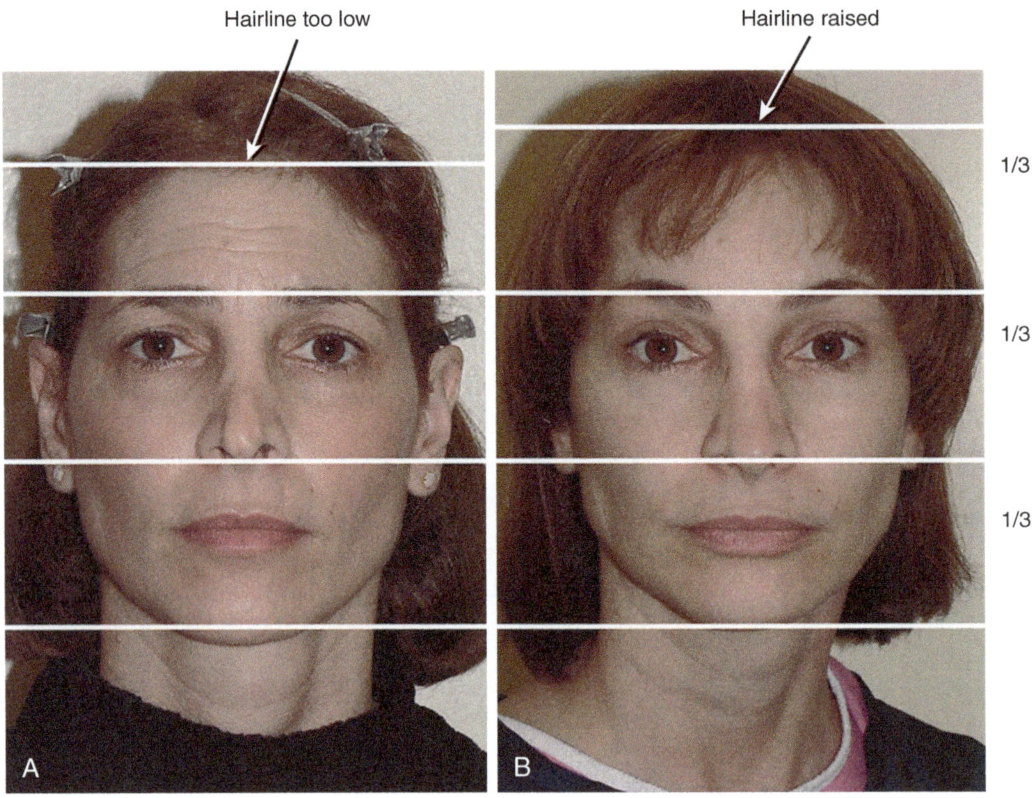

• **Fig. 63.25** Idealization of hairline position using coronal technique. Analysis of the patient's face shown in Fig. 63.23 using the artist's canon of equal facial thirds shows that (A) preoperatively her hairline is too low. (B) Postoperatively it can be seen that her hairline has been raised and that the component parts of her facial relationships fall into an equal facial thirds arrangement. This is typically viewed as more esthetically balanced, harmonious, and artistically appropriate. (Courtesy Timothy Marten, MD, FACS and the Marten Clinic of Plastic Surgery, San Francisco, CA; with permission.)

eyebrow elevation or (if corrugator myetomy is performed) frown-line reduction (see Fig. 63.28).

A key aspect of a successful outcome in hairline-lowering foreheadplasty lies in proper planning of the incision and meticulous execution of the technical procedure. The part of the incision situated along the frontal hairline should be made as a meandering, wavy, random line just within fine hair at the anteriormost portion of the hairline, parallel to hair follicles, or beveled slightly posteriorly (Fig. 63.29).

It is not necessary to exaggerate the incision bevel into the hairline to obtain hair growth through the scar, and the incision is best made just within the fine hair along the existing hairline, and not more posteriorly within coarser scalp hair ("pretrichial" is not literally accurate and a misnomer). If the incision is made too far within the hairline, fine hair will be eliminated and a less natural appearing hairline with abrupt transition from forehead skin to coarse scalp hair will result postoperatively.

As the pretrichial incision continues laterally it should travel through the finer hair in the temporal triangles, rather that more posteriorly against coarser scalp hair. This prevents unnatural transitions at these areas as outlined above. The remaining portion of the incision over the temporal scalp is made as a straight line precisely parallel to hair follicles as is done when a coronal incision is employed. It is not necessary or productive to make wavy, "zig-zag" or other types of irregular incisions in areas where the incision is situated within scalp hair.

Although the use of a pretrichial ("hairline") incision will prevent hairline retrodisplacement, it results in forehead *shortening*, not true hairline lowering (that is the distance between the eyebrow and hairline diminishes, but the hairline is not actually lowered). A pretrichial incision, when combined with mobilization of the posterior scalp flap and release of galeal tethering, however, allows scalp to be advanced and the hairline to be actually lowered, when indicated (see Fig. 63.1, 63.26–63.28).

When only a modest amount of frontal hairline lowering is needed, the posterior scalp flap is undermined in a subgaleal plane until the desired degree of advancement is obtained. In certain instances this entails extending posterior scalp flap undermining well over the occiput. When a greater degree of frontal hairline lowering is needed and scalp undermining alone is insufficient, transverse incision of the galea (galeotomy) to release its tethering effect is planned. This will produce variable degrees of scalp expansion and further advancement in the hairline (Fig. 63.30).

Good candidates for the hairline-lowering foreheadplasty include the patient with a high hairline, good scalp mobility, healthy hair, and no scalp disease who has had no prior scalp surgery and is accepting of the resultant scar. Suboptimal candidates include those with poorly mobile scalps and

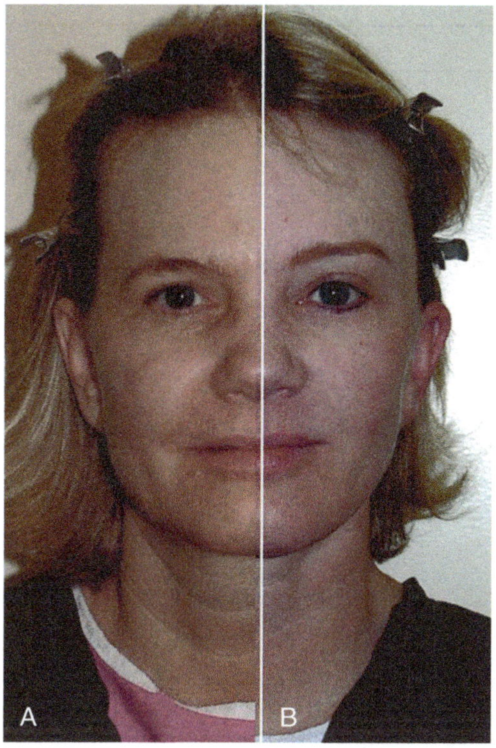

Before After

• **Fig. 63.26** Hairline lowering and forehead shortening. A composite of facial half splits from the left half of a patient's face (A) before and (B) after "hairline" forehead lift (the before side is the patient's left side before photo flipped horizontally) employing an incision along the frontal hairline. (A) Preoperatively it can be seen that the patient's eyebrow is in low position and flat configuration more typical of male eyebrow position. The frontal hairline can also be seen to be high and to have a more rectangular masculine shape. (B) Postoperatively it can be seen that the eyebrow has been raised and placed in an arched configuration more typical of that regarded to be optimal for the female face. Note that the hairline has been lowered and moved into a more rounded and less rectangular shape more consistent with an ideal female appearance. When considered together, eyebrow elevation and hairline lowering can be seen to result in shortening of the forehead (decreased distance between the eyebrow and hairline). Hairline lowering and forehead shortening are not possible when coronal or endoscopic techniques are used. (The patient has also had a facelift, necklift and facial fat grafting.) (Courtesy Timothy Marten, MD, FACS and the Marten Clinic of Plastic Surgery, San Francisco, CA; with permission.)

thin or fragile hair or those who have had prior scalp surgery (hair transplants, hair flaps, and foreheadplasty). The procedure should be recommended with caution to heavy smokers, those with significant scalp disease, a history of stress-induced or unexplained hair loss, or any patient reluctant or unwilling to accept the tradeoff of a scar along their frontal hairline.

It is convenient but not necessary to anchor the posterior scalp flap once mobilized and released in its advanced position on the cranium to unicortical converging drill holes on by other cranial anchoring technique. This stabilizes the posterior scalp flap and facilitates trimming and tailoring of the forehead flap against it. A facelift flap marker should be used to carefully gauge forehead flap redundancy and only forehead flap skin that is truly redundant should be excised. The key to obtaining an inconspicuous scar is closure of the wound under no tension. If desired eyebrow position and configuration cannot be obtained without the application of tension to the wound the forehead flap has been inadequately mobilized and released and additional time should be spent until proper release has been obtained.

Closure along the frontal hairline is made with a combination of half-buried vertical mattress sutures of 4-0 nylon with the knots tied on the scalp side and simple interrupted sutures of 6-0 nylon. The half-buried vertical mattress sutures of 4-0 nylon provide support of the wound without causing cross-hatched scars (suture marks) while the simple interrupted sutures of 6-0 nylon are used to insure meticulous wound edge alignment. The 6-0 sutures are removed in 5 days and the 4-0 sutures are removed in 7–9 days. No deep (galeal) sutures are required or used.

Partial Hairline Forehead Lift Plan

A useful variation of the full hairline forehead lift is a partial hairline plan (Fig. 63.31). These procedures are very useful in older patients with poor lamination of their forehead tissues layers with temporal recession of their hairlines whose central hairline is well situated and in whom the idea of avoiding a scar along the central hairline has merit. Often these patients have had previous corrugator myectomy or are using neuromodulators to control corrugator hyperfunction and there is not a need to create a full open flap to access the corrugator muscles. Alternatively, this approach can be combined with transpalpebral (through the eyelid) or endoscopic corrugator myectomy when surgical treatment of the corrugators is desired.

Planning Treatment of the Corrugator Supercilii Muscles in Open Foreheadplasty Procedures

The corrugator supercilii muscles exert a complex action on the medial aspect of the eyebrow and the inferior central forehead resulting in medial movement of the brows and vertical glabellar wrinkling. As such, their action is the underlying cause of vertical glabellar creases and the principle agent of a pained, sad, and melancholic appearance that typically occurs with age. Near total myectomy of the corrugators will effectively soften these expressions and was traditionally performed as part of most foreheadplasty procedures. Over time, however, management of corrugator supercilii muscle hyperfunction has largely been supplanted by treatment by the use of neuromodulators (botulinum toxins) or by transpalpebral corrugator myectomy/myoplasty (see discussion later in this chapter) and in our practices open corrugator muscle surgery (myectomy through a coronal or hairline incision) is only occasionally now performed.

Supraciliary and Forehead Crease Incision Techniques

In addition to improving eyebrow position and configuration using a bicoronal or hairline incision, like improvements

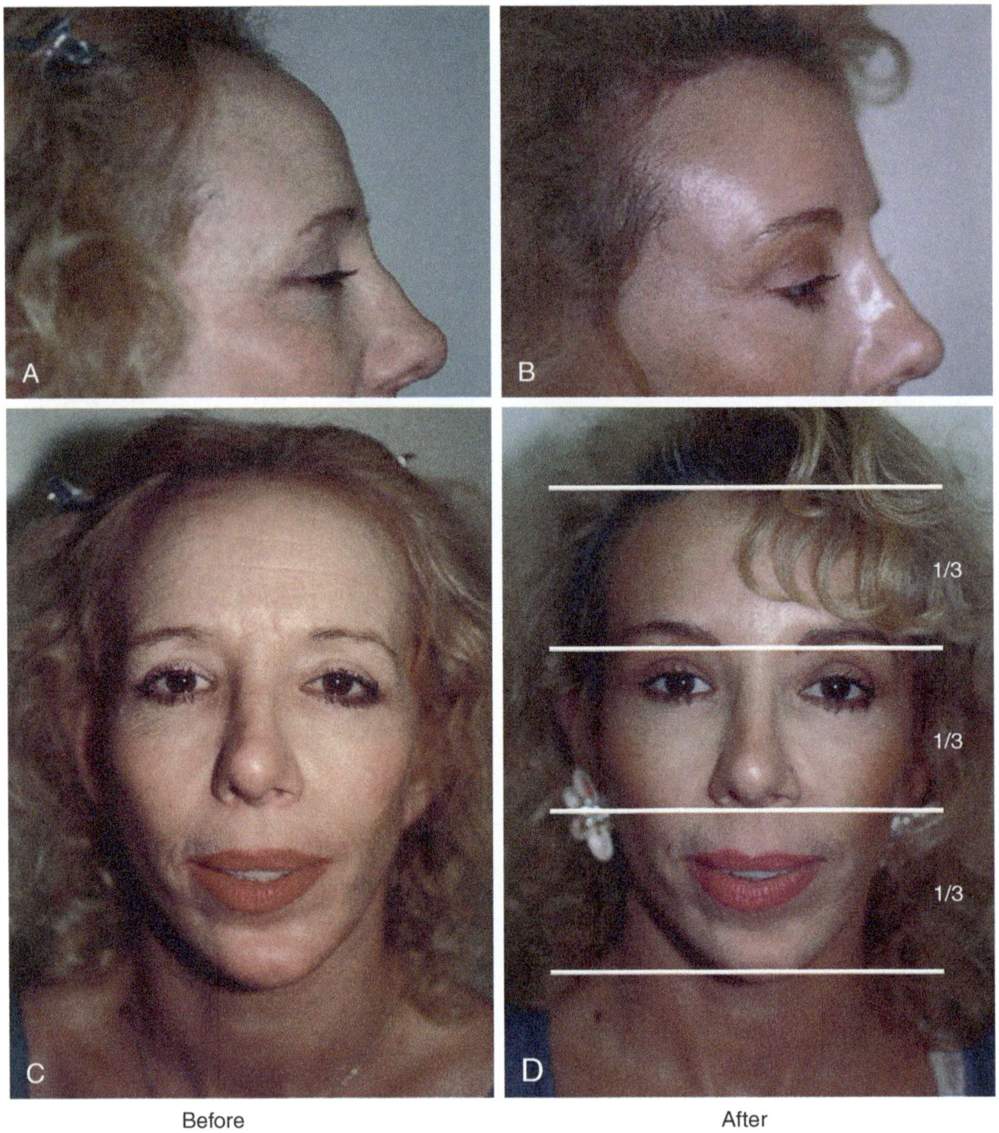

• **Fig. 63.27** Hairline lowering and forehead shortening. (A,B) Patient shown in Fig. 63.26 seen preoperatively in lateral view. Note that the hairline not only appears elevated in the anteroposterior view but elevated and retrodisplaced (posteriorly situated) in this view. A coronal or endoscopic forehead lift would make both problems worse. (C,D) Same patient as shown in Fig. 63.1 seen postoperatively in lateral view following hairline-lowering forehead lift using an incision along the hairline. Note that not only has the hairline been lowered (as seen in AP view), but that retrodisplacement has also been improved (hairline moved further forward anteriorly). (Courtesy Timothy Marten, MD, FACS and the Marten Clinic of Plastic Surgery, San Francisco, CA; with permission.)

can be made using supraciliary or forehead crease incisions. These incision plans are useful in bald or balding men, men with very short hair, men with shaved heads, men who have previously undergone hair transplants (who fear injury to expensive hair grafts (bicoronal or endoscopic) or drawing attention to their hairlines (hairline incision)), older women with thin hair or who are concerned with hair loss, and men or women seeking upper eyelid surgery who have brow ptosis but object to traditional forehead lift procedures. Both procedures can readily be performed under local anesthesia and thus are particularly useful in the latter category of patients mentioned above.

A supraciliary incision plan (Fig. 63.32) is useful in both men and women, but is typically used in older age groups. It is a simple and effective way to raise and shape the eyebrow and will result in a well-concealed scar in properly selected patients. This plan also arguably provides the most predictable and effective lift in patients with poor lamination of their forehead tissues and marked forehead tissue redundancy (older patients), and a very durable correction, as correction is made in close proximity to the eyebrow rather than distant to it. A supraciliary incision has the significant drawback that it does not lift the temple and cannot compensate for excess skin pushed into the temple area when

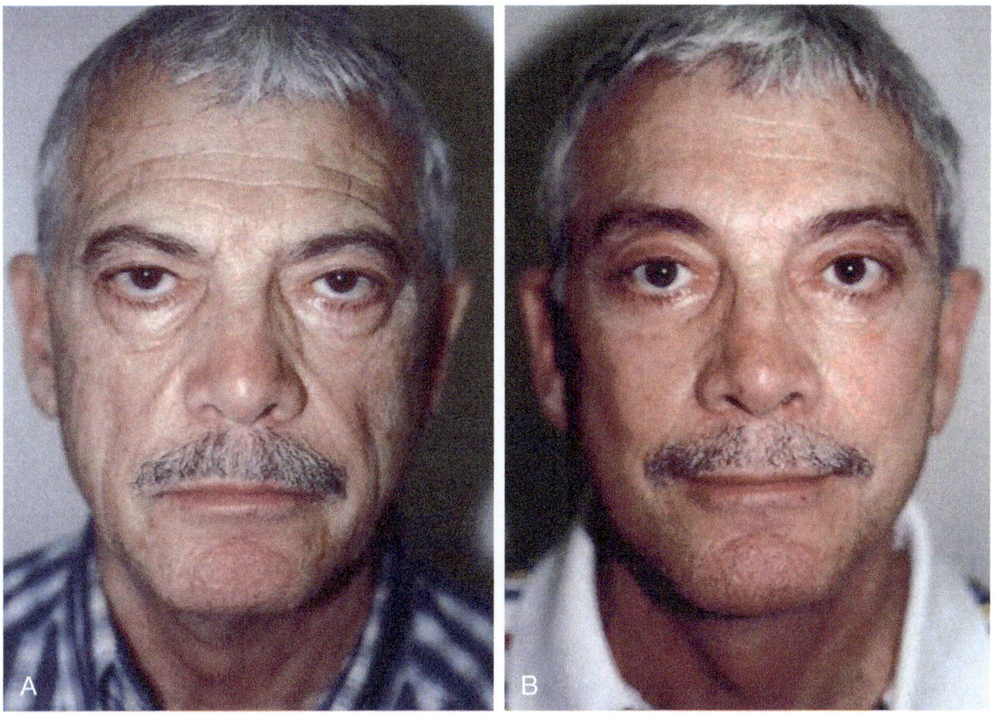

• **Fig. 63.28** Hairline forehead lift. (A) Male patient age 63 seen preoperatively. Note suboptimal eyebrow position and high forehead. A bicoronal or endoscopic forehead lift would make his hairline higher. (B) Same patient following hairline-lowering forehead lift using an incision along the hairline. The poor eyebrow position and shape seen before surgery has been corrected and the hairline has been lowered. (The patient has also undergone a facelift, necklift, lower blepharoplasty and facial fat grafting.) (Courtesy Timothy Marten, MD, FACS and the Marten Clinic of Plastic Surgery, San Francisco, CA; with permission.)

a facelift is performed, unlike all three other categories of eyebrow lift procedures.

A forehead crease incision (Fig. 63.33) is conceptually similar to a supraciliary incision, but finds greater utility in male patients in whom forehead creases are often deep and more consistent with a male appearance. Typically, these can be extended further laterally than a supraciliary incision allowing a greater lift of redundancy in the temple area while still remaining well concealed, with the resulting scar mimicking the existing forehead crease.

Closed, Short-Scar Foreheadplasty Procedures

"Closed" foreheadplasty techniques, including endoscopic foreheadplasty, limited-incision forehead lift, and short-scar foreheadplasty employing transpalpebral corrugator myectomy, have found their earliest and widest applications in younger patients with low or low–normal hairlines who had minimal or modest frontalis hyperfunction and transverse forehead wrinkling and who were undergoing isolated forehead or forehead and eyelid surgery. Typically, these patients have tight lamination of the tissue layers of their forehead and minimal "slide" between them, and "pull" placed on the periosteum or galea. In these situations, a full bicoronal incision and scalp excision is not necessary, if the surgeon can improve eyebrow position and configuration and perform muscle modification with a near equal degree of precision

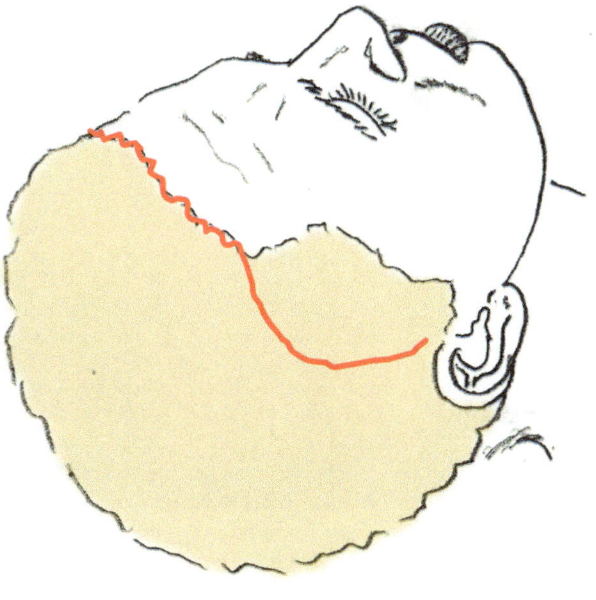

• **Fig. 63.29** Plan for "pretrichial" forehead lift. The part of the incision situated along the frontal hairline should be made as a meandering, wavy, random line just within fine hair at the anteriormost portion of the hairline, and beveled slightly posteriorly. As the incision continues laterally it should travel through the finer hair in the temporal triangles, rather that more posteriorly against coarser scalp hair. The remaining portion of the incision over the temporal scalp is made as a straight line precisely parallel to hair follicles. (Courtesy Timothy Marten, MD, FACS and the Marten Clinic of Plastic Surgery, San Francisco, CA; with permission.)

as in an "open" technique. Indeed, experience has shown that it is not necessary to remove scalp in many patients to produce an attractive and sustained improvement in upper facial appearance (Fig. 63.34).

Experience has also shown that an endoscope is not required to mobilize and release the forehead and treat the corrugator supercilii muscles if forehead anatomy is understood, the operation is correctly planned, and a transpalpebral approach to treat the corrugators is used. While an endoscope can be used for these purposes if desired, designing a procedure in which it is not necessary saves time, avoids problems related to the device itself (fogging, mechanical failure, etc.), and avoids the costs of purchasing, leasing, and maintaining expensive needed equipment and (in some circumstances) obtaining hospital credentialing to use endoscopic equipment.

A number of strong arguments can in fact be made against the use of an endoscope for corrugator muscle modification, however, even though this is considered by many to be a breakthrough application of the technology and something many find technical gratification in doing. First, it is exceedingly easy to over-elevate the medial brow in forehead lift procedures, but deceptively difficult to raise the lateral eyebrow. Because the corrugator muscles act as partial depressors of the medial brow, simple muscle excision, regardless of technique, can result in some medial brow elevation. The obligatory undermining of the glabella and dividing the periosteum that is necessary to gain access to the corrugator muscles endoscopically also disrupts the ligaments and attachments that hold the medial brow in an esthetically optimal low position and predictably results in additional undesirable central brow elevation and this has been the "Achilles heel" of the endoscopic procedure since its inception. Modifying the corrugators transpalpebrally through an upper eyelid incision preserves ligaments and periosteal attachments in the glabellar area, however, and helps keep the medial brow in a more natural-appearing and attractive lower position consistent with a younger appearance. As a practical matter, endoscopic access to the

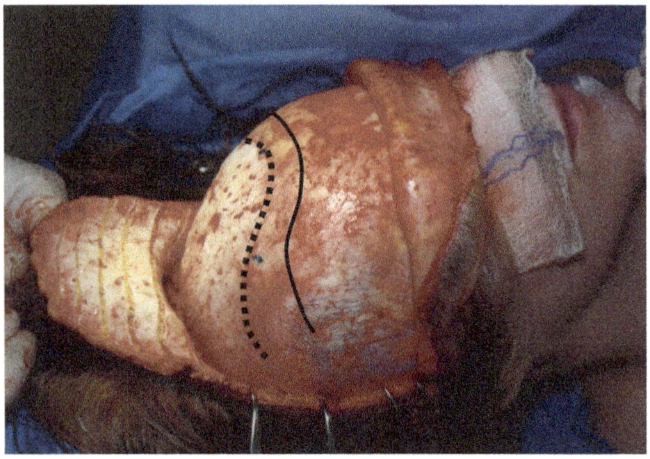

• **Fig. 63.30** Overview of hairline-lowering technique. An undulating "pretrichial" incision has been made along the frontal hairline and continued inferiorly onto the temporal scalp to the root of the ear. A forehead flap was subsequently elevated and traditional foreheadplasty maneuvers (corrugator excision, etc.) performed. A parieto-occipital scalp flap has been elevated posteriorly in a subgaleal plane up to the occipital protuberance and the galea multiply incised to allow flap expansion. The black dashed line marks the original position of the hairline on the cranium. The unbroken black line marks the position of the hairline on the cranium after scalp flap mobilization, galeotomy, and flap advancement. The distance between the two lines represents the amount of hairline lowering. (Courtesy Timothy Marten, MD, FACS and the Marten Clinic of Plastic Surgery, San Francisco, CA; with permission.)

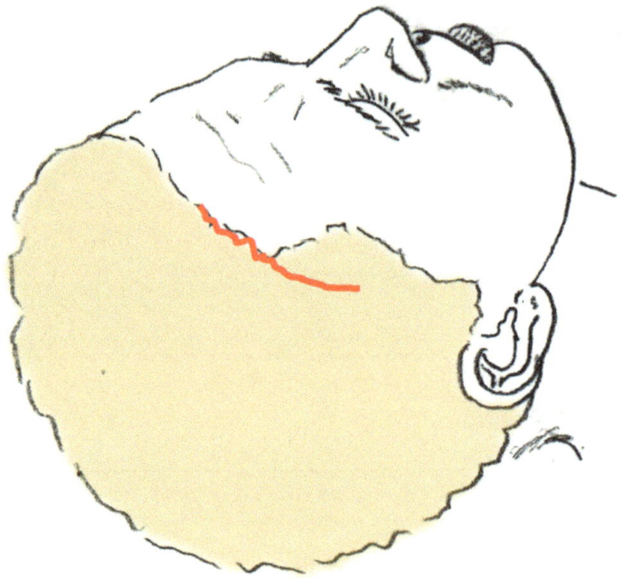

• **Fig. 63.31** Plan for "partial hairline" forehead lift. This variation is useful in older patients with poor lamination of their forehead tissue layers with temporal recession of their hairline whose central hairline is well situated and in whom the idea of avoiding a scar along the central hairline has merit. (Courtesy Timothy Marten, MD, FACS and the Marten Clinic of Plastic Surgery, San Francisco, CA; with permission.)

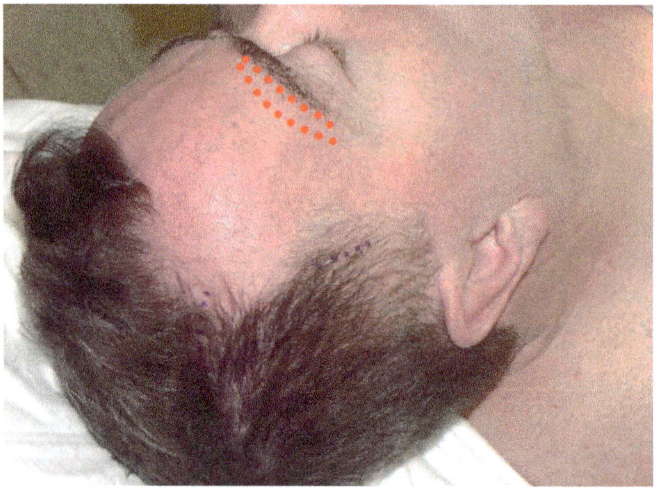

• **Fig. 63.32** Plan for supraciliary eyebrow lift. A supraciliary incision plan is useful in both men and women and is typically used in older age groups. It is a simple and effective way to raise and shape the eyebrow and will result in a well-concealed scar in properly selected patients. (Courtesy Timothy Marten, MD, FACS and the Marten Clinic of Plastic Surgery, San Francisco, CA; with permission.)

corrugators can also often be difficult in the patient with a high hairline or curved, sloping forehead, because of the endoscope's straight design. In such situations, a nonendoscopic approach using a transpalpebral approach to the corrugators is arguably a superior one.

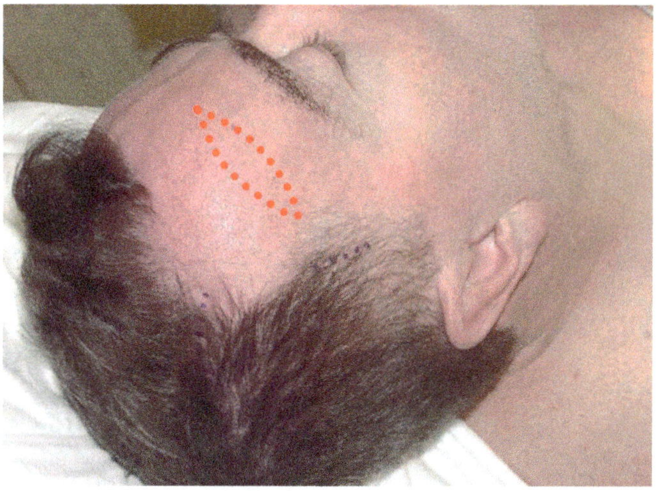

• **Fig. 63.33** Plan for superciliary eyebrow lift. A forehead crease incision is conceptually similar to a supraciliary incision but finds greater utility in male patients in whom forehead creases are often deep and more consistent with a male appearance. This plan is also useful in patients (mostly male) seeking upper eyelid surgery who have brow ptosis but object to traditional forehead lift procedures. (Courtesy Timothy Marten, MD, FACS and the Marten Clinic of Plastic Surgery, San Francisco, CA; with permission.)

Transpalpebral corrugator myectomy, when used in conjunction with closed mobilization and resuspension of the forehead, not only provides a method for performing a closed, short-scar foreheadplasty without the need for an endoscope, but also provides a means by which medial brow elevation can be minimized or avoided.

The method of corrugator modification also has an impact on the procedure's outcome and can reduce the frequency of patient complaints following surgery. In endoscopic procedures, a near-total corrugator myectomy is generally performed in which the majority of the corrugator muscle is removed and the supratrochlear nerves are skeletonized. This, however, can result in paresthesias and dysesthesias, that can be disturbing to patients. When a transpalpebral modification of the corrugator is performed, the muscle can simply be divided (myotomy) between the supraorbital and supratrochelar nerves (or only partially resected) and an interposition fat graft taken from elsewhere on the face can be placed between the cut ends of the muscle. When this is done, muscle function is usually significantly reduced, but sensory nerves need not be formally dissected. Typically, this results in fewer disturbing sensations and dysesthesias in the forehead area. It should be noted that despite the assertion by some surgeons to the contrary, a simple corrugator myotomy (dividing the corrugator) rarely results in a sustained reduction in corrugator supercilii muscle function in and of itself. In most such cases, the cut ends of the muscle heal together and the muscle regains function.

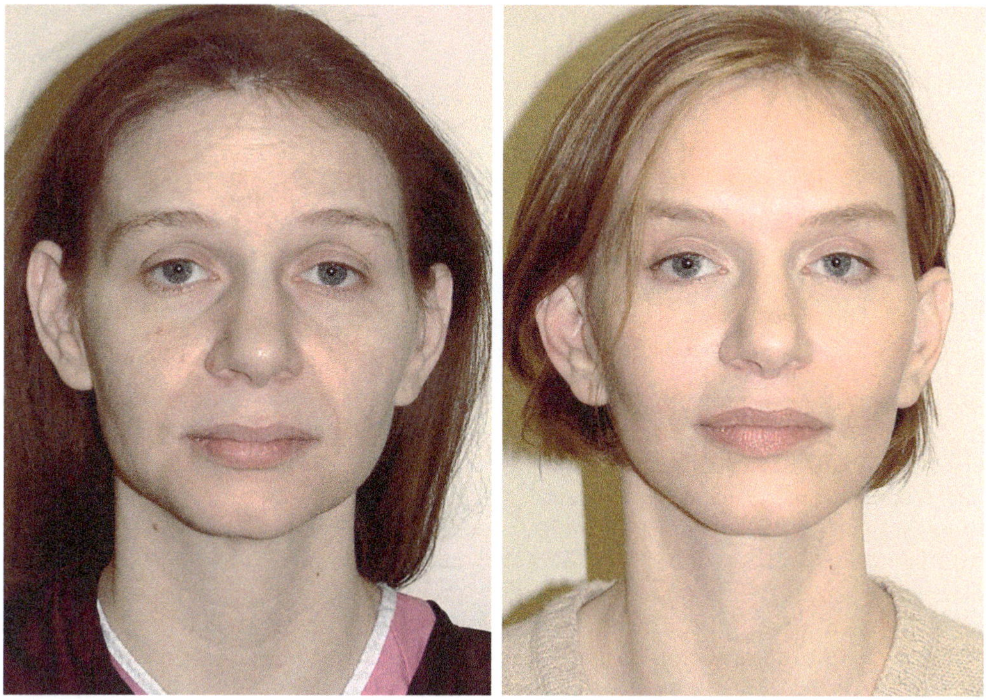

• **Fig. 63.34** Closed, short-scar, nonendoscopic forehead lift. (A) Patient, age 42, seen preoperatively. Note suboptimal eyebrow position and shape. Some would claim that this degree of brow abnormality would be best treated with an "open" foreheadplasty technique. (B) Same patient 13 months following closed, short-scar, nonendoscopic forehead lift. The poor eyebrow position and shape seen before surgery has been corrected with minimal elevation of the hairline. (The patient has also undergone facelift, necklift, upper and lower blepharoplasty, partial facial fat injections, and an upper lip lift.) (Courtesy Timothy Marten, MD, FACS and the Marten Clinic of Plastic Surgery, San Francisco, CA; with permission.)

A final and initially unexpected benefit of closed techniques, including the nonendoscopic one described here, is that hairline retrodisplacement is reduced in comparison to bicoronal procedures. This is because the majority of the forehead flap elevated in a closed dissection is elevated in a subperiosteal plane, and the flap is thus relatively inelastic as compared with a flap dissected through a coronal incision and elevated in a subgaleal plane. In all, the closed, short-scar, nonendoscopic forehead lift procedure provides the potential for an overall reduction in incision length, less hairline elevation, decreased operating time, better improvement in eyebrow shape, and possible reduction in forehead and scalp neurosensory disturbance.

Anesthesia

Most foreheadplasties performed in the authors' clinic are performed under local anesthesia with heavy sedation using a laryngeal mask airway, but any skillfully administered anesthetic is adequate. After sedation has been administered or anesthesia established, supraorbital, supratrochlear, and lacrimal nerve blocks are performed with 0.25% bupivicaine with 1:200,000 epinephrine. Proposed sites for incisions are subsequently infiltrated with the same solution. "Hyperinflating" incision sites with additional (and typically more dilute) local anesthetic solution (0.1% lidocaine with 1:1,000,000 epinephrine) immediately before incisions are made helps reduce bleeding by establishing a partial hydrostatic tamponade. Local anesthesia should be administered even if general anesthesia is used, to reduce bleeding and lower the overall amount of narcotics and anesthetics required. Upon completion of the procedure but before the patient is awake, nerve blocks should be readministered to minimize patient discomfort in the postoperative period.

Operative Technique for Closed, Nonendoscopic Forehead Lift

The closed, short-scar, nonendoscopic forehead lift technique is a very commonly performed procedure for forehead lifting in our practices and is performed through four (or occasionally five) small scalp incisions made just posterior to the hairline, and consists of a blind subperiosteal mobilization of a forehead flap centrally and a subgaleal dissection laterally, a release of the temporal line and periosteum over the lateral brow, flap suspension with permanent suture to converging unicortical bony tunnels (or other method of direct cranial suspension of choice), and transpalpebral modification of the corrugator supercilii muscles (if indicated and desired) (Box 63.1).

• BOX 63.1 Overview of Closed, Nonendoscopic, Foreheadplasty Technique

1. Four small scalp incisions
2. Blind mobilization of forehead in a subgaleal plane laterally and a subperiosteal plane centrally
3. Release of the temporal line
4. Release of periosteum beneath the lateral brow
5. Suture suspension to unicortical bony tunnels
6. Transpalpebral (through eyelid incision) corrugator excision (if indicated)

Marking Incisions

Incisions should be marked after anesthesia has been administered, but before prepping and draping is performed. Four incisions approximately 2 cm in length just within existing hairlines are required. In patients with large foreheads and higher hairlines, a central incision is occasionally made to facilitate subperiosteal undermining in the upper central forehead, though this is seldom needed if proper instruments are available.

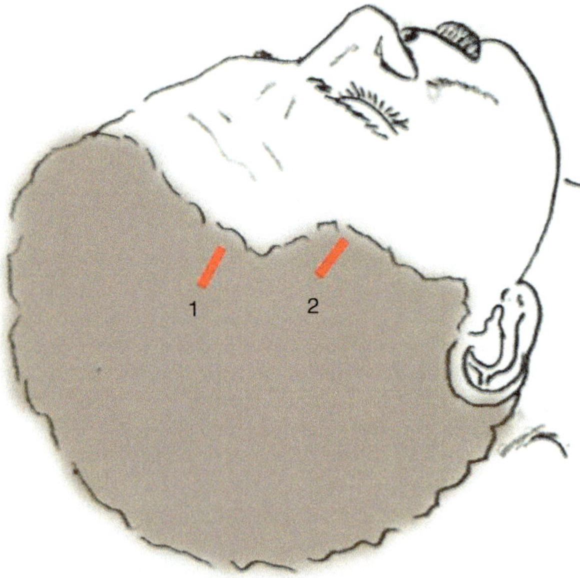

• Fig. 63.35 Incision plan for closed, nonendoscopic forehead lift. The two most superior incisions (*1*) are marked radially near the junction of the frontal and fronto-temporal hairlines. The two temporal incisions (*2*) are marked just within the temporal tuft of hair behind the frontotemporal hairline. (Courtesy Timothy Marten, MD, FACS and the Marten Clinic of Plastic Surgery, San Francisco, CA; with permission.)

The two most superior incisions (see *1* in Fig. 63.35 below) are marked radially near the junction of the frontal and frontotemporal hairlines (Figs. 63.35 and 63.36).

In bald or balding men, the superiormost incisions may be placed more laterally along the anterior margin of the temporal tuft of hair in the same approximate location. In either case, the incisions should lie just medial to the temporal line and are used to provide access for subperiosteal undermining of the ipsilateral forehead (Fig. 63.37). They also are used as points for flap fixation. Making these incisions radially facilitates closure and results in a scar that is less conspicuous than when incisions are made in transverse fashion or placed along the hairline.

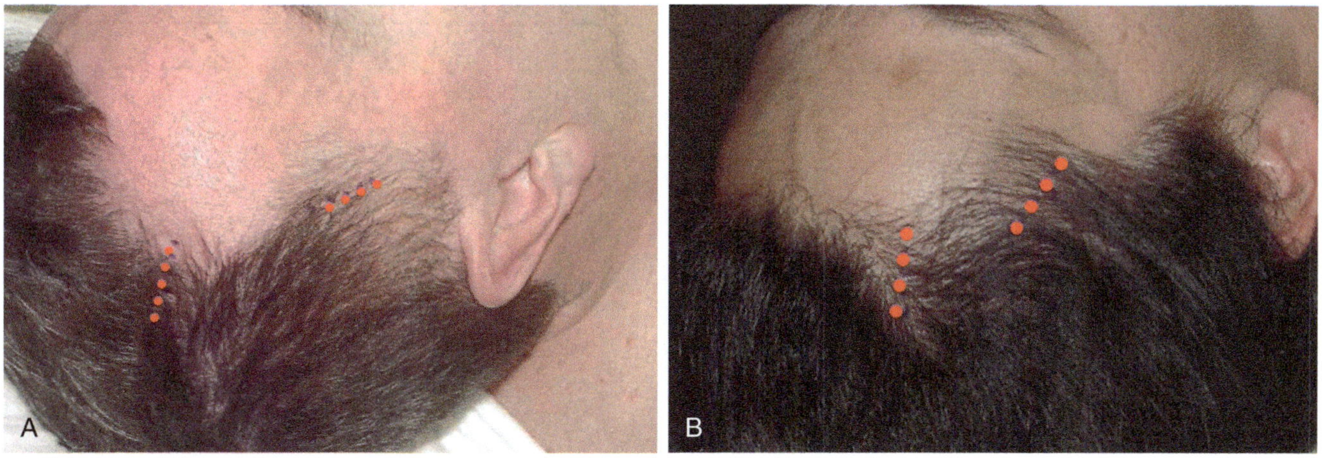

• **Fig. 63.36** Incision plan for closed, nonendoscopic forehead lift marked on patients. (A) Markings for incisions for closed, nonendoscopic forehead lift in a male patient. (B) Markings for incisions for closed, nonendoscopic forehead lift in a female patient. (Courtesy Timothy Marten, MD, FACS and the Marten Clinic of Plastic Surgery, San Francisco, CA; with permission.)

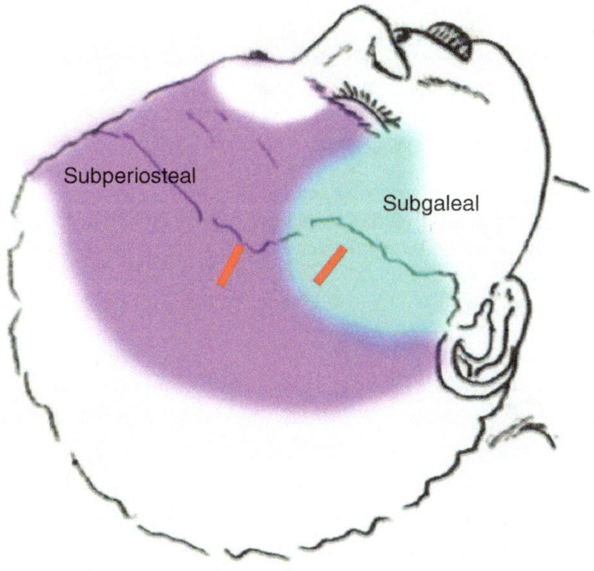

• **Fig. 63.37** Flap undermining in closed, nonendoscopic forehead lift. The incision on the temporal scalp (see *2* in Fig. 63.35) is used to undermine the lateral forehead in a subgaleal plane (light-green shaded area). The superior incision at the junction of the frontal and frontotemporal hairlines (see *1* in Fig. 63.35) is used to undermine the central forehead in a subperiosteal plane (violet shaded area). Note that subperiosteal undermining is carried posteriorly to accommodate flap advancement, but that the inferiocentral forehead and glabellar region is not released. The interface between the lateral subgaleal and the medial subperiosteal planes is the temporal line of fusion or "temporal line." (Courtesy Timothy Marten, MD, FACS and the Marten Clinic of Plastic Surgery, San Francisco, CA; with permission.)

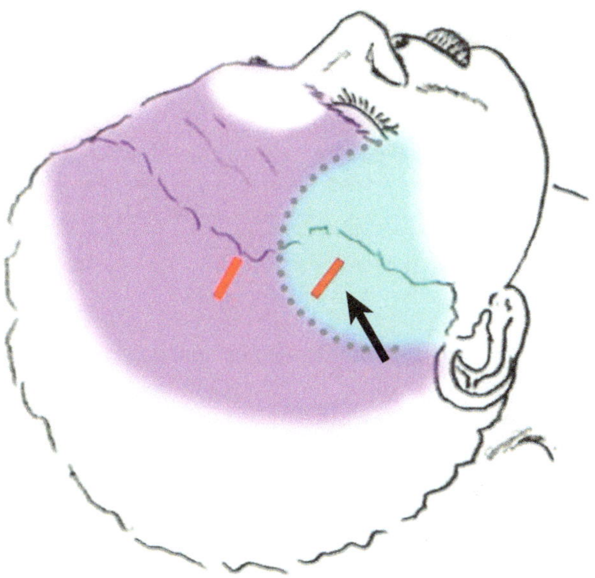

• **Fig. 63.38** Releasing the temporal line. The lateral incision on the temporal scalp is used to divide the bridge of tissue along the temporal line (*dotted line*) between the central subperiosteal dissection of the forehead and the lateral subgaleal dissection. This can be done without an endoscope under direct vision with a Metzenbaum scissors and small retractor if the patient's head is turned, the table is elevated to eye level, and a fiberoptic headlight is worn. (Courtesy Timothy Marten, MD, FACS and the Marten Clinic of Plastic Surgery, San Francisco, CA; with permission.)

The two temporal incisions are marked just within the temporal tuft of hair behind the frontotemporal hairline (see Fig. 63.35). These incisions lie lateral to the temporal line and are used to provide access for subgaleal undermining of the ipsilateral temple and lateral orbital regions (see Fig. 63.36). These incisions also provide access for dividing the bridge of tissue along the temporal line between the central subperiosteal dissection of the forehead and the subgaleal dissection of the temple and lateral forehead (Fig. 63.38), and for dividing the periosteum beneath the lateral two-thirds of the ipsilateral eyebrow under direct vision (Fig. 63.39). If a facelift is performed at the same time as closed foreheadplasty and the temporal part of the facelift incisions are on the temporal scalp, the upper portion of the facelift incisions may be used to undermine the temporal forehead, divide the bridge of tissue between the subgaleal and subperiosteal planes, and to release the periosteum beneath the lateral two-thirds of the eyebrows. In

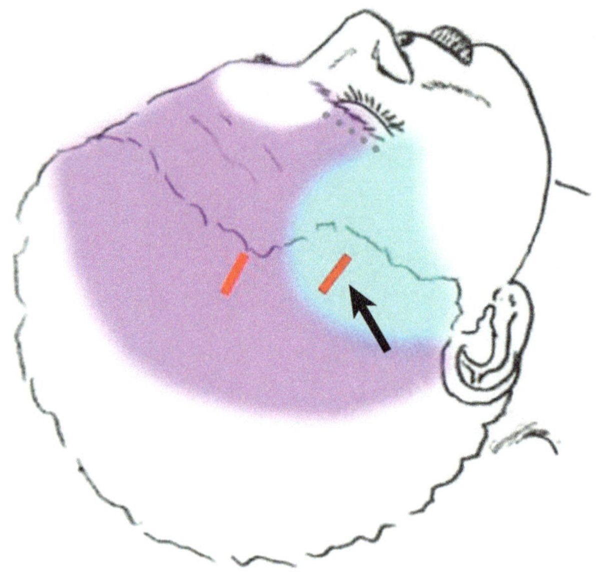

• **Fig. 63.39** Releasing the periosteum over the lateral brow. The lateral incision on the temporal scalp is used to divide the periosteum beneath the lateral eyebrow (*dotted line*) to mobilize and release the forehead flap. This can be done without an endoscope under direct vision with pistol grip endoscopic scissors (or even Metzenbaum scissors) and small retractor if the patient's head is turned, the table is elevated to eye level, and a fiberoptic headlight is worn. *Red lines* indicate sites of incisions. Light-green shaded area is area of subgaleal dissection. Violet shaded area is area of subperiosteal dissection. (Courtesy Timothy Marten, MD, FACS and the Marten Clinic of Plastic Surgery, San Francisco, CA; with permission.)

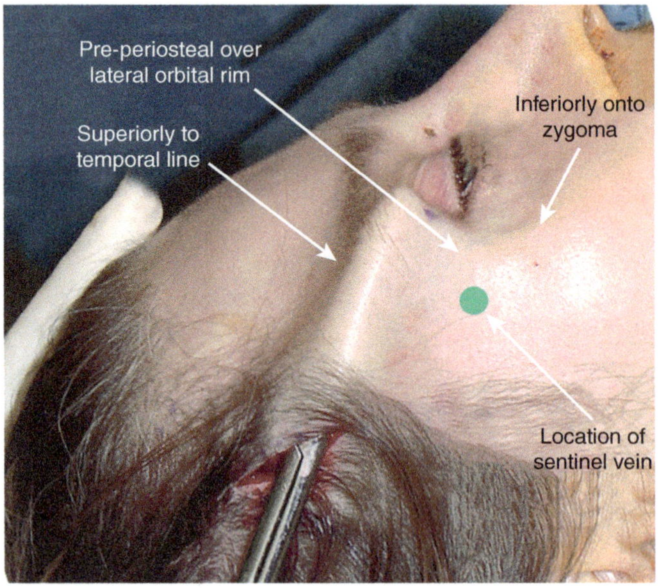

• **Fig. 63.40** Subgaleal dissection of temple. Forehead undermining and release is usually begun in the temple regions. Wound edges are retracted, the galea incised, and the subgaleal plane entered. Typically this is a loose areolar plane that is dissected bluntly with closed Metzenbaum scissors (as shown), and dissection proceeds up to and over the lateral orbital rim in subgaleal/preperiosteal plane. The dissection is then blindly and bluntly extended superiorly to the temporal line, and inferiorly over the lateral orbit through somewhat thicker attachments onto the upper zygoma. Due to the location of the access incision, and the fact that dissection is made bluntly with a blunt instrument, this can be accomplished without injuring the sentinel vein. (Courtesy Timothy Marten, MD, FACS and the Marten Clinic of Plastic Surgery, San Francisco, CA; with permission.)

such cases, the separate temporal incisions described above are not necessary.

Making Incisions

Incising the scalp is a key step in forehead lift surgery in which the surgeon exercises direct influence over the quality of the resulting scar. All incisions on the scalp, including the small "closed" ports used in these procedures, must be made precisely parallel with hair follicles to avoid injury to them. An incision made carelessly or other than in this manner will injure hair follicles and result in peri-incisional alopecia.

After each incision is made, the wound edges are retracted and vessels traversing the wound in the deep subcutaneous plane are grasped and cauterized. Care is taken to avoid thermal injury to the more superficially situated hair follicles, and no cauterization is performed in the plane in which the hair follicles are present. Superiorly, incisions are carried down through the galea and the periosteum is incised. Laterally, dissection is deepened through the galea and the temporalis muscle fascia exposed.

Forehead Flap Elevation

The plane beneath which the forehead flap is raised in "closed" foreheadplasty procedures has been the subject of debate and surgeons have advocated both subgaleal and subperiosteal dissections. Most surgeons now seem to prefer the subperiosteal plane, owing to its safety, ease of dissection, and the protection it affords the deep branch of the supraorbital nerve. It should be noted that when a "subperiosteal" technique is used, the entire flap dissection is not in a subperiosteal plane. Medial to the temporal line, the dissection is subperioseal. Lateral to the temporal line, the dissection is in a subgaleal plane.

Forehead undermining and release usually begins in the temple regions. Wound edges are retracted, the galea incised, and the subgaleal plane entered. Typically, this is a loose areolar plane that is dissected bluntly with closed Metzenbaum scissors, a Boise nasal elevator, or like blunt instrument, and dissection generally proceeds easily up to and over the lateral orbital rim in subgaleal/preperiosteal plane in this manner (Fig. 63.40). The dissection is then blindly and bluntly extended superiorly to the temporal line, and inferiorly over the lateral orbit through somewhat thicker attachments onto the upper zygoma. Due to the location of the access incision, and the fact that dissection is made bluntly with a blunt instrument, this can be accomplished without injuring the sentinel vein.

Once the lateral forehead has been dissected, attention shifts to the most superiorly situated incision located above the junction of the frontal and frontotemporal hairlines (see *1* in Fig. 63.35). Wound edges are retracted, the galea and periosteum are incised, and the central–lateral forehead undermined in a subperiosteal plane (Fig. 63.41). This

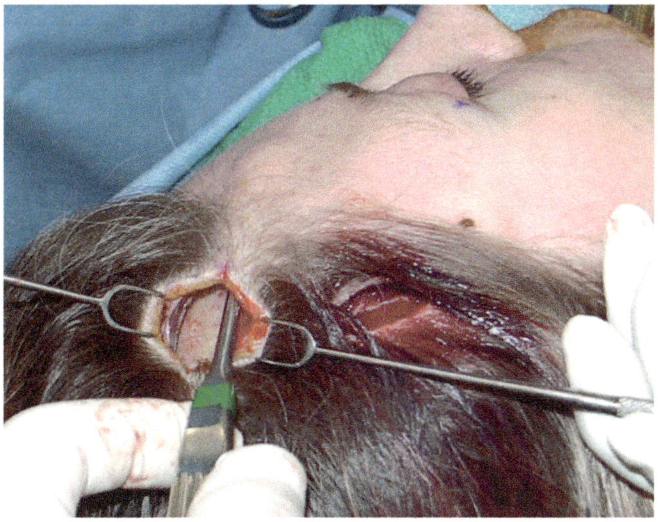

• **Fig. 63.41** Subperiosteal dissection of forehead. Wound edges are retracted, the galea and periosteum are incised, and the central-lateral forehead undermined in a subperiosteal plane. This dissection can be quickly made without the aid of an endoscope from temporal line extending posteriorly using an Obwegeser or similar periosteal elevator. Some posterior dissection is required to allow the flap to redistribute itself after it is advanced, and to avoid puckering and gathering posterior to the suspension points when the flap is anchored. (Courtesy Timothy Marten, MD, FACS and the Marten Clinic of Plastic Surgery, San Francisco, CA; with permission.)

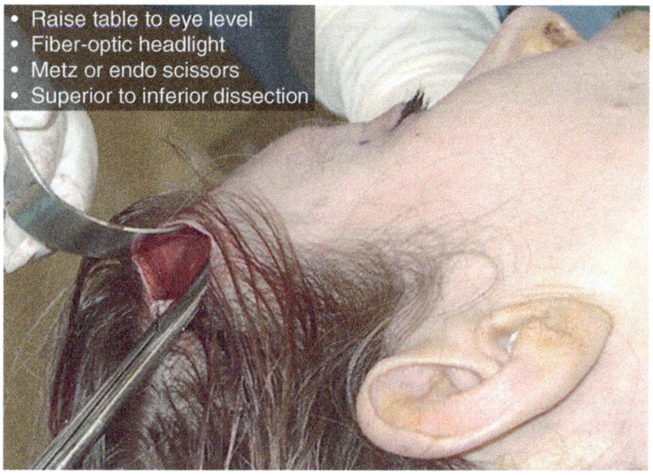

• **Fig. 63.42** Releasing the adherence along the temporal line. Mobilization of the forehead flap continues by dividing the bridge of tissue along the temporal line of fusion between the subperiosteal dissection in the lateral forehead and the lateral subgaleal dissection in the temple beginning superiorly and extending inferiorly to the lateral orbital rim. As experience is gained, this can be done without an endoscope through the incision on the temporal scalp under direct vision using a fiberoptic headlight and Metzenbaum scissors by raising the table to eye level, turning the patient's head, and retracting the flap with a small malleable ribbon retractor or similar instrument as shown. (Courtesy Timothy Marten, MD, FACS and the Marten Clinic of Plastic Surgery, San Francisco, CA; with permission.)

dissection can be quickly made without the aid of an endoscope from temporal line to temporal line extending posteriorly to the approximate location of the coronal suture using an Obwegeser or similar periosteal elevator. Some posterior dissection is required to allow the flap to redistribute itself after it is advanced, and to avoid puckering and gathering posterior to the suspension points when the flap is anchored.

As the mid-inferior brow is approached, the inferior aspect of the supraorbital rims should be palpated through infra-brow skin and the location of the foramen or notch from which the supraorbital nerve exits identified. This maneuver helps avoid dissection of these areas, which can vary somewhat anatomically from patient to patient. In the majority of cases, a notch ("frontal notch") is palpable on the inferior aspect of the supraorbital rim along a vertical line passing through the medial limbus. In patients with no palpable notch, the nerve usually exits through a foramen, which often is not palpable, more superiorly. Additional care in dissection is taken under these circumstances or an endoscope can be used.

When corrugator resection is planned through an eyelid incision ("transpalpebral corrugator myectomy"), the centroinferior forehead and glabella should not be undermined. Indeed, this is a significant advantage of this technique because it limits central forehead dissection and minimizes the possibility that the medial brow will be elevated.

Mobilization of the forehead flap continues by dividing the bridge of tissue along the temporal line of fusion between the central subperiosteal dissection and the lateral subgaleal dissection beginning superiorly and extending inferiorly to the lateral orbital rim (see Fig. 63.37; see Chapter 62 for details of anatomical spaces). As experience is gained, this can be done without an endoscope through the incision on the temporal scalp under direct vision using a fiberoptic headlight and Metzenbaum scissors by raising the table to eye level, turning the patient's head, and retracting the flap with a small malleable ribbon retractor or similar instrument (Fig. 63.42). If facelift is being performed concurrently and the temporal portion of the facelift incision is in the temporal scalp this maneuver will be even easier.

Releasing and Mobilizing the Lateral Brow

To fully mobilize the lateral forehead and obtain optimal elevation of the lateral brow, the periosteum beneath the lateral two-thirds of the eyebrow must be divided (see Fig. 63.39). As experience is gained, this can be done without the aid of the endoscope through the incision on the temporal scalp under direct vision using a fiberoptic headlight and Metzenbaum or a pistol grip endoscopic scissors by raising the table to eye level, turning the patient's head, and retracting the flap with a small malleable ribbon retractor or similar instrument (Fig. 63.43). This maneuver will be easier in patients with anteriorly situated hairlines where the access incision is closer to the area to be incised, and more difficult in patients with more posteriorly situated hairlines where the access incision is farther away.

When the flap is retracted, the periosteum is visible as a dense white fascial layer, and its lateral margin corresponds to the release made previously along the temporal line. Division of the periosteum beneath the lateral brow begins by confirming one's position beneath the flap by pushing up

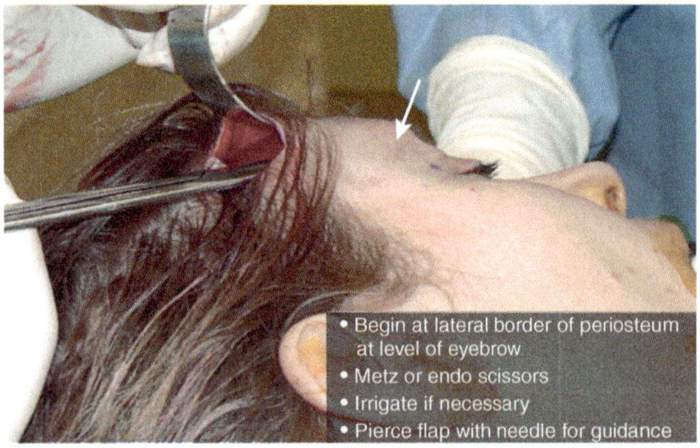

• **Fig. 63.43** Releasing the lateral brow. To fully mobilize the lateral forehead and obtain optimal elevation of the lateral brow, the periosteum beneath the lateral two-thirds of the eyebrow must be divided (see Fig. 63.39). As experience is gained, this can be done without the aid of the endoscope through the incision on the temporal scalp under direct vision using a fiberoptic headlight and Metzenbaum or a pistol grip endoscopic scissors by raising the table to eye level, turning the patient's head, and retracting the flap with a small malleable ribbon retractor or similar instrument. (Courtesy Timothy Marten, MD, FACS and the Marten Clinic of Plastic Surgery, San Francisco, CA; with permission.)

upon it with the closed scissors and visually confirming on the skin surface that one is starting in the proper location. The periosteum only is divided in small increments beginning laterally and working medially to avoid possible injury to the deep branch or the supraorbital nerve that lies several centimeters medially and more superficially, but in near proximity to the periosteum. Division of the periosteum continues medially over the lateral two-thirds of the brow just at the level of the eyebrow. The superficial (main) branch of the supraorbital nerve should remain well medial to the dissection and should not be seen. If facelift is being performed concurrently and the temporal portion of the facelift incision is in the temporal scalp this maneuver will be even easier.

After the periosteum of the lateral orbit has been divided, a Boise (or similar) blunt elevator is used to complete the release of the lateral forehead by applying gentle upward and outward pressure to the upper lateral orbital area. Typically, this maneuver provides additional flap mobilization that would not be obtained if the periosteum was only divided. Care must be taken, however, even when blunt elevation is made in the lateral orbital and temporal areas, because delicate terminal fibers of the frontal branch of the facial nerve travel through them. Dissection in this manner continues until adequate and symmetric release of the right and left lateral forehead is obtained. This is determined by returning the flap to the forehead, advancing it superiorly by placing gentle traction on the two most superior scalp incisions, and noting the effect on the eyebrows and brows.

While it is deceptively easy to elevate the lateral eyebrow preoperatively by pulling superiorly on the supra-brow skin, it is in reality much more difficult to do so intraoperatively by pulling from a point more superiorly on a composite forehead flap dissected in a subgaleal or subperiosteal plane. This is particularly true of thick-skinned individuals with advanced brow ptosis in whom standard flap undermining and release often proves inadequate in releasing the lateral brow and providing adequate elevation of the lateral eyebrow. In these cases, additional lateral brow elevation can be obtained by extended undermining of the temple and lateral face.

The procedure is summarized in Box 63.2.

• **BOX 63.2 Overview of Flap Mobilization in Closed Forehead Lift**

- Blind mobilization of temple in a subgaleal plane laterally
- Blind mobilization in subperiosteal plane in lateral and upper central forehead
- Release of the temporal line (interface of subgaleal and subperiosteal dissections at temporal line of fusion)
- Release of periosteum beneath the lateral brow
- Blunt mobilization of lateral brow

Drain Placement

Experience has shown that a drain, while not absolutely necessary, helps close down dead space beneath the parietal scalp behind forehead flap suspension points, reduce fluid collections in this area, and limits the amount of postoperative periorbital edema and ecchymosis experienced by patients, and as such, drains are used routinely in most procedures. Drain placement must be performed properly however if a beneficial effect is expected and problems are to be avoided. Careless drain placement can result in alopecia, slough, pain, paresthesias, and other problems.

A 7-F round multiperforated soft Silastic Jackson–Pratt closed suction drain is placed through a central–lateral site of insertion approximately 1 to 2 fingerbreadths posterior to the hairline and 1 to 2 fingerbreadths medial to the right superior incision (Fig. 63.44). The stab incision for drain insertion should be made carefully parallel to hair follicles to avoid injury to them. The drain should then be pulled through in a retrograde inside-to-outside fashion to avoid pulling hair into the wound and anchored with a 4-0 nylon suture tied loosely to the scalp but securely to the drain itself. Loosely tying the suture to the scalp allows for scalp swelling without hair follicle injury and facilitates drain removal. Overtightening the drain suture to the scalp can result in postoperative discomfort, difficulty in suture removal, and peri-incisional alopecia.

After the drain has been properly secured at its exit site, its perforated portion is cut to appropriate length and inserted subperiosteally and directed inferiomedially across the mid forehead to the opposite side. After incisions have been closed, the drain tube is attached to a small bulb suction reservoir. This provides continuous low vacuum and is easily managed by most patients while in place.

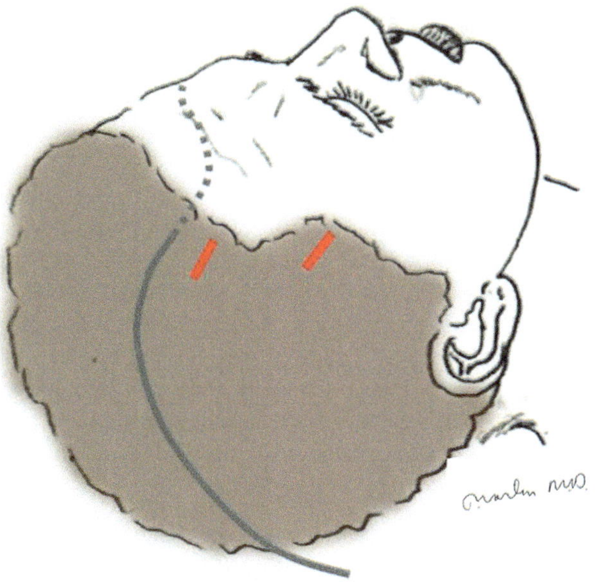

• **Fig. 63.44** Drain placement. A 7-F round multiperforated soft Silastic Jackson–Pratt closed suction drain is placed through a central-lateral site of insertion approximately 1 to 2 fingerbreadths posterior to the hairline and 1 to 2 fingerbreadths medial to the right superior incision. The drain is then directed across the forehead to the opposite side. *Red lines* indicate sites of incisions. *Solid line* indicates external part of drain. *Dotted line* shows approximate path of internal portion of the drain. (Courtesy Timothy Marten, MD, FACS and the Marten Clinic of Plastic Surgery, San Francisco, CA; with permission.)

Flap Repositioning

Once the drain has been inserted and secured, the forehead flap is elevated by pulling superiorly and medially on the two most superior incisions as the surgeon's goal is largely to tilt the eyebrow and rotate its lateral portion up, not to raise the entire eyebrow. Correct eyebrow position and configuration should then be confirmed. For most women, this should be in a soft arch with the lateral portion of the eyebrow lying several millimeters above its medialmost portion (see Fig. 63.21A). For men, the eyebrow should be horizontal or near horizontal, with the medial and lateral portions lying at the same level (see Fig. 63.21B). In thick-skinned individuals with heavy forehead tissues and brows, some overcorrection laterally is usually required.

In closed procedures, the amount of eyebrow elevation obtained is determined by the extent of flap release, and there is no contribution obtained from scalp excision as is the case in open approaches.

If inadequate brow elevation is seen to be present, or if asymmetry is noted, additional undermining and release are indicated and should be continued until the desired effect is obtained. Tying anchoring sutures tightly cannot compensate for incomplete flap release and will predictably result in hair loss at the anchoring point.

There should be no lateral component of shift when repositioning the forehead flap in foreheadplasty procedures, and the best biomechanical effect on the brow is obtained when the forehead flap is elevated along a vertical or slightly vertical–*medial* vector. Many surgeons mistakenly add a lateral component of shift in a conceptually and technically flawed attempt to smooth glabellar frown lines. Pulling laterally on the forehead will not correct glabellar frown lines, as proper and effective treatment of these requires attenuation or elimination of corrugator supercilii muscle action. Pulling laterally on the forehead flap also is not the optimal vector to reposition and shape it.

Flap Anchoring

Various methods of forehead flap anchoring have been advocated for use in closed foreheadplasty procedures but it should be recognized that the means by which the forehead flap is anchored is not the definitive step in the procedure and that there is no special "magic" in any one particular method. How the flap is anchored is unimportant as long as it achieves the intended purpose, and success or failure lies largely in the adequate *mobilization* of the flap – not the particular method of anchoring used.

Methods of forehead flap anchoring that have been described and reported include, but are not limited to, cranial flap fixation using internal microscrews, flap fixation using a microscrew and pledget of Gortex (polytetrafluoroethylene), flap fixation using prethreaded metallic anchors (Mitec anchor), flap fixation using an absorbable polyglycolic acid (PGA) cranial peg (Endotine) or PGA (Lactcosorb) screw, and suture fixation to converging unicortical bony tunnels. Other flap anchoring strategies include suspension using a removable transcutaneous cranial post (large, removable, externalized screw), an external bolster, and tissue glues. The use of small "T" to "V" excisions of scalp at endoscopic entry ports has also been reported. Each of these methods has advantages and disadvantages that should be considered including, but not limited to, poor patient acceptance (external bolsters, external removable screws, internal metallic screws), palpability (PGA pegs and screws), expense (Endotine, Mitec), poor healing and hair loss ("T" to "V" excisions and other attempts to excise scalp), and concerns regarding disease transmission (pooled plasma-derived tissue glues).

Experience has shown that the effectiveness and longevity of closed forehead lift procedures are significantly improved when some sort of secure and permanent direct cranial fixation of the flap is performed, and suturing the galea and periosteum at the leading edge of the superiorly situated incisions (see *1* in Fig. 63.35) to converging unicortical bony tunnels made in the outer cortex of the calvarium with a 3-0 braided polyester (Mersilene) suture has proven to be a convenient and reliable way to accomplish this. This method, unlike many of the others noted above, is easy to perform, reliably results in excellent healing, and is readily acceptable to most patients owing to the fact that no metal screws are used and the fixation is low profile, nonpalpable, noninflammatory, long-lasting, and inexpensive (Fig. 63.45).

Once balanced and symmetric release of the forehead flap has been confirmed and the flap advanced, the edge of each superior incision is retracted and a mark made in the center of each on the cranium in water-soluble surgical ink (methylene blue). These spots mark the sites at which the flap will be anchored. A Desmarres retractor is then used to protect the wound edge on the side being drilled and converging unicortical drill holes made at approximately 30- to 45-degree angles. Care must be taken to ensure that minimal pressure on the drill handpiece is applied while holes are being drilled, and that only the outer cortex is penetrated (Fig. 63.46).

After converging holes have been drilled in the outer calvarial cortex at marked sites, a 3-0 braided polyester (Mersilene) suture is passed through each drill hole by bending the needle and passing it in a retrograde fashion through each, or by drawing the back end of the suture through the hole by applying a Frazier-tipped suction to one side. At first, this step can prove to be a bit cumbersome, but, as experience is acquired, it can be performed quickly and easily. The suture is then passed through the galea and periosteum just at the inferior aspect of each incision and tied under modest tension only.

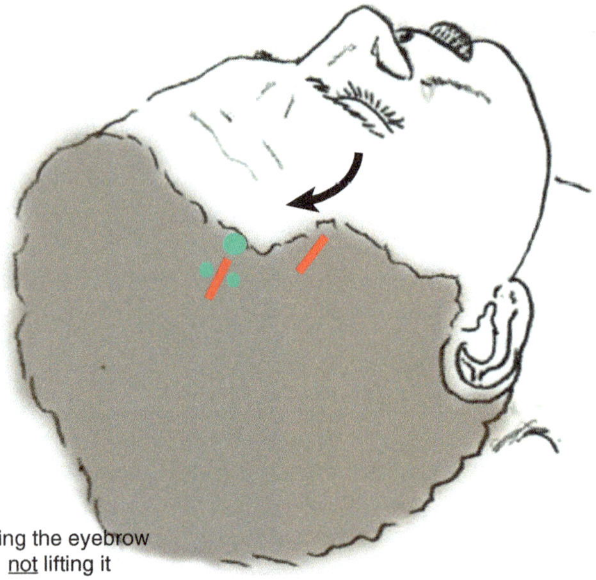

• **Fig. 63.45** Flap repositioning and anchoring. The galea and periosteal of the closed forehead flap situated just inferior to the inferior-most extent of the superior incision (*large dot*) is anchored to converging unicortical bony tunnels in the outer calvarial cortex *(small dots)* with a 3-0 braided polyester (Mersilene) suture. Arrow shows proper (superiorly directed or slightly superior-medial) direction of flap shift. *Red lines* indicate sites of incisions. (Courtesy Timothy Marten, MD, FACS and the Marten Clinic of Plastic Surgery, San Francisco, CA; with permission.)

Anchoring the flap superiorly provides the needed and the adequate mechanical effect on the brow and it is typically not necessary or productive to anchor the flap at the temporal (lateral) incision sites. It is also not necessary, and will make any secondary procedure more difficult, if temporalis muscle fascia is excised in an effort to create suspensory adhesions in the lateral temporal areas.

Incision Closure

After flap-anchoring sutures have been placed, irrigation is performed with antibiotic solution and scalp incisions are closed in one layer with simple interrupted sutures of 4-0 nylon (Fig. 63.47). No deep suture is required. If closure is performed meticulously and in a way that provides good wound edge alignment without overly tight sutures, an inconspicuous scar will be obtained.

Staples are generally inadequate for closing scalp incisions in both open and closed foreheadplasty procedures in that a properly-made incision on the scalp is typically beveled to some extent so as to remain parallel to hair follicles and avoid injury to them, and staples are designed to close wounds with perpendicular edges. Attempting to staple an incision with bevel edges often results in overriding of wound edges and poor wound edge alignment. The use of staples is also frequently uncomfortable and disturbing to patients. A ratcheting staple and external screw technique should not be used to suspend the flap in closed foreheadplasty procedures. Such a plan places excessive tension on the scalp tissue in the plane of the hair follicles and commonly results in hair loss.

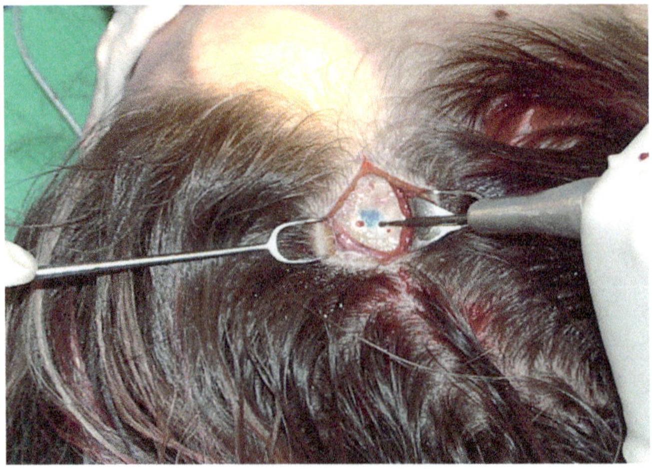

• **Fig. 63.46** Flap anchoring to converging unicortical drill holes. A Desmarres retractor is then used to protect the wound edge on the side being drilled and converging unicortical drill holes made at approximately 30- to 45-degree angles. Care must be taken to ensure that minimal pressure is applied to the drill handpiece while holes are being drilled, and that only the outer cortex is penetrated. (Courtesy Timothy Marten, MD, FACS and the Marten Clinic of Plastic Surgery, San Francisco, CA; with permission.)

Corrugator Myoplasty

While corrugator muscle surgery was a routine part of foreheadplasty surgery a little over a decade ago, the widespread use of neuromodulators has gradually and largely supplanted the need for this procedure. Neurotoxin usually produces a superior suppression of muscle hyperfunction with few problems and complications, and it is generally a mistake to give the impression to a patient that corrugator myectomy can produce an equivalent permanent result. Typically, myectomy results in a reduction in corrugator hyperfunction, but not a complete elimination of all glabellar movement that patients using neuromodulator agents have come to expect.

Once flap mobilization, repositioning, anchoring, and incision closure is complete, attention turns to the corrugator myoplasty, if indicated and/or desired by the patient. We have found the demand for corrugator surgery to be continually diminishing and have noted an increasing preference in patients to manage corrugator hyperfunction with neuromodulators. Nonetheless, we feel there still is a place for corrugator myectomy/myoplasty.

Surgically, attenuating corrugator hyperfunction forms the basis of the surgical treatment of glabellar frown lines and is adequate for many patients with mild to moderate problems. The expectations of patients with marked muscle hyperfunction and deep lines must be properly set, however, and all patients must be made aware that the goal of surgical treatment of corrugator hyperfunction and glabellar frown lines is a reduction in frown-line intensity, and not complete elimination of all glabellar movement. Patients should also be made aware that they may want or need to undergo neurotoxin (botulinum toxin) injections, even after correctly performed procedures.

Correct management of the corrugator supercilii muscles requires a detailed understanding of their anatomy, and their relationship with adjacent agonists and antagonists muscles. The corrugators are obliquely oriented muscles that originate on the medialmost portion of the supraorbital ridge. The muscles traverse superiolaterally to and insert on the skin overlying the medial and mid-brow. The corrugators are intimately associated with a group of important agonists and antagonists that together are responsible for the expression of a wide range of human emotions. These include the procerus, frontalis, orbicularis oculi, and the depressor supercilii muscles. The limits of these neighboring muscles are not always easily defined, and as the corrugators are followed laterally toward their insertion they are seen to overlap, override, intermingle, and merge with them, and these relationships allow for complex interactions and are important when contemplating surgical modification of muscle action.

A careful consideration of the anatomical arrangement of the corrugator supercilii muscles makes clear their effect on the eyebrow and the bulges and lines that develop upon their contraction. Each muscle is arranged so that its fibers exert action in several directions, and as such, they exert different effects at various locations along the brow. Over the medial third of the eyebrow, the corrugator acts as an antagonist to the frontalis and an agonist to the procerus and superior medial portion of the orbicularis oculi. There is no specific antagonism to medially directed contraction of the corrugator, however, and thus no opposing force to its medially directed pull on the brow. This explains why, upon cursory consideration, vertical glabellar wrinkling seems to be the overriding effect of corrugator action. It also explains why resecting the corrugator, in and of itself, can result in medial brow elevation, even if no undermining and advancement of a forehead flap is made.

The corrugator muscle action results in a complex action on the medial aspect of the eyebrow and the inferior central forehead, resulting in vertical glabellar wrinkling and an angry or disapproving appearance. Traditionally, near-total corrugator myectomy was performed to diminish these expressions using an open or endoscopic technique, and when properly performed was effective in doing so. Traditional myectomy, performed using either of these techniques, has several disadvantages, however, including disruption of attachments and ligaments that hold the medial brow and eyebrow inferiorly. Traditional open or

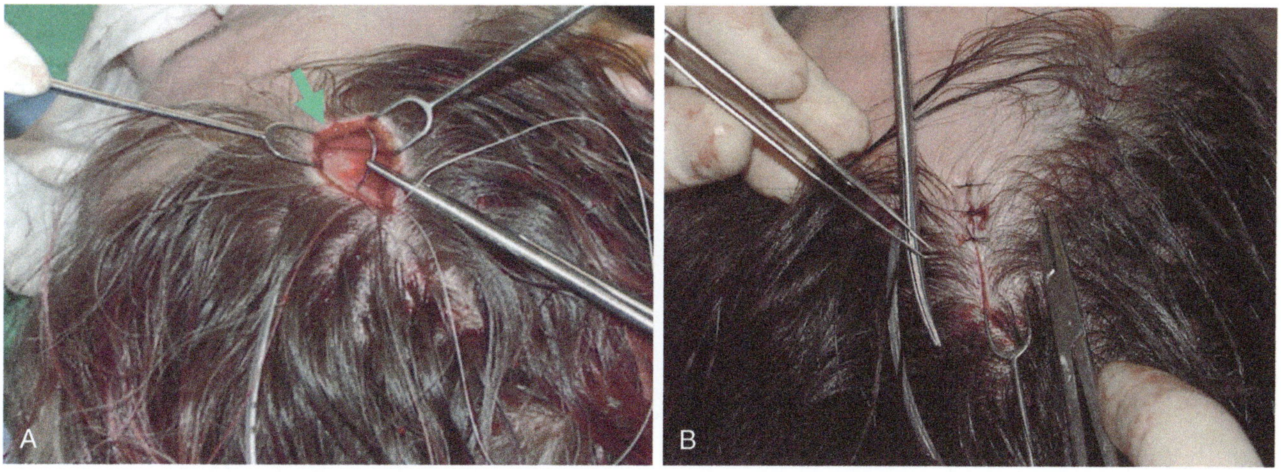

• **Fig. 63.47** Incision closure. (A) After flap-anchoring sutures have been placed, (B) scalp incisions are closed in one layer with simple interrupted sutures of 4-0 nylon. (Note that incision on temple scalp had already been closed.) (Courtesy Timothy Marten, MD, FACS and the Marten Clinic of Plastic Surgery, San Francisco, CA; with permission.)

endoscopic myectomy also typically produces some temporary and occasionally permanent paresthesias and dysesthesias due to dissection of the supratrochlear nerves. These problems can often be diminished or avoided if a modified technique and transpalpebral approach is used in which the corrugator muscle is divided or divided and partially resected lateral to the supratrochlear nerve branches, and a fat graft is interposed to defunctionalize the muscle by preventing the divided segments from reattaching upon healing. This approach will hereafter be referred to as "corrugator myoplasty" and the involved steps are described in the following paragraphs.

Dissection of the corrugator supercilii muscles is facilitated and bleeding is diminished if the medial brow is hyperinflated by injecting a dilute local anesthetic–epinephrine solution and an adequate time is allowed for a proper anesthetic and hemostatic effect. The surgeon should also wear a headlight, and a fine-tipped cautery, Ragnell retractor, and Frazier-tipped suction should be available.

Upper blepharoplasty incisions are made according to the preoperative plan and need not be modified when transpalpebral corrugator myoplasty is being performed. If a patient does not need upper blepharoplasty but desires frown line reduction, consent is obtained to make an incision along the upper lid tarsal crease to provide access to the corrugator muscle and to allow corrugator muscle myoplasty to be performed. When the advantages of the technique are explained to patients, most will allow an eyelid incision to be made in such situations and, if it is closed properly, the scar will usually be difficult to find once healed. If patients do not wish to have an upper eyelid incision, the muscles can be treated in a traditional endoscopic fashion, or by other means.

The superior margin of the blepharoplasty incision is retracted by the assistant using two 10-mm double-pronged skin hook retractors and dissection is carried down to the orbital septum using needle-tipped cautery and low electrocautery current (Fig. 63.48A). Dissection is then continued superiorly superficial to the septum up to the supraorbital rim in a preseptal plane. Typically this dissection is made in a loose areolar plane and as the medial aspect of the supraorbital rim is approached, the outline of the inferior portion of the corrugator supercilii muscle will be seen (Fig. 63.48B).

Once the corrugator is identified in this fashion, the tips of a tenotomy scissors are introduced between the underside of the muscle and the brow bone, and they are used to bluntly dissect the plane between the muscle and the bony periosteum (Fig. 63.48C). This dissection is performed well medial to the supraorbital nerve, which is typically not seen and need not be specifically identified during the procedure. If the glabella has been hyperinflated with local anesthetic–epinephrine solution before muscle dissection, minimal bleeding is usually encountered. If bleeding is encountered, however, it is best controlled by placing firm direct pressure on the skin overlying the region against the boney brow for several minutes or until it stops.

Next, the tips of the tenotomy scissors are introduced between the anterior surface of the muscle and the brow skin, and they are used to bluntly dissect the plane between them (Fig. 63.48D). If the brow has been hyperinflated with local anesthetic–epinephrine solution before its dissection, little bleeding will typically be encountered during this part of the dissection as well. If bleeding is encountered, it is best controlled as previously described by placing direct pressure on the skin overlying the region until it stops. Once this maneuver is complete, the corrugator is isolated and can be grasped with a forceps or a similar instrument (Fig. 63.48E).

Once the corrugator has been isolated and separated from adjacent structures, it is divided or a small segment is resected (Fig. 63.48F).

This is accomplished by introducing one blade of the tenotomy scissors between the corrugator muscle and the brow bone, and the other between the muscle and the skin. The scissors are then turned parallel to the supraorbital and supratrochlear nerves and the muscle divided between them. If the brow has been hyperinflated with local anesthetic–epinephrine solution before its dissection, little bleeding will typically be encountered when the muscle is divided. If bleeding is encountered following this maneuver, it is best controlled by packing the wound with the corner of a sponge and placing direct pressure on the skin overlying the region until it stops. Alternatively, bleeding can often be controlled directly in some cases by placing a Ragnelle-type retractor in the wound, applying suction with a small Frazier suction, and cauterizing oozing areas with a fine-tipped cautery under direction vision. This, when necessary, is most readily accomplished when a fiberoptic headlight is worn.

Once the corrugator has been divided and hemostasis obtained (if necessary), the cut edges of the muscle retract and a gap between the cut edges will be seen (Fig. 63.48G). If fat is available from elsewhere in the face (e.g., from a blepharoplasty, facelift, or neck lift procedure), it is used as an interposition graft to defunctionalize the muscle and to ensure that smooth brow contours will be present once healing is complete (Fig. 63.48H). If this is not done, the muscles will predictably heal back together and minimal improvement will typically be obtained. If fat is not available from the face, the small amount needed can be harvested through a small incision in the suprapubic or other concealed area where adequate fat is present. Alternatively, the head of the muscle can be subtotally resected by carefully picking it out from between the supratrochlear nerves with a fine-tipped hemostat. When this is done, more forehead dysesthesias and upper eyelid ecchymosis will be more likely to occur and should be expected.

Fat grafts are trimmed to fit the defect and typically measure approximately 10×10×10 mm. Fat grafts are most easily secured using a transcutaneous pullout suture of 6-0 nylon (Fig. 63.48H, I). This is placed while the wound is held open with a Ragnell retractor and 10-mm double pronged skin hook, and is introduced through the brow skin just at

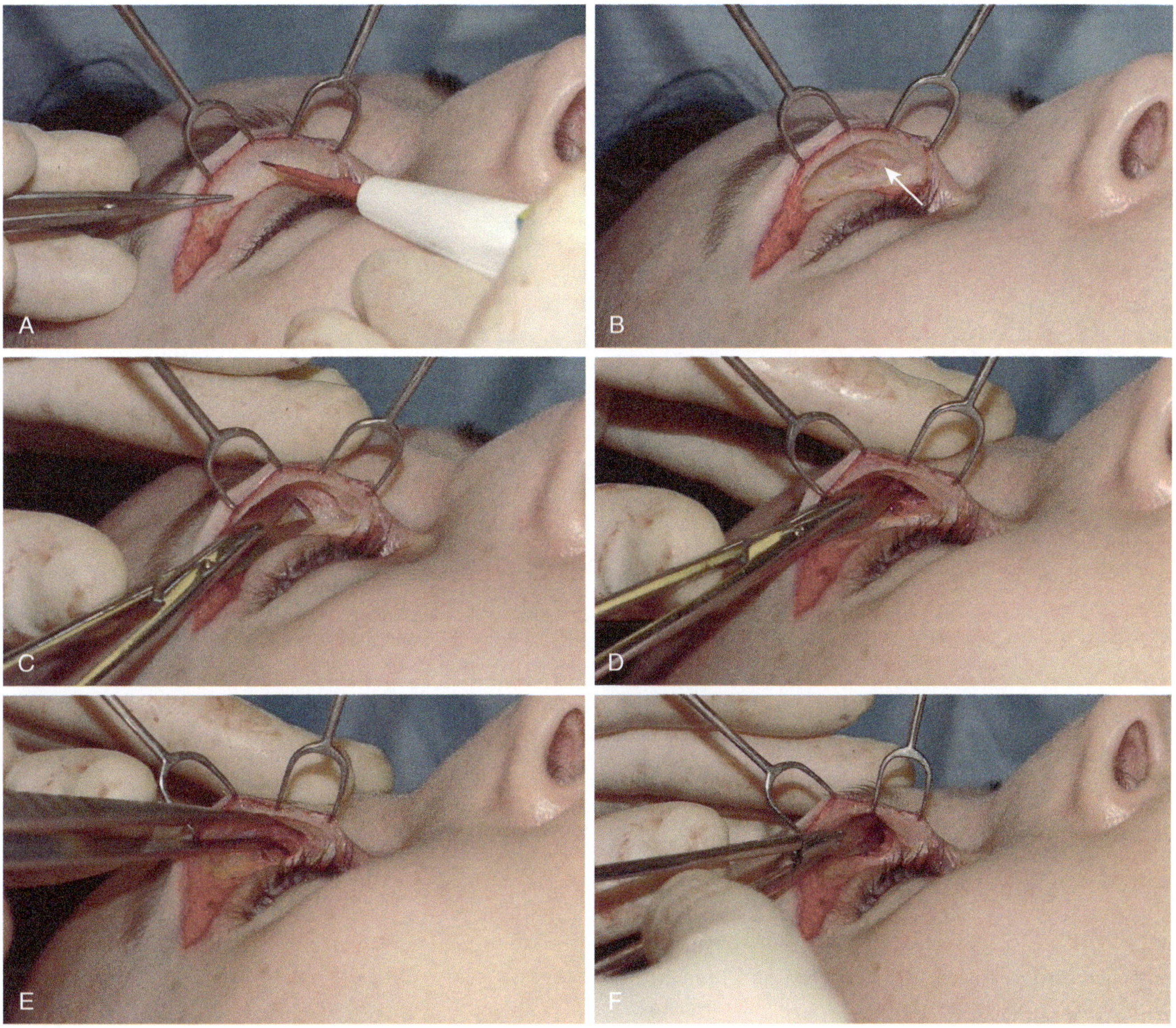

• **Fig. 63.48** Transpalpebral approach to the corrugator supercilii muscle. (A) The superior margin of the blepharoplasty incision is retracted by the assistant and dissection made superiorly superficial to the septum up to the supraorbital rim using needle-tipped cautery and low cautery current in a preseptal plane. (B) As dissection is made superiorly on top of the orbital septum to the supraorbital rim, the inferior part of the corrugator supercilii muscle (*arrow*) becomes visible. (C) Once the corrugator is identified, the tips of a pair of tenotomy scissors are introduced between the underside of the muscle and the brow, and they are used to bluntly dissect the plane between the muscle and the bony periosteum. (D) After the deep side of the muscle has been dissected, the tips of the tenotomy scissors are introduced between the anterior surface of the muscle and the brow skin. They are then used to dissect the plane between them. (E) Once the superficial and deep surface of the corrugator has been dissected, its central portion will be isolated separated from adjacent structures and can be grasped with a DeBakey forceps or a similar instrument. It can then be divided (see Fig. 63.14) or subtotally resected as desired. (F) Dividing the corrugator supercilii muscle. Once the corrugator has been isolated, one blade of the tenotomy scissors is inserted between the corrugator muscle and the brow bone, and the other between the muscle and the skin. The scissors are then turned parallel to the supraorbital and supratrochlear nerves and the muscle is divided between them.

Continued

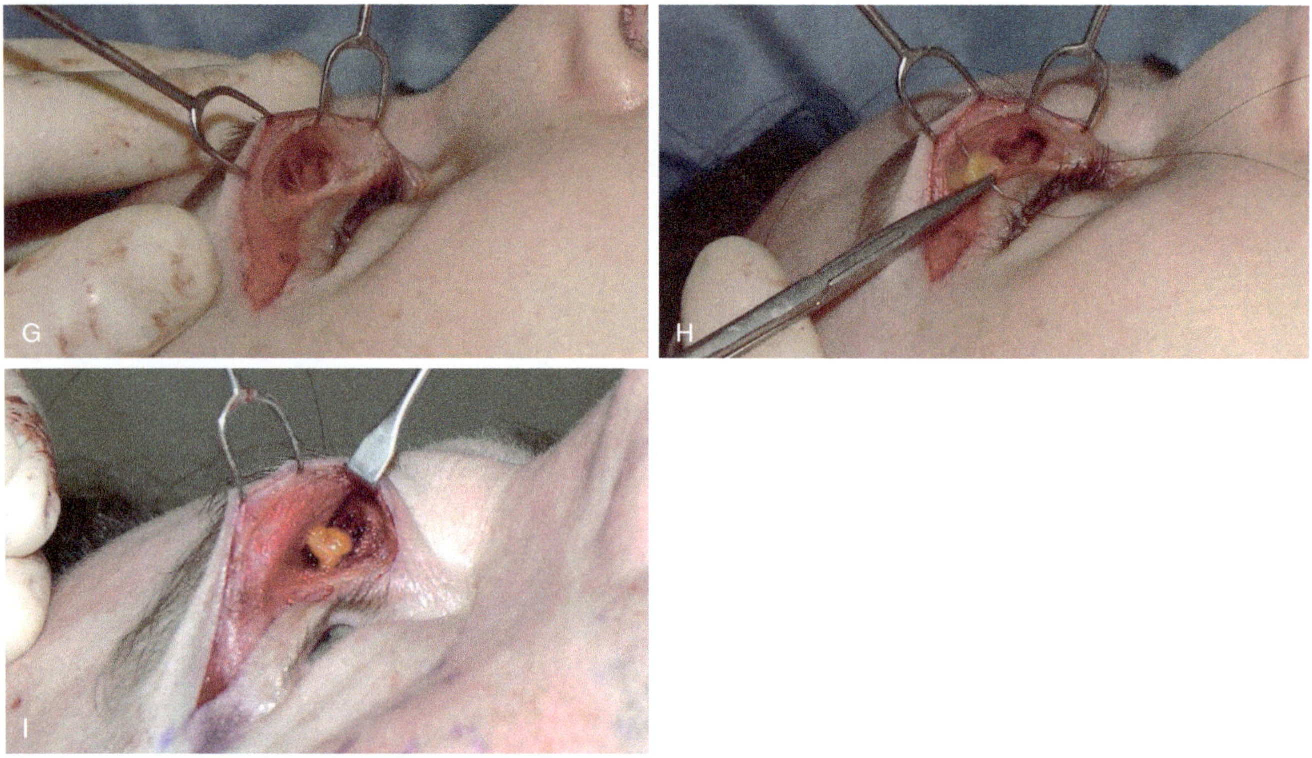

• **Fig. 63.48 cont'd** (G) Completed transpalpebral division of the corrugator supercilii muscle. Once the corrugator has been divided and the cut edges of the muscle retract and a gap appears. (H) Transpalpebral placement of interposition fat graft. Fat obtained from elsewhere in the face (e.g., from a blepharoplasty, facelift, or neck lift procedure) is used as an interposition graft to prevent the cut muscle edges from readhering to each other and to defunctionalize the muscle. The fat graft also ensures that brow contours will be smooth once healing is complete. (I) Securing the interposition fat graft. Fat grafts are most easily secured using a transcutaneous 6-0 nylon pull-out suture. Placed while the wound is held open with a Ragnell retractor as shown, the suture is introduced through the brow skin just at the superomedial aspect of the eyebrow and brought out through the eyelid incision between the divided muscle segments. The needle is then passed through the fat graft and then back through the eyelid incision between the muscle segments and out the skin near the spot it entered. As the suture is pulled up and tied, the fat graft is drawn up into the incision and held between the divided muscle segments. (Courtesy Timothy Marten, MD, FACS and the Marten Clinic of Plastic Surgery, San Francisco, CA; with permission.)

the superomedial aspect of the eyebrow and brought out through the eyelid incision between the divided segments of corrugator muscle. The needle is then passed through the fat graft, and then back through the eyelid incision between the muscle segments and out the skin near the spot it entered. As the suture is pulled up and tied, the fat graft is drawn up into the incision and held between the divided muscle segments (see Fig. 63.48I).

Because the knot is small and sits at the superior edge of the eyebrow, it is often not noticed by patients during the recovery process (Fig. 63.49). The eyelid incision is then closed with a simple running suture of 6-0 polypropylene (Prolene) or another suture of choice.

Not all patients today will need or want corrugator muscle modification surgery that was in one form or another more or less a routine part of foreheadplasty procedures performed in the past. Many patients will now be encountered who are using neuromodulators (botulinum toxin) to control corrugator hyperfunction who are happy with the improvement they obtain

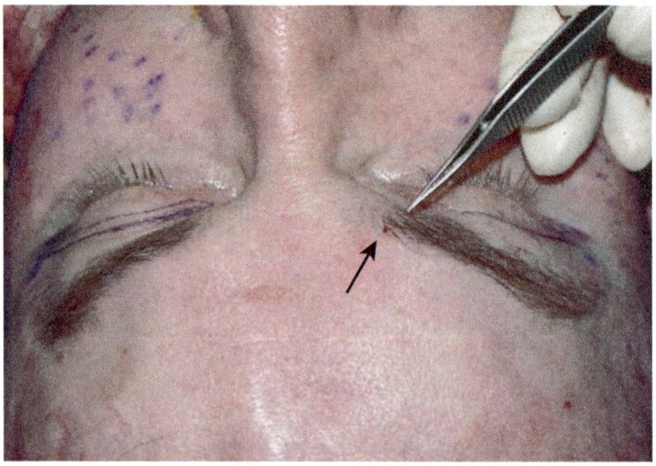

• **Fig. 63.49** Completed transcutaneous anchoring of the interposition fat graft. Because the suture knot is small and sits at the superior edge of the eyebrow (*arrow*), it is typically not noticed by patients during the recovery process. (Courtesy of the Timothy Marten, MD, FACS and the Marten Clinic of Plastic Surgery, San Francisco, CA; with permission.)

from it (albeit a temporary one) and who wish to continue to use it. Indeed, in many instances it could be argued that neuromodulators produce a more predictable, complete, and trouble free improvement than surgical muscle modification, and that its use has largely supplanted muscle surgery for treatment of glabellar frown lines. In these cases transpalpebral myoplasty (or other forms for corrugator muscle modification) need not be performed and the foreheadplasty procedure is undertaken to optimize eyebrow position and configuration only (tilt the lateral eyebrow up), and it is referred to in our practices as a "temple lift" to distinguish it from more comprehensive "forehead lift" and/or "brow lift" procedures. It is important that the patient has a clear understanding of whether or not corrugator muscle surgery will be performed, however, and when corrugator muscle modification is planned in the authors' clinic "corrugator muscle modification" is typically listed on the patient's informed consent document and procedure price quote, and additional charges are applied for the additional time and materials involved in carrying out the procedure.

Dressings

After all planned procedures have been completed and all incisions have been closed, the patient's hair is washed with shampoo and conditioner and if long it is placed in a soft braid. The hair is then allowed to dry or is blown dry in the recovery room. No dressing is required or applied. Patients are typically discharged with a hat, scarf, and sunglasses following the procedure.

Postoperative Care

Correct postoperative care of the foreheadplasty patient ensures the best result with the fewest problems and complications. Although most patients are treated as outpatients unless a facelift or related procedures are simultaneously performed, all are discharged to the care of a responsible adult third party with a specific set of written aftercare instructions.

Patients are asked to rest quietly and apply cold compresses to their forehead and eyes for 15–20 minutes of every hour they are awake for the first 3 days after surgery. For most patients, edema peaks at about this time. It is not necessary or productive to apply ice compresses continually throughout the day or at night.

The forehead drain is removed the morning after surgery if the patient stays overnight in our aftercare facility, or at the first postoperative visit.

Case Example (Fig. 63.50)*

The 55-year-old female patient is shown preoperatively in (A). Note that she has a somewhat tired, stern, and angry appearance even though her face is in repose. She has had no prior plastic surgery.

Photograph (B) shows the patient at 18 months following short-scar nonendoscopic forehead lift. Note that her eyebrow position and configuration has been improved and that she has a more rested and agreeable appearance. A facelift, neck lift, upper and lower eye lifts, chin augmentation, and fat transfer to the cheeks and lips have also been performed.

A preoperative view of the same patient frowning is shown in (C). Note that she has strong frown muscles that produce deep creases and an intense angry appearance.

Photograph (D) shows the patient at 18 months following short-scar nonendoscopic forehead lift with transpalpebral corrugator myoplasty. Note that she is trying to frown but frown intensity is markedly reduced.

(*All procedures were performed by Timothy Marten, MD, FACS. Case and illustrations courtesy of Timothy Marten, MD, FACS and the Marten Clinic of Plastic Surgery, San Francisco, CA; with permission.)

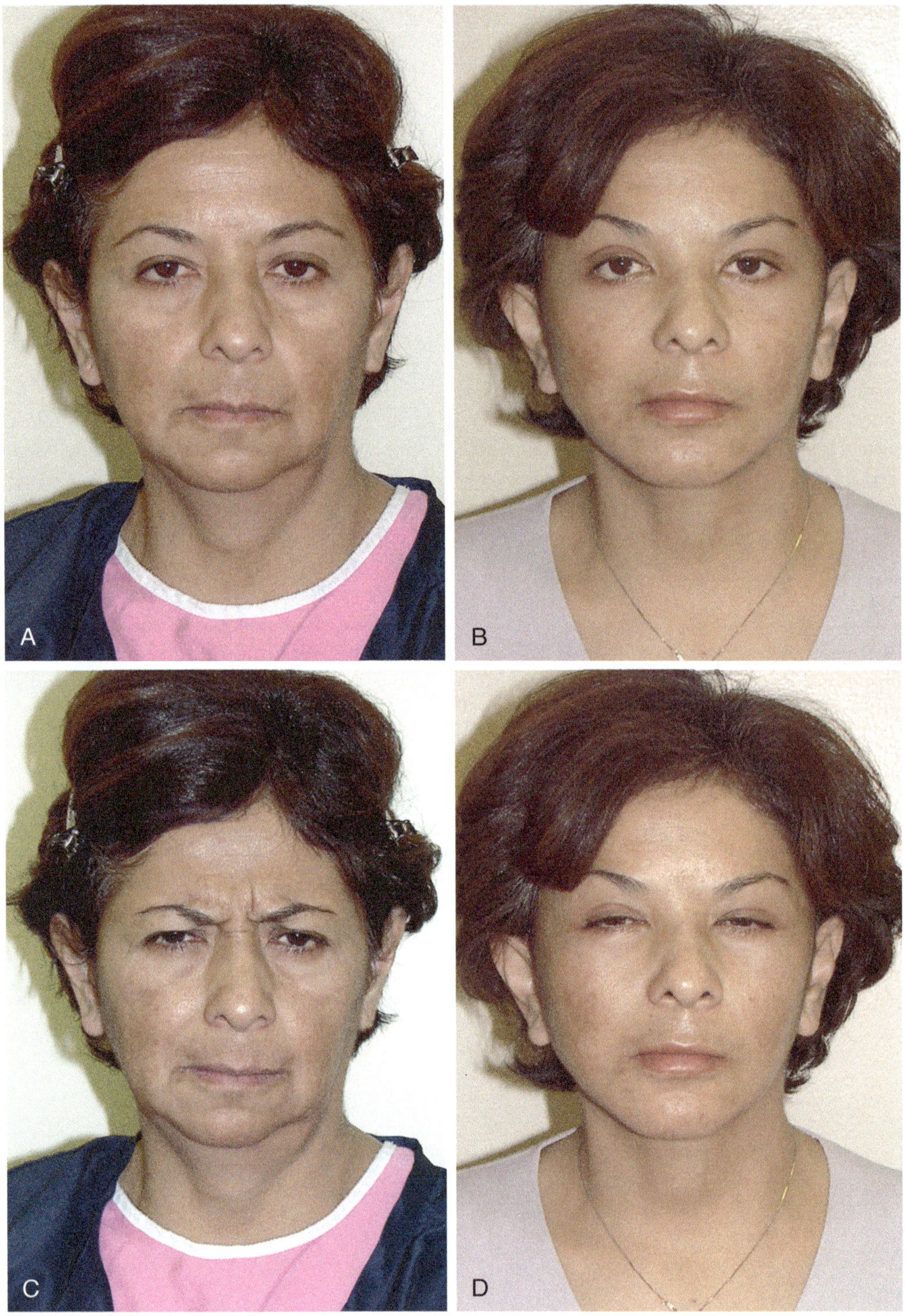

• **Fig. 63.50** Case study of a patient who had foreheadplasty. See text for details.

Further Reading

Connell BF, Lambros VS, Neurohr GH. The forehead-lift: techniques to avoid complications and produce optimal results. *Aesthetic Plast Surg*. 1989;19:217.

Connell BF, Marten TJ. Foreheadplasty: recognizing and treating aging in the upper face. *Clin Plast Surg*. 1991;18:653.

Faigin G. *The Artist's Complete Guide to Facial Expression*. New York: Watson–Guptill Publications; 1990.

Huntley HE. *The Divine Proportion*. New York: Dover; 1970.

Knize DM. A study of the supraorbital nerve. *Plast Reconstr Surg*. 1995;96:564.

Knize DM. Limited incision forehead lift. In: Knize DM, ed. *The Forehead and Temporal Fossa: Anatomy and Technique*. Philadelphia: Lippincott Williams and Wilkins; 2001.

Marten TJ. Hairline lowering foreheadplasty. *Plast Reconstr Surg*. 1999;103:224–236.

Marten TJ. Forehead aesthetics and pre-operative assessment of the foreheadplasty patient. In: Knize DM, ed. *The Forehead and Temporal Fossa: Anatomy and Technique*. Philadelphia: Lippincott Williams and Wilkins; 2001.

Marten TJ. Open foreheadplasty. In: Knize DM, ed. *The Forehead and Temporal Fossa: Anatomy and Technique*. Philadelphia: Lippincott Williams and Wilkins; 2001.

Marten TJ. Closed, non-endoscopic, small-incision forehead lift. *Clin Plast Surg*. 2008;35(3):363–378; discussion 361.

Powell H, Humphrieys B. *Proportions of the Aesthetic Face*. New York: Thieme–Stratton; 1984.

Rickets RM. Divine proportion in facial aesthetics. *Clin Plast Surg*. 1982;9:401.

Sullivan P, Salomon JA, Woo S, et al. The importance of the retaining ligamentous attachments of the fore-head for selective eyebrow reshaping and forehead rejuvenation. *Plast Reconstr Surg*. 2006;117:95–104.

Tolleth H. Concepts for the plastic surgeon from art and sculpture. *Clin Plast Surg*. 1987;14:585.

64

Upper Eyelid Rejuvenation

JULIA L. KEROLUS, GRACE LEE PENG, AND PAUL S. NASSIF

For videos accompanying this chapter see ExpertConsult.com. See inside cover for access details.

Introduction

The human mind instinctively examines another's eyes before any other facial feature. Trustworthiness, aggression, and even fertility are conveyed by the appearance of the eyes. The periorbital region influences facial harmony and is the most powerful tool for nonverbal communication and expression.[1] For these reasons, esthetic enhancement of the upper eyelid has been sought after for centuries and is one of the most commonly performed cosmetic operations today.[2]

Patients seek correction of excess skin, tired or sad-looking eyes, and droopy eyelids, which can often be achieved with upper blepharoplasty. Other rejuvenation techniques, including brow and midface lift, skin resurfacing, and volume restoration with fat or dermal fillers may also be utilized. Upper eyelid blepharoplasty is often perceived as technically simple with high reward and relatively low risk. This can subsequently translate to surgeon complacency and universal application of the same techniques to all patients. An improved understanding of periorbital aging and evolving patient expectations have led to the development of more effective surgical approaches in upper blepharoplasty.[3]

Periorbital Aging

Aged appearance of the upper lid is influenced by skin quality, volume of the eyelid and position of the brow and periorbita. The youthful upper eyelid is voluminous and smooth with a crisp upper lid crease.[4] The relationship of the brow to the upper eyelid has been described by Goldgerg and is emphasized when examining the esthetics of the periorbital region. The term *brow fat span* (BFS) represents the distance between the brow and upper lid crease; *tarsal platform show* (TPS) is the distance from the lid crease to the upper eyelid margin. Studies have identified that a youthful TPS:BFS ratio is 1:1.5 medially and 1:3 laterally[5] (Fig. 64.1).

Signs of aging result from environmental factors including sun exposure and smoking but also from genetic characteristics such as familial fat pseudoherniation which may be apparent in the teen years.[6] With age, patients experience soft tissue ptosis and loss of orbital bony support. Dermatochalasis is caused by loss of skin elasticity. Thinning of the orbicularis oculi and weakening of the orbital septum lead to pseudoherination of orbital fat resulting in a heavy appearance to the upper lid. Hooding of the lid is caused by atrophy of temple, brow, and eyelid fat. Brow ptosis is more significantly impacted by volume loss rather than actual decent of the brow.[7]

Anatomy

The upper eyelid is composed of anterior and posterior lamellae. From superficial to deep, the layers include: skin and orbicularis oculi muscle (which make up the anterior lamella), retro-orbicularis oculi fat (ROOF), orbital septum, orbital fat, levator palpebrae muscle superiorly and levator aponeurosis inferiorly, Müller's muscle inserting to tarsal plate and conjunctiva (the latter two forming the posterior lamella)[8] (Fig. 64.2).

The upper lid skin is the thinnest in the body and is intimately associated with the underlying orbicularis oculi muscle. The orbicularis oculi contains voluntary and involuntary muscle and is innervated by the temporal branch of the facial nerve. It is composed of orbital, preseptal, and pretarsal components, named for the underlying structures. Pretarsal orbicularis oculi forms the medial and lateral canthal tendons.[8]

The orbital septum is an extension of orbital periosteum and originates at the arcus marginalis. It separates eyelid (preseptal) from orbital (postseptal) contents and confines the orbital fat. The upper eyelid contains two fat compartments, one medial and one central, which are separated by the trochlea.[9] The lacrimal gland lies laterally in the same plane as the orbital fat and appears pink and firm, compared to the soft yellow fat compartments.

The levator muscle is located deep to the orbital fat and is the major retractor of the lid. The upper lid crease is formed by the insertion of the levator aponeurosis and orbital septum into the orbicularis oculi and skin. The lid crease is 7–9 mm superior to the lid margin in women and 5–7 mm in men. In the occidental eyelid, this fusion occurs superior to

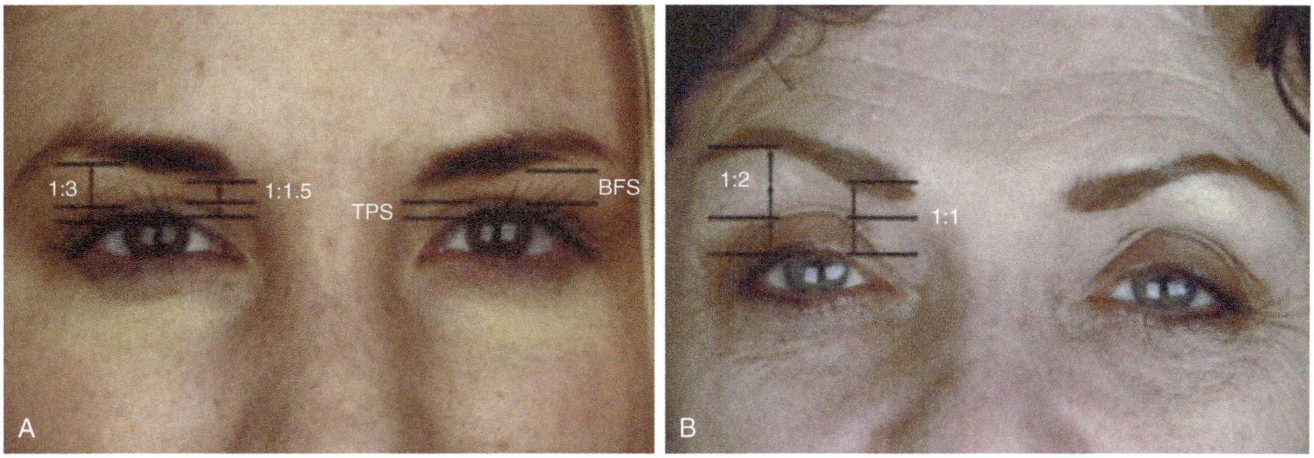

• **Fig. 64.1** (A) The tarsal platform show (TPS) is the distance from the lash line to the upper lid crease. The brow–fat span (BFS) is the distance between the lid crease and inferior edge of the brow. The youthful TPS to BFS ratio is 1:1.5 medially and 1:3 laterally. (B) With age, bone, and soft tissue loss around the eye increases the amount of TPS and decreases the BFS. In some patients, this can give the illusion of brow ptosis, when in fact the actual distance of the brow from the lash line is the same or even increased.

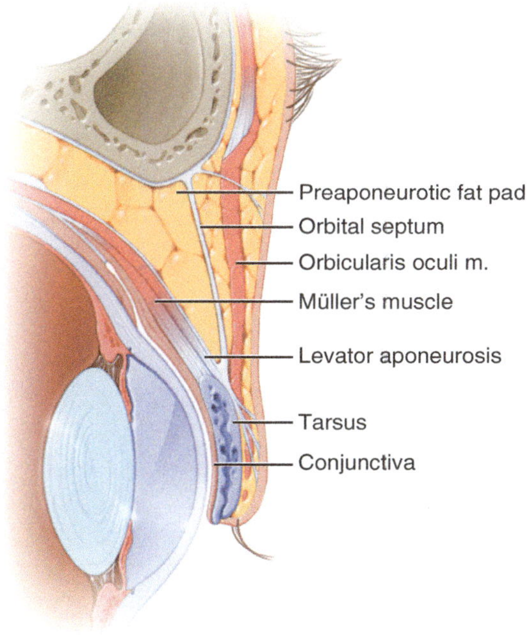

• **Fig. 64.2** Sagittal view of the upper eyelid demonstrating important anatomic layers. m., muscle. (From Briceno CA, Massry GG. Minimally invasive complementary adjuncts to upper blepharoplasty. In: Azizzadeh B, Murphy M, Johnson C, et al. *Master Techniques in Facial Rejuventation*. 2nd edn. Elsevier; 2018.)

the tarsal border. In the Asian eyelid, the levator aponeurosis and orbital septum attach further inferiorly and anterior to the tarsus. This creates fullness of the upper lid and prevents crease formation[10] (Fig. 64.3). Whitnall's ligament is formed by a thickening of the levator aponeurosis and suspends the levator muscle from the trochlea to the lacrimal gland fossa. Müller's muscle arises from the undersurface of the levator aponeurosis and attaches to the superior tarsal plate. It has sympathetic innervation and produces 2–3 mm of eyelid retraction.[9]

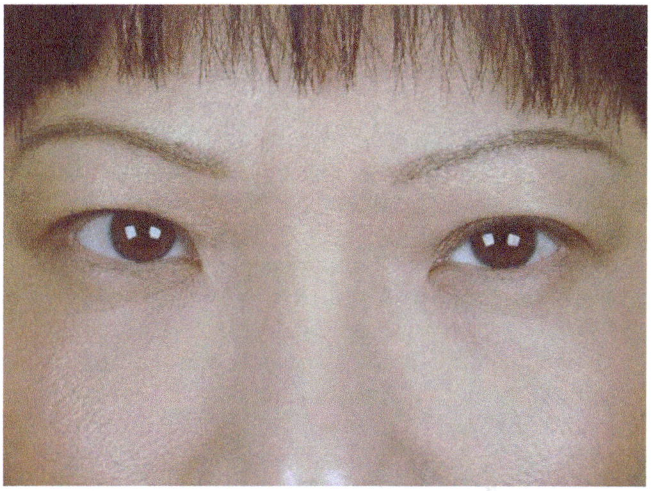

• **Fig. 64.3** Asian patient with a full upper lid and absent crease.

Patient Evaluation

As with any cosmetic procedure, diligent patient evaluation and selection in upper blepharoplasty is critical to successful outcomes. Preoperative documentation should include full medical history, medications, and dedicated ophthalmological history. Specifically, the patient is questioned regarding vision, use of corrective lenses, esthetic concerns, symptoms of dry eye or excess tearing, history of ocular disease (trauma, glaucoma, Grave's ophthalmopathy), and previous facial surgeries.[11] Upper blepharoplasty should be delayed at least 6 months following refractive corneal surgery.

The examination begins with obtaining standard preoperative photographs including:

- Full face frontal, oblique, lateral
- Close-up frontal with eyes in neutral gaze, upward gaze, and eyes closed
- Close-up lateral and oblique of each eye.

The patient is then examined in a sitting position and facial repose. When determining candidacy for upper eyelid surgery, specific anatomical and physiological factors should be evaluated. They include:

- Skin elasticity and texture
- Frontal and temporal hairline position
- Eyebrow shape, position, mobility, texture, and symmetry
  - Position may be influenced by involuntary contraction of the frontalis muscle in patients with lateral hooding. To eliminate this, patients should close their eyes and the surgeon stabilizes the brow as the eyes are opened
- Forehead and lateral canthal (crow's feet) rhytids
- Deep set orbits or upper lid hollowing
- Upper lid dermatochalasis, tone, hooding and presence of herniated fat pads
- Evidence of prior surgery or scarring
- Presence of lagophthalmos (inability to close the palpebral fissure completely) and ptosis

Visual acuity and visual field testing should be performed, especially if there are functional concerns. Severity of dry eye can be assessed with Schirmer's test and patients should be counseled that upper blepharoplasty may worsen symptoms of dry eye.[12]

The patient's expectations and motivations for seeking plastic surgery must also be carefully analyzed and discussed during the initial consultation. Patient dissatisfaction frequently arises secondary to poor communication regarding the surgical goals and unrealistic patient expectations.[12] A patient seeking a blepharoplasty who is found to have significant brow ptosis and little dermatochalasis should be counseled that a brow lift may be the best option. It is the responsibility of the surgeon to guide the patient toward the approach that will best address their concerns. Following the education process, candidates for upper eyelid rejuvenation must give informed consent after the possible adverse outcomes and risks of the selected surgical procedure are discussed.

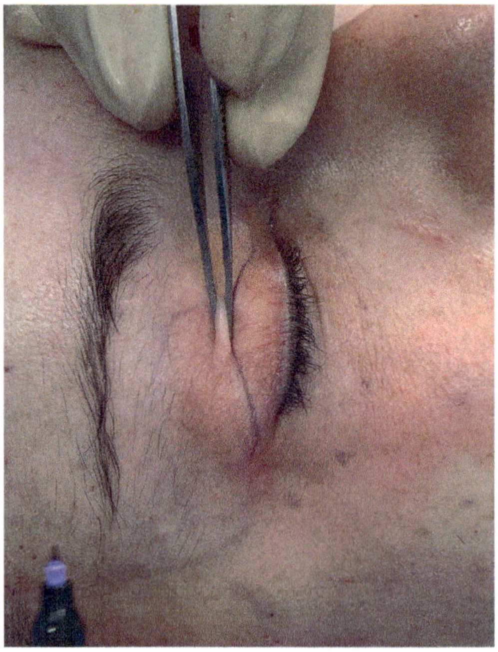

• **Fig. 64.4** The skin is pinched gently with non-toothed forceps to estimate the appropriate amount of skin to be excised.

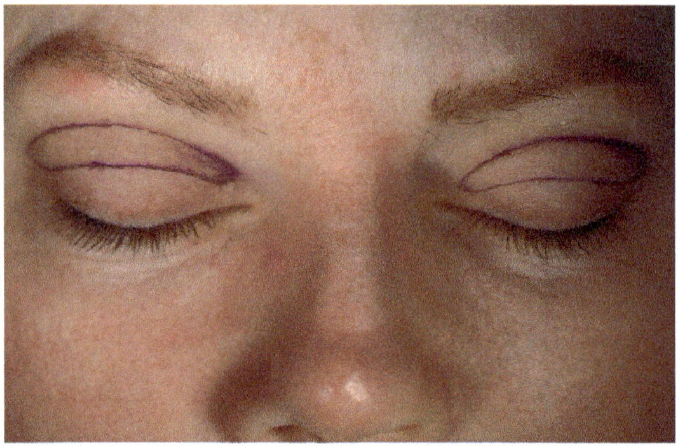

• **Fig. 64.5** The proposed incision does not pass the medial canthus. The lateral incision does not extend past an imaginary line drawn from the lateral canthus to the tail of the brow.

Surgical Techniques

Generally, brow elevation procedures are performed prior to upper blepharoplasty to allow for the appropriate amount of upper eyelid skin to be removed. This helps to prevent excessive elevation of the brow–lid complex and subsequent lagophthalmos.

Marking

Many surgeons prefer marking of the upper lid to be done with the patient in a seated position, however it is the practice of the authors to mark the patient while supine. The natural upper lid crease is marked as the inferior limb of the incision, approximately 6–9 mm above the lid margin. A caliper is used, and exact measurements are recorded. It is imperative to mark the skin with a fine-tip marking pen with the lid skin under tension. The amount of skin to be excised is estimated with a pinch technique (Fig. 64.4). The lateral marking is curved superiorly and should not extend lateral to an imaginary line drawn from the lateral canthus to the tail of the brow (Fig. 64.5). More skin is taken laterally to address lateral hooding. It is important to maintain a minimum of 20 mm of lid height to guarantee normal lid closure. The superior marking should be at least 10 mm from the inferior border of the brow to maintain an appropriate *brow–fat span* distance. Fat pseudoherniation is also identified and marked preoperatively.

Anesthesia

Upper blepharoplasty may be performed with the patient under general anesthesia, using intravenous or oral sedation or local anesthetic alone. Regardless of the mechanism of anesthesia, the upper lid is infiltrated in the subcutaneous

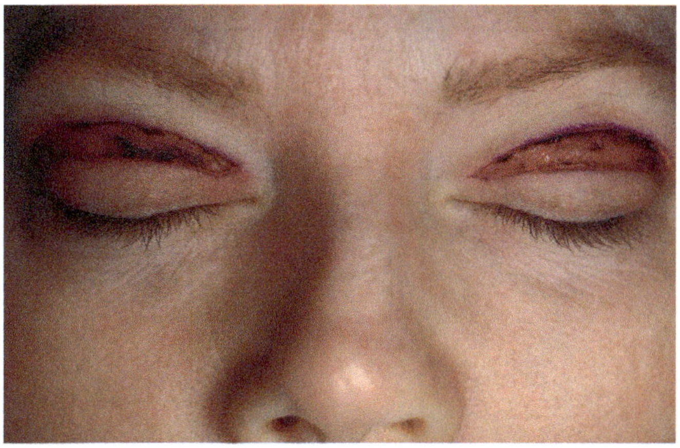

• **Fig. 64.6** Following skin removal, the orbicularis oculi muscle remains intact. Monopolar cautery has been applied to the lower aspect of the incision to aid in crease definition.

plane with 1% lidocaine with 1:100,000 epinephrine on a 27G needle. This aids with hydrodissection and hemostasis prior to skin incision.

Skin Incision and Excision

The incision is made with a number 15 blade scalpel, then excised leaving the orbicularis oculi muscle intact. Hemostasis is achieved with monopolar cautery. Application of cautery at the inferior edge of the wound creates a site for transorbicularis fibrosis and crease formation (Fig. 64.6). This maneuver has largely replaced the reductive technique of excision of orbicularis oculi muscle. Excision of muscle should be reserved for those with orbicularis redundancy and relative hypertrophy.

Orbital Fat

In select candidates, conservative fat excision or repositioning may be performed. After skin removal, a small septotomy is made at the superior aspect of the skin excision (Fig. 64.7). Gentle pressure on the globe helps to identify any redundant fat. Only the fat that comes easily into the wound should be manipulated. The nasal compartment contains white fat which can be excised very conservatively using cautery or repositioned centrally (Fig. 64.8). The central fat pad is yellow and easily repositioned to fill the superior sulcus. Aggressive fat excision can lead to hollowing and A-frame deformity that gives an operated look.

Additional Procedures

At this point, ptosis repair can be performed if indicated. Additionally, brow–fat pad repositioning can be added to restore eyebrow volume.

Skin Closure

The skin is reapproximated with simple interrupted key sutures centrally and laterally to decrease tension and prevent dog-ear formation. The incision is then closed with a running 6-0 Prolene suture (Fig. 64.9).

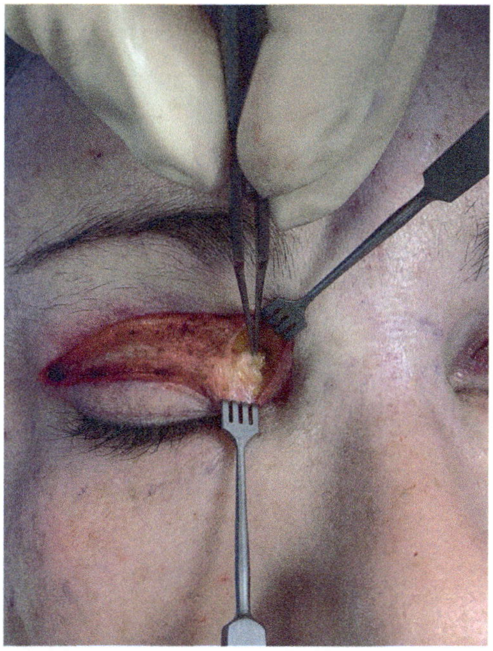

• **Fig. 64.7** The orbicularis and septum are entered medially with the edges of the wound raised to prevent inadvertent injury to the levator.

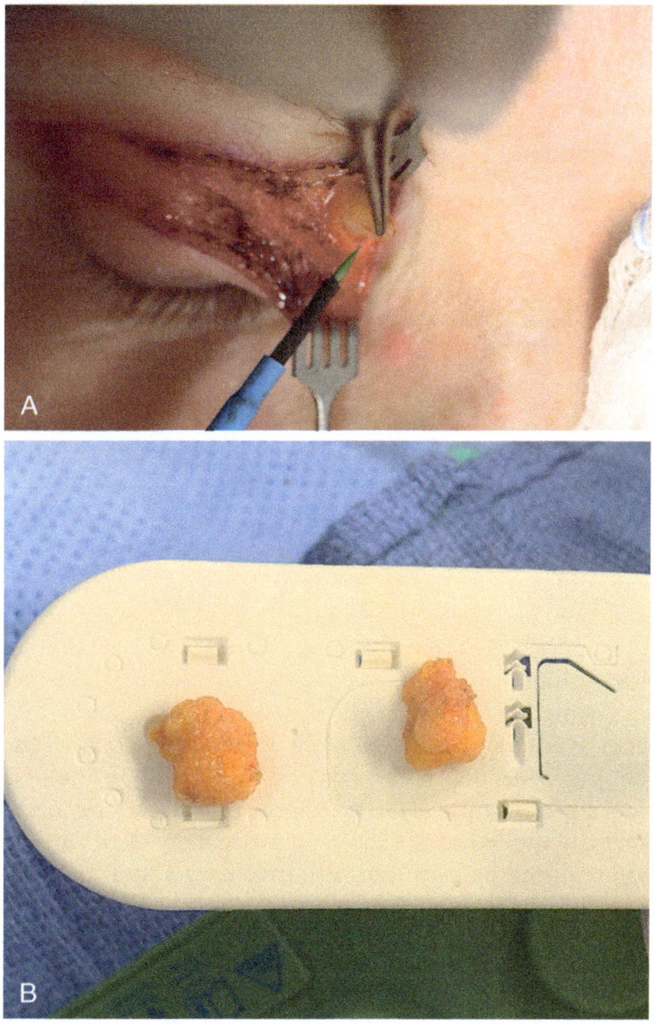

• **Fig. 64.8** (A) Nasal fat is removed conservatively. Care is taken to completely cauterize the fat to prevent retraction of any vessels into the post-septal area. (B) Excised fat pads.

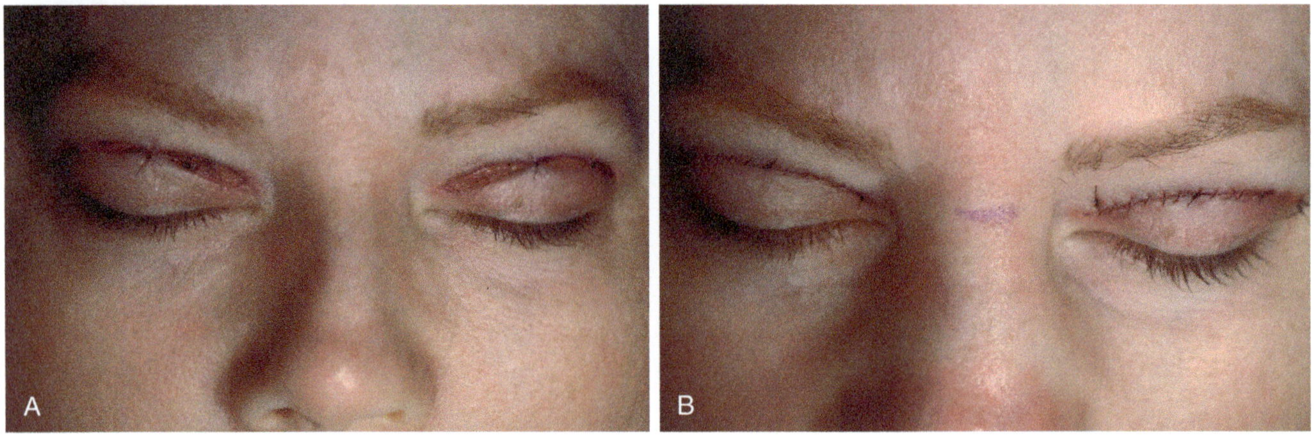

• **Fig. 64.9** (A) Simple interrupted sutures are placed centrally and laterally to decrease wound tension. (B) Skin closure with running nylon suture.

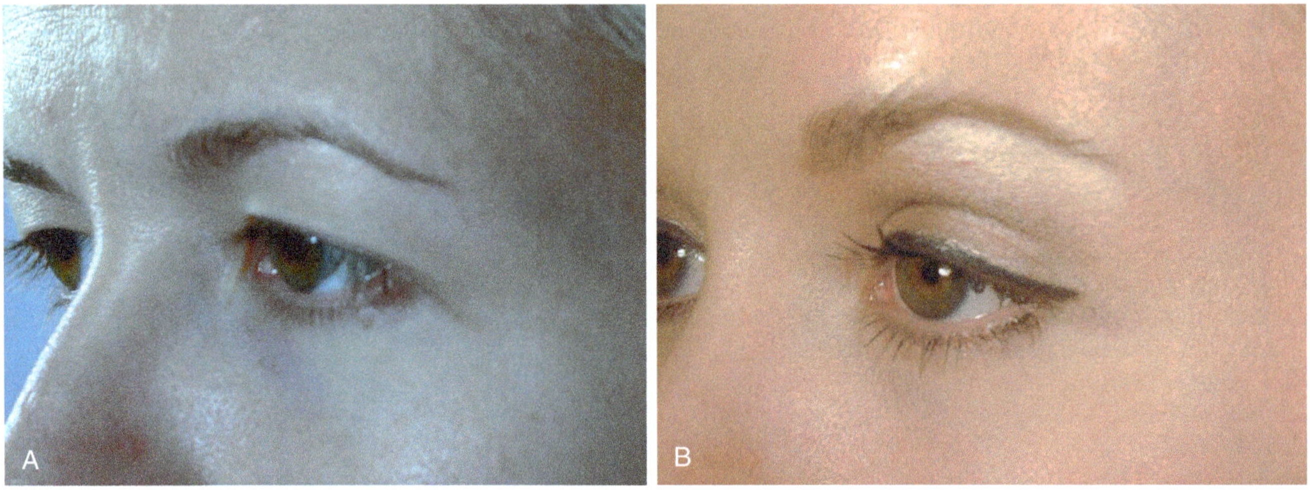

• **Fig. 64.10** (A) Before and (B) 10 months after endoscopic brow lift and upper blepharoplasty.

Postoperative Care

Immediately following the procedure, the eyes are gently covered with ice-soaked gauze and kept in place continuously until the patient goes to sleep. Compressive bandages are not routinely used but cold compresses are recommended every hour for the next 48 hours to diminish swelling.

Artificial tears are used as needed and ocular lubricant is recommended at night given the potential for temporary lagophthalmos caused by swelling in the first few days. A thin layer of ophthalmic antibiotic ointment is applied to the incisions twice daily until sutures are removed between postoperative days 5 and 7. Hand hygiene is encouraged prior to touching the face or the incisions. Pain is minimal and usually well controlled with acetaminophen.

Head elevation to 45° is recommended for the first 14 days following surgery to minimize edema. The use of makeup is permitted after one week. Intense physical activity is limited for 3 weeks as exercise could contribute to bleeding or worsened swelling or bruising. Alcohol, caffeine, and blood-thinning products are avoided for 2 weeks before and 2 weeks following the operation. All incisions are protected from sun exposure for a minimum of 3 months postoperatively. Figs. 64.10–64.14 demonstrate examples of patients before and after upper eyelid surgery.

Complications

Complications following upper blepharoplasty are much less common compared to lower blepharoplasty and can often be prevented with appropriate patient selection and careful surgical planning. The development of a complication requires prompt recognition, counseling, and appropriate management to mitigate permanent sequalae.

Retrobulbar Hematoma

Retrobulbar hematoma is the most dreaded and devastating complication of upper blepharoplasty and can progress to permanent vision loss. It is caused by retraction of a bleeding vessel into the orbit that may be unrecognized or

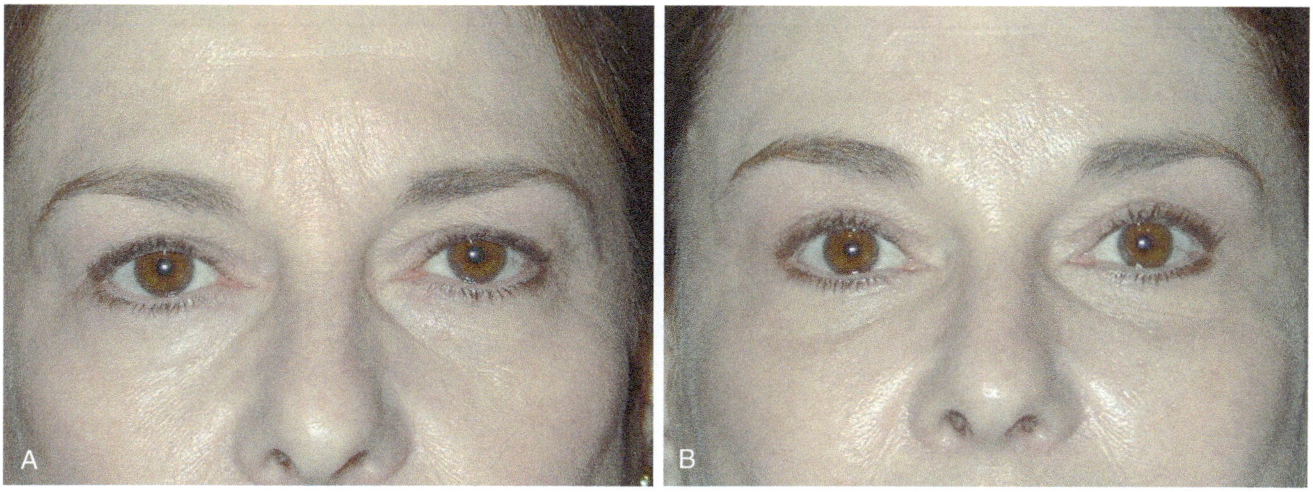

• **Fig. 64.11** (A) Before and (B) 2 months after temporal brow lift and upper blepharoplasty.

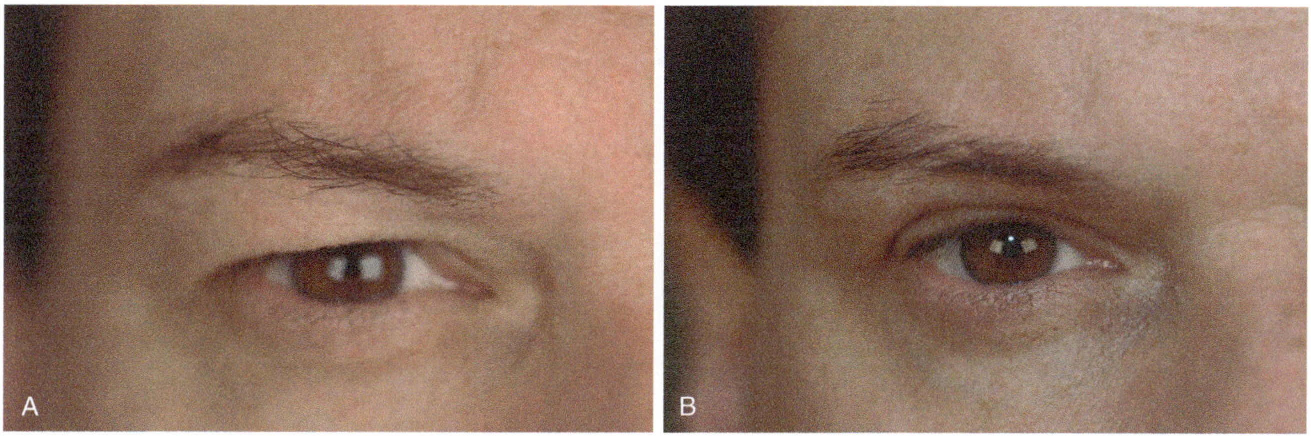

• **Fig. 64.12** (A) Before and (B) 3 months after upper blepharoplasty.

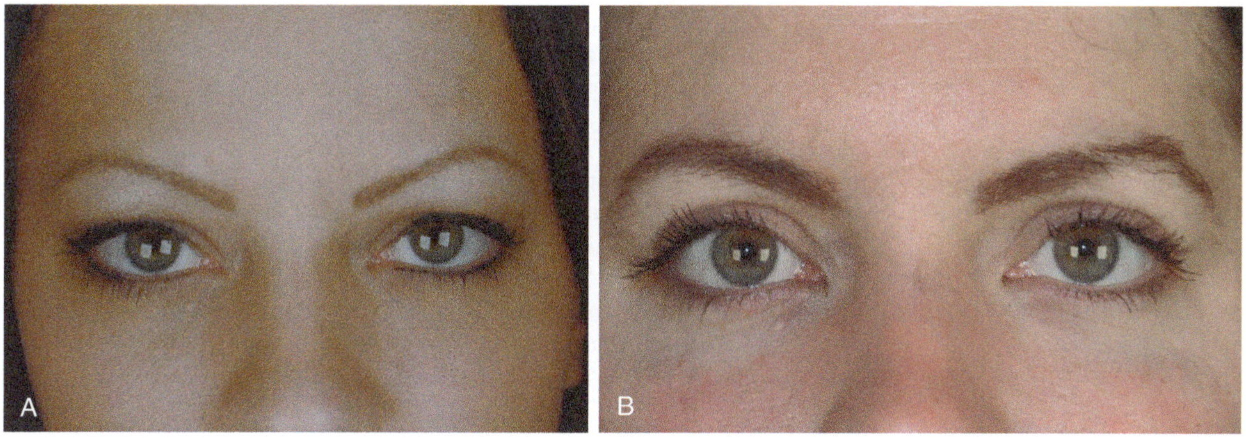

• **Fig. 64.13** (A) Before and (B) 5 years after upper blepharoplasty.

difficult to control given its location. Symptoms include decreased visual acuity, diminished extraocular movement, pain, nausea, and vomiting. The patient develops proptosis and firmness of the globe and lid, loss of pupillary response, and scleral hematoma. Treatment involves immediate recognition and return to the operating room for lateral canthotomy and release of orbital ligaments to relieve intraocular pressure. Adjunct therapy includes administration of mannitol, diuretics, and intravenous steroids.

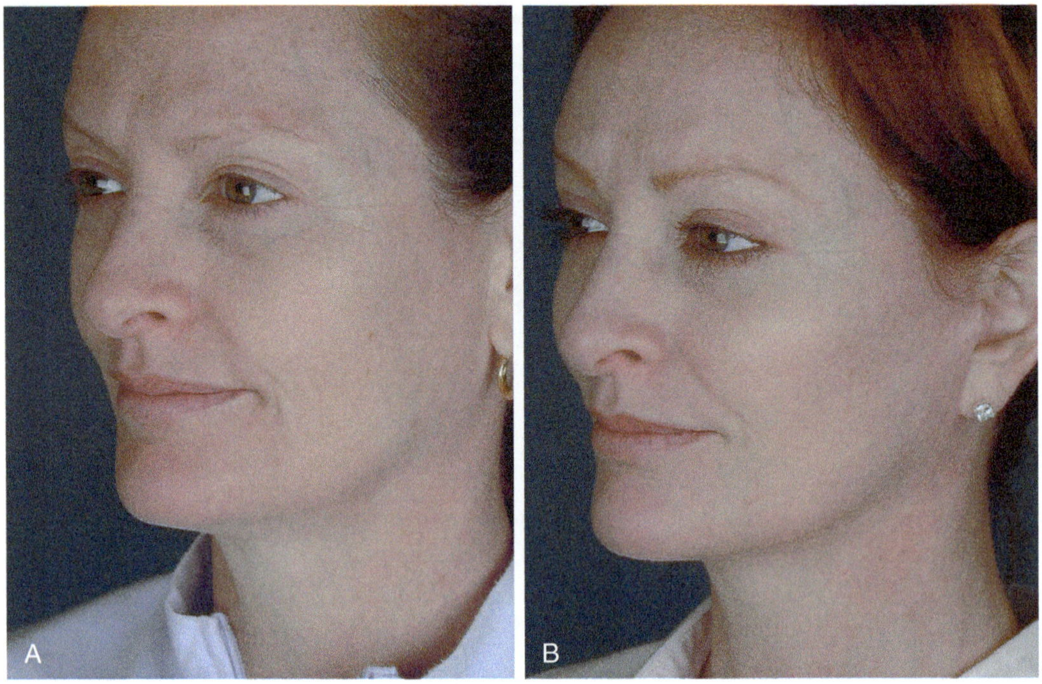

• **Fig. 64.14** (A) Before and (B) 5 months temporal brow lift and upper blepharoplasty.

Lagophthalmos

Incomplete lid closure following upper blepharoplasty is often temporary and secondary to postoperative edema. Causes of persistent lagophthalmos include over-resection of skin, scarring, a weakened orbicularis oculi muscle or paralysis of the temporal branch of the facial nerve. This condition may be managed conservatively with massage to stretch the lid and ocular lubrication to prevent corneal injury. Full thickness skin grafting may be necessary to restore lid height in severe lagophthalmos.

Blepharoptosis

Temporary ptosis is usually a result of upper lid edema and resolves spontaneously. The most common cause of postoperative ptosis is undiagnosed ptosis preoperatively. The presence of any degree of ptosis preoperatively should be clearly documented and discussed with the patient. Interruption of the levator mechanism can occur during deep fat dissection or excision of orbicularis muscle (Fig. 64.15). If ptosis persists, repair should be delayed until blepharoplasty healing is complete.

Medial Canthal Webbing

Webbing of the upper lid incision results from extension of the medial incision beyond the medial canthus. Careful marking and conservative resection of skin medially will prevent webbing. It may be corrected with Z, W, or V to Y-plasty as indicated.

Conjunctivitis/Chemosis

Conjunctival inflammation can result from infection, corneal abrasion or disruption of eyelid lymphatics. Infection is rare but should be recognized and treated appropriately with culture-directed antibiotic therapy. Corneal abrasion often presents with pain and severe light sensitivity. It is treated with eye patch or contact lens placement. Chemosis is managed conservatively with lubrication and massage. Chemosis may last several months. Severe cases can require suture tarsorrhaphy and patching.

Oversculpting/Hallowed Appearance

The shift toward fat conservation and repositioning has helped to decrease the incidence of hallowing the orbit. Careful preoperative assessment and conservative fat removal, if any, can prevent this unnatural result. If needed, improvement can be achieved with dermal fillers or fat transfer.

Epiphora/Dry Eye

Both excess tearing and dryness can be consequences of lagophthalmos. Lid margin malposition and disruption of the lacrimal system will lead to dryness. Symptoms of preexisting dry eye can be exacerbated after blepharoplasty. Ocular protection and addressing the underlying causes is the mainstay of treatment.

Conclusion

Upper blepharoplasty is a vital aspect of facial rejuvenation. Modern trends toward natural cosmetic goals have propelled surgeons to convert from a subtractive surgical approach to one of volume restoration. When executed by a mindful surgeon in an ideal candidate, upper blepharoplasty can restore youth and enhance beauty of the upper third of the face.

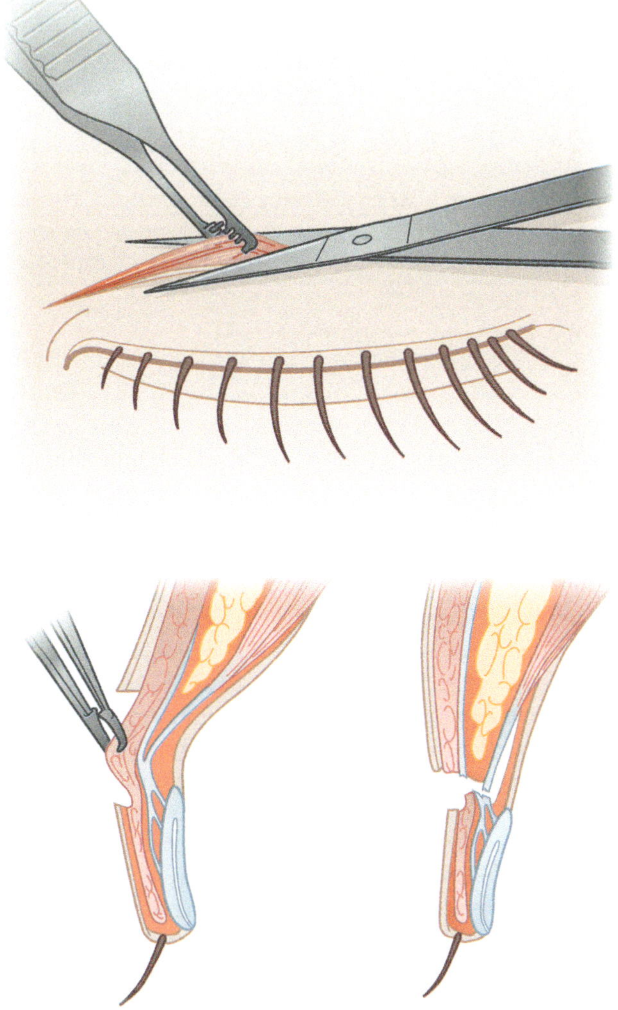

• **Fig. 64.15** Risk of inadvertent injury to the levator aponeurosis during resection of orbicularis oculi muscle.

References

1. Bhattacharjee K, Misra DK, Deori N. Updates on upper eyelid blepharoplasty. *Indian J Ophthalmol.* 2017;65:551–558.
2. Castro E, Foster JA. Upper lid blepharoplasty. *Facial Plast Surg.* 1999;15:173–181.
3. Romeo F. Upper eyelid filling approach (U.E.F.A.) technique: state of the art after 500 consecutive patients. *Aesthetic Plast Surg.* 2019;43(3):663–672.
4. Rohrich RJ, Villanueva NL, Afrooz PN. Refinements in upper blepharoplasty: the five-step technique. *Plast Reconstr Surg.* 2018;141:1144–1146.
5. Goldberg RA, Lew H. Cosmetic outcome of posterior approach ptosis surgery (an American Ophthalmologic Society thesis). *Trans Am Ophthalmol Soc.* 2011;109:157–167.
6. Drolet BC, Sullivan PK. Evidence-based medicine: blepharoplasty. *Plast Reconstr Surg.* 2014;133:1195–1205.
7. DeBiasio F, Miotti G, Zingaretti NM, et al. Study on the aging dynamics of the periorbital region: from observation to knowledge of physiopathology. et al. *Ophthalmic Plast Reconstr Surg.* 2019;35(4):333–341.
8. Leatherbarrow B. *Oculoplastic Surgery.* London: Informa Healthcare; 2011.
9. Spinelli HM. *Atlas of Aesthetic Eyelid and Periocular Surgery.* Philadelphia: Saunders; 2004.
10. Doxanas MT, Anderson RL. Oriental eyelids: an anatomic study. *Arch Ophthalmol.* 1984;102:1232–1235.
11. Holt JE, Holt GR. Blepharoplasty: indications and preoperative assessment. *Arch Otolaryngol Head Neck Surg.* 1985;111:394–397.
12. Weissman JD, Most SP. Upper lid blepharoplasty. *Facial Plast Surg.* 2013;29:16–21.

65 Lower Eyelid and Midcheek Rejuvenation

CHIN HO WONG AND BRYAN MENDELSON

For videos accompanying this chapter see ExpertConsult.com. See inside cover for access details.

Introduction

The lower eyelid and midcheek are areas that patients commonly present with, usually with the complaint of eye bags or just "looking tired." Intuitively, it should be appreciated that these patients are actually looking for rejuvenation of the midcheek and to look more youthful, not merely for the elimination of the eye bags. The eye bags – bulging of the preseptal segment of the lower lid – is perhaps one of the earliest signs of facial aging, accordingly the patients come in complaining of the deformity. It is, however, certainly not the sole physical change responsible for the features of the aging midcheek. Collectively, these changes result in the "tired" look.[1–5] Accordingly, removal of the eye bags alone, without concomitantly addressing other aspects of the aging midcheek, will lead to disappointment for the patient and the surgeon. In order to rejuvenate the midcheek, each component that changes with aging has to be addressed. Accordingly, technique selection depends on the specific aging changes needing to be addressed for the individual patient. Understanding the surgical anatomy is the key to the development of anatomically sound surgical approaches, that are effective, while minimizing trauma from the surgery and thereby reducing downtime and complications.[6,7]

The Youthful Midcheek

The principles of the construction of the facial soft tissues and the key concepts of facial gliding planes, called facial soft tissue spaces, and facial retaining ligaments have been discussed in our chapter on facial aging (Chapter 62). The youthful midcheek is full and firm located high on the cheeks. The contour is smooth, without surface grooves or bulges. The pretarsal bulge, anatomically the pretarsal part of the orbicularis oculi, may be prominent relative to the preseptal part, and is the visual location of the junction of the lower eyelid and cheek – the so-called lid–cheek junction. What is called the youthful lid–cheek junction is high and actually on the lid itself, above the midcheek! This high lid–cheek junction appearance is so profound that it dominates over other aging areas of the face for the overall perception of youth and vigor.

Changes of the Midcheek with Aging

With aging, changes occur at the two fundamental levels: the *midcheek skeleton* and the overlying *soft tissues*. The midcheek skeleton, especially the maxilla medially, retrudes significantly with aging (Fig. 65.1).[1,2] The resultant loss of projection and support for the overlying soft tissues predisposes to sagging of the tissue, which gives the visual impression of loss of soft tissue volume. Where the soft tissues overlie retaining ligaments the skin remains firmly attached to the underlying skeleton and manifests as surface grooves, given different names at different locations on the face. These include the nasojugal groove, so-called tear trough deformity, medially and midcheek furrow more laterally, whereas over the facial soft tissue spaces laxity in the roof of the space manifests as a surface bulge. In the lower eyelid, bulging over the preseptal space results in the development of eye bags. Laxity over the roof of the prezygomatic space is the anatomical basis for malar mounds or bags. This combination of relatively strong fixation in areas directly overlying retaining ligaments contrasted with laxity of tissue in the roof of adjacent soft tissue spaces results in segmentation of the midcheek into three segments – the lid–cheek, malar, and nasolabial segments (Fig. 65.2).[5] The visual location of the lid–cheek junction moves inferiorly to the groove formed by the tear trough ligament and the orbicularis retaining ligament, resulting in a lowered lid–cheek junction, which is a feature of aging.

Surgical Anatomy and Dissection Planes

This combination of skeletal retrusion with the resulting weakening of the support for the overlying soft tissues and the propensity for the midcheek soft tissue to develop specific areas of laxity results in the prototypical and predictable changes seen with aging in the midcheek. To restore and rejuvenate the midcheek soft tissues, the logical approach is to surgically address these aging changes directly at the level

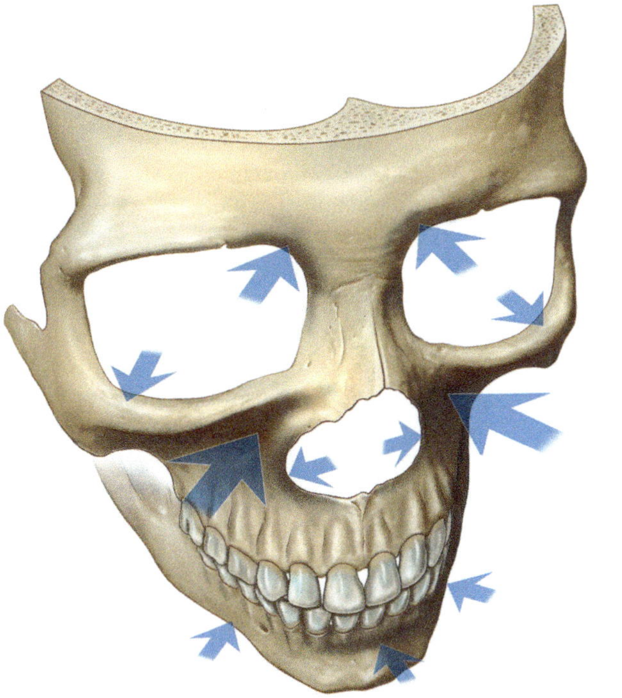

• **Fig. 65.1** The areas of the facial skeleton documented in the literature that selectively resorb with aging. The arrow size indicates the relative tendency for bone loss. Note the strong tendency for the medial midcheek (the maxilla) to resorb with aging, resulting in significant loss of projection of the overlying soft tissues. (From Mendelson B, Wong C-H. Facelift: Facial anatomy and aging. In Rubin JP, Neligan PC, eds. *Plastic Surgery*. Volume 2: *Aesthetic Surgery*. 4th edn. Elsevier; 2018: Fig. 6.1.17. © Dr. Levent Efe, CMI.)

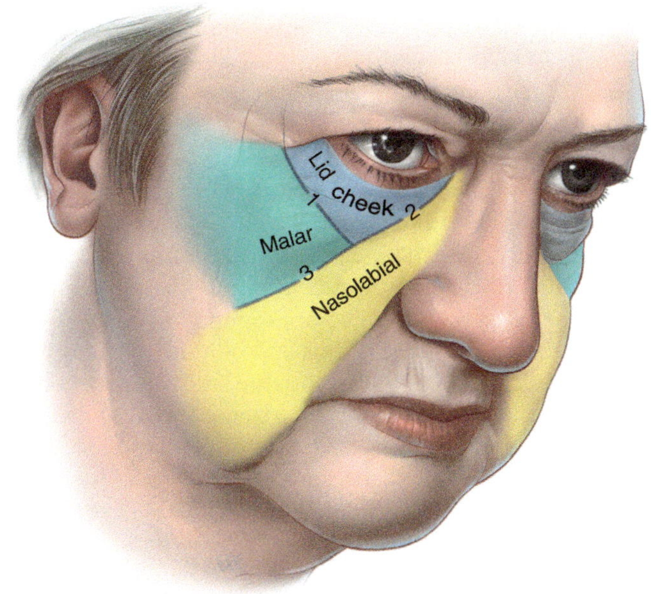

• **Fig. 65.2** In youth, the spaces are tight, being more potential than real. The retaining ligaments are stout and the transition between spaces is not discernible. With aging, the spaces expand to a greater extent than the laxity that develops in the ligaments within their boundaries, resulting in bulges between areas of relative fixation. This results in the "segmentation" of the midcheek into three characteristic segments; the lid–cheek, malar, and nasolabial segments. (From Mendelson B, Wong C-H. Facelift: Facial anatomy and aging. In: Rubin JP, Neligan PC, eds. *Plastic Surgery.* Volume 2: *Aesthetic Surgery*. 4th edn. Elsevier; 2018: Fig. 6.1.19. © Dr. Levent Efe, CMI.)

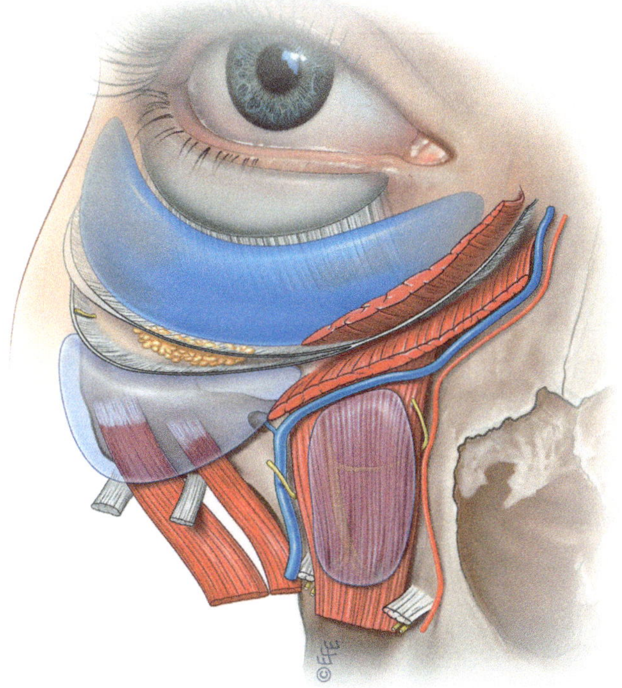

• **Fig. 65.3** The midcheek soft tissue spaces and facial retaining ligaments. (From Mendelson B, Wong C-H. Facelift: Facial anatomy and aging. In: Rubin JP, Neligan PC, eds. *Plastic Surgery*. Volume 2: *Aesthetic Surgery*. 4th edn. Elsevier; 2018: Fig. 6.1.11. © Dr. Levent Efe, CMI.)

these changes are occurring. To produce natural results and minimize downtime associated with surgical dissection, the key is to utilize the midcheek facial soft tissue spaces, which are preexisting gliding planes that are avascular with no vital structures traversing within (Fig. 65.3).[8–10] To access these spaces, the retaining ligaments in the boundary of the spaces must be sharply released. Once released, the surgeon will note the profound mobility of the roof with traction. This approach may be summarized as "through the facial soft tissues spaces with precise release of intervening retaining ligaments approach."[3] In terms of dissection plane, this is a sub-SMAS (superficial musculoaponeurotic system) dissection. This concept will be detailed in the surgical techniques below. Aging of the facial skeleton[2] may be addressed by skeletal augmentation, using either hydroxyapatite bone substitute, structural fat grafting or facial fillers.

Patient Selection

Patient selection is key in ensuring the delivery of results that are gratifying for the patient and surgeon. In general, patient with early aging changes may be treated with nonsurgical methods with good results.[1] While noninvasive methods are appealing, it is a camouflage technique that provides no correction of the underlying anatomy for a long-term solution to rejuvenate the patient, and requires repeated treatments with associated risks. Modern advanced minimally invasive techniques (extended transconjunctival approach) are indicated for the majority of patients that one would consider for treatment with facial fillers. Significantly, the transconjunctival approach provides a long-term result compared with the use of fillers. It is up to the individual patient and plastic surgeon to decide on the approach to be used. For patients with more significant aging changes, a more aggressive approach incorporating some form of midcheek tightening is required to deliver a more profound rejuvenation.

Nonsurgical Techniques

A nonsurgical approach has become extremely popular with doctors of various expertise levels performing these procedures.[2] Nonsurgical technique for rejuvenation of the midcheek is primarily delivered via the use of fillers. Fillers may be broadly classified into synthetic and autologous materials. The most commonly used synthetic fillers are hyaluronic acid (HA)-based. A variety of semi-permanent and permanent fillers are available in different markets. The authors recommend the use of HA-based fillers only as in the event of adverse outcomes or complications an antidote (Hylase) is available to dissolve and remove the unwanted filler material. Fat grafts are an autologous filler. The benefits of autologous tissues are they integrate with the facial soft tissue, are long lasting (when done correctly), and give benefits beyond volumization from mesenchymal stem cells in the transferred fat. The disadvantages are that harvesting of the fat is required and the procedure is more technically demanding. Fat grating, however, is usually used as an adjunct to surgical treatment and the discussion below pertains specifically to the use of HA-based fillers.

As discussed, aging is a multifactorial process, involving retrusion of the midcheek skeleton and laxity/sagging of the tissues. Fillers work by providing volume/support that to a certain degree compensates for the retrusion of the facial skeleton thus providing a subtle rejuvenating effect. Used in combination, fillers and neurotoxins soften the tear trough (TT) deformity in appropriately selected patients, in general, patients with early aging changes looking to have a little freshening up. Fig. 65.4 illustrates patient classification for treatment with injectables. This degree of "softening" is usually sufficient and may *even* be very satisfying for grades 1 and 2 TT deformity. As the tear trough ligament cannot be released or divided with nonsurgical techniques, the correction achievable in more advanced tear trough deformities (grades 3 and 4 TT) is generally insufficient and a surgical approach is needed.

Filler for the correction of the tear trough deformity and camouflaging mild eye bags may be placed deep and/or superficial. Deep placement of the filler should be placed caudal to the tear trough ligament on the anterior maxilla (Fig. 65.5). Fillers here function to correct the skeletal/maxillary retrusion (which may be congenital in some patients or as a result of anterior maxillary resorption with aging in older patients) as well as the deflation that occurs with aging. This correction restores the soft tissue support inferior to the tear trough ligament and prevents the soft tissues from "dragging" on the tear trough ligament. The tethering effect is thus reduced and in some patients eliminated, resulting in a smoother lid–cheek junction. As the placement is deep and for the purpose of skeletal augmentation, the volume of filler material needed is relatively large; depending on the degree of maxillary retrusion, generally 0.1–0.5 mL per side over the anterior maxilla. Either blunt cannulas or needles may be used for deep injections. As for the type of product, a softer product should be used due to the very thin soft tissues in this area (Fig. 65.6). *Fillers should not be placed above the tear trough ligament* as placement here will worsen the tear trough deformity, similar to the effect eye bags have on the tear trough deformity. Superficial placement, in contrast, is for a different purpose. It is to correct the superficial wrinkling that is seen in some patients. As the skin is very thin and delicate at the tear trough, the amount of filler material needed (or can be injected) is very little, no more than 0.05–0.2 mL per side. As for the type of product, only very thin or fluid material should be used.

Neurotoxins complement the use of fillers in the correction of the tear trough deformity, by relaxing the orbicularis oculi located above the tear trough ligament. The microbotox technique is preferred in the tear trough (about 2–4 units in 0.3 mL of saline) injected in a very superficial level raising blebs above and below the tear trough ligament to give a more even relaxation of the muscles.

Complications of Injectables in the Midcheek

The use of fillers and botox in the tear trough is technically difficult. Potential complications include bruising from injuring the angular vein (more commonly) or the angular artery, prolonged swelling, lumpiness (that results from too much filler being injected or, over the long term, granuloma formation), surface irregularity (from placement of the product too superficially), and bluish discoloration over the medial midcheek. The bluish discoloration is the result of the Tyndall effect from placement of too much product too superficially. More severe complications included vascular compromise with skin necrosis and blindness due to intravascular injection and embolization of the filler materials.

Significantly, and perhaps not commonly discussed, are the undesirable effects of filler overuse. Filling is beneficial only up to a degree. Fillers cannot be used to address laxity or sagging that logically should be addressed with some form of tightening/lift. Accordingly, when more significant aging has manifest, surgical intervention is indicated. Attempting to correct the laxity by injecting more filler in the erroneous belief that filling the cheeks out would take up the laxity is flawed thinking. All plastic surgeons have seen the unnatural appearance of the "overfilled syndrome" that has resulted from this misguided approach.

A further adverse effect of the use of fillers is the relatively high incidence of granuloma formation in the long term. This present a problem for the surgeon as many patients these days would have some fillers injected. When

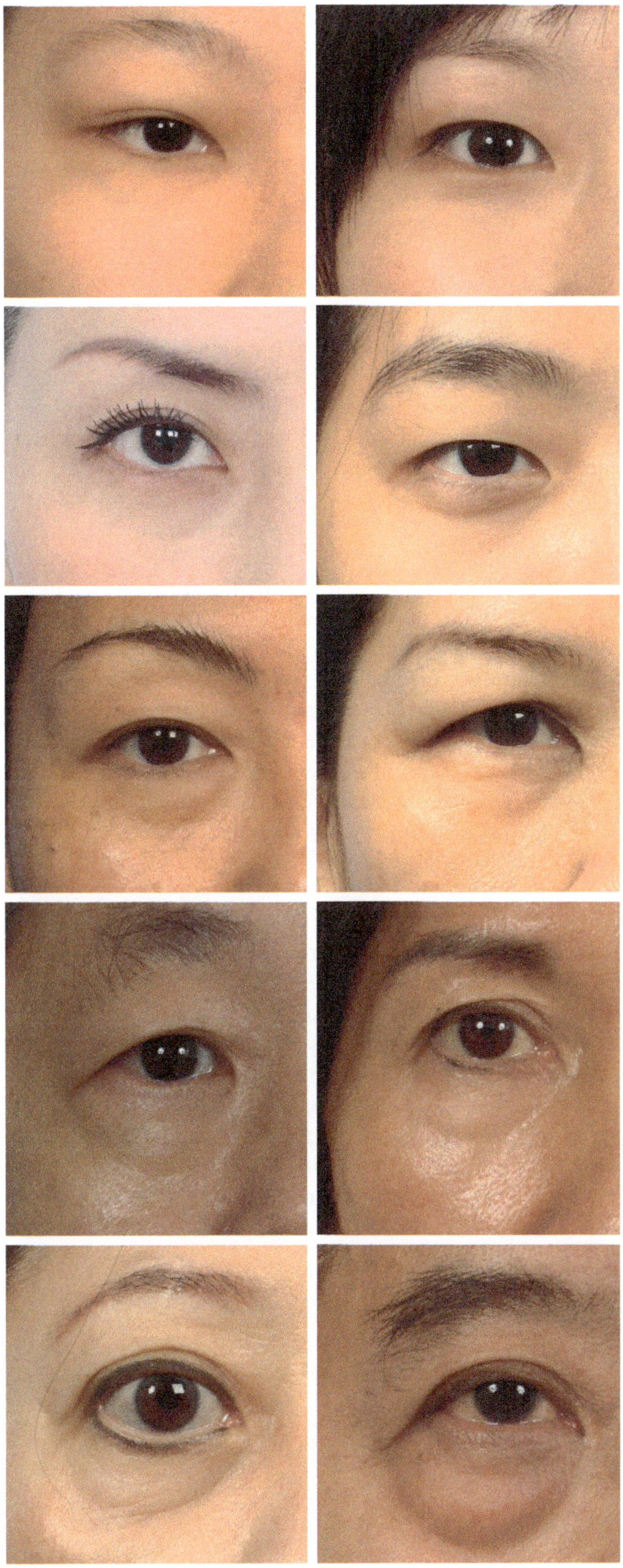

• **Fig. 65.4** A grading system for the tear trough (TT) deformity. Top row: Grade 0 TT: This is a youthful lower eyelid. The lid–cheek junction is high with no evident tethering seen from the tear trough ligament. A pretarsal bulge (from a hypertrophic orbicularis oculi) may (right image) or may not (left image) be present. Second row: Grade 1 TT: The tear trough is seen in repose as a shallow groove extending from just below the medial canthus to (but not extending beyond) the medial pupil line. Eye bags are absent and a pretarsal bulge may (right image) or may not (left image) be present. Third row: Grade 2 TT: The clinical findings are similar to Grade 1 TT but with the addition of the presence of eye bags. Fourth row: Grade 3 TT: The tear trough becomes continuous with the palpebromalar groove with a visually distinct (and low) lid–cheek junction (or separation). Eye bags are seen and midcheek retrusion and ptosis seen below this. Fifth row: Grade 4 TT: A sharply demarcated and continuous lid–cheek junction is seen. Prominent eye bags above and midcheek descent and retrusion is seen below the lid–cheek junction.

these patients present for surgery, it is best to dissolve these granulomas with a mixture of Hylase (if these were HA-based fillers) and steroids at least 1 week prior to surgery. If this is not feasible, then it must be done immediately before the surgery in combination with the administration of local anesthetic.

Surgical Correction of Midcheek Aging

Surgery remains the gold standard for natural and lasting rejuvenation of the midcheek. Two main approaches to midcheek and eye bags may be used: the transconjunctival approach or the subciliary (transcutaneous) approach. Each has its specific indication, benefits, and risks. Correction of the midcheek skeletal retrusion with fat grafting or skeletal augmentation may be used as adjunctive procedures with either approach. The selection of the approach depends primarily on the extent of aging changes present and the patient's specific requests.

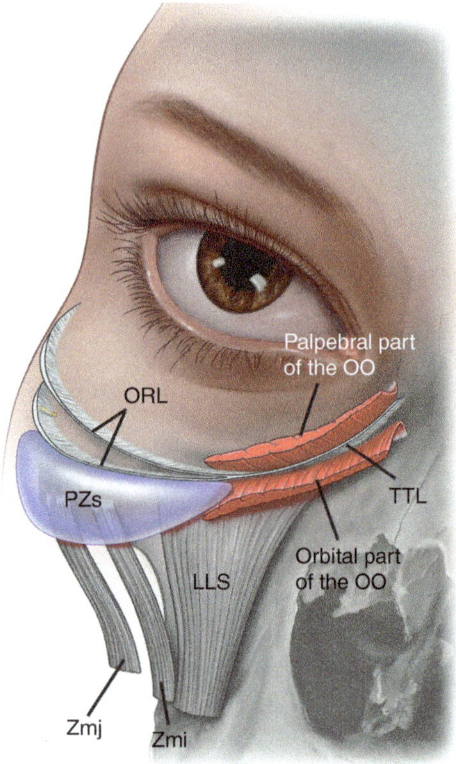

• **Fig. 65.5** The anatomy of the tear trough ligament. (From Mendelson B, Wong C-H. Facelift: Facial anatomy and aging. In: Rubin JP, Neligan PC, eds. *Plastic Surgery*. Volume 2: *Aesthetic Surgery*. 4th edn. Elsevier; 2018: Fig 6.1.14. © Dr. Levent Efe, CMI.)

Extended Transconjunctival Lower Eyelid Blepharoplasty

The transconjunctival lower eyelid blepharoplasty offers an advantageous access to the lower eyelid and midcheek because of its safety (by avoiding trauma to the anterior lamella of the lower eyelid) and its quick recovery.[11] The transconjunctival fat removal only type of procedures are very popular, effective for patients with true lower eyelid fat pad excesses, and easy to perform. The benefit of the procedure is limited to the lid–cheek segment of the midcheek due to the limited nature of the dissection. However, for more profound rejuvenation via the transconjunctival approach, it is necessary to take the dissection significantly caudal to the orbital rim.[9,10,12,13] This type of procedure, called the extended transconjunctival approach, as described below, is more versatile and powerful to address aging changes of the midcheek. This approach is good for patients with prominent eye bags, with tear trough deformity with minimal laxity of the midcheek soft tissues. In patients with midcheek loss of projection, structural fat grafting may be performed at the same time.

Markings and Preparation

Preoperatively, with the patient upright, the location and amount of fat pads to be removed are determined and marked. A mental image of the expected fat to be excised should be visualized as the key component to good results is precise removal of fat. The midcheek groove, anatomically formed by the tear trough ligament and orbicularis retaining ligament, that needs to be released is also marked. The procedure can be performed either under local or general anesthesia. The cornea is anaesthetized with 2 drops of Alcaine 0.5% eye drops (Alcon-Couvreur, Belgium). The

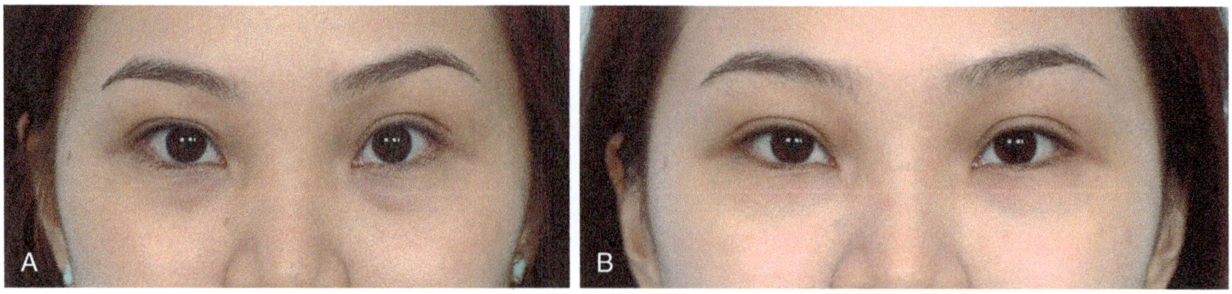

• **Fig. 65.6** (A,B) This 26-year-old woman presented with eye bags and looking tired. She had congenitally retruded maxillae with inadequate skeletal support, which resulted in the premature appearance of eye bags. She has Grade 2 tear trough, no laxity of her soft tissue, and small eye bags, and is a good candidate for filler injections. Correction was achieved by preperiosteal (deep) placement of a soft hyaluronic acid filler (1 mL) inferior to the tear trough ligament to enhance the skeleton. A soft filler is preferred for correction of the tear troughs to reduce palpability in this area of thin soft tissues.

cornea is lubricated with some Duratears (Alcon-Couvreur) and protective corneal eye shield placed. The conjunctiva, lower eyelid, and midcheek are anaesthetized with a mixture of 10 mL of 1% ropivacaine, 10 mL 1% lidocaine and 0.25 mL of 1:1000 adrenaline. The lower lid, midcheek and lateral orbital rim is infiltrated with a total of 3 mL of the local anesthetic mixture each side.

Surgical Technique

See Video 65.1 for demonstration of the authors' surgical technique. With two fine skin hooks applying gentle upward traction on the lower eyelids, an approximately 15-mm transconjunctival incision is made about 2 mm inferior to the lower edge of the tarsus using a sharp point diathermy, incising through the conjunctival and lower eyelid retractors. The skin hooks are replaced by a small, insulated Desmarres retractor. The preseptal space is bluntly entered with a tenotomy scissors. The orbital septum is then opened directly over the areas where the fat pads would be removed. The orbital fat pads are excised as indicated and meticulous hemostasis performed.

The Desmarres is replaced with the blunt end of a cat's paw retractor and the preseptal space then bluntly developed to its boundaries with a gentle sweeping motion with a cotton bud, carefully looking for the white line that defines the location of the arcus marginalis. A key landmark, the origin of the palpebral part of the orbicularis oculi is located slightly caudal to the arcus marginalis. With the assistant holding the retractor upwards and the surgeon pushing the orbital septum down with the cotton bud, the orbicularis oculi is sharply released with cutting cautery at its bony origin. The palpebral part of the orbicularis oculi, tear trough ligament, and the orbital part of the orbicularis oculi are sequentially released, taking care that the dissection stays close to the anterior maxilla. The end point of the release is the visualization of muscular fibers of the levator labii superioris. This heralds the entrance into the premaxillary space and, accordingly, the complete release of the tear trough ligament (Fig. 65.7). More laterally, the medial part of the orbicularis retaining ligament is also released.

The excised fat is then placed under the tear trough ligament as free fat grafts and secured with Vicryl 6-0 percutaneous sutures. These are secured with Steristrips. The

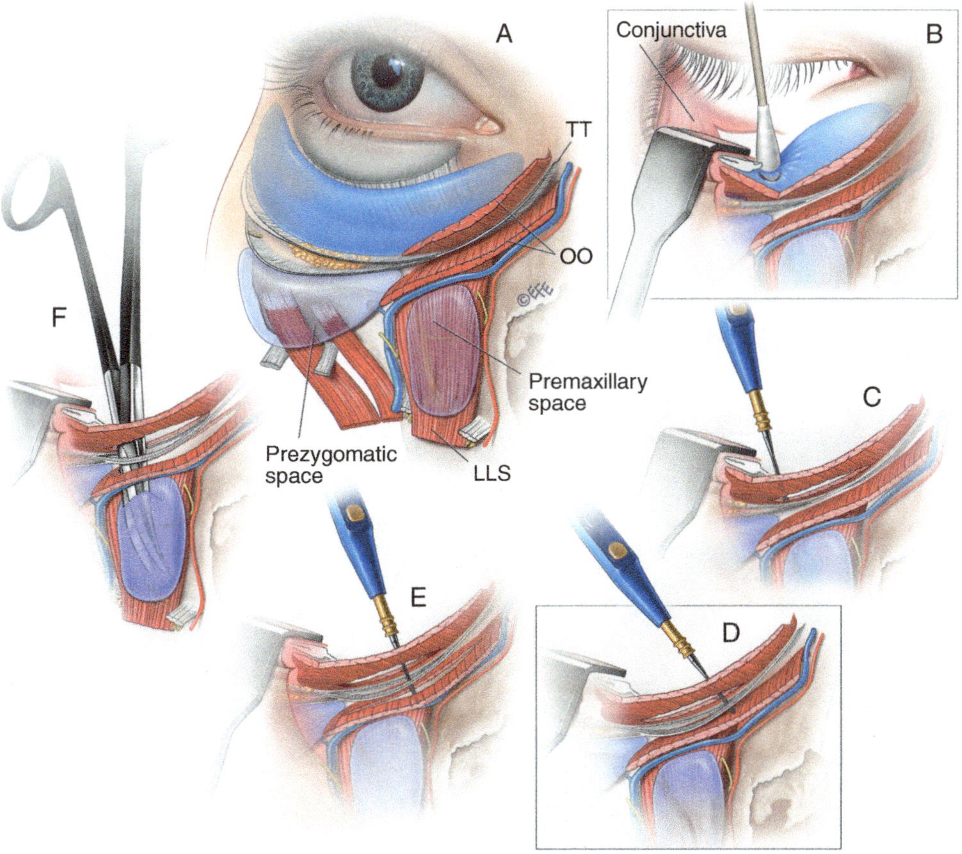

• **Fig. 65.7** (A) Facial soft tissue spaces and retaining ligaments of the midcheek. (B) Bluntly opening the preseptal space. Sharp release of (C) the palpebral part of the orbicularis oculi, (D) the tear trough ligament, and (E) the orbital part of the orbicularis oculi. (F) Bluntly opening the premaxillary space with tenotomy scissors. This is the concept of atraumatic dissection by dissecting in the facial soft tissue spaces and precisely releasing the retaining ligaments that separate the spaces. (From Wong CH, Mendelson B. Long-term static and dynamic effects of the release of the tear trough ligament and origins of the orbicularis oculi in lower eyelid blepharoplasty. *Plast Reconstr Surg*. 2019;144(3):583–591. © Dr. Levent Efe, CMI.)

conjunctival incision is closed with two or three buried 6-0 plain catgut sutures. Fig. 65.8 illustrates the correction achieved after completion of the procedure with release of the tear trough ligament and fat redistribution. Midcheek structural fat grafting, if indicated, is then performed using the Coleman technique.

The benefit of the transconjunctical approach is its relative safety. By avoiding trauma to the middle lamella of the lower lid the risk of middle lamella contracture that may result in lower eyelid malposition, scleral show, and ectropion is minimized. The surgical trauma associated with the surgical access is minimized by utilizing this "through the spaces approach" as detailed above; this would minimize downtime of the procedure (Fig. 65.9). Figs. 65.10 and 65.11 show the long-term result of this technique. This technique has consistently been effective in eliminating the tired look, with long-term correction of the tear trough deformity and in rejuvenating the midcheek. The long-term safety and efficacy of release of the tear trough ligament and its associated release of the orbicularis oculi origins has been demonstrated. The lower eyelid remains stable with no increased incidence of scleral show or ectropion.

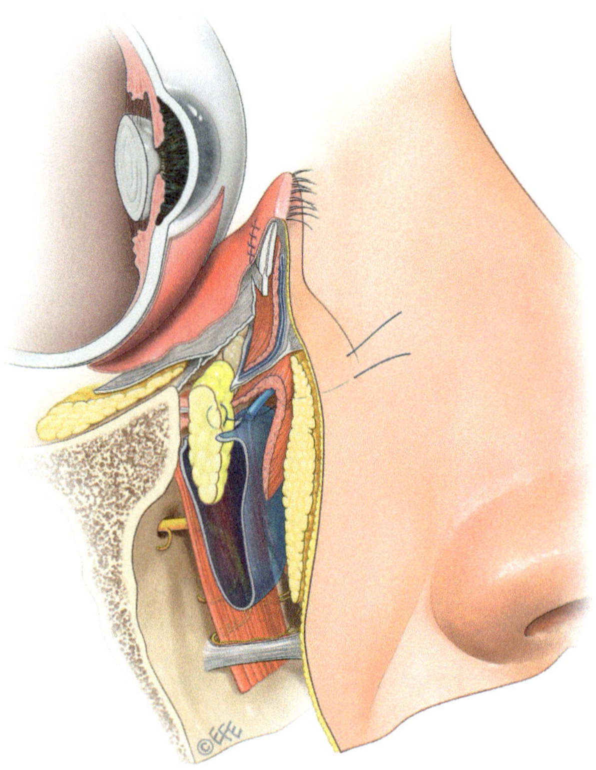

• **Fig. 65.8** Surgical correction achieved at the completion of the procedure with elimination of the eye bags and released tear trough ligament and interpositional fat grafting to revent reattachment of the tear trough ligament and augmentation of the anterior maxilla with the excised orbital fat. (From Wong CH, Mendelson B. Extended transconjunctival lower eyelid blepharoplasty with release of the tear trough ligament and fat redistribution. *Plast Reconstr Surg*. 2017;140:273–282. © Dr. Levent Efe, CMI.)

Complications

The complications of this procedure are relatively minor and infrequent. These are mostly technical. These include inadequate fat pad removal requiring revision in less than 5%, significant bruising specifically from injury to the angular vein, prolonged swelling in some patients, and transient chemosis usually lasting less than a few days. Of note, chemosis is rare with the transconjunctival approach. More serious complications reported in the literature include

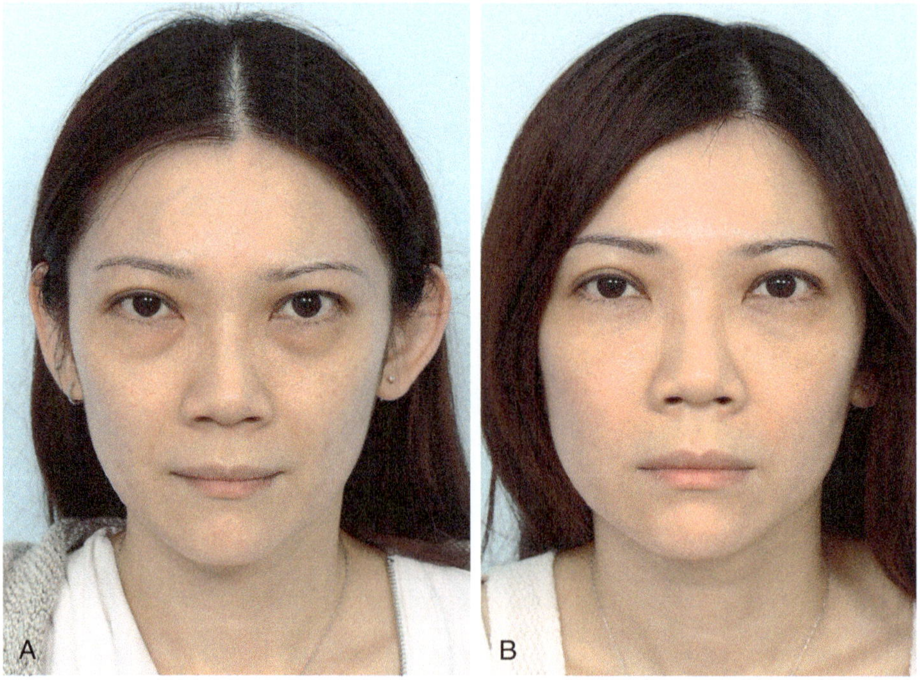

• **Fig. 65.9** (A,B) A 40-year-old woman presented with a very tired look. She underwent transconjunctival lower blepharoplasty with tear tough ligament release and fat redistribution. Shown here 7 days post surgery.

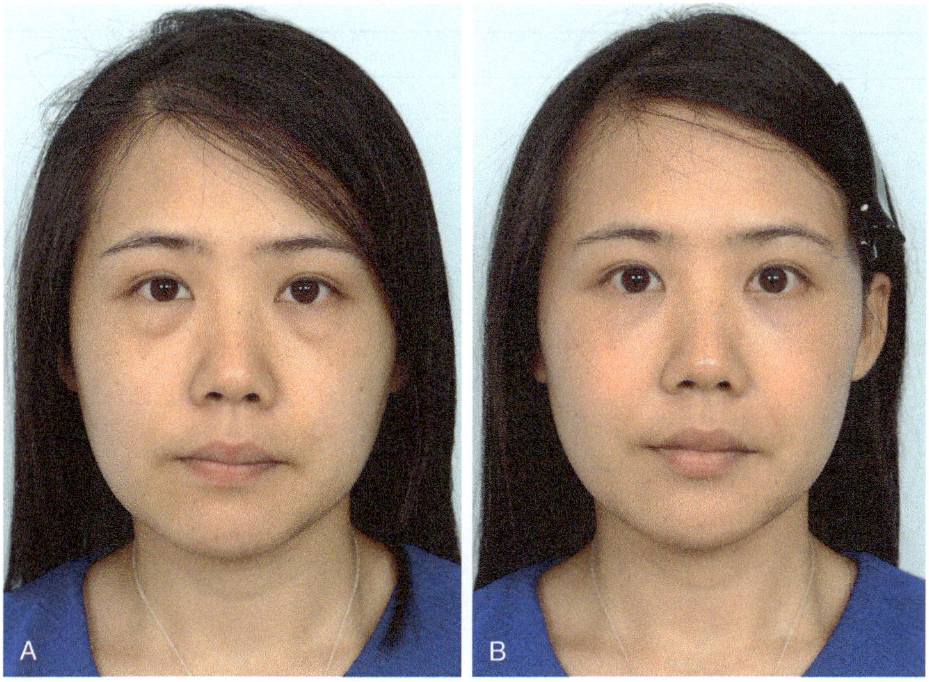

• **Fig. 65.10** (A,B) A 31-year-old woman presented with eye bags and prominent tear trough deformity. An extended transconjunctival lower blepharoplasty with tear tough ligament release and fat redistribution was performed. Shown 1-year post surgery.

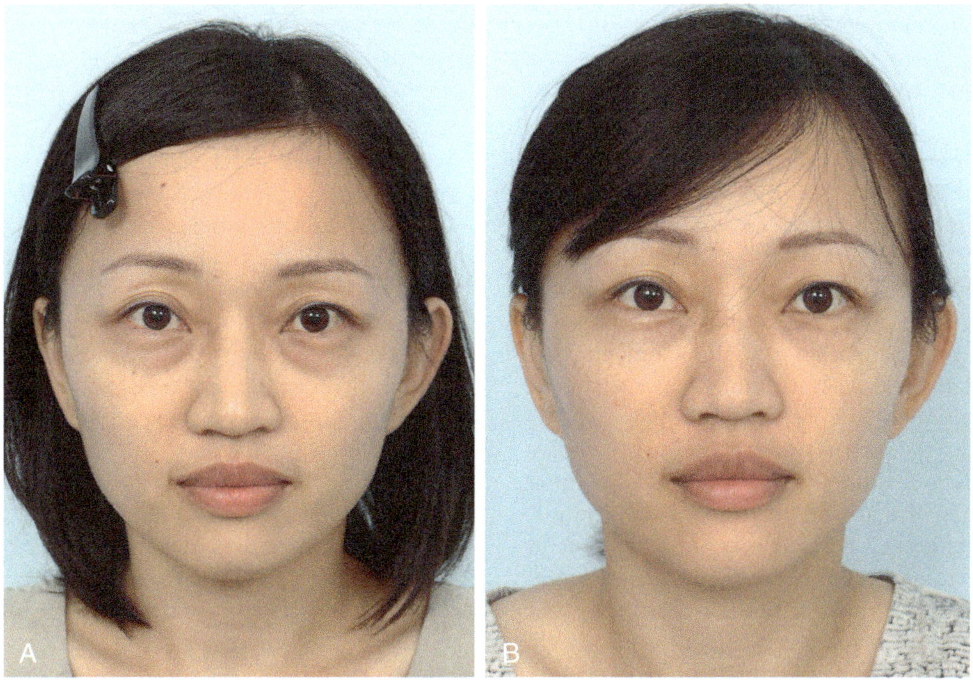

• **Fig. 65.11** (A,B) A 34-year-old woman presented with eye bags and a "tired look." She underwent transconjunctival lower blepharoplasty with tear tough ligament release and fat redistribution; also, fat grafting of the midcheek and upper eyelid. Sharp needle intradermal fat grafting (SNIF) was also performed. Shown 1-year post operation. Note the improvement of the tear trough deformity with elimination of the lid–cheek junction and also the improvement of the dark eye circles, giving a fresher and more youthful appearance.

corneal abrasions, lid retraction, diplopia from injury to the inferior oblique muscle, and dreaded retrobulbar bleed. Of note, these are rare when the technique is done correctly and is the reason for the preference of many surgeons for this technique, for its safety and quicker recovery.

Long-Term Effects of the Release of the Tear Trough Ligament and Its Associated Orbicularis Oculi Origins

A recent long-term study on the effect of release of the tear trough ligament and associated origins of the orbicularis

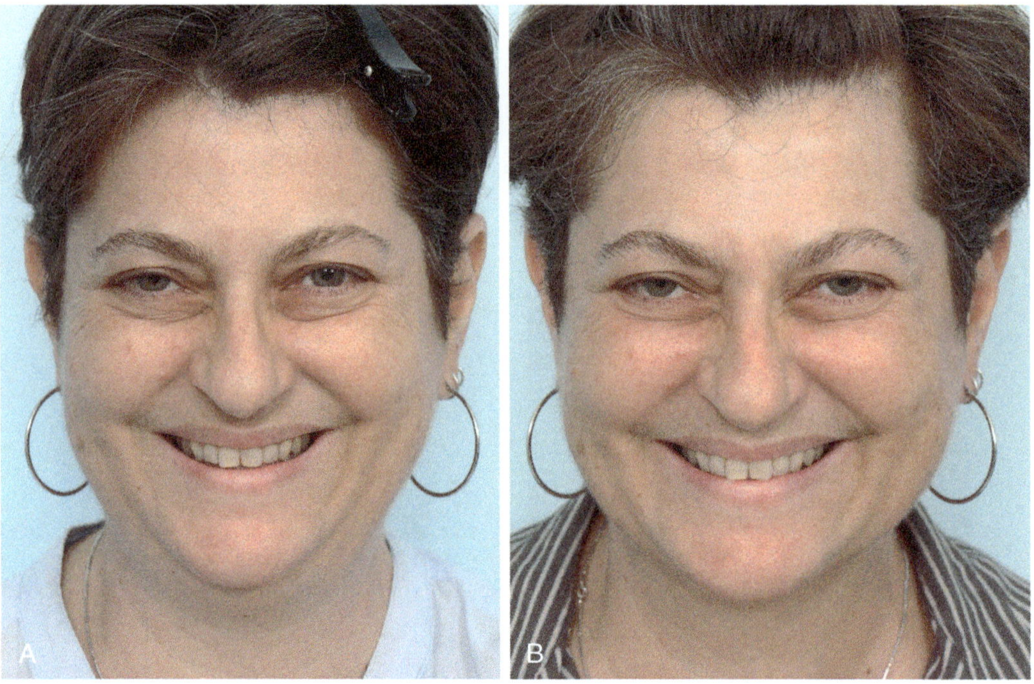

• **Fig. 65.12** (A,B) A 48-year-old woman underwent extended transconjunctival eye bag removal with release of the tear trough ligament. She is shown in (B) 24 months post surgery. Note the profound change in the esthetics of the smile. The lid–cheek junction was eliminated and "elevation" of the lid–cheek junction with smiling gives a more pleasant and youthful smile. With less efficient contraction of the orbicularis, wrinkling was visibly less. While this effect was not as powerful as that achievable with botox, it is nonetheless beneficial and is permanent, not needing repeated procedures.

documented the safety of this maneuver in the long term as well as noted the esthetic benefits of this release.[14] With release of the ligament, the following long-term changes were evident. First, the tethering with smiling was eliminated. Second, the vector of contraction of the orbicularis oculi changed to a more upward and outward direction. In combination with the elimination of the blocking effect of the tear trough ligament on elevation of cheek soft tissues with smiling, elevation of the visual location of the lid–cheek junction when the patient smiles gives the impression of a more youthful and pleasant smile (Fig. 65.12). Third, with release of the orbicularis origins, the muscle contraction becomes less efficient. This has two potential benefits on the esthetics of the smile. For patients who have a prominent pretarsal bulge due to orbicularis hypertrophy, the bulge on smiling becomes less prominent postoperatively, resulting in a more esthetic appearance. The reduced efficiency of contraction also resulted in slightly fewer crow's feet with smiling (Fig. 65.13).

Subciliary/Transcutaneous Approach

In patients with more advanced aging changes, with sagging of the midcheek, malar bags, and prominent nasolabial folds, it is important to incorporate tightening of the midcheek soft tissue into the surgical procedure.[15–17] As discussed, with recent advances in anatomical understanding, many advanced steps such as release of the tear trough ligament, septal reset, fat redistribution, and midcheek augmentation may be achieved using the transconjunctival approach, with its quicker recovery and perhaps less complications than the transcutaneous approach. The advantage provided by the subciliary approach is the opportunity it provides for a midcheek lift.[18] Accordingly, the subciliary (transcutaneous) approach is indicated for patients with cheek laxity, sagging, malar bags,and heavy nasolabial folds, while any skin excess may be addressed at the same time.

Preoperative Preparation

The areas of fat excess, and the extent of the tear trough to be corrected are marked. A mental quantitation of fat redistribution and/or removal is made. Precise planning of this aspect is crucial for effective blending of the lid–cheek junction. The procedure can be performed under local or general anesthesia. The lower eyelid, midcheek, and lateral orbital rim are anesthetized with 4–5 mL of the previously described local anesthetic mixture each side.

Surgical Technique

Our surgical technique is demonstrated in Video 65.2. A subciliary incision is made with a Beaver blade precisely elevating a skin only flap. The skin is raised off the orbicularis oculi for about 15 mm below the lateral canthus and10 mm. below the mid-pupil. This is to provide a significant cuff of orbicularis oculi as a handle on which to elevate the midcheek and to facilitate later skin redraping and excision following

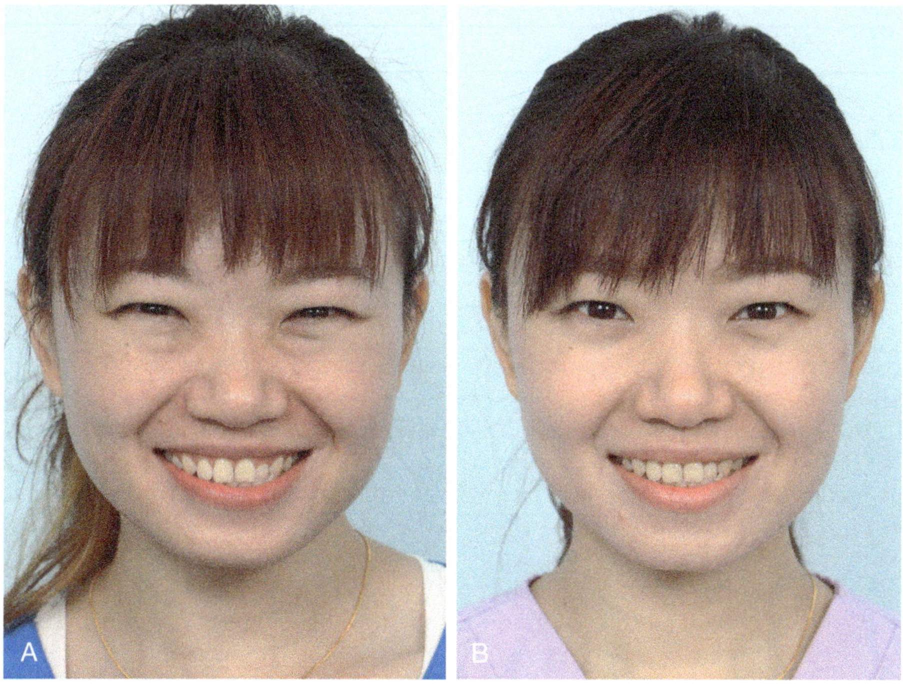

• **Fig. 65.13** (A) A 33-year-old woman presented with the primary concern of prominent eye bags when smiling. An extended transconjunctival lower eyelid blepharoplasty was performed. (B) At 6 months post surgery, note the elimination of the eye bags and augmentation of the anterior maxilla with good survival of the free fat grafts. The benefit of releasing the tear trough ligament is evident when the patient smiles. Elimination of the tethering and scrunching centered at the tear trough ligament results in a more relaxed and beautiful smile.

elevation of the cheek. At about the level of the lateral canthus with the orbicularis oculi tented up with skin hooks, a window is created in the muscle with cutting cautery. A blunt tenotomy scissor is then introduced into the suborbicularis plane and the preseptal space opened with gentle spreading of the blades. The orbicularis oculi is then tented up and cut with cautery to approximately the level of the medial corneoscleral limbus, ensuring preservation of about 5–7 mm of pretarsal orbicularis oculi. The preseptal space is a bloodless plane that can be fully developed bluntly using a cotton tip to its boundary, which is the orbicularis oculi origin medially and the orbicularis retaining ligament (ORL) laterally. Medially, over the maxilla, the origin of the orbicularis oculi (the palpebral and orbital parts of the orbicularis oculi) and the tear trough ligament located between them is sharply released with cutting cautery. Complete release then brings the dissection into the premaxillary space, heralded by the visualization of the suborbicularis oculi fat (SOOF) adherent to the underside of the orbicularis oculi muscle fascia in the roof and the levator labii superioris muscle in the floor (Fig. 65.14). This ensures the tear trough ligament is completely released. This maneuver eliminates the tear trough deformity as well as allowing mobilization of the midcheek with the concomitant release of the ORL. The ORL is completely released with cutting cautery in the preperiosteal plane. The ORL is bilamella with a distance of 5–7 mm between the upper and lower lamellae. Complete release of the ORL laterally, over the body of the zygoma, takes the dissection into the prezygomatic space. The zygomaticofacial nerve (and its associated vessels), emerge from a foramen in the body of the zygoma, closely associated with the inferior lamella of the ORL. Accordingly, visualizing this nerve heralds the entrance into the prezygomatic space and the complete release of the

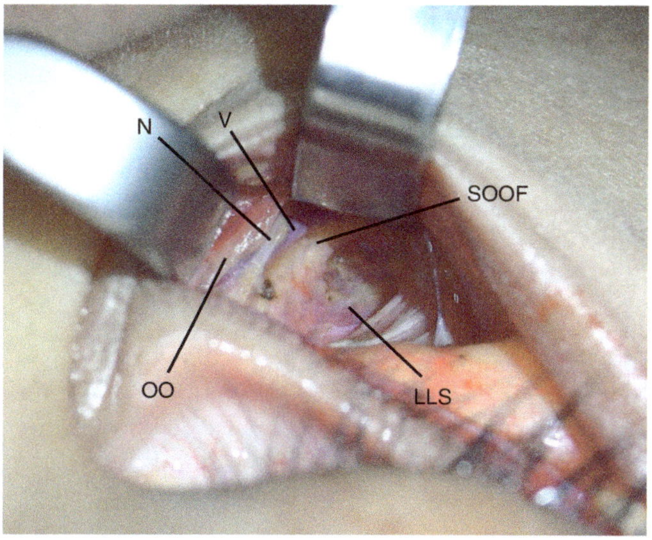

• **Fig. 65.14** Entrance into the premaxillary space is achieved by complete release of the orbicularis origin (OO) (with concomitant release of the tear trough ligament). This is confirmed by the visualization of the levator labii superioris (LLS) in the floor and the suborbicularis oculi fat (SOOF) in the roof. Note the close association of the angular vein (V) and terminal branches of the zygomatic nerve (N) with the orbicularis oculi muscle medially. Injury to these structures is avoided during the preperiosteal release of the muscle by staying close to the bone.

ORL. More laterally, the ORL continues as the lateral orbital thickening (LOT), the inferior part of which needs to be released, up to the level of the lateral canthus, to allow free elevation of the midcheek. With this release (surgically connecting the three facial soft tissue spaces of the midcheek, the preseptal, premaxillary, and prezygomatic), upward traction on the orbicularis oculi allows free and unhindered elevation of the entire midcheek. The end-point for surgical release of the midcheek ligaments is the free elevation of the upper part of the nasolabial fold as well as the malar fat pad with traction on the orbicularis oculi.

To address the eye bags and tear trough deformity, depending on the patient's anatomy, one of two maneuvers may be selected. In patients with a tear trough deformity without a significant palpebromalar groove, transposition of the medial and middle fat pads over the medial orbital rim, onto the anterior maxilla is performed. The orbital septum is opened and the fat pads transposed over the rim and secured with Vicryl 6-0 sutures. In patients presenting with more advanced aging changes with a deep lid–cheek junction, a septal reset is done. Fat removal is done conservatively, only in patients with a true excess of retro-orbital fat, usually from the lateral compartment. A canthopexy is routinely performed for all patients with a 4-0 double-arm Mersilene suture, generally at the level of the inferior edge of the pupil for patients with normal eye prominence but carefully adjusted superiorly or inferiorly depending on eye prominence as well as ensuring symmetry and good lower eyelid posture and position after tying the suture.

The midcheek lift is achieved by orbicularis suspension. This is performed in a more superior vector with Ethibond 3-0 sutures secured to the lateral orbit periosteum at or just slightly below the level of the canthopexy. Two of these sutures are placed. This achieves the midcheek lift, ensuring that the malar eminence and the upper nasolabial fold lifts sufficiently with tightening of the sutures. Excess orbicularis is trimmed laterally. Bunching of the skin below the lateral canthus is usually observed with this maneuver, and addressed by further mobilizing the skin off the orbicularis and redraping the skin in a more vertical direction. The excess skin is then conservatively trimmed and the incision closed. Midcheek fat grafting is then performed using the Coleman technique in selected patients to correct deflation of the midcheeks. The fat is placed in tiny aliquots in a multiplanar manner. The volume of fat injected ranges from 1.5 mL to 3.5 mL per side depending on the degree of deflation present.

Postoperative Care

Commitment to meticulous postoperative care is crucial in subciliary techniques. The midcheek is taped with Steristrips for 5 days and sutures removed after about 6 days. Lower eyelid massaging is started 2 weeks after the operation. This is done by gently pushing the lower lid superomedially against the globe and holding it in position for 1 minute, for up to five times a day. This is generally continued for about 1 month. Patients are seen weekly in the initial postoperative period to check on the lower eyelid position and healing in general. Long-term results of the midcheek lift are shown in Figs. 65.15 and 65.16.

Complication

Patients with certain anatomy such as a negative vector orbit, preexisting scleral show (the so-called "polar bear syndrome") with laxity and poor recoil of the lower eyelids, are at greater risk of complications. Particular care should be taken to ensure the lower eyelid is supported in a good position and posture at the end of the procedure with correct placement of the canthopexy suture. To support the lower eyelid in the early recovery period, canthopexies were routinely done for all patients with the subciliary approach. Reported complications include prolonged swelling, midcheek edema, and prolonged chemosis. Prolonged chemosis (more than 1 month) is one of the more problematic and common complications with more aggressive subciliary surgery. Chemosis, reported to occur in up to 10%–15% and is due to disruption of the lymphatic of the lower eyelid in *anatomically predisposed patient*. Chemosis usually resolves with conservative treatment of eye lubrication and lower eyelid massaging. In very symptomatic patients, a temporary tarsorrhaphy to relieve symptoms and promote resolution of the chemosis should be considered. As a technical pearl, consider doing a tarsorrhaphy if chemosis is noted at the end of the surgery and maintain it for several days. One of the feared complications of the subciliary approach is lower eyelid positional issues. These include scleral show, lid retraction, ectropion. These problems may arise anytime between immediate post operation to 6 weeks after the surgery. Accordingly, it is important to follow patients closely in the early postoperative period. Even a hint of lower eyelid malposition, demands an immediate proactive approach. Rigorous lower eyelid massaging as described above should be started. Early tightening in the middle lamella requires injection of small amounts of a mixture of triamcinolone and 5-fluouoracil into the orbital septum, which is effective to prevent and reduce early scar formation and should be repeated weekly as needed to resolve the situation. In refractory cases, it would be advisable to wait for at least 4 (preferably 6) months before attempting correction. Techniques to correct scleral show include tarsal strip canthoplasty, and dermal pennant flap. Correction of ectropion is more complicated, depending of severity and location of the contracture, in addition to canthoplasty or tarsal strip, a posterior lamella spacer graft (for posterior lamella shortage), and a midcheek lift (for anterior lamella shortage) will be needed. If the lower eyelid is stiffened and is unable to elevate freely, reconstruction of the posterior lamella spacer would be needed. Material used may be autologous tissue (hard palate or ear cartilage) or acellular dermal matrix (ADM).

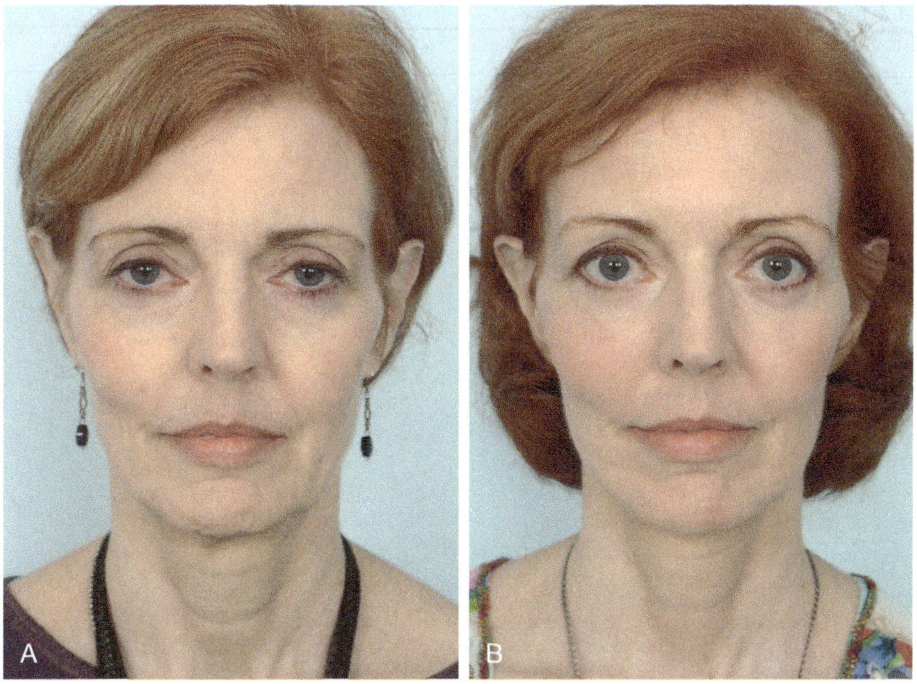

• **Fig. 65.15** (A,B) A 59-year-old woman presented for facial rejuvenation. The lower blepharoplasty with midcheek lift via the facial soft tissue spaces was used to address the midcheek aging. Concomitantly, a composite facelift was performed with facial fat grafting. She is shown 1 year post surgery.

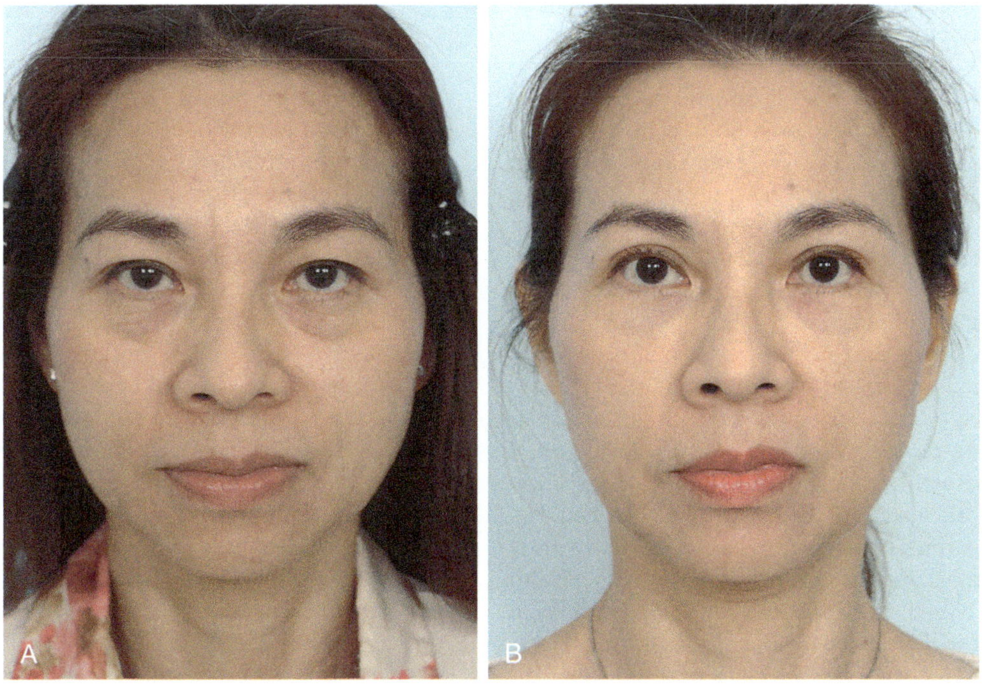

• **Fig. 65.16** (A,B) A 53-year-old woman presented with the complaints of looking tired and difficulty opening her upper eyelids. A midcheek lift and upper eyelid blepharoplasty with levator advancement was performed. The medial and central fat pads were transposed over the orbital rim and the lateral fat pad excess conservatively excised. Excised fat from the upper blepharoplasty and lower lid bags was grafted into the premaxillary space. Midcheek fat grafting was also performed. She is shown 1 year post surgery.

Discussion

With current understanding, midcheek aging may be conceptualized as several components: retrusion of the facial skeleton, predisposing to loss of support of soft tissues resulting in laxity or sagging, primarily over the roof of facial soft tissue spaces in contrast to the tethering of the retaining ligaments resulting in surface grooves.[2,3] To effectively rejuvenate patients with significant midcheek aging, three aspects of the aging midcheek need to be addressed:

first, the prominent eye bags, second the sagging and laxity of the cheeks, and finally, the deflation or volume loss that occurs with aging. Depending on the pathology present, these individual aspects need to be specifically targeted to achieve natural and harmonious rejuvenation of the midcheek. These may be achieved via transconjunctival or subciliary approaches to the midcheek.

Release of the tear trough ligament is a key maneuver in rejuvenation of the midcheek. To prevent reattachment of the ligament to the anterior maxilla and to correct retrusion of the maxilla here, interpositional fat is needed, either transposed as a flap or as free fat grafts of the excised orbital fat.[6,7,11,18] The importance of this maneuver can be clearly demonstrated in patients whose appearance becomes "less attractive" when they smile.[14] These are typically patients with hypertrophic orbicularis oculi, small eye bags at rest, and maxillary retrusion. With animation, strong contraction of the periorbital muscles squeezes the retro-orbital fat pads forward and medially against the tightly fixed tear trough ligament, increasing the bulging of the eye bags and prominence of the tear trough deformity. Removal of the eye bags alone, which has the effect of reducing the bulge, provides only a partial solution. With release of the tear trough ligament and orbicularis origins, the tethering effect is eliminated and the *dynamics* of the smile changed. This change in *vectoring* of the action of the orbicularis oculi gives a more relaxed and beautiful smile (see Figs. 65.12 and 65.13).

The midcheek is an area of compaction of structures, as described in Chapter 62. Safe dissection may be done with good technique. This may be achieved with the application of retraction to move vital structures out of the dissection. From the lower eyelid, the preseptal space is opened, with traction on the origins of the orbicularis oculi under tension, the muscle (and the closely associated tear trough ligament) is released, staying close to the anterior maxilla while applying upward retraction on the tear trough ligament. This is important as the blood vessels (the angular vein and artery) are located in close relation, on the underside of the orbital part of the orbicularis oculi close to its origin, and therefore need to be lifted out of the way of the dissection (see Fig. 65.14). The extent of the release is determined preoperatively, by marking the indent of tear trough deformity and its lateral extension as the palpebromalar groove. With the right eye as reference, this release usually extends from the 4 o'clock to the 8 o'clock positions. Medially, the release should not extend medial to the 4 o'clock position, as in this area the angular nerve (which innervates the inner canthal orbicularis, glabella, and procerus) and the angular artery and vein become very closely associated with the tear trough ligament and are at risk of injury.[19] Laterally, the release may be done as needed depending on the preoperative plan. For a lift of the midcheek, however, the orbicularis retaining ligament and the inferior part of the lateral orbital thickening need to be released to mobilize the midcheek (Fig. 65.17).

When considering midcheek lifts via the lower eyelid, two planes of dissections are used, the subperiosteal and

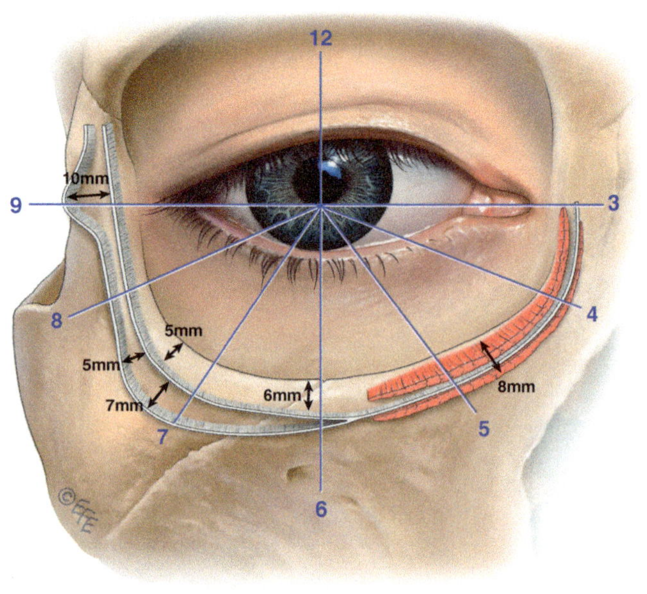

• **Fig. 65.17** Extent of the release of the tear trough–orbicularis retaining ligament (TTL–ORL) complex generally extends from the 4 o'clock to the 8 o'clock position for treatment of the tear trough deformity and from 4 o'clock to 12 o'clock for midcheek lift. (From Wong CH, Mendelson B. Extended transconjunctival lower eyelid blepharoplasty with release of the tear trough ligament and fat redistribution. *Plast Reconstr Surg*. 2017;140:273–282. Figure 12. © Dr. Levent Efe, CMI.)

the preperiosteal planes. The subperiosteal plane is popular for its simplicity and when properly applied is effective in lifting the midcheek. However, the subperiosteal plane has the problem of prolonged swelling and has significant potential complications. The preperiosteal approach has been used by several authors, but the anatomy is complicated and not well described, hence the exact dissection approach was poorly understood. With recent advances in the understanding of the midcheek anatomy, particularly the anatomy medially, that of the tear trough ligament and the premaxillary space, we can now harness this knowledge in safely and effectively mobilizing the midcheek. The preperiosteal plane offers some advantages over the subperiosteal technique in that, firstly, division of the ligament at the preperiosteal level allows the entire superficial fascia (composing the composite of skin, subcutaneous tissue, and orbicularis oculi) to redrape and lift more effectively to tighten the superficial fascia. Secondly, recurrence is less likely, as the release permanently separates the superficial fascia from the deep fascia (in contrast to the subperiosteal dissection which, in essence, leaves the tear trough–orbicularis retaining ligament complex, intact). Finally, swelling and bruising is much less than with the subperiosteal dissection.

Summary

Utilizing the midcheek facial soft tissue spaces to release the tear trough ligament and mobilize the midcheek is a safe and effective technique. As the spaces are anatomical glide planes, dissection is easy, atraumatic, and bloodless. The key is the precise release of the retaining ligaments that separate the spaces. Utilizing this anatomy, recovery is quick and the results lasting, with low complication rates.

References

1. Wong CH, Mendelson B. Newer understanding of specific anatomic targets in the aging face as applied to injectables: aging changes in the craniofacial skeleton and facial ligaments. *Plast Reconstr Surg*. 2015;136(suppl 5):44S–48S.
2. Mendelson B, Wong CH. Changes in the facial skeleton with aging: implications and clinical applications in facial rejuvenation. *Aesthetic Plast Surg*. 2012;36(4):753–760.
3. Mendelson BC, Wong CH. Anatomy of the aging face. In: 3rd ed. Warren RJ, Neligan PC, eds. *Plastic Surgery*. Vol. 2. *Aesthetic*. Philadelphia: Saunders; 2012:78–92.
4. Mendelson BC. Facelift anatomy, SMAS, retaining ligaments and facial spaces. In: Aston SJ, Steinbrech DS, Walden JL, eds. *Aesthetic Plastic Surgery*. London: Saunders; 2009.
5. Mendelson BC, Jacobson SR. Surgical anatomy of the midcheek: facial layers, spaces, and the midcheek segments. *Clin Plast Surg*. 2008;35:395–404; discussion 393.
6. Wong CH, Hsieh MK, Mendelson B. The tear trough ligament: anatomical basis for the tear trough deformity. *Plast Reconstr Surg*. 2012;129(6):1392–1402.
7. Wong CH, Mendelson B. Facial soft-tissue spaces and retaining ligaments of the midcheek: defining the premaxillary space. *Plast Reconstr Surg*. 2013;132(1):49–56.
8. Mendelson BC, Muzaffar AR, Adams Jr WP. Surgical anatomy of the midcheek and malar mounds. *Plast Reconstr Surg*. 2002;110(3):885–896; discussion 897–911.
9. Muzaffar AR, Mendelson BC, Adams WP. Surgical anatomy of the ligamentous attachments of the lower lid and lateral canthus. *J Plast Reconstr Surg*. 2002;110(3):873–884; discussion 897–911.
10. Jelks GW, Jelks EB. The "no touch" lower blepharoplasty. *Can J Plast Surg*. 2009;17:102–103.
11. Wong CH, Mendelson B. Extended transconjunctival lower eyelid blepharoplasty with release of the tear trough ligament and fat redistribution. *Plast Reconstr Surg*. 2017;140:273–282.
12. Sullivan PK, Drolet BC. Extended lower lid blepharoplasty for eyelid and midface rejuvenation. *Plast Reconstr Surg*. 2013;132:1093–1101.
13. Goldberg RA. Transconjunctival orbital fat repositioning: transposition of orbital fat pedicles into a subperiosteal pocket. *Plast Reconstr Surg*. 2000;105:743.
14. Wong CH, Mendelson B. Long-term static and dynamic effects of the release of the tear trough ligament and origins of the orbicularis oculi in lower eyelid blepharoplastry. *Plast Reconstr Surg*. 2019;144(3):583–591.
15. Codner MA, Wolfli JN, Anzarut A. Primary transcutaneous lower blepharoplasty with routine lateral canthal support: a comprehensive 10-year review. *Plast Reconstr Surg*. 2008;121:241–250.
16. Schiller JD. Lysis of the Orbicularis retaining ligament and orbicularis oculi insertion: a powerful modality for lower eyelid and cheek rejuvenation. *Plast Reconstr Surg*. 2012;129(4):692e–700e.
17. Hidalgo DA. An integrated approach to lower blepharoplasty. *Plast Reconstr Surg*. 2011;127(1):386–395.
18. Wong CH, Mendelson B. Midcheek lift using facial soft-tissue spaces of the midcheek. *Plast Reconstr Surg*. 2015;136(6):1155–1165.
19. Caminer DM, Newman MI, Boyd JB. Angular nerve: new insights on innervation of the corrugator supercilii and procerus muscles. *J Plast Reconstr Aesthet Surg*. 2006;59(4):366–372.

66

Facelift

BRYAN MENDELSON AND ROSTAM D. FARHADIEH

For video accompanying this chapter see ExpertConsult.com. See inside cover for access details.

Introduction

Our face is our most inextricable sense of self. A person's self-image and self-esteem are powerfully influenced by their appearance. People requesting a facelift are aware of loss of confidence as a result of their altered "look." The way people are "judged" and treated by others, whether supportive or discriminatory, is largely determined by others' perception of their character and personality, so often fallaciously based on first impressions from their facial appearance. This aspect places a significant responsibility for the facelift patient's future psychological wellbeing in the hands of the surgeon, an added dimension, for which trainees are usually not prepared, but which they must quickly appreciate.

The myriad of possible facelift surgery techniques reflects two separate considerations in the evolution of the field. First, the unique subjective, esthetic, and artistic elements that distinguish surgery of the face from more objective measures-riven fields, such as microsurgical patency. Second, and more importantly, the lagging understanding of the anatomical basis of facelift technique. By contrast, the anatomy of the hand, recognized by plastic surgeons as being complex, is more overtly functional and most of the detail was defined during the classical era of anatomy. In facelift surgery the empirical techniques preceded, what is only now becoming, an almost complete and nuanced understanding of the functional anatomy, as well as the anatomicopathological basis of the aging face. Skoog's insightful advance into anatomically-based rejuvenation along with the description of the superficial musculoaponeurotic system (SMAS) were the start of this journey.[1,2] The work on the functional, as well as anatomical, basis of the more recently defined sub-SMAS spaces of the face and role of the facial ligaments as well as aging of its skeletal foundations has created a detailed surgical roadmap to safe, natural, and lasting facelift surgery outcomes.[3–7] This is the holy grail of facial rejuvenation and this clarification in thinking around the anatomical basis of facelift surgery is being reflected in the availability of cadaver dissection courses and the training of the younger generation of plastic surgeons.

Considerations of esthetics in appearance are paramount. While facelift surgery is inherently a technical exercise, the importance of the surgeon's esthetic eye cannot be overlooked as it is a critical, although intangible, factor in the outcome (Fig. 66.1). Facelift patients in general have a more advanced visual esthetic than the young technical surgeon, who does not intuitively have, or yet developed, this level of esthetic appreciation. Just as a young musician learns by listening to music, the young plastic surgeon must cultivate the habit of analysing faces. Without nuanced understanding of what looks attractive and why, the practitioner of esthetic surgery does not have an appreciation of the specific outcome to be aimed for.

This chapter will give the reader an overview of the subject. Overlapping aspects are covered in the relevant preceding chapters on facial aging and lower eyelid rejuvenation. The senior author's evolved approach to facelift surgery is laid out.

The Aging Face

The face is a complex three-dimensional structure based on a solid skeleton containing three large apertures (the orbits and the extensive oral cavity). The openings of these cavities are closed by the dynamic sphincter muscles of the eyelids and lips, whose effect is modified by ancillary levator muscles of the lids and brows, and by the levator and depressor lip muscles. Supporting soft tissue volumes are held together by visible and invisible ligamentous extensions upon which our interaction in life, emotions, and expressions is played out. Genetics and time take their toll on our appearance modified by environment, lifestyle, and ultimately, gravity. A tired look with wrinkles, a changed shape of the face with sagging into jowls, and a loose hanging neck are the exacting toll of life's vectors on the face. The logical way to start thinking about the face is that its aging is related to its function based around the skeletal apertures, located on the front of the face. The same muscles are used for communication by voice or facial expression. The lateral part of the face by contrast, being remote from the cavities, is more a platform for the structures of mastication, and has less aging as it is relatively fixed, requiring less mobility.

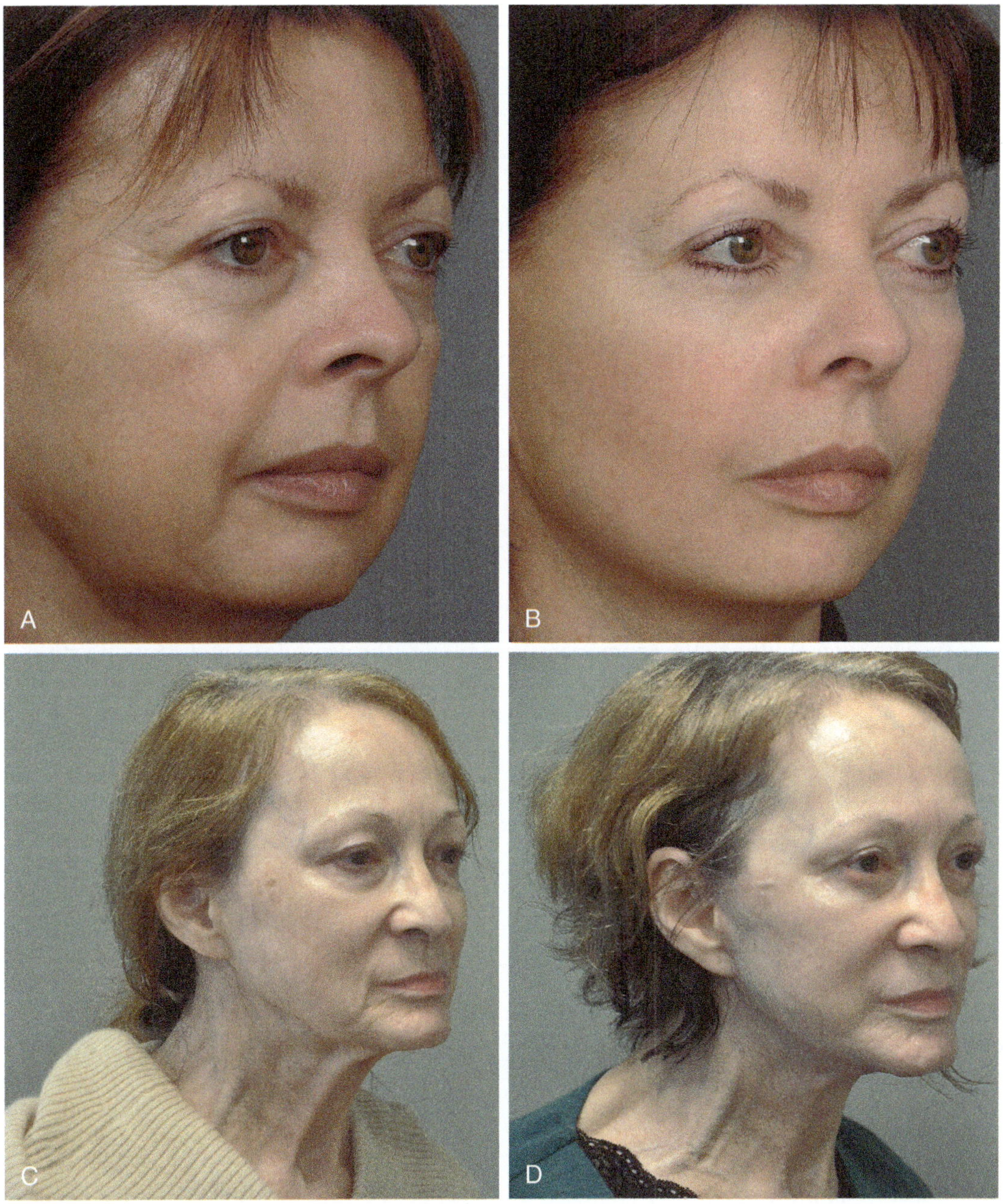

• **Fig. 66.1** The objective of a modern facelift is to restore youthful shape to the face. (A) A 56-year-old woman with significant cheek laxity. (B) One year following a composite facelift, which emphasizes tightening of SMAS laxity of the anterior face. The patient's look is refreshened and the typical facelift pulled look avoided. (C) A 72-year-old woman with significant aging of the face. (D) One year following a composite facelift without lipoinfiltration which demonstrates the significant change in the older patient group. (A,B Courtesy Dr. Bryan Mendelson and C,D Courtesy Dr. Rostam D. Farhadieh.)

The original surgical techniques, from the early 1900s, were limited to the skin envelope. The improvements in a person's aging look seemed remarkable because such a change had not been possible before this time. To be tackling facial appearance was bold surgery, even if addressing laxity of the facial skin was not. With success, the procedures evolved over the years with progressively more undermining and redraping of the facial skin. The risks were few, mainly to do with bleeding, skin circulation, and visible scars.

Deeper contouring surgery commenced only in the 1960s, with direct submental lipectomy introduced by Millard.[8] Profound results were obtained in this era preceding liposuction. The modern facelift era commenced in the mid 1970s with Skoog's revolutionary "anatomical" approach in which the flap is in a deeper plane.[1] Then, Mitz and Peyronie's seminal 1976 paper on the anatomical details of the superficial fascia introduced the important concept of the superficial musculoaponeurotic system (SMAS).[2] Skoog's was the first sub-SMAS dissection plane facelift. It took over a full decade after the SMAS description before the potential benefit of the SMAS was to be realized by mobilizing the SMAS of the anterior face. This required the release of the strong attachment of the SMAS to the zygoma. Furnas later described these attachments as part of a system of named retaining ligaments, that attach the facial soft tissues to the skeleton in between areas of mobility.[9] Even now, 30 years on, understanding how to use the SMAS and retaining ligaments to best advantage is ongoing.[7,10–14]

The soft tissue volume changes reflect the atrophy of normal aging, possibly accelerated by weight loss as well as "shrinkage" of skeletal projection, particularly of the perioral "dental" bones and dentition. The recent advent of soft tissue fillers and lipofilling has turned attention towards the role of correcting soft tissue atrophy of both subcutaneous fat compartments, and deeper sub-SMAS spaces, as an alternative to surgical lifting.[15] The recent history of adding volume mirrors the earlier era of subcutaneous hydrocarbon (paraffin) injections, from the early 1900s, whose popularity well exceeded surgical correction for a time. Volume addition can achieve tissue tightening according to the location on the face, e.g., directly on the skeleton, and in proportion to the volume placed. To lift sagging tissue by this form of tightening is a greater challenge, although in the midcheek it may compete with surgical lifting. The appropriate method of correcting a person's aging tissue laxity, must be individualized.

Subcutaneous Facelift

The earliest facial rejuvenation surgery, at the beginning of the 20th century, consisted of the simple excision of carefully-located and shaped ellipses or half-moons of skin at the back of the face (hairline, pretragal). These were performed under local anesthesia without undermining and direct closure was performed with controlled skin tension. Multiple sessions were often involved. By the late 1920s the additional benefit of undermining the skin for a short distance was appreciated. Interestingly, even then with this small advance in technique a pattern was emerging, acknowledging the advance as being "too much for the would-be surgeon." Similarly, poor facelift results were being seen, with an unnatural appearance resulting from tightly stretched skin.[16]

Modern subcutaneous lifting commenced in the 1930s as a result of linking the multiple skin excisions with a continuous incision, along with the release of subcutaneous attachments. These tentative first steps in facelifting progressed with surgical experience. Increased demand resulted from the increased social affluence of the post-World War Two years and general medical progress, with the advent of antibiotics and improved anesthesia. A rather standard technique evolved consisting of the dissection of large, random pattern skin flaps of the cheek and jowls with redraping in a superolateral suspension vector and resection of excess skin.[16] To improve the cheek correction, the extent of skin flap dissection was progressively extended towards the nasolabial fold, usually, but not always, stopping a few centimeters short of this landmark. The extension of undermining over the lower zygoma has been more of a challenge, due to the difficulty of subcutaneous dissection in this area along with more bleeding. The reason was subsequently found to be due to the fibrous extensions of the zygomaticocutaneous ligament, the strongest of the osteocutaneous ligaments, which continue through the SMAS and divide in the subcutaneous layer as they extend to the dermal attachments. Below the mandible the extent of undermining has continued into the neck towards the midline to a variable extent without this ligamentous difficulty.

Following satisfactory hemostasis, with appropriate tension applied to the skin flaps, the excess skin is marked and key sutures placed before trimming the redundant skin and closure of the incisions, with or without drains. A thin face with modest skin laxity and/or excess, and indeed revision facelifts, may be appropriate cases where a subcutaneous technique can still be considered.

There are innumerable variations in the extent of subcutaneous undermining. The dermal attachments are not uniform across the face as first assumed, but reflect the underlying pattern of facial ligamentous attachment. This is the rational basis for deciding the extent of surgical release. The depth level of dissection within the subcutaneous layer is also varied according to the surgical objective. A superficial subcutaneous dissection has the advantage of being the most remote from the facial nerve branches, hence minimizing the risk of facial nerve damage. This can be important where the subcutaneous layer is thin, as over the temple, particularly in the elderly, where there may be less than usual protection of the underlying temporal branches of the facial nerve. The nerves are at greater risk in secondary facelifts, due to their fixation by fibrosis from previous surgical intervention, and especially when this is more than usual, for example, as a result of previous hematoma.

When a separate SMAS flap is planned, it is beneficial to leave most of the retinacula cutis (in the subcutaneous layer) attached to the SMAS, as this fibrous component reinforces the strength of the SMAS flap.[17] A meticulous dissection technique is required with superficial subcutaneous dissection to avoid visible irregularities and damage to the dermal circulation.

Otherwise, a deep level of subcutaneous dissection is preferred, especially when the surface of the SMAS is to be exposed preliminary to superficial SMAS, platysma manipulation techniques. It is considerably easier to perform the dissection at the deep subcutaneous level and with less bleeding, although the plane is closer to the nerves. This level of dissection has been named the superficial musculo-aponeurotic plane (SMAP).[9] When this plane of dissection is continued in front of the zygoma, directly on the surface of orbicularis oculi, direct access is provided to the malar fat pad. The malar fat pad is the discrete mass of thicker subcutaneous fat of the anterior cheek, whose inferior descent forms the volume of the nasolabial fold. Specific suture suspension of the malar fat pad provides a controlled correction of the medial cheek/nasolabial fold contour, but at the expense of prolonged postoperative edema.[18]

The skin flap technique remains popular with some surgeons owing to its surgical "simplicity," and safety, being remote from the structure of the face. The benefits are touted as short operative time with relatively speedy recovery, and relatively satisfactory early postoperative results. There are inherent long-term shortcomings with the technique as a consequence of the viscoelastic properties of skin, making it less than ideal for taking tension. As a consequence, facial shape cannot be maintained by tightening the skin envelope alone. Additional manipulation of the underlying parenchyma is required, as in other plastic surgery procedures, most notably breast reductions. Other inherent limitations when depending on direct skin tightening include a propensity to skin flap necrosis, traction effect on the pinna, and scar widening.

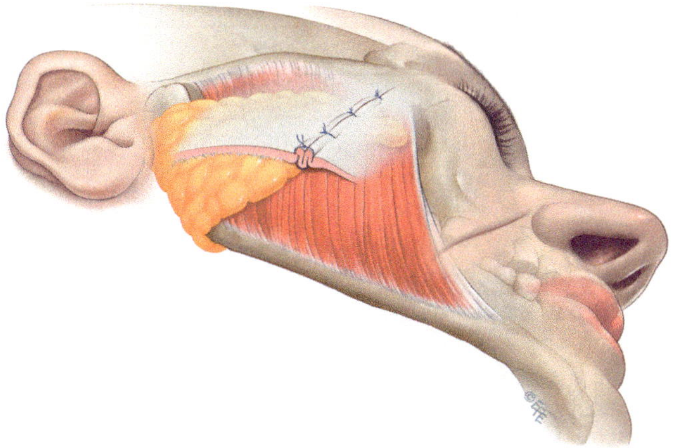

• **Fig. 66.2** SMAS imbrication.

SMAS Manipulation Techniques

Originating with Skoog's technique and the subsequent anatomical description of the SMAS by Mitz and Peyronie, it became evident that utilization of the underlying SMAS was the key to controlling the tension on the skin closure.[2] This was the first accepted benefit of SMAS surgery. It took many years, with further anatomical studies and improved understanding of the potential of the SMAS, along with multiple evolutions of the technique of SMAS correction, for it to be appreciated as the tool for reshaping the face as well as for providing more lasting outcomes.[7,11–14,18]

SMAS Plication/Imbrication

The original version of this technique was to first perform a standard, skin-only facelift dissection and then perform a SMAS incision located directly beneath the facelift incision to mobilize the SMAS, as a completely separate layer. However, dissection of the thin SMAS flap in the preauricular area is inherently difficult due to the absence of a natural cleavage plane as the SMAS has a strong adherence to the parotid capsule (*fixed SMAS*), which Furnas named the platysma auricular fascia. The early SMAS mobilizations were limited in extent to the anterior border of the parotid, as advised by Mitz and Peyronie, the focus being on avoiding the risk of damage to the facial nerve branches as they emerge from the parotid. It became appreciated that to satisfactorily tighten the medial cheek and jowl it is necessary to extend the SMAS release into the mobile SMAS forward of the parotid capsule and release the SMAS from the restraining effect of the vertical line of masseteric cutaneous ligaments (Fig. 66.2).

On completion of the SMAS dissection, the subsequent handling of the SMAS is varied according to the individual facial morphology, specifically the SMAS thickness. The options include plication (simple infolding of the lax SMAS) and imbrication (undermining of the SMAS and subsequent overlapping). Tightening is performed perpendicular to the nasolabial fold using buried sutures to reduce laxity and fullness. Thereafter, the redundant pre- and post-auricular skin is managed as in a standard skin facelift.

Variations of this technique continue to have wide popularity. The advantages include relative safety in relation to the sub-SMAS facial nerve branches, while providing a degree of effective manipulation of the mobile SMAS, combined with a reasonably fast postoperative recovery, yielding a more lasting improvement than skin-only rhytidectomies. Superolateral traction on the SMAS without release of its more anterior retaining ligaments (masseteric cutaneous) is a limitation as this restricts the tightening of the more anterior laxity towards the nasolabial fold and oral commissure, which explains why correction of the anterior midface had traditionally been limited.

The Deep Plane and Composite Rhytidectomy

The role of the SMAS was the major topic of discussion in facelifts through the late 1980s and 1990s. In this context the newly introduced deep plane and then composite facelift techniques, introduced by Hamra, became hot topics.[11,19] These were an evolution of the original Skoog operation. Skoog did not describe his operation as being sub-SMAS as it preceded the introduction of the term. Skoog described the plane of dissection used in his revolutionary facelift, in correct anatomical terms, as being under the superficial fascia.[1] For surgeons of the time, for whom considerations of anatomy were not usual in the context of facelifts, this concept was not readily accepted until the surgical term the "deep plane" was later introduced. Hamra's deep plane concept, being clearly descriptive of the dissection plane, was less anatomically confusing and the term became widely adopted and remains in use to this day, although Hamra's surgical plane of dissection transitioned from being sub-SMAS to become more superficial, as the dissection continued medially over zygomaticus major.

Some clarification regarding use of the term "composite" is required, as two different, yet similar, meanings are attributed to it. In the context of flaps, a composite flap is one in which the several concentric tissue layers in a compound flap remain in their natural fused anatomical relationship. A scalp flap is the archetypal composite flap, consisting of the outer three tissue layers, skin (layer 1), subcutaneous layer (layer 2), and galea aponeurotica (layer 3), that form a vertical composite. Elevation of a scalp flap involves dissection through the subgaleal areolar tissue glide plane (layer 4) beneath the composite flap, allowing it to be separated from the underlying fixed deep fascia, the periosteum. (layer 5).

In Hamra's composite facelift, described in 1990, the term composite was used to denote the surgical extension medially of the same SMAS layer to incorporate the orbicularis oculi within the flap. According to Hamra's description, it is the inclusion of the lower lid orbicularis in the flap (elevation and repositioning) and its (horizontal) continuity with the sub-SMAS cheek flap that determines Hamra's composite. Otherwise, a deep plane facelift does not impact the lower eyelid in spite of obtaining vertical cheek movement. Hamra's composite concept evolved to include a package of procedures: elevation of the lower lid deep to the orbicularis in layer 4, i.e., an extended submuscular flap, using a "zygorbicular" dissection and redraping the lid cheek in a superomedial vector after performing a septal reset procedure.[20] This results in a powerful correction of the lid and upper cheek, as well as direct benefit to the midcheek and nasolabial fold.

A standard facelift incision is used, with 2–3 cm subcutaneous skin flap dissection. The fixed SMAS is incised over the parotid and the sub-SMAS dissection continued superiorly to the malar eminence, dividing the zygomaticocutaneous and relevant masseteric ligaments. Dissection is continued medially over the surface of zygomaticus major muscle towards the nasolabial fold, while the remaining zygomaticocutaneous ligaments are divided to provide access to the malar fat pad. The musculocutaneous flap, once developed, is advanced and rotated superiorly. For the neck, the anterior neck is opened and the medial upper platysma edges approximated following excision of redundant medial platysma in the lower neck. This communicates with a superficial, preplatysmal dissection plane from the lateral approach with dissection carried 8–10 cm below the mandibular angle, with defatting of the flap where indicated. This leaves separate dissection pockets in the face and the neck, which do not communicate anatomically. Closure is performed with tension on the SMAS applied in the temporal fixation.[11]

Hamra addressed a limitation of previous facelifts, being the failure to correct the upper cheek. He appreciated the importance of correcting aging changes of the lid–cheek junction (the lowering of the position of the upper cheek with lengthening of the lower lid) for complete facial rejuvenation. He further observed the benefit of correcting orbicularis oculi laxity in the roof of the prezygomatic space, which contributes to the appearance of malar mounds (crescent, bags) and modified his facelift to address this. To correct laxity of the orbicularis oculi of the upper cheek required an inferior extension of the submuscular lower lid blepharoplasty dissection, with communication through into the pocket of the, previously dissected, deep plane facelift. It was necessary to release the restraining effect of the

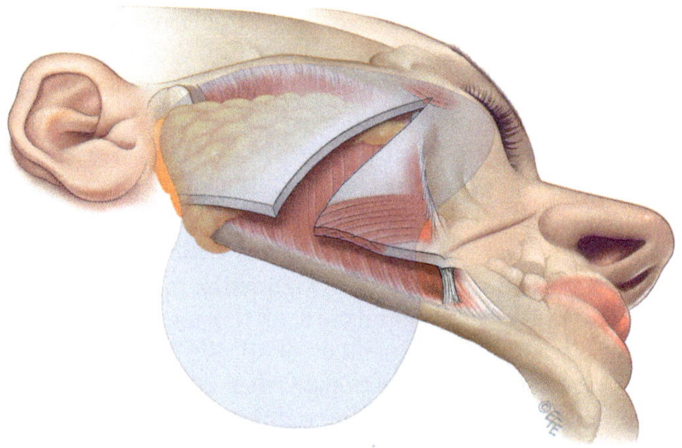

• **Fig. 66.3** SMASectomy.

ligamentous attachments along the orbital rim (later recognized to be the orbicularis retaining ligament) for this to occur.[20] In contrast to the superolateral vector usually used in redraping a lower lid blepharoplasty flap, a superomedial vector is used to oppose the inferolateral vectors of upper cheek aging. The tightening is achieved at the completion of the facelift by suspension of the orbicularis flap to the lateral orbital rim.[19,21]

Hamra's composite facelift clinical series demonstrated impressive results as a result of the anatomically composite musculocutanenous flap that provides robust vascularity with reduced tension on the skin closure. In addition, the surgically composite access to the malar fat pad and superomedial cheeklift vector corrects the lid cheek area more effectively than do the extended and high SMAS counterparts. Similar to these techniques, potential damage to facial nerve branches in the dissection field and higher operative technical requirements with longer postoperative recovery are disadvantages that have limited usage of this specific technique (Fig. 66.3).

Lateral SMASectomy

Dr. Daniel Baker developed this SMAS technique. On the basis of its simplicity and predictability, it became extremely popular, usually in association with a "short-scar" (i.e., shorter skin incision) technique. Baker recognized the real benefit came from tightening the mobile SMAS over the anterior masseter area. So, the SMAS incision was moved logically forward to where the excess was excised to tighten the SMAS.[14]

Accordingly, the tedious lateral sub-SMAS dissection over the parotid could be avoided, especially as it provided no specific benefit.

Baker also popularized the "short-scar" technique by minimising the postauricular skin incision and undermining behind the ear. Of course, this is successful in proportion to the amount of neck skin redundancy and the degree of its correction. The standard SMASectomy begins with the subcutaneous dissection of a lateral cheek skin flap to within 2–3 cm of the nasolabial fold, and 5–6 cm below the level of the mandible into the neck. The mobile SMAS anterior to the parotid is identified and depending on the individual patient's facial morphology, a strip of redundant SMAS is either resected or simply plicated. Where a resection is planned, the mobile anterior SMAS is manipulated in a vector perpendicular to the nasolabial fold from the angle of the mandible to the lateral malar eminence. The redundant SMAS is marked and excised before the mobile anterior SMAS is secured against the fixed lateral SMAS overlying the parotid, commencing inferiorly and moving superiorly. In a thinner face this technique allows for "stacking" of the SMAS to augment the lateral cheek. Various modifications of the technique have been reported.[22]

This technique corrects the lateral cheek and jowls, and provides for resection of redundant SMAS where indicated. The limitation is the failure to address the deep ligamentous attachments of the mobile SMAS along the anterior masseter border. While relative simplicity is its attraction, by design this technique does not fully address the midface (Fig. 66.4).

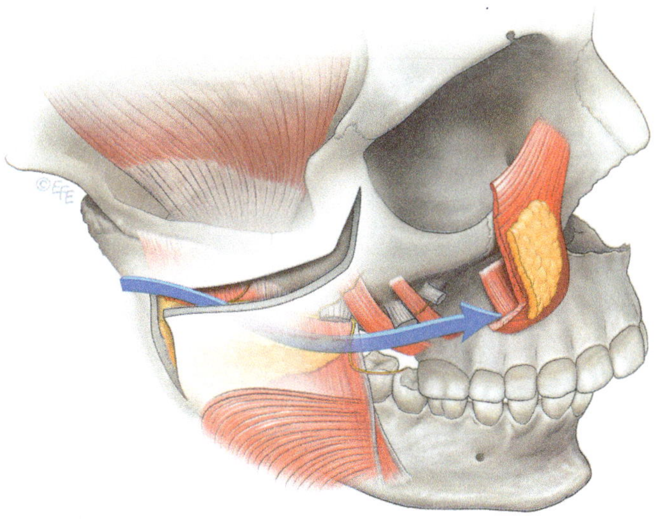

• **Fig. 66.4** Extended SMAS facelift.

Extended SMAS

This is an early SMAS technique that evolved to incorporate understanding of the ligamentous anatomy on the zygoma and its relationship with the SMAS of the anterior face.[13] Visible contour changes of the cheek are a key part of the aging process, particularly the reduction of prominence over the zygoma and loss of the contrasting infrazygomatic (submalar) youthful concavity over the buccal recess. The zygomatic ligaments are recognized as suspending the cheek soft tissues including the malar fat pad from the zygoma.[6,23] Descent of this facial fat has been the explanation for these contour changes and presumed to be secondary to attenuation of the zygomatic ligaments with age. In reality, given the stout nature of these ligaments, the weakening more likely occurs in the SMAS attachments of the ligaments.

The principles of this technique are based on the anatomical details of the retaining ligaments of the face, as well as consideration to vectors of facial and neck rejuvenation originating from the pioneering work of Dr. Bruce Connell.[24] A bidirectional manipulation of skin and SMAS is advocated. A standard facelift skin incision is used; the skin is dissected widely in standard fashion to a few centimeters short of the nasolabial fold and below the mandible. The skin overlying the lateral two-thirds of the zygoma is mobilized. It is imperative to leave some fat on the SMAS, especially medially as it thins out to reduce proneness to tearing during the subsequent SMAS dissection and elevation. Following the standard posterior dissection of the fixed SMAS over the parotid up to the zygomatic arch a forward extension of the SMAS incision, commencing 1 cm below the arch (to protect the frontal branch of the facial nerve) and continues forward to the junction of the arch and body of the zygoma. From there the incision is angled towards the lateral canthus for a distance of about 3 cm, following which the SMAS incision angled down at 90 degrees, away from the lower lid towards the superior nasolabial fold.[13] The SMAS dissection provides access to the zygomatico-cutaneous ligaments, including the strong medial ligament just medial to zygomaticus minor that extends from the zygomatico-maxillary suture. The preauricular SMAS incision is extended below the mandibular border for 5-6 cm along the posterior border of the platysma. In the malar region the flap is elevated superficial to the orbicularis oculi as well as superficial to the zygomaticus major and minor muscles. Mobility of the SMAS flap is obtained by freeing it from the zygomatic prominence along with release of the masseteric ligaments. Often some extended dissection of the SMAS is undertaken medial to the zygomaticus minor, beyond the boundaries of the subcutaneous dissection, in the plane between the malar fat pad and levator labii superioris.

The malar SMAS flap is redraped in a superolateral vector parallel to zygomaticus major and fixed to the zygomatic prominence. The excess tissue is either excised or used as a soft tissue autoaugmentation over the zygoma. The remaining cheek SMAS flap is rotated perpendicular to the mandible to contour the jowl area. To accentuate the jawline and contrasting submental and neck concavity, a strong posterior vector is obtained, using an inferiorly-based flap of a preauricular SMAS as a strip transposed behind the ear securing to the mastoid. Drains are usually required on account of the extensive subcutaneous dissection.

This SMAS rejuvenation technique is based on sound anatomical principles of releasing the SMAS from its deep fixation by key retaining ligaments. Its advantage over the other SMAS techniques discussed so far is the access to the malar fat pad and improvement of the anterior part of the midface (Fig. 66.5).

The High SMAS Facelift

The "high SMAS facelift" was conceived by Barton in the early 1980s and also advocated by Owsley, another pioneer

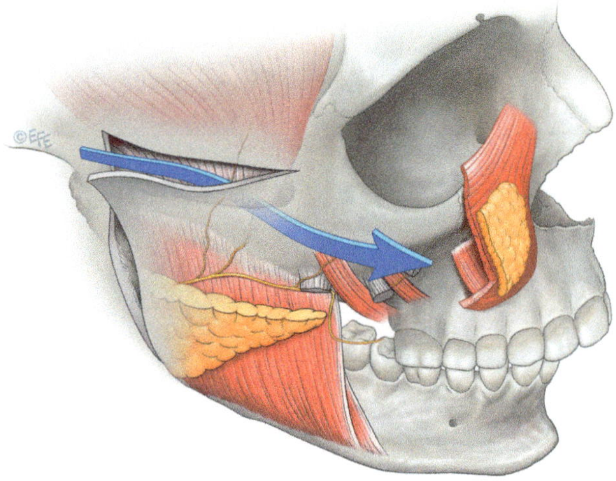

• **Fig. 66.5** The high SMAS facelift.

in the application of SMAS anatomy, is popular among experienced plastic surgeons.[18] It is not dissimilar to the extended SMAS but obtains a simpler, higher approach to the upper SMAS and provides a greater benefit of SMAS redraping over the body of the zygoma and into the area of the lid cheek.

This area is not addressed with standard SMAS operations (imbrication/plication and lateral SMASectomy). Leverage of the upper SMAS over the zygoma results from raising the level of the transverse SMAS incision to just above the zygomatic arch. While a standard facelift incision is used, the skin undermining is minimized to 4–5 cm in the preauricular area and continues above the zygomatic arch and forward to the lateral border of the orbicularis oculi. To establish the correct plane, the fixed SMAS dissection commences over the parotid, then at the anterior border of the parotid the mobile SMAS is undermined using blunt dissection, protecting the facial nerve branches. The risk of damage to the frontal branches of the facial nerve is avoided by keeping the transverse SMAS incision superficial, just above the zygomatic arch where the nerves are deeper on the periosteum. The lateral edge of orbicularis oculi is used as a guide to the origin of zygomaticus major. A thin layer of fat is left over this muscle to protect those zygomatic facial nerve branches passing superficially to innervate the lateral orbicularis oculi. The pattern of nerve supply and anatomical boundaries of the prezygomatic space are detailed by Mendelson et al.[6] Releasing the SMAS from the fixation of the zygomatico-cutaneous retaining ligaments and accessing the subcutaneous plane over zygomaticus major allows mobilization of the midface cheek mass including the malar fat pad. The flap is strong as it is reinforced by the multiple ramifications of the zygomatic ligament and is lifted in a vertical direction and secured to the deep temporal fascia above the arch, where it not only suspends the cheek but also provides supports to the lower eyelid.[12]

The advantage of this technique, similar to its extended counterpart, is that it incorporates midface rejuvenation in addition to the jowls and neck. Elevation of an anatomically composite skin–SMAS flap provides a better vascularized flap than separate skin and SMAS flaps, with less bruising, induration, and hematoma risk. The reluctance over the years to use a high SMAS incision had been the concern about the risk of damage to the temporal nerve branches as they cross the zygomatic arch. However, this has been strongly repudiated by good anatomical descriptions and the combined results from Owsley and Barton of 3000 cases with no permanent temporal branch injury.[25,26] The traditional concern about not being able to redrape the skin and SMAS in different vectors is not a realistic shortcoming.[25]

Subperiosteal Facelift

Given that advances in facelifts were associated with increasing anatomical challenges with the facial nerve, advent of the subperiosteal facelift as a spin off from craniofacial surgery seemed logical and enjoyed a short era in facelifting preceding the endoscopic era and until understanding of the facial anatomy further evolved. In 1980, Tessier extended his craniofacial approach to facial rejuvenation. Utilizing a bicoronal or temporal hairline approach, and subperiosteal dissection plane, the lateral and midface was detached from the zygoma and maxilla. The origins of the superficial muscles, zygomaticus major and minor, levator labii superioris, levator anguli oris, as well as orbicularis occuli and related ligaments, are inherently detached with this dissection and are repositioned. In the lateral cheek the dissection continues with detachment of the overlying masseteric fascial layer from the zygomatic insertion, but is limited by its masseteric attachments. A frontoglabellar dissection, if used, can continue to the tip of the nose preserving the medial canthal ligament. The entire facial soft tissue is thus freed from its underlying skeletal attachment, is advanced 2–3 cm in the superior direction, and is fixed against the deep temporal fascia.

Initial reports of this technique reported unacceptably high rates of frontal facial nerve (up to 20%), as well as zygomatic branches palsies. The injuries were sustained over the zygomatic arch and body respectively, where the zygomatic branch may be caught in suspending sutures.[27] An extended technique was developed after further anatomical studies addressing these concerns. The vital dissection over the zygomatic arch where facial fascial layers coalesce, was modified. About 2 cm above the zygomatic arch an incision is made in the continuation of the subperiosteal pocket into the superficial layer of the deep temporal fascia breaching the superficial temporal fat pad to protect the overlying temporoparietal fascia and frontal nerve branch. A periosteal incision at the superomedial margin of the zygomatic arch along its length allows access to the lateral cheek where the masseteric fascia is detached from its zygomatic origin. This is combined with a minimal preauricular subcutaneous dissection. The redundant skin is excised, after suspension of the face and the wounds closed.[28]

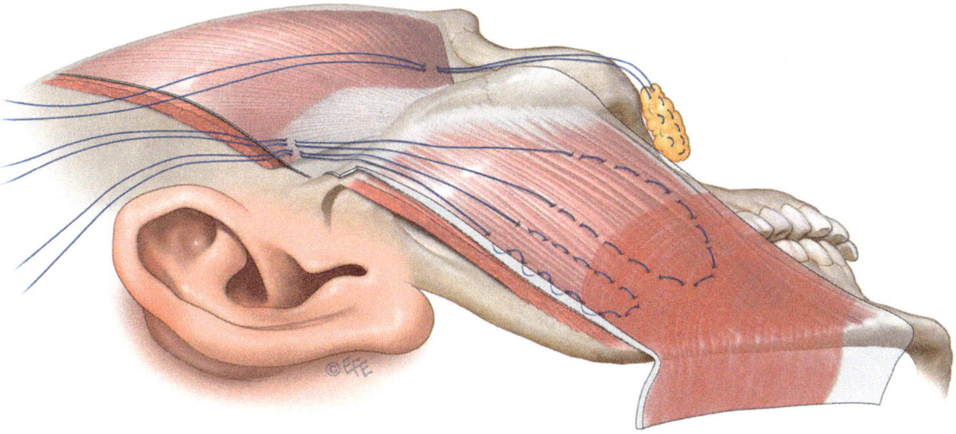

• **Fig. 66.6** The MACS lift.

The disadvantages of this technique include the steep learning curve and need for increased familiarity with craniofacial principles, but most significantly, the prolonged swelling leading to longer postoperative recovery times. The periosteum strongly reattaches to the bone, carrying the facial soft tissues including the retaining ligament and muscle origins previously detached. Studies demonstrate that origins and insertion of the facial muscles do not attenuate with aging.[29] In relocating the origins of these mimetic muscles, unnatural vectors of facial animation are an inherent consequence, which may account for the name "mask lift." While effective, interest in this procedure diminished with the advances in anatomical understanding. The original attraction had been the quality of correction obtainable over the zygoma, while avoiding the nerve risks of sub-SMAS dissection in this area, at the time when this lack of anatomical understanding was prohibitive (Fig. 66.6).

Minimal Access Cranial Suspension (MACS) Lift

This technique was developed by Tonnard and Verpaele, at a time when each advance in facelifting seemed to be further anatomically complicated. The original attractions of the MACS lift were its simplicity and safety, with short operating time, the use of local anesthesia and short postoperative recovery. It reverted to a simple subcutaneous dissection with unusual short scar, utilizing a technically simple SMAS manipulation using only vertical looped suspension sutures. The original MACS lift addressed the lower third of the face, the jowls, marionette lines, and neck.[30] Subsequent modifications of the technique were introduced to address insufficient correction of the midface and malar fat pad and named the extended MACS lift.[31,32] These have complicated a previously simple operation to bring the results in line with current expectations. Well performed, the results are surprisingly good for such a noninvasive technique, making it an excellent facelift procedure for the occasional facelift surgeon. Selection of the technique is based on a personal risk–benefit analysis, where an extensive skin undermining is considered preferable to more involved SMAS techniques. The shorter operative time advantage has diminished due to the requirement to enhance the result with further suspension sutures, yet the safe plane of dissection and reduced risk of major complications are the real advantages of this technique. It is often performed under local anesthetic and sedation; patients are frequently discharged home the same day.

A zigzag temporal pre-hairline incision is made from the level of the lateral canthus and the lower end of the incision finishes at the ear lobe, not extending postauricularly. In the extended variant the temporal incision is extended 1–2 cm cephalad. Wide skin undermining is performed for 5–6 cm extending to approximately 2 cm below the mandibular angle until the posterior platysma border is visualized. The facial shaping is achieved by a pair of U-shaped loop sutures anchored above to the deep temporal fascia above the zygomatic arch, 1 cm anterior to the helical root and weaved into the SMAS below. A posterior loop suture extends down to the posterosuperior border of the platysma and because of the mobility of the platysma, as the purse string suture is tied the platysma laxity is displaced. This tightens the contours of the cervicomental angle and the pre-liposuctioned neck. A second more open O-shaped suture originating from the same site is angled at 30 degrees towards the jowls. Tightening the second suture places the mobile SMAS under concentric tension reducing the laxity that contributes to the jowls and marionette lines. Where an extended technique is performed, a third U-shaped suture is placed in the furthest anterior limit of the deep temporal fascia and is directed towards the malar fat pad suspending it with an oblique vector. The redundant skin is then excised in a purely vertical vector. The redundant subcilliary skin at the lower lid is excised (4–8 mm on average) through a lower lid blepharoplasty incision.[30,32]

The focus on a purely vertical preauricular lift, which is considerable, is designed to avoid the skin redundancy behind the ears that results from neck correction and instead transfers the skin excess to the temple, where it is removed without displacement of the temporal hair. The necessity for a pre-hairline scar is considered a disadvantage compared to the usual postauricular scar and is debated. The location of the loop sutures avoids a "flat" facelift look. While the technique does not require any release of the facial retaining ligaments at the sub-SMAS level (with its attendant drawbacks), the procedure does cleverly take advantage of the innate anatomical areas of mobility of the platysma and the midcheek SMAS. Its critics consider the disadvantages of the technique manifold. The results are relatively lasting as the SMAS plication suture provides multiple small imbrications with fibrosis induced around the suture, whose benefit is maintained after the suture has resorbed.

Complications

Hematoma

This remains the most common early postoperative complication of facelifts. Correct treatment of hematomas is required to avoid secondary consequences of skin necrosis, prolonged facial edema, and pigmentation. Large series have reported rates of 0.01%–4.5% and as high as 8% in males.[19,33–36] In general, bleeding is much less with dissection in the avascular sub-SMAS plane compared to subcutaneous dissection with the hematoma risk considerably reduced. In their series of 1078 consecutive facelifts Waterhouse and Jones reported a 4.5% hematoma rate requiring evacuation. Statistically significant risk factors identified were systolic blood pressure, male gender, anterior plastysmaplasty, smoking and consumption of nonsteroidal antiinflammatory drugs (NSAIDs).[35]

Nerve Injury

The sensory innervation of the facial skin flap is always damaged from subcutaneous dissection, the extent of numbness being in proportion to the extent of dissection. This usually resolves in 15–18 months. The great auricular nerve branches are at risk during the neck dissection where they are superficial above McKinney's point, 6.5 cm below the external auditory canal.

All facial motor nerve branches are considered at risk during facelifts. Traction neurapraxia is the most frequent injury leading to temporary muscle paresis that resolves with time. A major neurapraxia may be evident for 12–16 weeks. The buccal branch is thought to be the most commonly affected, but fortunately, owing to having multiple interconnecting branches with intraneural overlap, clinical significance is diminished. Frontal and marginal mandibular branch injuries are more clinically significant as these are terminal branches. Permanent facial nerve injury is a major complication and fortunately rare, being reported in several large series with a range of 0–0.3%. Most nerve injuries recover during the postoperative months.[19,28,36]

Skin Loss

Traditional facelift techniques utilize large, random pattern, and often thin, flaps that are sutured under tension. This predisposes to areas of skin loss, from circulatory deficiency. These are most often postauricular. Conservative management is recommended to allow secondary healing. Skin loss is an avoidable complication with recognized predisposing risk factors, smoking being the major risk. Smoking was implicated in 74% of patients with skin loss in a major retrospective analysis by Rees et al, and smokers are estimated to be 12.5 times more likely to suffer skin necrosis.[37] Another prospective series estimated skin necrosis in 19.5% of smokers and only 5% of non-smokers.[38]

Unsatisfactory Scars

Skin hyper- or hypopigmentation may occur with any scar. Widened visible scars from skin tension, even small, are an ever-present risk, while hypertrophic and keloid scarring are possible complications in thick-skin individuals due to tension or delayed healing. Temporal hairline deformities and earlobe distortion are consequence of incision design error and traction from excess skin tension, as are loss of hair and scar widening.

Infection

Infections are not a problem in facelift surgery and occur in well less than 1% of cases.[14]

Senior Author's Limited Dissection Composite Facelift Technique

The evolution of facelift technique has largely been the result of the application of further anatomical understanding. As a result, aspects of the surgery that had previously been hailed as an advance, may not remain important. One such previous significant advance, which had been introduced to overcome the difficult dissection of the posterior SMAS from the parotid capsule, was to effectively avoid it, by instead continuing the initial subcutaneous dissection over this part of the SMAS.[14,36] The SMAS entry point incision was made only after the mobile anterior SMAS was reached, as this part of the SMAS inherently dissects more easily (Fig. 66.7).

The reality is that the posterior SMAS dissection was made difficult by weakening of the SMAS layer as a result of dissecting it as a separate layer. By contrast, when a composite flap is used, the structural fibrous reinforcement of the SMAS remains intact, and the elevation of the reinforced posterior SMAS is not difficult.

This information provides an additional benefit, of liberating the location of the SMAS "entry point." Rather than the priority for the SMAS entry point being for the benefit of the dissection, its location can now be used for the benefit of the fixation and patient recovery. This is the rationale underlying the "limited dissection composite facelift."

There are several advantages in limiting the subcutaneous undermining. In addition to having less bleeding during sub-SMAS dissection and a dramatically lower hematoma rate, limiting the skin undermining to only the area of excess skin that will be removed completely avoids residual

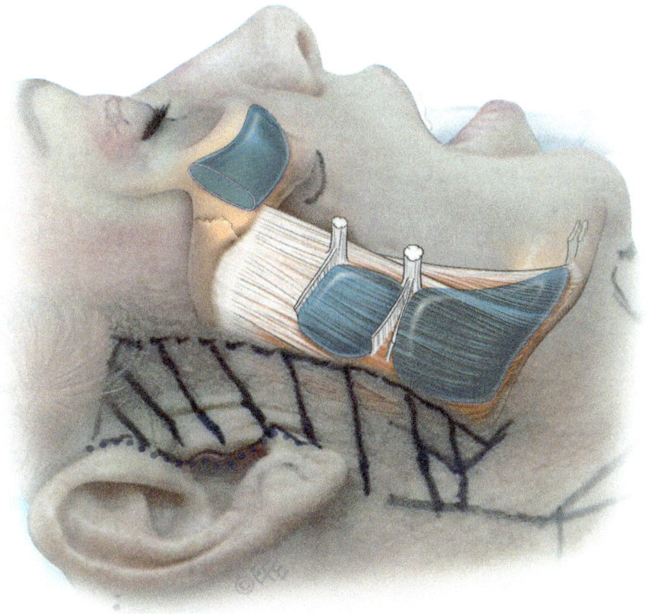

• **Fig. 66.7** Limited dissection composite facelift. The cross-hatch skin marking outlines the limited extent of subcutaneous undermining. After the skin flap has been raised, the adequacy of the extent of this is confirmed. Then, the incision through the SMAS is performed at this level. All further undermining is performed by sub-SMAS dissection, initially into the premasseter spaces (blue). The sub-SMAS dissection over the masseter is also limited, not extending forward of the vertical ligament boundary near the anterior masseter. Over the zygoma, the sub-SMAS dissection extends into the prezygomatic space.

subcutaneous dead space. The result is minimal postoperative ecchymosis, without the need for drains. It is a positive early contribution to patient satisfaction with the outcome having a less traumatized-looking face.

The stronger composite flap inherently provides a more powerful lift that includes an element of soft tissue shaping, paradoxically, with less skin tension. The fixation of a composite flap is central, where the natural ligamentous fixation is located, rather than at the periphery of the SMAS. Central fixation provides for multiple vectors to suit the redraping needs of each part of the face. Furthermore, the traditional requirement for bilaminar (separate skin and SMAS) flaps is avoided with proper mobilization of the composite flap. The skin viability of the edge of a composite flap is robust, negating skin edge necrosis risk.

References

1. Skoog T. *Plastic Surgery: New Methods and Refinements*. Philadelphia: Saunders; 1974.
2. Mitz V, Peyronie M. The superficial musculoaponeurotic system (SMAS) in parotid and cheek area. *Plast Reconstr Surg*. 1976;58:80–88.
3. Mendelson BC, Freeman ME, Wu W, et al. Surgical anatomy of the lower face: the premasseter space, the jowl, and the labiomandibular fold. *Aesthetic Plast Surg*. 2008;32(2):185–195.
4. Mendelson BC, Hartley W, Scott M, et al. Age-related changes of the orbit and midcheek and the implications for facial rejuvenation. *Aesthetic Plast Surg*. 2007;31(5):419–423.
5. Mendelson BC, Jacobson SR. Surgical anatomy of the midcheek: facial layers, spaces, and the midcheek segments. *Clin Plast Surg*. 2008;35(3):395–404; discussion 393.
6. Mendelson BC, Muzaffar AR, Adams Jr WP. Surgical anatomy of the midcheek and malar mounds. *Plast Reconstr Surg*. 2002;110(3):885–896; discussion 97–911.
7. Mendelson BC. Surgery of the superficial musculoaponeurotic system: principles of release, vectors, and fixation. *Plast Reconstr Surg*. 2001;107:1545–1552; discussion 1553–1555, 1556–1557, 1558–1561.
8. Millard DR, Pigott RW, Hedo A. Submandibular lipectomy. *Plast Reconstr Surg*. 1968;41(6):513–522.
9. Furnas DW. The superficial musculoaponeurotic plane and the retaining ligaments of the face. In: Psillakis JM, ed. *Deep Facelifting Techniques*. New York: Thieme Medical Publishers; 1994.
10. Hamra ST. Composite rhytidectomy. Finesse and refinements in technique. *Clin Plast Surg*. 1997;24(2):337–346.
11. Hamra ST. The deep-plane rhytidectomy. *Plast Reconstr Surg*. 1990;86(1):53–61; discussion 2–3.
12. Barton FE, Hunt J. The high-superficial aponeurotic system technique in facial rejuvenation. *Plast Reconstr Surg*. 2003;112:1910–1917.
13. Stuzin JM, Baker TJ, Gordon HL, et al. Extended SMAS dissection as an approach to midface rejuvenation. *Clin Plast Surg*. 1995;22(2):295–311.
14. Baker DC. Lateral SMASectomy, plication and short scar facelifts: indications and techniques. *Clin Plast Surg*. 2008;35:533–550.
15. Lambros V. Models of facial aging and implications for treatment. *Clin Plast Surg*. 2008;35:319–327.
16. Bettman AG. Plastic and cosmetic surgery of the face. *Northwest Med*. 1920;91:205–209.
17. Connell BF. Neck contour deformities. The art, engineering, anatomic diagnosis, architectural planning and aesthetics of surgical correction. *Clin Plast Surg*. 1987;14(4):683–692.
18. Owsley JQ. Lifting the malar fat pad for correction of prominent nasolabial folds. *Plast Reconstr Surg*. 1993;3:463–474.
19. Hamra ST. Composite rhytidectomy. *Plast Reconstr Surg*. 1992;90(1):1–13.
20. Hamra ST. The zygorbicular dissection in composite rhytidectomy: an ideal midface plane. *Plast Reconstr Surg*. 1998;102(5):1646–1657.
21. Hamra ST. Repositioning the orbicularis oculi muscle in the composite rhytidectomy. *Plast Reconstr Surg*. 1992;90(1):14–22.
22. Waterhouse N, Vesely M, Bulstrode NW. Modified lateral SMASectomy. *Plast Reconstr Surg*. 2007;119(3):1021–1026.
23. Furnas DW. The retaining ligaments of the cheek. *Plast Reconstr Surg*. 1989;83:11–16.
24. Connell BF, Marten TJ. The trifurcated SMAS flap: three part segmentation of the conventional flap for improved in the midface, cheek and neck *Aesthetic*. *Plast Surg*. 1995;19:415–420.
25. Agarwal CA, Mendenhall 3rd SD, Foreman KB, et al. The course of the frontal branch of the facial nerve in relation to fascial planes: an anatomic study. *Plast Reconstr Surg*. 2010;125(2):532–537.
26. Trussler AP, Stephan P, Hatef D, et al. The frontal branch of the facial nerve across the zygomatic arch: anatomical relevance of the high-SMAS technique. *Plast Reconstr Surg*. 2010;125(4):1221–1229.
27. Psillakis JM, Rumley TO, Camargos A. Subperiosteal approach as an improved concept for correction of the aging face. *Plast Reconstr Surg*. 1988;82:383–394.

28. Ramirez OM, Maillard GF, Musolas A. The extended subperiosteal facelift: a definitive soft tissue remodelling for facial rejuvenation. *Plast Reconstr Surg*. 1991;88(2):227–236.
29. Gosain AK, Amarante MT, Hyde JS, et al. A dynamic analysis of changes in the nasolabial fold using magnetic resonance imaging: implications for facial rejuvenation and facial animation surgery. *Plast Reconstr Surg*. 1996;98:622–636.
30. Tonnard P, Verpaele A, Monstrey S, et al. Minimal access cranial suspension lift: a modified S lift. *Plast Reconsrt Surg*. 2002;109(6):2074–2086.
31. Tonnard P, Verpaele A, Sibila G. Optimising results from minimal access cranial suspension lifting. *Aesthetic Plast Surg*. 2005;29:213–220.
32. Verpaele A, Tonnard P, Gaia S, et al. The third suture in MACS-lifting: making midface-lifting simple and safe. *J Plast Reconstr Aesthet Surg*. 2007;60(12):1287–1295.
33. Baker DC, Aston SJ, Guy CL, et al. The male rhytidectomy. *Plast Reconsrt Surg*. 1977;50:514–522.
34. Lemmon ML, Hamra ST. Skoog rhytidectomy: a five year experience with 577 patients. *Plast Reconstr Surg*. 1980;65(3):283–297.
35. Grover R, Jones BM, Waterhouse N. The prevention of haematoma following rhytidectomy: a review of 1078 consecutive facelifts. *Br J Plast Surg*. 2001;54(6).
36. Baker DC. Minimal incision rhytidectomy (short scar face lift) with lateral SMASectomy; evolution and application. *Aesthet Surg J*. 2001;21(1):14–26.
37. Rees TD, Liverett DM, Guy CL. The effect of cigarette smoking on skin-flap survival in the face lift patient. *Plast Reconstr Surg*. 1984;73(6):911–915.
38. Riefkohl R, Wolfe JA, Cox EB, et al. Association between cutaneous occlusive vascular disease, cigarette smoking, and skin slough after rhytidectomy. *Plast Reconstr Surg*. 1986;77(4):592–595.

67
Neck Lift

TIMOTHY J. MARTEN AND DINO ELYASSNIA

For video accompanying this chapter see ExpertConsult.com. See inside cover for access details.

Introduction

Why Perform a Neck Lift?

Why perform a neck lift? Why not just lift the cheeks and jawline or perform other procedures that rejuvenate the eyes or upper face? The simple answer is that a well-contoured neck is an artistic imperative to an attractive and appealing appearance. A good neckline conveys a sense of youth, health, fitness, and vitality, and lends an appearance of decisiveness, sensuality, and beauty (Fig. 67.1). Neck improvement is of high priority to almost every patient seeking facial rejuvenation, and the results of our "facelift" procedures are largely judged by the outcome we achieve in the neck. If the neck is not sufficiently improved our patients will feel we have failed them.

How Should a Neck Lift be Performed?

It is unlikely there will ever be a consensus on how a neck lift should be performed and it is a fact that no one procedure will be best for all patients. The technique used cannot be arbitrary, will depend on deformities present, and will necessarily vary from patient to patient. Success or failure in treating the neck, like the nose, breast, and body, lies in the diagnosis of problems and the application of a logical surgical plan, and any surgeon capable of identifying the anatomic basis of patient problems and forming a sound plan for their correction can achieve excellent outcomes.

So how should one perform a neck lift? Perhaps it is easiest to start by stating what not to do. Despite the fact that it is the traditional approach and remains a common practice, it is not enough to perform submental liposuction and tighten the skin in most patients. This approach ignores a number of anatomical problems present in many patients seeking neck improvement, including platysmal laxity, platysmal bands, excess subplatysmal fat, large submandibular glands, digastric muscle hypertrophy, and developmental factors such as the size and shape of the bony jaw and chin. Removing subcutaneous fat and tightening skin over these problems does not correct them, and the presence or absence of each must be looked for in order to create and apply an appropriate surgical plan (Fig. 67.2).

Strategies for Neck Lift

Patients seeking neck improvement have a range of options available to them depending on the problems present, the degree of improvement they seek, and the time, trouble, and expense they are willing to undergo to obtain the improvement they desire. And while it is incumbent upon us to discuss these options and the advantages and disadvantages of each, patients are also seeking our guidance as to what is possible, what is practical, and what is really best. It is not enough to steer patients to procedures we are comfortable with. We are professionally bound and ethically obliged to refer patients for the care they need and desire if we are not able to provide it ourselves.

Submental Liposuction

Submental liposuction (and arguably "noninvasive" treatments including cryolipolysis, deoxycholic acid injections, and radiofrequency and ultrasound "skin shrinking" treatments) is the simplest and likely the most commonly performed procedure to improve neck contour in the range of options available to patients. It does not constitute a true neck lift, however, and only occasionally produces optimal outcomes. Patients and surgeons are predictably drawn into a sense of denial of this, however, by the fact that submental liposuction will occasionally produce worthwhile improvement in some cases, and it is these atypical outcomes that are predictably displayed in offices, placed in advertisements, shown on TV and websites, published in the beauty press, and even included in presentations at plastic surgery symposia. Adding to the deception is the fact that these photographs have usually been taken in the early postoperative period when swelling is still present that obscures irregularities and underlying but untreated deep layer problems.

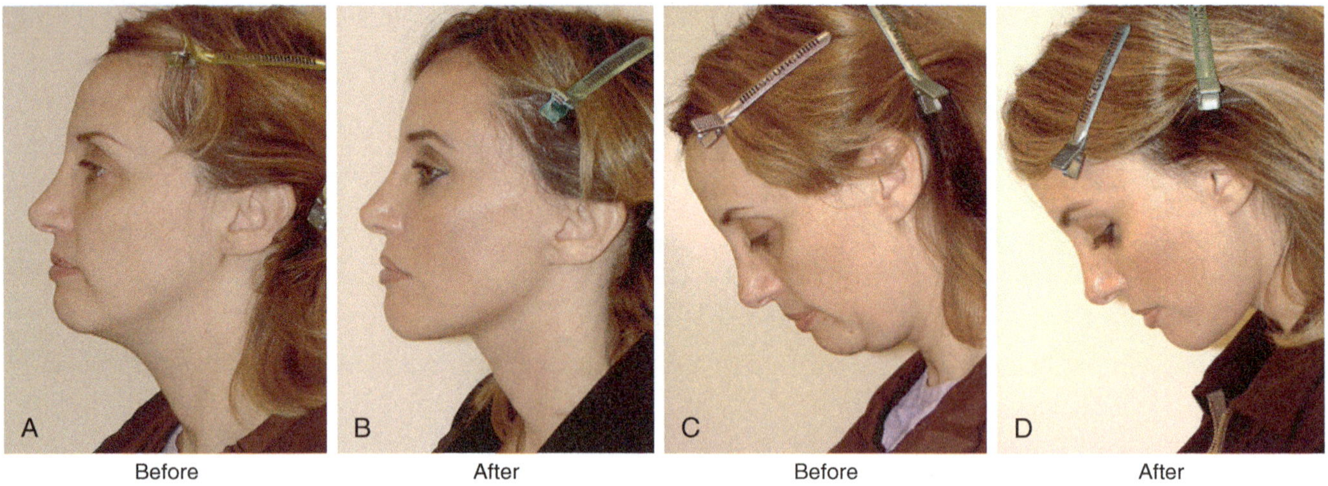

• **Fig. 67.1** Patient seen before and after neck lift. A good neckline conveys a sense of youth, health, fitness, confidence, vitality, decisiveness, sensuality, and beauty. The patient is seen (A,C) before and (B,D) 1 year and 3 months after facelift, temple lift, lower eyelid surgery, and facial fat injections. (Courtesy Timothy Marten, MD, FACS and the Marten Clinic of Plastic Surgery, San Francisco, CA; with permission. All procedures performed by Timothy Marten, MD, FACS.)

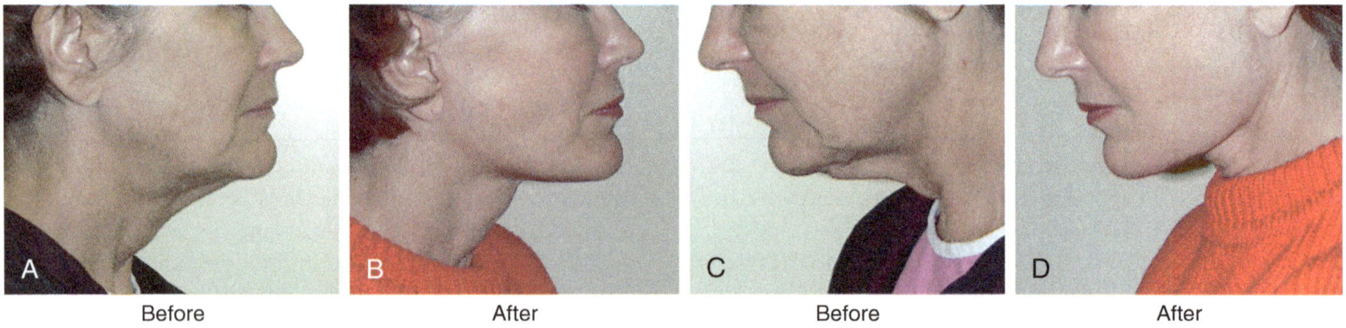

• **Fig. 67.2** Patient seen before and after neck lift. It is not enough to perform submental liposuction and tighten the skin in most patients. Such an approach ignores anatomical problems present in many patients seeking neck improvement. (A,C) A careful evaluation shows the patient preoperatively to be troubled by platysmal laxity, platysma bands, excess subplatysmal fat, large submandibular glands, digastric muscle hypertrophy. (B,D) Removing subcutaneous fat and tightening skin over these problems does not correct them, and cannot produce the type of improvement shown. (Courtesy Timothy Marten, MD, FACS and the Marten Clinic of Plastic Surgery, San Francisco, CA; with permission. All procedures performed by Timothy Marten, MD, FACS.)

In reality, submental liposuction (and noninvasive procedures that target subcutaneous neck fat) is an incomplete solution to neck problems for most patients. As a standalone treatment it suffers the significant drawback that it falsely assumes poor neck contour to be solely the result of the accumulation of subcutaneous fat only, and it is conceptually flawed in that it does not address platysma laxity and other deep layer problems which together typically play a much larger and more important role in the aging neck and neck contour deformities. As a result, most patients undergoing this procedure arguably achieve marginal improvement, but not comprehensive correction of their neck problems, and ultimately relying on this technique as the only method to obtain improved neck contour will seldom be consistently successful (Fig. 67.3).

Submental liposuction is also a frequent cause of many vexing patient problems and complications as it often leads to unintended but inappropriate removal of subcutaneous fat essential to a natural and youthful appearance, and this can, in turn, expose underlying problems of deep layer origin. Misapplied and overused, or when aggressive "ultrasonic" and "laser" techniques and other "power tools" are over-zealously employed, submental liposuction can all too commonly result in extreme overresection of precious subcutaneous fat and very unnatural and objectionable appearances. These problems are typically not evident in the operating room or in the early postoperative period when cervicosubmental tissues are swollen, but appear later, and once present, are very difficult to correct (Fig. 67.4).

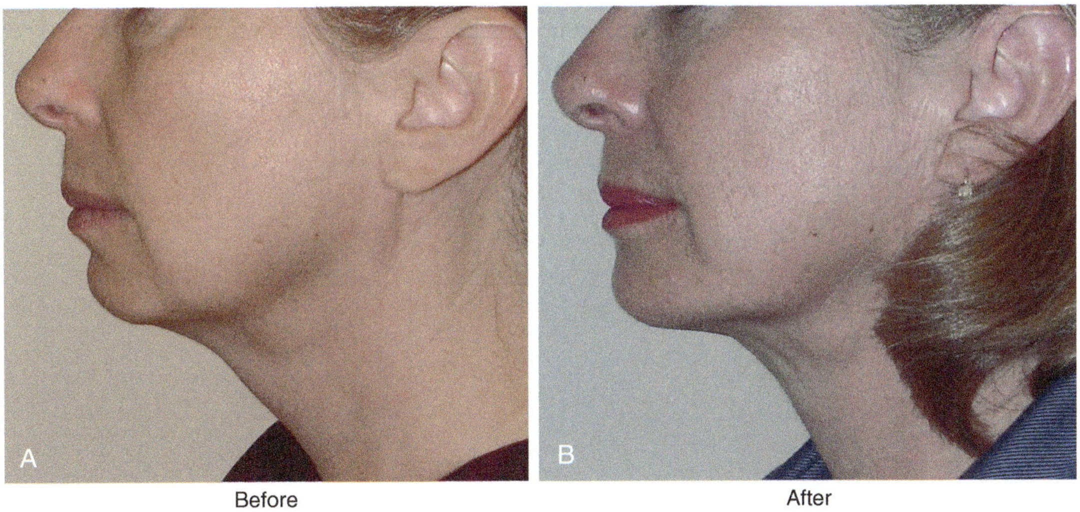

• **Fig. 67.3** (A,B) Typical outcome seen with submental liposuction. Submental liposuction is an incomplete solution to neck problems for most patients as it falsely assumes that poor neck contour is solely the result of the accumulation of subcutaneous fat, and it does *not* address platysma laxity and other deep layer problems which usually play a much larger role in the aging neck. Note that the large submandibular salivary gland is still present, platysma laxity has not been corrected, and aggressive fat removal has made platysma bands more obvious. (Courtesy Timothy Marten, MD, FACS and the Marten Clinic of Plastic Surgery, San Francisco, CA; with permission.)

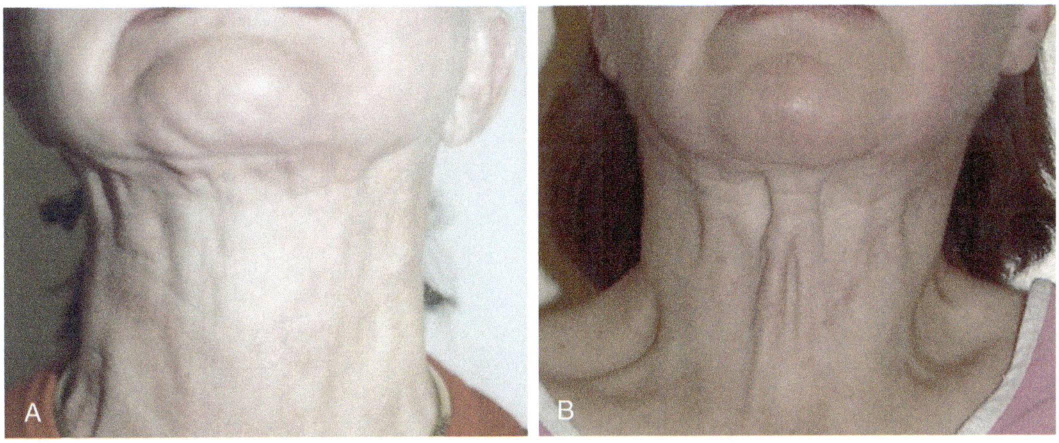

• **Fig. 67.4** Overexcision of subcutaneous fat with liposuction. (A) The patient has had aggressive "small cannula micro-liposculpture" by an unknown surgeon, which resulted in too much fat being removed. The neck and submental region are irregular, unnatural, and unattractive. (B) A different patient has had "laser liposuction" performed by an unknown surgeon. Inappropriate overresection of fat has resulted in harsh and unnatural contours along with unattractive exposure of platysmal bands. (Courtesy Timothy Marten, MD, FACS and the Marten Clinic of Plastic Surgery, San Francisco, CA; with permission. All procedures performed by unknown surgeons.)

Liposuction, in combination with ill-conceived overtightening of neck skin, can add the additional objectionable problems of hairline displacement and wide postauricular scars, and compound the overall deformity (Fig. 67.5).

Despite its many drawbacks and propensity to precipitate troublesome and difficult-to-treat problems, the conceptual and comparative technical simplicity of submental liposuction is particularly appealing to inexperienced surgeons and nonsurgeons performing esthetic surgery procedures. Indeed, these characteristics of the technique almost guarantee that, effective or not, it will continue to be overused and inappropriately recommended to patients who are not good candidates for the procedure for the foreseeable future.

"Short-Scar" Neck Lift (Neck Lift with Submental Incision Only)

Although submental liposuction alone will rarely produce optimal neck improvement, a neck lift performed through a submental incision without any removal of skin can create attractive cervical contour in many patients (Fig. 67.6).

This is due to the fact that, unlike liposuction, a neck lift performed through a submental incision allows deep layer problems (subplatysmal fat excess and submandibular gland enlargement) and platysmal laxity typically present in the majority of patients seeking neck improvement to be

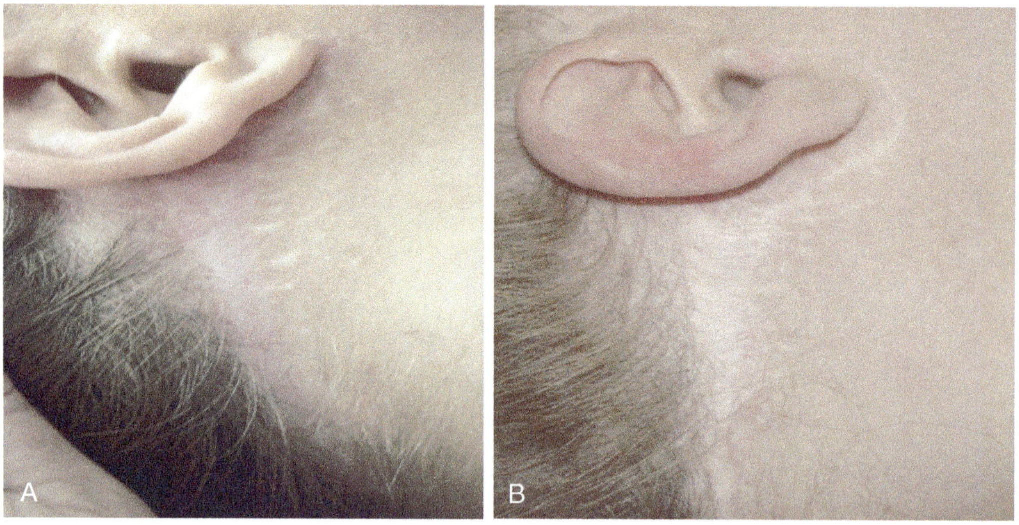

• **Fig. 67.5** (A,B) Overexcision of postauricular skin. It is a common error to attempt to lift the neck by tightening neck skin. It is not possible, however, to create a sustained improvement in neck contour in this manner and ill-conceived over-tightening of neck skin will result in wide post-auricular scars (and if the incision is planned poorly, hairline displacement). Neck contour is properly created by modification of deep layer structures and only skin that is truly redundant should be removed. In some case no skin at all needs be removed (see Fig. 67.6). (Courtesy Timothy Marten, MD, FACS and the Marten Clinic of Plastic Surgery, San Francisco, CA; with permission. All procedures performed by unknown surgeons.)

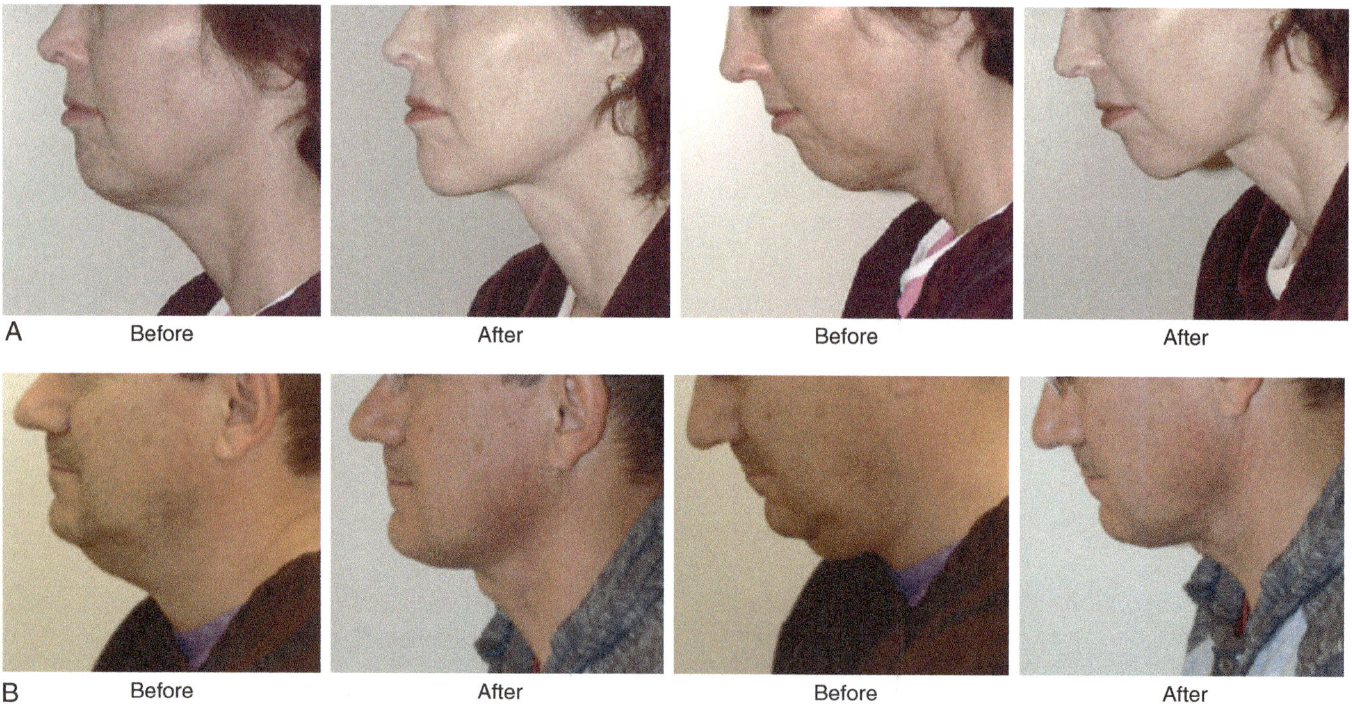

• **Fig. 67.6** Neck lift with a submental incision only. Although submental liposuction alone will rarely produce optimal neck improvement, a neck lift performed through a submental incision without any removal of skin can create attractive cervical contour in many patients. These patients had their procedures performed through a submental incision only. No incisions were made in the periauricular areas and there are no periauricular scars. Improvement in neck contour was achieved by modifying and reducing subplatysmal structures, not by tightening the skin, removing subcutaneous fat, or by tightening the platysma. (Courtesy Timothy Marten, MD, FACS and the Marten Clinic of Plastic Surgery, San Francisco, CA; with permission. A, Procedure performed by Timothy J. Marten, MD, FACS. B, Procedure performed by Dino Elyassnia, MD, FACS – Courtesy Dino Elyassnia, MD.)

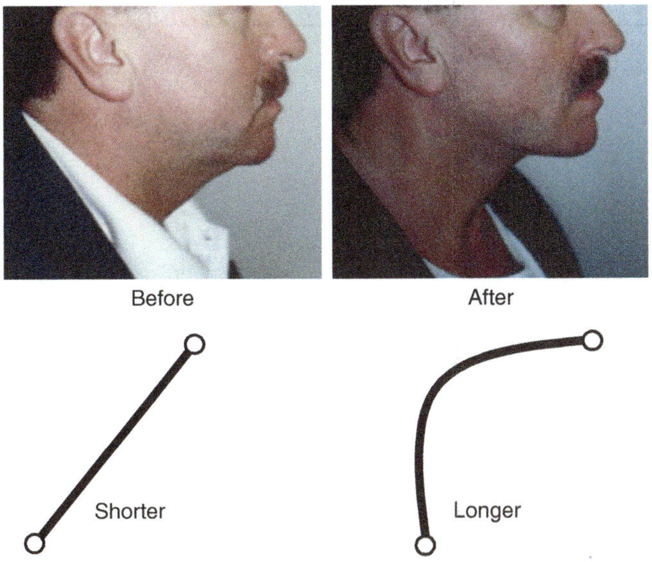

• **Fig. 67.7** Redistribution of "excess" skin in short-scar neck lift. In the preoperative condition (*left*) subplatysmal fullness (subplatysmal fat and large submandibular glands) has resulted in an oblique neck and the neck skin is distributed over a straight surface between the chin and the sternum. This straight line comprises the shortest distance between the two points and to the eye excess skin appears to be present. In the postoperative condition (*right*) subplatysmal fullness has been eliminated and a deeper, more concave, and geometrically larger and longer neck surface has been created. The skin is redistributed over a curved line that takes a longer path between the two points. (Courtesy Timothy Marten, MD, FACS and the Marten Clinic of Plastic Surgery, San Francisco, CA; with permission. Procedure performed by Timothy J. Marten, MD, FACS.)

addressed. This, however, begs the question, how can good neck contour be created without removing and tightening the skin, and what happens to the "excess" skin if only the deeper layer treatment is made and no skin is excised? The answer to this question is twofold. First, is the simple but often difficult to accept concept that in a properly performed neck lift contour is created by modification of deep layers of the neck and *not* by tightening of the skin, the covering layer. Skin stretches and relaxes, as we move and express ourselves; it is not intended to be a structural supporting layer, to hold up sagging muscle, fat and/or lift hypertrophied structures lying beneath it. The second part of the answer lies in the increase in neck surface area that occurs when deep neck contour is improved. Improving neck contour by excising redundant subplatysmal fat and performing other deep layer maneuvers as indicated, followed by the removal of lax platysma, will result in a deepened cervicomental angle, a longer curvilinear distance from the mentum to the sternal notch, a more concave, geometrically larger and longer neck surface (Fig. 67.7). When neck skin is redraped and redistributed over the deeper, more concave surface, "excess" skin is absorbed and none need be removed.

These simple but not intuitive or immediately obvious facts underlie the reason that skin excision need not be performed in patients with good skin quality and mild to moderate skin excess to obtain a good result. In female patients good results can be obtained from short-scar neck lifts in patients up to their late thirties. In male patients satisfactory outcomes can be achieved in patients up to their late fifties.

It is therefore clear why it is counterproductive to excise any skin from the submental incision, as this can create a "bow-string" effect and actually blunts the cervicomental angle. The submental skin incision is used for access to the neck only in a correctly performed neck lift, and if skin excision is necessary it is more practically, effectively, and logically removed from the postauricular area (extended neck lift or a facelift procedure) along a more appropriately directed lateral vector (Fig. 67.8).

The results that can be obtained with a short-scar neck lift stand as compelling confirmation of the supremacy of the "deep layer" approach over more traditional procedures that mistakenly focused on skin excision, subcutaneous fat removal, and platysmal tightening.

There is a limit to the amount of neck skin that can be absorbed and managed by the short-scar neck lift technique, however, and an isolated neck lift performed through a submental incision only is typically best for male patients and younger women with mild to moderate skin excess, good skin elasticity, and minimal or modest aging in the midface, cheek, and jowl.

Neck Lift with a Chin Implant

The difference between the presence of poor neck contour and microgenia is commonly misunderstood, and it is a common misconception that placement of a chin implant improves neck contour. A chin implant is a treatment for microgenia – not a poor neckline – and the presence or absence of microgenia and the need for a chin implant is a cephalometric determination that is independent of the condition of the neck. Placement of a chin implant when microgenia is not present is a conceptual and artistic error that will create unnatural appearances.

When true microgenia is present however, placing a chin implant in combination with a neck lift will produce a more harmonious and balanced profile and a more esthetic and attractive cervicofacial profile (Fig. 67.9).

"Extended" Neck Lift

If a significant amount of redundant skin is present, it must be excised to obtain the best result, and in such situations it is most logically and effectively excised in the postauricular areas using periauricular skin incisions. Skin excision can be combined with treatment of the neck through the submental incision as an "extended" or "long-scar" neck lift, or as part of a facelift procedure (Figs. 67.10–67.12).

Neck Lift with Facelift

Practically speaking, most patients in need of a neck lift with skin excision also need a facelift. It is unusual to

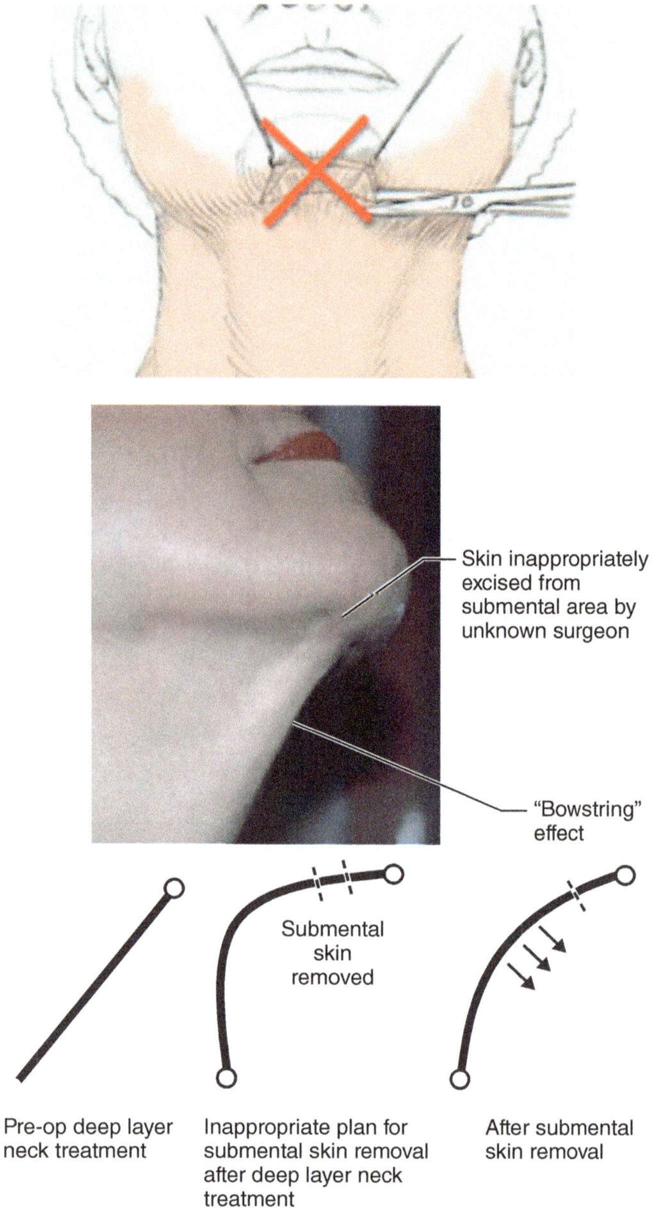

• **Fig. 67.8** Incorrect excision of skin from the submental incision and "bowstring effect." Once it is recognized that increased neck surface area and deepening the cervicomental angle is created by treatment of subplatysmal neck problems it becomes clear why it is counter-productive to excise any skin from the submental incision as this can create a "bowstring" effect and actually blunt the cervicomental angle. This maneuver will also result in objectionable "dog-ears" at each end of the incision that spoil cervicosubmental contour. If skin excision is necessary it is more practically, effectively, and logically removed from the postauricular area. (Courtesy Timothy Marten, MD, FACS and the Marten Clinic of Plastic Surgery, San Francisco, CA; with permission.)

encounter patients with excess skin in the neck but not elsewhere on the face. This is particularly true in women and it is esthetically inappropriate to perform an isolated neck lift in most women who present for facial rejuvenation. Lifting only the neck but not the cheeks, jowls, and jawline can create an unnatural and unfeminine appearance.

Combining a facelift with a neck lift is almost always the best approach to obtain a balanced, natural, and harmonious rejuvenation of the female face, although not all patients will recognize or accept this (see Fig. 67.12). Performing a facelift in combination with a neck lift also allows for more complete and comprehensive removal of neck skin. And while many men will be put off by the idea of a "facelift," they will readily agree to undergo the more palatable sounding "extended neck lift" procedure.

Surgical Planning in Neck Lift

Planning the Submental Incision

Whether performing a neck lift alone or in combination with a facelift, optimal improvement in the neck cannot generally be obtained in most patients without a submental incision. Traditionally, this incision is placed directly in and along the submental crease in a well-intended but counterproductive attempt to conceal the resulting scar (Fig. 67.13).

This, however, will surgically reinforce the crease and accentuate a "double chin" or "witch's chin" deformity. Exposure of the submental region will also be compromised, and difficulty will be encountered when suturing or dissecting low in the neck. A more posterior placement of this incision will eliminate these problems, but still result in an inconspicuous and well-concealed scar (Figs. 67.14–67.16).

The incision should be approximately 3–3.5 cm in length, but may be made longer, as long as neither end will be advanced up upon a visible portion of the face when skin flaps are shifted. Healing will be best, and the scar will be best concealed, if it is made as a straight, and not as a curved line (Fig. 67.17).

Planning Treatment of the Platysma

As surgeons have pursued improved outcomes in treating the neck, our understanding of the origin of platysma muscle irregularities has improved and platysma muscle treatment techniques have evolved. Experience has shown that the traditional notion that platysma tightening will correct deep layer, neck problems, including accumulations of subplatysmal fat and the presence of large submandibular glands and protruding digastric muscles, was misguided, and that correct treatment of these problems will require "deep layer" procedures that address the actual anatomical problems present. Over time, thoughtful surgeons have come to understand and accept that a sustained improvement in neck contour is not created by platysma tightening, but by these deep layer maneuvers (subplatysmal fat excision, submandibular gland reduction, and partial digastric myectomy) that specifically target these problems.

Experience has also confirmed that traditional platysma tightening will not universally correct "platysma bands," and that our traditional view that all platysma bands were a homogenous problem and simply a product of age-associated horizontal platysmal laxity was conceptually flawed and the underlying cause of many decades of failed treatments. In reality "platysma bands" comprise a heterogeneous group

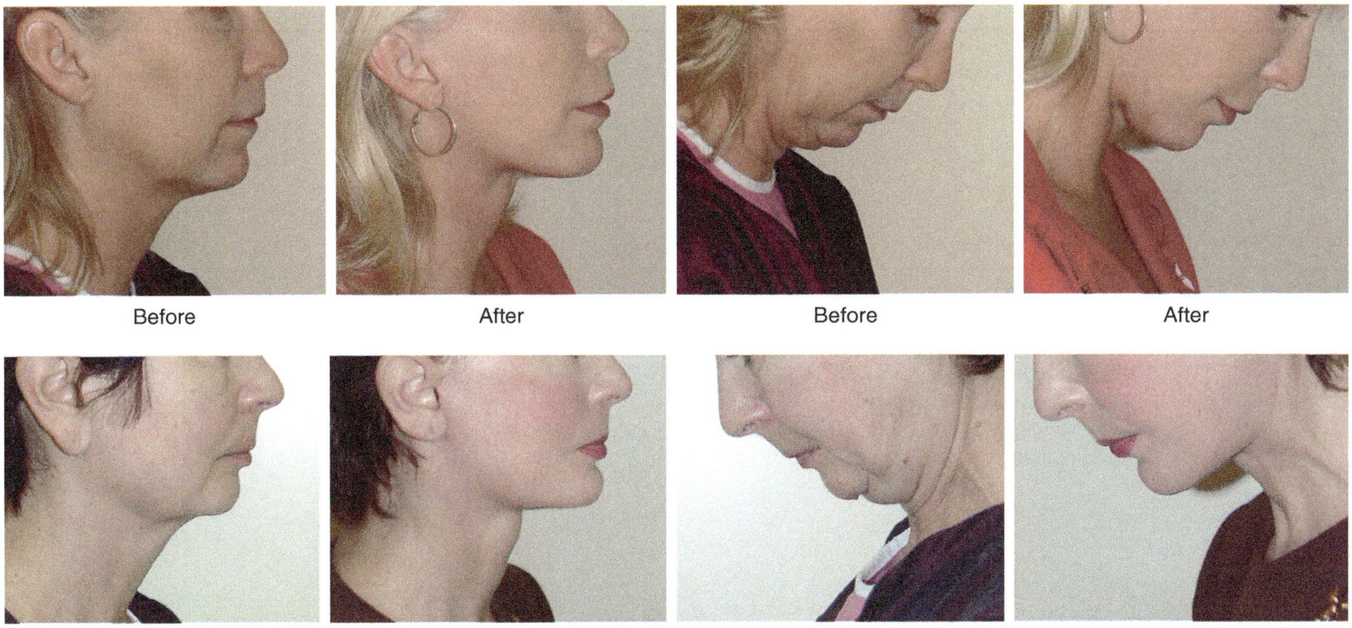

• **Fig. 67.9** Neck lift with a chin implant. The difference between the presence of poor neck contour and microgenia is commonly misunderstood, and it is a common misconception that placement of a chin implant improves neck contour. When true microgenia is present, however, placing a chin implant in combination with a neck lift will produce a more harmonious and balanced profile and a more esthetic and attractive cervicofacial profile (Courtesy Timothy Marten, MD, FACS and the Marten Clinic of Plastic Surgery, San Francisco, CA; with permission. Procedures performed by Timothy J. Marten, MD, FACS.)

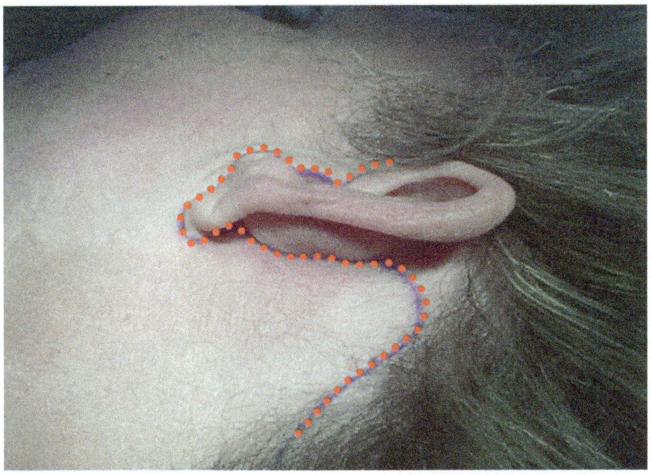

• **Fig. 67.10** Incision lift plan for a long scar or "extended" neck. If a significant amount of redundant skin is present on the neck it must be excised to obtain the best result, and in such situations it is most logically and effectively excised in the postauricular areas using a peri-auricular skin incision rather than one under the chin. This incision plan avoids a temporal incision that is of concern to some patients but provides for significant skin removal from the neck. (Courtesy Timothy Marten, MD, FACS and the Marten Clinic of Plastic Surgery, San Francisco, CA; with permission.)

of distinct problems, and for many patients platysma bands can be seen to be the product of not only horizontal laxity but *longitudinal platysmal hyperfunction*, and as such, refractory to traditional horizontal lifting and pulling procedures. Correct treatment of these problems requires horizontal platysma transection to disrupt longitudinal hyperfunction, or treatment by other like means.

Assessing Platysma Deformity

The cervicosubmental region of each patient must be carefully examined both at rest and *during platysmal activation* if complete assessment of platysmal deformity is to be made. This is best accomplished by asking the patient to "push the jaw forward and tighten the neck." It is often helpful if the surgeon demonstrates this maneuver first for the patient to be sure it is correctly performed. Frequently, an insignificant appearing deformity at rest will be obvious upon muscle activation (Fig. 67.18). Failure to recognize and appropriately correct these "*dynamic deformities*" is the reason too many facelift patients appear improved in repose but unnatural or bizarre in conversation, animation, and during other activities that result in platysma muscle activation.

Examination of the cervicosubmental region with and without platysmal activation allows one to distinguish between "hard" dynamic and "soft" *a*dynamic cervical bands. Soft, adynamic bands change little during platysma activation and are predominantly a problem of loose skin or horizontal platysmal laxity. Hard dynamic bands become tight or exaggerated upon platysmal activation and indicate a problem of *longitudinal platysmal hyperfunction.*

If submental support is poor due to horizontal platysmal laxity or platysmal diastasis and optimal improvement in the anterior neck is desired, *anterior platysmaplasty* is planned (Fig. 67.19). In this procedure, the medial borders of the platysma muscle are sutured together to help consolidate the neck, reduce horizontal platysmal laxity, and improve neck appearance when the patient flexes the neck and looks down

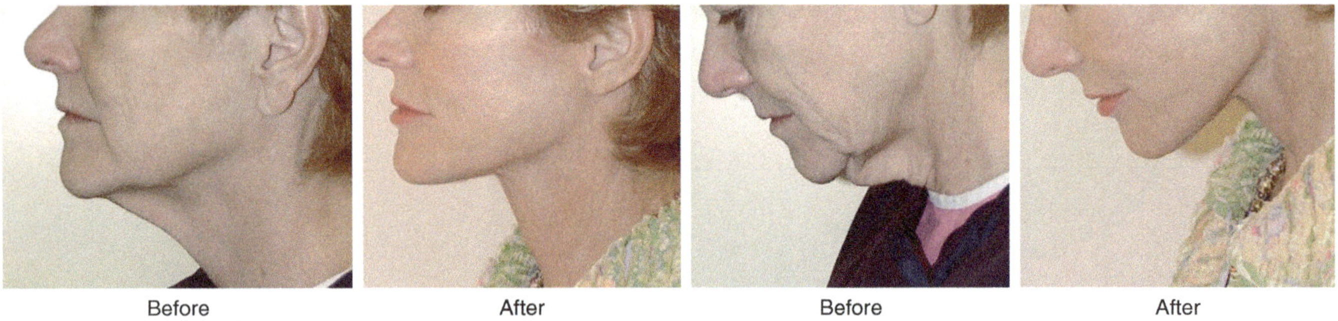

• **Fig. 67.11** Extended neck lift. Skin excision can be combined with treatment of the neck through the submental incision as an "extended" or "long-scar" neck lift, or as part of a facelift procedure. The patient had skin excised as part of the procedures, and an incision was made in the periauricular area. (Courtesy Timothy Marten, MD, FACS and the Marten Clinic of Plastic Surgery, San Francisco, CA; with permission. Procedures performed by Timothy J. Marten, MD, FACS.)

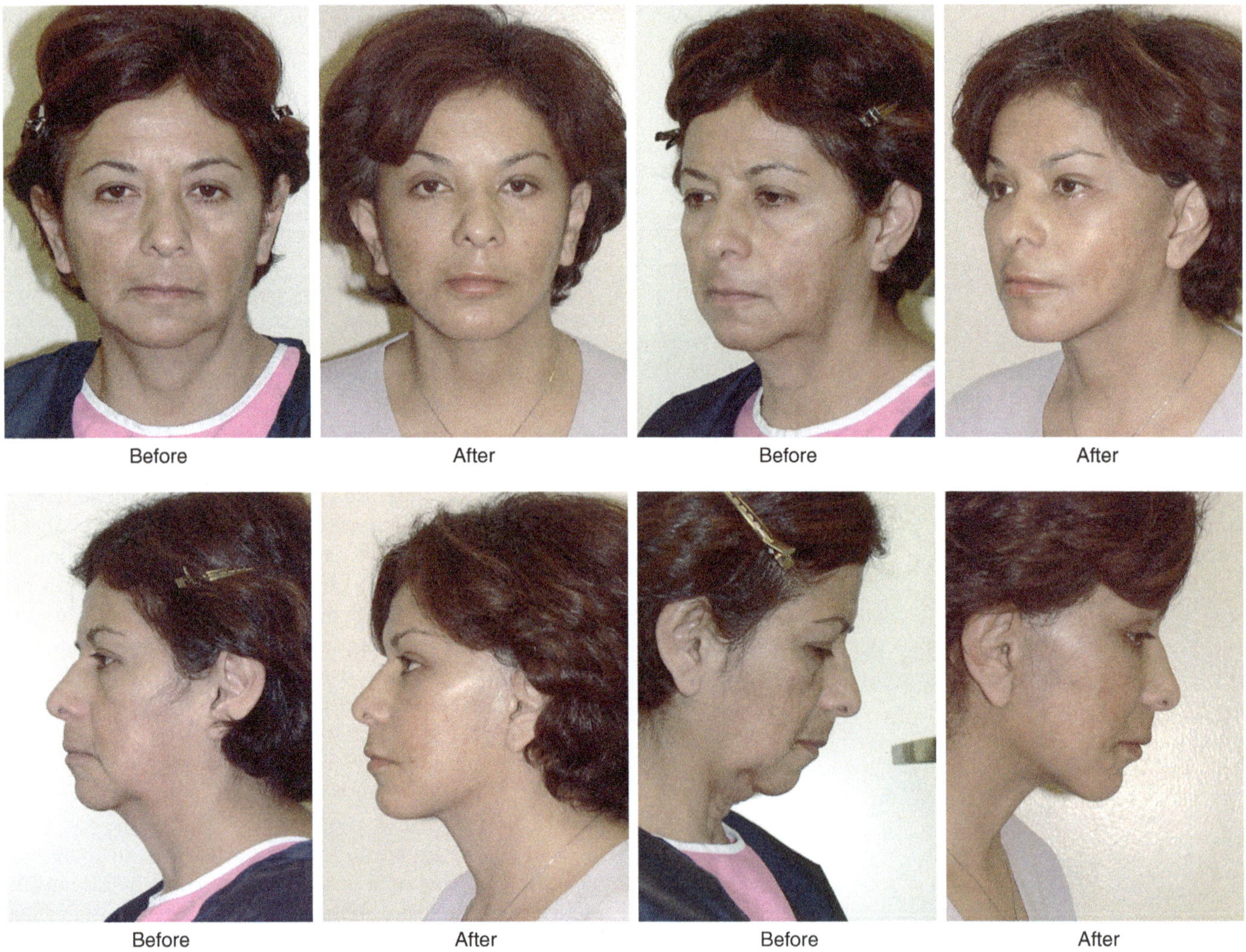

• **Fig. 67.12** Comprehensive rejuvenation of the face. Combining a neck lift with a facelift and related procedures is almost always the best approach to obtain a balanced, natural, and harmonious rejuvenation of the female face, although not all patients will recognize or accept this. This 55-year-old woman underwent facelift, neck lift, limited-incision ("short-scar") forehead lift, upper and lower blepharoplasties, chin augmentation, and fat transfer to the lips and cheeks. Addressing all regions of the face has produced a natural balanced outcome, and a far better result than neck lift alone (see also Fig. 67.1). (Courtesy Timothy Marten, MD, FACS and the Marten Clinic of Plastic Surgery, San Francisco, CA; with permission. Procedures performed by Timothy J. Marten, MD, FACS.)

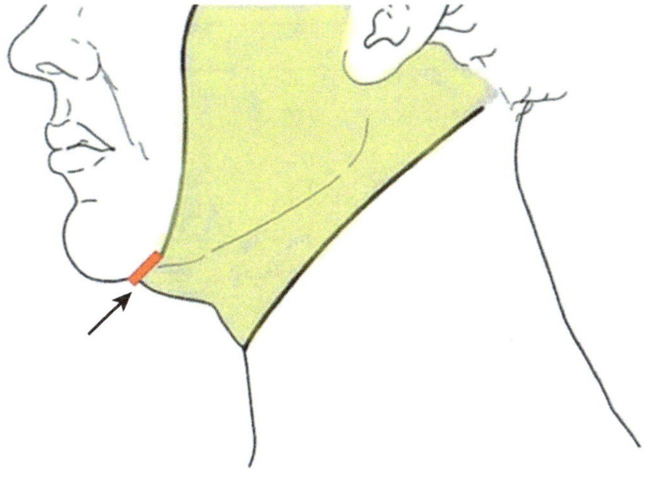

• **Fig. 67.13** Traditional, but *incorrect* plan for the submental incision. The incision should not be placed directly along the submental crease (*arrow*) as this will reinforce the submental retaining ligaments and accentuate the "double chin" appearance. Note that typical plan of skin undermining (yellow area) also promotes a "double chin" appearance because the crease is not undermined, retaining ligaments are not released, and the fat of the chin and the neck cannot be readily blended to create a smooth transition between them. (Courtesy Timothy Marten, MD, FACS and the Marten Clinic of Plastic Surgery, San Francisco, CA; with permission.)

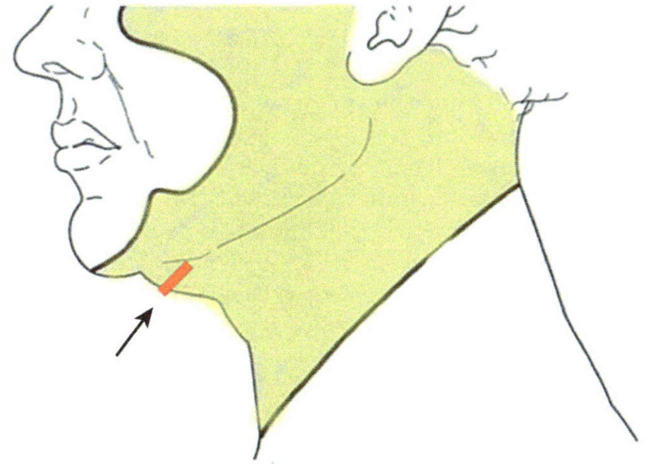

• **Fig. 67.14** Correct location for the submental incision. Placing the submental incision 1.5 cm *posterior* to the submental crease (*arrow*) prevents accentuation of the "double chin" and "witch's chin" deformities and provides for easier dissection and suturing in the anterior neck (compare with Fig. 67.10). Note that this incision plan allows the submental crease to be undermined and submental retaining ligaments to be released, and the fat of the chin pad and neck to be blended to create a smooth transition between them (see Fig. 67.15). (Courtesy Timothy Marten, MD, FACS and the Marten Clinic of Plastic Surgery, San Francisco, CA; with permission.)

(see Fig. 67.11). It is *not*, however, adequate or effective in the treatment of excess subplatysmal fat, prominent submandibular glands, hypertrophy of the anterior bellies of the digastric muscles, or the treatment of "hard" dynamic platysmal bands. Not recognizing and acknowledging this fact, and well-intended but misguided attempts to treat these problems by medial or lateral platysmal pulling and tightening, has led to frustration for many surgeons treating the aging neck. Treatment of these problems will require that other maneuvers discussed elsewhere in this chapter be performed.

It is important to distinguish between "soft" adynamic playsmal bands and "hard" dynamic bands as treatment will vary depending on the type present. Patients with soft bands are usually adequately treated with skin excision or skin excision and platysmaplasty alone. Patients with "hard" bands however require *transverse platysma myotomy* or some other procedure that disrupts *longitudinal platysma muscle hyperfunction* and prevents the muscle from contracting upon itself. Much like when a dancer ruptures their Achilles tendon they cannot point their toe, dividing the platysma transversely prevents it from pulling itself away from the anterior surface of the neck. The result of platysma myotomy when correctly performed is dramatic, long-lasting, and superior to any suture, suture suspension, lateral suspension of the platysmal border, or "corset" platysmal tightening technique (Fig. 67.20). The length of transection required can be varied depending on the location and configuration of bands present, and may thus differ from patient to patient. *The key to success in treating hard, dynamic bands is to recognize that they are the product of longitudinal platysma muscle hyperfunction and not one of horizontal platysma laxity, and employing a plan of treatment that recognizes this fact. Pulling medially or laterally on the platysma muscle borders as commonly advocated does not address the origin of dynamic platysma bands, and is not a logical or effective treatment of them.* Likewise, attempts to vertically excise dynamic platysma bands along the length of the muscle fibers is not a logical or effective treatment, as the band is not fixed in location and any such a maneuver does not address overall longitudinal muscle hyperfunction.

Platysmal bands are generally seen to lie in medial and lateral locations and are often referred to as *anterior* and *lateral* platysma bands (see Fig. 67.18D). Each band is situated near the medial and lateral platysma muscle borders, but does not usually correlate precisely with them and is not specifically fixed in location. Patients with *anterior* platysmal bands only can be treated with a partial transverse platysma myotomy by dividing the muscle medially and subtotally through and beyond the section of it in which the band is present low in the neck at the level of the *cricoid* cartilage (Fig. 67.21). The platysma muscles need not be completely transected when an anterior band only is present, just the region where the platysmal band is located.

If *lateral*, as well as anterior bands are present, the myotomy is carried more laterally to include them as well (Fig. 67.22). If poor definition is present over the lateral mandibular border, in addition to anterior and lateral neck bands, or if comprehensive improvement is desired, platysmal myotomy is planned to continue "full width" superior-laterally up to the anterior border of the sternocleidomastoid muscle (Fig. 67.23). A similar full-width myotomy of this type is also indicated in a firm obtuse neck with a "short platysma" and poor definition over the mandibular angle, but no bands.

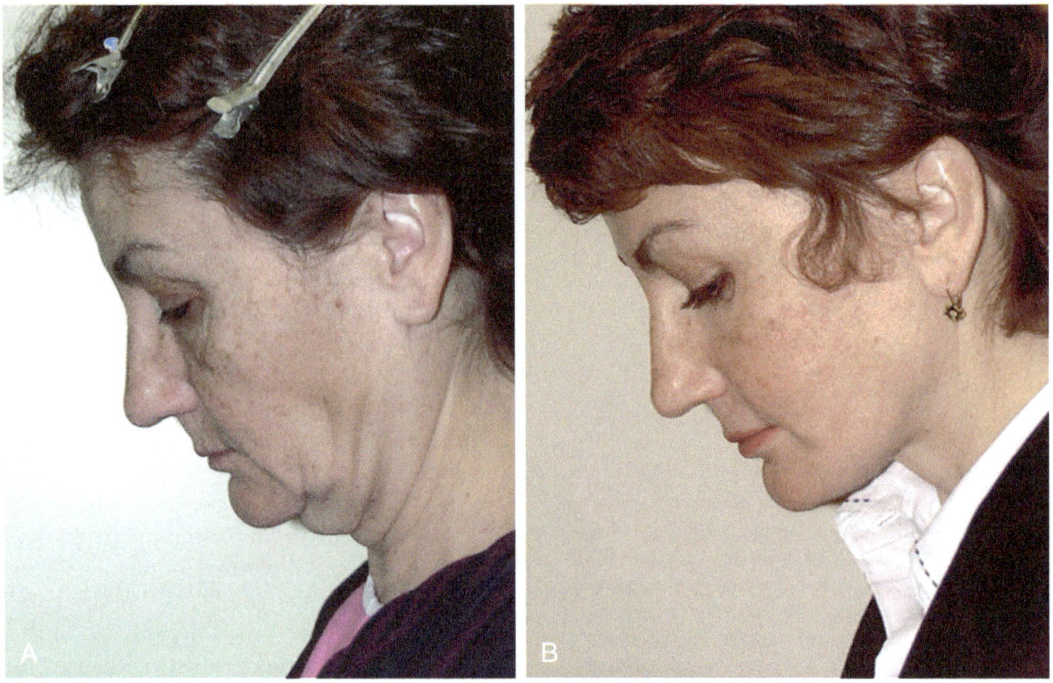

• **Fig. 67.15** Correction of the "double chin" deformity. (A) Patient with "double chin" seen preoperatively. (B) Same patient seen after face and neck lift. The submental incision was made posterior to the submental crease to allow undermining and release on the submental retaining ligaments and blending of chin and neck fat to create a smooth and esthetically pleasing transition between them. (Courtesy Timothy Marten, MD, FACS and the Marten Clinic of Plastic Surgery, San Francisco, CA; with permission. Procedures performed by Timothy J. Marten, MD, FACS.)

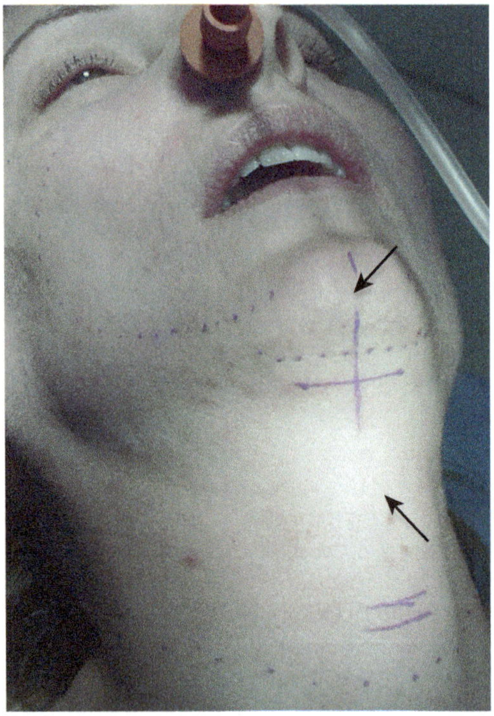

• **Fig. 67.16** Plan for the submental incision. The submental portion of the facelift incision (*solid line*) should be placed posterior to the submental crease (*dotted line*), approximately one-half the distance between the mentum and hyoid (*arrows*). Usually this corresponds to a point about 1.5 cm posterior to the submental crease. (Courtesy Timothy Marten, MD, FACS and the Marten Clinic of Plastic Surgery, San Francisco, CA; with permission.)

In theory and principle, in many necks a subtotal myotomy only is indicated and need be performed. As a practical matter, however, complete transection of the platysma is typically performed in most of our patients when any form of myotomy is indicated to limit the possibility of band reoccurrence in areas of muscle that were not divided, or that residual platysma bands will be present. Despite assertions to the contrary, full-width platysma myotomy will not result in an overly thin appearing neck ("lollipop neck"), or "reduced support" of the submandibular glands when correctly performed. These are merely false assertions put forth by surgeons who do not perform the procedure and do not want to take the time and trouble of learning and performing it.

Medial wedge resections of platysma at the hyoid and vertical excisions of platysma bands, while shown in many textbooks, are not typically effective in treating dynamic platysma bands in that a large segment of adjacent and more laterally situated muscle remains untreated. Vertical excision of platysma bands while still advocated by some has proven to be an ineffective treatment that has been abandoned by experienced surgeons. Trying to isolate and specifically excise the responsible muscle segment is difficult at best since the band is not specifically fixed in its location, and a partial excision along a vertical axis typically allows or incites new bands to form in an adjacent untreated area.

Medial wedge resections of platysma at the hyoid can result in unesthetic exposure of underlying cervical anatomy, a harsh transition from the submental region to the neck, as well as lower lip dysfunction and asymmetric smile.

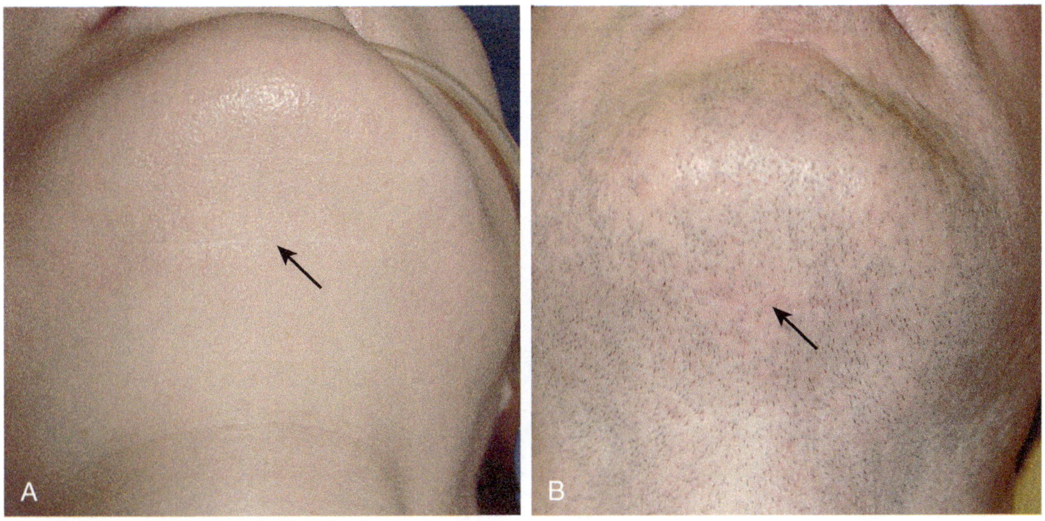

• **Fig. 67.17** Healed submental incisions. (A,B) Placement of the submental incision posterior to the submental crease will still result in an inconspicuous, well-concealed scar and simultaneously provide better access and exposure when working in the deep layers of the neck. (Courtesy Timothy Marten, MD, FACS and the Marten Clinic of Plastic Surgery, San Francisco, CA; with permission. Procedures performed by Timothy J. Marten, MD, FACS.)

These procedures are not recommended in routine treatment of platysmal bands although they may be useful in certain secondary cases and in situations where there has been fibrosis and scarring of the platysma in that area. These problems can result from noninvasive treatment of the neck with radiofrequency, ultrasound, internal tissue heating, cryolipolysis, chemolipolysis, laser liposuction, and the use of inflammatory fillers in the neck area. When these problems are present a "high" myotomy (division at the level of the thyroid cartilage rather than the cricoid), or even a partial myectomy (excising damaged platysma muscle from the anterior neck at the level of the thyroid cartilage) may be indicated.

Similarly, attempts to place rigid support across the cervicomental angle in the form of a mastoid to mastoid "noose" of suture or commercially available straps to lift platysmal bands is conceptually flawed and practically problematic. Experience has shown that these maneuvers do not work and are the source of many patient problems.

Assessing the Anatomical Basis of Neck Problems

Planning the Modification of the Submental Region

Traditional neck lift techniques do not adequately address many aspects of aging in the submental region and it is not enough in most situations to limit treatment of the neck to preplatysmal lipectomy alone or with postauricular skin excision. For many patients subplatysmal fat accumulation, submandibular salivary gland "ptosis" (enlargement), and digastric muscle hypertrophy will contribute significantly to the neck deformity present and necessitate additional treatment if optimal improvement is to be obtained (Fig. 67.24).

It must be acknowledged and accepted that simply tightening the platysma and creating a tight platysma "corset" over these problems will not correct them and will not produce a sustained improvement in neck contour if underlying deep layer problems are not addressed.

Identifying the Neck with Excess Subplatysmal Volume

The presence of abnormal fullness in the submental space can be demonstrated preoperatively by taking and examining a lateral-looking down view photograph (Connell's view) of the patient's neck (Fig. 67.25). Often a neck that looks reasonably good in the straight lateral view will be revealed to be unexpectedly full when the patient looks down as they would when looking at work on their desk, a menu at a restaurant, or their phone screen. Failure to appreciate subplatysmal fullness preoperatively and treat it appropriately intraoperatively will result in compromised outcomes.

Fullness in the subplatysmal space and the need to explore and treat the "deep neck" is indicated when the neck is full in Connell's view and this picture should be taken and examined by any surgeon performing neck surgery. If this view is not taken before and after surgery the analysis of the patient's neck was incomplete and the documentation that the procedure was well performed is inadequate.

Understanding the Distribution of Fat in the Neck

A key element to obtaining good outcomes in the neck lies in understanding the distribution of fat in the cervicosubmental region and choosing a treatment plan accordingly. Cervical fat is present in three distinct anatomic layers: (1) preplatysmal (subcutaneous), (2) subplatysmal, and (3) deep

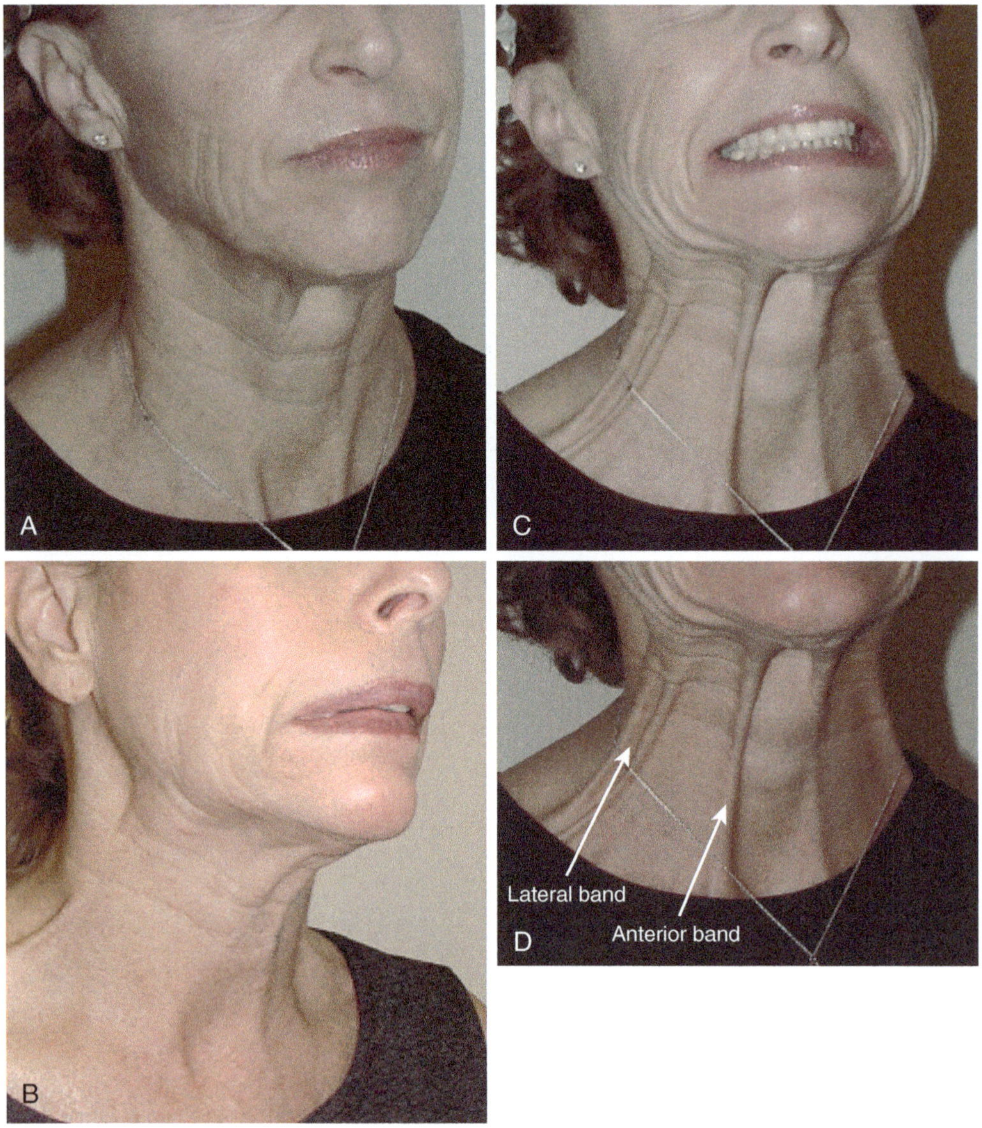

• **Fig. 67.18** Dynamic assessment of the cervicosubmental region. (A) A patient's neck is seen in repose. (B) A patient's neck during platysma activation. Soft, adynamic bands change little during platysma activation and are predominantly a problem of loose skin or horizontal platysmal laxity. (C) Dynamic platysma muscle irregularities are often referred to as "platysma bands." Hard dynamic bands become tight or exaggerated upon platysma activation and indicate a problem of longitudinal platysma hyperfunction. (D) Platysma bands are generally seen to lie in medial and lateral locations and are often referred to as *anterior* and *lateral* platysma bands. Each band is situated near the medial and lateral platysma muscle borders, but does not usually correlate precisely with them. (Courtesy Timothy Marten, MD, FACS and the Marten Clinic of Plastic Surgery, San Francisco, CA; with permission.)

cervicosubmuscular ("interdigastric"). While our traditional focus has been the preplatysmal layer (which all too often ended up overresected), the secret to good outcomes in the neck is aggressively treating the subplatysmal layer to create contour (typically in conjunction with prominent submandibular glands and digastric muscle hypertrophy – the "deep neck triad"), and fighting to preserve subcutaneous fat to maintain a youthful, healthy, and soft appearance. As such, contemporary neck lift requires many surgeons to rethink what they have been taught and the techniques that they are using. In all cases it should be the aim of the surgeon to produce a youthful, attractive, and healthy-appearing neck, and not simply one devoid of fat.

In all but the unusual or young patient, the majority of cervical fat accumulation in patients seeking neck lifts and facelifts will be present in a *sub*platysmal location, and little if any will need to be removed from the preplatysmal layer. Indeed, as patients age, fat stores generally shift from a preplatysmal location to a subplatysmal one, and the small amount of subcutaneous fat present in the typical patient presenting for a facelift or neck lift is necessary and must be preserved if a soft, youthful, natural, "nonsurgical," and attractive appearance is to be obtained. Although the necks of patients undergoing liposuction (or like procedures that target subcutaneous fat) may look good initially when swelling is present, once it resolves, they typically display an unnatural and unesthetic

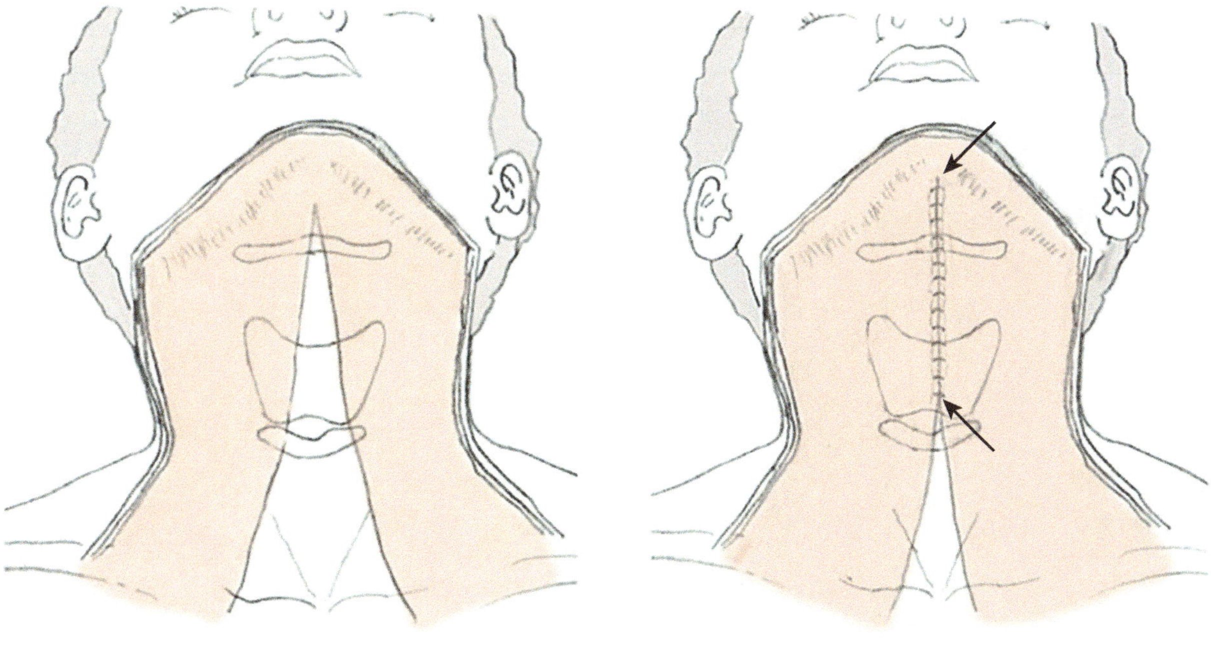

• **Fig. 67.19** Anterior platysmaplasty. Anterior platysmaplasty reduces horizontal platysma laxity, improves submental support, consolidates the neck and enhances appearance when the patient looks down (see Fig. 67.11), and is the primary treatment of "soft" platysma bands. It is *not* adequate or effective treatment of dynamic "hard" platysma bands or excess subplatysmal fat, prominent submandibular glands, and protrusion of the anterior bellies of the digastric muscles. (Courtesy of the Timothy Marten, MD, FACS and the Marten Clinic of Plastic Surgery, San Francisco, CA; with permission.)

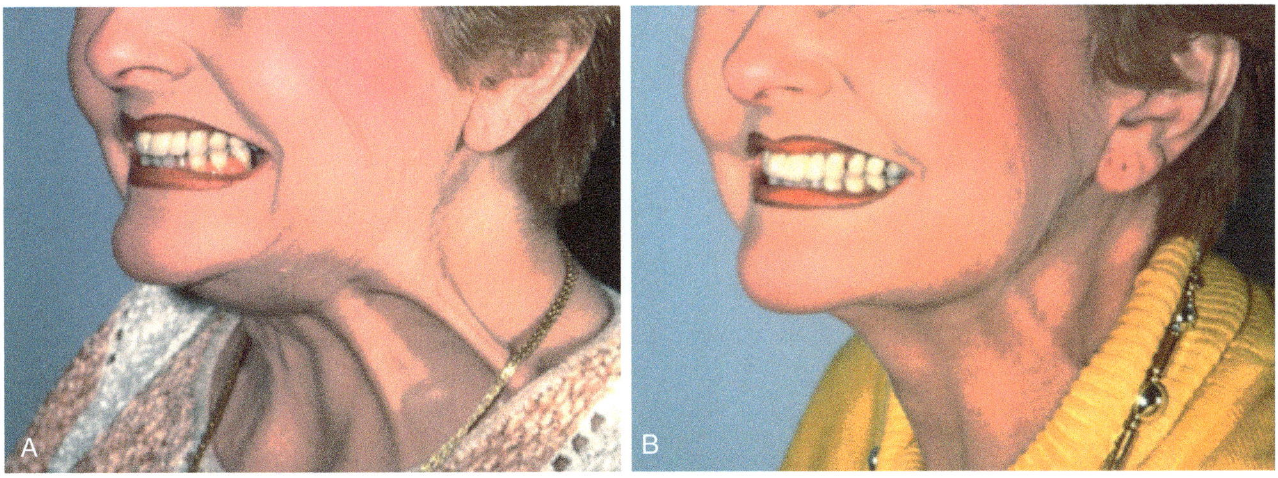

• **Fig. 67.20** Platysma myotomy. (A) Patient seen preoperatively with objectionable-appearing "hard" dynamic platysma bands. (B) The patient after platysma myotomy. The result of platysma myotomy is typically dramatic, long-lasting, and superior to any suture, suture suspension, lateral suspension of the lateral platysmal border, or "corset" platysma-tightening technique. (Courtesy Timothy Marten, MD, FACS and the Marten Clinic of Plastic Surgery, San Francisco, CA; with permission.)

"overresected" or "gutted" appearance. Once one acknowledges these facts, the futility and undesirability of cervicosubmental liposuction in most patients becomes obvious.

Often just taking a moment to look carefully at the oblique neck of a patient presenting for neck lift surgery will reveal that despite oblique contour a paucity of *sub*cutaneous fat is actually present (see Fig. 67.24). In many circumstances the majority of deeper anatomy can be easily seen beneath the skin lending an "old" appearance to the neck. This is in stark contrast to the plushly padded necks of young people where little if any deep neck anatomy can be seen.

The presence or absence of preplatysmal fat can also be assessed by examining the neck with and without platysma activation. In necks where little preplatysmal fat is present the bands will be clearly visible along their entire course and a "skin on muscle" appearance will be seen

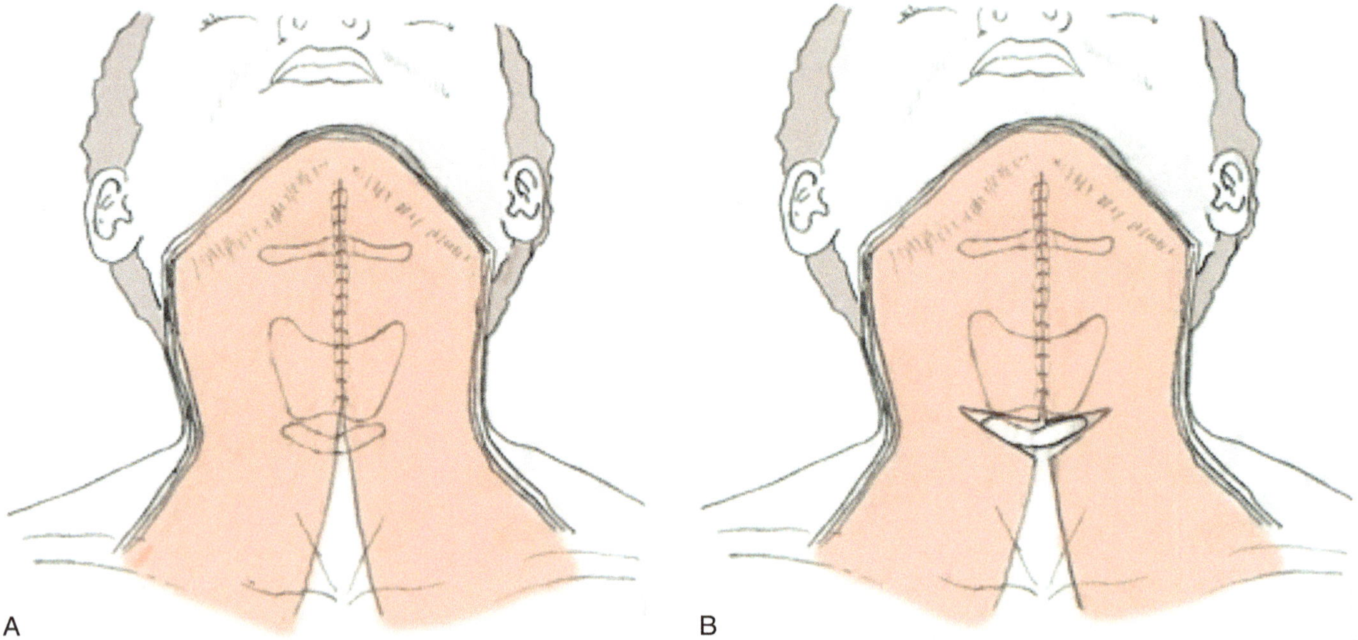

A B

• **Fig. 67.21** Plan for treatment of "anterior" dynamic "hard" platysmal bands. Transverse platysma myotomy is performed in the region of the platysma muscle where the platysmal band is present. (A) Anterior neck after platysmaplasty but before anterior platysma myotomy. (B) After anterior platysma myotomy. (Note: Myotomy is most easily and effectively performed after platysmaplasty has been completed. Also, because uninterrupted muscle is present laterally the potential for new band formation in that area is possible.) (Courtesy Timothy Marten, MD, FACS and the Marten Clinic of Plastic Surgery, San Francisco, CA; with permission.)

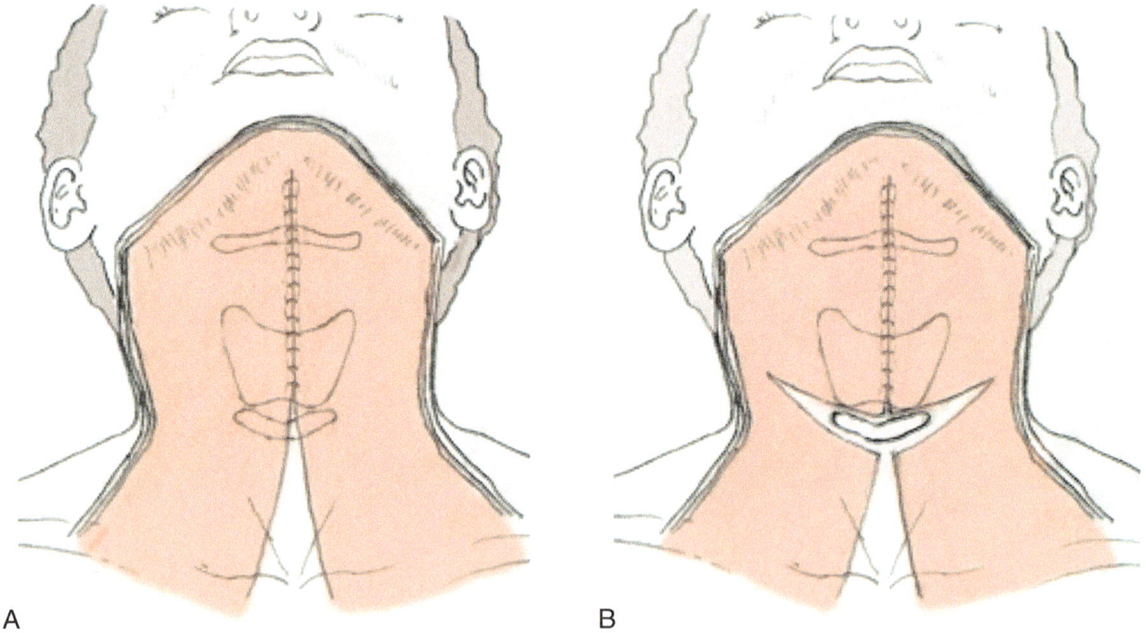

A B

• **Fig. 67.22** Pan for treatment of "anterior" and "lateral" platysmal bands. If *lateral* bands are present, the myotomy is carried more laterally to include them as well. (A) Anterior neck after platysmaplasty but before anterolateral platysmal myotomy. (B) After anterolateral myotomy. (Note: Myotomy is most easily and effectively performed after platysmaplasty has been completed. Also, because uninterrupted muscle is present laterally the potential for new band formation in that area is possible.) (Courtesy Timothy Marten, MD, FACS and the Marten Clinic of Plastic Surgery, San Francisco, CA; with permission.)

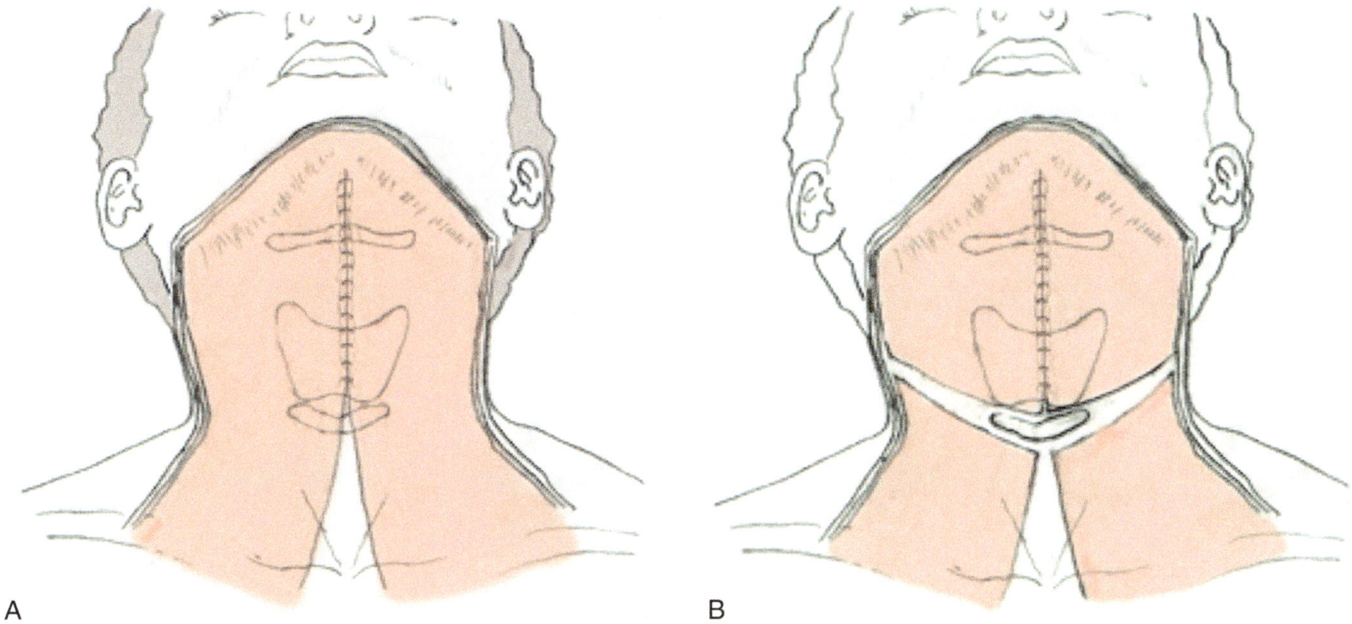

A B

• **Fig. 67.23** Plan for "full-width" platysmal transection. Full-width myotomy corrects not only anterior and lateral bands, but provides improved definition over the lateral mandibular border. (A) Anterior neck after platysmaplasty but before full-width platysmal myotomy. (B) After full-width platysmal myotomy. (Note: Myotomy is most easily and effectively performed after platysmaplasty has been completed.) (Courtesy Timothy Marten, MD, FACS and the Marten Clinic of Plastic Surgery, San Francisco, CA; with permission.)

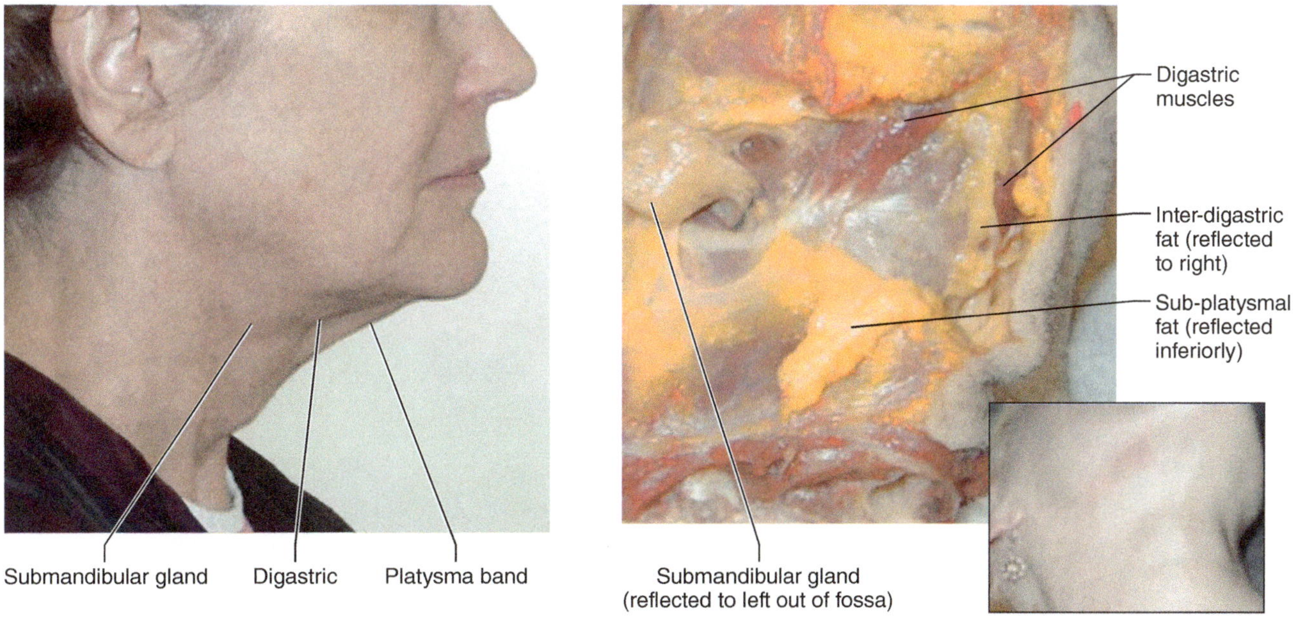

• **Fig. 67.24** Recognizing the origin of neck problems in the submental region. For many patients subplatysmal fat accumulation, submandibular salivary gland "ptosis" (enlargement), and digastric muscle hypertrophy will contribute significantly to the neck deformity present and necessitate specific treatment. Simply tightening the platysma over these problems will not correct them. Specific additional treatment is necessary if these problems are to be improved. (Note that the presence of submandibular gland and digastric muscle problems can be diagnosed simply by looking at this patient.) (Courtesy Timothy Marten, MD, FACS and the Marten Clinic of Plastic Surgery, San Francisco, CA; with permission.)

(see Figs. 67.18A–C, 67.20). When preplatysmal fat is present however, the bands will be partially obscured, usually predominantly in the submental area, and the presence of subcutaneous fat overlying them, lying between the skin and the platysma, can be seen (Fig. 67.26).

Abnormal collections of subplatysmal fat can be identified by preoperative palpation of the neck "wattle" with and without platysmal activation. Fat lying predominantly in a preplatysmal position will generally feel "soft" and will remain in the examiner's grasp upon platysmal muscle

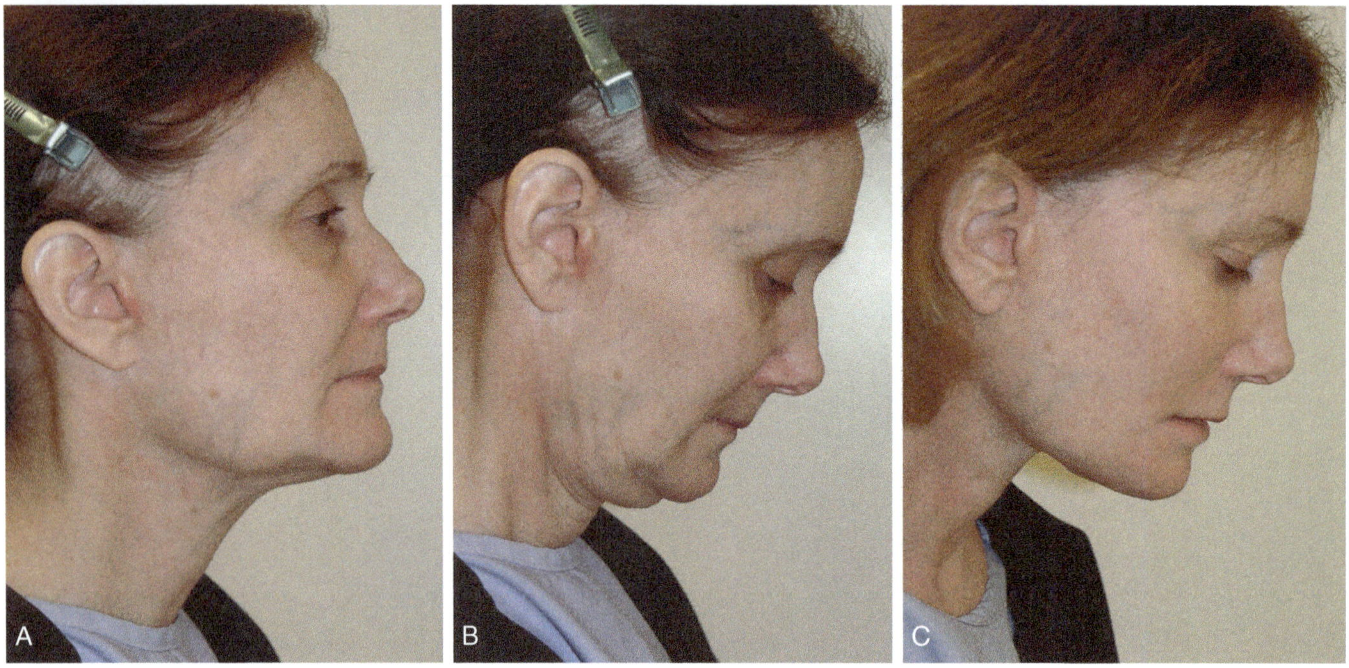

Before Before – Connell's view After

• **Fig. 67.25** Assessing the presence of fullness in the subplatysmal space. (A) Patient seen following traditional neck lift procedure in the standard lateral view. The result appears ostensibly good. (B) Same patient seen after traditional neck lift procedure in lateral flex view ("Connell's view"). Inadequate treatment of the subplatysmal space is evident and the resulting objectionable submental fullness can be seen. (C) Same patient after secondary face and neck lift that included treatment of irregularities in the subplatysmal space (subplatysmal fat, large submandibular salivary glands, and protruding anterior belly of the digastric muscle). Proper treatment of the deep neck has provided an improved outcome. (Courtesy Timothy Marten, MD, FACS and the Marten Clinic of Plastic Surgery, San Francisco, CA; with permission. A and B, Procedures performed by an unknown surgeon. C, Procedure performed by Timothy J. Marten, MD, FACS.)

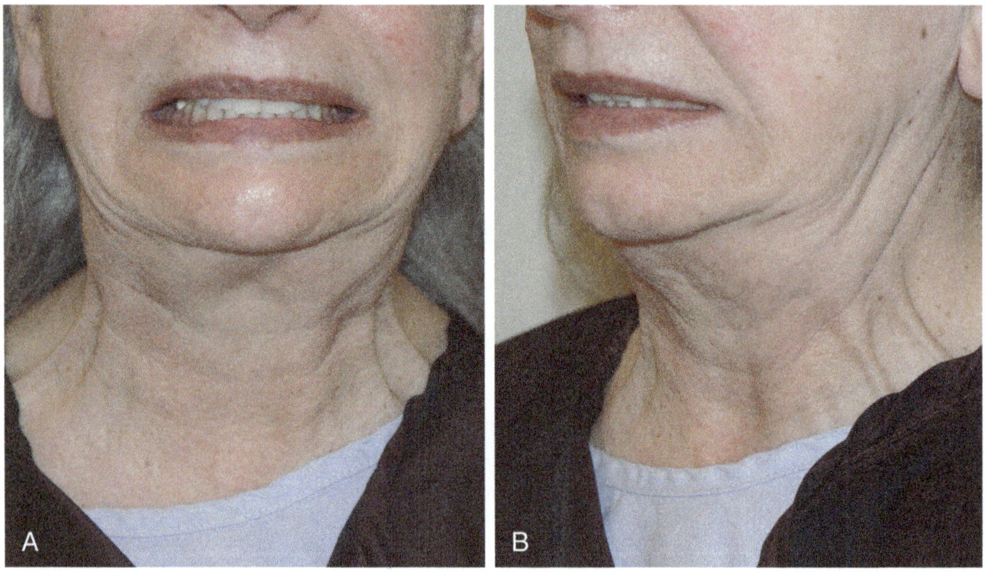

• **Fig. 67.26** (A,B) Recognizing the presence of *pre*platysmal fat. The presence of preplatysmal fat can be identified by examining the neck with the platysma contracted. When preplatysmal fat is present the platysmal bands will be partially obscured, usually predominantly in the submental area, and the presence of subcutaneous fat overlying them, lying between the skin and the platysma, can be seen. Note how in this patient platysma bands can be seen clearly in the inferior neck where little subcutaneous fat is present, while they are hidden and lost more superiorly in the submental region where preplatysmal fat is present (compare to Figs. 67.18 and 67.20). It should be noted that it is relatively rare to find excess preplatysmal fat to be present in most patients in this age group and presenting for facelift surgery. (Courtesy Timothy Marten, MD, FACS and the Marten Clinic of Plastic Surgery, San Francisco, CA; with permission.)

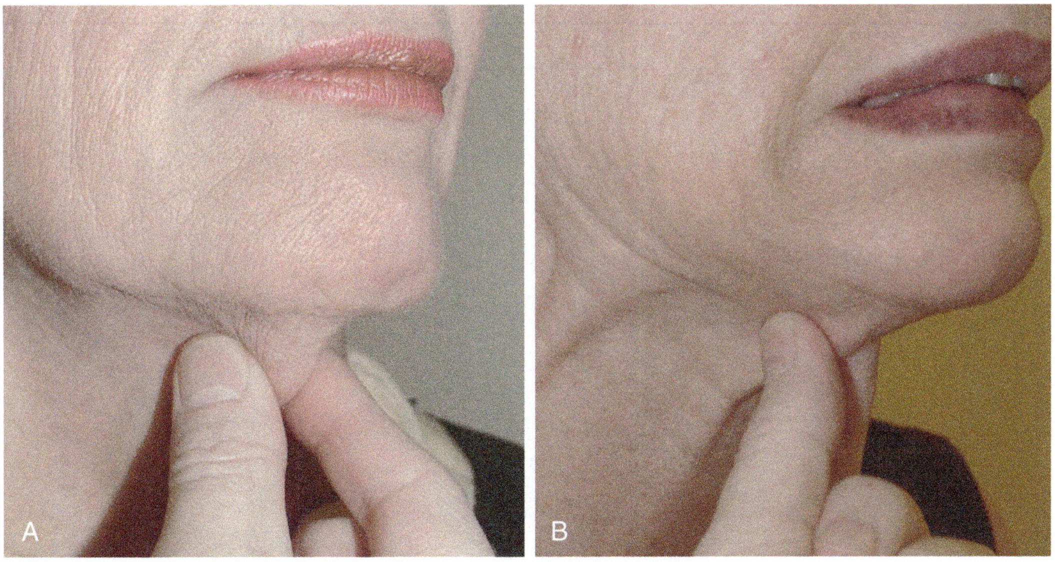

• **Fig. 67.27** Assessing the location of cervicosubmental fat. (A) Submental “waddle” is grasped with the face and neck in repose and the platysma muscle relaxed. (B) The patient is then asked to activate the platysma muscle. In this example fat is pulled superiorly from the examiner’s grasp indicating a predominantly *sub*platysmal position. Fat lying predominantly in a subcutaneous, *pre*platysmal position would tend to remain within the examiner’s grasp when the platysma is activated. (Courtesy Timothy Marten, MD, FACS and the Marten Clinic of Plastic Surgery, San Francisco, CA; with permission.)

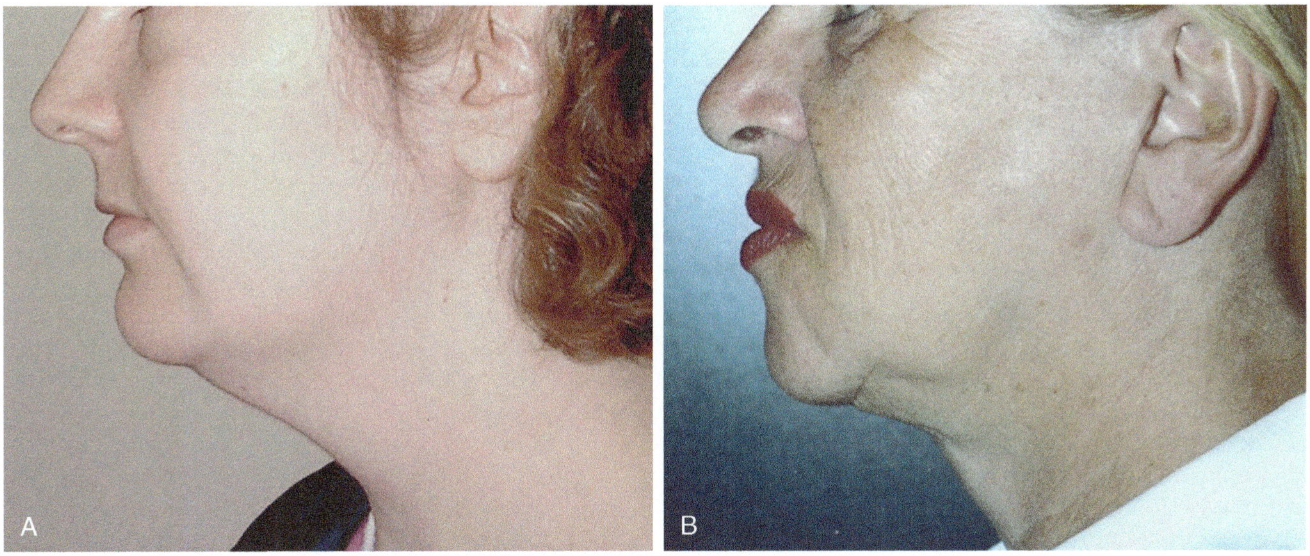

• **Fig. 67.28** Patients likely to have *sub*platysmal fat accumulation. (A) Young patient with firm, obtuse neck who has been troubled by lifelong cervicomental fullness. These patients typically have large collections of subplatysmal fat and are suboptimal candidates for submental liposuction. (B) Patient presenting for secondary surgery (primary procedure performed by unknown surgeon) who has poor cervical contour. It can be seen that superficial subcutaneous fat has been stripped out at the primary procedure and the remaining fat is almost completely in a subplatysmal location. Note the harsh appearance of the neck compared to the plushly padded appearance of the face. (Courtesy Timothy Marten, MD, FACS and the Marten Clinic of Plastic Surgery, San Francisco, CA; with permission.)

activation. Fat lying in a subplatysmal position, however, will have a firmer feel, and will tend to be pulled superiorly out of the examiner’s grasp when the platysma is contracted (Fig. 67.27). This test can be performed by the patient on himself or herself under the surgeon’s supervision as means of helping them understand why liposuction will not properly address their problem and why a submental incision must be made and subplatysmal fat removed.

Two typical scenarios where subplatysmal fat is likely to be present is in patients with firm, obtuse necks who have been troubled by lifelong cervicomental fullness and patients presenting for secondary surgery who have poor cervical contour (Fig. 67.28). In these individuals, partial subplatysmal lipectomy will likely be required.

Not all fat should arbitrarily be removed from the deep neck, however, and deep cervical fat (interdigastric fat)

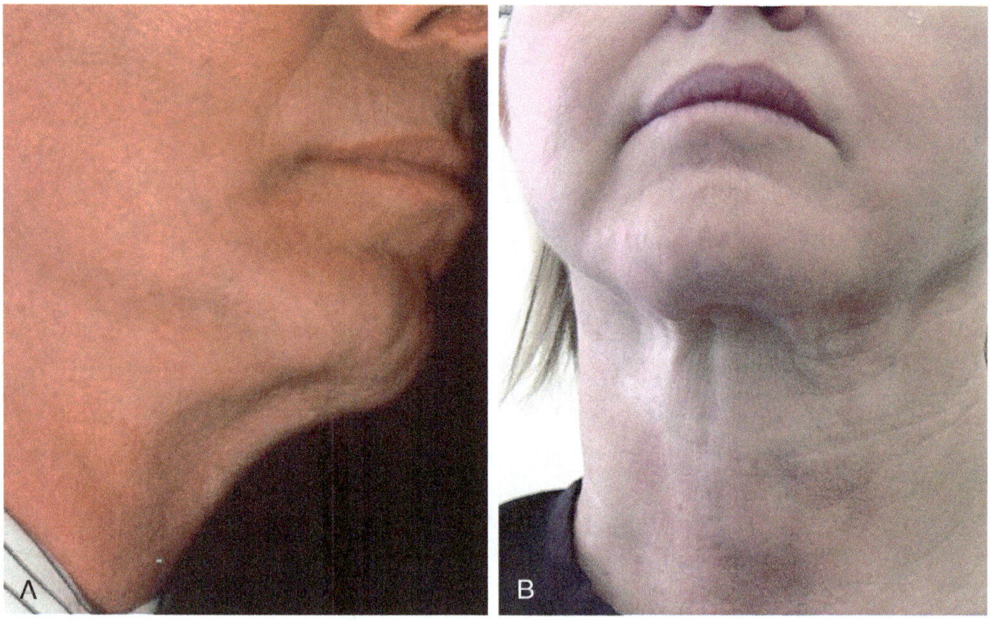

• **Fig. 67.29** (A,B) The "dug out neck" or "cobra neck" deformity is a term used to describe situations in which too much deep cervical fat (interdigastric fat) has been erroneously excised resulting in an objectionable depression in the submental region. A similar appearance can also occur when subplatysmal fat is aggressively excised but large submandibular glands and hypertrophic anterior bellies of the digastric muscles are not reduced. (Courtesy Timothy Marten, MD, FACS and the Marten Clinic of Plastic Surgery, San Francisco, CA; with permission.)

should not be removed. When deep cervical fat is erroneously excised, an objectionable depression in the submental region may result, commonly referred to as the "dug out neck" or "cobra-neck" deformity (Fig. 67.29). Typically this depression is more evident when the neck is flexed somewhat or when the patient swallows.

Planning Treatment of the Prominent Submandibular Gland

Preoperative assessment of the submandibular glands must be made in patients seeking improvement in neck contour as they often contribute to the appearance of a full, "obtuse," and "lumpy" neck. Large submandibular glands are most easily seen in the upper lateral neck in the secondary facelift patient who has had prior aggressive cervicosubmental lipectomy (Fig. 67.30).

However, large glands are frequently hidden by submental fat or lax platysma muscle in the patient with a full neck presenting for a primary procedure, and a plan that does not recognize this fact will lead to disappointing and unexpected bulges in the lateral submental regions postoperatively (Fig. 67.31).

Submandibular glands are usually palpable as firm, smooth, discrete, mobile masses in the lateral submental triangle, lateral to the anterior belly of the digastric muscle and medial to the inner aspect of the ipsilateral mandibular border. Submandibular glands lying superior to the plane tangent to the inferior border of the mandible and the ipsilateral anterior belly of the digastric muscle do *not* disrupt neck contour and will usually *not* require treatment. Glands protruding *inferior* to this plane are likely to be problematic, however, if excess cervical fat is removed, the platysma muscles are reapproximated, and redundant skin is excised. These glands demand treatment if optimal improvement in neck contour is to be obtained.

Despite various claims to the contrary, experience has shown that prominent submandibular glands are actually large, *not* ptotic, and that the platysma contributes little to their position or support. Attempts at tightening the platysma when a prominent gland is present usually results in modest improvement that is short lived. The same is true with various conceptually flawed suture suspension methods that have been proposed and tried in the past that had purported to lift the "ptotic" glands that have now been largely abandoned. Careful sculpting of the periglandular fat will sometimes allow "small" prominent glands to remain relatively disguised, but large, prominent glands will require that the *protruding portion* be resected if optimal improvement is to be obtained (Fig. 67.32).

It is prudent that the decision to perform submandibular gland reduction be made in conjunction with the patient after appropriate discussion of the advantages and disadvantages of the procedure have been made. Patients should know that the procedure may prolong submental induration and edema, and carries a small theoretical but unlikely risk of resulting in bleeding, sialoma, salivary fistula, and dry mouth symptoms. Patients should also be aware, however, that such problems are uncommon, and they should understand that the protruding portion of the gland only is excised, and that the majority of the gland is left in place and is not removed.

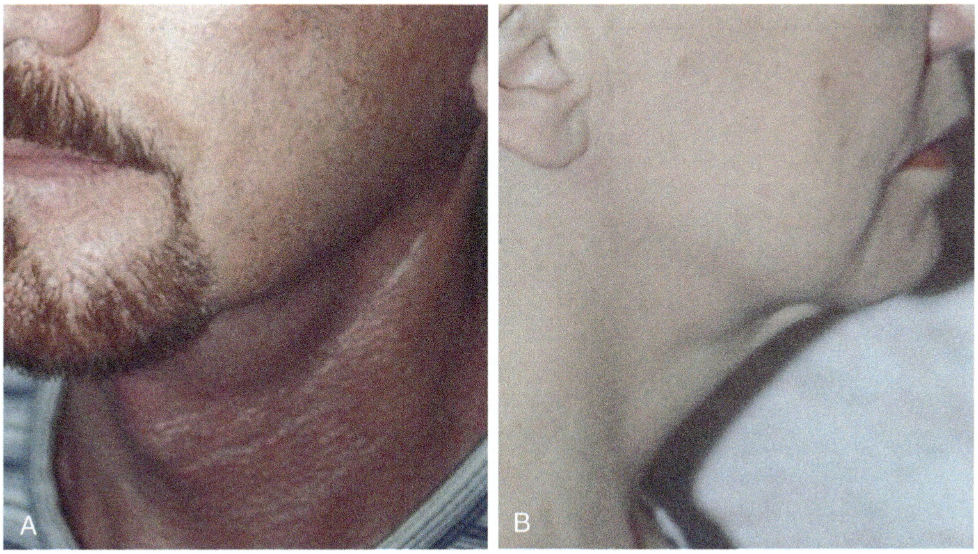

• **Fig. 67.30** Prominent submandibular glands. Large submandibular glands are usually evident as protruding masses in the lateral submental triangle, lateral to the anterior belly of the ipsilateral digastric muscle and medial to the mandibular border. (A) Patient with residual prominent submandibular gland after facelift and submental liposuction. His prior procedure has made the prominent glands more obvious. (B) Patient with residual prominent submandibular gland after "weekend neck lift." Aggressive resection of subcutaneous fat has exposed the prominent gland, which was not treated. (Courtesy Timothy Marten, MD, FACS and the Marten Clinic of Plastic Surgery, San Francisco, CA; with permission.)

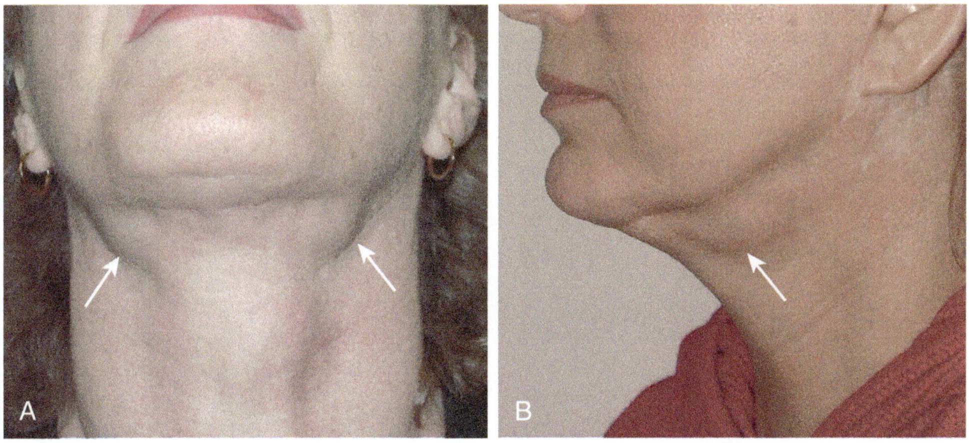

• **Fig. 67.31** Failure of platysma tightening to improve prominent submandibular glands. It is a common misconception that tightening the platysma will lift "ptotic" submandibular glands. Clinical evaluation of prominent glands has shown them to be large, not ptotic, and clinical experience has demonstrated that an attempt to lift them by platysmaplasty is conceptually flawed and will predictably fail. A plan that does not recognize this fact will lead to disappointing and unexpected bulges in the lateral submental regions postoperatively. (A) Patient with prominent submandibular salivary glands after "platysma plication." Too much subcutaneous fat has been removed and platysma tightening has failed to conceal the protruding part of each gland (*arrows*). (B) Patient with prominent submandibular gland after "corset platysmaplasty." The traditional "corset" tightening of the platysma muscles has failed to conceal the protruding gland (*arrow*). (Courtesy Timothy Marten, MD, FACS and the Marten Clinic of Plastic Surgery, San Francisco, CA; with permission. Procedures performed by unknown surgeons.)

A subgroup of patients will present with large, bulky anterior bellies of their digastric muscles that are evident as *linear paramedian submental fullness* (Fig. 67.33).

Large anterior bellies of the digastric muscles are most easily seen in the secondary facelift patient who has had prior aggressive cervicosubmental lipectomy. However, large muscles are frequently hidden by excess submental fat or lax platysma muscle in the patient presenting for primary procedures, and failure to identify them may lead to unexpected and objectionable submental bulges postoperatively. When large, prominent digastric muscles are identified subtotal *superficial digastric myectomy* (excising the protruding portion of the muscle) should be considered. In unclear cases the final decision as to whether partial digastric myectomy

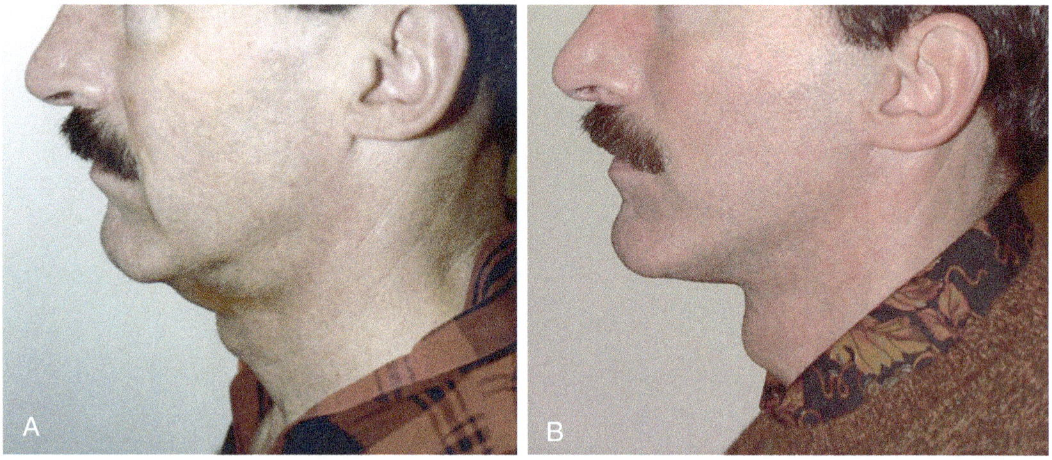

• **Fig. 67.32** Prominent submandibular glands are actually large and not "ptotic" and will require that the protruding portion be resected if optimal improvement is to be obtained. (A) Patient with prominent submandibular gland that contributes significantly to poor neck contour. (B) Same patient seen after neck lift that included submandibular gland reduction. (Courtesy Timothy Marten, MD, FACS and the Marten Clinic of Plastic Surgery, San Francisco, CA; with permission. Procedures performed by Timothy J. Marten, MD, FACS.)

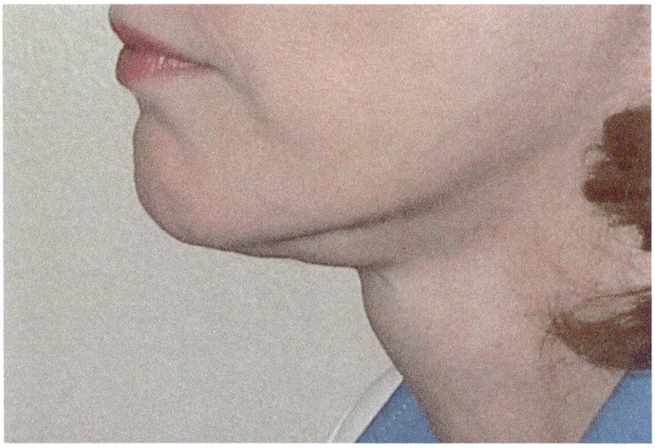

• **Fig. 67.33** Prominent anterior belly of the digastric muscle. The anterior belly of the digastric muscle can be seen as objectionable linear paramedian fullness in the submental region. Prominent digastric muscles often go unnoticed at the time of the primary procedure due to the fact that they are frequently hidden by cervical fat and lax platysma muscle. (Courtesy Timothy Marten, MD, FACS and the Marten Clinic of Plastic Surgery, San Francisco, CA; with permission.)

should be performed is often best deferred until the day of surgery and the improvement produced by other modifications of the deep neck (subplatysmal fat excision and submandibular gland reduction) can be assessed, and digastric muscle reduction is usually performed as the third step in treatment of these three structures ("deep neck triad").

Preoperative Preparations and Care

All patients undergo a preoperative physical evaluation and all those over 50 years old and any with significant medical problems must be cleared by their internist or personal physician before their procedure is performed. Each patient is required to avoid agents known to cause platelet dysfunction for 2 weeks prior to surgery and a list of products that contain aspirin and other medications and products that have antiplatelet activity is provided.

Smokers and Former Smokers

All patients who smoke are asked to quit 4 weeks before their procedure and are required to avoid smoking and all secondhand smoke for 2 weeks after. Patients who smoke, or have a significant history of smoking but have quit, are advised in writing that their risk of serious complications, including poor healing, flap necrosis, skin slough, and thromboembolic phenomena, is significantly higher than in nonsmokers. It is generally assumed, however, that most patients will not cease smoking and extra care should be taken to be sure informed consent is complete in this regard.

Fortunately, flap viability is dependent upon a variety of factors other than smoking that are under the surgeon's control and that are minimized by the high SMAS (superficial musculoaponeurotic system) procedure design (see Chapter 66, Facelift). These factors include the amount of tissue trauma during dissection, the extent of skin undermining, and the amount of tension of the skin flap. Because deep neck lifting procedures create contour by modifying deep neck structures and not by placing tension on delicate cervicofacial skin flaps, a careful surgeon employing correct technique can operate with acceptable risk on smokers. *Smokers should always be approached with caution, however, and it should be recognized these patients are suboptimal candidates for surgery and at increased risk for serious local and systemic complications.*

Ultrasonic and Radiofrequency "Skin Shrinking" Treatments

Patients should be questioned carefully about previous noninvasive radiofrequency and ultrasonic "skin shrinking" procedures (Ulthera, Thermage, Thermi, etc) as these treatments appear to damage skin subdermal microcirculation and compromise superficial microlymphatic vessels, and patients who have undergone these treatments seem to be compromised candidates for neck lift procedures.

The patient who has undergone facial ultrasonic and radiofrequency "skin shrinking" treatments is part of a growing body of patients who seem to sustain clinically significant compromise of their skin microcirculation as a result of these and like treatments that puts them at greater risk of slough and healing-related problems following facelift and neck lift procedures. Unlike when laser resurfacing is performed, in "skin shrinking" procedures energy is directed and dissipated *under* the skin, rather than on its surface, and energy meant to "tighten" the face appears to damage both subdermal microcirculation and adjacent superficial microlymphatic vessels. The incidence of problems seems to parallel the number and intensity of treatments the patient has undergone, which one would expect to parallel the degree of compromise to their tissues. These patients also seem to experience prolonged edema and a longer period of recovery following facelift and neck lift surgery when they have previously undergone these procedures.

Consideration should be given to advising patients who have undergone previous ultrasonic and radiofrequency "skin shrinking" treatments in writing that their risk of serious complications, including poor healing, flap necrosis, and skin slough, is significantly higher than in patients who have not undergone these procedures, especially if they have undergone multiple previous treatments. From the surgeon's standpoint, these patients should be regarded, approached, and treated as similar to smokers.

Allocating Operating Room Time

It is important that adequate OR time be allotted for contemporary facelift and neck lift procedures as they are deceptively time-consuming when compared to traditional techniques. A neck lift when performed in conjunction with facelift, foreheadplasty, eyelid surgery, fat injections, skin resurfacing, and other procedures will often encompass up to 6–8 hours or more, even when performed by a "fast" surgeon working with a well-organized and experienced operating room team. Most surgeons we know who perform these complicated combined procedures on a regular basis have resigned themselves to this fact, and have made appropriate adjustments in their surgery schedules. Usually this means allotting an entire day for the procedure. For difficult procedures, or when additional surgery is requested (e.g., rhinoplasty), it is recommended that the procedures be staged over two separate days.

Anesthesia

Although surgeons have their own anesthesia preferences for surgeries they carry out, performance of this surgery under local anesthetic compromises the very foundations of modern neck lift surgery – access and treatment of the deep neck structures. The majority of our neck lifts are now performed under deep sedation administered by an anesthetist using a laryngeal mask airway. The use of a laryngeal mask allows the patient to be heavily sedated without compromise of their airway, but the patient need not receive muscle relaxants and can be allowed to breathe spontaneously. A laryngeal mask airway is also less likely to become dislodged during the procedure than an endotracheal tube, and will not trigger coughing and bucking when the patient's head is turned during surgery or when they emerge from their anesthetic.

Surgical Technique

The patient is placed supine on a warmed and well-padded, slightly flexed operating table and a special effort is made to insure and document that the elbows, heels, and other potential pressure points are well protected. Standard care including sequential calf compressors (SCUDS), indwelling catheter (surgery >4 hours), antibiotic cover, and sterile field is instituted.

Local anesthetic is administered even if deep sedation or general anesthesia is used (Fig. 67.34). This limits stimulation of the patient and the overall amount of anesthetic needed, and significantly reduces or often eliminates the need for intraoperative narcotics. A significant and helpful hemostatic effect is also obtained when epinephrine/tranexamic acid-containing solutions are used.

The submental incision should be made 1.5 cm or more posterior to the submental crease approximately half-way between the mentum and hyoid. Making the incision in this location helps conceal it in the shadow of the mandible, avoids surgical reinforcement of the crease and accentuation of the "double chin" and "witch's chin" deformities, and provides better exposure of the deep neck (see Figs. 67.13–67.16).

Once the submental incision has been made the surgeon should stand at the head of the table during dissection of the submental region, while the assistant retracts the edges of the incision with a pair of 10-mm double-pronged skin hooks. Having one's assistant retract frees up the surgeon's nondominant hand to apply counter traction to the skin being elevated and to assess flap thickness, and provides for optimal teamwork. Skin undermining should be made using a medium curved Metzenbaum scissors and the dissection should be made subcutaneously leaving the majority of the subcutaneous/preplatysmal fat on the platysma surface. This makes fat excision and sculpting easier later in the procedure if required, and precludes the need for difficult and tedious excision of fat from the undersurface of the cervical skin flap. Unlike the dissection of the facelift skin flap in which a conscious effort must be made to prevent the flap from becoming too thick and the SMAS for being compromised, a slightly deeper dissection should be made in the neck to preserve a slightly thicker layer of subcutaneous fat. Preservation of a thicker layer of fat helps avoid a hard or overresected appearance in the cervicosubmental area, and objectionable overexposure of underlying neck anatomy postoperatively. In many necks only subplatysmal fat will be removed, and little if any subcutaneous fat will be excised.

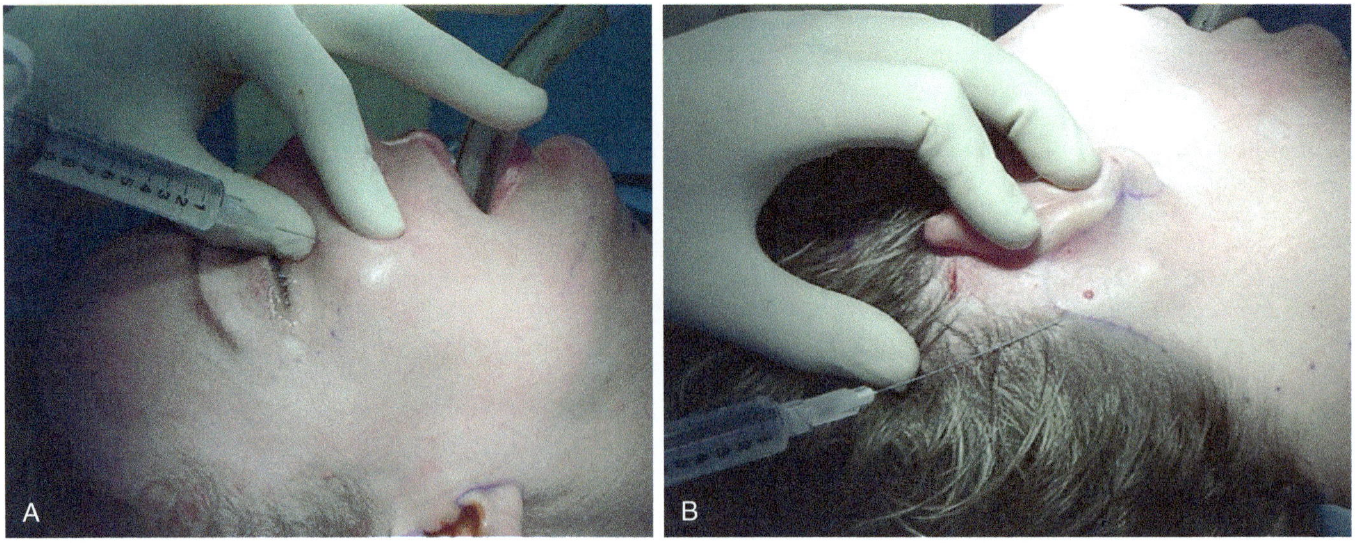

• **Fig. 67.34** (A,B) Local anesthetic solutions infiltration. See text for make up. (Courtesy Timothy Marten, MD, FACS and the Marten Clinic of Plastic Surgery, San Francisco, CA; with permission.)

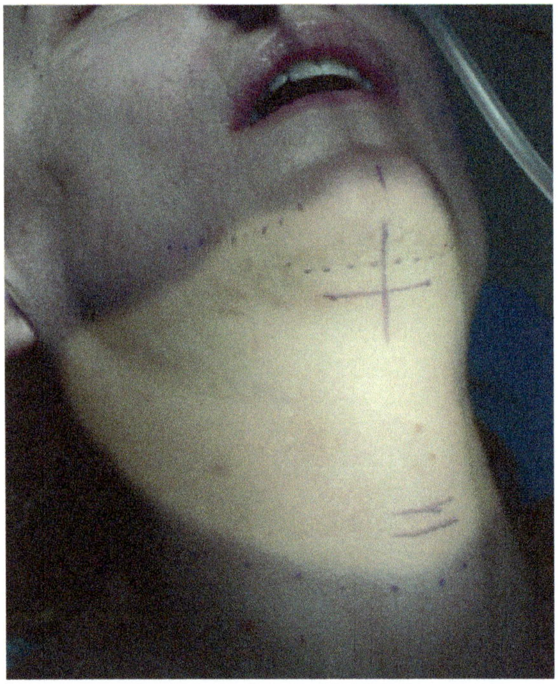

• **Fig. 67.35** Extent of skin undermining in short-scar neck lift. Skin undermining is carried inferiorly below the level of the cricoid cartilage (*double solid lines*), laterally to the anterior border of the sternocleidomastoid muscle, and superiorly beneath the submental crease (*dotted line*) and through the submental and mandibular retaining ligaments. Undermining and releasing the submental crease, and carrying the dissection retrograde up onto the chin allows the fat of the chin and submental area to be seamlessly blended. *Solid line* shown posterior to the submental cease is the site for the submental skin incision. (Courtesy Timothy Marten, MD, FACS and the Marten Clinic of Plastic Surgery, San Francisco, CA; with permission.)

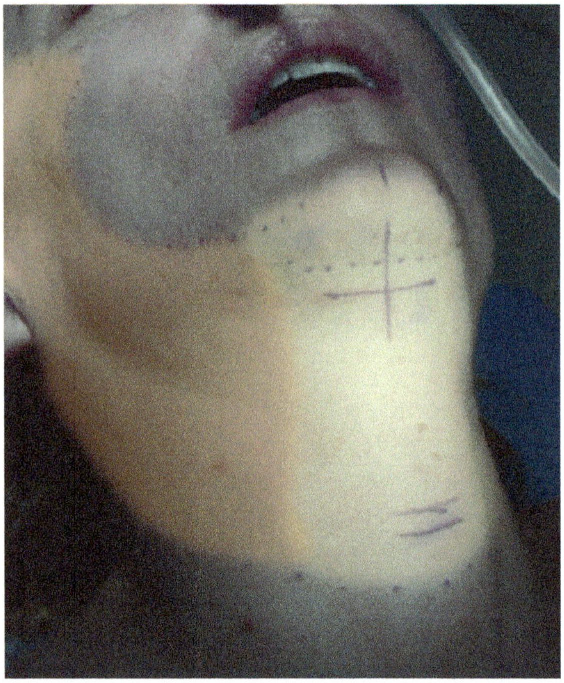

• **Fig. 67.36** Subcutaneous skin undermining in neck lift. Orange shaded area shows subcutaneous skin undermining that is performed through the periauricular incisions when a neck lift is performed with a facelift (or during an extended neck lift procedure). Submental skin undermining (yellow shaded area) is then completed through the submental incision (*solid line* in submental area). (Courtesy Timothy Marten, MD, FACS and the Marten Clinic of Plastic Surgery, San Francisco, CA; with permission.)

Submental dissection is continued inferiorly and laterally. If a "short-scar" neck lift is being performed the dissection is extended laterally to the anterior border of the sternocleidomastiod muscle and up into the postlobular area (Fig. 67.35).

If an "extended ('long-scar') neck lift" or concomitant facelift is being performed, this dissection will join the upper lateral neck dissection made through postauricular and perilobular incisions (Fig. 67.36).

Upon completion of subcutaneous undermining of the anterior neck and submental regions, a retrograde dissection should be made subcutaneously up onto the inferior chin. This will ensure the submental restraining ligaments have been divided and that the submental crease has been released from its bony attachments and provides for subsequent blending of chin and submental fat after other neck maneuvers have been completed to obtain a visually smooth and optimally seamless, esthetic transition for chin to submental region. Some bleeding from perforating vessels that accompany ligaments in this region is usually encountered during this maneuver, but this should not prevent one from completing this important step.

If a facelift or "extended" neck lift is being performed and the upper lateral neck is being approached from a postauricular incision, care must be taken to avoid injury to the great auricular nerve. This nerve provides sensation to the lower two-thirds of the ear and travels superficially superiorly in the upper lateral neck over the sternocleidomastoid muscle fascia. The most superficial portion of the nerve is anatomically constant and lies approximately 6.5 cm inferior to the auditory meatus midway between the anterior and posterior borders of the sternocleidomastoid muscle and it is helpful to mark this spot preoperatively on the neck skin surface to guide one during dissection. If the dissection is performed in the correct plane, however, the nerve will lie deep to the plane of skin flap elevation and will be covered by a layer of varying thickness of subcutaneous fat. It is prudent, however, that all dissection made over the great auricular nerve through the "great auricular corridor" is made under direct vision and not blindly. It is neither necessary nor advisable to attempt to specifically identify or isolate this nerve through additional dissection.

Patients with thin faces, or those undergoing secondary facelifts, will not uncommonly have little subcutaneous fat between the superficially situated portion of the great auricular nerve and the skin, however. For this reason, extra caution must be taken in these patients if elevating the skin flap in this area, and a clear knowledge of nerve anatomy is required.

As stated above, understanding the distribution of the three distinct anatomical layers of fat in the cervicosubmental region – preplatysmal (subcutaneous), subplatysmal, and deep cervicosubmuscular ("interdigastric") and choosing a treatment plan accordingly is key to obtaining good outcomes in the neck.

Cervical lipectomy is a technically demanding maneuver that requires patience, perseverance, and artistic sensitivity. It should be the aim of the surgeon to produce an attractive neck, and not simply one devoid of fat. Contrary to what is traditionally practiced, if a facelift is being performed in conjunction with the neck lift, subcutaneous lipectomy (including liposuction), if indicated, should be performed after deep neck maneuvers and shifting and suturing of the SMAS and platysma, and not at the beginning of the procedure. If subcutaneous lipectomy and/or submental liposuction is performed at the beginning of the procedure fat will be mistakenly excised from regions of the neck that will be raised onto the face when SMAS flaps are advanced and suspended, and can result in inadvertent creation of harsh or irregular mandibular contours (Fig. 67.37). In almost all cases it is best to leave the subcutaneous fat layer untouched until all other maneuvers are completed and improvements obtained which can then be assessed. Only then should fat be removed from the subcutaneous layer. Typically what appeared to be excess fat initially will be seen to not be so after deep layer maneuvers have been completed.

Exploration of the subplatysmal space is indicated if preoperative assessment suggests a significant collection of subplatysmal fat is present, large digastric muscles are detected, large submandibular glands are identified, or if uncertainty exists as to any aspect of the subplatysmal condition. The presence of excess volume in the submental space can be demonstrated preoperatively by examining a lateral-looking down view photograph (Connell's view) of the patient's neck (see Fig. 67.25). Significant accumulations of *subplatysmal* fat and the presence of abnormal fullness in the subplatysmal space can also be demonstrated intraoperatively by Connell's test. This consists of placing gentle superior traction on the cheek flaps (if facelift) or cheeks (isolated neck lift) and flexing the neck. If the neck appears full upon this maneuver, consideration should be given to exploration of the subplatysmal space and the removal of redundant subplatysmal fat and/or protruding portions of other enlarged structures.

Subplatysmal exploration is performed through the submental incision and after skin flaps have been elevated and hemostasis achieved. The subplatysmal space is entered by incising the superficially-situated fascia between the medial platysma muscle borders using a Metzenbaum scissors or electrocautery. A combination of blunt and sharp scissors technique is used to isolate each muscle edge. The muscle edge is then grasped and retracted by the assistant. The dissection is subsequently carried laterally, over the anterior belly of the digastric muscle hugging the underside of the platysma. If this dissection is carefully made a well-defined and relatively avascular plane can usually be identified. Small communicating vessels are not infrequently encountered, however, especially near the medial muscle borders. These should be carefully cauterized and divided as required. Subplatysmal fat should be left on the deep surface of the neck and *not* raised with the platysma flap. This will facilitate fat removal, as it is technically more difficult to resect fat from the undersurface of the muscle.

The plane tangent to the anterior bellies of the digastric muscles with the neck in neutral or slightly flexed position should be used as the landmark for subplatysmal fat removal. Fat deep to this plane is deep cervicosubmental fat (interdigastric fat) that should not be removed if a "dug out neck"/"cobra neck deformity" is to be avoided. All fat lying superficial to this plane consists of subplatysmal fat that should theoretically be removed if optimal contour is to be obtained. If fat excision is made with the neck flexed inadvertent overexcision of interdigastric fat can occur.

As a practical matter, overall neck contour must be considered, as it is the curvilinear plane across the submental region tangent to the borders of the mandible and

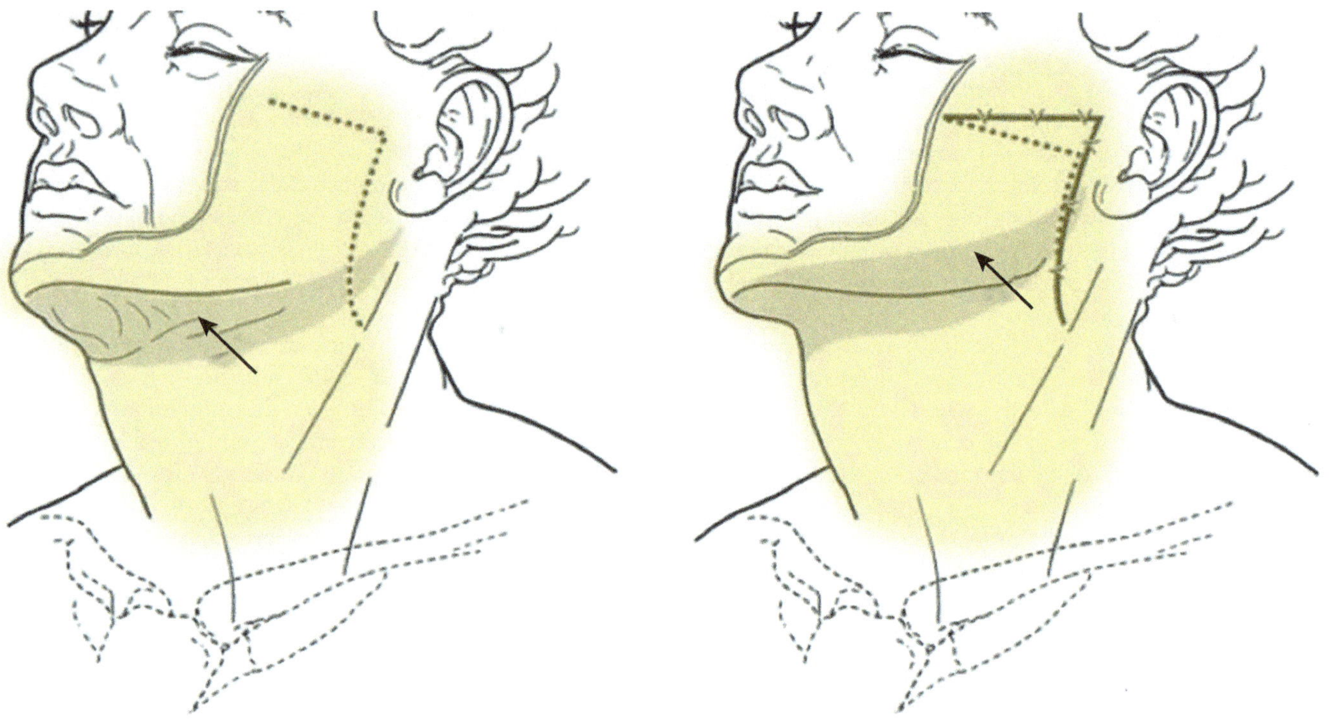

• **Fig. 67.37** Sequencing excision of preplatysmal fat when simultaneous facelift and necklift are performed. If submental liposuction is performed *before* the SMAS is elevated, denuded areas will be subsequently advanced onto the lower face. This can result in a harsh mandibular contour. To avoid this problem, preplatysmal fat should be removed, if indicated, *after* the SMAS flap has been raised. (A) Incorrect plan for preplatysmal fat excision (gray shaded area). Submental liposuction is performed at the beginning of the procedure before SMAS flap is raised. (B) After SMAS elevation, areas stripped of fat (gray shaded area) are moved up onto the lower face. (Courtesy Timothy Marten, MD, FACS and the Marten Clinic of Plastic Surgery, San Francisco, CA; with permission.)

the anterior bellies of the digastric muscles that ultimately determines attractive neck contour (Fig. 67.38).

If large submandibular glands and/or anterior bellies of the digastric muscles are present and it is elected that they not be treated, subplatysmal fat removal should be more conservative if accentuation of these problems is to be avoided. Fibrous fat in the prehyoid region should also not be arbitrarily removed, especially in women, as accentuation and masculinization of the larynx can occur. If prominent submandibular glands and digastric muscles are appropriately treated, however, more aggressive resection of subplatysmal fat can be made.

Subplatysmal fat will be evident as a centrally situated triangular-shaped fat pad with its base lying at the hyoid and tip near the mentum (Fig. 67.39). It should be removed incrementally, as appropriate, and as determined by the position and size of the digastric muscles and the size of the submandibular glands. Fat removal should not be arbitrary, and close attention must be paid to the new contours created. Subplatysmal fat excision often results in division of tributaries of small pretracheal vessels and a long shielded cautery forceps and good suction should be available to obtain adequate hemostasis when required.

Fat situated deep to the plane tangent to anterior bellies of the digastric muscles and beneath the deep cervical fascia (deep cervical or "interdigastric" fat) should not be removed and the

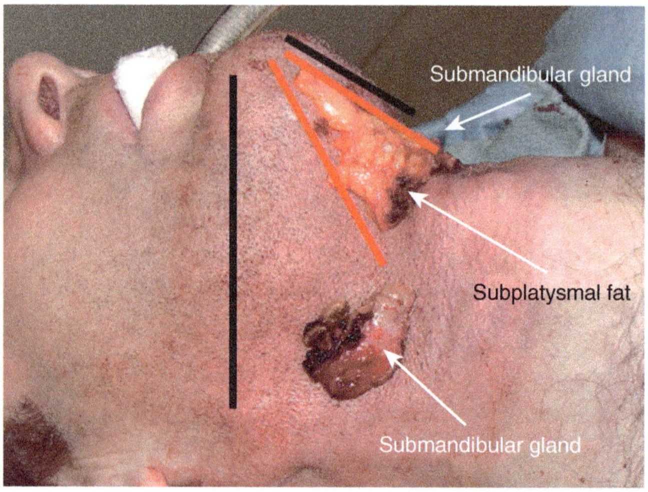

• **Fig. 67.38** Anatomy of optimal neck contour. The curvilinear plane across the submental region tangent to the borders of the mandible (*near black line*) to the ipsilateral anterior belly of the digastric muscle (*near red line*) to the contralateral digastric (*far red line*), to the contralateral mandibular border (*far black line*) ultimately defines attractive neck contour. Between the border of the mandible and the ipsilateral digastric poor contour is due to protruding submandibular glands. Between the digastric muscle bellies the problem is the subplatysmal fat. Additional improvement can be obtained after subplatysmal fat removal and submandibular salivary gland reduction by reducing the anterior digastric muscle bellies themselves. (Courtesy Timothy Marten, MD, FACS and the Marten Clinic of Plastic Surgery, San Francisco, CA; with permission. Procedures performed by Timothy J. Marten, MD, FACS.)

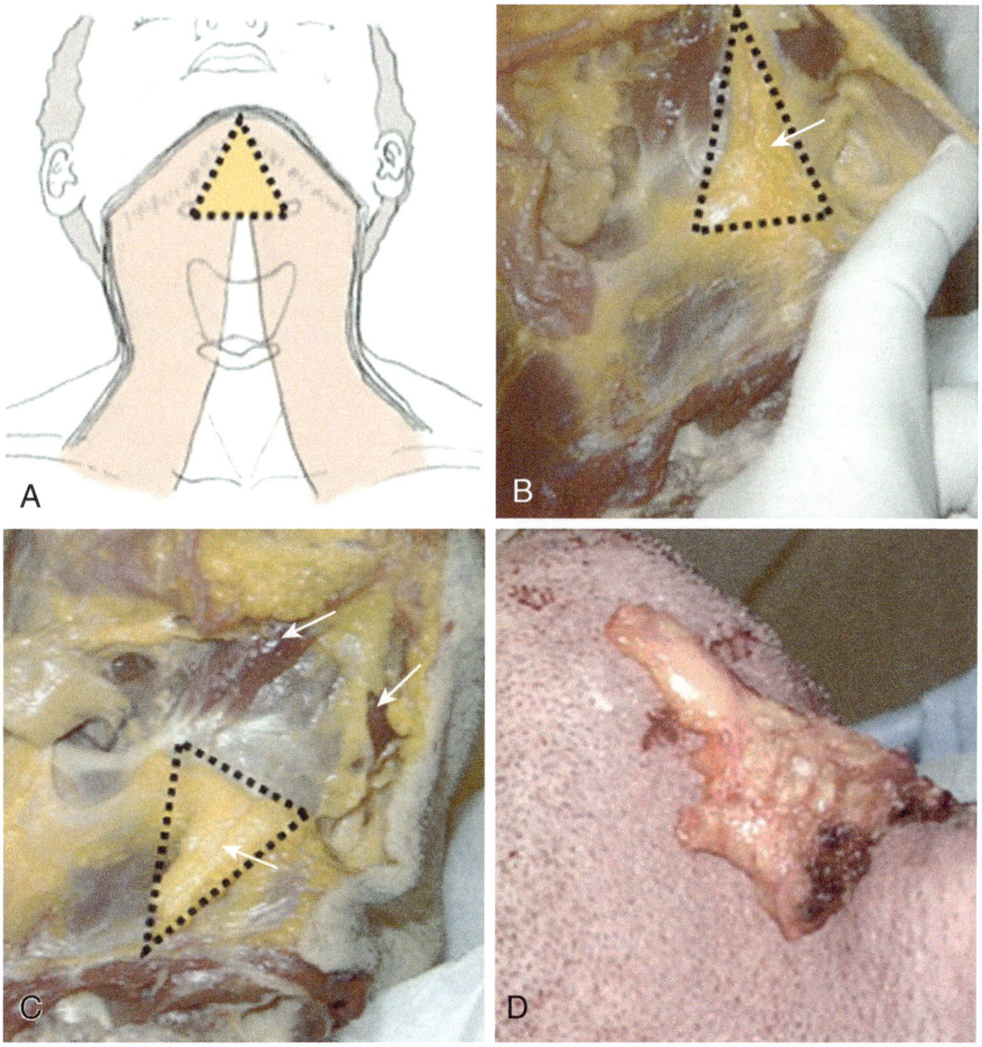

• **Fig. 67.39** (A) Illustration showing the position of the triangular-shaped subplatysmal fat pad located in the submental space with its tip near the mentum and base at the hyoid bone. (B) Cadaver view of the submental region and subplatysmal fat similar to that shown in (A). The arrow is pointing to the subplatysmal fat, which has been outlined (*dashed line*). The right and left borders of the platysma have been elevated showing the contents of the submental space. The subplatysmal fat pad can be seen overlying the digastric muscles to the upper right and left of the triangle. The hyoid bone is at the base of the triangle. (C) Cadaver demonstration of subplatysmal fat. The head is slightly turned to the viewer's right and the chin is at the upper right-hand corner of the photo. The two upper arrows point to the anterior bellies of the right and left digastric muscles and the lower arrow to the subplatysmal fat pad. In this photo, the fat pad has been reflected inferiorly but is still attached at its base. The hyoid is now visible along with the interdigastric space. There is a small amount of deep cervical fat (interdigastric fat) visible (*between arrows*) that has been reflected to the right. (D) Intraoperative demonstration of the subplatysmal fat specimen lying over the submental space from which it was removed. The patient's chin is pointing superiorly and is in the upper left corner of the photo. The neck is in the lower right corner of the photo. (Courtesy Timothy Marten, MD, FACS and the Marten Clinic of Plastic Surgery, San Francisco, CA; with permission.)

overwhelming temptation to "clean out" the deep cervical space resisted. Platysmaplasty, invaginating platysma in a "corset" fashion, suturing the anterior bellies of the digastric muscles together, and other like maneuvers cannot compensate for overzealous excision of deep fat and, in time, an objectionable submental depression will appear in the necks of patients so treated (see Fig. 67.29).

Once the platysma muscles have been raised and prominent submanbibular glands have been identified and mobilized in their capsules (see discussion that follows), the subplatysmal fat pad is most easily isolated and removed by identifying each anterior belly of the digastric muscle near its insertion at the chin by making a small incision with scissors in the overlying fat and fascia. Once the muscle belly is identified in that location the dissection is carried down inferiorly and laterally on its anterior (inferior) surface to its insertion at the lateral hyoid. If the submandibular glands have been previously mobilized inside their capsules, the dissection along the surface of each digastric muscle can be taken into the submandibular capsule. This dissection along the anterior surface of each digastric anterior muscle belly defines the lateral border of the subplatysmal fat pad.

Fat overlaying each anterior digastric muscle belly is then divided with electrocautery due to the predictable presence of a branch vein. Once the lateral borders of the fat pad have been dissected the right and left inferior corners are dissected up off the underlying muscle fascia towards the midline. The plane tangent to each digastric muscle anterior belly is then imagined and all fat lying inferior (superficial) to that plane is removed using electrocautery leaving the interdigastric fat between the digastric muscles intact and in place. Typically, a vein will be encountered and require cautery in the prehyoid region.

Submandibular Gland Reduction

If large submandibular glands are present they can usually be seen and palpated lateral to the ipsilateral belly of the anterior digastric muscle on each side within its respective submandibular triangle protruding inferiorly to a plane tangent to the digastric belly and the mandibular border. The protruding portion can be incrementally resected through the submental incision before submental platysmaplasty is performed to improve neck contour, if indicated (see Fig. 67.30 and Case Examples).

Prominent submandibular glands will be encountered as subplatysmal dissection is carried over the anterior belly of the ipsilateral digastric muscle (Fig. 67.40). The prominent gland will appear as a smooth pink to tan-colored mass covered by a smooth capsule. Reduction is begun by incising the capsule overlying the gland inferomedially just lateral to the anterior belly of the digastric muscle. The submandibular gland will be evident once exposed in this manner due to its distinctive lobulated appearance. Its inferior portion can be grasped with an atraumatic forceps (DeBakey or similar) and easily separated from adjacent tissue inside its capsule using a gentle blunt scissors spreading technique. Although all vital structures are outside the glandular capsule, care should be taken when mobilizing the gland superior-laterally as both the retromandibular vein and the marginal mandibular branch of the facial nerve are in proximity in that area.

An examination of the gland once mobilized inside its capsule will show it to be large, and not merely "ptotic," and this observation forms the basis of the recommendation that partial resection of the protruding portion be performed. Examination of the exposed gland will also clearly demonstrate that attempts to reposition it more superiorly by suture suspension, or by tightening overlying platysma muscle, will ultimately be fruitless.

A key step in the safe performance of the procedure is adequate mobilization of the gland, and a modest overmobilization will make both gland resection and the control of any intraglandular bleeding that might be encountered much easier.

Once adequately mobilized inside its capsule, the inferior portion of the gland is grasped, and pulled gently inferiorly and medially out of its fossa and away from adjacent structures. The redundant portion is subsequently excised incrementally under direct vision in a medial to lateral direction along the planned line of resection with coagulating current cautery. Excision of the excess part of the gland should be performed in such a manner that the portion protruding inferior to the plane tangent to the ipsilateral anterior belly of the digastric muscle and the ipsilateral mandibular border will be resected. It is usually best that initial resection is conservative and that the gland is incrementally reduced thereafter as required. Never is it necessary or appropriate to remove an entire gland. This may result in an objectionable-appearing depression or other contour abnormality, and is arguably more likely to precipitate "dry mouth" condition.

Excision of the redundant and protruding portion of the submandibular gland should be performed using an extended flat-tipped cautery and a long, high-quality pair of atraumatic (DeBakey or similar) forceps. Experience has shown flat-tipped, extended cautery is superior for controlling bleeding of an intraglandular vessel should it be encountered than is a needlepoint cautery tip. A pair of long, high-quality, insulated coagulation forceps is also required.

As in all surgery of the neck and submental region, a fiberoptic headlight or retractor is mandatory, as is a competent assistant and a second scrubbed team member to pass instruments and sutures as needed. One person cannot safely perform both these roles. A suction cannula or smoke-evacuating retractor should also be placed, and the position of the cautery tip relative to vital adjacent structures must be known at all times during the resection. If a smoke evacuating retractor is used a second suction set-up for a Yanchor suction should be available in the event that bleeding is encountered during the resection and suction is needed to obtain hemostasis.

Submandibular gland reduction must not be performed without good light, correct instruments, requisite exposure, adequate suction, sufficient personnel, and considered caution as intraglandular vessels may be encountered. These vessels are more commonly encountered when larger resections are necessary and are most easily managed by immediate and thorough fulguration before further dissection is made. Typically, bleeding will occur from both the gland and the specimen side and this is usually best controlled by quickly moving the cautery back and forth between each end of the cut vessel. If only the gland side is cauterized, bleeding will often continue from the specimen side obscuring the surgical field.

If bleeding cannot be readily controlled by direct cauterization of each side of the cut vessel, suction should be applied and an insulated forceps used to directly grasp the bleeding point and the point subsequently cauterized by application of coagulating cautery current to the instrument. If bleeding is brisk and not easily controlled by cauterization as described above, the gland should be pulled inferiorly and the entire cut edge of it should be compressed proximally with a second pair of forceps. Once bleeding is controlled in this manner the wound can be irrigated and suctioned to clear the field

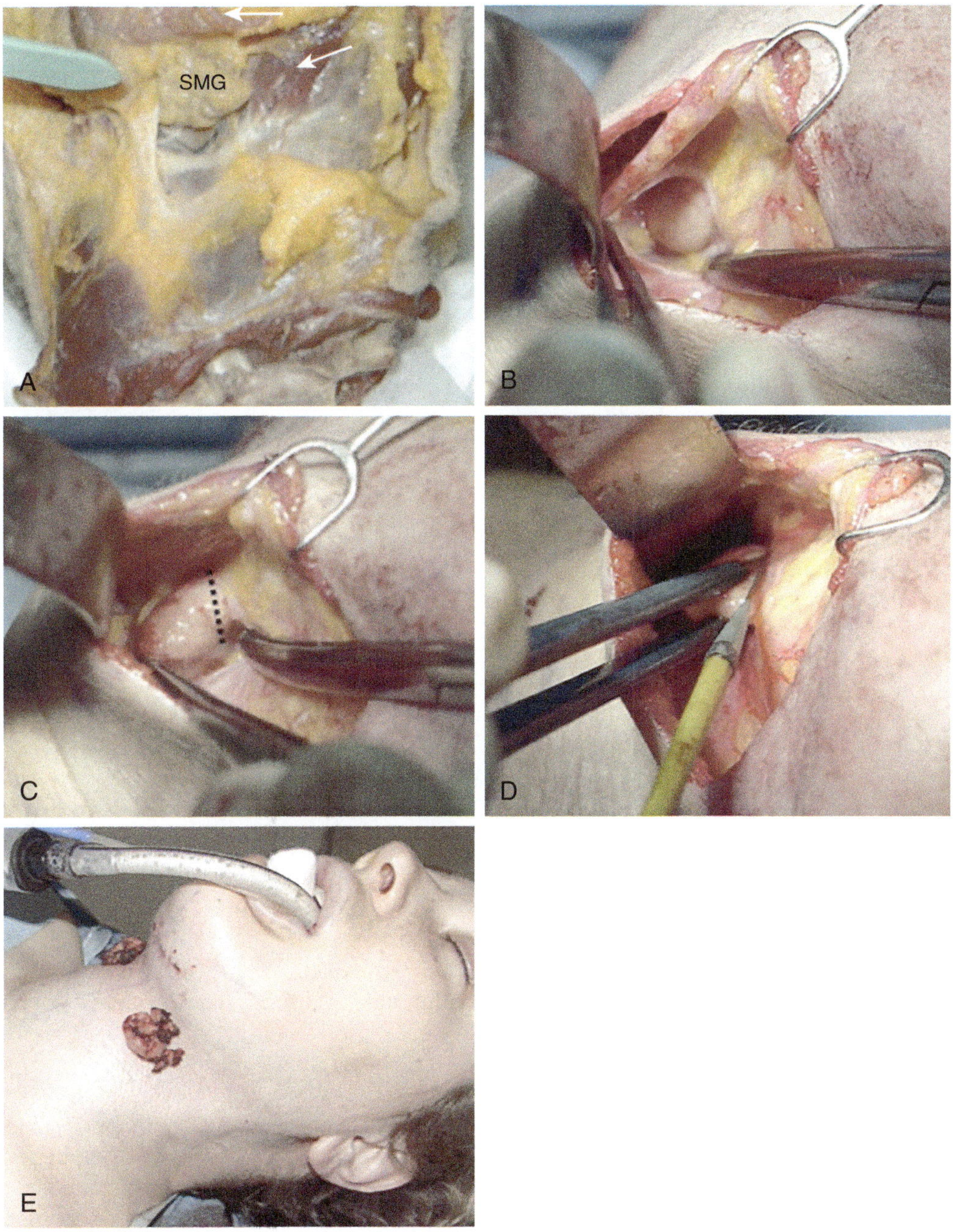

• **Fig. 67.40** Surgical approach to submandibular gland reduction. (A) Cadaver demonstration of submandibular triangle. The chin is in the upper right corner of the photo. The excessive portion of the submandibular gland (*SMG*) is found protruding inferiorly to a plane tangent to the digastric (*lower arrow*) and the mandibular border (*small upper arrow*). (B) Intraoperative photo demonstrating exposure of the submandibular gland. A submental incision has been made approximately 1 cm posterior to the submental crease and the neck subcutaneously undermined. The right platysma muscle has been elevated and is retracted with a double-pronged skin hook and a malleable retractor. The capsule of the gland has been opened and the gland mobilized within it. The gland can be seen inside its capsule just lateral to the ipsilateral anterior belly of the digastric (digastric muscle lies under tip of scissors). (C) Intraoperative photo prior to resection of the excess portion of the gland. The gland has been mobilized and gently pulled inferiorly. *Dotted line* represents the level at which the inferior portion of the gland will be excised and represents the plane tangent to the ipsilateral mandibular border and anterior belly of the digastric muscle. (D) Intraoperative photo just prior to excision of the protruding part of the gland. This should be performed incrementally with electrocautery in such a manner that the portion protruding inferior to the plane tangent to the ipsilateral anterior belly of the digastric muscle and the ipsilateral mandibular border will be resected. (E) Patient seen immediately after neck lift that included partial submandibular gland reduction but no skin resection. The photo shows the excellent contour created without skin tightening. The excised portions of the submandibular glands are also demonstrated on both the right and left sides (subplatysmal fat was also removed and digastric muscles reduced). (Courtesy Timothy Marten, MD, FACS and the Marten Clinic of Plastic Surgery, San Francisco, CA; with permission. Procedures performed by Timothy J. Marten, MD, FACS.)

and the vessel then carefully identified. It can then be grasped with a second instrument and cautery applied.

In the unlikely event that bleeding cannot be controlled by these maneuvers the submandibular fossae should be packed with a gauze sponge and digital pressure firmly applied for several minutes pressing the gland against the inner aspect of the mandible and the floor of the mouth. In most cases when the gauze is carefully removed the bleeding will be seen to have stopped, the subplatysmal space can be irrigated and suctioned to clear the operative field of any blood, and a search for the bleeding point can be made and any suspicious areas cauterized.

The submandibular artery enters the submandibular gland superolaterally and will not be directly and specifically encountered when performing conservative resections typically made for esthetic purposes and only its terminal branches extending into the gland itself will be encountered. Dissection should always be made carefully in this area, however, and as one becomes more practiced in the procedure and more comprehensive resections as a result are made, this vessel will often be seen as a discrete branch of the much larger submental artery. In many cases, if care is exercised, resection of the most superolateral portion of the protruding portion of the gland can be made without injuring it and it can be isolated and grasped with a hemostatic (Schnitz) forceps and ligated.

Once excision of the protruding portion of the gland is complete, the submental region is irrigated and a check for hemostasis along the gland's cut edge is made. It is not necessary or productive to attempt to oversew the cut edge of the gland, or close the glandular capsule. These maneuvers are not only technically difficult, but could result in injury to nearby neurovascular structures. It is also not necessary or productive to overcauterize the cut edge of the gland in an attempt to shrink or seal it. This typically results in more pain and swelling, and prolonged submental induration. Subtotal submandibular gland excision to date has not resulted in any cases of hematoma, airway compromise, salivary fistula, or gustatory sweating in our practices.

Experience has shown that when submandibular gland reduction is performed a drain should be placed in the subplatysmal space for at least several days after the procedure to reduce edema and induration in the submental area and to speed the patient's overall recovery. It is safest to perform the platysmaplasty before drain placement, and then to thread the drain into place. If the drain is placed before platysmaplasty is performed there is a chance that the drain could be caught in one of the sutures, making its removal problematic.

Submandibular gland reduction, although important in the rejuvenation of many necks, will not in and of itself result in attractive neck contour. Other problems must be identified and addressed if optimal results are to be obtained.

Submandibular reduction should be regarded as an advanced technique. It should be undertaken by surgeons well versed in cervical anatomy and experienced in more basic maneuvers used to rejuvenate the neck, and the operating surgeon must at all times have the specific algorithm for managing bleeding clearly in mind. It is highly recommended that any surgeon uncertain of the anatomy of the submental triangle or the exact relationships of important structures in this area review them carefully before undertaking this dissection.

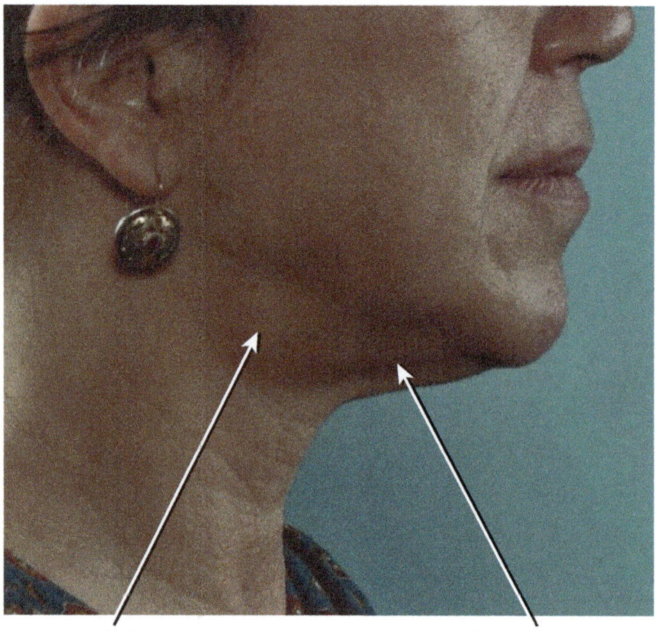

• **Fig. 67.41** Surface expression of large digastric muscle. Typically large digastric muscles will appear as a linear paramedian fullness lying medial to the rounder and more laterally situated submandibular gland fullness and the difference in appearance of the two problems is a reflection of their differing anatomical origins. In can be seen that in many cases the diagnosis of both problems can be made by simply looking at the patient's neck. (Courtesy Timothy Marten, MD, FACS and the Marten Clinic of Plastic Surgery, San Francisco, CA; with permission.)

Partial Digastric Myectomy

After subplatysmal lipectomy and submandibular gland reduction have been performed assessment should be made of the anterior bellies of the digastric muscles and whether partial digastric myectomy would produce further improvement in neck contour. In most cases, additional improvement in neck contour can be obtained by performing this procedure.

Typically, large digastric muscles will appear as a linear paramedian fullness lying medial to the rounder and more laterally situated submandibular gland fullness and the difference in appearance of the two problems is a reflection of their differing anatomical origins: the anterior belly of the digastric muscles is a linear paramedian structure and the submandibular gland is a rounder more laterally-situated structure (Fig. 67.41).

Typically, the presence of digastric muscle excess is most readily identified after subplatysmal lipectomy and submandibular gland reduction has been performed, but in some cases it may be evident preoperatively in patients seeking secondary, and less commonly, primary surgery. In these situations additional improvement in neck contour may be obtained by performing superficial, subtotal anterior *digastric myectomy* (excising the protruding portion of the muscle).

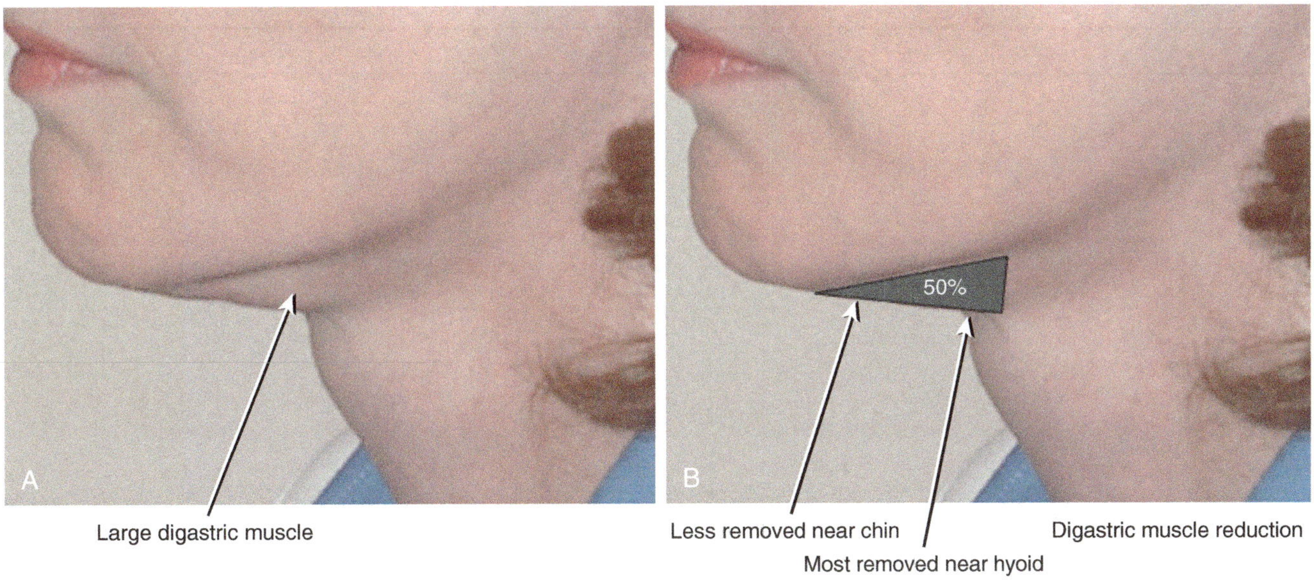

• **Fig. 67.42** Digastric muscle reduction strategy. (A) Typical appearance of a large anterior belly of the digastric muscle. (B) Digastric muscle fullness is treated in a manner that optimizes submental contour. Approximately 50% of the muscle is removed in the typical case with more muscle removed near the hyoid and less near the chin. (Courtesy Timothy Marten, MD, FACS and the Marten Clinic of Plastic Surgery, San Francisco, CA; with permission.)

A subset of patients will be encountered who will be identified as having objectionably large anterior digastric muscle bellies. Usually these are most evident after subplatysmal lipectomy and submandibular gland reduction has been performed, but they may sometimes be evident preoperatively in patients seeking secondary, and occasionally, primary surgery. In these situations additional improvement in neck contour may be obtained by performing superficial, subtotal anterior *digastric myectomy*.

Superficial, subtotal anterior digastric myectomy is performed under direct vision, through the submental incision after the subplatysmal space has been opened, the platysma muscle mobilized, and subplatysmal fat and protruding portions of the submandibular gland resected, if indicated. The redundant portion of muscle can be excised by either a tangential strip excision technique or by a partial division and excision technique. While both are reliable and effective, in most cases tangential strip excision provides the simplest and most intuitive and straightforward means of removing the protruding portion of the muscle belly.

Tangential strip excision is performed by visually gauging the muscle redundancy, grasping the redundant portion with a DeBakey or similar forceps, and tangentially excising a strip of muscle longitudinally from the muscle belly with a Metzenbaum or, more commonly, with elecrocuatery using coagulating current. Typically, tangential excision will result in modest bleeding from the excised area that is easily controlled with cautery once muscle reduction is complete if a Metzenbaum scissors is used.

Excision is begun near the muscle origin at the mentum and continuing to the muscle belly insertion at the lateral hyoid. The muscle is then reassessed and the action repeated until the protruding portion is fully removed and optimal contour has been established. Approximately 50% of the muscle is removed in the typical case with the most muscle removed near the hyoid and the least near the chin (Fig. 67.42).

In the partial division and excision technique of digastric muscle reduction the excess muscle present is gauged and isolated on a tonsil forceps by pushing the tips of the instrument through the mid-muscle belly at the level of optimal contour and spreading to split the muscle along the length of its fibers. The isolated muscle segment resting on the instrument consisting of the superficial, protruding portion of it is then excised with scissors or cautery by dividing it near the mandible and the hyoid (Fig. 67.43). The neck is re-examined and the maneuver repeated if necessary until an improved contour is obtained. Usually this entails the excision of the superficial-most half or less of each muscle, with more muscle excised near the hyoid and less near the chin, as is the case when the tangential excision technique is used.

It should be noted that the myectomy, regardless of how it is performed, is a partial and subtotal reduction of the protruding portion of the digastric muscle only, and not an arbitrary exenteration of the entire muscle belly. It must also be understood that optimal contour is achieved when more muscle is resected near the hyoid and less near the chin. In addition, partial, superficial digastric myectomy, although an important maneuver in the rejuvenation of many necks, will not in and of itself produce attractive neck contour. Other problems must be identified and treated if optimal results are to be obtained. Finally, it should be noted that partial, superficial digastric myectomy, although straightforward and conceptually simple, should be regarded as an advanced technique. It should be undertaken by surgeons familiar with cervical anatomy and experienced in more basic maneuvers used to rejuvenate the neck.

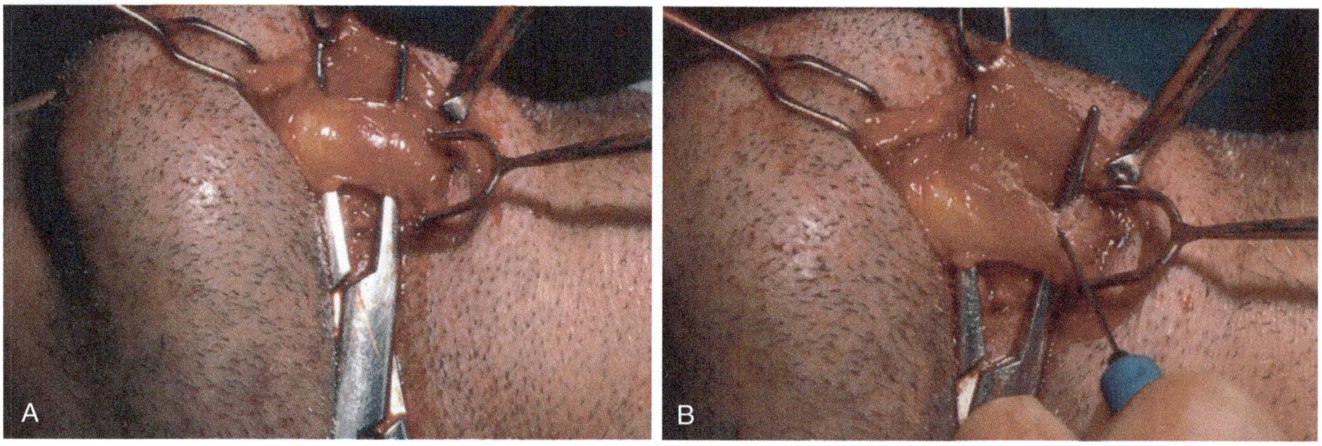

• **Fig. 67.43** Partial division and excision technique of digastric muscle reduction. (A) Excess muscle present is gauged and isolated on a tonsil forceps by pushing the tips of the instrument through the mid-muscle belly at the level of optimal contour and spreading to split the muscle along the length of its fibers. (View from patient's right of right digastric muscle through submental incision. Patient's chin is at the left upper corner of the photo and the neck is on right). (B) The isolated muscle segment resting on the instrument consisting of the superficial, protruding portion of it is then excised with scissors or cautery by dividing it near the mandible and the hyoid. The neck is re-examined and the maneuver repeated if necessary until an improved contour is obtained. (Courtesy Timothy Marten, MD, FACS and the Marten Clinic of Plastic Surgery, San Francisco, CA; with permission.)

Anterior Platysmaplasty

Once subplatysmal fat excision, submandibular gland reduction, and partial digastric myectomy have been performed as indicated and treatment of the subplatysmal space is complete, anterior platysmaplasty is performed. Anterior platysmaplasty is the procedure in which the medial borders of the platysma muscle are sutured together to help consolidate the neck, reduce horizontal platysma laxity, and improve neck appearance when patients flex their neck and look down (see Figs. 67.11 and 67.19).

Platysmaplasty is performed by suturing the medial muscle borders of the platysma muscles together from mentum to thyroid cartilage. If redundant muscle is present medially, it is excised and discarded before suturing is performed so that a smooth, edge-to-edge approximation of the medial muscle borders can be made without inversion, invagination, or imbrication (Fig. 67.44). Experience has shown that this produces a better and more consistent outcome and reduces the likelihood that objectionable midline fullness or bands will result after healing and relaxation of tissues has occurred than when excess muscle is invaginated and a multilayer "plication" or "corset" is performed.

Typically, platysmaplasty is performed by suturing the medial muscle borders together with interrupted sutures beginning at the mentum and proceeding inferiorly to the hyoid and then down to the level of the midthyroid cartilage. Alternatively, approximation can be started at the hyoid and then extended superiorly to the mentum and then from hyoid to midthyroid level. The approach is not as important as is creating a smooth, well-tailored approximation and reconstitution of the platysmal layer.

When performing a face and neck lift, together platysmaplasty should be performed *after* cheek SMAS flap dissection and suspension to prevent an accentuation of the effects of aging and gravity and compromised improvement on the face (Fig. 67.45). Although raising and suspending cheek SMAS flaps first makes platysmaplasty suture placement more difficult, it allows optimal repositioning of the cheek and jowl, and provides for the best overall improvement. *If platysmaplasty is performed first the cheeks and jowls will be pulled inferiorly towards and into the neck, and the effectiveness of the SMAS flap will be significantly diminished* (Fig. 67.46). *Platysmaplasty should be performed with the neck in a neutral position.* If the closure is made with the neck extended, excessive tightness may result when the patient looks down after surgery. This is particularly the case if platysmaplasty is performed in conjunction with a postauricular transposition flap of cheek SMAS ("postauricular transposition flap").

Management of the Lateral Platysmal Border

If a "short-scar" neck lift is performed there is no access to, or option for, lateral platysma suspension. If a neck lift is performed in conjunction with a facelift, or if an extended neck lift is being performed, lateral platysmapexy (Fig. 67.47) can be performed, or more typically a postauricular transposition flap is created (Fig. 67.48).

When mild horizontal platysma muscle redundancy is present in the neck, *lateral platysmapexy* is performed (see Fig. 67.47). Lateral platysmapexy insures that the platysma is draped smoothly and snugly along the cervicomental angle and helps to further consolidate the neck, especially when the patient looks down. It is usually effective only when suturing is performed over the upper one-fourth of the sternocleidomastoid muscle where its fascia is less mobile. In thin necks the cut muscle edges can be overlapped. In fuller

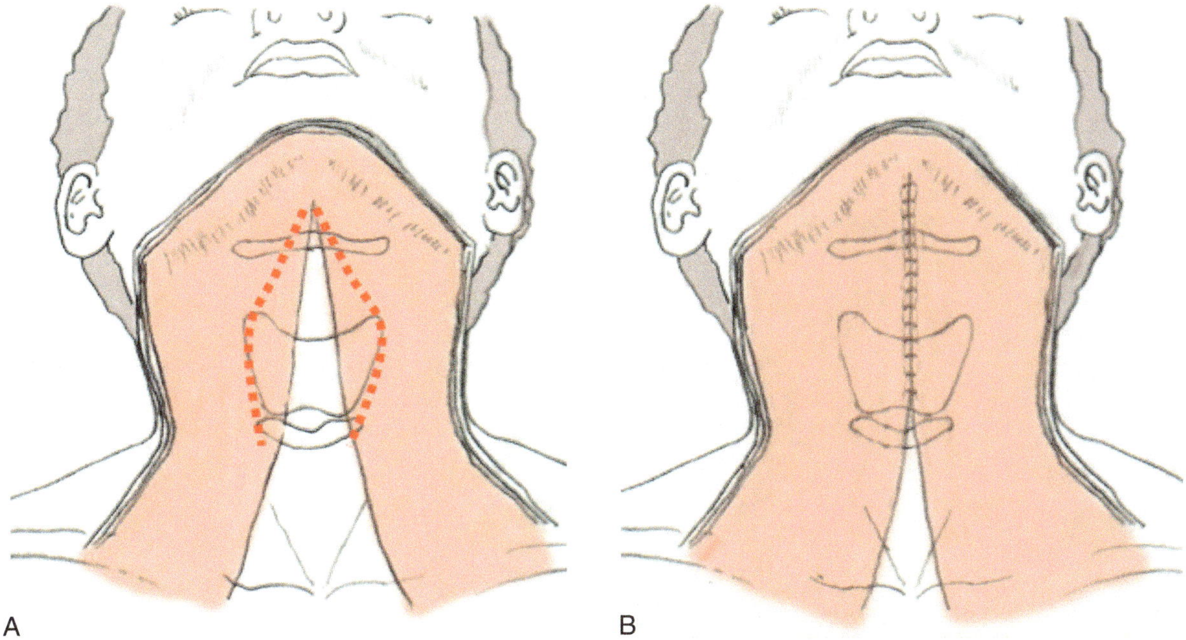

A B

• **Fig. 67.44** Anterior platysmaplasty. (A) If redundant muscle is present medially (*dashed red line* in A), it is gauged and excised before suturing is performed so that (B) a smooth, edge-to-edge approximation of the medial muscle borders can be made. This produces a better outcome and reduces the likelihood that objectionable midline fullness or bands will result after healing has occurred than when excess muscle is invaginated and a multilayer "plication" or "corset" is performed. (Courtesy Timothy Marten, MD, FACS and the Marten Clinic of Plastic Surgery, San Francisco, CA; with permission.)

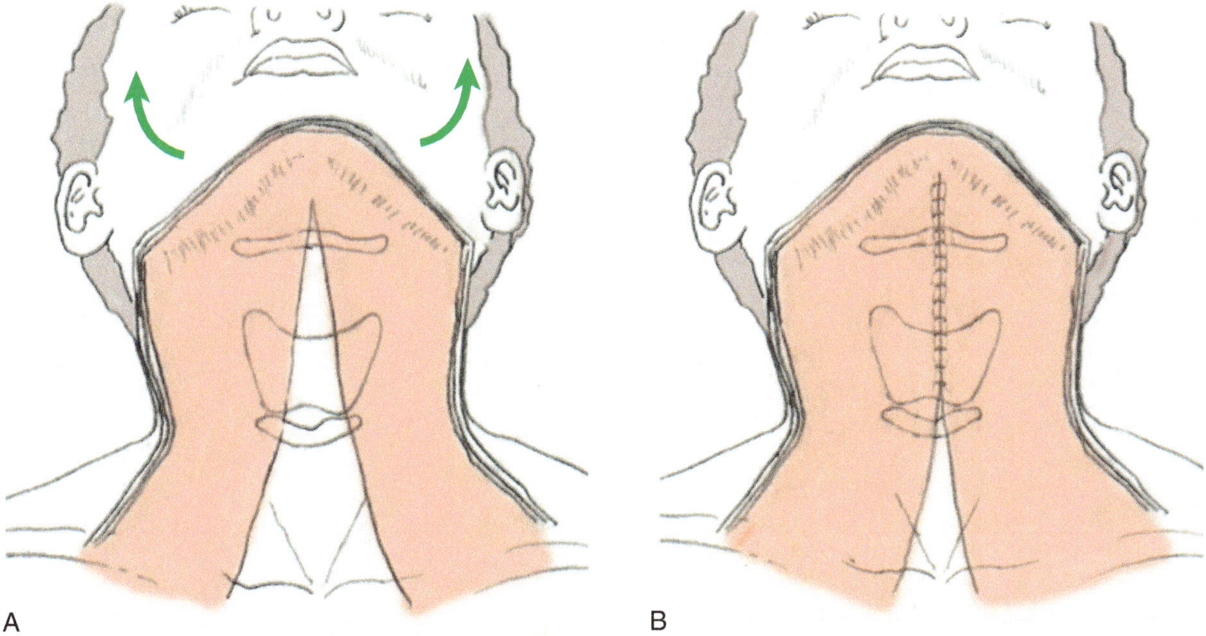

A B

• **Fig. 67.45** (A,B) SMAS flaps should be raised before platysmaplasty is performed. If the neck lift is done with a facelift the cheek SMAS should be suspended *before* platysmaplasty is performed. (Courtesy Timothy Marten, MD, FACS and the Marten Clinic of Plastic Surgery, San Francisco, CA; with permission.)

necks redundant muscle can be trimmed and the muscle segments sutured edge-to edge. Due to the overall mobility of sternocleidomastoid fascia, however, limited support can be obtained by these maneuvers.

When horizontal platysma muscle redundancy is large, or optimal improvement in cervicomental contour is desired, a postauricular transposition flap (PATF) of cheek SMAS is planned (see Figs. 67.48 and 67.49). The PATF is created by splitting off redundant tissue from the posterior margin of the cheek SMAS flap, but leaving it attached inferiorly to the cervicosubmental platysma. If properly constructed and secured, this flap will provide for optimal reduction in

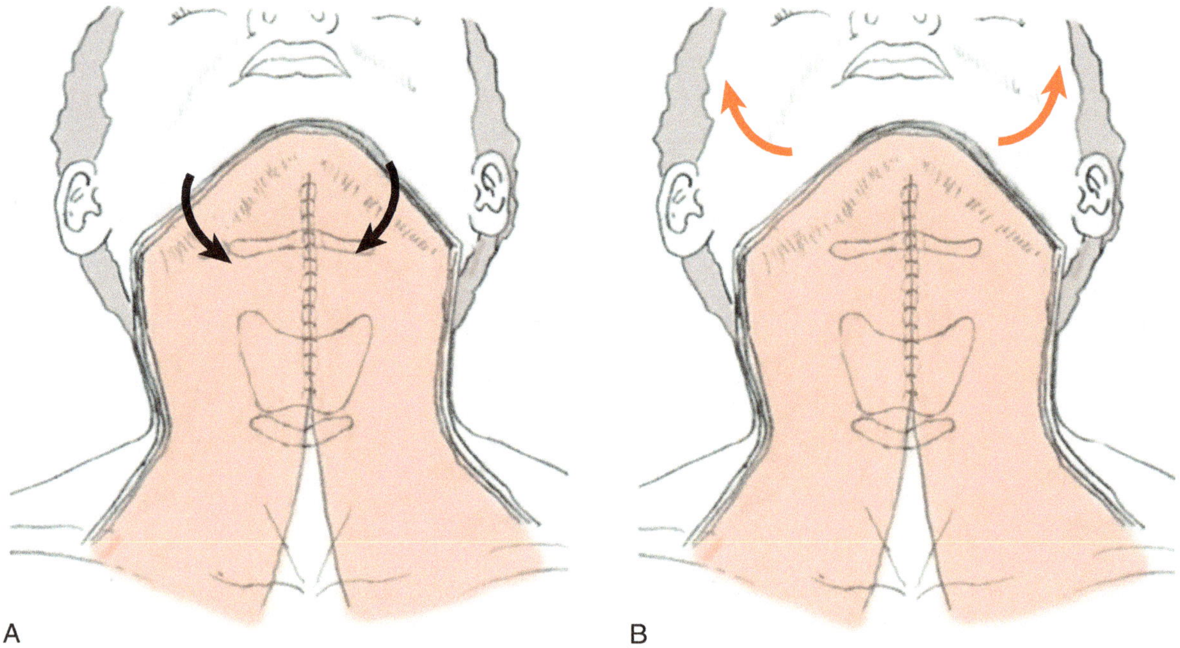

• **Fig. 67.46** If platysmaplasty is performed before cheek SMAS suspension (*black arrows* in A), elevation of the cheek SMAS flaps and improvement in the face will be compromised (*red arrows* in B). (Courtesy Timothy Marten, MD, FACS and the Marten Clinic of Plastic Surgery, San Francisco, CA; with permission.)

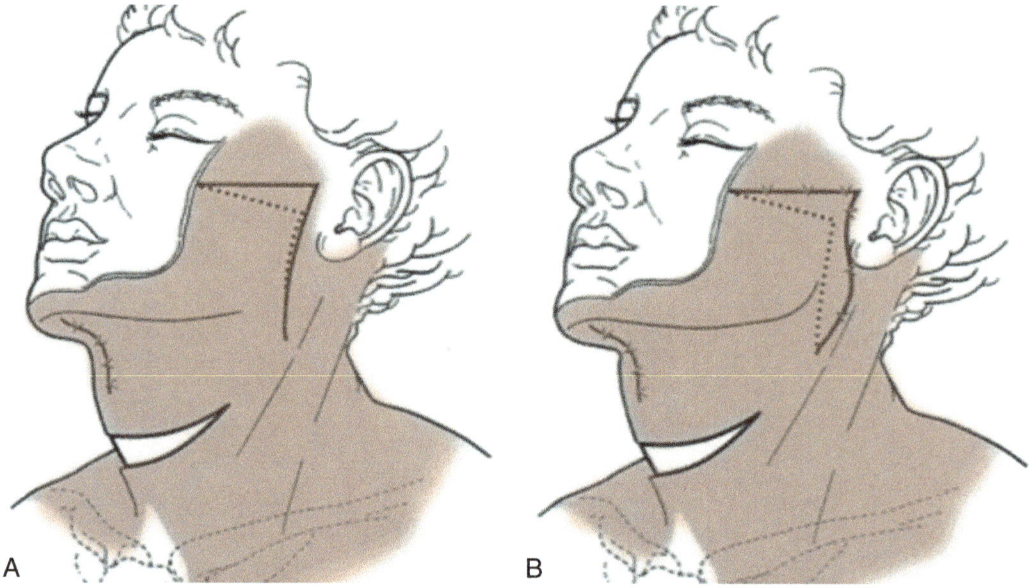

• **Fig. 67.47** When mild horizontal platysma muscle redundancy is present in the neck, lateral platysmapexy may suffice. (A) Before lateral platysmapexy. (B) After lateral platysmapexy. The inferior border of the posterior margin of the SMAS flap is advanced laterally and posteriorly and sutured to the upper sternocleidomastoid fascia in a manner that tightens the platysma under the mandibular border and along the cervicomental angle. Lateral platysmapexy should be performed *after* anterior platysmaplasty. (Courtesy Timothy Marten, MD, FACS and the Marten Clinic of Plastic Surgery, San Francisco, CA; with permission.)

horizontial platysma laxity and dynamic reinforcement of the upper neck and submental areas when the patient looks down. When used in conjunction with an anterior platysmaplasty, PATFs result in a continuous mastoid-to-mastoid sling of muscle across the upper neck along the cervicomental angle and optimal improvement in neck contour.

If an extended neck lift is performed a limited periauricular incision will be present but a PATF can still be created and a low SMAS flap can be used to effect improvement in the lower face and along the jawline that otherwise would not be obtained if platysmaplasty alone, or platysmaplasty and lateral platysmapexy, were performed (see Fig. 67.48).

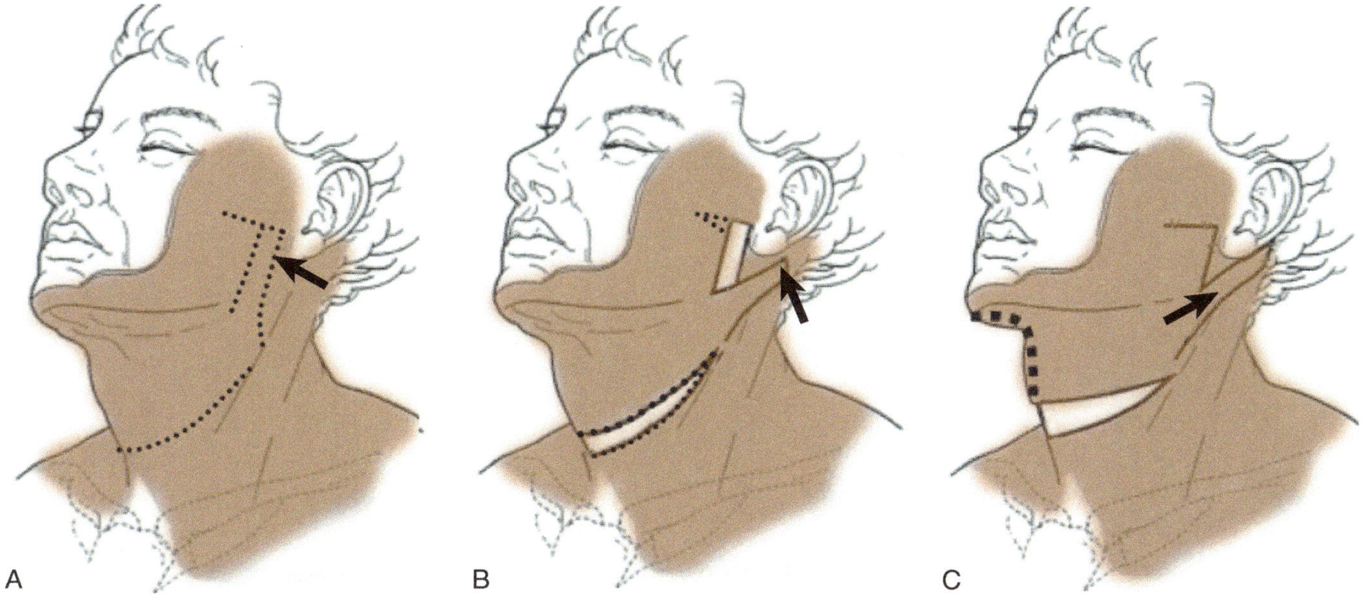

• **Fig. 67.48** If an extended neck lift is performed, a limited periauricular incision will be present but a postauricular transposition flap (PATF) can still be created and a "low" SMAS flap can be used to effect improvement in the lower face and along the jawline that otherwise would not be obtained. (A) Plan for PATF with low SMAS flap. (B) After flap creation and transposition to the postauricular area. (C) After elevation and suturing of low SMAS flap and suturing of PATF to the mastoid fascia. In combination with anterior platysmaplasty (*dashed line*) a mastoid-to-mastoid sling of autologous tissue that defines the cervicomental angle is created. The low SMAS flap provides improvement in the lower face and along the jawline that would not be otherwise obtained if platysmaplasty alone, or platysmaplasty and lateral platysmapexy, were performed. (Courtesy Timothy Marten, MD, FACS and the Marten Clinic of Plastic Surgery, San Francisco, CA; with permission.)

As high SMAS flap has been elevated and its superior margin anchored over the zygomatic arch. Because the SMAS flap is properly advanced along a vector parallel to the long axis of the zygomaticus major muscle some redundancy is present along the posterior margin of the flap. This is excised in a manner such that when the posterior margin of the flap is sutured to the preauricular SMAS remnant it is closed under no tension, but it is left attached to the cervical platysma *below* the mandibular border. This allows suspension of the lateral platysma border to the fixed mastoid fascia.

If PATFs are planned, suspension of the flaps to the mastoid should be performed *after* anterior platysmaplasty has been performed. If the transposition flaps are suspended first, the platysma muscles can be shifted laterally and it may be difficult to join them in the midline (Fig. 67.50). Suspension to the mastoid is performed with interrupted sutures of 4-0 polyglactin (Vicryl) (or other suture of choice). The more proximal portions of the flap are secured to the underlying fascia with a simple running suture of the same material. This consolidates the deep layer repair in the perilobular area and prevents the flap from bunching up or rolling up upon itself.

If suspension of the lateral platysmal borders (lateral platysmapexy or PATF) is performed *before* anterior platysmaplasty (*black arrows*), the plastysma muscles may be laterally displaced and approximation of the medial plastysmal borders (platysmaplasty) may not be possible (*red arrows* in Fig. 67.50B).

For the PATF to be effective it must be properly designed and constructed and its intended purpose kept in mind. A common error is for the surgeon to construct it too timidly and superiorly and in a manner that its pull is placed over and along the mandibular border (Fig. 67.51A). Such a design pulls on the lateral face and does not improve the neck and cervicomental angle. Properly constructed, the flap should exert its pull *below and inferior* to the mandible and along the cervicomental angle (Fig. 67.51B).

Transverse Platysma Myotomy

Although anterior platysmaplasty will often result in an attractive neck at rest and on the operating table, objectionable-appearing dynamic platysma bands and muscle striations will often still be evident in conversation and during animation after surgery if additional steps are not taken. These problems can be minimized by performing *transverse platysma myotomy* (see Figs. 67.20–67.23). The extent of platysma transection will depend upon the muscle irregularities present and thus will vary from patient to patient.

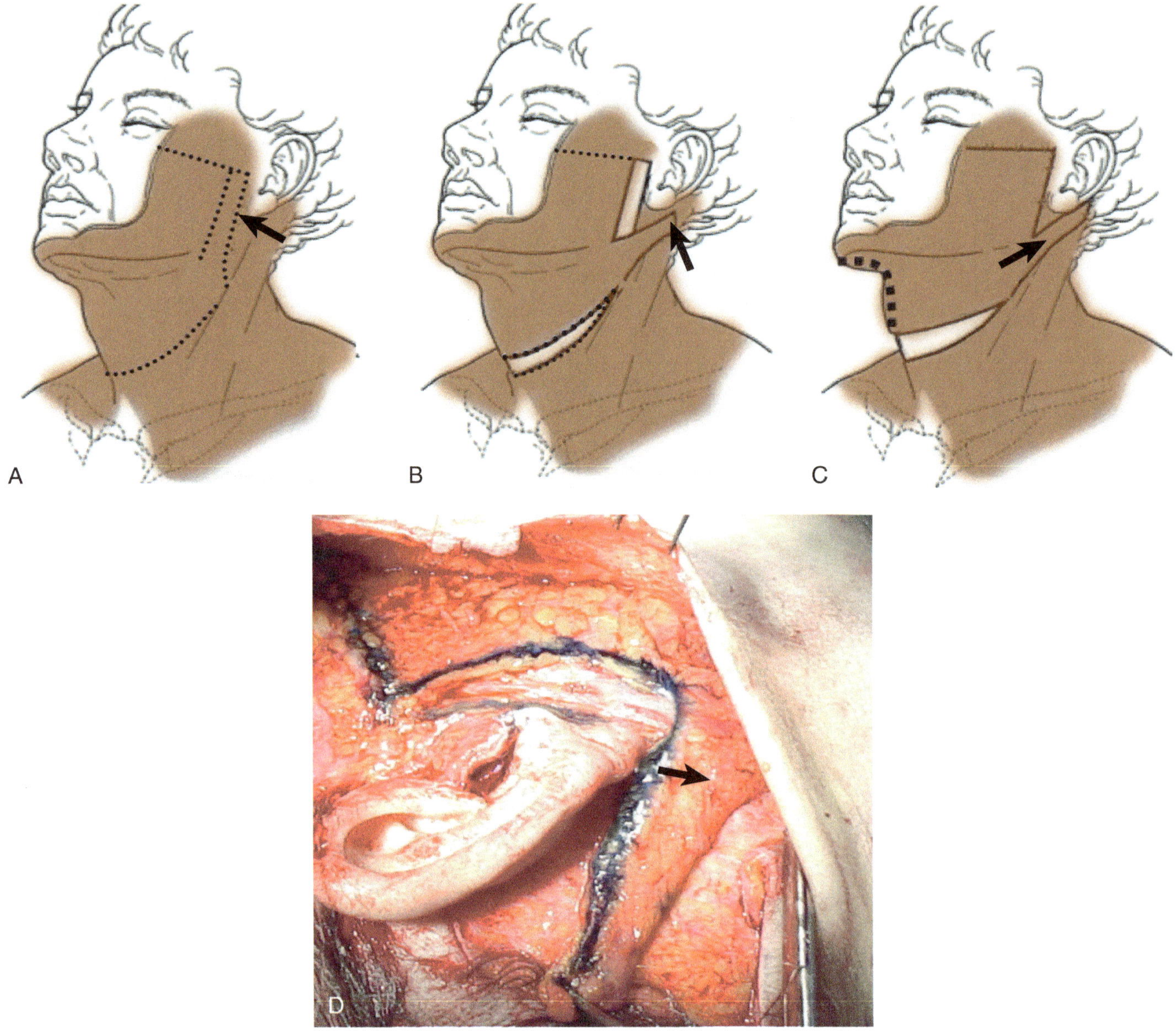

• **Fig. 67.49** If a facelift is performed a postauricular transposition flap (PATF) can be created from the posterior margin of a "high" SMAS flap and the high SMAS flap can be used to effect improvement in the cheek and midface region. (A) Plan for PATF with high SMAS flap (superior margin of SMAS flap planned at level of zygomatic arch). (B) After flap creation and transposition to the postauricular area. (C) After elevation and suturing of high SMAS flap and suturing of PATF to the mastoid fascia (typically some shortening of the flap is performed). In combination with anterior platysmaplasty (*dashed line*) a mastoid-to-mastoid sling of autologous tissue that defines the cervicomental angle is created. The high SMAS flap provides improvement in the upper face and midface that would not be otherwise obtained if platysmaplasty alone, or platysmaplasty and lateral platysmapexy, or platysmaplasty and low SMAS lift was performed. (D) Partially completed PATF seen in a facelift patient. (Courtesy Timothy Marten, MD, FACS and the Marten Clinic of Plastic Surgery, San Francisco, CA; with permission.)

Platysma myotomy should be performed after anterior platysmaplasty and lateral platysmal suspension (lateral platysmapexy or PATF) has been completed as the platysma muscle will be uniformly distributed over the anterior neck and under slight tension. Myotomy should be performed low in the neck at the level of the *cricoid* cartilage and extended slightly superiorly as it is extended laterally (Fig. 67.52A). At this level the muscle is thin and will bleed less, and the cut edges are less likely to be visible postoperatively but muscle action will nonetheless be interrupted. In addition, a smooth transition across the cervicomental angle is maintained and lower lip dysfunction is avoided. If transection is made higher, these benefits can be lost (Fig. 67.52B). This is particularly true when myotomy is performed at the level of the hyoid along the cervicomental angle or when wedges of

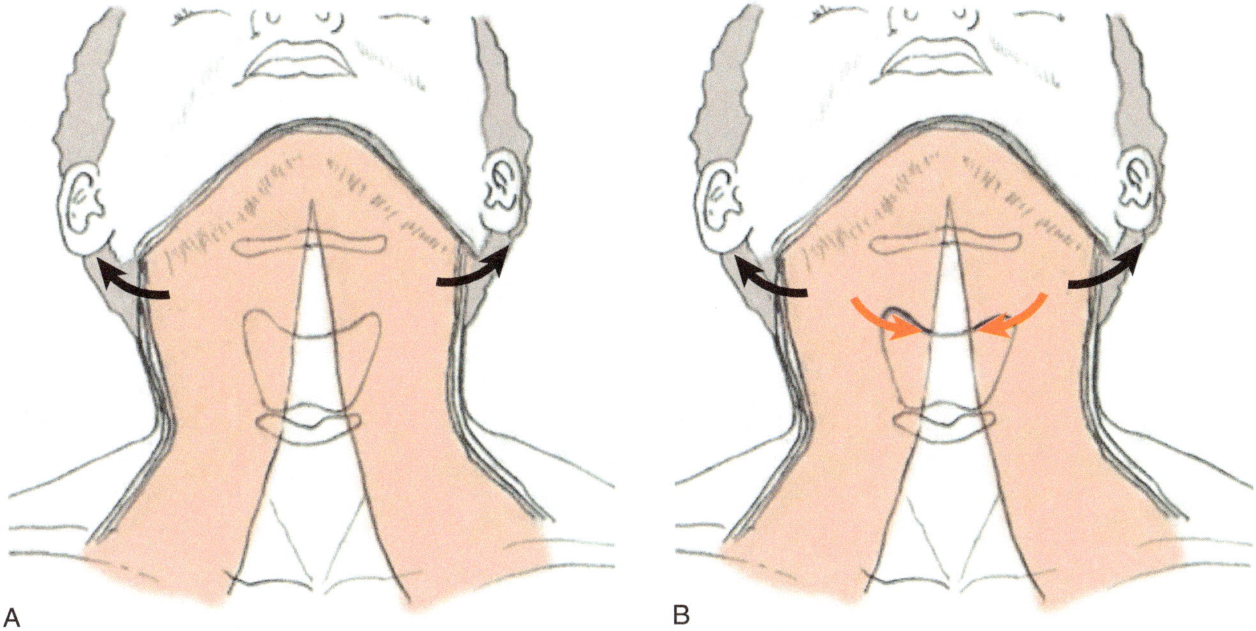

A B

• **Fig. 67.50** (A,B) Anterior platysmaplasty should be performed before lateral platysma suspension. (Courtesy Timothy Marten, MD, FACS and the Marten Clinic of Plastic Surgery, San Francisco, CA; with permission.)

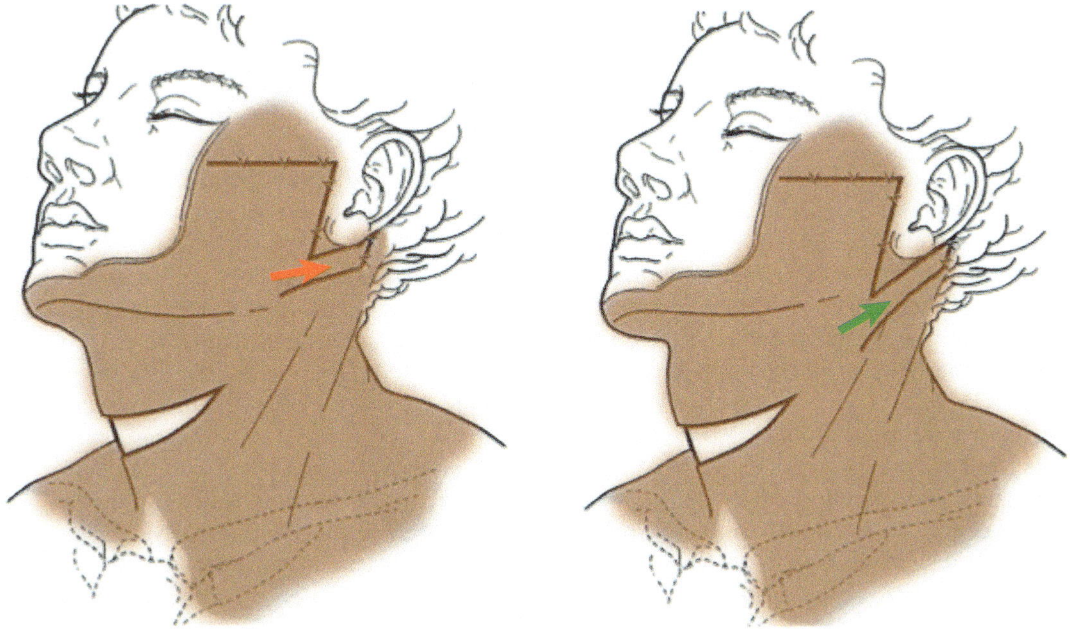

A Incorrect B Correct

• **Fig. 67.51** Incorrect and correct construction of the postauricular transposition flap (PATF). (A) *Improper* design and construction of the PATF. The flap has been designed and constructed too superiorly and pulls along the lower face and lateral mandibular border (*red arrow*). Such a construction does little to improve the neck. (B) Correct design and construction of the PATF. The flap has been designed and constructed more inferiorly so that its resultant pull is below the mandible and along the cervicomental angle (*green arrow*). Such a design optimizes cervicosubmental contour. (Courtesy Timothy Marten, MD, FACS and the Marten Clinic of Plastic Surgery, San Francisco, CA; with permission.)

platysma muscle are removed at that location as is shown in many plastic surgery textbooks. The platysma muscle is much thicker at that level, the cut edges are more likely to bleed and/or be visible after surgery. In addition, a high transection or resection of this sort can result in a severe and unesthetic transition for the submental region to the neck, and adversely effect platysma action and result in asymmetrical movement of the lower lip during speaking and expression. Transecting the platysma high along the cervicomental angle laterally also puts both the

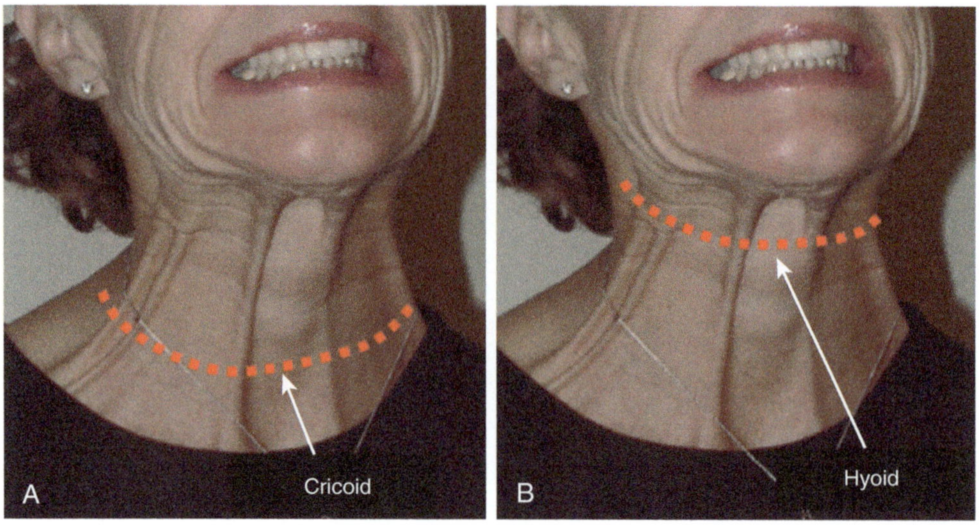

• **Fig. 67.52** Correct and incorrect level for plastysma myotomy. (A) *Correct* level (level of cricoid cartilage) for platysma myotomy. Myotomy should be performed low in the neck at the level of the *cricoid* cartilage and extended slightly superiorly as it is extended laterally. At this level the muscle is thin and will bleed less, and the cut edges are less likely to be visible postoperatively. In addition, a smooth transition across the cervicomental angle is maintained and lower lip dysfunction is avoided. (B) *Incorrect* level (level of hyoid cartilage) for platysma myotomy. The platysma muscle is much thicker, the cut edges are more likely to bleed and be visible after surgery. In addition, a high transection or resection can result in an unesthetic transition from the submental region to the neck, and result in asymmetrical movement of the lower lip. (Courtesy Timothy Marten, MD, FACS and the Marten Clinic of Plastic Surgery, San Francisco, CA; with permission.)

cervical and marginal mandibular branches of the facial nerve at risk.

Serrated and "super-sharp" scissors should not be used as they tend to pick up and cut adjacent tissue, and can result in injury to the anterior jugular vein. Unintended injury to the anterior jugular vein will result in annoying bleeding that can be difficult to control. Gentle spreading with scissors tips before each cut is made helps separate the platysma from underlying cervical fascia and facilitates dissection.

Myotomy is continued laterally and slightly superiorly according to the preoperative plan. If a "full width" division of the platysma is planned, the lateral-most portion of the transection (lateral half of the muscle) is completed through the postauricular incisions by identifying the lateral muscle border, incising it, and incrementally extending the incision until it is brought into continuity with the incision made in the muscle anteriorly through the submental incision using the method previously described.

Once correction of deep layer neck problems has been made and platysmaplasty, platysma myotomy, and suspension of postauricular transposition flaps have been performed as indicated, final contouring of subcutaneous superficial cervicofacial fat should be performed. This can be done under direct vision using Metzenbaum scissors or a small suction cannula. Final fat sculpting should be continued until all contours are smooth and regular, but *it is essential that not all fat be removed if an attractive appearance is to be obtained.* In addition, if a "double chin" or "witch's chin" is present, an extended dissection of the perimental area and chin pad should be made and fat contributing to these problems sculpted and excised, and the two regions seamlessly blended to insure a smooth transition for the chin to the submental area. In full necks where a true excess or preplatysmal fat is present, preplatysmal lipectomy can be performed with a suction cannula using an "open" liposuction technique by placing the cannula hole down under the skin flap and holding the skin flap down as resection is made. In thin necks, and in most of our cases, excision is made using a scissors technique.

Drains are used routinely and our experience has shown that they reduce postoperative ecchymosis and seromas, and allow patients to return to their work and social lives sooner. As a practical matter drains are generally necessary when aggressive deep neck maneuvers (subplatysmal fat excision and submandibular gland reduction) are performed, and "tissue glues" advocated by some surgeons to consolidate the subcutaneous plane cannot be expected to prevent collections in the subplatysmal area. It should be acknowledged that drains will not substitute for poor hemostasis in either plane, however, and will not prevent hematoma formation.

Experience has shown that when subplatysmal fat excision and submandibular gland reduction is performed it is prudent to place a drain in both the subcutaneous and the subplatysmal space for at least several days after the procedure to reduce edema and induration in the submental area to reduce the chance of a fluid collection (lymphatic fluid leakage from the division of lymphatic vessels during subplatysmal fat excision, and saliva leakage from the cut edge of the submandibular gland) and to speed the patient's overall recovery. The vacuum force applied by the subplatysmal drain will capture and remove lymphatic fluid and saliva, close down the subplatysmal space, and pull the underside of the platysmal muscle against the cut edge of each gland. It is convenient to place the exit site of the *subcutaneous* drain on the opposite side of the neck (opposite the exit site of the subplatysmal drain) so that it is clear which drain is which and output from each can readily be monitored. In a male face, or in a large female face, two subcutaneous drains may be required to adequately drain the subcutaneous space. The vacuum force applied by the subcutaneous drain captures and removes fluid from the subcutaneous space of both the face and neck and no drains are needed in the face.

Incision Closure

If a "short-scar" neck lift has been performed a submental incision only will be present and this can be conveniently closed in two layers. Prior to closure it is important to confirm that the wound edge thickness and amount of subcutaneous fat present on each side of the incision is similar. Typically the would edge of the cervical side will have a thinner edge and have less subcutaneous fat due to contact with instruments and retractors during preceding steps in the procedure and the mental, superior side will be thicker and have more fat. If a discrepancy is present, as it often will be, fat is carefully removed from the thicker superior side. The first layer of closure consists of several subcutaneous sutures of 5-0 Monocryl (or other suture of choice) to ensure that an equal amount of fat is present behind the closed wound and so that a depressed or irregular scar is avoided. Final approximation is then made with simple interrupted sutures of 6-0 nylon (or other suture of choice).

If an "extended" neck lift is performed, or a facelift is performed in conjunction with a neck lift procedure, skin will be excised from the postauricular area. The postauricular flap is shifted posteriorly and somewhat superiorly, roughly parallel to transverse neck creases and the mandibular border, in such a manner that skin is suspended under minimal or no tension and that *little or no skin need be trimmed from the anterior (postauricular) flap border*. Excessive trimming of skin from the anterior border of the postauricular skin flap will require the flap to be shifted along an incorrect superiorly directed vector, and this will produce a compromised result. The first point of suspension is located in the postauricular area at the anterior–superior aspect of the occipitomastoid incision. The flap is secured at this point with a simple interrupted suture of 4-0 nylon. No incision into the flap is necessary and no deep suture is used.

Once this suspension suture has been placed, the flap overlying the inferior portion of the ear should be carefully divided and the lobule exteriorized. *This is a key step in the procedure that must be performed incrementally and with great care if a visible scar, lobular malposition, and objectionable "pixy earlobe" is to be avoided.* If the incision to exteriorize the lobule is made correctly, the apex of the incision should rest snugly against the inferiormost portion of the conchal cartilage. If the incision into the cheek flap is made too far anteriorly or inferiorly, however, artistically appropriate resetting of the lobule will not be possible, and the outcome of the overall procedure significantly compromised.

Postauricular closure along the auriculomastoid sulcus is performed next, and should be completed before trimming and closure of the occipital portion of the incision and resetting of the lobule. It is begun by conservatively trimming the anterior border of the postauricular skin flap into a soft curve to match the curve of the incision made in the auriculomastiod sulcus. The incision is then closed with several interrupted sutures of 4-0 nylon. No deep suture is necessary or used.

It is a significant error and conceptually flawed concept to excise any skin over (superior to) the apex of the occipitomastoid incision and to shorten the postauricular flap along the long axis of the sternocleidomastoid muscle as commonly practiced and shown in many plastic surgery textbooks. Despite an apparent redundancy in this area when the patient is supine on the operating table, there is never any true skin excess at this location. This pseudo-excess of skin is present only because of the patient's high shoulder position in the supine position. It will vanish when she or he sits up and the shoulders drop to a normal position. Skin along the axis of the sternocleidomastoid muscle is also needed for side-to-side head tilt. Inappropriate excision of skin over the apex of the occipitomastoid defect is the ultimate underlying cause of hypertrophic healing in the postauricular region, and of a wide postauricular scar.

Trimming and closure of the occipital portion of the incision should be performed after closure of the postauricular area and suspension without trimming along the transmastoid portion of the postauricular incision. A facelift marker should be used to gauge skin flap redundancy along the occipital incision, and all points along the flap should be intentionally trimmed with 2–3 mm of redundancy. It must be remembered that the goal of skin excision is to remove redundancy, and not to tighten the cervical skin flap. If trimming is performed correctly wound edges should abut one another, and no gaps should be present, *before* sutures are placed. The incision is then closed in one layer with multiple half-buried vertical mattress sutures of 4-0 nylon with the knots tied on the scalp side and simple interrupted sutures of 6-0 nylon. No deep sutures are required and staples should not be used. This plan will provide precise wound edge alignment and prevent cross-hatched scars (suture marks). In addition, if the incision is closed under no tension as described an inconspicuous scar will be obtained.

If the postauricular skin flap has been shifted along a proper vector, and tissue distributed appropriately under no tension over the occipital area, a precise fit should be obtained. If neck skin redundancy is large, or if the postauricular flap has been suspended under tension, a dog-ear will often be present at the inferior-most portion of the occipital incision. This should not be chased down the occipital hairline as an obvious scar will result in the fine hair on the nape of the neck. A better result is obtained under these circumstances if the dog-ear is inset *posteriorly* into the occipital scalp, above the junction of thick and fine hair, and secured with simple interrupted sutures of 4-0 nylon. This requires that a small ellipse of *scalp* be excised from the *scalp side of the incision*, but moves the end of the incision into dense hair where it is well concealed. *No dressing is required or applied.* Patients are typically discharged with a hat, scarf, and sunglasses following the procedure.

Postoperative Care

Performance of the procedure itself only fulfills part of our obligation to the patient and the care they receive postoperatively is arguably as important as the surgery itself. Diligent postoperative care will also ensure the best result and limit the likelihood that problems and complications will occur.

Patients are discharged with specific written instructions as to how they are to care for themselves, and the surgeon should always be available to answer questions and see any patient, if needed.

Sleeping and Head Position

All patients are instructed to sleep flat on their backs without a pillow. A small cylindrical neck roll is permitted if the patient requests or requires it. This posture assures a "chin up" open cervicomental angle and averts dangerous folding of the neck skin flap and obstruction of regional cervical lymphatics that inevitably occurs if the patient is allowed to "elevate their head on pillows" as is commonly recommended after head and neck surgery. If patients are allowed to elevate their head on pillows, their neck will inevitably end up flexed and their skin bunched and folded. In addition, a flat-in-bed position encourages swelling to drain posteriorly to the back of the head instead of inferiorly to the anterior neck, where it is not harmful, less noticeable, and more rapidly transmitted away from the head and neck area when the patient sits upright. This is particularly helpful if a facelift has been performed as part of the procedure.

Patients are asked to rest quietly and apply cold compresses to their face and neck for 15–20 minutes of every hour they are awake for the first 3 days after surgery. For most patients, edema peaks at about this time. It is not necessary or productive to apply cool compresses continually throughout the day or at night. Ice and "ice packs" should never be applied directly to the skin.

Patients undergoing neck lift are placed on a "salivary rest" diet consisting of soft, wet, easy to swallow foods and are encouraged to avoid sweet, salty, sour, dry, and difficult to chew foods and citrus for several weeks. It is particularly important to avoid these sorts of foods that stimulate salivation for 7–10 days if submandibular gland reduction has been performed if fluid collections and neck induration is to be avoided. Patients are asked to abstain from the intake of alcohol for 2 weeks after surgery.

Patients are instructed to begin a daily routine of showering and shampooing no later than 3 days after surgery. Patients are allowed to shower even if their drains are still in place. This helps remove crusting about the suture lines, keeps incisions clean, and usually improves the patient's general outlook and well-being.

Drain Removal

Drains are usually left in the neck until the patient's first clinic visit for suture removal 5 days following their surgery. This is because drain output often quickly falls on the first or second day after surgery during the time the patient is mostly supine and resting, but then typically picks up again when the patient begins to spend more time upright, starts to move their head about more, and begins to eat more. Leaving the neck drains in longer, for 5–7 days, will reduce the likelihood that small collections will form and it will speed the overall resolution of edema, ecchymosis, and induration in the neck area. At the patient's first suture removal visit 5 days after surgery their progress and drain output is accessed. If healing is progressing well, drain output is minimal and no fluid collections are present, and if it appears that the patient is following dietary and other instructions, drains are removed at that time. It is prudent to release suction before drain removal and to have the patient on an assistant hold pressure over their anterior neck as the drain is removed for several minutes to avoid inducing the formation of a hematoma.

If a patient's neck appears congested at their 5th postoperative day, if drain output is still significant, or if the patient appears to not be following dietary and other instructions, drains are not removed and are left in place until the patient's second suture removal visit 7 days after surgery. In almost all cases, drains, if still present, are removed at that time.

Case Examples

Case 1

This woman, age 65, had had prior upper and lower eye lifts by an unknown surgeon. In the *Before* views note the lax skin, obtuse cervicosubmental contour, paucity of subcutaneous neck fat, and "double chin" appearance when the patient looks down. A large submandibular salivary gland is clearly visible in the lateral submental triangle in the lateral view, and the patient appears to have a "low hyoid." A facelift, neck lift, forehead lift, upper and lower eye lifts, perioral dermabrasion, and fat transfer to cheeks and lips were performed. The neck lift procedure included excision of excess subplatysmal fat, submandibular salivary gland reduction, superficial digastric myectomy, anterior platysmaplasty, and full-width platysma myotomy. In the *After* views at 13 months post surgery note the well-defined jawline and attractive, youthful-appearing neckline even when the patient looks down. Comprehensive neck surgery has corrected problems that are commonly misinterpreted as a low hyoid position.

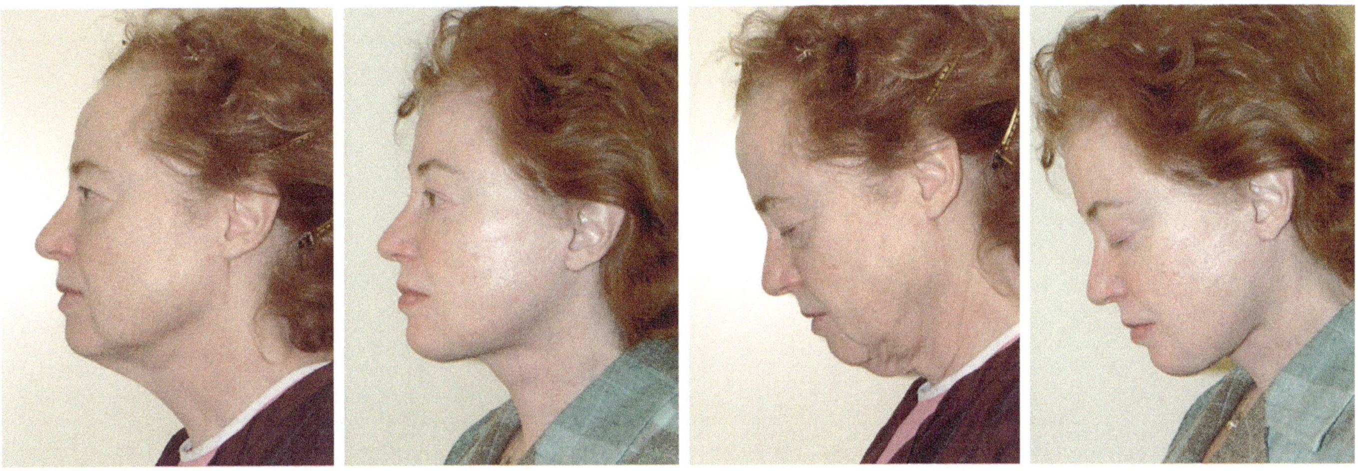

Before After Before After

Case 1 (Courtesy Timothy Marten, MD, FACS and the Marten Clinic of Plastic Surgery, San Francisco, CA; with permission. Procedures performed by Timothy J. Marten, MD, FACS.)

Case 2

This 46-year-old woman had had no prior surgery. In the *Before* views note the full neck, obtuse cervicosubmental contour, and "double chin" appearance when the patient looks down. Palpation of the lateral submental triangle revealed a firm mobile mass consistent with an enlarged submandibular salivary gland. Her preoperative appearance suggests the presence of a "low hyoid."

Facelift, neck lift, forehead lift, lower eye lifts, and facial fat injections were performed. The neck lift procedure included excision of subplatysmal fat, submanbibular salivary gland reduction, superficial digastric myectomy, anterior platysmaplasty, and full-width platysmal myotomy. In the *After* views at 11 months post surgery note the attractive, youthful-appearing neckline even when the patient looks down. Comprehensive neck surgery has corrected problems that are commonly misinterpreted as a low hyoid position. The "double chin" deformity has also been corrected.

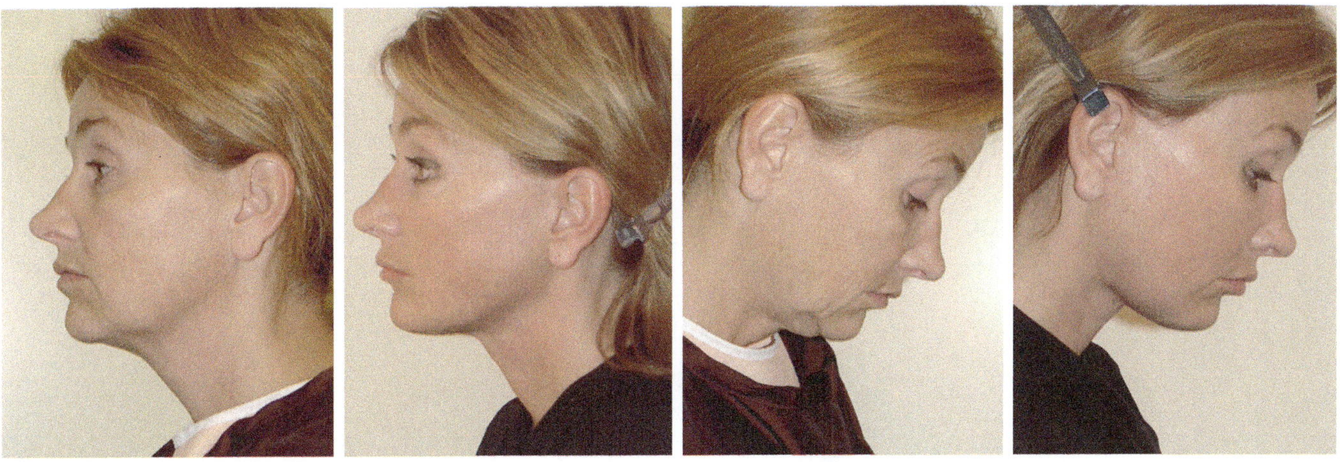

Before After Before After

Case 2 (Courtesy Timothy Marten, MD, FACS and the Marten Clinic of Plastic Surgery, San Francisco, CA; with permission. Procedures performed by Timothy J. Marten, MD, FACS.)

Case 3

This woman, age 55, had had prior eye lifts and a perioral chemical peel performed by an unknown surgeon. In the *Before* views note the full neck, obtuse cervicosubmental contour, and "double chin" appearance that is exacerbated when the patient looks down. Palpation of the lateral submental triangle revealed a firm mobile mass consistent with an enlarged submandibular salivary gland. Note paucity of subcutaneous neck fat, suggesting submental liposuction had been performed at her previous procedure.

The *After* views show the patient 1 year and 4 months after facelift, neck lift, forehead lift, upper and lower eye lifts, perioral dermabrasion, and facial fat injections. The neck lift procedure included excision of a large amount of subplatysmal fat, submanbibular salivary gland reduction, superficial digastric myectomy, anterior platysmaplasty, and full-width platysma myotomy. Note the well-defined jawline and attractive, youthful-appearing neckline even when the patient looks down. The "double chin" deformity has been corrected by releasing the submental-retaining ligaments and blending the fat of the chin and the submental area.

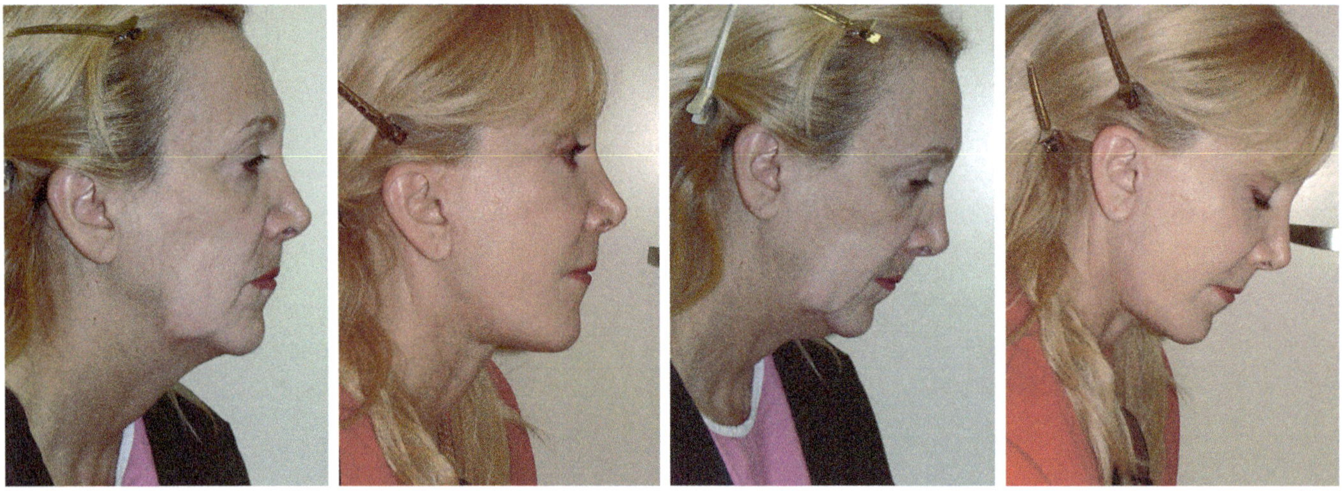

Before After Before After

Case 3 (Courtesy Timothy Marten, MD, FACS and the Marten Clinic of Plastic Surgery, San Francisco, CA; with permission. Procedures performed by Timothy J. Marten, MD, FACS.)

Case 4

This woman, age 55, had had prior eye lifts and a perioral chemical peel performed by an unknown surgeon. In the *Before* views note the full neck, obtuse cervicosubmental contour, and "double chin" appearance that is exacerbated when the patient looks down. Palpation of the lateral submental triangle revealed a firm mobile mass consistent with an enlarged submandibular salivary gland. Note paucity of subcutaneous neck fat suggesting submental liposuction had been performed at her previous procedure.

Facelift, neck lift, forehead lift, upper and lower eye lifts, perioral dermabrasion, and facial fat injections were performed. The neck lift procedure included excision of a large amount of subplatysmal fat, submanbibular salivary gland reduction, superficial digastric myectomy, anterior platysmaplasty, and full-width platysma myotomy. The *After* views show the patient at 1 year and 4 months after surgery. Note the well-defined jawline and attractive, youthful-appearing neckline even when the patient looks down. The "double chin" deformity has been corrected by releasing the submental retaining ligaments and blending the fat of the chin and the submental area.

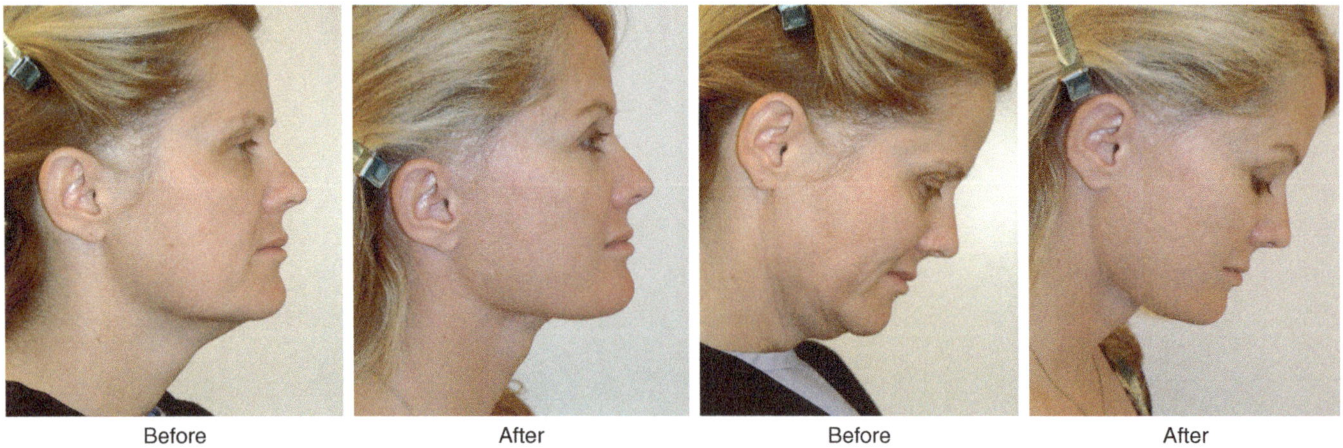

Before After Before After

Case 4 (Courtesy Timothy Marten, MD, FACS and the Marten Clinic of Plastic Surgery, San Francisco, CA; with permission. Procedures performed by Timothy J. Marten, MD, FACS.)

Case 5

This 68-year-old man had had no prior plastic surgery. In the *Before* views note the poor cervicosubmental contour and "double chin" appearance when the patient looks down. An enlarged submandibular salivary gland can be seen beneath the skin in the left lateral view and confirmed on palpation. Note the paucity of subcutaneous neck fat that is typical for patients in older age groups. Platysma bands are visible in the anterior neck.

Facelift, neck lift, forehead lift, upper and lower eye lifts, partial facial fat transfer, and ear lobe reduction were performed. The neck lift procedure included excision of a large amount of subplatysmal fat, submanbibular salivary gland reduction, superficial digastric myectomy, anterior platysmaplasty, and full-width platysma myotomy. In the *After* views at 1 year and 9 months post surgery note the well-defined jawline and masculine-appearing neckline even when the patient looks down.

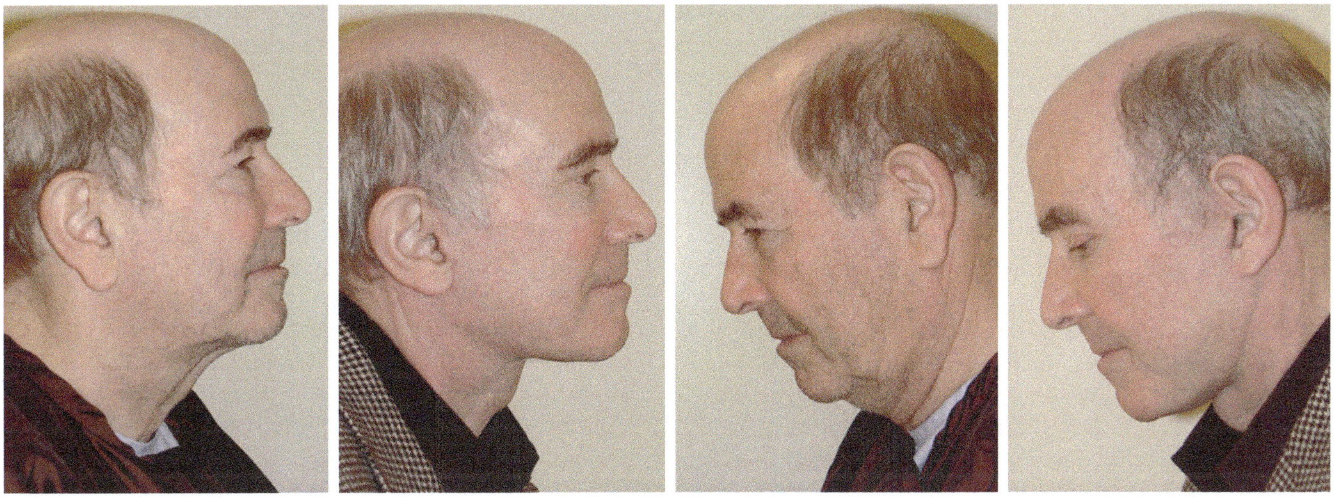

Before After Before After

Case 5 (Courtesy Timothy Marten, MD, FACS and the Marten Clinic of Plastic Surgery, San Francisco, CA; with permission. Procedures performed by Timothy J. Marten, MD, FACS.)

Acknowledgment

All photographs, illustrations, descriptions, and text contained in this chapter are property of the Marten Clinic of Plastic Surgery, San Francisco, CA, and are used with permission.

Further Reading

Marten T. Secondary facelift. In: Mathes S, ed. *Plastic Surgery*. Volume 2: *The Head and Neck*. Philadelphia: Saunders; 2005.

Marten TJ. High SMAS facelift: combined single flap lifting of the jawline, cheek, and midface. *Clin Plast Surg*. 2008;35(4):569–603.

Marten T. Lamellar high SMAS face and mid-lift: improved design of the SMAS facelift for better results in the mid-face and infra-orbital region. In: Nahai F, ed. *The Art of Aesthetic Surgery*. Volume 2. 2nd edn. Boca Raton, FL: CRC Press; 2011:1525–1621.

Marten T. Male facelift. In: Rubin JP, Neligan PC, eds. *Plastic Surgery*. Volume 2: *Aesthetic Surgery*. 4th edn. Elsevier; 2018. Ch. 6.9.

Marten T. Secondary facelift. In: Rubin JP, Neligan PC, eds. *Plastic Surgery*. Volume 2: *Aesthetic Surgery*. 4th edn. Elsevier; 2018. Ch. 6.10.

Marten TJ. Facelift: planning and technique. *Clin Plast Surg*. 1997;24(2):269–308.

Marten T, Elyassnia D. Management of the platysma in neck lift. *Clin Plast Surg*. 2018;45(4):555–570.

Marten T, Elyassnia D. Neck lift: defining anatomic problems and choosing appropriate treatment strategies. *Clin Plast Surg*. 2018;45(4):455–484.

Marten T, Elyassnia D. Short-scar neck lift: neck lift using a submental incision only. *Clin Plast Surg*. 2018;45(4):585–600.

68 Rhinoplasty

ALI TOTONCHI AND BAHMAN GUYURON

For videos accompanying this chapter see ExpertConsult.com. See inside cover for access details.

Introduction

The nose is a multifarious structure with critical mechanical and functional roles, which by virtue of its position, serves as the central and salient component of the face. Its relationship to surrounding structures is in part responsible for a harmonious, pleasing form as a whole. Functionally, the nose provides an airway and acts to warm, filter, and humidify air passing through it. Noses that deviate from ideal structural proportions – whether subtle variations of normal or more dramatic posttraumatic or neoplastic deformities – have motivated rhinoplasty surgeons since ancient India 800 BCE.

Anatomy

A thorough appreciation and understanding of relevant anatomy is crucial for all surgery. Obviously, recognition of the nuances and subtle variations of nasal anatomy is absolutely vital for execution of a successful rhinoplasty.

Skin

A thorough rhinoplasty evaluation must assess skin type and thickness. The surgeon must anticipate the advantages and limitations afforded by a particular skin type. In general, thin skin is unlikely to camouflage even minor irregularities in the underlying cartilaginous and osseous structures, particularly with grafting. In contrast, thick skin conceals imperfections in the nasal skeleton and may hide surgical flaws or reduce the desired definition intended from alteration of underlying cartilage and bone.[1] Sebaceous skin can give the tip a bulbous appearance. The skin is thickest at the nasion. More caudally, the remaining upper half of nose tends to have skin that is thinner and more mobile than the lower half. In the tip area, there tend to be more sebaceous glands. However, in the infratip region, the columella and ala again are usually covered with thinner skin.[2,3]

Cartilaginous and Bony Support

An understanding of the bony and cartilaginous structural components of the nose should be complemented by correlation with landmarks of the surface anatomy (Fig. 68.1). Caudal to the glabellar protrusion, the deepest point of the surface of the nose is referred to as the radix. The root of the nose, just caudal to the nasofrontal suture line, is referred to as the nasion, minor adjustments of which can change the overall character of the nose. The rhinion describes the position along the dorsum where the nasal bones articulate with the upper lateral cartilages and the pronasale refers to the region extending from the supratip break, including the tip and infratip lobule, to the anterior-most aspect of the columella. The tip-defining points are the anterior-most points of the nose corresponding to the intermediate crura of the lower lateral cartilages.

Nasal Bones

The bony vault is pyramidal in shape and comprises the paired nasal bones that articulate with the frontal bone superiorly and the ascending maxillary processes laterally. The bony pyramid is narrowest at the level of the intercanthal line and widens inferiorly.[2] The nasal bones are thickest cephalically and become thinner caudally.[2,4] The nasal bones are supported superiorly at the nasofrontal suture line, laterally at their articulation with the ascending process of the maxilla, and dorsally at their fusion with the perpendicular plate of the ethmoid. The junction between the upper third and lower two-thirds of the nose where the cartilaginous septum meets the nasal bones is referred to as the "keystone area," as this area is essential for structural support, and stabilizing the nasal dorsum for height and projection.[3]

Upper Lateral Cartilages

The upper lateral cartilages articulate with the septum and extend cephalically and laterally. The upper lateral cartilages are supported primarily by their connection with the nasal bones and frontal process of maxilla. On their deep surface, they are lined by perichondrium that is continuous with the septal perichondrium.[3] Their articulation with the septum forms the internal nasal valve; the angle should be between 9 and 15 degrees.[5]

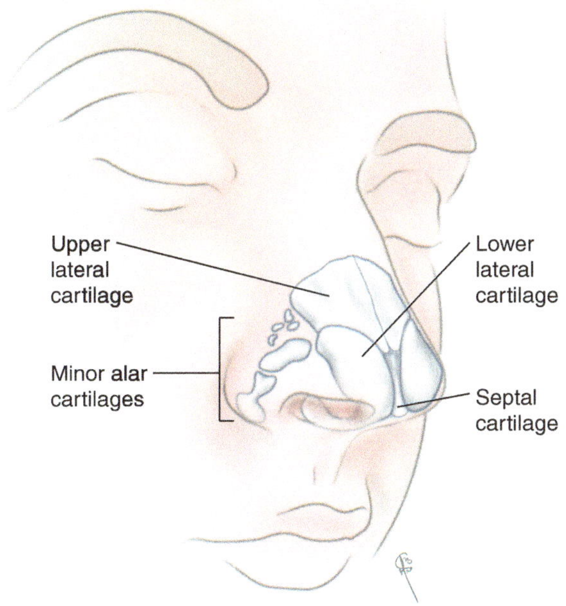

• **Fig. 68.1** The cartilaginous components of the nose in relation to surface anatomy.

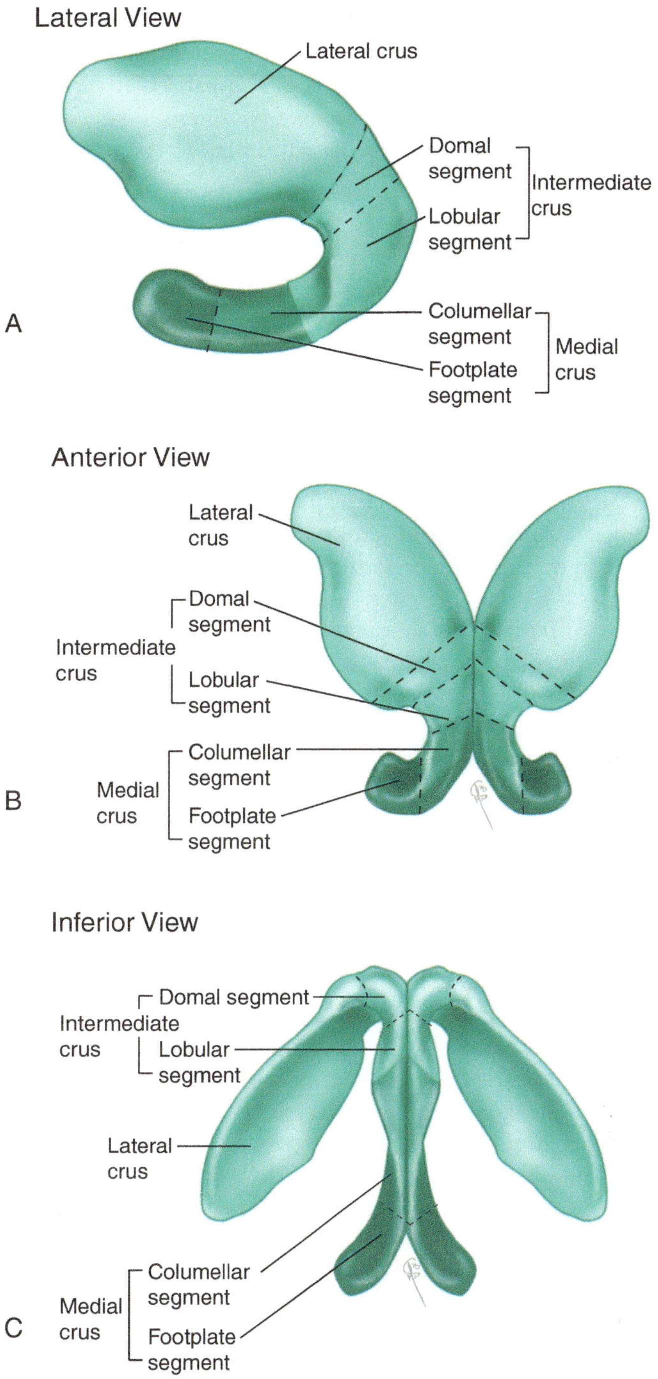

• **Fig. 68.2** Lateral, anterior, and inferior views of the lower lateral cartilages (LLC).

Lower Lateral Cartilages

The lower lateral cartilages (LLC) are paired structures in the caudal third of the nose that can be subdivided into three segments: the lateral, intermediate/middle, and medial crura (Fig. 68.2). The lateral crus supports the alar rim. The scroll area is the region where the superior edge of the lower lateral cartilage curls downward as it meets the inferior edge of the upper lateral cartilage. This area provides some support for the internal nasal valve. Superior and lateral to the scroll area, one can find several small sesamoid cartilages connected by fibrous tissue that wraps around the alae laterally.[2,3] The intermediate crus has the most variability in shape and may be convex, boxy, broad or concave; it forms the tip-defining point. It should be noted that skin over this region is particularly delicate as there is a deficiency of subcutaneous tissue: the skin directly abuts the perichondrium necessitating meticulous dissection.[3] The medial crura sit next to each other in the columella. The footplate is the area closest to the nasal spine where variable degrees of divergence exist. The columellar segment, the middle portion of the columella, extends towards the intermediate crura where the cartilages may diverge again to reach the tip-defining points.

Several analogies have been proposed to describe the dynamics of tip rhinoplasty, relating the medial and lateral crura of the lower lateral cartilages and their attachment to the caudal septum to tip support, projection, and rotation. The "tripod concept" of the nasal base is the most popular analogy for understanding the interdependent relationships of the nasal base structures. This theory proposes that the nasal base structurally functions like a tripod with the paired medial crura acting as one leg of the tripod and each of the lateral crura acting as one of the other two tripod legs. Altering the length or strength of the legs will result in changes of the rotation and projection of the tip. While the tripod theory has ample utility in the understanding and planning of surgery,[6,7] it has limitations in that it may not be the most accurate predictor of the true forces on the nasal tip. Westreich et al. proposed an alternate model, which extrapolates on the tripod concept described as a "cantilevered spring tripod." They measured stiffness and elastic modulus of the different cartilages and found that the septal cartilage had the greatest tensile strength. They also found that the strength and support of the nasal tip depended greatly on the thickness of the cartilage and perichondrial attachments more than the elastic modulus of the particular cartilage. With these findings, they proposed considering the nasal tip as a cantilever from the caudal septum.[8]

Septum

The septum is comprised of bony and cartilaginous portions. The bony septum is made up of the perpendicular plate of the ethmoid bone superiorly, the vomer inferiorly and posteriorly, and the maxillary crest, which forms the caudal-most projection of the premaxilla, anteriorly and inferiorly. The cartilaginous septum is composed of a single continuous quadrangular cartilage that articulates with the vomer and the perpendicular plate of the ethmoid posteriorly and superiorly and is supported inferiorly by the maxillary crest. The anterior aspect of the quadrangular cartilage supports the nasal dorsum and provides tip projection. The anterior septal angle supports the nasal tip with attachments to the medial crura of the lower lateral cartilages. The posterior septal angle articulates with the anterior-most portion of the maxillary crest. The amount of cartilage in the quadrangular cartilage varies among patients and is typically less robust in non-Caucasian patients.[3]

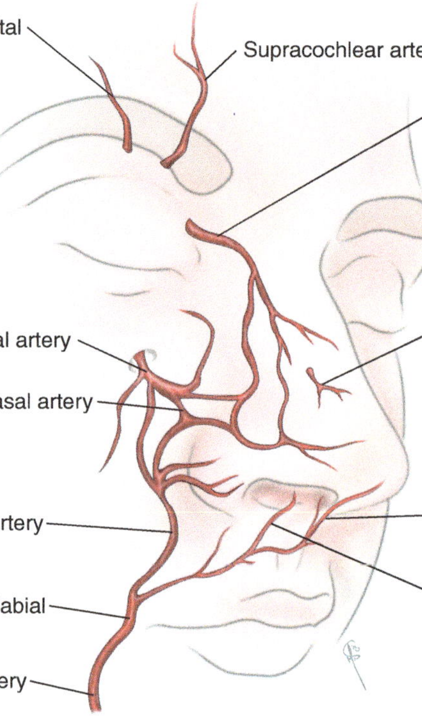

• **Fig. 68.3** Blood supply of the external nose.

SMAS

In the nose, the SMAS is a continuation of the subcutaneous musculoaponeurotic system, which is contiguous from the galea to platysma. Muscles associated with the nose within the SMAS can be categorized into elevators and depressors of the nasal tip. The elevator muscle group includes the procerus, levator labii superioris, alaque nasi, and the anomalous nasi. Depressors include the alar and transverse portions of the nasalis, the dilator naris posterior, depressor septi nasi, and compressor narium.

Blood Supply

Understanding the blood supply of the nose is important in order to avoid ischemic consequences if this rich blood supply is inadvertently and sufficiently disrupted. The dorsal nasal artery, a branch of the ophthalmic artery, penetrates the orbital septum above the medial palpebral ligament and courses along the side of the nose, providing robust blood supply to the dorsal nasal skin. It ultimately anastomoses with the lateral nasal artery, a branch of the angular artery (itself the terminal branch of the facial artery), with numerous branches that enter the subdermal plexus thereby supplying the lateral surface of the caudal nose. The tip of the nose is supplied both by the external nasal branch of the anterior ethmoid artery (a branch of the ophthalmic artery), the columellar artery (a branch of the superior labial artery), and branches of the lateral nasal artery. The external nasal branch of the anterior ethmoid artery passes between the nasal bone and the upper lateral cartilage to supply skin of the nasal tip. Branches of the superior labial artery supply the nostril sill and columellar base (Fig. 68.3). Intranasal blood supply is from branches of the anterior and posterior ethmoid arteries, the superior labial and greater palatine arteries, and the maxillary artery.

Venous drainage of the external nose generally consists of veins with names that correspond to the associated arteries, which veins drain through the facial vein, the pterygoid plexus, and ophthalmic veins, the pterygoid plexus and the facial vein. Lymphatic drainage of the nasal tip follows the same path and appears to be limited to the lateral walls, sparing the columella.[9]

Nerve Supply

Branches of the second and third divisions of the trigeminal nerves provide sensory innervation of the nose while motor innervation is supplied by the zygomatic branch of the facial nerve. From V_2, the ophthalmic nerve gives off the supratrochlear and infratrochlear nerves to supply sensation to the rhinion, radix sidewalls. The anterior ethmoid nerve gives off external branches that travel within the SMAS layer to supply sensation to the tip; therefore, careful dissection beneath the SMAS over the tip will preserve tip sensation. From V_3, the maxillary nerve branches and supplies sensation to the lateral vestibule and columella (Fig. 68.4).

Patient Assessment

The process of rhinoplasty begins with patient evaluation. Arguably, the foundation of a successful rhinoplasty is

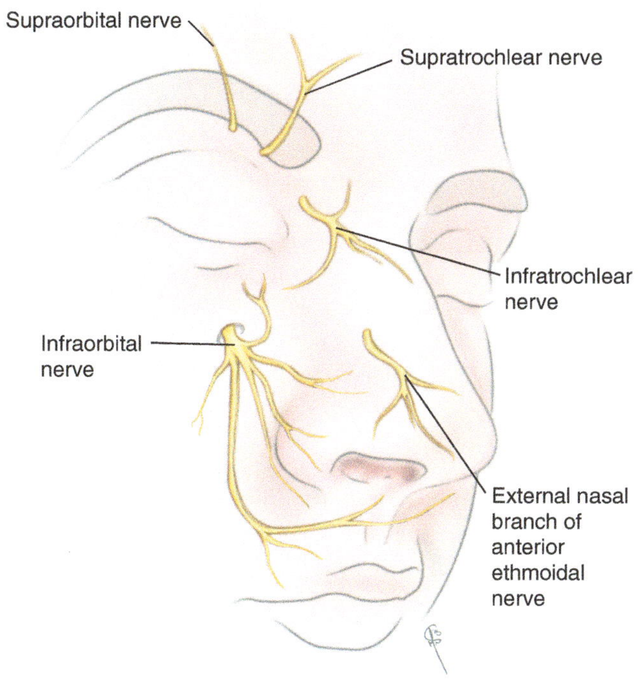

• **Fig. 68.4** Sensory nerve supply of the external nose.

established at the initial patient visit including a thorough, accurate evaluation of the nose; its relation to the rest of the patient's face; identification of appropriate and realistic goals given the patient's anatomy; clear communication; and mutual understanding and agreement of surgical goals between the patient and the surgeon. A vital part of any successful rhinoplasty is the detection of the functional abnormalities. This begins with keen observation of mouth breathing, which often is unbeknown to the patients, and ends with circumspect examination of the internal and external nasal valves, septal deviation, and enlargement of the turbinates. Meticulous preoperative photodocumentation is crucial and life-size based planning or computer generated images of potential postoperative goals may be helpful in facilitating patient–surgeon discussion and establishing matching and achievable operative goals.

History

Important components of a complete history include medical, surgical, family, and social history as well as thorough review of all prescription and nonprescription medications. Of particular interest is whether there has been any previous nasal trauma or surgery. A history of diabetes, connective tissue disease, anticoagulation, or a bleeding or clotting disorder should be noted. Smoking significantly impedes healing and can lead to scarring, skin necrosis, and a poor outcome. A psychiatric history may help the surgeon understand a patient's motivation for cosmetic surgery. If a patient's motives are self-driven rather than driven by pressure from peers or a significant other, the patient is more likely to be satisfied with the ultimate surgical outcome. In addition to motivation, it is important to elicit a clear picture of the patient's desires and expectations from rhinoplasty. This should be considered in the surgeon's nasal analysis and proposal of surgical goals and limitations with thorough counselling and establishment of reasonable goals. History of sinus infections, sinus headaches or migraine headaches should be documented in depth.

Physical Examination

Physical exam should include a thorough facial analysis characterizing the nasal structures themselves and their relationship to the face as a whole. A careful intranasal exam should also be performed, including inspection of the septum, turbinates, nasal valves, and an assessment of nasal breathing. Finger palpation is an essential component of the exam.

Only in idealized drawings is the face completely symmetric, and strict symmetry of the nose and the face should not be anticipated. The nose should occupy the middle third of the face horizontally and the middle fifth of the face vertically. The nose itself may be divided into thirds vertically. Generally, the upper third is comprised of the nasal bones, the middle third is comprised of the upper lateral cartilages, and the lower third is comprised of the tip and the lower lateral cartilages. Deviations from the ideal should be accurately localized and surgical correction of these variations should address the appropriate structures.

An important feature is the smooth, unbroken, and symmetric brow-tip esthetic line, which is described as a "gentle sweeping line from the medial brow to the lateral nasal wall to the tip-defining point;" the ideal shape of this esthetic line in a female nose is that of an hourglass, narrowing in the middle and flaring at the top and bottom.[1]

Numerous proportions and relationships have been described to characterize the ideal nose. In the frontal view, the ideal nasal length is two-thirds that of the midface, measured from the glabella to the alar base, and equal to the vertical length of the chin, measured from the stomion to the menton.[10] The width of the alar base should approximate the intercanthal distance and may be up to but not more than 2 mm wider,[1] so long as the intercanthal distance is normal. The radix should be at the level of the supratarsal crease.

In the lateral view, the nasofrontal angle should be approximately 115–130 degrees[4] and the radix should be 4–6 mm deep. In females, the dorsum should extend as a straight line until reaching the supratip break, which esthetically separates the dorsum from the tip unit. Ideally, the nasolabial angle should be 93–98 degrees for men and 95–100 degrees for women, although this angle varies somewhat based on the height of the patient. In general, shorter individuals may have a more obtuse angle while taller individuals may have a more acute angle. In the lateral view, the alar base should be 2 mm above the line between the lower and middle third of the nose.[11] The lateral tip projection can be measured from the alar–cheek junction to the tip-defining point.[10]

The alar–columellar relationship should be carefully evaluated from the lateral view. When viewed from this aspect, the upper border of the nostril is formed by the alar rim and the lower border is formed by the columellar rim. Gunter described a method of analysing this relationship. A line is drawn which approximates the long axis of the nostril: the ala should be 1–2 mm above this line and the columella 1–2 mm below this line. If the columellar rim is less than 1–2 mm from this line, the columella is considered to be retracted; conversely, if the distance is greater than 1–2 mm, the columella is considered to be "hanging." If the ala is less than 1–2 mm from this axis, it is considered to be a hanging ala; if it is greater than 1–2 mm from this axis it is considered a retracted ala.[12,13]

The alar–columellar relationship and alar rim deformities should also include analysis from the alar base view. The ideal base view is an equilateral triangle with each ala forming the sides of the triangle and the alar base width forming the remaining side. A concave ala is present when the lateral border of the ala is medial to the line of the equilateral triangle whereas when it extends lateral to the line of the triangle, it should be considered convex.[14]

The ideal nostril is oval-shaped, wider than the columella, and should be almost parallel to the vertical axis of the columella in the Caucasian nose. The length of the columella should be twice the height of the infratip lobule. The alae should insert at a soft angle to the cheek with a slight curve medially. Disharmonies of the alar base can be in either the vertical or horizontal plane, and careful analysis is critical, as surgical correction of these deformities differ depending on the nature of the deformity.[11]

The relationship of the nose to surrounding facial structures affects the perception of nasal features. A sloping forehead may give the illusion of overprojection of the nasal tip whereas a flattened forehead may give the illusion of an underprojected nasal tip. Similarly, an underprojected chin may make the nose appear relatively overprojected and vice versa.

The esthetics of the nasal tip may be defined by a number of relationships, many of which are quite subtle. The angle at which the lateral and medial crura of the lower lateral cartilages meet should be about 30 degrees on either side. The ideal nasal tip should be well defined. Subtle variations in anatomy may make it appear boxy or bulbous. Wide lateral crura may blunt dome definition, resulting in a boxy tip. A greater than 30-degree angle between the lateral and medial crura or divergent domes can result in a bulbous-appearing tip.[1]

Physical examination should include palpation of the bony and cartilaginous components of the nasal dorsum to understand the relationships between them. The tip recoil test is performed by placing gentle pressure on the tip to assess the strength of the lower lateral cartilages. An intranasal exam should be performed to identify deviations of the nasal septum, turbinate hypertrophy, and any internal causes of nasal obstruction. The Cottle or modified Cottle maneuver is performed to assess nasal valve collapse.

Although the most thoroughly studied and well-described ideal nasal esthetics pertain to the Caucasian nose, much individual variety exists and these ideals cannot be indiscriminately applied to all noses, particularly in different ethnicities such as the African, Asian, Middle Eastern or Hispanic noses.[15]

The African nose has a wide base and low, flattened-appearing dorsum. The ascending maxillary process often lacks vertical projection, which contributes to the low dorsum. The nasal bones are short. Increased distance at alar insertion and alar flaring both contribute to the increased interalar distance.[16] There also tends to be increased fibrofatty tissue and thicker sebaceous skin at the tip, both of which contribute to lack of tip and soft tissue triangle definition.[15]

The Asian nose has typical characteristics somewhere in between the Caucasian and African nose. There is typically a low dorsum that begins more caudally. Again, the skin at the tip and supratip region is thicker than the Caucasian nose but not quite to the extent of the African nose. The alar width is slightly wider than the Caucasian nose. Characteristically, in the Asian nose, there is paucity of septal cartilage leading to a less projected tip and occasionally retracted-appearing columella. This should be anticipated in Asian rhinoplasty and consideration of other sources of cartilage grafts should be explored and discussed. There also tends to be weaker lower lateral cartilage.[17]

The Middle Eastern and Indian nose share some characteristics with the Caucasian nose,with similar height of the dorsum.[15] However, they also frequently have overprojection of the dorsum resulting in a high dorsal hump. There is mild alar flaring, and thick skin around the tip region. There is variable skin thickness of tip and alar flaring. Dorsal height also varies between the norms of Caucasian and Asian nose.[18]

Photography

The standard approach to photography for rhinoplasty is to obtain realistic preoperative photography using a digital single lens reflex (SLR) camera. Photos should be taken with a standard blue background with appropriate lighting. Many surgeons will have a dedicated space for photography in their office. Standardization of patient positioning, lighting, and angles should be maintained. This will facilitate the surgeon's study of the patient's nasal anatomy and facial harmony for surgical planning. Moreover, it permits accurate pre- and postoperative comparison thereby facilitating the surgeon's self-assessment and critique allowing continual refinement of surgical technique (Fig. 68.5).

An important aspect of successful photography is the lighting and positioning for rhinoplasty portraits. The simplest lighting setup is a single mounted flash on top of the camera itself; however, this can result in harsh and uneven shadows. There are several established, sophisticated lighting arrangements that have been described.[19] The key light system, developed for portrait photography, positions the

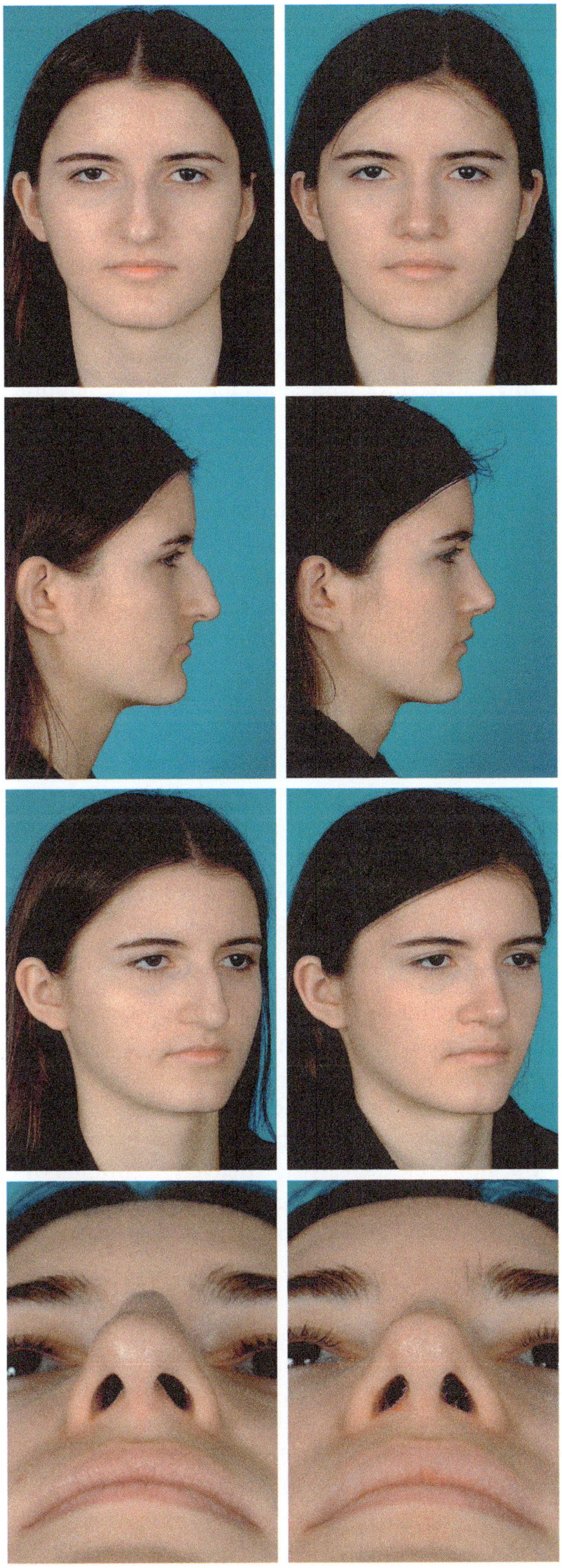

• **Fig. 68.5** Photographic standardization assists surgical planning and allows accurate pre- and postoperative comparison, thereby facilitating the surgeon's self-assessment and critique allowing continual refinement of surgical technique.

main light at a 45-degree angle from the patient, casting a shadow from the nasal tip to the oral commissure. A second fill light is placed at nearly the same angle on the opposite side in a position that it fills the shadow cast from the main light. Then, two backlights are placed behind the patient to separate him/her from the background. The quarter system places two lights equally at 45-degree angles from the patient.

The traditional six standard photographic views taken for rhinoplasty are the frontal anteroposterior (AP), right and left lateral, right and left oblique, and base view.[20,21] A top view is a useful addition that can be used to better characterize and understand deviations in the crooked nose, especially for patients with dorsal deviation.[5] Some surgeons routinely obtain a smiling view. Proper positioning in both frontal and lateral views requires alignment along the Frankfort horizontal plane, defined by a line that connects the top of the tragus to the infraorbital rim; this line should be truly horizontal and parallel to the ground.[20]

Rhinoplasty Dynamics

The nose is a 3-dimensional centerpiece on the face with critical structural and functional roles. There are many variables and dimensions that can be adjusted to alter the esthetic appearance, structural components, and functional role of the nose. There are many tools and maneuvers available to the rhinoplasty surgeon to adjust these numerous variables. While each adjustment may have a primary anticipated effect, such as increasing tip projection or reducing a dorsal hump, it will invariably have consequences, desirable or undesirable, to another variable nasal dimension.[22]

Adjusting the height at the radix or the caudal aspect of the dorsum will have different effects on a number of facial dimensions. Lowering the radix will frequently result in the appearance of increased intercanthal distance and increased nasal length. Augmenting the dorsum at the radix will appear to reduce the intercanthal distance and shorten the nose. In contrast, reducing the height of the dorsum more caudally can have the opposite effect, giving the nose a shorter appearance and the illusion of greater cephalic rotation of the tip. Similarly, reduction of the caudal dorsum will cause the intercanthal distance to appear wider, while augmenting the dorsum will cause the intercanthal distance to appear more narrow. Reducing the caudal dorsum may also reduce the tip projection as the caudal septum has an important role in supporting tip projection. Osteotomies can result in a narrower-appearing nose and intercanthal distance.[22]

Numerous procedures may be used to adjust tip projection and width; however, not every procedure is appropriate for every patient. For example, an overprojected tip can be reduced with a cephalic trim of the lower lateral cartilages only if the cephalic portions of the lower lateral cartilages are actually the highest projecting part of the caudal tip. If this is not the case, securing the footplate of the medial crura to the caudal septum can decrease or increase tip projection depending on the location on the septum to which they are secured. Reducing tip projection may result in the appearance of a relatively widened alar base and bowed columella. A number of maneuvers are frequently used to both increase tip projection and increase the angle of cephalic tip rotation. Placement of a columellar strut, anchoring the medial crura to the caudal septum, approximating the medial crura foot plates, and advancing the nasal spine can all result in the appearance of increased cephalic rotation and projection. Advancing the nasal spine may also shorten the upper lip. Care must be taken to choose the appropriate procedure for the anatomical constraints presented by each patient.[22]

The astute nasal surgeon will be aware of these effects in planning for rhinoplasty to anticipate the most appropriate and effective maneuvers for a specific patient's anatomy, during surgery to make adjustments when needed, and postoperatively to assess the results of their adjustments.

Operative Approach

For several decades, surgeons have debated the merits of "open" or the "external approach" versus endonasal rhinoplasty. In the USA, most rhinoplasty was performed endonasally in the latter decades of the 20th century, whereas today, open approach rhinoplasty is the technique of choice for most patients by the majority of rhinoplasty surgeons including the authors, who reserve the endonasal approach for certain patients needing only minor revisions One cannot definitively say that one approach is better than the other for all surgeons, as good results can be achieved by some surgeons using one method whereas equally good results can be achieved by others using the other technique. Some criticize external approach rhinoplasty with the assertion that by opening the skin–soft tissue envelope, some of the strength and support of the tip are lost when the soft tissue attachments are separated from the cartilaginous support. Proponents of the external approach feel there is better visualization and understanding of the anatomy, especially for the novice rhinoplasty surgeon and in the teaching setting. Cartilages are observed in their natural anatomical position and can thus be manipulated "in situ" as opposed to delivering them to make changes. Endonasal rhinoplasty may be more suitable for noses that may require a limited cephalic trim but otherwise have a well-defined tip and symmetric base requiring minimal if any intervention in these areas.[23]

While the primary difference between the two approaches appears to be the midcolumellar incision which connects the bilateral marginal incisions also used in the endonasal approach, we believe that the more important difference is the ability to directly visualize the underlying structures and their relationships to one another in their resting position. Indeed, most of the trimming, suture, and grafting techniques performed are more easily performed with the exposure provided by the external approach.

Endonasal Rhinoplasty

A very brief discussion of endonasal rhinoplasty is warranted, although not our preferred approach. Endonasal rhinoplasty is performed using one of several incisions: a marginal incision (at the lower border of the lower lateral cartilage), an intercartilaginous incision (between the upper and lower lateral cartilages), a transcartilaginous incision, or a rim incision (largely abandoned because of predictable alar notching). To modify the nasal tip with the endonasal technique, the lower lateral cartilages are typically brought out of the nostrils, or "delivered." The bilateral marginal and intercartilaginous incisions allow the development of bipedicled chondromucosal flaps consisting of the lower lateral cartilages and the underlying mucosa. The cartilages are delivered through the nostril from which they came or can be delivered through a single nostril and then modified as required. The main drawback of cartilage delivery with the endonasal approach is that it requires retraction of the lower lateral cartilages from their normal anatomic position; adjustments are then made with the cartilages out of their normal resting positions.

The plane of dissection is similar to that of the external approach: above the perichondrium and periosteum of the nasal cartilages and bones. Concurrent septoplasty is well described and routinely performed with good outcome, although it is performed through a hemitransfixion incision or a Killian incision as opposed to from above. Dorsal hump reduction can be achieved using an osteotome or rasps, albeit with less direct visual control to make fine adjustments compared to the external approach.[7]

Many surgeons feel that a primary limitation of the endonasal technique when combined with septoplasty is if there is deviation of the L-strut requiring stabilization with spreader grafts, as this can be difficult to accomplish. Many surgeons also feel that the endonasal technique is more limited in its ability to allow adjustments of the alar rim, base and tip; however, the cartilage delivery technique of endonasal rhinoplasty can provide access to perform cephalic trim of the lower lateral crura as well as a variety of dome sutures.

External Approach (Open) Rhinoplasty

Although every rhinoplasty operation should be individualized to each patient's particular anatomic indications, a systematic order and algorithm may be helpful in operative planning as well as establishing a logical progression of steps and maintaining stability. Local anesthesia using lidocaine with epinephrine should be carefully but judiciously infiltrated into all of the areas of the nose to be dissected, but not adding so much volume that the features and subtle nuances of anatomy are masked. We prefer the administration of 1 in 200,000 epinephrine solution in lidocaine to minimize the systemic effects of the epinephrine followed after 5 minutes with 1 in 100,000 epinephrine solution to maximize the local vasoconstriction. Between the injections we also place Oxymetazoline-soaked packings inside the nostrils and around the septum to boost the effects of epinephrine.

Numerous variations of the columellar incision exist. The authors use a midcolumellar stair-step incision while other surgeons might prefer an inverted-V or 5-cornered incision which is connected with bilateral marginal incisions placed at the caudal border of the lower lateral cartilages. Care is taken not to violate the soft tissue triangles. Dissection of the skin–soft tissue envelope is performed in the subperichondrial avascular plane directly over the cartilage of the lower lateral cartilages, then the upper lateral cartilages; keeping the dissection in this plane will allow the surgeon to avoid the neurovascular structures near the nasal tip.[9] The dissection is then continued cephalically to the caudal aspect of the nasal bones at which point a periosteal elevator is used to elevate the periosteum of the nasal bones in the nasion region.

As previously noted, each operation should be individualized to address each patient's anatomy. As required, the radix is addressed first, either by reducing it with a guarded bur if it is overprojected or by placing radix grafts if it is underprojected.

Next, the bony and cartilaginous dorsum is addressed. Preoperative evaluation of the dorsum should have identified whether there is an excess or deficiency of the dorsum. The skin is thinnest at the rhinion or bony-cartilaginous junction and becomes thicker cephalically towards the radix and caudally towards the nasal tip. Therefore, a slight prominence should exist at the upper portion of the upper lateral cartilage in order to compensate for the thinner skin to create a straight profile. Any cartilage or bony hump in excess of this should be removed.[3]

The upper lateral cartilages are released from the septum, preserving the underlying mucoperichondrium thereby minimizing chances of postoperative internal valve narrowing. Any significant prominence of the cartilaginous and bony dorsum is addressed together using sharp dissection and an osteotome or a rasp. For a larger dorsal hump, a Rubin osteotome may be used to reduce the bony hump en bloc.[23,24] The bony dorsum can be further reduced or smoothed with rasping.[23] Precise cartilage reduction can be achieved by removing consecutive thin slices with a 15 blade until reaching the desired profile. After dorsal hump reduction, the patient may be left with an "open roof deformity" where the lateral nasal bones and upper lateral cartilages are no longer touching the septum. This deformity is corrected later in the procedure with osteotomies and spreader grafts. When the dorsum is deficient, grafts can be placed to create a pleasing esthetic.

If there is significant septal deviation, the septum is addressed at this time either from the dorsal/open approach or intranasally through a hemitransfixion or Killian incision. Also at this time, if cartilage grafting is anticipated, septal cartilage can be harvested. As the old adage wisely professes: "Where the septum goes so goes the nose ...".

Several indications exist for septoplasty in septorhinoplasty: obstructed nasal breathing associated with septal deviation, dorsal deviation associated with deviation of the anterior septum, and for harvest of graft material for other aspects of the rhinoplasty.

When septoplasty is performed from the dorsal approach, the anterior septal angle is identified: the lower lateral cartilages are retracted laterally and downward and the septum is identified caudal to its attachment to the upper lateral cartilage. The perichondrial envelope is dissected from the septal cartilage in the subperichondrial plane and if not already performed or as dissection proceeds, the upper lateral cartilages are released from the septum to provide adequate visualization of the more posterior septum. Preservation of the mucoperichondrium provides support and ultimately reduces internal valve collapse.

Once the septal cartilage and bone is exposed, it is assessed to determine which portion of the septal cartilage must be resected or weakened in order to relieve the deviation. One should also consider how much cartilage grafting material should be harvested. An important principle guiding septoplasty or septorhinoplasty is to maintain the structurally supportive "L-strut" comprised of dorsal and caudal septum. We recommend leaving at least a 1.5 cm, preferably 2–2.5 cm, dorsal strut to maximize the degree of support. If significant deviation exists in the L-strut, this may be corrected and stabilized with unilateral or bilateral spreader grafts[5] or septal rotations suture (an effectively placed horizontal mattress suture (e.g., 4-0 PDS) may correct mild deviations of the L-strut). Gruber et al demonstrated that a 10-mm wide, 0.5-mm thick piece of cartilage with a curvature may be adequately straightened with a horizontal mattress suture placed with an 8-mm longitudinal spacing with the knot on the convex side.[25]

If there is a spur or deviation involving the bony septum either superiorly in the perpendicular plate of the ethmoid or posteriorly in the vomer, these may be addressed by resecting the deviated portions. Caution should be exercised during resection of the perpendicular plate, avoiding rocking motions, as cerebrospinal fluid (CSF) leak may occur as a rare complication of septorhinoplasty.

If the inferior edge of the caudal L-strut has been released from the maxillary crest, it can be repositioned in the midline and sutured to the maxillary crest periosteum to secure it. Alternatively a piece of cartilage may be secured with a permanent suture as bridge between the caudal septum and the nasal spine if there is not enough length for adequate projection.[5]

If the septorhinoplasty is being performed to improve nasal airway obstruction, inferior turbinate hypertrophy should be addressed with submucosal resection, inferior turbinate outfracture, and/or conservative resection of the hypertrophic portions of the turbinate, being careful not to be overzealous, possibly causing atrophic rhinitis or empty nose syndrome.

Once satisfactory dorsal projection is achieved, osteotomies are planned and executed as necessary. Osteotomies are performed to narrow the bony dorsum, to close an open roof deformity created by dorsal hump reduction, or to straighten a crooked bony dorsum. Recalling anatomic considerations, the ideal width of the bony dorsum is about two-thirds that of the alar base width. The nasal bones and ascending maxilla tend to be thicker cephalically; therefore, planning osteotomies higher may help to minimize the narrowing effect on the internal nasal valve and nasal breathing. However, if the osteotomy is carried too high or if the medial and lateral osteotomies do not meet, a rocker deformity may result. Another anatomical consideration in osteotomy is the patient age: younger patients tend to have more flexible bone while older patients have more brittle and easily fractured bone. Interrupted "postage stamp style" osteotomies in younger patients may be less effective if they result in greenstick fracture and their nasal bones spring back into place.[4]

It is important to perform effective injection of local anesthetic containing epinephrine prior to the osteotomies in order to minimize bleeding and postoperative swelling. The periosteum of the nasal bones is elevated medially while the lateral periosteum is left attached to bone in order to provide stability to the segment of bone after lateral osteotomy during the healing period. If significant hump reduction has been performed, a formal medial osteotomy may be unnecessary.

In general, medial osteotomies should be performed first, followed by vertical osteotomies, then the lateral osteotomies, in order to maintain stability of the remaining lateral portions of the nasal bones for each succeeding osteotomy. Medial osteotomies are usually performed intranasally by seating the osteotome between the septum and the upper lateral cartilage at the caudal edge of the nasal bone. Since the upper lateral cartilages obtain their structural support from their connection to the underside of the nasal bones, this relationship must not be interrupted[4] if narrowing of the bony dorsum is part of the preoperative plan, a second medial osteotomy is performed to remove the excess bone as a wedge. Medial osteotomy is followed with vertical (anteroposterior) osteotomy at the level of the medial canthal ligament (the deepest part of frontonasal suture laterally) to connect the lateral osteotomy with medial osteotomy and mobilize the bony segment.[2] Vertical osteotomies should be performed below the level of the canthus to minimize risk of lacrimal system injury, and if performed correctly can provide more precise control of nasal bone positioning.[22]

The lateral osteotomy is performed in a continuous fashion in a caudal to cephalic direction through nostril incisions and using a guarded osteotome. With this approach, the inferior limit of the lateral osteotomy should be just above the level of the inferior turbinate insertion in the ascending process of the maxilla and care must be taken to preserve the bony triangle at the level of the piriform aperture at the caudal aspect of the maxillary bone. Staying above the inferior turbinate, as in a high-to-low osteotomy will minimize risk of nasal airway compromise and address a wide bony base at the same time, the alternative way is to infracture the inferior turbinate to minimize the chance of airway compromise.

Tip and Lower Lateral Cartilages

The ideal nasal tip should be well projected, supported, not over- or underrotated, and well defined without being bulbous or have skin that is so tightly pulled over the cartilage that the tip appears bifid. Appropriate tip projection may vary in different ethnicities. This should be considered in ethnic rhinoplasty as overprojection may result in racial incongruity[15,17] and disharmony with the rest of the patient's face.

Various cartilaginous trimming, grafting, and suture techniques may achieve nasal tip definition and correct mild tip deviations. Conservative trimming of the lateral crus may be performed to even out asymmetries. It is imperative to leave a minimum of 6 mm strip of the lateral crus to preserve enough strength to prevent buckling.[25]

The domes should about 4.5 mm wide and the width of overall tip should be around 8–11 mm, with the average being 9 mm. The thicker the soft tissues of the tip, the narrower the tip should be. A lateral crural mattress suture may be used to strengthen the lateral crus or to straighten convexities of the ala, either after overresection or in the setting of weak cartilage. For the lower lateral cartilage, typically about 6 mm wide and 0.5 mm thick, a mattress suture may be placed with 6 mm spacing between the two loops of the stitch. Multiple stitches may be placed along the length of the lower lateral cartilage for added strength.[25] The same concept may be used to provide a subtle increase in strength for the columella. A columellar–septal suture strengthens the columella when only a mild weakness is present that does not require grafting.[25]

Dome stitches may be used to not only create more definition of the nasal tip but also to correct mild deviations or asymmetries by bringing together divergent intermediate crura.[5] If there is any chance of knots protruding into the skin, absorbable monofilament PDS is preferred. If sutures are placed deep in a location with no risk of extrusion or visibility, nylon is also a viable option.[25] A hemitransdomal stitch is placed through the vestibular skin and traverses the most cephalic end of the dome and attempts to evert the lateral crus. A transdomal suture is a horizontal mattress suture that brings together the medial and lateral crura of one of the lower lateral cartilage.[26] When placing this stitch, care must be taken to avoid causing the lateral crus to invert as it may result in concavity of the ala. Also, if the lateral bite of the stitch is not placed laterally enough, it may result in counterrotation and decrease in projection. A transdomal stitch placed appropriately laterally should increase tip rotation, projection, and definition.[23] An interdomal stitch approximates the medial crura together and is set back from the tip several millimeters.[25]

In profile the domes should rise about 6 mm beyond the dorsum. This projection should be increased to 8 mm or even more on noses with thick skin. As previously described, in the ideal profile view of the nose, the ala sits 1–2 mm above the long axis of the nostril and the columella 1–2 mm below it. It is vital to identify the correct anatomical problem: when a hanging ala is present, this should be correctly distinguished from retracted columella so that the appropriate problem is addressed.[13] If a mild alar retraction exists (<2 mm from the long axis of the nostril), an alar rim graft will not only correct this deformity, it will also correct the concavity commonly associated with the retraction. On noses with wide bases and mild alar retraction, a small wedge of alar skin may be resected and the remaining ala repositioned inferiorly. If greater than 2 mm of retraction exists, a V–Y advancement, a composite graft, or an intercartilagenous graft may be required between the upper and lower lateral cartilages on that side.[22] These maneuvers can lower the ala 4–8 mm. A hanging ala may be corrected by excising a small wedge of vestibular skin intranasally or by resecting a strip of cartilage at the caudal edge of the lateral crus of the lower lateral cartilage. A hanging columella can be corrected by resecting a thin strip of the caudal cartilaginous septum or by securing the medial crura to the caudal septum in a tongue-in-groove configuration.[27]. Columellar retraction can be addressed by columellar strut or septal extension grafting.[13]

The base view of the nose should approximate an equilateral triangle. If there is convex ala protruding from the triangle, debulking of soft tissue, trimming lateral crura, or placing dome-spanning sutures may correct this. Concave ala may be corrected by alar rim or strut grafting with cartilaginous grafts on top of or deep to the lateral crus respectively, depending on the severity of the concavity.[14]

Grafts

Autologous graft material is preferable to alloplastic implants, as the latter is significantly more prone to infection and extrusion. Common choices of graft material include septal cartilage, conchal cartilage, rib cartilage, and temporalis fascia. Cadaveric irradiated cartilage and alloplastic materials such as Medpore, silicone, and Gortex are used by some surgeons. For most primary rhinoplasties, septal cartilage is preferred and has several advantages: it is readily accessible and in the same operative field, abundant (in patients who have not undergone septoplasty), and strong, which is ideal for supportive grafts. Auricular conchal cartilage can be harvested without additional prep if its use is anticipated and the ear is prepped into the operative field. Some surgeons prefer a preauricular incision whereas others prefer a postauricular incision for graft harvest. A significant amount of cartilage may be harvested without compromising the structural or esthetic appearance of the ear as long as a few millimeters of rim is left in place along the conchal wall. Conchal cartilage is curved and significantly weaker than septal cartilage thus making it less suited for supportive strut grafts and better for alar reconstruction. Potential donor site morbidity includes auricular hematoma or perichondritis, although their risk can be minimized by the use of antibiotics and a bolster dressing.

Rib cartilage may be necessary for significant nasal reconstructive procedures. The rib provides an abundant source of graft material but it carries the minor disadvantage of requiring a second harvest site and potentially causing a pneumothorax. The most common source of costal cartilage for grafting in females is the sixth and seventh rib cartilages, as the incision can be hidden in the inframammary crease. Costal cartilage carries the risk of warping once it is in place. The effect of warping can be minimized by keeping the cartilage in saline for 30–60 minutes after harvest, determining in which direction twist will occur, and anticipating warp when carving the cartilage. A warping prevention suture described by us could be used to minimize the potential for a revision surgery. After deciphering the direction of the warping following placing the cartilage in saline solution, a 4-0 or 5-0 PDS suture is passed back and forth on the convex side of the cartilage from one end to the other end and tied tight enough to straighten the warped cartilage. This suture negates the need for the use of Kirschner-wire (K-wire). Perichondrium, native fascia or temporal–parietal fascia harvested from the patient can be laid over cartilage grafts to camouflage irregularities. Multiple layers of fascia can be laid on top of each other with each layer of fascia resulting in 0.5 mm of augmentation[28] although additional layers of fascia may prolong postoperative swelling. For bulk, any of the above cartilages can be diced and wrapped in fascia. These fascia-wrapped cartilage grafts can add volume in areas such as the dorsum but have little utility as supportive grafts.[28] We prefer placement of diced cartilage using a 1-mL insulin syringe in an ideally prepared pocket without fascia. Alloplastic material such as Medpore, a high-density polyethylene, is theoretically biocompatible and intentionally placed pores allow fibrovascular ingrowth which serves to prevent graft migration. However, the risks of extrusion and infection and the fact that it is often difficult to remove because of the fibrovascular ingrowth make it less ideal than autologous graft materials.[29]

Spreader Grafts

Spreader grafts may be indicated when there is midvault nasal obstruction to widen the internal nasal valve, to augment an overly narrow dorsum, to support a deviated L-strut, to fill a defect from dorsal hump reduction, or when there is an inverted-V deformity. We believe that any time a large enough hump is removed to create an open roof the use of spreader grafts becomes mandatory, otherwise an inverted-V deformity will ensue months or years later. The ideal material for a spreader graft is septal cartilage. Costal cartilage, layered or folded conchal cartilage, or the medial edge of the upper lateral cartilages (spreader flap) may also be used. Typically the cartilage is cut into strips approximately 5 mm high and 30 mm long, spanning the cartilaginous dorsum. If there is a curve in the graft cartilage, it can be scored and oriented so that the two pieces counteract the other's curve. The graft is secured with at least two mattress sutures. The mattress sutures each traverse five layers securing both pieces to the septum medially and the upper lateral cartilages laterally.[5]

Supportive Grafts

The columellar strut graft is the most commonly used graft. The ideal material for a columellar strut is septal cartilage. It can be placed to help support the tip and overcome ptosis and overrotation of the tip. The medial crura of the LLC can be secured to the graft to prevent hanging columella.[10]

For dorsal augmentation and increased tip projection with adequate support, onlay grafting may be performed. Adequate healthy skin must be present at the tip, as this graft may stretch the skin increasing the risk of skin necrosis. The ideal graft material is either septal cartilage or a straight segment of rib.[10]

A lateral crural strut graft can be placed to correct a prior concavity of the base view of the ala or to counteract the effect of dome sutures that may lead to concavity. A pocket is dissected on the deep surface of the lateral crus of the LLC beneath the vestibular skin intranasally. The graft cartilage is placed in the pocket and secured to the lateral crura using mattress sutures.

Alar rim grafts, fashioned from septal or costal cartilage, may be used to support the nasal valve or cosmetic purpose, it is ideally placed in a pocket at the lowest part of the alar rim. Cephalic placement on the lower lateral cartilage will stent open the internal nasal valve while caudal placement on the lower lateral cartilage will stent open the external nasal valve.[29] Once the appropriate placement is done, the graft is secured with a suture that will be used to repair the rim incision.

The ideal alar rim smoothly transitions from the tip-defining point to the nasofacial insertion, the contour and strength of which are determined by the lateral crus of the LLC. The LLC is in a position close to the rim more medially but laterally is in a more cephalic position as it moves away from the alar margin: this lack of rigid support can lead to scarring, retraction, and/or unpredictable asymmetry. The alar rim graft, placed along the alar margin, is a powerful graft capable of directly altering the contour and strength of the alar margin. Indications include correction of alar flare, cephalic malposition and inadequate alar support, and correction of dynamic margin collapse.[30] On patients with cephalically oriented LLC, the lateral crura are dissected and transposed caudally.

Several types of tip grafts can be used to create a more defined-appearing tip and/or to achieve slight increase in projection of the nasal tip. A shield or onlay graft is cut or prepared using the tip punch device designed by our group and placed as an onlay graft on top of the LLC or as a shield graft.[31] A tip graft is created from a horizontal piece of cartilage that crosses both domes with beveled edges laterally. The tip graft can be used to correct minor tip asymmetries. An infralobular graft can be attached to the septal cartilage in order to increase columellar show in noses with a retracted columella. After placement of a columellar strut, an onlay to the nasal tip is supported by the columellar strut and overlies both domes. A subdomal graft can be used to correct a pinched dome appearance or set the distance between the domes. The subdomal graft is placed after dissecting a tunnel under the domes and secured with 6-0 Vicryl suture; septum is the ideal location for donor site and graft is around 1×1×8 mm.[32]

Alar Base Adjustments

Alar adjustments should be reserved for the last step after all the tip refinement and supportive grafts have been completed. An overprojected nasal tip or hypoplastic maxilla may give the illusion of narrowed alar width. Similarly an underprojected tip or protruding maxilla may give the illusion of widened alar width. These issues must be ruled out before considering adjusting the alar base positions.[11] Ala that are displaced cephalically can be repositioned by resecting an ellipse of skin around the alar base and repositioning the ala medially; this will bring it to a more medial and caudal position. Wedge excisions according to the appropriate abnormality can remove part of nasal sill, ala, or both. V–Y advancement and inverted-T excision for wide and thick alae are other maneuvers that can be useful in certain patients.[11]

Final Steps

Typically, if septoplasty has been performed and there is a mucosal incision, it is closed with interrupted 5-0 chromic sutures and intranasal Silastic or Doyle splints are placed. Some surgeons prefer quilting sutures to reapproximate the apposing mucoperichondrial flaps in the absence of the removed septal cartilage. The columellar incision is closed with interrupted 6-0 fast-absorbing catgut sutures. Marginal incisions are closed with interrupted 6-0 fast-absorbing catgut sutures.

The dorsum is taped with Steri-Strips (3M). If osteotomies were performed, the dorsum is splinted with a Denver Splint or a thermoplastic splint. If a rib graft has been used for dorsal grafts, it may have been secured in place with K-wires: these are pulled through the splint and secured in place until they are removed 2–3 weeks postoperatively.

Postoperative Care

Postoperative care varies among surgeons. Patients are counseled about the potential for postoperative bleeding, which can be self-limited and treated with oxymetazoline spray. In the immediate postoperative period (24–48 hours), patients should to keep their head elevated to minimize swelling. Patients should avoid exercise or strenuous activity for 2–4 weeks postoperatively. Postoperative antibiotic prophylaxis may be considered if intranasal splints have been placed or an ear bolster is used after conchal cartilage harvest. Sutures and splints are removed 1 week postoperatively. Although it is not always necessary or indicated, postoperative steroids have been observed to be effective in decreasing swelling.[33] Perioperative steroids have been shown to decrease periorbital edema in the immediate postoperative period.[34]

Complications

After rhinoplasty, the normal postoperative course has some expected inconveniences that the patient should be made aware of preoperatively and should not be considered as complications. Pain, bruising, and postoperative swelling are to be expected. If the swelling is excessive or prolonged, postoperative oral steroids may help to speed resolution. Taping the nose may be helpful in decreasing swelling and may be continued by the patient on a nightly basis even weeks after surgery.[15] Gryskiewicz et al feel that after 14 days, Kenalog injections may be considered every 2–4 weeks for up to six injections.[35]

Intraoperative complications should be identified and addressed prior to completion of surgery. These include excessive bleeding, iatrogenic injury to the nasal skin or underlying cartilages, lack of dorsal support as a result of fracture of the L-strut, septal fracture; inward displacement or collapse of the nasal bones; "rocker deformity;" and cribriform plate fracture. The risk of bleeding can be minimized by counseling the patient to avoid not only anticoagulants and nonsteroidal anti-inflammatory drugs (NSAIDs), but also supplements that may have anticoagulative effects. Bleeding can also be minimized with control of hypertension, topical intranasal vasoconstrictors, adequate preoperative injection of a local anesthetic combined with epinephrine, dissection in the proper plane, and careful but judicious use of bipolar cautery. Hypertension is the most common reason for intraoperative bleeding and should be appropriately controlled by the anesthesiologist. Von Willebrand disease is more common than many realize and patients are treated with desmopressin (DDAVP) or tranexamic acid, also useful in patients who have taken NSAIDs. Obviously, iatrogenic injury to the nasal cartilages or nasal skin should be avoided, but careful repair should be performed if such an injury occurs. The septum can be fractured in about 1% of septorhinoplasty cases. This is more likely to occur if there has been previous septal cartilage harvest or significant dorsal hump reduction, deficient nasal bones or a severely deviated septum. A fractured L-strut can be addressed with suture fixation to spreader grafts and/or by fixation of the strut to the nasal bones. Intraoperative complications associated with osteotomies can be identified immediately after the osteotomies are completed. A collapsed or unstable displaced nasal bone can be suspended from the septum if still attached to the upper lateral cartilages. Sutures, or infrequently, K-wires can be used to stabilize the bones or, one can place a Merocel pack intranasally for 1 week to hold the bone(s) in position. A rocker deformity may occur if the lateral osteotomy is carried too far upward and laterally beyond the radix. With a rocker deformity, inward displacement of the nasal bone will result in outward and lateral displacement of the frontal bone segment. This is corrected by an additional osteotomy in the appropriate position.[4] If a CSF leak is observed, it should be managed immediately. Nasal packing and lumbar drainage may be necessary.[35]

In the immediate postoperative period, complications may include bleeding, erythema related to vascular congestion, infection, skin loss or necrosis, and early patient dissatisfaction. While mild bleeding may be expected after rhinoplasty, excessive postoperative bleeding is rare (0.9%).[35] In cases of troublesome or excessive bleeding, hypertension should be controlled, topical vasoconstrictors should be used, and DDAVP may be infused without the need for additional intervention.[36] Packing should be avoided. Early postoperative erythema may be a sign of vascular congestion (more common in revision cases), contact dermatitis, or early infection. When erythema appears to be of infectious etiology, early initiation of aggressive oral antibiotic treatment is indicated. The skin over the nasal tip is delicate and at risk for necrosis, especially if the patient is a smoker. Its vascular supply can be compromised by excessive soft tissue trimming or cauterization over the ala, which may disrupt the lateral nasal artery, or with grafts that exert too much stretch or tension on the skin.

In the intermediate postoperative period (2 weeks to 2 months), additional complications may be noted such as prolonged edema, delayed healing, patient concern/dissatisfaction, synechiae, osseous overgrowth, septal perforation, anosmia or "late" presentation of a CSF leak. As the initial postoperative swelling subsides, subtle defects or irregularities may be noticed; more obvious abnormalities such as graft migration may be recognized and will likely need to be addressed surgically.[35] Patients may voice concern about the appearance of the nose because they cannot anticipate its final shape. Osseous overgrowths may occur at the site of bony resections or torn perichondrium and can be addressed with conservative rasping in a revision procedure. Septal perforations may occur, more commonly if bilateral septal tears were created and not repaired. Anosmia that continues after splints are removed and expected postoperative swelling has diminished may be the result of cribriform plate injury. Clear rhinorrhea that begins in the later postoperative period can be a late presentation of CSF leakage. CSF leaks are rare after rhinoplasty (1.17%) and usually seal on their own; however, patients with suspected leaks should be counselled to be vigilant in watching for signs of meningitis.

Late complications from rhinoplasty include nasal airway obstruction; various irregularities and deformities; implant exposure, extrusion, or migration; scarring, silent sinus syndrome; enophthalmos; and mucocele formation. Nasal obstruction may result from nasal valve collapse due to overexcision of the lateral crura of the LLC, mid-vault collapse, aggressive medialization of the bony pyramid, or intranasal scarring in the form of synechiae. Saddle nose deformity may result from overresection of the septum or bony dorsum. Open roof deformity results from failure to fill the midline defect created from dorsal hump resection with osteotomies and spreader grafts. Unsightly scarring may occur at the columellar incision with notching. Scarring may also occur at the site of percutaneous osteotomies with hyperpigmentation or tethering of the skin. Ethnic incongruity may occur by inappropriate planning in ethnic rhinoplasty. Autologous implants may become infected, migrate, extrude, or be associated with skin contracture which must be addressed by removal and replacement with an autologous graft, if appropriate.[35]

Secondary and Tertiary Rhinoplasty

It is not uncommon for the rhinoplasty surgeon to be presented with a patient who has had a prior rhinoplasty. It is estimated that between 2% and 30% of rhinoplasties result in secondary rhinoplasty.[37] The preoperative assessment described above for primary rhinoplasty, for the most part, applies in revision rhinoplasty. Of particular importance is the patient's previous surgical history, the nature of their concerns or dissatisfaction, the patient's social history and psychiatric history, and of course, a thorough objective evaluation of the patient's anatomy.

Evaluation

Operative History

It is important to attempt to obtain the operative record of any and all previous nasal surgeries as part of the preoperative evaluation of a patient presenting for revision rhinoplasty. The most common reasons for revision rhinoplasty are underresection or overresection of the structural cartilages. Consequently, eliciting information from the operative record and comparing it with the patient's physical examination may help the surgeon clarify whether the remaining cartilages need to be trimmed further or reinforced with grafts. Also, the extent of previous septoplasty or septal cartilage removed may help the revision rhinoplasty surgeon anticipate the need for various alternative cartilage grafting sources such as conchal or costal cartilage and whether these sources have previously been used.[37]

Patient Reported Issues

The surgeon needs to have a very clear and specific understanding of the source of the patient's dissatisfaction. Perhaps even more than with primary rhinoplasty, realistic expectations must be established. If the patient's expectations are judged to be unrealistic, it should be made clear and documented whether the surgeon believes that their desired results are attainable.[37] A number of patient-reported issues may be unique in the setting of prior surgery. Most of these relate to postoperative complications such as an inappropriately placed graft, graft migration, pain, infection or extrusion of implants, or nasal airflow obstruction secondary to nasal valve collapse from excessive cartilage resection.

Objective Issues

A full examination and facial analysis should be performed. The height, width, and symmetry of the nose should be assessed. The nasofrontal angle location and angulation should be noted. The dorsum should be visually examined and palpated for irregularity. The bony pyramid should be examined noting its width, any asymmetries, and whether there is an inverted-V deformity. The supratip area should be assessed for pollybeak deformity. Adequacy of tip projection and rotation should be assessed. Assessment of the LLC should include evaluation for symmetry, bossae, alar rim collapse, the tip-defining points, width, position, and columellar angle. Intranasal examination can identify valve narrowing or weakness, synechiae, or septal perforation from prior surgery and give the revision surgeon clues as to how much septal cartilage may be available for grafting.[37]

Skin

Skin examination in the patient who has had a previous rhinoplasty is important as it can be thinned or scarred from previous surgery, perhaps more often with external approach or with extensive dissection. Also, previously placed alloplastic graft material may have resulted in scarring. The presence of scarring may increase the risk of skin necrosis and poor outcome. When the skin is extremely thin and scarring seems highly likely, it may be prudent to stage the revision procedure by placing a dermal graft and allowing it to heal prior to performing revision rhinoplasty so that a healthy skin flap can be elevated and redraped with a good chance of healing at the time of surgery.[28]

Structural Support

The full nasal examination and analysis as described above will provide insight about the structural support remaining in the previously operated nose. Often due to prior cartilage removal, there may be a lack of support to the tip and alae that may require grafting.

Operative Principles and Approach

One can argue that for revision rhinoplasty cases, the external approach is particularly advantageous, allowing full examination of the anatomy and assessment of what has been done in the previous surgery unless the revision surgery is minor, which can be done through a closed technique. In revision cases, it is wise to err on the side of minimal resection, as the structural support has already been compromised by prior dissection and resection. Sources of cartilage for grafting should be considered and planned out prior to surgery. When autologous septal cartilage is not available, the authors prefer to utilize other autogenous materials like rib or conchal cartilage.

When possible, the nose should be entered through the previous incision unless it has been poorly designed. This can avoid leaving the patient with an additional scar and allow the surgeon to resect and revise an unsightly scar. Dissection on the cartilage should proceed with caution, anticipating scarring from previous dissection. If a dorsal onlay graft is deemed necessary, the recipient surface should be flattened with a rasp to minimize irregularity. If costal cartilage is used, securing it with K-wire can limit warping and migration.[37] The septum is addressed as described previously. If the L-strut is significantly weakened, it can be reinforced with spreader grafts.

Tip reconstruction is performed, as described for primary rhinoplasty. If supportive grafts are necessary, one should begin by supporting the columella. Grafts can be secured in various ways including by drilling a K-wire into the maxilla just lateral to the maxillary crest and securing the graft to the wire. Occasionally, when there has been excessive resection of the lateral crura, supportive grafts may not be enough and alar replacement is required. Conchal cartilage has a natural curve that mimics the curve of the lower lateral cartilages and is a good choice for this indication. The soft tissue is dissected creating a tissue pocket at the pyriform aperture and the graft is placed in this pocket. An anchor graft may be used in revision cases for alar retraction: conchal cartilage is shaped to look like an upside-down anchor with the sides at each lower lateral cartilage and the middle secured to the septum or a columellar graft. Previous rhinoplasty may create a pinched dome appearance. A dome spreader graft may address this by securing a small piece of cartilage between the medial crura.[29]

Complications

The spectrum of complications that may occur after revision rhinoplasty is essentially the same as that for primary rhinoplasty, although postoperative edema may take longer to resolve and there may be a higher risk of skin necrosis in previously dissected tissue.

References

1. Woodard CR, Park SS. Nasal and facial analysis. *Clin Plast Surg.* 2010;37(2):181–189.
2. Lessard ML, Daniel RK. Surgical anatomy of septorhinoplasty. *Arch Otolaryngol.* 1985;111(1):25–29.
3. Oneal RM, Beil RJ. Surgical anatomy of the nose. *Clin Plast Surg.* 2010;37(2):191–211.
4. Dobratz EJ, Hilger PA. Osteotomies. *Clin Plast Surg.* 2010;37(2):301–311.
5. Stepnick D, Guyuron B. Surgical treatment of the crooked nose. *Clin Plast Surg.* 2010;37(2):313–325.
6. Petroff MA, McCullough EG, Hom D, et al. Nasal tip projection. Quantitative changes following rhinoplasty. *Arch Otolaryngol Head Neck Surg.* 1991;117(7):783–788.
7. Tebbets JB. 2006. Open and closed rhinoplasty (minus the "versus"): analyzing processes. *Aesthet Surg J.* 2006;26(4):456–459.
8. Westreich RW, Courtland HW, Nasser P, et al. Defining nasal cartilage elasticity: biomechanical testing of the tripod theory based on a cantilevered model. *Arch Facial Plast Surg.* 2007;9(4):264–270.
9. Toriumi DM, Mueller RA, Grosch T, et al. Vascular anatomy of the nose and the external rhinoplasty approach. *Arch Otolaryngol Head Neck Surg.* 1996;122(1):24–34.
10. Hobar PC, Adams WP, Mitchell CA. Lengthening the short nose. *Clin Plast Surg.* 2010;37(2):327–333.
11. Ponsky D, Guyuron B. Alar base disharmonies. *Clin Plast Surg.* 2010;37(2):245–251.
12. Gunter JP, Rohrich RJ, Friedman RM. Classification and correction of alar-columellar discrepancies in rhinoplasty. *Plast Reconstr Surg.* 1996;97(3):643–648.
13. Hackney FL. Diagnosis and correction of alar rim deformities in rhinoplasty. *Clin Plast Surg.* 2010;37(2):223–229.
14. Guyuron B. Alar rim deformities. *Plast Reconstr Surg.* 2001;107(3):856–863.
15. Rohrich RJ, Bolden K. Ethnic rhinoplasty. *Clin Plast Surg.* 2010;37(2):353–370.
16. Porter JP, Olson KL. Analysis of the African American female nose. *Plast Reconstr Surg.* 2003;111(2):620–626.
17. Toriumi DM, Pero CD. Asian rhinoplasty. *Clin Plast Surg.* 2010;37(2):335–352.
18. Milgrim LM, Lawson W, Cohen AF. Anthropometric analysis of the female Latino nose. Revised aesthetic concepts and their surgical implications. *Arch Otolaryngol Head Neck Surg.* 1996;122(10):1079–1086.
19. Galdino GM, DaSilva And D, Gunter JP. Digital photography for rhinoplasty. *Plast Reconstr Surg.* 2002;109(4):1421–1434.
20. Swamy RS, Sykes JM, Most SP. Principles of photography in rhinoplasty for the digital photographer. *Clin Plast Surg.* 2010;37(2):213–221.
21. Henderson JL, Larrabee Jr WF, Krieger BD. Photographic standards for facial plastic surgery. *Arch Facial Plast Surg.* 2005;7(5):331–333.
22. Guyuron B. Dynamics of rhinoplasty. In: Guyuron B, ed. *Rhinoplasty.* Philadelphia: Saunders; 2012:61–102.
23. Toriumi DM. Structural approach to primary rhinoplasty. *Aesthet Surg J.* 2002;22(1):72–84.
24. Simons RL, Greene RM. Rhinoplasty pearls: value of the endonasal approach and vertical dome division. *Clin Plast Surg.* 2010;37(2):265–283.
25. Gruber RP, Chang E, Buchanan E. Suture techniques in rhinoplasty. *Clin Plast Surg.* 2010;37(2):231–243.
26. Guyuron B, Behmand RA. Nasal tip sutures part II: the interplays. *Plast Reconstr Surg.* 2003;112(4):1130–1145.
27. Kridel RW, Scott BA, Foda HM. The tongue-in-groove technique in septorhinoplasty. A 10-year experience. *Arch Facial Plast Surg.* 1999;(4):246–256.
28. Daniel RK. Rhinoplasty: dorsal grafts and the designer dorsum. *Clin Plast Surg.* 2010;37(2):293–300.
29. Weber SM, Baker SR. Alar cartilage grafts. *Clin Plast Surg.* 37(2):253–264.
30. Boahene KDO, Hilger PA. Alar rim grafting in rhinoplasty: indications, technique, and outcomes. *Arch Facial Plast Surg.* 2009;11(5):285–289.
31. Guyuron B, Jackowe D. Modified tip grafts and tip punch devices. *Plast Reconstr Surg.* 2007;120(7):2004–2010.
32. Guyuron B, Poggi JT, Michelow BJ. The subdomal graft. *Plast Reconstr Surg.* 2004;113(3):1037–1040.
33. Gurlek A, Fariz A, Aydogan H, et al. Effects of different corticosteroids on edema and ecchymosis in open rhinoplasty. *Aesthetic Plast Surg.* 2006;30(2):150–154.
34. Kara CO, Gokalan I. Effects of single-dose steroid usage on edema, ecchymosis, and intraoperative bleeding in rhinoplasty. *Plast Reconstr Surg.* 1999;104(7):2213–2218.
35. Gryskiewicz JM, Hatef DA, Bullocks JM, et al. Problems in rhinoplasty. *Clin Plast Surg.* 2010;37(2):389–399.
36. Faber C, Larson K, Amirlak B, et al. Use of desmopressin for unremitting epistaxis following septorhinoplasty and turbinectomy. *Plast Reconstr Surg.* 2011;128(6):728e–732e.
37. Cochran CS, Gunter JP. Secondary rhinoplasty and the use of autogenous rib cartilage grafts. *Clin Plast Surg.* 37(2):371–382.

69

Blepharoptosis

ALAN A. McNAB

Definition

Blepharoptosis is defined as a lower than normal position of the upper eyelid in relation to the globe and pupil. The term is often abbreviated to ptosis.

The upper eyelid normally covers the upper 1–2 mm of the cornea, but this tends to increase slightly in old age. As the cornea has a diameter of 11 mm, the distance from the upper eyelid margin to the inferior corneoscleral limbus is therefore normally 9–10 mm. This distance can be used as a means of measuring the amount of ptosis but, conventionally, the distance from the upper eyelid margin to a reflection of a point source of light shone directly at the patient is used. This distance is called the Margin Reflex Distance 1 or MRD1. This is normally 3–4 mm. (The MRD2 is the distance from the light reflex to the lower lid margin.) The disadvantage of using the MRD1 over a simple measure from the upper lid margin to the inferior limbus is that when the upper eyelid margin is lower than the position of the light reflex on the cornea, the lid must be lifted up to then get an indirect measure of how far below the light reflex the lid margin sits. If it is lower than the light reflex it is expressed as a negative value in millimeters.

Anatomy

Knowledge of the anatomy relevant to ptosis is vital in understanding the etiology and mechanisms of ptosis, and the clinical signs and surgery of ptosis.

The main surface anatomy marking of relevance is the upper eyelid crease or eyelid fold. In Caucasians this lies about 6–10 mm above the eyelash line. In Asian eyelids there is much more variability, with the crease being absent or often much lower than in Caucasian eyelids, with an associated fullness of the upper eyelid. This is because the orbital septum attaches much lower in most Asian eyelids with the preaponeurotic fat pad extending more inferiorly giving the eyelid a fuller appearance.

The upper eyelid retractor, the levator palpebrae superioris (LPS), is innervated by the third cranial nerve (oculomotor nerve). The muscle belly arises from the apex of the orbit on the lesser wing of the sphenoid, just above the optic canal. It travels anteriorly in the orbit below the orbital roof, partly overlapping the superior rectus muscle, which lies immediately below it. As it reaches the anterior orbit, it turns more inferiorly towards the tarsal plate of the eyelid. About 8–10 mm above the superior border of the tarsus, it broadens out into a tendinous aponeurosis. This aponeurosis attaches onto the anterior surface of the tarsal plate, and also sends fibers to attach between bundles of the orbicularis oculi muscle just under the eyelid skin to form the upper eyelid skin crease (Fig. 69.1).

The levator aponeurosis expands medially and laterally as its medial and lateral horns. The lateral horn is much stronger and attaches on to Whitnall's tubercle just inside the lateral orbital rim. The lateral horn also partially divides the lacrimal gland into orbital and palpebral lobes, with the two lobes continuous behind the posterior edge of the lateral horn. The medial horn is less well defined and becomes weaker with age. It attaches to the superior border of the medial canthal tendon.[1]

There is a smooth muscle component of the levator apparatus, called Müller's muscle, which is innervated by sympathetic nerve fibers. This is a sheet of smooth muscle fibers with a rich blood supply that arises from the undersurface of the levator muscle and extends downwards under the levator aponeurosis to attach to the superior border of the tarsal plate. It is about 10 mm in length.

There is a strong transverse band of connective tissue running from the region of the trochlea to the lacrimal gland, which runs over the superior surface of the levator muscle near the point where it turns more inferiorly towards the tarsal plate. This is called the superior transverse ligament or Whitnall's ligament. There is a less well-defined portion of this structure which passes under the levator muscle, called the transverse superior fascial expansion.[2]

The antagonist muscle of the LPS is the orbicularis oculi muscle, innervated by branches of the facial nerve. It runs circumferentially around the eyelids, divided into parts called pretarsal, preseptal and orbital. The orbicularis oculi muscle lies immediately below the skin of the upper eyelid, which is extremely thin.

The orbital septum in the upper eyelid extends from the superior orbital rim downwards to attach to the anterior surface of the levator aponeurosis. Behind the orbital septum and lying over the levator aponeuroris and anterior

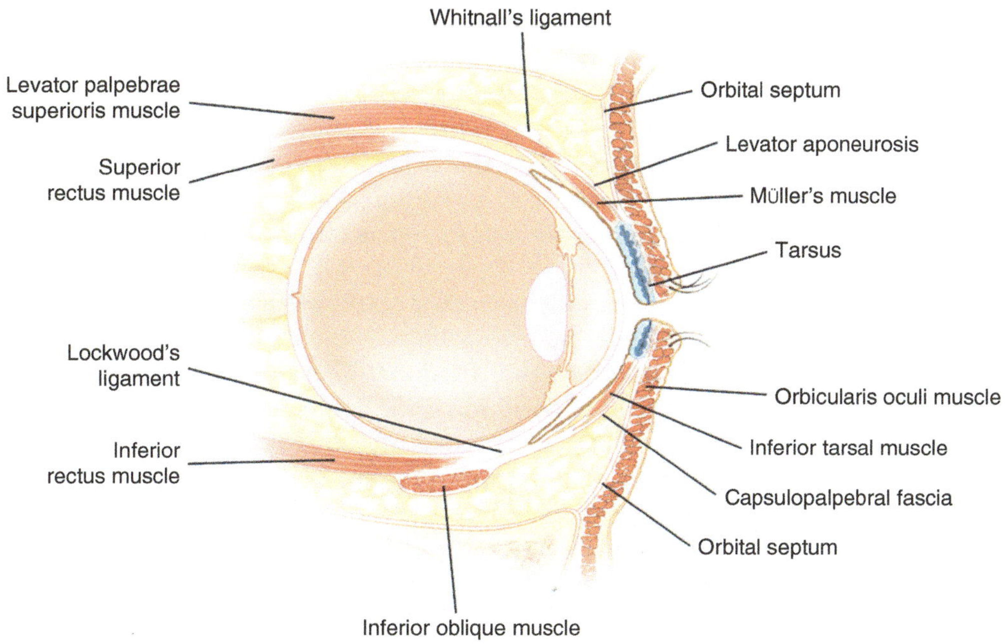

• **Fig. 69.1** A sagittal section through the eyelids to show the relationship between the levator apparatus, tarsal plate, and orbital septum.

portion of the levator muscle belly is the preaponeurotic fat pad, a vital landmark in levator aponeurosis and muscle surgery. Laterally, in the same retroseptal space, the orbital lobe of the lacrimal gland is located. Medially, there is a medial upper fat pad. The tendon of the superior oblique muscle partially separates the central preaponeurotic and medial fat pads as it extends down to attach to the globe medial to the medial edge of the levator muscle belly.

The tarsal plate of the upper eyelid is a semilunar-shaped semi-rigid structure made up of meibomian glands set in a fibrous stroma with the conjunctiva firmly adherent to its undersurface. It attaches via the upper limbs of the medial and lateral canthal tendons to Whitnall's tubercle laterally and the frontal process of the maxilla just anterior to the anterior lacrimal crest (anterior limb of the medial canthal tendon) and to the posterior lacrimal crest (posterior limb). The upper tarsal plate is about 9–10 mm in vertical height centrally and about 1 mm thick.

There is a vascular arcade overlying Müller's muscle at its lower edge, and under the levator aponeurosis, just above the superior border of the tarsal plate. A smaller vascular arcade runs just above the lash bulbs near the margin of the eyelid, within fibers of orbicularis oculi.

Etiological Factors

When considering the causes of blepharoptosis, it is conventional to divide them into congenital and acquired. However, there is some overlap in these two groups.[3]

The following classification is useful:

A. Congenital Ptosis
- 1. Congenital neurogenic ptosis
  - 1a. Congenital third nerve palsy
  - 1b. Congenital Horner's syndrome
- 2. Congenital myogenic ptosis (sometimes called congenital dystrophic ptosis)
  - 2a. Isolated congenital dystrophic ptosis
  - 2b. Congenital dystrophic ptosis with associated weak globe elevator(s)
  - 2c. Congenital dystrophic ptosis as part of a syndrome
    - i. Blepharophimosis syndrome
    - ii. Other syndromes (e.g., Noonan's, Saethre Chotzen)
- 3. Congenital ptosis with synkinesis (jaw-winking ptosis, others)
- 4. Congenital aponeurotic ptosis (rare)

B. Acquired Ptosis
- 1. Neurogenic ptosis
  - 1a. Third nerve palsy
  - 1b. Horner's syndrome
- 2. Myogenic ptosis
  - 2a. Myopathic ptosis
    - i. Mitochondrial cytopathies (chronic progressive external ophthalmoplegia (CPEO) and its variants)
    - ii. Myotonic dystrophy
    - iii. Oculopharyngeal muscular dystrophy
    - iv. Other myopathies
  - 2b. Myasthenia
    - i. Ocular myasthenia
    - ii. Myasthenia gravis
- 3. Involutional ptosis
  - 3a. Involutional aponeurotic ptosis
  - 3b. Involutional myogenic ptosis
- 4. Mechanical ptosis (lumps and swellings of the eyelid)
- 5. Traumatic ptosis (may be multiple factors)

C. Pseudoptosis
1. Globe hypotropia
2. Enophthalmos, or a small eye
3. Blepharospasm
4. Dermatochalasis.

Congenital and acquired neurogenic ptosis can be considered together in terms of investigation and management. Third nerve palsies may be partial or complete, and there may be aberrant regeneration complicating the clinical picture. Congenital aponeurotic ptosis is rare, but can also be managed in the same way as acquired aponeurotic ptosis.

Congenital myogenic or dystrophic ptosis may be unilateral or bilateral (symmetric or asymmetric) and is due to a maldevelopment of the levator muscle, which is variably replaced by fatty and fibrous tissue. The muscle contracts and relaxes less than normally. This type of ptosis often occurs with a positive family history and there are a number of genetic defects that continue to be identified. Whilst it is usually an isolated abnormality, there are well-recognized associations, including poor functioning of the superior rectus muscle and double elevator palsy. Children with these additional muscle problems will usually have a vertical strabismus with the globe pointing downwards (hypotropia).

Congenital myogenic ptosis may be part of a more extensive syndrome. The best known of these is blepharophimosis or BPES (blepharophimosis, ptosis, epicanthus inversus syndrome). Numerous other less common syndromes may have ptosis as one manifestation of the condition and Noonan's and Saethre Chotzen syndrome are two examples.

Congenital ptosis with synkinesis is a special subcategory of congenital ptosis. The best recognized form is Marcus Gunn jaw-winking ptosis. The child will have unilateral ptosis and with contraction of the ipsilateral lateral pterygoid muscle, the levator muscle is stimulated and the lid rises, sometimes higher than its normal position. Synkinesis with other muscles is less common but well described. These include lid elevation with contraction of the medial pterygoid, digastric, the lateral rectus muscle, and with swallowing.

Acquired myogenic ptosis is an important diagnosis to make because of the significant general health aspects of these conditions.

Involutional or age-related ptosis is by far the commonest form of ptosis seen in clinical practice. A mild degree of ptosis is common in the elderly, but more advanced degrees may occur and impact on visual function. Traditionally, the majority of involutional ptosis has been attributed to dehiscence and/or stretching of the levator aponeurosis, but in a significant proportion of older patients with acquired ptosis, the levator muscle itself appears to be abnormal with infiltration by fatty tissue into the muscle belly.

Some lumps on the upper eyelid may induce ptosis by their weight alone, and this is the classic cause of so-called mechanical ptosis. Other mechanical factors may be at play in some cases of ptosis, including scarring or adhesion between parts of the muscle and other structures such as the orbital roof after fractures, or adhesions between the eyelid and the globe.

Traumatic ptosis is often multifactorial. Traumatic nerve injuries may lead to ptosis, as may injuries to the muscle belly or aponeurosis. Some patients will develop ptosis after episodes of eyelid bruising or swelling and it is thought that such swelling may lead to dehiscence of the levator aponeurosis. Other forms of ocular surgery may sometimes lead to ptosis. The mechanism is not always clear.

Repeated minor trauma may also lead to ptosis. This is thought to be the cause in patients who develop ptosis after many years of wearing hard or rigid gas permeable contact lenses, who often remove the lenses by applying traction at the lateral canthus to remove the lens.

Pseudoptosis has a number of causes. An important one to recognize is hypotropia. With the globe looking down compared to its fellow eye, the lid will also be lower than normal because the lid follows the eye downwards. If the normal eye is covered and the patient takes up fixation with the hypotropic eye, the lid will usually rise at least partially as well. This uncovers the element of the ptosis which is due to "pseudoptosis." Ideally, the hypotropia should be corrected first to eliminate any element of pseudoptosis.

A small or enophthalmic eye will often have a narrower than normal palpebral fissure, due to inadequate posterior support of the eyelid, but this is not due to any abnormality of the levator apparatus or eyelid and is classified as a form of pseudoptosis.

Patients with increased tone in the orbicularis oculi muscle will often have a narrowed palpebral fissure also. This may be due to increased tone with or without an element of aberrant reinnervation after a facial palsy. The lid fissure may narrow further when muscles in the lower face contract. Similarly patients with hemifacial spasm will display episodic narrowing of the palpebral fissure associated with spasm of other facial muscles on the same side.

Finally, marked dermatochalasis will often look like true ptosis but if the hood of abnormal skin is lifted out of the way, the lid position can then be properly assessed. Many cases of true involutional ptosis will of course also have a degree of dermatochalasis.

Preoperative Assessment

As in any medical condition, a proper history and examination is essential. The history will usually easily separate congenital from acquired ptosis. Questions should be asked about time and rapidity of onset and variability of the ptosis, associated diplopia, other neuromuscular problems, any history of trauma, lid swelling or contact lens wear. A family history of ptosis or muscle problems should be sought. Older patients should be asked about a history of dry eye problems as elevating the eyelid in a patient with dry eyes may exacerbate the dry eye problem.

A standard sequence of examination steps will usually give an answer, in addition to the details of the history, as to what has caused the ptosis, and make surgical planning safer. The examination steps may seem arduous, but with experience, a targeted ptosis examination can be performed in a few minutes. The steps should include the following:

1. *Measure and record the patient's vision.* This is especially important in children in the amblyogenic age group (less than 10 years of age). There is a strong association between ptosis and amblyopia.
2. *Measure the degree of ptosis.* This can be done by measuring the MRD1 (upper lid to corneal light reflex), or the distance from upper lid to lower limbus (normal is 9–10 mm). The degree of ptosis should be measured with the brow held in a neutral position to eliminate any elevation of the lid by the brow.
3. *Measure the levator excursion or "levator function."* This is the distance the lid moves between extreme up- and downgaze. Normal should be about 13–15 mm.
4. *Look at the position of the ptotic lid on downgaze.* In congenital myogenic ptosis, because the levator relaxes less well, the lid does not drop as much as normal on downgaze. With involutional aponeurotic ptosis, the lid will drop more than normal on downgaze.
5. *Measure the position of the eyelid crease.* This helps in diagnosis and surgical planning. The crease is usually elevated compared to the normal side in aponeurotic ptosis. The crease may be absent in more severe congenital ptosis.
6. *Examine the patient's eye movements.* This is a vital part of the examination. Patients with myogenic ptosis will usually have signs of abnormal eye movements, which may be subtle at the first presentation. The range of eye movements, rapidity of eye movements (tested by examining saccadic eye movement), and presence or absence of strabismus in any position of gaze by performing a cover test, should all be performed.
7. *Examine the pupils.* The pupil will be enlarged in many third nerve palsies, and in Horner's syndrome the pupil will be smaller on the affected side. This difference is more obvious in dim light where the normal side dilates more.
8. *Examine eyelid closure.* Gentle eyelid closure should be tested first, looking for lagophthalmos, indicating orbicularis weakness. Forced closure should be tested also, looking for weakness.
9. *Examine for Bell's phenomenon.* This is where the eye rolls upwards on forced lid closure. If absent, the risk of corneal exposure problems is increased with ptosis surgery.
10. *Evert the upper eyelid and examine the conjunctival fornices.* The tarsal surface of the lid may be abnormal after previous ptosis surgery, and the conjunctival fornices may be hiding rare disorders such as subconjunctival lymphoma (seen as a salmon patch) or conjunctival amyloidosis.
11. *Look for associated clinical signs.* These include brow position (the frontalis muscle on the side of a unilateral ptosis will be usually overacting, elevating the brow), the presence of synkinetic movements (ask the patient to open the mouth and move the jaw side-to-side), and evidence of other features of myopathies or myasthenia (frontal balding in myotonic dystrophy, muscle weakness elsewhere, fatigability with myasthenia on sustained upgaze, a twitch of the upper eyelid on upward saccades of the eyes, known as Cogan's lid twitch, and occurring with myasthenia).
12. *Check that corneal sensation is normal.* This can be done with a strand of cotton teased from the end of a cotton tip. Reduced corneal sensation is rarely seen in ptosis patients, but if present, it markedly increases the risk of corneal complications after ptosis surgery.
13. *Examine the ocular surface.* This is best done with a slit-lamp after placing a drop of fluorescein in the eye. Alternatively, a direct ophthalmoscope with a cobalt blue filter can be used. The adequacy of the tear film should be assessed as well as the presence of corneal drying. A Schirmer's test can be helpful. If the tear film is deficient or the cornea stains with fluorescein, there is a significant risk of worsening corneal drying or even ulceration with ptosis surgery.

At the end of the history and examination, a confident diagnosis of the cause of the ptosis can be made in most patients. If there is doubt, or certain diagnoses are suspected, then further investigations or referral to other specialists may be appropriate. The following scenarios deserve further investigation or referral:

1. Acquired 3rd nerve palsy. Should be referred for neurological assessment and imaging.
2. Acquired Horner's syndrome. Neurological referral.
3. Suspected myasthenia. An ice-test is a simple investigation that can help establish a diagnosis of myasthenia. An ice pack is placed over the eye with ptosis for 3–5 minutes. In myasthenia, the lid should elevate by at least 2 mm, and in patients with diplopia, this may temporarily resolve or reduce. All suspected myasthenics should be referred for neurological assessment and investigation.
4. Suspected myopathic ptosis. Neurological referral. Most myasthenics are managed medically. Occasionally, myasthenic ptosis may resist medical therapy and in some cases, surgery can be cautiously offered.
5. Reduced vision in a child under 10. Should be referred to an ophthalmologist.
6. Presence of strabismus. Referral to an ophthalmologist.

There may be other scenarios requiring further investigation or referral and if in doubt about the cause of the ptosis, then assessment by an ocular plastics specialist ophthalmologist or neuro-ophthalmologist is appropriate.

Treatment Principles

The principles of surgical and other forms of management of ptosis can be divided into the following groups:

1. Congenital ptosis
2. Blepharophimosis syndrome
3. Jaw-winking ptosis
4. Myopathic ptosis
5. Involutional ptosis

TABLE 69.1 Amount of Levator Resection According to Degree of Ptosis and Levator Function in Congenital Ptosis

Amount of Ptosis	Levator Function	Levator Function	Levator Resection
2 mm or less	Good	10 mm plus	10–13 mm
3 mm	Good	10 mm plus	14–17 mm
3 mm	Fair	7–10 mm	18–22 mm
4 mm or more	Fair	7–10 mm	23 mm
4 mm or more	Poor	6 mm or less	23 mm or more

Adapted from Callahan M, Beard C. *Beard's Ptosis*. 4th edn. Birmingham, AL: Aesculapius; 1990.

Congenital Ptosis

The management of congenital ptosis can be divided into several steps.

1. Refer all congenital ptosis for ophthalmological assessment at first diagnosis. Ideally this should be as soon as the diagnosis is made, shortly after birth. The ophthalmologist will assess the infant for refractive error and amblyopia and initiate appropriate treatment. If the ptosis is severe and the vision is not developing normally despite amblyopia therapy (glasses, patching or atropine penalization with drops), then early surgery may be indicated. Otherwise, the surgery can be delayed until accurate measurements of the degree of ptosis and levator function can be made, allowing proper surgical planning.
2. If there is a squint present, then the patient should also be referred as early as possible to an ophthalmologist. The commonest squint present with unilateral congenital ptosis is a hypotropia. If present, the hypotropia should be corrected before any ptosis surgery, because there will often be an element of pseudoptosis present which will be reduced by correcting the hypotropia. Additionally, correcting the hypotropia will reduce the risk of corneal exposure problems by improving globe elevation and the Bell's phenomenon.
3. If the vision is developing normally and there is no strabismus, then ptosis surgery can be planned around the age of 3–5 years, when good measurements can be obtained that help in the planning of ptosis surgery.

Surgery for Congenital Ptosis

If early intervention is required because of the presence of amblyopia, then normally a brow suspension is performed using non-autogenous material such as silicone. This allows for later removal and more definitive ptosis surgery at a later age if required. The technique for brow suspension is discussed later.

If the ptosis surgery is performed electively at or after the age of about 4 years, when good and reproducible measurements of the degree of ptosis and levator function can be obtained, then the choice of procedure will be determined principally by the degree of ptosis and levator function. If the levator function is poor (5–6 mm or less), then performing a levator resection or shortening procedure will lead inevitably to undercorrection. In this setting a brow suspension is preferred.

For congenital ptosis with 7 mm or more of levator function, a levator shortening or resection is preferred. The amount of resection is determined by the degree of ptosis and levator function. Complex tables are published, and the best known of these is that of Beard.[4] In general, levator function can be divided into poor, moderate, and good. "Good" levator function in congenital ptosis is 8 mm or more. Moderate is 6–8 mm. The range of shortening or resection for congenital ptosis is of the order of 10–25 mm. For genuine congenital ptosis with a myogenic cause, a resection of less than 10 mm is likely to lead to undercorrection. Within the group of patients with moderate levator function, the amount of resection will depend on the degree of ptosis (Table 69.1). An additional useful guide for the amount to resect the levator is Berke's rule of 7s. Under general anesthesia, if the levator function is 7 mm then the lid should be set to the desired level (usually 2 mm below the superior limbus). If more than 7 mm, it is set lower, and of less than 7 mm, it is set higher.

Additional factors which may influence the amount to resect the levator muscle include:

1. The presence of milder ptosis on the other side. Smaller resections may be performed to try to achieve symmetrical bilateral mild ptosis.
2. The presence of poor superior rectus function – an additional 4 mm is resected.
3. The decision to preserve Müller's muscle or not – an additional 2 mm is resected.

For very mild congenital ptosis (1–2 mm) with near normal levator function (13 mm or more), a posterior approach with resection of conjunctiva and Müller's muscle, or conjunctiva, Müller's muscle and tarsus (Fasanella–Servat procedure) can be performed (see below).

Techniques

Levator Resection

The amount to resect the muscle will have been determined preoperatively. The patient will usually be under general anesthesia. The following steps will be performed:

1. **Mark the upper lid skin crease.** This will be generally marked to match the other (normal) side and should

have been measured preoperatively, as it is not always obvious under general anesthesia.
2. **Inject local anesthetic.** Inject some local anesthetic with adrenaline into the eyelid. 1–2 mL is injected under the skin in the region of the planned incision. A very small bleb can also be injected subconjunctivally in the superior formix after everting the upper eyelid.
3. **Make an incision.** Make an incision in the marked crease through skin. The wound is then deepened through orbicularis muscle (Fig. 69.2A).
4. **Expose the tarsal plate.** Dissect downwards onto the anterior surface of the tarsal plate. As the tarsal plate is exposed, the lower end of the levator aponeurosis will be transected giving it a free lower edge. The tarsus should be exposed for most of its width and over its upper 3–4 mm (Fig. 69.2B).
5. **Open the orbital septum** (Fig. 69.2C). To do this, the upper edge of the wound is grasped and pulled upwards. An assistant grasps the lower edge of the levator aponeurosis. Sharp dissection is performed between the orbicularis muscle and levator aponeurosis, extending under the orbicularis. As the septum is opened, the anterior part of the levator muscle is exposed. A key landmark is the preaponerotic fat pad, a mobile, bright yellow pad of fat that overlies the anterior portion of the levator muscle belly. Once exposed, the fat pad is pulled upwards and the dissection of the muscle belly is extended into the superior orbit. The transverse or Whitnall's ligament will be seen. The dissection can proceed beyond this if a larger resection is required.
6. **Separate the levator from the tarsus and conjunctiva** (Figs. 69.2D,E) The aim here is to isolate the levator aponeurosis and muscle on its under surface to allow it to be resected. The initial separation is at the upper border of the tarsal plate. There is a vascular arcade here that bleeds. Müller's muscle lies on the conjunctiva and can be separated by initial sharp dissection, then blunt dissection. As the dissection proceeds, a thicker layer of connective tissue that is white in color is seen. This is the layer known as the common sheath or suspensory ligament of the fornix, and is the layer of connective tissue that extends forwards between the levator and superior rectus muscles. If damaged, prolapse of the superior conjunctival fornix can occur.
7. **Divide the medial and lateral horns** (Fig. 69.2F). If the resection is larger (>14–16 mm), then the medial and lateral horns should be divided to allow the muscle belly to advance more easily. The cuts should be made towards the belly of the muscle to avoid injury to the superior oblique tendon medially, and the lacrimal gland laterally. Once these cuts are made, the levator aponeurosis and muscle are able to be shortened or resected the desired amount. In some cases Whitnall's ligament may need to be separated from the LPS to allow it to advance (Fig. 69.2G).
8. **Place a central suture** (Fig. 69.2H). Use a nonabsorbable or long-acting absorbable double-armed suture such as 5-0 polyester or Vicryl. Pass one needle partial thickness through the tarsus about 2 mm below its superior border at a point just medial to the pupil line, where the peak of the lid contour will be. Pass both needles up under the belly of the muscle to emerge through the muscle 2–3 mm apart at a point determined preoperatively by reference to Table 69.1. Have an assistant hold the muscle on tension and tie a bow in the suture and assess the lid height. Using Berke's rule of 7s, the suture can be adjusted if necessary. Undo the bow once the lid height is satisfactory.
9. **Place medial and lateral sutures** (Fig. 69.2I). Sutures are then passed in a similar fashion medially and laterally. The central suture can be tied, then the medial and lateral sutures put on a bow to assess the lid contour. Adjustments are made as needed to achieve a satisfactory lid contour, then both are also tied.
10. **Trim the muscle.** The levator muscle and aponeurosis and Müller's muscle are then trimmed below the sutures.
11. **Reform the lid crease** (Fig. 69.2J). This can be done by using an absorbable 6-0 suture from the orbicularis of the lower wound edge to the cut edge of the levator muscle at three or more points. This gives a more natural "soft" crease. Alternatively, a suture from skin to levator to skin can be used to create a harder crease.
12. **Suture the skin.** Absorbable sutures can be used.
13. **Apply ointment.** In children, copious ointment is inserted into the eye and over the wound without an eyepad. In older patients, a temporary Frost suture can be used in the first 24 hours for corneal protection, with a double eyepad.

Tarsoconjunctival Resection (Fasanella–Servat Procedure)[5]

For very mild congenital ptosis with near normal levator function, a tarsoconjunctival resection can be performed. This is an uncommon clinical scenario and the large majority of congenital ptosis will require levator resection or brow suspension surgery.

1. **Evert the upper eyelid.** This is most easily done after placing a 4-0 traction suture in the lid margin and using a Desmarres retractor.
2. **Inject local anesthetic.** Anesthetic with adrenaline is injected subconjunctivally just above the superior border of the tarsus.
3. **Mark the area of tarsus and conjunctiva to resect.** This will be 3–4 mm of tarsus centrally (leaving at least 4 mm of tarsus from the margin), tapering medially and laterally. A similar amount of conjunctiva is marked.
4. **Resect the tarsus and conjunctiva/Müller's muscle.** Obtain hemostasis.
5. **Suture the wound.** This can be done by passing a nonabsorbable suture such as 6-0 prolene or nylon from the external surface of the lid to emerge at one end of the wound, then suturing continuously with a small number of bites and emerging externally at the other end of

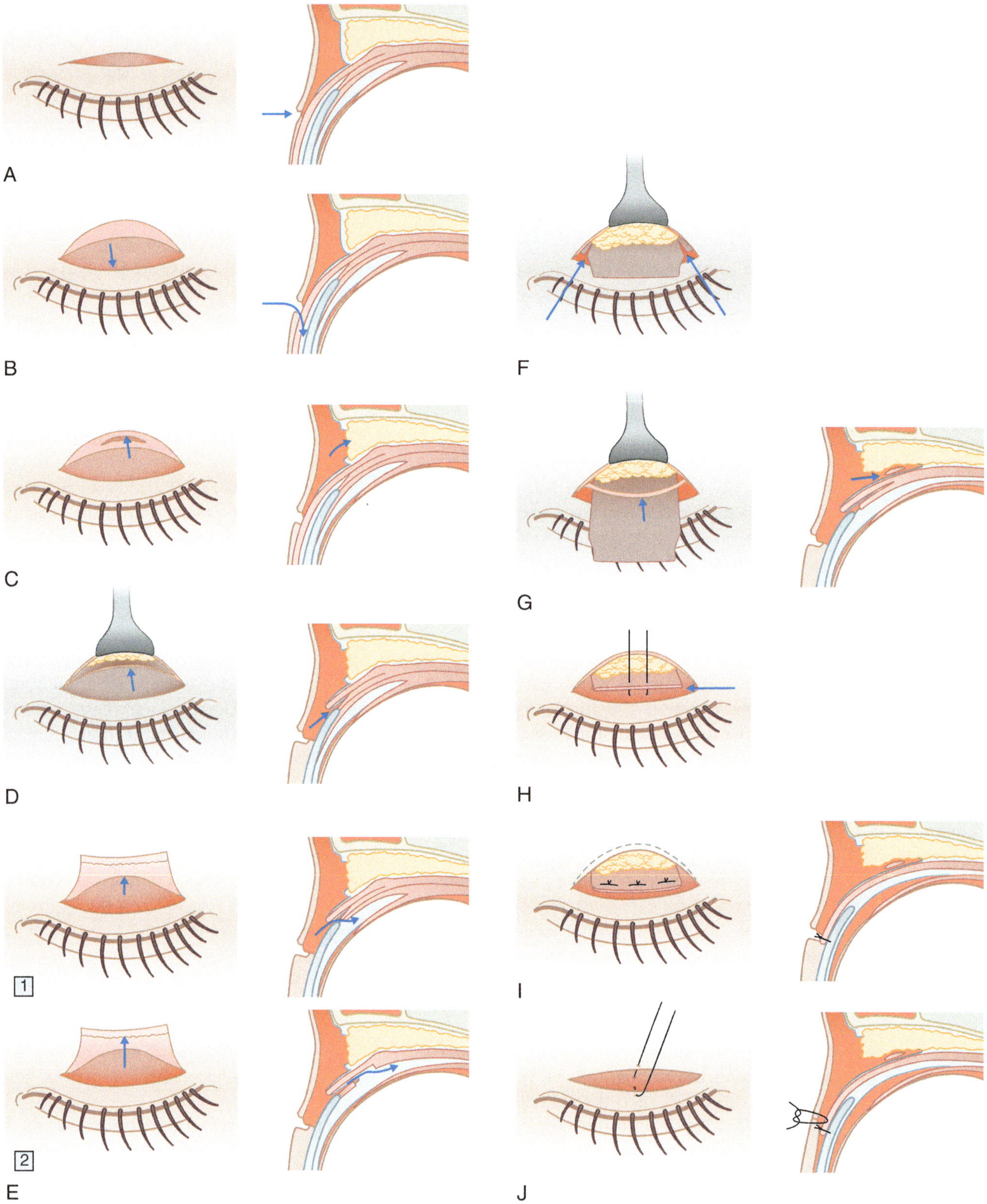

• **Fig. 69.2** A levator resection procedure for congenital dystrophic ptosis. (From Collin JRO. Ptosis. In: JRO Collin. *A Manual of Systematic Eyelid Surgery.* 3rd edn. Oxford: Butterworth–Heinemann; 2006: 85–114. Reproduced with permission of Elsevier.)

the lid. The suture is pulled tight to minimize the risk of corneal abrasion, and the ends tied together over the skin. It is removed at 1 week. In very young patients, an absorbable suture can be used with the knots tied on the skin surface.

6. **Apply ointment.**

Brow Suspension

A brow suspension procedure is indicated when the levator muscle function is poor (5–6 mm or less). If there is bilateral symmetrical ptosis with poor levator function, then the procedure is performed bilateral. If there is bilateral asymmetric ptosis and one side has poor levator function, and the other side has moderate function, then again, a bilateral brow suspension is preferred so as to give better symmetry both in primary position and in downgaze.

If the brow suspension is being done in a young infant because of the development or risk of amblyopia, then a nonautogenous material can be used, such as a silicone sling or a strong suture such as 2-0 Prolene.

For elective brow suspension beyond the age of about 3 years, then fascia lata is the most widely used material. Alternatively, if present, plantaris tendon can be used.

1. **Harvest the fascia lata.** There are strong transverse fibers on the fascia lata, which can be stripped off bluntly with toothed forceps to reveal the parallel longitudinal fibers that are to be harvested. For a bilateral procedure, the strip should be about 12–15 mm wide. Less is taken for a unilateral brow suspension. A blunt curved artery forceps can be used to split the fibers and begin the dissection. A length is isolated in the wound and clamped. It is divided at the lower end of the wound and the end then passed into the mouth of the fascial stripper which is then pushed up the thigh, bluntly separating the strip of fascia. Once the stripper is in the upper part of the thigh, the strip is cut and retrieved, and the wound sutured.
2. **Divide the fascia into strips.** The strips should be 3–4 mm wide. Wider strips produce large knots that are harder to bury. The strips can be made by dividing the large strip near one end for a few millimeters, grasping that part and pulling it away from the remainder to make a thin strip. Sharp dissection should not be needed.
3. **Mark the incisions in the lid and brow.** The brow suspension can be performed in a "closed" or open sky technique. A closed technique works well for fascia lata. For redo procedures or if silicone or Prolene is used, an open sky method works better. For an open sky method, the tarsus is exposed as for a levator resection and the material sutured to the tarsal plate before completing the brow suspension (see below under Myopathic Ptosis). For a closed brow suspension, three small marks are made at a level about 2 mm below the desired level of the skin crease, centrally, medially (just lateral to a point above the punctum), and laterally (2–3 mm medial to the lateral canthus). Two small incisions (about 4–5 mm in length) are marked almost directly above the medial and lateral marks at the upper border of the eyebrow and the third brow incision placed in the forehead to form an equilateral triangle with the two brow incisions.
4. **Make the incisions.** In the eyelid, these are made as small stab incisions with the end of an No. 11 blade. In the brow and forehead, they are longer to allow the knots in the fascia to be buried, and should be down to pericranium.
5. **Insert the fascial strips in the eyelid (Crawford pattern).**[6] Using a Wright's fascial needle, a pass is made from the medial eyelid wound to the central wound, passing deep to orbicularis and anterior to tarsus, across the lid. Place one strip in the eye of the needle and pull it back through the wound. Place another strip similarly from the central to the lateral lid wound. Then pass the fascial needle from the medial brow wound, at a depth just superficial to pericranium, and beneath the orbicularis in the eyelid, being careful to avoid passing the needle through the lid into the fornix or eye. An eye shield should be used. One end of the medial loop is retrieved, then the other so both ends emerge from the medial brow wound. The same is done from the lateral brow wound with the other loop.
6. **Tie the knots in the brow wounds.** The fascial strips are pulled up, leaving one end longer (for later passage to the forehead wound). The lid should rise to the desired level about 2 mm below the upper limbus. If the lid pulls away from the globe before this point is reached, stop at the point just before the lid pulls off the globe. A single throw is made and the square knot completed with a second single throw. The fascial knot should be reinforced with a suture such as 6-0 Vicryl passed through the fascial knot.
7. **Pass the strips to the forehead wound and tie.** The longer ends of the fascial strips are then passed to the forehead wound. They should be tied with some tension to maintain the desired lid level and reinforced.
8. **Suture the brow and forehead wounds.** The eyelid punctures do not need sutures.
9. **Apply copious ointment in the eye(s).**

Surgery for Blepharophimosis Syndrome

Children (or adults) with BPES syndrome have poor levator function and will need brow suspension surgery. It is customary to correct the telecanthus and epicanthic folds initially, usually at the age of 3–4 years, and then perform the brow suspension about 6 months later. Some patients with BPES will benefit from lateral ectropion surgery.

Medial Canthoplasty

A variety of techniques has been described for the management of telecanthus and epicanthic folds in BPES. These include Mustarde's technique,[7] its variation, the 5-flap technique of Anderson,[8] a Y–V plasty, and transnasal wire. The author's preference is for the Anderson 5-flap technique, which better addresses the epicanthic folds. The detail of these procedures is beyond the scope of this chapter and the reader is directed towards the appropriate references listed below.

Brow Suspension

The technique is the same as described for poor levator function congenital ptosis (above).

Surgery for Jaw-Winking Ptosis

The surgical management of jaw-winking ptosis is complex and several options are available, depending on the desire to abolish (or ignore) the wink, the desire to achieve symmetry, and any concerns held by the patient or their parents about operating on the contralateral (normal) side.

If the main concern is with the ptosis (almost always unilateral) only, and the wink is of less concern, then a simple levator resection can be performed. The amount to resect the levator muscle is determined in a similar way to simple dystrophic myogenic congenital ptosis, but a slightly larger resection is often needed to achieve good symmetry in primary position.

If it is desired to abolish the wink, the only reliable way to achieve this is to ablate the levator muscle, creating complete ptosis with no levator function, and then perform a brow suspension procedure. If this is done unilaterally, there will be asymmetry, often in primary position, with a degree of undercorrection, and more marked asymmetry in downgaze, with hang-up of the upper lid on downgaze on the operated side. This is the reason that some surgeons recommend bilateral surgery in this scenario. The levator can be ablated on the affected side, then a bilateral brow suspension is performed, so that there is better symmetry in downgaze. Further improvement in symmetry can be achieved by ablating the levator muscle on both sides and performing bilateral brow suspension surgery (the Beard procedure). However, many patients and their parents are reluctant to consider surgery on the normal side, which converts a normal eyelid into one with limited excursion and potential complications in later life from incomplete closure and corneal exposure complications.

Levator Ablation

If levator ablation is chosen (either unilateral or bilateral), it is most easily achieved via an anterior skin crease approach.

1. **Make an upper eyelid skin crease incision.**
2. **Open the orbital septum** and expose the anterior portion of the belly of the levator muscle.
3. **Dissect superiorly** to expose the belly of the muscle above Whitnall's suspensory ligament. Pass two squint hooks under the belly of the muscle and resect several millimeters of the muscle belly making sure all fibers and the muscle sheath are divided, otherwise the wink will not be abolished.
4. **Proceed with brow suspension surgery**, with the fascial strips sutured directly to the tarsal plate (see above).

Surgery for Myopathic Ptosis

Surgery for myopathic ptosis will depend on several critical factors which include:

1. The diagnosis
2. The expected long-term progression of the disease
3. The levator muscle function
4. Eye movements
5. Orbicularis oculi muscle strength.

The exact diagnosis of myopathic ptosis should generally be pursued before any surgical correction, because different forms of myopathic ptosis have different natural histories, different relative involvement of extraocular muscles and orbicularis oculi, and some are better treated medically (myasthenia). Additionally, there may be genetic counseling issues in many of these patients.

Myotonic dystrophy often carries a worse prognosis than some other forms of myopathic ptosis as orbicularis oculi is more severely affected. Oculopharyngeal muscular dystrophy generally does well with brow suspension surgery, as orbicularis oculi tends to be better preserved, and eye movements are less severely affected, reducing the risk of corneal exposure. CPEO varies in its severity, depending on the subset. Early onset CPEO in the form of Kearns–Sayre syndrome is more severe and more rapidly progressive. Systemic problems are also commoner and include cardiac disease, generalized severe myopathy, and early onset diabetes.

If there is any suspicion of a myopathic form of ptosis, appropriate referral should be made to a neurologist with expertise in neuromuscular diseases.

Myasthenia

Surgery is not usually indicated for myasthenic ptosis, which should be treated medically. However, in some longstanding patients, surgery may be indicated for stable ptosis which does not respond to medical therapies. The surgery should be performed cautiously, bearing in mind the increased risk of inducing corneal exposure problems.

Levator Muscle Surgery in Myopathic Ptosis

Caution should be exercised in performing levator muscle surgery in myopathic ptosis. It should only ever be used where the levator muscle function is good. Often larger degrees of muscle shortening are required to elevate the lid sufficiently despite the apparently good levator muscle function and this leads to an increased risk in later life of corneal exposure problems. If performing levator muscle surgery (or brow suspension surgery) in these patients, lifelong follow-up is required as these diseases progress and ocular surface complications increase. The surgeon should be prepared to reverse the ptosis surgery if the cornea is at significant risk.

Brow Suspension Surgery for Myopathic Ptosis

Often, a more conservative brow suspension procedure is safer in these patients than a levator shortening procedure. The lid can be lifted by the often well-preserved frontalis muscle to a point just above the visual axis, allowing the patient to function reasonably well, and at the same time allowing reasonable eyelid closure and minimizing corneal exposure.

The choice of material used for the brow suspension surgery will depend on personal preference as well as other factors such as the ease of reversibility or adjustment later, and the requirement of general anesthesia if harvesting fascia lata. For oculopharyngeal muscular dystrophy, which carries a relatively good prognosis, fascia lata brow suspension surgery is preferable. Under general anesthesia, the eyelids should be set open just 2–3 mm, and when awake and the frontalis muscle is activated, the lids will generally rise above the visual axis, and eyelid closure will be reasonably well preserved.

For the more severe forms of myopathic ptosis, many surgeons prefer to use nonautogenous material such as silicone, Gore-Tex, or heavy Prolene suture. Local anesthetic can be used for this procedure also. If using these materials, an open-sky technique is preferred with the sling material sutured directly to the tarsal plate with nonabsorbable sutures. The material is inserted in a pentagonal shape (Fox pentagon), with the final knot tied in the forehead. Again, the lid should be set just open, about 2 mm.

Surgery for Involutional Ptosis

The majority of surgical procedures for ptosis will be for involutional ptosis. The same techniques are used for involutional ptosis as for aponeurotic ptosis that may occur with long-term hard contact lens wear, after some cases of trauma or lid swelling, or in the rare blepharochalasis syndrome.

The surgical steps can be broken down into the following.

1. **Mark the proposed incision(s) in the upper eyelid.** The placement of the incision will be determined by the desired height of the eyelid crease, which will be made to match the opposite side in unilateral cases. In many cases of involutional ptosis, excess upper eyelid skin will be excised also, not just for appearance, but to reduce the increased overhang of skin that would otherwise occur if the lid alone is elevated. The amount of skin to be excised should be judged carefully in each patient, and is more easily determined in bilateral cases. Removing too much skin should be clearly avoided, as the risk of corneal exposure is increased when ptosis is corrected at the same time.
2. **Inject the local anesthetic.** This should be kept to a minimum volume, and 1–1.5 mL is usually adequate. An excess volume may cause a mechanical ptosis, and a larger volume is more likely to spread deep to the orbital septum and partially paralyse the levator muscle fibers, making the assessment of the lid height more difficult. Recheck the lid height and levator function before proceeding.
3. **Make the skin incisions.** Excess skin is removed at this stage. If the surgery is bilateral, each step can be performed on each side so that the surgery advances in parallel. This makes achieving symmetry easier.
4. **Expose the anterior surface of the tarsal plate.** This is achieved by sharp dissection below the orbicularis muscle at the inferior edge of the incision, heading obliquely towards the tarsal plate. As the tarsal plate is exposed, the fibers of the levator aponeurosis that are destined for the tarsal plate, are divided, creating an inferior edge on the aponeurosis which can be used later for attachment or advancement on the tarsal plate.
5. **Open the orbital septum.** Sharp dissection proceeds under the orbicularis muscle superiorly, with an assistant holding the inferior edge of the levator aponeurosis downwards. Dissection proceeds until the preaponeurotic fat is exposed, which is then dissected gently off the underlying levator muscle and aponeurosis.
6. **Recheck the eyelid levels.** Sometimes the lid may elevate without advancing the aponeurosis possibly by epinephrine in the local anesthetic stimulating the Müller's muscle, or the lid may drop because the aponeurosis has been detached from the tarsus.
7. **Pass a double-armed 5-0 or 6-0 nonabsorbable suture** partial thickness through the tarsal plate about 2 mm below its superior border, at a point where the peak of the arch of the lid contour should lie. This will usually be just medial to the mid-pupil. Pass each needle superiorly under the levator aponeurosis, between it and the Müller's muscle, to emerge through the aponeurosis. The level at which the sutures pass will be based on several factors, including the appearance of the muscle (is there fatty infiltration and degeneration?), and the length and appearance of the aponeurosis. In any event, the level of the initial pass is by trial and error. Once both ends are passed, a bow is tied and the lid height assessed. In most cases, the aim will be to set the lid at or just below the superior limbus (bilateral cases) or 1–2 mm higher than the unoperated side (unilateral cases). Some surgeons assess lid height with the patient lying down, some sitting up. Either is acceptable and each surgeon should be consistent to better achieve more predictable outcomes. If the lid height is not correct, withdraw and reposition the sutures until the desired height is achieved.
8. **Insert medial and lateral sutures** once the desired lid height is achieved. The central suture is untied, and similar sutures are passed medially and laterally. The central suture is then tied, and the medial and lateral sutures are secured with a bow. The lid contour is checked and any adjustments made that might be required.
9. **Reform the upper eyelid skin crease.** Pass an absorbable suture from the orbicularis muscle adjacent to the inferior skin incision, onto the levator aponeurosis, making sure that the anterior lamella of the eyelid is draped over the tarsus without it being too tight or too loose. Three sutures are sufficient. The skin is then sutured separately.
10. **Apply antibiotic ointment.** Dressings can be applied if desired, and ice packs also.

Complications

The potential complications of ptosis surgery are many, but the commonest will be addressed here. These are:

1. Undercorrection
2. Overcorrection
3. Poor lid contour
4. Poor eyelid closure with corneal exposure.

Undercorrection

This is common. In many instances, the surgeon may aim for "undercorrection," particularly in older patients with poor tear film and dry eyes, or in patients with myopathic ptosis where the risk of corneal exposure is much higher.

If undercorrection is present at the first postoperative visit, it is usually better to wait for any swelling or possible underaction of the levator or Müller's muscle due to hematoma to settle before reoperating. This usually means waiting 6 weeks or more.

Overcorrection

Mild initial overcorrection is common and should be expected in unilateral cases. There is loss of function of the pretarsal orbicularis muscle, that will recover over about 8 weeks, by which time the lid will drop about 1 mm, occasionally a little more.

More significant overcorrection should be corrected early. The wound can be reopened under local anesthetic and the sutures released. The levator aponeurosis (in involutional ptosis cases) will recess by a small amount only usually. More formal recessions may be required in more severe cases, with "hang-back" sutures from the tarsus to the free edge of the aponeurosis.

Poor Lid Contour

This will not resolve with time and should be corrected. This can be performed early or late. One or more sutures may need to be replaced, higher or lower.

Poor Eyelid Closure with Corneal Exposure

This is commoner in the early weeks after ptosis surgery, and can often be managed with increased ocular lubricants including ointment, especially at night when the lid may be open during sleep. Eyelid closure improves in the first 8 weeks after surgery, and if after that time the corneal exposure does not settle, then consideration should be given to lowering the lid.

References

1. Kakizaki H, Zako M, Nakano T, et al. The medial horn and capsulopalpebral fascia in the medial canthus are significant antagonists of the orbicularis oculi muscle for lacrimal drainage. *Ophthalmologica*. 2004;218:419–423.
2. Ettl A, Priglinger S, Kramer J, et al. Functional anatomy of the levator palpebrae superioris muscle and its connective tissue system. *Br J Ophthalmol.* 1996;80:702–707.
3. Collin JRO. Ptosis. In: Collin JRO, ed. *A Manual of Systematic Eyelid Surgery*. 3rd edn. Oxford: Butterworth–Heinemann; 2006:85–114.
4. Callahan M. *Beard's Ptosis.* 4th edn. Ophthalmic Leasing Company; 1990.
5. Fasanella RM, Servat J. Levator resection for minimal ptosis: another simplified operation. *Arch Ophthalmol.* 1961;65:493–496.
6. Crawford JS. Repair of ptosis using frontalis muscle and fascia lata: a 20 year review. *Ophthalmic Surg*. 1977;8:31–40.
7. Mustardé JC. Epicanthus, telecanthus, blepharophimosis and related conditions. In: Mustardé JC, ed. *Repair and Reconstruction in the Orbital Region*. 3rd edn. Edinburgh: Churchill Livingstone; 1991:474–478.
8. Anderson RL, Nowinski TS. The five-flap technique for blepharophimosis. *Arch Ophthalmol.* 1989;107:448–452.

70

Liposuction and Liposculpture

FRANCESCO M. EGRO, NATHANIEL A. BLECHER, J. PETER RUBIN, AND SYDNEY R. COLEMAN

Introduction

Liposuction and liposculpture represent the evolution of minimally invasive plastic surgery techniques developed in an attempt at restoring shape and form. Liposuction was first described in the 1920s but it was not until the 1970s that the technique was popularized in Europe by Illouz, Fournier, and Otteni whereby fat was harvested using a blunt cannula and aspirated using negative pressure. Prior to liposuction, fat was directly excised leaving unsightly scars and increased morbidity. The effect of liposuction on the body has been extensively studied and it has been shown to be safe and effective. Other than producing improved contour cosmesis, liposuction was shown to reduce body weight, BMI, waist circumference, body fat, plasma leptin, and insulin levels. Although fat grafting was first described back in 1893 by Neuber, it was Coleman who popularized free fat transfer in a minimally traumatic fashion leading to a consistently higher graft retention compared to prior techniques.[1] As research in the field increased, the indications and quoted graft retention rates also increased (20%–90%). Part of the reason for the wide variation in the results is the sheer amount of factors involved in graft survival. Though the Coleman technique is often accepted as the standard, in the nascent field of fat grafting, multiple strategies for liposuction, fat processing, and grafting have evolved, which makes standardization and optimization challenging. This chapter critically appraises each step in the process of liposuction and fat grafting, from harvesting to processing to injecting, to provide a detailed overview for the plastic surgeon of the 21st century.

Harvest Site

Liposuction for body sculpting or for fat harvesting purposes can be performed anywhere around the body as long as there is sufficient adiposity. The most common sites include the abdomen, flanks, and thighs. However, both animal and human studies have shown that donor site does not influence the quality of the lipoaspirate and the graft survival.[2] In fact, in a murine model Ullmann et al found no significant differences based on thigh, abdomen, and breast donor sites in graft retention or histology after 16 weeks.[2] Li et al repeated and expanded upon these animal findings, finding no difference in retention from five separate donor sites (flank, upper and lower abdomen, and lateral and inner thigh) after 12 weeks.[2] Human studies have also found no difference based on comparative symmetry scores of craniofacial patients grafted with fat from the abdomen versus other areas (medial thigh, suprapubic).[2] Similarly, in breast reconstruction Small et al found no significant difference in graft retention after 140 days in fat harvested from the abdomen versus the thighs.[2] There is currently no evidence to support that harvest site independently influences graft survival. However, this parity has not been proven with higher-level prospective cohorts or randomized control trials, and further research is needed.

Donor Site Preparation

Liposuction can be performed dry (no wetting solution), wet (200 mL/area), superwet (1 mL infiltrate per 1 mL of aspirate), or tumescent (2–3 mL infiltrate per 1 mL of aspirate). The wetting solution may contain lidocaine, epinephrine, and/or sodium bicarbonate depending on surgeon's preference. The benefit of using a superwet or tumescent solution is the significant decrease in blood loss down to 1%. Other benefits of using a wetting solution is the analgesic effect provided by lidocaine, volume replacement, and enhanced cavitation and heat dissipation in ultrasound-assisted liposuction. The concern of the use of wetting solutions in the setting of fat grafting is the potential effect on adipocyte viability and blood flow reduction to grafts.[2] However, as early as 2005 Shoshani et al demonstrated no significant difference in weight and volume retention at 15 weeks between xenografts harvested with lidocaine and epinephrine versus a control of saline.[2] Livaoğlu et al further proved the safety of local anesthesia showing no significant difference in retention at 180 days between control, lidocaine plus epinephrine, or prilocaine groups in an autologous murine model.[2]

Lastly, Rohrich et al found no significant differences in adipocyte viability among four donor sites (abdomen, flank, thigh, knee) determined on an in vitro colorimetric assay of cell proliferation.[2] Overall, despite theoretical concerns for the use of local anesthesia, graft survival does not seem to be greatly affected by its use in animal models. This finding should be further investigated in human studies.

Harvest Technique

Depth of Liposuction

Fat can be aspirated at different depths of the subcutaneous layer but one has to be aware of potential risks and variation in quality of the fat (relevant if used for fat grafting). The superficial subcutaneous layer contains dense fat, which is adherent to overlying skin. The intermediate subcutaneous layer is the safest and most commonly aspirated layer. The deep subcutaneous layer contains looser and less compact fat, and can be safely aspirated in most areas except the buttocks. Ideally, the surgeon should avoid violating the superficial plane above the superficial fascia to ensure preservation of subdermal structures, and prevent surface irregularities. A variety of zones of adherence have been described, which should not be violated during liposuction because of the risk of contour deformity. These zones include the gluteal crease, middle medial thigh, lateral gluteal depression, distal posterior thigh, and distal iliotibial tract.

Cannula Size

The use of single-bore blunt-tip harvesting cannula has been standard practice since the description of the technique by Coleman. There are very few studies examining the impact of different parameter in cannula such as bore size and single versus multiple perforation.[3]

To determine the impact of bore size, Erdim et al compared fatty aspirate obtained from 2-mm, 4-mm, and 6-mm blunt cannulas and found significantly higher in vitro adipocyte survival in the 6-mm group compared to both the 2-mm and 4-mm groups. However, this viability assessment was only based on brilliant cresyl blue supravital stained adipocyte counts after collagenase digestion and centrifuging.[3] A similar in vitro study by Alharbi et al comparing 3-mm single-bore and 2-mm multiperforated St'rim cannulas (Thiebaud Biomedical Devices), found no significant difference in cell viability between the groups when measured by alamarBlue (ThermoFischer) reagent.[3] Lastly, Kirkham et al compared 3-mm and 5-mm Coleman cannulas in a murine model using a dry technique, and found significantly higher graft retention and histologically healthier grafts in the larger cannula group at 6 weeks.[3] These findings suggest that, generally, larger bore cannulas produce more viable cells leading to better graft retention. However, we must balance these results with data on parcel size discussed below. Given the limited data on graft survival, further longer-term, in vivo research with more modern viability assays is justified.

Parcel Size

The importance of parcel size in fat graft survival is based on the same general theories of imbibition and neovascularization that are vital to survival of all tissue grafts. Early research theorized on how graft shape could affect percentage of graft that was more than 1.5 mm from the edge and how this would impact survival. This theory was expanded upon by Eto et al, who identified three distinct zones of adipocyte survival. Outer surviving zone with cells located within 300 μm of the graft edge; middle regenerating zone with cells undergo necrosis but are replaced by adipose-derived stem cells (ASCs); and central necrotic zone where no viable fat survives.[4] The same group published further evidence of the behavior of grafts based on distance from the edge, showing adipogenesis via $CD34^+/Ki67^+$ ASCs in the regenerating zone (600–1200 μm thick) peaked at 4 weeks and concluded by 12 weeks, while stabilization via $MAC2^+/CD206^-$ M1 macrophages $MAC2^+/CD206^+$ M2 macrophages in the central necrotic zone persisted through 12 weeks.[4] The importance of the relation between graft and surrounding tissue has been further demonstrated in injected fat. Our group demonstrated that as the total fat volume transferred increases, grafted deposits coalesce to form larger globules (especially at ratios beyond 1:4). Therefore, increasing the likelihood of central necrosis and subsequent graft loss.[5] Our group also showed that larger grafts contain central cores that could not be cleared appropriately by macrophages, allowing for persistent necrosis that skew retention as a measure of survival.[6] The architecture of fat grafts is clearly important, with the principles of different survival zones based on distance to the vascularized edge providing insight into how parcel size may affect graft survival. The research using cannula size surrogates has not been conclusive and no research exists to date directly examining lobule size in vivo. Further research must be performed to determine the relationship between parcel size and graft survival in vivo.

Aspiration Technique

The amount of liposuction performed depends on the level of lipodystrophy, desired result, and amount of fat needed for grafting. Large-volume liposuction is usually considered to be anything above 5 liters of fat aspiration. These cases should be performed in an acute care hospital or an accredited facility because of the increased complication rates associated with larger volume liposuction. To ensure safety, vital signs, urine output, overnight monitoring, and appropriate fluid replacement are required.

Various aspiration techniques have been developed over the years, including suction-assisted, ultrasound-assisted, water-assisted, and laser-assisted liposuction.[7–10] Use of either hand aspiration or machine-assisted liposuction is a compromise between efficiency and the risk of adipocyte damage. Early studies in aspiration pressure were based on cell viability with varying pressures. Pu et al found that there was a significantly greater number of viable adipocytes harvested via hand aspiration compared to machine aspiration at no greater than 20 cmH_2O.[8] In contrary, Lee et al found that there was no difference in graft weight retention or histology between −15 mmHg handheld aspirate and −25 mmHg machine-harvested fat.[2]

Ultrasound-assisted liposuction (UAL) was first described by Zocchi, and it is a result of alternating currents that cause piezoelectric crystals to expand and contract, releasing ultrasonic waves that emulsify fat by micromechanical, thermal, and cavitation action. Our group showed no difference in graft retention in a murine model between UAL and traditional suction-assisted liposuction at 430 mmHg in graft retention or histology.[7] Yin et al compared graft survival between xenografts harvested via water-jet assisted liposuction and traditional liposuction set to −0.5 bar and found significantly improved graft retention and adipocyte viability in the water-jet assisted liposuction group.[9] Laser-assisted liposuction (LAL) uses a laser fiber to disrupt fat cell membranes and emulsifying fat. The most common wavelengths in LAL include 924/975 nm, 1064 nm, 1319/1320 nm, and 1450 nm. Prado et al showed no major differences between SAL and LAL, other than higher concentrations of free-fatty acids after LAL. However, limited conclusions can be drawn given the small sample size.[10]

In the current literature, increased pressure from machine-assisted liposuction does not appear to impact actual graft survival though it may affect cell viability. While many of these studies discuss graft survival, none compares techniques based on esthetic outcomes. Thus the assertion of superiority of nonvacuum techniques on esthetic outcomes is not yet defined. With limited studies, more research should be pursued comparing graft retention based on aspiration method potential comparing hand, machine, ultrasound, water-jet, and laser-assisted liposuction.

Processing Technique

Centrifugation, Filtration, Decanting, and Rolling Techniques

Four primary processing methods have been used clinically to process fat graft: centrifugation, filtration, decanting, and rolling techniques.

Centrifuging has been a mainstay in fat processing as a method of separating viable adipocytes from additional, undesirable lipoaspirate. As a commonly utilized technique, it has been more highly researched with investigation into ideal centrifuge speeds and how the method compares to other processing techniques.[2,6,7,11–13] Early research into the utility of centrifuging for improving fat graft survival in humans by Butterwick showed that, when compared to noncentrifuged fat, centrifuged grafts to the hand were rated by both patients and physicians as having better retention and more visual improvement as long as months after the procedure.[2] Ferraro et al also utilized digital photography to compare resorption rates in patients grafted with fat centrifuged at 3000 rpm (1500 *g*) for 3 minutes, 1300 rpm (250 *g*) for 5 minutes, or uncentrifuged and decanted fat injected in the gluteal region and found the lowest resorption rates in the slow centrifuge group and highest in decantation after 12 months.[2] Quantitative research to evaluate the effect of centrifuging speeds on graft survival has been completed in murine models. Using percent oil extracted after centrifuging as a surrogate for adipocyte damage, Hoareau et al determined speeds up to 400 *g* had little effect on harvested fat whereas a speed of 900 *g* had significantly damaged adipocytes.[2] On the other hand, higher centrifuge speeds produced more concentrated adipocyte fractions with maximal concentration being achieved at 5000 *g*.[11] Thus, in determining the ideal speed, concentrating power and cell damage must be balanced to produce optimal graft survival. Kurita et al compared grafts either not centrifuged or centrifuged at 400 *g*, 700 *g*, 1200 *g*, 3000 *g*, or 4200 *g* for 3 minutes and found significantly improved retention up to 3000 *g*, but when balanced with ASC concentration and volume compaction, suggested 1200 *g* was the ideal speed.[2] Additionally, the group suggested that increased oil isolated above 400 *g* was due to separation of existing oil rather than cell damage as grafts up to 4200 *g* were histologically intact. Other studies have suggested the ideal speed to be as low as 698.75 *g* or as high as 5000 *g*.[7,13] Centrifuging at any speed creates multiple layers of density, which Allen et al compared to determine if the density of the processed fat affected survival. They found that the highest density fraction had significantly higher retention and improved architecture at 2 and 10 weeks.[2]

Centrifuging has also been compared to other methods of processing such as sieves and gauze rolling. When comparing these three methods in a murine model, Minn et al found no significant differences in graft retention or necrosis at 12 weeks, but did find significantly lower in vitro cell viability in the metal sieve group based on XTT metabolization.[2] These results were echoed by Salinas et al when they found centrifuging at 1200 *g* and mesh/gauze processing produced equivalent graft retention and histology scores in mice at 4 weeks, noting the result was expecting as the two methods achieved the same level of adipocyte concentration.[11] However, Canizares et al found that when compared to centrifuging at 1200 *g*, telfa rolling produced superior graft retention at 2 and 10 weeks in a murine model as well as adipocyte functionality as determined by glycerol-3-phosphate dehydrogenase assay.[12] Fisher et al similarly found that xenograft retention at 6 weeks for the telfa roll method was superior to both centrifuging via the Coleman method and Tissu-Trans Filtron filtration.[7]

The current evidence suggests that fat should be processed using centrifugation or rolling techniques. However, one must consider the practical aspect of fat processing technique, which must allow feasible workflow in the operating room. For this reason, a surgeon might need to tailor the processing technique based on the volume of fat that needs to be grafted. For instance, smaller volumes can be processed with either centrifugation or rolling techniques;

whereas, larger volumes may be more efficiently processed with filtering or decantation.

Washing

Washing serves as another method of processing and purifying lipoaspirate, which is performed often in isolation rather than as an adjunct, by adding and removing solutions.[2,14] Girard et al showed improved fat graft retention in immunodeficient mice at 4 weeks, by combining centrifugation with Ringer's lactate washing.[14] Khater et al found better esthetic results when lipoaspirate was washed 1:1 with physiological serum instead of centrifugation, which they attributed to the noncentrifuged graft's higher leptin expression and number of preadipocytes as identified by morphology.[2] In a similar study, Botti et al found no difference between centrifuging and washing with normal saline.[2] Condé-Green et al showed that while washing lipoaspirate with normal saline three times in a 1:1 ratio leads to high histological fat graft viability, cell assisted lipotransfer and centrifuged fat graft had significantly more consistent volume retention of 0.3 mL grafts at 12 weeks in immunodeficient mice.[2]

Taken as a whole, current data seems to suggest washing provides comparable retention to other methods of processing but may provide benefits to cell viability. However, further research is needed to determine its superiority.

Pharmacological Additives

A multitude of individual additives have been tested to improve graft retention including IL-8, PDGF, VEGF-loaded microspheres, botulinum toxin-A, M2 macrophages, N-acetylcysteine, phosphodiesterase inhibitors, insulin, EGF, anti-TNF-α improved autograft, bone marrow aspirate or concentrate. These pharmacological additives show promising results. However, the majority of these studies utilize non-ideal methods in their processing and assessment of viability of their grafts. Whereas among those studies that do, the heterogeneity in methodology makes comparison of additives impossible. To determine the true benefits and superiority of additives in the clinical setting, further standardized studies using methods that reduce spurious retention and demonstrate viability must first be pursued.

Injection Technique

The technique employed to inject fat is crucial to optimize the esthetics and retention of the graft. Injection of the processed fat into the recipient site requires significant care to produce long-lasting desirable outcomes. The original technique described by Dr. Coleman uses Luer lock syringes connected to a 17G blunt cannula to inject the processed lipoaspirate. The cannula is withdrawn as the lipoaspirate is injected, in order to allow the grafted fat to fall into the natural tissue planes as the cannula is removed. A fan injection pattern is also recommended because as described by our group the distribution of the injected fat is of utmost importance to survival.[6,15] Given the impact of injection pattern on survival, other aspects of injection method have also been researched.[2,16–18]

Much as with harvesting, a focus on injection technique has been needle size. Erdim et al found no difference in in vitro adipocyte count between 14G, 16G, and 20G injection needle gauges.[2] Their findings were reinforced by Nguyen et al, who found no significant differences in graft retention or histology when comparing injections of 0.7 mL of fat with 17G, 20G, 23G, or 25G needles.[16] Contrarily, Luan et al suggest injection cannula does impact survival, finding that injection of 0.2 mL xenograft through a 14G 8-cm cannula led to significantly better histology than fat injected through longer or narrower cannulas, and that volume retention was significantly better than a 18G 8-cm cannula.[18] Possible differences in outcomes with different injection cannulas have been attributed to shear stress during injection. Lee et al proposed that the increase in shear stress with fast injection rate (3–5 mL/second) over slow injection rate (0.5–1 mL/second) was the cause of decreased retention and histology scores in their - mL xenografts at 4 weeks.[2] Chung et al investigated how a low shear, automated adipose tissue injector device affected grafts, finding a significant increase in in vitro viability and proliferation, and improved in vivo retention and histology at 12 weeks.[17]

While early studies suggested no effect, later investigation using more ideal models demonstrated clear preference toward low-shear stress injection methods. Further research pursuing these methods should be completed in clinical trials to confirm their success.

Recipient Site

Researchers have suggested differences in retention due to recipient site may be due to factors such as site mobility, existing vascularity, and injection effect on architecture.[19–21] Fat graft retention depends on revascularization among many factors, which means that lipoaspirate injection into a vascularized bed is essential. Karacaoglu et al tested optimal recipient bed by comparing fat grafting in the subcutaneous, supramuscular, and submuscular layer of the buccomandibular area of rabbits, and found that grafting into the supramuscular layer had significantly improved retention and histopathological scores.[21] Shi et al showed that 0.1-mL allografts to the fat pad had the highest weight retention compared to the intramuscular and subcutaneous layers. However, angiogenesis and vascularized connective tissue were more prominent in fat injected in the intramuscular layer, likely being the reason for the highest survival rates among the three recipient sites.[20]

A potential factor impacting graft retention is the degree of mobility of the underlying tissue. The face is a prime example with areas like the glabella and lips that are less amenable to correction, compared to less mobile areas like the malar and lateral cheek.

Denadai et al demonstrated radiologically that fat graft retention was better in the cheek unit at 12 months compared to the forehead or the chin units.[22] Furthermore, Mojallal et al showed in their clinical trial that fat injected to the malar region had significantly better esthetic result than grafts to the temporal and lip areas.[2]

The manipulation of recipient site offers the chance to enhance graft survival and predictability. Much of the research in the area has been dedicated to preexpansion, where the mechanotransduction properties of preexpansion lead to conversion of mechanical tension into growth-promoting signals creating a vascularized scaffold that allows for larger graft volumes and better retention rates.[2] The BRAVA (Brava, LLC, Miami, FL) preexpansion device is a prime example and the benefit of this technology was demonstrated in a prospective multicenter study highlighting the significant improvement in weighted mean graft retention rate and the ability to inject much larger volumes of fat graft.[2] Lee et al used posttransplant negative external pressure on 1-g en bloc autografts, finding a significant improvement at 3 months in the experimental group's weight retention and viability.[23] Sezgin et al examined the effect of microneedling prior to fat grafting and found that it had significantly better retention and histopathological scores at 15 weeks of 100-mg grafts, but did not find a significant difference in the grafts triglyceride content.[24] By housing posttransplant mice in oxygen-enriched environments, Kato et al investigated the effect of normobaric hyperoxygenation on a perilipin staining and weight retention calculated engraftment score for 0.2-mg murine autografts, proving that this pretreatment significantly increased survival at 12 weeks by increasing the surviving and regeneration zones over the central necrotic zone of grafts.[25]

These techniques are promising strategies to support the recipient bed and should be further explored in human trials.

Intrinsic Patient Variability in Adipose Tissue

The unpredictability of fat graft retention remains a major issue and intrinsic patient factors are likely to play a role. Much of the research into the efficacy of fat grafting has focused on how technique affects graft survival, and only few papers have directly examined the effect of different patient characteristics on the grafts they receive.[2,16,19,22,26–30] Commonly, patient factors will be reported in studies to show standardization between study groups but will not be subject to analysis for potential significance. Furthermore, while some studies have performed patient factor analysis, this is rarely the primary focus of the paper, rather being a secondary finding. Geissler et al examined the fat of 24 female patients harvested from the flanks, lower abdomen, and inner thigh and showed that younger patients had greater adipocyte viability in the lower abdomen than in the flank, whereas older patients did not show any differences. Younger lower abdominal fat showed superior adipocyte viability compared to older patients. However, flank fat had higher adipocyte viability in older patients. Patient weight did not appear to affect adipocyte viability.[30] In the only prospective study found specifically designed to examine the effect of patient factors on graft survival, Dendai et al identified several factors which impacted fat graft survival in patients with unilateral craniofacial contour deformities. The authors identified Parry–Romberg syndrome, previous craniofacial bone surgery, forehead unit, grafted volume, and older age as independently negative predictors of fat graft retention, whereas injection in the cheek unit was an independently positive predictor.[22] It therefore appears that age and underlying pathology of the recipient play a role in adipocyte viability and retention. Another factor that has been studied is exposure to radiation. Choi et al and Small et al found that prior radiation exposure did not significantly affect graft retention over time in breast reconstruction.[2,28] However, when radiation exposure was examined in a murine case–control trial by Garza et al, they found radiation to be significantly detrimental to graft survival.[27] Due to this discrepancy, further clinical trials specifically examining radiation exposure are warranted. The role of other factors like gender, smoking, obesity, diabetes, and hypertension on the impact of graft retention and adipocyte viability remains uncertain. Özalp and Çakmakoğlu looked into the impact of smoking on facial fat grafting in their 18-patient retrospective cohort study, and highlighted a low fat graft survival rate and reduced skin quality improvement; however, no controls were included.[19] Jung et al demonstrated in their murine model the negative impact of diabetes on graft retention and histological quality.[26] Whereas Herly et al showed in their long-term retention study that the only factor having a significant positive impact on graft retention was male gender.[29] Among the current literature, there is discrepancy of the impact of variables such as radiation exposure, age, and gender. Larger-scale, prospective human studies specifically examining multiple patient factors are required for the different applications of fat grafting.

Volume Retention Over Time

Animal studies have shown that active remodeling, resorption, and adipogenesis stabilize around the 12-week mark.[4,25] How this process of stabilization effects long-term volume retention has been observed in various clinical trials.[2,26,29,31,32]

Early photographic assessment supports the later observed laboratory kinetics, with facial grafting generally stabilizing around 3–4 months and breast grafting around 4–6 months, though there may be subtle volume decreases out to a year.[31,32] Denadai et al confirmed these findings in their study, showing with ultrasound measurements a steady decrease of soft tissue thickness over 3 months with no significant decrease after that point out to a year.[22]

Counter to these studies, Herly et al reached steady state point much later, as demonstrated by MRI analysis that loss of <5% original volume per year was not reached until 806 days after grafting.[29] However, this study was performed with en bloc fat grafted to the postauricular region, making it less applicable to routine clinical practice. On the other

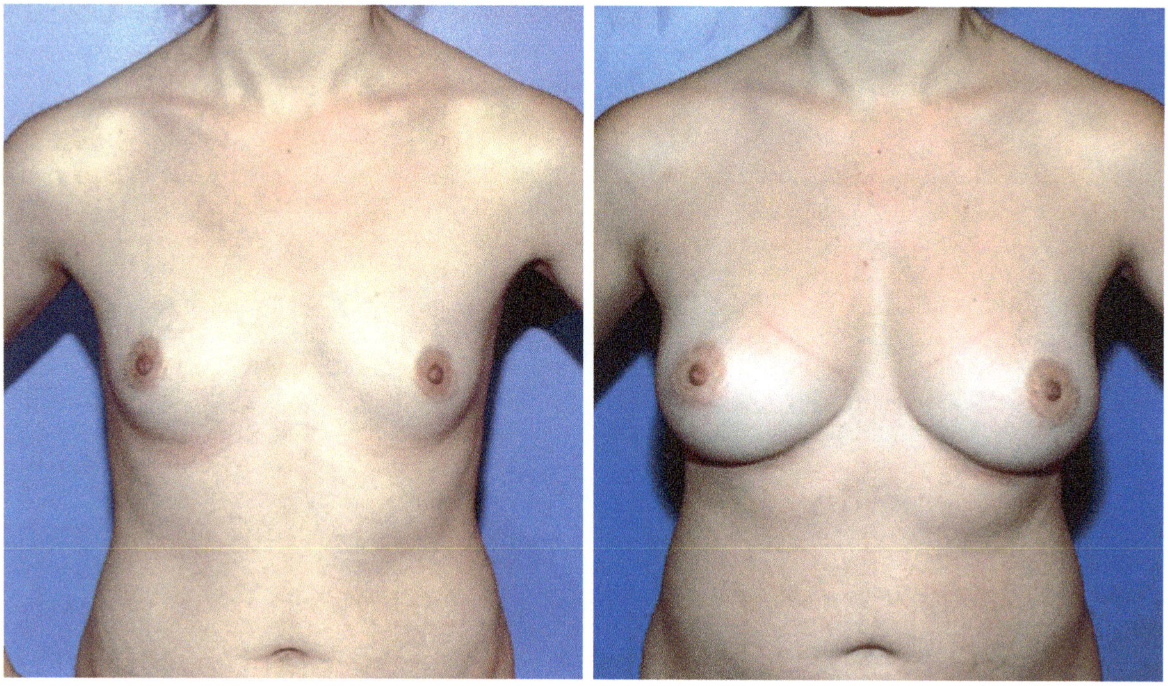

• **Fig. 70.1** Preoperative and 2.5 years postoperative photographs of bilateral breast augmentation using two rounds of fat grafting. Fat was harvested from the patient's abdomen, and bilateral thighs using 10-mL syringes and Coleman harvesting cannulas. The fat was processed in the standard manner using the Coleman technique. The first round required 232 mL of fat graft for the right breast and 230 mL for the left breast. The second round required 237.5 mL of fat graft for the right breast and 287 mL for the left breast. The patient has a lasting result of breast augmentation with improved breast contour.

hand, Choi et al's fat grafting results reached steady state sooner with larger volume breast grafts nearing stability closer to 49 days while small volumes continued to rapidly shrink out to 140 days.[28] All of the studies that qualified long-term retention found optimal results ranging from 51% to 68%.[19,29] These discrepancies in results require clarification with larger-scale prospective trials using lipofilling techniques.

Impact of Serial Fat Grafting

With the uncertainty of graft retention, varying use of multiple injections have been implemented.[2,33-35]

Serial fat grafting is often needed to correct deformities. A prime example is fat grafting for breast augmentation or reconstruction either with or without the use of a preexpansion device (Fig. 70.1). Khouri et al report using between 1 and 10 rounds of fat grafting at a minimum of 8-week intervals to achieve satisfactory results, noting needing more injections in delayed reconstruction and post-radiation patients, and higher volumes injected in later procedures.[34] Kim et al used fat grafting for secondary breast reconstruction, reporting about a quarter of their patients required reinjection due to inadequate volume.[33]

The ideal interval between grafting procedures remains unclear. Lim et al found no significant difference in symmetry outcomes when comparing patients undergoing serial fat grafting with short versus long intervals, though this result was obtained by comparing facial symmetry using 2D facial analysis.[2] Jiang et al used a 3D laser scanner to compare volume retention of serial grafts and found significantly higher retention in the second graft over the first in a pilot study of 13 patients.[35] While serial grafting is a frequently employed technique, information regarding its efficacy and predictability remain uncertain. Further information on who is a good candidate and respondent for serial fat grafting is crucial to ensure the appropriate technique is employed.

Role of ASCs in Fat Graft Survival

ASCs reside in the perivascular compartments of the stroma of adipose tissue and is part of the stromal vascular fraction (SVF), which contains various progenitor cells other than ASCs including pericytes, transit amplifying cells, and endothelial progenitor cells. Whether supplementing the lipoaspirate with SVF or ASCs or enriching these cells through centrifugation, all of these methods have enhanced fat graft retention and improved clinical outcomes by providing sites of adipogenesis in zones in which the graft would otherwise not survive as well as improving vascular support via endothelial cell proliferation.[4,36,37] Very strong preclinical and clinical evidence supports the benefit of ASC-enriched fat grafting. In a landmark study, Yoshimura et al introduced cell-assisted lipotransfer (CAL) or SVF-enriched fat grafting, and reported a very high graft retention in 40 patients undergoing breast augmentation with CAL.[37] Kølle et al conducted a triple-blinded randomized controlled trial of 10 patients receiving ASC-enriched or nonenriched fat grafting and showed improved graft retention, enhanced formation of connective tissue and reduced fat graft necrosis in ASC-enriched fat graft.[2] Tanikawa et al conducted a randomized controlled trial of 14 patients with craniofacial microsomia and ASC-enriched graft significantly improved volume retention at 6 months.[38] Koh et al found similar results in hemifacial atrophy secondary to Parry–Romberg disease though with ASCs that were derived by culture expansion.[39] The benefits of ASC-enriched fat graft are increasingly highlighted in the literature. However, before stem cell therapies can become mainstream, a higher level of scrutiny and regulation needs to take place to protect the safety of our patients.

Complications and Emerging Safety Concerns

Liposuction and fat grafting are usually well tolerated and very safe. Complications are very infrequent and most commonly minor in nature. Liposuction can lead to ecchymosis, edema, pain, and mild oozing, which normally are self-resolving. As mentioned above, inappropriate liposuction technique may lead to contour irregularities due to excessive and/or heterogenous aspiration. These can be prevented by careful and frequent reassessment of the harvested area. Fat grafting may also lead to minor complications like undercorrection, overcorrection, visible irregularities, graft resorption, migration of injected fat. More serious complications can infrequently occur, like infection or injury of underlying structures (e.g., muscle, nerve, glands) during the harvesting and grafting processes. Lastly, the most dreaded complication is embolization after intravascular injections which can lead to blindness (injections to the face), respiratory compromise or death (injection in the buttocks).

Gluteal fat grafting (GFG) for gluteal augmentation has become one of the fastest growing fields in cosmetic surgery, with its popularity growing dramatically in the USA over the past seven years, from 7382 procedures in 2011 to 23,115 procedures in 2017 (American Society for Aesthetic Plastic Surgeons statistics). This trend can be explained by an increased understanding of the female form, a growing role of the female buttocks as a secondary sexual characteristic in popular culture, and an evolving ethnic variation in the USA. Fat grafting is a technically challenging procedure and complication rates may increase if performed by inexperienced physicians. Along with this rise in number of GFG procedures, serious safety issues are evolving, with severe morbidity and mortality events publicized in the media. Although GFG has been performed across the globe for decades without safety concerns raised, the more recent expansion in case volume broadens the range of surgeons performing this procedure. Moreover, clinicians not trained in plastic surgery are performing GFG. It is estimated that as many as 25% more of these procedures are performed by practitioners other than plastic surgeons, facial plastic surgeons or dermatologists, resulting in a total of approximately 23,774 procedures performed in 2017 in the USA.[40] GFG can lead to serious complications, including death, which was found by the Aesthetic Surgery Education and Research Foundation (ASERF) Task Force to be between 1:2351 and 1:6241, many times higher than other plastic surgery procedures.[40] Autopsy findings indicate that the key technical problem is fat grafting material being introduced into major blood vessels (including the iliac veins) following tearing of the vessels with the cannulas. These fat parcels then travel around the body leading to fat embolism syndrome or pulmonary fat emboli. For this reason, understanding the location and relationship of the major vessels to the port sites and gluteal muscles is imperative. The superior and inferior gluteal veins drain into the internal iliac vein and can be 4 mm or more in diameter as they cross the glutei maximus and medius towards the iliac wing. Larger diameter veins (6 mm or more) may also be present near the sciatic notch, which divide into smaller perforators at the level of the gluteal muscle fascia to supply the subcutaneous tissue and skin.[40] Given the life-threatening association with GFG, the Multi-Society Gluteal Fat Grafting Task Force was created under the direction of Dan Mills, J. Peter Rubin and Renato Saltz, and found that all examined autopsies of deceased GFG patients shared common findings: (1) fat in the gluteal muscles; (2) fat beneath the muscles; (3) damage to the superior or inferior gluteal vein; (4) massive fat emboli in the heart and/or lungs. No post mortem has yet shown a cause of death with fat only in the subcutaneous space; this means that surgeons have injected more deeply than they had intended. The mechanism of death is presumed to be high pressure extravascular grafted fat entering the circulation via tears in the large gluteal veins with subsequent embolization to the heart and lungs. The Task Force proposed several recommendations to minimize morbidity and mortality, which are summarized in Table 70.1, but significant caution should be taken when performing this procedure to ensure patient safety.[41]

Conclusion

Liposuction and liposculpture has revolutionized how challenging contour irregularities and facial rejuvenation are tackled. Fat is an ideal filler given its biocompatibility, ease of harvest, and regenerative properties. A wide spectrum of studies explored the various facets of fat grafting from harvesting to injection technique. However, the surgeon should be mindful of the current literature to optimize adipocyte survival and graft retention, and should be aware of the emerging safety concerns. Many unanswered questions still remain, mostly due to the lack of coherence in surgical methodology, making interpretation of outcomes very challenging. Fat grafting is a common procedure performed by most surgeons and thus a methodical approach is needed to ensure patient safety and excellent outcomes.

TABLE 70.1 Multi-Society Gluteal Fat Grafting Task Force Recommendations on Gluteal Fat Grafting[41]

1.	Stay as far away from the gluteal veins and sciatic nerve as possible. Fat should only be grafted into the superficial planes, with the subcutaneous space considered safest. If the esthetic goal requires more fat than can be placed in the subcutaneous layer the surgeon should consider staging the procedure rather than injecting deep
2.	Concentrate on the position of the cannula tip throughout every stroke to assure there is no unintended deeper pass, particularly in the medial half of the buttock overlying the critical structures
3.	Use access incisions that best allow a superficial trajectory for each part of the buttock; avoid deep angulation of the cannula; and palpate externally with the nondominant hand to assure the cannula tip remains superficial
4.	Use instrumentation that offers control of the cannula; avoid bendable cannulas and mobile Luer connections. Vibrating injection cannulas may provide additional tactile feedback
5.	Injection should only be done while the cannula is in motion in order to avoid high pressure bolus injections
6.	The risk of death should be discussed with every prospective [GFG] patient

References

1. Coleman SR. The technique of periorbital lipoinfiltration. *Oper Tech Plast Reconstr Surg.* 1994;1:20–26.
2. Strong AL, Cederna PS, Rubin JP, et al. The current state of fat grafting: a review of harvesting, processing, and injection techniques. *Plast Reconstr Surg.* 2015;136(4):897–912.
3. Gause TM, Kling RE, Sivak WN, et al. Particle size in fat graft retention: a review on the impact of harvesting technique in lipofilling surgical outcomes. *Adipocyte.* 2014;3(4):273–279.
4. Kato H, Mineda K, Eto H, et al. Degeneration, regeneration, and cicatrization after fat grafting: dynamic total tissue remodeling during the first 3 months. *Plast Reconstr Surg.* 2014;133(3):303e–313e.
5. Bourne DA, James IB, Wang SS, et al. The architecture of fat grafting: what lies beneath the surface. *Plast Reconstr Surg.* 2016;137(3):1072–1079.
6. Kokai LE, Jones TL, Silowash R, et al. Optimization and standardization of the immunodeficient mouse model for assessing fat grafting outcomes. *Plast Reconstr Surg.* 2017;140(6):1185–1194.
7. Fisher C, Grahovac TL, Schafer ME, et al. Comparison of harvest and processing techniques for fat grafting and adipose stem cell isolation. *Plast Reconstr Surg.* 2013;132(2):351–361.
8. Pu LLQ, Coleman SR, Cui X, et al. Autologous fat grafts harvested and refined by the Coleman technique: a comparative study. *Plast Reconstr Surg.* 2008;122(3):932–937.
9. Yin S, Luan J, Fu S, et al. Does water-jet force make a difference in fat grafting? In vitro and in vivo evidence of improved lipoaspirate viability and fat graft survival. *Plast Reconstr Surg.* 2015;135(1):127–138.
10. Prado A, Andrades P, Danilla S, et al. A prospective, randomized, double-blind, controlled clinical trial comparing laser-assisted lipoplasty with suction-assisted lipoplasty. *Plast Reconstr Surg.* 2006;118(4):1032–1045.
11. Salinas HM, Broelsch GF, Fernandes JR, et al. Comparative analysis of processing methods in fat grafting. *Plast Reconstr Surg.* 2014;134(4):675–683.
12. Canizares OJ, Thomson JE, Allen RJJ, et al. The effect of processing technique on fat graft survival. *Plast Reconstr Surg.* 2017;140(5):933–943.
13. Bozkurt M, Kapı E, Şirinoğlu H, et al. The effects of the centrifugation speed on the survival of autogenous fat grafts in a rat model. *J Plast Surg Hand Surg.* 2016;50(3):161–166.
14. Girard A-C, Mirbeau S, Gence L, et al. Effect of washes and centrifugation on the efficacy of lipofilling with or without local anesthetic. *Plast Reconstr Surg Glob Open.* 2015;3(8):e496.
15. Coleman SR. Long-term survival of fat transplants: controlled demonstrations. *Aesthetic Plast Surg.* 1995;19(5):421–425.
16. Nguyen PSA, Desouches C, Gay AM, et al. Development of micro-injection as an innovative autologous fat graft technique: the use of adipose tissue as dermal filler. *J Plast Reconstr Aesthet Surg.* 2012;65(12):1692–1699.
17. Chung MT, Paik KJ, Atashroo DA, et al. Studies in fat grafting: part I. Effects of injection technique on in vitro fat viability and in vivo volume retention. *Plast Reconstr Surg.* 2014;134(1):29–38.
18. Luan A, Zielins ER, Wearda T, et al. Dynamic rheology for the prediction of surgical outcomes in autologous fat grafting. *Plast Reconstr Surg.* 2017;140(3):517–524.
19. Özalp B, Çakmakoğlu Ç. The effect of smoking on facial fat grafting surgery. *J Craniofac Surg.* 2017;28(2):449–453.
20. Shi Y, Yuan Y, Dong Z, et al. The fate of fat grafts in different recipient areas: subcutaneous plane, fat pad, and muscle. *Dermatol Surg.* 2016;42(4):535–542.
21. Karacaoglu E, Kizilkaya E, Cermik H, et al. The role of recipient sites in fat-graft survival: experimental study. *Ann Plast Surg.* 2005;55(1):63–68; discussion 68.
22. Denadai R, Raposo-Amaral CA, Pinho AS, et al. Predictors of autologous free fat graft retention in the management of craniofacial contour deformities. *Plast Reconstr Surg.* 2017;140(1):50e–61e.
23. Lee JW, Han YS, Kim SR, et al. A rabbit model of fat graft recipient site preconditioning using external negative pressure. *Arch Plast Surg.* 2015;42(2):150–158.
24. Sezgin B, Ozmen S, Bulam H, et al. Improving fat graft survival through preconditioning of the recipient site with microneedling. *J Plast Reconstr Aesthet Surg.* 2014;67(5):712–720.
25. Kato H, Araki J, Doi K, et al. Normobaric hyperoxygenation enhances initial survival, regeneration, and final retention in fat grafting. *Plast Reconstr Surg.* 2014;134(5):951–959.
26. Jung JA, Kim YW, Cheon YW, et al. Effects of the diabetic condition on grafted fat survival: an experimental study using streptozotocin-induced diabetic rats. *Arch Plast Surg.* 2014;41(3):241–247.
27. Garza RM, Paik KJ, Chung MT, et al. Studies in fat grafting: part III. Fat grafting irradiated tissue: improved skin quality and decreased fat graft retention. *Plast Reconstr Surg.* 2014;134(2):249–257.
28. Choi M, Small K, Levovitz C, et al. The volumetric analysis of fat graft survival in breast reconstruction. *Plast Reconstr Surg.* 2013;131(2):185–191.

29. Herly M, Ørholt M, Glovinski PV, et al. Quantifying long-term retention of excised fat grafts: a longitudinal, retrospective cohort study of 108 patients followed for up to 8.4 years. *Plast Reconstr Surg.* 2017;139(5):1223–1232.
30. Geissler PJ, Davis K, Roostaeian J, et al. Improving fat transfer viability: the role of aging, body mass index, and harvest site. *Plast Reconstr Surg.* 2014;134(2):227–232.
31. Coleman SR. Structural fat grafting: more than a permanent filler. *Plast Reconstr Surg.* 2006;118(suppl 3):108S–120S.
32. Coleman SR, Saboeiro AP. Fat grafting to the breast revisited: safety and efficacy. *Plast Reconstr Surg.* 2007;119(3):775–785.
33. Kim HY, Jung BK, Lew DH, et al. Autologous fat graft in the reconstructed breast: fat absorption rate and safety based on sonographic identification. *Arch Plast Surg.* 2014;41(6):740–747.
34. Khouri RK, Rigotti G, Khouri RK, et al. Tissue-engineered breast reconstruction with Brava-assisted fat grafting: a 7-year, 488-patient, multicenter experience. *Plast Reconstr Surg.* 2015;135(3):643–658.
35. Jiang T, Xie Y, Zhu M, et al. The second fat graft has significantly better outcome than the first fat graft for Romberg syndrome: a study of three-dimensional volumetric analysis. *J Plast Reconstr Aesthet Surg.* 2016;69(12):1621–1626.
36. James IB, Coleman SR, Rubin JP. Fat, stem cells, and platelet-rich plasma. *Clin Plast Surg.* 2016;43(3):473–488.
37. Yoshimura K, Sato K, Aoi N, et al. Cell-assisted lipotransfer for cosmetic breast augmentation: supportive use of adipose-derived stem/stromal cells. *Aesthetic Plast Surg.* 2008;32(1):48–55; discussion 56–57.
38. Tanikawa DYS, Aguena M, Bueno DF, et al. Fat grafts supplemented with adipose-derived stromal cells in the rehabilitation of patients with craniofacial microsomia. *Plast Reconstr Surg.* 2013;132(1):141–152.
39. Koh KS, Oh TS, Kim H, et al. Clinical application of human adipose tissue-derived mesenchymal stem cells in progressive hemifacial atrophy (Parry–Romberg disease) with microfat grafting techniques using 3-dimensional computed tomography and 3-dimensional camera. *Ann Plast Surg.* 2012;69(3):331–337.
40. Mofid MM, Teitelbaum S, Suissa D, et al. Report on mortality from gluteal fat grafting: recommendations from the ASERF Task Force. *Aesthet Surg J.* 2017;37(7):796–806.
41. Inter-Society Gluteal Fat Grafting Task Force. Multi-Society Gluteal Fat Grafting Task Force issues safety advisory urging practitioners to reevaluate technique. [Internet] https://www.surgery.org/sites/default/files/Gluteal-Fat-Grafting-02-06-18_0.pdf.

71 Abdominoplasty and Body Contouring

DIRK F. RICHTER AND TOBIAS HEUFT

Anatomy

An excellent knowledge of the entire anatomy of the lower trunk and extremities is essential for esthetic and reconstructive skin-tightening procedures. In addition to knowledge of the main perforating vessels, the course of important nerves is mandatory to avoid postoperative complications. Furthermore, the knowledge of Langer's lines (relaxed skin tension lines) is crucial for the best possible scar development.[1]

Skin

Abdominal skin and fat tend to become distributed in the lower abdomen with aging and pregnancy. Striae also become common, especially as a result of multiple pregnancies, resulting in a rupture and separation of dermal collagen with consequent skin thinning. Following postbariatric weight loss, patients have been shown to have damaged skin in recent studies evaluating the content and structure of collagen and elastin when compared to nonbariatric patients.[2]

The skin of the abdomen has areas of increased adherence to the underlying fascia ("zones of adherence") in the vertical midline area, and occasionally in a horizontal direction just superior to the umbilicus (supraumbilical skin fold), as well as in a horizontal direction above the anterior superior iliac crest.

Fascia

The abdominal subcutaneous tissue is divided by two layers of fascia: the superficial Camper's fascia and the deep Scarpa's fascia, a strong fibrous layer of connective tissue which is continuous with the fascia lata of the thigh.

Fat

The superficial fat layer has a more compact character with smaller lobules and a rich vascularization, while the deeper fat stains larger lobules with a more scattered pattern.[3]

The Umbilicus

In most patients, the umbilicus is the most important landmark on the abdominal wall. It is normally situated in the midline, approximately 9–12 cm above the upper border of the mons pubis region. A round or ellipsoid shape may characterize it. The abdominal fascia in this region can present as weak with an increased incidence for hernias. The blood supply derives from branches of the subdermal plexus, from both deep inferior epigastric arteries, as well as a blood supply from the median umbilical ligament. In general, the umbilical stalk is blunted and dissociated from the surrounding fat tissue.

Musculoaponeurotic System

The abdominal musculature includes four paired muscles: the rectus abdominis, connected in the median linea alba, the external oblique and internal oblique, and the transversus abdominis muscle, which incorporate into the anterior and posterior rectus sheath at the linea semilunaris. The rectus abdominis muscles are enclosed by an anterior and posterior sheath, originating at the infracostal margin and attaching at the symphysis pubis. Above the arcuate line (situated approximately midway between umbilicus and pubic symphysis), the anterior rectus sheath is formed by the external oblique and internal oblique aponeurosis, whereas the posterior rectus sheath is formed by the internal oblique and transversus aponeurosis. Below the arcuate line, the posterior rectus sheath is absent, except for the transversus fascia and the peritoneum. At the inferior aspect of the rectus muscles, the pyramidalis muscles are present in 80%–90% of patients (Fig. 71.1).

Lymphatic Drainage

The abdominal lymphatic system is divided into supraumbilical drainage to the ipsilateral axillary lymph nodes and an infraumbilical drainage into the superficial inguinal lymph nodes. The lymph vessels in the infraumbilical area pass through the sub-Scarpal plane, emphasizing the importance of Scarpa's fascia preservation in abdominal wall surgery.

Blood Supply

The blood supply to the abdominal wall is derived from numerous major arteries of the thorax and pelvic region; these

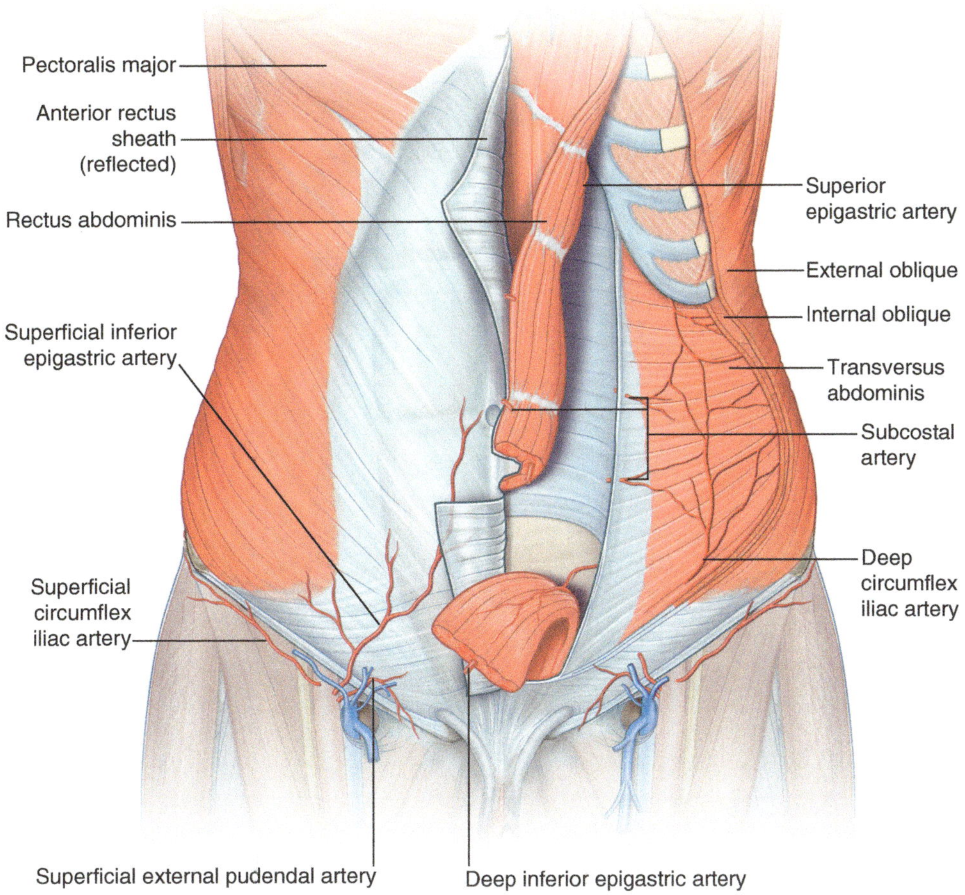

• **Fig. 71.1** Anatomy of the abdominal musculature with abdominal blood supply. (From Richter DF, Schwaiger N. Abdominoplasty procedures. In: Rubin JP, Neligan PC, eds. *Plastic Surgery*. Volume 2: *Aesthetic Surgery*, 4th edn. Philadelphia: Elsevier; 2018: Fig. 23.2A.)

communicate through many anastomotic interconnections. Two types of cutaneous blood supply are known: direct vessels that supply the skin directly and indirect perforating vessels that emerge from the deep fascia as terminal spent branches of arteries whose main purpose is to supply the muscles and other deep tissues. Moon and Taylor were able to demonstrate connections between the deep superior and deep inferior epigastric systems and their relationship to the cutaneous circulation.[4–6]

A detailed knowledge of the arterial supply of the abdominal wall is crucial to abdominal wall surgery, especially in cases of prior abdominal wall surgery. Huger described different zones of the abdominal blood supply which should guide the surgeon in planning and performing a safe operation.[4] Huger defined zone I of the abdominal wall as the area that is fed anteriorly by the vertically oriented deep epigastric arcade. Zone III was defined as the lateral aspect of the abdominal wall (flanks) that are fed by the six lateral intercostal and four lumbar arteries. The lower abdominal circulation is provided by the superficial epigastric, superficial external pudendal, and superficial circumflex iliac systems (zone II). A rich plexus between these systems allows collateral flow (see Fig. 71.1, Fig. 71.2).

In standard abdominoplasty procedures, the blood supply to zone I and main parts of zone II is disrupted after flap mobilization, resulting in an abdominal flap perfusion mainly supplied by zone III. The lateral perforating branches from the lateral intercostals and lumbar arteries are essential for the remaining flap perfusion. Therefore, it is crucial to study any preoperative existing scar, such as subcostal cholecystectomy incisions (see Fig. 71.2).

Nerve Supply

The sensibility of the abdominal wall derives from the anterior and lateral cutaneous branches of the eight to twelfth intercostal nerves, which reach the skin and fascia by passing between the internal oblique and transversus abdominis muscles and finally through the rectus abdominis muscle. The lateral cutaneous branches penetrate the intercostal muscles in the midaxillary line, ending in the subcutaneous layer.

The motor branches of the rectus abdominis muscle derive from lateral branches of the fifth to twelfth intercostal nerves, which pass behind the rectus muscles and enter the muscles at the junction of the lateral third and medial two-thirds. The oblique and transversus abdominis muscle are innervated by branches from the lower thoracic and lumbar dorsal nerves (Fig. 71.3).[5]

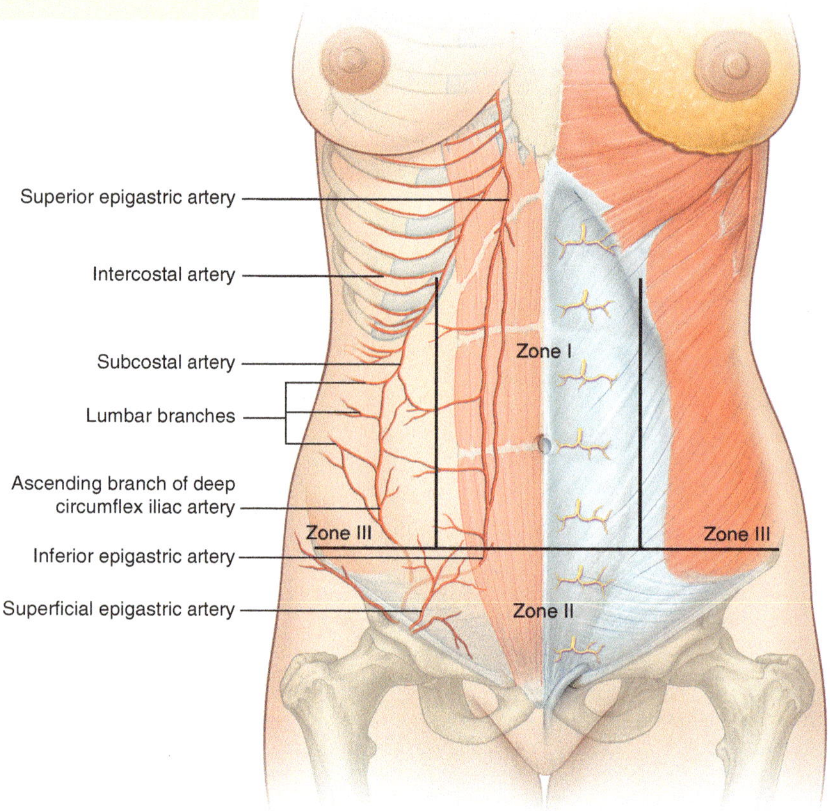

• **Fig. 71.2** Huge's zones of superficial abdominal blood supply. (From Richter DF, Schwaiger N. Abdominoplasty procedures. In: Rubin JP, Neligan PC, eds. *Plastic Surgery.* Volume 2: *Aesthetic Surgery*, 4th edn. Philadelphia: Elsevier, 2018: Fig. 23.4.)

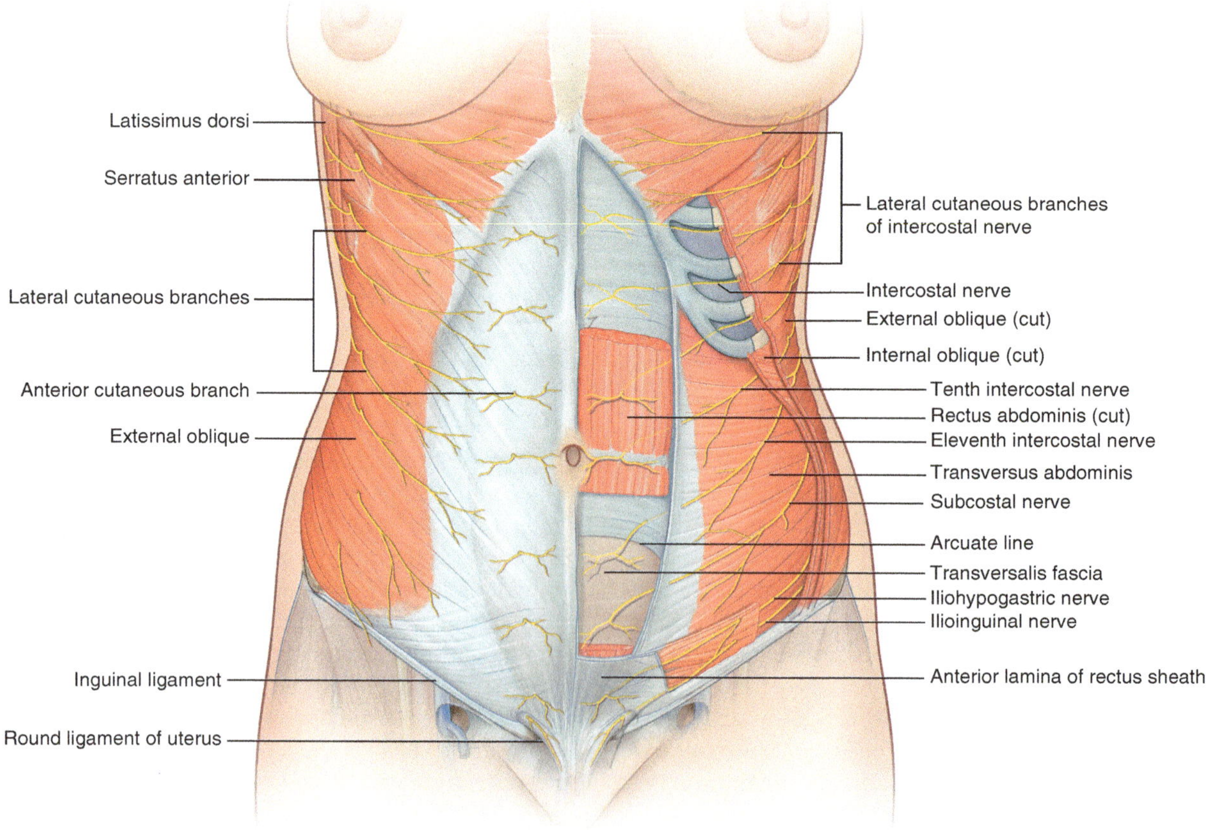

• **Fig. 71.3** Anatomical nerve supply. (From Richter DF, Schwaiger N. Abdominoplasty procedures. In: Rubin JP, Neligan PC, eds. *Plastic Surgery*. Volume 2: *Aesthetic Surgery*, 4th edn. Philadelphia: Elsevier; 2018: Fig. 23.5.)

Peripheral nerves such as the iliohypogastric and ilioinguinal must be noted, as they may be injured in lateral transverse lower abdominal incisions, resulting in consistent loss of sensory in the area of the groin and medioventral thigh.

Anatomical Landmarks

Normal abdominal anatomical proportions (Fig. 71.4):

- The umbilicus is located in line with the most superior point of the iliac crest in 99% of patients.
- Distance between the top of mons and anterior valvar commissure (*A*): average height is 5–7 cm.
- Distance between umbilicus and top of mons (*A*+*B*): average height is 11–13 cm.
- Distance between umbilicus and top of anterior and vulvar commissure (*C*=*D*).

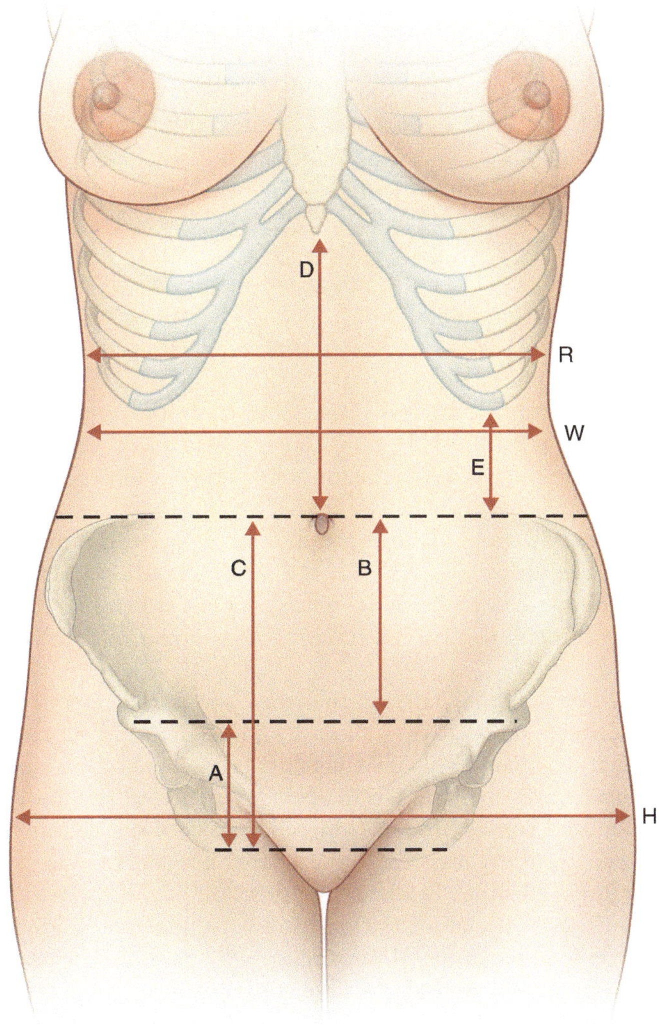

• **Fig. 71.4** Anatomical landmarks (see text) with normal anatomical proportions. (From Richter DF, Schwaiger N. Abdominoplasty procedures. In: Rubin JP, Neligan PC, eds. *Plastic Surgery*. Volume 2: *Aesthetic Surgery*, 4th edn. Philadelphia: Elsevier; 2018: Fig. 23.1.)

- Distance between the costal marginal and the iliac crest (*E*). The proportion of this distance to the width of the base of the rib cage (*R*) determines whether the patient is long-waisted or short-waisted. The normal proportion (*E*:*R*) is roughly 1:3 (long-waisted approaches 1:2, short-waisted approaches 1:3).
- The rib cage tapers inferiorly. A narrower lower rib cage relative to the width under the armpits helps to emphasize the waist by creating a subtle V.
- Hip width (*H*). A wider pelvis than rib cage emphasizes the waist; the waist is more defined when *R*<*H*.
- Natural waist (*W*) – the narrowest point of the torso. (Note that the umbilicus usually sits below the natural waist by about 1–4 cm.) Relative to the hips, this waist-to-hip (*W*:*H*) ratio in healthy women is roughly 0.72:1; in healthy men, it is roughly 0.83:1. Note that the natural contour of the healthy abdomen reveals a subtle epigastric sagittal depression transitioning to a mild infraumbilical convexity. A subtle vertical sulcus at the lateral rectus border, which is more distinct in a muscular person, may also be seen (see Fig. 71.4).[7]

Esthetic Assessment

Abdominal Wall

The esthetic assessment of the abdominal wall includes:

- Regions of local adipose tissue and their thickness in centimeters
- Local adipose tissue in the upper and central abdominal region
- Regions of local skin excess
- Local skin excess in the upper and central abdominal region
- Presence of skin folds and their depths
- Areas of maximal looseness and adherence
- Local adipose tissue in the adjoining regions of the flanks, hips and breasts
- Local adipose tissue in the mons pubis region
- Skin laxity in the mons pubis region
- Any asymmetric aspects
- Any bulginess
- Any preexisting scars and their quality
- Presence and degree of striae.

Umbilicus

The esthetic assessment of the umbilicus includes:

- Shape and depth of the umbilical stalk
- Position of the umbilical basis on the abdominal wall (to be demonstrated to the patient)
- Height of umbilical descent
- Any existing umbilical herniation or adipose tumor
- Any existing eczema, hyperpigmentation or preexisting scars
- Any prior operation in the umbilical region has to be clarified, since impaired perfusion after dissection may occur in these cases.

Back, Thighs, and Buttocks

The esthetic assessment of the back, thigh, and buttocks includes:

- Regions of local adipose tissue and their thickness in centimeters in the back
- Mobility of the dorsal skin in the lower back region
- Local skin excess m the back region
- Presence of dorsal skin folds and their depth
- Local adipose tissue in the gluteal region
- Regions of local skin excess, measured by pinching in vertical distance in the gluteal and flank region
- Presence of gluteal skin folds and their depths
- Areas of maximal looseness and adherence
- Local adipose tissue in the anterior, posterior, lateral and inner thigh region
- Skin laxity in all thigh regions
- Presence of skin folds in the thigh region (e.g., inner thigh, distal anterior)
- Any asymmetric aspects
- Any bulginess
- Any preexisting scars and their quality
- Any existing eczema or hyperpigmentations
- Presence and degree of striae.

Patient Assessment

History

During the first consultation a review of the patient's medical history is mandatory. We recommend a review of this prior to surgery, when it is performed with a delay from the first consultation and at least annually. The assessment of medical history includes the current weight, the ABSI (a body shape index) and body mass index (BMI), the weight history with weight fluctuations and constancy periods, the frequency of exercises, former bariatric procedures, nutritional disorders, medication, the number of pregnancies and children, history of cesarean section, abdominal surgeries and abdominal hernias, gastrointestinal, cardiac, and pulmonary history, a smoking history, and any existing coagulation disorder. Patients should be asked specifically about previous liposuction in the abdominal area, often overlooked by patients in past surgical history.

Physical Examination

Physical examination is part of every medical history assessment. It evaluates the entire region the patient is concerned about. An examination of the skin tissue and the different fat layers is performed by pinching and measuring the subcutaneous layer thickness. Skin quality with the presence of striae should be noted, clarifying with the patient that supraumbilical striae will not be resected in abdominoplasty procedures (except for fleur-de-lis procedures). In this context, it is helpful to handout of studies on skin quality in postbariatric patients who have demonstrated damage to collagen structures.[8,9]

It is important to assess and measure the lower and upper abdominal pannus, documenting any existing eczema or consequent hyperpigmentation. The entire skin excess in the areas inferior to the lower abdominal fold, in the area of the lateral and upper abdomen, the waist, hips and thighs, as well as the lower chest, have to be included in the preoperative assessment, during upright standing, supine, as well as sitting positions. Any preexisting scars (subcostal, midline, horizontal) in the abdominal area have to be documented, since they can impair the blood supply. Furthermore, the status of the abdominal musculature should be assessed and any existing rectus diastasis, incisional, epigastric or umbilical hernia excluded. Supportive CT or MRI scans may be considered.

In this context, it is mandatory to evaluate intraabdominal pressure to avoid any postoperative pressure increase or abdominal compartment syndrome. In cases of elevated intraabdominal pressure, in the supine position, the abdominal wall elevates above the costal margin and the level of the iliac crest. Abdominoplasty procedures, especially with fascial reconstruction, have to be performed cautiously in such cases. In these cases, it is mandatory to wear a compression girdle for at least 8–12 weeks prior to surgery to improve and adapt the body to the postoperative situation and to prevent respiratory difficulties.

Documentation

It is mandatory to ensure a complete medical photographic documentation pre- and postoperatively, consisting of different views (anterior, oblique, side, and posterior). Postoperative photo documentation should be made at 3, 9, and 12 months. In individual cases it is recommended to perform additional photo documentation of standard arm and thigh positions, tissue characteristics with relaxed and contracted muscles, the patient in sitting position to demonstrate redundant upper abdominal laxity and tissue excess, additional views with the patient holding up and pinching excess tissue in the specific region or bending forward to demonstrate skin excess in the upper abdominal region.

Informing the patients in detail about the operative procedure, alternative techniques, and the general and operation-related risks and benefits is an essential part of preoperative documentation. Besides standard and individualized consent forms, which have to be reviewed and signed by the patient at the earliest opportunity and at the latest 24 hours prior to the operation, we recommend an audiovisual demonstration for exact understanding. In general, we recommend informing every patient transparently about any and all possible complications. Moreover, patients have to be informed about their postoperative care, including their expected level of activity, and the limitations of the surgical result in cases of existing variables of bone structure, fat distribution, and any existing scars.[10–12]

Esthetics

The preoperative esthetic status of the body region of concern has to be well documented in written and photographic format after a precise physical examination. For a classification of the different deformities, we found the Pittsburgh Rating Scale to be helpful for patient demonstration and selection of the best operative approach.[13] However, we have experienced a wider indication for the combined technique of liposuction and excisional procedures in all body regions.

General

Patients are advised to stabilize their weight for at least 6–12 months preoperatively; any desired weight loss should be completed prior to the surgery. Smokers should stop smoking at least 6 weeks prior to surgery and continue for 6 weeks after surgery.

Where a postoperative blood transfusion is considered (e.g., body lifts), patients have to be informed preoperatively, as this requires a blood typing and informed consent and the possibility of an autologous blood transfusion should be discussed. Anticoagulant drugs and supplements must be avoided 14 days prior to surgery. In cases of a planned abdominal procedure, we advise patients to perform bowel purgation the night before surgery. In some cases, patients can be restricted to a fluid diet for 24 hours prior to surgery.

Patients have to be informed about the intraoperative procedures, including any change of position with the risks of postoperative complication, antithrombotic prophylaxis, urinary catheter, drains, and garment placement, as well as patient-controlled analgesia (PCA). Moreover, they have to be instructed about the postoperative course, regarding thromboembolism prevention (we administer dalteparin 5000 IU perioperatively and daily for at least 2 weeks), respiratory exercises, early mobilization, avoidance of high abdominal pressure maneuvers, the estimated time point for drain and/or suture removal, as well as the minimum time required off work and abstinence from exercise. Length of inpatient admission must be discussed with patients where surgery cannot be performed in an outpatient setting, Diabetes may be considered a relative contraindication to this procedure, especially in poorly controlled patients. Staging procedures may be necessary to improve patient safety and to improve outcomes. An inspection of the abdominal skin and umbilicus areas for local skin irritation during consultation, and immediately prior to the operation, is strongly advisable.

Prophylaxis for deep venous thrombosis (DVT) and pulmonary embolus (PE) is an essential consideration in all patients, especially in smokers and patients taking birth control medications or hormone replacement therapy.[14] We inform patients that this specific risk will be decreased if hormonal therapy is discontinued 3–4 weeks prior to surgery and until at least 14 days after surgery.

In cases of an existing extended diastasis or hernia, the reconstruction of the fascia results in an increased intraabdominal pressure, which may be a source of respiratory difficulties. Therefore, we advise preoperative breathing exercises (utilizing an incentive spirometer) beginning 1–2 weeks prior to and continuing for 2 weeks after the surgery or, as described above, the application of a compression girdle for 8–12 weeks prior to surgery. A cold, dry cough or any kind of respiratory infections should lead to postponement of surgery, since fits of coughing may provoke a rupture of the fascial sutures with consequent secondary bleeding.[9,10,15]

Operative Principles and Approach

Various procedures are available with various indications as listed in Table 71.1.

Liposuction

The indication for sole liposuction of the abdomen is seen very rarely. In patients with an abdominal contour impaired by an irregular and solely thickened abdominal fat layer, liposuction may improve the abdominal shape dramatically.

TABLE 71.1 Indication for Different Techniques Dependent on Redundant Adipose Tissue

	Mini	Standard	HLT	Fleur-de-Lis	Bodylift	Reverse
Lower abdomen	+	+++	+++	+++	+++	0
Periumbilical	(+)	++	++	+++	++	(+)
Upper abdomen	0	++	++	+++	++	+++
Diastasis/hernia	(+)	++	++	+++	++	(+)
Flanks/hips/thighs	0	(+)	+	++	+++	0

From Moon HK, Taylor GL. The vascular anatomy of rectus abdominis musculocutaneous taps based on the deep superior epigastric System. *Plast Reconstr Surg*. 1988;82(5):815–832.

Nevertheless, as soon as a patient highlights his or her frustration due to a laxity of skin, it will not be worthwhile to perform liposuction without simultaneous skin excision. Ideal cases for liposuction are patients with localized adipose tissue in the flank/hip region, the infra- and/or supraumbilical region. They can be optimally treated by liposuction under local anesthesia as an outpatient. For achievement of maximum outcomes, it could be reasonable to acquire one of the assisted liposuction techniques nowadays available (e.g., laser-, ultrasonic- or radiofrequency-assisted liposuction), which allow simultaneous skin tightening. It should be clarified with patients that such a procedure can result in a higher risk of complications if an abdominoplasty is performed afterwards.

In all cases of liposuction in the abdominal region it is mandatory to exclude any existing rectus diastasis or abdominal hernia. If required, diagnostics may include an ultrasonic scan, CT or MRI (Fig. 71.5).

Any adjunctive liposuction of the abdominal wall should be performed at the beginning of the abdominoplasty procedure in order to sufficiently thin out the different layers, including the subfascial and, carefully, the epifascial layer.[16] It is important to assess the relation of excess skin and fatty tissue, since in cases of extensive skin excess in the upper and midabdominal region a fleur-de-lis procedure may be indicated. In these cases, there is usually no necessity for liposuction in the abdominal region, since a maximal amount of abdominal tissue is resected.

Adjoining regions (e.g., the flanks and hips) may be treated by liposuction during the abdominoplasty procedure, preferably at the end of the operation. Infiltration of tumescence solution should be performed at the beginning of the procedure and liposuction can then be performed after a sufficient time of exposure during the abdominoplasty procedure.[6,11]

Standard Abdominoplasty

The standard abdominoplasty is one of the most common procedures in plastic surgery. It enables the simultaneous treatment of the upper abdomen, periumbilical area, and lower abdomen, with optimally concealable scars.

Traditional abdominoplasty procedures involved wide mobilization of the abdominal wall up to the costal arch in order to ensure a tension-free wound closure. Multiple studies have since demonstrated that circulatory disturbance of the abdominal skin flap is the result of extensive undermining and destruction of the lateral perforators of Huger's zone III. In modern abdominoplasty, undermining cranially to the umbilicus is mainly performed in the midline area anterior to the linea alba and both rectus muscles, including the zones of

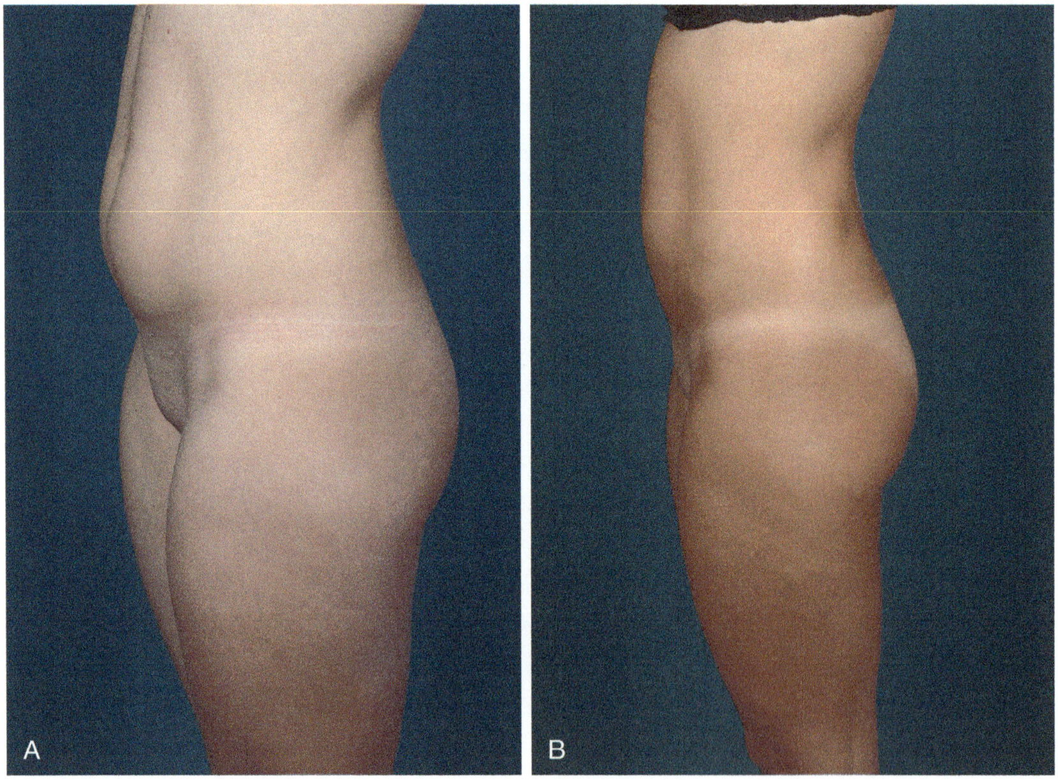

• **Fig. 71.5** (A) A 30-year-old woman with preoperative local adipose tissue in the lower abdomen without significant skin surplus. (B) Six months after water-jet-assisted liposuction of 750 mL fat tissue.

adhesion described by Lockwood and specified by Aly. The lateral abdominal flap may be securely released by additional liposuction or the Lockwood dissector for discontinuous undermining, preserving the lateral perforators and the lateral attachment to the rectus abdominus muscles.[17–20]

The standard abdominoplasty is indicated in patients that typically demonstrate a localized and diet-resistant adiposity of the abdominal wall in combination with coexisting slack and atonic skin, such as patients after multiple pregnancies, patients with weakness of the connective tissue or patients after weight loss (Fig. 71.6).

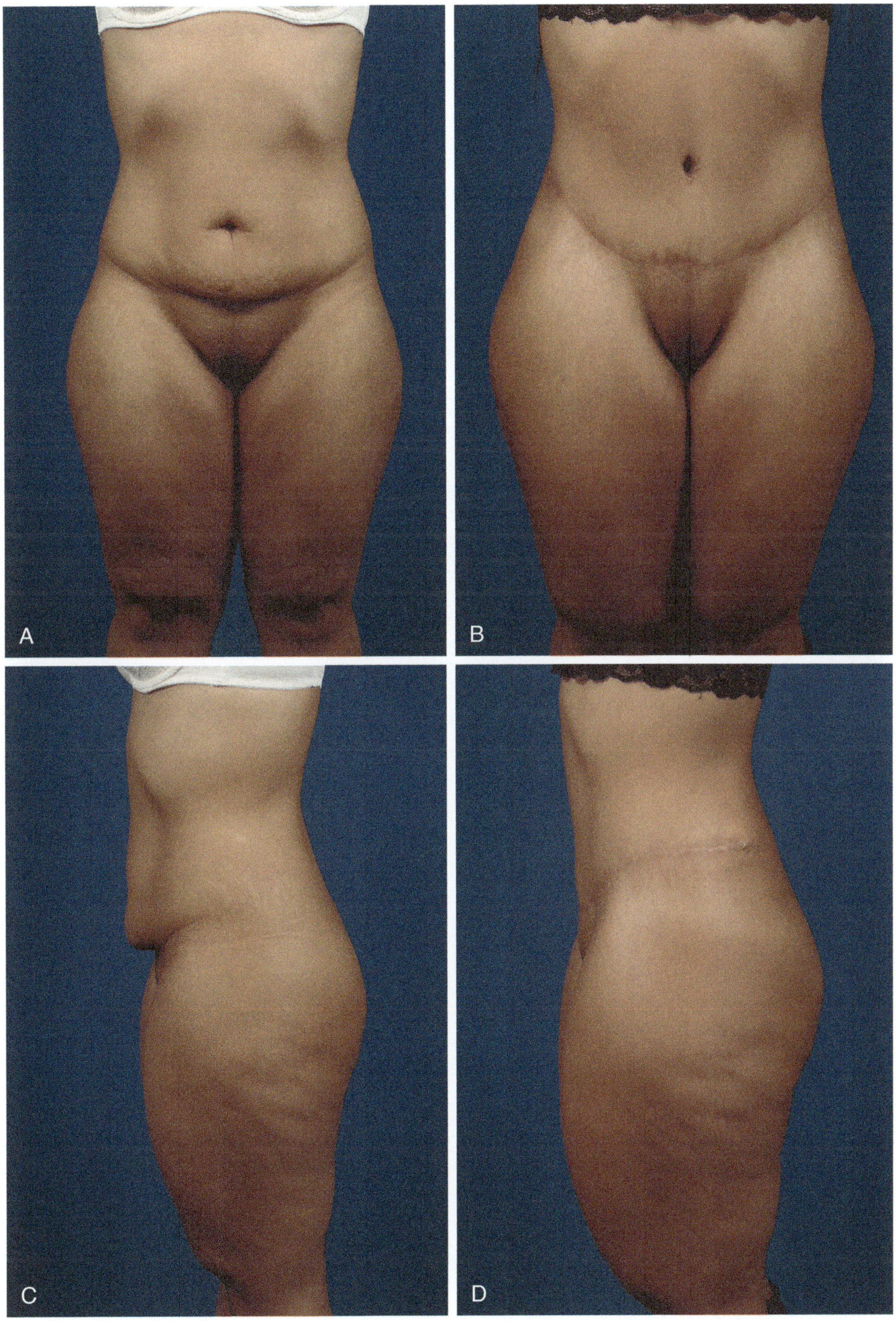

• **Fig. 71.6** (A,C) A 27-year-old woman with significant abdominal pannus after 60 kg weight loss. (B,D) One year after a standard abdominoplasty with a good contouring of the umbilical region.

Markings

The markings are started in the upright position with the midline, the borders of the patient's underwear and the expected and desired scar position. Next, the patient is asked to elevate the redundant abdominal tissue for identification of the abdominal fold. A vertical distance of 6 cm is measured from the upper vulvar commissure to the lower incision, followed by marking of the lower incision line parallel to the abdominal fold. By pinching of the abdominal tissue, the upper incision line is marked next, which can be checked in supine position. It is advisable to mark parallel lines at various heights to ensure a symmetric resection. The patient should always be informed about the risk of an inverted T-scar in the midline if the resection does not completely include the umbilical incision.

Evaluation of possible preexisting hernias and diastasis should be performed and marked in the supine position. Furthermore, the length of the scar line may be measured bilaterally starting from the midline to ensure symmetry. In this context the surgeon has to be aware that a longer inferior incision will lead to a gently curved upward course of the scar (Baroudi) and a longer superior incision will cause a straighter or downward course of the scar (Pitanguy).[21,22]

Technique

The operation is started with a repetitive check and trace of the markings. It has to be ensured that the umbilical stalk is thoroughly cleaned. Perioperative antibiotic prophylaxis should be given to all patients with longer operations such as abdominoplastys, lower bodylifts or thigh lifts, as well as sequential calf compressors and DVT prophylaxis.

The lower incision line is infiltrated with local anesthetics to reduce postoperative pain and the consequent risk of blood pressure increase. The lower incision line is carried down to Scarpa's fascia with ligation of superficial epigastric vessels. For adequate preparation of Scarpa's fascia, we recommend use of the Colorado Microneedle (Stryker CMF) and to ensure a sufficient upward pull of the abdominal flap. By preservation of Scarpa's fascia, the subjacent lymphatic vessels are preserved. In general, we find a thin fat layer below Scarpa's fascia. Continuous dissection superficial to Scarpa's fascia is performed cranially up to a level as wide as 3–4 fingerbreadths inferior to the umbilicus. At this level, Scarpa's fascia is incised, and dissection continues down the anterior rectus sheath.

At the umbilical level, the abdominal flap is incised in the midline and the umbilical stalk is completely mobilized (skeletonized without any remaining fat tissue) from the abdominal flap. In patients after massive weight loss, the umbilical stalk has to be shortened and fixated to the anterior rectus fascia retaining the stalk's base, preferably with absorbable sutures at 3, 6, 9, and 12 o'clock positions. Further dissection continues superiorly on the anterior rectus fascia strictly over the rectus abdominus muscles up to the xiphoid. The linea alba can easily be identified as it is distinctively connected to Scarpa's fascia. In the area of the costal margin, it is essential to preserve the lateral perforators for sufficient flap perfusion. The abdominal flap is now sufficiently mobilized in cases of concomitant rectus diastasis, the plication of the anterior rectus sheath from the xiphoid to the symphysis is accomplished using nonabsorbable or absorbable suture material in any preferred technique. In case of a diastasis at the lower abdomen, Scarpa's fascia and underlying tissue may be bluntly mobilized to allow for further midline fascial plication (Fig. 71.7). For cases of asymmetrically located umbilical stalk or for further accentuation of waist tightening, an additional paramedian plication of the anterior rectus sheath may be facilitated. Since lateral dissection is avoided up to the costal arch for preservation of the lateral perforators, a discontinuous separation of lateral adhesions using Lockwood's dissector may improve flap mobilization.

In selected patients with a pronounced abdominal fat layer the fatty tissue beneath Scarpa's fascia should be resected in the entire mobilized area. This may avoid postoperative complications due to infected fat necrosis. After repeated meticulous hemostasis, Scarpa's fascia is sutured down to the anterior rectus fascia with absorbable progressive tension sutures, starting superior to the umbilicus. Alternatively, the supraumbilical subcutaneous tissue may be sutured in the midline to the anterior rectus fascia to accentuate a midline depression for superior esthetics. The new umbilical position is estimated and marked. Several umbilical incision patterns have been described; we prefer the superior-based inverted V or U incision. This umbilical section of the abdominal flap is then circumferentially defatted for a circular umbilical depression. The supraumbilical midline may also be reduced through midline liposuction or open excision. After the umbilical stalk is pulled through the new umbilical tunnel, additional progressive tension sutures are placed in the lower flap area. For tissue resection, bullet forceps or a Pitanguy tissue demarcator can support the estimation of the upper resection line. Further evaluation of the amount of resection may be facilitated by additional vertical flap incisions and temporary wound closure utilizing bullet forceps or skin staples. The upper incision line is then marked and the resection is performed oblique to the wound edge in a 45-degree angle to enable a more precise adaptation of varyingly thick layers.

Finally, the patient is bent into the beach-chair position and temporary wound closure is performed with bullet forceps, starting lateral to medial. To avoid dog-ears, the longer superior wound edge is shifted slightly medially to adapt to the shorter inferior. After the placement of 2–3 drains the final wound closure is performed for all layers, starting with a reconstruction of the superficial fascial layer with absorbable sutures, followed by the subcutaneous layer and completed with intradermal running sutures. To reduce operating time in wound closure we recommend the use of absorbable barbed sutures (e.g., Quill; Surgical Specialties) such as PDO 2×0 for fascial and subcutaneous closure and Monoderm 3×0 for intradermal closure. Alternatively, skin closure time can be drastically reduced by closing the deeper wound layers and applying the two-component skin closure

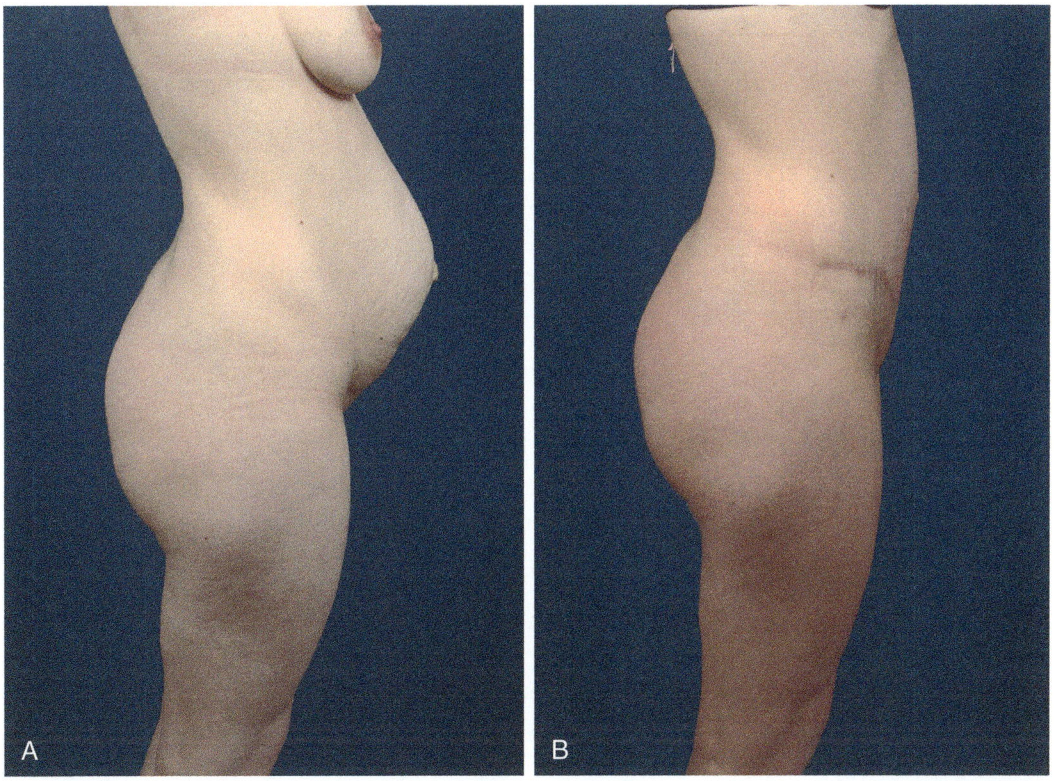

• **Fig. 71.7** (A) A 36-year-old woman after a twin-pregnancy and a subsequent rectus diastasis. (B) Six months after a fascial tightening and standard abdominoplasty.

system PRINEO (Ethicon) (consisting of 2-octyl cyanoacrylate glue and self-adhering mesh) without the need of dermal stiches.[23]

After a final wound antiseptic cleaning, Steri-Strips (3M) are affixed longitudinally to the scar. These supportive dressings should remain for 3 weeks postoperatively. Finally, a sterile wound dressing and an adjustable compression girdle are applied.

We prefer to perform the standard abdominoplasty procedure on an inpatient basis with a minimum 1–3 nights hospital stay. A slight postoperative discoloration of the umbilicus is usually not a cause for alarm, especially when there was no previous surgery of the umbilicus. A complete necrosis of the umbilical stalk is seen very seldom and may be treated conservatively with satisfying results.

Patient satisfaction after standard abdominoplasty is usually high due to a possible treatment of the entire abdomen.

The legacy of a long scar with limited treatment effects to the hips and the back region is an unavoidable aspect of this procedure for a certain patient groups. In cases of a fascial midline plication a tissue gathering may result in the epigastric region. This tissue excess may be easily and safely reduced by open excision or additional liposuction.[6,11]

Mini-abdominoplasty

The mini-abdominoplasty procedure differs from a standard abdominoplasty with a shorter resulting scar and limited skin resection. The results of the short-scar technique are limited to the lower abdominal wall and have the best results if there is no herniation or diastasis of the rectus muscles above the umbilical stalk. If such is present in the upper abdominal wall a free-floating umbilicus abdominoplasty is a better choice (Fig. 71.8).

Mini-abdominoplasty is indicated in patients with a mild to moderate skin laxity and tissue excess of the lower infraumbilical abdomen, together with a sufficient distance between the umbilicus and symphysis, mostly more than 12 cm or for patients who already have a cesarean section scar. Liposuction of the upper abdomen and flanks has a supportive effect by improving the abdominal contour. With respect to vascular anatomy, the mini-abdominoplasty is a safe procedure since a single Huger's zone (zone II) is compromised.

Markings

Markings are performed with the patient in the upright standing position. The distance between the umbilicus and the upper incision line should be a minimum distance of 9 cm to avoid an unesthetic appearance. For cases with redundant tissue in the lower abdomen and a relatively high position of the umbilicus (approximately 14–18 cm above the pubic symphysis), the lower incision line is marked 6 cm above the labial commissure and the upper incision line 9 cm below the umbilicus. In cases of a distance less than 9 cm after skin resection, an inverse T-scar with umbilical transposition should be preferred.

In relation to the required scar length, the fat distribution in the region of the iliac crest should be evaluated

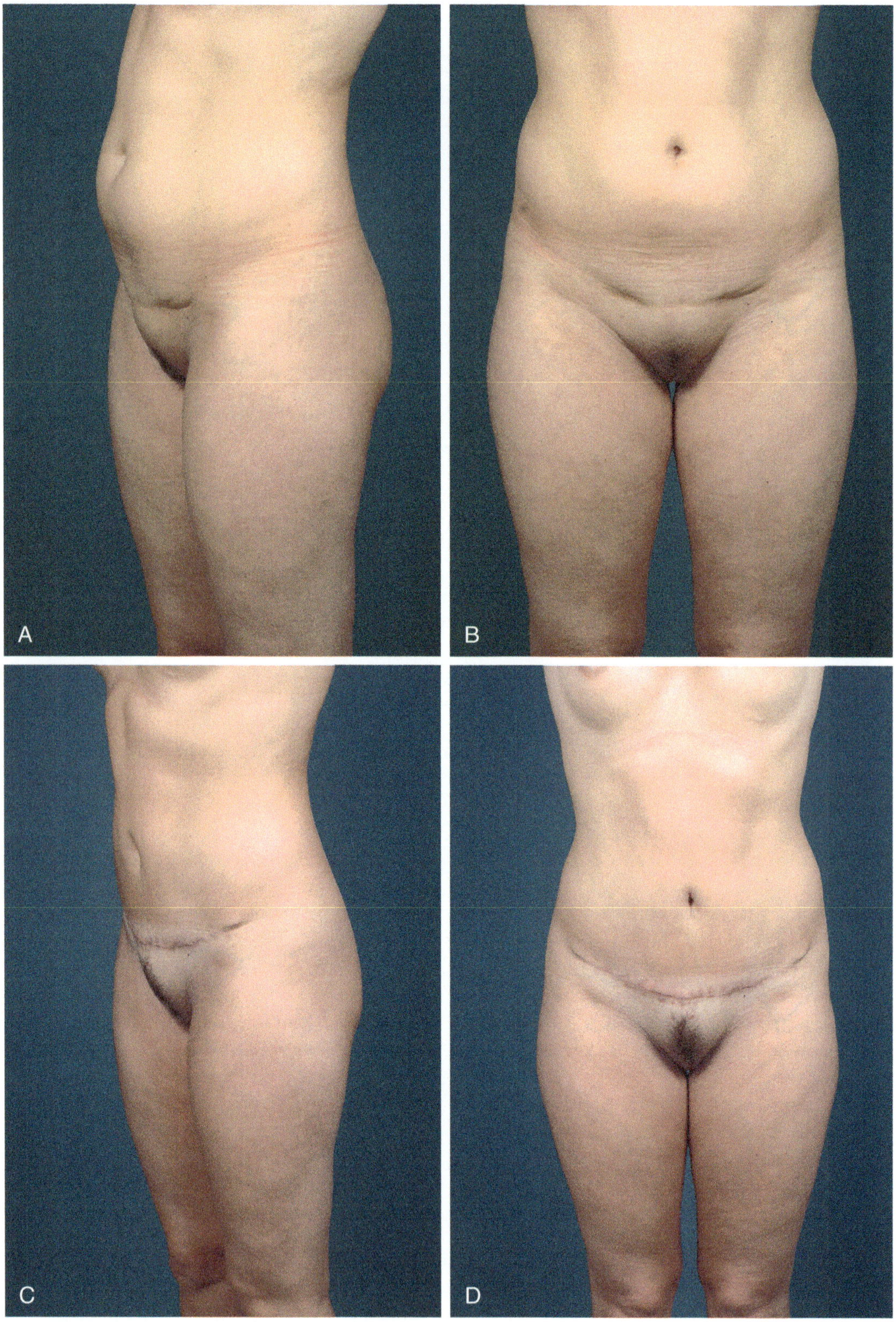

• **Fig. 71.8** A 44-year-old woman after three pregnancies with two cesarean sections. (A,B) Pre- and (C,D) postoperative oblique and front views of a free-floating abdominoplasty with fascial reconstruction. Note the high-riding umbilicus in the preoperative pictures.

preoperatively and the patients has to be informed about an optimized cosmetic outcome despite a prolonged final scar length.

Technique

This procedure may be performed under local anesthesia and adjuvant sedation. If a reconstruction of the anterior rectus sheath is required, we recommend general anesthesia or spinal anesthesia.

Any supportive liposuction of the abdominal wall and flanks should be performed at the beginning of the abdominoplasty procedure in order to sufficiently reduce the epi- and subfascial layer. Techniques such as radiofrequency- or ultrasonic-assisted liposuction may generate shrinking of the skin for additional skin tightening effect. In young patients with an elastic skin tone and a long distance between the umbilicus and symphysis an umbilical transposition may be avoided.

The operative technique is similar to a standard abdominoplasty, although abdominal flap mobilization is performed and adjusted to local tissue characteristics. In all cases, tissue dissection is performed above Scarpa's fascia. The abdominal flap is mobilized cranially up to the level of the umbilical stalk. The abdominal flap is drawn caudally and the umbilical range of motion can be assessed. Markings should always be done on stretched skin and adhere to a distance of minimum 9 cm between umbilicus and upper incision line.

The estimation of the amount of tissue resection and wound closure are always performed in the same manner as described above. If there is no excessive bleeding, drains may be dispensable.

Free-Floating Umbilicus Abdominoplasty

In contrast to the mini-abdominoplasty ,the free-floating umbilicus abdominoplasty is a very powerful technique for patients with a moderate laxity of the entire abdominal wall with or without a diastasis recti and for patients who complain about periumbilical wrinkles combined with a relatively high position of the umbilical stalk (corresponding to the mini-abdominoplasty approximately 14–18 cm above the pubic symphysis). Care must be taken by patients who have previously had surgical interventions at or nearby the umbilicus. Those interventions should be at least one year prior to the planned operation.

Markings

The markings are as described above with a minimum distance of 9 cm between the upper resection line and the umbilical stalk to avoid a poor esthetic appearance. In cases of a distance less than 9 cm, skin resection with this technique is not recommendable.

Technique

The operative technique is similar to a standard abdominoplasty. The abdominal flap is mobilized cranially up to the level of the umbilical stalk. The umbilical base should be marked for its refixation. Then after inspection for hidden and small periumbilical herniation and transection of the umbilical stalk from the rectus muscle fascia, the dissection is continued to the xiphoid and costal margins. After plication of the anterior rectus fascia, the abdominal flap is drawn caudally and with the help of progressive tension sutures the umbilical range of motion can be assessed. Markings should always be done on stretched skin and adhere to a distance of minimum 9 cm between umbilicus and upper incision line. Before resection of the skin flap the umbilical stalk is fixated to the abdominal wall and infraumbilical progressive tension sutures should be placed to ensure a tension-free wound closure. For this maneuver nonabsorbable or absorbable suture material can be used. Before wound closure, drains should be inserted if a plication of the anterior rectus sheath was performed.

High Lateral Tension (HLT) Abdominoplasty

In the 1990s Ted Lockwood presented this modified abdominoplasty procedure, which allows a full treatment of the abdomen and limited treatment of the hips and the lateral thigh in terms of a modified incision pattern.[16] Lockwood enumerated several surgical principles that were in many ways diametrically opposed to the ones of a standard abdominoplasty, namely, an extensive discontinuous undermining and a more conservative resection centrally with wider excision of the lateral skin. Separately, due to new insurance guidelines locally, in our practice even though the circumferential tissue resection would be the best treatment for some of our patients the HLT abdominoplasty has regained importance in treatment of publicly funded patients.

Female patients usually suffer from an additional skin laxity in the lateral thigh region, whereas male patients complain about the typical fat distribution in terms of "love handles." The experienced surgeon may, however, be confronted with a HLT abdominoplasty procedure that results with lateral dog-ears, despite the extent of lateral tissue excision and scar elongation. Additional liposuction may be supportive, although often insufficient due to a surplus of lateral skin.

Markings

Preoperative markings are similar to those for standard abdominoplasty markings. The inferior incision line is continued laterally to the anterior axillary line and runs upwards to the midaxillary line at an angle of 45 degrees. The upper incision line starts at the highest point of the umbilicus, continuing parallel to the lower incision line until the anterior axillary line, then turning downwards at an angle of 45 degrees to meet the lower line in the midaxillary line to form an angle of 90 degrees.

Technique

For this procedure it is helpful to position the patient on an additional cushion in the gluteal area for elevation of the flanks and lateral thighs and optimal access to these regions. Alternatively, the patient may be changed into a lateral position. The operative technique is similar to that for standard abdominoplasty, although central abdominal flap mobilization is more limited and only as far laterally as necessary for a required rectus plication. Additional flap advancement can be achieved through vertical discontinuous undermining, utilizing the Lockwood dissector. The lateral skin resection pattern with significant lateral resection is performed with a subsequent high-tension wound closure. For the lateral wound edges a reduction of subdermal fat and, if necessary, a lengthening of the incision may be performed in order to avoid dog-ears. A lateral elongation of the scar has to be acceptable for a satisfactory result; this is generally well accepted by the patients. Since the lateral abdominal perforators are preserved, stable blood supply is achieved.[16]

Fleur-de-Lis Abdominoplasty

Fleur-de-lis abdominoplasty is the most powerful procedure for maximal tightening of the entire abdomen and reshaping the lower body. It was popularized in 1985, and derives from techniques previously described by Regnault (classic W technique) or Kelly (1910) and Babcock (1916).[24–27] The procedure enables the elimination of vertical and horizontal tissue excess on the lower and upper abdomen. Using this approach, a maximum improvement of body shape and reduction of waist circumference is achievable. In cases of large abdominal pannus or patients with existing medical handicap, it can be performed as a two-stage procedure. In general, we advise refraining from lateral undermining for maximal preservation of perforators. Furthermore, we recommend a check of the markings intraoperatively prior to resection to avoid postoperative complications.

The suitable indication for this technique is an adequate, mainly horizontal tissue surplus of the lower and, in particular, the upper abdomen, usually in patients after moderate to massive weight loss. Any patient who presents with a preexisting midline scar may be considered primarily for this technique. Because of the improved overall outcome, the midline scar is generally good accepted by our patients.

In patients with a vertical tissue surplus in the upper abdomen and a request for a breast procedure requiring a submammary incision, an additional reverse upper abdominoplasty may be considered.

Many patients in whom a fleur-de-lis abdominoplasty is indicated need a circumferential tissue resection as well. However, we often see that, due to a wide range of reasons, the patients choose an abdominal procedure only. These patients have to be informed that such a procedure will most certainly result in an accentuation of the waist-to-hip ratio with the impression of a postoperatively worse saddlebag region.

Markings

Preoperative markings should be performed while the patient is standing upright. In the supine position, the lateral tissues move backwards and make an accurate estimation of tissue excess difficult.

First, the midline is marked, then the patient is asked to pull up their entire lower abdominal tissue in a symmetric manner. A distance of 6 cm to the upper vulvar commissure is marked. Next the tissue surplus is estimated through precise pinching of the skin and marked in an elliptical pattern. With the patient in supine position the distance from each line to the midline should be measured and equalized if necessary, since any small mismatch may result in an uneven midline scar. Next, the upper horizontal incision line is marked. This line should generally run 3–5 cm inferior to the umbilicus. Finalized markings usually result in an omega-like figure (Fig. 71.9). We recommend limiting the superior extent of the scar line primarily by local superficial liposuction rather than a further superior excision. Finally, all vertical and horizontal markings should be checked and measured in upright and supine positions.

Technique

Abdominal flap mobilization is performed as in standard abdominoplasty procedures, except that the lateral flap mobilization should strictly be limited to the height of the upper incision line to preserve maximal perfusion of the lower medial apex of the flap. As soon as the mobilization of the umbilical stalk has been completed, the entire estimated vertical and transverse resection area is temporarily closed using bullet forceps and the required marking adjustments performed. Next, the incision lines are incised and the redundant tissue excised in a monobloc fashion. After hemostasis the flaps are temporarily approximated and drains inserted.

The umbilicus has to be integrated into the vertical scar, and this should be performed in straight and not bent position. At the appropriate umbilical height a limited transverse incision is made on both abdominal flaps with reserved circular fat excision in the periumbilical region. The umbilical stalk is then integrated into the abdominal flaps, allowing skin excisions for optimal incorporation. A secondary esthetically unpleasing trumpet-like widening of the umbilicus may result from extensive periumbilical skin removal. Therefore, we recommend a step-by-step excision with observation of any transverse tensile forces. In general, we insert three or four drains (including the upper abdomen) during subcuticular and intradermal wound closure.

If flap mobilization in the lateral aspect is limited to the resection lines only a maximal preservation of perforators, flap perfusion, and dermal wound healing should be uncomplicated. Despite the long scar formation, the esthetic improvements to the hip and waist are dramatic and not comparable to any other abdominoplasty technique. It is worth noting the back and flank folds may be improved due to maximal recruitment of lateral skin (see Fig. 71.9).

Postoperative Care

The different operations can be performed as outpatient or inpatient surgery. If the hospital offers an intensive or

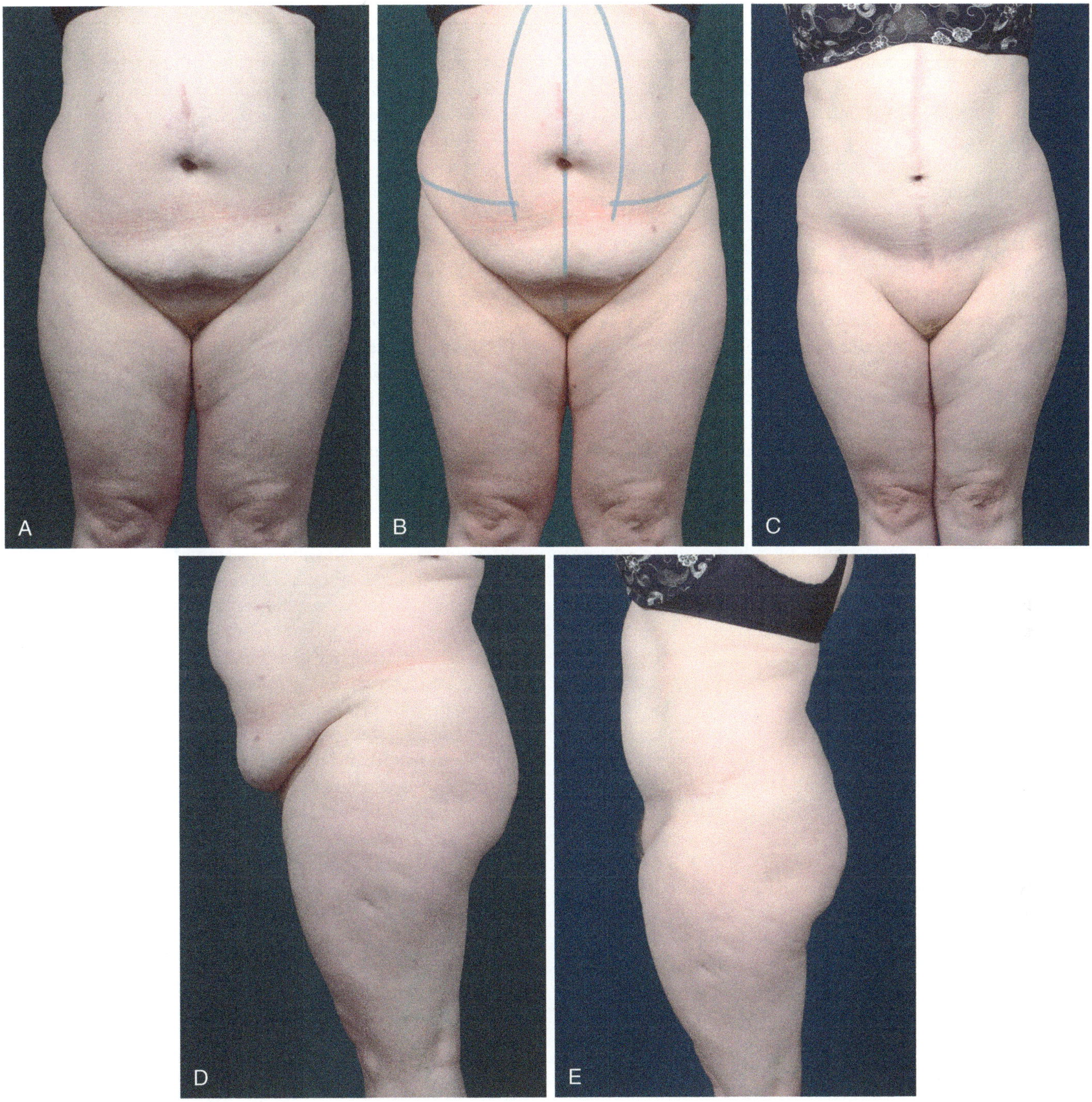

• **Fig. 71.9** (A,D) A 42-year-old woman with significant abdominal pannus combined with rectus diastasis after massive weight loss. (C,E) Two years postoperatively after fleur-de-lis abdominoplasty. (B) Markings.

intermediate care unit, patients may be monitored after circumferential procedures for the initial 24 hours postoperatively. For reduction of superficial wound tension, we intraoperatively apply longitudinally vectored Steri-Strips for the first 3 weeks. During the initial 48 hours postoperatively, laboratory checks for electrolytes and hemoglobin are performed routinely after abdominoplasty and circumferential procedures, patients are positioned in the beach-chair position, where available on an air mattress, with electronically adjustable positions. DVT prophylaxis is administered using low-molecular-weight heparins in regular doses for patients with a high perioperative risk of thrombosis (e.g., enoxaparin 40 mg or dalteparin 5000 IU), compression stockings and sequential calf compressors. Initial wound care includes an absorbent dressing, in abdominoplasty and body lift cases two compression girdles, in breast cases a zip sports bra, and in arm and thigh cases a circumferential compression gown. The immediate postoperative compression therapy reduces shearing forces supporting the adhesion of different tissue layers. In this context, drains may be kept for a minimum of 4 days postoperatively. They are removed when drainage is less then 30 mL in 24 hours.

Patients are instructed to move their feet frequently and not to cross their legs.

Because of the extended scars we offer an individualized PCA to all our patients during the initial 48 hours postoperatively. Patients are mobilized on the first postoperative day and instructed to do deep breathing exercises to prevent pneumonia. The urinary catheter, which is indicated in any prolonged procedure such as circumferential or combined procedures and thigh liftings, is removed after 2–3 days to help with patient mobilization.

Showering is generally permitted after drain removal. Postoperative clinical examination should investigate the possibility of seromas. In cases of hernia or diastasis rectus repair, patients should be asked about bowel habits; abdominal auscultation, percussion and ultrasound may be indicated. Any nonresorbable sutures or wound closure material is removed at the latest 3 weeks postoperatively. For at least 3 months postoperatively we recommend our patients to cover the entire scars with silicone sheets for improved scar formation.

Sporting activities should not be resumed for 8 weeks postoperatively. Patients should be advised to avoid saunas and tanning beds. Before patients are discharged, we individually adapt a compression garment for 8 weeks postoperatively.

Complications

General symptoms after skin-tightening procedures include postoperative pain, numbness of the abdominal flap, bruising, general fatigue and discomfort due to increased skin tension for many weeks.

Local complications in all regions include hematoma (approximately 3% incidence), seroma (approximately 17%), wound infection (approximately 4%), fat necrosis, wound dehiscence (approximately 33%), paresthesia, and persisting numbness. Seromas are a very common problem in the abdominal region and usually handled with serial punctures and drainage. Persistent seromas may require a secondary surgical procedure. In general, seromas should be detected in time and treated by simple aspiration to avoid superinfection or any consequent wound separation.

Minor wound dehiscences are common and self-limiting. Significant dehiscences may be caused by increased tension or marginal wound necrosis (approximately 10%). Appropriate treatment of wound necrosis is initial conservative wound care, until the area of necrosis has been demarcated for surgical revision. Additional flap advancement may allow optimal secondary wound closure. Further local complications include dog-ears, hypertrophic or malpositioned scars, and in the abdominal region cosmetic problems related to the umbilicus. Most of these issues can be avoided with good preoperative planning and attention to surgical detail.

Treatment by liposuction may lead to postoperative contour irregularities and dermal tethering. Further swelling may occur in cases of circular liposuction of the extremities.

Systemic complications include DVT (2%), PE (ca. 1%), fat embolism, respiratory compromise due to increased intraabdominal pressure in abdominal cases with fascial tightening, and systemic infections including toxic shock syndrome are rare but reported. In general, abdominoplasty procedures have a higher systemic complication rate than any other type of routine cosmetic surgical procedures.[6,9,10,11,19,28]

Body Contouring after Massive Weight Loss

Reconstructive procedures after massive weight loss resulting from bariatric surgeries or diet therapy include abdominoplasty, lower body lift, upper body lift, breast lift, upper lateral thoracic lift, bra-lift, thigh lift, lower leg lift, upper arm lift, lower arm lift, and facelift/neck lift.

Preoperative Management

A patient's first consultation should include a detailed description of all procedures planned for reconstruction. It is essential, that the patient be informed about the number of surgical stages that will be necessary for the desired changes, including any secondary skin-tightening procedures. We recommend clarification of all important issues using a digital presentation with all available images, including medical record photo documented complications. The patient should be informed about all possible complications.

Prior to the surgery, the patient should consult the surgeon for a second time to discuss any remaining issues. At this time, the patient can reconfirm the informed consent. We recommend schematizing all discussed scar courses and important tissue displacements. The patient has to be informed about the placement of drains, urinary catheter, and type and placement of suture material. Furthermore, any additional proposed maneuvers (e.g., fascial reconstruction or Scarpa's lift) should be clarified.[29] Since patients having bariatric procedures may suffer from nutritional deficiency due to a disturbance of nutrient uptake, we ask all patients to have a current blood test during their first consultation as well as prior to the surgery to avoid any late failures regarding the operative scheduling. Any coagulant dysfunction has to be evaluated and excluded preoperatively, where necessary by way of consultation with a hematologist. We routinely advise all patients about the supplement of all necessary nutrients (including zinc, selenium, vitamin C) 4 weeks prior to and 4 weeks after the surgery.

The sequence of surgical procedures may be discussed with the patient and adapted between the single steps. We favor starting the reconstructive process with the lower body lift, followed by any further indicated procedures. In patients with excessive remaining subdermal tissue in the thighs, it might be sensible to start with a thigh lift to prevent excessive traction on the circumferential scar tissues with a consequent early descent of the tissue. The time frame between each stage should be at least 2–3 months to allow for sufficient recovery.[9,10,19]

Circumferential Lower Truncal Dermatolipectomy

A lower body lift (circumferential lower truncal dermatolipectomy, CLTD, our modification of a lower body lift) is indicated in almost every patient after weight loss. The patient should be informed about the pros and cons of abdominoplasty versus circular procedures.[9,10]

Markings

Markings are performed in upright standing position. First, the midline is marked, then the patient is asked to pull up their entire lower abdominal tissue in a symmetric manner. Meanwhile a distance of 6 cm to the upper vulvar commissure is marked. At this height an almost horizontal lower incision line is marked to both flanks, followed by the upper horizontal incision line at the height of the umbilicus. Next, the patient has to turn and the posterior markings are performed. The upper incision line is marked, starting at the highest point of the gluteal cleft and running upwards in a round curved shape to the lateral end of the anterior upper incision line. Finally, the lower incision line is assessed and marked by pinching and connected to the lower anterior incision line.

Technique

Dorsal Surgery

The initial skin incision is made along the superior marking line and is carried down to the level of the underlying superficial fascia, which is exposed using the Colorado Microdissection needle. This easily separates the superficial lamellar from the subfascial lobular fat. Next, the dissection is continued inferiorly just above the superficial fascia. The preservation of fascia to the deep gluteal fat as the "gluteal superficial muscular aponeurotic system (SMAS)" is conceptually similar to the "facial SMAS" used in facelifts. The superficial fascia is dissected at the height of the inferior resection line, before flap mobilization is continued further caudally. Lateral gluteal adhesions are released bluntly down to the height of the gluteal fold, before dissection is continued to the lateral thigh, where preparation level is above the tensor fascia lata muscle. Further distal mobilization of the lateral thigh can be carried out bluntly using the Lockwood dissectors, but is no longer recommended due to excessive seroma occurrence. With completion of dissection, the waist and gluteal fatty tissue is widely mobilized and covered with robust superficial fascia. This is particularly suited for autologous gluteal augmentations, since patients after massive weight loss frequently have flattened buttocks. For this purpose, 2–3 1×0 threads are sutured from lateral to medial, grasping the stable fascia and consequently displacing the gluteal fatty tissue to the middle of the buttocks. For cranial repositioning 3–4 1×0 nonabsorbable threads are sutured from caudal to cranial at the medial aspect of the buttocks. Reconstruction and tightening of the gluteal adipose tissues lift the gluteal flaps cranially with a subsequent final skin closure under less tension. Furthermore, this maneuver improves the shape of the waist.

Detachment in the zones of adherence combined with extended mobilization allows an enormous tightening of skin. A symmetrical resection is then undertaken. We advise use of bullet forceps for determination of the amount of resection. Next, the flap is incised laterally and adjusted for maximum tension. The redundant gluteal flap arising in this way with its lower incision line is measured precisely in the tensed condition for symmetry before the resection of the flap is performed.

In general, the superficial fascial system (SFS) is extremely stable and allows a sufficient suturing for reconstructive purpose. After reshaping the SFS, wound closure is performed in multiple layers with resorbable suture material (see above). Two suction drains are placed in each gluteal/back and lateral thigh region. Before patients are turned into supine position, we perform a temporary closure of the lateral skin excess using a stapler and an occlusive dressing.

Anterior Surgery

The inferior incision is checked and re-marked, adjusting the initial inferior line to the laterally ending gluteal incision line. With all techniques, the dissection level is performed above Scarpa's fascia (see above), which has a number of key advantages: long-lasting swellings can be prevented because the underlying lymphatic vessels are preserved, and the tightening of the SFS craniomedially provides an additional inner traction on the deep penetrating fascial system of the thigh (Colles' fascia). The SFS may then be fixed with 1-0 nonabsorbable sutures to the anterior rectus fascia. Approximately three fingerbreadths below the umbilicus, Scarpa's fascia is dissected and further mobilization of the abdominal flap is performed cranially above the rectus fascia. The central supraumbilical adhesion zone is sharply dissected between both rectus muscles, preserving the laterally-incoming perforator vessels.

Further dissection is performed as in the abdominoplasty procedure described above. After meticulous hemostasis, the patient is bent and several progressive tension sutures are placed superior to the umbilicus, the umbilical stalk is pulled through the abdominal flap and further progressive tension sutures are placed for reduction of the dead space and the superficial tension. Next, temporary wound closure is performed with bullet forceps or skin staples. Superficial fascial reconstruction, wound and skin closure may then be performed alternatively with barbed sutures or the two-component skin closure system as described previously (Figs. 71.10–71.12).[9,10]

Therapy of "Love Handles" in Male Patients

Male patients frequently complain of local fat distributions in the hip and dorsal region, commonly known as "love handles." In the past, these were treated by liposuction. However, patients often complained about a local

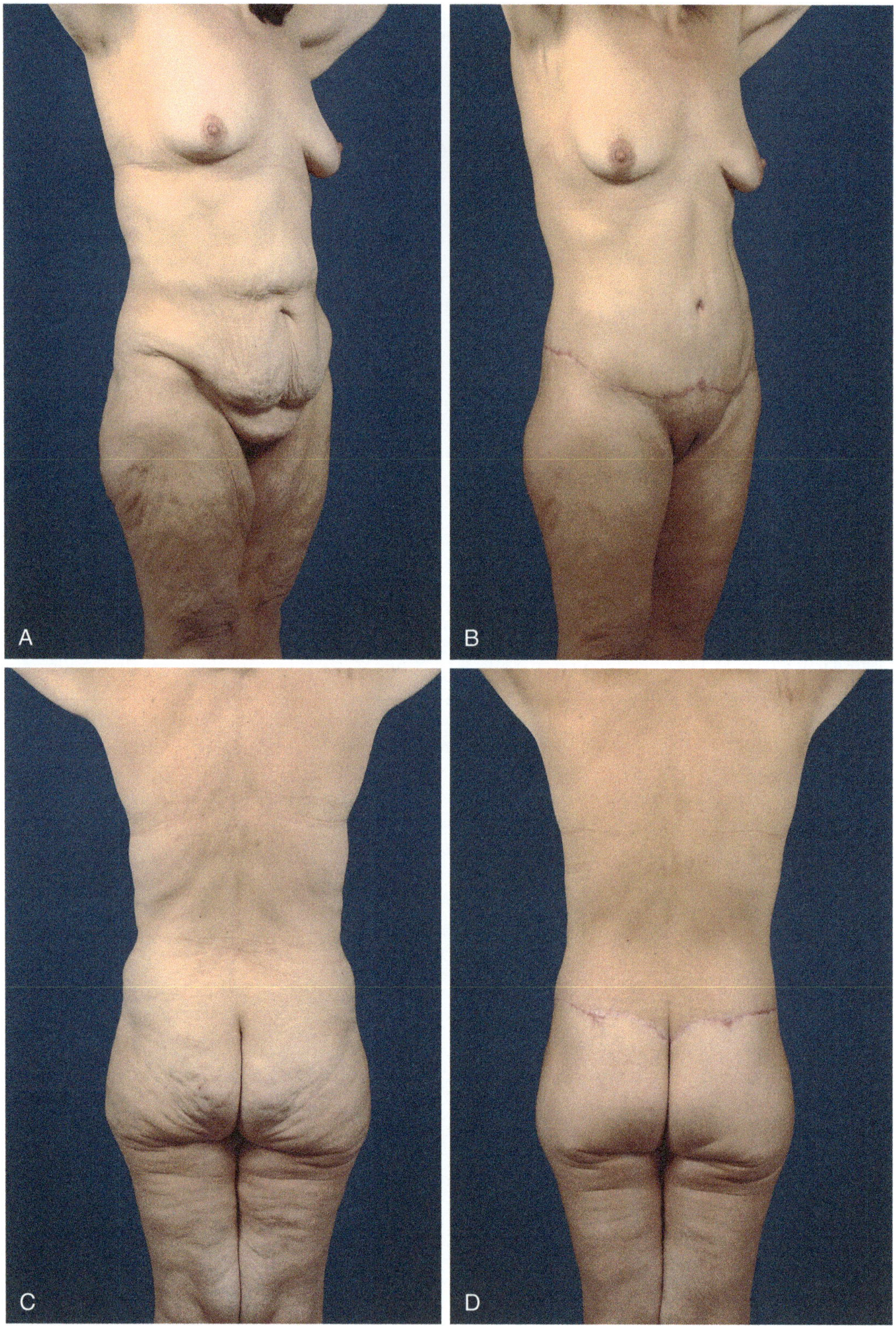

• **Fig. 71.10** (A,C) A 54-year-old woman with a weight loss of 65 kg following diet and sportive action. (B,D) Six months postoperatively after circumferential lower truncal dermatolipectomy (CLTD).

recurrence with a minimal weight increase. During circumferential preparation, these isolated fat pads can be easily identified and excised (see Fig. 71.11). A meticulous hemostasis is mandatory since large vessels are generally observed for their isolated blood supply.

Thigh Lift

Thigh lifts are an essential part of body-contouring procedures and may be performed through different approaches. Preferentially, the scar is placed at the inner thigh region in

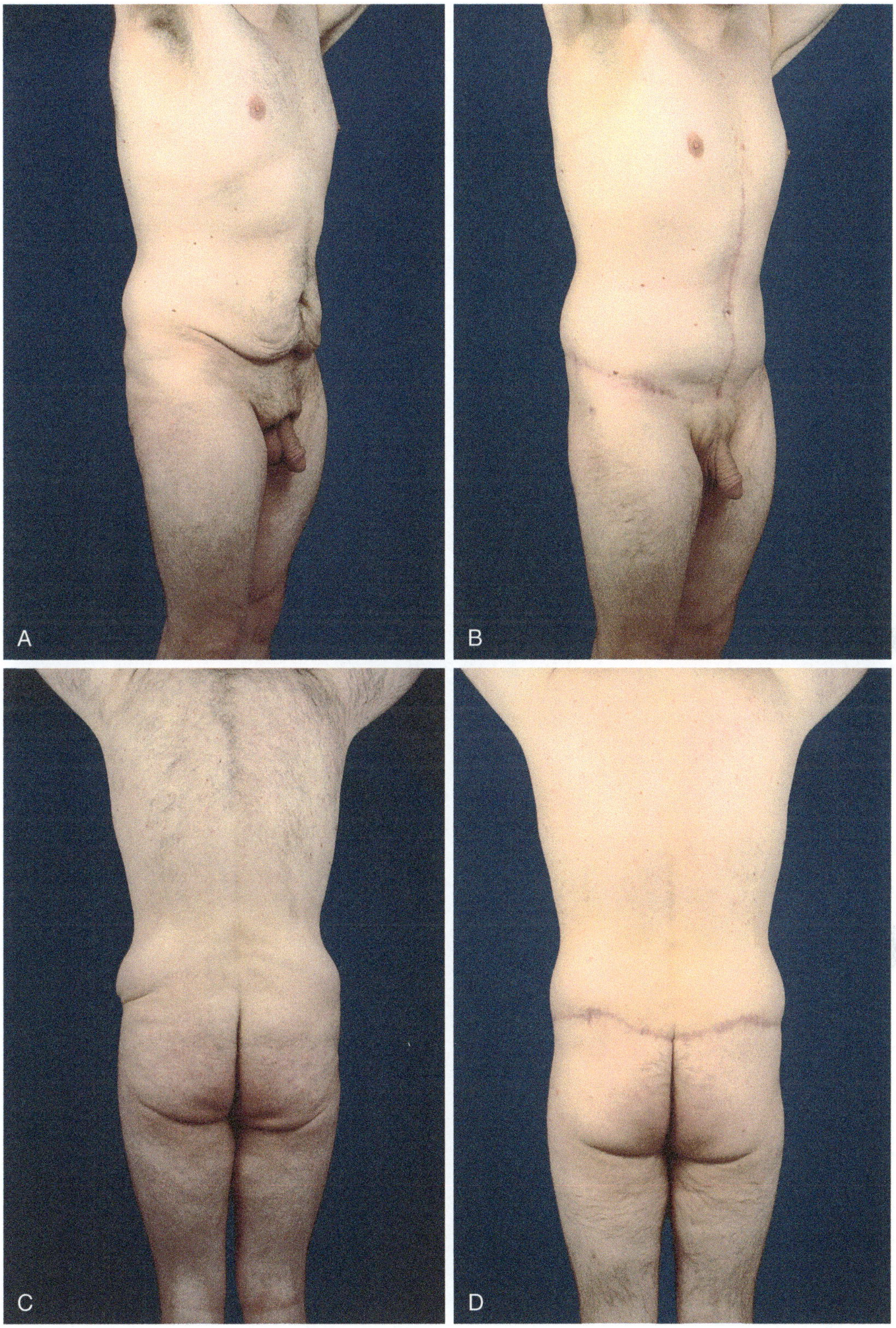

• **Fig. 71.11** (A,C) A 36-year-old man with a weight loss of 72 kg following diet and sportive action. (B,D) Eighteen months postoperatively after circumferential lower truncal dermatolipectomy (CLTD) with anterior fleur-de-lis excision.

a vertical direction, in a horizontal direction in the groin region or in a combination of the vertical and horizontal scars (T- or J-shaped). We do not recommend a horizontal thigh lift because of the high risk of scar migration combined with labial spreading.

In very rare cases additional scar placements may be required, such as a horizontal scar just superior to the knee. The staging of the procedure should be discussed with the patient. In general, abdominoplasty or lower circular procedures should be staged prior to a thigh lift, since they enable

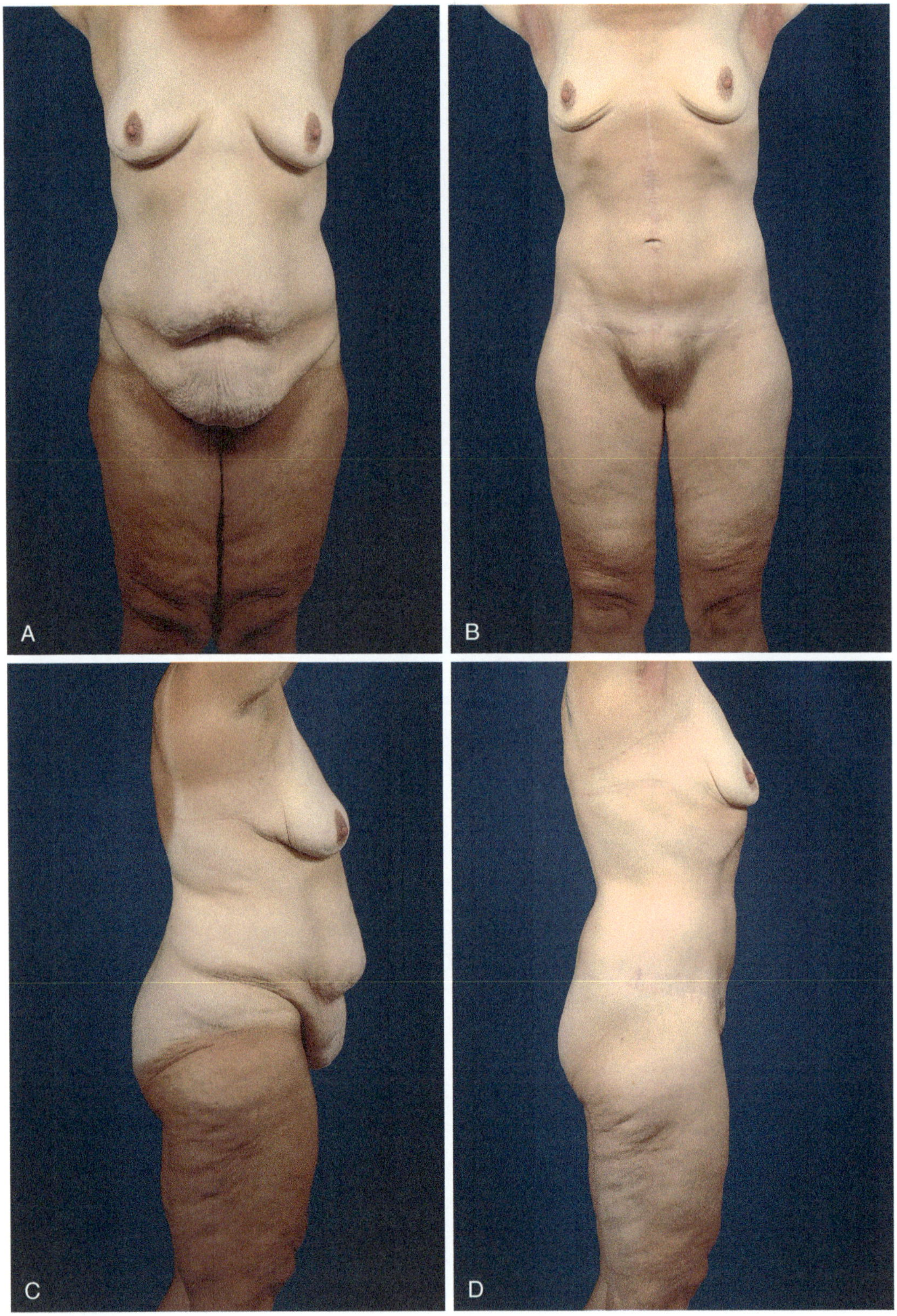

• **Fig. 71.12** (A,C) A 44-year-old woman with a weight loss of 64 kg following diet and sportive action. (B,D) Two years postoperatively after circumferential lower truncal dermatolipectomy (CLTD) with anterior fleur-de-lis excision and inner thigh lift.

an improvement in vertical direction to the thigh region. If, as described above, the subcutaneous tissue remains very prominent, starting with a thigh lift may have a better outcome for a following lower circular procedure.

Preoperative Assessment

Prior to thigh lift surgery, all patients should have an examination of their deep vein system and should have had any necessary therapy of varicose veins.

The preoperative evaluation includes the skin quality (e.g., thickness, laxity, presence of striae) as well as the thickness of the subcutaneous tissue in all thigh regions. The circumference has to be measured from the ankle in 5-cm increments to the top of the thigh to record comparable results. The thighs should be documented with photographs in different views (front, side, back, inner side, and in an abducted position). With the patient standing and the thigh in a 60-degree abducted position the overhanging redundant skin should be measured. All existing eczemas and hyperpigmentation should be assessed and photo documented. Since the range of varying adipose distributions is wide, every patient has to be evaluated and plans for an individualized therapy regime prepared. Male patients generally present with skin and adipose excess in the upper inner thigh regions only without any redundant tissue in the other thigh regions. They very seldom complain about a local adipose tissue in either the outer and front thigh. Female patients, on the other hand, are characterized by minimum subcutaneous tissue in most parts of the thigh (except for the inner thigh). Some female patients complain about a massive adipose tissue surplus in the thigh region, which is totally resistant to any weight loss. In some female patients the weight may have settled in an acceptable range with maximal reduced adipose tissue in the entire upper and lower body but not in the entire thigh region, where they present with subcutaneous tissue several centimeters thick accompanied with pain and tendency to bruising (DD: lipedema). In those cases a staged liposuction of the thigh prior to the lifting procedure is mandatory.

Markings

The marking is performed in the upright position first. The desired scar course is marked bilaterally and demonstrated to the patient. The symmetry can be easily checked while the patient is standing upright with legs together. The groin crease should be marked precisely to avoid any dislocation or vertical lengthening of the scar, which can be easily observed in vertical procedures. This groin crease line demonstrates the highest point of incision in either vertical, all horizontal or combined procedures.

Depending on the tissue characteristic and any asymmetries, the resection lines are marked next. This can be initially performed in upright and checked for modifications in supine position. It has proven to be helpful to mark these lines in relation to the proposed scar line.

A helpful tool is the double-ellipse marking technique of Aly, which allows safer and more precise marking. After marking an outer ellipse based on existing skin excess a second inner ellipse is marked based on the outer ellipse reduced on each side by the thickness of subcutaneous fat to allow tension-free wound closure.

Technique

Regardless of scar placement, we have standardized our technique for thigh lifts as a combination of liposuction and tissue resection. Because of postoperative swelling of the treated tissue it is mandatory to perform liposuction in the area of skin resection. This area in the inner thigh is extensively treated by liposuction (5 mm cannula), removing any detectable fat tissue. Next, the marked resection area is checked using bullet forceps for a temporary approximation. After confirmation of the resection lines the skin is incised and excised by a scalpel or electrocautery-assisted avulsion from proximal to distal. It has been shown to be important to remove the skin in a combination of sharp and blunt resection, as this allows the sectioning of all vessels, including lymphatic vessels, at the weakest point, reducing the risk of lymphocele, and avoids the development of heat-induced seromas.

After meticulous hemostasis the wound is temporarily closed with bullet forceps, subsequently replaced by staples. It is important to perform the temporary closure as soon as possible to avoid wound closure problems due to increasing tissue swelling. At this time point any required adjustments may be performed for any surplus skin and fat tissue in the groin or adjoining regions. These may easily be treated through limited liposuction. No undermining is performed to minimize impairment of the wound edge perfusion.

In cases of a sole or additional horizontal incision placed in the groin crease we recommend fixing the distal skin flap to Colles' fascia of the pubic region to avoid any distal displacement of the final scar.

In general, we do not place drains for this procedure, however in case of excessive bleeding they may be placed before final wound closure commences. Wound closure is performed in the subcuticular and deep layers, using absorbable sutures in single knot or with barbed sutures in running manner as described above. Final application of Steri-Strips (transversely to the wound) and a sterile wound dressing is followed by a circular compression dressing which includes the feet and hips. During the first postoperative days, this compression winding is then changed to a custom-tailored compression garment. Postoperatively, lymph drainage therapy may be of some help (Fig. 71.13).

Arm Lift (Brachioplasty)

Arm lifts (brachioplasty) are commonly indicated in patients after weight loss to remove skin and fat excess and achieve pleasing and youthful upper and lower arm contours. Furthermore, the aging patient may suffer from loose and flabby skin in the inner upper arm region. Plastic surgeons will consult with patients about undergoing surgery for an arm lift if they wish to tighten this skin to look and feel more youthful. The incision extends from the elbow to the axillary crease, and sometimes extending on to the side of the chest. In some instances, liposuction may be used alone or in conjunction with an arm lift to remove excess fat in the upper arms.

In patients after massive weight loss, the redundant upper arm skin frequently crosses the axillary crease and extends onto the lateral thoracic region. This has to be demonstrated and marked with the patient. In a few individual cases, the

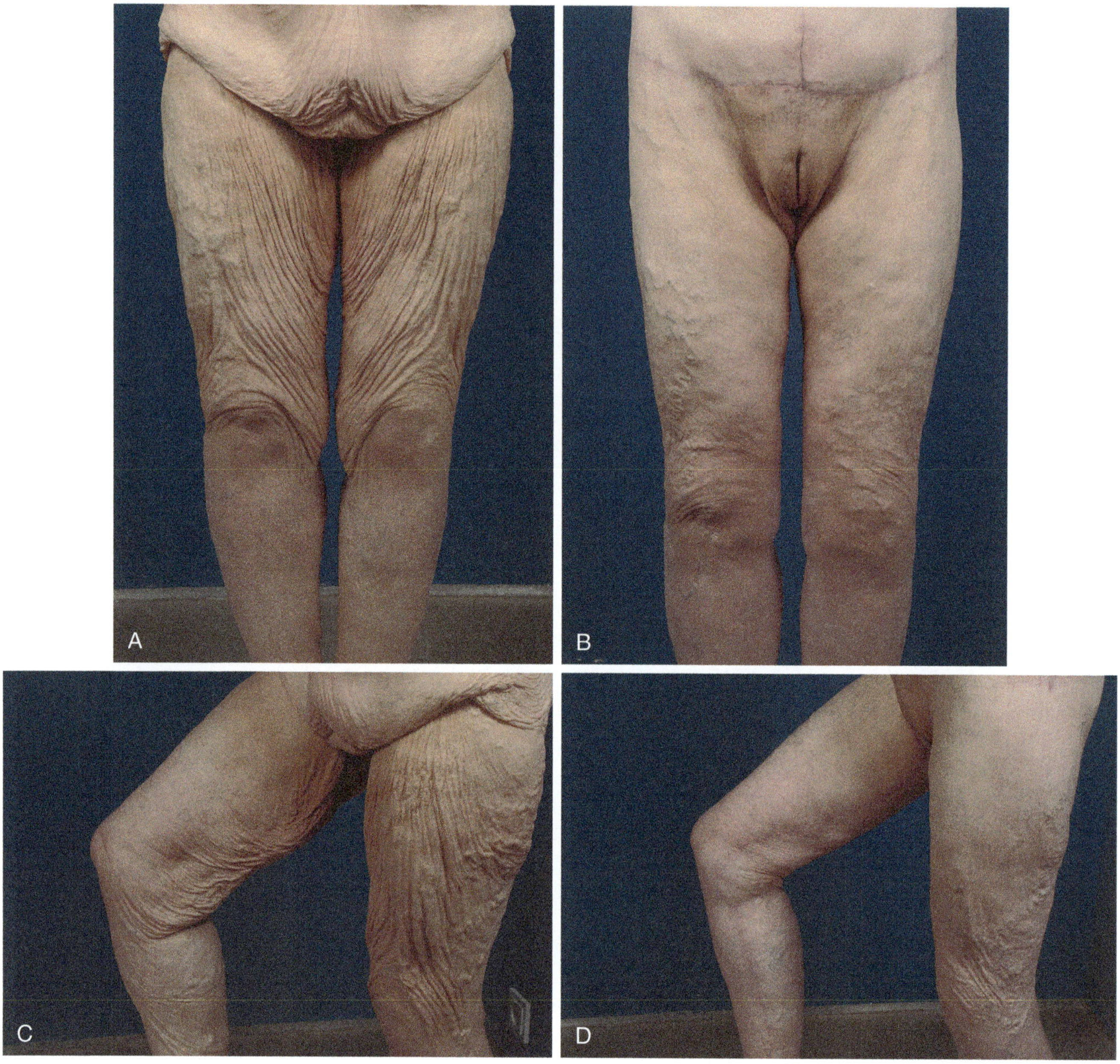

• **Fig. 71.13** (A,C) A 43-year-old woman after 93 kg of weight loss following diet and sportive action. (B,D) Eight months postoperatively after inner thigh lift and lower bodylift surgery.

skin excess extends to the lower arms. This has to be clarified to the patient, since this redundancy will be more conspicuous after an isolated upper arm lift.

Preoperative Assessment

Skin laxity (presence of striae) and skin excess has to evaluated in the entire upper and lower arm with the adjoining lateral chest region. The circular and vertical skin excess can easily be measured on the extended arm. Furthermore, especially in weight loss patients, local adipose tissue may be assessed in the entire arm.

Markings

The positioning of the incision lines depends on surgeon preference and should be demonstrated to the patient. In general, patients have to be informed preoperatively that the scar is either visible over the medial bicipital groove or on the hanging arm in a dorsal view. There are several techniques, from which the ideal one can be chosen for the patient. In many cases a dorsal scar is not inevitable if the patient has excess subdermal fat tissue left.

We perform markings while the patient is standing and elevating his or her straight arm in a 90° position. We establish whether there is a difference in surplus tissue between the sides. The first line marked should be the anterior line, just at the top of the medial bicipital groove. From this line the posterior line is evaluated through pinching. Alternatively, the double-ellipse technique described by Aly can be used. This technique may ensure a more accurate marking, especially for the novice surgeon. Finally, while the patient stretches both arms straight in front, a check of symmetry may be performed. In cases of tissue excess in the lower arm, the markings should extend over the elbow to the lower arm.

Technique

Our technique of arm lifts is performed similar to the thigh lift procedure as described previously, a combination of liposuction and tissue resection. In general, patients present with adipose tissue excess in the inner and dorsal arm region. The preoperatively marked area of resection at the inner arm is extensively thinned out by liposuction, removing any detectable fat tissue. This can ideally be performed with a 2–3 mm-cannula. After completion, the marked resection area is checked using bullet forceps for a temporary approximation, before the confirmed resection lines are incised and excised by a scalpel or electrocautery-assisted avulsion from proximal to distal. This has been shown to be important to tear off the skin without any mechanical transection, as this allows the sectioning of all vessels including lymphatic vessels at their weakest point. Once meticulous hemostasis is completed, the wound is closed temporarily in the same manner as thigh procedures. Again, as in thigh procedures, it is important to perform the temporary closure as soon as possible to avoid wound closure problems due to tissue edema. At this point any required changes may be performed regarding excess skin and fatty tissue in the axillary, elbow region or obvious adipose excess in adjoining regions, which may easily be treated through liposuction.

In cases of a sole or additional horizontal incision placed in the axillary crease we recommend fixation of the crease with fastening sutures.

Drains are uncommon but may be placed before wound closure, which is performed in the same way as described for the thigh lift. Final application of Steri-Strips, a sterile wound dressing, and a circular compression dressing including the hands is performed in all cases. A custom-made compression garment may be adjusted prior to surgery and dressed intraoperatively. In those patients lymph drainage therapy may be of some help as well (Fig. 71.14).[30–35]

Complications

The variety of complications in massive weight loss patients is similar to those of normal weight patients. The most important difference is the quality of the skin after massive weight loss, this explains almost all the differences. One of the most important complications, especially in massive weight loss patients, is relaxation of the skin shortly after the intervention. This is due to the experienced excess of expansion during weight gain which damaged the collagen tissue and altered the elasticity of the skin.

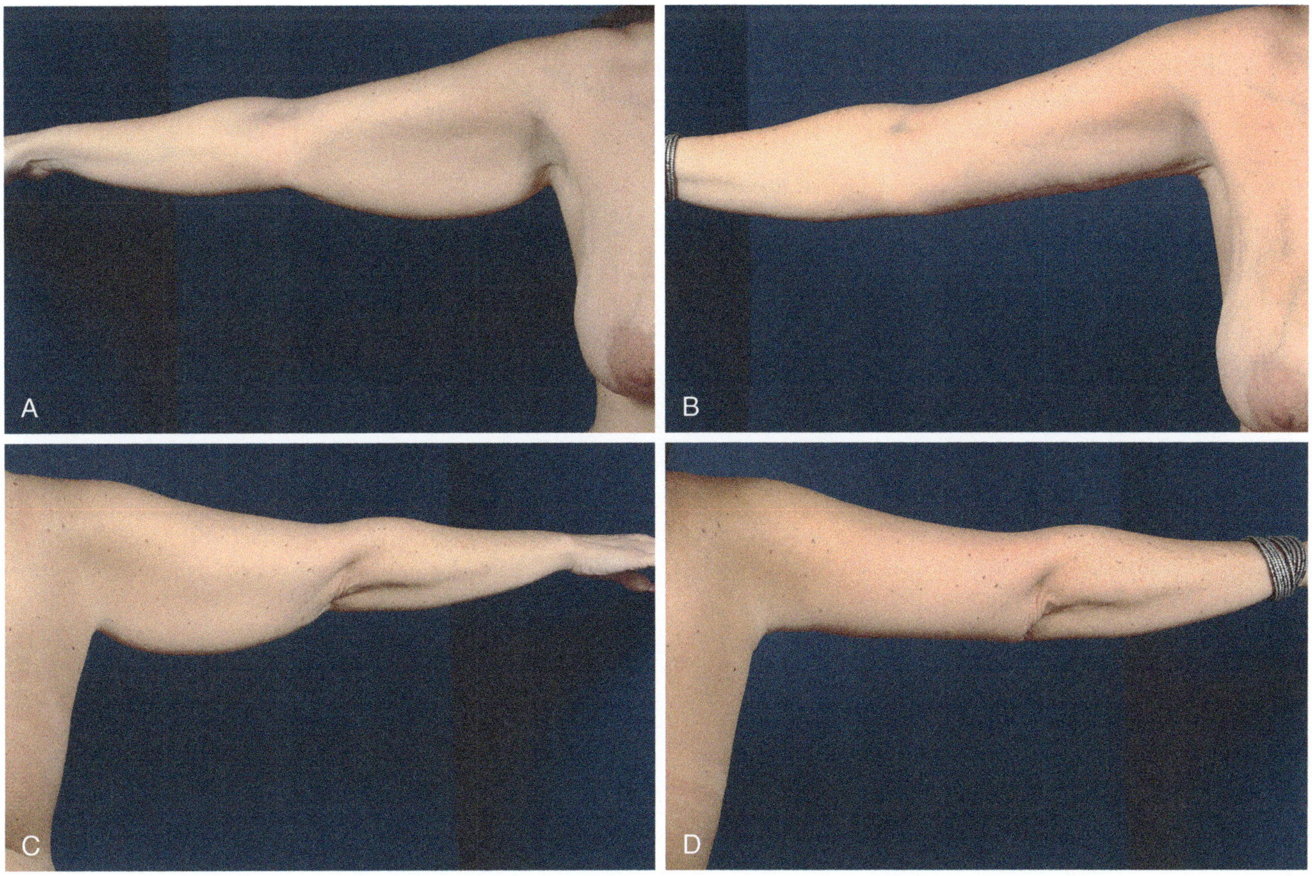

• **Fig. 71.14** (A,C) A 38-year-old woman after 48 kg of weight loss following diet and sportive action. (B,D) Three months postoperatively after lipoassisted arm lift.

Other common complications are seroma, which tend to correlate with the amount of weight loss and wound dehiscences. Both complications are related at least in part to the relative malnutrition that is ubiquitous in postbariatric patients. All patients with skin tightening procedures should have a diet including sufficient vitamins and proteins.

Summary

Body contouring operations are essential tools in patients after massive weight loss, multiple pregnancies or in patients with weakness of the connective tissue. The surgeon executing those procedures should be able to distinguish between the different types of deformities and tailor a treatment plan for each individual patient matching to their personal circumstance, including medical history, amount of weight loss, region of skin excess, personal circumstances, etc.

The surgeon must not always choose the most efficient technique, but the one that combines highest patient safety with the best esthetic outcome achievable in each patient.

References

1. Borges AF, Alexander JE. Relaxed skin tension lines, Z-plasties on scars, and fusiform excision of lesions. *Br J Plast Surg.* 1962;15:242–254.
2. Orpheu SC, Coltro PS, Scopel GP, et al. Collagen and elastic content of abdominal skin after surgical weight loss. *Obesity Surg.* 2010;20(4):480–486.
3. Mitz V, Elbaz JS, Vilde F. Study of dermal elastic fibers during plastic surgery of the trunk. *Ann Chir Plast.* 1975;20(l):3l–43.
4. Costa-Ferreira A, Rebelo M, Vásconez LO, et al. Scarpa fascia preservation during abdominoplasty: a prospective study. *Plast Reconstr Surg.* 2010;125(4):1232–1239.
5. Huger Jr WE. The anatomic rationale for abdominal lipectomy. *Am Surg.* 1979;45(9):612–617.
6. Moon HK, Taylor GL. The vascular anatomy of rectus abdominis musculocutaneous taps based on the deep superior epigastric system. *Plast Reconstr Surg.* 1988;82(5):815–832.
7. Richter DF, Stoff A. Abdominoplasty procedures. In: Warren R, Neligan P, eds. *Plastic Surgery.* Volume 2: *Aesthetic Surgery.* 3rd edn. St. Louis, MO: Saunders; 2012.
8. Orpheu SC, Coltro PS, Scopel GP, et al. Collagen and elastic content of abdominal skin after surgical weight loss. *Obesity Surg.* 2010;20(4):480–486.
9. Light D, Arvanitis GM, Abramson D, et al. Effect of weight loss after bariatric surgery on skin and the extracellular matrix. *Plast Reconstr Surg.* 2010;125(1):343–351.
10. Richter DF, Stoff A. Lower body lift. In: Rubin P, Jewell M, Richler DF, eds. *Body Contouring and Liposuction.* St. Louis, MO: Saunders; 2012.
11. Richter DF, Stoff A, Velasco FJ, et al. Circumferential lower truncal dermato-lipectomy. *Clin Plast Surg.* 2008;35(1):53–71.
12. Hunstad JP, Repta R. *Atlas of Abdominoplasty.* St. Louis, MO: Saunders; 2009.
13. Song AY, Jean RD, Hurwitz DJ, et al. A classification of contour deformities after bariatric weight loss: the Pittsburgh Rating Scale. *Plast Reconstr Surg.* 2006;116(5):1535–1544.
14. Krueger JK, Rohrich RJ. Clearing the smoke: the scientific rationale for tobacco abstention with plastic surgery. *Plast Reconstr Surg.* 2001;108(4):1063–1073; discussion 1074–1077.
15. Rubin JP, Nguyen V, Schwentker A. Perioperative management of the post-gastric-bypass patient presenting for body contour surgery. *Clin Plast Surg.* 2004;31(4):601–610, vi.
16. Matarasso A. Abdominolipoplasty: a system of classification and treatment for combined abdominoplasty and suction-assisted lipectomy. *Aesthetic Plast Surg.* 1991;15(2):111–121.
17. Lockwood TE. Superficial fascial system (SFS) of the trunk and extremities; a new concept. *Plast Reconstr Surg.* 1991;87(6):1009–1018.
18. Lockwood TE. Maximizing aesthetics in lateral-tension abdominoplasty and body lifts. *Clin Plast Surg.* 2004;31(4):523–537.
19. Aly AS, Cram AE, Chao M, et al. Belt lipectomy for circumferential truncal excess: the University of Iowa experience. *Plast Reconstr Surg.* 2003;111:398.
20. Aly AS. *Body Contouring after Massive Weight Loss.* St. Louis, MO: Quality Medical Publishing; 2006.
21. Baroudi R, Moraes M. Philosophy, technical principles, selection, and indications in body contouring surgery. *Aesthetic Plast Surg.* 1991;15:1–18.
22. Pitanguy I. Abdominolipectomy. An approach to it through an analysis of 300 consecutive cases. *Plast Reconstr Surg.* 1967;40:384.
23. Richter DF, Stoff A, Ramakrishnan V, et al. A comparison of a new skin closure device and intradermal sutures in the closure of full-thickness surgical incisions. *Plast Reconstr Surg.* 2012;130(4):843–850.
24. Dellon AL. Fleur-de-lis abdominoplasty. *Aesthetic Plast Surg.* 1985;9:27.
25. Regnault P. *Abdominal Lipectomy, A Low "W" Incision.* New York: New York International Society of Aesthetic Plastic Surgery; 1972.
26. Kelly HA. Excision of fat of the abdominal wall lipectomy. *Surg Gynecol Obstet.* 1910;10:229.
27. Babcock WW. The correction of the obese and relaxed abdominal wall with special reference to the use of buried silver chain. *Am J Obstet Gynecol.* 1916;74:596.
28. Nemerofsky RB, Oliak DA, Capella JF. Body lift: an account of 200 consecutive cases in the massive weight loss patient. *Plast Reconstr Surg.* 2006;117(2):414–430.
29. Richter DF, Stoff A. The Scarpa-lift – a novel technique for minimal invasive medial thigh lifts. *Obesity Surg.* 2011;21(12):1975–1980.
30. Richter DF, Stoff A. [Lower body contouring procedures]. *Chirurg.* 2011;82(9):797–800, 802–806 [in German].
31. Hurwitz DJ. Single-staged total body lift after massive weight loss. *Ann Plast Surg.* 2004;52(5):435–441; discussion 441.
32. Kenkel JM. Body contouring surgery after massive weight loss. *Plast Reconstr Surg.* 2006;suppl 117:1–86.
33. Rohrich RJ, Gosman AA, Conrad MH, et al. Simplifying circumferential body contouring: the central body lift evolution. *Plast Reconstr Surg.* 2006;118(2):525–535; discussion 536–538.
34. Strauch B, Herman C, Rohde C, et al. Mid-body contouring in the post-bariatric surgery patient. *Plast Reconstr Surg.* 2006;117(7):2200–2211.
35. Richter DF, Stoff A. Circumferential body contouring: the lower body lift. *Clin Plast Surg.* 2014;41(4):775–788.

72 Board and Fellowships Exams

DANIEL P. BUTLER, DONALD W. BUCK II, SABRINA CUGNO, KRISHNA RAO, AND ROSTAM D. FARHADIEH

Introduction

The fellowship or boards of plastic surgery equivalent exams are the final trial by ordeal for most trainees, who will have faced exams over a large portion of their adult lives. Their respective examining boards put together the general structure of all four exams with the aim of presenting a safe surgeon who has adequately covered the entire plastic surgery curriculum. This is perhaps the most stressful academic period in a prospective surgeon's training career. All exams have their own unique quirks of technique and reflect examiners' habits or favorite topics. In recent years the various boards have attempted to provide a more standardized format to ensure reproducibility and fairness. As they begin to prepare for the final exam each candidate finds their favored study modality. Group study with a long-term timetable, regular tutorials from recently passed surgeons and more experienced senior surgeons together form the basis of most trainees' approach to the exams. The structure of the FRACS(Plast), FRCS(Plast), FRCSC, the American Board of Plastic Surgery, and the European Board of Plastic Reconstructive and Aesthetic Surgery (EBOPRAS) exams is described below, with reflections by the authors on their personal experiences of their individual examination process.

FRACS(Plast)/EBOPRAS Exams

The Australasian College of Surgeons invites final year trainees from a 5-year specialist training program conducted by the Royal Australasian College of Surgeons to sit the fellowship exams. All candidates must have passed a PRSSPE (PRS Science and Principle Examination) multiple-choice exam usually as a SET 2 candidate. The final fellowship has the following components:

(I) Two written papers: each of 2 hours' duration, 2 questions in each paper and multiple parts in each question
(II) Clinical – long cases: 2 cases, each of 30 minutes
(III) Clinical – short cases: 6 cases, each of 5 minutes
(IV) Surgical Pathology and Operative Surgery (SPOS) 1 – viva: 2 scenarios, each of 12.5 minutes
(V) SPOS 2 – viva: 6 slides, each of 5 minutes
(VI) Anatomy – viva: 25 minutes.

The scoring is a Closed Marking system – 8, 8.5, 9, 9.5. Support can be given in each of the marks: 9 is a clear pass, 8.5 is borderline fail, 8 is a clear fail. Any candidate can be failed on one critical error irrespective of the marks. Critical errors are considered those decisions that may be life- or limb-threatening. Although all seven segments are considered equal in value, during court of examiner discussions more emphasis is placed on clinical components, in particular long cases. These exams are held twice a year.

The EBOPRAS exam is divided into written and viva components. The written exam is a multiple-choice exam covering clinical as well as basic sciences. The viva component is divided into two 25-minute sections; clinical scenarios covering congenital, trauma, tumor management, esthetic and general reconstruction are conducted by two examiners.

As a candidate, I (Rostam D. Farhadieh) had the dubious pleasure of sitting three of the five exams discussed in this chapter (FRACS(Plast), FRCS(Plast), EBOPRAS). Each had its own strengths and weaknesses, however the common theme is that the examiners were not intent on failing the candidates, but to discover what their knowledge limits and more critically where their clinical limits lay. The FRACS is the most rigorous of these exams in terms of expected depth of knowledge, however it is not necessarily the broadest exam. The written form is significantly more detailed and in my opinion more in line with expectations of a specialist surgeon. The FRCS exam is the broadest exam; each candidate is assured that a series of congenital, trauma, esthetic and general reconstructive viva questions will be asked. The arrays of short cases were undoubtedly the best outpatients clinic not only I but also all candidates are likely ever to attend. The EBOPRAS exams similarly seek to cover the same broad base. The candidates are often, however, qualified surgeons and as such the exam format may seem more like a semi-formal discussion amongst colleagues than tutor to pupil format of the FRACS and FRCS exams.

The most pertinent advice for a prospective candidate is a broad formal clinical experience. This experience is best gathered in the trenches of interminable dressings and initial consultation clinics. Formal long case, short case practice and presentation is essential not only to success but also to a crisp and succinct decision-making process. This will become less formal, but nevertheless form the crux of your clinical practice for years to come. The examiners are destined to have more clinical experience than the candidates and this is where the candidate can compensate by depth and breadth of knowledge. The more a candidate reads and knows around a topic, the more confident and systematic they will become in replying to questions and putting clinical scenarios into a correct perspective. Review CME articles from the journals *Plastic and Reconstructive Surgery*, *Clinics in Plastic Surgery*, and *Hand Clinics* formed the basis of my own reading, in addition to the standard single-volume texts, although the latter I often found inadequate. Revision and complete command of surgical anatomy is mandatory in clinical practice of plastic surgery. Unfortunately, neither the FRCS nor the EBOPRAS exam stresses this component. This results in what is often perceived to be a deficit in many of the British and European candidates' knowledge base.

FRACS(Plast): The IMG (International Medical Graduate) Perspective

The common theme from an IMG perspective with recent experiences of FRACS(Plast) and FRCS(Plast) is that in both exams the examiners were not intent on failing the candidates, but to discover what their knowledge limits were and, more critically, where their clinical limits lay. The FRACS significantly differs from the FRCS in having a written component. The written form is significantly more detailed and requires careful tactful organization in addition to knowledge. It helps to practice answer-writing and the previous question papers may be obtained from RACS itself. During practice runs, one must stay within the allotted time. The time allotted to each component of a question is clearly mentioned and serves as a useful guide to the detail required. It was easier to utilize bullet point answers to lend a structure to replies, whilst reducing the size. The most pertinent advice for a prospective candidate is broad formal clinical experience. This experience is best gathered in review and initial consultation clinics. Formal long case, short case practice and presentation is essential not only to success but also to a crisp and succinct decision-making process. At the same time, it is better to have concise but clear, rather than extensive but haphazard, knowledge. Every candidate has their own way of covering the syllabus and gaining requisite knowledge. This could be in the form of personal notes, standard textbooks, concise revision books, selected review articles or a combination of these.

My personal feeling after the exams was that failure is rarely from lack of sufficient knowledge. The Australian exam in being drawn out over 3 days is good at testing the examinee's stamina and resolve. A good night's sleep is much better than last minute cramming. Being part of a cohort of examinees is very useful. Revision and complete command of surgical anatomy is mandatory in clinical practice of plastic surgery. Although the common feeling was that *Last's Anatomy* is the reference text, it is best to use a text whose figures make the most sense. Regular practice sessions with fellows and especially past examiners are very useful. Several opportunities are available in Australia and New Zealand to attend mock exams and one of these is readily available at the SET conference. Practicing with a cohort of examinees provides good opportunity to improve upon presentation skills.

FRCS(Plast) Exams

UK plastic surgery trainees are required to complete the FRCS(Plast) examination as part of the portfolio of evidence required to be awarded a Certificate of Completion of Training (CCT). The examination is administered and regulated by the Joint Committee on Intercollegiate Examinations (www.jcie.org.uk) on the behalf of the four Royal Colleges of Surgeons within the British Isles (England, Edinburgh, and Ireland, and the Royal College of Physicians and Surgeons, Glasgow).

Trainees should aim to complete the examination within the last two years of training. This allows adequate exposure to the breadth of the plastic surgery curriculum during the earlier years of training. There are two sittings for each section of the examination per year, which gives some flexibility in planning the optimal time to sit the exam.

The FRCS(Plast) is composed of two sections. Both aim to cover the full breadth of the syllabus and therefore cover clinical, basic science, ethics, consent, and statistics relevant to plastic surgery.

Section 1 consists of two written papers: Single Best Answer paper (2 hours) and Extended Matching Question paper (2.5 hours). Both papers are completed on the same day at a Pearson VUE computer-based examination center. In the past few years there has been a move to make the examination more clinically-focused. As a result, basic science and ethical topics are often incorporated into a clinical scenario. This has the benefit of making the examination more relevant to the candidate's day-to-day practice, but it becomes more important to identify the theme being assessed to help determine the correct answer. The pass mark is determined by a standard-setting exercise completed by experienced FRCS(Plast) examiners. This varies with each exam sitting but is typically between 60% and 70%.

Section 2 is the verbal component and consists of both a clinical and oral exam. These are held over two days at a single hospital in the UK. The clinical examination comprises both short and long cases with the candidate being taken through the exam by three different pairs of examiners. The short cases are completed in two 30-minute periods with candidates examining five patients within each block.

Examiners will guide the candidate on which aspect(s) of history, examination, and diagnostic study interpretation they want to focus upon. Following this, a discussion on the management of the patient typically follows. The long cases involve assessing two patients with each lasting 15 minutes. This allows ample time for a detailed evaluation of the patient, interpretation of relevant diagnostic investigations, and in-depth discussion of subsequent management.

The oral exam is viva-based and involves the candidate sitting with two examiners at each station to discuss a broad spectrum of clinical cases. No patients are present for this part of the exam. There are three viva stations each of which contain three core subject areas:

1. Hand trauma, other trauma (lower limb, maxillofacial), and wounds (pressure sores, wound care), burns.
2. Head and neck tumors, cleft and craniofacial, trunk, and urogenital.
3. Basic sciences, ethics and consent, esthetics.

At each viva station the candidate will be asked questions relating to six cases with at least one question from each core subject area. Clinical questions are usually based around a brief history and clinical photograph. Typical follow-on questions may relate to the results of diagnostic tests, drawing a diagram or explaining the reasoning behind the management proposed.

Performance in Section 2 of the exam is judged against the standard expected of a newly-appointed consultant in the National Health Service (NHS).

The marking is structured. Each constituent part of Section 2, the short cases, the long cases, and the oral exam, contains a certain number of marking events which are each given a score between 4 and 8 (6 is a pass). At each marking event, two examiners will score the candidate. It should also be noted that the long cases are weighted in such a way that each case, scored by two examiners, contributes six marking events. An average score of 6 is required to pass and, therefore, an overall score of at least 408 is required. No one score is able to result in an immediate fail, instead, the overall performance throughout Section 2 of the examination is considered.

Weighting of scores for the different parts is as follows:

Long cases: 2 cases, 12 marking events (pass mark = 72)
Short cases A: 5 cases, 10 marking events (pass mark = 60)
Short cases B: 5 cases, 10 marking events (pass mark = 60)
Viva 1: 6 scenarios, 12 marking events (pass mark = 72)
Viva 2: 6 scenarios, 12 marking events (pass mark = 72)
Viva 3: 6 scenarios, 12 marking events (pass mark = 72)

When attributing a score, the examiners take the following areas of a candidate's performance into consideration:

1. Overall professional capability/patient care
2. Knowledge and judgement
3. Quality of response and 'bedside manner'.

A copy of the marking descriptors that will be used by the examiners is sent to candidates in advance with their examination pack and there is also an up-to-date copy on the JCIE website (http://www.jcie.org.uk). It is advisable for candidates to check this for any changes to the marking scheme that may subsequently occur.

Each candidate has a maximum of four attempts over a 2-year period for Section 1 and four attempts at Section 2. The whole exam process must be completed within 7 years. Once Section 1 is complete, the candidate is not required to complete this part again should they fail Section 2.

Preparation is a personal approach, however general principles apply. At this stage of medical training, every candidate will have their own particular way of preparing for an examination. To ensure an adequate depth of knowledge is acquired, a detailed text such as this textbook should be used from the outset. This will also help guide further reading of appropriate journal articles, as single-volume textbooks often do not provide adequate detail in the core topics of hands, breast, burns, and head and neck. As the exam approaches, a more succinct textbook allows for quick revision of the key topics. Specific to Section 1 is the need to practice both Single Best Answer and Extended Matching Questions and a number of books are available that facilitate this. The JCIE also provide a small selection of past questions to help demonstrate the standard required.

The candidates should be familiar with the current UK guidelines, especially for skin cancers (produced jointly by the British Association of Dermatologists (BAD) and the British Association of Plastic Reconstructive and Aesthetic Surgeons (BAPRAS)) and lower limb trauma (produced jointly by the BAPRAS and the British Orthopaedic Association). The latter can be downloaded from the BAPRAS website. The National Institute for Health and Care Excellence (NICE; www.nice.org.uk) also produces a range of clinical guidelines (in addition to evaluating new interventions or technologies and cost/benefit analysis), some of which are particularly relevant to plastic surgery (e.g., pressure sore management, fat grafting, venous thromboembolism prophylaxis), and candidates should be familiar with these. It is helpful to go through summaries of guidance on consent and ethics from the General Medical Council website (www.gmc%2duk.org) under the section entitled Good Medical Practice.

When preparing for Section 2 it is essential to practice discussing clinical cases and evaluating patients. Although day-to-day clinical activities provide ample exposure, a modified technique is required for the exam to allow for the time constraints and format. Practice should ideally be undertaken with others sitting the exam as well as both newly-appointed and senior consultants. Another very useful resource are senior trainees who have recently sat the examination and are, therefore, familiar with the examination format and standard. Although the main emphasis should be on the candidate answering questions, the value of watching others answer questions should not be ignored.

Here are my tips for the exams. Exam technique is an essential component when preparing for Section 2. The following are some pointers that were of particular help.

- Speak like a consultant. The FRCS(Plast) is the first time the majority of candidates will be completing an examination that expects them to interact with the examiners in the role of a fellow consultant. An answer should, therefore, focus on succinctly describing the key aspects in the history and examination and follow-on with a clear management plan that describes what will be done rather than what options are available. The examiners will critique your proposed management, so be prepared to explain the reasoning behind the decisions made.

- Prepare an opening statement. This is particularly relevant to the viva where the breadth of topics covered allows for preparation prior to the exam. A focused opening statement allows the candidate to demonstrate a good understanding of the key aspects of the case and its initial management. Further time can then be spent demonstrating higher-order thinking and, hopefully, scoring beyond the pass mark. An example for a head and neck cancer case would be: "My initial management will comprise obtaining a tissue diagnosis with HPV status, determining the local and distant extent of the disease and identifying the patient factors that will impact on any treatment proposed to allow me to generate a plan I can take to the head and neck oncology MDT."
- Say what you would do in real life. It can be tempting to pick a treatment option or procedure that might demonstrate a high level of knowledge. This is a risky strategy, as the examiners may press you to explain the details of this intervention. A safer approach is to keep the treatment chosen simple and in line with things you have directly experienced. Allow the examiners to push you for further treatment options later in the case discussion.
- Show good clinical judgment before quoting papers. A concern of many candidates preparing for the exam relates to the level of knowledge of the existing evidence base required. Although being able to reference a relevant paper supporting the management pathway chosen is one aspect of demonstrating higher-order thinking, candidates should first aim to demonstrate robust clinical judgment grounded upon their own clinical experience. The reality of the exam is that there is often little time to discuss the evidence base and so it is often best to be guided by the examiners' questioning to decide if quoting a paper would be appropriate (e.g., "What is the evidence for that?").
- Keep going. No one score is able to cause an automatic fail, so aim to avoid lingering on cases gone before and instead keep motivated and focused on the present topic.
- Don't forget the importance of a succinct, focused history. This is of particular importance in the long cases. Done well, these are easy to score on given the additional weighting they carry. History-taking should be quick and with some patients it may be necessary to take control. Some omissions can be a fail, for example skipping family history in breast cancer, and it is wise to remember these. It is important to reach a definitive plan in the long case with at least a backup plan. The examiner may try to streamline the examination in order to reach the discussion stage and it is important to take hints and yet not skip on important things.
- Focus on the case in hand. Short cases can be compromised if the candidate starts thinking about the previous short cases. Evaluating five short cases in 30 minutes requires alertness and full concentration on the present case. Many of the short cases may have complex problems but the evaluation may be on only one of the components. Always answer exactly what the examiner is asking without second guessing.
- It is acceptable to say "I don't know" when asked a difficult question. It is better to take a hint and accept a wrong answer early rather than proceed along the wrong path.
- Answers should be succinct and to the point. This way the candidate gets to move on to the next question. It is good to aim high and answer well as this can compensate for a borderline poor performance elsewhere. Sometimes if a scenario is not going well, the examiner may ask a standard default question like stages of graft take. These questions have almost standardized answers with buzzwords and these questions have to be answered well.
- If you feel comfortable with a technique that differs from an examiner's, do not change. This scenario is common when asked for cleft lip marking in which examiners rarely are comfortable with a repair other than Millard's. Be prepared to mark and explain your technique well. Trying to change marking technique for exams may end badly.
- Just as the focus of any clinical encounter is the patient, the exams are no different. It is important to put the patient at ease and treat them with dignity and respect. Always ask for tenderness before palpation, ensure you have a chaperone and thank the patient at the end. These are things we do in our daily lives and exams are no different.

FRCSC Exams

At the end of plastic surgery training in Canada, candidates are invited to sit the Canadian Plastic Surgery Royal College examination. The title Fellow of the Royal College of Surgeons of Canada (FRCSC) – Plastic and Reconstructive Surgery is awarded following successful completion of this examination. The FRCSC is a renowned designation recognized worldwide and is usually a requirement for specialty licensure in Canadian jurisdictions. This final certification exam consists of two components: a written section and an oral examination approximately 2 weeks later. Candidates are required to pass both the written and the oral components in order to successfully complete the exam. The examination addresses all facets of plastic and reconstructive surgery, including basic science, basic principles and techniques, pediatric plastic surgery, craniofacial surgery, burns and wound care, head and neck reconstruction, esthetic surgery, trunk and lower extremity reconstruction, breast and hand surgery. A more detailed description of the plastic surgery curriculum can be found at www.royalcollege.ca.

Although this examination is stressful and comes at the end of a long and arduous residency training, it is considered to be a fair exam. There is an enormous quantity of information to master (as evidenced by the content of this book), but in the end, review and critical appraisal of the material while preparing for the exam will make any potential candidate a better plastic surgeon.

Failure is usually a function of two primary deficiencies: lack of knowledge and lack of examination-taking skills. The former shortcoming, a lack of knowledge, occurs simply because candidates did not read enough. Some may be more proficient at memorizing the material, but ultimately, with weeks, months and years of commitment, everyone should be able to learn the required knowledge. There are no excuses. Preparation for the Plastic Surgery Royal College exam does not begin a few weeks or months before the exam, it starts at the beginning of the candidate's residency. The latter point cannot be emphasized enough. It is of the utmost importance that early on residents read around their cases and on the topics relevant to their current rotation. Consistent and continued acquisition of information throughout residency is key. A strong knowledge base is a function of discipline and dedication to acquisition of the material. It is simple: if one does not have sufficient knowledge, one will not pass this exam. So, the secret to success? Read, read, and re-read.

It remains an unfortunate truth that even when armed with the knowledge required to pass the exam, failure may ensue due to a lack of examination-taking skills. However, as the word "skill" implies, this can be gained through experience and training. With regard to the oral examination, very often anxiety can overshadow one's ability to relay information in a proficient and succinct fashion. In like manner, for the written component, failure to pace oneself can often result in falling short of completing the entire series of questions. The latter limitations can be improved with continued practice. Indeed, preparation for the exam can be likened to training for a marathon, and as any seasoned runner can attest, in order to achieve the objective of a long run, one must first devise a practice plan of shorter runs. Likewise, at the outset of one's final year of residency, formulation of a good reading and oral exam practice plan is essential. Training is always easier in a group, and organizing a study group of 3–4 residents with whom one can review the material, questions, cases and articles is recommended. Each member is likely to have a particular strength, which would assist the other residents in the group in gaining a better understanding on that topic.

Remember, the objective of the exam is not to impress the examiners nor is it a platform to exhibit innovative solutions to common clinical problems. Rather, it is to demonstrate that once in practice, without the direct guidance and supervision of senior colleagues, one has the necessary competence and will exercise the safety requisite to independent practice.

The written examination, which can be taken in French or English, consists of two 3-hour sessions of short answer questions (approximately 40 questions per session). The questions cover the entire breadth of plastic and reconstructive surgery, including basic science, embryology, anatomy, classifications, etc. The questions are prepared by plastic surgeons across Canada and submitted to the Examination Board of Plastic Surgery. Following a rigorous review process, a final set of questions is selected to appropriately assess candidates' competence. These questions vary in complexity, from listing a series of answers to completing a number of questions relating to a specific clinical scenario or particular pathology.

Here are my tips for the exam:

1. Do not be late.
2. Pay attention to the instructions provided by the invigilators and outlined in the booklet.
3. In order to answer all the questions, manage the allotted time thoughtfully. For instance, if there are 40 questions worth 10 marks each to be completed in 3 hours, approximately 5 minutes should be allocated to each question.
4. Answer the question in a clear and concise manner. If, for example, the question is to "list three risk factors," then provide three, not four or five. Extra credit is not given for any additional answers provided.
5. Make an effort to write legibly. If the examiner cannot read the answer, then credit will not be granted.
6. Answer all the questions to accumulate the maximum number of points.

As an adjunct to point 6, it is highly recommended not to linger on those questions where the answers are not straightforward. Rather, mark these more difficult questions with sticky notes so that they can easily be identified and come back to answer them once the rest of the exam is completed.

The oral examination can also be taken in French or English. It consists of two 1-hour sessions, each session consisting of nine clinical scenarios with associated questions. The objective of the oral component of the exam is to assess the candidate's application of theoretical knowledge and clinical judgment. More importantly, the examiner seeks to ascertain that the candidate is safe with regard to clinical decision-making.

The examinee is permitted 15 minutes prior to the start of the examination to review the series of clinical scenarios. Typically, two examiners will independently evaluate each candidate. Upon entering the room, the examiners will introduce themselves and give the candidate a short explanation about the oral exam. The clinical vignettes, illustrated with photographs, radiological imaging, etc., cover all areas of plastic and reconstructive surgery and with questions related to each. The aim of a scenario may be to evaluate a clinical problem, design a treatment plan, manage a complication, etc. Ultimately, it is important to understand that the examiners want candidates to pass the exam, and as such, they will guide you through the scenarios when necessary in an effort to elicit all information critical to passing the question. Examiners are instructed to not lead the candidate, so one should not expect any positive or negative reinforcement for responses given. Examiners may, however, redirect the candidate if responses are completely erroneous. At the end of each session, the candidate is allotted time for so-called sober second thoughts, where modifications or clarifications of any answers can be made.

My tips for the oral exam are as follows:

1. Practice, practice, and practice oral examinations. Whereas the written component of the exam is a reflection of knowledge acquired, the oral exam is, in principle, a skill that requires much practice to master. The latter also pertains to drawings and/or markings.
2. Answers are an indication of the candidate's thought process, and so structured and succinct answers demonstrate that the candidate's approach to a clinical problem is organized. It exhibits experience and preparedness for clinical practice.
3. As a corollary to point 2, it is important to listen carefully to the question and answer the question specifically. For instance, if asked for a specific investigation, do not elaborate on history and physical exam. Likewise, if asked about "your preferred flap option for the given defect," do not list a number of potential reconstructive options. Instead, state your surgical plan.
4. Show confidence, but avoid arrogance.
5. In the event you do not know the answer, it is acceptable to state it, rather than present a guess. In like manner, pausing (briefly) to reflect and properly formulate a response is appropriate.
6. Pertinent and selective consultation of other subspecialties is advisable. However, referral of every problem and/or every patient is inappropriate and demonstrates a lack of knowledge, judgment and/or confidence.
7. The Royal College exam is not the time to conceive of a new treatment option or suggest an innovative operation. Be safe and provide a well-established solution for the clinical problem at hand, and preferably, one seen or done during your training. If presented with a controversial topic, begin by explaining that this is an area of controversy and exercise caution when stating your response. Remember, ultimately, the examiners want to ensure you are a *safe* surgeon.
8. Stay positive and focused. If one question/scenario did not go well, do not dwell on it and instead concentrate on the next question. Do not let one question disturb your focus or confidence for the following questions. Keep in mind that at the end of the session, there will be time for any sober second thoughts.
9. Remember, the examiners ask the questions, not the examinee. By asking for more than the occasional clarification, the candidate may give the examiner the impression that they lack knowledge or confidence. Moreover, this is a waste of time, time which should be maximized to answer the question.
10. Formulating a standard template for each potential topic is useful as the type of cases tend to be repeated.
11. Finally, approach each case as though confronted with the clinical scenario in actual practice.

To conclude, it is indeed a difficult process, but with the right approach and adequate preparation, a passing result is an achievable task. Ultimately, review and critical appraisal of the material while preparing for the exam will make any potential candidate a better plastic surgeon. These are all fair exams, and most graduating residents are well prepared to pass. Candidates would do well to remember that the objective is not to impress the examiners, but to demonstrate that once in practice, without the direct guidance and supervision of senior colleagues, one has the necessary competence and will exercise the safety requisite to independent practice.

Plastic Surgery Fellowships in the United States

Many plastic surgery residents elect to augment their surgical training by completing additional time in a subspecialty focus area of interest following their residency training experiences. While most of these fellowship training programs are completed following graduation from residency, some residents may elect to complete research-related fellowships at various time points during their residencies.

Fellowship programs in the United States are available in nearly every possible subspecialty focus area within the full spectrum of plastic surgery, including burn/critical care, microsurgery, esthetic surgery, hand surgery, breast surgery, peripheral nerve surgery, craniofacial surgery, pediatric plastic surgery, oculoplastic surgery, and body contouring. Most fellowship programs are 1 year in length, although there may be some that offer supplemental training in the 3–6-month range.

Many of the fellowship programs in major subspecialty focus areas, such as microsurgery, hand surgery, esthetic surgery, and craniofacial surgery, require a formal application, interview, and match process that is not too different from the process graduating medical students must endure prior to beginning their residency training. Some of these programs will also be recognized and accredited by the Accreditation Council for Graduate Medical Education (ACGME), which will affect the formality of the process, the timing of the application, interview, and residency matching period, as well as certain program requirements surrounding educational and training aspects.

While some fellowships may not be formal ACGME accredited programs, in general they all require some form of an application, interview, and selection process. For this reason, it is imperative that trainees interested in pursuing fellowship training meet regularly, and early, with their Program Director and faculty mentors to discuss their interests so they will meet application deadlines. Although many programs will conduct their interview and match in the PGY-5 and/or PGY-6 years, beginning this process early, as soon as a specialty area of focus is identified, cannot be underscored as some fellowship programs can be filled nearly 2 years in advance (e.g., esthetic surgery).

For a detailed listing of available fellowship programs, including updated contact information, residents are encouraged to review the fellowship clearinghouse page located on the American Council of Academic Plastic Surgeons (ACAPS) website (http://acaplasticsurgeons.org/fellowship-listing/). Although this list may not contain every possible fellowship program, it is updated annually and is generally thought to be the most detailed list of programs available. Additional fellowship program information may also be found on individual institutional, or program, websites and through specialty societies, such as the American Society of Reconstructive Microsurgery (ASRM) fellowship page (https://www.microsurg.org/fellowships/match/).

The American Board of Plastic Surgery (ABPS) was first organized in 1937 by Vilray Blair, and other surgical colleagues across the United States, who were interested in a new subspecialty of surgery that focused on the repair, reconstruction, or replacement of physical deficits in human form or function. Prior to this establishment, Plastic Surgery was not recognized as its own major specialty within the field of American surgery. In 1938 the American Board of Surgery (ABS) recognized the ABPS as a subsidiary of General Surgery. And in 1941, the ABPS was awarded status as an independent major specialty board within the United States.[1]

As stated in the annual ABPS booklet of information, the mission of the ABPS is to "promote safe, ethical, efficacious plastic surgery to the public by maintaining high standards for the education, examination, certification, and maintenance of certification of plastic surgeons as specialists and subspecialists."[1] In an effort to fulfil this mission, the Board has established several requirements for the qualifications of applicants requesting certification. Once all applicant qualifications have been met, the board then conducts examinations for certification. The examination process, which will be discussed in more depth below, occurs in two phases – a written examination, followed by an oral examination once the written portion is completed successfully.

In addition to the above objective criteria for obtaining board certification, the ABPS also encourages a culture of ethics within plastic surgery that begins in residency training and extends throughout the professional career of the surgeon. For instance, the Board does not allow fraudulent, or unethical, advertising or marketing practices. They also prohibit marketing events where injectables, procedures, or operations are provided in a social or educational setting where alcohol is served. Such practices, if brought to the attention of the board, can result in inadmissibility to examinations, disciplinary action, and/or revocation of a certification. Likewise, the Board is strict in preventing surgeons in training from conducting themselves in any manner that could be misrepresentative of their trainee status to the public (i.e., personal practice websites, etc.).

Once certification is obtained, the ABPS certified surgeon must continue to maintain an ethical practice as well as complete various maintenance of certification (MOC) milestones, to be eligible for re-certification every 10 years.

To be eligible for ABPS certification, applicants must have graduated from a medical school in the United States that is accredited by the Liaison Committee for Medical Education (LCME), a Canadian Medical School accredited by the Committee on Accreditation of Canadian Medical Schools (CACMS), or from a United States school of osteopathic medicine accredited by the American Osteopathic Association (AOA). Graduates of schools outside of the above, and accepted into an ACGME approved plastic surgery residency program, must have a valid certificate from the Educational Commission for Foreign Medical Graduates (ECFMG) or have completed a Fifth Pathway program in an accredited school of medicine in the United States. Graduates of schools outside of the above who have been accepted into a Canadian Plastic Surgery residency program must match through the Canadian Resident Matching Service (CaRMS).

There are two approved residency training models for plastic surgery that must be completed prior to admissibility to the board examination phase by the ABPS: the Integrated Model and the Independent Model. Regardless of the model, the board requires that residents acquire basic surgical science knowledge in 10 essential content areas, and advance knowledge in plastic surgery principles and practice. A list of the critical content areas can be found on the ABPS website and within the ABPS booklet of information (https://www.abplasticsurgery.org/).

While residents may be accepted into plastic surgery residency training programs directly from medical school, there are two alternative pathways which are considered to be acceptable prerequisite training experiences prior to plastic surgery residency: completion of an American Board of Medical Specialties (ABMS) training program in General Surgery, Vascular Surgery, Neurological Surgery, Orthopedic Surgery, Otolaryngology, Thoracic Surgery, or Urology; completion of a residency program in Oral and Maxillofacial Surgery approved by the American Dental Association (ADA).

For requisite training, the ABPS requires a minimum of 3 years of plastic surgery training in an Independent program or 6 years of plastic surgery training in an Integrated program. To be eligible for certification, the training in plastic surgery must be obtained in either the United States or Canada. For US training programs, the board will only accept training which has been completed in a program that is accredited by the ACGME. Likewise, for Canadian programs, training must be completed in a program accredited by the Royal College of Physicians and Surgeons of Canada (RCPSC).

Upon completion of the above requisite education and training in Plastic Surgery, graduates may apply for admissibility to complete the official board examination process. Candidates for ABPS certification have 8 years to complete certification following the completion of training. If certification is not obtained after the first 5 years of admissibility, the candidate will be required to submit additional reapplication materials.

Candidates who have successfully met the above requirements and passed both the written and oral examination will be issued official ABPS certificates attesting to their qualifications in plastic surgery. The certificate is valid for 10 years. Per the ABPS, the certification process is a "lifelong commitment to continued education, professionalism, and ethical behavior."[1]

The purpose of the written examination is to evaluate the knowledge base and overall training of the candidate. The written exam is completed via a computer-based test offered at a specific testing center. The examination is given on only one day annually throughout the United States and Canada.

To sit for the written examination, candidates must have a current, valid medical license to practice medicine, and hold admitting privileges in plastic surgery in the United States or Canada unless the candidate is a graduating resident or in fellowship training. All candidates take the entire written examination on the same date. Beginning in 2020, the written exam is planned to be administered in June, immediately prior to graduation for residents in their final year of training. Prior to this date, the written exam was typically administered in the fall.

The examination consists of 350 multiple-choice questions formatted in three blocks of 100 questions and one block of 50 questions. Candidates are allowed a total, optional, break-time of 60 minutes. The candidates have 7 hours to complete the 350 questions. Each test item consists of a case history or situation, a question, followed by a list of possible answers. Subjects covered can be found on the ABPS website, or in the ABPS booklet of information, and include anatomy, embryology, basic pathology, basic techniques, trauma/resuscitation, preoperative and postoperative care, anesthesia, cosmetic and reconstructive surgery, hand surgery, craniofacial surgery, congenital anomalies and pediatric plastic surgery, and psychiatry and legal medicine.

The examination is graded on a pass/fail system. Candidates who pass the written examination are eligible to sit for the oral examination. Candidates who fail the written exam are eligible to re-take the examination the following year.

For the oral exam, once the candidate has successfully passed the written examination, they may submit a 9-month case list for admissibility to the oral examination. The case collection period normally begins on July 1 and continues until March 31. Case lists of less than 9-months are allowed if they meet the board criteria regarding quality, complexity, and variety of cases. Case collection cannot occur during fellowship training.

Candidates must perform a minimum of 50 major operative cases to be considered admissible for the oral boards. The cast list must include all operative procedures performed by the candidate, including those in the inpatient, outpatient, or office setting, all patients hospitalized by the candidate as the admitting physician, all emergency room patients who require an operation, co-surgeon cases if the candidate is the surgeon of record, cases performed by a resident with the candidate as the responsible attending surgeon, skin resurfacing laser procedures of the head and neck, laser ablation of congenital malformations greater than 5 cm^2, and any office-based procedures.

Each case submitted must include specific patient information, the healthcare setting, admission status, date of the procedure, duration of the procedure, anesthesia type, diagnosis, procedure description, CPT codes plus modifiers used for billing, outcome information including adverse events/complications, and case classification including category and anatomy. The category classification includes congenital, cosmetic, general reconstructive, hand, skin, and trauma. The anatomy classification includes breast, hand/upper extremity, head and neck, lower extremity, and trunk/genitalia.

In addition to case submission, all candidates eligible for the oral exam must submit one copy of all advertising and marketing materials, as well as pertinent website content including the candidate's homepage, profile page, any page with candidate qualifications/credentials, and any page that includes any board or society emblem.

Once finalized, the board will review the candidate's case list to determine if the list has an acceptable diversity and complexity to allow admission to the oral examination. If the candidate is deemed to have an inadequate case list, they will not be allowed to take the oral examination and must submit another case list for the following year. If the case list is acceptable, the Board will select five cases from the list and the candidate must prepare detailed case reports for these "known" or selected cases.

The case reports for the five selected cases will be uploaded online and must include a narrative summary of the case and outcome, all pertinent preoperative, operative, and postoperative documentation, anesthetic reports, laboratory data, pathology reports, radiology reports, consent forms, billing information, as well as one preoperative and postoperative photograph.

Once the cases are uploaded and submitted online, the board will review each case for completeness. If a case report is deemed incomplete, the candidate will have a limited opportunity to provide additional requested, or missing, information. If the board request is not satisfied, the candidate will not be admissible to the exam.

The oral exam consists of three exam sessions, each 45 minutes in length, spread out over 2 days. It is typically administered in the fall. Candidates are graded by trained, certified board examiners within each of these sessions, however, the overall pass/fail grade is dependent upon the combined performance on all three sessions. The three sessions are split up into two theory and practice sessions (also called the "unknown" sessions), and one case report session (also called the "known" session). The "unknown" sessions consist of general discussion of 6 "cases" or clinical scenarios that span the spectrum of plastic surgery. The "known" session consists of a discussion about the candidate's five selected cases.

Performance in each of the exam sessions follows the following standardized guidelines: diagnosis/planning, management/treatment, complications/outcome, clinical judgment/limitations. In the known examination/case report session, candidates will also be scored on safety (practicing within the acceptable standard of care and avoiding excessive risk), and ethics/professionalism (honest, ethical, and professional in practice).

Per the ABPS booklet of information, a passing performance on the oral exam requires the following criteria:

1. A reasonable analysis of the problem.
2. An acceptable plan of treatment that has a reasonable chance for success.
3. Recognition of possible complications of the initial plan with understanding of methods to avoid and/or manage these complications.
4. Knowledge of a "back-up" plan in the event the first plan fails.

The oral examination is also graded on a pass/fail system. Candidates who pass the oral examination will be issued an official board certification, and recognized as a diplomate of the ABPS. Candidates who fail the oral exam are eligible to re-submit cases the following year, so long as they are within the 8-year window.

Here is my advice for examination preparation. It is imperative that candidates for board certification have an accurate understanding of how they best prepare for an examination, and follow these techniques during test preparation. While the individual preparation techniques for the written exam and oral exam may differ, they both share a common denominator: time. There is no substitute for adequate time spent preparing for each exam. Candidates *must* put in the time to prepare for each step in the certification process if they wish to be successful; after all, these examinations are, without question, the most important examinations of the candidate's career. Therefore, they must be taken seriously and approached with adequate and thorough preparation. In addition, the booklet of information published directly by the ABPS and the ABPS website have detailed information on the common, or important testing topics covered in the examination process. A review of these topics should guide the candidate's study focus.

The written examination is designed to test the candidate's general fund of knowledge regarding the full spectrum of plastic surgery. Like any standardized test, there will be certain test nuances, which require good testmanship to overcome. Familiarizing oneself with the computer-based exam by completing the tutorial is a great way to understand and be comfortable with the electronic format of the exam. Likewise, tests such as these will often cover general concepts as well as the minutiae. Therefore, review of an adequate depth of knowledge of general plastic surgery is required. To obtain this fund of knowledge, review of several sources should be considered. It is good to utilize a general, detailed, plastic surgery textbook, such as this one, to establish a baseline fundamental knowledge. In addition, utilizing review books and/or high-yield focused textbooks, such as *Core Procedures in Plastic Surgery*[2] or *Review of Plastic* Surgery,[3] will help to drive home key concepts in a quick, bulleted fashion. Lastly, completion of practice exams, review of past in-service examinations, and review of frequent questions will help the candidate familiarize themselves with the test environment and overall format of clinical scenario and multiple-choice answers.

The oral exam is quite different from the written exam, thus it is no surprise that it requires a different type of preparation. While the oral exam will also test knowledge, more importantly, it will test the candidate's ability to communicate effectively, think on their toes, and communicate under pressure. Similar to an actor preparing for a play or scene, candidates preparing for the oral exam must prepare out loud, that is to say they should either practice discussing plastic surgery topics and cases by speaking to themselves in a mirror, or more commonly, practicing with a colleague so they can improve the effectiveness and efficiency of their communication. Due to the recent standardization of the oral exam, a candidate's performance is graded more as a collection of checkboxes and buzzwords, rather than based on the subjective feeling of the examiner regarding the candidate's competence. As such, if the candidate is not talking during the exam, or cannot communicate efficiently and effectively, then they are not likely orating the critical buzzwords required to check the boxes, receive credit, and ultimately score points; thus the oral exam is more of a performance, and requires practice, rather than rote memorization of facts.

One key difference between the oral exam and the written exam, is that one-third of the oral exam is "open book." By that I mean the case report session should be the easiest session for which to prepare (although it is often the most common session that results in failure of the exam). Candidates should know their cases inside and out. They must be able to communicate the indication and justification for their surgical intervention, the steps taken during their operation, and the plausible reasons for their outcome. Likewise, having an understanding of how one could have, or should have, done things differently is helpful.

For the unknown sessions, the best way to prepare is to review as many cases as possible. Again, the ABPS website and booklet of information will detail common topics tested during these sessions. However, utilizing review books such as *Core Procedures in Plastic Surgery* and *Review of Plastic Surgery*, are helpful in understanding all of the nuances for the most common plastic surgery conditions and operations. Likewise, working with colleagues, peers, and partners to review as many cases as possible will not only improve your knowledge, but will also help you generate a script to effectively communicate the diagnosis, preoperative considerations, operative plans and details, and postoperative care and considerations for these topics. Adequate preparation and practice cannot be overstated. Additional tips listed in this chapter will also help you prepare for the oral examination.

References

1. The American Board of Plastic Surgery, Inc. *ABPS Booklet of Information, 2019–2020*. https://www.abplasticsurgery.org/about-us/publications-requirements/.
2. Neligan PC, Buck DW, eds. *Core Procedures in Plastic Surgery*. 2nd edn. Elsevier; 2019.
3. Buck DW, ed. *Review of Plastic Surgery*. Elsevier; 2017.

Index

Page numbers followed by "*f*" indicate figures, "*t*" indicate tables, and "*b*" indicate boxes.

D

G

I

N

T